INGENIX®

Physician Solutions

FOR PRICING DETAILS

Visit **www.ingenix.com/ physicians**

Call toll-free **1.800.765.6704** and mention source code **FB11F**

Have a Fully Integrated Practice.

More companies rely on our medical coding expertise than anyone in the industry. That first-hand knowledge of all the stakeholders gives us unique insight, and we use it to create integrated information, technology and consulting solutions that address the range of financial and clinical challenges practices face.

← **Payers** – Connect with thousands of payers to verify eligibility and manage referral requirements, remittances and claims

← **Clinical partners** – Work with real-time clinical data from labs, pharmacies, radiologists, hospitals and other key partners

← **Patients** – Automate your appointment confirms, electronic statements, collect payments online, letters and inbound patient calls

Powerful solutions that work as one.

Start with your practice management platform or ours. Then plug in the powerful applications you need to enhance care or optimize your revenue cycle.

- **Electronic health records (EHR).**
  Low-cost, web-based EHR that puts your practice and your patients first. Ingenix CareTracker integrates with all the operational functions of the practice, improves quality and reduces costs

- **Practice management.**
  Next-generation, web-based practice management with today's financial and administrative productivity. Our automated billing process electronically connects to more than 1,000 national insurance plans and submits your claims for you, overnight

- **Coding tools.**
  The industry's broadest and most preferred coding tools. Our ever-evolving coding solutions are available in multiple formats to meet your needs

- **Claims editing.**
  Powerful claims software that leverages our information and your rules. The industry's average resubmission cost is $25 per claim—our solutions help you get paid faster

- **Electronic data interchange (EDI).**
  The way to navigate EDI your way, through clearinghouse connections, direct connections or both. Our connectivity solutions are HIPAA compliant, easy-to-use, efficient and affordable

- **Contract monitoring.**
  Organizing and managing your payer agreements for automated reimbursement and compliance. If your total claims value is underpaid by 5%, you're losing about a day's worth of earnings every month

INGENIX®

ICD-9-CM

for Physicians – Volumes 1 & 2

2011 | Professional

International Classification of Diseases
9th Revision
Clinical Modification
Sixth Edition

Edited by:
Anita C. Hart, RHIA, CCS, CCS-P
Melinda S. Stegman, MBA, CCS
Beth Ford, RHIT, CCS

Ingenix is committed to providing you with the ICD-9-CM code update information you need to code accurately and to be in compliance with HIPAA regulations. In case of adoption of additional ICD-9-CM code changes effective April 1, 2011, Ingenix will provide these code changes to you at no additional cost! Just check back at www.shopingenix.com/productalerts to review the latest information concerning any new code changes.

Codes Valid October 1, 2010, through September 30, 2011

Publisher's Notice

All codes, indexes, and other material in the ICD-9-CM are compiled from official ICD-9-CM codes and instructions as well as the Medicare regulations and manuals issued or authorized by the Centers for Medicare and Medicaid Services. The code book is designed to provide accurate and authoritative information in regard to the subject covered, and every reasonable effort has been made to ensure the accuracy of the information within these pages. However, the ultimate responsibility for correct coding lies with the provider of services.

Ingenix, its employees, agents and staff make no representation, warranty or guarantee that this compilation of codes and narratives is error-free or that the use of this code book will prevent differences of opinion or disputes with Medicare or other third-party payers as to the codes that are accepted or the amounts that will be paid to providers for services, and will bear no responsibility or liability for the results or consequences of the use of this code book.

Our Commitment to Accuracy

Ingenix is committed to producing accurate and reliable materials. To report corrections, please visit www.ingenixonline.com/accuracy or email accuracy@ingenix.com. You can also reach customer service by calling 1.800.INGENIX (464.3649), option 1.

Preface

ICD-9-CM for Physicians has been designed with the physician office professional in mind. The most recent official government versions of volumes 1 and 2 have been combined to provide physicians and their office staff with an ICD-9-CM book that is easy to use.

In addition, our technical experts have drawn upon their extensive hands-on experience to enhance the government's official version with valuable features essential to correct coding and reimbursement. With these enhancements, physician office health information professionals will increase the efficiency and timeliness of claim submission for both Medicare and other third-party payers.

As you review the content, you'll find the following:

- All the official ICD-9-CM codes, indexes, notes, footnotes and symbols
- Complete official coding guidelines
- Our exclusive color coding, symbols, and footnotes that alert coders to coding and reimbursement issues. Medicare outpatient code edits, such as invalid fourth or fifth digit for diagnosis codes are identified.
- Illustrations and clinically oriented definitions to aid in correct code assignment
- Coding tips based upon the official coding guidelines and advice found in AHA's *Coding Clinic for ICD-9-CM*
- Symbols identifying new codes and text revisions; pages are dated to indicate when the changes were made
- Exclusive QuickFlip Color Tabs for quick, easy location of terms and codes in the Alphabetic Index and Tabular List

Use of Official Sources

This *ICD-9-CM for Physicians* contains the official U.S. Department of Health and Human Services, ICD-9-CM codes, effective for the current year.

The color coding, footnotes and symbols, which identify coding and reimbursement issues, are derived from official federal government sources, including the Medicare Outpatient Code Editor as well as the knowledge of our technical experts.

The American Hospital Association's (AHA) *Coding Clinic for ICD-9-CM* references are used with permission of the AHA.

Important Information About Your Subscription Service

If you have purchased the updateable *ICD-9-CM for Physicians*, your subscription includes an updating service throughout the year to keep the code book current and accurate. Whenever CMS issues changes or corrections to the ICD-9-CM codes, We will issue an update to the book. In July you will receive a list of all new, revised, and invalid codes for the upcoming year.

Technical Editors

Anita C. Hart, RHIA, CCS, CCS-P, *Product Manager, Ingenix*
Ms. Hart's experience includes conducting and publishing research in clinical medicine and human genetics for Yale University, Massachusetts General Hospital, and Massachusetts Institute of Technology. In addition, Ms. Hart has supervised medical records management, health information management, coding and reimbursement, and worker's compensation issues as the office manager for a large physical therapy rehabilitation practice. Ms. Hart is an expert in physician and facility coding, reimbursement systems, and compliance issues. Ms. Hart has developed and has served as technical consultant for numerous other publications for hospital and physician practices. Currrently, Ms. Hart is the Product Manager and Technical Editor for the ICD-9-CM and ICD-10-CM/PCS product lines.

Melinda S. Stegman, MBA, CCS, *Clinical/Technical Editor, Ingenix*
Ms. Stegman has more than 25 years of experience in the HIM profession and has been responsible for managing the clinical aspects of the HSS/Ingenix HIM consulting practice in the Washington, D.C., area office. Her areas of specialization include training on inpatient and DRG coding, outpatient coding, and ambulatory payment classifications (APCs) for HIM professionals, software developers, and other clients; developing an outpatient billing/coding compliance tool for a major accounting firm; and managing HIM consulting practices. Ms. Stegman is a regular contributing author for *Advance for Health Information Management Professionals* and for the *Journal of Health Care Compliance*. She has performed coding assessments and educational sessions throughout the country. Ms. Stegman is credentialed by the American Health Information Management Association (AHIMA) as a Certified Coding Specialist (CCS) and holds a Master of Business Administration degree with a concentration in health care management from the University of New Mexico—Albuquerque.

Beth Ford, RHIT, CCS, *Clinical/Technical Editor, Ingenix*
Ms. Ford is a clinical/technical editor for Ingenix. She has extensive background in both physician and facility ICD-9-CM and CPT/HCPCS coding. Ms. Ford has served as a coding specialist, coding manager, coding trainer/educator and coding consultant, as well as a health information management director. She is an active member of the American Heath Information Management Association (AHIMA).

In addition to the editors, the following people have contributed to this book:

Stacy Perry, *Manager, Desktop Publishing*
Tracy Betzler, *Desktop Publishing Specialist*
Hope Dunn, *Desktop Publishing Specialist*
Toni Stewart, *Desktop Publishing Specialist*
Kate Holden, *Editor*

What to Do If You Have Questions

If you have any questions call our customer service department toll-free at 800-INGENIX (464-3649), option 1.

If you have comments on the content of this book, please e-mail them to customerservice@ingenix.com or fax to 801-982-4033.

Additional Copies

Contact the customer service order department toll-free at 800-INGENIX (464-3649), option 1.

Introduction

History and Future of ICD-9

The International Classification of Diseases, Ninth Revision, Clinical Modification (ICD-9-CM) is based on the official version of the World Health Organization's Ninth Revision, International Classification of Diseases (ICD-9). ICD-9-CM classifies morbidity and mortality information for statistical purposes, indexing of hospital records by disease and operations, data storage, and retrieval.

This modification of ICD-9 supplants the Eighth Revision International Classification of Diseases, Adapted for Use in the United States (ICDA-8) and the Hospital Adaptation of ICDA (H-ICDA).

The concept of extending the International Classification of Diseases for use in hospital indexing was originally developed in response to a need for a more efficient basis for storage and retrieval of diagnostic data. In 1950, the U.S. Public Health Service and the Veterans Administration began independent tests of the International Classification of Diseases for hospital indexing purposes. The following year, the Columbia Presbyterian Medical Center in New York City adopted the International Classification of Diseases, Sixth Revision, with some modifications for use in its medical record department. A few years later, the Commission on Professional and Hospital Activities (CPHA) in Ann Arbor, Mich., adopted the International Classification of Diseases with similar modifications for use in hospitals participating in the Professional Activity Study.

The problem of adapting ICD for indexing hospital records was addressed by the U.S. National Committee on Vital and Health Statistics through its subcommittee on hospital statistics. The subcommittee reviewed the modifications made by the various users of ICD and proposed that uniform changes be made. This was done by a small working party.

In view of the growing interest in the use of the International Classification of Diseases for hospital indexing, a study was undertaken in 1956 by the American Hospital Association and the American Medical Record Association (then the American Association of Medical Record Librarians) of the relative efficiencies of coding systems for diagnostic indexing. This study indicated the International Classification of Diseases provided a suitable and efficient framework for indexing hospital records. The major users of the International Classification of Diseases for hospital indexing purposes then consolidated their experiences, and an adaptation was first published in December 1959. A revision was issued in 1962 and the first "Classification of Operations and Treatments" was included.

In 1966, the international conference for revising the International Classification of Diseases noted the eighth revision of ICD had been constructed with hospital indexing in mind and considered the revised classification suitable, in itself, for hospital use in some countries. However, it was recognized that the basic classification might provide inadequate detail for diagnostic indexing in other countries. A group of consultants was asked to study the eighth revision of ICD (ICD-8) for applicability to various users in the United States. This group recommended that further detail be provided for coding of hospital and morbidity data. The American Hospital Association was requested to develop the needed adaptation proposals. This was done by an advisory committee (the Advisory Committee to the Central Office on ICDA). In 1968 the United States Public Health Service published the product, Eighth Revision International Classification of Diseases, Adapted for Use in the United States. This became commonly known as ICDA-8, and beginning in 1968 it served as the basis for coding diagnostic data for both official morbidity and mortality statistics in the United States.

In 1968, the CPHA published the Hospital Adaptation of ICDA (H-ICDA) based on both the original ICD-8 and ICDA-8. In 1973, CPHA published a revision of H-ICDA, referred to as H-ICDA-2. Hospitals throughout the United States were divided in their use of these classifications until January 1979, when ICD-9-CM was made the single classification intended primarily for use in the United States, replacing these earlier related, but somewhat dissimilar, classifications.

Physicians have been required by law to submit diagnosis codes for Medicare reimbursement since the passage of the Medicare Catastrophic Coverage Act of 1988. This act requires physician offices to include the appropriate diagnosis codes when billing for services provided to Medicare beneficiaries on or after April 1, 1989. The Centers for Medicare and Medicaid Services (CMS) designated ICD-9-CM as the coding system physicians must use.

In 1993 the World Health Organization published the newest version of International Classification of Diseases, Tenth Revision, ICD-10. This version contains the greatest number of changes in the history of ICD. There are more codes (5,500 more than ICD-9) to allow more specific reporting of diseases and newly recognized conditions. ICD-10 consists of three volumes; Tabular List (volume I), instructions (volume 2) and the Alphabetic Index (volume 3). It contains 21 chapters including two supplementary ones. The codes are alphanumeric (A00–T88, V00–Y99 and Z00–Z99). Currently ICD-10 is being used in some European countries with an implementation date of October 1, 2013, in the United States.

ICD-9-CM Background

In February 1977, a steering committee was convened by the National Center for Health Statistics to provide advice and counsel in developing a clinical modification of ICD-9. The organizations represented on the steering committee included the following:

- American Association of Health Data Systems
- American Hospital Association
- American Medical Record Association
- Association for Health Records
- Council on Clinical Classifications
- Centers for Medicare and Medicaid Services, Department of Health and Human Services
- WHO Center for Classification of Diseases for North America, sponsored by the National Center for Health Statistics, Department of Health and Human Services

The Council on Clinical Classifications was sponsored by the following:

- American Academy of Pediatrics
- American College of Obstetricians and Gynecologists
- American College of Physicians
- American College of Surgeons
- American Psychiatric Association
- Commission on Professional and Hospital Activities

The steering committee met periodically in 1977. Clinical guidance and technical input were provided by task forces on classification from the Council on Clinical Classification's sponsoring organizations.

ICD-9-CM is a clinical modification of the World Health Organization's ICD-9. The term "clinical" is used to emphasize the modification's intent: to serve as a useful tool to classify morbidity data for indexing medical records, medical care review, and ambulatory and other medical care programs, as well as for basic health statistics. To describe the clinical picture of the patient, the codes must be more precise than those needed only for statistical groupings and trend analysis.

Characteristics of ICD-9-CM

ICD-9-CM far exceeds its predecessors in the number of codes provided. The disease classification has been expanded to include health-related conditions and to provide greater specificity at the fifth-digit level of detail. These fifth digits are not optional; they are intended for use in recording the information substantiated in the clinical record.

Volume I (Tabular List) of ICD-9-CM contains four appendixes:

Appendix A: Morphology of Neoplasms

Appendix B: Deleted effective October 1, 2004

Appendix C: Classification of Drugs by American Hospital Formulary Service List Number and Their ICD-9-CM Equivalents

These appendixes are included as a reference to provide further information about the patient's clinical picture, to further define a diagnostic statement, to aid in classifying new drugs or to reference three-digit categories.

Volume 2 (Alphabetic Index) of ICD-9-CM contains many diagnostic terms that do not appear in volume I since the index includes most diagnostic terms currently in use.

The Disease Classification

ICD-9-CM is totally compatible with its parent system, ICD-9, thus meeting the need for comparability of morbidity and mortality statistics at the international level. A few fourth-digit codes were created in existing three-digit rubrics only when the necessary detail could not be accommodated by the use of a fifth-digit subclassification. To ensure that each rubric of ICD-9-CM collapses back to its ICD-9 counterpart the following specifications governed the ICD-9-CM disease classification:

Specifications for the Tabular List:

1. Three-digit rubrics and their contents are unchanged from ICD-9.

2. The sequence of three-digit rubrics is unchanged from ICD-9.

3. Three-digit rubrics are not added to the main body of the classification.

4. Unsubdivided three-digit rubrics are subdivided where necessary to
   - add clinical detail
   - isolate terms for clinical accuracy

5. The modification in ICD-9-CM is accomplished by adding a fifth digit to existing ICD-9 rubrics, except as noted under #7 below.

6. The optional dual classification in ICD-9 is modified.
   - Duplicate rubrics are deleted:
     – four-digit manifestation categories duplicating etiology entries
     – manifestation inclusion terms duplicating etiology entries[2]
   - Manifestations of disease are identified, to the extent possible, by creating five-digit codes in the etiology rubrics.
   - When the manifestation of a disease cannot be included in the etiology rubrics, provision for its identification is made by retaining the ICD-9 rubrics used for classifying manifestations of disease.

7. The format of ICD-9-CM is revised from that used in ICD-9.
   - American spelling of medical terms is used.
   - Inclusion terms are indented beneath the titles of codes.
   - Codes not to be used for primary tabulation of disease are printed in italics with the notation, "code first underlying disease."

Specifications for the Alphabetic Index:

1. The format of the Alphabetic Index follows that of ICD-9.

2. When two codes are required to indicate etiology and manifestation, the manifestation code appears in brackets (e.g., diabetic cataract 250.5 [*366.41*]).

The ICD-9-CM Coordination and Maintenance Committee

The ICD-9-CM Coordination and Maintenance Committee, a federal committee, was created as a forum for proposals to update International Classification of Diseases, Ninth Revision, Clinical Modification, Sixth Edition (ICD-9-CM). A representative from the National Center for Health Statistics (NCHS) and one from the Centers for Medicare and Medicaid Services (CMS) co-chair the ICD-9-CM Coordination and Maintenance Committee meetings. Responsibility for maintaining ICD-9-CM is divided between the two agencies, with NCHS classifying diagnoses (volumes 1 and 2) and CMS classifying procedures (volume 3).

Proposals for changes to the ICD-9-CM classification system are submitted and discussed in open forum meetings held in March and September of each year at the headquarters of CMS in Baltimore. Comments received during or after the meetings are then reviewed and evaluated. All final decisions are made by the director of NCHS and the administrator of CMS. The complete official document of changes to the classification system is released as the Addenda for the International Classification of Disease, Ninth Revision, Clinical Modification, Sixth Edition, Volume 1, 2, & 3.

The *ICD-9-CM for Physicians, Volumes 1 & 2,* is based on the official version of the International Classification of Diseases, Ninth Revision, Clinical Modification, Sixth Edition, issued by the U.S. Department of Health and Human Services. Annual code changes are implemented by the government and are effective October 1 and valid through September 30 of the following year. If a convincing case is made that requires a new code to capture new technology or an emerging disease, this new code may be implemented on April 1 of the following year.

How to Use the ICD-9-CM for Physicians (Volumes 1 & 2)

ICD-9-CM for Physicians is based on the official version of the International Classification of Diseases, Ninth Revision, Clinical Modification, Sixth Edition, issued by the U.S. Department of Health and Human Services. Annual code changes are implemented by the government and are effective Oct. 1 and valid through Sept. 30 of the following year.

To accommodate the coder's approach to coding, the Alphabetic Index (Volume 2) has been placed before the Tabular List (Volume 1). This allows the user to locate the term in the index, then confirm the accuracy of the code in the Tabular List.

10 Steps to Correct Coding

To code accurately, it is necessary to have a working knowledge of medical terminology and to understand the characteristics, terminology and conventions of ICD-9-CM. Transforming descriptions of diseases, injuries, conditions and procedures into numerical designations (coding) is a complex activity and should not be undertaken without proper training.

Originally, coding allowed retrieval of medical information by diagnoses and operations for medical research, education and administration. Coding today is used to describe the medical necessity of a procedure and facilitate payment of health services, to evaluate utilization patterns and to study the appropriateness of health care costs. Coding provides the basis for epidemiological studies and research into the quality of health care. Incorrect or inaccurate coding can lead to investigations of fraud and abuse. Therefore, coding must be performed correctly and consistently to produce meaningful statistics to aid in planning for the health needs of the nation.

Follow the steps below to code correctly:

Step 1: Identify the reason for the visit (e.g., sign, symptom, diagnosis, condition to be coded).

Physicians describe the patient's condition using terminology that includes specific diagnoses as well as symptoms, problems or reasons for the encounter. If symptoms are present but a definitive diagnosis has not yet been determined, code the symptoms. Do not code conditions that are referred to as "rule out," "suspected," "probable" or "questionable."

Step 2: Always consult the Alphabetic Index, Volume 2, before turning to the Tabular List.

The most critical rule is to begin a code search in the index. Never turn first to the Tabular List (Volume 1), as this will lead to coding errors and less specificity in code assignments. To prevent coding errors, use both the Alphabetic Index and the Tabular List when locating and assigning a code.

Step 3: Locate the main entry term.

The Alphabetic Index is arranged by condition. Conditions may be expressed as nouns, adjectives and eponyms. Some conditions have multiple entries under their synonyms. Main terms are identified using boldface type.

Step 4: Read and interpret any notes listed with the main term

Notes are identified using italicized type.

Step 5: Review entries for modifiers

Nonessential modifiers are in parentheses. These parenthetical terms are supplementary words or explanatory information that may either be present or absent in the diagnostic statement and do not affect code assignment.

Step 6: Interpret abbreviations, cross-references, symbols and brackets

Cross-references used are "*see*," "*see category*," or "*see also*." The abbreviation NEC may follow main terms or subterms. NEC (not elsewhere classified) indicates that there is no specific code for the condition even though the medical documentation may be very specific. The ☑ box indicates the code requires an additional digit. If the appropriate digits are not found in the index, in a box beneath the main term, you MUST refer to the Tabular List. Italicized brackets [ ], are used to enclose a second code number that must be used with the code immediately preceding it and in that sequence.

Step 7: Choose a tentative code and locate it in the Tabular List.

Be guided by any inclusion or exclusion terms, notes or other instructions, such as "*code first*" and "use additional code," that would direct the use of a different or additional code from that selected in the index for a particular diagnosis, condition or disease.

Step 8: Determine whether the code is at the highest level of specificity.

Assign three-digit codes (category codes) if there are no four-digit codes within the code category. Assign four-digit codes (subcategory codes) if there are no five-digit codes for that category. Assign five-digit codes (fifth-digit subclassification codes) for those categories where they are available.

Step 9: Consult the color coding and reimbursement prompts, including the age and sex edits.

Consult the official ICD-9-CM guidelines for coding and reporting, and refer to the AHA's *Coding Clinic for ICD-9-CM* for coding guidelines governing the use of specific codes.

Step 10: Assign the code.

Organization

Introduction

The introductory material in this book includes the history and future of ICD-9-CM as well as an overview of the classification system

Official ICD-9-CM Conventions

This section provides a full explanation of all the official footnotes, symbols, instructional notes, and conventions found in the official government version

Additional Conventions

Exclusive color-coding, symbols, and notations have been included in the *ICD-9-CM for Physicians, Volumes 1 and 2* to alert coders to important coding and reimbursement issues. This section provides a full explanation of the additional conventions used throughout this book.

Summary of Code Changes

This section includes a complete listing of all code changes for the current year.

Summary of AHA's *Coding Clinic for ICD-9-CM* Topics

This is a brief summary of the official advice concerning coding topics covered in the latest issues of AHA's *Coding Clinic for ICD-9-CM* and is found **ONLY** in the *ICD-9-CM Expert for Physicians* updateable edition.

ICD-9-CM Code Changes for 2010: An Insider's View

Chapter-by-chapter detailed clinical and coding information with coding scenarios for all new codes adopted for 2010 located in one resource for quick reference and training. This section is found **only** in the Expert editions.

Coding Guidelines

Included in this book are the official ICD-9-CM coding guidelines as approved by the four cooperating parties of the ICD-9-CM Coordination and Maintenance Committee. Failure to comply with these official coding guidelines may result in denied or delayed claims.

Disease Classification: Alphabetic Index to Diseases

The Alphabetic Index to Diseases is separated by tabs labeled with the letters of the alphabet, contains diagnostic terms for illnesses, injuries and reasons for encounters with health care professionals. Both the Table of Drugs and Chemicals and the Alphabetic Index to External Causes of Injury and Poisoning are easily located with the tabs in this section.

The warning statement at the bottom of every page of the index, ▽ Subterms under main terms may continue to next column or page, is a reminder to always check for additional subterms before making final selection.

Disease Classification: Tabular List of Diseases

The Tabular List of Diseases arranges the ICD-9-CM codes and descriptors numerically. Tabs divide this section into chapters, identified by the code range on the tab.

The Tabular List includes two supplementary classifications:

- V Codes–Supplementary Classification of Factors Influencing Health Status and Contact with Health Services (V01–V91)
- E Codes–Supplementary Classification of External Causes of Injury and Poisoning (E000–E999)

ICD-9-CM includes four official appendixes.

- Appendix A   Morphology of Neoplasms
- Appendix B   Deleted effective October 1, 2004
- Appendix C   Classification of Drugs by AHFS List
- Appendix D   Classification of Industrial Accidents According to Agency
- Appendix E   List of Three-digit Categories

These appendixes are included as a reference to provide further Information about the patient's circumstances, help further define a diagnostic statement, maintain a tumor registry and aid in classifying new drugs.

Resources

Listed below are the exclusive resources found **ONLY** in the *ICD-9-CM Expert for Physicians, Volumes 1 & 2.*

10 Steps to Correct Coding

This is a valuable resource that takes the coder step by step through the coding process with detailed explanations accompanied by coding examples that demonstrate the practical application of ICD-9-CM conventions and coding guidelines in 10 steps.

Valid Three-digit Code Table

ICD-9-CM is composed of codes with either 3, 4, or 5 digits. A code is invalid if it has not been coded to the full number of digits required for that code. There are a certain number codes that are valid for reporting as three digit codes. A list of these valid three-digit code is included as a convenient reference when auditing claims.

Code Tables

Exclusive coding tables covering abortion, burns, complications, diabetes, hernia, pregnancy, and others are provided to simplify those complex coding issues.

ICD-9-CM Official Conventions

ICD-9-CM Footnotes, Symbols, Instructional Notes and Conventions

This *ICD-9-CM for Physicians* preserves all the footnotes, symbols, instructional notes and conventions found in the government's official version. Accurate coding depends upon understanding the meaning of these elements.

The following appear in the disease Tabular List, unless otherwise noted.

Official Government Symbols

§   The section mark preceding a code denotes a footnote on the page. This symbol is used in the Tabular List of Diseases.

ICD-9-CM Conventions Used in the Tabular List

In addition to the symbols and footnotes above, the ICD-9-CM disease tabular has certain abbreviations, punctuation, symbols and other conventions. Our *ICD-9-CM for Physicians* preserves these conventions. Proper use of the conventions will lead to efficient and accurate coding.

Abbreviations

NEC   Not elsewhere classifiable

This abbreviation is used when the ICD-9-CM system does not provide a code specific for the patient's condition.

NOS   Not otherwise specified

This abbreviation is the equivalent of "unspecified" and is used only when the coder lacks the information necessary to code to a more specific four-digit subcategory.

[ ]   Brackets enclose synonyms, alternative terminology or explanatory phrases:

482.2   Pneumonia due to Hemophilus influenzae [H. influenzae]

Brackets that appear beneath a code indicate the fifth digits that are considered valid fifth digits for the code. This convention is applied for those instances in ICD-9-CM where not all common fifth digits are considered valid for each subcategory within a category.

715.0   Osteoarthrosis, generalized
[0,4,9]

Generalized arthrosis can only be assigned in cases for which the degenerative joint disease involves multiple joints. Therefore, this code is considered for arthrosis in the sites described as unspecified, hand (which consists of multiple joints), or multiple sites. Therefore, only fifth digits 0, 4, and 9 are valid with subcategory 715.0.

[ ]   Slanted brackets that appear in the Alphabetic Index indicate mandatory multiple coding. Both codes must be assigned to fully describe the condition and are sequenced in the order listed.

Tachycardia
ventricular (paroxysmal)
psychogenic 316 *[427.1]*

Psychogenic paroxysmal tachycardia is reported using both 316, Psychogenic factors associated with diseases classified elsewhere, and 427.1, Paroxysmal ventricular tachydcardia.

( )   Parentheses enclose supplementary words, called nonessential modifiers, that may be present in the narrative description of a disease without affecting the code assignment:

198.4   Other parts of nervous system
Meninges (cerebral) (spinal)

:   Colons are used in the Tabular List after an incomplete term that needs one or more of the modifiers that follow in order to make it assignable to a given category:

021.1   Enteric tularemia
Tularemia:
cryptogenic
intestinal
typhoidal

}   Braces enclose a series of terms, each of which is modified by the statement appearing to the right of the brace:

560.2   Volvulus
Knotting
Strangulation   } of intestine, bowel, or
Torsion   colon
Twist

Other Conventions

Boldface   Boldface type is used for all codes and titles in the Tabular List.

Italicized   Italicized type is used for all exclusion notes and to identify codes that should not be used for describing the primary diagnosis.

General Notes Used in the Tabular List

These notes appear only in the Tabular List of Diseases:

Includes   An includes note further defines or clarifies the content of the chapter, subchapter, category, subcategory or subclassification. The includes note in the example below applies only to category 461.

Excludes   following the word "Excludes" are not classified to the chapter, subchapter, category, subcategory or specific subclassification code under which it is found. The note also may provide the location of the excluded diagnosis. Excludes notes are italicized.

461   Acute sinusitis
     INCLUDES   abscess
              empyema   } acute, of sinus
              infection   (accessory)
              inflammation   (nasal)
              suppuration
     EXCLUDES   *chronic or unspecified sinusitis (473.0-473.9)*

Instructional Notes

The following official instructional notes are critical to correct coding practices. The instructional notes appear in red type in the Tabular List.

Use additional code:

This instruction signals the coder that an additional code should be used if the information is available to provide a more complete picture of that diagnosis.

362.13 Changes in vascular appearance
Vascular sheathing of retina

Use additional code for any associated atherosclerosis (440.8)

For emphasis this instructional note appears in red type in the tabular section.

There are coding circumstances outside of the etiology/ manifestation convention when multiple coding for a single condition is required. The "Use additional code" note will be found under the associated condition code in the tabular. In the index, the multiple coding requirement is indicated by the use of the slanted bracket. The two codes are to be sequenced as listed in the index. For example, retinal arteriosclerosis must be coded using two codes sequenced as listed in the index.

Arteriosclerosis, arteriosclerotic
retinal (vascular) 440.8 *[362.13]*

Code first underlying disease:

The *"Code first underlying"* instructional note found under certain codes is a sequencing rule. Most often this sequencing rule applies to the etiology/manifestation convention and is found under the manifestation code. The manifestation code may never be used alone or as a primary diagnosis (i.e., sequenced first). The instructional note, the code and its descriptor appear in italics in the Tabular List.

> **590.81 *Pyelitis or pyelonephritis in diseases classified elsewhere***
>> *Code first underlying disease as:*
>> tuberculosis (016.0)

Not all codes with a "Code first underlying disease" instructional note are part of the etiology/manifestation convention. The `Code first' note will appear, but the title of the code and the instructional note are not in italics. These codes may be reported alone or as the secondary diagnosis. For example, disseminated chorioretinitis may be reported as a principal or first-listed diagnosis. However, if the underlying condition that caused disseminated chorioretinitis is known, such as tuberculous disseminated chorioretinitis, two codes are required and sequenced as listed in the index.

> **363.13 Disseminated choroiditis and chorioretinitis, generalized**
>> *Code first underlying disease as:*
>> tuberculosis (017.3)

For emphasis this instructional note appears in red type in the tabular section.

Code, if applicable, any causal condition first:

A code with this note indicates that this code may be assigned as a principal diagnosis when the causal condition is unknown or not applicable. If a causal condition is known, then the code for that condition should be sequenced as the principal or first-listed diagnosis.

> **590.0 Chronic pyelonephritis**
>> Chronic pyelitis
>> Chronic pyonephrosis
>> Code, if applicable, any causal condition first

For emphasis this instructional note appears in red type in the tabular section.

Instructional Notes Used in the Index

Omit code:

"Omit code" is used to instruct the coder that no code is to be assigned. When this instruction is found in the Alphabetic Index to Diseases the medical term should not be coded as a diagnosis.

> **Metaplasia**
>> cervix — *omit code*

See Condition:

The "see condition" note found in the Alphabetic Index to Disease instructs the coder to refer to a main term for the condition. This note will follow index terms that are nouns for anatomical sites or adjectival forms of disease term. In the example below, the index terms "Cervix" and "Diffuse" are followed by the — see condition. Coders should search the index using a condition term such as atrophy or prolapse.

> **Cervix** — *see* condition
> **Diffuse** — *see* condition

Morphology Codes:

For each neoplastic disease listed in the index, a morphology code is provided that identifies histological type and behavior.

> *Example:*

> **Myelolipoma** (M8870/0) — *see* Neoplasm, by site, benign

The histology is identified by the first four digits and the behavior is identified by the digit following the slash. Appendix A of Volume 1 contains a listing of morphology codes. This appendix is helpful when the pathology report identifies the neoplasm by using an M code. The coder may refer to Appendix A to determine the nomenclature of the neoplasm that will be the main term to search in the Index. The behavior classification is as follows:

- · 0 Benign
- · 1 Uncertain behavior
- · 2 Carcinoma in situ
- · 3 Malignant, primary site
- · 6 Malignant, secondary site.

Additional Conventions

Symbols and Notations

New and Revised Text Symbols

●   A bullet at a code or line of text indicates that the entry is new.

▲   A triangle in the Tabular List indicates that the code title is revised. In the Alphabetic Index the triangle indicates that a code has changed.

►◄   These symbols appear at the beginning and at the end of a section of new or revised text.

When these symbols appear on a page there will be a date on the lower outside corner of the page indicating the date of the change, (e.g., October 2010).

Additional Digits Required

✓4ᵗʰ   This symbol indicates that the code requires a fourth digit.

✓5ᵗʰ   This symbol indicates that a code requires a fifth digit.

☑   This symbol found only in the Alphabetic Index sections and the Table of Drugs and Chemicals indicates that an additional digit is required. Referring to the tabular section is essential to locate the appropriate additional digit.

AHA's *Coding Clinic for ICD-9-CM* References

The four cooperating parties have designated the AHA's *Coding Clinic for ICD-9-CM* as the official publication for coding guidelines. The references are identified by the notation **AHA:** followed by the issue, year and page number.

In the example below, AHA's *Coding Clinic for ICD-9-CM*, third quarter 1991, page 15, contains a discussion on code assignment for vitreous hemorrhage:

> **379.23 Vitreous hemorrhage**
> **AHA:** 3Q, '91, 15

The table below explains the abbreviations in the *Coding Clinic* references:

J-F	January/February
M-A	March/April
M-J	May/June
J-A	July/August
S-O	September/October
N-D	November/December
1Q	First quarter
2Q	Second quarter
3Q	Third quarter
4Q	Fourth quarter

AHA's *Coding Clinic for ICD-9-CM* references appear in blue type in the Tabular List.

Age and Sex Edit Symbols

The age edits below address OCE edits and are used to detect inconsistencies between the patient's age and diagnosis. They appear in the Tabular List of Diseases to the right of the code description.

Newborn Age: 0   **N**
These diagnoses are intended for newborns and neonates and the patient's age must be 0 years.

Pediatric Age: 0-17   **P**
These diagnoses are intended for children and the patient's age must between 0 and 17 years.

Maternity Age: 12-55   **M**
These diagnoses are intended for the patients between the age of 12 and 55 years.

Adult Age: 15-124   **A**
These diagnoses are intended for the patients between the age of 15 and 124 years.

The sex symbols below address OCE edits and are used to detect inconsistencies between the patient's sex and diagnosis. They appear in the Tabular List of Diseases to the right of the code description:

♂   **Male diagnosis only**
This symbol appears to the right of the code description. This reference appears in the disease Tabular List.

♀   **Female diagnosis only**
This symbol appears to the right of the code description. This reference appears in the disease Tabular List.

Color Coding

To alert the coder to Medicare outpatient code edits and other important reimbursement issues, color bars have been added over the code descriptors in the Tabular List. Some codes carry more than one color.

Carriers use the Medicare Outpatient Code Editor (OCE) to examine claims for coding and billing accuracy and completeness. Color codes in this book signify Medicare code edits for manifestation codes not to be reported as a primary diagnosis, and when a more specific diagnosis code should be used.

Manifestation Code

These codes will appear in italic type as well as with a blue color bar over the code title. A manifestation code is not allowed to be reported as a first-listed diagnosis because each describes a manifestation of some other underlying disease, not the disease itself. This is referred to as mandatory multiple coding of etiology and manifestation. Code the underlying disease first. A *Code first underlying disease* instructional note will appear with underlying disease codes identified. In the Alphabetic Index these codes are listed as the secondary code in slanted brackets with the code for the underlying disease listed first.

Other Specified Code

These codes will appear with a gray color bar over the code title. Use these codes when the documentation indicates a specified diagnosis, but the ICD-9-CM system does not have a specific code that describes the diagnosis. These codes are may be stated as "Other" or "Not elsewhere classified (NEC)."

Unspecified Code

These codes will have a yellow color bar over the code title. Use these codes when the neither the diagnostic statement nor the documentation provides enough information to assign a more specified diagnosis code. These codes may be stated as "Unspecified" or "Not otherwise specified (NOS)." Note: Do not assign these codes when a more specific diagnosis has been determined.

Other Notations

DEF: This symbol indicates a definition of disease term. The definition will appear in blue type in the Disease Tabular Lists.

TIPS: This symbol precedes official coding advice found in the official coding guidelines and AHA's *Coding Clinic for ICD-9-CM*. Coding tips appear in blue type in the Tabular List.

I-10   In preparation for the transition to coding using the ICD-10-CM classification system, examples of ICD-10-CM codes have been provided for selected ICD-9-CM diagnosis codes. This symbol indicates that the code provided is an ICD-10-CM code to which the selected ICD-9-CM code is mapped.

Note: Coding professionals should keep in mind the following points when referring to the ICD-10-CM codes provided:

- ICD-10-CM codes are not currently valid for reporting purposes.
- The ICD-10-CM code may represent only one possible coding option. Since mappings between ICD-9-CM and ICD-10-CM are not always straightforward one-to-one correspondences due to the differences in terminology and clinical concepts, the mapping may result in a one-to-many code option. Not all code options for a particular ICD-9-CM

code are provided. For cases in which many code alternatives are possible in ICD-10-CM, only one example is provided.

- The ICD-10-CM code examples are provided only for the most frequently reported ICD-9-CM codes in each chapter.
- The ICD-10-CM codes are examples only and are provided to ease the transition to the new classification system.

PDx This symbol identifies a V code that generally is for use as a first listed diagnosis only but may be used as an additional diagnosis if the patient has more than one encounter on one day or there is more than one reason for the encounter.

Note: A V code without a symbol may be used as either a primary or secondary diagnosis.

Note: Please note that the symbols indicating the V code "principal or first-listed only" designation and the V codes that may be principal or first listed diagnoses included in the official coding guidelines [Section 1.C.18.e] are consistent with reporting guidelines for health care encounters *excluding acute care inpatient admissions*. These V code edits are often in conflict with the inpatient prospective payment system (IPPS) edits. For example, V22.0 Encounter for supervision of a normal first pregnancy, may be an appropriate primary reason for an outpatient encounter. However, supervision for a normal pregnancy is not an acceptable principal diagnosis for an inpatient admission and will have an unacceptable principal diagnosis edit under IPPS.

Medicare as Secondary Payer (MSP)

Note: This edit is no longer included in the official Medicare Code Editor (MCE).

Wrong Surgery Edit

When a particular surgical or other invasive procedure is indicated to treat a medical condition and the wrong procedure is performed, the procedure is not considered reasonable and necessary. Assign E codes to report these wrong surgery incidents. A Wrong Surgery edit associated with the E code will be triggered and the claim will be denied and returned to the provider. The wrong surgery E codes are identified with an asterisk (*) and a footnote.

Alphabetic Indexes

⏷ **Subterms under main terms may continue to next column/page.** This warning statement is a reminder to always check for additional subterms and information that may continue on to the next page or column before making a final selection.

Summary of Code Changes

● 786.30	Hemoptysis, unspecified Inclusion note added	
● 786.31	Acute idiopathic pulmonary hemorrhage in infants [AIPHI] Inclusion note added Exclusion note added	
● 786.39	Other hemoptysis Inclusion note added	
● 787.60	Full incontinence of feces Inclusion note added	
● 787.61	Incomplete defecation Exclusion note added	
● 787.62	Fecal smearing Inclusion note added	
● 787.63	Fecal urgency	
796.0	Use additional code note added	
● 799.5	Signs and symptoms involving cognition Exclusion note added	
● 799.51	Attention or concentration deficit	
● 799.52	Cognitive communication deficit	
● 799.53	Visuospatial deficit	
● 799.54	Psychomotor deficit	
● 799.55	Frontal lobe and executive function deficit	
● 799.59	Other signs and symptoms involving cognition	
799.82	Code first note added Use additional code note revised Exclusion term deleted	
800-999	INJURY AND POISONING Use additional code note added	
836.51	Inclusion term revised	
836.52	Inclusion term revised	
836.61	Inclusion note added	
836.62	Inclusion note added	
● 970.81	Cocaine Inclusion note added	
● 970.89	Other central nervous system stimulants	
980-989	TOXIC EFFECTS OF SUBSTANCES CHIEFLY NONMEDICINAL AS TO SOURCE Use additional code added	
992.0	Use additional code added	
▲ 995.2	Other and unspecified adverse effect of drug, medicinal and biological substance (due) to correct medicina substance properly administered Inclusion note deleted	
995.20	Inclusion note added	
995.27	Inclusion note added	
995.29	Inclusion note added	
995.94	Code first term added	
998	Exclusion note added	
▲ 999.6	ABO incompatibility reaction ▶due to transfusion of blood or blood products◀ Inclusion note deleted	
● 999.60	ABO incompatibility reaction, unspecified Inclusion note added	
● 999.61	ABO incompatibility with hemolytic transfusion reaction not specified as acute or delayed Inclusion note added	
● 999.62	ABO incompatibility with acute hemolytic transfusion reaction Inclusion note added	

● 999.63	ABO incompatibility with delayed hemolytic transfusion reaction Inclusion note added
● 999.69	Other ABO incompatibility reaction Inclusion note added
▲ 999.7	Rh ▶and other non-ABO◀ incompatibility reaction ▶due to transfusion of blood or blood products◀ Inclusion note deleted
● 999.70	Rh incompatibility reaction, unspecified Inclusion note added
● 999.71	Rh incompatibility with hemolytic transfusion reaction not specified as acute or delayed Inclusion note added
● 999.72	Rh incompatibility with acute hemolytic transfusion reaction Inclusion note added
● 999.73	Rh incompatibility with delayed hemolytic transfusion reaction Inclusion note added
● 999.74	Other Rh incompatibility reaction Inclusion note added
● 999.75	Non-ABO incompatibility reaction, unspecified Inclusion note added
● 999.76	Non-ABO incompatibility with hemolytic transfusion reaction not specified as acute or delayed Inclusion note added
● 999.77	Non-ABO incompatibility with acute hemolytic transfusion reaction Inclusion note added
● 999.78	Non-ABO incompatibility with delayed hemolytic transfusion reaction Inclusion note added
● 999.79	Other non-ABO incompatibility reaction Inclusion note added
▲ 999.8	Other ▶and unspecified◀ infusion and transfusion reaction Exclusion terms added
● 999.80	Transfusion reaction, unspecified Inclusion note added
● 999.83	Hemolytic transfusion reaction, incompatibility unspecified Inclusion note added
● 999.84	Acute hemolytic transfusion reaction, incompatibility unspecified Inclusion note added
● 999.85	Delayed hemolytic transfusion reaction, incompatibility unspecified Inclusion note added
999.89	Inclusion term added Inclusion term deleted
V01-V91	SUPPLEMENTARY CLASSIFICATION OF FACTORS INFLUENCING HEALTH STATUS AND CONTACT WITH HEALTH SERVICES ▶(V01-V91)◀
▲ V07	Need for isolation and other prophylactic ▶or treatment◀ measures Exclusion term added
▲ V07.5	Prophylactic uUse of agents affecting estrogen receptors and estrogen levels

▲ V07.51	Prophylactic uUse of selective estrogen receptor modulators (SERMs) Inclusion term revised
▲ V07.52	Prophylactic uUse of aromatase inhibitors Inclusion term revised
▲ V07.59	Prophylactic uUse of other agents affecting estrogen receptors and estrogen levels Inclusion term revised
▲ V07.8	Other specified prophylactic ▶or treatment◀ measure
▲ V07.9	Unspecified prophylactic ▶or treatment◀ measure
V10.5	Exclusion note added
● V11.4	Combat and operational stress reaction
V13.2	Exclusion term revised
● V13.23	Personal history of vaginal dysplasia Inclusion note added Exclusion note added`
● V13.24	Personal history of vulvar dysplasia Inclusion note added Exclusion note added
▲ V13.6	Congenital ▶(corrected)◀ malformations
▲ V13.61	Personal history of ▶(corrected) ◀ hHypospadias Hhypospadias
● V13.62	Personal history of other (corrected) congenital malformations of genitourinary system
● V13.63	Personal history of (corrected) congenital malformations of nervous system
● V13.64	Personal history of (corrected) congenital malformations of eye, ear, face and neck Inclusion note added
● V13.65	Personal history of (corrected) congenital malformations of heart and circulatory system
● V13.66	Personal history of (corrected) congenital malformations of respiratory system
● V13.67	Personal history of (corrected) congenital malformations of digestive system
● V13.68	Personal history of (corrected) congenital malformations of integument, limbs, and musculoskeletal systems
▲ V13.69	Personal history of other ▶(corrected) ◀ congenital malformations
● V15.53	Personal history of retained foreign body fully removed
V23.2	Exclusion terms revised
▲ V25.1	▶Encounter for insertion or removal◀ of intrauterine contraceptive device Exclusion note added
● V25.11	Encounter for insertion of intrauterine contraceptive device
● V25.12	Encounter for removal of intrauterine contraceptive device
● V25.13	Encounter for removal and reinsertion of intrauterine contraceptive device Inclusion note added
V25.4	Exclusion note deleted

V25.42	Inclusion term revised
	Exclusion note added
V26.32	Use additional code note revised
V26.35	Encounter for testing of male partner of ~~habitual aborter~~ ▶female with recurrent pregnancy loss◀
V45.01	Exclusion note added
V45.02	Inclusion note added
V45.5	Exclusion note deleted
V45.51	Exclusion note added
V45.79	Exclusion note added
V46.3	Code first note revised
● V49.86	Do not resuscitate status
● V49.87	Physical restraints status
	Exclusion note added
V53.31	Exclusion terms added
V53.32	Inclusion note added
V55	Exclusion term revised
V58.6	Inclusion terms added
	Exclusion term revised
● V62.85	Homicidal ideation
V76.51	Inclusion note added
● V85.41	Body Mass Index 40.0-44.9, adult
● V85.42	Body Mass Index 45.0-49.9, adult
● V85.43	Body Mass Index 50.0-59.9, adult
● V85.44	Body Mass Index 60.0-69.9, adult
● V85.45	Body Mass Index 70 and over, adult
V87.3	Exclusion term added
● V88.1	Acquired absence of pancreas
	Use additional code note added
● V88.11	Acquired total absence of pancreas
	Inclusion note added
● V88.12	Acquired partial absence of pancreas
●	RETAINED FOREIGN BODY (V90)
● V90	Retained foreign body
	Inclusion note added
	Exclusion note added
● V90.0	Retained radioactive fragment
● V90.01	Retained depleted uranium fragments
● V90.09	Other retained radioactive fragments
	Inclusion note added
● V90.1	Retained metal fragments
	Exclusion note added

● V90.10	Retained metal fragments, unspecified
	Inclusion note added
● V90.11	Retained magnetic metal fragments
● V90.12	Retained nonmagnetic metal fragments
● V90.2	Retained plastic fragments
	Inclusion note added
● V90.3	Retained organic fragments
● V90.31	Retained animal quills or spines
● V90.32	Retained tooth
● V90.33	Retained wood fragments
● V90.39	Other retained organic fragments
● V90.8	Other specified retained foreign body
● V90.81	Retained glass fragments
● V90.83	Retained stone or crystalline fragments
	Inclusion note added
● V90.89	Other specified retained foreign body
● V90.9	Retained foreign body, unspecified material
●	MULTIPLE GESTATION PLACENTA STATUS (V91)
● V91	Multiple gestation placenta status
	Code first note added
● V91.0	Twin gestation placenta status
● V91.00	Twin gestation, unspecified number of placenta, unspecified number of amniotic sacs
● V91.01	Twin gestation, monochorionic/monoamniotic (one placenta, one amniotic sac)
● V91.02	Twin gestation, monochorionic/diamniotic (one placenta, two amniotic sacs)
● V91.03	Twin gestation, dichorionic/diamniotic (two placentae, two amniotic sacs)
● V91.09	Twin gestation, unable to determine number of placenta and number of amniotic sacs
● V91.1	Triplet gestation placenta status
● V91.10	Triplet gestation, unspecified number of placenta and unspecified number of amniotic sacs

● V91.11	Triplet gestation, with two or more monochorionic fetuses
● V91.12	Triplet gestation, with two or more monoamniotic fetuses
● V91.19	Triplet gestation, unable to determine number of placenta and number of amniotic sacs
● V91.2	Quadruplet gestation placenta status
● V91.20	Quadruplet gestation, unspecified number of placenta and unspecified number of amniotic sacs
● V91.21	Quadruplet gestation, with two or more monochorionic fetuses
● V91.22	Quadruplet gestation, with two or more monoamniotic fetuses
● V91.29	Quadruplet gestation, unable to determine number of placenta and number of amniotic sacs
● V91.9	Other specified multiple gestation placenta status
	Inclusion note added
● V91.90	Other specified multiple gestation, unspecified number of placenta and unspecified number of amniotic sacs
● V91.91	Other specified multiple gestation, with two or more monochorionic fetuses
● V91.92	Other specified multiple gestation, with two or more monoamniotic fetuses
● V91.99	Other specified multiple gestation, unable to determine number of placenta and number of amniotic sacs
● E000.2	Volunteer activity
	Exclusion note added
E000.8	Inclusion term added
	Inclusion term deleted
E865	Exclusion term revised
E800-E848	Inclusion term added
	Inclusion term revised
E884.3	Inclusion note added
E885.0	Exclusion note added

Official ICD-9-CM Guidelines for Coding and Reporting

> **Note:** Revisions to these guidelines effective for October 1, 2010 were not available in time to be included in this edition. Once the revised guidelines are released, Ingenix will post the complete revised guidelines along with a summary of the changes on our web site. Log on to www.shopingenix.com/productalerts to review, download and print the documents.

Effective October 1, 2009
Narrative changes appear in bold text. Items underlined have been moved within the guidelines since October 1, 2008.

The Centers for Medicare and Medicaid Services (CMS) and the National Center for Health Statistics (NCHS), two departments within the U.S. Federal Government's Department of Health and Human Services (DHHS) provide the following guidelines for coding and reporting using the International Classification of Diseases, 9th Revision, Clinical Modification (ICD-9-CM). These guidelines should be used as a companion document to the official version of the ICD-9-CM as published on CD-ROM by the U.S. Government Printing Office (GPO).

These guidelines have been approved by the four organizations that make up the Cooperating Parties for the ICD-9-CM: the American Hospital Association (AHA), the American Health Information Management Association (AHIMA), CMS, and NCHS. These guidelines are included on the official government version of the ICD-9-CM, and also appear in *Coding Clinic for ICD-9-CM* published by the AHA.

These guidelines are a set of rules that have been developed to accompany and complement the official conventions and instructions provided within the ICD-9-CM itself. **The instructions and conventions of the classification take precedence over guidelines.** These guidelines are based on the coding and sequencing instructions in Volumes I, II and III of ICD-9-CM, but provide additional instruction. Adherence to these guidelines when assigning ICD-9-CM diagnosis and procedure codes is required under the Health Insurance Portability and Accountability Act (HIPAA). The diagnosis codes (Volumes 1-2) have been adopted under HIPAA for all healthcare settings. Volume 3 procedure codes have been adopted for inpatient procedures reported by hospitals. A joint effort between the healthcare provider and the coder is essential to achieve complete and accurate documentation, code assignment, and reporting of diagnoses and procedures. These guidelines have been developed to assist both the healthcare provider and the coder in identifying those diagnoses and procedures that are to be reported. The importance of consistent, complete documentation in the medical record cannot be overemphasized. Without such documentation accurate coding cannot be achieved. The entire record should be reviewed to determine the specific reason for the encounter and the conditions treated.

The term encounter is used for all settings, including hospital admissions. In the context of these guidelines, the term provider is used throughout the guidelines to mean physician or any qualified health care practitioner who is legally accountable for establishing the patient's diagnosis. Only this set of guidelines, approved by the Cooperating Parties, is official.

The guidelines are organized into sections. Section I includes the structure and conventions of the classification and general guidelines that apply to the entire classification, and chapter-specific guidelines that correspond to the chapters as they are arranged in the classification. Section II includes guidelines for selection of principal diagnosis for non-outpatient settings. Section III includes guidelines for reporting additional diagnoses in non-outpatient settings. Section IV is for outpatient coding and reporting.

Section I. Conventions, general coding guidelines and chapter specific guidelines

A. Conventions for the ICD-9-CM
  1. Format:
  2. Abbreviations
      a. Index abbreviations
      b. Tabular abbreviations
  3. Punctuation
  4. Includes and Excludes Notes and Inclusion terms
  5. Other and Unspecified codes
      a. "Other" codes
      b. "Unspecified" codes
  6. Etiology/manifestation convention ("code first", "use additional code" and "in diseases classified elsewhere" notes)
  7. "And"
  8. "With"
  9. "See" and "See Also"

B. General Coding Guidelines
  1. Use of Both Alphabetic Index and Tabular List
  2. Locate each term in the Alphabetic Index
  3. Level of Detail in Coding
  4. Code or codes from 001.0 through V91.99
  5. Selection of codes 001.0 through 999.9
  6. Signs and symptoms
  7. Conditions that are an integral part of a disease process
  8. Conditions that are not an integral part of a disease process
  9. Multiple coding for a single condition
  10. Acute and Chronic Conditions
  11. Combination Code
  12. Late Effects
  13. Impending or Threatened Condition
  14. Reporting Same Diagnosis Code More than Once
  15. Admissions/Encounters for Rehabilitation
  16. Documentation for BMI and Pressure Ulcer Stages
  17. **Syndromes**

C. Chapter-Specific Coding Guidelines
  1. Chapter 1: Infectious and Parasitic Diseases (001-139)
      a. Human Immunodeficiency Virus (HIV) Infections
      b. Septicemia, Systemic Inflammatory Response Syndrome (SIRS), Sepsis, Severe Sepsis and Septic Shock
      c. Methicillin Resistant *Staphylococcus aureus* (MRSA) Conditions
  2. Chapter 2: Neoplasms (140-239)
      a. Treatment directed at the malignancy
      b. Treatment of secondary site
      c. Coding and sequencing of complications
      d. Primary malignancy previously excised
      e. Admissions/Encounters involving chemotherapy, immunotherapy and radiation therapy
      f. Admission/encounter to determine extent of malignancy
      g. Symptoms, signs, and ill-defined conditions listed in Chapter 16 associated with neoplasms
      h. Admission/encounter for pain control/management
      i. Malignant neoplasm associated with transplanted organ

Section II. Selection of Principal Diagnosis

A.   Codes for symptoms, signs, and ill-defined conditions

B.   Two or more interrelated conditions, each potentially meeting the definition for principal diagnosis

C.   Two or more diagnoses that equally meet the definition for principal diagnosis

D.   Two or more comparative or contrasting conditions

E.   A symptom(s) followed by contrasting/comparative diagnoses

F.   Original treatment plan not carried out

G.   Complications of surgery and other medical care

H.   Uncertain Diagnosis

I.   Admission from Observation Unit

    1.   Admission Following Medical Observation

    2.   Admission Following Post-Operative Observation

J.   Admission from Outpatient Surgery

Section III. Reporting Additional Diagnoses

A.   Previous conditions

B.   Abnormal findings

C.   Uncertain diagnosis

Section IV. Diagnostic Coding and Reporting Guidelines for Outpatient Services

A.   Selection of first-listed condition

    1.   Outpatient Surgery

    2.   Observation Stay

B.   Codes from 001.0 through V89.09

C.   Accurate reporting of ICD-9-CM diagnosis codes

D.   Selection of codes 001.0 through 999.9

E.   Codes that describe symptoms and signs

F.   Encounters for circumstances other than a disease or injury

G.   Level of Detail in Coding

    1.   ICD-9-CM codes with 3, 4, or 5 digits

    2.   Use of full number of digits required for a code

H.   ICD-9-CM code for the diagnosis, condition, problem, or other reason for encounter/visit

I.   Uncertain diagnosis

J.   Chronic diseases

K.   Code all documented conditions that coexist

L.   Patients receiving diagnostic services only

M.   Patients receiving therapeutic services only

N.   Patients receiving preoperative evaluations only

O.   Ambulatory surgery

P.   Routine outpatient prenatal visits

Appendix I: Present on Admission Reporting Guidelines

SECTION I. CONVENTIONS, GENERAL CODING GUIDELINES AND CHAPTER SPECIFIC GUIDELINES

The conventions, general guidelines and chapter-specific guidelines are applicable to all health care settings unless otherwise indicated. **The conventions and instructions of the classification take precedence over guidelines.**

A.   Conventions for the ICD-9-CM

The conventions for the ICD-9-CM are the general rules for use of the classification independent of the guidelines. These conventions are incorporated within the index and tabular of the ICD-9-CM as instructional notes. The conventions are as follows:

    1.   Format:

        The ICD-9-CM uses an indented format for ease in reference

    2.   Abbreviations

        a.   Index abbreviations

            NEC " Not elsewhere classifiable"
            This abbreviation in the index represents "other specified" when a specific code is not available for a condition the index directs the coder to the "other specified" code in the tabular.

        b.   Tabular abbreviations

            NEC "Not elsewhere classifiable"
            This abbreviation in the tabular represents "other specified". When a specific code is not available for a condition the tabular includes an NEC entry under a code to identify the code as the "other specified" code.

            See Section I.A.5.a. "Other" codes"

            NOS "Not otherwise specified"
            This abbreviation is the equivalent of unspecified.
            See Section I.A.5.b., "Unspecified" codes

    3.   Punctuation

        [ ]   Brackets are used in the tabular list to enclose synonyms, alternative wording or explanatory phrases. Brackets are used in the index to identify manifestation codes.

            See Section I.A.6. "Etiology/manifestations"

        ( )   Parentheses are used in both the index and tabular to enclose supplementary words that may be present or absent in the statement of a disease or procedure without affecting the code number to which it is assigned. The terms within the parentheses are referred to as nonessential modifiers.

        :   Colons are used in the Tabular list after an incomplete term which needs one or more of the modifiers following the colon to make it assignable to a given category.

    4.   Includes and Excludes Notes and Inclusion terms

        Includes: This note appears immediately under a three-digit code title to further define, or give examples of, the content of the category.

        Excludes: An excludes note under a code indicates that the terms excluded from the code are to be coded elsewhere. In some cases the codes for the excluded terms should not be used in conjunction with the code from which it is excluded. An example of this is a congenital condition excluded from an acquired form of the same condition. The congenital and acquired codes should not be used together. In other cases, the excluded terms may be used together with an excluded code. An example of this is when fractures of different bones are coded to different codes. Both codes may be used together if both types of fractures are present.

        Inclusion terms: List of terms is included under certain four and five digit codes. These terms are the conditions for which that code number is to be used. The terms may be synonyms of the code title, or, in the case of "other specified" codes, the terms are a list of the various conditions assigned to that code. The inclusion terms are not necessarily exhaustive. Additional terms found only in the index may also be assigned to a code.

    5.   Other and Unspecified codes

        a.   "Other" codes
            Codes titled "other" or "other specified" (usually a code with a 4th digit 8 or fifth-digit 9 for diagnosis codes) are for use when the information in the medical record provides detail for which a specific code does not exist. Index entries with NEC in the line designate "other" codes in the tabular. These index entries represent specific disease entities for which no specific code exists so the term is included within an "other" code.

        b.   "Unspecified" codes
            Codes (usually a code with a 4th digit 9 or 5th digit 0 for diagnosis codes) titled "unspecified" are for use when the information in the medical record is insufficient to assign a more specific code.

    6.   Etiology/manifestation convention ("Code first," "Use additional code" and "In diseases classified elsewhere" notes)

        Certain conditions have both an underlying etiology and multiple body system manifestations due to the underlying etiology. For such conditions, the ICD-9-CM has a coding convention that requires the underlying condition be sequenced first followed by the manifestation. Wherever such a combination exists, there is a "Use additional code" note at the etiology code, and a "Code first" note at the manifestation code. These instructional notes indicate the proper sequencing order of the codes, etiology followed by manifestation.

In most cases the manifestation codes will have in the code title, "In diseases classified elsewhere." Codes with this title are a component of the etiology/ manifestation convention. The code title indicates that it is a manifestation code. "In diseases classified elsewhere" codes are never permitted to be used as first listed or principal diagnosis codes. They must be used in conjunction with an underlying condition code and they must be listed following the underlying condition.

There are manifestation codes that do not have "In diseases classified elsewhere" in the title. For such codes a "Use additional code" note will still be present and the rules for sequencing apply.

In addition to the notes in the tabular, these conditions also have a specific index entry structure. In the index both conditions are listed together with the etiology code first followed by the manifestation codes in brackets. The code in brackets is always to be sequenced second.

The most commonly used etiology/manifestation combinations are the codes for Diabetes mellitus, category 250. For each code under category 250 there is a use additional code note for the manifestation that is specific for that particular diabetic manifestation. Should a patient have more than one manifestation of diabetes, more than one code from category 250 may be used with as many manifestation codes as are needed to fully describe the patient's complete diabetic condition. The category 250 diabetes codes should be sequenced first, followed by the manifestation codes.

"Code first" and "Use additional code" notes are also used as sequencing rules in the classification for certain codes that are not part of an etiology/ manifestation combination.

See - Section I.B.9. "Multiple coding for a single condition."

7. **"And"**
   The word "and" should be interpreted to mean either "and" or "or" when it appears in a title.

8. **"With"**
   The word "with" in the alphabetic index is sequenced immediately following the main term, not in alphabetical order.

9. **"See" and "See Also"**
   The "see" instruction following a main term in the index indicates that another term should be referenced. It is necessary to go to the main term referenced with the "see" note to locate the correct code.

   A "see also" instruction following a main term in the index instructs that there is another main term that may also be referenced that may provide additional index entries that may be useful. It is not necessary to follow the "see also" note when the original main term provides the necessary code.

B. **General Coding Guidelines**

1. **Use of Both Alphabetic Index and Tabular List**
   Use both the Alphabetic Index and the Tabular List when locating and assigning a code. Reliance on only the Alphabetic Index or the Tabular List leads to errors in code assignments and less specificity in code selection.

2. **Locate each term in the Alphabetic Index**
   Locate each term in the Alphabetic Index and verify the code selected in the Tabular List. Read and be guided by instructional notations that appear in both the Alphabetic Index and the Tabular List.

3. **Level of Detail in Coding**
   Diagnosis and procedure codes are to be used at their highest number of digits available.

   ICD-9-CM diagnosis codes are composed of codes with 3, 4, or 5 digits. Codes with three digits are included in ICD-9-CM as the heading of a category of codes that may be further subdivided by the use of fourth and/or fifth-digits, which provide greater detail.

A three-digit code is to be used only if it is not further subdivided. Where fourth-digit subcategories and/or fifth-digit subclassifications are provided, they must be assigned. A code is invalid if it has not been coded to the full number of digits required for that code. For example, Acute myocardial infarction, code 410, has fourth-digits that describe the location of the infarction (e.g., 410.2, Of inferolateral wall), and fifth-digits that identify the episode of care. It would be incorrect to report a code in category 410 without a fourth and fifth-digit.

ICD-9-CM Volume 3 procedure codes are composed of codes with either 3 or 4 digits. Codes with two digits are included in ICD-9-CM as the heading of a category of codes that may be further subdivided by the use of third and/or fourth-digits, which provide greater detail.

4. **Code or codes from 001.0 through V91.99**
   The appropriate code or codes from 001.0 through V89.09 must be used to identify diagnoses, symptoms, conditions, problems, complaints or other reason(s) for the encounter/visit.

5. **Selection of codes 001.0 through 999.9**
   The selection of codes 001.0 through 999.9 will frequently be used to describe the reason for the admission/encounter. These codes are from the section of ICD-9-CM for the classification of diseases and injuries (e.g., infectious and parasitic diseases; neoplasms; symptoms, signs, and ill-defined conditions, etc.).

6. **Signs and symptoms**
   Codes that describe symptoms and signs, as opposed to diagnoses, are acceptable for reporting purposes when a related definitive diagnosis has not been established (confirmed) by the provider. Chapter 16 of ICD-9-CM, Symptoms, Signs, and Ill-Defined conditions (codes 780.0 - 799.9) contain many, but not all codes for symptoms.

7. **Conditions that are an integral part of a disease process**
   Signs and symptoms that are associated routinely with a disease process should not be assigned as additional codes, unless otherwise instructed by the classification.

8. **Conditions that are not an integral part of a disease process**
   Additional signs and symptoms that may not be associated routinely with a disease process should be coded when present.

9. **Multiple coding for a single condition**
   In addition to the etiology/manifestation convention that requires two codes to fully describe a single condition that affects multiple body systems, there are other single conditions that also require more than one code. "Use additional code" notes are found in the tabular at codes that are not part of an etiology/manifestation pair where a secondary code is useful to fully describe a condition. The sequencing rule is the same as the etiology/manifestation pair, the "Use additional code" indicates that a secondary code should be added.

   For example, for infections that are not included in chapter 1, a secondary code from category 041, Bacterial infection in conditions classified elsewhere and of unspecified site, may be required to identify the bacterial organism causing the infection. A "Use additional code" note will normally be found at the infectious disease code, indicating a need for the organism code to be added as a secondary code.

   "Code first" notes are also under certain codes that are not specifically manifestation codes but may be due to an underlying cause. When a "Code first" note is present and an underlying condition is present the underlying condition should be sequenced first.

   "Code, if applicable, any causal condition first", notes indicate that this code may be assigned as a principal diagnosis when the causal condition is unknown or not applicable. If a causal condition is known, then the code for that condition should be sequenced as the principal or first-listed diagnosis.

   Multiple coding may be needed for late effects, complication codes and obstetric codes to more fully describe a condition. See the specific guidelines for these conditions for further instruction.

10. **Acute and Chronic Conditions**
    If the same condition is described as both acute (subacute) and chronic, and separate subentries exist in the Alphabetic Index at the same indentation level, code both and sequence the acute (subacute) code first.

11. Combination Code
A combination code is a single code used to classify:

- Two diagnoses, or

- A diagnosis with an associated secondary process (manifestation)

- A diagnosis with an associated complication

Combination codes are identified by referring to subterm entries in the Alphabetic Index and by reading the inclusion and exclusion notes in the Tabular List.

Assign only the combination code when that code fully identifies the diagnostic conditions involved or when the Alphabetic Index so directs. Multiple coding should not be used when the classification provides a combination code that clearly identifies all of the elements documented in the diagnosis. When the combination code lacks necessary specificity in describing the manifestation or complication, an additional code should be used as a secondary code.

12. Late Effects
A late effect is the residual effect (condition produced) after the acute phase of an illness or injury has terminated. There is no time limit on when a late effect code can be used. The residual may be apparent early, such as in cerebrovascular accident cases, or it may occur months or years later, such as that due to a previous injury. Coding of late effects generally requires two codes sequenced in the following order: The condition or nature of the late effect is sequenced first. The late effect code is sequenced second.

An exception to the above guidelines are those instances where the code for late effect is followed by a manifestation code identified in the Tabular List and title, or the late effect code has been expanded (at the fourth and fifth-digit levels) to include the manifestation(s). The code for the acute phase of an illness or injury that led to the late effect is never used with a code for the late effect.

13. Impending or Threatened Condition
Code any condition described at the time of discharge as "impending" or "threatened" as follows:

If it did occur, code as confirmed diagnosis. If it did not occur, reference the Alphabetic Index to determine if the condition has a subentry term for "impending" or "threatened" and also reference main term entries for "Impending" and for "Threatened." If the subterms are listed, assign the given code. If the subterms are not listed, code the existing underlying condition(s) and not the condition described as impending or threatened.

14. Reporting Same Diagnosis Code More than Once
Each unique ICD-9-CM diagnosis code may be reported only once for an encounter. This applies to bilateral conditions or two different conditions classified to the same ICD-9-CM diagnosis code.

15. Admissions/Encounters for Rehabilitation
When the purpose for the admission/encounter is rehabilitation, sequence the appropriate V code from category V57, Care involving use of rehabilitation procedures, as the principal/first-listed diagnosis. The code for the condition for which the service is being performed should be reported as an additional diagnosis.

Only one code from category V57 is required. Code V57.89, Other specified rehabilitation procedures, should be assigned if more than one type of rehabilitation is performed during a single encounter. A procedure code should be reported to identify each type of rehabilitation therapy actually performed.

16. Documentation for BMI and Pressure Ulcer Stages
For the Body Mass Index (BMI) and pressure ulcer stage codes, code assignment may be based on medical record documentation from clinicians who are not the patient's provider (i.e., physician or other qualified healthcare practitioner legally accountable for establishing the patient's diagnosis), since this information is typically documented by other clinicians involved in the care of the patient (e.g., a dietitian often documents the BMI and nurses often documents the pressure ulcer

stages). However, the associated diagnosis (such as overweight, obesity, or pressure ulcer) must be documented by the patient's provider. If there is conflicting medical record documentation, either from the same clinician or different clinicians, the patient's attending provider should be queried for clarification.

The BMI and pressure ulcer stage codes should only be reported as secondary diagnoses. As with all other secondary diagnosis codes, the BMI and pressure ulcer stage codes should only be assigned when they meet the definition of a reportable additional diagnosis.

See Section III, Reporting Additional Diagnoses.

17. Syndromes
Follow the Alphabetic Index guidance when coding syndromes. In the absence of index guidance, assign codes for the documented manifestations of the syndrome.

C. Chapter-Specific Coding Guidelines
In addition to general coding guidelines, there are guidelines for specific diagnoses and/or conditions in the classification. Unless otherwise indicated, these guidelines apply to all health care settings. Please refer to Section II for guidelines on the selection of principal diagnosis.

1. Chapter 1: Infectious and Parasitic Diseases (001-139)

a. Human Immunodeficiency Virus (HIV) Infections

1) Code only confirmed cases
Code only confirmed cases of HIV infection/illness. This is an exception to the hospital inpatient guideline Section II, H.

In this context, "confirmation" does not require documentation of positive serology or culture for HIV; the provider's diagnostic statement that the patient is HIV positive, or has an HIV-related illness is sufficient.

2) Selection and sequencing of HIV codes

(a) Patient admitted for HIV-related condition
If a patient is admitted for an HIV-related condition, the principal diagnosis should be 042, followed by additional diagnosis codes for all reported HIV-related conditions.

(b) Patient with HIV disease admitted for unrelated condition
If a patient with HIV disease is admitted for an unrelated condition (such as a traumatic injury), the code for the unrelated condition (e.g., the nature of injury code) should be the principal diagnosis. Other diagnoses would be 042 followed by additional diagnosis codes for all reported HIV-related conditions.

(c) Whether the patient is newly diagnosed
Whether the patient is newly diagnosed or has had previous admissions/encounters for HIV conditions is irrelevant to the sequencing decision.

(d) Asymptomatic human immunodeficiency virus
V08 Asymptomatic human immunodeficiency virus [HIV] infection, is to be applied when the patient without any documentation of symptoms is listed as being "HIV positive," "known HIV," "HIV test positive," or similar terminology. Do not use this code if the term "AIDS" is used or if the patient is treated for any HIV-related illness or is described as having any condition(s) resulting from his/her HIV positive status; use 042 in these cases.

(e) Patients with inconclusive HIV serology
Patients with inconclusive HIV serology, but no definitive diagnosis or manifestations of the illness, may be assigned code 795.71, Inconclusive serologic test for Human Immunodeficiency Virus [HIV].

(f) Previously diagnosed HIV-related illness
Patients with any known prior diagnosis of an HIV-related illness should be coded to 042. Once a patient has developed an HIV-related illness, the patient should always

be assigned code 042 on every subsequent admission/encounter. Patients previously diagnosed with any HIV illness (042) should never be assigned to 795.71 or V08.

(g) HIV Infection in Pregnancy, Childbirth and the Puerperium
During pregnancy, childbirth or the puerperium, a patient admitted (or presenting for a health care encounter) because of an HIV-related illness should receive a principal diagnosis code of 647.6x, Other specified infectious and parasitic diseases in the mother classifiable elsewhere, but complicating the pregnancy, childbirth or the puerperium, followed by 042 and the code(s) for the HIV-related illness(es). Codes from Chapter 15 always take sequencing priority.

Patients with asymptomatic HIV infection status admitted (or presenting for a health care encounter) during pregnancy, childbirth, or the puerperium should receive codes of 647.6x and V08.

(h) Encounters for testing for HIV If a patient is being seen to determine his/her HIV status, use code V73.89, Screening for other specified viral disease. Use code V69.8, Other problems related to lifestyle, as a secondary code if an asymptomatic patient is in a known high risk group for HIV. Should a patient with signs or symptoms or illness, or a confirmed HIV related diagnosis be tested for HIV, code the signs and symptoms or the diagnosis. An additional counseling code V65.44 may be used if counseling is provided during the encounter for the test.

When a patient returns to be informed of his/her HIV test results use code V65.44, HIV counseling, if the results of the test are negative.

If the results are positive but the patient is asymptomatic use code V08, Asymptomatic HIV infection. If the results are positive and the patient is symptomatic use code 042, HIV infection, with codes for the HIV related symptoms or diagnosis. The HIV counseling code may also be used if counseling is provided for patients with positive test results.

b. Septicemia, Systemic Inflammatory Response Syndrome (SIRS), Sepsis, Severe Sepsis, and Septic Shock

1) SIRS, Septicemia, and Sepsis

(a) The terms *septicemia* and *sepsis* are often used interchangeably by providers, however they are not considered synonymous terms. The following descriptions are provided for reference but do not preclude querying the provider for clarification about terms used in the documentation:

(i) Septicemia generally refers to a systemic disease associated with the presence of pathological microorganisms or toxins in the blood, which can include bacteria, viruses, fungi or other organisms.

(ii) Systemic inflammatory response syndrome (SIRS) generally refers to the systemic response to infection, trauma/burns, or other insult (such as cancer) with symptoms including fever, tachycardia, tachypnea, and leukocytosis.

(iii) Sepsis generally refers to SIRS due to infection.

(iv) Severe sepsis generally refers to sepsis with associated acute organ dysfunction.

(b) The coding of SIRS, sepsis and severe sepsis
The coding of SIRS, sepsis and severe sepsis requires a minimum of 2 codes: a code for the underlying cause (such as infection or trauma) and a code from subcategory 995.9 Systemic inflammatory response syndrome (SIRS).

(i) The code for the underlying cause (such as infection or trauma) must be sequenced before the code from subcategory 995.9 Systemic inflammatory response syndrome (SIRS).

(ii) Sepsis and severe sepsis require a code for the systemic infection (038.xx, 112.5, etc.) and either code 995.91, Sepsis, or 995.92, Severe sepsis. If the causal organism is not documented, assign code 038.9, Unspecified septicemia.

(iii) Severe sepsis requires additional code(s) for the associated acute organ dysfunction(s).

(iv) If a patient has sepsis with multiple organ dysfunctions, follow the instructions for coding severe sepsis.

(v) Either the term sepsis or SIRS must be documented to assign a code from subcategory 995.9.

See Section I.C.17.g, Injury and poisoning, for information regarding systemic inflammatory response syndrome (SIRS) due to trauma/burns and other non-infectious processes.

(c) Due to the complex nature of sepsis and severe sepsis, some cases may require querying the provider prior to assignment of the codes.

2) Sequencing sepsis and severe sepsis

(a) Sepsis and severe sepsis as principal diagnosis
If sepsis or severe sepsis is present on admission, and meets the definition of principal diagnosis, the systemic infection code (e.g., 038.xx, 112.5, etc) should be assigned as the principal diagnosis, followed by code 995.91, Sepsis, or 995.92, Severe sepsis, as required by the sequencing rules in the Tabular List. Codes from subcategory 995.9 can never be assigned as a principal diagnosis. A code should also be assigned for any localized infection, if present.

If the sepsis or severe sepsis is due to a postprocedural infection, *see Section I.C.10 for guidelines related to sepsis due to postprocedural infection.*

(b) Sepsis and severe sepsis as secondary diagnoses
When sepsis or severe sepsis develops during the encounter (it was not present on admission), the systemic infection code and code 995.91 or 995.92 should be assigned as secondary diagnoses.

(c) Documentation unclear as to whether sepsis or severe sepsis is present on admission
Sepsis or severe sepsis may be present on admission but the diagnosis may not be confirmed until sometime after admission. If the documentation is not clear whether the sepsis or severe sepsis was present on admission, the provider should be queried.

3) Sepsis/SIRS with Localized Infection
If the reason for admission is both sepsis, severe sepsis, or SIRS and a localized infection, such as pneumonia or cellulitis, a code for the systemic infection (038.xx, 112.5, etc) should be assigned first, then code 995.91 or 995.92, followed by the code for the localized infection. If the patient is admitted with a localized infection, such as pneumonia, and sepsis/SIRS doesn't develop until after admission, see guideline I.C.1.b.2.b.

If the localized infection is postprocedural, *see Section I.C.10 for guidelines related to sepsis due to postprocedural infection.*

Note: The term urosepsis is a nonspecific term. If that is the only term documented then only code 599.0 should be assigned based on the default for the term in the ICD-9-CM index, in addition to the code for the causal organism if known.

4) Bacterial Sepsis and Septicemia

In most cases, it will be a code from category 038, Septicemia, that will be used in conjunction with a code from subcategory 995.9 such as the following:

(a) Streptococcal sepsis

If the documentation in the record states streptococcal sepsis, codes 038.0, Streptococcal septicemia, and code 995.91 should be used, in that sequence.

(b) Streptococcal septicemia

If the documentation states streptococcal septicemia, only code 038.0 should be assigned, however, the provider should be queried whether the patient has sepsis, an infection with SIRS.

5) Acute organ dysfunction that is not clearly associated with the sepsis

If a patient has sepsis and an acute organ dysfunction, but the medical record documentation indicates that the acute organ dysfunction is related to a medical condition other than the sepsis, do not assign code 995.92, Severe sepsis. An acute organ dysfunction must be associated with the sepsis in order to assign the severe sepsis code. If the documentation is not clear as to whether an acute organ dysfunction is related to the sepsis or another medical condition, query the provider.

6) Septic shock

(a) Sequencing of septic shock

Septic shock generally refers to circulatory failure associated with severe sepsis, and, therefore, it represents a type of acute organ dysfunction.

For all cases of septic shock, the code for the systemic infection should be sequenced first, followed by codes 995.92 and 785.52. Any additional codes for other acute organ dysfunctions should also be assigned. As noted in the sequencing instructions in the Tabular List, the code for septic shock cannot be assigned as a principal diagnosis.

(b) Septic Shock without documentation of severe sepsis

Septic shock indicates the presence of severe sepsis.

Code 995.92, Severe sepsis, must be assigned with code 785.52, Septic shock, even if the term severe sepsis is not documented in the record. The "Use additional code" note and the "Code first" note in the tabular support this guideline.

7) Sepsis and septic shock complicating abortion and pregnancy

Sepsis and septic shock complicating abortion, ectopic pregnancy, and molar pregnancy are classified to category codes in Chapter 11 (630-639).

See section I.C.11.i.7. for information on the coding of puerperal sepsis.

8) Negative or inconclusive blood cultures

Negative or inconclusive blood cultures do not preclude a diagnosis of septicemia or sepsis in patients with clinical evidence of the condition, however, the provider should be queried.

9) Newborn sepsis

See Section I.C.15.j for information on the coding of newborn sepsis.

10) Sepsis due to a postprocedural infection

(a) Documentation of causal relationship

As with all postprocedural complications, code assignment is based on the provider's documentation of the relationship between the infection and the procedure.

(b) Sepsis due to postprocedural infection

In cases of postprocedural sepsis, the complication code, such as code 998.59, Other postoperative infection, or 674.3x, Other complications of obstetrical surgical wounds

should be coded first followed by the appropriate sepsis codes (systemic infection code and either code 995.91 or 995.92). An additional code(s) for any acute organ dysfunction should also be assigned for cases of severe sepsis.

11) External cause of injury codes with SIRS

Refer to Section I.C.19.a.7 for instruction on the use of external cause of injury codes with codes for SIRS resulting from trauma.

12) Sepsis and severe sepsis associated with noninfectious process

In some cases, a non-infectious process, such as trauma, may lead to an infection which can result in sepsis or severe sepsis. If sepsis or severe sepsis is documented as associated with a non-infectious condition, such as a burn or serious injury, and this condition meets the definition for principal diagnosis, the code for the noninfectious condition should be sequenced first, followed by the code for the systemic infection and either code 995.91, Sepsis, or 995.92, Severe sepsis. Additional codes for any associated acute organ dysfunction(s) should also be assigned for cases of severe sepsis. If the sepsis or severe sepsis meets the definition of principal diagnosis, the systemic infection and sepsis codes should be sequenced before the non-infectious condition. When both the associated non-infectious condition and the sepsis or severe sepsis meet the definition of principal diagnosis, either may be assigned as principal diagnosis.

See Section I.C.1.b.2) (a) for guidelines pertaining to sepsis or severe sepsis as the principal diagnosis.

Only one code from subcategory 995.9 should be assigned. Therefore, when a non-infectious condition leads to an infection resulting in sepsis or severe sepsis, assign either code 995.91 or 995.92. Do not additionally assign code 995.93, Systemic inflammatory response syndrome due to non-infectious process without acute organ dysfunction, or 995.94, Systemic inflammatory response syndrome with acute organ dysfunction.

See Section I.C.17.g for information on the coding of SIRS due to trauma/burns or other non-infectious disease processes.

c. Methicillin Resistant *Staphylococcus aureus* (MRSA) Conditions

1) Selection and sequencing of MRSA codes

(a) Combination codes for MRSA infection

When a patient is diagnosed with an infection that is due to methicillin resistant *Staphylococcus aureus* (MRSA), and that infection has a combination code that includes the causal organism (e.g., septicemia, pneumonia) assign the appropriate code for the condition (e.g., code 038.12, Methicillin resistant *Staphylococcus aureus* septicemia or code 482.42, Methicillin resistant pneumonia due to *Staphylococcus aureus*). Do not assign code 041.12, Methicillin resistant *Staphylococcus aureus*, as an additional code because the code includes the type of infection and the MRSA organism. Do not assign a code from subcategory V09.0, Infection with microorganisms resistant to penicillins, as an additional diagnosis.

See Section C.1.b.1 for instructions on coding and sequencing of septicemia.

(b) Other codes for MRSA infection

When there is documentation of a current infection (e.g., wound infection, stitch abscess, urinary tract infection) due to MRSA, and that infection does not have a combination code that includes the causal organism, select the appropriate code to identify the condition along with code 041.12, Methicillin resistant *Staphylococcus aureus*, for the MRSA infection. Do not assign a code from subcategory V09.0, Infection with microorganisms resistant to penicillins.

(c) **Methicillin susceptible *Staphylococcus aureus* (MSSA) and MRSA colonization**
The condition or state of being colonized or carrying MSSA or MRSA is called colonization or carriage, while an individual person is described as being colonized or being a carrier. Colonization means that MSSA or MSRA is present on or in the body without necessarily causing illness. A positive MRSA colonization test might be documented by the provider as "MRSA screen positive" or "MRSA nasal swab positive".

Assign code V02.54, Carrier or suspected carrier, Methicillin resistant *Staphylococcus aureus*, for patients documented as having MRSA colonization. Assign code V02.53, Carrier or suspected carrier, Methicillin susceptible *Staphylococcus aureus*, for patient documented as having MSSA colonization. Colonization is not necessarily indicative of a disease process or as the cause of a specific condition the patient may have unless documented as such by the provider.

Code V02.59, Other specified bacterial diseases, should be assigned for other types of staphylococcal colonization (e.g., S. epidermidis, S. saprophyticus). Code V02.59 should not be assigned for colonization with any type of *Staphylococcus aureus* (MRSA, MSSA).

(d) **MRSA colonization and infection**
If a patient is documented as having both MRSA colonization and infection during a hospital admission, code V02.54, Carrier or suspected carrier, Methicillin resistant *Staphylococcus aureus*, and a code for the MRSA infection may both be assigned.

2. Chapter 2: Neoplasms (140-239)

General guidelines
Chapter 2 of the ICD-9-CM contains the codes for most benign and all malignant neoplasms. Certain benign neoplasms, such as prostatic adenomas, may be found in the specific body system chapters. To properly code a neoplasm it is necessary to determine from the record if the neoplasm is benign, in-situ, malignant, or of uncertain histologic behavior. If malignant, any secondary (metastatic) sites should also be determined.

The neoplasm table in the Alphabetic Index should be referenced first. However, if the histological term is documented, that term should be referenced first, rather than going immediately to the Neoplasm Table, in order to determine which column in the Neoplasm Table is appropriate. For example, if the documentation indicates "adenoma," refer to the term in the Alphabetic Index to review the entries under this term and the instructional note to "see also neoplasm, by site, benign." The table provides the proper code based on the type of neoplasm and the site. It is important to select the proper column in the table that corresponds to the type of neoplasm. The tabular should then be referenced to verify that the correct code has been selected from the table and that a more specific site code does not exist.

See Section I. C. 18.d.4. for information regarding V codes for genetic susceptibility to cancer.

a. **Treatment directed at the malignancy**
If the treatment is directed at the malignancy, designate the malignancy as the principal diagnosis.

The only exception to this guideline is if a patient admission/encounter is solely for the administration of

chemotherapy, immunotherapy or radiation therapy, assign the appropriate V58.x code as the first-listed or principal diagnosis, and the diagnosis or problem for which the service is being performed as a secondary diagnosis.

b. **Treatment of secondary site**
When a patient is admitted because of a primary neoplasm with metastasis and treatment is directed toward the secondary site only, the secondary neoplasm is designated as the principal diagnosis even though the primary malignancy is still present.

c. **Coding and sequencing of complications**
Coding and sequencing of complications associated with the malignancies or with the therapy thereof are subject to the following guidelines:

1) **Anemia associated with malignancy**
When admission/encounter is for management of an anemia associated with the malignancy, and the treatment is only for anemia, the appropriate anemia code (such as code 285.22, Anemia in neoplastic disease) is designated as the principal diagnosis and is followed by the appropriate code(s) for the malignancy.

Code 285.22 may also be used as a secondary code if the patient suffers from anemia and is being treated for the malignancy.

Code 285.22, Anemia in neoplastic disease, and code 285.3, Antineoplastic chemotherapy induced anemia, may both be assigned if anemia in neoplastic disease and anemia due to antineoplastic chemotherapy are both documented.

2) **Anemia associated with chemotherapy, immunotherapy and radiation therapy**
When the admission/encounter is for management of an anemia associated with chemotherapy, immunotherapy or radiotherapy and the only treatment is for the anemia, the anemia is sequenced first. The appropriate neoplasm code should be assigned as an additional code.

3) **Management of dehydration due to the malignancy**
When the admission/encounter is for management of dehydration due to the malignancy or the therapy, or a combination of both, and only the dehydration is being treated (intravenous rehydration), the dehydration is sequenced first, followed by the code(s) for the malignancy.

4) **Treatment of a complication resulting from a surgical procedure**
When the admission/encounter is for treatment of a complication resulting from a surgical procedure, designate the complication as the principal or first-listed diagnosis if treatment is directed at resolving the complication.

d. **Primary malignancy previously excised**
When a primary malignancy has been previously excised or eradicated from its site and there is no further treatment directed to that site and there is no evidence of any existing primary malignancy, a code from category V10, Personal history of malignant neoplasm, should be used to indicate the former site of the malignancy. Any mention of extension, invasion, or metastasis to another site is coded as a secondary malignant neoplasm to that site. The secondary site may be the principal or first-listed with the V10 code used as a secondary code.

e. **Admissions/Encounters involving chemotherapy, immunotherapy and radiation therapy**

1) **Episode of care involves surgical removal of neoplasm**
When an episode of care involves the surgical removal of a neoplasm, primary or secondary site, followed by adjunct chemotherapy or radiation treatment during the same episode of care, the neoplasm code should be assigned as principal or first-listed diagnosis, using codes in the 140-198 series or where appropriate in the 200-203 series.

2) Patient admission/encounter solely for administration of chemotherapy, immunotherapy and radiation therapy

If a patient admission/encounter is solely for the administration of chemotherapy, immunotherapy or radiation therapy assign code V58.0, Encounter for radiation therapy, or V58.11, Encounter for antineoplastic chemotherapy, or V58.12, Encounter for antineoplastic immunotherapy as the first-listed or principal diagnosis. If a patient receives more than one of these therapies during the same admission more than one of these codes may be assigned, in any sequence.

The malignancy for which the therapy is being administered should be assigned as a secondary diagnosis.

3) Patient admitted for radiotherapy/chemotherapy and immunotherapy and develops complications

When a patient is admitted for the purpose of radiotherapy, immunotherapy or chemotherapy and develops complications such as uncontrolled nausea and vomiting or dehydration, the principal or first-listed diagnosis is V58.0, Encounter for radiotherapy, or V58.11, Encounter for antineoplastic chemotherapy, or V58.12, Encounter for antineoplastic immunotherapy followed by any codes for the complications.

f. Admission/encounter to determine extent of malignancy

When the reason for admission/encounter is to determine the extent of the malignancy, or for a procedure such as paracentesis or thoracentesis, the primary malignancy or appropriate metastatic site is designated as the principal or first-listed diagnosis, even though chemotherapy or radiotherapy is administered.

g. Symptoms, signs, and ill-defined conditions listed in Chapter 16 associated with neoplasms

Symptoms, signs, and ill-defined conditions listed in Chapter 16 characteristic of, or associated with, an existing primary or secondary site malignancy cannot be used to replace the malignancy as principal or first-listed diagnosis, regardless of the number of admissions or encounters for treatment and care of the neoplasm.

h. Admission/encounter for pain control/management

See Section I.C.6.a.5 for information on coding admission/encounter for pain control/management.

i. Malignant neoplasm associated with transplanted organ

A malignant neoplasm of a transplanted organ should be coded as a transplant complication. Assign first the appropriate code from subcategory 996.8, Complications of transplanted organ, followed by code 199.2, Malignant neoplasm associated with transplanted organ. Use an additional code for the specific malignancy.

3. Chapter 3: Endocrine, Nutritional, and Metabolic Diseases and Immunity Disorders (240-279)

a. Diabetes mellitus

Codes under category 250, Diabetes mellitus, identify complications/manifestations associated with diabetes mellitus. A fifth-digit is required for all category 250 codes to identify the type of diabetes mellitus and whether the diabetes is controlled or uncontrolled.

See Section I.C.3.a.7 for secondary diabetes

1) Fifth-digits for category 250:

The following are the fifth-digits for the codes under category 250:

0   type II or unspecified type, not stated as uncontrolled

1   type I, [juvenile type], not stated as uncontrolled

2   type II or unspecified type, uncontrolled

3   type I, [juvenile type], uncontrolled

The age of a patient is not the sole determining factor, though most type I diabetics develop the condition before reaching puberty. For this reason type I diabetes mellitus is also referred to as juvenile diabetes.

2) Type of diabetes mellitus not documented

If the type of diabetes mellitus is not documented in the medical record the default is type II.

3) Diabetes mellitus and the use of insulin

All type I diabetics must use insulin to replace what their bodies do not produce. However, the use of insulin does not mean that a patient is a type I diabetic. Some patients with type II diabetes mellitus are unable to control their blood sugar through diet and oral medication alone and do require insulin.

If the documentation in a medical record does not indicate the type of diabetes but does indicate that the patient uses insulin, the appropriate fifth-digit for type II must be used. For type II patients who routinely use insulin, code V58.67, Long-term (current) use of insulin, should also be assigned to indicate that the patient uses insulin. Code V58.67 should not be assigned if insulin is given temporarily to bring a type II patient's blood sugar under control during an encounter.

4) Assigning and sequencing diabetes codes and associated conditions

When assigning codes for diabetes and its associated conditions, the code(s) from category 250 must be sequenced before the codes for the associated conditions. The diabetes codes and the secondary codes that correspond to them are paired codes that follow the etiology/manifestation convention of the classification *(See Section I.A.6., Etiology/manifestation convention)*. Assign as many codes from category 250 as needed to identify all of the associated conditions that the patient has. The corresponding secondary codes are listed under each of the diabetes codes.

(a) Diabetic retinopathy/ diabetic macular edema

Diabetic macular edema, code 362.07, is only present with diabetic retinopathy. Another code from subcategory 362.0, Diabetic retinopathy, must be used with code 362.07. Codes under subcategory 362.0 are diabetes manifestation codes, so they must be used following the appropriate diabetes code.

5) Diabetes mellitus in pregnancy and gestational diabetes

(a) For diabetes mellitus complicating pregnancy, *see Section I.C.11.f., Diabetes mellitus in pregnancy.*

(b) For gestational diabetes, *see Section I.C.11, g., Gestational diabetes.*

6) Insulin pump malfunction

(a) Underdose of insulin due insulin pump failure

An underdose of insulin due to an insulin pump failure should be assigned 996.57, Mechanical complication due to insulin pump, as the principal or first listed code, followed by the appropriate diabetes mellitus code based on documentation.

(b) Overdose of insulin due to insulin pump failure

The principal or first listed code for an encounter due to an insulin pump malfunction resulting in an overdose of insulin, should also be 996.57, Mechanical complication due to insulin pump, followed by code 962.3, Poisoning by insulins and antidiabetic agents, and the appropriate diabetes mellitus code based on documentation.

7) Secondary Diabetes Mellitus

Codes under category 249, Secondary diabetes mellitus, identify complications/ manifestations associated with secondary diabetes mellitus. Secondary diabetes is always caused by another condition or event (e.g., cystic fibrosis, malignant neoplasm of pancreas, pancreatectomy, adverse effect of drug, or poisoning).

(a) Fifth-digits for category 249:

A fifth-digit is required for all category 249 codes to identify whether the diabetes is controlled or uncontrolled.

(b) Secondary diabetes mellitus and the use of insulin

For patients who routinely use insulin, code V58.67, Long-term (current) use of insulin, should also be assigned. Code V58.67 should not be assigned if insulin is given temporarily to bring a patient's blood sugar under control during an encounter.

(c) Assigning and sequencing secondary diabetes codes and associated conditions

When assigning codes for secondary diabetes and its associated conditions (e.g. renal manifestations), the code(s) from category 249 must be sequenced before the codes for the associated conditions. The secondary diabetes codes and the diabetic manifestation codes that correspond to them are paired codes that follow the etiology/manifestation convention of the classification. Assign as many codes from category 249 as needed to identify all of the associated conditions that the patient has. The corresponding codes for the associated conditions are listed under each of the secondary diabetes codes. For example, secondary diabetes with diabetic nephrosis is assigned to code 249.40, followed by 581.81.

(d) Assigning and sequencing secondary diabetes codes and its causes

The sequencing of the secondary diabetes codes in relationship to codes for the cause of the diabetes is based on the reason for the encounter, applicable ICD-9-CM sequencing conventions, and chapter-specific guidelines.

If a patient is seen for treatment of the secondary diabetes or one of its associated conditions, a code from category 249 is sequenced as the principal or first-listed diagnosis, with the cause of the secondary diabetes (e.g. cystic fibrosis) sequenced as an additional diagnosis.

If, however, the patient is seen for the treatment of the condition causing the secondary diabetes (e.g., malignant neoplasm of pancreas), the code for the cause of the secondary diabetes should be sequenced as the principal or first-listed diagnosis followed by a code from category 249.

(i) Secondary diabetes mellitus due to pancreatectomy

For postpancreatectomy diabetes mellitus (lack of insulin due to the surgical removal of all or part of the pancreas), assign code 251.3, Postsurgical hypoinsulinemia. **Assign a code from subcategory 249 and a code from V88.1x, Acquired absence of pancreas as additional codes.** Code also any diabetic manifestations (e.g. diabetic nephrosis 581.81).

(ii) Secondary diabetes due to drugs

Secondary diabetes may be caused by an adverse effect of correctly administered medications, poisoning or late effect of poisoning.

See Section I.C.17.e for coding of adverse effects and poisoning, and section I.C.19 for E code reporting.

4. Chapter 4: Diseases of Blood and Blood Forming Organs (280-289)

a. Anemia of chronic disease

Subcategory 285.2, Anemia in chronic illness, has codes for anemia in chronic kidney disease, code 285.21; anemia in neoplastic disease, code 285.22; and anemia in other chronic illness, code 285.29. These codes can be used as the principal/first listed code if the reason for the encounter is to treat the anemia. They may also be used as secondary codes if treatment of the anemia is a component of an encounter, but not the primary reason for the encounter. When using a code from subcategory 285 it is also necessary to use the code for the chronic condition causing the anemia.

1) Anemia in chronic kidney disease

When assigning code 285.21, Anemia in chronic kidney disease, it is also necessary to assign a code from category 585, Chronic kidney disease, to indicate the stage of chronic kidney disease.

See I.C.10.a. Chronic kidney disease (CKD).

2) Anemia in neoplastic disease

When assigning code 285.22, Anemia in neoplastic disease, it is also necessary to assign the neoplasm code that is responsible for the anemia. Code 285.22 is for use for anemia that is due to the malignancy, not for anemia due to antineoplastic chemotherapy drugs. **Assign code 285.3 for anemia due to antineoplastic chemotherapy.**

See Section I.C.2.c.1 Anemia associated with malignancy. See Section I.C.2.c.2 Anemia associated with chemotherapy, immunotherapy and radiation therapy.

5. Chapter 5: Mental Disorders (290-319)

Reserved for future guideline expansion

6. Chapter 6: Diseases of Nervous System and Sense Organs (320-389)

a. Pain - Category 338

1) General coding information

Codes in category 338 may be used in conjunction with codes from other categories and chapters to provide more detail about acute or chronic pain and neoplasm- related pain, unless otherwise indicated below.

If the pain is not specified as acute or chronic, do not assign codes from category 338, except for post-thoracotomy pain, postoperative pain, neoplasm related pain, or central pain syndrome.

A code from subcategories 338.1 and 338.2 should not be assigned if the underlying (definitive) diagnosis is known, unless the reason for the encounter is pain control/ management and not management of the underlying condition.

(a) Category 338 codes as principal or first-listed diagnosis

Category 338 codes are acceptable as principal diagnosis or the first-listed code:

- When pain control or pain management is the reason for the admission/encounter (e.g., a patient with displaced intervertebral disc, nerve impingement and severe back pain presents for injection of steroid into the spinal canal). The underlying cause of the pain should be reported as an additional diagnosis, if known.

- When an admission or encounter is for a procedure aimed at treating the underlying condition (e.g., spinal fusion, kyphoplasty), a code for the underlying condition (e.g., vertebral fracture, spinal stenosis) should be assigned as the principal diagnosis. No code from category 338 should be assigned.

- When a patient is admitted for the insertion of a neurostimulator for pain control, assign the appropriate pain code as the principal or first listed diagnosis. When an admission or encounter is for a procedure aimed at treating the underlying condition and a neurostimulator is inserted for pain control during the same admission/encounter, a code for the underlying condition should be assigned as the principal diagnosis and the appropriate pain code should be assigned as a secondary diagnosis.

(b) Use of category 338 codes in conjunction with site specific pain codes

(i) Assigning category 338 codes and site-specific pain codes

Codes from category 338 may be used in conjunction with codes that identify the site of pain (including codes from chapter 16) if the category 338 code provides additional information. For example, if the code describes the site of the pain, but does not fully describe whether the pain is acute or chronic, then both codes should be assigned.

(ii) Sequencing of category 338 codes with site-specific pain codes

The sequencing of category 338 codes with site-specific pain codes (including chapter 16 codes), is dependent on the circumstances of the encounter/admission as follows:

- If the encounter is for pain control or pain management, assign the code from category 338 followed by the code identifying the specific site of pain (e.g., encounter for pain management for acute neck pain from trauma is assigned code 338.11, Acute pain due to trauma, followed by code 723.1, Cervicalgia, to identify the site of pain).

- If the encounter is for any other reason except pain control or pain management, and a related definitive diagnosis has not been established (confirmed) by the provider, assign the code for the specific site of pain first, followed by the appropriate code from category 338.

2) Pain due to devices, implants and grafts

Pain associated with devices, implants or grafts left in a surgical site (for example painful hip prosthesis) is assigned to the appropriate code(s) found in Chapter 17, Injury and Poisoning. Use additional code(s) from category 338 to identify acute or chronic pain due to presence of the device, implant or graft (338.18- 338.19 or 338.28-338.29).

3) Postoperative pain

Post-thoracotomy pain and other postoperative pain are classified to subcategories 338.1 and 338.2, depending on whether the pain is acute or chronic. The default for post-thoracotomy and other postoperative pain not specified as acute or chronic is the code for the acute form.

Routine or expected postoperative pain immediately after surgery should not be coded.

(a) Postoperative pain not associated with specific postoperative complication

Postoperative pain not associated with a specific postoperative complication is assigned to the appropriate postoperative pain code in category 338.

(b) Postoperative pain associated with specific postoperative complication

Postoperative pain associated with a specific postoperative complication (such as painful wire sutures) is assigned to the appropriate code(s) found in Chapter 17, Injury and Poisoning. If appropriate, use additional code(s) from category 338 to identify acute or chronic pain (338.18 or 338.28). If pain control/management is the reason for the encounter, a code from category 338 should be assigned as the principal or first-listed diagnosis in accordance with *Section I.C.6.a.1.a above.*

(c) Postoperative pain as principal or first-listed diagnosis

Postoperative pain may be reported as the principal or first-listed diagnosis when the stated reason for the admission/encounter is documented as postoperative pain control/management.

(d) Postoperative pain as secondary diagnosis

Postoperative pain may be reported as a secondary diagnosis code when a patient presents for outpatient surgery and develops an unusual or inordinate amount of postoperative pain.

The provider's documentation should be used to guide the coding of postoperative pain, as well as *Section III. Reporting Additional Diagnoses* and *Section IV. Diagnostic Coding and Reporting in the Outpatient Setting.*

See Section II.I.2 for information on sequencing of diagnoses for patients admitted to hospital inpatient care following post-operative observation.

See Section II.J for information on sequencing of diagnoses for patients admitted to hospital inpatient care from outpatient surgery.

See Section IV.A.2 for information on sequencing of diagnoses for patients admitted for observation.

4) Chronic pain

Chronic pain is classified to subcategory 338.2. There is no time frame defining when pain becomes chronic pain. The provider's documentation should be used to guide use of these codes.

5) Neoplasm related pain

Code 338.3 is assigned to pain documented as being related, associated or due to cancer, primary or secondary malignancy, or tumor. This code is assigned regardless of whether the pain is acute or chronic.

This code may be assigned as the principal or first-listed code when the stated reason for the admission/encounter is documented as pain control/pain management. The underlying neoplasm should be reported as an additional diagnosis.

When the reason for the admission/encounter is management of the neoplasm and the pain associated with the neoplasm is also documented, code 338.3 may be assigned as an additional diagnosis.

See Section I.C.2 for instructions on the sequencing of neoplasms for all other stated reasons for the admission/encounter (except for pain control/pain management).

6) Chronic pain syndrome

This condition is different than the term "chronic pain," and therefore this code should only be used when the provider has specifically documented this condition.

7. Chapter 7: Diseases of Circulatory System (390-459)

a. Hypertension
Hypertension Table
The Hypertension Table, found under the main term, "Hypertension," in the Alphabetic Index, contains a complete listing of all conditions due to or associated with hypertension and classifies them according to malignant, benign, and unspecified.

1) Hypertension, essential, or NOS
Assign hypertension (arterial) (essential) (primary) (systemic) (NOS) to category code 401 with the appropriate fourth-digit to indicate malignant (.0), benign (.1), or unspecified (.9). Do not use either .0 malignant or .1 benign unless medical record documentation supports such a designation.

2) Hypertension with heart disease
Heart conditions (425.8, 429.0-429.3, 429.8, 429.9) are assigned to a code from category 402 when a causal relationship is stated (due to hypertension) or implied (hypertensive). Use an additional code from category 428 to identify the type of heart failure in those patients with heart failure. More than one code from category 428 may be assigned if the patient has systolic or diastolic failure and congestive heart failure.

The same heart conditions (425.8, 429.0-429.3, 429.8, 429.9) with hypertension, but without a stated causal relationship, are coded separately. Sequence according to the circumstances of the admission/encounter.

3) Hypertensive chronic kidney disease
Assign codes from category 403, Hypertensive chronic kidney disease, when conditions classified to categories 585 are present. Unlike hypertension with heart disease, ICD-9-CM presumes a cause-and-effect relationship and classifies chronic kidney disease (CKD) with hypertension as hypertensive chronic kidney disease.

Fifth-digits for category 403 should be assigned as follows:

- 0 with CKD stage I through stage IV, or unspecified.

- 1 with CKD stage V or end stage renal disease.

The appropriate code from category 585, Chronic kidney disease, should be used as a secondary code with a code from category 403 to identify the stage of chronic kidney disease.

See Section I.C.10.a for information on the coding of chronic kidney disease.

4) Hypertensive heart and chronic kidney disease
Assign codes from combination category 404, Hypertensive heart and chronic kidney disease, when both hypertensive kidney disease and hypertensive heart disease are stated in the diagnosis. Assume a relationship between the hypertension and the chronic kidney disease, whether or not the condition is so designated. Assign an additional code from category 428, to identify the type of heart failure. More than one code from category 428 may be assigned if the patient has systolic or diastolic failure and congestive heart failure.

Fifth-digits for category 404 should be assigned as follows:

- 0 without heart failure and with chronic kidney disease (CKD) stage I through stage IV, or unspecified

- 1 with heart failure and with CKD stage I through stage IV, or unspecified

- 2 without heart failure and with CKD stage V or end stage renal disease

- 3 with heart failure and with CKD stage V or end stage renal disease

The appropriate code from category 585, Chronic kidney disease, should be used as a secondary code with a code from category 404 to identify the stage of kidney disease.

See Section I.C.10.a for information on the coding of chronic kidney disease.

5) Hypertensive cerebrovascular disease
First assign codes from 430-438, Cerebrovascular disease, then the appropriate hypertension code from categories 401-405.

6) Hypertensive retinopathy
Two codes are necessary to identify the condition. First assign the code from subcategory 362.11, Hypertensive retinopathy, then the appropriate code from categories 401-405 to indicate the type of hypertension.

7) Hypertension, secondary
Two codes are required: one to identify the underlying etiology and one from category 405 to identify the hypertension. Sequencing of codes is determined by the reason for admission/encounter.

8) Hypertension, transient
Assign code 796.2, Elevated blood pressure reading without diagnosis of hypertension, unless patient has an established diagnosis of hypertension. Assign code 642.3x for transient hypertension of pregnancy.

9) Hypertension, controlled
Assign appropriate code from categories 401-405. This diagnostic statement usually refers to an existing state of hypertension under control by therapy.

10) Hypertension, uncontrolled
Uncontrolled hypertension may refer to untreated hypertension or hypertension not responding to current therapeutic regimen. In either case, assign the appropriate code from categories 401-405 to designate the stage and type of hypertension. Code to the type of hypertension.

11) Elevated blood pressure
For a statement of elevated blood pressure without further specificity, assign code 796.2, Elevated blood pressure reading without diagnosis of hypertension, rather than a code from category 401.

b. Cerebral infarction/stroke/cerebrovascular accident (CVA)
The terms stroke and CVA are often used interchangeably to refer to a cerebral infarction. The terms stroke, CVA, and cerebral infarction NOS are all indexed to the default code 434.91, Cerebral artery occlusion, unspecified, with infarction. Code 436, Acute, but ill-defined, cerebrovascular disease, should not be used when the documentation states stroke or CVA.

See Section I.C.18.d.3 for information on coding status post administration of tPA in a different facility within the last 24 hours.

c. Postoperative cerebrovascular accident
A cerebrovascular hemorrhage or infarction that occurs as a result of medical intervention is coded to 997.02, Iatrogenic cerebrovascular infarction or hemorrhage. Medical record documentation should clearly specify the cause- and-effect relationship between the medical intervention and the cerebrovascular accident in order to assign this code. A secondary code from the code range 430-432 or from a code from subcategories 433 or 434 with a fifth-digit of "1" should also be used to identify the type of hemorrhage or infarct.

This guideline conforms to the use additional code note instruction at category 997. Code 436, Acute, but ill-defined, cerebrovascular disease, should not be used as a secondary code with code 997.02.

d. Late Effects of cerebrovascular disease

1) Category 438, late effects of cerebrovascular disease
Category 438 is used to indicate conditions classifiable to categories 430-437 as the causes of late effects (neurologic deficits), themselves classified elsewhere. These "late effects" include neurologic deficits that persist after initial onset of conditions classifiable to 430-437. The neurologic deficits caused by cerebrovascular disease may be present from the onset or may arise at any time after the onset of the condition classifiable to 430-437.

2) Codes from category 438 with codes from 430-437
Codes from category 438 may be assigned on a health care record with codes from 430-437, if the patient has a current cerebrovascular accident (CVA) and deficits from an old CVA.

3) Code V12.54
Assign code V12.54, Transient ischemic attack (TIA), and cerebral infarction without residual deficits (and not a code from category 438) as an additional code for history of cerebrovascular disease when no neurologic deficits are present.

e. Acute myocardial infarction (AMI)

1) ST elevation myocardial infarction (STEMI) and non ST elevation myocardial infarction (NSTEMI)
The ICD-9-CM codes for acute myocardial infarction (AMI) identify the site, such as anterolateral wall or true posterior wall. Subcategories 410.0-410.6 and 410.8 are used for ST elevation myocardial infarction (STEMI). Subcategory 410.7, Subendocardial infarction, is used for non ST elevation myocardial infarction (NSTEMI) and nontransmural MIs.

2) Acute myocardial infarction, unspecified
Subcategory 410.9 is the default for the unspecified term acute myocardial infarction. If only STEMI or transmural MI without the site is documented, query the provider as to the site, or assign a code from subcategory 410.9.

3) AMI documented as nontransmural or subendocardial but site provided
If an AMI is documented as nontransmural or subendocardial, but the site is provided, it is still coded as a subendocardial AMI. If NSTEMI evolves to STEMI, assign the STEMI code. If STEMI converts to NSTEMI due to thrombolytic therapy, it is still coded as STEMI.

See Section I.C.18.d.3 for information on coding status post administration of tPA in a different facility within the last 24 hours.

8. **Chapter 8: Diseases of Respiratory System (460-519)**

See I.C.17.f. for ventilator-associated pneumonia.

a. **Chronic obstructive pulmonary disease [COPD] and asthma**

1) Conditions that comprise COPD and asthma
The conditions that comprise COPD are obstructive chronic bronchitis, subcategory 491.2, and emphysema, category 492. All asthma codes are under category 493, Asthma. Code 496, Chronic airway obstruction, not elsewhere classified, is a nonspecific code that should only be used when the documentation in a medical record does not specify the type of COPD being treated.

2) Acute exacerbation of chronic obstructive bronchitis and asthma
The codes for chronic obstructive bronchitis and asthma distinguish between uncomplicated cases and those in acute exacerbation. An acute exacerbation is a worsening or a decompensation of a chronic condition. An acute exacerbation is not equivalent to an infection superimposed on a chronic condition, though an exacerbation may be triggered by an infection.

3) Overlapping nature of the conditions that comprise COPD and asthma
Due to the overlapping nature of the conditions that make up COPD and asthma, there are many variations in the way these conditions are documented. Code selection must be based on the terms as documented. When selecting the correct code for the documented type of COPD and asthma, it is essential to first review the index, and then verify the code in the tabular list. There are many instructional notes under the different COPD subcategories and codes. It is important that all such notes be reviewed to assure correct code assignment.

4) Acute exacerbation of asthma and status asthmaticus
An acute exacerbation of asthma is an increased severity of the asthma symptoms, such as wheezing and shortness of breath. Status asthmaticus refers to a patient's failure to respond to therapy administered during an asthmatic episode and is a life threatening complication that requires emergency care. If status asthmaticus is documented by the provider with any type of COPD or with acute bronchitis, the status asthmaticus should be sequenced first. It supersedes any type of COPD including that with acute exacerbation or acute bronchitis. It is inappropriate to assign an asthma code with 5th digit 2, with acute exacerbation, together with an asthma code with 5th digit 1, with status asthmatics. Only the 5th digit 1 should be assigned.

b. **Chronic obstructive pulmonary disease [COPD] and bronchitis**

1) Acute bronchitis with COPD
Acute bronchitis, code 466.0, is due to an infectious organism. When acute bronchitis is documented with COPD, code 491.22, Obstructive chronic bronchitis with acute bronchitis, should be assigned. It is not necessary to also assign code 466.0. If a medical record documents acute bronchitis with COPD with

acute exacerbation, only code 491.22 should be assigned. The acute bronchitis included in code 491.22 supersedes the acute exacerbation. If a medical record documents COPD with acute exacerbation without mention of acute bronchitis, only code 491.21 should be assigned.

c. **Acute Respiratory Failure**

1) Acute respiratory failure as principal diagnosis
Code 518.81, Acute respiratory failure, may be assigned as a principal diagnosis when it is the condition established after study to be chiefly responsible for occasioning the admission to the hospital, and the selection is supported by the Alphabetic Index and Tabular List. However, chapter-specific coding guidelines (such as obstetrics, poisoning, HIV, newborn) that provide sequencing direction take precedence.

2) Acute respiratory failure as secondary diagnosis
Respiratory failure may be listed as a secondary diagnosis if it occurs after admission, or if it is present on admission, but does not meet the definition of principal diagnosis.

3) Sequencing of acute respiratory failure and another acute condition
When a patient is admitted with respiratory failure and another acute condition, (e.g., myocardial infarction, cerebrovascular accident, aspiration pneumonia), the principal diagnosis will not be the same in every situation. This applies whether the other acute condition is a respiratory or nonrespiratory condition. Selection of the principal diagnosis will be dependent on the circumstances of admission. If both the respiratory failure and the other acute condition are equally responsible for occasioning the admission to the hospital, and there are no chapter-specific sequencing rules, the guideline regarding two or more diagnoses that equally meet the definition for principal diagnosis *(Section II, C.)* may be applied in these situations.

If the documentation is not clear as to whether acute respiratory failure and another condition are equally responsible for occasioning the admission, query the provider for clarification.

d. **Influenza due to *certain* identified *viruses***
Code only confirmed cases of avian influenza **(code 488.0, Influenza due to identified avian influenza virus)** or novel **H1N1 influenza virus (H1N1 or swine flu, code 488.1).** This is an exception to the hospital inpatient guideline Section II, H. (Uncertain Diagnosis).

In this context, "confirmation" does not require documentation of positive laboratory testing specific for avian **or novel H1N1** influenza. However, coding should be based on the provider's diagnostic statement that the patient has avian **or novel H1N1 (H1N1 or swine flu)** influenza.

If the provider records "suspected or possible or probable avian **or novel H1N1** influenza **(H1N1 or swine flu),**" the appropriate influenza code from category 487 should be assigned. **A code from category** 488, Influenza due to **certain** identified **viruses**, should not be assigned.

9. **Chapter 9: Diseases of Digestive System (520-579)**

Reserved for future guideline expansion

10. **Chapter 10: Diseases of Genitourinary System (580-629)**

a. **Chronic kidney disease**

1) Stages of chronic kidney disease (CKD)
The ICD-9-CM classifies CKD based on severity. The severity of CKD is designated by stages I-V. Stage II, code 585.2, equates to mild CKD; stage III, code 585.3, equates to moderate CKD; and stage IV, code 585.4, equates to severe CKD. Code 585.6, End stage renal disease (ESRD), is assigned when the provider has documented end-stage-renal disease (ESRD).

If both a stage of CKD and ESRD are documented, assign code 585.6 only.

2) Chronic kidney disease and kidney transplant status

Patients who have undergone kidney transplant may still have some form of CKD, because the kidney transplant may not fully restore kidney function. Therefore, the presence of CKD alone does not constitute a transplant complication. Assign the appropriate 585 code for the patient's stage of CKD and code V42.0. If a transplant complication such as failure or rejection is documented, see section I.C.17.f.**2**.b for information on coding complications of a kidney transplant. If the documentation is unclear as to whether the patient has a complication of the transplant, query the provider.

3) Chronic kidney disease with other conditions

Patients with CKD may also suffer from other serious conditions, most commonly diabetes mellitus and hypertension. The sequencing of the CKD code in relationship to codes for other contributing conditions is based on the conventions in the tabular list.

See Section I.C.3.a.4 for sequencing instructions for diabetes.
See Section I.C.4.a.1 for anemia in CKD.
See Section I.C.7.a.3 for hypertensive chronic kidney disease.
See Section I.C.17.f.2.b, Kidney transplant complications, for instructions on coding of documented rejection or failure.

11. Chapter 11: Complications of Pregnancy, Childbirth, and the Puerperium (630-679)

a. General Rules for Obstetric Cases

1) Codes from chapter 11 and sequencing priority

Obstetric cases require codes from chapter 11, codes in the range 630-679, Complications of Pregnancy, Childbirth, and the Puerperium. Chapter 11 codes have sequencing priority over codes from other chapters. Additional codes from other chapters may be used in conjunction with chapter 11 codes to further specify conditions. Should the provider document that the pregnancy is incidental to the encounter, then code V22.2 should be used in place of any chapter 11 codes. It is the provider's responsibility to state that the condition being treated is not affecting the pregnancy.

2) Chapter 11 codes used only on the maternal record

Chapter 11 codes are to be used only on the maternal record, never on the record of the newborn.

3) Chapter 11 fifth-digits

Categories 640-648, 651-676 have required fifth-digits, which indicate whether the encounter is antepartum, postpartum and whether a delivery has also occurred.

4) Fifth-digits, appropriate for each code

The fifth-digits, which are appropriate for each code number, are listed in brackets under each code. The fifth-digits on each code should all be consistent with each other. That is, should a delivery occur all of the fifth-digits should indicate the delivery.

b. Selection of OB Principal or First-listed Diagnosis

1) Routine outpatient prenatal visits

For routine outpatient prenatal visits when no complications are present codes V22.0, Supervision of normal first pregnancy, and V22.1, Supervision of other normal pregnancy, should be used as the first-listed diagnoses. These codes should not be used in conjunction with chapter 11 codes.

2) Prenatal outpatient visits for high-risk patients

For prenatal outpatient visits for patients with high-risk pregnancies, a code from category V23, Supervision of high-risk pregnancy, should be used as the first-listed diagnosis. Secondary Chapter 11 codes may be used in conjunction with these codes if appropriate.

3) Episodes when no delivery occurs

In episodes when no delivery occurs, the principal diagnosis should correspond to the principal complication of the pregnancy, which necessitated the encounter. Should more than one complication exist, all of which are treated or monitored, any of the complications codes may be sequenced first.

4) When a delivery occurs

When a delivery occurs, the principal diagnosis should correspond to the main circumstances or complication of the delivery. In cases of cesarean delivery, the selection of the principal diagnosis **should be the condition established after study that was responsible for the patient's admission. If the patient was admitted with a condition that resulted in the performance of a cesarean procedure, that condition should be selected as the principal diagnosis. If** the reason for **the** admission/encounter was unrelated to the condition resulting in the cesarean delivery, **the condition related to the reason for the admission/encounter should be selected as the principal diagnosis, even if a cesarean was performed.**

5) Outcome of delivery

An outcome of delivery code, V27.0-V27.9, should be included on every maternal record when a delivery has occurred. These codes are not to be used on subsequent records or on the newborn record.

c. Fetal conditions affecting the management of the mother

1) Codes from category 655

Known or suspected fetal abnormality affecting management of the mother, and category 656, Other fetal and placental problems affecting the management of the mother, are assigned only when the fetal condition is actually responsible for modifying the management of the mother, i.e., by requiring diagnostic studies, additional observation, special care, or termination of pregnancy. The fact that the fetal condition exists does not justify assigning a code from this series to the mother's record.

See Section I.C.18.d. for suspected maternal and fetal conditions not found

2) In utero surgery

In cases when surgery is performed on the fetus, a diagnosis code from category 655, Known or suspected fetal abnormalities affecting management of the mother, should be assigned identifying the fetal condition. Procedure code 75.36, Correction of fetal defect, should be assigned on the hospital inpatient record.

No code from Chapter 15, the perinatal codes, should be used on the mother's record to identify fetal conditions. Surgery performed in utero on a fetus is still to be coded as an obstetric encounter.

d. HIV infection in pregnancy, childbirth and the puerperium

During pregnancy, childbirth or the puerperium, a patient admitted because of an HIV-related illness should receive a principal diagnosis of 647.6x, Other specified infectious and parasitic diseases in the mother classifiable elsewhere, but complicating the pregnancy, childbirth or the puerperium, followed by 042 and the code(s) for the HIV-related illness(es).

Patients with asymptomatic HIV infection status admitted during pregnancy, childbirth, or the puerperium should receive codes of 647.6x and V08.

e. Current conditions complicating pregnancy

Assign a code from subcategory 648.x for patients that have current conditions when the condition affects the management of the pregnancy, childbirth, or the puerperium. Use additional secondary codes from other chapters to identify the conditions, as appropriate.

f.   Diabetes mellitus in pregnancy

Diabetes mellitus is a significant complicating factor in pregnancy. Pregnant women who are diabetic should be assigned code 648.0x, Diabetes mellitus complicating pregnancy, and a secondary code from category 250, Diabetes mellitus, or category 249, Secondary diabetes to identify the type of diabetes.

Code V58.67, Long-term (current) use of insulin, should also be assigned if the diabetes mellitus is being treated with insulin.

g.   Gestational diabetes

Gestational diabetes can occur during the second and third trimester of pregnancy in women who were not diabetic prior to pregnancy. Gestational diabetes can cause complications in the pregnancy similar to those of pre-existing diabetes mellitus. It also puts the woman at greater risk of developing diabetes after the pregnancy. Gestational diabetes is coded to 648.8x, Abnormal glucose tolerance. Codes 648.0x and 648.8x should never be used together on the same record.

Code V58.67, Long-term (current) use of insulin, should also be assigned if the gestational diabetes is being treated with insulin.

h.   Normal delivery, Code 650

1)   Normal delivery

Code 650 is for use in cases when a woman is admitted for a full-term normal delivery and delivers a single, healthy infant without any complications antepartum, during the delivery, or postpartum during the delivery episode. Code 650 is always a principal diagnosis. It is not to be used if any other code from chapter 11 is needed to describe a current complication of the antenatal, delivery, or perinatal period. Additional codes from other chapters may be used with code 650 if they are not related to or are in any way complicating the pregnancy.

2)   Normal delivery with resolved antepartum complication

Code 650 may be used if the patient had a complication at some point during her pregnancy, but the complication is not present at the time of the admission for delivery.

3)   V27.0, Single liveborn, outcome of delivery

V27.0, Single liveborn, is the only outcome of delivery code appropriate for use with 650.

i.   The postpartum and peripartum periods

1)   Postpartum and peripartum periods

The postpartum period begins immediately after delivery and continues for six weeks following delivery. The peripartum period is defined as the last month of pregnancy to five months postpartum.

2)   Postpartum complication

A postpartum complication is any complication occurring within the six-week period.

3)   Pregnancy-related complications after 6 week period

Chapter 11 codes may also be used to describe pregnancy-related complications after the six-week period should the provider document that a condition is pregnancy related.

4)   Postpartum complications occurring during the same admission as delivery

Postpartum complications that occur during the same admission as the delivery are identified with a fifth-digit of "2." Subsequent admissions/encounters for postpartum complications should be identified with a fifth-digit of "4."

5)   Admission for routine postpartum care following delivery outside hospital

When the mother delivers outside the hospital prior to admission and is admitted for routine postpartum care and no complications are noted, code V24.0, Postpartum care and examination immediately after delivery, should be assigned as the principal diagnosis.

6)   Admission following delivery outside hospital with postpartum conditions

A delivery diagnosis code should not be used for a woman who has delivered prior to admission to the hospital. Any postpartum conditions and/or postpartum procedures should be coded.

7)   Puerperal sepsis

Code 670.2x, Puerperal sepsis, should be assigned with a secondary code to identify the causal organism (e.g., for a bacterial infection, assign a code from category 041, Bacterial infections in conditions classified elsewhere and of unspecified site). A code from category 038, Septicemia, should not be used for puerperal sepsis. Do not assign code 995.91, Sepsis, as code 670.2x describes the sepsis. If applicable, use additional codes to identify severe sepsis (995.92) and any associated acute organ dysfunction.

j.   Code 677, Late effect of complication of pregnancy

1)   Code 677

Code 677, Late effect of complication of pregnancy, childbirth, and the puerperium is for use in those cases when an initial complication of a pregnancy develops a sequelae requiring care or treatment at a future date.

2)   After the initial postpartum period

This code may be used at any time after the initial postpartum period.

3)   Sequencing of Code 677

This code, like all late effect codes, is to be sequenced following the code describing the sequelae of the complication.

k.   Abortions

1)   Fifth-digits required for abortion categories

Fifth-digits are required for abortion categories 634-637. **Fifth digit assignment is based on the status of the patient at the beginning (or start) of the encounter.** Fifth-digit 1, incomplete, indicates that all of the products of conception have not been expelled from the uterus. fifth-digit 2, complete, indicates that all products of conception have been expelled from the uterus prior to the episode of care.

2)   Code from categories 640-648 and 651-659

A code from categories 640-648 and 651-659 may be used as additional codes with an abortion code to indicate the complication leading to the abortion.

Fifth-digit 3 is assigned with codes from these categories when used with an abortion code because the other fifth-digits will not apply. Codes from the 660-669 series are not to be used for complications of abortion.

3)   Code 639 for complications

Code 639 is to be used for all complications following abortion. Code 639 cannot be assigned with codes from categories 634-638.

4)   Abortion with liveborn fetus

When an attempted termination of pregnancy results in a liveborn fetus assign code 644.21, Early onset of delivery, with an appropriate code from category V27, Outcome of Delivery. The procedure code for the attempted termination of pregnancy should also be assigned.

5)   Retained products of conception following an abortion

Subsequent admissions for retained products of conception following a spontaneous or legally induced abortion are assigned the appropriate code from category 634, Spontaneous abortion, or 635, Legally induced abortion, with a fifth-digit of "1" (incomplete). This advice is appropriate even when the patient was discharged previously with a discharge diagnosis of complete abortion.

12. Chapter 12: Diseases of Skin and Subcutaneous Tissue (680-709)

a. Pressure ulcer stage codes

1) Pressure ulcer stages

Two codes are needed to completely describe a pressure ulcer: A code from subcategory 707.0, Pressure ulcer, to identify the site of the pressure ulcer and a code from subcategory 707.2, Pressure ulcer stages.

The codes in subcategory 707.2, Pressure ulcer stages, are to be used as an additional diagnosis with a code(s) from subcategory 707.0, Pressure Ulcer. Codes from 707.2, Pressure ulcer stages, may not be assigned as a principal or first-listed diagnosis. The pressure ulcer stage codes should only be used with pressure ulcers and not with other types of ulcers (e.g., stasis ulcer).

The ICD-9-CM classifies pressure ulcer stages based on severity, which is designated by stages I-IV and unstageable.

2) Unstageable pressure ulcers

Assignment of code 707.25, Pressure ulcer, unstageable, should be based on the clinical documentation. Code 707.25 is used for pressure ulcers whose stage cannot be clinically determined (e.g., the ulcer is covered by eschar or has been treated with a skin or muscle graft) and pressure ulcers that are documented as deep tissue injury but not documented as due to trauma. This code should not be confused with code 707.20, Pressure ulcer, stage unspecified. Code 707.20 should be assigned when there is no documentation regarding the stage of the pressure ulcer.

3) Documented pressure ulcer stage

Assignment of the pressure ulcer stage code should be guided by clinical documentation of the stage or documentation of the terms found in the index. For clinical terms describing the stage that are not found in the index, and there is no documentation of the stage, the provider should be queried.

4) Bilateral pressure ulcers with same stage

When a patient has bilateral pressure ulcers (e.g., both buttocks) and both pressure ulcers are documented as being the same stage, only the code for the site and one code for the stage should be reported.

5) Bilateral pressure ulcers with different stages

When a patient has bilateral pressure ulcers at the same site (e.g., both buttocks) and each pressure ulcer is documented as being at a different stage, assign one code for the site and the appropriate codes for the pressure ulcer stage.

6) Multiple pressure ulcers of different sites and stages

When a patient has multiple pressure ulcers at different sites (e.g., buttock, heel, shoulder) and each pressure ulcer is documented as being at different stages (e.g., stage 3 and stage 4), assign the appropriate codes for each different site and a code for each different pressure ulcer stage.

7) Patients admitted with pressure ulcers documented as healed

No code is assigned if the documentation states that the pressure ulcer is completely healed.

8) Patients admitted with pressure ulcers documented as healing

Pressure ulcers described as healing should be assigned the appropriate pressure ulcer stage code based on the documentation in the medical record. If the documentation does not provide information about the stage of the healing pressure ulcer, assign code 707.20, Pressure ulcer stage, unspecified.

If the documentation is unclear as to whether the patient has a current (new) pressure ulcer or if the patient is being treated for a healing pressure ulcer, query the provider.

9) Patient admitted with pressure ulcer evolving into another stage during the admission

If a patient is admitted with a pressure ulcer at one stage and it progresses to a higher stage, assign the code for highest stage reported for that site.

13. Chapter 13: Diseases of Musculoskeletal and Connective Tissue (710-739)

a. Coding of pathologic fractures

1) Acute fractures vs. aftercare

Pathologic fractures are reported using subcategory 733.1, when the fracture is newly diagnosed. Subcategory 733.1 may be used while the patient is receiving active treatment for the fracture. Examples of active treatment are: surgical treatment, emergency department encounter, evaluation and treatment by a new physician.

Fractures are coded using the aftercare codes (subcategories V54.0, V54.2, V54.8 or V54.9) for encounters after the patient has completed active treatment of the fracture and is receiving routine care for the fracture during the healing or recovery phase. Examples of fracture aftercare are: cast change or removal, removal of external or internal fixation device, medication adjustment, and follow up visits following fracture treatment.

Care for complications of surgical treatment for fracture repairs during the healing or recovery phase should be coded with the appropriate complication codes.

Care of complications of fractures, such as malunion and nonunion, should be reported with the appropriate codes.

See Section I. C. 17.b for information on the coding of traumatic fractures.

14. Chapter 14: Congenital Anomalies (740-759)

a. Codes in categories 740-759, congenital anomalies

Assign an appropriate code(s) from categories 740-759, Congenital Anomalies, when an anomaly is documented. A congenital anomaly may be the principal/first listed diagnosis on a record or a secondary diagnosis.

When a congenital anomaly does not have a unique code assignment, assign additional code(s) for any manifestations that may be present.

When the code assignment specifically identifies the congenital anomaly, manifestations that are an inherent component of the anomaly should not be coded separately. Additional codes should be assigned for manifestations that are not an inherent component.

Codes from Chapter 14 may be used throughout the life of the patient. If a congenital anomaly has been corrected, a personal history code should be used to identify the history of the anomaly. Although present at birth, a congenital anomaly may not be identified until later in life. Whenever the condition is diagnosed by the physician, it is appropriate to assign a code from codes 740-759.

For the birth admission, the appropriate code from category V30, Liveborn infants, according to type of birth should be sequenced as the principal diagnosis, followed by any congenital anomaly codes, 740-759.

15. Chapter 15: Newborn (Perinatal) Guidelines (760-779)

For coding and reporting purposes the perinatal period is defined as before birth through the 28th day following birth. The following guidelines are provided for reporting purposes. Hospitals may record other diagnoses as needed for internal data use.

a. General perinatal rules

1) Chapter 15 Codes
They are <u>never</u> for use on the maternal record. Codes from Chapter 11, the obstetric chapter, are never permitted on the newborn record. Chapter 15 code may be used throughout the life of the patient if the condition is still present.

2) Sequencing of perinatal codes
Generally, codes from Chapter 15 should be sequenced as the principal/first-listed diagnosis on the newborn record, with the exception of the appropriate V30 code for the birth episode, followed by codes from any other chapter that provide additional detail. The "use additional code" note at the beginning of the chapter supports this guideline. If the index does not provide a specific code for a perinatal condition, assign code 779.89, Other specified conditions originating in the perinatal period, followed by the code from another chapter that specifies the condition. Codes for signs and symptoms may be assigned when a definitive diagnosis has not been established.

3) Birth process or community acquired conditions
If a newborn has a condition that may be either due to the birth process or community acquired and the documentation does not indicate which it is, the default is due to the birth process and the code from Chapter 15 should be used. If the condition is community-acquired, a code from Chapter 15 should not be assigned.

4) Code all clinically significant conditions
All clinically significant conditions noted on routine newborn examination should be coded. A condition is clinically significant if it requires:

- clinical evaluation; or
- therapeutic treatment; or
- diagnostic procedures; or
- extended length of hospital stay; or
- increased nursing care and/or monitoring; or
- has implications for future health care needs

Note: The perinatal guidelines listed above are the same as the general coding guidelines for "additional diagnoses", except for the final point regarding implications for future health care needs. Codes should be assigned for conditions that have been specified by the provider as having implications for future health care needs. Codes from the perinatal chapter should not be assigned unless the provider has established a definitive diagnosis.

b. Use of codes V30-V39
When coding the birth of an infant, assign a code from categories V30-V39, according to the type of birth. A code from this series is assigned as a principal diagnosis, and assigned only once to a newborn at the time of birth.

c. Newborn transfers
If the newborn is transferred to another institution, the V30 series is not used at the receiving hospital.

d. Use of category V29

1) Assigning a code from category V29
Assign a code from category V29, Observation and evaluation of newborns and infants for suspected conditions not found, to identify those instances when a healthy newborn is evaluated for a suspected condition that is determined after study not to

be present. Do not use a code from category V29 when the patient has identified signs or symptoms of a suspected problem; in such cases, code the sign or symptom.

A code from category V29 may also be assigned as a principal code for readmissions or encounters when the V30 code no longer applies. Codes from category V29 are for use only for healthy newborns and infants for which no condition after study is found to be present.

2) V29 code on a birth record
A V29 code is to be used as a secondary code after the V30, Outcome of delivery, code.

e. Use of other V codes on perinatal records
V codes other than V30 and V29 may be assigned on a perinatal or newborn record code. The codes may be used as a principal or first-listed diagnosis for specific types of encounters or for readmissions or encounters when the V30 code no longer applies.

See Section I.C.18 for information regarding the assignment of V codes.

f. Maternal causes of perinatal morbidity
Codes from categories 760-763, Maternal causes of perinatal morbidity and mortality, are assigned only when the maternal condition has actually affected the fetus or newborn. The fact that the mother has an associated medical condition or experiences some complication of pregnancy, labor or delivery does not justify the routine assignment of codes from these categories to the newborn record.

g. Congenital anomalies in newborns
For the birth admission, the appropriate code from category V30, Liveborn infants according to type of birth, should be used, followed by any congenital anomaly codes, categories 740-759. Use additional secondary codes from other chapters to specify conditions associated with the anomaly, if applicable.

Also, see Section I.C.14 for information on the coding of congenital anomalies.

h. Coding additional perinatal diagnoses

1) Assigning codes for conditions that require treatment
Assign codes for conditions that require treatment or further investigation, prolong the length of stay, or require resource utilization.

2) Codes for conditions specified as having implications for future health care needs
Assign codes for conditions that have been specified by the provider as having implications for future health care needs.

Note: This guideline should not be used for adult patients.

3) Codes for newborn conditions originating in the perinatal period
Assign a code for newborn conditions originating in the perinatal period (categories 760-779), as well as complications arising during the current episode of care classified in other chapters, only if the diagnoses have been documented by the responsible provider at the time of transfer or discharge as having affected the fetus or newborn.

i. Prematurity and fetal growth retardation
Providers utilize different criteria in determining prematurity. A code for prematurity should not be assigned unless it is documented. The 5th digit assignment for codes from category 764 and subcategories 765.0 and 765.1 should be based on the recorded birth weight and estimated gestational age.

A code from subcategory 765.2, Weeks of gestation, should be assigned as an additional code with category 764 and codes from 765.0 and 765.1 to specify weeks of gestation as documented by the provider in the record.

j. Newborn sepsis
Code 771.81, Septicemia [sepsis] of newborn, should be assigned with a secondary code from category 041, Bacterial infections in conditions classified elsewhere and of unspecified site, to identify

the organism. A code from category 038, Septicemia, should not be recorded on a newborn record. Do not assign code 995.91, Sepsis, as code 771.81 describes the sepsis. If applicable, use additional codes to identify severe sepsis (995.92) and any associated acute organ dysfunction.

16. Chapter 16: Signs, Symptoms and Ill-Defined Conditions (780-799)

Reserved for future guideline expansion

17. Chapter 17: Injury and Poisoning (800-999)

a. Coding of injuries

When coding injuries, assign separate codes for each injury unless a combination code is provided, in which case the combination code is assigned. Multiple injury codes are provided in ICD-9-CM, but should not be assigned unless information for a more specific code is not available. These **traumatic injury** codes are not to be used for normal, healing surgical wounds or to identify complications of surgical wounds.

The code for the most serious injury, as determined by the provider and the focus of treatment, is sequenced first.

1) Superficial injuries

Superficial injuries such as abrasions or contusions are not coded when associated with more severe injuries of the same site.

2) Primary injury with damage to nerves/blood vessels

When a primary injury results in minor damage to peripheral nerves or blood vessels, the primary injury is sequenced first with additional code(s) from categories 950-957, Injury to nerves and spinal cord, and/or 900-904, Injury to blood vessels. When the primary injury is to the blood vessels or nerves, that injury should be sequenced first.

b. Coding of traumatic fractures

The principles of multiple coding of injuries should be followed in coding fractures. Fractures of specified sites are coded individually by site in accordance with both the provisions within categories 800-829 and the level of detail furnished by medical record content. Combination categories for multiple fractures are provided for use when there is insufficient detail in the medical record (such as trauma cases transferred to another hospital), when the reporting form limits the number of codes that can be used in reporting pertinent clinical data, or when there is insufficient specificity at the fourth-digit or fifth-digit level. More specific guidelines are as follows:

1) Acute fractures vs. aftercare

Traumatic fractures are coded using the acute fracture codes (800-829) while the patient is receiving active treatment for the fracture. Examples of active treatment are: surgical treatment, emergency department encounter, and evaluation and treatment by a new physician.

Fractures are coded using the aftercare codes (subcategories V54.0, V54.1, V54.8, or V54.9) for encounters after the patient has completed active treatment of the fracture and is receiving routine care for the fracture during the healing or recovery phase. Examples of fracture aftercare are: cast change or removal, removal of external or internal fixation device, medication adjustment, and follow up visits following fracture treatment.

Care for complications of surgical treatment for fracture repairs during the healing or recovery phase should be coded with the appropriate complication codes.

Care of complications of fractures, such as malunion and nonunion, should be reported with the appropriate codes.

Pathologic fractures are not coded in the 800-829 range, but instead are assigned to subcategory 733.1. *See Section I.C.13.a for additional information.*

2) Multiple fractures of same limb

Multiple fractures of same limb classifiable to the same three-digit or four-digit category are coded to that category.

3) Multiple unilateral or bilateral fractures of same bone

Multiple unilateral or bilateral fractures of same bone(s) but classified to different fourth-digit subdivisions (bone part) within the same three-digit category are coded individually by site.

4) Multiple fracture categories 819 and 828

Multiple fracture categories 819 and 828 classify bilateral fractures of both upper limbs (819) and both lower limbs (828), but without any detail at the fourth-digit level other than open and closed type of fractures.

5) Multiple fractures sequencing

Multiple fractures are sequenced in accordance with the severity of the fracture. The provider should be asked to list the fracture diagnoses in the order of severity.

c. Coding of burns

Current burns (940-948) are classified by depth, extent and by agent (E code). Burns are classified by depth as first degree (erythema), second degree (blistering), and third degree (full-thickness involvement).

1) Sequencing of burn and related condition codes

Sequence first the code that reflects the highest degree of burn when more than one burn is present.

a. When the reason for the admission or encounter is for treatment of external multiple burns, sequence first the code that reflects the burn of the highest degree.

b. When a patient has both internal and external burns, the circumstances of admission govern the selection of the principal diagnosis or first-listed diagnosis.

c. When a patient is admitted for burn injuries and other related conditions such as smoke inhalation and/or respiratory failure, the circumstances of admission govern the selection of the principal or first-listed diagnosis.

2) Burns of the same local site

Classify burns of the same local site (three-digit category level, 940-947) but of different degrees to the subcategory identifying the highest degree recorded in the diagnosis.

3) Non-healing burns

Non-healing burns are coded as acute burns.

Necrosis of burned skin should be coded as a non-healed burn.

4) Code 958.3, posttraumatic wound infection

Assign code 958.3, Posttraumatic wound infection, not elsewhere classified, as an additional code for any documented infected burn site.

5) Assign separate codes for each burn site

When coding burns, assign separate codes for each burn site. Category 946, Burns of Multiple specified sites, should only be used if the location of the burns are not documented.

Category 949, Burn, unspecified, is extremely vague and should rarely be used.

6) Assign codes from category 948, burns

Burns classified according to extent of body surface involved, when the site of the burn is not specified or when there is a need for additional data. It is advisable to use category 948 as additional coding when needed to provide data for evaluating burn mortality, such as that needed by burn units. It is also advisable to use category 948 as an additional code for reporting purposes when there is mention of a third-degree burn involving 20 percent or more of the body surface.

In assigning a code from category 948:

Fourth-digit codes are used to identify the percentage of total body surface involved in a burn (all degree).

Fifth-digits are assigned to identify the percentage of body surface involved in third-degree burn.

Fifth-digit zero (0) is assigned when less than 10 percent or when no body surface is involved in a third-degree burn.

Category 948 is based on the classic "rule of nines" in estimating body surface involved: head and neck are assigned nine percent, each arm nine percent, each leg 18 percent, the anterior trunk 18 percent, posterior trunk 18 percent, and genitalia one percent. Providers may change these percentage assignments where necessary to accommodate infants and children who have proportionately larger heads than adults and patients who have large buttocks, thighs, or abdomen that involve burns.

7) Encounters for treatment of late effects of burns
Encounters for the treatment of the late effects of burns (i.e., scars or joint contractures) should be coded to the residual condition (sequelae) followed by the appropriate late effect code (906.5-906.9). A late effect E code may also be used, if desired.

8) Sequelae with a late effect code and current burn
When appropriate, both a sequelae with a late effect code, and a current burn code may be assigned on the same record (when both a current burn and sequelae of an old burn exist).

d. Coding of debridement of wound, infection, or burn
Excisional debridement involves surgical removal or cutting away, as opposed to a mechanical (brushing, scrubbing, washing) debridement.

For coding purposes, excisional debridement is assigned to code 86.22.

Nonexcisional debridement is assigned to code 86.28.

e. Adverse effects, poisoning and toxic effects
The properties of certain drugs, medicinal and biological substances or combinations of such substances, may cause toxic reactions. The occurrence of drug toxicity is classified in ICD-9-CM as follows:

1) Adverse effect
When the drug was correctly prescribed and properly administered, code the reaction plus the appropriate code from the E930-E949 series. Codes from the E930-E949 series must be used to identify the causative substance for an adverse effect of drug, medicinal and biological substances, correctly prescribed and properly administered. The effect, such as tachycardia, delirium, gastrointestinal hemorrhaging, vomiting, hypokalemia, hepatitis, renal failure, or respiratory failure, is coded and followed by the appropriate code from the E930-E949 series.

Adverse effects of therapeutic substances correctly prescribed and properly administered (toxicity, synergistic reaction, side effect, and idiosyncratic reaction) may be due to (1) differences among patients, such as age, sex, disease, and genetic factors, and (2) drug-related factors, such as type of drug, route of administration, duration of therapy, dosage, and bioavailability.

2) Poisoning

(a) Error was made in drug prescription
Errors made in drug prescription or in the administration of the drug by provider, nurse, patient, or other person, use the appropriate poisoning code from the 960-979 series.

(b) Overdose of a drug intentionally taken
If an overdose of a drug was intentionally taken or administered and resulted in drug toxicity, it would be coded as a poisoning (960-979 series).

(c) Nonprescribed drug taken with correctly prescribed and properly administered drug
If a nonprescribed drug or medicinal agent was taken in combination with a correctly prescribed and properly administered drug, any drug toxicity or other reaction resulting from the interaction of the two drugs would be classified as a poisoning.

(d) Interaction of drug(s) and alcohol
When a reaction results from the interaction of a drug(s) and alcohol, this would be classified as poisoning.

(e) Sequencing of poisoning
When coding a poisoning or reaction to the improper use of a medication (e.g., wrong dose, wrong substance, wrong route of administration) the poisoning code is sequenced first, followed by a code for the manifestation. If there is also a diagnosis of drug abuse or dependence to the substance, the abuse or dependence is coded as an additional code.

See Section I.C.3.a.6.b. if poisoning is the result of insulin pump malfunctions and Section I.C.19 for general use of E-codes.

3) Toxic effects

(a) Toxic effect codes
When a harmful substance is ingested or comes in contact with a person, this is classified as a toxic effect. The toxic effect codes are in categories 980-989.

(b) Sequencing toxic effect codes
A toxic effect code should be sequenced first, followed by the code(s) that identify the result of the toxic effect.

(c) External cause codes for toxic effects
An external cause code from categories E860-E869 for accidental exposure, codes E950.6 or E950.7 for intentional self-harm, category E962 for assault, or categories E980-E982, for undetermined, should also be assigned to indicate intent.

f. Complications of care

1) Complications of care

(a) Documentation of complications of care
As with all procedural or postprocedural complications, code assignment is based on the provider's documentation of the relationship between the condition and the procedure.

2) Transplant complications

(a) Transplant complications other than kidney
Codes under subcategory 996.8, Complications of transplanted organ, are for use for both complications and rejection of transplanted organs. A transplant complication code is only assigned if the complication affects the function of the transplanted organ. Two codes are required to fully describe a transplant complication, the appropriate code from subcategory 996.8 and a secondary code that identifies the complication.

Pre-existing conditions or conditions that develop after the transplant are not coded as complications unless they affect the function of the transplanted organs.

See I.C.18.d.3) for transplant organ removal status

See I.C.2.i for malignant neoplasm associated with transplanted organ.

(b) Chronic kidney disease and kidney transplant complications

Patients who have undergone kidney transplant may still have some form of chronic kidney disease (CKD) because the kidney transplant may not fully restore kidney function. Code 996.81 should be assigned for documented complications of a kidney transplant, such as transplant failure or rejection or other transplant complication. Code 996.81 should not be assigned for post kidney transplant patients who have chronic kidney (CKD) unless a transplant complication such as transplant failure or rejection is documented. If the documentation is unclear as to whether the patient has a complication of the transplant, query the provider.

For patients with CKD following a kidney transplant, but who do not have a complication such as failure or rejection, *see section I.C.10.a.2, Chronic kidney disease and kidney transplant status.*

3) Ventilator associated pneumonia

(a) Documentation of Ventilator associated Pneumonia

As with all procedural or postprocedural complications, code assignment is based on the provider's documentation of the relationship between the condition and the procedure.

Code 997.31, Ventilator associated pneumonia, should be assigned only when the provider has documented ventilator associated pneumonia (VAP). An additional code to identify the organism (e.g., Pseudomonas aeruginosa, code 041.7) should also be assigned. Do not assign an additional code from categories 480-484 to identify the type of pneumonia.

Code 997.31 should not be assigned for cases where the patient has pneumonia and is on a mechanical ventilator but the provider has not specifically stated that the pneumonia is ventilator-associated pneumonia.

If the documentation is unclear as to whether the patient has a pneumonia that is a complication attributable to the mechanical ventilator, query the provider.

(b) Patient admitted with pneumonia and develops VAP

A patient may be admitted with one type of pneumonia (e.g., code 481, Pneumococcal pneumonia) and subsequently develop VAP. In this instance, the principal diagnosis would be the appropriate code from categories 480-484 for the pneumonia diagnosed at the time of admission. Code 997.31, Ventilator associated pneumonia, would be assigned as an additional diagnosis when the provider has also documented the presence of ventilator associated pneumonia.

g. SIRS due to non-infectious process

The systemic inflammatory response syndrome (SIRS) can develop as a result of certain non-infectious disease processes, such as trauma, malignant neoplasm, or pancreatitis. When SIRS is documented with a noninfectious condition, and no subsequent infection is documented, the code for the underlying condition, such as an injury, should be assigned, followed by code 995.93, Systemic inflammatory response syndrome due to noninfectious process without acute organ dysfunction, or 995.94, Systemic inflammatory response syndrome due to non-infectious process with acute organ dysfunction. If an acute organ dysfunction is documented, the appropriate code(s) for the associated acute organ dysfunction(s) should be assigned in addition to code 995.94. If acute organ dysfunction is documented, but it cannot be determined if the acute organ dysfunction is associated with SIRS or due to another condition (e.g., directly due to the trauma), the provider should be queried.

When the non-infectious condition has led to an infection that results in SIRS, *see Section I.C.1.b.12 for the guideline for sepsis and severe sepsis associated with a non-infectious process.*

18. Classification of Factors Influencing Health Status and Contact with Health Service (Supplemental V01-V91)

Note: The chapter specific guidelines provide additional information about the use of V codes for specified encounters.

a. Introduction

ICD-9-CM provides codes to deal with encounters for circumstances other than a disease or injury. The Supplementary Classification of Factors Influencing Health Status and Contact with Health Services (V01.0 - V89.09) is provided to deal with occasions when circumstances other than a disease or injury (codes 001-999) are recorded as a diagnosis or problem.

There are four primary circumstances for the use of V codes:

1) A person who is not currently sick encounters the health services for some specific reason, such as to act as an organ donor, to receive prophylactic care, such as inoculations or health screenings, or to receive counseling on health related issues.

2) A person with a resolving disease or injury, or a chronic, long-term condition requiring continuous care, encounters the health care system for specific aftercare of that disease or injury (e.g., dialysis for renal disease; chemotherapy for malignancy; cast change). A diagnosis/symptom code should be used whenever a current, acute, diagnosis is being treated or a sign or symptom is being studied.

3) Circumstances or problems influence a person's health status but are not in themselves a current illness or injury.

4) Newborns, to indicate birth status

b. V codes use in any healthcare setting

V codes are for use in any healthcare setting. V codes may be used as either a first listed (principal diagnosis code in the inpatient setting) or secondary code, depending on the circumstances of the encounter. Certain V codes may only be used as first listed, others only as secondary codes.

See Section I.C.18.e, **V Codes That May Only be Principal/ First-Listed Diagnosis.**

c. V Codes indicate a reason for an encounter

They are not procedure codes. A corresponding procedure code must accompany a V code to describe the procedure performed.

d. Categories of V codes

1) Contact/exposure

Category V01 indicates contact with or exposure to communicable diseases. These codes are for patients who do not show any sign or symptom of a disease but have been exposed to it by close personal contact with an infected individual or are in an area where a disease is epidemic. These codes may be used as a first listed code to explain an encounter for testing, or, more commonly, as a secondary code to identify a potential risk.

2) Inoculations and vaccinations

Categories V03-V06 are for encounters for inoculations and vaccinations. They indicate that a patient is being seen to receive a prophylactic inoculation against a disease. The injection itself must be represented by the appropriate procedure code. A code from V03-V06 may be used as a secondary code if the inoculation is given as a routine part of preventive health care, such as a well-baby visit.

3) Status

Status codes indicate that a patient is either a carrier of a disease or has the sequelae or residual of a past disease or condition. This includes such things as the presence of prosthetic or mechanical devices resulting from past treatment. A status code is informative, because the status may affect the course of treatment and its outcome. A status code is distinct from a history code. The history code indicates that the patient no longer has the condition.

A status code should not be used with a diagnosis code from one of the body system chapters, if the diagnosis code includes the information provided by the status code. For example, code V42.1, Heart transplant status, should not be used with code 996.83, Complications of transplanted heart. The status code does not provide additional information. The complication code indicates that the patient is a heart transplant patient.

The status V codes/categories are:

V02   Carrier or suspected carrier of infectious diseases

Carrier status indicates that a person harbors the specific organisms of a disease without manifest symptoms and is capable of transmitting the infection.

V07.5x   Use of agents affecting estrogen receptors and estrogen level

This code indicates when a patient is receiving a drug that affects estrogen receptors and estrogen levels for prevention of cancer.

V08   Asymptomatic HIV infection status

This code indicates that a patient has tested positive for HIV but has manifested no signs or symptoms of the disease.

V09   Infection with drug-resistant microorganisms

This category indicates that a patient has an infection that is resistant to drug treatment. Sequence the infection code first.

V21   Constitutional states in development

V22.2   Pregnant state, incidental

This code is a secondary code only for use when the pregnancy is in no way complicating the reason for visit. Otherwise, a code from the obstetric chapter is required.

V26.5x   Sterilization status

V42   Organ or tissue replaced by transplant

V43   Organ or tissue replaced by other means

V44   Artificial opening status

V45   Other postsurgical states

Assign code V45.87, Transplant organ removal status, to indicate that a transplanted organ has been previously removed. This code should not be assigned for the encounter in which the transplanted organ is removed. The complication necessitating removal of the transplant organ should be assigned for that encounter.

See section I.C17.f.2. for information on the coding of organ transplant complications.

Assign code V45.88, Status post administration of tPA (rtPA) in a different facility within the last 24 hours prior to admission to the current facility, as a secondary diagnosis when a patient is received by transfer into a facility and documentation indicates they were administered tissue plasminogen activator (tPA) within the last 24 hours prior to admission to the current facility.

This guideline applies even if the patient is still receiving the tPA at the time they are received into the current facility.

The appropriate code for the condition for which the tPA was administered (such as cerebrovascular disease or myocardial infarction) should be assigned first.

Code V45.88 is only applicable to the receiving facility record and not to the transferring facility record.

V46   Other dependence on machines

V49.6   Upper limb amputation status

V49.7   Lower limb amputation status

Note: Categories V42-V46, and subcategories V49.6, V49.7 are for use only if there are no complications or malfunctions of the organ or tissue replaced, the amputation site or the equipment on which the patient is dependent.

V49.81   Postmenopausal status

V49.82   Dental sealant status

V49.83   Awaiting organ transplant status

V58.6x   Long-term (current) drug use

Codes from this subcategory indicate a patient's continuous use of a prescribed drug (including such things as aspirin therapy) for the long-term treatment of a condition or for prophylactic use. It is not for use for patients who have addictions to drugs. This subcategory is not for use of medications for detoxification or maintenance programs to prevent withdrawal symptoms in patients with drug dependence (e.g., methadone maintenance for opiate dependence). Assign the appropriate code for the drug dependence instead.

Assign a code from subcategory V58.6, Long-term (current) drug use, if the patient is receiving a medication for an extended period as a prophylactic measure (such as for the prevention of deep vein thrombosis) or as treatment of a chronic condition (such as arthritis) or a disease requiring a lengthy course of treatment (such as cancer). Do not assign a code from subcategory V58.6 for medication being administered for a brief period of time to treat an acute illness or injury (such as a course of antibiotics to treat acute bronchitis).

V83   Genetic carrier status

Genetic carrier status indicates that a person carries a gene, associated with a particular disease, which may be passed to offspring who may develop that disease. The person does not have the disease and is not at risk of developing the disease.

V84   Genetic susceptibility status

Genetic susceptibility indicates that a person has a gene that increases the risk of that person developing the disease.

Codes from category V84, Genetic susceptibility to disease, should not be used as principal or first-listed codes. If the patient has the condition to which he/she is susceptible, and that condition is the reason for the encounter, the code for the current condition should be sequenced first. If the patient is being seen for follow-up after completed treatment for this condition, and the condition no longer exists, a follow-up code should be sequenced first, followed by the appropriate personal history and genetic susceptibility codes. If the purpose of the encounter is genetic counseling associated with procreative management, a code from subcategory V26.3, Genetic counseling and testing, should be assigned as the first-listed code, followed by a code from category V84. Additional codes should be assigned for any applicable family or personal history.

See Section I.C. 18.d.14 for information on prophylactic organ removal due to a genetic susceptibility.

V85   Body Mass Index (BMI)

V86   Estrogen receptor status

V88   Acquired absence of other organs and tissue

4) **History (of)**

There are two types of history V codes, personal and family. Personal history codes explain a patient's past medical condition that no longer exists and is not receiving any treatment, but that has the potential for recurrence, and therefore may require continued monitoring. The exceptions to this general rule are category V14, Personal history of allergy to medicinal agents, and subcategory V15.0, Allergy, other than to medicinal agents. A person who has had an allergic episode to a substance or food in the past should always be considered allergic to the substance.

Family history codes are for use when a patient has a family member(s) who has had a particular disease that causes the patient to be at higher risk of also contracting the disease.

Personal history codes may be used in conjunction with follow-up codes and family history codes may be used in conjunction with screening codes to explain the need for a test or procedure. History codes are also acceptable on any medical record regardless of the reason for visit. A history of an illness, even if no longer present, is important information that may alter the type of treatment ordered.

The history V code categories are:

V10	Personal history of malignant neoplasm
V12	Personal history of certain other diseases
V13	Personal history of other diseases
	Except: V13.4, Personal history of arthritis, and V13.6, Personal history of congenital malformations. These conditions are life-long so are not true history codes.
V14	Personal history of allergy to medicinal agents
V15	Other personal history presenting hazards to health Except: V15.7, Personal history of contraception.
V16	Family history of malignant neoplasm
V17	Family history of certain chronic disabling diseases
V18	Family history of certain other specific diseases
V19	Family history of other conditions
V87	Other specified personal exposures and history presenting hazards to health

5) Screening

Screening is the testing for disease or disease precursors in seemingly well individuals so that early detection and treatment can be provided for those who test positive for the disease. Screenings that are recommended for many subgroups in a population include: routine mammograms for women over 40, a fecal occult blood test for everyone over 50, an amniocentesis to rule out a fetal anomaly for pregnant women over 35, because the incidence of breast cancer and colon cancer in these subgroups is higher than in the general population, as is the incidence of Down's syndrome in older mothers.

The testing of a person to rule out or confirm a suspected diagnosis because the patient has some sign or symptom is a diagnostic examination, not a screening. In these cases, the sign or symptom is used to explain the reason for the test.

A screening code may be a first listed code if the reason for the visit is specifically the screening exam. It may also be used as an additional code if the screening is done during an office visit for other health problems. A screening code is not necessary if the screening is inherent to a routine examination, such as a pap smear done during a routine pelvic examination.

Should a condition be discovered during the screening then the code for the condition may be assigned as an additional diagnosis.

The V code indicates that a screening exam is planned. A procedure code is required to confirm that the screening was performed.

The screening V code categories:

V28	Antenatal screening
V73-V82	Special screening examinations

6) Observation

There are three observation V code categories. They are for use in very limited circumstances when a person is being observed for a suspected condition that is ruled out. The observation codes are not for use if an injury or illness or any signs or symptoms related to the suspected condition are present. In such cases the diagnosis/symptom code is used with the corresponding E code to identify any external cause.

The observation codes are to be used as principal diagnosis only. The only exception to this is when the principal diagnosis is required to be a code from the V30, Live born infant, category. Then the V29 observation code is sequenced after the V30 code. Additional codes may be used in addition to the observation code but only if they are unrelated to the suspected condition being observed.

Codes from subcategory V89.0, Suspected maternal and fetal conditions not found, may either be used as a first listed or as an additional code assignment depending on the case. They are for use in very limited circumstances on a maternal record when an encounter is for a suspected maternal or fetal condition that is ruled out during that encounter (for example, a maternal or fetal condition may be suspected due to an abnormal test result). These codes should not be used when the condition is confirmed. In those cases, the confirmed condition should be coded. In addition, these codes are not for use if an illness or any signs or symptoms related to the suspected condition or problem are present. In such cases the diagnosis/symptom code is used.

Additional codes may be used in addition to the code from subcategory V89.0, but only if they are unrelated to the suspected condition being evaluated.

Codes from subcategory V89.0 may not be used for encounters for antenatal screening of mother.
See Section I.C.18.d., Screening.

For encounters for suspected fetal condition that are inconclusive following testing and evaluation, assign the appropriate code from category 655, 656, 657 or 658.

The observation V code categories:

V29	Observation and evaluation of newborns for suspected condition not found For the birth encounter, a code from category V30 should be sequenced before the V29 code.
V71	Observation and evaluation for suspected condition not found
V89	Suspected maternal and fetal conditions not found

7) Aftercare

Aftercare visit codes cover situations when the initial treatment of a disease or injury has been performed and the patient requires continued care during the healing or recovery phase, or for the long-term consequences of the disease. The aftercare V code should not be used if treatment is directed at a current, acute disease or injury. The diagnosis code is to be used in these cases. Exceptions to this rule are codes V58.0, Radiotherapy, and codes from subcategory V58.1, Encounter for chemotherapy and immunotherapy for neoplastic conditions. These codes are to be first listed, followed by the diagnosis code when a patient's encounter is solely to receive radiation therapy or chemotherapy for the treatment of a neoplasm. Should a patient receive both chemotherapy and radiation therapy during the same encounter code V58.0 and V58.1 may be used together on a record with either one being sequenced first.

The aftercare codes are generally first listed to explain the specific reason for the encounter. An aftercare code may be used as an additional code when some type of aftercare is provided in addition to the reason for admission and no diagnosis code is applicable. An example of this would be the closure of a colostomy during an encounter for treatment of another condition.

Aftercare codes should be used in conjunction with any other aftercare codes or other diagnosis codes to provide better detail on the specifics of an aftercare encounter visit, unless otherwise directed by the classification. The sequencing of multiple aftercare codes is discretionary.

Certain aftercare V code categories need a secondary diagnosis code to describe the resolving condition or sequelae, for others, the condition is inherent in the code title.

Additional V code aftercare category terms include, fitting and adjustment, and attention to artificial openings.

Status V codes may be used with aftercare V codes to indicate the nature of the aftercare. For example code V45.81, Aortocoronary bypass status, may be used with code V58.73, Aftercare following surgery of the circulatory system, NEC, to indicate the surgery for which the aftercare is being performed. Also, a transplant status code may be used following code V58.44, Aftercare following organ transplant, to identify the organ transplanted. A status code should not be used when the aftercare code indicates the type of status, such as using V55.0, Attention to tracheostomy with V44.0, Tracheostomy status. *See Section I. B.15 Admissions/Encounter for Rehabilitation*

The aftercare V category/codes:

V51.0	Encounter for breast reconstruction following mastectomy
V52	Fitting and adjustment of prosthetic device and implant
V53	Fitting and adjustment of other device
V54	Other orthopedic aftercare
V55	Attention to artificial openings
V56	Encounter for dialysis and dialysis catheter care
V57	Care involving the use of rehabilitation procedures
V58.0	Radiotherapy
V58.11	Encounter for antineoplastic chemotherapy
V58.12	Encounter for antineoplastic immunotherapy
V58.3x	Attention to dressings and sutures
V58.41	Encounter for planned post-operative wound closure
V58.42	Aftercare, surgery, neoplasm
V58.43	Aftercare, surgery, trauma
V58.44	Aftercare involving organ transplant
V58.49	Other specified aftercare following surgery
V58.7x	Aftercare following surgery
V58.81	Fitting and adjustment of vascular catheter
V58.82	Fitting and adjustment of non-vascular catheter
V58.83	Monitoring therapeutic drug
V58.89	Other specified aftercare

8) Follow-up

The follow-up codes are used to explain continuing surveillance following completed treatment of a disease, condition, or injury. They imply that the condition has been fully treated and no longer exists. They should not be confused with aftercare codes that explain current treatment for a healing condition or its sequelae. Follow-up codes may be used in conjunction with history codes to provide the full picture of the healed condition and its treatment. The follow-up code is sequenced first, followed by the history code.

A follow-up code may be used to explain repeated visits. Should a condition be found to have recurred on the follow-up visit, then the diagnosis code should be used in place of the follow-up code.

The follow-up V code categories:

V24	Postpartum care and evaluation
V67	Follow-up examination

9) Donor

Category V59 is the donor codes. They are used for living individuals who are donating blood or other body tissue. These codes are only for individuals donating for others, not for self donations. They are not for use to identify cadaveric donations.

10) Counseling

Counseling V codes are used when a patient or family member receives assistance in the aftermath of an illness or injury, or when support is required in coping with family or social problems. They are not necessary for use in conjunction with a diagnosis code when the counseling component of care is considered integral to standard treatment.

The counseling V categories/codes:

V25.0	General counseling and advice for contraceptive management
V26.3	Genetic counseling
V26.4	General counseling and advice for procreative management
V61.**x**	Other family circumstances
V65.1	Person consulted on behalf of another person
V65.3	Dietary surveillance and counseling
V65.4	Other counseling, not elsewhere classified

11) Obstetrics and related conditions

See Section I.C.11., the Obstetrics guidelines for further instruction on the use of these codes.

V codes for pregnancy are for use in those circumstances when none of the problems or complications included in the codes from the Obstetrics chapter exist (a routine prenatal visit or postpartum care). Codes V22.0, Supervision of normal first pregnancy, and V22.1, Supervision of other normal pregnancy, are always first listed and are not to be used with any other code from the OB chapter.

The outcome of delivery, category V27, should be included on all maternal delivery records. It is always a secondary code.

V codes for family planning (contraceptive) or procreative management and counseling should be included on an obstetric record either during the pregnancy or the postpartum stage, if applicable.

Obstetrics and related conditions V code categories:

V22	Normal pregnancy
V23	Supervision of high-risk pregnancy Except: V23.2, Pregnancy with history of abortion. Code 646.3, Habitual aborter, from the OB chapter is required to indicate a history of abortion during a pregnancy.
V24	Postpartum care and evaluation
V25	Encounter for contraceptive management Except V25.0x *See Section I.C.18.d.11, Counseling*
V26	Procreative management Except V26.5x, Sterilization status, V26.3 and V26.4 *See Section I.C.18.d.11., Counseling*
V27	Outcome of delivery
V28	Antenatal screening *See Section I.C.18.d.6., Screening*

12) Newborn, infant and child

See Section I.C.15, the Newborn guidelines for further instruction on the use of these codes.

Newborn V code categories:

V20	Health supervision of infant or child
V29	Observation and evaluation of newborns for suspected condition not found *See Section I.C.18.d.7, Observation*
V30-V39	Liveborn infant according to type of birth

13) Routine and administrative examinations

The V codes allow for the description of encounters for routine examinations, such as, a general check-up, or, examinations for administrative purposes, such as, a pre-employment physical.

The codes are not to be used if the examination is for diagnosis of a suspected condition or for treatment purposes. In such cases the diagnosis code is used. During a routine exam, should a diagnosis or condition be discovered, it should be coded as an additional code. Pre-existing and chronic conditions and history codes may also be included as additional codes as long as the examination is for administrative purposes and not focused on any particular condition.

Pre-operative examination **and pre-procedural laboratory examination** V codes are for use only in those situations when a patient is being cleared for **a procedure or** surgery and no treatment is given.

The V codes categories/code for routine and administrative examinations:

V20.2   Routine infant or child health check
         Any injections given should have a corresponding procedure code.

V70   General medical examination

V72   Special investigations and examinations
         Codes V72.5 **and V72.62** may be used if the reason for the patient encounter is for routine laboratory/radiology testing in the absence of any signs, symptoms, or associated diagnosis. If routine testing is performed during the same encounter as a test to evaluate a sign, symptom, or diagnosis, it is appropriate to assign both the V code and the code describing the reason for the non-routine test.

14) Miscellaneous V codes

The miscellaneous V codes capture a number of other health care encounters that do not fall into one of the other categories. Certain of these codes identify the reason for the encounter, others are for use as additional codes that provide useful information on circumstances that may affect a patient's care and treatment.

Prophylactic organ removal

For encounters specifically for prophylactic removal of breasts, ovaries, or another organ due to a genetic susceptibility to cancer or a family history of cancer, the principal or first listed code should be a code from subcategory V50.4, Prophylactic organ removal, followed by the appropriate genetic susceptibility code and the appropriate family history code.

If the patient has a malignancy of one site and is having prophylactic removal at another site to prevent either a new primary malignancy or metastatic disease, a code for the malignancy should also be assigned in addition to a code from subcategory V50.4. A V50.4 code should not be assigned if the patient is having organ removal for treatment of a malignancy, such as the removal of the testes for the treatment of prostate cancer.

Miscellaneous V code categories/codes:

V07   Need for isolation and other prophylactic or treatment measures
         Except V07.5, Use of agents affecting estrogen receptors and estrogen levels

V50   Elective surgery for purposes other than remedying health states

V58.5   Orthodontics

V60   Housing, household, and economic circumstances

V62   Other psychosocial circumstances

V63   Unavailability of other medical facilities for care

V64   Persons encountering health services for specific procedures, not carried out

V66   Convalescence and palliative care

V68   Encounters for administrative purposes

V69   Problems related to lifestyle

15) Nonspecific V codes

Certain V codes are so non-specific, or potentially redundant with other codes in the classification, that there can be little justification for their use in the inpatient setting. Their use in the outpatient setting should be limited to those instances when there is no further documentation to permit more precise coding. Otherwise, any sign or symptom or any other reason for visit that is captured in another code should be used.

Nonspecific V code categories/codes:

V11   Personal history of mental disorder A code from the mental disorders chapter, with an in remission fifth-digit, should be used.

V13.4   Personal history of arthritis

V13.6   Personal history of congenital malformations

V15.7   Personal history of contraception

V23.2   Pregnancy with history of abortion

V40   Mental and behavioral problems

V41   Problems with special senses and other special functions

V47   Other problems with internal organs

V48   Problems with head, neck, and trunk

V49   Problems with limbs and other problems
         Exceptions:
         V49.6   Upper limb amputation status
         V49.7   Lower limb amputation status
         V49.81   Postmenopausal status
         V49.82   Dental sealant status
         V49.83   Awaiting organ transplant status

V51.8   Other aftercare involving the use of plastic surgery

V58.2   Blood transfusion, without reported diagnosis

V58.9   Unspecified aftercare
         See Section IV.K. and Section IV.L. of the Outpatient guidelines.

e. V Codes That May Only be Principal/First-Listed Diagnosis

The list of V codes/categories below may only be reported as the principal/first-listed diagnosis, except when there are multiple encounters on the same day and the medical records for the encounters are combined or when there is more than one V code that meets the definition of principal diagnosis (e.g., a patient is admitted to home healthcare for both aftercare and rehabilitation and they equally meet the definition of principal diagnosis). These codes should not be reported if they do not meet the definition of principal or first-listed diagnosis.

See Section II and Section IV.A for information on selection of principal and first-listed diagnosis.

See Section II.C for information on two or more diagnoses that equally meet the definition for principal diagnosis.

V20.x   Health supervision of infant or child

V22.0   Supervision of normal first pregnancy

V22.1   Supervision of other normal pregnancy

V24.x   Postpartum care and examination

V26.81   Encounter for assisted reproductive fertility procedure cycle

V26.82   Encounter for fertility preservation procedure

V30.x   Single liveborn

V31.x   Twin, mate liveborn

V32.x   Twin, mate stillborn

V33.x   Twin, unspecified

V34.x   Other multiple, mates all liveborn

V35.x   Other multiple, mates all stillborn

V36.x   Other multiple, mates live- and stillborn

V37.x	Other multiple, unspecified
V39.x	Unspecified
V46.12	Encounter for respirator dependence during power failure
V46.13	Encounter for weaning from respirator [ventilator]
V51.0	Encounter for breast reconstruction following mastectomy
V56.0	Extracorporeal dialysis
V57.x	Care involving use of rehabilitation procedures
V58.0	Radiotherapy
V58.11	Encounter for antineoplastic chemotherapy
V58.12	Encounter for antineoplastic immunotherapy
V59.x	Donors
V66.0	Convalescence and palliative care following surgery
V66.1	Convalescence and palliative care following radiotherapy
V66.2	Convalescence and palliative care following chemotherapy
V66.3	Convalescence and palliative care following psychotherapy and other treatment for mental disorder
V66.4	Convalescence and palliative care following treatment of fracture
V66.5	Convalescence and palliative care following other treatment
V66.6	Convalescence and palliative care following combined treatment
V66.9	Unspecified convalescence
V68.x	Encounters for administrative purposes
V70.0	Routine general medical examination at a health care facility
V70.1	General psychiatric examination, requested by the authority
V70.2	General psychiatric examination, other and unspecified
V70.3	Other medical examination for administrative purposes
V70.4	Examination for medicolegal reasons
V70.5	Health examination of defined subpopulations
V70.6	Health examination in population surveys
V70.8	Other specified general medical examinations
V70.9	Unspecified general medical examination
V71.x	Observation and evaluation for suspected conditions not found

19. **Supplemental Classification of External Causes of Injury and Poisoning (E codes, E000-E999)**
Introduction: These guidelines are provided for those who are currently collecting E codes in order that there will be standardization in the process. If your institution plans to begin collecting E codes, these guidelines are to be applied. The use of E codes is supplemental to the application of ICD-9-CM diagnosis codes.

External causes of injury and poisoning codes (**categories E000 and E800-E999**) are intended to provide data for injury research and evaluation of injury prevention strategies. **Activity codes (categories E001-E030) are intended to be used to describe the activity of a person seeking care for injuries as well as other health conditions, when the injury or other health condition resulted from an activity or the activity contributed to a condition.** E codes capture how the injury, **poisoning, or adverse effect** happened (cause), the intent (unintentional or accidental; or intentional, such as suicide or assault), **the person's status (e.g. civilian, military), the associated activity** and the place where the event occurred.

Some major categories of E codes include:

- transport accidents
- poisoning and adverse effects of drugs, medicinal substances and biologicals
- accidental falls
- accidents caused by fire and flames
- accidents due to natural and environmental factors
- late effects of accidents, assaults or self injury
- assaults or purposely inflicted injury
- suicide or self inflicted injury

These guidelines apply for the coding and collection of E codes from records in hospitals, outpatient clinics, emergency departments, other ambulatory care settings and provider offices, and nonacute care settings, except when other specific guidelines apply.

a. **General E code coding guidelines**

1) **Used with any code in the range of 001-V89**
An E code **from categories E800-E999** may be used with any code in the range of 001-V89, which indicates an injury, poisoning, or adverse effect due to an external cause.

An activity E code (categories E001-E030) may be used with any code in the range of 001-V89 that indicates an injury, or other health condition that resulted from an activity, or the activity contributed to a condition.

2) **Assign the appropriate E code for all initial treatments**
Assign the appropriate E code for the initial encounter of an injury, poisoning, or adverse effect of drugs, not for subsequent treatment.

External cause of injury codes (E-codes) may be assigned while the acute fracture codes are still applicable.

See Section I.C.17.b.1 for coding of acute fractures.

3) **Use the full range of E codes**
Use the full range of E codes (**E800-E999**) to completely describe the cause, the intent and the place of occurrence, if applicable, for all injuries, poisonings, and adverse effects of drugs.

See a.1.), j.), and k.) in this section for information on the use of status and activity E codes.

4) **Assign as many E codes as necessary**
Assign as many E codes as necessary to fully explain each cause.

5) **The selection of the appropriate E code**
The selection of the appropriate E code is guided by the Index to External Causes, which is located after the alphabetical index to diseases and by Inclusion and Exclusion notes in the Tabular List.

6) **E code can never be a principal diagnosis**
An E code can never be a principal (first listed) diagnosis.

7) **External cause code(s) with systemic inflammatory response syndrome (SIRS)**
An external cause code is not appropriate with a code from subcategory 995.9, unless the patient also has **another condition for which an E code would be appropriate (such as** an injury, poisoning, or adverse effect of drugs).

8. **Multiple Cause E Code Coding Guidelines**
More than one E-code is required to fully describe the external cause of an illness, injury or poisoning. The assignment of E-codes should be sequenced in the following priority:

If two or more events cause separate injuries, an E code should be assigned for each cause. The first listed E code will be selected in the following order:

E codes for child and adult abuse take priority over all other E codes.

See Section I.C.19.e., Child and Adult abuse guidelines.

E codes for terrorism events take priority over all other E codes except child and adult abuse.

E codes for cataclysmic events take priority over all other E codes except child and adult abuse and terrorism.

E codes for transport accidents take priority over all other E codes except cataclysmic events, child and adult abuse and terrorism.

Activity and external cause status codes are assigned following all causal (intent) E codes.

The first-listed E code should correspond to the cause of the most serious diagnosis due to an assault, accident, or self-harm, following the order of hierarchy listed above.

9. **If the reporting format limits the number of E codes**
   If the reporting format limits the number of E codes that can be used in reporting clinical data, report the code for the cause/intent most related to the principal diagnosis. If the format permits capture of additional E codes, the cause/intent, including medical misadventures, of the additional events should be reported rather than the codes for place, activity or external status.

b. **Place of occurrence guideline**
   Use an additional code from category E849 to indicate the Place of Occurrence for injuries and poisonings. The Place of Occurrence describes the place where the event occurred and not the patient's activity at the time of the event.
   Do not use E849.9 if the place of occurrence is not stated.

c. **Adverse effects of drugs, medicinal and biological substances guidelines**

   1) **Do not code directly from the Table of Drugs**
      Do not code directly from the Table of Drugs and Chemicals. Always refer back to the Tabular List.

   2) **Use as many codes as necessary to describe**
      Use as many codes as necessary to describe completely all drugs, medicinal or biological substances.

      If the reporting format limits the number of E codes, and there are different fourth digit codes in the same three digit category, use the code for "Other specified" of that category of drugs, medicinal or biological substances. If there is no "Other specified" code in that category, use the appropriate "Unspecified" code in that category.

      If the reporting format limits the number of E codes, and the codes are in different three digit categories, assign the appropriate E code for other multiple drugs and medicinal substances.

   3) **If the same E code would describe the causative agent**
      If the same E code would describe the causative agent for more than one adverse reaction, assign the code only once.

   4) **If two or more drugs, medicinal or biological substances**
      If two or more drugs, medicinal or biological substances are reported, code each individually unless the combination code is listed in the Table of Drugs and Chemicals. In that case, assign the E code for the combination.

   5) **When a reaction results from the interaction of a drug(s)**
      When a reaction results from the interaction of a drug(s) and alcohol, use poisoning codes and E codes for both.

   6) **Codes from the E930-E949 series**
      Codes from the E930-E949 series must be used to identify the causative substance for an adverse effect of drug, medicinal and biological substances, correctly prescribed and properly administered. The effect, such as tachycardia, delirium, gastrointestinal hemorrhaging, vomiting, hypokalemia, hepatitis, renal failure, or respiratory failure, is coded and followed by the appropriate code from the E930-E949 series.

d. **Child and adult abuse guideline**

   1) **Intentional injury**
      When the cause of an injury or neglect is intentional child or adult abuse, the first listed E code should be assigned from categories E960-E968, Homicide and injury purposely inflicted by other persons, (except category E967). An E code from category E967, Child and adult battering and other maltreatment, should be added as an additional code to identify the perpetrator, if known.

   2) **Accidental intent**
      In cases of neglect when the intent is determined to be accidental E code E904.0, Abandonment or neglect of infant and helpless person, should be the first listed E code.

e. **Unknown or suspected intent guideline**

   1) **If the intent (accident, self-harm, assault) of the cause of an injury or poisoning is unknown**
      If the intent (accident, self-harm, assault) of the cause of an injury or poisoning is unknown or unspecified, code the intent as undetermined E980-E989.

   2) **If the intent (accident, self-harm, assault) of the cause of an injury or poisoning is questionable**
      If the intent (accident, self-harm, assault) of the cause of an injury or poisoning is questionable, probable or suspected, code the intent as undetermined E980-E989.

f. **Undetermined cause**
   When the intent of an injury or poisoning is known, but the cause is unknown, use codes: E928.9, Unspecified accident, E958.9, Suicide and self-inflicted injury by unspecified means, and E968.9, Assault by unspecified means.

   These E codes should rarely be used, as the documentation in the medical record, in both the inpatient, outpatient and other settings, should normally provide sufficient detail to determine the cause of the injury.

g. **Late effects of external cause guidelines**

   1) **Late effect E codes**
      Late effect E codes exist for injuries and poisonings but not for adverse effects of drugs, misadventures and surgical complications.

   2) **Late effect E codes (E929, E959, E969, E977, E989, or E999.1)**
      A late effect E code (E929, E959, E969, E977, E989, or E999.1) should be used with any report of a late effect or sequela resulting from a previous injury or poisoning (905-909).

   3) **Late effect E code with a related current injury**
      A late effect E code should never be used with a related current nature of injury code.

   4) **Use of late effect E codes for subsequent visits**
      Use a late effect E code for subsequent visits when a late effect of the initial injury or poisoning is being treated. There is no late effect E code for adverse effects of drugs. Do not use a late effect E code for subsequent visits for follow-up care (e.g., to assess healing, to receive rehabilitative therapy) of the injury or poisoning when no late effect of the injury has been documented.

h. **Misadventures and complications of care guidelines**

   1) **Code range E870-E876**
      Assign a code in the range of E870-E876 if misadventures are stated by the provider. **When applying the E code guidelines pertaining to sequencing, these E codes are considered causal codes.**

2) **Code range E878-E879**

Assign a code in the range of E878-E879 if the provider attributes an abnormal reaction or later complication to a surgical or medical procedure, but does not mention misadventure at the time of the procedure as the cause of the reaction.

i. **Terrorism guidelines**

1) **Cause of injury identified by the Federal Government (FBI) as terrorism**

When the cause of an injury is identified by the Federal Government (FBI) as terrorism, the first-listed E-code should be a code from category E979, Terrorism. The definition of terrorism employed by the FBI is found at the inclusion note at E979. The terrorism E-code is the only E-code that should be assigned. Additional E codes from the assault categories should not be assigned.

2) **Cause of an injury is suspected to be the result of terrorism**

When the cause of an injury is suspected to be the result of terrorism a code from category E979 should not be assigned. Assign a code in the range of E codes based circumstances on the documentation of intent and mechanism.

3) **Code E979.9, Terrorism, secondary effects**

Assign code E979.9, Terrorism, secondary effects, for conditions occurring subsequent to the terrorist event. This code should not be assigned for conditions that are due to the initial terrorist act.

4) **Statistical tabulation of terrorism codes**

For statistical purposes these codes will be tabulated within the category for assault, expanding the current category from E960-E969 to include E979 and E999.1.

j. **Activity Code Guidelines**

Assign a code from category E001-E030 to describe the activity that caused or contributed to the injury or other health condition.

Unlike other E codes, activity E codes may be assigned to indicate a health condition (not just injuries) resulted from an activity, or the activity contributed to the condition.

The activity codes are not applicable to poisonings, adverse effects, misadventures or late effects.

k. **External cause status**

A code from category E000, External cause status, should be assigned whenever any other E code is assigned for an encounter, including an Activity E code, except for the events noted below. Assign a code from category E000, External cause status, to indicate the work status of the person at the time the event occurred. The status code indicates whether the event occurred during military activity, whether a non-military person was at work, whether an individual including a student or volunteer was involved in a non-work activity at the time of the causal event.

A code from E000, External cause status, should be assigned, when applicable, with other external cause codes, such as transport accidents and falls. The external cause status codes are not applicable to poisonings, adverse effects, misadventures or late effects.

Do not assign a code from category E000 if no other E codes (cause, activity) are applicable for the encounter.

Do not assign code E000.9, Unspecified external cause status, if the status is not stated.

Section II. Selection of Principal Diagnosis

The circumstances of inpatient admission always govern the selection of principal diagnosis. The principal diagnosis is defined in the Uniform Hospital Discharge Data Set (UHDDS) as "that condition established after study to be chiefly responsible for occasioning the admission of the patient to the hospital for care."

The UHDDS definitions are used by hospitals to report inpatient data elements in a standardized manner. These data elements and their definitions can be found in the July 31, 1985, Federal Register (Vol. 50, No, 147), pp. 31038-40.

Since that time the application of the UHDDS definitions has been expanded to include all non-outpatient settings (acute care, short term, long term care and psychiatric hospitals; home health agencies; rehab facilities; nursing homes, etc.).

In determining principal diagnosis the coding conventions in the ICD-9-CM, Volumes I and II take precedence over these official coding guidelines.

(See Section I.A., Conventions for the ICD-9-CM)

The importance of consistent, complete documentation in the medical record cannot be overemphasized. Without such documentation the application of all coding guidelines is a difficult, if not impossible, task.

A. **Codes for symptoms, signs, and ill-defined conditions**

Codes for symptoms, signs, and ill-defined conditions from Chapter 16 are not to be used as principal diagnosis when a related definitive diagnosis has been established.

B. **Two or more interrelated conditions, each potentially meeting the definition for principal diagnosis**

When there are two or more interrelated conditions (such as diseases in the same ICD-9-CM chapter or manifestations characteristically associated with a certain disease) potentially meeting the definition of principal diagnosis, either condition may be sequenced first, unless the circumstances of the admission, the therapy provided, the Tabular List, or the Alphabetic Index indicate otherwise.

C. **Two or more diagnoses that equally meet the definition for principal diagnosis**

In the unusual instance when two or more diagnoses equally meet the criteria for principal diagnosis as determined by the circumstances of admission, diagnostic workup and/or therapy provided, and the Alphabetic Index, Tabular List, or another coding guidelines does not provide sequencing direction, any one of the diagnoses may be sequenced first.

D. **Two or more comparative or contrasting conditions**

In those rare instances when two or more contrasting or comparative diagnoses are documented as "either/or" (or similar terminology), they are coded as if the diagnoses were confirmed and the diagnoses are sequenced according to the circumstances of the admission. If no further determination can be made as to which diagnosis should be principal, either diagnosis may be sequenced first.

E. **A symptom(s) followed by contrasting/comparative diagnoses**

When a symptom(s) is followed by contrasting/comparative diagnoses, the symptom code is sequenced first. All the contrasting/comparative diagnoses should be coded as additional diagnoses.

F. **Original treatment plan not carried out**

Sequence as the principal diagnosis the condition, which after study occasioned the admission to the hospital, even though treatment may not have been carried out due to unforeseen circumstances.

G. **Complications of surgery and other medical care**

When the admission is for treatment of a complication resulting from surgery or other medical care, the complication code is sequenced as the principal diagnosis. If the complication is classified to the 996-999 series and the code lacks the necessary specificity in describing the complication, an additional code for the specific complication should be assigned.

H. **Uncertain diagnosis**

If the diagnosis documented at the time of discharge is qualified as "probable", "suspected", "likely", "questionable", "possible", or "still to be ruled out", or other similar terms indicating uncertainty, code the condition as if it existed or was established. The bases for these guidelines are the diagnostic workup, arrangements for further workup or observation, and initial therapeutic approach that correspond most closely with the established diagnosis.

Note: This guideline is applicable only to inpatient admissions to short-term, acute, long-term care and psychiatric hospitals.

I.   Admission from observation unit

1.   Admission following medical observation

When a patient is admitted to an observation unit for a medical condition, which either worsens or does not improve, and is subsequently admitted as an inpatient of the same hospital for this same medical condition, the principal diagnosis would be the medical condition which led to the hospital admission.

2.   Admission following post-operative observation

When a patient is admitted to an observation unit to monitor a condition (or complication) that develops following outpatient surgery, and then is subsequently admitted as an inpatient of the same hospital, hospitals should apply the Uniform Hospital Discharge Data Set (UHDDS) definition of principal diagnosis as "that condition established after study to be chiefly responsible for occasioning the admission of the patient to the hospital for care."

J.   Admission from outpatient surgery

When a patient receives surgery in the hospital's outpatient surgery department and is subsequently admitted for continuing inpatient care at the same hospital, the following guidelines should be followed in selecting the principal diagnosis for the inpatient admission:

- If the reason for the inpatient admission is a complication, assign the complication as the principal diagnosis.

- If no complication, or other condition, is documented as the reason for the inpatient admission, assign the reason for the outpatient surgery as the principal diagnosis.

- If the reason for the inpatient admission is another condition unrelated to the surgery, assign the unrelated condition as the principal diagnosis.

SECTION III. REPORTING ADDITIONAL DIAGNOSES
GENERAL RULES FOR OTHER (ADDITIONAL) DIAGNOSES

For reporting purposes the definition for "other diagnoses" is interpreted as additional conditions that affect patient care in terms of requiring:

clinical evaluation; or
therapeutic treatment; or
diagnostic procedures; or
extended length of hospital stay; or
increased nursing care and/or monitoring.

The UHDDS item #11-b defines Other Diagnoses as "all conditions that coexist at the time of admission, that develop subsequently, or that affect the treatment received and/or the length of stay. Diagnoses that relate to an earlier episode which have no bearing on the current hospital stay are to be excluded." UHDDS definitions apply to inpatients in acute care, short-term, long term care and psychiatric hospital setting. The UHDDS definitions are used by acute care short-term hospitals to report inpatient data elements in a standardized manner. These data elements and their definitions can be found in the July 31, 1985, Federal Register (Vol. 50, No, 147), pp. 31038-40.

Since that time the application of the UHDDS definitions has been expanded to include all non-outpatient settings (acute care, short term, long term care and psychiatric hospitals; home health agencies; rehab facilities; nursing homes, etc).

The following guidelines are to be applied in designating "other diagnoses" when neither the Alphabetic Index nor the Tabular List in ICD-9-CM provide direction. The listing of the diagnoses in the patient record is the responsibility of the attending provider.

A.   Previous conditions

If the provider has included a diagnosis in the final diagnostic statement, such as the discharge summary or the face sheet, it should ordinarily be coded. Some providers include in the diagnostic statement resolved conditions or diagnoses and status-post procedures from previous admission that have no bearing on the current stay. Such conditions are not to be reported and are coded only if required by hospital policy.

However, history codes (V10-V19) may be used as secondary codes if the historical condition or family history has an impact on current care or influences treatment.

B.   Abnormal findings

Abnormal findings (laboratory, x-ray, pathologic, and other diagnostic results) are not coded and reported unless the provider indicates their clinical significance. If the findings are outside the normal range and the attending provider has ordered other tests to evaluate the condition or prescribed treatment, it is appropriate to ask the provider whether the abnormal finding should be added.

Please note: This differs from the coding practices in the outpatient setting for coding encounters for diagnostic tests that have been interpreted by a provider.

C.   Uncertain diagnosis

If the diagnosis documented at the time of discharge is qualified as "probable", "suspected", "likely", "questionable", "possible", or "still to be ruled out" or other similar terms indicating uncertainty, code the condition as if it existed or was established. The bases for these guidelines are the diagnostic workup, arrangements for further workup or observation, and initial therapeutic approach that correspond most closely with the established diagnosis.

Note: This guideline is applicable only to inpatient admissions to short-term, acute, long-term care and psychiatric hospitals.

SECTION IV. DIAGNOSTIC CODING AND REPORTING GUIDELINES FOR OUTPATIENT SERVICES

These coding guidelines for outpatient diagnoses have been approved for use by hospitals/ providers in coding and reporting hospital-based outpatient services and provider-based office visits.

Information about the use of certain abbreviations, punctuation, symbols, and other conventions used in the ICD-9-CM Tabular List (code numbers and titles), can be found in Section IA of these guidelines, under "Conventions Used in the Tabular List." Information about the correct sequence to use in finding a code is also described in Section I.

The terms encounter and visit are often used interchangeably in describing outpatient service contacts and, therefore, appear together in these guidelines without distinguishing one from the other.

Though the conventions and general guidelines apply to all settings, coding guidelines for outpatient and provider reporting of diagnoses will vary in a number of instances from those for inpatient diagnoses, recognizing that:

The Uniform Hospital Discharge Data Set (UHDDS) definition of principal diagnosis applies only to inpatients in acute, short-term, long-term care and psychiatric hospitals.

Coding guidelines for inconclusive diagnoses (probable, suspected, rule out, etc.) were developed for inpatient reporting and do not apply to outpatients.

A.   Selection of first-listed condition

In the outpatient setting, the term first-listed diagnosis is used in lieu of principal diagnosis.

In determining the first-listed diagnosis the coding conventions of ICD-9-CM, as well as the general and disease specific guidelines take precedence over the outpatient guidelines.

Diagnoses often are not established at the time of the initial encounter/visit. It may take two or more visits before the diagnosis is confirmed.

The most critical rule involves beginning the search for the correct code assignment through the Alphabetic Index. Never begin searching initially in the Tabular List as this will lead to coding errors.

1.   Outpatient surgery

When a patient presents for outpatient surgery, code the reason for the surgery as the first-listed diagnosis (reason for the encounter), even if the surgery is not performed due to a contraindication.

2.   Observation stay

When a patient is admitted for observation for a medical condition, assign a code for the medical condition as the first-listed diagnosis.

When a patient presents for outpatient surgery and develops complications requiring admission to observation, code the reason for the surgery as the first reported diagnosis (reason for the encounter), followed by codes for the complications as secondary diagnoses.

B.   Codes from 001.0 through V89

The appropriate code or codes from 001.0 through V89 must be used to identify diagnoses, symptoms, conditions, problems, complaints, or other reason(s) for the encounter/visit.

C.   Accurate reporting of ICD-9-CM diagnosis codes

For accurate reporting of ICD-9-CM diagnosis codes, the documentation should describe the patient's condition, using terminology which includes specific diagnoses as well as symptoms, problems, or reasons for the encounter. There are ICD-9-CM codes to describe all of these.

D.   Selection of codes 001.0 through 999.9

The selection of codes 001.0 through 999.9 will frequently be used to describe the reason for the encounter. These codes are from the section of ICD-9-CM for the classification of diseases and injuries (e.g. infectious and parasitic diseases; neoplasms; symptoms, signs, and ill-defined conditions, etc.).

E.   Codes that describe symptoms and signs

Codes that describe symptoms and signs, as opposed to diagnoses, are acceptable for reporting purposes when a diagnosis has not been established (confirmed) by the provider. Chapter 16 of ICD-9-CM, Symptoms, Signs, and Ill-defined conditions (codes 780.0-799.9) contain many, but not all codes for symptoms.

F.   Encounters for circumstances other than a disease or injury

ICD-9-CM provides codes to deal with encounters for circumstances other than a disease or injury. The Supplementary Classification of factors Influencing Health Status and Contact with Health Services (V01.0-V89) is provided to deal with occasions when circumstances other than a disease or injury are recorded as diagnosis or problems. *See Section I.C. 18 for information on V-codes*

G.   Level of detail in coding

1.   ICD-9-CM codes with 3, 4, or 5 digits

ICD-9-CM is composed of codes with either 3, 4, or 5 digits. Codes with three digits are included in ICD-9-CM as the heading of a category of codes that may be further subdivided by the use of fourth and/or fifth-digits, which provide greater specificity.

2.   Use of full number of digits required for a code

A three-digit code is to be used only if it is not further subdivided. Where fourth-digit subcategories and/or fifth-digit subclassifications are provided, they must be assigned. A code is invalid if it has not been coded to the full number of digits required for that code.

See also discussion under Section I.b.3., General Coding Guidelines, Level of Detail in Coding.

H.   ICD-9-CM code for the diagnosis, condition, problem, or other reason for encounter/visit

List first the ICD-9-CM code for the diagnosis, condition, problem, or other reason for encounter/visit shown in the medical record to be chiefly responsible for the services provided. List additional codes that describe any coexisting conditions. In some cases the first-listed diagnosis may be a symptom when a diagnosis has not been established (confirmed) by the physician.

I.   Uncertain diagnosis

Do not code diagnoses documented as "probable", "suspected," "questionable," "rule out," or "working diagnosis" or other similar terms indicating uncertainty. Rather, code the condition(s) to the highest degree of certainty for that encounter/visit, such as symptoms, signs, abnormal test results, or other reason for the visit.

Please note: This differs from the coding practices used by short-term, acute care, long-term care and psychiatric hospitals.

J.   Chronic diseases

Chronic diseases treated on an ongoing basis may be coded and reported as many times as the patient receives treatment and care for the condition(s)

K.   Code all documented conditions that coexist

Code all documented conditions that coexist at the time of the

encounter/visit, and require or affect patient care treatment or management. Do not code conditions that were previously treated and no longer exist. However, history codes (V10-V19) may be used as secondary codes if the historical condition or family history has an impact on current care or influences treatment.

L.   Patients receiving diagnostic services only

For patients receiving diagnostic services only during an encounter/visit, sequence first the diagnosis, condition, problem, or other reason for encounter/visit shown in the medical record to be chiefly responsible for the outpatient services provided during the encounter/visit. Codes for other diagnoses (e.g., chronic conditions) may be sequenced as additional diagnoses.

For encounters for routine laboratory/radiology testing in the absence of any signs, symptoms, or associated diagnosis, assign V72.5 and **a code from the subcategory** V72.6. If routine testing is performed during the same encounter as a test to evaluate a sign, symptom, or diagnosis, it is appropriate to assign both the V code and the code describing the reason for the non-routine test.

For outpatient encounters for diagnostic tests that have been interpreted by a physician, and the final report is available at the time of coding, code any confirmed or definitive diagnosis(es) documented in the interpretation. Do not code related signs and symptoms as additional diagnoses.

Please note: This differs from the coding practice in the hospital inpatient setting regarding abnormal findings on test results.

M.   Patients receiving therapeutic services only

For patients receiving therapeutic services only during an encounter/visit, sequence first the diagnosis, condition, problem, or other reason for encounter/visit shown in the medical record to be chiefly responsible for the outpatient services provided during the encounter/visit. Codes for other diagnoses (e.g., chronic conditions) may be sequenced as additional diagnoses.

The only exception to this rule is that when the primary reason for the admission/encounter is chemotherapy, radiation therapy, or rehabilitation, the appropriate V code for the service is listed first, and the diagnosis or problem for which the service is being performed listed second.

N.   Patients receiving preoperative evaluations only

For patients receiving preoperative evaluations only, sequence first a code from category V72.8, Other specified examinations, to describe the pre-op consultations. Assign a code for the condition to describe the reason for the surgery as an additional diagnosis. Code also any findings related to the pre-op evaluation.

O.   Ambulatory surgery

For ambulatory surgery, code the diagnosis for which the surgery was performed. If the postoperative diagnosis is known to be different from the preoperative diagnosis at the time the diagnosis is confirmed, select the postoperative diagnosis for coding, since it is the most definitive.

P.   Routine outpatient prenatal visits

For routine outpatient prenatal visits when no complications are present, codes V22.0, Supervision of normal first pregnancy, or V22.1, Supervision of other normal pregnancy, should be used as the principal diagnosis. These codes should not be used in conjunction with chapter 11 codes.

APPENDIX I. PRESENT ON ADMISSION REPORTING GUIDELINES

Introduction

These guidelines are to be used as a supplement to the *ICD-9-CM Official Guidelines for Coding and Reporting* to facilitate the assignment of the Present on Admission (POA) indicator for each diagnosis and external cause of injury code reported on claim forms (UB-04 and 837 Institutional).

These guidelines are not intended to replace any guidelines in the main body of the *ICD-9-CM Official Guidelines for Coding and Reporting.* The POA guidelines are not intended to provide guidance on when a condition should be coded, but rather, how to apply the POA indicator to the final set of diagnosis codes that have been assigned in accordance with Sections I, II, and III of the official coding guidelines. Subsequent to the assignment of the ICD-9-CM codes, the POA indicator should then be assigned to those conditions that have been coded.

As stated in the Introduction to the ICD-9-CM Official Guidelines for Coding and Reporting, a joint effort between the healthcare provider and the coder is essential to achieve complete and accurate documentation, code assignment, and reporting of diagnoses and procedures. The importance of consistent, complete documentation in the medical record cannot be overemphasized. Medical record documentation from any provider involved in the care and treatment of the patient may be used to support the determination of whether a condition was present on admission or not. In the context of the official coding guidelines, the term "provider" means a physician or any qualified healthcare practitioner who is legally accountable for establishing the patient's diagnosis.

These guidelines are not a substitute for the provider's clinical judgment as to the determination of whether a condition was/was not present on admission. The provider should be queried regarding issues related to the linking of signs/symptoms, timing of test results, and the timing of findings.

General Reporting Requirements

All claims involving inpatient admissions to general acute care hospitals or other facilities that are subject to a law or regulation mandating collection of present on admission information.

Present on admission is defined as present at the time the order for inpatient admission occurs. Conditions that develop during an outpatient encounter, including emergency department, observation, or outpatient surgery, are considered as present on admission.

POA indicator is assigned to principal and secondary diagnoses (as defined in Section II of the Official Guidelines for Coding and Reporting) and the external cause of injury codes.

Issues related to inconsistent, missing, conflicting or unclear documentation must still be resolved by the provider.

If a condition would not be coded and reported based on UHDDS definitions and current official coding guidelines, then the POA indicator would not be reported.

Reporting Options

Y - Yes

N - No

U - Unknown

W – Clinically undetermined

Unreported/Not used (or "1" for Medicare usage) – (Exempt from POA reporting)

Reporting Definitions

Y = present at the time of inpatient admission

N = not present at the time of inpatient admission

U = documentation is insufficient to determine if condition is present on admission

W = provider is unable to clinically determine whether condition was present on admission or not

Timeframe for POA Identification and Documentation

There is no required timeframe as to when a provider (per the definition of "provider" used in these guidelines) must identify or document a condition to be present on admission. In some clinical situations, it may not be possible for a provider to make a definitive diagnosis (or a condition may not be recognized or reported by the patient) for a period of time after admission. In some cases it may be several days before the provider arrives at a definitive diagnosis. This does not mean that the condition was not present on admission. Determination of whether the condition was present on admission or not will be based on the applicable POA guideline as identified in this document, or on the provider's best clinical judgment.

If at the time of code assignment the documentation is unclear as to whether a condition was present on admission or not, it is appropriate to query the provider for clarification.

Assigning the POA Indicator

Condition is on the "Exempt from Reporting" list

Leave the "present on admission" field blank if the condition is on the list of ICD-9-CM codes for which this field is not applicable. This is the only circumstance in which the field may be left blank.

POA explicitly documented

Assign Y for any condition the provider explicitly documents as being present on admission.

Assign N for any condition the provider explicitly documents as not present at the time of admission.

Conditions diagnosed prior to inpatient admission

Assign "Y" for conditions that were diagnosed prior to admission (example: hypertension, diabetes mellitus, asthma)

Conditions diagnosed during the admission but clearly present before admission

Assign "Y" for conditions diagnosed during the admission that were clearly present but not diagnosed until after admission occurred.

Diagnoses subsequently confirmed after admission are considered present on admission if at the time of admission they are documented as suspected, possible, rule out, differential diagnosis, or constitute an underlying cause of a symptom that is present at the time of admission.

Condition develops during outpatient encounter prior to inpatient admission

Assign Y for any condition that develops during an outpatient encounter prior to a written order for inpatient admission.

Documentation does not indicate whether condition was present on admission

Assign "U" when the medical record documentation is unclear as to whether the condition was present on admission. "U" should not be routinely assigned and used only in very limited circumstances. Coders are encouraged to query the providers when the documentation is unclear.

Documentation states that it cannot be determined whether the condition was or was not present on admission

Assign "W" when the medical record documentation indicates that it cannot be clinically determined whether or not the condition was present on admission.

Chronic condition with acute exacerbation during the admission

If the code is a combination code that identifies both the chronic condition and the acute exacerbation, see POA guidelines pertaining to combination codes.

If the combination code only identifies the chronic condition and not the acute exacerbation (e.g., acute exacerbation of CHF), assign "Y."

Conditions documented as possible, probable, suspected, or rule out at the time of discharge

If the final diagnosis contains a possible, probable, suspected, or rule out diagnosis, and this diagnosis was **based on signs, symptoms or clinical findings** suspected at the time of inpatient admission, assign "Y."

If the final diagnosis contains a possible, probable, suspected, or rule out diagnosis, and this diagnosis was based on **signs,** symptoms or clinical findings that were not present on admission, assign "N".

Conditions documented as impending or threatened at the time of discharge

If the final diagnosis contains an impending or threatened diagnosis, and this diagnosis is based on symptoms or clinical findings that were present on admission, assign "Y".

If the final diagnosis contains an impending or threatened diagnosis, and this diagnosis is based on symptoms or clinical findings that were not present on admission, assign "N".

Acute and chronic conditions

Assign "Y" for acute conditions that are present at time of admission and N for acute conditions that are not present at time of admission.

Assign "Y" for chronic conditions, even though the condition may not be diagnosed until after admission.

If a single code identifies both an acute and chronic condition, see the POA guidelines for combination codes.

Combination codes

Assign "N" if any part of the combination code was not present on admission (e.g., obstructive chronic bronchitis with acute exacerbation and the exacerbation was not present on admission; gastric ulcer that does not start bleeding until after admission; asthma patient develops status asthmaticus after admission)

Assign "Y" if all parts of the combination code were present on admission (e.g., patient with diabetic nephropathy is admitted with uncontrolled diabetes)

If the final diagnosis includes comparative or contrasting diagnoses, and both were present, or suspected, at the time of admission, assign "Y".

For infection codes that include the causal organism, assign "Y" if the infection (or signs of the infection) was present on admission, even though the culture results may not be known until after admission (e.g., patient is admitted with pneumonia and the provider documents pseudomonas as the causal organism a few days later).

Same diagnosis code for two or more conditions

When the same ICD-9-CM diagnosis code applies to two or more conditions during the same encounter (e.g. bilateral condition, or two separate conditions classified to the same ICD-9-CM diagnosis code):

Assign "Y" if all conditions represented by the single ICD-9-CM code were present on admission (e.g. bilateral fracture of the same bone, same site, and both fractures were present on admission)

Assign "N" if any of the conditions represented by the single ICD-9-CM code was not present on admission (e.g. dehydration with hyponatremia is assigned to code 276.1, but only one of these conditions was present on admission).

Obstetrical conditions

Whether or not the patient delivers during the current hospitalization does not affect assignment of the POA indicator. The determining factor for POA assignment is whether the pregnancy complication or obstetrical condition described by the code was present at the time of admission or not.

If the pregnancy complication or obstetrical condition was present on admission (e.g., patient admitted in preterm labor), assign "Y".

If the pregnancy complication or obstetrical condition was not present on admission (e.g., 2nd degree laceration during delivery, postpartum hemorrhage that occurred during current hospitalization, fetal distress develops after admission), assign "N".

If the obstetrical code includes more than one diagnosis and any of the diagnoses identified by the code were not present on admission (e.g., Code 642.7, Pre-eclampsia or eclampsia superimposed on preexisting hypertension) assign "N".

If the obstetrical code includes information that is not a diagnosis, do not consider that information in the POA determination. Example, code 652.1x, Breech or other malpresentation successfully converted to cephalic presentation, should be reported as present on admission if the fetus was breech on admission but was converted to cephalic presentation after admission. Since the conversion to cephalic presentation does not represent a diagnosis, the fact that the conversion occurred after admission has no bearing on the POA determination.

Perinatal conditions

Newborns are not considered to be admitted until after birth. Therefore, any condition present at birth or that developed in utero is considered present at admission and should be assigned "Y". This includes conditions that occur during delivery (e.g., injury during delivery, meconium aspiration, exposure to streptococcus B in the vaginal canal).

Congenital conditions and anomalies

Assign "Y" for congenital conditions and anomalies. Congenital conditions are always considered present on admission.

External cause of injury codes

Assign "Y" for any E code representing an external cause of injury or poisoning that occurred prior to inpatient admission (e.g., patient fell out of bed at home, patient fell out of bed in emergency room prior to admission)

Assign "N" for any E code representing an external cause of injury or poisoning that occurred during inpatient hospitalization (e.g., patient fell out of hospital bed during hospital stay, patient experienced an adverse reaction to a medication administered after inpatient admission)

CATEGORIES AND CODES EXEMPT FROM DIAGNOSIS PRESENT ON ADMISSION REQUIREMENT

Note: "Diagnosis present on admission" for these code categories are exempt because they represent circumstances regarding the healthcare encounter or factors influencing health status that do not represent a current disease or injury or are always present on admission

137-139	Late effects of infectious and parasitic diseases
268.1	Rickets, late effect
326	Late effects of intracranial abscess or pyogenic infection
412	Old myocardial infarction
438	Late effects of cerebrovascular disease
650	Normal delivery
660.7	Failed forceps or vacuum extractor, unspecified
677	Late effect of complication of pregnancy, childbirth, and the puerperium
905-909	Late effects of injuries, poisonings, toxic effects, and other external causes
V02	Carrier or suspected carrier of infectious diseases
V03	Need for prophylactic vaccination and inoculation against bacterial diseases
V04	Need for prophylactic vaccination and inoculation against certain viral diseases
V05	Need for other prophylactic vaccination and inoculation against single diseases
V06	Need for prophylactic vaccination and inoculation against combinations of diseases
V07	Need for isolation and other prophylactic or treatment measures
V10	Personal history of malignant neoplasm
V11	Personal history of mental disorder
V12	Personal history of certain other diseases
V13	Personal history of other diseases
V14	Personal history of allergy to medicinal agents
V15.01-V15.09	Other personal history, Allergy, other than to medicinal agents
V15.1	Other personal history, Surgery to heart and great vessels
V15.2	Other personal history, Surgery to other major organs
V15.3	Other personal history, Irradiation
V15.4	Other personal history, Psychological trauma
V15.5	Other personal history, Injury
V15.6	Other personal history, Poisoning
V15.7	Other personal history, Contraception

V15.80	**Other personal history, History of failed moderate sedation**	V60	Housing, household, and economic circumstances
V15.81	Other personal history, Noncompliance with medical treatment	V61	Other family circumstances
V15.82	Other personal history, History of tobacco use	V62	Other psychosocial circumstances
V15.83	**Other personal history, Underimmunization status**	V64	Persons encountering health services for specific procedures, not carried out
V15.84	**Other personal history, Contact with and (suspected) exposure to asbestos**	V65	Other persons seeking consultation
V15.85	**Other personal history, Contact with and (suspected) exposure to potentially hazardous body fluids**	V66	Convalescence and palliative care
		V67	Follow-up examination
V15.86	**Other personal history, Contact with and (suspected) exposure to lead**	V68	Encounters for administrative purposes
V15.88	Other personal history, History of fall	V69	Problems related to lifestyle
V15.89	Other personal history, Other	V70	General medical examination
V15.9	Unspecified personal history presenting hazards to health	V71	Observation and evaluation for suspected condition not found
V16	Family history of malignant neoplasm	V72	Special investigations and examinations
V17	Family history of certain chronic disabling diseases	V73	Special screening examination for viral and chlamydial diseases
V18	Family history of certain other specific conditions	V74	Special screening examination for bacterial and spirochetal diseases
V19	Family history of other conditions	V75	Special screening examination for other infectious diseases
V20	Health supervision of infant or child	V76	Special screening for malignant neoplasms
V21	Constitutional states in development	V77	Special screening for endocrine, nutritional, metabolic, and immunity disorders
V22	Normal pregnancy	V78	Special screening for disorders of blood and blood-forming organs
V23	Supervision of high-risk pregnancy		
V24	Postpartum care and examination	V79	Special screening for mental disorders and developmental handicaps
V25	Encounter for contraceptive management		
V26	Procreative management	V80	Special screening for neurological, eye, and ear diseases
V27	Outcome of delivery	V81	Special screening for cardiovascular, respiratory, and genitourinary diseases
V28	Antenatal screening		
V29	Observation and evaluation of newborns for suspected condition not found	V82	Special screening for other conditions
		V83	Genetic carrier status
V30-V39	Liveborn infants according to type of birth	V84	Genetic susceptibility to disease
V42	Organ or tissue replaced by transplant	V85	Body Mass Index
V43	Organ or tissue replaced by other means	V86	Estrogen receptor status
V44	Artificial opening status	**V87.32**	**Contact with and (suspected) exposure to algae bloom**
V45	Other postprocedural states	V87.4	Personal history of drug therapy
V46	Other dependence on machines	V88	Acquired absence of cervix and uterus
V49.60-V49.77	Upper and lower limb amputation status	V89	Suspected maternal and fetal conditions not found
V49.81-V49.84	Other specified conditions influencing health status	**E000**	**External cause status**
V50	Elective surgery for purposes other than remedying health states	**E001-E030**	**Activity**
V51	Aftercare involving the use of plastic surgery	E800-E807	Railway accidents
V52	Fitting and adjustment of prosthetic device and implant	E810-E819	Motor vehicle traffic accidents
V53	Fitting and adjustment of other device	E820-E825	Motor vehicle nontraffic accidents E826-E829, Other road vehicle accidents
V54	Other orthopedic aftercare		
V55	Attention to artificial openings	E830-E838	Water transport accidents
V56	Encounter for dialysis and dialysis catheter care	E840-E845	Air and space transport accidents
V57	Care involving use of rehabilitation procedures	E846-E848	Vehicle accidents not elsewhere classifiable
V58	Encounter for other and unspecified procedures and aftercare	E849.0-E849.6	Place of occurrence
		E849.8-E849.9	Place of occurrence
V59	Donors	E883.1	Accidental fall into well

E883.2	Accidental fall into storm drain or manhole
E884.0	Fall from playground equipment
E884.1	Fall from cliff
E885.0	Fall from (nonmotorized) scooter
E885.1	Fall from roller skates
E885.2	Fall from skateboard
E885.3	Fall from skis
E885.4	Fall from snowboard
E886.0	Fall on same level from collision, pushing, or shoving, by or with other person, In sports
E890.0-E890.9	Conflagration in private dwelling
E893.0	Accident caused by ignition of clothing, from controlled fire in private dwelling
E893.2	Accident caused by ignition of clothing, from controlled fire not in building or structure
E894	Ignition of highly inflammable material
E895	Accident caused by controlled fire in private dwelling
E897	Accident caused by controlled fire not in building or structure
E898.0-E898.1	Accident caused by other specified fire and flames
E917.0	Striking against or struck accidentally by objects or persons, in sports without subsequent fall
E917.1	Striking against or struck accidentally by objects or persons, caused by a crowd, by collective fear or panic without subsequent fall
E917.2	Striking against or struck accidentally by objects or persons, in running water without subsequent fall
E917.5	Striking against or struck accidentally by objects or persons, object in sports with subsequent fall
E917.6	Striking against or struck accidentally by objects or persons, caused by a crowd, by collective fear or panic with subsequent fall

E919.0-E919.1	Accidents caused by machinery
E919.3-E919.9	Accidents caused by machinery
E921.0-E921.9	Accident caused by explosion of pressure vessel
E922.0-E922.9	Accident caused by firearm and air gun missile
E924.1	Caustic and corrosive substances
E926.2	Visible and ultraviolet light sources
E928.0-E928.8	Other and unspecified environmental and accidental causes
E929.0-E929.9	Late effects of accidental injury
E959	Late effects of self-inflicted injury
E970-E978	Legal intervention
E979	Terrorism
E981.0-E981.8	Poisoning by gases in domestic use, undetermined whether accidentally or purposely inflicted
E982.0-E982.9	Poisoning by other gases, undetermined whether accidentally or purposely inflicted
E985.0-E985.7	Injury by firearms, air guns and explosives, undetermined whether accidentally or purposely inflicted
E987.0	Falling from high place, undetermined whether accidentally or purposely inflicted, residential premises
E987.2	Falling from high place, undetermined whether accidentally or purposely inflicted, natural sites
E989	Late effects of injury, undetermined whether accidentally or purposely inflicted
E990-E999	Injury resulting from operations of war

POA EXAMPLES
The POA examples have been removed from the guidelines.

A

AAT (alpha-1 antitrypsin) deficiency 273.4
AAV (disease) (illness) (infection) — *see* Human immunodeficiency virus (disease) (illness) (infection)
Abactio — *see* Abortion, induced
Abactus venter — *see* Abortion, induced
Abarognosis 781.99
Abasia (-astasia) 307.9
    atactica 781.3
    choreic 781.3
    hysterical 300.11
    paroxysmal trepidant 781.3
    spastic 781.3
    trembling 781.3
    trepidans 781.3
Abderhalden-Kaufmann-Lignac syndrome (cystinosis) 270.0
Abdomen, abdominal — *see also* condition
    accordion 306.4
    acute 789.0 ☑
    angina 557.1
    burst 868.00
    convulsive equivalent (*see also* Epilepsy) 345.5 ☑
    heart 746.87
    muscle deficiency syndrome 756.79
    obstipum 756.79
Abdominalgia 789.0 ☑
    periodic 277.31
Abduction contracture, hip or other joint — *see* Contraction, joint
Abercrombie's syndrome (amyloid degeneration) 277.39
Aberrant (congenital) — *see also* Malposition, congenital
    adrenal gland 759.1
    blood vessel NEC 747.60
        arteriovenous NEC 747.60
        cerebrovascular 747.81
        gastrointestinal 747.61
        lower limb 747.64
        renal 747.62
        spinal 747.82
        upper limb 747.63
    breast 757.6
    endocrine gland NEC 759.2
    gastrointestinal vessel (peripheral) 747.61
    hepatic duct 751.69
    lower limb vessel (peripheral) 747.64
    pancreas 751.7
    parathyroid gland 759.2
    peripheral vascular vessel NEC 747.60
    pituitary gland (pharyngeal) 759.2
    renal blood vessel 747.62
    sebaceous glands, mucous membrane, mouth 750.26
    spinal vessel 747.82
    spleen 759.0
    testis (descent) 752.51
    thymus gland 759.2
    thyroid gland 759.2
    upper limb vessel (peripheral) 747.63
Aberratio
    lactis 757.6
    testis 752.51
Aberration — *see also* Anomaly
    chromosome — *see* Anomaly, chromosome(s)
    distantial 368.9
    mental (*see also* Disorder, mental, nonpsychotic) 300.9
Abetalipoproteinemia 272.5
Abionarce 780.79
Abiotrophy 799.89
Ablatio
    placentae — *see* Placenta, ablatio
    retinae (*see also* Detachment, retina) 361.9
Ablation
    pituitary (gland) (with hypofunction) 253.7
    placenta — *see* Placenta, ablatio
    uterus 621.8
Ablepharia, ablepharon, ablephary 743.62
Ablepsia — *see* Blindness
Ablepsy — *see* Blindness

Ablutomania 300.3
Abnormal, abnormality, abnormalities — *see also* Anomaly
    acid-base balance 276.4
        fetus or newborn — *see* Distress, fetal
    adaptation curve, dark 368.63
    alveolar ridge 525.9
    amnion 658.9 ☑
        affecting fetus or newborn 762.9
    anatomical relationship NEC 759.9
    apertures, congenital, diaphragm 756.6
    auditory perception NEC 388.40
    autosomes NEC 758.5
        13 758.1
        18 758.2
        21 or 22 758.0
        D₁ 758.1
        E₃ 758.2
        G 758.0
    ballistocardiogram 794.39
    basal metabolic rate (BMR) 794.7
    biosynthesis, testicular androgen 257.2
    blood level (of)
        cobalt 790.6
        copper 790.6
        iron 790.6
        lead 790.6
        lithium 790.6
        magnesium 790.6
        mineral 790.6
        zinc 790.6
    blood pressure
        elevated (without diagnosis of hypertension) 796.2
        low (*see also* Hypotension) 458.9
            reading (incidental) (isolated) (nonspecific) 796.3
    blood sugar 790.29
    bowel sounds 787.5
    breathing behavior — *see* Respiration
    caloric test 794.19
    cervix (acquired) NEC 622.9
        congenital 752.40
        in pregnancy or childbirth 654.6 ☑
            causing obstructed labor 660.2 ☑
                affecting fetus or newborn 763.1
    chemistry, blood NEC 790.6
    chest sounds 786.7
    chorion 658.9 ☑
        affecting fetus or newborn 762.9
    chromosomal NEC 758.89
        analysis, nonspecific result 795.2
        autosomes (*see also* Abnormal, autosomes NEC) 758.5
        fetal, (suspected) affecting management of pregnancy 655.1 ☑
        sex 758.81
    clinical findings NEC 796.4
    communication — *see* Fistula
    configuration of pupils 379.49
    coronary
        artery 746.85
        vein 746.9
    cortisol-binding globulin 255.8
    course, Eustachian tube 744.24
    creatinine clearance 794.4
    dentofacial NEC 524.9
        functional 524.50
        specified type NEC 524.89
    development, developmental NEC 759.9
        bone 756.9
        central nervous system 742.9
    direction, teeth 524.30
    Dynia (*see also* Defect, coagulation) 286.9
    Ebstein 746.2
    echocardiogram 793.2
    echoencephalogram 794.01
    echogram NEC — *see* Findings, abnormal, structure
    electrocardiogram (ECG) (EKG) 794.31
    electroencephalogram (EEG) 794.02
    electromyogram (EMG) 794.17
        ocular 794.14
    electro-oculogram (EOG) 794.12
    electroretinogram (ERG) 794.11
    erythrocytes 289.9

Abnormal, abnormality, abnormalities — *see also* Anomaly — *continued*
    erythrocytes — *continued*
        congenital, with perinatal jaundice 282.9 [774.0]
    Eustachian valve 746.9
    excitability under minor stress 301.9
    fat distribution 782.9
    feces 787.7
    fetal heart rate — *see* Distress, fetal
    fetus NEC
        affecting management of pregnancy — *see* Pregnancy, management affected by, fetal
        causing disproportion 653.7 ☑
            affecting fetus or newborn 763.1
            causing obstructed labor 660.1 ☑
                affecting fetus or newborn 763.1
    findings without manifest disease — *see* Findings, abnormal
    fluid
        amniotic 792.3
        cerebrospinal 792.0
        peritoneal 792.9
        pleural 792.9
        synovial 792.9
        vaginal 792.9
    forces of labor NEC 661.9 ☑
        affecting fetus or newborn 763.7
    form, teeth 520.2
    function studies
        auditory 794.15
        bladder 794.9
        brain 794.00
        cardiovascular 794.30
        endocrine NEC 794.6
        kidney 794.4
        liver 794.8
        nervous system
            central 794.00
            peripheral 794.19
        oculomotor 794.14
        pancreas 794.9
        placenta 794.9
        pulmonary 794.2
        retina 794.11
        special senses 794.19
        spleen 794.9
        thyroid 794.5
        vestibular 794.16
    gait 781.2
        hysterical 300.11
    gastrin secretion 251.5
    globulin
        cortisol-binding 255.8
        thyroid-binding 246.8
    glucagon secretion 251.4
    glucose 790.29
        in pregnancy, childbirth, or puerperium 648.8 ☑
            fetus or newborn 775.0
        non-fasting 790.29
    gravitational (G) forces or states 994.9
    hair NEC 704.2
    hard tissue formation in pulp 522.3
    head movement 781.0
    heart
        rate
            fetus, affecting liveborn infant
                before the onset of labor 763.81
                during labor 763.82
                unspecified as to time of onset 763.83
            intrauterine
                before the onset of labor 763.81
                during labor 763.82
                unspecified as to time of onset 763.83
            newborn
                before the onset of labor 763.81
                during labor 763.82
                unspecified as to time of onset 763.83
        shadow 793.2
        sounds NEC 785.3

Abnormal, abnormality, abnormalities — *see also* Anomaly — *continued*
    hemoglobin (*see also* Disease, hemoglobin) 282.7
        trait — *see* Hemoglobin, abnormal
    hemorrhage, uterus — *see* Hemorrhage, uterus
    histology NEC
    increase
        in
            appetite
            develop...
    involuntary movement 781.0
    jaw closure 524.51
    karyotype 795.2
    knee jerk 796.1
    labor NEC 661.9 ☑
        affecting fetus or newborn 763.7
    laboratory findings — *see* Findings, abnormal
    length, organ or site, congenital — *see* Distortion
    liver function test 790.6
    loss of height 781.91
    loss of weight 783.21
    lung shadow 793.1
    mammogram 793.80
        calcification 793.89
        calculus 793.89
        microcalcification 793.81
    Mantoux test 795.5
    membranes (fetal)
        affecting fetus or newborn 762.9
        complicating pregnancy 658.8 ☑
    menstruation — *see* Menstruation
    metabolism (*see also* condition) 783.9
    movement 781.0
        disorder NEC 333.90
            sleep related, unspecified 780.58
            specified NEC 333.99
        head 781.0
        involuntary 781.0
        specified type NEC 333.99
    muscle contraction, localized 728.85
    myoglobin (Aberdeen) (Annapolis) 289.9
    narrowness, eyelid 743.62
    optokinetic response 379.57
    organs or tissues of pelvis NEC
        in pregnancy or childbirth 654.9 ☑
            affecting fetus or newborn 763.89
            causing obstructed labor 660.2 ☑
                affecting fetus or newborn 763.1
    origin — *see* Malposition, congenital
    palmar creases 757.2
    Papanicolaou (smear)
        anus 796.70
            with
                atypical squamous cells
                    cannot exclude high grade squamous intraepithelial lesion (ASC-H) 796.72
                    of undetermined significance (ASC-US) 796.71
                cytologic evidence of malignancy 796.76
                high grade squamous intraepithelial lesion (HGSIL) 796.74
                low grade squamous intraepithelial lesion (LGSIL) 796.73
                glandular 796.70
                specified finding NEC 796.79
        cervix 795.00
            with
                atypical squamous cells
                    cannot exclude high grade squamous intraepithelial lesion (ASC-H) 795.02
                    of undetermined significance (ASC-US) 795.01
                cytologic evidence of malignancy 795.06
                high grade squamous intraepithelial lesion (HGSIL) 795.04

☑ **Additional Digit Required** — Refer to the Tabular List for Digit Selection   ▽ **Subterms under main terms may continue to next column or page**

2011 ICD-9-CM   ▶◀ Revised Text   ● New Line   ▲ Revised Code   Volume 2 — 1

Abnormal, abnormality, abnormalities —
see also Anomaly — continued
Papanicolaou — continued
   cervix — continued
      with — continued
         low grade squamous intraepithe-
            lial lesion (LGSIL) 795.03
         nonspecific finding NEC 795.09
      other site 796.9
      vagina 795.10
         with
            atypical squamous cells
               cannot exclude high grade
                  squamous intraepithe-
                  lial lesion (ASC-H)
                  795.12
               of undetermined significance
                  (ASC-US) 795.11
            cytologic evidence of malignancy
               795.16
            high grade squamous intraepithe-
               lial lesion (HGSIL) 795.14
            low grade squamous intraepithe-
               lial lesion (LGSIL) 795.13
         glandular 795.10
         specified finding NEC 795.19
parturition
   affecting fetus or newborn 763.9
   mother — see Delivery, complicated
pelvis (bony) — see Deformity, pelvis
percussion, chest 786.7
periods (grossly) (see also Menstruation)
   626.9
phonocardiogram 794.39
placenta — see Placenta, abnormal
plantar reflex 796.1
plasma protein — see Deficiency, plasma,
   protein
pleural folds 748.8
position (see also Malposition)
   gravid uterus 654.4 ☑
      causing obstructed labor 660.2 ☑
         affecting fetus or newborn 763.1
posture NEC 781.92
presentation (fetus) — see Presentation,
   fetus, abnormal
product of conception NEC 631
puberty — see Puberty
pulmonary
   artery 747.3
   function, newborn 770.89
   test results 794.2
   ventilation, newborn 770.89
      hyperventilation 786.01
pulsations in neck 785.1
pupil reflexes 379.40
quality of milk 676.8 ☑
radiological examination 793.99
   abdomen NEC 793.6
   biliary tract 793.3
   breast 793.89
      mammogram NOS 793.80
      mammographic
         calcification 793.89
         calculus 793.89
         microcalcification 793.81
   gastrointestinal tract 793.4
   genitourinary organs 793.5
   head 793.0
   image test inconclusive due to excess
      body fat 793.91
   intrathoracic organ NEC 793.2
   lung (field) 793.1
   musculoskeletal system 793.7
   retroperitoneum 793.6
   skin and subcutaneous tissue 793.99
   skull 793.0
red blood cells 790.09
   morphology 790.09
   volume 790.09
reflex NEC 796.1
renal function test 794.4
respiration signs — see Respiration
response to nerve stimulation 794.10
retinal correspondence 368.34
rhythm, heart (see also Arrhythmia)

Abnormal, abnormality, abnormalities —
see also Anomaly — continued
rhythm, heart (see also Arrhythmia) — continued
   fetus — see Distress, fetal
saliva 792.4
scan
   brain 794.09
   kidney 794.4
   liver 794.8
   lung 794.2
   thyroid 794.5
secretion
   gastrin 251.5
   glucagon 251.4
semen 792.2
serum level (of)
   acid phosphatase 790.5
   alkaline phosphatase 790.5
   amylase 790.5
   enzymes NEC 790.5
   lipase 790.5
shape
   cornea 743.41
   gallbladder 751.69
   gravid uterus 654.4 ☑
      affecting fetus or newborn 763.89
      causing obstructed labor 660.2 ☑
         affecting fetus or newborn 763.1
   head (see also Anomaly, skull) 756.0
   organ or site, congenital NEC — see
      Distortion
sinus venosus 747.40
size
   fetus, complicating delivery 653.5 ☑
      causing obstructed labor 660.1 ☑
   gallbladder 751.69
   head (see also Anomaly, skull) 756.0
   organ or site, congenital NEC — see
      Distortion
   teeth 520.2
skin and appendages, congenital NEC 757.9
soft parts of pelvis — see Abnormal, organs
   or tissues of pelvis
spermatozoa 792.2
sputum (amount) (color) (excessive) (odor)
   (purulent) 786.4
stool NEC 787.7
   bloody 578.1
      occult 792.1
   bulky 787.7
   color (dark) (light) 792.1
   content (fat) (mucus) (pus) 792.1
   occult blood 792.1
synchondrosis 756.9
test results without manifest disease — see
   Findings, abnormal
thebesian valve 746.9
thermography — see Findings, abnormal,
   structure
threshold, cones or rods (eye) 368.63
thyroid-binding globulin 246.8
thyroid product 246.8
toxicology (findings) NEC 796.0
tracheal cartilage (congenital) 748.3
transport protein 273.8
ultrasound results — see Findings, abnormal, structure
umbilical cord
   affecting fetus or newborn 762.6
   complicating delivery 663.9 ☑
   specified NEC 663.8 ☑
union
   cricoid cartilage and thyroid cartilage
      748.3
   larynx and trachea 748.3
   thyroid cartilage and hyoid bone 748.3
urination NEC 788.69
   psychogenic 306.53
   stream
      intermittent 788.61
      slowing 788.62
      splitting 788.61
      weak 788.62
   urgency 788.63
urine (constituents) NEC 791.9

Abnormal, abnormality, abnormalities —
see also Anomaly — continued
uterine hemorrhage (see also Hemorrhage,
   uterus) 626.9
   climacteric 627.0
   postmenopausal 627.1
vagina (acquired) (congenital)
   in pregnancy or childbirth 654.7 ☑
      affecting fetus or newborn 763.89
      causing obstructed labor 660.2 ☑
         affecting fetus or newborn 763.1
vascular sounds 785.9
vectorcardiogram 794.39
visually evoked potential (VEP) 794.13
vulva (acquired) (congenital)
   in pregnancy or childbirth 654.8 ☑
      affecting fetus or newborn 763.89
      causing obstructed labor 660.2 ☑
         affecting fetus or newborn 763.1
weight
   gain 783.1
      of pregnancy 646.1 ☑
         with hypertension — see Tox-
            emia, of pregnancy
   loss 783.21
x-ray examination — see Abnormal, radiological examination
Abnormally formed uterus — see Anomaly,
   uterus
Abnormity (any organ or part) — see Anomaly
ABO
   hemolytic disease 773.1
   incompatibility ▶(due to transfusion of
      blood or blood products)◀
      with hemolytic transfusion reaction ●
         (HTR) (not specified as acute or ●
         delayed) 999.61
      24 hours or more after transfusion ●
         999.63
      acute 999.62   ●
      delayed 999.63   ●
      less than 24 hours after transfusion ●
         999.62
      unspecified time after transfusion ●
         999.61
   reaction 999.60   ●
   specified NEC 999.69   ●
Abocclusion 524.20
Abolition, language 784.69
Aborter, habitual or recurrent NEC
   without current pregnancy 629.81
   current abortion (see also Abortion, sponta-
      neous) 634.9 ☑
      affecting fetus or newborn 761.8
   observation in current pregnancy 646.3 ☑
Abortion (complete) (incomplete) (inevitable)
   (with retained products of conception)
   637.9 ☑

┌───┐
│ Note — Use the following fifth-digit   │
│ subclassification with categories   │
│ 634–637:   │
│   │
│ 0   unspecified   │
│   │
│ 1   incomplete   │
│   │
│ 2   complete   │
└───┘

   with
      complication(s) (any) following previous
         abortion — see category 639 ☑
      damage to pelvic organ (laceration)
         (rupture) (tear) 637.2 ☑
      embolism (air) (amniotic fluid) (blood
         clot) (pulmonary) (pyemic) (sep-
         tic) (soap) 637.6 ☑
      genital tract and pelvic infection
         637.0 ☑
      hemorrhage, delayed or excessive
         637.1 ☑
      metabolic disorder 637.4 ☑
      renal failure (acute) 637.3 ☑
      sepsis (genital tract) (pelvic organ)
         637.0 ☑
         urinary tract 637.7 ☑
      shock (postoperative) (septic) 637.5 ☑
      specified complication NEC 637.7 ☑

Abortion — continued
   with — continued
      toxemia 637.3 ☑
      unspecified complication(s) 637.8 ☑
      urinary tract infection 637.7 ☑
   accidental — see Abortion, spontaneous
   artificial — see Abortion, induced
   attempted (failed) — see Abortion, failed
   criminal — see Abortion, illegal
   early — see Abortion, spontaneous
   elective — see Abortion, legal
   failed (legal) 638.9
      with
         damage to pelvic organ (laceration)
            (rupture) (tear) 638.2
         embolism (air) (amniotic fluid) (blood
            clot) (pulmonary) (pyemic)
            (septic) (soap) 638.6
         genital tract and pelvic infection
            638.0
         hemorrhage, delayed or excessive
            638.1
         metabolic disorder 638.4
         renal failure (acute) 638.3
         sepsis (genital tract) (pelvic organ)
            638.0
            urinary tract 638.7
         shock (postoperative) (septic) 638.5
         specified complication NEC 638.7
         toxemia 638.3
         unspecified complication(s) 638.8
         urinary tract infection 638.7
   fetal indication — see Abortion, legal
   fetus 779.6
   following threatened abortion — see Abor-
      tion, by type
   habitual or recurrent (care during pregnan-
      cy) 646.3 ☑
      with current abortion (see also Abortion,
         spontaneous) 634.9 ☑
         affecting fetus or newborn 761.8
      without current pregnancy 629.81
   homicidal — see Abortion, illegal
   illegal 636.9 ☑
      with
         damage to pelvic organ (laceration)
            (rupture) (tear) 636.2 ☑
         embolism (air) (amniotic fluid) (blood
            clot) (pulmonary) (pyemic)
            (septic) (soap) 636.6 ☑
         genital tract and pelvic infection
            636.0 ☑
         hemorrhage, delayed or excessive
            636.1 ☑
         metabolic disorder 636.4 ☑
         renal failure 636.3 ☑
         sepsis (genital tract) (pelvic organ)
            636.0 ☑
            urinary tract 636.7 ☑
         shock (postoperative) (septic)
            636.5 ☑
         specified complication NEC 636.7 ☑
         toxemia 636.3 ☑
         unspecified complication(s) 636.8 ☑
         urinary tract infection 636.7 ☑
   fetus 779.6
   induced 637.9 ☑
      illegal — see Abortion, illegal
      legal indications — see Abortion, legal
      medical indications — see Abortion, le-
         gal
      therapeutic — see Abortion, legal
   late — see Abortion, spontaneous
   legal (legal indication) (medical indication)
      (under medical supervision) 635.9 ☑
      with
         damage to pelvic organ (laceration)
            (rupture) (tear) 635.2 ☑
         embolism (air) (amniotic fluid) (blood
            clot) (pulmonary) (pyemic)
            (septic) (soap) 635.6 ☑
         genital tract and pelvic infection
            635.0 ☑
         hemorrhage, delayed or excessive
            635.1 ☑

☑ **Additional Digit Required** — Refer to the Tabular List for Digit Selection   ▽ **Subterms under main terms may continue to next column or page**

2 — Volume 2 • October 2010   ▶◀ **Revised Text**   ● **New Line**   ▲ **Revised Code**   **2011 ICD-9-CM**

Abortion — *continued*
  legal — *continued*
    with — *continued*
      metabolic disorder 635.4 ☑
      renal failure (acute) 635.3 ☑
      sepsis (genital tract) (pelvic organ) 635.0 ☑
      urinary tract 635.7 ☑
      shock (postoperative) (septic) 635.5 ☑
      specified complication NEC 635.7 ☑
      toxemia 635.3 ☑
      unspecified complication(s) 635.8 ☑
      urinary tract infection 635.7 ☑
    fetus 779.6
  medical indication — *see* Abortion, legal
  mental hygiene problem — *see* Abortion, legal
  missed 632
  operative — *see* Abortion, legal
  psychiatric indication — *see* Abortion, legal
  recurrent — *see* Abortion, spontaneous
  self-induced — *see* Abortion, illegal
  septic — *see* Abortion, by type, with sepsis
  spontaneous 634.9 ☑
    with
      damage to pelvic organ (laceration) (rupture) (tear) 634.2 ☑
      embolism (air) (amniotic fluid) (blood clot) (pulmonary) (pyemic) (septic) (soap) 634.6 ☑
      genital tract and pelvic infection 634.0 ☑
      hemorrhage, delayed or excessive 634.1 ☑
      metabolic disorder 634.4 ☑
      renal failure 634.3 ☑
      sepsis (genital tract) (pelvic organ) 634.0 ☑
        urinary tract 634.7 ☑
      shock (postoperative) (septic) 634.5 ☑
      specified complication NEC 634.7 ☑
      toxemia 634.3 ☑
      unspecified complication(s) 634.8 ☑
      urinary tract infection 634.7 ☑
    fetus 761.8
    threatened 640.0 ☑
      affecting fetus or newborn 762.1
  surgical — *see* Abortion, legal
  therapeutic — *see* Abortion, legal
  threatened 640.0 ☑
    affecting fetus or newborn 762.1
  tubal — *see* Pregnancy, tubal
  voluntary — *see* Abortion, legal
Abortus fever 023.9
Aboulomania 301.6
Abrachia 755.20
Abrachiatism 755.20
Abrachiocephalia 759.89
Abrachiocephalus 759.89
Abrami's disease (acquired hemolytic jaundice) 283.9
Abramov-Fiedler myocarditis (acute isolated myocarditis) 422.91
Abrasion — *see also* Injury, superficial, by site
  cornea 918.1
  dental 521.20
    extending into
      dentine 521.22
      pulp 521.23
    generalized 521.25
    limited to enamel 521.21
    localized 521.24
  teeth, tooth (dentifrice) (habitual) (hard tissues) (occupational) (ritual) (traditional) (wedge defect) (*see also* Abrasion, dental) 521.20
Abrikossov's tumor (M9580/0) — *see also* Neoplasm, connective tissue, benign
  malignant (M9580/3) — *see* Neoplasm, connective tissue, malignant
Abrism 988.8
Abruption, placenta — *see* Placenta, abruptio
Abruptio placentae — *see* Placenta, abruptio

Abscess (acute) (chronic) (infectional) (lymphangitic) (metastatic) (multiple) (pyogenic) (septic) (with lymphangitis) — *see also* Cellulitis 682.9
  abdomen, abdominal
    cavity 567.22
    wall 682.2
  abdominopelvic 567.22
  accessory sinus (chronic) (*see also* Sinusitis) 473.9
  adrenal (capsule) (gland) 255.8
  alveolar 522.5
    with sinus 522.7
  ambic 006.3
    bladder 006.8
    brain (with liver or lung abscess) 006.5
    liver (without mention of brain or lung abscess) 006.3
      with
        brain abscess (and lung abscess) 006.5
        lung abscess 006.4
    lung (with liver abscess) 006.4
      with brain abscess 006.5
    seminal vesicle 006.8
    specified site NEC 006.8
    spleen 006.8
  anaerobic 040.0
  ankle 682.6
  anorectal 566
  antecubital space 682.3
  antrum (chronic) (Highmore) (*see also* Sinusitis, maxillary) 473.0
  anus 566
  apical (tooth) 522.5
    with sinus (alveolar) 522.7
  appendix 540.1
  areola (acute) (chronic) (nonpuerperal) 611.0
    puerperal, postpartum 675.1 ☑
  arm (any part, above wrist) 682.3
  artery (wall) 447.2
  atheromatous 447.2
  auditory canal (external) 380.10
  auricle (ear) (staphylococcal) (streptococcal) 380.10
  axilla, axillary (region) 682.3
    lymph gland or node 683
  back (any part) 682.2
  Bartholin's gland 616.3
    with
      abortion — *see* Abortion, by type, with sepsis
      ectopic pregnancy (*see also* categories 633.0–633.9) 639.0
      molar pregnancy (*see also* categories 630–632) 639.0
    complicating pregnancy or puerperium 646.6 ☑
    following
      abortion 639.0
      ectopic or molar pregnancy 639.0
  bartholinian 616.3
  Bezold's 383.01
  bile, biliary, duct or tract (*see also* Cholecystitis) 576.8
  bilharziasis 120.1
  bladder (wall) 595.89
    amebic 006.8
  bone (subperiosteal) (*see also* Osteomyelitis) 730.0 ☑
    accessory sinus (chronic) (*see also* Sinusitis) 473.9
    acute 730.0 ☑
    chronic or old 730.1 ☑
    jaw (lower) (upper) 526.4
    mastoid — *see* Mastoiditis, acute
    petrous (*see also* Petrositis) 383.20
    spinal (tuberculous) (*see also* Tuberculosis) 015.0 ☑ *[730.88]*
      nontuberculous 730.08
  bowel 569.5
  brain (any part) 324.0
    amebic (with liver or lung abscess) 006.5
    cystic 324.0
    late effect — *see* category 326

Abscess — *see also* Cellulitis — *continued*
  brain — *continued*
    otogenic 324.0
    tuberculous (*see also* Tuberculosis) 013.3 ☑
  breast (acute) (chronic) (nonpuerperal) 611.0
    newborn 771.5
    puerperal, postpartum 675.1 ☑
    tuberculous (*see also* Tuberculosis) 017.9 ☑
  broad ligament (chronic) (*see also* Disease, pelvis, inflammatory) 614.4
    acute 614.3
  Brodie's (chronic) (localized) (*see also* Osteomyelitis) 730.1 ☑
  bronchus 519.19
  buccal cavity 528.3
  bulbourethral gland 597.0
  bursa 727.89
    pharyngeal 478.29
  buttock 682.5
  canaliculus, breast 611.0
  canthus 372.20
  cartilage 733.99
  cecum 569.5
    with appendicitis 540.1
  cerebellum, cerebellar 324.0
    late effect — *see* category 326
  cerebral (embolic) 324.0
    late effect — *see* category 326
  cervical (neck region) 682.1
    lymph gland or node 683
    stump (*see also* Cervicitis) 616.0
  cervix (stump) (uteri) (*see also* Cervicitis) 616.0
  cheek, external 682.0
    inner 528.3
  chest 510.9
    with fistula 510.0
    wall 682.2
  chin 682.0
  choroid 363.00
  ciliary body 364.3
  circumtonsillar 475
  cold (tuberculous) (*see also* Tuberculosis, abscess)
    articular — *see* Tuberculosis, joint
  colon (wall) 569.5
  colostomy or enterostomy 569.61
  conjunctiva 372.00
  connective tissue NEC 682.9
  cornea 370.55
    with ulcer 370.00
  corpus
    cavernosum 607.2
    luteum (*see also* Salpingo-oophoritis) 614.2
  Cowper's gland 597.0
  cranium 324.0
  cul-de-sac (Douglas') (posterior) (*see also* Disease, pelvis, inflammatory) 614.4
    acute 614.3
  dental 522.5
    with sinus (alveolar) 522.7
  dentoalveolar 522.5
    with sinus (alveolar) 522.7
  diaphragm, diaphragmatic 567.22
  digit NEC 681.9
  Douglas' cul-de-sac or pouch (*see also* Disease, pelvis, inflammatory) 614.4
    acute 614.3
  Dubois' 090.5
  ductless gland 259.8
  ear
    acute 382.00
    external 380.10
    inner 386.30
    middle — *see* Otitis media
  elbow 682.3
  endamebic — *see* Abscess, amebic
  entamebic — *see* Abscess, amebic
  enterostomy 569.61
  epididymis 604.0
  epidural 324.9
    brain 324.0

Abscess — *see also* Cellulitis — *continued*
  epidural — *continued*
    late effect — *see* category 326
    spinal cord 324.1
  epiglottis 478.79
  epiploon, epiploic 567.22
  erysipelatous (*see also* Erysipelas) 035
  esophagostomy 530.86
  esophagus 530.19
  ethmoid (bone) (chronic) (sinus) (*see also* Sinusitis, ethmoidal) 473.2
  external auditory canal 380.10
  extradural 324.9
    brain 324.0
    late effect — *see* category 326
    spinal cord 324.1
  extraperitoneal — *see* Abscess, peritoneum
  eye 360.00
  eyelid 373.13
  face (any part, except eye) 682.0
  fallopian tube (*see also* Salpingo-oophoritis) 614.2
  fascia 728.89
  fauces 478.29
  fecal 569.5
  femoral (region) 682.6
  filaria, filarial (*see also* Infestation, filarial) 125.9
  finger (any) (intrathecal) (periosteal) (subcutaneous) (subcuticular) 681.00
  fistulous NEC 682.9
  flank 682.2
  foot (except toe) 682.7
  forearm 682.3
  forehead 682.0
  frontal (sinus) (chronic) (*see also* Sinusitis, frontal) 473.1
  gallbladder (*see also* Cholecystitis, acute) 575.0
  gastric 535.0 ☑
  genital organ or tract NEC
    female 616.9
      with
        abortion — *see* Abortion, by type, with sepsis
        ectopic pregnancy (*see also* categories 633.0–633.9) 639.0
        molar pregnancy (*see also* categories 630–632) 639.0
      following
        abortion 639.0
        ectopic or molar pregnancy 639.0
      puerperal, postpartum, childbirth 670.8 ☑
    male 608.4
  genitourinary system, tuberculous (*see also* Tuberculosis) 016.9 ☑
  gingival 523.30
  gland, glandular (lymph) (acute) NEC 683
  glottis 478.79
  gluteal (region) 682.5
  gonorrheal NEC (*see also* Gonococcus) 098.0
  groin 682.2
  gum 523.30
  hand (except finger or thumb) 682.4
  head (except face) 682.8
  heart 429.89
  heel 682.7
  helminthic (*see also* Infestation, by specific parasite) 128.9
  hepatic 572.0
    amebic (*see also* Abscess, liver, amebic) 006.3
    duct 576.8
  hip 682.6
    tuberculous (active) (*see also* Tuberculosis) 015.1 ☑
  ileocecal 540.1
  ileostomy (bud) 569.61
  iliac (region) 682.2
    fossa 540.1
  iliopsoas 567.31
    nontuberculous 728.89
    tuberculous (*see also* Tuberculosis) 015.0 ☑ *[730.88]*
  infraclavicular (fossa) 682.3

☑ **Additional Digit Required** — Refer to the Tabular List for Digit Selection   ▽ **Subterms under main terms may continue to next column or page**

2011 ICD-9-CM   ►◄ Revised Text   ● New Line   ▲ Revised Code   **Volume 2 — 3**

Abortion — Abscess

Index

Abscess — Abscess

Abscess — see also Cellulitis — continued
inguinal (region) 682.2
lymph gland or node 683
intersphincteric (anus) 566
intestine, intestinal 569.5
rectal 566
intra-abdominal (see also Abscess, peritoneum) 567.22
postoperative 998.59
intracranial 324.0
late effect — see category 326
intramammary — see Abscess, breast
intramastoid (see also Mastoiditis, acute) 383.00
intraorbital 376.01
intraperitoneal 567.22
intraspinal 324.1
late effect — see category 326
intratonsillar 475
iris 364.3
ischiorectal 566
jaw (bone) (lower) (upper) 526.4
skin 682.0
joint (see also Arthritis, pyogenic) 711.0 ☑
vertebral (tuberculous) (see also Tuberculosis) 015.0 ☑ [730.88]
nontuberculous 724.8
kidney 590.2
with
abortion — see Abortion, by type, with urinary tract infection
calculus 592.0
ectopic pregnancy (see also categories 633.0–633.9) 639.8
molar pregnancy (see also categories 630–632) 639.8
complicating pregnancy or puerperium 646.6 ☑
affecting fetus or newborn 760.1
following
abortion 639.8
ectopic or molar pregnancy 639.8
knee 682.6
joint 711.06
tuberculous (active) (see also Tuberculosis) 015.2 ☑
labium (majus) (minus) 616.4
complicating pregnancy, childbirth, or puerperium 646.6 ☑
lacrimal (passages) (sac) (see also Dacryocystitis) 375.30
caruncle 375.30
gland (see also Dacryoadenitis) 375.00
lacunar 597.0
larynx 478.79
lateral (alveolar) 522.5
with sinus 522.7
leg, except foot 682.6
lens 360.00
lid 373.13
lingual 529.0
tonsil 475
lip 528.5
Littre's gland 597.0
liver 572.0
amebic 006.3
with
brain abscess (and lung abscess) 006.5
lung abscess 006.4
due to Entamoeba histolytica 006.3
dysenteric (see also Abscess, liver, amebic) 006.3
pyogenic 572.0
tropical (see also Abscess, liver, amebic) 006.3
loin (region) 682.2
lumbar (tuberculous) (see also Tuberculosis) 015.0 ☑ [730.88]
nontuberculous 682.2
lung (miliary) (putrid) 513.0
amebic (with liver abscess) 006.4
with brain abscess 006.5
lymphangitic, acute — see Cellulitis
lymph, lymphatic, gland or node (acute) 683
any site, except mesenteric 683

Abscess — see also Cellulitis — continued
lymph, lymphatic, gland or node — continued
mesentery 289.2
malar 526.4
mammary gland — see Abscess, breast
marginal (anus) 566
mastoid (process) (see also Mastoiditis, acute) 383.00
subperiosteal 383.01
maxilla, maxillary 526.4
molar (tooth) 522.5
with sinus 522.7
premolar 522.5
sinus (chronic) (see also Sinusitis, maxillary) 473.0
mediastinum 513.1
meibomian gland 373.12
meninges (see also Meningitis) 320.9
mesentery, mesenteric 567.22
mesosalpinx (see also Salpingo-oophoritis) 614.2
milk 675.1 ☑
Monro's (psoriasis) 696.1
mons pubis 682.2
mouth (floor) 528.3
multiple sites NEC 682.9
mural 682.2
muscle 728.89
psoas 567.31
myocardium 422.92
nabothian (follicle) (see also Cervicitis) 616.0
nail (chronic) (with lymphangitis) 681.9
finger 681.02
toe 681.11
nasal (fossa) (septum) 478.19
sinus (chronic) (see also Sinusitis) 473.9
nasopharyngeal 478.29
nates 682.5
navel 682.2
newborn NEC 771.4
neck (region) 682.1
lymph gland or node 683
nephritic (see also Abscess, kidney) 590.2
nipple 611.0
puerperal, postpartum 675.0 ☑
nose (septum) 478.19
external 682.0
omentum 567.22
operative wound 998.59
orbit, orbital 376.01
ossifluent — see Abscess, bone
ovary, ovarian (corpus luteum) (see also Salpingo-oophoritis) 614.2
oviduct (see also Salpingo-oophoritis) 614.2
palate (soft) 528.3
hard 526.4
palmar (space) 682.4
pancreas (duct) 577.0
paradontal 523.30
parafrenal 607.2
parametric, parametrium (chronic) (see also Disease, pelvis, inflammatory) 614.4
acute 614.3
paranephric 590.2
parapancreatic 577.0
parapharyngeal 478.22
pararectal 566
parasinus (see also Sinusitis) 473.9
parauterine (see also Disease, pelvis, inflammatory) 614.4
acute 614.3
paravaginal (see also Vaginitis) 616.10
parietal region 682.8
parodontal 523.30
parotid (duct) (gland) 527.3
region 528.3
parumbilical 682.2
newborn 771.4
pectoral (region) 682.2
pelvirectal 567.22
pelvis, pelvic
female (chronic) (see also Disease, pelvis, inflammatory) 614.4
acute 614.3

Abscess — see also Cellulitis — continued
pelvis, pelvic — continued
male, peritoneal (cellular tissue) — see Abscess, peritoneum
tuberculous (see also Tuberculosis) 016.9 ☑
penis 607.2
gonococcal (acute) 098.0
chronic or duration of 2 months or over 098.2
perianal 566
periapical 522.5
with sinus (alveolar) 522.7
periappendiceal 540.1
pericardial 420.99
pericecal 540.1
pericemental 523.30
pericholecystic (see also Cholecystitis, acute) 575.0
pericoronal 523.30
peridental 523.30
perigastric 535.0 ☑
perimetric (see also Disease, pelvis, inflammatory) 614.4
acute 614.3
perinephric, perinephritic (see also Abscess, kidney) 590.2
perineum, perineal (superficial) 682.2
deep (with urethral involvement) 597.0
urethra 597.0
periodontal (parietal) 523.31
apical 522.5
periosteum, periosteal (see also Periostitis) 730.3 ☑
with osteomyelitis (see also Osteomyelitis) 730.2 ☑
acute or subacute 730.0 ☑
chronic or old 730.1 ☑
peripleuritic 510.9
with fistula 510.0
periproctic 566
periprostatic 601.2
perirectal (staphylococcal) 566
perirenal (tissue) (see also Abscess, kidney) 590.2
perisinuous (nose) (see also Sinusitis) 473.9
peritoneum, peritoneal (perforated) (ruptured) 567.22
with
abortion — see Abortion, by type, with sepsis
appendicitis 540.1
ectopic pregnancy (see also categories 633.0–633.9) 639.0
molar pregnancy (see also categories 630–632) 639.0
following
abortion 639.0
ectopic or molar pregnancy 639.0
pelvic, female (see also Disease, pelvis, inflammatory) 614.4
acute 614.3
postoperative 998.59
puerperal, postpartum, childbirth 670.8 ☑
tuberculous (see also Tuberculosis) 014.0 ☑
peritonsillar 475
perityphlic 540.1
periureteral 593.89
periurethral 597.0
gonococcal (acute) 098.0
chronic or duration of 2 months or over 098.2
periuterine (see also Disease, pelvis, inflammatory) 614.4
acute 614.3
perivesical 595.89
pernicious NEC 682.9
petrous bone — see Petrositis
phagedenic NEC 682.9
chancroid 099.0
pharynx, pharyngeal (lateral) 478.29
phlegmonous NEC 682.9
pilonidal 685.0
pituitary (gland) 253.8

Abscess — see also Cellulitis — continued
pleura 510.9
with fistula 510.0
popliteal 682.6
postanal 566
postcecal 540.1
postlaryngeal 478.79
postnasal 478.19
postpharyngeal 478.24
posttonsillar 475
posttyphoid 002.0
Pott's (see also Tuberculosis) 015.0 ☑ [730.88]
pouch of Douglas (chronic) (see also Disease, pelvis, inflammatory) 614.4
premammary — see Abscess, breast
prepatellar 682.6
prostate (see also Prostatitis) 601.2
gonococcal (acute) 098.12
chronic or duration of 2 months or over 098.32
psoas 567.31
nontuberculous 728.89
tuberculous (see also Tuberculosis) 015.0 ☑ [730.88]
pterygopalatine fossa 682.8
pubis 682.2
puerperal — see Puerperal, abscess, by site
pulmonary — see Abscess, lung
pulp, pulpal (dental) 522.0
finger 681.01
toe 681.10
pyemic — see Septicemia
pyloric valve 535.0 ☑
rectovaginal septum 569.5
rectovesical 595.89
rectum 566
regional NEC 682.9
renal (see also Abscess, kidney) 590.2
retina 363.00
retrobulbar 376.01
retrocecal 567.22
retrolaryngeal 478.79
retromammary — see Abscess, breast
retroperineal 682.2
retroperitoneal 567.38
postprocedural 998.59
retropharyngeal 478.24
tuberculous (see also Tuberculosis) 012.8 ☑
retrorectal 566
retrouterine (see also Disease, pelvis, inflammatory) 614.4
acute 614.3
retrovesical 595.89
root, tooth 522.5
with sinus (alveolar) 522.7
round ligament (see also Disease, pelvis, inflammatory) 614.4
acute 614.3
rupture (spontaneous) NEC 682.9
sacrum (tuberculous) (see also Tuberculosis) 015.0 ☑ [730.88]
nontuberculous 730.08
salivary duct or gland 527.3
scalp (any part) 682.8
scapular 730.01
sclera 379.09
scrofulous (see also Tuberculosis) 017.2 ☑
scrotum 608.4
seminal vesicle 608.0
amebic 006.8
septal, dental 522.5
with sinus (alveolar) 522.7
septum (nasal) 478.19
serous (see also Periostitis) 730.3 ☑
shoulder 682.3
side 682.2
sigmoid 569.5
sinus (accessory) (chronic) (nasal) (see also Sinusitis) 473.9
intracranial venous (any) 324.0
late effect — see category 326
Skene's duct or gland 597.0
skin NEC 682.9

Abscess — *see also* Cellulitis — *continued*
skin — *continued*
tuberculous (primary) (*see also* Tuberculosis) 017.0 ☑
sloughing NEC 682.9
specified site NEC 682.8
amebic 006.8
spermatic cord 608.4
sphenoidal (sinus) (*see also* Sinusitis, sphenoidal) 473.3
spinal
cord (any part) (staphylococcal) 324.1
tuberculous (*see also* Tuberculosis) 013.5 ☑
epidural 324.1
spine (column) (tuberculous) (*see also* Tuberculosis) 015.0 ☑ [730.88]
nontuberculous 730.08
spleen 289.59
amebic 006.8
staphylococcal NEC 682.9
stitch 998.59
stomach (wall) 535.0 ☑
strumous (tuberculous) (*see also* Tuberculosis) 017.2 ☑
subarachnoid 324.9
brain 324.0
cerebral 324.0
late effect — *see* category 326
spinal cord 324.1
subareolar (*see also* Abscess, breast)
puerperal, postpartum 675.1 ☑
subcecal 540.1
subcutaneous NEC 682.9
subdiaphragmatic 567.22
subdorsal 682.2
subdural 324.9
brain 324.0
late effect — *see* category 326
spinal cord 324.1
subgaleal 682.8
subhepatic 567.22
sublingual 528.3
gland 527.3
submammary — *see* Abscess, breast
submandibular (region) (space) (triangle) 682.0
gland 527.3
submaxillary (region) 682.0
gland 527.3
submental (pyogenic) 682.0
gland 527.3
subpectoral 682.2
subperiosteal — *see* Abscess, bone
subperitoneal 567.22
subphrenic (*see also* Abscess, peritoneum) 567.22
postoperative 998.59
subscapular 682.2
subungual 681.9
suburethral 597.0
sudoriparous 705.89
suppurative NEC 682.9
supraclavicular (fossa) 682.3
suprahepatic 567.22
suprapelvic (*see also* Disease, pelvis, inflammatory) 614.4
acute 614.3
suprapubic 682.2
suprarenal (capsule) (gland) 255.8
sweat gland 705.89
syphilitic 095.8
teeth, tooth (root) 522.5
with sinus (alveolar) 522.7
supporting structures NEC 523.30
temple 682.0
temporal region 682.0
temporosphenoidal 324.0
late effect — *see* category 326
tendon (sheath) 727.89
testicle — *see* Orchitis
thecal 728.89
thigh (acquired) 682.6
thorax 510.9
with fistula 510.0
throat 478.29

Abscess — *see also* Cellulitis — *continued*
thumb (intrathecal) (periosteal) (subcutaneous) (subcuticular) 681.00
thymus (gland) 254.1
thyroid (gland) 245.0
toe (any) (intrathecal) (periosteal) (subcutaneous) (subcuticular) 681.10
tongue (staphylococcal) 529.0
tonsil(s) (lingual) 475
tonsillopharyngeal 475
tooth, teeth (root) 522.5
with sinus (alveolar) 522.7
supporting structure NEC 523.30
trachea 478.9
trunk 682.2
tubal (*see also* Salpingo-oophoritis) 614.2
tuberculous — *see* Tuberculosis, abscess
tubo-ovarian (*see also* Salpingo-oophoritis) 614.2
tunica vaginalis 608.4
umbilicus NEC 682.2
newborn 771.4
upper arm 682.3
upper respiratory 478.9
urachus 682.2
urethra (gland) 597.0
urinary 597.0
uterus, uterine (wall) (*see also* Endometritis) 615.9
ligament (*see also* Disease, pelvis, inflammatory) 614.4
acute 614.3
neck (*see also* Cervicitis) 616.0
uvula 528.3
vagina (wall) (*see also* Vaginitis) 616.10
vaginorectal (*see also* Vaginitis) 616.10
vas deferens 608.4
vermiform appendix 540.1
vertebra (column) (tuberculous) (*see also* Tuberculosis) 015.0 ☑ [730.88]
nontuberculous 730.0 ☑
vesical 595.89
vesicouterine pouch (*see also* Disease, pelvis, inflammatory) 614.4
vitreous (humor) (pneumococcal) 360.04
vocal cord 478.5
von Bezold's 383.01
vulva 616.4
complicating pregnancy, childbirth, or puerperium 646.6 ☑
vulvovaginal gland (*see also* Vaginitis) 616.3
web-space 682.4
wrist 682.4

Absence (organ or part) (complete or partial)
acoustic nerve 742.8
adrenal (gland) (congenital) 759.1
acquired V45.79
albumin (blood) 273.8
alimentary tract (complete) (congenital) (partial) 751.8
lower 751.5
upper 750.8
alpha-fucosidase 271.8
alveolar process (acquired) 525.8
congenital 750.26
anus, anal (canal) (congenital) 751.2
aorta (congenital) 747.22
aortic valve (congenital) 746.89
appendix, congenital 751.2
arm (acquired) V49.60
above elbow V49.66
below elbow V49.65
congenital (*see also* Deformity, reduction, upper limb) 755.20
lower — *see* Absence, forearm, congenital
upper (complete) (partial) (with absence of distal elements, incomplete) 755.24
with
complete absence of distal elements 755.21
forearm (incomplete) 755.23
artery (congenital) (peripheral) NEC (*see also* Anomaly, peripheral vascular system) 747.60

Absence — *continued*
artery (*see also* Anomaly, peripheral vascular system) — *continued*
brain 747.81
cerebral 747.81
coronary 746.85
pulmonary 747.3
umbilical 747.5
atrial septum 745.69
auditory canal (congenital) (external) 744.01
auricle (ear) (with stenosis or atresia of auditory canal), congenital 744.01
bile, biliary duct (common) or passage (congenital) 751.61
bladder (acquired) V45.74
congenital 753.8
bone (congenital) NEC 756.9
marrow 284.9
acquired (secondary) 284.89
congenital 284.09
hereditary 284.09
idiopathic 284.9
skull 756.0
bowel sounds 787.5
brain 740.0
specified part 742.2
breast(s) (acquired) V45.71
congenital 757.6
broad ligament (congenital) 752.19
bronchus (congenital) 748.3
calvarium, calvaria (skull) 756.0
canaliculus lacrimalis, congenital 743.65
carpal(s) (congenital) (complete) (partial) (with absence of distal elements, incomplete) (*see also* Deformity, reduction, upper limb) 755.28
with complete absence of distal elements 755.21
cartilage 756.9
caudal spine 756.13
cecum (acquired) (postoperative) (posttraumatic) V45.72
congenital 751.2
cementum 520.4
cerebellum (congenital) (vermis) 742.2
cervix (acquired) (uteri) V88.01
with remaining uterus V88.03
and uterus V88.01
congenital 752.43 ▲
chin, congenital 744.89
cilia (congenital) 743.63
acquired 374.89
circulatory system, part NEC 747.89
clavicle 755.51
clitoris (congenital) 752.49
coccyx, congenital 756.13
cold sense (*see also* Disturbance, sensation) 782.0
colon (acquired) (postoperative) V45.72
congenital 751.2
congenital
lumen — *see* Atresia
organ or site NEC — *see* Agenesis
septum — *see* Imperfect, closure
corpus callosum (congenital) 742.2
cricoid cartilage 748.3
diaphragm (congenital) (with hernia) 756.6
with obstruction 756.6
digestive organ(s) or tract, congenital (complete) (partial) 751.8
acquired V45.79
lower 751.5
upper 750.8
ductus arteriosus 747.89
duodenum (acquired) (postoperative) V45.72
congenital 751.1
ear, congenital 744.09
acquired V45.79
auricle 744.01
external 744.01
inner 744.05
lobe, lobule 744.21
middle, except ossicles 744.03
ossicles 744.04
ossicles 744.04

Absence — *continued*
ejaculatory duct (congenital) 752.89
endocrine gland NEC (congenital) 759.2
epididymis (congenital) 752.89
acquired V45.77
epiglottis, congenital 748.3
epileptic (atonic) (typical) (*see also* Epilepsy) 345.0 ☑
erythrocyte 284.9
erythropoiesis 284.9
congenital 284.01
esophagus (congenital) 750.3
Eustachian tube (congenital) 744.24
extremity (acquired)
congenital (*see also* Deformity, reduction) 755.4
lower V49.70
upper V49.60
extrinsic muscle, eye 743.69
eye (acquired) V45.78
adnexa (congenital) 743.69
congenital 743.00
muscle (congenital) 743.69
eyelid (fold), congenital 743.62
acquired 374.89
face
bones NEC 756.0
specified part NEC 744.89
fallopian tube(s) (acquired) V45.77
congenital 752.19
femur, congenital (complete) (partial) (with absence of distal elements, incomplete) (*see also* Deformity, reduction, lower limb) 755.34
with
complete absence of distal elements 755.31
tibia and fibula (incomplete) 755.33
fibrin 790.92
fibrinogen (congenital) 286.3
acquired 286.6
fibula, congenital (complete) (partial) (with absence of distal elements, incomplete) (*see also* Deformity, reduction, lower limb) 755.37
with
complete absence of distal elements 755.31
tibia 755.35
with
complete absence of distal elements 755.31
femur (incomplete) 755.33
with complete absence of distal elements 755.31
finger (acquired) V49.62
congenital (complete) (partial) (*see also* Deformity, reduction, upper limb) 755.29
meaning all fingers (complete) (partial) 755.21
transverse 755.21
fissures of lungs (congenital) 748.5
foot (acquired) V49.73
congenital (complete) 755.31
forearm (acquired) V49.65
congenital (complete) (partial) (with absence of distal elements, incomplete) (*see also* Deformity, reduction, upper limb) 755.25
with
complete absence of distal elements (hand and fingers) 755.21
humerus (incomplete) 755.23
fovea centralis 743.55
fucosidase 271.8
gallbladder (acquired) V45.79
congenital 751.69
gamma globulin (blood) 279.00
genital organs
acquired V45.77
congenital
female 752.89
external 752.49

☑ Additional Digit Required — Refer to the Tabular List for Digit Selection   ⌐ Subterms under main terms may continue to next column or page

2011 ICD-9-CM   ▶◀ Revised Text   ● New Line   ▲ Revised Code   October 2010 · Volume 2 — 5

Absence — *continued*
genital organs — *continued*
  congenital — *continued*
    female — *continued*
      internal NEC 752.89
     male 752.89
      penis 752.69
genitourinary organs, congenital NEC 752.89
glottis 748.3
gonadal, congenital NEC 758.6
hair (congenital) 757.4
  acquired — *see* Alopecia
hand (acquired) V49.63
  congenital (complete) (*see also* Deformity, reduction, upper limb) 755.21
heart (congenital) 759.89
  acquired — *see* Status, organ replacement
heat sense (*see also* Disturbance, sensation) 782.0
humerus, congenital (complete) (partial) (with absence of distal elements, incomplete) (*see also* Deformity, reduction, upper limb) 755.24
  with
    complete absence of distal elements 755.21
    radius and ulna (incomplete) 755.23
hymen (congenital) 752.49
ileum (acquired) (postoperative) (posttraumatic) V45.72
  congenital 751.1
immunoglobulin, isolated NEC 279.03
  IgA 279.01
  IgG 279.03
  IgM 279.02
incus (acquired) 385.24
  congenital 744.04
internal ear (congenital) 744.05
intestine (acquired) (small) V45.72
  congenital 751.1
    large 751.2
  large V45.72
    congenital 751.2
iris (congenital) 743.45
jaw — *see* Absence, mandible
jejunum (acquired) V45.72
  congenital 751.1
joint, congenital NEC 755.8
kidney(s) (acquired) V45.73
  congenital 753.0
labium (congenital) (majus) (minus) 752.49
labyrinth, membranous 744.05
lacrimal apparatus (congenital) 743.65
larynx (congenital) 748.3
leg (acquired) V49.70
  above knee V49.76
  below knee V49.75
  congenital (partial) (unilateral) (*see also* Deformity, reduction, lower limb) 755.31
    lower (complete) (partial) (with absence of distal elements, incomplete) 755.35
      with
        complete absence of distal elements (foot and toes) 755.31
        thigh (incomplete) 755.33
          with complete absence of distal elements 755.31
    upper — *see* Absence, femur
lens (congenital) 743.35
  acquired 379.31
ligament, broad (congenital) 752.19
limb (acquired)
  congenital (complete) (partial) (*see also* Deformity, reduction) 755.4
    lower 755.30
      complete 755.31
      incomplete 755.32
      longitudinal — *see* Deficiency, lower limb, longitudinal
      transverse 755.31
    upper 755.20

Absence — *continued*
limb — *continued*
  congenital (*see also* Deformity, reduction) — *continued*
    upper — *continued*
      complete 755.21
      incomplete 755.22
      longitudinal — *see* Deficiency, upper limb, longitudinal
      transverse 755.21
    lower NEC V49.70
    upper NEC V49.60
lip 750.26
liver (congenital) (lobe) 751.69
lumbar (congenital) (vertebra) 756.13
  isthmus 756.11
  pars articularis 756.11
lumen — *see* Atresia
lung (bilateral) (congenital) (fissure) (lobe) (unilateral) 748.5
  acquired (any part) V45.76
mandible (congenital) 524.09
maxilla (congenital) 524.09
menstruation 626.0
metacarpal(s), congenital (complete) (partial) (with absence of distal elements, incomplete) (*see also* Deformity, reduction, upper limb) 755.28
  with all fingers, complete 755.21
metatarsal(s), congenital (complete) (partial) (with absence of distal elements, incomplete) (*see also* Deformity, reduction, lower limb) 755.38
  with complete absence of distal elements 755.31
muscle (congenital) (pectoral) 756.81
  ocular 743.69
musculoskeletal system (congenital) NEC 756.9
nail(s) (congenital) 757.5
neck, part 744.89
nerve 742.8
nervous system, part NEC 742.8
neutrophil 288.00
nipple (congenital) 757.6
  acquired V45.71
nose (congenital) 748.1
  acquired 738.0
nuclear 742.8
ocular muscle (congenital) 743.69
organ
  of Corti (congenital) 744.05
  or site
    acquired V45.79
    congenital NEC 759.89
osseous meatus (ear) 744.03
ovary (acquired) V45.77
  congenital 752.0
oviduct (acquired) V45.77
  congenital 752.19
pancreas (congenital) 751.7
  acquired (postoperative) (posttraumatic) V88.11   ▲
    partial V88.12   ●
    total V88.11   ●
parathyroid gland (congenital) 759.2
parotid gland(s) (congenital) 750.21
patella, congenital 755.64
pelvic girdle (congenital) 755.69
penis (congenital) 752.69
  acquired V45.77
pericardium (congenital) 746.89
perineal body (congenital) 756.81
phalange(s), congenital 755.4
  lower limb (complete) (intercalary) (partial) (terminal) (*see also* Deformity, reduction, lower limb) 755.39
    meaning all toes (complete) (partial) 755.31
    transverse 755.31
  upper limb (complete) (intercalary) (partial) (terminal) (*see also* Deformity, reduction, upper limb) 755.29

Absence — *continued*
phalange(s), congenital — *continued*
  upper limb (*see also* Deformity, reduction, upper limb) — *continued*
    meaning all digits (complete) (partial) 755.21
    transverse 755.21
pituitary gland (congenital) 759.2
postoperative — *see* Absence, by site, acquired
prostate (congenital) 752.89
  acquired V45.77
pulmonary
  artery 747.3
  trunk 747.3
  valve (congenital) 746.01
  vein 747.49
punctum lacrimale (congenital) 743.65
radius, congenital (complete) (partial) (with absence of distal elements, incomplete) 755.26
  with
    complete absence of distal elements 755.21
    ulna 755.25
      with
        complete absence of distal elements 755.21
        humerus (incomplete) 755.23
ray, congenital 755.4
  lower limb (complete) (partial) (*see also* Deformity, reduction, lower limb) 755.38
    meaning all rays 755.31
    transverse 755.31
  upper limb (complete) (partial) (*see also* Deformity, reduction, upper limb) 755.28
    meaning all rays 755.21
    transverse 755.21
rectum (congenital) 751.2
  acquired V45.79
red cell 284.9
  acquired (secondary) 284.81
  congenital 284.01
  hereditary 284.01
  idiopathic 284.9
respiratory organ (congenital) NEC 748.9
rib (acquired) 738.3
  congenital 756.3
roof of orbit (congenital) 742.0
round ligament (congenital) 752.89
sacrum, congenital 756.13
salivary gland(s) (congenital) 750.21
scapula 755.59
scrotum, congenital 752.89
seminal tract or duct (congenital) 752.89
  acquired V45.77
septum (congenital) (*see also* Imperfect, closure, septum)
  atrial 745.69
    and ventricular 745.7
  between aorta and pulmonary artery 745.0
  ventricular 745.3
    and atrial 745.7
sex chromosomes 758.81
shoulder girdle, congenital (complete) (partial) 755.59
skin (congenital) 757.39
skull bone 756.0
  with
    anencephalus 740.0
    encephalocele 742.0
    hydrocephalus 742.3
      with spina bifida (*see also* Spina bifida) 741.0 ☑
    microcephalus 742.1
spermatic cord (congenital) 752.89
spinal cord 742.59
spine, congenital 756.13
spleen (congenital) 759.0
  acquired V45.79
sternum, congenital 756.3

Absence — *continued*
stomach (acquired) (partial) (postoperative) V45.75
  with postgastric surgery syndrome 564.2
  congenital 750.7
submaxillary gland(s) (congenital) 750.21
superior vena cava (congenital) 747.49
tarsal(s), congenital (complete) (partial) (with absence of distal elements, incomplete) (*see also* Deformity, reduction, lower limb) 755.38
teeth, tooth (congenital) 520.0
  with abnormal spacing 524.30
  acquired 525.10
    with malocclusion 524.30
    due to
      caries 525.13
      extraction 525.10
      periodontal disease 525.12
      trauma 525.11
tendon (congenital) 756.81
testis (congenital) 752.89
  acquired V45.77
thigh (acquired) 736.89
thumb (acquired) V49.61
  congenital 755.29
thymus gland (congenital) 759.2
thyroid (gland) (surgical) 246.8
  with hypothyroidism 244.0
  cartilage, congenital 748.3
  congenital 243
tibia, congenital (complete) (partial) (with absence of distal elements, incomplete) (*see also* Deformity, reduction, lower limb) 755.36
  with
    complete absence of distal elements 755.31
    fibula 755.35
      with
        complete absence of distal elements 755.31
        femur (incomplete) 755.33
          with complete absence of distal elements 755.31
toe (acquired) V49.72
  congenital (complete) (partial) 755.39
    meaning all toes 755.31
    transverse 755.31
  great V49.71
tongue (congenital) 750.11
tooth, teeth (congenital) 520.0
  with abnormal spacing 524.30
  acquired 525.10
    with malocclusion 524.30
    due to
      caries 525.13
      extraction 525.10
      periodontal disease 525.12
      trauma 525.11
trachea (cartilage) (congenital) (rings) 748.3
transverse aortic arch (congenital) 747.21
tricuspid valve 746.1
ulna, congenital (complete) (partial) (with absence of distal elements, incomplete) (*see also* Deformity, reduction, upper limb) 755.27
  with
    complete absence of distal elements 755.21
    radius 755.25
      with
        complete absence of distal elements 755.21
        humerus (incomplete) 755.23
umbilical artery (congenital) 747.5
ureter (congenital) 753.4
  acquired V45.74
urethra, congenital 753.8
  acquired V45.74
urinary system, part NEC, congenital 753.8
  acquired V45.74
uterus (acquired) V88.01
  with remaining cervical stump V88.02
    and cervix V88.01

☑ Additional Digit Required — Refer to the Tabular List for Digit Selection   ▽ Subterms under main terms may continue to next column or page

6 — Volume 2 · October 2010   ▶◀ Revised Text   ● New Line   ▲ Revised Code   **2011 ICD-9-CM**

Absence — continued
  uterus — continued
    congenital 752.31 ▲
    uvula (congenital) 750.26
  vagina, congenital 752.45 ▲
    acquired V45.77
  vas deferens (congenital) 752.89
    acquired V45.77
  vein (congenital) (peripheral) NEC (see also
      Anomaly, peripheral vascular system)
      747.60
    brain 747.81
    great 747.49
    portal 747.49
    pulmonary 747.49
  vena cava (congenital) (inferior) (superior)
      747.49
  ventral horn cell 742.59
  ventricular septum 745.3
  vermis of cerebellum 742.2
  vertebra, congenital 756.13
  vulva, congenital 752.49
Absentia epileptica — see also Epilepsy
    345.0 ☑
Absinthemia — see also Dependence 304.6 ☑
Absinthism — see also Dependence 304.6 ☑
Absorbent system disease 459.89
Absorption
  alcohol, through placenta or breast milk
      760.71
  antibiotics, through placenta or breast milk
      760.74
  anticonvulsants, through placenta or breast
      milk 760.77
  antifungals, through placenta or breast milk
      760.74
  anti-infective, through placenta or breast
      milk 760.74
  antimetabolics, through placenta or breast
      milk 760.78
  chemical NEC 989.9
    specified chemical or substance — see
        Table of Drugs and Chemicals
    through placenta or breast milk (fetus
        or newborn) 760.70
      alcohol 760.71
      anticonvulsants 760.77
      antifungals 760.74
      anti-infective agents 760.74
      antimetabolics 760.78
      cocaine 760.75
      "crack" 760.75
      diethylstilbestrol [DES] 760.76
      hallucinogenic agents 760.73
      medicinal agents NEC 760.79
      narcotics 760.72
      obstetric anesthetic or analgesic drug
          763.5
      specified agent NEC 760.79
      suspected, affecting management of
          pregnancy 655.5 ☑
  cocaine, through placenta or breast milk
      760.75
  drug NEC (see also Reaction, drug)
    through placenta or breast milk (fetus
        or newborn) 760.70
      alcohol 760.71
      anticonvulsants 760.77
      antifungals 760.74
      anti-infective agents 760.74
      antimetabolics 760.78
      cocaine 760.75
      "crack" 760.75
      diethylstilbestrol [DES] 760.76
      hallucinogenic agents 760.73
      medicinal agents NEC 760.79
      narcotics 760.72
      obstetric anesthetic or analgesic drug
          763.5
      specified agent NEC 760.79
      suspected, affecting management of
          pregnancy 655.5 ☑
  fat, disturbance 579.8
  hallucinogenic agents, through placenta or
      breast milk 760.73

Absorption — continued
  immune sera, through placenta or breast
      milk 760.79
  lactose defect 271.3
  medicinal agents NEC, through placenta or
      breast milk 760.79
  narcotics, through placenta or breast milk
      760.72
  noxious substance — see Absorption,
      chemical
  protein, disturbance 579.8
  pus or septic, general — see Septicemia
  quinine, through placenta or breast milk
      760.74
  toxic substance — see Absorption, chemical
  uremic — see Uremia
Abstinence symptoms or syndrome
  alcohol 291.81
  drug 292.0
  neonatal 779.5
Abt-Letterer-Siwe syndrome (acute histiocy-
    tosis X) (M9722/3) 202.5 ☑
Abulia 799.89
Abulomania 301.6
Abuse
  adult 995.80
    emotional 995.82
    multiple forms 995.85
    neglect (nutritional) 995.84
    physical 995.81
    psychological 995.82
    sexual 995.83
  alcohol — see also Alcoholism 305.0 ☑
    dependent 303.9 ☑
    non-dependent 305.0 ☑
  child 995.50
    counseling
      perpetrator
        non-parent V62.83
        parent V61.22
      victim V61.21
    emotional 995.51
    multiple forms 995.59
    neglect (nutritional) 995.52
    physical 995.54
      shaken infant syndrome 995.55
    psychological 995.51
    sexual 995.53
  drugs, nondependent 305.9 ☑

> Note — Use the following fifth-digit
> subclassification with the following
> codes: 305.0, 305.2–305.9:
>
> 0   unspecified
>
> 1   continuous
>
> 2   episodic
>
> 3   in remission

      amphetamine type 305.7 ☑
      antidepressants 305.8 ☑
      anxiolytic 305.4 ☑
      barbiturates 305.4 ☑
      caffeine 305.9 ☑
      cannabis 305.2 ☑
      cocaine type 305.6 ☑
      hallucinogens 305.3 ☑
      hashish 305.2 ☑
      hypnotic 305.4 ☑
      inhalant 305.9 ☑
      LSD 305.3 ☑
      marijuana 305.2 ☑
      mixed 305.9 ☑
      morphine type 305.5 ☑
      opioid type 305.5 ☑
      phencyclidine (PCP) 305.9 ☑
      sedative 305.4 ☑
      specified NEC 305.9 ☑
      tranquilizers 305.4 ☑
  spouse 995.80
  tobacco 305.1
Acalcerosis 275.40
Acalcicosis 275.40
Acalculia 784.69
  developmental 315.1
Acanthocheilonemiasis 125.4

Acanthocytosis 272.5
Acanthokeratodermia 701.1
Acantholysis 701.8
  bullosa 757.39
Acanthoma (benign) (M8070/0) — see also
    Neoplasm, by site, benign
  malignant (M8070/3) — see Neoplasm, by
      site, malignant
Acanthosis (acquired) (nigricans) 701.2
  adult 701.2
  benign (congenital) 757.39
  congenital 757.39
  glycogenic
    esophagus 530.89
  juvenile 701.2
  tongue 529.8
Acanthrocytosis 272.5
Acapnia 276.3
Acarbia 276.2
Acardia 759.89
Acardiacus amorphus 759.89
Acardiotrophia 429.1
Acardius 759.89
Acariasis 133.9
  sarcoptic 133.0
Acaridiasis 133.9
Acarinosis 133.9
Acariosis 133.9
Acarodermatitis 133.9
  urticarioides 133.9
Acarophobia 300.29
Acatalasemia 277.89
Acatalasia 277.89
Acatamathesia 784.69
Acataphasia 784.59
Acathisia 781.0
  due to drugs 333.99
Acceleration, accelerated
  atrioventricular conduction 426.7
  idioventricular rhythm 427.89
Accessory (congenital)
  adrenal gland 759.1
  anus 751.5
  appendix 751.5
  atrioventricular conduction 426.7
  auditory ossicles 744.04
  auricle (ear) 744.1
  autosome(s) NEC 758.5
    21 or 22 758.0
  biliary duct or passage 751.69
  bladder 753.8
  blood vessels (peripheral) (congenital) NEC
      (see also Anomaly, peripheral vascu-
      lar system) 747.60
    cerebral 747.81
    coronary 746.85
  bone NEC 756.9
    foot 755.67
  breast tissue, axilla 757.6
  carpal bones 755.56
  cecum 751.5
  cervix 752.44 ▲
  chromosome(s) NEC 758.5
    13-15 758.1
    16-18 758.2
    21 or 22 758.0
    autosome(s) NEC 758.5
    D_1 758.1
    E_3 758.2
    G 758.0
    sex 758.81
  coronary artery 746.85
  cusp(s), heart valve NEC 746.89
    pulmonary 746.09
  cystic duct 751.69
  digits 755.00
  ear (auricle) (lobe) 744.1
  endocrine gland NEC 759.2
  external os 752.44 ▲
  eyelid 743.62
  eye muscle 743.69
  face bone(s) 756.0
  fallopian tube (fimbria) (ostium) 752.19
  fingers 755.01
  foreskin 605
  frontonasal process 756.0

Accessory — continued
  gallbladder 751.69
  genital organ(s)
    female 752.89
      external 752.49
      internal NEC 752.89
    male NEC 752.89
      penis 752.69
  genitourinary organs NEC 752.89
  heart 746.89
    valve NEC 746.89
      pulmonary 746.09
  hepatic ducts 751.69
  hymen 752.49
  intestine (large) (small) 751.5
  kidney 753.3
  lacrimal canal 743.65
  leaflet, heart valve NEC 746.89
    pulmonary 746.09
  ligament, broad 752.19
  liver (duct) 751.69
  lobule (ear) 744.1
  lung (lobe) 748.69
  muscle 756.82
  navicular of carpus 755.56
  nervous system, part NEC 742.8
  nipple 757.6
  nose 748.1
  organ or site NEC — see Anomaly, specified
      type NEC
  ovary 752.0
  oviduct 752.19
  pancreas 751.7
  parathyroid gland 759.2
  parotid gland (and duct) 750.22
  pituitary gland 759.2
  placental lobe — see Placenta, abnormal
  preauricular appendage 744.1
  prepuce 605
  renal arteries (multiple) 747.62
  rib 756.3
    cervical 756.2
  roots (teeth) 520.2
  salivary gland 750.22
  sesamoids 755.8
  sinus — see condition
  skin tags 757.39
  spleen 759.0
  sternum 756.3
  submaxillary gland 750.22
  tarsal bones 755.67
  teeth, tooth 520.1
    causing crowding 524.31
  tendon 756.89
  thumb 755.01
  thymus gland 759.2
  thyroid gland 759.2
  toes 755.02
  tongue 750.13
  tragus 744.1
  ureter 753.4
  urethra 753.8
  urinary organ or tract NEC 753.8
  uterus 752.2
  vagina 752.49
  valve, heart NEC 746.89
    pulmonary 746.09
  vertebra 756.19
  vocal cords 748.3
  vulva 752.49
Accident, accidental — see also condition
  birth NEC 767.9
  cardiovascular (see also Disease, cardiovas-
      cular) 429.2
  cerebral (see also Disease, cerebrovascular,
      acute) 434.91
  cerebrovascular (current) (CVA) (see also
      Disease, cerebrovascular, acute)
      434.91
    aborted 434.91
    embolic 434.11
    healed or old V12.54
    hemorrhagic — see Hemorrhage, brain
    impending 435.9
    ischemic 434.91

☑ Additional Digit Required — Refer to the Tabular List for Digit Selection   ⬐ Subterms under main terms may continue to next column or page

2011 ICD-9-CM   ▶◀ Revised Text   ● New Line   ▲ Revised Code   October 2010 · Volume 2 — 7

Accident, accidental — see also condition — continued
  cerebrovascular (see also Disease, cerebrovascular, acute) — continued
    late effect — see Late effect(s) (of) cerebrovascular disease
    postoperative 997.02
    thrombotic 434.01
  coronary (see also Infarct, myocardium) 410.9 ☑
  craniovascular (see also Disease, cerebrovascular, acute) 436
  during pregnancy, to mother, affecting fetus or newborn 760.5
  heart, cardiac (see also Infarct, myocardium) 410.9 ☑
  intrauterine 779.89
  vascular — see Disease, cerebrovascular, acute
Accommodation
  disorder of 367.51
    drug-induced 367.89
    toxic 367.89
  insufficiency of 367.4
  paralysis of 367.51
    hysterical 300.11
  spasm of 367.53
Accouchement — see Delivery
Accreta placenta (without hemorrhage) 667.0 ☑
  with hemorrhage 666.0 ☑
Accretio cordis (nonrheumatic) 423.1
Accretions on teeth 523.6
Accumulation secretion, prostate 602.8
Acephalia, acephalism, acephaly 740.0
Acephalic 740.0
Acephalobrachia 759.89
Acephalocardia 759.89
Acephalocardius 759.89
Acephalochiria 759.89
Acephalochirus 759.89
Acephalogaster 759.89
Acephalostomus 759.89
Acephalothorax 759.89
Acephalus 740.0
Acetonemia 790.6
  diabetic 250.1 ☑
    due to secondary diabetes 249.1 ☑
Acetonglycosuria 982.8
Acetonuria 791.6
Achalasia 530.0
  cardia 530.0
  digestive organs congenital NEC 751.8
  esophagus 530.0
  pelvirectal 751.3
  psychogenic 306.4
  pylorus 750.5
  sphincteral NEC 564.89
Achard-Thiers syndrome (adrenogenital) 255.2
Ache(s) — see Pain
Acheilia 750.26
Acheiria 755.21
Achil[]bursitis 726.71
Achillodynia 726.71
Achlorhydria, achlorhydric 536.0
  anemia 280.9
  diarrhea 536.0
  neurogenic 536.0
  postvagotomy 564.2
  psychogenic 306.4
  secondary to vagotomy 564.2
Achloroblepsia 368.52
Achloropsia 368.52
Acholia 575.8
Acholuric jaundice (familial) (splenomegalic) — see also Spherocytosis 282.0
  acquired 283.9
Achondroplasia 756.4
Achrestic anemia 281.8
Achroacytosis, lacrimal gland 375.00
  tuberculous (see also Tuberculosis) 017.3 ☑
Achroma, cutis 709.00
Achromate (congenital) 368.54
Achromatopia 368.54
Achromatopsia (congenital) 368.54

Achromia
  congenital 270.2
  parasitica 111.0
  unguium 703.8
Achylia
  gastrica 536.8
    neurogenic 536.3
    psychogenic 306.4
  pancreatica 577.1
Achylosis 536.8
Acid
  burn (see also Burn, by site)
    from swallowing acid — see Burn, internal organs
  deficiency
    amide nicotinic 265.2
    amino 270.9
    ascorbic 267
    folic 266.2
    nicotinic (amide) 265.2
    pantothenic 266.2
  intoxication 276.2
  peptic disease 536.8
  stomach 536.8
    psychogenic 306.4
Acidemia 276.2
  arginosuccinic 270.6
  fetal
    affecting management of pregnancy 656.3 ☑
    before onset of labor, in liveborn infant 768.2
    during labor and delivery in liveborn infant 768.3
    intrauterine 656.3 ☑
    unspecified as to time of onset, in liveborn infant 768.4
  newborn 775.81
  pipecolic 270.7
Acidity, gastric (high) (low) 536.8
  psychogenic 306.4
Acidocytopenia 288.59
Acidocytosis 288.3
Acidopenia 288.59
Acidosis 276.2
  diabetic 250.1 ☑
    due to secondary diabetes 249.1 ☑
  fetal, affecting management of pregnancy 756.8 ☑
  fetal, affecting newborn 775.81
  kidney tubular 588.89
    newborn 775.81
  lactic 276.2
  metabolic NEC 276.2
    with respiratory acidosis 276.4
      of newborn 775.81
    late, of newborn 775.7
  newborn 775.81
  renal
    hyperchloremic 588.89
    tubular (distal) (proximal) 588.89
  respiratory 276.2
    complicated by
      metabolic acidosis 276.4
        of newborn 775.81
      metabolic alkalosis 276.4
Aciduria 791.9
  arginosuccinic 270.6
  beta-aminoisobutyric (BAIB) 277.2
  glutaric
    type I 270.7
    type II (type IIA, IIB, IIC) 277.85
    type III 277.86
  glycolic 271.8
  methylmalonic 270.3
    with glycinemia 270.7
  organic 270.9
  orotic (congenital) (hereditary) (pyrimidine deficiency) 281.4
Acladiosis 111.8
  skin 111.8
Aclasis
  diaphyseal 756.4
  tarsoepiphyseal 756.59
Acleistocardia 745.5
Aclusion 524.4

Acmesthesia 782.0
Acne (pustular) (vulgaris) 706.1
  agminata (see also Tuberculosis) 017.0 ☑
  artificialis 706.1
  atrophica 706.0
  cachecticorum (Hebra) 706.1
  conglobata 706.1
  conjunctiva 706.1
  cystic 706.1
  decalvans 704.09
  erythematosa 695.3
  eyelid 706.1
  frontalis 706.0
  indurata 706.1
  keloid 706.1
  lupoid 706.0
  necrotic, necrotica 706.0
    miliaris 704.8
  neonatal 706.1
  nodular 706.1
  occupational 706.1
  papulosa 706.1
  rodens 706.0
  rosacea 695.3
  scorbutica 267
  scrofulosorum (Bazin) (see also Tuberculosis) 017.0 ☑
  summer 692.72
  tropical 706.1
  varioliformis 706.0
Acneiform drug eruptions 692.3
Acnitis (primary) — see also Tuberculosis 017.0 ☑
Acomia 704.00
Acontractile bladder 344.61
Aconuresis — see also Incontinence 788.30
Acosta's disease 993.2
Acousma 780.1
Acoustic — see condition
Acousticophobia 300.29
Acquired — see condition
Acquired immune deficiency syndrome — see Human immunodeficiency virus (disease) (illness) (infection)
Acquired immunodeficiency syndrome — see Human immunodeficiency virus (disease) (illness) (infection)
Acragnosis 781.99
Acrania 740.0
Acroagnosis 781.99
Acroasphyxia, chronic 443.89
Acrobrachycephaly 756.0
Acrobystiolith 608.89
Acrobystitis 607.2
Acrocephalopolysyndactyly 755.55
Acrocephalosyndactyly 755.55
Acrocephaly 756.0
Acrochondrohyperplasia 759.82
Acrocyanosis 443.89
  newborn 770.83
    meaning transient blue hands and feet — omit code
Acrodermatitis 686.8
  atrophicans (chronica) 701.8
  continua (Hallopeau) 696.1
  enteropathica 686.8
  Hallopeau's 696.1
  perstans 696.1
  pustulosa continua 696.1
  recalcitrant pustular 696.1
Acrodynia 985.0
Acrodysplasia 755.55
Acrohyperhidrosis — see also Hyperhidrosis 780.8
Acrokeratosis verruciformis 757.39
Acromastitis 611.0
Acromegaly, acromegalia (skin) 253.0
Acromelalgia 443.82
Acromicria, acromikria 756.59
Acronyx 703.0
Acropachyderma 757.39
Acropachy, thyroid — see also Thyrotoxicosis 242.9 ☑
Acroparesthesia 443.89
  simple (Schultz's type) 443.89
  vasomotor (Nothnagel's type) 443.89

Acropathy thyroid — see also Thyrotoxicosis 242.9 ☑
Acrophobia 300.29
Acroposthitis 607.2
Acroscleriasis — see also Scleroderma 710.1
Acroscleroderma — see also Scleroderma 710.1
Acrosclerosis — see also Scleroderma 710.1
Acrosphacelus 785.4
Acrosphenosyndactylia 755.55
Acrospiroma, eccrine (M8402/0) — see Neoplasm, skin, benign
Acrostealgia 732.9
Acrosyndactyly — see also Syndactylism 755.10
Acrotrophodynia 991.4
Actinic — see also condition
  cheilitis (due to sun) 692.72
    chronic NEC 692.74
    due to radiation, except from sun 692.82
  conjunctivitis 370.24
  dermatitis (due to sun) (see also Dermatitis, actinic) 692.70
  due to
    roentgen rays or radioactive substance 692.82
    ultraviolet radiation, except from sun 692.82
    sun NEC 692.70
  elastosis solare 692.74
  granuloma 692.73
  keratitis 370.24
  ophthalmia 370.24
  reticuloid 692.73
Actinobacillosis, general 027.8
Actinobacillus
  lignieresii 027.8
  mallei 024
  muris 026.1
Actinocutitis NEC — see also Dermatitis, actinic 692.70
Actinodermatitis NEC — see also Dermatitis, actinic 692.70
Actinomyces
  israelii (infection) — see Actinomycosis
  muris-ratti (infection) 026.1
Actinomycosis, actinomycotic 039.9
  with
    pneumonia 039.1
  abdominal 039.2
  cervicofacial 039.3
  cutaneous 039.0
  pulmonary 039.1
  specified site NEC 039.8
  thoracic 039.1
Actinoneuritis 357.89
Action, heart
  disorder 427.9
    postoperative 997.1
  irregular 427.9
    postoperative 997.1
    psychogenic 306.2
Active — see condition
Activity decrease, functional 780.99
Acute — see also condition
  abdomen NEC 789.0 ☑
  gallbladder (see also Cholecystitis, acute) 575.0
Acyanoblepsia 368.53
Acyanopsia 368.53
Acystia 753.8
Acystinervia — see Neurogenic, bladder
Acystineuria — see Neurogenic, bladder
Adactylia, adactyly (congenital) 755.4
  lower limb (complete) (intercalary) (partial) (terminal) (see also Deformity, reduction, lower limb) 755.39
    meaning all digits (complete) (partial) 755.31
    transverse (complete) (partial) 755.31
  upper limb (complete) (intercalary) (partial) (terminal) (see also Deformity, reduction, upper limb) 755.29
    meaning all digits (complete) (partial) 755.21
    transverse (complete) (partial) 755.21

☑ Additional Digit Required — Refer to the Tabular List for Digit Selection   ⬙ Subterms under main terms may continue to next column or page

8 — Volume 2   ▶◀ Revised Text   ● New Line   ▲ Revised Code   2011 ICD-9-CM

Adair-Dighton syndrome (brittle bones and blue sclera, deafness) 756.51
Adamantinoblastoma (M9310/0) — *see* Ameloblastoma
Adamantinoma (M9310/0) — *see* Ameloblastoma
Adamantoblastoma (M9310/0) — *see* Ameloblastoma
Adams-Stokes (-Morgagni) disease or syndrome (syncope with heart block) 426.9
Adaptation reaction — *see also* Reaction, adjustment 309.9
Addiction — *see also* Dependence
   absinthe 304.6 ☑
   alcoholic (ethyl) (methyl) (wood) 303.9 ☑
      complicating pregnancy, childbirth, or puerperium 648.4 ☑
         affecting fetus or newborn 760.71
         suspected damage to fetus affecting management of pregnancy 655.4 ☑
   drug (*see also* Dependence) 304.9 ☑
   ethyl alcohol 303.9 ☑
   heroin 304.0 ☑
   hospital 301.51
   methyl alcohol 303.9 ☑
   methylated spirit 303.9 ☑
   morphine (-like substances) 304.0 ☑
   nicotine 305.1
   opium 304.0 ☑
   tobacco 305.1
   wine 303.9 ☑
Addison's
   anemia (pernicious) 281.0
   disease (bronze) (primary adrenal insufficiency) 255.41
      tuberculous (*see also* Tuberculosis) 017.6 ☑
   keloid (morphea) 701.0
   melanoderma (adrenal cortical hypofunction) 255.41
Addison-Biermer anemia (pernicious) 281.0
Addison-Gull disease — *see* Xanthoma
Addisonian crisis or melanosis (acute adrenocortical insufficiency) 255.41
Additional — *see also* Accessory
   chromosome(s) 758.5
      13-15 758.1
      16-18 758.2
      21 758.0
      autosome(s) NEC 758.5
      sex 758.81
Adduction contracture, hip or other joint — *see* Contraction, joint
ADEM (acute disseminated encephalomyelitis) (postinfectious) 136.9 *[323.61]*
   infectious 136.9 *[323.61]*
   noninfectious 323.81
Adenasthenia gastrica 536.0
Aden fever 061
Adenitis — *see also* Lymphadenitis 289.3
   acute, unspecified site 683
      epidemic infectious 075
   axillary 289.3
      acute 683
      chronic or subacute 289.1
   Bartholin's gland 616.89
   bulbourethral gland (*see also* Urethritis) 597.89
   cervical 289.3
      acute 683
      chronic or subacute 289.1
   chancroid (Ducrey's bacillus) 099.0
   chronic (any lymph node, except mesenteric) 289.1
      mesenteric 289.2
   Cowper's gland (*see also* Urethritis) 597.89
   epidemic, acute 075
   gangrenous 683
   gonorrheal NEC 098.89
   groin 289.3
      acute 683
      chronic or subacute 289.1
   infectious 075
   inguinal (region) 289.3
      acute 683

Adenitis — *see also* Lymphadenitis — *continued*
   inguinal — *continued*
      chronic or subacute 289.1
   lymph gland or node, except mesenteric 289.3
      acute 683
      chronic or subacute 289.1
   mesenteric (acute) (chronic) (nonspecific) (subacute) 289.2
      due to Pasteurella multocida (P. septica) 027.2
   parotid gland (suppurative) 527.2
   phlegmonous 683
   salivary duct or gland (any) (recurring) (suppurative) 527.2
   scrofulous (*see also* Tuberculosis) 017.2 ☑
   septic 289.3
   Skene's duct or gland (*see also* Urethritis) 597.89
   strumous, tuberculous (*see also* Tuberculosis) 017.2 ☑
   subacute, unspecified site 289.1
   sublingual gland (suppurative) 527.2
   submandibular gland (suppurative) 527.2
   submaxillary gland (suppurative) 527.2
   suppurative 683
   tuberculous — *see* Tuberculosis, lymph gland
   urethral gland (*see also* Urethritis) 597.89
   venereal NEC 099.8
   Wharton's duct (suppurative) 527.2
Adenoacanthoma (M8570/3) — *see* Neoplasm, by site, malignant
Adenoameloblastoma (M9300/0) 213.1
   upper jaw (bone) 213.0
Adenocarcinoma (M8140/3) — *see also* Neoplasm, by site, malignant

Note — The list of adjectival modifiers below is not exhaustive. A description of adenocarcinoma that does not appear in this list should be coded in the same manner as carcinoma with that description. Thus, "mixed acidophil-basophil adenocarcinoma," should be coded in the same manner as "mixed acidophil-basophil carcinoma," which appears in the list under "Carcinoma."

Except where otherwise indicated, the morphological varieties of adenocarcinoma in the list below should be coded by site as for "Neoplasm, malignant."

   with
      apocrine metaplasia (M8573/3)
      cartilaginous (and osseous) metaplasia (M8571/3)
      osseous (and cartilaginous) metaplasia (M8571/3)
      spindle cell metaplasia (M8572/3)
      squamous metaplasia (M8570/3)
   acidophil (M8280/3)
      specified site — *see* Neoplasm, by site, malignant
      unspecified site 194.3
   acinar (M8550/3)
   acinic cell (M8550/3)
   adrenal cortical (M8370/3) 194.0
   alveolar (M8251/3)
      and
         epidermoid carcinoma, mixed (M8560/3)
         squamous cell carcinoma, mixed (M8560/3)
   apocrine (M8401/3)
      breast — *see* Neoplasm, breast, malignant
      specified site NEC — *see* Neoplasm, skin, malignant
      unspecified site 173.9
   basophil (M8300/3)
      specified site — *see* Neoplasm, by site, malignant
      unspecified site 194.3

Adenocarcinoma — *see also* Neoplasm, by site, malignant — *continued*
   bile duct type (M8160/3)
      liver 155.1
      specified site NEC — *see* Neoplasm, by site, malignant
      unspecified site 155.1
   bronchiolar (M8250/3) — *see* Neoplasm, lung, malignant
   ceruminous (M8420/3) 173.2
   chromophobe (M8270/3)
      specified site — *see* Neoplasm, by site, malignant
      unspecified site 194.3
   clear cell (mesonephroid type) (M8310/3)
   colloid (M8480/3)
   cylindroid type (M8200/3)
   diffuse type (M8145/3)
      specified site — *see* Neoplasm, by site, malignant
      unspecified site 151.9
   duct (infiltrating) (M8500/3)
      with Paget's disease (M8541/3) — *see* Neoplasm, breast, malignant
      specified site — *see* Neoplasm, by site, malignant
      unspecified site 174.9
   embryonal (M9070/3)
   endometrioid (M8380/3) — *see* Neoplasm, by site, malignant
   eosinophil (M8280/3)
      specified site — *see* Neoplasm, by site, malignant
      unspecified site 194.3
   follicular (M8330/3)
      and papillary (M8340/3) 193
      moderately differentiated type (M8332/3) 193
      pure follicle type (M8331/3) 193
      specified site — *see* Neoplasm, by site, malignant
      trabecular type (M8332/3) 193
      unspecified type 193
      well differentiated type (M8331/3) 193
   gelatinous (M8480/3)
   granular cell (M8320/3)
   Hürthle cell (M8290/3) 193
   in
      adenomatous
         polyp (M8210/3)
         polyposis coli (M8220/3) 153.9
      polypoid adenoma (M8210/3)
      tubular adenoma (M8210/3)
      villous adenoma (M8261/3)
   infiltrating duct (M8500/3)
      with Paget's disease (M8541/3) — *see* Neoplasm, breast, malignant
      specified site — *see* Neoplasm, by site, malignant
      unspecified site 174.9
   inflammatory (M8530/3)
      specified site — *see* Neoplasm, by site, malignant
      unspecified site 174.9
   in situ (M8140/2) — *see* Neoplasm, by site, in situ
   intestinal type (M8144/3)
      specified site — *see* Neoplasm, by site, malignant
      unspecified site 151.9
   intraductal (noninfiltrating) (M8500/2)
      papillary (M8503/2)
         specified site — *see* Neoplasm, by site, in situ
         unspecified site 233.0
      specified site — *see* Neoplasm, by site, in situ
      unspecified site 233.0
   islet cell (M8150/3)
      and exocrine, mixed (M8154/3)
         specified site — *see* Neoplasm, by site, malignant
         unspecified site 157.9
      pancreas 157.4
      specified site NEC — *see* Neoplasm, by site, malignant

Adenocarcinoma — *see also* Neoplasm, by site, malignant — *continued*
   islet cell — *continued*
      unspecified site 157.4
   lobular (M8520/3)
      specified site — *see* Neoplasm, by site, malignant
      unspecified site 174.9
   medullary (M8510/3)
   mesonephric (M9110/3)
   mixed cell (M8323/3)
   mucinous (M8480/3)
   mucin-producing (M8481/3)
   mucoid (M8480/3) (*see also* Neoplasm, by site, malignant)
      cell (M8300/3)
         specified site — *see* Neoplasm, by site, malignant
         unspecified site 194.3
   nonencapsulated sclerosing (M8350/3) 193
   oncocytic (M8290/3)
   oxyphilic (M8290/3)
   papillary (M8260/3)
      and follicular (M8340/3) 193
      intraductal (noninfiltrating) (M8503/2)
         specified site — *see* Neoplasm, by site, in situ
         unspecified site 233.0
      serous (M8460/3)
         specified site — *see* Neoplasm, by site, malignant
         unspecified site 183.0
   papillocystic (M8450/3)
      specified site — *see* Neoplasm, by site, malignant
      unspecified site 183.0
   pseudomucinous (M8470/3)
      specified site — *see* Neoplasm, by site, malignant
      unspecified site 183.0
   renal cell (M8312/3) 189.0
   sebaceous (M8410/3)
   serous (M8441/3) (*see also* Neoplasm, by site, malignant)
      papillary
         specified site — *see* Neoplasm, by site, malignant
         unspecified site 183.0
   signet ring cell (M8490/3)
   superficial spreading (M8143/3)
   sweat gland (M8400/3) — *see* Neoplasm, skin, malignant
   trabecular (M8190/3)
   tubular (M8211/3)
   villous (M8262/3)
   water-clear cell (M8322/3) 194.1
Adenofibroma (M9013/0)
   clear cell (M8313/0) — *see* Neoplasm, by site, benign
   endometrioid (M8381/0) 220
      borderline malignancy (M8381/1) 236.2
      malignant (M8381/3) 183.0
   mucinous (M9015/0)
      specified site — *see* Neoplasm, by site, benign
      unspecified site 220
   prostate 600.20
      with
         other lower urinary tract symptoms (LUTS) 600.21
         urinary
            obstruction 600.21
            retention 600.21
   serous (M9014/0)
      specified site — *see* Neoplasm, by site, benign
      unspecified site 220
   specified site — *see* Neoplasm, by site, benign
   unspecified site 220
Adenofibrosis
   breast 610.2
   endometrioid 617.0
Adenoiditis 474.01
   acute 463
   chronic 474.01

☑ Additional Digit Required — Refer to the Tabular List for Digit Selection   ▽ Subterms under main terms may continue to next column or page

2011 ICD-9-CM   ▶◀ Revised Text   ● New Line   ▲ Revised Code   Volume 2 — 9

Adenoiditis — *continued*
  chronic — *continued*
    with chronic tonsillitis 474.02
Adenoids (congenital) (of nasal fossa) 474.9
  hypertrophy 474.12
  vegetations 474.2
Adenolipomatosis (symmetrical) 272.8
Adenolymphoma (M8561/0)
  specified site — *see* Neoplasm, by site, benign
  unspecified 210.2
Adenomatosis (M8220/0)
  endocrine (multiple) (M8360/1)
    single specified site — *see* Neoplasm, by site, uncertain behavior
    two or more specified sites 237.4
    unspecified site 237.4
  erosive of nipple (M8506/0) 217
  pluriendocrine — *see* Adenomatosis, endocrine
  pulmonary (M8250/1) 235.7
    malignant (M8250/3) — *see* Neoplasm, lung, malignant
  specified site — *see* Neoplasm, by site, benign
  unspecified site 211.3
Adenomatous
  cyst, thyroid (gland) — *see* Goiter, nodular
  goiter (nontoxic) (*see also* Goiter, nodular) 241.9
    toxic or with hyperthyroidism 242.3 ☑
Adenoma (sessile) (M8140/0) — *see also* Neoplasm, by site, benign

Note — Except where otherwise indicated, the morphological varieties of adenoma in the list below should be coded by site as for "Neoplasm, benign."

  acidophil (M8280/0)
    specified site — *see* Neoplasm, by site, benign
    unspecified site 227.3
  acinar (cell) (M8550/0)
  acinic cell (M8550/0)
  adrenal (cortex) (cortical) (functioning) (M8370/0) 227.0
    clear cell type (M8373/0) 227.0
    compact cell type (M8371/0) 227.0
    glomerulosa cell type (M8374/0) 227.0
    heavily pigmented variant (M8372/0) 227.0
    mixed cell type (M8375/0) 227.0
  alpha cell (M8152/0)
    pancreas 211.7
    specified site NEC — *see* Neoplasm, by site, benign
    unspecified site 211.7
  alveolar (M8251/0)
  apocrine (M8401/0)
    breast 217
    specified site NEC — *see* Neoplasm, skin, benign
    unspecified site 216.9
  basal cell (M8147/0)
  basophil (M8300/0)
    specified site — *see* Neoplasm, by site, benign
    unspecified site 227.3
  beta cell (M8151/0)
    pancreas 211.7
    specified site NEC — *see* Neoplasm, by site, benign
    unspecified site 211.7
  bile duct (M8160/0) 211.5
  black (M8372/0) 227.0
  bronchial (M8140/1) 235.7
    carcinoid type (M8240/3) — *see* Neoplasm, lung, malignant
    cylindroid type (M8200/3) — *see* Neoplasm, lung, malignant
  ceruminous (M8420/0) 216.2
  chief cell (M8321/0) 227.1
  chromophobe (M8270/0)
    specified site — *see* Neoplasm, by site, benign
    unspecified site 227.3

Adenoma — *see also* Neoplasm, by site, benign — *continued*
  clear cell (M8310/0)
  colloid (M8334/0)
    specified site — *see* Neoplasm, by site, benign
    unspecified site 226
  cylindroid type, bronchus (M8200/3) — *see* Neoplasm, lung, malignant
  duct (M8503/0)
  embryonal (M8191/0)
  endocrine, multiple (M8360/1)
    single specified site — *see* Neoplasm, by site, uncertain behavior
    two or more specified sites 237.4
    unspecified site 237.4
  endometrioid (M8380/0) (*see also* Neoplasm, by site, benign)
    borderline malignancy (M8380/1) — *see* Neoplasm, by site, uncertain behavior
  eosinophil (M8280/0)
    specified site — *see* Neoplasm, by site, benign
    unspecified site 227.3
  fetal (M8333/0)
    specified site — *see* Neoplasm, by site, benign
    unspecified site 226
  follicular (M8330/0)
    specified site — *see* Neoplasm, by site, benign
    unspecified site 226
  hepatocellular (M8170/0) 211.5
  Hürthle cell (M8290/0) 226
  intracystic papillary (M8504/0)
  islet cell (functioning) (M8150/0)
    pancreas 211.7
    specified site NEC — *see* Neoplasm, by site, benign
    unspecified site 211.7
  liver cell (M8170/0) 211.5
  macrofollicular (M8334/0)
    specified site NEC — *see* Neoplasm, by site, benign
    unspecified site 226
  malignant, malignum (M8140/3) — *see* Neoplasm, by site, malignant
  mesonephric (M9110/0)
  microfollicular (M8333/0)
    specified site — *see* Neoplasm, by site, benign
    unspecified site 226
  mixed cell (M8323/0)
  monomorphic (M8146/0)
  mucinous (M8480/0)
  mucoid cell (M8300/0)
    specified site — *see* Neoplasm, by site, benign
    unspecified site 227.3
  multiple endocrine (M8360/1)
    single specified site — *see* Neoplasm, by site, uncertain behavior
    two or more specified sites 237.4
    unspecified site 237.4
  nipple (M8506/0) 217
  oncocytic (M8290/0)
  oxyphilic (M8290/0)
  papillary (M8260/0) (*see also* Neoplasm, by site, benign)
    intracystic (M8504/0)
  papillotubular (M8263/0)
  Pick's tubular (M8640/0)
    specified site — *see* Neoplasm, by site, benign
    unspecified site
      female 220
      male 222.0
  pleomorphic (M8940/0)
  polypoid (M8210/0)
  prostate (benign) (600.20)
    with
      other lower urinary tract symptoms (LUTS) 600.21
      urinary
        obstruction 600.21

Adenoma — *see also* Neoplasm, by site, benign — *continued*
  prostate — *continued*
    with — *continued*
      urinary — *continued*
        retention 600.21
  rete cell 222.0
  sebaceous, sebaceum (gland) (senile) (M8410/0) (*see also* Neoplasm, skin, benign)
    disseminata 759.5
  Sertoli cell (M8640/0)
    specified site — *see* Neoplasm, by site, benign
    unspecified site
      female 220
      male 222.0
  skin appendage (M8390/0) — *see* Neoplasm, skin, benign
  sudoriferous gland (M8400/0) — *see* Neoplasm, skin, benign
  sweat gland or duct (M8400/0) — *see* Neoplasm, skin, benign
  testicular (M8640/0)
    specified site — *see* Neoplasm, by site, benign
    unspecified site
      female 220
      male 222.0
  thyroid 226
  trabecular (M8190/0)
  tubular (M8211/0) (*see also* Neoplasm, by site, benign)
    papillary (M8460/3)
    Pick's (M8640/0)
      specified site — *see* Neoplasm, by site, benign
      unspecified site
        female 220
        male 222.0
  tubulovillous (M8263/0)
  villoglandular (M8263/0)
  villous (M8261/1) — *see* Neoplasm, by site, uncertain behavior
  water-clear cell (M8322/0) 227.1
  wolffian duct (M9110/0)
Adenomyoma (M8932/0) — *see also* Neoplasm, by site, benign
  prostate 600.20
    with
      other lower urinary tract symptoms (LUTS) 600.21
      urinary
        obstruction 600.21
        retention 600.21
Adenomyometritis 617.0
Adenomyosis (uterus) (internal) 617.0
Adenopathy (lymph gland) 785.6
  inguinal 785.6
  mediastinal 785.6
  mesentery 785.6
  syphilitic (secondary) 091.4
  tracheobronchial 785.6
    tuberculous (*see also* Tuberculosis) 012.1 ☑
      primary, progressive 010.8 ☑
  tuberculous (*see also* Tuberculosis, lymph gland) 017.2 ☑
    tracheobronchial 012.1 ☑
      primary, progressive 010.8 ☑
Adenopharyngitis 462
Adenophlegmon 683
Adenosalpingitis 614.1
Adenosarcoma (M8960/3) 189.0
Adenosclerosis 289.3
Adenosis
  breast (sclerosing) 610.2
  vagina, congenital 752.49
Adentia (complete) (partial) — *see also* Absence, teeth 520.0
Adherent
  labium (minus) 624.4
  pericardium (nonrheumatic) 423.1
    rheumatic 393
  placenta 667.0 ☑
    with hemorrhage 666.0 ☑

Adherent — *continued*
  prepuce 605
  scar (skin) NEC 709.2
  tendon in scar 709.2
Adhesion(s), adhesive (postinfectional) (postoperative)
  abdominal (wall) (*see also* Adhesions, peritoneum) 568.0
  amnion to fetus 658.8 ☑
    affecting fetus or newborn 762.8
  appendix 543.9
  arachnoiditis — *see* Meningitis
  auditory tube (Eustachian) 381.89
  bands (*see also* Adhesions, peritoneum)
    cervix 622.3
    uterus 621.5
  bile duct (any) 576.8
  bladder (sphincter) 596.8
  bowel (*see also* Adhesions, peritoneum) 568.0
  cardiac 423.1
    rheumatic 398.99
  cecum (*see also* Adhesions, peritoneum) 568.0
  cervicovaginal 622.3
    congenital 752.49
    postpartal 674.8 ☑
    old 622.3
  cervix 622.3
  clitoris 624.4
  colon (*see also* Adhesions, peritoneum) 568.0
  common duct 576.8
  congenital (*see also* Anomaly, specified type NEC)
    fingers (*see also* Syndactylism, fingers) 755.11
    labium (majus) (minus) 752.49
    omental, anomalous 751.4
    ovary 752.0
    peritoneal 751.4
    toes (*see also* Syndactylism, toes) 755.13
    tongue (to gum or roof of mouth) 750.12
  conjunctiva (acquired) (localized) 372.62
    congenital 743.63
    extensive 372.63
  cornea — *see* Opacity, cornea
  cystic duct 575.8
  diaphragm (*see also* Adhesions, peritoneum) 568.0
  due to foreign body — *see* Foreign body
  duodenum (*see also* Adhesions, peritoneum) 568.0
    with obstruction 537.3
  ear, middle — *see* Adhesions, middle ear
  epididymis 608.89
  epidural — *see* Adhesions, meninges
  epiglottis 478.79
  Eustachian tube 381.89
  eyelid 374.46
    postoperative 997.99
      surgically created V45.69
  gallbladder (*see also* Disease, gallbladder) 575.8
  globe 360.89
  heart 423.1
    rheumatic 398.99
  ileocecal (coil) (*see also* Adhesions, peritoneum) 568.0
  ileum (*see also* Adhesions, peritoneum) 568.0
  intestine (postoperative) (*see also* Adhesions, peritoneum) 568.0
    with obstruction 560.81
      with hernia (*see also* Hernia, by site, with obstruction)
        gangrenous — *see* Hernia, by site, with gangrene
  intra-abdominal (*see also* Adhesions, peritoneum) 568.0
  iris 364.70
    to corneal graft 996.79
  joint (*see also* Ankylosis) 718.5 ☑
  kidney 593.89
  labium (majus) (minus), congenital 752.49
  liver 572.8

☑ **Additional Digit Required** — Refer to the Tabular List for Digit Selection   ▽ **Subterms under main terms may continue to next column or page**

10 — Volume 2   ▶◀ Revised Text   ● New Line   ▲ Revised Code   **2011 ICD-9-CM**

Adhesion(s), adhesive — *continued*
  lung 511.0
  mediastinum 519.3
  meninges 349.2
    cerebral (any) 349.2
      congenital 742.4
    congenital 742.8
    spinal (any) 349.2
      congenital 742.59
    tuberculous (cerebral) (spinal) (*see also*
      Tuberculosis, meninges) 013.0 ☑
  mesenteric (*see also* Adhesions, peritoneum)
    568.0
  middle ear (fibrous) 385.10
    drum head 385.19
      to
        incus 385.11
        promontorium 385.13
        stapes 385.12
    specified NEC 385.19
  nasal (septum) (to turbinates) 478.19
  nerve NEC 355.9
    spinal 355.9
      root 724.9
        cervical NEC 723.4
        lumbar NEC 724.4
        lumbosacral 724.4
        thoracic 724.4
  ocular muscle 378.60
  omentum (*see also* Adhesions, peritoneum)
    568.0
  organ or site, congenital NEC — *see*
    Anomaly, specified type NEC
  ovary 614.6
    congenital (to cecum, kidney, or omen-
      tum) 752.0
  parauterine 614.6
  parovarian 614.6
  pelvic (peritoneal)
    female (postoperative) (postinfection)
      614.6
    male (postoperative) (postinfection) (*see*
      also Adhesions, peritoneum)
      568.0
    postpartal (old) 614.6
    tuberculous (*see also* Tuberculosis)
      016.9 ☑
  penis to scrotum (congenital) 752.69
  periappendiceal (*see also* Adhesions, peri-
    toneum) 568.0
  pericardium (nonrheumatic) 423.1
    rheumatic 393
    tuberculous (*see also* Tuberculosis)
      017.9 ☑ *[420.0]*
  pericholecystic 575.8
  perigastric (*see also* Adhesions, peritoneum)
    568.0
  periovarian 614.6
  periprostatic 602.8
  perirectal (*see also* Adhesions, peritoneum)
    568.0
  perirenal 593.89
  peritoneum, peritoneal (fibrous) (postoper-
    ative) 568.0
    with obstruction (intestinal) 560.81
      with hernia (*see also* Hernia, by site,
        with obstruction)
        gangrenous — *see* Hernia, by site,
          with gangrene
    duodenum 537.3
    congenital 751.4
    female (postoperative) (postinfective)
      614.6
    pelvic, female 614.6
    pelvic, male 568.0
    postpartal, pelvic 614.6
    to uterus 614.6
  peritubal 614.6
  periureteral 593.89
  periuterine 621.5
  perivesical 596.8
  perivesicular (seminal vesicle) 608.89
  pleura, pleuritic 511.0
    tuberculous (*see also* Tuberculosis,
      pleura) 012.0 ☑
  pleuropericardial 511.0

Adhesion(s), adhesive — *continued*
  postoperative (gastrointestinal tract) (*see*
    also Adhesions, peritoneum) 568.0
    eyelid 997.99
      surgically created V45.69
    pelvic female 614.9
    pelvic male 568.0
    urethra 598.2
  postpartal, old 624.4
  preputial, prepuce 605
  pulmonary 511.0
  pylorus (*see also* Adhesions, peritoneum)
    568.0
  Rosenmüller's fossa 478.29
  sciatic nerve 355.0
  seminal vesicle 608.89
  shoulder (joint) 726.0
  sigmoid flexure (*see also* Adhesions, peri-
    toneum) 568.0
  spermatic cord (acquired) 608.89
    congenital 752.89
  spinal canal 349.2
    nerve 355.9
      root 724.9
        cervical NEC 723.4
        lumbar NEC 724.4
        lumbosacral 724.4
        thoracic 724.4
  stomach (*see also* Adhesions, peritoneum)
    568.0
  subscapular 726.2
  tendonitis 726.90
    shoulder 726.0
  testicle 608.89
  tongue (congenital) (to gum or roof of
    mouth) 750.12
    acquired 529.8
  trachea 519.19
  tubo-ovarian 614.6
  tunica vaginalis 608.89
  ureter 593.89
  uterus 621.5
    to abdominal wall 614.6
      in pregnancy or childbirth 654.4 ☑
        affecting fetus or newborn 763.89
  vagina (chronic) (postoperative) (postradia-
    tion) 623.2
  vaginitis (congenital) 752.49
  vesical 596.8
  vitreous 379.29
Adie (-Holmes) syndrome (tonic pupillary reaction) 379.46
Adiponecrosis neonatorum 778.1
Adiposa dolorosa 272.8
Adiposalgia 272.8
Adiposis
  cerebralis 253.8
  dolorosa 272.8
  tuberosa simplex 272.8
Adiposity 278.02
  heart (*see also* Degeneration, myocardial)
    429.1
  localized 278.1
Adiposogenital dystrophy 253.8
Adjustment
  prosthesis or other device — *see* Fitting of
  reaction — *see* Reaction, adjustment
Administration, prophylactic
  antibiotics, ►long-term◄ V58.62   ▲
    short-term use — *omit code*   ●
  antitoxin, any V07.2
  antivenin V07.2
  chemotherapeutic agent NEC V07.39
  chemotherapy NEC V07.39
  diphtheria antitoxin V07.2
  fluoride V07.31
  gamma globulin V07.2
  immune sera (gamma globulin) V07.2
  passive immunization agent V07.2
  RhoGAM V07.2
Admission (encounter)
  as organ donor — *see* Donor
  by mistake V68.9
  for
    adequacy testing (for)
      hemodialysis V56.31

Admission — *continued*
  for — *continued*
    adequacy testing — *continued*
      peritoneal dialysis V56.32
    adjustment (of)
      artificial
        arm (complete) (partial) V52.0
        eye V52.2
        leg (complete) (partial) V52.1
      brain neuropacemaker V53.02
      breast
        implant V52.4
          exchange (different material)
            (different size) V52.4
        prosthesis V52.4
      cardiac device V53.39
        defibrillator, automatic im-
          plantable ►(with syn-
          chronous cardiac pacemak-
          er)◄ V53.32
        pacemaker V53.31
          carotid sinus V53.39
      catheter
        non-vascular V58.82
        vascular V58.81
      cerebral ventricle (communicating)
        shunt V53.01
      colostomy belt V55.3
      contact lenses V53.1
      cystostomy device V53.6
      dental prosthesis V52.3
      device, unspecified type V53.90
        abdominal V53.59
        cardiac V53.39
          defibrillator, automatic im-
            plantable ►(with syn-
            chronous cardiac pace-
            maker◄ V53.32
          pacemaker V53.31
        carotid sinus V53.39
        cerebral ventricle (communicat-
          ing) shunt V53.01
        gastrointestinal NEC V53.59
        insulin pump V53.91
        intestinal V53.50
        nervous system V53.09
        orthodontic V53.4
        other device V53.99
        prosthetic V52.9
          breast V52.4
          dental V52.3
          eye V52.2
          specified type NEC V52.8
        special senses V53.09
        substitution
          auditory V53.09
          nervous system V53.09
          visual V53.09
        urinary V53.6
      dialysis catheter
        extracorporeal V56.1
        peritoneal V56.2
      diaphragm (contraceptive) V25.02
      gastric lap band V53.51
      gastrointestinal appliance and device
        NEC V53.59
      growth rod V54.02
      hearing aid V53.2
      ileostomy device V55.2
      intestinal appliance and device
        V53.50
      neuropacemaker (brain) (peripheral
        nerve) (spinal cord) V53.02
      orthodontic device V53.4
      orthopedic (device) V53.7
        brace V53.7
        cast V53.7
        shoes V53.7
      pacemaker
        brain V53.02
        cardiac V53.31
        carotid sinus V53.39
        peripheral nerve V53.02
        spinal cord V53.02
      prosthesis V52.9
        arm (complete) (partial) V52.0

Admission — *continued*
  for — *continued*
    adjustment — *continued*
      prosthesis — *continued*
        breast V52.4
        dental V52.3
        eye V52.2
        leg (complete) (partial) V52.1
        specified type NEC V52.8
        spectacles V53.1
        wheelchair V53.8
    adoption referral or proceedings V68.89
    aftercare (*see also* Aftercare) V58.9
      cardiac pacemaker V53.31
      chemotherapy (oral) (intravenous)
        V58.11
      dialysis
        extracorporeal (renal) V56.0
        peritoneal V56.8
        renal V56.0
      fracture (*see also* Aftercare, fracture)
        V54.9
      medical V58.89
      organ transplant V58.44
      orthopedic V54.9
        specified care NEC V54.89
      pacemaker device
        brain V53.02
        cardiac V53.31
        carotid sinus V53.39
        nervous system V53.02
        spinal cord V53.02
      postoperative NEC V58.49
        wound closure, planned V58.41
      postpartum
        immediately after delivery V24.0
        routine follow-up V24.2
      postradiation V58.0
      radiation therapy V58.0
      removal of
        non-vascular catheter V58.82
        vascular catheter V58.81
      specified NEC V58.89
      surgical NEC V58.49
        wound closure, planned V58.41
    antineoplastic
      chemotherapy (oral) (intravenous)
        V58.11
      immunotherapy V58.12
    artificial insemination V26.1
    assisted reproductive fertility procedure
      cycle V26.81
    attention to artificial opening (of) V55.9
      artificial vagina V55.7
      colostomy V55.3
      cystostomy V55.5
      enterostomy V55.4
      gastrostomy V55.1
      ileostomy V55.2
      jejunostomy V55.4
      nephrostomy V55.6
      specified site NEC V55.8
        intestinal tract V55.4
        urinary tract V55.6
      tracheostomy V55.0
      ureterostomy V55.6
      urethrostomy V55.6
    battery replacement
      cardiac pacemaker V53.31
    blood typing V72.86
      Rh typing V72.86
    boarding V65.0
    breast
      augmentation or reduction V50.1
      implant exchange (different material)
        (different size) V52.4
      reconstruction following mastectomy
        V51.0
      removal
        prophylactic V50.41
        tissue expander without syn-
          chronous insertion of per-
          manent implant V52.4
    change of
      cardiac pacemaker (battery) V53.31
      carotid sinus pacemaker V53.39

☑ **Additional Digit Required** — Refer to the Tabular List for Digit Selection   ᵂ **Subterms under main terms may continue to next column or page**

2011 ICD-9-CM   ►◄ Revised Text   ● New Line   ▲ Revised Code   October 2010 · Volume 2 — 11

Index

Admission — Admission

Admission — *continued*
  for — *continued*
    change of — *continued*
      catheter in artificial opening — *see*
        Attention to, artificial, open-
        ing
      drains V58.49
      dressing
        wound V58.30
          nonsurgical V58.30
          surgical V58.31
      fixation device
        external V54.89
        internal V54.01
      Kirschner wire V54.89
      neuropacemaker device (brain) (pe-
        ripheral nerve) (spinal cord)
        V53.02
      nonsurgical wound dressing V58.30
      pacemaker device
        brain V53.02
        cardiac V53.31
        carotid sinus V53.39
        nervous system V53.02
      plaster cast V54.89
      splint, external V54.89
      Steinmann pin V54.89
      surgical wound dressing V58.31
      traction device V54.89
      wound packing V58.30
        nonsurgical V58.30
        surgical V58.31
    checkup only V70.0
    chemotherapy, (oral) (intravenous) anti-
      neoplastic V58.11
    circumcision, ritual or routine (in ab-
      sence of medical indication)
      V50.2
    clinical research investigation (control)
      (normal comparison) (participant)
      V70.7
    closure of artificial opening — *see* Atten-
      tion to, artificial, opening
    contraceptive
      counseling V25.09
        emergency V25.03
        postcoital V25.03
      management V25.9
        specified type NEC V25.8
    convalescence following V66.9
      chemotherapy V66.2
      psychotherapy V66.3
      radiotherapy V66.1
      surgery V66.0
      treatment (for) V66.5
        combined V66.6
        fracture V66.4
        mental disorder NEC V66.3
        specified condition NEC V66.5
    cosmetic surgery NEC V50.1
      breast reconstruction following
        mastectomy V51.0
      following healed injury or operation
        V51.8
    counseling (*see also* Counseling) V65.40
      without complaint or sickness V65.49
      contraceptive management V25.09
        emergency V25.03
        postcoital V25.03
      dietary V65.3
      exercise V65.41
      fertility preservation (prior to cancer
        therapy) (prior to surgical re-
        moval of gonads) V26.42
      for
        nonattending third party V65.19
        pediatric
          pre-adoption visit for adop-
            tive parent(s) V65.11
          pre-birth visit for expectant
            parent(s) V65.11
      victim of abuse
        child V61.21
        partner or spouse V61.11
      genetic V26.33
      gonorrhea V65.45

Admission — *continued*
  for — *continued*
    counseling (*see also* Counseling) — con-
      tinued
      HIV V65.44
      human immunodeficiency virus
        V65.44
      injury prevention V65.43
      insulin pump training V65.46
      natural family planning
        procreative V26.41
        to avoid pregnancy V25.04
      procreative management V26.49
        using natural family planning
        V26.41
      sexually transmitted disease NEC
        V65.45
        HIV V65.44
      specified reason NEC V65.49
      substance use and abuse V65.42
      syphilis V65.45
      victim of abuse
        child V61.21
        partner or spouse V61.11
    desensitization to allergens V07.1
    dialysis V56.0
      catheter
        fitting and adjustment
          extracorporeal V56.1
          peritoneal V56.2
        removal or replacement
          extracorporeal V56.1
          peritoneal V56.2
      extracorporeal (renal) V56.0
      peritoneal V56.8
      renal V56.0
    dietary surveillance and counseling
      V65.3
    drug monitoring, therapeutic V58.83
    ear piercing V50.3
    elective surgery V50.9
      breast
        augmentation or reduction V50.1
        reconstruction following mastec-
          tomy V51.0
        removal, prophylactic V50.41
      circumcision, ritual or routine (in ab-
        sence of medical indication)
        V50.2
      cosmetic NEC V50.1
        breast reconstruction following
          mastectomy V51.0
        following healed injury or opera-
          tion V51.8
      ear piercing V50.3
      face-lift V50.1
      hair transplant V50.0
      plastic
        breast reconstruction following
          mastectomy V51.0
        cosmetic NEC V50.1
        following healed injury or opera-
          tion V51.8
      prophylactic organ removal V50.49
        breast V50.41
        ovary V50.42
      repair of scarred tissue (following
        healed injury or operation)
        V51.8
      specified type NEC V50.8
    end-of-life care V66.7
    examination (*see also* Examination)
      V70.9
      administrative purpose NEC V70.3
      adoption V70.3
      allergy V72.7
      antibody response V72.61
      at health care facility V70.0
      athletic team V70.3
      camp V70.3
      cardiovascular, preoperative V72.81
      clinical research investigation (con-
        trol) (participant) V70.7
      dental V72.2
      developmental testing (child) (infant)
        V20.2

Admission — *continued*
  for — *continued*
    examination (*see also* Examination) —
      continued
      donor (potential) V70.8
      driver's license V70.3
      ear V72.19
      employment V70.5
      eye V72.0
      fertility preservation (prior to cancer
        therapy) (prior to surgical re-
        moval of gonads) V26.82
      follow-up (routine) — *see* Examina-
        tion, follow-up
      for admission to
        old age home V70.3
        school V70.3
      general V70.9
        specified reason NEC V70.8
      gynecological V72.31
      health supervision
        child (over 28 days old) V20.2
        infant (over 28 days old) V20.2
        newborn
          8 to 28 days old V20.32
          under 8 days old V20.31
      hearing V72.19
        following failed hearing screen-
          ing V72.11
      immigration V70.3
      infant
        8 to 28 days old V20.32
        over 28 days old, routine V20.2
        under 8 days old V20.31
      insurance certification V70.3
      laboratory V72.60
        ordered as part of a routine gen-
          eral medical examination
          V72.62
        pre-operative V72.63
        pre-procedural V72.63
        specified NEC V72.69
      marriage license V70.3
      medical (general) (*see also* Examina-
        tion, medical) V70.9
      medicolegal reasons V70.4
      naturalization V70.3
      pelvic (annual) (periodic) V72.31
      postpartum checkup V24.2
      pregnancy (possible) (unconfirmed)
        V72.40
        negative result V72.41
        positive result V72.42
      preoperative V72.84
        cardiovascular V72.81
        respiratory V72.82
        specified NEC V72.83
      preprocedural V72.84
        cardiovascular V72.81
        general physical V72.83
        respiratory V72.82
        specified NEC V72.83
      prior to chemotherapy V72.83
      prison V70.3
      psychiatric (general) V70.2
        requested by authority V70.1
      radiological NEC V72.5
      respiratory, preoperative V72.82
      school V70.3
      screening — *see* Screening
      skin hypersensitivity V72.7
      specified type NEC V72.85
      sport competition V70.3
      vision V72.0
      well baby and child care V20.2
    exercise therapy V57.1
    face-lift, cosmetic reason V50.1
    fertility preservation (prior to cancer
      therapy) (prior to surgical re-
      moval of gonads) V26.82
    fitting (of)
      artificial
        arm (complete) (partial) V52.0
        eye V52.2
        leg (complete) (partial) V52.1
      biliary drainage tube V58.82

Admission — *continued*
  for — *continued*
    fitting — *continued*
      brain neuropacemaker V53.02
      breast V52.4
        implant V52.4
        prosthesis V52.4
      cardiac pacemaker V53.31
      catheter
        non-vascular V58.82
        vascular V58.81
      cerebral ventricle (communicating)
        shunt V53.01
      chest tube V58.82
      colostomy belt V55.2
      contact lenses V53.1
      cystostomy device V53.6
      dental prosthesis V52.3
      device, unspecified type V53.90
        abdominal V53.59
        cerebral ventricle (communicat-
          ing) shunt V53.01
        gastrointestinal NEC V53.59
        insulin pump V53.91
        intestinal V53.50
        intrauterine contraceptive
          insertion V25.11   ●
          removal V25.12   ●
            and reinsertion V25.13 ●
          replacement V25.13   ●
        nervous system V53.09
        orthodontic V53.4
        other device V53.99
        prosthetic V52.9
          breast V52.4
          dental V52.3
          eye V52.2
        special senses V53.09
        substitution
          auditory V53.09
          nervous system V53.09
          visual V53.09
      diaphragm (contraceptive) V25.02
      fistula (sinus tract) drainage tube
        V58.82
      gastric lap band V53.51
      gastrointestinal appliance and device
        NEC V53.59
      growth rod V54.02
      hearing aid V53.2
      ileostomy device V55.2
      intestinal appliance and device
        V53.50
      intrauterine contraceptive device
        insertion V25.11   ●
        removal V25.12   ●
          and reinsertion V25.13 ●
        replacement V25.13   ●
      neuropacemaker (brain) (peripheral
        nerve) (spinal cord) V53.02
      orthodontic device V53.4
      orthopedic (device) V53.7
        brace V53.7
        cast V53.7
        shoes V53.7
      pacemaker
        brain V53.02
        cardiac V53.31
        carotid sinus V53.39
        spinal cord V53.02
      pleural drainage tube V58.82
      portacath V58.81
      prosthesis V52.9
        arm (complete) (partial) V52.0
        breast V52.4
        dental V52.3
        eye V52.2
        leg (complete) (partial) V52.1
        specified type NEC V52.8
      spectacles V53.1
      wheelchair V53.8
    follow-up examination (routine) (follow-
      ing) V67.9
      cancer chemotherapy V67.2
      chemotherapy V67.2
      high-risk medication NEC V67.51

☑ Additional Digit Required — Refer to the Tabular List for Digit Selection   𝖵𝖾𝖻 Subterms under main terms may continue to next column or page

Admission — *continued*
  for — *continued*
    follow-up examination — *continued*
      injury NEC V67.59
      psychiatric V67.3
      psychotherapy V67.3
      radiotherapy V67.1
      specified surgery NEC V67.09
      surgery V67.00
        vaginal pap smear V67.01
      treatment (for) V67.9
        combined V67.6
        fracture V67.4
        involving high-risk medication
          NEC V67.51
        mental disorder V67.3
        specified NEC V67.59
    hair transplant, for cosmetic reason
      V50.0
    health advice, education, or instruction
      V65.4 ☑
    hearing conservation and treatment
      V72.12
    hormone replacement therapy (post-
      menopausal) V07.4
    hospice care V66.7
    immunizations (childhood) appropriate
      for age V20.2
    immunotherapy, antineoplastic V58.12
    insertion (of)
      intrauterine contraceptive device ●
        V25.11   ●
      subdermal implantable contracep-
        tive V25.5
    insulin pump titration V53.91
    insulin pump training V65.46
    intrauterine device
      insertion V25.11   ▲
      management V25.42
      removal V25.12   ●
        and reinsertion V25.13   ●
      replacement V25.13   ●
    investigation to determine further dispo-
      sition V63.8
    in vitro fertilization cycle V26.81
    isolation V07.0
    issue of
      disability examination certificate
        V68.01
      medical certificate NEC V68.09
      repeat prescription NEC V68.1
        contraceptive device NEC V25.49
    kidney dialysis V56.0
    lengthening of growth rod V54.02
    mental health evaluation V70.2
      requested by authority V70.1
    natural family planning counseling and
      advice
      procreative V26.41
      to avoid pregnancy V25.04
    nonmedical reason NEC V68.89
    nursing care evaluation V63.8
    observation (without need for further
      medical care) (*see also* Observa-
      tion) V71.9
      accident V71.4
      alleged rape or seduction V71.5
      criminal assault V71.6
      following accident V71.4
        at work V71.3
      foreign body ingestion V71.89
      growth and development variations,
        childhood V21.0
      inflicted injury NEC V71.6
      ingestion of deleterious agent or
        foreign body V71.89
      injury V71.6
      malignant neoplasm V71.1
      mental disorder V71.09
      newborn — *see* Observation, suspect-
        ed, condition, newborn
      rape V71.5
      specified NEC V71.89
      suspected
        abuse V71.81
        accident V71.4

Admission — *continued*
  for — *continued*
    observation (*see also* Observation) —
      continued
      suspected — *continued*
        accident — *continued*
          at work V71.3
        benign neoplasm V71.89
        cardiovascular V71.7
        disorder V71.9
        exposure
          anthrax V71.82
          biological agent NEC V71.83
          SARS V71.83
        heart V71.7
        inflicted injury NEC V71.6
        malignant neoplasm V71.1
        maternal and fetal problem not
          found
          amniotic cavity and mem-
            brane V89.01
          cervical shortening V89.05
          fetal anomaly V89.03
          fetal growth V89.04
          oligohydramnios V89.01
          other specified NEC V89.09
          placenta V89.02
          polyhydramnios V89.01
        mental NEC V71.09
        neglect V71.81
        specified condition NEC V71.89
        tuberculosis V71.2
      tuberculosis V71.2
    occupational therapy V57.21
    organ transplant, donor — *see* Donor
    ovary, ovarian removal, prophylactic
      V50.42
    palliative care V66.7
    Papanicolaou smear
      cervix V76.2
        for suspected malignant neo-
          plasm V76.2
        no disease found V71.1
        routine, as part of gynecological
          examination V72.31
        to confirm findings of recent nor-
          mal smear following initial
          abnormal smear V72.32
      vaginal V76.47
        following hysterectomy for malig-
          nant condition V67.01
    passage of sounds or bougie in artificial
      opening — *see* Attention to, arti-
      ficial, opening
    paternity testing V70.4
    peritoneal dialysis V56.32
    physical therapy NEC V57.1
    plastic surgery
      breast reconstruction following
        mastectomy V51.0
      cosmetic NEC V50.1
      following healed injury or operation
        V51.8
    postmenopausal hormone replacement
      therapy V07.4
    postpartum observation
      immediately after delivery V24.0
      routine follow-up V24.2
    poststerilization (for restoration) V26.0
    procreative management V26.9
      assisted reproductive fertility proce-
        dure cycle V26.81
      in vitro fertilization cycle V26.81
      specified type NEC V26.89
    prophylactic
      administration of
        antibiotics, ▶long-term◀
          V58.62   ▲
          short-term use — *omit code* ●
        antitoxin, any V07.2
        antivenin V07.2
        chemotherapeutic agent NEC
          V07.39
        chemotherapy NEC V07.39
        diphtheria antitoxin V07.2
        fluoride V07.31

Admission — *continued*
  for — *continued*
    prophylactic — *continued*
      administration of — *continued*
        gamma globulin V07.2
        immune sera (gamma globulin)
          V07.2
        RhoGAM V07.2
        tetanus antitoxin V07.2
      breathing exercises V57.0
      chemotherapy NEC V07.39
        fluoride V07.31
      measure V07.9
        specified type NEC V07.8
      organ removal V50.49
        breast V50.41
        ovary V50.42
    psychiatric examination (general) V70.2
      requested by authority V70.1
    radiation management V58.0
    radiotherapy V58.0
    reconstruction following mastectomy
      V51.0
    reforming of artificial opening — *see*
      Attention to, artificial, opening
    rehabilitation V57.9
      multiple types V57.89
      occupational V57.21
      orthoptic V57.4
      orthotic V57.81
      physical NEC V57.1
      specified type NEC V57.89
      speech (-language) V57.3
      vocational V57.22
    removal of
      breast tissue expander without syn-
        chronous insertion of perma-
        nent implant V52.4
      cardiac pacemaker V53.31
      cast (plaster) V54.89
      catheter from artificial opening —
        see Attention to, artificial,
        opening
      cerebral ventricle (communicating)
        shunt V53.01
      cystostomy catheter V55.5
      device
        cerebral ventricle (communicat-
          ing) shunt V53.01
        fixation
          external V54.89
          internal V54.01
        intrauterine contraceptive
          V25.12   ▲
        traction, external V54.89
      drains V58.49
      dressing
        wound V58.30
          nonsurgical V58.30
          surgical V58.31
      fixation device
        external V54.89
        internal V54.01
      intrauterine contraceptive device
        V25.12   ▲
      Kirschner wire V54.89
      neuropacemaker (brain) (peripheral
        nerve) (spinal cord) V53.02
      nonsurgical wound dressing V58.30
      orthopedic fixation device
        external V54.89
        internal V54.01
      pacemaker device
        brain V53.02
        cardiac V53.31
        carotid sinus V53.39
        nervous system V53.02
      plaster cast V54.89
      plate (fracture) V54.01
      rod V54.01
      screw (fracture) V54.01
      splint, traction V54.89
      staples V58.32
      Steinmann pin V54.89
      subdermal implantable contracep-
        tive V25.43

Admission — *continued*
  for — *continued*
    removal of — *continued*
      surgical wound dressing V58.31
      sutures V58.32
      traction device, external V54.89
      ureteral stent V53.6
      wound packing V58.30
        nonsurgical V58.30
        surgical V58.31
    repair of scarred tissue (following healed
      injury or operation) V51.8
    replacement of intrauterine contracep- ●
      tive device V25.13   ●
    reprogramming of cardiac pacemaker
      V53.31
    respirator [ventilator] dependence
      during
        mechanical failure V46.14
        power failure V46.12
      for weaning V46.13
    restoration of organ continuity (postster-
      ilization) (tuboplasty) (vasoplasty)
      V26.0
    Rh typing V72.86
    routine infant and child vision and
      hearing testing V20.2
    sensitivity test (*see also* Test, skin)
      allergy NEC V72.7
      bacterial disease NEC V74.9
      Dick V74.8
      Kveim V82.89
      Mantoux V74.1
      mycotic infection NEC V75.4
      parasitic disease NEC V75.8
      Schick V74.3
      Schultz-Charlton V74.8
    social service (agency) referral or evalua-
      tion V63.8
    speech (-language) therapy V57.3
    sterilization V25.2
    suspected disorder (ruled out) (without
      need for further care) — *see* Ob-
      servation
    terminal care V66.7
    tests only — *see* Test
    therapeutic drug monitoring V58.83
    therapy
      blood transfusion, without reported
        diagnosis V58.2
      breathing exercises V57.0
      chemotherapy, antineoplastic V58.11
        prophylactic NEC V07.39
          fluoride V07.31
      dialysis (intermittent) (treatment)
        extracorporeal V56.0
        peritoneal V56.8
        renal V56.0
        specified type NEC V56.8
      exercise (remedial) NEC V57.1
        breathing V57.0
      immunotherapy, antineoplastic
        V58.12
      long-term (current) ▶(prophylac-
        tic)◀ drug use NEC V58.69
        antibiotics V58.62
          short-term use — *omit code* ●
        anticoagulants V58.61
        anti-inflammatories, non-
          steroidal (NSAID) V58.64
        antiplatelets V58.63
        antithrombotics V58.63
        aspirin V58.66
        high-risk medications NEC V58.69
        insulin V58.67
        methadone V58.69
        opiate analgesic V58.69
        steroids V58.65
      occupational V57.21
      orthoptic V57.4
      physical NEC V57.1
      radiation V58.0
      speech (-language) V57.3
      vocational V57.22

Index

Admission — Aftercare

Admission — *continued*
for — *continued*
toilet or cleaning
of artificial opening — *see* Attention to, artificial, opening
of non-vascular catheter V58.82
of vascular catheter V58.81
treatment ●
measure V07.9 ●
specified type NEC V07.8 ●
tubal ligation V25.2
tuboplasty for previous sterilization V26.0
ultrasound, routine fetal V28.3
vaccination, prophylactic (against)
arthropod-borne virus, viral NEC V05.1
disease NEC V05.1
encephalitis V05.0
Bacille Calmette Guérin (BCG) V03.2
BCG V03.2
chickenpox V05.4
cholera alone V03.0
with typhoid-paratyphoid (cholera + TAB) V06.0
common cold V04.7
dengue V05.1
diphtheria alone V03.5
diphtheria-tetanus-pertussis (DTP) (DTaP) V06.1
with
poliomyelitis (DTP + polio) V06.3
typhoid-paratyphoid (DTP + TAB) V06.2
diphtheria-tetanus [Td] [DT] without pertussis V06.5
disease (single) NEC V05.9
bacterial NEC V03.9
specified type NEC V03.89
combinations NEC V06.9
specified type NEC V06.8
specified type NEC V05.8
viral NEC V04.89
encephalitis, viral, arthropod-borne V05.0
Hemophilus influenzae, type B [Hib] V03.81
hepatitis, viral V05.3
human papillomavirus (HPV) V04.89
immune sera (gamma globulin) V07.2
influenza V04.81
with
Streptococcus pneumoniae [pneumococcus] V06.6
Leishmaniasis V05.2
measles alone V04.2
measles-mumps-rubella (MMR) V06.4
mumps alone V04.6
with measles and rubella (MMR) V06.4
not done because of contraindication V64.09
pertussis alone V03.6
plague V03.3
pneumonia V03.82
poliomyelitis V04.0
with diphtheria-tetanus-pertussis (DTP+ polio) V06.3
rabies V04.5
respiratory syncytial virus (RSV) V04.82
rubella alone V04.3
with measles and mumps (MMR) V06.4
smallpox V04.1
specified type NEC V05.8
Streptococcus pneumoniae [pneumococcus] V03.82
with
influenza V06.6
tetanus toxoid alone V03.7
with diphtheria [Td] [DT] V06.5
and pertussis (DTP) (DTaP) V06.1

Admission — *continued*
for — *continued*
vaccination, prophylactic — *continued*
tuberculosis (BCG) V03.2
tularemia V03.4
typhoid alone V03.1
with diphtheria-tetanus-pertussis (TAB + DTP) V06.2
typhoid-paratyphoid alone (TAB) V03.1
typhus V05.8
varicella (chicken pox) V05.4
viral encephalitis, arthropod-borne V05.0
viral hepatitis V05.3
yellow fever V04.4
vasectomy V25.2
vasoplasty for previous sterilization V26.0
vision examination V72.0
vocational therapy V57.22
waiting period for admission to other facility V63.2
undergoing social agency investigation V63.8
well baby and child care V20.2
x-ray of chest
for suspected tuberculosis V71.2
routine V72.5
Adnexitis (suppurative) — *see also* Salpingo-oophoritis 614.2
Adolescence NEC V21.2
Adoption
agency referral V68.89
examination V70.3
held for V68.89
Adrenal gland — *see* condition
Adrenalism 255.9
tuberculous (*see also* Tuberculosis) 017.6 ☑
Adrenalitis, adrenitis 255.8
meningococcal hemorrhagic 036.3
Adrenarche, precocious 259.1
Adrenocortical syndrome 255.2
Adrenogenital syndrome (acquired) (congenital) 255.2
iatrogenic, fetus or newborn 760.79
Adrenoleukodystrophy 277.86
neonatal 277.86
x-linked 277.86
Adrenomyeloneuropathy 277.86
Adventitious bursa — *see* Bursitis
Adynamia (episodica) (hereditary) (periodic) 359.3
Adynamic
ileus or intestine (*see also* Ileus) 560.1
ureter 753.22
Aeration lung, imperfect, newborn 770.5
Aerobullosis 993.3
Aerocele — *see* Embolism, air
Aerodermectasia
subcutaneous (traumatic) 958.7
surgical 998.81
surgical 998.81
Aerodontalgia 993.2
Aeroembolism 993.3
Aerogenes capsulatus infection — *see also* Gangrene, gas 040.0
Aero-otitis media 993.0
Aerophagy, aerophagia 306.4
psychogenic 306.4
Aerosinusitis 993.1
Aerotitis 993.0
Affection, affections — *see also* Disease
sacroiliac (joint), old 724.6
shoulder region NEC 726.2
Afibrinogenemia 286.3
acquired 286.6
congenital 286.3
postpartum 666.3 ☑
African
sleeping sickness 086.5
tick fever 087.1
trypanosomiasis 086.5
Gambian 086.3
Rhodesian 086.4

Aftercare V58.9
amputation stump V54.89
artificial openings — *see* Attention to, artificial, opening
blood transfusion without reported diagnosis V58.2
breathing exercise V57.0
cardiac device V53.39
defibrillator, automatic implantable
▶(with synchronous cardiac pacemaker)◀ V53.32
pacemaker V53.31
carotid sinus V53.39
carotid sinus pacemaker V53.39
cerebral ventricle (communicating) shunt V53.01
chemotherapy (oral) (intravenous) session (adjunctive) (maintenance) V58.11
defibrillator, automatic implantable cardiac
▶(with synchronous cardiac pacemaker)◀ V53.32
exercise (remedial) (therapeutic) V57.1
breathing V57.0
extracorporeal dialysis (intermittent) (treatment) V56.0
following surgery NEC V58.49
for
injury V58.43
neoplasm V58.42
organ transplant V58.44
trauma V58.43
joint replacement V54.81
of
circulatory system V58.73
digestive system V58.75
genital organs V58.76
genitourinary system V58.76
musculoskeletal system V58.78
nervous system V58.72
oral cavity V58.75
respiratory system V58.74
sense organs V58.71
skin V58.77
subcutaneous tissue V58.77
teeth V58.75
urinary system V58.76
spinal — *see* Aftercare, following surgery, of, specified body system
wound closure, planned V58.41
fracture V54.9
healing V54.89
pathologic
ankle V54.29
arm V54.20
lower V54.22
upper V54.21
finger V54.29
foot V54.29
hand V54.29
hip V54.23
leg V54.24
lower V54.26
upper V54.25
pelvis V54.29
specified site NEC V54.29
toe(s) V54.29
vertebrae V54.27
wrist V54.29
traumatic
ankle V54.19
arm V54.10
lower V54.12
upper V54.11
finger V54.19
foot V54.19
hand V54.19
hip V54.13
leg V54.14
lower V54.16
upper V54.15
pelvis V54.19
specified site NEC V54.19
toe(s) V54.19
vertebrae V54.17
wrist V54.19

Aftercare — *continued*
fracture — *continued*
removal of
external fixation device V54.89
internal fixation device V54.01
specified care NEC V54.89
gait training V57.1
for use of artificial limb(s) V57.81
internal fixation device V54.09
involving
dialysis (intermittent) (treatment)
extracorporeal V56.0
peritoneal V56.8
renal V56.0
gait training V57.1
for use of artificial limb(s) V57.81
growth rod
adjustment V54.02
lengthening V54.02
internal fixation device V54.09
orthoptic training V57.4
orthotic training V57.81
radiotherapy session V58.0
removal of
drains V58.49
dressings
wound V58.30
nonsurgical V58.30
surgical V58.31
fixation device
external V54.89
internal V54.01
fracture plate V54.01
nonsurgical wound dressing V58.30
pins V54.01
plaster cast V54.89
rods V54.01
screws V58.32
staples V58.32
surgical wound dressings V58.31
sutures V58.32
traction device, external V54.89
wound packing V58.30
nonsurgical V58.30
surgical V58.31
neuropacemaker (brain) (peripheral nerve) (spinal cord) V53.02
occupational therapy V57.21
orthodontic V58.5
orthopedic V54.9
change of external fixation or traction device V54.89
following joint replacement V54.81
internal fixation device V54.09
removal of fixation device
external V54.89
internal V54.01
specified care NEC V54.89
orthoptic training V57.4
orthotic training V57.81
pacemaker
brain V53.02
cardiac V53.31
carotid sinus V53.39
peripheral nerve V53.02
spinal cord V53.02
peritoneal dialysis (intermittent) (treatment) V56.8
physical therapy NEC V57.1
breathing exercises V57.0
radiotherapy session V58.0
rehabilitation procedure V57.9
breathing exercises V57.0
multiple types V57.89
occupational V57.21
orthoptic V57.4
orthotic V57.81
physical therapy NEC V57.1
remedial exercises V57.1
specified type NEC V57.89
speech (-language) V57.3
therapeutic exercises V57.1
vocational V57.22
renal dialysis (intermittent) (treatment) V56.0
specified type NEC V58.89

Aftercare — *continued*
  specified type — *continued*
    removal of non-vascular catheter V58.82
    removal of vascular catheter V58.81
  speech (-language) therapy V57.3
  stump, amputation V54.89
  vocational rehabilitation V57.22
After-cataract 366.50
  obscuring vision 366.53
  specified type, not obscuring vision 366.52
Agalactia 676.4 ☑
Agammaglobulinemia 279.00
  with lymphopenia 279.2
  acquired (primary) (secondary) 279.06
  Bruton's X-linked 279.04
  infantile sex-linked (Bruton's) (congenital) 279.04
  Swiss-type 279.2
Aganglionosis (bowel) (colon) 751.3
Age (old) — *see also* Senile 797
Agenesis — *see also* Absence, by site, congenital
  acoustic nerve 742.8
  adrenal (gland) 759.1
  alimentary tract (complete) (partial) NEC 751.8
    lower 751.2
    upper 750.8
  anus, anal (canal) 751.2
  aorta 747.22
  appendix 751.2
  arm (complete) (partial) (*see also* Deformity, reduction, upper limb) 755.20
  artery (peripheral) NEC (*see also* Anomaly, peripheral vascular system) 747.60
    brain 747.81
    coronary 746.85
    pulmonary 747.3
    umbilical 747.5
  auditory (canal) (external) 744.01
  auricle (ear) 744.01
  bile, biliary duct or passage 751.61
  bone NEC 756.9
  brain 740.0
    specified part 742.2
  breast 757.6
  bronchus 748.3
  canaliculus lacrimalis 743.65
  carpus NEC (*see also* Deformity, reduction, upper limb) 755.28
  cartilage 756.9
  cecum 751.2
  cerebellum 742.2
  cervix 752.43   ▲
  chin 744.89
  cilia 743.63
  circulatory system, part NEC 747.89
  clavicle 755.51
  clitoris 752.49
  coccyx 756.13
  colon 751.2
  corpus callosum 742.2
  cricoid cartilage 748.3
  diaphragm (with hernia) 756.6
  digestive organ(s) or tract (complete) (partial) NEC 751.8
    lower 751.2
    upper 750.8
  ductus arteriosus 747.89
  duodenum 751.1
  ear NEC 744.09
    auricle 744.01
    lobe 744.21
  ejaculatory duct 752.89
  endocrine (gland) NEC 759.2
  epiglottis 748.3
  esophagus 750.3
  Eustachian tube 744.24
  extrinsic muscle, eye 743.69
  eye 743.00
    adnexa 743.69
  eyelid (fold) 743.62
  face
    bones NEC 756.0
    specified part NEC 744.89
  fallopian tube 752.19

Agenesis — *see also* Absence, by site, congenital — *continued*
  femur NEC (*see also* Absence, femur, congenital) 755.34
  fibula NEC (*see also* Absence, fibula, congenital) 755.37
  finger NEC (*see also* Absence, finger, congenital) 755.29
  foot (complete) (*see also* Deformity, reduction, lower limb) 755.31
  gallbladder 751.69
  gastric 750.8
  genitalia, genital (organ)
    female 752.89
      external 752.49
      internal NEC 752.89
    male 752.89
      penis 752.69
  glottis 748.3
  gonadal 758.6
  hair 757.4
  hand (complete) (*see also* Deformity, reduction, upper limb) 755.21
  heart 746.89
    valve NEC 746.89
      aortic 746.89
      mitral 746.89
      pulmonary 746.01
  hepatic 751.69
  humerus NEC (*see also* Absence, humerus, congenital) 755.24
  hymen 752.49
  ileum 751.1
  incus 744.04
  intestine (small) 751.1
    large 751.2
  iris (dilator fibers) 743.45
  jaw 524.09
  jejunum 751.1
  kidney(s) (partial) (unilateral) 753.0
  labium (majus) (minus) 752.49
  labyrinth, membranous 744.05
  lacrimal apparatus (congenital) 743.65
  larynx 748.3
  leg NEC (*see also* Deformity, reduction, lower limb) 755.30
  lens 743.35
  limb (complete) (partial) (*see also* Deformity, reduction) 755.4
    lower NEC 755.30
    upper 755.20
  lip 750.26
  liver 751.69
  lung (bilateral) (fissures) (lobe) (unilateral) 748.5
  mandible 524.09
  maxilla 524.09
  metacarpus NEC 755.28
  metatarsus NEC 755.38
  muscle (any) 756.81
  musculoskeletal system NEC 756.9
  nail(s) 757.5
  neck, part 744.89
  nerve 742.8
  nervous system, part NEC 742.8
  nipple 757.6
  nose 748.1
  nuclear 742.8
  organ
    of Corti 744.05
    or site not listed — *see* Anomaly, specified type NEC
  osseous meatus (ear) 744.03
  ovary 752.0
  oviduct 752.19
  pancreas 751.7
  parathyroid (gland) 759.2
  patella 755.64
  pelvic girdle (complete) (partial) 755.69
  penis 752.69
  pericardium 746.89
  perineal body 756.81
  pituitary (gland) 759.2
  prostate 752.89
  pulmonary
    artery 747.3

Agenesis — *see also* Absence, by site, congenital — *continued*
  pulmonary — *continued*
    trunk 747.3
    vein 747.49
  punctum lacrimale 743.65
  radioulnar NEC (*see also* Absence, forearm, congenital) 755.25
  radius NEC (*see also* Absence, radius, congenital) 755.26
  rectum 751.2
  renal 753.0
  respiratory organ NEC 748.9
  rib 756.3
  roof of orbit 742.0
  round ligament 752.89
  sacrum 756.13
  salivary gland 750.21
  scapula 755.59
  scrotum 752.89
  seminal duct or tract 752.89
  septum
    atrial 745.69
    between aorta and pulmonary artery 745.0
    ventricular 745.3
  shoulder girdle (complete) (partial) 755.59
  skull (bone) 756.0
    with
      anencephalus 740.0
      encephalocele 742.0
      hydrocephalus 742.3
        with spina bifida (*see also* Spina bifida) 741.0 ☑
      microcephalus 742.1
  spermatic cord 752.89
  spinal cord 742.59
  spine 756.13
    lumbar 756.13
      isthmus 756.11
      pars articularis 756.11
  spleen 759.0
  sternum 756.3
  stomach 750.7
  tarsus NEC 755.38
  tendon 756.81
  testicular 752.89
  testis 752.89
  thymus (gland) 759.2
  thyroid (gland) 243
    cartilage 748.3
  tibia NEC (*see also* Absence, tibia, congenital) 755.36
  tibiofibular NEC 755.35
  toe (complete) (partial) (*see also* Absence, toe, congenital) 755.39
  tongue 750.11
  trachea (cartilage) 748.3
  ulna NEC (*see also* Absence, ulna, congenital) 755.27
  ureter 753.4
  urethra 753.8
  urinary tract NEC 753.8
  uterus 752.31   ▲
  uvula 750.26
  vagina ▶(total)◀ (partial) 752.45   ▲
  vas deferens 752.89
  vein(s) (peripheral) NEC (*see also* Anomaly, peripheral vascular system) 747.60
    brain 747.81
    great 747.49
    portal 747.49
    pulmonary 747.49
  vena cava (inferior) (superior) 747.49
  vermis of cerebellum 742.2
  vertebra 756.13
    lumbar 756.13
      isthmus 756.11
      pars articularis 756.11
  vulva 752.49
Ageusia — *see also* Disturbance, sensation 781.1
Aggressiveness 301.3
Aggressive outburst — *see also* Disturbance, conduct 312.0 ☑
  in children or adolescents 313.9

Aging skin 701.8
Agitated — *see* condition
Agitation 307.9
  catatonic (*see also* Schizophrenia) 295.2 ☑
Aglossia (congenital) 750.11
Aglycogenosis 271.0
Agnail (finger) (with lymphangitis) 681.02
Agnosia (body image) (tactile) 784.69
  verbal 784.69
    auditory 784.69
      secondary to organic lesion 784.69
    developmental 315.8
    secondary to organic lesion 784.69
  visual 368.16
    object 368.16
Agoraphobia 300.22
  with panic disorder 300.21
Agrammatism 784.69
Agranulocytopenia — *see also* Agranulocytosis 288.09
Agranulocytosis — *see also* Neutropenia 288.09
  chronic 288.09
  cyclical 288.02
  due to infection 288.04
  genetic 288.01
  infantile 288.01
  periodic 288.02
  pernicious 288.09
Agraphia (absolute) 784.69
  with alexia 784.61
  developmental 315.39
Agrypnia — *see also* Insomnia 780.52
Ague — *see also* Malaria 084.6
  brass-founders' 985.8
  dumb 084.6
  tertian 084.1
Agyria 742.2
AHTR (acute hemolytic transfusion reaction) ●
  — *see* Complications, transfusion   ●
Ahumada-del Castillo syndrome (nonpuerperal galactorrhea and amenorrhea) 253.1
AIDS 042
AIDS-associated retrovirus (disease) (illness) 042
  infection — *see* Human immunodeficiency virus, infection
AIDS-associated virus (disease) (illness) 042
  infection — *see* Human immunodeficiency virus, infection
AIDS-like disease (illness) (syndrome) 042
AIDS-related complex 042
AIDS-related conditions 042
AIDS-related virus (disease) (illness) 042
  infection — *see* Human immunodeficiency virus, infection
AIDS virus (disease) (illness) 042
  infection — *see* Human immunodeficiency virus, infection
Ailment, heart — *see* Disease, heart
Ailurophobia 300.29
Ainhum (disease) 136.0
AIN I (anal intraepithelial neoplasia I) (histologically confirmed) 569.44
AIN II (anal intraepithelial neoplasia II) (histologically confirmed) 569.44
AIN III (anal intraepithelial neoplasia III) 230.6
  anal canal 230.5
AIPHI (acute idiopathic pulmonary hemorrhage in infants) (over 28 days old) ● ● ● 786.31
Air
  anterior mediastinum 518.1
  compressed, disease 993.3
  embolism (any site) (artery) (cerebral) 958.0
    with
      abortion — *see* Abortion, by type, with embolism
      ectopic pregnancy (*see also* categories 633.0–633.9) 639.6
      molar pregnancy (*see also* categories 630–632) 639.6

☑ **Additional Digit Required — Refer to the Tabular List for Digit Selection**   ▽ **Subterms under main terms may continue to next column or page**

2011 ICD-9-CM   ▶◀ Revised Text   ● New Line   ▲ Revised Code   October 2010 · Volume 2 — 15

Index

Air — Allocheiria, allochiria

Air — *continued*
  embolism — *continued*
    due to implanted device — *see* Complications, due to (presence of) any device, implant, or graft classified to 996.0–996.5 NEC
    following
      abortion 639.6
      ectopic or molar pregnancy 639.6
      infusion, perfusion, or transfusion 999.1
    in pregnancy, childbirth, or puerperium 673.0 ☑
    traumatic 958.0
  hunger 786.09
    psychogenic 306.1
  leak (lung) (pulmonary) (thorax) 512.8
    iatrogenic 512.1
    postoperative 512.1
  rarefied, effects of — *see* Effect, adverse, high altitude
  sickness 994.6
Airplane sickness 994.6
Akathisia, acathisia 781.0
  due to drugs 333.99
  neuroleptic-induced acute 333.99
Akinesia algeria 352.6
Akiyami 100.89
Akureyri disease (epidemic neuromyasthenia) 049.8
Alacrima (congenital) 743.65
Alactasia (hereditary) 271.3
Alagille syndrome 759.89
Alalia 784.3
  developmental 315.31
    receptive-expressive 315.32
  secondary to organic lesion 784.3
Alaninemia 270.8
Alastrim 050.1
Albarrán's disease (colibacilluria) 791.9
Albers-Schönberg's disease (marble bones) 756.52
Albert's disease 726.71
Albinism, albino (choroid) (cutaneous) (eye) (generalized) (isolated) (ocular) (oculocutaneous) (partial) 270.2
Albinismus 270.2
Albright (-Martin) (-Bantam) disease (pseudohypoparathyroidism) 275.49
Albright (-McCune) (-Sternberg) syndrome (osteitis fibrosa disseminata) 756.59
Albuminous — *see* condition
Albuminuria, albuminuric (acute) (chronic) (subacute) 791.0
  Bence-Jones 791.0
  cardiac 785.9
  complicating pregnancy, childbirth, or puerperium 646.2 ☑
    with hypertension — *see* Toxemia, of pregnancy
    affecting fetus or newborn 760.1
  cyclic 593.6
  gestational 646.2 ☑
  gravidarum 646.2 ☑
    with hypertension — *see* Toxemia, of pregnancy
    affecting fetus or newborn 760.1
  heart 785.9
  idiopathic 593.6
  orthostatic 593.6
  postural 593.6
  pre-eclamptic (mild) 642.4 ☑
    affecting fetus or newborn 760.0
    severe 642.5 ☑
      affecting fetus or newborn 760.0
  recurrent physiologic 593.6
  scarlatinal 034.1
Albumosuria 791.0
  Bence-Jones 791.0
  myelopathic (M9730/3) 203.0 ☑
Alcaptonuria 270.2
Alcohol, alcoholic
  abstinence 291.81
  acute intoxication 305.0 ☑
    with dependence 303.0 ☑
  addiction (*see also* Alcoholism) 303.9 ☑

Alcohol, alcoholic — *continued*
  addiction (*see also* Alcoholism) — *continued*
    maternal
      with suspected fetal damage affecting management of pregnancy 655.4 ☑
      affecting fetus or newborn 760.71
  amnestic disorder, persisting 291.1
  anxiety 291.89
  brain syndrome, chronic 291.2
  cardiopathy 425.5
  chronic (*see also* Alcoholism) 303.9 ☑
  cirrhosis (liver) 571.2
  delirium 291.0
    acute 291.0
    chronic 291.1
    tremens 291.0
    withdrawal 291.0
  dementia NEC 291.2
  deterioration 291.2
  drunkenness (simple) 305.0 ☑
  hallucinosis (acute) 291.3
  induced
    circadian rhythm sleep disorder 291.82
    hypersomnia 291.82
    insomnia 291.82
    mental disorder 291.9
      anxiety 291.89
      mood 291.89
      sexual 291.89
      sleep 291.82
      specified type 291.89
    parasomnia 291.82
    persisting
      amnestic disorder 291.1
      dementia 291.2
    psychotic disorder
      with
        delusions 291.5
        hallucinations 291.3
    sleep disorder 291.82
  insanity 291.9
  intoxication (acute) 305.0 ☑
    with dependence 303.0 ☑
    pathological 291.4
  jealousy 291.5
  Korsakoff's, Korsakov's, Korsakow's 291.1
  liver NEC 571.3
    acute 571.1
    chronic 571.2
  mania (acute) (chronic) 291.9
  mood 291.89
  paranoia 291.5
  paranoid (type) psychosis 291.5
  pellagra 265.2
  poisoning, accidental (acute) NEC 980.9
    specified type of alcohol — *see* Table of Drugs and Chemicals
  psychosis (*see also* Psychosis, alcoholic) 291.9
    Korsakoff's, Korsakov's, Korsakow's 291.1
    polyneuritic 291.1
    with
      delusions 291.5
      hallucinations 291.3
  related disorder 291.9
  withdrawal symptoms, syndrome NEC 291.81
    delirium 291.0
    hallucinosis 291.3
Alcoholism 303.9 ☑

> **Note** — Use the following fifth-digit subclassification with category 303:
>
> 0   unspecified
>
> 1   continuous
>
> 2   episodic
>
> 3   in remission

  with psychosis (*see also* Psychosis, alcoholic) 291.9
  acute 303.0 ☑
  chronic 303.9 ☑
    with psychosis 291.9

Alcoholism — *continued*
  complicating pregnancy, childbirth, or puerperium 648.4 ☑
    affecting fetus or newborn 760.71
  history V11.3
  Korsakoff's, Korsakov's, Korsakow's 291.1
  suspected damage to fetus affecting management of pregnancy 655.4 ☑
Alder's anomaly or syndrome (leukocyte granulation anomaly) 288.2
Alder-Reilly anomaly (leukocyte granulation) 288.2
Aldosteronism (primary) 255.10
  congenital 255.10
  familial type I 255.11
  glucocorticoid-remediable 255.11
  secondary 255.14
Aldosteronoma (M8370/1) 237.2
Aldrich (-Wiskott) syndrome (eczema-thrombocytopenia) 279.12
Aleppo boil 085.1
Aleukemic — *see* condition
Aleukia
  congenital 288.09
  hemorrhagica 284.9
    acquired (secondary) 284.89
    congenital 284.09
    idiopathic 284.9
  splenica 289.4
Alexia (congenital) (developmental) 315.01
  secondary to organic lesion 784.61
Algoneurodystrophy 733.7
Algophobia 300.29
Alibert-Bazin disease (M9700/3) 202.1 ☑
Alibert's disease (mycosis fungoides) (M9700/3) 202.1 ☑
Alice in Wonderland syndrome 293.89
Alienation, mental — *see also* Psychosis 298.9
Alkalemia 276.3
Alkalosis 276.3
  metabolic 276.3
    with respiratory acidosis 276.4
  respiratory 276.3
Alkaptonuria 270.2
Alkalosis 276.3
Allen-Masters syndrome 620.6
Allergic bronchopulmonary aspergillosis 518.6
Allergy, allergic (reaction) 995.3
  air-borne substance — *see also* Fever, hay 477.9
    specified allergen NEC 477.8
  alveolitis (extrinsic) 495.9
    due to
      Aspergillus clavatus 495.4
      cryptostroma corticale 495.6
      organisms (fungal, thermophilic actinomycete, other) growing in ventilation (air conditioning systems) 495.7
    specified type NEC 495.8
  anaphylactic shock 995.0   ▲
    due to food — *see* Anaphylactic shock, due to, food
  angioneurotic edema 995.1
  animal (cat) (dog) (epidermal) 477.8
    dander 477.2
    hair 477.2
  arthritis (*see also* Arthritis, allergic) 716.2 ☑
  asthma — *see* Asthma
  bee sting (anaphylactic shock) 989.5
  biological — *see* Allergy, drug
  bronchial asthma — *see* Asthma
  conjunctivitis (eczematous) 372.14
  dander, animal (cat) (dog) 477.2
  dandruff 477.8
  dermatitis (venenata) — *see* Dermatitis
  diathesis V15.09
  drug, medicinal substance, and biological (any) (correct medicinal substance properly administered) (external) (internal) 995.27
    wrong substance given or taken NEC 977.9
      specified drug or substance — *see* Table of Drugs and Chemicals
  dust (house) (stock) 477.8

Allergy, allergic — *continued*
  eczema — *see* Eczema
  endophthalmitis 360.19
  epidermal (animal) 477.8
  existing dental restorative material 525.66
  feathers 477.8
  food (any) (ingested) 693.1
    atopic 691.8
    in contact with skin 692.5
  gastritis 535.4 ☑
  gastroenteritis 558.3
  gastrointestinal 558.3
  grain 477.0
  grass (pollen) 477.0
    asthma (*see also* Asthma) 493.0 ☑
    hay fever 477.0
  hair, animal (cat) (dog) 477.2
  hay fever (grass) (pollen) (ragweed) (tree) (*see also* Fever, hay) 477.9
  history (of) V15.09
    to
      arachnid bite V15.06
      eggs V15.03
      food additives V15.05
      insect bite V15.06
      latex V15.07
      milk products V15.02
      nuts V15.05
        peanuts V15.01
      radiographic dye V15.08
      seafood V15.04
      specified food NEC V15.05
      spider bite V15.06
  horse serum — *see* Allergy, serum
  inhalant 477.9
    dust 477.8
    pollen 477.0
    specified allergen other than pollen 477.8
  kapok 477.8
  medicine — *see* Allergy, drug
  migraine 339.00
  milk protein 558.3
  pannus 370.62
  pneumonia 518.3
  pollen (any) (hay fever) 477.0
    asthma (*see also* Asthma) 493.0 ☑
  primrose 477.0
  primula 477.0
  purpura 287.2
  ragweed (pollen) (Senecio jacobae) 477.0
    asthma (*see also* Asthma) 493.0 ☑
    hay fever 477.0
  respiratory (*see also* Allergy, inhalant) 477.9
    due to
      drug — *see* Allergy, drug
      food — *see* Allergy, food
  rhinitis (*see also* Fever, hay) 477.9
    due to food 477.1
  rose 477.0
  Senecio jacobae 477.0
  serum (prophylactic) (therapeutic) 999.5
    anaphylactic shock 999.4
  shock (anaphylactic) (due to adverse effect of correct medicinal substance properly administered) 995.0
    food — *see* Anaphylactic shock, due to, food
    from serum or immunization 999.5
      anaphylactic 999.4
  sinusitis (*see also* Fever, hay) 477.9
  skin reaction 692.9
    specified substance — *see* Dermatitis, due to
  tree (any) (hay fever) (pollen) 477.0
    asthma (*see also* Asthma) 493.0 ☑
  upper respiratory (*see also* Fever, hay) 477.9
  urethritis 597.89
  urticaria 708.0
  vaccine — *see* Allergy, serum
Allescheriosis 117.6
Alligator skin disease (ichthyosis congenita) 757.1
  acquired 701.1
Allocheiria, allochiria — *see also* Disturbance, sensation 782.0

☑ Additional Digit Required — Refer to the Tabular List for Digit Selection   ▽ Subterms under main terms may continue to next column or page

Almeida's disease (Brazilian blastomycosis) 116.1
Alopecia (atrophicans) (pregnancy) (premature) (senile) 704.00
  adnata 757.4
  areata 704.01
  celsi 704.01
  cicatrisata 704.09
  circumscripta 704.01
  congenital, congenitalis 757.4
  disseminata 704.01
  effluvium (telogen) 704.02
  febrile 704.09
  generalisata 704.09
  hereditaria 704.09
  marginalis 704.01
  mucinosa 704.09
  postinfectional 704.09
  seborrheica 704.09
  specific 091.82
  syphilitic (secondary) 091.82
  telogen effluvium 704.02
  totalis 704.09
  toxica 704.09
  universalis 704.09
  x-ray 704.09
Alpers' disease 330.8
Alpha-lipoproteinemia 272.4
Alpha thalassemia 282.49
Alphos 696.1
Alpine sickness 993.2
Alport's syndrome (hereditary hematuri-anephropathy-deafness) 759.89
ALPS (autoimmune lymphoproliferative syndrome) 279.41
ALTE (apparent life threatening event) **in newborn and infant**) 799.82
Alteration (of), altered
  awareness 780.09
    transient 780.02
  consciousness 780.09
    persistent vegetative state 780.03
    transient 780.02
  mental status 780.97
    amnesia (retrograde) 780.93
    memory loss 780.93
Alternaria (infection) 118
Alternating — see condition
Altitude, high (effects) — see Effect, adverse, high altitude
Aluminosis (of lung) 503
Alvarez syndrome (transient cerebral ischemia) 435.9
Alveolar capillary block syndrome 516.3
Alveolitis
  allergic (extrinsic) 495.9
    due to organisms (fungal, thermophilic actinomycete, other) growing in ventilation (air conditioning systems) 495.7
    specified type NEC 495.8
  due to
    Aspergillus clavatus 495.4
    Cryptostroma corticale 495.6
  fibrosing (chronic) (cryptogenic) (lung) 516.3
    idiopathic 516.3
    rheumatoid 714.81
  jaw 526.5
  sicca dolorosa 526.5
Alveolus, alveolar — see condition
Alymphocytosis (pure) 279.2
Alymphoplasia, thymic 279.2
Alzheimer's
  dementia (senile)
    with behavioral disturbance 331.0 [294.11]
    without behavioral disturbance 331.0 [294.10]
  disease or sclerosis 331.0
    with dementia — see Alzheimer's, dementia
Amastia — see also Absence, breast 611.89
Amaurosis (acquired) (congenital) — see also Blindness 369.00
  fugax 362.34

Amaurosis — see also Blindness — continued
  hysterical 300.11
  Leber's (congenital) 362.76
  tobacco 377.34
  uremic — see Uremia
Amaurotic familial idiocy (infantile) (juvenile) (late) 330.1
Ambisexual 752.7
Amblyopia (acquired) (congenital) (partial) 368.00
  color 368.59
    acquired 368.55
  deprivation 368.02
  ex anopsia 368.00
  hysterical 300.11
  nocturnal 368.60
    vitamin A deficiency 264.5
  refractive 368.03
  strabismic 368.01
  suppression 368.01
  tobacco 377.34
  toxic NEC 377.34
  uremic — see Uremia
Ameba, amebic (histolytica) — see also Amebiasis
  abscess 006.3
    bladder 006.8
    brain (with liver and lung abscess) 006.5
    liver 006.3
      with
        brain abscess (and lung abscess) 006.5
        lung abscess 006.4
    lung (with liver abscess) 006.4
      with brain abscess 006.5
    seminal vesicle 006.8
    spleen 006.8
  carrier (suspected of) V02.2
  meningoencephalitis
    due to Naegleria (gruberi) 136.29
    primary 136.29
Amebiasis NEC 006.9
  with
    brain abscess (with liver or lung abscess) 006.5
    liver abscess (without mention of brain or lung abscess) 006.3
    lung abscess (with liver abscess) 006.4
      with brain abscess 006.5
  acute 006.0
  bladder 006.8
  chronic 006.1
  cutaneous 006.6
  cutis 006.6
  due to organism other than Entamoeba histolytica 007.8
  hepatic (see also Abscess, liver, amebic) 006.3
  nondysenteric 006.2
  seminal vesicle 006.8
  specified
    organism NEC 007.8
    site NEC 006.8
Ameboma 006.8
Amelia 755.4
  lower limb 755.31
  upper limb 755.21
Ameloblastoma (M9310/0) 213.1
  jaw (bone) (lower) 213.1
    upper 213.0
  long bones (M9261/3) — see Neoplasm, bone, malignant
  malignant (M9310/3) 170.1
    jaw (bone) (lower) 170.1
      upper 170.0
  mandible 213.1
  tibial (M9261/3) 170.7
Amelogenesis imperfecta 520.5
  nonhereditaria (segmentalis) 520.4
Amenorrhea (primary) (secondary) 626.0
  due to ovarian dysfunction 256.8
  hyperhormonal 256.8
Amentia — see also Retardation, mental 319
  Meynert's (nonalcoholic) 294.0
    alcoholic 291.1

Amentia — see also Retardation, mental — continued
  nevoid 759.6
American
  leishmaniasis 085.5
  mountain tick fever 066.1
  trypanosomiasis — see Trypanosomiasis, American
Ametropia — see also Disorder, accommodation 367.9
Amianthosis 501
Amimia 784.69
Amino acid
  deficiency 270.9
    anemia 281.4
  metabolic disorder (see also Disorder, amino acid) 270.9
Aminoaciduria 270.9
  imidazole 270.5
Amnesia (retrograde) 780.93
  auditory 784.69
    developmental 315.31
    secondary to organic lesion 784.69
  dissociative 300.12
  hysterical or dissociative type 300.12
  psychogenic 300.12
  transient global 437.7
Amnestic (confabulatory) **syndrome** 294.0
  alcohol-induced persisting 291.1
  drug-induced persisting 292.83
  posttraumatic 294.0
Amniocentesis screening (for) V28.2
  alphafetoprotein level, raised V28.1
  chromosomal anomalies V28.0
Amnion, amniotic — see also condition
  nodosum 658.8 ☑
Amnionitis (complicating pregnancy) 658.4 ☑
  affecting fetus or newborn 762.7
Amoral trends 301.7
Amotio retinae — see also Detachment, retina 361.9
Ampulla
  lower esophagus 530.89
  phrenic 530.89
Amputation
  any part of fetus, to facilitate delivery 763.89
  cervix (supravaginal) (uteri) 622.8
    in pregnancy or childbirth 654.6 ☑
      affecting fetus or newborn 763.89
  clitoris — see Wound, open, clitoris
  congenital
    lower limb 755.31
    upper limb 755.21
  neuroma (traumatic) (see also Injury, nerve, by site)
    surgical complication (late) 997.61
  penis — see Amputation, traumatic, penis
  status (without complication) — see Absence, by site, acquired
  stump (surgical) (posttraumatic)
    abnormal, painful, or with complication (late) 997.60
    healed or old NEC (see also Absence, by site, acquired)
      lower V49.70
      upper V49.60
  traumatic (complete) (partial)

Note — "Complicated" includes traumatic amputation with delayed healing, delayed treatment, foreign body, or infection.

    arm 887.4
      at or above elbow 887.2
        complicated 887.3
      below elbow 887.0
        complicated 887.1
      both (bilateral) (any level(s)) 887.6
        complicated 887.7
      complicated 887.5
      finger(s) (one or both hands) 886.0
        with thumb(s) 885.0
          complicated 885.1
        complicated 886.1
      foot (except toe(s) only) 896.0
        and other leg 897.6
          complicated 897.7

Amputation — continued
  traumatic — continued
    foot(s only) — continued
      both (bilateral) 896.2
        complicated 896.3
      complicated 896.1
      toe(s) only (one or both feet) 895.0
        complicated 895.1
    genital organ(s) (external) NEC 878.8
      complicated 878.9
    hand (except finger(s) only) 887.0
      and other arm 887.6
        complicated 887.7
      both (bilateral) 887.6
        complicated 887.7
      complicated 887.1
      finger(s) (one or both hands) 886.0
        with thumb(s) 885.0
          complicated 885.1
        complicated 886.1
      thumb(s) (with fingers of either hand) 885.0
        complicated 885.1
    head 874.9
    late effect — see Late, effects (of), amputation
    leg 897.4
      and other foot 897.6
        complicated 897.7
      at or above knee 897.2
        complicated 897.3
      below knee 897.0
        complicated 897.1
      both (bilateral) 897.6
        complicated 897.7
      complicated 897.5
    lower limb(s) except toe(s) — see Amputation, traumatic, leg
    nose — see Wound, open, nose
    penis 878.0
      complicated 878.1
    sites other than limbs — see Wound, open, by site
    thumb(s) (with finger(s) of either hand) 885.0
      complicated 885.1
    toe(s) (one or both feet) 895.0
      complicated 895.1
    upper limb(s) — see Amputation, traumatic, arm
Amputee (bilateral) (old) — see also Absence, by site, acquired V49.70
Amusia 784.69
  developmental 315.39
  secondary to organic lesion 784.69
Amyelencephalus 740.0
Amyelia 742.59
Amygdalitis — see Tonsillitis
Amygdalolith 474.8
Amyloid disease or degeneration 277.30
  heart 277.39 [425.7]
Amyloidosis (familial) (general) (generalized) (genetic) (primary) 277.30
  with lung involvement 277.39 [517.8]
  cardiac, hereditary 277.39
  heart 277.39 [425.7]
  nephropathic 277.39 [583.81]
  neuropathic (Portuguese) (Swiss) 277.39 [357.4]
  pulmonary 277.39 [517.8]
  secondary 277.39
  systemic, inherited 277.39
Amylopectinosis (brancher enzyme deficiency) 271.0
Amylophagia 307.52
Amyoplasia, congenita 756.89
Amyotonia 728.2
  congenita 358.8
Amyotrophia, amyotrophy, amyotrophic 728.2
  congenita 756.89
  diabetic 250.6 ☑ [353.5]
    due to secondary diabetes 249.6 ☑ [353.5]
  lateral sclerosis (syndrome) 335.20
  neuralgic 353.5

☑ **Additional Digit Required — Refer to the Tabular List for Digit Selection**   ▽ **Subterms under main terms may continue to next column or page**

2011 ICD-9-CM   ▶◀ **Revised Text**   ● **New Line**   ▲ **Revised Code**   **Volume 2 — 17**

Amyotrophia, amyotrophy, amyotrophic — *continued*
  sclerosis (lateral) 335.20
  spinal progressive 335.21
Anacidity, gastric 536.0
  psychogenic 306.4
Anaerosis of newborn 770.88
Analbuminemia 273.8
Analgesia — *see also* Anesthesia 782.0
Analphalipoproteinemia 272.5
Anaphylactic shock or reaction (correct substance properly administered) 995.0
  due to
    food 995.60
      additives 995.66
      crustaceans 995.62
      eggs 995.68
      fish 995.65
      fruits 995.63
      milk products 995.67
      nuts (tree) 995.64
      peanuts 995.61
      seeds 995.64
      specified NEC 995.69
      tree nuts 995.64
      vegetables 995.63
    immunization 999.4
    overdose or wrong substance given or taken 977.9
      specified drug — *see* Table of Drugs and Chemicals
    serum 999.4
  following sting(s) 989.5
  purpura 287.0
  serum 999.4
Anaphylactoid shock or reaction — *see* Anaphylactic shock
Anaphylaxis — *see* Anaphylactic shock
Anaplasia, cervix 622.10
Anarthria 784.51
Anarthritic rheumatoid disease 446.5
Anasarca 782.3
  cardiac (*see also* Failure, heart) 428.0
  fetus or newborn 778.0
  lung 514
  nutritional 262
  pulmonary 514
  renal (*see also* Nephrosis) 581.9
Anaspadias 752.62
Anastomosis
  aneurysmal — *see* Aneurysm
  arteriovenous, congenital NEC (*see also* Anomaly, arteriovenous) 747.60
    ruptured, of brain (*see also* Hemorrhage, subarachnoid) 430
  intestinal 569.89
    complicated NEC 997.4
      involving urinary tract 997.5
  retinal and choroidal vessels 743.58
    acquired 362.17
Anatomical narrow angle (glaucoma) 365.02
Ancylostoma (infection) (infestation) 126.9
  americanus 126.1
  braziliense 126.2
  caninum 126.8
  ceylanicum 126.3
  duodenale 126.0
  Necator americanus 126.1
Ancylostomiasis (intestinal) 126.9
  ancylostoma
    americanus 126.1
    caninum 126.8
    ceylanicum 126.3
    duodenale 126.0
  braziliense 126.2
  Necator americanus 126.1
Anders' disease or syndrome (adiposis tuberosa simplex) 272.8
Andersen's glycogen storage disease 271.0
Anderson's disease 272.7
Andes disease 993.2
Andrews' disease (bacterid) 686.8
Androblastoma (M8630/1)
  benign (M8630/0)
    specified site — *see* Neoplasm, by site, benign

Androblastoma — *continued*
  benign — *continued*
    unspecified site
      female 220
      male 222.0
  malignant (M8630/3)
    specified site — *see* Neoplasm, by site, malignant
    unspecified site
      female 183.0
      male 186.9
  specified site — *see* Neoplasm, by site, uncertain behavior
  tubular (M8640/0)
    with lipid storage (M8641/0)
      specified site — *see* Neoplasm, by site, benign
      unspecified site
        female 220
        male 222.0
    specified site — *see* Neoplasm, by site, benign
    unspecified site
      female 220
      male 222.0
  unspecified site
    female 236.2
    male 236.4
Android pelvis 755.69
  with disproportion (fetopelvic) 653.3 ☑
    affecting fetus or newborn 763.1
    causing obstructed labor 660.1 ☑
      affecting fetus or newborn 763.1
Anectasis, pulmonary (newborn or fetus) 770.5
Anemia 285.9
  with
    disorder of
      anaerobic glycolysis 282.3
      pentose phosphate pathway 282.2
    koilonychia 280.9
  6-phosphogluconic dehydrogenase deficiency 282.2
  achlorhydric 280.9
  achrestic 281.8
  Addison's (pernicious) 281.0
  Addison-Biermer (pernicious) 281.0
  agranulocytic 288.09
  amino acid deficiency 281.4
  antineoplastic chemotherapy induced 285.3
  aplastic 284.9
    acquired (secondary) 284.89
    congenital 284.01
    constitutional 284.01
    due to
      antineoplastic chemotherapy 284.89
      chronic systemic disease 284.89
      drugs 284.89
      infection 284.89
      radiation 284.89
    idiopathic 284.9
    myxedema 244.9
    of or complicating pregnancy 648.2 ☑
    red cell (acquired) (adult) (with thymoma) 284.81
      congenital 284.01
      pure 284.01
    specified type NEC 284.89
    toxic (paralytic) 284.89
  aregenerative 284.9
    congenital 284.01
  asiderotic 280.9
  atypical (primary) 285.9
  autohemolysis of Selwyn and Dacie (type I) 282.2
  autoimmune hemolytic 283.0
  Baghdad Spring 282.2
  Balantidium coli 007.0
  Biermer's (pernicious) 281.0
  blood loss (chronic) 280.0
    acute 285.1
  bothriocephalus 123.4
  brickmakers' (*see also* Ancylostomiasis) 126.9
  cerebral 437.8
  childhood 282.9

Anemia — *continued*
  chlorotic 280.9
  chronica congenita aregenerativa 284.01
  chronic simple 281.9
  combined system disease NEC 281.0 *[336.2]*
    due to dietary deficiency 281.1 *[336.2]*
  complicating pregnancy or childbirth 648.2 ☑
  congenital (following fetal blood loss) 776.5
    aplastic 284.01
    due to isoimmunization NEC 773.2
    Heinz-body 282.7
    hereditary hemolytic NEC 282.9
    nonspherocytic
      Type I 282.2
      Type II 282.3
    pernicious 281.0
    spherocytic (*see also* Spherocytosis) 282.0
  Cooley's (erythroblastic) 282.49
  crescent — *see* Disease, sickle-cell
  cytogenic 281.0
  Dacie's (nonspherocytic)
    type I 282.2
    type II 282.3
  Davidson's (refractory) 284.9
  deficiency 281.9
    2, 3 diphosphoglycurate mutase 282.3
    2, 3 PG 282.3
    6-PGD 282.2
    6-phosphogluronic dehydrogenase 282.2
    amino acid 281.4
    combined B_{12} and folate 281.3
    enzyme, drug-induced (hemolytic) 282.2
    erythrocytic glutathione 282.2
    folate 281.2
      dietary 281.2
      drug-induced 281.2
    folic acid 281.2
      dietary 281.2
      drug-induced 281.2
    G-6-PD 282.2
    GGS-R 282.2
    glucose-6-phosphate dehydrogenase (G-6-PD) 282.2
    glucose-phosphate isomerase 282.3
    glutathione peroxidase 282.2
    glutathione reductase 282.2
    glyceraldehyde phosphate dehydrogenase 282.3
    GPI 282.3
    G SH 282.2
    hexokinase 282.3
    iron (Fe) 280.9
      specified NEC 280.8
    nutritional 281.9
      with
        poor iron absorption 280.9
        specified deficiency NEC 281.8
      due to inadequate dietary iron intake 280.1
      specified type NEC 281.8
    of or complicating pregnancy 648.2 ☑
    pentose phosphate pathway 282.2
    PFK 282.3
    phosphofructo-aldolase 282.3
    phosphofructokinase 282.3
    phosphoglycerate kinase 282.3
    PK 282.3
    protein 281.4
    pyruvate kinase (PK) 282.3
    TPI 282.3
    triosephosphate isomerase 282.3
    vitamin B_{12} NEC 281.1
      dietary 281.1
      pernicious 281.0
  Diamond-Blackfan (congenital hypoplastic) 284.01
  dibothriocephalus 123.4
  dimorphic 281.9
  diphasic 281.8
  diphtheritic 032.89
  Diphyllobothrium 123.4
  drepanocytic (*see also* Disease, sickle-cell) 282.60

Anemia — *continued*
  due to
    antineoplastic chemotherapy 285.3
    blood loss (chronic) 280.0
      acute 285.1
    chemotherapy, antineoplastic 285.3
    defect of Embden-Meyerhof pathway glycolysis 282.3
    disorder of glutathione metabolism 282.2
    drug — *see* Anemia, by type (*see also* Table of Drugs and Chemicals)
      chemotherapy, antineoplastic 285.3
    fetal blood loss 776.5
    fish tapeworm (D. latum) infestation 123.4
    glutathione metabolism disorder 282.2
    hemorrhage (chronic) 280.0
      acute 285.1
    hexose monophosphate (HMP) shunt deficiency 282.2
    impaired absorption 280.9
    loss of blood (chronic) 280.0
      acute 285.1
    myxedema 244.9
    Necator americanus 126.1
    prematurity 776.6
    selective vitamin B_{12} malabsorption with proteinuria 281.1
  Dyke-Young type (secondary) (symptomatic) 283.9
  dyserythropoietic (congenital) (types I, II, III) 285.8
  dyshemopoietic (congenital) 285.8
  Egypt (*see also* Ancylostomiasis) 126.9
  elliptocytosis (*see also* Elliptocytosis) 282.1
  enzyme deficiency, drug-induced 282.2
  epidemic (*see also* Ancylostomiasis) 126.9
  EPO resistant 285.21
  erythroblastic
    familial 282.49
    fetus or newborn (*see also* Disease, hemolytic) 773.2
    late 773.5
  erythrocytic glutathione deficiency 282.2
  erythropoietin-resistant (EPO resistant anemia) 285.21
  essential 285.9
  Faber's (achlorhydric anemia) 280.9
  factitious (self-induced blood letting) 280.0
  familial erythroblastic (microcytic) 282.49
  Fanconi's (congenital pancytopenia) 284.09
  favism 282.2
  fetal 678.0 ☑
    following blood loss, affecting newborn 776.5
  fetus or newborn
    due to
      ABO
        antibodies 773.1
        incompatibility, maternal/fetal 773.1
        isoimmunization 773.1
      Rh
        antibodies 773.0
        incompatibility, maternal/fetal 773.0
        isoimmunization 773.0
    following fetal blood loss 776.5
  fish tapeworm (D. latum) infestation 123.4
  folate (folic acid) deficiency 281.2
    dietary 281.2
    drug-induced 281.2
  folate malabsorption, congenital 281.2
  folic acid deficiency 281.2
    dietary 281.2
    drug-induced 281.2
  G-6-PD 282.2
  general 285.9
  glucose-6-phosphate dehydrogenase deficiency 282.2
  glutathione-reductase deficiency 282.2
  goat's milk 281.2
  granulocytic 288.09
  Heinz-body, congenital 282.7
  hemoglobin deficiency 285.9

Anemia — *continued*
- hemolytic 283.9
  - acquired 283.9
    - with hemoglobinuria NEC 283.2
    - autoimmune (cold type) (idiopathic) (primary) (secondary) (symptomatic) (warm type) 283.0
    - due to
      - cold reactive antibodies 283.0
      - drug exposure 283.0
      - warm reactive antibodies 283.0
    - fragmentation 283.19
    - idiopathic (chronic) 283.9
    - infectious 283.19
      - autoimmune 283.0
    - non-autoimmune 283.10
    - toxic 283.19
    - traumatic cardiac 283.19
  - acute 283.9
    - due to enzyme deficiency NEC 282.3
    - fetus or newborn (*see also* Disease, hemolytic) 773.2
      - late 773.5
    - Lederer's (acquired infectious hemolytic anemia) 283.19
  - autoimmune (acquired) 283.0
  - chronic 282.9
    - idiopathic 283.9
  - cold type (secondary) (symptomatic) 283.0
  - congenital (spherocytic) (*see also* Spherocytosis) 282.0
    - nonspherocytic — *see* Anemia, hemolytic, nonspherocytic, congenital
  - drug-induced 283.0
    - enzyme deficiency 282.2
  - due to
    - cardiac conditions 283.19
    - drugs 283.0
    - enzyme deficiency NEC 282.3
      - drug-induced 282.2
    - presence of shunt or other internal prosthetic device 283.19
    - thrombotic thrombocytopenic purpura 446.6
  - elliptocytotic (*see also* Elliptocytosis) 282.1
  - familial 282.9
  - hereditary 282.9
    - due to enzyme deficiency NEC 282.3
    - specified NEC 282.8
  - idiopathic (chronic) 283.9
  - infectious (acquired) 283.19
  - mechanical 283.19
  - microangiopathic 283.19
  - non-autoimmune NEC 283.10
  - nonspherocytic
    - congenital or hereditary NEC 282.3
      - glucose-6-phosphate dehydrogenase deficiency 282.2
      - pyruvate kinase (PK) deficiency 282.3
      - type I 282.2
      - type II 282.3
    - type I 282.2
    - type II 282.3
  - of or complicating pregnancy 648.2 ☑
  - resulting from presence of shunt or other internal prosthetic device 283.19
  - secondary 283.19
    - autoimmune 283.0
  - sickle-cell — *see* Disease, sickle-cell
  - Stransky-Regala type (Hb-E) (*see also* Disease, hemoglobin) 282.7
  - symptomatic 283.19
    - autoimmune 283.0
  - toxic (acquired) 283.19
  - uremic (adult) (child) 283.11
  - warm type (secondary) (symptomatic) 283.0
- hemorrhagic (chronic) 280.0
  - acute 285.1
- HEMPAS 285.8

Anemia — *continued*
- hereditary erythroblast multinuclearity-positive acidified serum test 285.8
- Herrick's (hemoglobin S disease) 282.61
- hexokinase deficiency 282.3
- high A₂ 282.49
- hookworm (*see also* Ancylostomiasis) 126.9
- hypochromic (idiopathic) (microcytic) (normoblastic) 280.9
  - with iron loading 285.0
  - due to blood loss (chronic) 280.0
    - acute 285.1
  - familial sex linked 285.0
  - pyridoxine-responsive 285.0
- hypoplasia, red blood cells 284.81
  - congenital or familial 284.01
- hypoplastic (idiopathic) 284.9
  - congenital 284.01
  - familial 284.01
  - of childhood 284.09
- idiopathic 285.9
  - hemolytic, chronic 283.9
- in (due to) (with)
  - chronic illness NEC 285.29
  - chronic kidney disease 285.21
  - end-stage renal disease 285.21
  - neoplastic disease 285.22
- infantile 285.9
- infective, infectional 285.9
- intertropical (*see also* Ancylostomiasis) 126.9
- iron (Fe) deficiency 280.9
  - due to blood loss (chronic) 280.0
    - acute 285.1
  - of or complicating pregnancy 648.2 ☑
  - specified NEC 280.8
- Jaksch's (pseudoleukemia infantum) 285.8
- Joseph-Diamond-Blackfan (congenital hypoplastic) 284.01
- labyrinth 386.50
- Lederer's (acquired infectious hemolytic anemia) 283.19
- leptocytosis (hereditary) 282.49
- leukoerythroblastic 284.2
- macrocytic 281.9
  - nutritional 281.2
  - of or complicating pregnancy 648.2 ☑
  - tropical 281.2
- malabsorption (familial), selective B₁₂ with proteinuria 281.1
- malarial (*see also* Malaria) 084.6
- malignant (progressive) 281.0
- malnutrition 281.9
- marsh (*see also* Malaria) 084.6
- Mediterranean (with hemoglobinopathy) 282.49
- megaloblastic 281.9
  - combined B₁₂ and folate deficiency 281.3
  - nutritional (of infancy) 281.2
  - of infancy 281.2
  - of or complicating pregnancy 648.2 ☑
  - refractory 281.3
  - specified NEC 281.3
- megalocytic 281.9
- microangiopathic hemolytic 283.19
- microcytic (hypochromic) 280.9
  - due to blood loss (chronic) 280.0
    - acute 285.1
  - familial 282.49
  - hypochromic 280.9
- microdrepanocytosis 282.49
- miners' (*see also* Ancylostomiasis) 126.9
- myelopathic 285.8
- myelophthisic (normocytic) 284.2
- newborn (*see also* Disease, hemolytic) 773.2
  - due to isoimmunization (*see also* Disease, hemolytic) 773.2
  - late, due to isoimmunization 773.5
  - posthemorrhagic 776.5
- nonregenerative 284.9
- nonspherocytic hemolytic — *see* Anemia, hemolytic, nonspherocytic
- normocytic (infectional) (not due to blood loss) 285.9
  - due to blood loss (chronic) 280.0
    - acute 285.1

Anemia — *continued*
- normocytic — *continued*
  - myelophthisic 284.2
- nutritional (deficiency) 281.9
  - with
    - poor iron absorption 280.9
    - specified deficiency NEC 281.8
  - due to inadequate dietary iron intake 280.1
  - megaloblastic (of infancy) 281.2
- of childhood 282.9
- of chronic
  - disease NEC 285.29
  - illness NEC 285.29
- of or complicating pregnancy 648.2 ☑
  - affecting fetus or newborn 760.8
- of prematurity 776.6
- orotic aciduric (congenital) (hereditary) 281.4
- osteosclerotic 289.89
- ovalocytosis (hereditary) (*see also* Elliptocytosis) 282.1
- paludal (*see also* Malaria) 084.6
- pentose phosphate pathway deficiency 282.2
- pernicious (combined system disease) (congenital) (dorsolateral spinal degeneration) (juvenile) (myelopathy) (neuropathy) (posterior sclerosis) (primary) (progressive) (spleen) 281.0
  - of or complicating pregnancy 648.2 ☑
- pleochromic 285.9
  - of sprue 281.8
- portal 285.8
- posthemorrhagic (chronic) 280.0
  - acute 285.1
  - newborn 776.5
- postoperative
  - due to (acute) blood loss 285.1
    - chronic blood loss 280.0
  - other 285.9
- postpartum 648.2 ☑
- pressure 285.9
- primary 285.9
- profound 285.9
- progressive 285.9
  - malignant 281.0
  - pernicious 281.0
- protein-deficiency 281.4
- pseudoleukemica infantum 285.8
- puerperal 648.2 ☑
- pure red cell 284.81
  - congenital 284.01
- pyridoxine-responsive (hypochromic) 285.0
- pyruvate kinase (PK) deficiency 282.3
- refractoria sideroblastica 238.72
- refractory (primary) 238.72
  - with
    - excess
      - blasts-1 (RAEB-1) 238.72
      - blasts-2 (RAEB-2) 238.73
    - hemochromatosis 238.72
    - ringed sideroblasts (RARS) 238.72
  - due to
    - drug 285.0
    - myelodysplastic syndrome 238.72
    - toxin 285.0
  - hereditary 285.0
  - idiopathic 238.72
  - megaloblastic 281.3
  - sideroblastic 238.72
    - hereditary 285.0
  - sideropenic 280.9
- Rietti-Greppi-Micheli (thalassemia minor) 282.49
- scorbutic 281.8
- secondary (to) 285.9
  - blood loss (chronic) 280.0
    - acute 285.1
  - hemorrhage 280.0
    - acute 285.1
  - inadequate dietary iron intake 280.1
- semiplastic 284.9
- septic 285.9
- sickle-cell (*see also* Disease, sickle-cell) 282.60

Anemia — *continued*
- sideroachrestic 285.0
- sideroblastic (acquired) (any type) (congenital) (drug-induced) (due to disease) (hereditary) (primary) (secondary) (sex-linked hypochromic) (vitamin B₆ responsive) 285.0
  - refractory 238.72
  - congenital 285.0
  - drug-induced 285.0
  - hereditary 285.0
  - sex-linked hypochromic 285.0
  - vitamin B₆-responsive 285.0
- sideropenic (refractory) 280.9
  - due to blood loss (chronic) 280.0
    - acute 285.1
- simple chronic 281.9
- specified type NEC 285.8
- spherocytic (hereditary) (*see also* Spherocytosis) 282.0
- splenic 285.8
  - familial (Gaucher's) 272.7
- splenomegalic 285.8
- stomatocytosis 282.8
- syphilitic 095.8
- target cell (oval) 282.49
- thalassemia 282.49
- thrombocytopenic (*see also* Thrombocytopenia) 287.5
- toxic 284.89
- triosephosphate isomerase deficiency 282.3
- tropical, macrocytic 281.2
- tuberculous (*see also* Tuberculosis) 017.9 ☑
- vegan's 281.1
- vitamin
  - B₆-responsive 285.0
  - B₁₂ deficiency (dietary) 281.1
    - pernicious 281.0
- von Jaksch's (pseudoleukemia infantum) 285.8
- Witts' (achlorhydric anemia) 280.9
- Zuelzer (-Ogden) (nutritional megaloblastic anemia) 281.2

Anencephalus, anencephaly 740.0
- fetal, affecting management of pregnancy 655.0 ☑

Anergasia — *see also* Psychosis, organic 294.9
- senile 290.0

Anesthesia, anesthetic 782.0
- complication or reaction NEC 995.22
  - due to
    - correct substance properly administered 995.22
    - overdose or wrong substance given 968.4
      - specified anesthetic — *see* Table of Drugs and Chemicals
- cornea 371.81
- death from
  - correct substance properly administered 995.4
  - during delivery 668.9 ☑
  - overdose or wrong substance given 968.4
  - specified anesthetic — *see* Table of Drugs and Chemicals
- eye 371.81
- functional 300.11
- hyperesthetic, thalamic 338.0
- hysterical 300.11
- local skin lesion 782.0
- olfactory 781.1
- sexual (psychogenic) 302.72
- shock
  - due to
    - correct substance properly administered 995.4
    - overdose or wrong substance given 968.4
    - specified anesthetic — *see* Table of Drugs and Chemicals
- skin 782.0
- tactile 782.0
- testicular 608.9
- thermal 782.0

☑ **Additional Digit Required** — Refer to the Tabular List for Digit Selection   ⑩ **Subterms under main terms may continue to next column or page**

2011 ICD-9-CM   ▶◀ **Revised Text**   ● **New Line**   ▲ **Revised Code**   **Volume 2 — 19**

Index

Anetoderma — Angiodysplasia

Anetoderma (maculosum) 701.3
Aneuploidy NEC 758.5
Aneurin deficiency 265.1
Aneurysm (anastomotic) (artery) (cirsoid) (diffuse) (false) (fusiform) (multiple) (ruptured) (saccular) (varicose) 442.9
 abdominal (aorta) 441.4
  ruptured 441.3
  syphilitic 093.0
 aorta, aortic (nonsyphilitic) 441.9
  abdominal 441.4
   dissecting 441.02
   ruptured 441.3
   syphilitic 093.0
  arch 441.2
   ruptured 441.1
  arteriosclerotic NEC 441.9
   ruptured 441.5
  ascending 441.2
   ruptured 441.1
  congenital 747.29
  descending 441.9
   abdominal 441.4
    ruptured 441.3
   ruptured 441.5
   thoracic 441.2
    ruptured 441.1
  dissecting 441.00
   abdominal 441.02
   thoracic 441.01
   thoracoabdominal 441.03
  due to coarctation (aorta) 747.10
  ruptured 441.5
  sinus, right 747.29
  syphilitic 093.0
  thoracoabdominal 441.7
   ruptured 441.6
  thorax, thoracic (arch) (nonsyphilitic) 441.2
   dissecting 441.01
   ruptured 441.1
   syphilitic 093.0
  transverse 441.2
   ruptured 441.1
  valve (heart) (see also Endocarditis, aortic) 424.1
 arteriosclerotic NEC 442.9
  cerebral 437.3
   ruptured (see also Hemorrhage, subarachnoid) 430
 arteriovenous (congenital) (peripheral) NEC (see also Anomaly, arteriovenous) 747.60
  acquired NEC 447.0
   brain 437.3
    ruptured (see also Hemorrhage, subarachnoid) 430
   coronary 414.11
   pulmonary 417.0
  brain (cerebral) 747.81
   ruptured (see also Hemorrhage, subarachnoid) 430
  coronary 746.85
  pulmonary 747.3
  retina 743.58
  specified site NEC 747.89
   acquired 447.0
  traumatic (see also Injury, blood vessel, by site) 904.9
 basal — see Aneurysm, brain
 berry (congenital) (ruptured) (see also Hemorrhage, subarachnoid) 430
 brain 437.3
  arteriosclerotic 437.3
   ruptured (see also Hemorrhage, subarachnoid) 430
  arteriovenous 747.81
   acquired 437.3
    ruptured (see also Hemorrhage, subarachnoid) 430
   ruptured (see also Hemorrhage, subarachnoid) 430
  berry (congenital) (ruptured) (see also Hemorrhage, subarachnoid) 430
  congenital 747.81

Aneurysm — continued
 brain — continued
  congenital — continued
   ruptured (see also Hemorrhage, subarachnoid) 430
  meninges 437.3
   ruptured (see also Hemorrhage, subarachnoid) 430
  miliary (congenital) (ruptured) (see also Hemorrhage, subarachnoid) 430
  mycotic 421.0
   ruptured (see also Hemorrhage, subarachnoid) 430
  nonruptured 437.3
  ruptured (see also Hemorrhage, subarachnoid) 430
  syphilitic 094.87
  syphilitic (hemorrhage) 094.87
  traumatic — see Injury, intracranial
 cardiac (false) (see also Aneurysm, heart) 414.10
 carotid artery (common) (external) 442.81
  internal (intracranial portion) 437.3
   extracranial portion 442.81
   ruptured into brain (see also Hemorrhage, subarachnoid) 430
  syphilitic 093.89
   intracranial 094.87
 cavernous sinus (see also Aneurysm, brain) 437.3
  arteriovenous 747.81
   ruptured (see also Hemorrhage, subarachnoid) 430
  congenital 747.81
   ruptured (see also Hemorrhage, subarachnoid) 430
 celiac 442.84
 central nervous system, syphilitic 094.89
 cerebral — see Aneurysm, brain
 chest — see Aneurysm, thorax
 circle of Willis (see also Aneurysm, brain) 437.3
  congenital 747.81
   ruptured (see also Hemorrhage, subarachnoid) 430
   ruptured (see also Hemorrhage, subarachnoid) 430
 common iliac artery 442.2
 congenital (peripheral) NEC 747.60
  brain 747.81
   ruptured (see also Hemorrhage, subarachnoid) 430
  cerebral — see Aneurysm, brain, congenital
  coronary 746.85
  gastrointestinal 747.61
  lower limb 747.64
  pulmonary 747.3
  renal 747.62
  retina 743.58
  specified site NEC 747.89
  spinal 747.82
  upper limb 747.63
 conjunctiva 372.74
 conus arteriosus (see also Aneurysm, heart) 414.10
 coronary (arteriosclerotic) (artery) (vein) (see also Aneurysm, heart) 414.11
  arteriovenous 746.85
  congenital 746.85
  syphilitic 093.89
 cylindrical 441.9
  ruptured 441.5
  syphilitic 093.9
 dissecting 442.9
  aorta 441.00
   abdominal 441.02
   thoracic 441.01
   thoracoabdominal 441.03
  syphilitic 093.9
 ductus arteriosus 747.0
 embolic — see Embolism, artery
 endocardial, infective (any valve) 421.0
 femoral 442.3
 gastroduodenal 442.84
 gastroepiploic 442.84

Aneurysm — continued
 heart (chronic or with a stated duration of over 8 weeks) (infectional) (wall) 414.10
  acute or with a stated duration of 8 weeks or less (see also Infarct, myocardium) 410.9 ☑
  congenital 746.89
  valve — see Endocarditis
 hepatic 442.84
 iliac (common) 442.2
 infective (any valve) 421.0
 innominate (nonsyphilitic) 442.89
  syphilitic 093.89
 interauricular septum (see also Aneurysm, heart) 414.10
 interventricular septum (see also Aneurysm, heart) 414.10
 intracranial — see Aneurysm, brain
 intrathoracic (nonsyphilitic) 441.2
  ruptured 441.1
  syphilitic 093.0
 jugular vein ▶(acute)◀ 453.89
  chronic 453.76   ●
 lower extremity 442.3
 lung (pulmonary artery) 417.1
 malignant 093.9
 mediastinal (nonsyphilitic) 442.89
  syphilitic 093.89
 miliary (congenital) (ruptured) (see also Hemorrhage, subarachnoid) 430
 mitral (heart) (valve) 424.0
 mural (arteriovenous) (heart) (see also Aneurysm, heart) 414.10
 mycotic, any site 421.0
  without endocarditis — see Aneurysm by site
  ruptured, brain (see also Hemorrhage, subarachnoid) 430
 myocardium (see also Aneurysm, heart) 414.10
 neck 442.81
 pancreaticoduodenal 442.84
 patent ductus arteriosus 747.0
 peripheral NEC 442.89
  congenital NEC (see also Aneurysm, congenital) 747.60
 popliteal 442.3
 pulmonary 417.1
  arteriovenous 747.3
   acquired 417.0
  syphilitic 093.89
  valve (heart) (see also Endocarditis, pulmonary) 424.3
 racemose 442.9
  congenital (peripheral) NEC 747.60
 radial 442.0
 Rasmussen's (see also Tuberculosis) 011.2 ☑
 renal 442.1
 retinal (acquired) 362.17
  congenital 743.58
  diabetic 250.5 ☑ [362.01]
   due to secondary diabetes 249.5 ☑ [362.01]
 sinus, aortic (of Valsalva) 747.29
 specified site NEC 442.89
 spinal (cord) 442.89
  congenital 747.82
  syphilitic (hemorrhage) 094.89
 spleen, splenic 442.83
 subclavian 442.82
  syphilitic 093.89
 superior mesenteric 442.84
 syphilitic 093.9
  aorta 093.0
  central nervous system 094.89
  congenital 090.5
  spine, spinal 094.89
 thoracoabdominal 441.7
  ruptured 441.6
 thorax, thoracic (arch) (nonsyphilitic) 441.2
  dissecting 441.01
  ruptured 441.1
  syphilitic 093.0
 traumatic (complication) (early) — see Injury, blood vessel, by site

Aneurysm — continued
 tricuspid (heart) (valve) — see Endocarditis, tricuspid
 ulnar 442.0
 upper extremity 442.0
 valve, valvular — see Endocarditis
 venous 456.8
  congenital NEC (see also Aneurysm, congenital) 747.60
 ventricle (arteriovenous) (see also Aneurysm, heart) 414.10
 visceral artery NEC 442.84
Angiectasis 459.89
Angiectopia 459.9
Angiitis 447.6
 allergic granulomatous 446.4
 hypersensitivity 446.20
  Goodpasture's syndrome 446.21
  specified NEC 446.29
 necrotizing 446.0
 Wegener's (necrotizing respiratory granulomatosis) 446.4
Angina (attack) (cardiac) (chest) (effort) (heart) (pectoris) (syndrome) (vasomotor) 413.9
 abdominal 557.1
 accelerated 411.1
 agranulocytic 288.03
 aphthous 074.0
 catarrhal 462
 crescendo 411.1
 croupous 464.4
 cruris 443.9
  due to atherosclerosis NEC (see also Arteriosclerosis, extremities) 440.20
 decubitus 413.0
 diphtheritic (membranous) 032.0
 equivalent 413.9
 erysipelatous 034.0
 erythematous 462
 exudative, chronic 476.0
 faucium 478.29
 gangrenous 462
  diphtheritic 032.0
 infectious 462
 initial 411.1
 intestinal 557.1
 ludovici 528.3
 Ludwig's 528.3
 malignant 462
  diphtheritic 032.0
 membranous 464.4
  diphtheritic 032.0
 mesenteric 557.1
 monocytic 075
 nocturnal 413.0
 phlegmonous 475
  diphtheritic 032.0
 preinfarctional 411.1
 Prinzmetal's 413.1
 progressive 411.1
 pseudomembranous 101
 psychogenic 306.2
 pultaceous, diphtheritic 032.0
 scarlatinal 034.1
 septic 034.0
 simple 462
 stable NEC 413.9
 staphylococcal 462
 streptococcal 034.0
 stridulous, diphtheritic 032.3
 syphilitic 093.9
  congenital 090.5
 tonsil 475
 trachealis 464.4
 unstable 411.1
 variant 413.1
 Vincent's 101
Angioblastoma (M9161/1) — see Neoplasm, connective tissue, uncertain behavior
Angiocholecystitis — see also Cholecystitis, acute 575.0
Angiocholitis — see also Cholecystitis, acute 576.1
Angiodysgensis spinalis 336.1
Angiodysplasia (intestinalis) (intestine) 569.84
 with hemorrhage 569.85

☑ Additional Digit Required — Refer to the Tabular List for Digit Selection   ▽ Subterms under main terms may continue to next column or page

20 — Volume 2 · October 2010   ▶◀ Revised Text   ● New Line   ▲ Revised Code   2011 ICD-9-CM

Angiodysplasia — continued
  duodenum 537.82
    with hemorrhage 537.83
  stomach 537.82
    with hemorrhage 537.83
Angioedema (allergic) (any site) (with urticaria) 995.1
  hereditary 277.6
Angioendothelioma (M9130/1) — see also Neoplasm, by site, uncertain behavior
  benign (M9130/0) (see also Hemangioma, by site) 228.00
  bone (M9260/3) — see Neoplasm, bone, malignant
  Ewing's (M9260/3) — see Neoplasm, bone, malignant
  nervous system (M9130/0) 228.09
Angiofibroma (M9160/0) — see also Neoplasm, by site, benign
  juvenile (M9160/0) 210.7
    specified site — see Neoplasm, by site, benign
    unspecified site 210.7
Angiohemophilia (A) (B) 286.4
Angioid streaks (choroid) (retina) 363.43
Angiokeratoma (M9141/0) — see also Neoplasm, skin, benign
  corporis diffusum 272.7
Angiokeratosis
  diffuse 272.7
Angioleiomyoma (M8894/0) — see Neoplasm, connective tissue, benign
Angioleucitis 683
Angiolipoma (M8861/0) — see also Lipoma, by site 214.9
  infiltrating (M8861/1) — see Neoplasm, connective tissue, uncertain behavior
Angioma (M9120/0) — see also Hemangioma, by site 228.00
  capillary 448.1
  hemorrhagicum hereditaria 448.0
  malignant (M9120/3) — see Neoplasm, connective tissue, malignant
  pigmentosum et atrophicum 757.33
  placenta — see Placenta, abnormal
  plexiform (M9131/0) — see Hemangioma, by site
  senile 448.1
  serpiginosum 709.1
  spider 448.1
  stellate 448.1
Angiomatosis 757.32
  bacillary 083.8
  corporis diffusum universale 272.7
  cutaneocerebral 759.6
  encephalocutaneous 759.6
  encephalofacial 759.6
  encephalotrigeminal 759.6
  hemorrhagic familial 448.0
  hereditary familial 448.0
  heredofamilial 448.0
  meningo-oculofacial 759.6
  multiple sites 228.09
  neuro-oculocutaneous 759.6
  retina (Hippel's disease) 759.6
  retinocerebellosa 759.6
  retinocerebral 759.6
  systemic 228.09
Angiomyolipoma (M8860/0)
  specified site — see Neoplasm, connective tissue, benign
  unspecified site 223.0
Angiomyoliposarcoma (M8860/3) — see Neoplasm, connective tissue, malignant
Angiomyoma (M8894/0) — see Neoplasm, connective tissue, benign
Angiomyosarcoma (M8894/3) — see Neoplasm, connective tissue, malignant
Angioneurosis 306.2
Angioneurotic edema (allergic) (any site) (with urticaria) 995.1
  hereditary 277.6
Angiopathia, angiopathy 459.9
  diabetic (peripheral) 250.7 ☑ [443.81]
    due to secondary diabetes
      249.7 ☑ [443.81]

Angiopathia, angiopathy — continued
  peripheral 443.9
    diabetic 250.7 ☑ [443.81]
      due to secondary diabetes
        249.7 ☑ [443.81]
    specified type NEC 443.89
  retinae syphilitica 093.89
  retinalis (juvenilis) 362.18
    background 362.10
    diabetic 250.5 ☑ [362.01]
      due to secondary diabetes
        249.5 ☑ [362.01]
    proliferative 362.29
    tuberculous (see also Tuberculosis)
      017.3 ☑ [362.18]
Angiosarcoma (M9120/3) — see Neoplasm, connective tissue, malignant
Angiosclerosis — see Arteriosclerosis
Angioscotoma, enlarged 368.42
Angiospasm 443.9
  brachial plexus 353.0
  cerebral 435.9
  cervical plexus 353.2
  nerve
    arm 354.9
      axillary 353.0
      median 354.1
      ulnar 354.2
    autonomic (see also Neuropathy, peripheral, autonomic) 337.9
    axillary 353.0
    leg 355.8
      plantar 355.6
    lower extremity — see Angiospasm, nerve, leg
    median 354.1
    peripheral NEC 355.9
    spinal NEC 355.9
    sympathetic (see also Neuropathy, peripheral, autonomic) 337.9
    ulnar 354.2
    upper extremity — see Angiospasm, nerve, arm
  peripheral NEC 443.9
  traumatic 443.9
    foot 443.9
    leg 443.9
    vessel 443.9
Angiospastic disease or edema 443.9
Angle's
  class I 524.21
  class II 524.22
  class III 524.23
Anguillulosis 127.2
Angulation
  cecum (see also Obstruction, intestine) 560.9
  coccyx (acquired) 738.6
    congenital 756.19
  femur (acquired) 736.39
    congenital 755.69
  intestine (large) (small) (see also Obstruction, intestine) 560.9
  sacrum (acquired) 738.5
    congenital 756.19
  sigmoid (flexure) (see also Obstruction, intestine) 560.9
  spine (see also Curvature, spine) 737.9
  tibia (acquired) 736.89
    congenital 755.69
  ureter 593.3
  wrist (acquired) 736.09
    congenital 755.59
Angulus infectiosus 686.8
Anhedonia 780.99
Anhidrosis (lid) (neurogenic) (thermogenic) 705.0
Anhydration 276.51
  with
    hypernatremia 276.0
    hyponatremia 276.1
Anhydremia 276.52
  with
    hypernatremia 276.0
    hyponatremia 276.1
Anidrosis 705.0
Aniridia (congenital) 743.45

Anisakiasis (infection) (infestation) 127.1
Anisakis larva infestation 127.1
Aniseikonia 367.32
Anisocoria (pupil) 379.41
  congenital 743.46
Anisocytosis 790.09
Anisometropia (congenital) 367.31
Ankle — see condition
Ankyloblepharon (acquired) (eyelid) 374.46
  filiforme (adnatum) (congenital) 743.62
  total 743.62
Ankylodactly — see also Syndactylism 755.10
Ankyloglossia 750.0
Ankylosis (fibrous) (osseous) 718.50
  ankle 718.57
  any joint, produced by surgical fusion V45.4
  cricoarytenoid (cartilage) (joint) (larynx) 478.79
  dental 521.6
  ear ossicle NEC 385.22
    malleus 385.21
  elbow 718.52
  finger 718.54
  hip 718.55
  incostapedial joint (infectional) 385.22
  joint, produced by surgical fusion NEC V45.4
  knee 718.56
  lumbosacral (joint) 724.6
  malleus 385.21
  multiple sites 718.59
  postoperative (status) V45.4
  sacroiliac (joint) 724.6
  shoulder 718.51
  specified site NEC 718.58
  spine NEC 724.9
  surgical V45.4
  teeth, tooth (hard tissues) 521.6
  temporomandibular joint 524.61
  wrist 718.53
Ankylostoma — see Ancylostoma
Ankylostomiasis (intestinal) — see Ancylostomiasis
Ankylurethria — see also Stricture, urethra 598.9
Annular — see also condition
  detachment, cervix 622.8
  organ or site, congenital NEC — see Distortion
  pancreas (congenital) 751.7
Anodontia (complete) (partial) (vera) 520.0
  with abnormal spacing 524.30
  acquired 525.10
    causing malocclusion 524.30
    due to
      caries 525.13
      extraction 525.10
      periodontal disease 525.12
      trauma 525.11
Anomaly, anomalous (congenital) (unspecified type) 759.9
  abdomen 759.9
  abdominal wall 756.70
  acoustic nerve 742.9
  adrenal (gland) 759.1
  Alder (-Reilly) (leukocyte granulation) 288.2
  alimentary tract 751.9
    lower 751.5
      specified type NEC 751.8
    upper (any part, except tongue) 750.9
      tongue 750.10
        specified type NEC 750.19
  alveolar 524.70
    ridge (process) 525.8
    specified NEC 524.79
  ankle (joint) 755.69
  anus, anal (canal) 751.5
  aorta, aortic 747.20
    arch 747.21
    coarctation (postductal) (preductal) 747.10
    cusp or valve NEC 746.9
    septum 745.0
    specified type NEC 747.29
  aorticopulmonary septum 745.0
  apertures, diaphragm 756.6
  appendix 751.5

Anomaly, anomalous — continued
  aqueduct of Sylvius 742.3
    with spina bifida (see also Spina bifida) 741.0 ☑
  arm 755.50
    reduction (see also Deformity, reduction, upper limb) 755.20
  arteriovenous (congenital) (peripheral) NEC 747.60
    brain 747.81
    cerebral 747.81
    coronary 746.85
    gastrointestinal 747.61
      acquired — see Angiodysplasia
    lower limb 747.64
    renal 747.62
    specified site NEC 747.69
    spinal 747.82
    upper limb 747.63
  artery (see also Anomaly, peripheral vascular system) NEC 747.60
    brain 747.81
    cerebral 747.81
    coronary 746.85
    eye 743.9
    pulmonary 747.3
    renal 747.62
    retina 743.9
    umbilical 747.5
  arytenoepiglottic folds 748.3
  atrial
    bands 746.9
    folds 746.9
    septa 745.5
  atrioventricular
    canal 745.69
    common 745.69
    conduction 426.7
    excitation 426.7
    septum 745.4
  atrium — see Anomaly, atrial
  auditory canal 744.3
    specified type NEC 744.29
      with hearing impairment 744.02
  auricle
    ear 744.3
      causing impairment of hearing 744.02
    heart 746.9
    septum 745.5
  autosomes, autosomal NEC 758.5
  Axenfeld's 743.44
  back 759.9
  band
    atrial 746.9
    heart 746.9
    ventricular 746.9
  Bartholin's duct 750.9
  biliary duct or passage 751.60
    atresia 751.61
  bladder (neck) (sphincter) (trigone) 753.9
    specified type NEC 753.8
  blood vessel 747.9
    artery — see Anomaly, artery
    peripheral vascular — see Anomaly, peripheral vascular system
    vein — see Anomaly, vein
  bone NEC 756.9
    ankle 755.69
    arm 755.50
    chest 756.3
    cranium 756.0
    face 756.0
    finger 755.50
    foot 755.67
    forearm 755.50
    frontal 756.0
    head 756.0
    hip 755.63
    leg 755.60
    lumbosacral 756.10
    nose 748.1
    pelvic girdle 755.60
    rachitic 756.4
    rib 756.3
    shoulder girdle 755.50

Index

Anomaly, anomalous — Anomaly, anomalous

Anomaly, anomalous — *continued*
 bone — *continued*
  skull 756.0
   with
    anencephalus 740.0
    encephalocele 742.0
    hydrocephalus 742.3
     with spina bifida (*see also*
      Spina bifida) 741.0 ☑
    microcephalus 742.1
  toe 755.66
 brain 742.9
  multiple 742.4
  reduction 742.2
  specified type NEC 742.4
  vessel 747.81
 branchial cleft NEC 744.49
  cyst 744.42
  fistula 744.41
  persistent 744.41
  sinus (external) (internal) 744.41
 breast 757.6
 broad ligament 752.10
  specified type NEC 752.19
 bronchus 748.3
 bulbar septum 745.0
 bulbus cordis 745.9
  persistent (in left ventricle) 745.8
 bursa 756.9
 canal of Nuck 752.9
 canthus 743.9
 capillary NEC (*see also* Anomaly, peripheral
   vascular system) 747.60
 cardiac 746.9
  septal closure 745.9
   acquired 429.71
  valve NEC 746.9
   pulmonary 746.00
   specified type NEC 746.89
 cardiovascular system 746.9
  complicating pregnancy, childbirth, or
    puerperium 648.5 ☑
 carpus 755.50
 cartilage, trachea 748.3
 cartilaginous 756.9
 caruncle, lacrimal, lachrymal 743.9
 cascade stomach 750.7
 cauda equina 742.59
 cecum 751.5
 cerebral (*see also* Anomaly, brain vessels)
   747.81
 cerebrovascular system 747.81
 cervix (uterus) 752.40
  with doubling of vagina and uterus
    752.2
  in pregnancy or childbirth 654.6 ☑
   affecting fetus or newborn 763.89
   causing obstructed labor 660.2 ☑
    affecting fetus or newborn 763.1
 Chédiak-Higashi (-Steinbrinck) (congenital
   gigantism of peroxidase granules)
   288.2
 cheek 744.9
 chest (wall) 756.3
 chin 744.9
  specified type NEC 744.89
 chordae tendineae 746.9
 choroid 743.9
  plexus 742.9
 chromosomes, chromosomal 758.9
  13 (13-15) 758.1
  18 (16-18) 758.2
  21 or 22 758.0
  autosomes NEC (*see also* Abnormal, au-
    tosomes) 758.5
   deletion 758.39
  Christchurch 758.39
  D₁ 758.1
  E₃ 758.2
  G 758.0
  mitochondrial 758.9
  mosaics 758.89
  sex 758.81
   complement, XO 758.6
   complement, XXX 758.81
   complement, XXY 758.7

Anomaly, anomalous — *continued*
 chromosomes, chromosomal — *continued*
  sex — *continued*
   complement, XYY 758.81
   gonadal dysgenesis 758.6
   Klinefelter's 758.7
   Turner's 758.6
   trisomy 21 758.0
 cilia 743.9
 circulatory system 747.9
  specified type NEC 747.89
 clavicle 755.51
 clitoris 752.40
 coccyx 756.10
 colon 751.5
 common duct 751.60
 communication
  coronary artery 746.85
  left ventricle with right atrium 745.4
 concha (ear) 744.3
 connection
  renal vessels with kidney 747.62
  total pulmonary venous 747.41
 connective tissue 756.9
  specified type NEC 756.89
 cornea 743.9
  shape 743.41
  size 743.41
  specified type NEC 743.49
 coronary
  artery 746.85
  vein 746.89
 cranium — *see* Anomaly, skull
 cricoid cartilage 748.3
 cushion, endocardial 745.60
  specified type NEC 745.69
 cystic duct 751.60
 dental arch 524.20
  specified NEC 524.29
 dental arch relationship 524.20
  angle's class I 524.21
  angle's class II 524.22
  angle's class III 524.23
  articulation
   anterior 524.27
   posterior 524.27
   reverse 524.27
  disto-occlusion 524.22
   division I 524.22
   division II 524.22
  excessive horizontal overlap 524.26
  interarch distance (excessive) (inade-
    quate) 524.28
  mesio-occlusion 524.23
  neutro-occlusion 524.21
  open
   anterior occlusal relationship 524.24
   posterior occlusal relationship 524.25
  specified NEC 524.29
 dentition 520.6
 dentofacial NEC 524.9
  functional 524.50
  specified type NEC 524.89
 dermatoglyphic 757.2
 Descemet's membrane 743.9
  specified type NEC 743.49
 development
  cervix 752.40
  vagina 752.40
  vulva 752.40
 diaphragm, diaphragmatic (apertures) NEC
   756.6
 digestive organ(s) or system 751.9
  lower 751.5
  specified type NEC 751.8
  upper 750.9
 distribution, coronary artery 746.85
 ductus
  arteriosus 747.0
  Botalli 747.0
 duodenum 751.5
 dura 742.9
  brain 742.4
  spinal cord 742.59
 ear 744.3

Anomaly, anomalous — *continued*
 ear — *continued*
  causing impairment of hearing 744.00
   specified type NEC 744.09
  external 744.3
   causing impairment of hearing
     744.02
   specified type NEC 744.29
  inner (causing impairment of hearing)
    744.05
  middle, except ossicles (causing impair-
    ment of hearing) 744.03
   ossicles 744.04
  ossicles 744.04
  prominent auricle 744.29
  specified type NEC 744.29
   with hearing impairment 744.09
 Ebstein's (heart) 746.2
  tricuspid valve 746.2
 ectodermal 757.9
 Eisenmenger's (ventricular septal defect)
   745.4
 ejaculatory duct 752.9
  specified type NEC 752.89
 elbow (joint) 755.50
 endocardial cushion 745.60
  specified type NEC 745.69
 endocrine gland NEC 759.2
 epididymis 752.9
 epiglottis 748.3
 esophagus 750.9
  specified type NEC 750.4
 Eustachian tube 744.3
  specified type NEC 744.24
 eye (any part) 743.9
  adnexa 743.9
   specified type NEC 743.69
  anophthalmos 743.00
  anterior
   chamber and related structures 743.9
    angle 743.9
     specified type NEC 743.44
    specified type NEC 743.44
   segment 743.9
    combined 743.48
    multiple 743.48
    specified type NEC 743.49
  cataract (*see also* Cataract) 743.30
  glaucoma (*see also* Buphthalmia) 743.20
  lid 743.9
   specified type NEC 743.63
  microphthalmos (*see also* Microphthal-
    mos) 743.10
  posterior segment 743.9
   specified type NEC 743.59
   vascular 743.58
   vitreous 743.9
    specified type NEC 743.51
  ptosis (eyelid) 743.61
  retina 743.9
   specified type NEC 743.59
  sclera 743.9
   specified type NEC 743.47
  specified type NEC 743.8
 eyebrow 744.89
 eyelid 743.9
  specified type NEC 743.63
 face (any part) 744.9
  bone(s) 756.0
  specified type NEC 744.89
 fallopian tube 752.10
  specified type NEC 752.19
 fascia 756.9
  specified type NEC 756.89
 femur 755.60
 fibula 755.60
 finger 755.50
  supernumerary 755.01
  webbed (*see also* Syndactylism, fingers)
    755.11
 fixation, intestine 751.4
 flexion (joint) 755.9
  hip or thigh (*see also* Dislocation, hip,
    congenital) 754.30
 folds, heart 746.9
 foot 755.67

Anomaly, anomalous — *continued*
 foramen
  Botalli 745.5
  ovale 745.5
 forearm 755.50
 forehead (*see also* Anomaly, skull) 756.0
 form, teeth 520.2
 fovea centralis 743.9
 frontal bone (*see also* Anomaly, skull) 756.0
 gallbladder 751.60
 Gartner's duct 752.41
 gastrointestinal tract 751.9
  specified type NEC 751.8
  vessel 747.61
 genitalia, genital organ(s) or system
  female 752.9
   external 752.40
    specified type NEC 752.49
   internal NEC 752.9
  male (external and internal) 752.9
   epispadias 752.62
   hidden penis 752.65
   hydrocele, congenital 778.6
   hypospadias 752.61
   micropenis 752.64
   testis, undescended 752.51
    retractile 752.52
  specified type NEC 752.89
 genitourinary NEC 752.9
 Gerbode 745.4
 globe (eye) 743.9
 glottis 748.3
 granulation or granulocyte, genetic 288.2
  constitutional 288.2
  leukocyte 288.2
 gum 750.9
 gyri 742.9
 hair 757.9
  specified type NEC 757.4
 hand 755.50
 hard tissue formation in pulp 522.3
 head (*see also* Anomaly, skull) 756.0
 heart 746.9
  auricle 746.9
  bands 746.9
  fibroelastosis cordis 425.3
  folds 746.9
  malposition 746.87
  maternal, affecting fetus or newborn
    760.3
  obstructive NEC 746.84
  patent ductus arteriosus (Botalli) 747.0
  septum 745.9
   acquired 429.71
   aortic 745.0
   aorticopulmonary 745.0
   atrial 745.5
   auricular 745.5
   between aorta and pulmonary artery
     745.0
   endocardial cushion type 745.60
    specified type NEC 745.69
   interatrial 745.5
   interventricular 745.4
    with pulmonary stenosis or atre-
      sia, dextraposition of aor-
      ta, and hypertrophy of
      right ventricle 745.2
    acquired 429.71
   specified type NEC 745.8
   ventricular 745.4
    with pulmonary stenosis or atre-
      sia, dextraposition of aor-
      ta, and hypertrophy of
      right ventricle 745.2
    acquired 429.71
  specified type NEC 746.89
  tetralogy of Fallot 745.2
  valve NEC 746.9
   aortic 746.9
    atresia 746.89
    bicuspid valve 746.4
    insufficiency 746.4
    specified type NEC 746.89
    stenosis 746.3
    subaortic 746.81

☑ **Additional Digit Required — Refer to the Tabular List for Digit Selection**   ▽ **Subterms under main terms may continue to next column or page**

Anomaly, anomalous — *continued*
  heart — *continued*
    valve — *continued*
      aortic — *continued*
        stenosis — *continued*
          supravalvular 747.22
      mitral 746.9
        atresia 746.89
        insufficiency 746.6
        specified type NEC 746.89
        stenosis 746.5
      pulmonary 746.00
        atresia 746.01
        insufficiency 746.09
        stenosis 746.02
          infundibular 746.83
          subvalvular 746.83
      tricuspid 746.9
        atresia 746.1
        stenosis 746.1
    ventricle 746.9
  heel 755.67
  Hegglin's 288.2
  hemianencephaly 740.0
  hemicephaly 740.0
  hemicrania 740.0
  hepatic duct 751.60
  hip (joint) 755.63
  hourglass
    bladder 753.8
    gallbladder 751.69
    stomach 750.7
  humerus 755.50
  hymen 752.40
  hypersegmentation of neutrophils, hereditary 288.2
  hypophyseal 759.2
  ileocecal (coil) (valve) 751.5
  ileum (intestine) 751.5
  ilium 755.60
  integument 757.9
    specified type NEC 757.8
  interarch distance (excessive) (inadequate) 524.28
  intervertebral cartilage or disc 756.10
  intestine (large) (small) 751.5
    fixational type 751.4
  iris 743.9
    specified type NEC 743.46
  ischium 755.60
  jaw NEC 524.9
    closure 524.51
    size (major) NEC 524.00
    specified type NEC 524.89
  jaw-cranial base relationship 524.10
    specified NEC 524.19
  jejunum 751.5
  joint 755.9
    hip
      dislocation (*see also* Dislocation, hip, congenital) 754.30
      predislocation (*see also* Subluxation, congenital, hip) 754.32
      preluxation (*see also* Subluxation, congenital, hip) 754.32
      subluxation (*see also* Subluxation, congenital, hip) 754.32
    lumbosacral 756.10
      spondylolisthesis 756.12
      spondylosis 756.11
    multiple arthrogryposis 754.89
    sacroiliac 755.69
  Jordan's 288.2
  kidney(s) (calyx) (pelvis) 753.9
    vessel 747.62
  Klippel-Feil (brevicollis) 756.16
  knee (joint) 755.64
  labium (majus) (minus) 752.40
  labyrinth, membranous (causing impairment of hearing) 744.05
  lacrimal
    apparatus, duct or passage 743.9
      specified type NEC 743.65
    gland 743.9
      specified type NEC 743.64
  Langdon Down (mongolism) 758.0

Anomaly, anomalous — *continued*
  larynx, laryngeal (muscle) 748.3
    web, webbed 748.2
  leg (lower) (upper) 755.60
    reduction NEC (*see also* Deformity, reduction, lower limb) 755.30
  lens 743.9
    shape 743.36
    specified type NEC 743.39
  leukocytes, genetic 288.2
    granulation (constitutional) 288.2
  lid (fold) 743.9
  ligament 756.9
    broad 752.10
    round 752.9
  limb, except reduction deformity 755.9
    lower 755.60
      reduction deformity (*see also* Deformity, reduction, lower limb) 755.30
      specified type NEC 755.69
    upper 755.50
      reduction deformity (*see also* Deformity, reduction, upper limb) 755.20
      specified type NEC 755.59
  lip 750.9
    harelip (*see also* Cleft, lip) 749.10
    specified type NEC 750.26
  liver (duct) 751.60
    atresia 751.69
  lower extremity 755.60
    vessel 747.64
  lumbosacral (joint) (region) 756.10
  lung (fissure) (lobe) NEC 748.60
    agenesis 748.5
    specified type NEC 748.69
  lymphatic system 759.9
  Madelung's (radius) 755.54
  mandible 524.9
    size NEC 524.00
  maxilla 524.9
    size NEC 524.00
  May (-Hegglin) 288.2
  meatus urinarius 753.9
    specified type NEC 753.8
  meningeal bands or folds, constriction of 742.8
  meninges 742.9
    brain 742.4
    spinal 742.59
  meningocele (*see also* Spina bifida) 741.9 ☑
    acquired 349.2
  mesentery 751.9
  metacarpus 755.50
  metatarsus 755.67
  middle ear, except ossicles (causing impairment of hearing) 744.03
    ossicles 744.04
  mitral (leaflets) (valve) 746.9
    atresia 746.89
    insufficiency 746.6
    specified type NEC 746.89
    stenosis 746.5
  mouth 750.9
    specified type NEC 750.26
  multiple NEC 759.7
    specified type NEC 759.89
  muscle 756.9
    eye 743.9
      specified type NEC 743.69
    specified type NEC 756.89
  musculoskeletal system, except limbs 756.9
    specified type NEC 756.9
  nail 757.9
    specified type NEC 757.5
  narrowness, eyelid 743.62
  nasal sinus or septum 748.1
  neck (any part) 744.9
    specified type NEC 744.89
  nerve 742.9
    acoustic 742.9
      specified type NEC 742.8
    optic 742.9
      specified type NEC 742.8
    specified type NEC 742.8

Anomaly, anomalous — *continued*
  nervous system NEC 742.9
    brain 742.9
      specified type NEC 742.4
    specified type NEC 742.8
  neurological 742.9
  nipple 757.6
  nonteratogenic NEC 754.89
  nose, nasal (bone) (cartilage) (septum) (sinus) 748.1
  ocular muscle 743.9
  omphalomesenteric duct 751.0
  opening, pulmonary veins 747.49
  optic
    disc 743.9
      specified type NEC 743.57
    nerve 742.9
  opticociliary vessels 743.9
  orbit (eye) 743.9
    specified type NEC 743.66
  organ
    of Corti (causing impairment of hearing) 744.05
    or site 759.9
      specified type NEC 759.89
  origin
    both great arteries from same ventricle 745.11
    coronary artery 746.85
    innominate artery 747.69
    left coronary artery from pulmonary artery 746.85
    pulmonary artery 747.3
    renal vessels 747.62
    subclavian artery (left) (right) 747.21
  osseous meatus (ear) 744.03
  ovary 752.0
  oviduct 752.10
  palate (hard) (soft) 750.9
    cleft (*see also* Cleft, palate) 749.00
  pancreas (duct) 751.7
  papillary muscles 746.9
  parathyroid gland 759.2
  paraurethral ducts 753.9
  parotid (gland) 750.9
  patella 755.64
  Pelger-Huët (hereditary hyposegmentation) 288.2
  pelvic girdle 755.60
    specified type NEC 755.69
  pelvis (bony) 755.60
    complicating delivery 653.0 ☑
    rachitic 268.1
      fetal 756.4
  penis (glans) 752.69
  pericardium 746.89
  peripheral vascular system NEC 747.60
    gastrointestinal 747.61
    lower limb 747.64
    renal 747.62
    specified site NEC 747.69
    spinal 747.82
    upper limb 747.63
  Peter's 743.44
  pharynx 750.9
    branchial cleft 744.41
    specified type NEC 750.29
  Pierre Robin 756.0
  pigmentation 709.00
    congenital 757.33
    specified NEC 709.09
  pituitary (gland) 759.2
  pleural folds 748.8
  portal vein 747.40
  position tooth, teeth 524.30
    crowding 524.31
    displacement 524.30
      horizontal 524.33
      vertical 524.34
    distance
      interocclusal
        excessive 524.37
        insufficient 524.36
    excessive spacing 524.32
    rotation 524.35
    specified NEC 524.39

Anomaly, anomalous — *continued*
  preauricular sinus 744.46
  prepuce 752.9
  prostate 752.9
  pulmonary 748.60
    artery 747.3
    circulation 747.3
    specified type NEC 748.69
    valve 746.00
      atresia 746.01
      insufficiency 746.09
      specified type NEC 746.09
      stenosis 746.02
        infundibular 746.83
        subvalvular 746.83
    vein 747.40
    venous
      connection 747.49
        partial 747.42
        total 747.41
      return 747.49
        partial 747.42
        total (TAPVR) (complete) (subdiaphragmatic) (supradiaphragmatic) 747.41
  pupil 743.9
  pylorus 750.9
    hypertrophy 750.5
    stenosis 750.5
  rachitic, fetal 756.4
  radius 755.50
  rectovaginal (septum) 752.40
  rectum 751.5
  refraction 367.9
  renal 753.9
    vessel 747.62
  respiratory system 748.9
    specified type NEC 748.8
  rib 756.3
    cervical 756.2
  Rieger's 743.44
  rings, trachea 748.3
  rotation (*see also* Malrotation)
    hip or thigh (*see also* Subluxation, congenital, hip) 754.32
  round ligament 752.9
  sacroiliac (joint) 755.69
  sacrum 756.10
  saddle
    back 754.2
    nose 754.0
      syphilitic 090.5
  salivary gland or duct 750.9
    specified type NEC 750.26
  scapula 755.50
  sclera 743.9
    specified type NEC 743.47
  scrotum 752.9
  sebaceous gland 757.9
  seminal duct or tract 752.9
  sense organs 742.9
    specified type NEC 742.8
  septum
    heart — *see* Anomaly, heart, septum
    nasal 748.1
  sex chromosomes NEC (*see also* Anomaly, chromosomes) 758.81
  shoulder (girdle) (joint) 755.50
    specified type NEC 755.59
  sigmoid (flexure) 751.5
  sinus of Valsalva 747.29
  site NEC 759.9
  skeleton generalized NEC 756.50
  skin (appendage) 757.9
    specified type NEC 757.39
  skull (bone) 756.0
    with
      anencephalus 740.0
      encephalocele 742.0
      hydrocephalus 742.3
        with spina bifida (*see also* Spina bifida) 741.0 ☑
      microcephalus 742.1
  specified type NEC
    adrenal (gland) 759.1

Anomaly, anomalous — *continued*
  specified type — *continued*
    alimentary tract (complete) (partial)
     751.8
     lower 751.5
     upper 750.8
    ankle 755.69
    anus, anal (canal) 751.5
    aorta, aortic 747.29
     arch 747.21
    appendix 751.5
    arm 755.59
    artery (peripheral) NEC (*see also*
     Anomaly, peripheral vascular
     system) 747.60
     brain 747.81
     coronary 746.85
     eye 743.58
     pulmonary 747.3
     retinal 743.58
     umbilical 747.5
    auditory canal 744.29
     causing impairment of hearing
      744.02
    bile duct or passage 751.69
    bladder 753.8
     neck 753.8
    bone(s) 756.9
     arm 755.59
     face 756.0
     leg 755.69
     pelvic girdle 755.69
     shoulder girdle 755.59
     skull 756.0
      with
       anencephalus 740.0
       encephalocele 742.0
       hydrocephalus 742.3
        with spina bifida (*see also*
         Spina bifida)
         741.0 ☑
       microcephalus 742.1
    brain 742.4
    breast 757.6
    broad ligament 752.19
    bronchus 748.3
    canal of Nuck 752.89
    cardiac septal closure 745.8
    carpus 755.59
    cartilaginous 756.9
    cecum 751.5
    cervix 752.49
    chest (wall) 756.3
    chin 744.89
    ciliary body 743.46
    circulatory system 747.89
    clavicle 755.51
    clitoris 752.49
    coccyx 756.19
    colon 751.5
    common duct 751.69
    connective tissue 756.89
    cricoid cartilage 748.3
    cystic duct 751.69
    diaphragm 756.6
    digestive organ(s) or tract 751.8
     lower 751.5
     upper 750.8
    duodenum 751.5
    ear 744.29
     auricle 744.29
      causing impairment of hearing
       744.02
     causing impairment of hearing
      744.09
     inner (causing impairment of hear-
      ing) 744.05
     middle, except ossicles 744.03
      ossicles 744.04
    ejaculatory duct 752.89
    endocrine 759.2
    epiglottis 748.3
    esophagus 750.4
    Eustachian tube 744.24
    eye 743.8
     lid 743.63

Anomaly, anomalous — *continued*
  specified type — *continued*
    eye — *continued*
     muscle 743.69
    face 744.89
     bone(s) 756.0
    fallopian tube 752.19
    fascia 756.89
    femur 755.69
    fibula 755.69
    finger 755.59
    foot 755.67
    fovea centralis 743.55
    gallbladder 751.69
    Gartner's duct 752.89
    gastrointestinal tract 751.8
    genitalia, genital organ(s)
     female 752.89
      external 752.49
      internal NEC 752.89
     male 752.89
      penis 752.69
      scrotal transposition 752.81
    genitourinary tract NEC 752.89
    glottis 748.3
    hair 757.4
    hand 755.59
    heart 746.89
     valve NEC 746.89
      pulmonary 746.09
    hepatic duct 751.69
    hydatid of Morgagni 752.89
    hymen 752.49
    integument 757.8
    intestine (large) (small) 751.5
     fixational type 751.4
    iris 743.46
    jejunum 751.5
    joint 755.8
    kidney 753.3
    knee 755.64
    labium (majus) (minus) 752.49
    labyrinth, membranous 744.05
    larynx 748.3
    leg 755.69
    lens 743.39
    limb, except reduction deformity 755.8
     lower 755.69
      reduction deformity (*see also* De-
       formity, reduction, lower
       limb) 755.30
     upper 755.59
      reduction deformity (*see also* De-
       formity, reduction, upper
       limb) 755.20
    lip 750.26
    liver 751.69
    lung (fissure) (lobe) 748.69
    meatus urinarius 753.8
    metacarpus 755.59
    mouth 750.26
    Müllerian   ●
     cervix 752.49   ●
     uterus 752.39   ●
     vagina 752.49   ●
    muscle 756.89
     eye 743.69
    musculoskeletal system, except limbs
     756.9
    nail 757.5
    neck 744.89
    nerve 742.8
     acoustic 742.8
     optic 742.8
    nervous system 742.8
    nipple 757.6
    nose 748.1
    organ NEC 759.89
     of Corti 744.05
    osseous meatus (ear) 744.03
    ovary 752.0
    oviduct 752.19
    pancreas 751.7
    parathyroid 759.2
    patella 755.64
    pelvic girdle 755.69

Anomaly, anomalous — *continued*
  specified type — *continued*
    penis 752.69
    pericardium 746.89
    peripheral vascular system NEC (*see also*
     Anomaly, peripheral vascular
     system) 747.60
    pharynx 750.29
    pituitary 759.2
    prostate 752.89
    radius 755.59
    rectum 751.5
    respiratory system 748.8
    rib 756.3
    round ligament 752.89
    sacrum 756.19
    salivary duct or gland 750.26
    scapula 755.59
    sclera 743.47
    scrotum 752.89
     transposition 752.81
    seminal duct or tract 752.89
    shoulder girdle 755.59
    site NEC 759.89
    skin 757.39
    skull (bone(s)) 756.0
     with
      anencephalus 740.0
      encephalocele 742.0
      hydrocephalus 742.3
       with spina bifida (*see also*
        Spina bifida) 741.0 ☑
      microcephalus 742.1
    specified organ or site NEC 759.89
    spermatic cord 752.89
    spinal cord 742.59
    spine 756.19
    spleen 759.0
    sternum 756.3
    stomach 750.7
    tarsus 755.67
    tendon 756.89
    testis 752.89
    thorax (wall) 756.3
    thymus 759.2
    thyroid (gland) 759.2
     cartilage 748.3
    tibia 755.69
    toe 755.66
    tongue 750.19
    trachea (cartilage) 748.3
    ulna 755.59
    urachus 753.7
    ureter 753.4
     obstructive 753.29
    urethra 753.8
     obstructive 753.6
    urinary tract 753.8
    uterus ▶(Müllerian)◀ 752.39   ▲
    uvula 750.26
    vagina 752.49
    vascular NEC (*see also* Anomaly, periph-
     eral vascular system) 747.60
     brain 747.81
    vas deferens 752.89
    vein(s) (peripheral) NEC (*see also*
     Anomaly, peripheral vascular
     system) 747.60
     brain 747.81
     great 747.49
     portal 747.49
     pulmonary 747.49
    vena cava (inferior) (superior) 747.49
    vertebra 756.19
    vulva 752.49
  spermatic cord 752.9
  spine, spinal 756.10
    column 756.10
    cord 742.9
     meningocele (*see also* Spina bifida)
      741.9 ☑
     specified type NEC 742.59
     spina bifida (*see also* Spina bifida)
      741.9 ☑
     vessel 747.82
    meninges 742.59

Anomaly, anomalous — *continued*
  spine, spinal — *continued*
    nerve root 742.9
  spleen 759.0
  Sprengel's 755.52
  sternum 756.3
  stomach 750.9
    specified type NEC 750.7
  submaxillary gland 750.9
  superior vena cava 747.40
  talipes — *see* Talipes
  tarsus 755.67
    with complete absence of distal ele-
     ments 755.31
  teeth, tooth NEC 520.9
    position 524.30
     crowding 524.31
     displacement 524.30
      horizontal 524.33
      vertical 524.34
     distance
      interocclusal
       excessive 524.37
       insufficient 524.36
     excessive spacing 524.32
     rotation 524.35
     specified NEC 524.39
     spacing 524.30
  tendon 756.9
    specified type NEC 756.89
  termination
    coronary artery 746.85
  testis 752.9
  thebesian valve 746.9
  thigh 755.60
    flexion (*see also* Subluxation, congenital,
     hip) 754.32
  thorax (wall) 756.3
  throat 750.9
  thumb 755.50
    supernumerary 755.01
  thymus gland 759.2
  thyroid (gland) 759.2
    cartilage 748.3
  tibia 755.60
    saber 090.5
  toe 755.66
    supernumerary 755.02
    webbed (*see also* Syndactylism, toes)
     755.13
  tongue 750.10
    specified type NEC 750.19
  trachea, tracheal 748.3
    cartilage 748.3
    rings 748.3
  tragus 744.3
  transverse aortic arch 747.21
  trichromata 368.59
  trichromatopsia 368.59
  tricuspid (leaflet) (valve) 746.9
    atresia 746.1
    Ebstein's 746.2
    specified type NEC 746.89
    stenosis 746.1
  trunk 759.9
  Uhl's (hypoplasia of myocardium, right
    ventricle) 746.84
  ulna 755.50
  umbilicus 759.9
    artery 747.5
  union, trachea with larynx 748.3
  unspecified site 759.9
  upper extremity 755.50
    vessel 747.63
  urachus 753.7
    specified type NEC 753.7
  ureter 753.9
    obstructive 753.20
    specified type NEC 753.4
     obstructive 753.29
  urethra (valve) 753.9
    obstructive 753.6
    specified type NEC 753.8
  urinary tract or system (any part, except
    urachus) 753.9
    specified type NEC 753.8

☑ **Additional Digit Required** — Refer to the Tabular List for Digit Selection   ▽ **Subterms under main terms may continue to next column or page**

24 — Volume 2 · October 2010   ▶◀ **Revised Text**   ● **New Line**   ▲ **Revised Code**   2011 ICD-9-CM

Anomaly, anomalous — *continued*
  urinary tract or system — *continued*
    urachus 753.7
    uterus 752.39 ▲
      with only one functioning horn
        752.33 ▲
      in pregnancy or childbirth 654.0 ☑
        affecting fetus or newborn 763.89
        causing obstructed labor 660.2 ☑
          affecting fetus or newborn 763.1
    uvula 750.9
    vagina 752.40
    valleculae 748.3
    valve (heart) NEC 746.9
      formation, ureter 753.29
      pulmonary 746.00
      specified type NEC 746.89
    vascular NEC (*see also* Anomaly, peripheral
      vascular system) 747.60
      ring 747.21
    vas deferens 752.9
    vein(s) (peripheral) NEC (*see also* Anomaly,
      peripheral vascular system) 747.60
      brain 747.81
      cerebral 747.81
      coronary 746.89
      great 747.40
        specified type NEC 747.49
      portal 747.40
      pulmonary 747.40
      retina 747.40
    vena cava (inferior) (superior) 747.40
    venous — *see* Anomaly, vein
    venous return (pulmonary) 747.49
      partial 747.42
      total 747.41
    ventricle, ventricular (heart) 746.9
      bands 746.9
      folds 746.9
      septa 745.4
    vertebra 756.10
    vesicourethral orifice 753.9
    vessels NEC (*see also* Anomaly, peripheral
      vascular system) 747.60
      optic papilla 743.9
    vitelline duct 751.0
    vitreous humor 743.9
      specified type NEC 743.51
    vulva 752.40
    wrist (joint) 755.50
Anomia 784.69
Anonychia 757.5
  acquired 703.8
Anophthalmos, anophthalmus (clinical)
  (congenital) (globe) 743.00
  acquired V45.78
Anopsia (altitudinal) (quadrant) 368.46
Anorchia 752.89
Anorchism, anorchidism 752.89
Anorexia 783.0
  hysterical 300.11
  nervosa 307.1
Anosmia — *see also* Disturbance, sensation
  781.1
  hysterical 300.11
  postinfectional 478.9
  psychogenic 306.7
  traumatic 951.8
Anosognosia 780.99
Anosphrasia 781.1
Anosteoplasia 756.50
Anotia 744.09
Anovulatory cycle 628.0
Anoxemia 799.02
  newborn 770.88
Anoxia 799.02
  altitude 993.2
  cerebral 348.1
    with
      abortion — *see* Abortion, by type,
        with specified complication
        NEC
      ectopic pregnancy (*see also* cate-
        gories 633.0–633.9) 639.8
      molar pregnancy (*see also* categories
        630–632) 639.8

Anoxia — *continued*
  cerebral — *continued*
    complicating
      delivery (cesarean) (instrumental)
        669.4 ☑
      ectopic or molar pregnancy 639.8
      obstetric anesthesia or sedation
        668.2 ☑
    during or resulting from a procedure
      997.01
    following
      abortion 639.8
      ectopic or molar pregnancy 639.8
    newborn (*see also* Distress, fetal, liveborn
      infant) 770.88
  due to drowning 994.1
  fetal, affecting newborn 770.88
  heart — *see* Insufficiency, coronary
  high altitude 993.2
  intrauterine
    fetal death (before onset of labor) 768.0
      during labor 768.1
    liveborn infant — *see* Distress, fetal,
      liveborn infant
  myocardial — *see* Insufficiency, coronary
  newborn 768.9
    mild or moderate 768.6
    severe 768.5
  pathological 799.02
Anteflexion — *see* Anteversion
Antenatal
  care, normal pregnancy V22.1
    first V22.0
  sampling
    chorionic villus V28.89
  screening of mother (for) V28.9
    based on amniocentesis NEC V28.2
      chromosomal anomalies V28.0
      raised alphafetoprotein levels V28.1
    chromosomal anomalies V28.0
    fetal growth retardation using ulatrason-
      ics V28.4
    genomic V28.89
    isoimmunization V28.5
    malformations using ulatrasonics V28.3
    proteomic V28.89
    raised alphafetoprotein levels in amniot-
      ic fluid V28.1
    risk
      pre-term labor V28.82
    specified condition NEC V28.89
    Streptococcus B V28.6
  survey
    fetal anatomic V28.81
  testing
    nuchal translucency V28.89
Antepartum — *see* condition
Anterior — *see also* condition
  spinal artery compression syndrome 721.1
Antero-occlusion 524.24
Anteversion
  cervix — *see* Anteversion, uterus
  femur (neck), congenital 755.63
  uterus, uterine (cervix) (postinfectional)
    (postpartal, old) 621.6
    congenital 752.39 ▲
    in pregnancy or childbirth 654.4 ☑
      affecting fetus or newborn 763.89
      causing obstructed labor 660.2 ☑
        affecting fetus or newborn 763.1
Anthracosilicosis (occupational) 500
Anthracosis (lung) (occupational) 500
  lingua 529.3
Anthrax 022.9
  with pneumonia 022.1 [484.5]
  colitis 022.2
  cutaneous 022.0
  gastrointestinal 022.2
  intestinal 022.2
  pulmonary 022.1
  respiratory 022.1
  septicemia 022.3
  specified manifestation NEC 022.8
Anthropoid pelvis 755.69
  with disproportion (fetopelvic) 653.2 ☑
    affecting fetus or newborn 763.1

Anthropoid pelvis — *continued*
  with disproportion — *continued*
    causing obstructed labor 660.1 ☑
    affecting fetus or newborn 763.1
Anthropophobia 300.29
Antibioma, breast 611.0
Antibodies
  maternal (blood group) (*see also* Incompat-
    ibility) 656.2 ☑
    anti-D, cord blood 656.1 ☑
      fetus or newborn 773.0
Antibody deficiency syndrome
  agammaglobulinemic 279.00
  congenital 279.04
  hypogammaglobulinemic 279.00
Anticoagulant, intrinsic, circulating, causing
  hemorrhagic disorder — *see also* Circu-
    lating anticoagulants 286.5
Antimongolism syndrome 758.39
Antimonial cholera 985.4
Antisocial personality 301.7
Antithrombinemia — *see also* Circulating an-
  ticoagulants 286.5
Antithromboplastinemia — *see also* Circulat-
  ing anticoagulants 286.5
Antithromboplastinogenemia — *see also*
  Circulating anticoagulants 286.5
Antitoxin complication or reaction — *see*
  Complications, vaccination
Anton (-Babinski) syndrome (hemiasomatog-
  nosia) 307.9
Antritis (chronic) 473.0
  maxilla 473.0
    acute 461.0
  stomach 535.4 ☑
Antrum, antral — *see* condition
Anuria 788.5
  with
    abortion — *see* Abortion, by type, with
      renal failure
    ectopic pregnancy (*see also* categories
      633.0–633.9) 639.3
    molar pregnancy (*see also* categories
      630–632) 639.3
  calculus (impacted) (recurrent) 592.9
    kidney 592.0
    ureter 592.1
  congenital 753.3
  due to a procedure 997.5
  following
    abortion 639.3
    ectopic or molar pregnancy 639.3
  newborn 753.3
  postrenal 593.4
  puerperal, postpartum, childbirth 669.3 ☑
  specified as due to a procedure 997.5
  sulfonamide
    correct substance properly administered
      788.5
    overdose or wrong substance given or
      taken 961.0
  traumatic (following crushing) 958.5
Anus, anal — *see also* condition
  high risk human papillomavirus (HPV) DNA
    test positive 796.75
  low risk human papillomavirus (HPV) DNA
    test positive 796.79
Anusitis 569.49
Anxiety (neurosis) (reaction) (state) 300.00
  alcohol-induced 291.89
  depression 300.4
  drug-induced 292.89
  due to or associated with physical condition
    293.84
  generalized 300.02
  hysteria 300.20
  in
    acute stress reaction 308.0
    transient adjustment reaction 309.24
  panic type 300.01
  separation, abnormal 309.21
  syndrome (organic) (transient) 293.84
Aorta, aortic — *see* condition
Aortectasia — *see also* Ectasia, aortic
  447.70 ▲
  with aneurysm 441.9 ●

Aortitis (nonsyphilitic) 447.6
  arteriosclerotic 440.0
  calcific 447.6
  Döhle-Heller 093.1
  luetic 093.1
  rheumatic (*see also* Endocarditis, acute,
    rheumatic) 391.1
  rheumatoid — *see* Arthritis, rheumatoid
  specific 093.1
  syphilitic 093.1
    congenital 090.5
Apathetic 799.25
  thyroid storm (*see also* Thyrotoxicosis)
    242.9 ☑
Apathy 799.25
Apepsia 536.8
  achlorhydric 536.0
  psychogenic 306.4
Aperistalsis, esophagus 530.0
Apert-Gallais syndrome (adrenogenital) 255.2
Apertognathia 524.20
Apert's syndrome (acrocephalosyndactyly)
  755.55
Aphagia 787.20
  psychogenic 307.1
Aphakia (acquired) (bilateral) (postoperative)
  (unilateral) 379.31
  congenital 743.35
Aphalangia (congenital) 755.4
  lower limb (complete) (intercalary) (partial)
    (terminal) 755.39
    meaning all digits (complete) (partial)
      755.31
    transverse 755.31
  upper limb (complete) (intercalary) (partial)
    (terminal) 755.29
    meaning all digits (complete) (partial)
      755.21
    transverse 755.21
Aphasia (amnestic) (ataxic) (auditory) (Broca's)
  (choreatic) (classic) (expressive) (global)
  (ideational) (ideokinetic) (ideomotor)
  (jargon) (motor) (nominal) (receptive)
  (semantic) (sensory) (syntactic) (verbal)
  (visual) (Wernicke's) 784.3
  developmental 315.31
  syphilis, tertiary 094.89
  uremic — *see* Uremia
Aphemia 784.3
  uremic — *see* Uremia
Aphonia 784.41
  clericorum 784.49
  hysterical 300.11
  organic 784.41
  psychogenic 306.1
Aphthae, aphthous — *see also* condition
  Bednar's 528.2
  cachectic 529.0
  epizootic 078.4
  fever 078.4
  oral 528.2
  stomatitis 528.2
  thrush 112.0
  ulcer (oral) (recurrent) 528.2
    genital organ(s) NEC
      female 616.50
      male 608.89
    larynx 478.79
Apical — *see* condition
Apical ballooning syndrome 429.83
Aplasia — *see also* Agenesis
  alveolar process (acquired) 525.8
    congenital 750.26
  aorta (congenital) 747.22
  aortic valve (congenital) 746.89
  axialis extracorticalis (congenital) 330.0
  bone marrow (myeloid) 284.9
    acquired (secondary) 284.89
    congenital 284.01
    idiopathic 284.9
  brain 740.0
    specified part 742.2
  breast 757.6
  bronchus 748.3
  cementum 520.4
  cerebellar 742.2

☑ **Additional Digit Required — Refer to the Tabular List for Digit Selection**

◥ **Subterms under main terms may continue to next column or page**

Aplasia — see also Agenesis — continued
  congenital (pure) red cell 284.01
  corpus callosum 742.2
  erythrocyte 284.81
    congenital 284.01
  extracortical axial 330.0
  eye (congenital) 743.00
  fovea centralis (congenital) 743.55
  germinal (cell) 606.0
  iris 743.45
  labyrinth, membranous 744.05
  limb (congenital) 755.4
    lower NEC 755.30
    upper NEC 755.20
  lung (bilateral) (congenital) (unilateral)
    748.5
  nervous system NEC 742.8
  nuclear 742.8
  ovary 752.0
  Pelizaeus-Merzbacher 330.0
  prostate (congenital) 752.89
  red cell (with thymoma) (adult) 284.81
    acquired (secondary) 284.81
    congenital 284.01
    hereditary 284.01
    of infants 284.01
    primary 284.01
    pure 284.01
  round ligament (congenital) 752.89
  salivary gland 750.21
  skin (congenital) 757.39
  spinal cord 742.59
  spleen 759.0
  testis (congenital) 752.89
  thymic, with immunodeficiency 279.2
  thyroid 243
  uterus 752.39   ▲
  ventral horn cell 742.59
Apleuria 756.3
Apnea, apneic (spells) 786.03
  newborn, neonatorum 770.81
    essential 770.81
    obstructive 770.82
    primary 770.81
    sleep 770.81
    specified NEC 770.82
  psychogenic 306.1
  sleep, unspecified 780.57
    with
      hypersomnia, unspecified 780.53
      hyposomnia, unspecified 780.51
      insomnia, unspecified 780.51
      sleep disturbance 780.57
    central, in conditions classified else-
      where 327.27
    obstructive (adult) (pediatric) 327.23
    organic 327.20
      other 327.29
    primary central 327.21
Apneumatosis newborn 770.4
Apodia 755.31
Aponeurosis 726.90
Apophysitis (bone) — see also Osteochondro-
    sis 732.9
  calcaneus 732.5
  juvenile 732.6
Apoplectiform convulsions — see also Dis-
    ease, cerebrovascular, acute 436
Apoplexia, apoplexy, apoplectic — see also
    Disease, cerebrovascular, acute 436
  abdominal 569.89
  adrenal 036.3
  attack 436
  basilar (see also Disease, cerebrovascular,
    acute) 436
  brain (see also Disease, cerebrovascular,
    acute) 436
  bulbar (see also Disease, cerebrovascular,
    acute) 436
  capillary (see also Disease, cerebrovascular,
    acute) 436
  cardiac (see also Infarct, myocardium)
    410.9 ☑
  cerebral (see also Disease, cerebrovascular,
    acute) 436

Apoplexia, apoplexy, apoplectic — see also
    Disease, cerebrovascular, acute —
    continued
  chorea (see also Disease, cerebrovascular,
    acute) 436
  congestive (see also Disease, cerebrovascu-
    lar, acute) 436
    newborn 767.4
  embolic (see also Embolism, brain) 434.1 ☑
  fetus 767.0
  fit (see also Disease, cerebrovascular, acute)
    436
  healed or old V12.54
  heart (auricle) (ventricle) (see also Infarct,
    myocardium) 410.9 ☑
  heat 992.0
  hemiplegia (see also Disease, cerebrovascu-
    lar, acute) 436
  hemorrhagic (stroke) (see also Hemorrhage,
    brain) 432.9
  ingravescent (see also Disease, cerebrovas-
    cular, acute) 436
  late effect — see Late effect(s) (of) cere-
    brovascular disease
  lung — see Embolism, pulmonary
  meninges, hemorrhagic (see also Hemor-
    rhage, subarachnoid) 430
  neonatorum 767.0
  newborn 767.0
  pancreatitis 577.0
  placenta 641.2 ☑
  progressive (see also Disease, cerebrovascu-
    lar, acute) 436
  pulmonary (artery) (vein) — see Embolism,
    pulmonary
  sanguineous (see also Disease, cerebrovas-
    cular, acute) 436
  seizure (see also Disease, cerebrovascular,
    acute) 436
  serous (see also Disease, cerebrovascular,
    acute) 436
  spleen 289.59
  stroke (see also Disease, cerebrovascular,
    acute) 436
  thrombotic (see also Thrombosis, brain)
    434.0 ☑
  uremic — see Uremia
  uteroplacental 641.2 ☑
Appendage
  fallopian tube (cyst of Morgagni) 752.11
  intestine (epiploic) 751.5
  preauricular 744.1
  testicular (organ of Morgagni) 752.89
Appendicitis 541
  with
    perforation, peritonitis (generalized), or
      rupture 540.0
      with peritoneal abscess 540.1
    peritoneal abscess 540.1
  acute (catarrhal) (fulminating) (gangrenous)
    (inflammatory) (obstructive) (retroce-
    cal) (suppurative) 540.9
    with
      perforation, peritonitis, or rupture
        540.0
        with peritoneal abscess 540.1
        peritoneal abscess 540.1
  amebic 006.8
  chronic (recurrent) 542
  exacerbation — see Appendicitis, acute
  fulminating — see Appendicitis, acute
  gangrenous — see Appendicitis, acute
  healed (obliterative) 542
  interval 542
  neurogenic 542
  obstructive 542
  pneumococcal 541
  recurrent 542
  relapsing 542
  retrocecal 541
  subacute (adhesive) 542
  subsiding 542
  suppurative — see Appendicitis, acute
  tuberculous (see also Tuberculosis) 014.8 ☑
Appendiclausis 543.9
Appendicolithiasis 543.9

Appendicopathia oxyurica 127.4
Appendix, appendicular — see also condition
  Morgagni (male) 752.89
    fallopian tube 752.11
Appetite
  depraved 307.52
  excessive 783.6
    psychogenic 307.51
  lack or loss (see also Anorexia) 783.0
    nonorganic origin 307.59
  perverted 307.52
    hysterical 300.11
Apprehension, apprehensiveness (abnormal)
    (state) 300.00
  specified type NEC 300.09
Approximal wear 521.10
Approximal wear 521.10
Apraxia (classic) (ideational) (ideokinetic)
    (ideomotor) (motor) 784.69
  oculomotor, congenital 379.51
  verbal 784.69
Aptyalism 527.7
Aqueous misdirection 365.83
Arabicum elephantiasis — see also Infesta-
    tion, filarial 125.9
Arachnidism 989.5
Arachnitis — see Meningitis
Arachnodactyly 759.82
Arachnoidism 989.5
Arachnoiditis (acute) (adhesive) (basic) (brain)
    (cerebrospinal) (chiasmal) (chronic)
    (spinal) — see also Meningitis 322.9
  meningococcal (chronic) 036.0
  syphilitic 094.2
  tuberculous (see also Tuberculosis,
    meninges) 013.0 ☑
Araneism 989.5
Arboencephalitis, Australian 062.4
Arborization block (heart) 426.6
Arbor virus, arbovirus (infection) NEC 066.9
ARC 042
Arches — see condition
Arcuate uterus 752.36   ●
Arcuatus uterus 752.36   ▲
Arcus (cornea)
  juvenilis 743.43
    interfering with vision 743.42
  senilis 371.41
Arc-welders' lung 503
Arc-welders' syndrome (photokeratitis) 370.24
Areflexia 796.1
Areola — see condition
Argentaffinoma (M8241/1) — see also Neo-
    plasm, by site, uncertain behavior
  benign (M8241/0) — see Neoplasm, by site,
    benign
  malignant (M8241/3) — see Neoplasm, by
    site, malignant
  syndrome 259.2
Argentinian hemorrhagic fever 078.7
Arginosuccinicaciduria 270.6
Argonz-Del Castillo syndrome (nonpuerperal
    galactorrhea and amenorrhea) 253.1
**Argyll-Robertson phenomenon, pupil, or
    syndrome** (syphilitic) 094.89
  atypical 379.45
  nonluetic 379.45
  nonsyphilitic 379.45
  reversed 379.45
Argyria, argyriasis NEC 985.8
  conjunctiva 372.55
  cornea 371.16
  from drug or medicinal agent
    correct substance properly administered
      709.09
    overdose or wrong substance given or
      taken 961.2
Arhinencephaly 742.2
Arias-Stella phenomenon 621.30
Ariboflavinosis 266.0
Arizona enteritis 008.1
Arm — see condition
Armenian disease 277.31
Arnold-Chiari obstruction or syndrome —
    see also Spina bifida 741.0 ☑
  type I 348.4
  type II (see also Spina bifida) 741.0 ☑

Arnold-Chiari obstruction or syndrome —
    see also Spina bifida — continued
  type III 742.0
  type IV 742.2
Arousals
  confusional 327.41
Arrest, arrested
  active phase of labor 661.1 ☑
    affecting fetus or newborn 763.7
  any plane in pelvis
    complicating delivery 660.1 ☑
      affecting fetus or newborn 763.1
  bone marrow (see also Anemia, aplastic)
    284.9
  cardiac 427.5
    with
      abortion — see Abortion, by type,
        with specified complication
        NEC
      ectopic pregnancy (see also cate-
        gories 633.0–633.9) 639.8
      molar pregnancy (see also categories
        630–632) 639.8
    complicating
      anesthesia
        correct substance properly admin-
          istered 427.5
        obstetric 668.1 ☑
        overdose or wrong substance
          given 968.4
        specified anesthetic — see
          Table of Drugs and
          Chemicals
      delivery (cesarean) (instrumental)
        669.4 ☑
      ectopic or molar pregnancy 639.8
      surgery (nontherapeutic) (therapeu-
        tic) 997.1
    fetus or newborn 779.85
    following
      abortion 639.8
      ectopic or molar pregnancy 639.8
    personal history, successfully resuscitat-
      ed V12.53
    postoperative (immediate) 997.1
      long-term effect of cardiac surgery
        429.4
  cardiorespiratory (see also Arrest, cardiac)
    427.5
  deep transverse 660.3 ☑
    affecting fetus or newborn 763.1
  development or growth
    bone 733.91
    child 783.40
    fetus 764.9 ☑
      affecting management of pregnancy
        656.5 ☑
    tracheal rings 748.3
  epiphyseal 733.91
  granulopoiesis 288.09
  heart — see Arrest, cardiac
  respiratory 799.1
    newborn 770.87
  sinus 426.6
  transverse (deep) 660.3 ☑
    affecting fetus or newborn 763.1
Arrhenoblastoma (M8630/1)
  benign (M8630/0)
    specified site — see Neoplasm, by site,
      benign
    unspecified site
      female 220
      male 222.0
  malignant (M8630/3)
    specified site — see Neoplasm, by site,
      malignant
    unspecified site
      female 183.0
      male 186.9
  specified site — see Neoplasm, by site, un-
    certain behavior
  unspecified site
    female 236.2
    male 236.4
Arrhinencephaly 742.2

☑ **Additional Digit Required** — Refer to the Tabular List for Digit Selection   ▽ **Subterms under main terms may continue to next column or page**

26 — Volume 2 · October 2010   ▶◀ **Revised Text**   ● **New Line**   ▲ **Revised Code**   **2011 ICD-9-CM**

Arrhinencephaly — *continued*
- due to
  - trisomy 13 (13-15) 758.1
  - trisomy 18 (16-18) 758.2

Arrhythmia (auricle) (cardiac) (cordis) (gallop rhythm) (juvenile) (nodal) (reflex) (sinus) (supraventricular) (transitory) (ventricle) 427.9
- bigeminal rhythm 427.89
- block 426.9
- bradycardia 427.89
- contractions, premature 427.60
- coronary sinus 427.89
- ectopic 427.89
- extrasystolic 427.60
- postoperative 997.1
- psychogenic 306.2
- vagal 780.2

Arrillaga-Ayerza syndrome (pulmonary artery sclerosis with pulmonary hypertension) 416.0

Arsenical
- dermatitis 692.4
- keratosis 692.4
- pigmentation 985.1
  - from drug or medicinal agent
    - correct substance properly administered 709.09
    - overdose or wrong substance given or taken 961.1

Arsenism 985.1
- from drug or medicinal agent
  - correct substance properly administered 692.4
  - overdose or wrong substance given or taken 961.1

Arterial — *see* condition

Arteriectasis 447.8

Arteriofibrosis — *see* Arteriosclerosis

Arteriolar sclerosis — *see* Arteriosclerosis

Arteriolith — *see* Arteriosclerosis

Arteriolitis 447.6
- necrotizing, kidney 447.5
- renal — *see* Hypertension, kidney

Arteriolosclerosis — *see* Arteriosclerosis

Arterionephrosclerosis — *see also* Hypertension, kidney 403.90

Arteriopathy 447.9

Arteriosclerosis, arteriosclerotic (artery) (deformans) (diffuse) (disease) (endarteritis) (general) (obliterans) (obliterative) (occlusive) (senile) (with calcification) 440.9
- with
  - gangrene 440.24
  - psychosis (*see also* Psychosis, arteriosclerotic) 290.40
  - ulceration 440.23
- aorta 440.0
- arteries of extremities — *see* Arteriosclerosis, extremities
- basilar (artery) (*see also* Occlusion, artery, basilar) 433.0 ☑
- brain 437.0
- bypass graft
  - coronary artery 414.05
    - autologous artery (gastroepiploic) (internal mammary) 414.04
    - autologous vein 414.02
    - nonautologous biological 414.03
    - of transplanted heart 414.07
  - extremity 440.30
    - autologous vein 440.31
    - nonautologous biological 440.32
- cardiac — *see* Arteriosclerosis, coronary
- cardiopathy — *see* Arteriosclerosis, coronary
- cardiorenal (*see also* Hypertension, cardiorenal) 404.90
- cardiovascular (*see also* Disease, cardiovascular) 429.2
- carotid (artery) (common) (internal) (*see also* Occlusion, artery, carotid) 433.1 ☑
- central nervous system 437.0
- cerebral 437.0
  - late effect — *see* Late effect(s) (of) cerebrovascular disease

Arteriosclerosis, arteriosclerotic — *continued*
- cerebrospinal 437.0
- cerebrovascular 437.0
- coronary (artery) 414.00
  - due to lipid rich plaque 414.3
  - graft — *see* Arteriosclerosis, bypass graft
  - native artery 414.01
    - of transplanted heart 414.06
- extremities (native artery) NEC 440.20
  - bypass graft 440.30
    - autologous vein 440.31
    - nonautologous biological 440.32
  - claudication (intermittent) 440.21
    - and
      - gangrene 440.24
      - rest pain 440.22
        - and
          - gangrene 440.24
          - ulceration 440.23
            - and gangrene 440.24
      - ulceration 440.23
        - and gangrene 440.24
  - gangrene 440.24
  - rest pain 440.22
    - and
      - gangrene 440.24
      - ulceration 440.23
        - and gangrene 440.24
  - specified site NEC 440.29
  - ulceration 440.23
    - and gangrene 440.24
- heart (disease) (*see also* Arteriosclerosis, coronary)
  - valve 424.99
    - aortic 424.1
    - mitral 424.0
    - pulmonary 424.3
    - tricuspid 424.2
- iliac 440.8 ●
- kidney (*see also* Hypertension, kidney) 403.90
- labyrinth, labyrinthine 388.00
- medial NEC (*see also* Arteriosclerosis, extremities) 440.20
- mesentery (artery) 557.1
- Mönckeberg's (*see also* Arteriosclerosis, extremities) 440.20
- myocarditis 429.0
- nephrosclerosis (*see also* Hypertension, kidney) 403.90
- peripheral (of extremities) — *see* Arteriosclerosis, extremities
- precerebral 433.9 ☑
  - specified artery NEC 433.8 ☑
- pulmonary (idiopathic) 416.0
- renal (*see also* Hypertension, kidney) 403.90
  - arterioles (*see also* Hypertension, kidney) 403.90
  - artery 440.1
- retinal (vascular) 440.8 [362.13]
- specified artery NEC 440.8
  - with gangrene 440.8 [785.4]
- spinal (cord) 437.0
- vertebral (artery) (*see also* Occlusion, artery, vertebral) 433.2 ☑

Arteriospasm 443.9

Arteriovenous — *see* condition

Arteritis 447.6
- allergic (*see also* Angiitis, hypersensitivity) 446.20
- aorta (nonsyphilitic) 447.6
  - syphilitic 093.1
- aortic arch 446.7
- brachiocephalica 446.7
- brain 437.4
  - syphilitic 094.89
- branchial 446.7
- cerebral 437.4
  - late effect — *see* Late effect(s) (of) cerebrovascular disease
  - syphilitic 094.89
- coronary (artery) (*see also* Arteriosclerosis, coronary)
  - rheumatic 391.9
    - chronic 398.99

Arteritis — *continued*
- coronary (*see also* Arteriosclerosis, coronary) — *continued*
  - syphilitic 093.89
- cranial (left) (right) 446.5
- deformans — *see* Arteriosclerosis
- giant cell 446.5
- necrosing or necrotizing 446.0
- nodosa 446.0
- obliterans (*see also* Arteriosclerosis)
  - subclaviocarotica 446.7
- pulmonary 417.8
- retina 362.18
- rheumatic — *see* Fever, rheumatic
- senile — *see* Arteriosclerosis
- suppurative 447.2
- syphilitic (general) 093.89
  - brain 094.89
  - coronary 093.89
  - spinal 094.89
- temporal 446.5
- young female, syndrome 446.7

Artery, arterial — *see* condition

Arthralgia — *see also* Pain, joint 719.4 ☑
- allergic (*see also* Pain, joint) 719.4 ☑
- in caisson disease 993.3
- psychogenic 307.89
- rubella 056.71
- Salmonella 003.23
- temporomandibular joint 524.62

Arthritis, arthritic (acute) (chronic) (subacute) 716.9 ☑
- meaning Osteoarthritis — *see* Osteoarthrosis

> *Note* — Use the following fifth-digit subclassification with categories 711–712, 715–716:
>
> 0   site unspecified
> 1   shoulder region
> 2   upper arm
> 3   forearm
> 4   hand
> 5   pelvic region and thigh
> 6   lower leg
> 7   ankle and foot
> 8   other specified sites
> 9   multiple sites

- allergic 716.2 ☑
- ankylosing (crippling) (spine) 720.0
  - sites other than spine 716.9 ☑
- atrophic 714.0
  - spine 720.9
- back (*see also* Arthritis, spine) 721.90
- Bechterew's (ankylosing spondylitis) 720.0
- blennorrhagic 098.50
- cervical, cervicodorsal (*see also* Spondylosis, cervical) 721.0
- Charcôt's 094.0 [713.5]
  - diabetic 250.6 ☑ [713.5]
    - due to secondary diabetes 249.6 ☑ [713.5]
  - syringomyelic 336.0 [713.5]
  - tabetic 094.0 [713.5]
- chylous (*see also* Filariasis) 125.9 [711.7] ☑
- climacteric NEC 716.3 ☑
- coccyx 721.8
- cricoarytenoid 478.79
- crystal (-induced) — *see* Arthritis, due to crystals
- deformans (*see also* Osteoarthrosis) 715.9 ☑
  - spine 721.90
    - with myelopathy 721.91
- degenerative (*see also* Osteoarthrosis) 715.9 ☑
  - idiopathic 715.09
  - polyarticular 715.09
  - spine 721.90
    - with myelopathy 721.91
- dermatoarthritis, lipoid 272.8 [713.0]
- due to or associated with
  - acromegaly 253.0 [713.0]

Arthritis, arthritic — *continued*
- due to or associated with — *continued*
  - actinomycosis 039.8 [711.4] ☑
  - amyloidosis 277.39 [713.7]
  - bacterial disease NEC 040.89 [711.4] ☑
  - Behçet's syndrome 136.1 [711.2] ☑
  - blastomycosis 116.0 [711.6] ☑
  - brucellosis (*see also* Brucellosis) 023.9 [711.4] ☑
  - caisson disease 993.3
  - coccidioidomycosis 114.3 [711.6] ☑
  - coliform (Escherichia coli) 711.0 ☑
  - colitis, ulcerative (*see also* Colitis, ulcerative) 556.9 [713.1]
  - cowpox 051.01 [711.5] ☑
  - crystals (*see also* Gout)
    - dicalcium phosphate 275.49 [712.1] ☑
    - pyrophosphate 275.49 [712.2] ☑
    - specified NEC 275.49 [712.8] ☑
  - dermatoarthritis, lipoid 272.8 [713.0]
  - dermatological disorder NEC 709.9 [713.3]
  - diabetes 250.6 ☑ [713.5]
    - due to secondary diabetes 249.6 ☑ [713.5]
  - diphtheria 032.89 [711.4] ☑
  - dracontiasis 125.7 [711.7] ☑
  - dysentery 009.0 [711.3] ☑
  - endocrine disorder NEC 259.9 [713.0]
  - enteritis NEC 009.1 [711.3] ☑
    - infectious (*see also* Enteritis, infectious) 009.0 [711.3] ☑
      - specified organism NEC 008.8 [711.3] ☑
    - regional (*see also* Enteritis, regional) 555.9 [713.1]
    - specified organism NEC 008.8 [711.3] ☑
  - epiphyseal slip, nontraumatic (old) 716.8 ☑
  - erysipelas 035 [711.4] ☑
  - erythema
    - epidemic 026.1
    - multiforme 695.10 [713.3]
    - nodosum 695.2 [713.3]
  - Escherichia coli 711.0 ☑
  - filariasis NEC 125.9 [711.7] ☑
  - gastrointestinal condition NEC 569.9 [713.1]
  - glanders 024 [711.4] ☑
  - Gonococcus 098.50
  - gout 274.00
  - helminthiasis NEC 128.9 [711.7] ☑
  - hematological disorder NEC 289.9 [713.2]
  - hemochromatosis 275.03 [713.0] ▲
  - hemoglobinopathy NEC (*see also* Disease, hemoglobin) 282.7 [713.2]
  - hemophilia (*see also* Hemophilia) 286.0 [713.2]
  - Hemophilus influenzae (H. influenzae) 711.0 ☑
  - Henoch (-Schönlein) purpura 287.0 [713.6]
  - H. influenzae 711.0 ☑
  - histoplasmosis NEC (*see also* Histoplasmosis) 115.99 [711.6] ☑
  - human parvovirus 079.83 [711.5] ☑
  - hyperparathyroidism 252.00 [713.0]
  - hypersensitivity reaction NEC 995.3 [713.6]
  - hypogammaglobulinemia (*see also* Hypogamma-globulinemia) 279.00 [713.0]
  - hypothyroidism NEC 244.9 [713.0]
  - infection (*see also* Arthritis, infectious) 711.9 ☑
  - infectious disease NEC 136.9 [711.8] ☑
  - leprosy (*see also* Leprosy) 030.9 [711.4] ☑
  - leukemia NEC (M9800/3) 208.9 [713.2]
  - lipoid dermatoarthritis 272.8 [713.0]
  - Lyme disease 088.81 [711.8] ☑
  - Mediterranean fever, familial 277.31 [713.7]

Index

Arthritis, arthritic — Ascites

Arthritis, arthritic — *continued*
  due to or associated with — *continued*
    meningococcal infection 036.82
    metabolic disorder NEC 277.9 *[713.0]*
    multiple myelomatosis (M9730/3) 203.0 *[713.2]*
    mumps 072.79 *[711.5]* ☑
    mycobacteria 031.8 *[711.4]* ☑
    mycosis NEC 117.9 *[711.6]* ☑
    neurological disorder NEC 349.9 *[713.5]*
    ochronosis 270.2 *[713.0]*
    O'Nyong Nyong 066.3 *[711.5]* ☑
    parasitic disease NEC 136.9 *[711.8]* ☑
    paratyphoid fever (*see also* Fever, paratyphoid) 002.9 *[711.3]* ☑
    parvovirus B19 079.83 *[711.5]* ☑
    Pneumococcus 711.0 ☑
    poliomyelitis (*see also* Poliomyelitis) 045.9 ☑ *[711.5]* ☑
    Pseudomonas 711.0 ☑
    psoriasis 696.0
    pyogenic organism (E. coli) (H. influenzae) (Pseudomonas) (Streptococcus) 711.0 ☑
    rat-bite fever 026.1 *[711.4]* ☑
    regional enteritis (*see also* Enteritis, regional) 555.9 *[713.1]*
    Reiter's disease 099.3 *[711.1]* ☑
    respiratory disorder NEC 519.9 *[713.4]*
    reticulosis, malignant (M9720/3) 202.3 *[713.2]*
    rubella 056.71
    salmonellosis 003.23
    sarcoidosis 135 *[713.7]*
    serum sickness 999.5 *[713.6]*
    Staphylococcus 711.0 ☑
    Streptococcus 711.0 ☑
    syphilis (*see also* Syphilis) 094.0 *[711.4]* ☑
    syringomyelia 336.0 *[713.5]*
    thalassemia 282.49 *[713.2]*
    tuberculosis (*see also* Tuberculosis, arthritis) 015.9 ☑ *[711.4]* ☑
    typhoid fever 002.0 *[711.3]* ☑
    ulcerative colitis (*see also* Colitis, ulcerative) 556.9 *[713.1]*
    urethritis
      nongonococcal (*see also* Urethritis, nongonococcal) 099.40 *[711.1]* ☑
      nonspecific (*see also* Urethritis, nongonococcal) 099.40 *[711.1]* ☑
      Reiter's 099.3
    viral disease NEC 079.99 *[711.5]* ☑
  erythema epidemic 026.1
  gonococcal 098.50
  gouty 274.00
    acute 274.01
  hypertrophic (*see also* Osteoarthrosis) 715.9 ☑
    spine 721.90
      with myelopathy 721.91
  idiopathic, blennorrheal 099.3
  in caisson disease 993.3 *[713.8]*
  infectious or infective (acute) (chronic) (subacute) NEC 711.9 ☑
    nonpyogenic 711.9 ☑
    spine 720.9
  inflammatory NEC 714.9
  juvenile rheumatoid (chronic) (polyarticular) 714.30
    acute 714.31
    monoarticular 714.33
    pauciarticular 714.32
  lumbar (*see also* Spondylosis, lumbar) 721.3
  meningococcal 036.82
  menopausal NEC 716.3 ☑
  migratory — *see* Fever, rheumatic
  neuropathic (Charcôt's) 094.0 *[713.5]*
    diabetic 250.6 ☑ *[713.5]*
      due to secondary diabetes 249.6 ☑ *[713.5]*
    nonsyphilitic NEC 349.9 *[713.5]*
    syringomyelic 336.0 *[713.5]*
    tabetic 094.0 *[713.5]*

Arthritis, arthritic — *continued*
  nodosa (*see also* Osteoarthrosis) 715.9 ☑
    spine 721.90
      with myelopathy 721.91
  nonpyogenic NEC 716.9 ☑
    spine 721.90
      with myelopathy 721.91
  ochronotic 270.2 *[713.0]*
  palindromic (see also Rheumatism, palindromic) 719.3
  pneumococcal 711.0 ☑
  postdysenteric 009.0 *[711.3]* ☑
  postrheumatic, chronic (Jaccoud's) 714.4
  primary progressive 714.0
    spine 720.9
  proliferative 714.0
    spine 720.0
  psoriatic 696.0
  purulent 711.0 ☑
  pyogenic or pyemic 711.0 ☑
  rheumatic 714.0
    acute or subacute — *see* Fever, rheumatic
    chronic 714.0
      spine 720.9
  rheumatoid (nodular) 714.0
    with
      splenoadenomegaly and leukopenia 714.1
      visceral or systemic involvement 714.2
    aortitis 714.89
    carditis 714.2
    heart disease 714.2
    juvenile (chronic) (polyarticular) 714.30
      acute 714.31
      monoarticular 714.33
      pauciarticular 714.32
    spine 720.0
  rubella 056.71
  sacral, sacroiliac, sacrococcygeal (*see also* Spondylosis, sacral) 721.3
  scorbutic 267
  senile or senescent (*see also* Osteoarthrosis) 715.9 ☑
    spine 721.90
      with myelopathy 721.91
  septic 711.0 ☑
  serum (nontherapeutic) (therapeutic) 999.5 *[713.6]*
  specified form NEC 716.8 ☑
  spine 721.90
    with myelopathy 721.91
    atrophic 720.9
    degenerative 721.90
      with myelopathy 721.91
    hypertrophic (with deformity) 721.90
      with myelopathy 721.91
    infectious or infective NEC 720.9
    Marie-Strümpell 720.0
    nonpyogenic 721.90
      with myelopathy 721.91
    pyogenic 720.9
    rheumatoid 720.0
    traumatic (old) 721.7
    tuberculous (*see also* Tuberculosis) 015.0 ☑ *[720.81]*
  staphylococcal 711.0 ☑
  streptococcal 711.0 ☑
  suppurative 711.0 ☑
  syphilitic 094.0 *[713.5]*
    congenital 090.49 *[713.5]*
  syphilitica deformans (Charcôt) 094.0 *[713.5]*
  temporomandibular joint 524.69
  thoracic (*see also* Spondylosis, thoracic) 721.2
  toxic of menopause 716.3 ☑
  transient 716.4 ☑
  traumatic (chronic) (old) (post) 716.1 ☑
    current injury — *see* nature of injury
  tuberculous (*see also* Tuberculosis, arthritis) 015.9 ☑ *[711.4]* ☑
  urethritica 099.3 *[711.1]* ☑
  urica, uratic 274.00
  venereal 099.3 *[711.1]* ☑
  vertebral (*see also* Arthritis, spine) 721.90

Arthritis, arthritic — *continued*
  villous 716.8 ☑
  von Bechterew's 720.0
Arthrocele — *see also* Effusion, joint 719.0 ☑
Arthrochondritis — *see* Arthritis
Arthrodesis status V45.4
Arthrodynia — *see also* Pain, joint 719.4 ☑
  psychogenic 307.89
Arthrodysplasia 755.9
Arthrofibrosis joint — *see also* Ankylosis 718.5 ☑
Arthrogryposis 728.3
  multiplex, congenita 754.89
Arthrokatadysis 715.35
Arthrolithiasis 274.00
Arthro-onychodysplasia 756.89
Arthro-osteo-onychodysplasia 756.89
Arthropathy — *see also* Arthritis 716.9 ☑

> *Note* — Use the following fifth-digit subclassification with categories 711–712, 716:
>
> 0   site unspecified
> 1   shoulder region
> 2   upper arm
> 3   forearm
> 4   hand
> 5   pelvic region and thigh
> 6   lower leg
> 7   ankle and foot
> 8   other specified sites
> 9   multiple sites

  Behçet's 136.1 *[711.2]* ☑
  Charcôt's 094.0 *[713.5]*
    diabetic 250.6 ☑ *[713.5]*
      due to secondary diabetes 249.6 ☑ *[713.5]*
    syringomyelic 336.0 *[713.5]*
    tabetic 094.0 *[713.5]*
  crystal (-induced) — *see* Arthritis, due to crystals
  gouty 274.00
    acute 274.01
    chronic (without mention of tophus (tophi)) 274.02
      with tophus (tophi) 274.03
  neurogenic, neuropathic (Charcôt's) (tabetic) 094.0 *[713.5]*
    diabetic 250.6 ☑ *[713.5]*
      due to secondary diabetes 249.6 ☑ *[713.5]*
    nonsyphilitic NEC 349.9 *[713.5]*
    syringomyelic 336.0 *[713.5]*
  postdysenteric NEC 009.0 *[711.3]* ☑
  postrheumatic, chronic (Jaccoud's) 714.4
  psoriatic 696.0
  pulmonary 731.2
  specified NEC 716.8 ☑
  syringomyelia 336.0 *[713.5]*
  tabes dorsalis 094.0 *[713.5]*
  tabetic 094.0 *[713.5]*
  transient 716.4 ☑
  traumatic 716.1 ☑
  uric acid 274.00
Arthrophyte — *see also* Loose, body, joint 718.1 ☑
Arthrophytis 719.80
  ankle 719.87
  elbow 719.82
  foot 719.87
  hand 719.84
  hip 719.85
  knee 719.86
  multiple sites 719.89
  pelvic region 719.85
  shoulder (region) 719.81
  specified site NEC 719.88
  wrist 719.83
Arthropyosis — *see also* Arthritis, pyogenic 711.0 ☑

Arthroscopic surgical procedure converted to open procedure V64.43
Arthrosis (deformans) (degenerative) — *see also* Osteoarthrosis 715.9 ☑
  Charcôt's 094.0 *[713.5]*
  polyarticular 715.09
  spine (*see also* Spondylosis) 721.90
Arthus phenomenon 995.21
  due to
    correct substance properly administered 995.21
    overdose or wrong substance given or taken 977.9
      specified drug — *see* Table of Drugs and Chemicals
    serum 999.5
Articular — *see also* condition
  disc disorder (reducing or non-reducing) 524.63
  spondylolisthesis 756.12
Articulation
  anterior 524.27
  posterior 524.27
  reverse 524.27
Artificial
  device (prosthetic) — *see* Fitting, device
  insemination V26.1
  menopause (states) (symptoms) (syndrome) 627.4
  opening status (functioning) (without complication) V44.9
    anus (colostomy) V44.3
    colostomy V44.3
    cystostomy V44.50
      appendico-vesicostomy V44.52
      cutaneous-vesicostomy V44.51
      specified type NEC V44.59
    enterostomy V44.4
    gastrostomy V44.1
    ileostomy V44.2
    intestinal tract NEC V44.4
    jejunostomy V44.4
    nephrostomy V44.6
    specified site NEC V44.8
    tracheostomy V44.0
    ureterostomy V44.6
    urethrostomy V44.6
    urinary tract NEC V44.6
    vagina V44.7
  vagina status V44.7
ARV (disease) (illness) (infection) — *see* Human immunodeficiency virus (disease) (illness) (infection)
Arytenoid — *see* condition
Asbestosis (occupational) 501
Asboe-Hansen's disease (incontinentia pigmenti) 757.33
Ascariasis (intestinal) (lung) 127.0
Ascaridiasis 127.0
Ascaridosis 127.0
Ascaris 127.0
  lumbricoides (infestation) 127.0
  pneumonia 127.0
Ascending — *see* condition
ASC-H (atypical squamous cells cannot exclude high grade squamous intraepithelial lesion)
  anus 796.72
  cervix 795.02
  vagina 795.12
Aschoff's bodies — *see also* Myocarditis, rheumatic 398.0
Ascites 789.59
  abdominal NEC 789.59
  cancerous (M8000/6) 789.51
  cardiac 428.0
  chylous (nonfilarial) 457.8
    filarial (*see also* Infestation, filarial) 125.9
  congenital 778.0
  due to S. japonicum 120.2
  fetal, causing fetopelvic disproportion 653.7 ☑
  heart 428.0
  joint (*see also* Effusion, joint) 719.0 ☑
  malignant (M8000/6) 789.51
  pseudochylous 789.59

☑ Additional Digit Required — Refer to the Tabular List for Digit Selection   ▼ Subterms under main terms may continue to next column or page

28 — Volume 2   ▶◀ Revised Text   ● New Line   ▲ Revised Code   **2011 ICD-9-CM**

Ascites — continued
syphilitic 095.2
tuberculous (see also Tuberculosis) 014.0 ☑
Ascorbic acid (vitamin C) **deficiency** (scurvy) 267
ASC-US (atypical squamous cells of undetermined significance)
anus 796.71
cervix 795.01
vagina 795.11
ASCVD (arteriosclerotic cardiovascular disease) 429.2
Aseptic — see condition
Asherman's syndrome 621.5
Asialia 527.7
Asiatic cholera — see also Cholera 001.9
Asocial personality or trends 301.7
Asomatognosia 781.8
Aspergillosis 117.3
with pneumonia 117.3 [484.6]
allergic bronchopulmonary 518.6
nonsyphilitic NEC 117.3
Aspergillus (flavus) (fumigatus) (infection) (terreus) 117.3
Aspermatogenesis 606.0
Aspermia (testis) 606.0
Asphyxia, asphyxiation (by) 799.01
antenatal — see Distress, fetal
bedclothes 994.7
birth (see also Asphyxia, newborn) 768.9
bunny bag 994.7
carbon monoxide 986
caul (see also Asphyxia, newborn) 768.9
cave-in 994.7
crushing — see Injury, internal, intrathoracic organs
constriction 994.7
crushing — see Injury, internal, intrathoracic organs
drowning 994.1
fetal, affecting newborn 768.9
food or foreign body (in larynx) 933.1
bronchioles 934.8
bronchus (main) 934.1
lung 934.8
nasopharynx 933.0
nose, nasal passages 932
pharynx 933.0
respiratory tract 934.9
specified part NEC 934.8
throat 933.0
trachea 934.0
gas, fumes, or vapor NEC 987.9
specified — see Table of Drugs and Chemicals
gravitational changes 994.7
hanging 994.7
inhalation — see Inhalation
intrauterine
fetal death (before onset of labor) 768.0
during labor 768.1
liveborn infant — see Distress, fetal, liveborn infant
local 443.0
mechanical 994.7
during birth (see also Distress, fetal) 768.9
mucus 933.1
bronchus (main) 934.1
larynx 933.1
lung 934.8
nasal passages 932
newborn 770.18
pharynx 933.0
respiratory tract 934.9
specified part NEC 934.8
throat 933.0
trachea 934.0
vaginal (fetus or newborn) 770.18
newborn 768.9
with neurologic involvement 768.5
blue 768.6
livida 768.6
mild or moderate 768.6
pallida 768.5
severe 768.5

Asphyxia, asphyxiation — continued
newborn — continued
white 768.5
pathological 799.01
plastic bag 994.7
postnatal (see also Asphyxia, newborn) 768.9
mechanical 994.7
pressure 994.7
reticularis 782.61
strangulation 994.7
submersion 994.1
traumatic NEC — see Injury, internal, intrathoracic organs
vomiting, vomitus — see Asphyxia, food or foreign body
Aspiration
acid pulmonary (syndrome) 997.39
obstetric 668.0 ☑
amniotic fluid 770.13
with respiratory symptoms 770.14
bronchitis 507.0
clear amniotic fluid 770.13
with
pneumonia 770.14
pneumonitis 770.14
respiratory symptoms 770.14
contents of birth canal 770.17
with respiratory symptoms 770.18
fetal 770.10
blood 770.15
with
pneumonia 770.16
pneumonitis 770.16
pneumonitis 770.18
food, foreign body, or gasoline (with asphyxiation) — see Asphyxia, food or foreign body
meconium 770.11
with
pneumonia 770.12
pneumonitis 770.12
respiratory symptoms 770.12
below vocal cords 770.11
with respiratory symptoms 770.12
mucus 933.1
into
bronchus (main) 934.1
lung 934.8
respiratory tract 934.9
specified part NEC 934.8
trachea 934.0
newborn 770.17
vaginal (fetus or newborn) 770.17
newborn 770.10
with respiratory symptoms 770.18
blood 770.15
with
pneumonia 770.16
pneumonitis 770.16
respiratory symptoms 770.16
pneumonia 507.0
fetus or newborn 770.18
meconium 770.12
pneumonitis 507.0
fetus or newborn 770.18
meconium 770.12
obstetric 668.0 ☑
postnatal stomach contents 770.85
with
pneumonia 770.86
pneumonitis 770.86
respiratory symptoms 770.86
syndrome of newborn (massive) 770.18
meconium 770.12
vernix caseosa 770.12
Asplenia 759.0
with mesocardia 746.87
Assam fever 085.0
Assimilation, pelvis
with disproportion 653.2 ☑
affecting fetus or newborn 763.1
causing obstructed labor 660.1 ☑
affecting fetus or newborn 763.1
Assmann's focus — see also Tuberculosis 011.0 ☑
Astasia (-abasia) 307.9

Astasia — continued
hysterical 300.11
Asteatosis 706.8
cutis 706.8
Astereognosis 780.99
Asterixis 781.3
in liver disease 572.8
Asteroid hyalitis 379.22
Asthenia, asthenic 780.79
cardiac (see also Failure, heart) 428.9
psychogenic 306.2
cardiovascular (see also Failure, heart) 428.9
psychogenic 306.2
heart (see also Failure, heart) 428.9
psychogenic 306.2
hysterical 300.11
myocardial (see also Failure, heart) 428.9
psychogenic 306.2
nervous 300.5
neurocirculatory 306.2
neurotic 300.5
psychogenic 300.5
psychoneurotic 300.5
psychophysiologic 300.5
reaction, psychoneurotic 300.5
senile 797
Stiller's 780.79
tropical anhidrotic 705.1
Asthenopia 368.13
accommodative 367.4
hysterical (muscular) 300.11
psychogenic 306.7
Asthenospermia 792.2
Asthma, asthmatic (bronchial) (catarrh) (spasmodic) 493.9 ☑

Note — Use the following fifth-digit subclassification with codes 493.0–493.2, 493.9:

0   without mention of status asthmaticus or acute exacerbation or unspecified

1   with status asthmaticus

2   with acute exacerbation

with
chronic obstructive pulmonary disease (COPD) 493.2 ☑
hay fever 493.0 ☑
rhinitis, allergic 493.0 ☑
allergic 493.9 ☑
stated cause (external allergen) 493.0 ☑
atopic 493.0 ☑
cardiac (see also Failure, ventricular, left) 428.1
cardiobronchial (see also Failure, ventricular, left) 428.1
cardiorenal (see also Hypertension, cardiorenal) 404.90
childhood 493.0 ☑
Colliers' 500
cough variant 493.82
croup 493.9 ☑
detergent 507.8
due to
detergent 507.8
inhalation of fumes 506.3
internal immunological process 493.0 ☑
endogenous (intrinsic) 493.1 ☑
eosinophilic 518.3
exercise induced bronchospasm 493.81
exogenous (cosmetics) (dander or dust) (drugs) (dust) (feathers) (food) (hay) (platinum) (pollen) 493.0 ☑
extrinsic 493.0 ☑
grinders' 502
hay 493.0 ☑
heart (see also Failure, ventricular, left) 428.1
IgE 493.0 ☑
infective 493.1 ☑
intrinsic 493.1 ☑
Kopp's 254.8
late-onset 493.1 ☑
meat-wrappers' 506.9
Millar's (laryngismus stridulus) 478.75

Asthma, asthmatic — continued
millstone makers' 502
miners' 500
Monday morning 504
New Orleans (epidemic) 493.0 ☑
platinum 493.0 ☑
pneumoconiotic (occupational) NEC 505
potters' 502
psychogenic 316 [493.9] ☑
pulmonary eosinophilic 518.3
red cedar 495.8
Rostan's (see also Failure, ventricular, left) 428.1
sandblasters' 502
sequoiosis 495.8
stonemasons' 502
thymic 254.8
tuberculous (see also Tuberculosis, pulmonary) 011.9 ☑
Wichmann's (laryngismus stridulus) 478.75
wood 495.8
Astigmatism (compound) (congenital) 367.20
irregular 367.22
regular 367.21
Astroblastoma (M9430/3)
nose 748.1
specified site — see Neoplasm, by site, malignant
unspecified site 191.9
Astrocytoma (cystic) (M9400/3)
anaplastic type (M9401/3)
specified site — see Neoplasm, by site, malignant
unspecified site 191.9
fibrillary (M9420/3)
specified site — see Neoplasm, by site, malignant
unspecified site 191.9
fibrous (M9420/3)
specified site — see Neoplasm, by site, malignant
unspecified site 191.9
gemistocytic (M9411/3)
specified site — see Neoplasm, by site, malignant
unspecified site 191.9
juvenile (M9421/3)
specified site — see Neoplasm, by site, malignant
unspecified site 191.9
nose 748.1
pilocytic (M9421/3)
specified site — see Neoplasm, by site, malignant
unspecified site 191.9
piloid (M9421/3)
specified site — see Neoplasm, by site, malignant
unspecified site 191.9
protoplasmic (M9410/3)
specified site — see Neoplasm, by site, malignant
unspecified site 191.9
specified site — see Neoplasm, by site, malignant
subependymal (M9383/1) 237.5
giant cell (M9384/1) 237.5
unspecified site 191.9
Astroglioma (M9400/3)
nose 748.1
specified site — see Neoplasm, by site, malignant
unspecified site 191.9
Asymbolia 784.60
Asymmetrical breathing 786.09
Asymmetry — see also Distortion
breast, between native and reconstructed 612.1
chest 786.9
face 754.0
jaw NEC 524.12
maxillary 524.11
pelvis with disproportion 653.0 ☑
affecting fetus or newborn 763.1
causing obstructed labor 660.1 ☑
affecting fetus or newborn 763.1

☑ Additional Digit Required — Refer to the Tabular List for Digit Selection   ⌐ Subterms under main terms may continue to next column or page

2011 ICD-9-CM   ▶◀ Revised Text   ● New Line   ▲ Revised Code   Volume 2 — 29

Asynergia 781.3
Asynergy 781.3
  ventricular 429.89
Asystole (heart) — *see also* Arrest, cardiac
  427.5
Ataxia, ataxy, ataxic 781.3
  acute 781.3
  brain 331.89
  cerebellar 334.3
    hereditary (Marie's) 334.2
    in
      alcoholism 303.9 ☑ *[334.4]*
      myxedema (*see also* Myxedema)
        244.9 *[334.4]*
      neoplastic disease NEC 239.9 *[334.4]*
  cerebral 331.89
  family, familial 334.2
    cerebral (Marie's) 334.2
    spinal (Friedreich's) 334.0
  Friedreich's (heredofamilial) (spinal) 334.0
  frontal lobe 781.3
  gait 781.2
    hysterical 300.11
  general 781.3
  hereditary NEC 334.2
    cerebellar 334.2
    spastic 334.1
    spinal 334.0
  heredofamilial (Marie's) 334.2
  hysterical 300.11
  locomotor (progressive) 094.0
    diabetic 250.6 ☑ *[337.1]*
      due to secondary diabetes
        249.6 ☑ *[337.1]*
  Marie's (cerebellar) (heredofamilial) 334.2
  nonorganic origin 307.9
  partial 094.0
  postchickenpox 052.7
  progressive locomotor 094.0
  psychogenic 307.9
  Sanger-Brown's 334.2
  spastic 094.0
    hereditary 334.1
    syphilitic 094.0
  spinal
    hereditary 334.0
    progressive locomotor 094.0
  telangiectasia 334.8
Ataxia-telangiectasia 334.8
Atelectasis (absorption collapse) (complete)
  (compression) (massive) (partial)
  (postinfective) (pressure collapse) (pulmonary) (relaxation) 518.0
  newborn (congenital) (partial) 770.5
    primary 770.4
  primary 770.4
  tuberculous (*see also* Tuberculosis, pul-
    monary) 011.9 ☑
Ateleiosis, ateliosis 253.3
Atelia — *see* Distortion
Ateliosis 253.3
Atelocardia 746.9
Atelomyelia 742.59
Athelia 757.6
Atheroembolism
  extremity
    lower 445.02
    upper 445.01
  kidney 445.81
  specified site NEC 445.89
Atheroma, atheromatous — *see also* Arteriosclerosis 440.9
  aorta, aortic 440.0
    valve (*see also* Endocarditis, aortic) 424.1
  artery — *see* Arteriosclerosis
  basilar (artery) (*see also* Occlusion, artery,
    basilar) 433.0 ☑
  carotid (artery) (common) (internal) (*see also*
    Occlusion, artery, carotid) 433.1 ☑
  cerebral (arteries) 437.0
  coronary (artery) — *see* Arteriosclerosis,
    coronary
  degeneration — *see* Arteriosclerosis
  heart, cardiac — *see* Arteriosclerosis, coro-
    nary
  mitral (valve) 424.0

Atheroma, atheromatous — *see also*
  Arteriosclerosis — *continued*
  myocardium, myocardial — *see* Arterioscle-
    rosis, coronary
  pulmonary valve (heart) (*see also* Endocardi-
    tis, pulmonary) 424.3
  skin 706.2
  tricuspid (heart) (valve) 424.2
  valve, valvular — *see* Endocarditis
  vertebral (artery) (*see also* Occlusion, artery,
    vertebral) 433.2 ☑
Atheromatosis — *see also* Arteriosclerosis
  arterial, congenital 272.8
Atherosclerosis — *see* Arteriosclerosis
Athetosis (acquired) 781.0
  bilateral 333.79
  congenital (bilateral) 333.6
  double 333.71
  unilateral 781.0
Athlete's
  foot 110.4
  heart 429.3
Athletic team examination V70.3
Athrepsia 261
Athyrea (acquired) — *see also* Hypothyroidism
  244.9
  congenital 243
Athyreosis (congenital) 243
  acquired — *see* Hypothyroidism
Athyroidism (acquired) — *see also* Hypothyroidism 244.9
  congenital 243
Atmospheric pyrexia 992.0
Atonia, atony, atonic
  abdominal wall 728.2
  bladder (sphincter) 596.4
    neurogenic NEC 596.54
      with cauda equina syndrome 344.61
  capillary 448.9
  cecum 564.89
    psychogenic 306.4
  colon 564.89
    psychogenic 306.4
  congenital 779.89
  dyspepsia 536.3
    psychogenic 306.4
  intestine 564.89
    psychogenic 306.4
  stomach 536.3
    neurotic or psychogenic 306.4
    psychogenic 306.4
  uterus 661.2 ☑
    with hemorrhage (postpartum) 666.1 ☑
    without hemorrhage
      intrapartum 661.2 ☑
      postpartum 669.8 ☑
  vesical 596.4
Atopy NEC V15.09
Atransferrinemia, congenital 273.8
Atresia, atretic (congenital) 759.89
  alimentary organ or tract NEC 751.8
    lower 751.2
    upper 750.8
  ani, anus, anal (canal) 751.2
  aorta 747.22
    with hypoplasia of ascending aorta and
      defective development of left
      ventricle (with mitral valve atre-
      sia) 746.7
    arch 747.11
    ring 747.21
  aortic (orifice) (valve) 746.89
    arch 747.11
  aqueduct of Sylvius 742.3
    with spina bifida (*see also* Spina bifida)
      741.0 ☑
  artery NEC (*see also* Atresia, blood vessel)
    747.60
    cerebral 747.81
    coronary 746.85
    eye 743.58
    pulmonary 747.3
    umbilical 747.5
  auditory canal (external) 744.02
  bile, biliary duct (common) or passage
    751.61

Atresia, atretic — *continued*
  bile, biliary duct or passage — *contin-
    ued*
    acquired (*see also* Obstruction, biliary)
      576.2
  bladder (neck) 753.6
  blood vessel (peripheral) NEC 747.60
    cerebral 747.81
    gastrointestinal 747.61
    lower limb 747.64
    pulmonary artery 747.3
    renal 747.62
    spinal 747.82
    upper limb 747.63
  bronchus 748.3
  canal, ear 744.02
  cardiac
    valve 746.89
      aortic 746.89
      mitral 746.89
      pulmonary 746.01
      tricuspid 746.1
  cecum 751.2
  cervix (acquired) 622.4
    congenital 752.43 ▲
    in pregnancy or childbirth 654.6 ☑
      affecting fetus or newborn 763.89
      causing obstructed labor 660.2 ☑
        affecting fetus or newborn 763.1
  choana 748.0
  colon 751.2
  cystic duct 751.61
    acquired 575.8
      with obstruction (*see also* Obstruc-
        tion, gallbladder) 575.2
  digestive organs NEC 751.8
  duodenum 751.1
  ear canal 744.02
  ejaculatory duct 752.89
  epiglottis 748.3
  esophagus 750.3
  Eustachian tube 744.24
  fallopian tube (acquired) 628.2
    congenital 752.19
  follicular cyst 620.0
  foramen of
    Luschka 742.3
      with spina bifida (*see also* Spina bifi-
        da) 741.0 ☑
    Magendie 742.3
      with spina bifida (*see also* Spina bifi-
        da) 741.0 ☑
  gallbladder 751.69
  genital organ
    external
      female 752.49
      male NEC 752.89
        penis 752.69
    internal
      female 752.89
      male 752.89
  glottis 748.3
  gullet 750.3
  heart
    valve NEC 746.89
      aortic 746.89
      mitral 746.89
      pulmonary 746.01
      tricuspid 746.1
  hymen 752.42
    acquired 623.3
    postinfective 623.3
  ileum 751.1
  intestine (small) 751.1
    large 751.2
  iris, filtration angle (*see also* Buphthalmia)
    743.20
  jejunum 751.1
  kidney 753.3
  lacrimal, apparatus 743.65
    acquired — *see* Stenosis, lacrimal
  larynx 748.3
  ligament, broad 752.19
  lung 748.5
  meatus urinarius 753.6
  mitral valve 746.89

Atresia, atretic — *continued*
  mitral valve — *continued*
    with atresia or hypoplasia of aortic ori-
      fice or valve, with hypoplasia of
      ascending aorta and defective
      development of left ventricle
      746.7
  nares (anterior) (posterior) 748.0
  nasolacrimal duct 743.65
  nasopharynx 748.8
  nose, nostril 748.0
    acquired 738.0
  organ or site NEC — *see* Anomaly, specified
    type NEC
  osseous meatus (ear) 744.03
  oviduct (acquired) 628.2
    congenital 752.19
  parotid duct 750.23
    acquired 527.8
  pulmonary (artery) 747.3
    valve 746.01
    vein 747.49
  pulmonic 746.01
  pupil 743.46
  rectum 751.2
  salivary duct or gland 750.23
    acquired 527.8
  sublingual duct 750.23
    acquired 527.8
  submaxillary duct or gland 750.23
    acquired 527.8
  trachea 748.3
  tricuspid valve 746.1
  ureter 753.29
  ureteropelvic junction 753.21
  ureterovesical orifice 753.22
  urethra (valvular) 753.6
  urinary tract NEC 753.29
  uterus 752.31 ▲
    acquired 621.8
  vagina (acquired) 623.2
    congenital ▶(total) (partial)◀
      752.45 ▲
    postgonococcal (old) 098.2
    postinfectional 623.2
    senile 623.2
  vascular NEC (*see also* Atresia, blood vessel)
    747.60
    cerebral 747.81
  vas deferens 752.89
  vein NEC (*see also* Atresia, blood vessel)
    747.60
    cardiac 746.89
    great 747.49
    portal 747.49
    pulmonary 747.49
  vena cava (inferior) (superior) 747.49
  vesicourethral orifice 753.6
  vulva 752.49
    acquired 624.8
Atrichia, atrichosis 704.00
  congenital (universal) 757.4
Atrioventricularis commune 745.69
At risk for falling V15.88
Atrophia — *see also* Atrophy
  alba 709.09
  cutis 701.8
    idiopathica progressiva 701.8
    senilis 701.8
  dermatological, diffuse (idiopathic) 701.8
  flava hepatis (acuta) (subacuta) (*see also*
    Necrosis, liver) 570
  gyrata of choroid and retina (central) 363.54
    generalized 363.57
  senilis 797
    dermatological 701.8
  unguium 703.8
    congenita 757.5
Atrophoderma, atrophodermia 701.9
  diffusum (idiopathic) 701.8
  maculatum 701.3
    et striatum 701.3
      due to syphilis 095.8
    syphilitic 091.3
  neuriticum 701.8
  pigmentosum 757.33

☑ **Additional Digit Required — Refer to the Tabular List for Digit Selection**

🔺 **Subterms under main terms may continue to next column or page**

▶◀ Revised Text   ● New Line   ▲ Revised Code

Atrophoderma, atrophodermia —
continued
reticulatum symmetricum faciei 701.8
senile 701.8
symmetrical 701.8
vermiculata 701.8
Atrophy, atrophic
adrenal (autoimmune) (capsule) (cortex)
(gland) 255.41
with hypofunction 255.41
alveolar process or ridge (edentulous)
525.20
mandible 525.20
minimal 525.21
moderate 525.22
severe 525.23
maxilla 525.20
minimal 525.24
moderate 525.25
severe 525.26
appendix 543.9
Aran-Duchenne muscular 335.21
arm 728.2
arteriosclerotic — *see* Arteriosclerosis
arthritis 714.0
spine 720.9
bile duct (any) 576.8
bladder 596.8
blanche (of Milian) 701.3
bone (senile) 733.99
due to
disuse 733.7
infection 733.99
tabes dorsalis (neurogenic) 094.0
posttraumatic 733.99
brain (cortex) (progressive) 331.9
with dementia 290.10
Alzheimer's 331.0
with dementia — *see* Alzheimer's,
dementia
circumscribed (Pick's) 331.11
with dementia
with behavioral disturbance
331.11 [294.11]
without behavioral disturbance
331.11 [294.10]
congenital 742.4
hereditary 331.9
senile 331.2
breast 611.4
puerperal, postpartum 676.3 ☑
buccal cavity 528.9
cardiac (brown) (senile) (*see also* Degeneration, myocardial) 429.1
cartilage (infectional) (joint) 733.99
cast, plaster of Paris 728.2
cerebellar — *see* Atrophy, brain
cerebral — *see* Atrophy, brain
cervix (endometrium) (mucosa) (myometrium) (senile) (uteri) 622.8
menopausal 627.8
Charcôt-Marie-Tooth 356.1
choroid 363.40
diffuse secondary 363.42
hereditary (*see also* Dystrophy, choroid)
363.50
gyrate
central 363.54
diffuse 363.57
generalized 363.57
senile 363.41
ciliary body 364.57
colloid, degenerative 701.3
conjunctiva (senile) 372.89
corpus cavernosum 607.89
cortical (*see also* Atrophy, brain) 331.9
Cruveilhier's 335.21
cystic duct 576.8
dacryosialadenopathy 710.2
degenerative
colloid 701.3
senile 701.3
Déjérine-Thomas 333.0
diffuse idiopathic, dermatological 701.8
disuse
bone 733.7

Atrophy, atrophic — *continued*
disuse — *continued*
muscle 728.2
pelvic muscles and anal sphincter 618.83
Duchenne-Aran 335.21
ear 388.9
edentulous alveolar ridge 525.20
mandible 525.20
minimal 525.21
moderate 525.22
severe 525.23
maxilla 525.20
minimal 525.24
moderate 525.25
severe 525.26
emphysema, lung 492.8
endometrium (senile) 621.8
cervix 622.8
enteric 569.89
epididymis 608.3
eyeball, cause unknown 360.41
eyelid (senile) 374.50
facial (skin) 701.9
facioscapulohumeral (Landouzy-Déjérine)
359.1
fallopian tube (senile), acquired 620.3
fatty, thymus (gland) 254.8
gallbladder 575.8
gastric 537.89
gastritis (chronic) 535.1 ☑
gastrointestinal 569.89
genital organ, male 608.89
glandular 289.3
globe (phthisis bulbi) 360.41
gum (*see also* Recession, gingival) 523.20
hair 704.2
heart (brown) (senile) (*see also* Degeneration, myocardial) 429.1
hemifacial 754.0
Romberg 349.89
hydronephrosis 591
infantile 261
paralysis, acute (*see also* Poliomyelitis,
with paralysis) 045.1 ☑
intestine 569.89
iris (generalized) (postinfectional) (sector
shaped) 364.59
essential 364.51
progressive 364.51
sphincter 364.54
kidney (senile) (*see also* Sclerosis, renal) 587
with hypertension (*see also* Hypertension, kidney) 403.90
congenital 753.0
hydronephrotic 591
infantile 753.0
lacrimal apparatus (primary) 375.13
secondary 375.14
Landouzy-Déjérine 359.1
laryngitis, infection 476.0
larynx 478.79
Leber's optic 377.16
lip 528.5
liver (acute) (subacute) (*see also* Necrosis,
liver) 570
chronic (yellow) 571.8
yellow (congenital) 570
with
abortion — *see* Abortion, by type,
with specified complica-
tion NEC
ectopic pregnancy (*see also* categories 633.0–633.9) 639.8
molar pregnancy (*see also* categories 630–632) 639.8
chronic 571.8
complicating pregnancy 646.7 ☑
following
abortion 639.8
ectopic or molar pregnancy 639.8
from injection, inoculation or transfusion (onset within 8 months
after administration) — *see*
Hepatitis, viral
healed 571.5
obstetric 646.7 ☑

Atrophy, atrophic — *continued*
liver (*see also* Necrosis, liver) — continued
yellow — *continued*
postabortal 639.8
postimmunization — *see* Hepatitis,
viral
posttransfusion — *see* Hepatitis, viral
puerperal, postpartum 674.8 ☑
lung (senile) 518.89
congenital 748.69
macular (dermatological) 701.3
syphilitic, skin 091.3
striated 095.8
muscle, muscular 728.2
disuse 728.2
Duchenne-Aran 335.21
extremity (lower) (upper) 728.2
familial spinal 335.11
general 728.2
idiopathic 728.2
infantile spinal 335.0
myelopathic (progressive) 335.10
myotonic 359.21
neuritic 356.1
neuropathic (peroneal) (progressive)
356.1
peroneal 356.1
primary (idiopathic) 728.2
progressive (familial) (hereditary) (pure)
335.21
adult (spinal) 335.19
infantile (spinal) 335.0
juvenile (spinal) 335.11
spinal 335.10
adult 335.19
hereditary or familial 335.11
infantile 335.0
pseudohypertrophic 359.1
spinal (progressive) 335.10
adult 335.19
Aran-Duchenne 335.21
familial 335.11
hereditary 335.11
infantile 335.0
juvenile 335.11
syphilitic 095.6
myocardium (*see also* Degeneration, myocardial) 429.1
myometrium (senile) 621.8
cervix 622.8
myotatic 728.2
myotonia 359.21
nail 703.8
congenital 757.5
nasopharynx 472.2
nerve (*see also* Disorder, nerve)
abducens 378.54
accessory 352.4
acoustic or auditory 388.5
cranial 352.9
first (olfactory) 352.0
second (optic) (*see also* Atrophy, optic nerve) 377.10
third (oculomotor) (partial) 378.51
total 378.52
fourth (trochlear) 378.53
fifth (trigeminal) 350.8
sixth (abducens) 378.54
seventh (facial) 351.8
eighth (auditory) 388.5
ninth (glossopharyngeal) 352.2
tenth (pneumogastric) (vagus) 352.3
eleventh (accessory) 352.4
twelfth (hypoglossal) 352.5
facial 351.8
glossopharyngeal 352.2
hypoglossal 352.5
oculomotor (partial) 378.51
total 378.52
olfactory 352.0
peripheral 355.9
pneumogastric 352.3
trigeminal 350.8
trochlear 378.53
vagus (pneumogastric) 352.3

Atrophy, atrophic — *continued*
nervous system, congenital 742.8
neuritic (*see also* Disorder, nerve) 355.9
neurogenic NEC 355.9
bone
tabetic 094.0
nutritional 261
old age 797
olivopontocerebellar 333.0
optic nerve (ascending) (descending) (infectional) (nonfamilial) (papillomacular
bundle) (postretinal) (secondary NEC)
(simple) 377.10
associated with retinal dystrophy 377.13
dominant hereditary 377.16
glaucomatous 377.14
hereditary (dominant) (Leber's) 377.16
Leber's (hereditary) 377.16
partial 377.15
postinflammatory 377.12
primary 377.11
syphilitic 094.84
congenital 090.49
tabes dorsalis 094.0
orbit 376.45
ovary (senile), acquired 620.3
oviduct (senile), acquired 620.3
palsy, diffuse 335.20
pancreas (duct) (senile) 577.8
papillary muscle 429.81
paralysis 355.9
parotid gland 527.0
patches skin 701.3
senile 701.8
penis 607.89
pharyngitis 472.1
pharynx 478.29
pluriglandular 258.8
polyarthritis 714.0
prostate 602.2
pseudohypertrophic 359.1
renal (*see also* Sclerosis, renal) 587
reticulata 701.8
retina (*see also* Degeneration, retina) 362.60
hereditary (*see also* Dystrophy, retina)
362.70
rhinitis 472.0
salivary duct or gland 527.0
scar NEC 709.2
sclerosis, lobar (of brain) 331.0
with dementia
with behavioral disturbance
331.0 [294.11]
without behavioral disturbance
331.0 [294.10]
scrotum 608.89
seminal vesicle 608.89
senile 797
degenerative, of skin 701.3
skin (patches) (senile) 701.8
spermatic cord 608.89
spinal (cord) 336.8
acute 336.8
muscular (chronic) 335.10
adult 335.19
familial 335.11
juvenile 335.10
paralysis 335.10
acute (*see also* Poliomyelitis, with
paralysis) 045.1 ☑
spine (column) 733.99
spleen (senile) 289.59
spots (skin) 701.3
senile 701.8
stomach 537.89
striate and macular 701.3
syphilitic 095.8
subcutaneous 701.9
due to injection 999.9
sublingual gland 527.0
submaxillary gland 527.0
Sudeck's 733.7
suprarenal (autoimmune) (capsule) (gland)
255.41
with hypofunction 255.41
tarso-orbital fascia, congenital 743.66

Atrophy, atrophic — *continued*
- testis 608.3
- thenar, partial 354.0
- throat 478.29
- thymus (fat) 254.8
- thyroid (gland) 246.8
  - with
    - cretinism 243
    - myxedema 244.9
  - congenital 243
- tongue (senile) 529.8
  - papillae 529.4
  - smooth 529.4
- trachea 519.19
- tunica vaginalis 608.89
- turbinate 733.99
- tympanic membrane (nonflaccid) 384.82
  - flaccid 384.81
- ulcer (*see also* Ulcer, skin) 707.9
- upper respiratory tract 478.9
- uterus, uterine (acquired) (senile) 621.8
  - cervix 622.8
  - due to radiation (intended effect) 621.8
- vagina (senile) 627.3
- vascular 459.89
- vas deferens 608.89
- vertebra (senile) 733.99
- vulva (primary) (senile) 624.1
- Werdnig-Hoffmann 335.0
- yellow (acute) (congenital) (liver) (subacute) (*see also* Necrosis, liver) 570
  - chronic 571.8
  - resulting from administration of blood, plasma, serum, or other biological substance (within 8 months of administration) — *see* Hepatitis, viral

Attack
- akinetic (*see also* Epilepsy) 345.0 ☑
- angina — *see* Angina
- apoplectic (*see also* Disease, cerebrovascular, acute) 436
- benign shuddering 333.93
- bilious — *see* Vomiting
- cataleptic 300.11
- cerebral (*see also* Disease, cerebrovascular, acute) 436
- coronary (*see also* Infarct, myocardium) 410.9 ☑
- cyanotic, newborn 770.83
- epileptic (*see also* Epilepsy) 345.9 ☑
- epileptiform 780.39
- heart (*see also* Infarct, myocardium) 410.9 ☑
- hemiplegia (*see also* Disease, cerebrovascular, acute) 436
- hysterical 300.11
- jacksonian (*see also* Epilepsy) 345.5 ☑
- myocardium, myocardial (*see also* Infarct, myocardium) 410.9 ☑
- myoclonic (*see also* Epilepsy) 345.1 ☑
- panic 300.01
- paralysis (*see also* Disease, cerebrovascular, acute) 436
- paroxysmal 780.39
- psychomotor (*see also* Epilepsy) 345.4 ☑
- salaam (*see also* Epilepsy) 345.6 ☑
- schizophreniform (*see also* Schizophrenia) 295.4 ☑
- sensory and motor 780.39
- syncope 780.2
- toxic, cerebral 780.39
- transient ischemic (TIA) 435.9
- unconsciousness 780.2
  - hysterical 300.11
- vasomotor 780.2
- vasovagal (idiopathic) (paroxysmal) 780.2

Attention to
- artificial opening (of) V55.9
  - digestive tract NEC V55.4
  - specified site NEC V55.8
  - urinary tract NEC V55.6
  - vagina V55.7
  - colostomy V55.3
  - cystostomy V55.5

Attention to — *continued*
- dressing
  - wound V58.30
    - nonsurgical V58.30
    - surgical V58.31
  - gastrostomy V55.1
  - ileostomy V55.2
  - jejunostomy V55.4
  - nephrostomy V55.6
  - surgical dressings V58.31
  - sutures V58.32
  - tracheostomy V55.0
  - ureterostomy V55.6
  - urethrostomy V55.6

Attrition
- gum (*see also* Recession, gingival) 523.20
- teeth (hard tissues) 521.10
  - excessive 521.10
    - extending into
      - dentine 521.12
      - pulp 521.13
    - generalized 521.15
    - limited to enamel 521.11
    - localized 521.14

Atypical — *see also* condition
- cells
  - endocervical 795.00
  - endometrial 795.00
  - glandular
    - anus 796.70
    - cervical 795.00
    - vaginal 795.10
  - distribution, vessel (congenital) (peripheral) NEC 747.60
  - endometrium 621.9
  - kidney 593.89

Atypism, cervix 622.10
Audible tinnitus — *see also* Tinnitus 388.30
Auditory — *see* condition
Audry's syndrome (acropachyderma) 757.39
Aujeszky's disease 078.89
Aura
- jacksonian (*see also* Epilepsy) 345.5 ☑
- persistent migraine 346.5 ☑
  - with cerebral infarction 346.6 ☑
  - without cerebral infarction 346.5 ☑

Aurantiasis, cutis 278.3
Auricle, auricular — *see* condition
Auriculotemporal syndrome 350.8
Australian
- Q fever 083.0
- X disease 062.4

Autism, autistic (child) (infantile) 299.0 ☑
Autodigestion 799.89
Autoerythrocyte sensitization 287.2
Autographism 708.3
Autoimmune
- cold sensitivity 283.0
- disease NEC 279.49
- hemolytic anemia 283.0
- lymphoproliferative syndrome (ALPS) 279.41
- thyroiditis 245.2

Autoinfection, septic — *see* Septicemia
Autointoxication 799.89
Automatism 348.89
- epileptic (*see also* Epilepsy) 345.4 ☑
- paroxysmal, idiopathic (*see also* Epilepsy) 345.4 ☑

Autonomic, autonomous
- bladder 596.54
  - neurogenic 596.54
    - with cauda equina 344.61
- dysreflexia 337.3
- faciocephalalgia (*see also* Neuropathy, peripheral, autonomic) 337.9
- hysterical seizure 300.11
- imbalance (*see also* Neuropathy, peripheral, autonomic) 337.9

Autophony 388.40
Autosensitivity, erythrocyte 287.2
Autotopagnosia 780.99
Autotoxemia 799.89
Autumn — *see* condition
Avellis' syndrome 344.89

Aviators
- disease or sickness (*see also* Effect, adverse, high altitude) 993.2
- ear 993.0
- effort syndrome 306.2

Avitaminosis (multiple NEC) — *see also* Deficiency, vitamin 269.2
- A 264.9
- B 266.9
  - with
    - beriberi 265.0
    - pellagra 265.2
- B$_1$ 265.1
- B$_2$ 266.0
- B$_6$ 266.1
- B$_{12}$ 266.2
- C (with scurvy) 267
- D 268.9
  - with
    - osteomalacia 268.2
    - rickets 268.0
- E 269.1
- G 266.0
- H 269.1
- K 269.0
- multiple 269.2
- nicotinic acid 265.2
- P 269.1

Avulsion (traumatic) 879.8
- blood vessel — *see* Injury, blood vessel, by site
- cartilage (*see also* Dislocation, by site)
  - knee, current (*see also* Tear, meniscus) 836.2
  - symphyseal (inner), complicating delivery 665.6 ☑
- complicated 879.9
- diaphragm — *see* Injury, internal, diaphragm
- ear — *see* Wound, open, ear
- epiphysis of bone — *see* Fracture, by site
- external site other than limb — *see* Wound, open, by site
- eye 871.3
- fingernail — *see* Wound, open, finger
- fracture — *see* Fracture, by site
- genital organs, external — *see* Wound, open, genital organs
- head (intracranial) NEC (*see also* Injury, intracranial, with open intracranial wound)
  - complete 874.9
  - external site NEC 873.8
    - complicated 873.9
- internal organ or site — *see* Injury, internal, by site
- joint (*see also* Dislocation, by site)
  - capsule — *see* Sprain, by site
  - ligament — *see* Sprain, by site
- limb (*see also* Amputation, traumatic, by site)
  - skin and subcutaneous tissue — *see* Wound, open, by site
- muscle — *see* Sprain, by site
- nerve (root) — *see* Injury, nerve, by site
- scalp — *see* Wound, open, scalp
- skin and subcutaneous tissue — *see* Wound, open, by site
- symphyseal cartilage (inner), complicating delivery 665.6 ☑
- tendon (*see also* Sprain, by site)
  - with open wound — *see* Wound, open, by site
- toenail — *see* Wound, open, toe(s)
- tooth 873.63
  - complicated 873.73

Awaiting organ transplant status V49.83
Awareness of heart beat 785.1
Axe grinders' disease 502
Axenfeld's anomaly or syndrome 743.44
Axilla, axillary — *see also* condition
- breast 757.6
Axonotmesis — *see* Injury, nerve, by site
Ayala's disease 756.89

Ayerza's disease or syndrome (pulmonary artery sclerosis with pulmonary hypertension) 416.0
Azoospermia 606.0
Azorean disease (of the nervous system) 334.8
Azotemia 790.6
- meaning uremia (*see also* Uremia) 586
Aztec ear 744.29
Azygos lobe, lung (fissure) 748.69

B

Baader's syndrome (erythema multiforme exudativum) 695.19
Baastrup's syndrome 721.5
Babesiasis 088.82
Babesiosis 088.82
Babington's disease (familial hemorrhagic telangiectasia) 448.0
Babinski-Fröhlich syndrome (adiposogenital dystrophy) 253.8
Babinski-Nageotte syndrome 344.89
Babinski's syndrome (cardiovascular syphilis) 093.89
Bacillary — *see* condition
Bacilluria 791.9
- asymptomatic, in pregnancy or puerperium 646.5 ☑
- tuberculous (*see also* Tuberculosis) 016.9 ☑
Bacillus — *see also* Infection, bacillus
- abortus infection 023.1
- anthracis infection 022.9
- coli
  - infection 041.4
    - generalized 038.42
    - intestinal 008.00
  - pyemia 038.42
  - septicemia 038.42
- Flexner's 004.1
- fusiformis infestation 101
- mallei infection 024
- Shiga's 004.0
- suipestifer infection (*see also* Infection, Salmonella) 003.9
Back — *see* condition
Backache (postural) 724.5
- psychogenic 307.89
- sacroiliac 724.6
Backflow (pyelovenous) — *see also* Disease, renal 593.9
Backknee — *see also* Genu, recurvatum 736.5
Bacteremia 790.7
- newborn 771.83
Bacteria
- in blood (*see also* Bacteremia) 790.7
- in urine (*see also* Bacteriuria) 599.0
Bacterial — *see* condition
Bactericholia — *see also* Cholecystitis, acute 575.0
Bacterid, bacteride (Andrews' pustular) 686.8
Bacteriuria, bacteruria 791.9
- with
  - urinary tract infection 599.0
- asymptomatic 791.9
  - in pregnancy or puerperium 646.5 ☑
    - affecting fetus or newborn 760.1
Bad
- breath 784.99
- heart — *see* Disease, heart
- trip (*see also* Abuse, drugs, nondependent) 305.3 ☑
Baehr-Schiffrin disease (thrombotic thrombocytopenic purpura) 446.6
Baelz's disease (cheilitis glandularis apostematosa) 528.5
Baerensprung's disease (eczema marginatum) 110.3
Bagassosis (occupational) 495.1
Baghdad boil 085.1
Bagratuni's syndrome (temporal arteritis) 446.5
Baker's
- cyst (knee) 727.51
  - tuberculous (*see also* Tuberculosis) 015.2 ☑
- itch 692.89

☑ **Additional Digit Required — Refer to the Tabular List for Digit Selection**   ▽ **Subterms under main terms may continue to next column or page**

32 — Volume 2   ▶◀ Revised Text   ● New Line   ▲ Revised Code   2011 ICD-9-CM

Bakwin-Krida syndrome (craniometaphyseal dysplasia) 756.89
Balanitis (circinata) (gangraenosa) (infectious) (vulgaris) 607.1
  amebic 006.8
  candidal 112.2
  chlamydial 099.53
  due to Ducrey's bacillus 099.0
  erosiva circinata et gangraenosa 607.1
  gangrenous 607.1
  gonococcal (acute) 098.0
    chronic or duration of 2 months or over 098.2
  nongonococcal 607.1
  phagedenic 607.1
  venereal NEC 099.8
  xerotica obliterans 607.81
Balanoposthitis 607.1
  chlamydial 099.53
  gonococcal (acute) 098.0
    chronic or duration of 2 months or over 098.2
  ulcerative NEC 099.8
Balanorrhagia — see Balanitis
Balantidiasis 007.0
Balantidiosis 007.0
Balbuties, balbutio ▶— see also Disorder, fluency◀ 315.35   ▲
Bald
  patches on scalp 704.00
  tongue 529.4
Baldness — see also Alopecia 704.00
Balfour's disease (chloroma) 205.3 ☑
Balint's syndrome (psychic paralysis of visual fixation) 368.16
Balkan grippe 083.0
Ball
  food 938
  hair 938
Ballantyne (-Runge) syndrome (postmaturity) 766.22
Balloon disease — see also Effect, adverse, high altitude 993.2
Ballooning posterior leaflet syndrome 424.0
Baló's disease or concentric sclerosis 341.1
Bamberger's disease (hypertrophic pulmonary osteoarthropathy) 731.2
Bamberger-Marie disease (hypertrophic pulmonary osteoarthropathy) 731.2
Bamboo spine 720.0
Bancroft's filariasis 125.0
Band(s)
  adhesive (see also Adhesions, peritoneum) 568.0
  amniotic 658.8 ☑
    affecting fetus or newborn 762.8
  anomalous or congenital (see also Anomaly, specified type NEC)
    atrial 746.9
    heart 746.9
    intestine 751.4
    omentum 751.4
    ventricular 746.9
  cervix 622.3
  gallbladder (congenital) 751.69
  intestinal (adhesive) (see also Adhesions, peritoneum) 568.0
    congenital 751.4
    obstructive (see also Obstruction, intestine) 560.81
  periappendiceal (congenital) 751.4
  peritoneal (adhesive) (see also Adhesions, peritoneum) 568.0
    with intestinal obstruction 560.81
    congenital 751.4
  uterus 621.5
  vagina 623.2
Bandemia (without diagnosis of specific infection) 288.66
Bandl's ring (contraction)
  complicating delivery 661.4 ☑
    affecting fetus or newborn 763.7
Bang's disease (Brucella abortus) 023.1
Bangkok hemorrhagic fever 065.4
Bannister's diseases 995.1

Bantam-Albright-Martin disease (pseudohypoparathyroidism) 275.49
Banti's disease or syndrome (with cirrhosis) (with portal hypertension) — see Cirrhosis, liver
Bar
  calcaneocuboid 755.67
  calcaneonavicular 755.67
  cubonavicular 755.67
  prostate 600.90
    with
        other lower urinary tract symptoms (LUTS) 600.91
      urinary
        obstruction 600.91
        retention 600.91
  talocalcaneal 755.67
Baragnosis 780.99
Barasheh, barashek 266.2
Barcoo disease or rot — see also Ulcer, skin 707.9
Bard-Pic syndrome (carcinoma, head of pancreas) 157.0
Bärensprung's disease (eczema marginatum) 110.3
Baritosis 503
Barium lung disease 503
Barlow (-Möller) disease or syndrome (meaning infantile scurvy) 267
Barlow's syndrome (meaning mitral valve prolapse) 424.0
Barodontalgia 993.2
Baron Münchausen syndrome 301.51
Barosinusitis 993.1
Barotitis 993.0
Barotrauma 993.2
  odontalgia 993.2
  otitic 993.0
  sinus 993.1
Barraquer's disease or syndrome (progressive lipodystrophy) 272.6
Barré-Guillain syndrome 357.0
Barrel chest 738.3
Barré-Liéou syndrome (posterior cervical sympathetic) 723.2
Barrett's esophagus 530.85
Barrett's syndrome or ulcer (chronic peptic ulcer of esophagus) 530.85
Bársony-Polgár syndrome (corkscrew esophagus) 530.5
Bársony-Teschendorf syndrome (corkscrew esophagus) 530.5
Bartholin's
  adenitis (see also Bartholinitis) 616.89
  gland — see condition
Bartholinitis (suppurating) 616.89
  gonococcal (acute) 098.0
    chronic or duration of 2 months or over 098.2
Barth syndrome 759.89
Bartonellosis 088.0
Bartter's syndrome (secondary hyperaldosteronism with juxtaglomerular hyperplasia) 255.13
Basal — see condition
Basan's (hidrotic) **ectodermal dysplasia** 757.31
Baseball finger 842.13
Basedow's disease or syndrome (exophthalmic goiter) 242.0 ☑
Basic — see condition
Basilar — see condition
Bason's (hidrotic) **ectodermal dysplasia** 757.31
Basopenia 288.59
Basophilia 288.65
Basophilism (corticoadrenal) (Cushing's) (pituitary) (thymic) 255.0
Bassen-Kornzweig syndrome (abetalipoproteinemia) 272.5
Bat ear 744.29
Bateman's
  disease 078.0
  purpura (senile) 287.2
Bathing cramp 994.1
Bathophobia 300.23

Batten's disease, retina 330.1 [362.71]
Batten-Mayou disease 330.1 [362.71]
Batten-Steinert syndrome 359.21
Battered
  adult (syndrome) 995.81
  baby or child (syndrome) 995.54
  spouse (syndrome) 995.81
Battey mycobacterium infection 031.0
Battledore placenta — see Placenta, abnormal
Battle exhaustion —see also Reaction, stress, acute 308.9
Baumgarten-Cruveilhier (cirrhosis) **disease, or syndrome** 571.5
Bauxite
  fibrosis (of lung) 503
  workers' disease 503
Bayle's disease (dementia paralytica) 094.1
Bazin's disease (primary) — see also Tuberculosis 017.1 ☑
Beach ear 380.12
Beaded hair (congenital) 757.4
Beals syndrome 759.82
Beard's disease (neurasthenia) 300.5
Bearn-Kunkel (-Slater) syndrome (lupoid hepatitis) 571.49
Beat
  elbow 727.2
  hand 727.2
  knee 727.2
Beats
  ectopic 427.60
  escaped, heart 427.60
    postoperative 997.1
  premature (nodal) 427.60
    atrial 427.61
    auricular 427.61
    postoperative 997.1
    specified type NEC 427.69
    supraventricular 427.61
    ventricular 427.69
Beau's
  disease or syndrome (see also Degeneration, myocardial) 429.1
  lines (transverse furrows on fingernails) 703.8
Bechterew's disease (ankylosing spondylitis) 720.0
Bechterew-Strümpell-Marie syndrome (ankylosing spondylitis) 720.0
Becker's
  disease
    idiopathic mural endomyocardial disease 425.2
    myotonia congenita, recessive form 359.22
  dystrophy 359.22
Beck's syndrome (anterior spinal artery occlusion) 433.8 ☑
Beckwith (-Wiedemann) syndrome 759.89
Bedbugs bite(s) — see Injury, superficial, by site
Bedclothes, asphyxiation or suffocation by 994.7
Bed confinement status V49.84
Bednar's aphthae 528.2
Bedsore (see also Ulcer, pressure) 707.00
  with gangrene 707.00 [785.4]
Bedwetting — see also Enuresis 788.36
Beer-drinkers' heart (disease) 425.5
Bee sting (with allergic or anaphylactic shock) 989.5
Begbie's disease (exophthalmic goiter) 242.0 ☑
Behavior disorder, disturbance — see also Disturbance, conduct
  antisocial, without manifest psychiatric disorder
    adolescent V71.02
    adult V71.01
    child V71.02
  dyssocial, without manifest psychiatric disorder
    adolescent V71.02
    adult V71.01
    child V71.02
  high risk — see Problem

Behçet's syndrome 136.1
Behr's disease 362.50
Beigel's disease or morbus (white piedra) 111.2
Bejel 104.0
Bekhterev's disease (ankylosing spondylitis) 720.0
Bekhterev-Strümpell-Marie syndrome (ankylosing spondylitis) 720.0
Belching — see also Eructation 787.3
Bell's
  disease (see also Psychosis, affective) 296.0 ☑
  mania (see also Psychosis, affective) 296.0 ☑
  palsy, paralysis 351.0
    infant 767.5
    newborn 767.5
    syphilitic 094.89
  spasm 351.0
Bence-Jones albuminuria, albuminosuria, or proteinuria 791.0
Bends 993.3
Benedikt's syndrome (paralysis) 344.89
Benign — see also condition
  cellular changes, cervix 795.09
  prostate
    with
        other lower urinary tract symptoms (LUTS) 600.21
      urinary
        obstruction 600.21
        retention 600.21
    hyperplasia 600.20
    neoplasm 222.2
Bennett's
  disease (leukemia) 208.9 ☑
  fracture (closed) 815.01
    open 815.11
Benson's disease 379.22
Bent
  back (hysterical) 300.11
  nose 738.0
    congenital 754.0
Bereavement V62.82
  as adjustment reaction 309.0
Bergeron's disease (hysteroepilepsy) 300.11
Berger's paresthesia (lower limb) 782.0
Beriberi (acute) (atrophic) (chronic) (dry) (subacute) (wet) 265.0
  with polyneuropathy 265.0 [357.4]
  heart (disease) 265.0 [425.7]
  leprosy 030.1
  neuritis 265.0 [357.4]
Berlin's disease or edema (traumatic) 921.3
Berloque dermatitis 692.72
Bernard-Horner syndrome — see also Neuropathy, peripheral, autonomic 337.9
Bernard-Sergent syndrome (acute adrenocortical insufficiency) 255.41
Bernard-Soulier disease or thrombopathy 287.1
Bernhardt's disease or paresthesia 355.1
Bernhardt-Roth disease or syndrome (paresthesia) 355.1
Bernheim's syndrome — see also Failure, heart 428.0
Bertielliasis 123.8
Bertolotti's syndrome (sacralization of fifth lumbar vertebra) 756.15
Berylliosis (acute) (chronic) (lung) (occupational) 503
Besnier's
  lupus pernio 135
  prurigo (atopic dermatitis) (infantile eczema) 691.8
Besnier-Boeck disease or sarcoid 135
Besnier-Boeck-Schaumann disease (sarcoidosis) 135
Best's disease 362.76
Bestiality 302.1
Beta-adrenergic hyperdynamic circulatory state 429.82
Beta-aminoisobutyric aciduria 277.2
Beta-mercaptolactate-cysteine disulfiduria 270.0

☑ **Additional Digit Required** — Refer to the Tabular List for Digit Selection   ▽ **Subterms under main terms may continue to next column or page**

2011 ICD-9-CM   ▶◀ **Revised Text**   ● **New Line**   ▲ **Revised Code**   **October 2010 · Volume 2 — 33**

Beta thalassemia (major) (minor) (mixed)
282.49
Beurmann's disease (sporotrichosis) 117.1
Bezoar 938
  intestine 936
  stomach 935.2
Bezold's abscess — see also Mastoiditis 383.01
Bianchi's syndrome (aphasia-apraxia-alexia)
  784.69
Bicornuate or bicornis uterus ▶(complete)
  (partial)◀ 752.34 ▲
  in pregnancy or childbirth 654.0 ☑
    with obstructed labor 660.2 ☑
      affecting fetus or newborn 763.1
    affecting fetus or newborn 763.89
Bicuspid aortic valve 746.4
Biedl-Bardet syndrome 759.89
Bielschowsky's disease 330.1
Bielschowsky-Jansky
  amaurotic familial idiocy 330.1
  disease 330.1
Biemond's syndrome (obesity, polydactyly,
  and mental retardation) 759.89
Biermer's anemia or disease (pernicious
  anemia) 281.0
Biett's disease 695.4
Bifid (congenital) — see also Imperfect, closure
  apex, heart 746.89
  clitoris 752.49
  epiglottis 748.3
  kidney 753.3
  nose 748.1
  patella 755.64
  scrotum 752.89
  toe 755.66
  tongue 750.13
  ureter 753.4
  uterus 752.34 ▲
  uvula 749.02
    with cleft lip (see also Cleft, palate, with
      cleft lip) 749.20
Biforis uterus (suprasimplex) 752.34 ▲
Bifurcation (congenital) — see also Imperfect,
  closure
  gallbladder 751.69
  kidney pelvis 753.3
  renal pelvis 753.3
  rib 756.3
  tongue 750.13
  trachea 748.3
  ureter 753.4
  urethra 753.8
  uvula 749.02
    with cleft lip (see also Cleft, palate, with
      cleft lip) 749.20
  vertebra 756.19
Bigeminal pulse 427.89
Bigeminy 427.89
Big spleen syndrome 289.4
Bilateral — see condition
Bile duct — see condition
Bile pigments in urine 791.4
Bilharziasis — see also Schistosomiasis 120.9
  chyluria 120.0
  cutaneous 120.3
  galacturia 120.0
  hematochyluria 120.0
  intestinal 120.1
  lipemia 120.9
  lipuria 120.0
  Oriental 120.2
  piarhemia 120.9
  pulmonary 120.2
  tropical hematuria 120.0
  vesical 120.0
Biliary — see condition
Bilious (attack) — see also Vomiting
  fever, hemoglobinuric 084.8
Bilirubinuria 791.4
Biliuria 791.4
Billroth's disease
  meningocele (see also Spina bifida) 741.9 ☑
Bilobate placenta — see Placenta, abnormal
Bilocular
  heart 745.7
  stomach 536.8

Bing-Horton syndrome (histamine cephalgia)
  339.00
Binswanger's disease or dementia 290.12
Biörck (-Thorson) syndrome (malignant carcinoid) 259.2
Biparta, bipartite — see also Imperfect, closure
  carpal scaphoid 755.59
  patella 755.64
  placenta — see Placenta, abnormal
  vagina 752.49
Bird
  face 756.0
  fanciers' lung or disease 495.2
  flu ▶— see also Influenza, avian◀
    488.02 ▲
Bird's disease (oxaluria) 271.8
Birth
  abnormal fetus or newborn 763.9
  accident, fetus or newborn — see Birth, in-
    jury
  complications in mother — see Delivery,
    complicated
  compression during NEC 767.9
  defect — see Anomaly
  delayed, fetus 763.9
  difficult NEC, affecting fetus or newborn
    763.9
  dry, affecting fetus or newborn 761.1
  forced, NEC, affecting fetus or newborn
    763.89
  forceps, affecting fetus or newborn 763.2
  hematoma of sternomastoid 767.8
  immature 765.1 ☑
    extremely 765.0 ☑
  inattention, after or at 995.52
  induced, affecting fetus or newborn 763.89
  infant — see Newborn
  injury NEC 767.9
    adrenal gland 767.8
    basal ganglia 767.0
    brachial plexus (paralysis) 767.6
    brain (compression) (pressure) 767.0
    cerebellum 767.0
    cerebral hemorrhage 767.0
    conjunctiva 767.8
    eye 767.8
    fracture
      bone, any except clavicle or spine
        767.3
      clavicle 767.2
      femur 767.3
      humerus 767.3
      long bone 767.3
      radius and ulna 767.3
      skeleton NEC 767.3
      skull 767.3
      spine 767.4
      tibia and fibula 767.3
    hematoma 767.8
      liver (subcapsular) 767.8
      mastoid 767.8
      skull 767.19
      sternomastoid 767.8
      testes 767.8
      vulva 767.8
    intracranial (edema) 767.0
    laceration
      brain 767.0
      by scalpel 767.8
      peripheral nerve 767.7
    liver 767.8
    meninges
      brain 767.0
      spinal cord 767.4
    nerves (cranial, peripheral) 767.7
      brachial plexus 767.6
      facial 767.5
    paralysis 767.7
      brachial plexus 767.6
      Erb (-Duchenne) 767.6
      facial nerve 767.5
      Klumpke (-Déjérine) 767.6
      radial nerve 767.6
      spinal (cord) (hemorrhage) (lacera-
        tion) (rupture) 767.4

Birth — continued
  injury — continued
    rupture
      intracranial 767.0
      liver 767.8
      spinal cord 767.4
      spleen 767.8
      viscera 767.8
    scalp 767.19
    scalpel wound 767.8
    skeleton NEC 767.3
    specified NEC 767.8
    spinal cord 767.4
    spleen 767.8
    subdural hemorrhage 767.0
    tentorial, tear 767.0
    testes 767.8
    vulva 767.8
  instrumental, NEC, affecting fetus or new-
    born 763.2
  lack of care, after or at 995.52
  multiple
    affected by maternal complications of
      pregnancy 761.5
    healthy liveborn — see Newborn, multi-
      ple
  neglect, after or at 995.52
  newborn — see Newborn
  palsy or paralysis NEC 767.7
  precipitate, fetus or newborn 763.6
  premature (infant) 765.1 ☑
  prolonged, affecting fetus or newborn 763.9
  retarded, fetus or newborn 763.9
  shock, newborn 779.89
  strangulation or suffocation
    due to aspiration of clear amniotic fluid
      770.13
      with respiratory symptoms 770.14
    mechanical 767.8
  trauma NEC 767.9
  triplet
    affected by maternal complications of
      pregnancy 761.5
    healthy liveborn — see Newborn, multi-
      ple
  twin
    affected by maternal complications of
      pregnancy 761.5
    healthy liveborn — see Newborn, twin
  ventouse, affecting fetus or newborn 763.3
Birthmark 757.32
Birt-Hogg-Dube syndrome 759.89
Bisalbuminemia 273.8
Biskra button 085.1
Bite(s)
  with intact skin surface — see Contusion
  animal — see Wound, open, by site
    intact skin surface — see Contusion
  bedbug — see Injury, superficial, by site
  centipede 989.5
  chigger 133.8
  fire ant 989.5
  flea — see Injury, superficial, by site
  human (open wound) (see also Wound,
    open, by site)
    intact skin surface — see Contusion
  insect
    nonvenomous — see Injury, superficial,
      by site
    venomous 989.5
  mad dog (death from) 071
  open
    anterior 524.24
    posterior 524.25
  poisonous 989.5
  red bug 133.8
  reptile 989.5
    nonvenomous — see Wound, open, by
      site
  snake 989.5
    nonvenomous — see Wound, open, by
      site
  spider (venomous) 989.5
    nonvenomous — see Injury, superficial,
      by site
  venomous 989.5

Biting
  cheek or lip 528.9
  nail 307.9
Black
  death 020.9
  eye NEC 921.0
  hairy tongue 529.3
  heel 924.20
  lung disease 500
  palm 923.20
Blackfan-Diamond anemia or syndrome
  (congenital hypoplastic anemia) 284.01
Blackhead 706.1
Blackout 780.2
Blackwater fever 084.8
Bladder — see condition
Blast
  blindness 921.3
  concussion — see Blast, injury
  injury 869.0
    with open wound into cavity 869.1
    abdomen or thorax — see Injury, inter-
      nal, by site
    brain (see also Concussion, brain) 850.9
      with skull fracture — see Fracture,
        skull
    ear (acoustic nerve trauma) 951.5
      with perforation, tympanic mem-
        brane — see Wound, open,
        ear, drum
    lung (see also Injury, internal, lung)
      861.20
    otitic (explosive) 388.11
Blastomycosis, blastomycotic (chronic) (cutaneous) (disseminated) (lung) (pulmonary) (systemic) 116.0
  Brazilian 116.1
  European 117.5
  keloidal 116.2
  North American 116.0
  primary pulmonary 116.0
  South American 116.1
Bleb(s) 709.8
  emphysematous (bullous) (diffuse) (lung)
    (ruptured) (solitary) 492.0
  filtering, eye (postglaucoma) (status) V45.69
    with complication 997.99
      postcataract extraction (complication)
        997.99
  lung (ruptured) 492.0
    congenital 770.5
  subpleural (emphysematous) 492.0
Bleeder (familial) (hereditary) — see also Defect, coagulation 286.9
  nonfamilial 286.9
Bleeding — see also Hemorrhage 459.0
  anal 569.3
  anovulatory 628.0
  atonic, following delivery 666.1 ☑
  capillary 448.9
  due to subinvolution 621.1
    puerperal 666.2 ☑
  ear 388.69
  excessive, associated with menopausal on-
    set 627.0
  familial (see also Defect, coagulation) 286.9
  following intercourse 626.7
  gastrointestinal 578.9
  gums 523.8
  hemorrhoids — see Hemorrhoids, bleeding
  intermenstrual
    irregular 626.6
    regular 626.5
  intraoperative 998.11
  irregular NEC 626.4
  menopausal 627.0
  mouth 528.9
  nipple 611.79
  nose 784.7
  ovulation 626.5
  postclimacteric 627.1
  postcoital 626.7
  postmenopausal 627.1
    following induced menopause 627.4
  postoperative 998.11
  preclimacteric 627.0

Bleeding — *see also* Hemorrhage —
   continued
   puberty 626.3
      excessive, with onset of menstrual peri-
         ods 626.3
   rectum, rectal 569.3
   tendencies (*see also* Defect, coagulation)
      286.9
   throat 784.8
   umbilical stump 772.3
   umbilicus 789.9
   unrelated to menstrual cycle 626.6
   uterus, uterine 626.9
      climacteric 627.0
      dysfunctional 626.8
      functional 626.8
      unrelated to menstrual cycle 626.6
   vagina, vaginal 623.8
      functional 626.8
   vicarious 625.8
Blennorrhagia, blennorrhagic — *see* Blennorrhea
Blennorrhea (acute) 098.0
   adultorum 098.40
   alveolaris 523.40
   chronic or duration of 2 months or over
      098.2
   gonococcal (neonatorum) 098.40
   inclusion (neonatal) (newborn) 771.6
   neonatorum 098.40
Blepharelosis — *see also* Entropion 374.00
Blepharitis (eyelid) 373.00
   angularis 373.01
   ciliaris 373.00
      with ulcer 373.01
   marginal 373.00
      with ulcer 373.01
   scrofulous (*see also* Tuberculosis)
      017.3 ☑ [373.00]
   squamous 373.02
   ulcerative 373.01
Blepharochalasis 374.34
   congenital 743.62
Blepharoclonus 333.81
Blepharoconjunctivitis — *see also* Conjunctivitis 372.20
   angular 372.21
   contact 372.22
Blepharophimosis (eyelid) 374.46
   congenital 743.62
Blepharoplegia 374.89
Blepharoptosis 374.30
   congenital 743.61
Blepharopyorrhea 098.49
Blepharospasm 333.81
   due to drugs 333.85
Blessig's cyst 362.62
Blighted ovum 631
Blind
   bronchus (congenital) 748.3
   eye (*see also* Blindness)
      hypertensive 360.42
      hypotensive 360.41
   loop syndrome (postoperative) 579.2
   sac, fallopian tube (congenital) 752.19
   spot, enlarged 368.42
   tract or tube (congenital) NEC — *see* Atresia
Blindness (acquired) (congenital) (both eyes)
   369.00
   with deafness V49.85
   blast 921.3
      with nerve injury — *see* Injury, nerve,
         optic
   Bright's — *see* Uremia
   color (congenital) 368.59
      acquired 368.55
      blue 368.53
      green 368.52
      red 368.51
      total 368.54
   concussion 950.9
   cortical 377.75
   day 368.10
      acquired 368.10
      congenital 368.10
      hereditary 368.10

Blindness — *continued*
   day — *continued*
      specified type NEC 368.10
   due to
      injury NEC 950.9
      refractive error — *see* Error, refractive
   eclipse (total) 363.31
   emotional 300.11
   face 368.16
   hysterical 300.11
   legal (both eyes) (USA definition) 369.4
      with impairment of better (less im-
         paired) eye
         near-total 369.02
            with
               lesser eye impairment 369.02
                  near-total 369.04
                  total 369.03
         profound 369.05
            with
               lesser eye impairment 369.05
                  near-total 369.07
                  profound 369.08
                  total 369.06
         severe 369.21
            with
               lesser eye impairment 369.21
                  blind 369.11
                  near-total 369.13
                  profound 369.14
                  severe 369.22
                  total 369.12
         total
            with lesser eye impairment
               total 369.01
   mind 784.69
   moderate
      both eyes 369.25
         with impairment of lesser eye (speci-
            fied as)
            blind, not further specified 369.15
            low vision, not further specified
               369.23
            near-total 369.17
            profound 369.18
            severe 369.24
            total 369.16
      one eye 369.74
         with vision of other eye (specified as)
            near-normal 369.75
            normal 369.76
   near-total
      both eyes 369.04
         with impairment of lesser eye (speci-
            fied as)
            blind, not further specified 369.02
            total 369.03
      one eye 369.64
         with vision of other eye (specified as)
            near-normal 369.65
            normal 369.66
   night 368.60
      acquired 368.62
      congenital (Japanese) 368.61
      hereditary 368.61
      specified type NEC 368.69
      vitamin A deficiency 264.5
   nocturnal — *see* Blindness, night
   one eye 369.60
      with low vision of other eye 369.10
   profound
      both eyes 369.08
         with impairment of lesser eye (speci-
            fied as)
            blind, not further specified 369.05
            near-total 369.07
            total 369.06
      one eye 369.67
         with vision of other eye (specified as)
            near-normal 369.68
            normal 369.69
   psychic 784.69
   severe
      both eyes 369.22

Blindness — *continued*
   severe — *continued*
      both eyes — *continued*
         with impairment of lesser eye (speci-
            fied as)
            blind, not further specified 369.11
            low vision, not further specified
               369.21
            near-total 369.13
            profound 369.14
            total 369.12
      one eye 369.71
         with vision of other eye (specified as)
            near-normal 369.72
            normal 369.73
   snow 370.24
   sun 363.31
   temporary 368.12
   total
      both eyes 369.01
      one eye 369.61
         with vision of other eye (specified as)
            near-normal 369.62
            normal 369.63
   transient 368.12
   traumatic NEC 950.9
   word (developmental) 315.01
      acquired 784.61
      secondary to organic lesion 784.61
Blister — *see also* Injury, superficial, by site
   beetle dermatitis 692.89
   due to burn — *see* Burn, by site, second
      degree
   fever 054.9
   fracture — *omit code*   ●
   multiple, skin, nontraumatic 709.8
Bloating 787.3
Bloch-Siemens syndrome (incontinentia pigmenti) 757.33
Bloch-Stauffer dyshormonal dermatosis
   757.33
Bloch-Sulzberger disease or syndrome (incontinentia pigmenti) (melanoblastosis)
   757.33
Block
   alveolar capillary 516.3
   arborization (heart) 426.6
   arrhythmic 426.9
   atrioventricular (AV) (incomplete) (partial)
      426.10
      with
         2:1 atrioventricular response block
            426.13
         atrioventricular dissociation 426.0
      first degree (incomplete) 426.11
      second dcgree (Mobitz type I) 426.13
         Mobitz (type) II 426.12
      third degree 426.0
      complete 426.0
         congenital 746.86
      congenital 746.86
      Mobitz (incomplete)
         type I (Wenckebach's) 426.13
         type II 426.12
      partial 426.13
   auriculoventricular (*see also* Block, atrioven-
      tricular) 426.10
      complete 426.0
         congenital 746.86
      congenital 746.86
   bifascicular (cardiac) 426.53
   bundle branch (complete) (false) (incom-
      plete) 426.50
      bilateral 426.53
      left (complete) (main stem) 426.3
         with right bundle branch block
            426.53
         anterior fascicular 426.2
            with
               posterior fascicular block
                  426.3
               right bundle branch block
                  426.52
         hemiblock 426.2
         incomplete 426.2

Block — *continued*
   bundle branch — *continued*
      left — *continued*
         incomplete — *continued*
            with right bundle branch block
               426.53
         posterior fascicular 426.2
            with
               anterior fascicular block 426.3
               right bundle branch block
                  426.51
      right 426.4
         with
            left bundle branch block (incom-
               plete) (main stem) 426.53
            left fascicular block 426.53
               anterior 426.52
               posterior 426.51
      Wilson's type 426.4
   cardiac 426.9
   conduction 426.9
      complete 426.0
   Eustachian tube (*see also* Obstruction, Eu-
      stachian tube) 381.60
   fascicular (left anterior) (left posterior) 426.2
   foramen Magendie (acquired) 331.3
      congenital 742.3
         with spina bifida (*see also* Spina bifi-
            da) 741.0 ☑
   heart 426.9
      first degree (atrioventricular) 426.11
      second degree (atrioventricular) 426.13
      third degree (atrioventricular) 426.0
      bundle branch (complete) (false) (incom-
         plete) 426.50
         bilateral 426.53
         left (*see also* Block, bundle branch,
            left) 426.3
         right (*see also* Block, bundle branch,
            right) 426.4
      complete (atrioventricular) 426.0
      congenital 746.86
      incomplete 426.13
      intra-atrial 426.6
      intraventricular NEC 426.6
      sinoatrial 426.6
      specified type NEC 426.6
   hepatic vein 453.0
   intraventricular (diffuse) (myofibrillar) 426.6
      bundle branch (complete) (false) (incom-
         plete) 426.50
         bilateral 426.53
         left (*see also* Block, bundle branch,
            left) 426.3
         right (*see also* Block, bundle branch,
            right) 426.4
   kidney (*see also* Disease, renal) 593.9
      postcystoscopic 997.5
   myocardial (*see also* Block, heart) 426.9
   nodal 426.10
   optic nerve 377.49
   organ or site (congenital) NEC — *see* Atresia
   parietal 426.6
   peri-infarction 426.6
   portal (vein) 452
   sinoatrial 426.6
   sinoauricular 426.6
   spinal cord 336.9
   trifascicular 426.54
   tubal 628.2
   vein NEC 453.9
Blocq's disease or syndrome (astasia-abasia)
   307.9
Blood
   constituents, abnormal NEC 790.6
   disease 289.9
      specified NEC 289.89
   donor V59.01
      other blood components V59.09
      stem cells V59.02
      whole blood V59.01
   dyscrasia 289.9
      with
         abortion — *see* Abortion, by type,
            with hemorrhage, delayed or
            excessive

☑ **Additional Digit Required** — Refer to the Tabular List for Digit Selection   ▽ **Subterms under main terms may continue to next column or page**

2011 ICD-9-CM   ▶◀ **Revised Text**   ● **New Line**   ▲ **Revised Code**   **October 2010 · Volume 2 — 35**

Blood — *continued*
  dyscrasia — *continued*
    with — *continued*
      ectopic pregnancy (*see also* categories 633.0–633.9) 639.1
      molar pregnancy (*see also* categories 630–632) 639.1
      following
        abortion 639.1
        ectopic or molar pregnancy 639.1
      newborn NEC 776.9
      puerperal, postpartum 666.3 ✅
  flukes NEC (*see also* Infestation, Schistosoma) 120.9
  in
    feces (*see also* Melena) 578.1
      occult 792.1
    urine (*see also* Hematuria) 599.70
  mole 631
  occult 792.1
  poisoning (*see also* Septicemia) 038.9
  pressure
    decreased, due to shock following injury 958.4
    fluctuating 796.4
    high (*see also* Hypertension) 401.9
      incidental reading (isolated) (nonspecific), without diagnosis of hypertension 796.2
    low (*see also* Hypotension) 458.9
      incidental reading (isolated) (nonspecific), without diagnosis of hypotension 796.3
  spitting (*see also* Hemoptysis) 786.30 ▲
  staining cornea 371.12
  transfusion
    without reported diagnosis V58.2
    donor V59.01
      stem cells V59.02
    reaction or complication — *see* Complications, transfusion
  tumor — *see* Hematoma
  vessel rupture — *see* Hemorrhage
  vomiting (*see also* Hematemesis) 578.0
Blood-forming organ disease 289.9
Bloodgood's disease 610.1
Bloodshot eye 379.93
Bloom (-Machacek) (-Torre) syndrome 757.39
Blotch, palpebral 372.55
Blount-Barber syndrome (tibia vara) 732.4
Blount's disease (tibia vara) 732.4
Blue
  baby 746.9
  bloater 491.20
    with
      acute bronchitis 491.22
      exacerbation (acute) 491.21
  diaper syndrome 270.0
  disease 746.9
  dome cyst 610.0
  drum syndrome 381.02
  sclera 743.47
    with fragility of bone and deafness 756.51
  toe syndrome 445.02
Blueness — *see also* Cyanosis 782.5
Blurring, visual 368.8
Blushing (abnormal) (excessive) 782.62
BMI (body mass index)
  adult
    25.0-25.9 V85.21
    26.0-26.9 V85.22
    27.0-27.9 V85.23
    28.0-28.9 V85.24
    29.0-29.9 V85.25
    30.0-30.9 V85.30
    31.0-31.9 V85.31
    32.0-32.9 V85.32
    33.0-33.9 V85.33
    34.0-34.9 V85.34
    35.0-35.9 V85.35
    36.0-36.9 V85.36
    37.0-37.9 V85.37
    38.0-38.9 V85.38
    39.0-39.9 V85.39
    ▶40.0-44.9◀ V85.41 ▲

BMI — *continued*
  adult — *continued*
    45.0-49.9 V85.42 ●
    50.0-59.9 V85.43 ●
    60.0-69.9 V85.44 ●
    70 and over V85.45 ●
    between 19-24 V85.1
    less than 19 V85.0
  pediatric
    5th percentile to less than 85th percentile for age V85.52
    85th percentile to less than 95th percentile for age V85.53
    greater than or equal to 95th percentile for age V85.54
    less than 5th percentile for age V85.51
Boarder, hospital V65.0
  infant V65.0
Bockhart's impetigo (superficial folliculitis) 704.8
Bodechtel-Guttmann disease (subacute sclerosing panencephalitis) 046.2
Boder-Sedgwick syndrome (ataxia-telangiectasia) 334.8
Body, bodies
  Aschoff (*see also* Myocarditis, rheumatic) 398.0
  asteroid, vitreous 379.22
  choroid, colloid (degenerative) 362.57
    hereditary 362.77
  cytoid (retina) 362.82
  drusen (retina) (*see also* Drusen) 362.57
    optic disc 377.21
  fibrin, pleura 511.0
  foreign — *see* Foreign body
  Hassall-Henle 371.41
  loose
    joint (*see also* Loose, body, joint) 718.1 ✅
      knee 717.6
    knee 717.6
    sheath, tendon 727.82
  Mallory's 034.1
  mass index (BMI)
    adult
      25.0-25.9 V85.21
      26.0-26.9 V85.22
      27.0-27.9 V85.23
      28.0-28.9 V85.24
      29.0-29.9 V85.25
      30.0-30.9 V85.30
      31.0-31.9 V85.31
      32.0-32.9 V85.32
      33.0-33.9 V85.33
      34.0-34.9 V85.34
      35.0-35.9 V85.35
      36.0-36.9 V85.36
      37.0-37.9 V85.37
      38.0-38.9 V85.38
      39.0-39.9 V85.39
      ▶40.0-44.9◀ V85.41 ▲
      45.0-49.9 V85.42 ●
      50.0-59.9 V85.43 ●
      60.0-69.9 V85.44 ●
      70 and over V85.45 ●
      between 19-24 V85.1
      less than 19 V85.0
    pediatric
      5th percentile to less than 85th percentile for age V85.52
      85th percentile to less than 95th percentile for age V85.53
      greater than or equal to 95th percentile for age V85.54
      less than 5th percentile for age V85.51
  Mooser 081.0
  Negri 071
  rice (joint) (*see also* Loose, body, joint) 718.1 ✅
    knee 717.6
  rocking 307.3
Boeck's
  disease (sarcoidosis) 135
  lupoid (miliary) 135
  sarcoid 135

Boerhaave's syndrome (spontaneous esophageal rupture) 530.4
●**Boggy**
  cervix 622.8 ●
  uterus 621.8 ●
Boil — *see also* Carbuncle 680.9
  abdominal wall 680.2
  Aleppo 085.1
  ankle 680.6
  anus 680.5
  arm (any part, above wrist) 680.3
  auditory canal, external 680.0
  axilla 680.3
  back (any part) 680.2
  Baghdad 085.1
  breast 680.2
  buttock 680.5
  chest wall 680.2
  corpus cavernosum 607.2
  Delhi 085.1
  ear (any part) 680.0
  eyelid 373.13
  face (any part, except eye) 680.0
  finger (any) 680.4
  flank 680.2
  foot (any part) 680.7
  forearm 680.3
  Gafsa 085.1
  genital organ, male 608.4
  gluteal (region) 680.5
  groin 680.2
  hand (any part) 680.4
  head (any part, except face) 680.8
  heel 680.7
  hip 680.6
  knee 680.6
  labia 616.4
  lacrimal (*see also* Dacryocystitis) 375.30
    gland (*see also* Dacryoadenitis) 375.00
    passages (duct) (sac) (*see also* Dacryocystitis) 375.30
  leg, any part, except foot 680.6
  multiple sites 680.9
  natal 085.1
  neck 680.1
  nose (external) (septum) 680.0
  orbit, orbital 376.01
  partes posteriores 680.5
  pectoral region 680.2
  penis 607.2
  perineum 680.2
  pinna 680.0
  scalp (any part) 680.8
  scrotum 608.4
  seminal vesicle 608.0
  shoulder 680.3
  skin NEC 680.9
  specified site NEC 680.8
  spermatic cord 608.4
  temple (region) 680.0
  testis 608.4
  thigh 680.6
  thumb 680.4
  toe (any) 680.7
  tropical 085.1
  trunk 680.2
  tunica vaginalis 608.4
  umbilicus 680.2
  upper arm 680.3
  vas deferens 608.4
  vulva 616.4
  wrist 680.4
Bold hives — *see also* Urticaria 708.9
Bolivian hemorrhagic fever 078.7
Bombé, iris 364.74
Bomford-Rhoads anemia (refractory) 238.72
Bone — *see* condition
Bonnevie-Ullrich syndrome 758.6
Bonnier's syndrome 386.19
Bonvale Dam fever 780.79
Bony block of joint 718.80
  ankle 718.87
  elbow 718.82
  foot 718.87
  hand 718.84
  hip 718.85

Bony block of joint — *continued*
  knee 718.86
  multiple sites 718.89
  pelvic region 718.85
  shoulder (region) 718.81
  specified site NEC 718.88
  wrist 718.83
BOOP (bronchiolitis obliterans organized pneumonia) 516.8
Borderline
  intellectual functioning V62.89
  osteopenia 733.90
  pelvis 653.1 ✅
    with obstruction during labor 660.1 ✅
      affecting fetus or newborn 763.1
  psychosis (*see also* Schizophrenia) 295.5 ✅
    of childhood (*see also* Psychosis, childhood) 299.8 ✅
  schizophrenia (*see also* Schizophrenia) 295.5 ✅
Borna disease 062.9
Bornholm disease (epidemic pleurodynia) 074.1
Borrelia vincentii (mouth) (pharynx) (tonsils) 101
Bostock's catarrh — *see also* Fever, hay 477.9
Boston exanthem 048
Botalli, ductus (patent) (persistent) 747.0
Bothriocephalus latus infestation 123.4
Botulism 005.1
  food poisoning 005.1
  infant 040.41
  non-foodborne 040.42
  wound 040.42
Bouba — *see also* Yaws 102.9
Bouffée délirante 298.3
Bouillaud's disease or syndrome (rheumatic heart disease) 391.9
Bourneville's disease (tuberous sclerosis) 759.5
Boutonneuse fever 082.1
Boutonniere
  deformity (finger) 736.21
  hand (intrinsic) 736.21
Bouveret (-Hoffmann) disease or syndrome (paroxysmal tachycardia) 427.2
Bovine heart — *see* Hypertrophy, cardiac
Bowel — *see* condition
Bowen's
  dermatosis (precancerous) (M8081/2) — *see* Neoplasm, skin, in situ
  disease (M8081/2) — *see* Neoplasm, skin, in situ
  epithelioma (M8081/2) — *see* Neoplasm, skin, in situ
  type
    epidermoid carcinoma in situ (M8081/2) — *see* Neoplasm, skin, in situ
    intraepidermal squamous cell carcinoma (M8081/2) — *see* Neoplasm, skin, in situ
Bowing
  femur 736.89
    congenital 754.42
  fibula 736.89
    congenital 754.43
  forearm 736.09
    away from midline (cubitus valgus) 736.01
    toward midline (cubitus varus) 736.02
  leg(s), long bones, congenital 754.44
  radius 736.09
    away from midline (cubitus valgus) 736.01
    toward midline (cubitus varus) 736.02
  tibia 736.89
    congenital 754.43
Bowleg(s) 736.42
  congenital 754.44
  rachitic 268.1
Boyd's dysentery 004.2
Brachial — *see* condition
Brachman-de Lange syndrome (Amsterdam dwarf, mental retardation, and brachycephaly) 759.89
Brachycardia 427.89

✅ Additional Digit Required — Refer to the Tabular List for Digit Selection   ▽ Subterms under main terms may continue to next column or page

36 — Volume 2 · October 2010   ▶◀ Revised Text   ● New Line   ▲ Revised Code   2011 ICD-9-CM

Brachycephaly 756.0
Brachymorphism and ectopia lentis 759.89
Bradley's disease (epidemic vomiting) 078.82
Bradycardia 427.89
  chronic (sinus) 427.81
  newborn 779.81
  nodal 427.89
  postoperative 997.1
  reflex 337.09
  sinoatrial 427.89
    with paroxysmal tachyarrhythmia or tachycardia 427.81
    chronic 427.81
  sinus 427.89
    with paroxysmal tachyarrhythmia or tachycardia 427.81
    chronic 427.81
    persistent 427.81
    severe 427.81
  tachycardia syndrome 427.81
  vagal 427.89
Bradykinesia 781.0
Bradypnea 786.09
Brailsford's disease 732.3
  radial head 732.3
  tarsal scaphoid 732.5
Brailsford-Morquio disease or syndrome (mucopolysaccharidosis IV) 277.5
Brain — *see also* condition
  death 348.89
  syndrome (acute) (chronic) (nonpsychotic) (organic) (with neurotic reaction) (with behavioral reaction) (*see also* Syndrome, brain) 310.9
    with
      presenile brain disease 290.10
      psychosis, psychotic reaction (*see also* Psychosis, organic) 294.9
    congenital (*see also* Retardation, mental) 319
Branched-chain amino-acid disease 270.3
Branchial — *see* condition
Brandt's syndrome (acrodermatitis enteropathica) 686.8
Brash (water) 787.1
Brass-founders' ague 985.8
Bravais-Jacksonian epilepsy — *see also* Epilepsy 345.5 ☑
Braxton Hicks contractions 644.1 ☑
Braziers' disease 985.8
Brazilian
  blastomycosis 116.1
  leishmaniasis 085.5
BRBPR (bright red blood per rectum) 569.3
Break
  cardiorenal — *see* Hypertension, cardiorenal
  retina (*see also* Defect, retina) 361.30
Breakbone fever 061
Breakdown
  device, implant, or graft — *see* Complications, mechanical
  nervous (*see also* Disorder, mental, nonpsychotic) 300.9
  perineum 674.2 ☑
Breast — *see also* condition
  buds 259.1
    in newborn 779.89
  dense 793.82
  nodule 793.89
Breast feeding difficulties 676.8 ☑
Breath
  foul 784.99
  holder, child 312.81
  holding spells 786.9
  shortness 786.05
Breathing
  asymmetrical 786.09
  bronchial 786.09
  exercises V57.0
  labored 786.09
  mouth 784.99
    causing malocclusion 524.59
  periodic 786.09
    high altitude 327.22
  tic 307.20
Breathlessness 786.09

Breda's disease — *see also* Yaws 102.9
Breech
  delivery, affecting fetus or newborn 763.0
  extraction, affecting fetus or newborn 763.0
  presentation (buttocks) (complete) (frank) 652.2 ☑
    with successful version 652.1 ☑
    before labor, affecting fetus or newborn 761.7
    during labor, affecting fetus or newborn 763.0
Breisky's disease (kraurosis vulvae) 624.09
Brennemann's syndrome (acute mesenteric lymphadenitis) 289.2
Brenner's
  tumor (benign) (M9000/0) 220
    borderline malignancy (M9000/1) 236.2
    malignant (M9000/3) 183.0
    proliferating (M9000/1) 236.2
Bretonneau's disease (diphtheritic malignant angina) 032.0
Breus' mole 631
Brevicollis 756.16
Bricklayers' itch 692.89
Brickmakers' anemia 126.9
Bridge
  myocardial 746.85
Bright's
  blindness — *see* Uremia
  disease (*see also* Nephritis) 583.9
    arteriosclerotic (*see also* Hypertension, kidney) 403.90
Bright red blood per rectum (BRBPR) 569.3
Brill's disease (recrudescent typhus) 081.1
  flea-borne 081.0
  louse-borne 081.1
Brill-Symmers disease (follicular lymphoma) (M9690/3) 202.0 ☑
Brill-Zinsser disease (recrudescent typhus) 081.1
Brinton's disease (linitis plastica) (M8142/3) 151.9
Brion-Kayser disease — *see also* Fever, paratyphoid 002.9
Briquet's disorder or syndrome 300.81
Brissaud's
  infantilism (infantile myxedema) 244.9
  motor-verbal tic 307.23
Brissaud-Meige syndrome (infantile myxedema) 244.9
Brittle
  bones (congenital) 756.51
  nails 703.8
    congenital 757.5
Broad — *see also* condition
  beta disease 272.2
  ligament laceration syndrome 620.6
Brock's syndrome (atelectasis due to enlarged lymph nodes) 518.0
Brocq's disease 691.8
  atopic (diffuse) neurodermatitis 691.8
  lichen simplex chronicus 698.3
  parakeratosis psoriasiformis 696.2
  parapsoriasis 696.2
Brocq-Duhring disease (dermatitis herpetiformis) 694.0
Brodie's
  abscess (localized) (chronic) (*see also* Osteomyelitis) 730.1 ☑
  disease (joint) (*see also* Osteomyelitis) 730.1 ☑
Broken
  arches 734
    congenital 755.67
  back — *see* Fracture, vertebra, by site
  bone — *see* Fracture, by site
  compensation — *see* Disease, heart
  heart syndrome 429.83
  implant or internal device — *see* listing under Complications, mechanical
  neck — *see* Fracture, vertebra, cervical
  nose 802.0
    open 802.1
  tooth, teeth 873.63
    complicated 873.73
Bromhidrosis 705.89

Bromidism, bromism
  acute 967.3
    correct substance properly administered 349.82
    overdose or wrong substance given or taken 967.3
  chronic (*see also* Dependence) 304.1 ☑
Bromidrosiphobia 300.23
Bromidrosis 705.89
Bronchi, bronchial — *see* condition
Bronchiectasis (cylindrical) (diffuse) (fusiform) (localized) (moniliform) (postinfectious) (recurrent) (saccular) 494.0
  with acute exacerbation 494.1
  congenital 748.61
  tuberculosis (*see also* Tuberculosis) 011.5 ☑
Bronchiolectasis — *see* Bronchiectasis
Bronchiolitis (acute) (infectious) (subacute) 466.19
  with
    bronchospasm or obstruction 466.19
    influenza, flu, or grippe ▶(*see also* Influenza)◀ 487.1
  catarrhal (acute) (subacute) 466.19
  chemical 506.0
    chronic 506.4
  chronic (obliterative) 491.8
  due to external agent — *see* Bronchitis, acute, due to
  fibrosa obliterans 491.8
  influenzal ▶(*see also* Influenza)◀ 487.1
  obliterans 491.8
    with organizing pneumonia (BOOP) 516.8
    status post lung transplant 996.84
  obliterative (chronic) (diffuse) (subacute) 491.8
    due to fumes or vapors 506.4
  respiratory syncytial virus 466.11
  vesicular — *see* Pneumonia, broncho-
Bronchitis (diffuse) (hypostatic) (infectious) (inflammatory) (simple) 490
  with
    emphysema — *see* Emphysema
    influenza, flu, or grippe ▶(*see also* Influenza)◀ 487.1
    obstruction airway, chronic 491.20
      with
        acute bronchitis 491.22
        exacerbation (acute) 491.21
    tracheitis 490
      acute or subacute 466.0
        with bronchospasm or obstruction 466.0
      chronic 491.8
  acute or subacute 466.0
    with
      bronchiectasis 494.1
      bronchospasm 466.0
      obstruction 466.0
      tracheitis 466.0
    chemical (due to fumes or vapors) 506.0
    due to
      fumes or vapors 506.0
      radiation 508.8
  allergic (acute) (*see also* Asthma) 493.9 ☑
  arachidic 934.1
  aspiration 507.0
    due to fumes or vapors 506.0
  asthmatic (acute) 493.90
    with
      acute exacerbation 493.92
      status asthmaticus 493.91
    chronic 493.2 ☑
  capillary 466.19
    with bronchospasm or obstruction 466.19
    chronic 491.8
  caseous (*see also* Tuberculosis) 011.3 ☑
  Castellani's 104.8
  catarrhal 490
    acute — *see* Bronchitis, acute
    chronic 491.0
  chemical (acute) (subacute) 506.0
    chronic 506.4

Bronchitis — *continued*
  chemical — *continued*
    due to fumes or vapors (acute) (subacute) 506.0
      chronic 506.4
  chronic 491.9
    with
      tracheitis (chronic) 491.8
    asthmatic 493.2 ☑
    catarrhal 491.0
    chemical (due to fumes and vapors) 506.4
    due to
      fumes or vapors (chemical) (inhalation) 506.4
      radiation 508.8
      tobacco smoking 491.0
    mucopurulent 491.1
    obstructive 491.20
      with
        acute bronchitis 491.22
        exacerbation (acute) 491.21
    purulent 491.1
    simple 491.0
    specified type NEC 491.8
  croupous 466.0
    with bronchospasm or obstruction 466.0
    due to fumes or vapors 506.0
  emphysematous 491.20
    with
      acute bronchitis 491.22
      exacerbation (acute) 491.21
  exudative 466.0
  fetid (chronic) (recurrent) 491.1
  fibrinous, acute or subacute 466.0
    with bronchospasm or obstruction 466.0
  grippal ▶(*see also* Influenza)◀ 487.1
  influenzal ▶(*see also* Influenza)◀ 487.1
  membranous, acute or subacute 466.0
    with bronchospasm or obstruction 466.0
  moulders' 502
  mucopurulent (chronic) (recurrent) 491.1
    acute or subacute 466.0
  obliterans 491.8
  obstructive (chronic) 491.20
    with
      acute bronchitis 491.22
      exacerbation (acute) 491.21
  pituitous 491.1
  plastic (inflammatory) 466.0
  pneumococcal, acute or subacute 466.0
    with bronchospasm or obstruction 466.0
  pseudomembranous 466.0
  purulent (chronic) (recurrent) 491.1
    acute or subacute 466.0
      with bronchospasm or obstruction 466.0
  putrid 491.1
  scrofulous (*see also* Tuberculosis) 011.3 ☑
  senile 491.9
  septic, acute or subacute 466.0
    with bronchospasm or obstruction 466.0
  smokers' 491.0
  spirochetal 104.8
  suffocative, acute or subacute 466.0
  summer (*see also* Asthma) 493.9 ☑
  suppurative (chronic) 491.1
    acute or subacute 466.0
  tuberculous (*see also* Tuberculosis) 011.3 ☑
  ulcerative 491.8
    Vincent's 101
  Vincent's 101
  viral, acute or subacute 466.0
Bronchoalveolitis 485
Bronchoaspergillosis 117.3
Bronchocele
  meaning
    dilatation of bronchus 519.19
    goiter 240.9
Bronchogenic carcinoma 162.9
Bronchohemisporosis 117.9
Broncholithiasis 518.89
  tuberculous (*see also* Tuberculosis) 011.3 ☑
Bronchomalacia 748.3
Bronchomoniliasis 112.89
Bronchomycosis 112.89

☑ **Additional Digit Required** — Refer to the Tabular List for Digit Selection   🔄 **Subterms under main terms may continue to next column or page**

2011 ICD-9-CM   ▶◀ **Revised Text**   ● **New Line**   ▲ **Revised Code**   October 2010 · Volume 2 — 37

Bronchonocardiosis 039.1
Bronchopleuropneumonia — *see* Pneumonia, broncho-
Bronchopneumonia — *see* Pneumonia, broncho-
Bronchopneumonitis — *see* Pneumonia, broncho-
Bronchopulmonary — *see* condition
Bronchopulmonitis — *see* Pneumonia, broncho-
Bronchorrhagia 786.30 ▲
  newborn 770.3
  tuberculous (*see also* Tuberculosis) 011.3 ☑
Bronchorrhea (chronic) (purulent) 491.0
  acute 466.0
Bronchospasm 519.11
  with
    asthma — *see* Asthma
    bronchiolitis, acute 466.19
      due to respiratory syncytial virus 466.11
    bronchitis — *see* Bronchitis
    chronic obstructive pulmonary disease (COPD) 496
    emphysema — *see* Emphysema
    due to external agent — *see* Condition, respiratory, acute, due to
  acute 519.11
  exercise induced 493.81
Bronchospirochetosis 104.8
Bronchostenosis 519.19
Bronchus — *see* condition
Bronze, bronzed
  diabetes 275.01 ▲
  disease (Addison's) (skin) 255.41
    tuberculous (*see also* Tuberculosis) 017.6 ☑
Brooke's disease or tumor (M8100/0) — *see* Neoplasm, skin, benign
Brown enamel of teeth (hereditary) 520.5
Brown-Séquard's paralysis (syndrome) 344.89
Brown's tendon sheath syndrome 378.61
Brow presentation complicating delivery 652.4 ☑
Brucella, brucellosis (infection) 023.9
  abortus 023.1
  canis 023.3
  dermatitis, skin 023.9
  melitensis 023.0
  mixed 023.8
  suis 023.2
Bruck-de Lange disease or syndrome (Amsterdam dwarf, mental retardation, and brachycephaly) 759.89
Bruck's disease 733.99
Brugada syndrome 746.89
Brug's filariasis 125.1
Brugsch's syndrome (acropachyderma) 757.39
Bruhl's disease (splenic anemia with fever) 285.8
Bruise (skin surface intact) — *see also* Contusion
  with
    fracture — *see* Fracture, by site
    open wound — *see* Wound, open, by site
    internal organ (abdomen, chest, or pelvis) — *see* Injury, internal, by site
  umbilical cord 663.6 ☑
    affecting fetus or newborn 762.6
Bruit 785.9
  arterial (abdominal) (carotid) 785.9
  supraclavicular 785.9
Brushburn — *see* Injury, superficial, by site
Bruton's X-linked agammaglobulinemia 279.04
Bruxism 306.8
  sleep related 327.53
Bubbly lung syndrome 770.7
Bubo 289.3
  blennorrhagic 098.89
  chancroidal 099.0
  climatic 099.1
  due to Hemophilus ducreyi 099.0
  gonococcal 098.89
  indolent NEC 099.8

Bubo — *continued*
  inguinal NEC 099.8
    chancroidal 099.0
    climatic 099.1
    due to H. ducreyi 099.0
  scrofulous (*see also* Tuberculosis) 017.2 ☑
  soft chancre 099.0
  suppurating 683
  syphilitic 091.0
    congenital 090.0
  tropical 099.1
  venereal NEC 099.8
  virulent 099.0
Bubonic plague 020.0
Bubonocele — *see* Hernia, inguinal
Buccal — *see* condition
Buchanan's disease (juvenile osteochondrosis of iliac crest) 732.1
Buchem's syndrome (hyperostosis corticalis) 733.3
Buchman's disease (osteochondrosis, juvenile) 732.1
Bucket handle fracture (semilunar cartilage) — *see also* Tear, meniscus 836.2
Budd-Chiari syndrome (hepatic vein thrombosis) 453.0
Budgerigar-fanciers' disease or lung 495.2
Büdinger-Ludloff-Läwen disease 717.89
Buds
  breast 259.1
  in newborn 779.89
Buerger's disease (thromboangiitis obliterans) 443.1
Bulbar — *see* condition
Bulbus cordis 745.9
  persistent (in left ventricle) 745.8
Bulging fontanels (congenital) 756.0
Bulimia 783.6
  nervosa 307.51
  nonorganic origin 307.51
Bulky uterus 621.2
Bulla(e) 709.8
  lung (emphysematous) (solitary) 492.0
Bullet wound — *see also* Wound, open, by site
  fracture — *see* Fracture, by site, open
  internal organ (abdomen, chest, or pelvis) — *see* Injury, internal, by site, with open wound
  intracranial — *see* Laceration, brain, with open wound
Bullis fever 082.8
Bullying — *see also* Disturbance, conduct 312.0 ☑
Bundle
  branch block (complete) (false) (incomplete) 426.50
    bilateral 426.53
    left (*see also* Block, bundle branch, left) 426.3
      hemiblock 426.2
    right (*see also* Block, bundle branch, right) 426.4
  of His — *see* condition
  of Kent syndrome (anomalous atrioventricular excitation) 426.7
Bungpagga 040.81
Bunion 727.1
Bunionette 727.1
Bunyamwera fever 066.3
Buphthalmia, buphthalmos (congenital) 743.20
  associated with
    keratoglobus, congenital 743.22
    megalocornea 743.22
    ocular anomalies NEC 743.22
  isolated 743.21
  simple 743.21
Bürger-Grütz disease or syndrome (essential familial hyperlipemia) 272.3
Buried roots 525.3
Burke's syndrome 577.8
Burkitt's
  tumor (M9750/3) 200.2 ☑

Burkitt's — *continued*
  type malignant, lymphoma, lymphoblastic, or undifferentiated (M9750/3) 200.2 ☑
Burn (acid) (cathode ray) (caustic) (chemical) (electric heating appliance) (electricity) (fire) (flame) (hot liquid or object) (irradiation) (lime) (radiation) (steam) (thermal) (x-ray) 949.0

Note — Use the following fifth-digit subclassification with category 948 to indicate the percent of body surface with third degree burn:

0	Less than 10% or unspecified
1	10–19%
2	20–29%
3	30–39%
4	40–49%
5	50–59%
6	60–69%
7	70–79%
8	80–89%
9	90% or more of body surface

  with
    blisters — *see* Burn, by site, second degree
    erythema — *see* Burn, by site, first degree
    skin loss (epidermal) (*see also* Burn, by site, second degree)
    full thickness (*see also* Burn, by site, third degree)
      with necrosis of underlying tissues — *see* Burn, by site, third degree, deep
  first degree — *see* Burn, by site, first degree
  second degree — *see* Burn, by site, second degree
  third degree — *see* Burn, by site, third degree
    deep — *see* Burn, by site, third degree, deep
  abdomen, abdominal (muscle) (wall) 942.03
    with
      trunk — *see* Burn, trunk, multiple sites
    first degree 942.13
    second degree 942.23
    third degree 942.33
      deep 942.43
        with loss of body part 942.53
  ankle 945.03
    with
      lower limb(s) — *see* Burn, leg, multiple sites
    first degree 945.13
    second degree 945.23
    third degree 945.33
      deep 945.43
        with loss of body part 945.53
  anus — *see* Burn, trunk, specified site NEC
  arm(s) 943.00
    first degree 943.10
    second degree 943.20
    third degree 943.30
      deep 943.40
        with loss of body part 943.50
    lower — *see* Burn, forearm(s)
    multiple sites, except hand(s) or wrist(s) 943.09
      first degree 943.19
      second degree 943.29
      third degree 943.39
        deep 943.49
          with loss of body part 943.59
    upper 943.03
      first degree 943.13
      second degree 943.23
      third degree 943.33
        deep 943.43
          with loss of body part 943.53

Burn — *continued*
  auditory canal (external) — *see* Burn, ear
  auricle (ear) — *see* Burn, ear
  axilla 943.04
    with
      upper limb(s), except hand(s) or wrist(s) — *see* Burn, arm(s), multiple sites
    first degree 943.14
    second degree 943.24
    third degree 943.34
      deep 943.44
        with loss of body part 943.54
  back 942.04
    with
      trunk — *see* Burn, trunk, multiple sites
    first degree 942.14
    second degree 942.24
    third degree 942.34
      deep 942.44
        with loss of body part 942.54
  biceps
    brachii — *see* Burn, arm(s), upper
    femoris — *see* Burn, thigh
  breast(s) 942.01
    with
      trunk — *see* Burn, trunk, multiple sites
    first degree 942.11
    second degree 942.21
    third degree 942.31
      deep 942.41
        with loss of body part 942.51
  brow — *see* Burn, forehead
  buttock(s) — *see* Burn, back
  canthus (eye) 940.1
    chemical 940.0
  cervix (uteri) 947.4
  cheek (cutaneous) 941.07
    with
      face or head — *see* Burn, head, multiple sites
    first degree 941.17
    second degree 941.27
    third degree 941.37
      deep 941.47
        with loss of body part 941.57
  chest wall (anterior) 942.02
    with
      trunk — *see* Burn, trunk, multiple sites
    first degree 942.12
    second degree 942.22
    third degree 942.32
      deep 942.42
        with loss of body part 942.52
  chin 941.04
    with
      face or head — *see* Burn, head, multiple sites
    first degree 941.14
    second degree 941.24
    third degree 941.34
      deep 941.44
        with loss of body part 941.54
  clitoris — *see* Burn, genitourinary organs, external
  colon 947.3
  conjunctiva (and cornea) 940.4
    chemical
      acid 940.3
      alkaline 940.2
  cornea (and conjunctiva) 940.4
    chemical
      acid 940.3
      alkaline 940.2
  costal region — *see* Burn, chest wall
  due to ingested chemical agent — *see* Burn, internal organs
  ear (auricle) (canal) (drum) (external) 941.01
    with
      face or head — *see* Burn, head, multiple sites
    first degree 941.11
    second degree 941.21

☑ **Additional Digit Required** — Refer to the Tabular List for Digit Selection   ▼ **Subterms under main terms may continue to next column or page**

38 — Volume 2 · October 2010   ▶◀ Revised Text   ● New Line   ▲ Revised Code   **2011 ICD-9-CM**

Burn — *continued*
ear — *continued*
third degree 941.31
deep 941.41
with loss of a body part 941.51
elbow 943.02
with
hand(s) and wrist(s) — *see* Burn, multiple specified sites
upper limb(s), except hand(s) or wrist(s) (*see also* Burn, arm(s), multiple sites)
first degree 943.12
second degree 943.22
third degree 943.32
deep 943.42
with loss of body part 943.52
electricity, electric current — *see* Burn, by site
entire body — *see* Burn, multiple, specified sites
epididymis — *see* Burn, genitourinary organs, external
epigastric region — *see* Burn, abdomen
epiglottis 947.1
esophagus 947.2
extent (percent of body surface)
less than 10 percent 948.0 ☑
10-19 percent 948.1 ☑
20-29 percent 948.2 ☑
30-39 percent 948.3 ☑
40-49 percent 948.4 ☑
50-59 percent 948.5 ☑
60-69 percent 948.6 ☑
70-79 percent 948.7 ☑
80-89 percent 948.8 ☑
90 percent or more 948.9 ☑
extremity
lower — *see* Burn, leg
upper — *see* Burn, arm(s)
eye(s) (and adnexa) (only) 940.9
with
face, head, or neck 941.02
first degree 941.12
second degree 941.22
third degree 941.32
deep 941.42
with loss of body part 941.52
other sites (classifiable to more than one category in 940–945) — *see* Burn, multiple, specified sites
resulting rupture and destruction of eyeball 940.5
specified part — *see* Burn, by site
eyeball (*see also* Burn, eye)
with resulting rupture and destruction of eyeball 940.5
eyelid(s) 940.1
chemical 940.0
face — *see* Burn, head
finger (nail) (subungual) 944.01
with
hand(s) — *see* Burn, hand(s), multiple sites
other sites — *see* Burn, multiple, specified sites
thumb 944.04
first degree 944.14
second degree 944.24
third degree 944.34
deep 944.44
with loss of body part 944.54
first degree 944.11
second degree 944.21
third degree 944.31
deep 944.41
with loss of body part 944.51
multiple (digits) 944.03
with thumb — *see* Burn, finger, with thumb
first degree 944.13
second degree 944.23
third degree 944.33

Burn — *continued*
finger — *continued*
multiple — *continued*
third degree — *continued*
deep 944.43
with loss of body part 944.53
flank — *see* Burn, abdomen
foot 945.02
with
lower limb(s) — *see* Burn, leg, multiple sites
first degree 945.12
second degree 945.22
third degree 945.32
deep 945.42
with loss of body part 945.52
forearm(s) 943.01
with
upper limb(s), except hand(s) or wrist(s) — *see* Burn, arm(s), multiple sites
first degree 943.11
second degree 943.21
third degree 943.31
deep 943.41
with loss of body part 943.51
forehead 941.07
with
face or head — *see* Burn, head, multiple sites
first degree 941.17
second degree 941.27
third degree 941.37
deep 941.47
with loss of body part 941.57
fourth degree — *see* Burn, by site, third degree, deep
friction — *see* Injury, superficial, by site
from swallowing caustic or corrosive substance NEC — *see* Burn, internal organs
full thickness — *see* Burn, by site, third degree
gastrointestinal tract 947.3
genitourinary organs
external 942.05
with
trunk — *see* Burn, trunk, multiple sites
first degree 942.15
second degree 942.25
third degree 942.35
deep 942.45
with loss of body part 942.55
internal 947.8
globe (eye) — *see* Burn, eyeball
groin — *see* Burn, abdomen
gum 947.0
hand(s) (phalanges) (and wrist) 944.00
first degree 944.10
second degree 944.20
third degree 944.30
deep 944.40
with loss of body part 944.50
back (dorsal surface) 944.06
first degree 944.16
second degree 944.26
third degree 944.36
deep 944.46
with loss of body part 944.56
multiple sites 944.08
first degree 944.18
second degree 944.28
third degree 944.38
deep 944.48
with loss of body part 944.58
head (and face) 941.00
first degree 941.10
second degree 941.20
third degree 941.30
deep 941.40
with loss of body part 941.50
eye(s) only 940.9
specified part — *see* Burn, by site
multiple sites 941.09

Burn — *continued*
head — *continued*
multiple sites — *continued*
with eyes — *see* Burn, eyes, with face, head, or neck
first degree 941.19
second degree 941.29
third degree 941.39
deep 941.49
with loss of body part 941.59
heel — *see* Burn, foot
hip — *see* Burn, trunk, specified site NEC
iliac region — *see* Burn, trunk, specified site NEC
infected 958.3
inhalation (*see also* Burn, internal organs) 947.9
internal organs 947.9
from caustic or corrosive substance (swallowing) NEC 947.9
specified NEC (*see also* Burn, by site) 947.8
interscapular region — *see* Burn, back
intestine (large) (small) 947.3
iris — *see* Burn, eyeball
knee 945.05
with
lower limb(s) — *see* Burn, leg, multiple sites
first degree 945.15
second degree 945.25
third degree 945.35
deep 945.45
with loss of body part 945.55
labium (majus) (minus) — *see* Burn, genitourinary organs, external
lacrimal apparatus, duct, gland, or sac 940.1
chemical 940.0
larynx 947.1
late effect — *see* Late, effects (of), burn
leg 945.00
first degree 945.10
second degree 945.20
third degree 945.30
deep 945.40
with loss of body part 945.50
lower 945.04
with other part(s) of lower limb(s) — *see* Burn, leg, multiple sites
first degree 945.14
second degree 945.24
third degree 945.34
deep 945.44
with loss of body part 945.54
multiple sites 945.09
first degree 945.19
second degree 945.29
third degree 945.39
deep 945.49
with loss of body part 945.59
upper — *see* Burn, thigh
lightning — *see* Burn, by site
limb(s)
lower (including foot or toe(s)) — *see* Burn, leg
upper (except wrist and hand) — *see* Burn, arm(s)
lip(s) 941.03
with
face or head — *see* Burn, head, multiple sites
first degree 941.13
second degree 941.23
third degree 941.33
deep 941.43
with loss of body part 941.53
lumbar region — *see* Burn, back
lung 947.1
malar region — *see* Burn, cheek
mastoid region — *see* Burn, scalp
membrane, tympanic — *see* Burn, ear
midthoracic region — *see* Burn, chest wall
mouth 947.0
multiple (*see also* Burn, unspecified) 949.0

Burn — *continued*
multiple (*see also* Burn, unspecified) — *continued*
specified sites classifiable to more than one category in 940-945 ☑, 946.0
first degree 946.1
second degree 946.2
third degree 946.3
deep 946.4
with loss of body part 946.5
muscle, abdominal — *see* Burn, abdomen
nasal (septum) — *see* Burn, nose
neck 941.08
with
face or head — *see* Burn, head, multiple sites
first degree 941.18
second degree 941.28
third degree 941.38
deep 941.48
with loss of body part 941.58
nose (septum) 941.05
with
face or head — *see* Burn, head, multiple sites
first degree 941.15
second degree 941.25
third degree 941.35
deep 941.45
with loss of body part 941.55
occipital region — *see* Burn, scalp
orbit region 940.1
chemical 940.0
oronasopharynx 947.0
palate 947.0
palm(s) 944.05
with
hand(s) and wrist(s) — *see* Burn, hand(s), multiple sites
first degree 944.15
second degree 944.25
third degree 944.35
deep 944.45
with loss of a body part 944.55
parietal region — *see* Burn, scalp
penis — *see* Burn, genitourinary organs, external
perineum — *see* Burn, genitourinary organs, external
periocular area 940.1
chemical 940.0
pharynx 947.0
pleura 947.1
popliteal space — *see* Burn, knee
prepuce — *see* Burn, genitourinary organs, external
pubic region — *see* Burn, genitourinary organs, external
pudenda — *see* Burn, genitourinary organs, external
rectum 947.3
sac, lacrimal 940.1
chemical 940.0
sacral region — *see* Burn, back
salivary (ducts) (glands) 947.0
scalp 941.06
with
face or neck — *see* Burn, head, multiple sites
first degree 941.16
second degree 941.26
third degree 941.36
deep 941.46
with loss of body part 941.56
scapular region 943.06
with
upper limb(s), except hand(s) or wrist(s) — *see* Burn, arm(s), multiple sites
first degree 943.16
second degree 943.26
third degree 943.36
deep 943.46
with loss of body part 943.56
sclera — *see* Burn, eyeball

☑ Additional Digit Required — Refer to the Tabular List for Digit Selection ▽ Subterms under main terms may continue to next column or page

2011 ICD-9-CM ▶◀ Revised Text ● New Line ▲ Revised Code Volume 2 — 39

Burn — *continued*
scrotum — *see* Burn, genitourinary organs, external
septum, nasal — *see* Burn, nose
shoulder(s) 943.05
  with
    hand(s) and wrist(s) — *see* Burn, multiple, specified sites
    upper limb(s), except hand(s) or wrist(s) — *see* Burn, arm(s), multiple sites
  first degree 943.15
  second degree 943.25
  third degree 943.35
    deep 943.45
      with loss of body part 943.55
skin NEC (*see also* Burn, unspecified) 949.0
skull — *see* Burn, head
small intestine 947.3
sternal region — *see* Burn, chest wall
stomach 947.3
subconjunctival — *see* Burn, conjunctiva
subcutaneous — *see* Burn, by site, third degree
submaxillary region — *see* Burn, head
submental region — *see* Burn, chin
sun — *see* Sunburn
supraclavicular fossa — *see* Burn, neck
supraorbital — *see* Burn, forehead
temple — *see* Burn, scalp
temporal region — *see* Burn, scalp
testicle — *see* Burn, genitourinary organs, external
testis — *see* Burn, genitourinary organs, external
thigh 945.06
  with
    lower limb(s) — *see* Burn, leg, multiple sites
  first degree 945.16
  second degree 945.26
  third degree 945.36
    deep 945.46
      with loss of body part 945.56
thorax (external) — *see* Burn, chest wall
throat 947.0
thumb(s) (nail) (subungual) 944.02
  with
    finger(s) — *see* Burn, finger, with other sites, thumb
    hand(s) and wrist(s) — *see* Burn, hand(s), multiple sites
  first degree 944.12
  second degree 944.22
  third degree 944.32
    deep 944.42
      with loss of body part 944.52
toe (nail) (subungual) 945.01
  with
    lower limb(s) — *see* Burn, leg, multiple sites
  first degree 945.11
  second degree 945.21
  third degree 945.31
    deep 945.41
      with loss of body part 945.51
tongue 947.0
tonsil 947.0
trachea 947.1
trunk 942.00
  first degree 942.10
  second degree 942.20
  third degree 942.30
    deep 942.40
      with loss of body part 942.50
  multiple sites 942.09
    first degree 942.19
    second degree 942.29
    third degree 942.39
      deep 942.49
        with loss of body part 942.59
  specified site NEC 942.09
    first degree 942.19
    second degree 942.29
    third degree 942.39
      deep 942.49

Burn — *continued*
trunk — *continued*
  specified site — *continued*
    third degree — *continued*
      deep — *continued*
        with loss of body part 942.59
tunica vaginalis — *see* Burn, genitourinary organs, external
tympanic membrane — *see* Burn, ear
tympanum — *see* Burn, ear
ultraviolet 692.82
unspecified site (multiple) 949.0
  with extent of body surface involved specified
    less than 10 percent 948.0 ☑
    10-19 percent 948.1 ☑
    20-29 percent 948.2 ☑
    30-39 percent 948.3 ☑
    40-49 percent 948.4 ☑
    50-59 percent 948.5 ☑
    60-69 percent 948.6 ☑
    70-79 percent 948.7 ☑
    80-89 percent 948.8 ☑
    90 percent or more 948.9 ☑
  first degree 949.1
  second degree 949.2
  third degree 949.3
    deep 949.4
      with loss of body part 949.5
uterus 947.4
uvula 947.0
vagina 947.4
vulva — *see* Burn, genitourinary organs, external
wrist(s) 944.07
  with
    hand(s) — *see* Burn, hand(s), multiple sites
  first degree 944.17
  second degree 944.27
  third degree 944.37
    deep 944.47
      with loss of body part 944.57
Burnett's syndrome (milk-alkali) 275.42
Burnier's syndrome (hypophyseal dwarfism) 253.3
Burning
feet syndrome 266.2
sensation (*see also* Disturbance, sensation) 782.0
tongue 529.6
Burns' disease (osteochondrosis, lower ulna) 732.3
Bursa — *see also* condition
pharynx 478.29
Bursitis NEC 727.3
Achilles tendon 726.71
adhesive 726.90
  shoulder 726.0
ankle 726.79
buttock 726.5
calcaneal 726.79
collateral ligament
  fibular 726.63
  tibial 726.62
Duplay's 726.2
elbow 726.33
finger 726.8
foot 726.79
gonococcal 098.52
hand 726.4
hip 726.5
infrapatellar 726.69
ischiogluteal 726.5
knee 726.60
occupational NEC 727.2
olecranon 726.33
pes anserinus 726.61
pharyngeal 478.29
popliteal 727.51
prepatellar 726.65
radiohumeral 727.3
scapulohumeral 726.19
  adhesive 726.0
shoulder 726.10
  adhesive 726.0

Bursitis — *continued*
subacromial 726.19
  adhesive 726.0
subcoracoid 726.19
subdeltoid 726.19
  adhesive 726.0
subpatellar 726.69
syphilitic 095.7
Thornwaldt's, Tornwaldt's (pharyngeal) 478.29
toe 726.79
trochanteric area 726.5
wrist 726.4
Burst stitches or sutures (complication of surgery) (external) (*see also* Dehiscence) 998.32
internal 998.31
Buruli ulcer 031.1
Bury's disease (erythema elevatum diutinum) 695.89
Buschke's disease or scleredema (adultorum) 710.1
Busquet's disease (osteoperiostitis) — *see also* Osteomyelitis 730.1 ☑
Busse-Buschke disease (cryptococcosis) 117.5
Buttock — *see* condition
Button
Biskra 085.1
Delhi 085.1
oriental 085.1
Buttonhole hand (intrinsic) 736.21
Bwamba fever (encephalitis) 066.3
Byssinosis (occupational) 504
Bywaters' syndrome 958.5

C

Cacergasia 300.9
Cachexia 799.4
cancerous (*see also* Neoplasm, by site, malignant) 799.4
cardiac — *see* Disease, heart
dehydration 276.51
  with
    hypernatremia 276.0
    hyponatremia 276.1
due to malnutrition 799.4
exophthalmic 242.0 ☑
heart — *see* Disease, heart
hypophyseal 253.2
hypopituitary 253.2
lead 984.9
  specified type of lead — *see* Table of Drugs and Chemicals
malaria 084.9
malignant (*see also* Neoplasm, by site, malignant) 799.4
marsh 084.9
nervous 300.5
old age 797
pachydermic — *see* Hypothyroidism
paludal 084.9
pituitary (postpartum) 253.2
renal (*see also* Disease, renal) 593.9
saturnine 984.9
  specified type of lead — *see* Table of Drugs and Chemicals
senile 797
Simmonds' (pituitary cachexia) 253.2
splenica 289.59
strumipriva (*see also* Hypothyroidism) 244.9
tuberculous NEC (*see also* Tuberculosis) 011.9 ☑
Café au lait spots 709.09
Caffey's disease or syndrome (infantile cortical hyperostosis) 756.59
Caisson disease 993.3
Caked breast (puerperal, postpartum) 676.2 ☑
Cake kidney 753.3
Calabar swelling 125.2
Calcaneal spur 726.73
Calcaneoapophysitis 732.5
Calcaneonavicular bar 755.67
Calcareous — *see* condition
Calcicosis (occupational) 502
Calciferol (vitamin D) **deficiency** 268.9

Calciferol (vitamin D) **deficiency** — *continued*
  with
    osteomalacia 268.2
    rickets (*see also* Rickets) 268.0
Calcification
adrenal (capsule) (gland) 255.41
  tuberculous (*see also* Tuberculosis) 017.6 ☑
aorta 440.0
artery (annular) — *see* Arteriosclerosis
auricle (ear) 380.89
bladder 596.8
  due to S. hematobium 120.0
brain (cortex) — *see* Calcification, cerebral
bronchus 519.19
bursa 727.82
cardiac (*see also* Degeneration, myocardial) 429.1
cartilage (postinfectional) 733.99
cerebral (cortex) 348.89
  artery 437.0
cervix (uteri) 622.8
choroid plexus 349.2
conjunctiva 372.54
corpora cavernosa (penis) 607.89
cortex (brain) — *see* Calcification, cerebral
dental pulp (nodular) 522.2
dentinal papilla 520.4
disc, intervertebral 722.90
  cervical, cervicothoracic 722.91
  lumbar, lumbosacral 722.93
  thoracic, thoracolumbar 722.92
fallopian tube 620.8
falx cerebri — *see* Calcification, cerebral
fascia 728.89
gallbladder 575.8
general 275.40
heart (*see also* Degeneration, myocardial) 429.1
  valve — *see* Endocarditis
intervertebral cartilage or disc (postinfectional) 722.90
  cervical, cervicothoracic 722.91
  lumbar, lumbosacral 722.93
  thoracic, thoracolumbar 722.92
intracranial — *see* Calcification, cerebral
intraspinal ligament 728.89
joint 719.80
  ankle 719.87
  elbow 719.82
  foot 719.87
  hand 719.84
  hip 719.85
  knee 719.86
  multiple sites 719.89
  pelvic region 719.85
  shoulder (region) 719.81
  specified site NEC 719.88
  wrist 719.83
kidney 593.89
  tuberculous (*see also* Tuberculosis) 016.0 ☑
larynx (senile) 478.79
lens 366.8
ligament 728.89
  intraspinal 728.89
  knee (medial collateral) 717.89
lung 518.89
  active 518.89
  postinfectional 518.89
  tuberculous (*see also* Tuberculosis, pulmonary) 011.9 ☑
lymph gland or node (postinfectional) 289.3
  tuberculous (*see also* Tuberculosis, lymph gland) 017.2 ☑
mammographic 793.89
massive (paraplegic) 728.10
medial NEC (*see also* Arteriosclerosis, extremities) 440.20
meninges (cerebral) 349.2
metastatic 275.40
Mönckeberg's — *see* Arteriosclerosis
muscle 728.10
  heterotopic, postoperative 728.13

☑ Additional Digit Required — Refer to the Tabular List for Digit Selection   ▽ Subterms under main terms may continue to next column or page

40 — Volume 2   ▶◀ Revised Text   ● New Line   ▲ Revised Code   2011 ICD-9-CM

Index

Burn — Calcification

Calcification — *continued*
- myocardium, myocardial (*see also* Degeneration, myocardial) 429.1
- ovary 620.8
- pancreas 577.8
- penis 607.89
- periarticular 728.89
- pericardium (*see also* Pericarditis) 423.8
- pineal gland 259.8
- pleura 511.0
  - postinfectional 518.89
  - tuberculous (*see also* Tuberculosis, pleura) 012.0 ☑
- pulp (dental) (nodular) 522.2
- renal 593.89
- Rider's bone 733.99
- sclera 379.16
- semilunar cartilage 717.89
- spleen 289.59
- subcutaneous 709.3
- suprarenal (capsule) (gland) 255.41
- tendon (sheath) 727.82
  - with bursitis, synovitis or tenosynovitis 727.82
- trachea 519.19
- ureter 593.89
- uterus 621.8
- vitreous 379.29

Calcified — *see also* Calcification
- hematoma NEC 959.9

Calcinosis (generalized) (interstitial) (tumoral) (universalis) 275.49
- circumscripta 709.3
- cutis 709.3
- intervertebralis 275.49 [722.90]
- Raynaud's phenomenonsclerodactylytelangiectasis (CRST) 710.1

Calciphylaxis — *see also* Calcification, by site 275.49

Calcium
- blood
  - high (*see also* Hypercalcemia) 275.42
  - low (*see also* Hypocalcemia) 275.41
- deposits (*see also* Calcification, by site)
  - in bursa 727.82
  - in tendon (sheath) 727.82
    - with bursitis, synovitis or tenosynovitis 727.82
- salts or soaps in vitreous 379.22

Calciuria 791.9

Calculi — *see* Calculus

Calculosis, intrahepatic — *see* Choledocholithiasis

Calculus, calculi, calculous 592.9
- ampulla of Vater — *see* Choledocholithiasis
- anuria (impacted) (recurrent) 592.0
- appendix 543.9
- bile duct (any) — *see* Choledocholithiasis
- biliary — *see* Cholelithiasis
- bilirubin, multiple — *see* Cholelithiasis
- bladder (encysted) (impacted) (urinary) 594.1
  - diverticulum 594.0
- bronchus 518.89
- calyx (kidney) (renal) 592.0
  - congenital 753.3
- cholesterol (pure) (solitary) — *see* Cholelithiasis
- common duct (bile) — *see* Choledocholithiasis
- conjunctiva 372.54
- cystic 594.1
  - duct — *see* Cholelithiasis
- dental 523.6
  - subgingival 523.6
  - supragingival 523.6
- epididymis 608.89
- gallbladder (*see also* Cholelithiasis)
  - congenital 751.69
- hepatic (duct) — *see* Choledocholithiasis
- intestine (impaction) (obstruction) 560.39
- kidney (impacted) (multiple) (pelvis) (recurrent) (staghorn) 592.0
  - congenital 753.3
- lacrimal (passages) 375.57
- liver (impacted) — *see* Choledocholithiasis

Calculus, calculi, calculous — *continued*
- lung 518.89
- mammographic 793.89
- nephritic (impacted) (recurrent) 592.0
- nose 478.19
- pancreas (duct) 577.8
- parotid gland 527.5
- pelvis, encysted 592.0
- prostate 602.0
- pulmonary 518.89
- renal (impacted) (recurrent) 592.0
  - congenital 753.3
- salivary (duct) (gland) 527.5
- seminal vesicle 608.89
- staghorn 592.0
- Stensen's duct 527.5
- sublingual duct or gland 527.5
  - congenital 750.26
- submaxillary duct, gland, or region 527.5
- suburethral 594.8
- tonsil 474.8
- tooth, teeth 523.6
- tunica vaginalis 608.89
- ureter (impacted) (recurrent) 592.1
- urethra (impacted) 594.2
- urinary (duct) (impacted) (passage) (tract) 592.9
  - lower tract NEC 594.9
    - specified site 594.8
- vagina 623.8
- vesical (impacted) 594.1
- Wharton's duct 527.5

Caliectasis 593.89

California
- disease 114.0
- encephalitis 062.5

Caligo cornea 371.03

Callositas, callosity (infected) 700

Callus (infected) 700
- bone 726.91
- excessive, following fracture (*see also* Late, effect (of), fracture)

Calvé (-Perthes) disease (osteochondrosis, femoral capital) 732.1

Calvities — *see also* Alopecia 704.00

Cameroon fever — *see also* Malaria 084.6

Camptocormia 300.11

Camptodactyly (congenital) 755.59

Camurati-Engelmann disease (diaphyseal sclerosis) 756.59

Canal — *see* condition

Canaliculitis (lacrimal) (acute) 375.31
- Actinomyces 039.8
- chronic 375.41

Canavan's disease 330.0

Cancer (M8000/3) — *see also* Neoplasm, by site, malignant

> Note — The term "cancer" when modified by an adjective or adjectival phrase indicating a morphological type should be coded in the same manner as "carcinoma" with that adjective or phrase. Thus, "squamous-cell cancer" should be coded in the same manner as "squamous-cell carcinoma," which appears in the list under "Carcinoma."

- bile duct type (M8160/3), liver 155.1
- hepatocellular (M8170/3) 155.0

Cancerous (M8000/3) — *see* Neoplasm, by site, malignant

Cancerphobia 300.29

Cancrum oris 528.1

Candidiasis, candidal 112.9
- with pneumonia 112.4
- balanitis 112.2
- congenital 771.7
- disseminated 112.5
- endocarditis 112.81
- esophagus 112.84
- intertrigo 112.3
- intestine 112.85
- lung 112.4
- meningitis 112.83
- mouth 112.0
- nails 112.3
- neonatal 771.7

Candidiasis, candidal — *continued*
- onychia 112.3
- otitis externa 112.82
- otomycosis 112.82
- paronychia 112.3
- perionyxis 112.3
- pneumonia 112.4
- pneumonitis 112.4
- skin 112.3
- specified site NEC 112.89
- systemic 112.5
- urogenital site NEC 112.2
- vagina 112.1
- vulva 112.1
- vulvovaginitis 112.1

Candidiosis — *see* Candidiasis

Candiru infection or infestation 136.8

Canities (premature) 704.3
- congenital 757.4

Canker (mouth) (sore) 528.2
- rash 034.1

Cannabinosis 504

Canton fever 081.9

Cap
- cradle 690.11

Capillariasis 127.5

Capillary — *see* condition

Caplan-Colinet syndrome 714.81

Caplan's syndrome 714.81

Capsule — *see* condition

Capsulitis (joint) 726.90
- adhesive (shoulder) 726.0
- hip 726.5
- knee 726.60
- labyrinthine 387.8
- thyroid 245.9
- wrist 726.4

Caput
- crepitus 756.0
- medusae 456.8
- succedaneum 767.19

Carapata disease 087.1

Carate — *see* Pinta

Carbohydrate-deficient glycoprotein syndrome (CGDS) 271.8

Carboxyhemoglobinemia 986

Carbuncle 680.9
- abdominal wall 680.2
- ankle 680.6
- anus 680.5
- arm (any part, above wrist) 680.3
- auditory canal, external 680.0
- axilla 680.3
- back (any part) 680.2
- breast 680.2
- buttock 680.5
- chest wall 680.2
- corpus cavernosum 607.2
- ear (any part) (external) 680.0
- eyelid 373.13
- face (any part, except eye) 680.0
- finger (any) 680.4
- flank 680.2
- foot (any part) 680.7
- forearm 680.3
- genital organ (male) 608.4
- gluteal (region) 680.5
- groin 680.2
- hand (any part) 680.4
- head (any part, except face) 680.8
- heel 680.7
- hip 680.6
- kidney (*see also* Abscess, kidney) 590.2
- knee 680.6
- labia 616.4
- lacrimal
  - gland (*see also* Dacryoadenitis) 375.00
  - passages (duct) (sac) (*see also* Dacryocystitis) 375.30
- leg, any part except foot 680.6
- lower extremity, any part except foot 680.6
- malignant 022.0
- multiple sites 680.9
- neck 680.1
- nose (external) (septum) 680.0
- orbit, orbital 376.01

Carbuncle — *continued*
- partes posteriores 680.5
- pectoral region 680.2
- penis 607.2
- perineum 680.2
- pinna 680.0
- scalp (any part) 680.8
- scrotum 608.4
- seminal vesicle 608.0
- shoulder 680.3
- skin NEC 680.9
- specified site NEC 680.8
- spermatic cord 608.4
- temple (region) 680.0
- testis 608.4
- thigh 680.6
- thumb 680.4
- toe (any) 680.7
- trunk 680.2
- tunica vaginalis 608.4
- umbilicus 680.2
- upper arm 680.3
- urethra 597.0
- vas deferens 608.4
- vulva 616.4
- wrist 680.4

Carbunculus — *see also* Carbuncle 680.9

Carcinoid (tumor) (M8240/1) — *see* Tumor, carcinoid

Carcinoidosis 259.2

Carcinomaphobia 300.29

Carcinomatosis
- peritonei (M8010/6) 197.6
- specified site NEC (M8010/3) — *see* Neoplasm, by site, malignant
- unspecified site (M8010/6) 199.0

Carcinoma (M8010/3) — *see also* Neoplasm, by site, malignant

> Note — Except where otherwise indicated, the morphological varieties of carcinoma in the list below should be coded by site as for "Neoplasm, malignant."

- with
  - apocrine metaplasia (M8573/3)
  - cartilaginous (and osseous) metaplasia (M8571/3)
  - osseous (and cartilaginous) metaplasia (M8571/3)
  - productive fibrosis (M8141/3)
  - spindle cell metaplasia (M8572/3)
  - squamous metaplasia (M8570/3)
- acidophil (M8280/3)
  - specified site — *see* Neoplasm, by site, malignant
  - unspecified site 194.3
- acidophil-basophil, mixed (M8281/3)
  - specified site — *see* Neoplasm, by site, malignant
  - unspecified site 194.3
- acinar (cell) (M8550/3)
- acinic cell (M8550/3)
- adenocystic (M8200/3)
- adenoid
  - cystic (M8200/3)
  - squamous cell (M8075/3)
- adenosquamous (M8560/3)
- adnexal (skin) (M8390/3) — *see* Neoplasm, skin, malignant
- adrenal cortical (M8370/3) 194.0
- alveolar (M8251/3)
  - cell (M8250/3) — *see* Neoplasm, lung, malignant
- anaplastic type (M8021/3)
- apocrine (M8401/3)
  - breast — *see* Neoplasm, breast, malignant
  - specified site NEC — *see* Neoplasm, skin, malignant
  - unspecified site 173.9
- basal cell (pigmented) (M8090/3) (*see also* Neoplasm, skin, malignant)
  - fibro-epithelial type (M8093/3) — *see* Neoplasm, skin, malignant
  - morphea type (M8092/3) — *see* Neoplasm, skin, malignant

☑ **Additional Digit Required** — Refer to the Tabular List for Digit Selection   ▽ **Subterms under main terms may continue to next column or page**

2011 ICD-9-CM   ▶◀ **Revised Text**   ● **New Line**   ▲ **Revised Code**   **Volume 2 — 41**

Index

Carcinoma — Carcinoma

Carcinoma — *see also* Neoplasm, by site, malignant — *continued*
  basal cell (*see also* Neoplasm, skin, malignant) — *continued*
    multicentric (M8091/3) — *see* Neoplasm, skin, malignant
  basaloid (M8123/3)
  basal-squamous cell, mixed (M8094/3) — *see* Neoplasm, skin, malignant
  basophil (M8300/3)
    specified site — *see* Neoplasm, by site, malignant
    unspecified site 194.3
  basophil-acidophil, mixed (M8281/3)
    specified site — *see* Neoplasm, by site, malignant
    unspecified site 194.3
  basosquamous (M8094/3) — *see* Neoplasm, skin, malignant
  bile duct type (M8160/3)
    and hepatocellular, mixed (M8180/3) 155.0
    liver 155.1
    specified site NEC — *see* Neoplasm, by site, malignant
    unspecified site 155.1
  branchial or branchiogenic 146.8
  bronchial or bronchogenic — *see* Neoplasm, lung, malignant
  bronchiolar (terminal) (M8250/3) — *see* Neoplasm, lung, malignant
  bronchiolo-alveolar (M8250/3) — *see* Neoplasm, lung, malignant
  bronchogenic (epidermoid) 162.9
  C cell (M8510/3)
    specified site — *see* Neoplasm, by site, malignant
    unspecified site 193
  ceruminous (M8420/3) 173.2
  chorionic (M9100/3)
    specified site — *see* Neoplasm, by site, malignant
    unspecified site
      female 181
      male 186.9
  chromophobe (M8270/3)
    specified site — *see* Neoplasm, by site, malignant
    unspecified site 194.3
  clear cell (mesonephroid type) (M8310/3)
  cloacogenic (M8124/3)
    specified site — *see* Neoplasm, by site, malignant
    unspecified site 154.8
  colloid (M8480/3)
  cribriform (M8201/3)
  cylindroid type (M8200/3)
  diffuse type (M8145/3)
    specified site — *see* Neoplasm, by site, malignant
    unspecified site 151.9
  duct (cell) (M8500/3)
    with Paget's disease (M8541/3) — *see* Neoplasm, breast, malignant
    infiltrating (M8500/3)
      specified site — *see* Neoplasm, by site, malignant
      unspecified site 174.9
  ductal (M8500/3)
  ductular, infiltrating (M8521/3)
  embryonal (M9070/3)
    and teratoma, mixed (M9081/3)
    combined with choriocarcinoma (M9101/3) — *see* Neoplasm, by site, malignant
    infantile type (M9071/3)
    liver 155.0
    polyembryonal type (M9072/3)
  endometrioid (M8380/3)
  eosinophil (M8280/3)
    specified site — *see* Neoplasm, by site, malignant
    unspecified site 194.3
  epidermoid (M8070/3) (*see also* Carcinoma, squamous cell)

Carcinoma — *see also* Neoplasm, by site, malignant — *continued*
  epidermoid (*see also* Carcinoma, squamous cell) — *continued*
    and adenocarcinoma, mixed (M8560/3)
    in situ, Bowen's type (M8081/2) — *see* Neoplasm, skin, in situ
    intradermal — *see* Neoplasm, skin, in situ
  fibroepithelial type basal cell (M8093/3) — *see* Neoplasm, skin, malignant
  follicular (M8330/3)
    and papillary (mixed) (M8340/3) 193
    moderately differentiated type (M8332/3) 193
    pure follicle type (M8331/3) 193
    specified site — *see* Neoplasm, by site, malignant
    trabecular type (M8332/3) 193
    unspecified site 193
    well differentiated type (M8331/3) 193
  gelatinous (M8480/3)
  giant cell (M8031/3)
    and spindle cell (M8030/3)
  granular cell (M8320/3)
  granulosa cell (M8620/3) 183.0
  hepatic cell (M8170/3) 155.0
  hepatocellular (M8170/3) 155.0
    and bile duct, mixed (M8180/3) 155.0
  hepatocholangiolitic (M8180/3) 155.0
  Hürthle cell (thyroid) 193
  hypernephroid (M8311/3)
  in
    adenomatous
      polyp (M8210/3)
      polyposis coli (M8220/3) 153.9
    pleomorphic adenoma (M8940/3)
    polypoid adenoma (M8210/3)
    situ (M8010/3) — *see* Carcinoma, in situ
    tubular adenoma (M8210/3)
    villous adenoma (M8261/3)
  infiltrating duct (M8500/3)
    with Paget's disease (M8541/3) — *see* Neoplasm, breast, malignant
    specified site — *see* Neoplasm, by site, malignant
    unspecified site 174.9
  inflammatory (M8530/3)
    specified site — *see* Neoplasm, by site, malignant
    unspecified site 174.9
  in situ (M8010/2) (*see also* Neoplasm, by site, in situ)
    epidermoid (M8070/2) (*see also* Neoplasm, by site, in situ)
      with questionable stromal invasion (M8076/2)
        specified site — *see* Neoplasm, by site, in situ
        unspecified site 233.1
      Bowen's type (M8081/2) — *see* Neoplasm, skin, in situ
    intraductal (M8500/2)
      specified site — *see* Neoplasm, by site, in situ
      unspecified site 233.0
    lobular (M8520/2)
      specified site — *see* Neoplasm, by site, in situ
      unspecified site 233.0
    papillary (M8050/2) — *see* Neoplasm, by site, in situ
    squamous cell (M8070/2) (*see also* Neoplasm, by site, in situ)
      with questionable stromal invasion (M8076/2)
        specified site — *see* Neoplasm, by site, in situ
        unspecified site 233.1
      transitional cell (M8120/2) — *see* Neoplasm, by site, in situ
    intestinal type (M8144/3)
      specified site — *see* Neoplasm, by site, malignant
      unspecified site 151.9

Carcinoma — *see also* Neoplasm, by site, malignant — *continued*
  intraductal (noninfiltrating) (M8500/2)
    papillary (M8503/2)
      specified site — *see* Neoplasm, by site, in situ
      unspecified site 233.0
    specified site — *see* Neoplasm, by site, in situ
    unspecified site 233.0
  intraepidermal (M8070/2) (*see also* Neoplasm, skin, in situ)
    squamous cell, Bowen's type (M8081/2) — *see* Neoplasm, skin, in situ
  intraepithelial (M8010/2) (*see also* Neoplasm, by site, in situ)
    squamous cell (M8072/2) — *see* Neoplasm, by site, in situ
  intraosseous (M9270/3) 170.1
    upper jaw (bone) 170.0
  islet cell (M8150/3)
    and exocrine, mixed (M8154/3)
      specified site — *see* Neoplasm, by site, malignant
      unspecified site 157.9
    pancreas 157.4
    specified site NEC — *see* Neoplasm, by site, malignant
    unspecified site 157.4
  juvenile, breast (M8502/3) — *see* Neoplasm, breast, malignant
  Kulchitsky's cell (carcinoid tumor of intestine) 259.2
  large cell (M8012/3)
    squamous cell, non-keratinizing type (M8072/3)
  Leydig cell (testis) (M8650/3)
    specified site — *see* Neoplasm, by site, malignant
    unspecified site 186.9
      female 183.0
      male 186.9
  liver cell (M8170/3) 155.0
  lobular (infiltrating) (M8520/3)
    non-infiltrating (M8520/3)
      specified site — *see* Neoplasm, by site, in situ
      unspecified site 233.0
    specified site — *see* Neoplasm, by site, malignant
    unspecified site 174.9
  lymphoepithelial (M8082/3)
  medullary (M8510/3)
    with
      amyloid stroma (M8511/3)
        specified site — *see* Neoplasm, by site, malignant
        unspecified site 193
      lymphoid stroma (M8512/3)
        specified site — *see* Neoplasm, by site, malignant
        unspecified site 174.9
  Merkel 209.36
    buttock 209.36
    ear 209.31
    eyelid, including canthus 209.31
    face 209.31
    genitals 209.36
    lip 209.31
    lower limb 209.34
    neck 209.32
    nodal presentation 209.75
    scalp 209.32
    secondary (any site) 209.75
    specified site NEC 209.36
    trunk 209.35
    unknown primary site 209.75
    upper limb 209.33
    visceral metastatic presentation 209.75
  mesometanephric (M9110/3)
  mesonephric (M9110/3)
  metastatic (M8010/6) — *see* Metastasis, cancer
  metatypical (M8095/3) — *see* Neoplasm, skin, malignant

Carcinoma — *see also* Neoplasm, by site, malignant — *continued*
  morphea type basal cell (M8092/3) — *see* Neoplasm, skin, malignant
  mucinous (M8480/3)
  mucin-producing (M8481/3)
  mucin-secreting (M8481/3)
  mucoepidermoid (M8430/3)
  mucoid (M8480/3)
    cell (M8300/3)
      specified site — *see* Neoplasm, by site, malignant
      unspecified site 194.3
  mucous (M8480/3)
  neuroendocrine
    high grade (M8240/3) 209.30
    malignant poorly differentiated (M8240/3) 209.30
  nonencapsulated sclerosing (M8350/3) 193
  noninfiltrating
    intracystic (M8504/2) — *see* Neoplasm, by site, in situ
    intraductal (M8500/2)
      papillary (M8503/2)
        specified site — *see* Neoplasm, by site, in situ
        unspecified site 233.0
      specified site — *see* Neoplasm, by site, in situ
      unspecified site 233.0
    lobular (M8520/2)
      specified site — *see* Neoplasm, by site, in situ
      unspecified site 233.0
  oat cell (M8042/3)
    specified site — *see* Neoplasm, by site, malignant
    unspecified site 162.9
  odontogenic (M9270/3) 170.1
    upper jaw (bone) 170.0
  onocytic (M8290/3)
  oxyphilic (M8290/3)
  papillary (M8050/3)
    and follicular (mixed) (M8340/3) 193
    epidermoid (M8052/3)
    intraductal (noninfiltrating) (M8503/2)
      specified site — *see* Neoplasm, by site, in situ
      unspecified site 233.0
    serous (M8460/3)
      specified site — *see* Neoplasm, by site, malignant
      surface (M8461/3)
        specified site — *see* Neoplasm, by site, malignant
        unspecified site 183.0
      unspecified site 183.0
    squamous cell (M8052/3)
    transitional cell (M8130/3)
  papillocystic (M8450/3)
    specified site — *see* Neoplasm, by site, malignant
    unspecified site 183.0
  parafollicular cell (M8510/3)
    specified site — *see* Neoplasm, by site, malignant
    unspecified site 193
  pleomorphic (M8022/3)
  polygonal cell (M8034/3)
  prickle cell (M8070/3)
  pseudoglandular, squamous cell (M8075/3)
  pseudomucinous (M8470/3)
    specified site — *see* Neoplasm, by site, malignant
    unspecified site 183.0
  pseudosarcomatous (M8033/3)
  regaud type (M8082/3) — *see* Neoplasm, nasopharynx, malignant
  renal cell (M8312/3) 189.0
  reserve cell (M8041/3)
  round cell (M8041/3)
  Schmincke (M8082/3) — *see* Neoplasm, nasopharynx, malignant
  Schneiderian (M8121/3)
    specified site — *see* Neoplasm, by site, malignant

☑ **Additional Digit Required** — Refer to the Tabular List for Digit Selection   ▽ **Subterms under main terms may continue to next column or page**

42 — Volume 2   ▶◀ **Revised Text**   ● **New Line**   ▲ **Revised Code**   **2011 ICD-9-CM**

Carcinoma — *see also* Neoplasm, by site, malignant — *continued*
  Schneiderian — *continued*
    unspecified site 160.0
  scirrhous (M8141/3)
  sebaceous (M8410/3) — *see* Neoplasm, skin, malignant
  secondary (M8010/6) — *see* Neoplasm, by site, malignant, secondary
  secretory, breast (M8502/3) — *see* Neoplasm, breast, malignant
  serous (M8441/3)
    papillary (M8460/3)
      specified site — *see* Neoplasm, by site, malignant
      unspecified site 183.0
    surface, papillary (M8461/3)
      specified site — *see* Neoplasm, by site, malignant
      unspecified site 183.0
  Sertoli cell (M8640/3)
    specified site — *see* Neoplasm, by site, malignant
    unspecified site 186.9
  signet ring cell (M8490/3)
    metastatic (M8490/6) — *see* Neoplasm, by site, secondary
  simplex (M8231/3)
  skin appendage (M8390/3) — *see* Neoplasm, skin, malignant
  small cell (M8041/3)
    fusiform cell type (M8043/3)
    squamous cell, non-keratinizing type (M8073/3)
  solid (M8230/3)
    with amyloid stroma (M8511/3)
      specified site — *see* Neoplasm, by site, malignant
      unspecified site 193
  spheroidal cell (M8035/3)
  spindle cell (M8032/3)
    and giant cell (M8030/3)
  spinous (M8070/3)
  squamous (cell) (M8070/3)
    adenoid type (M8075/3)
    and adenocarcinoma, mixed (M8560/3)
    intraepidermal, Bowen's type — *see* Neoplasm, skin, in situ
    keratinizing type (large cell) (M8071/3)
    large cell, non-keratinizing type (M8072/3)
    microinvasive (M8076/3)
      specified site — *see* Neoplasm, by site, malignant
      unspecified site 180.9
    non-keratinizing type (M8072/3)
    papillary (M8052/3)
    pseudoglandular (M8075/3)
    small cell, non-keratinizing type (M8073/3)
    spindle cell type (M8074/3)
    verrucous (M8051/3)
  superficial spreading (M8143/3)
  sweat gland (M8400/3) — *see* Neoplasm, skin, malignant
  theca cell (M8600/3) 183.0
  thymic (M8580/3) 164.0
  trabecular (M8190/3)
  transitional (cell) (M8120/3)
    papillary (M8130/3)
    spindle cell type (M8122/3)
  tubular (M8211/3)
  undifferentiated type (M8020/3)
  urothelial (M8120/3)
  ventriculi 151.9
  verrucous (epidermoid) (squamous cell) (M8051/3)
  villous (M8262/3)
  water-clear cell (M8322/3) 194.1
  wolffian duct (M9110/3)
Carcinosarcoma (M8980/3) — *see also* Neoplasm, by site, malignant
  embryonal type (M8981/3) — *see* Neoplasm, by site, malignant
Cardiac — *see also* condition
  death — *see* Disease, heart

Cardiac — *see also* condition — *continued*
  device
    defibrillator, automatic implantable
      ▶(with synchronous cardiac pacemaker)◀ V45.02
    in situ NEC V45.00
    pacemaker
      cardiac
        fitting or adjustment V53.31
        in situ V45.01
      carotid sinus
        fitting or adjustment V53.39
        in situ V45.09
  pacemaker — *see* Cardiac, device, pacemaker
  tamponade 423.3
Cardia, cardial — *see* condition
Cardialgia — *see also* Pain, precordial 786.51
Cardiectasis — *see* Hypertrophy, cardiac
Cardiochalasia 530.81
Cardiomalacia — *see also* Degeneration, myocardial 429.1
Cardiomegalia glycogenica diffusa 271.0
Cardiomegaly — *see also* Hypertrophy, cardiac 429.3
  congenital 746.89
  glycogen 271.0
  hypertensive (*see also* Hypertension, heart) 402.90
  idiopathic 429.3
Cardiomyoliposis — *see also* Degeneration, myocardial 429.1
Cardiomyopathy (congestive) (constrictive) (familial) (infiltrative) (obstructive) (restrictive) (sporadic) 425.4
  alcoholic 425.5
  amyloid 277.39 *[425.7]*
  beriberi 265.0 *[425.7]*
  cobalt-beer 425.5
  congenital 425.3
  due to
    amyloidosis 277.39 *[425.7]*
    beriberi 265.0 *[425.7]*
    cardiac glycogenosis 271.0 *[425.7]*
    Chagas' disease 086.0
    Friedreich's ataxia 334.0 *[425.8]*
    hypertension — *see* Hypertension, with, heart involvement
    mucopolysaccharidosis 277.5 *[425.7]*
    myotonia atrophica 359.21 *[425.8]*
    progressive muscular dystrophy 359.1 *[425.8]*
    sarcoidosis 135 *[425.8]*
  glycogen storage 271.0 *[425.7]*
  hypertensive — *see* Hypertension, with, heart involvement
  hypertrophic
    nonobstructive 425.4
    obstructive 425.1
      congenital 746.84
  idiopathic (concentric) 425.4
  in
    Chagas' disease 086.0
    sarcoidosis 135 *[425.8]*
  ischemic 414.8
  metabolic NEC 277.9 *[425.7]*
    amyloid 277.39 *[425.7]*
    thyrotoxic (*see also* Thyrotoxicosis) 242.9 ☑ *[425.7]*
    thyrotoxicosis (*see also* Thyrotoxicosis) 242.9 ☑ *[425.7]*
  newborn 425.4
    congenital 425.3
  nutritional 269.9 *[425.7]*
    beriberi 265.0 *[425.7]*
  obscure of Africa 425.2
  peripartum 674.5 ☑
  postpartum 674.5 ☑
  primary 425.4
  secondary 425.9
  stress induced 429.83
  takotsubo 429.83
  thyrotoxic (*see also* Thyrotoxicosis) 242.9 ☑ *[425.7]*
  toxic NEC 425.9

Cardiomyopathy — *continued*
  tuberculous (*see also* Tuberculosis) 017.9 ☑ *[425.8]*
Cardionephritis — *see* Hypertension, cardiorenal
Cardionephropathy — *see* Hypertension, cardiorenal
Cardionephrosis — *see* Hypertension, cardiorenal
Cardioneurosis 306.2
Cardiopathia nigra 416.0
Cardiopathy — *see also* Disease, heart 429.9
  hypertensive (*see also* Hypertension, heart) 402.90
  idiopathic 425.4
  mucopolysaccharidosis 277.5 *[425.7]*
Cardiopericarditis — *see also* Pericarditis 423.9
Cardiophobia 300.29
Cardioptosis 746.87
Cardiorenal — *see* condition
Cardiorrhexis — *see* Infarct, myocardium 410.9 ☑
Cardiosclerosis — *see* Arteriosclerosis, coronary
Cardiosis — *see* Disease, heart
Cardiospasm (esophagus) (reflex) (stomach) 530.0
  congenital 750.7
Cardiostenosis — *see* Disease, heart
Cardiosymphysis 423.1
Cardiothyrotoxicosis — *see* Hyperthyroidism
Cardiovascular — *see* condition
Carditis (acute) (bacterial) (chronic) (subacute) 429.89
  Coxsackie 074.20
  hypertensive (*see also* Hypertension, heart) 402.90
  meningococcal 036.40
  rheumatic — *see* Disease, heart, rheumatic
  rheumatoid 714.2
Care (of)
  child (routine) V20.1
  convalescent following V66.9
    chemotherapy V66.2
    medical NEC V66.5
    psychotherapy V66.3
    radiotherapy V66.1
    surgery V66.0
    surgical NEC V66.0
    treatment (for) V66.5
      combined V66.6
      fracture V66.4
      mental disorder NEC V66.3
      specified type NEC V66.5
  end-of-life V66.7
  family member (handicapped) (sick)
    creating problem for family V61.49
    provided away from home for holiday relief V60.5
    unavailable, due to
      absence (person rendering care) (sufferer) V60.4
      inability (any reason) of person rendering care V60.4
  holiday relief V60.5
  hospice V66.7
  lack of (at or after birth) (infant) (child) 995.52
    adult 995.84
  lactation of mother V24.1
  palliative V66.7
  postpartum
    immediately after delivery V24.0
    routine follow-up V24.2
  prenatal V22.1
    first pregnancy V22.0
    high-risk pregnancy V23.9
      specified problem NEC V23.89
  terminal V66.7
  unavailable, due to
    absence of person rendering care V60.4
    inability (any reason) of person rendering care V60.4
  well baby V20.1
Caries (bone) — *see also* Tuberculosis, bone 015.9 ☑ *[730.8]* ☑

Caries — *see also* Tuberculosis, bone — *continued*
  arrested 521.04
  cementum 521.03
  cerebrospinal (tuberculous) 015.0 ☑ *[730.88]*
  dental (acute) (chronic) (incipient) (infected) 521.00
    with pulp exposure 521.03
    extending to
      dentine 521.02
      pulp 521.03
    other specified NEC 521.09
    pit and fissure 521.06
    primary
      pit and fissure origin 521.06
      root surface 521.08
      smooth surface origin 521.07
    root surface 521.08
    smooth surface 521.07
  dentin (acute) (chronic) 521.02
  enamel (acute) (chronic) (incipient) 521.01
  external meatus 380.89
  hip (*see also* Tuberculosis) 015.1 ☑ *[730.85]*
  initial 521.01
  knee 015.2 ☑ *[730.86]*
  labyrinth 386.8
  limb NEC 015.7 ☑ *[730.88]*
  mastoid (chronic) (process) 383.1
  middle ear 385.89
  nose 015.7 ☑ *[730.88]*
  orbit 015.7 ☑ *[730.88]*
  ossicle 385.24
  petrous bone 383.20
  sacrum (tuberculous) 015.0 ☑ *[730.88]*
  spine, spinal (column) (tuberculous) 015.0 ☑ *[730.88]*
  syphilitic 095.5
    congenital 090.0 *[730.8]* ☑
  teeth (internal) 521.00
    initial 521.01
  vertebra (column) (tuberculous) 015.0 ☑ *[730.88]*
Carini's syndrome (ichthyosis congenita) 757.1
Carious teeth 521.00
Carneous mole 631
Carnosinemia 270.5
Carotid body or sinus syndrome 337.01
Carotidynia 337.01
Carotinemia (dietary) 278.3
Carotinosis (cutis) (skin) 278.3
Carpal tunnel syndrome 354.0
Carpenter's syndrome 759.89
Carpopedal spasm — *see also* Tetany 781.7
Carpoptosis 736.05
Carrier (suspected) of
  amebiasis V02.2
  bacterial disease (meningococcal, staphylococcal) NEC V02.59
  cholera V02.0
  cystic fibrosis gene V83.81
  defective gene V83.89
  diphtheria V02.4
  dysentery (bacillary) V02.3
    amebic V02.2
  Endamoeba histolytica V02.2
  gastrointestinal pathogens NEC V02.3
  genetic defect V83.89
  gonorrhea V02.7
  group B streptococcus V02.51
  HAA (hepatitis Australian-antigen) V02.61
  hemophilia A (asymptomatic) V83.01
    symptomatic V83.02
  hepatitis V02.60
    Australian-antigen (HAA) V02.61
    B V02.61
    C V02.62
    serum V02.61
    specified type NEC V02.69
    viral V02.60
  infective organism NEC V02.9
  malaria V02.9
  paratyphoid V02.3
  Salmonella V02.3
    typhosa V02.1
  serum hepatitis V02.61

☑ **Additional Digit Required — Refer to the Tabular List for Digit Selection**   ▽ **Subterms under main terms may continue to next column or page**

Carrier (suspected) **of** — continued
  Shigella V02.3
  Staphylococcus NEC V02.59
    methicillin
      resistant Staphylococcus aureus
        V02.54
      susceptible Staphylococcus aureus
        V02.53
  Streptococcus NEC V02.52
    group B V02.51
  typhoid V02.1
  venereal disease NEC V02.8
Carrión's disease (Bartonellosis) 088.0
Car sickness 994.6
Carter's
  relapsing fever (Asiatic) 087.0
Cartilage — see condition
Caruncle (inflamed)
  abscess, lacrimal (see also Dacryocystitis)
    375.30
  conjunctiva 372.00
    acute 372.00
  eyelid 373.00
  labium (majus) (minus) 616.89
  lacrimal 375.30
  urethra (benign) 599.3
  vagina (wall) 616.89
Cascade stomach 537.6
Caseation lymphatic gland — see also Tuberculosis 017.2 ☑
Caseous
  bronchitis — see Tuberculosis, pulmonary
  meningitis 013.0 ☑
  pneumonia — see Tuberculosis, pulmonary
Cassidy (-Scholte) syndrome (malignant carcinoid) 259.2
Castellani's bronchitis 104.8
Castleman's tumor or lymphoma (mediastinal lymph node hyperplasia) 785.6
Castration, traumatic 878.2
  complicated 878.3
Casts in urine 791.7
Catalepsy 300.11
  catatonic (acute) (see also Schizophrenia)
    295.2 ☑
  hysterical 300.11
  schizophrenic (see also Schizophrenia)
    295.2 ☑
Cataphasia ▶— see also Disorder, fluency◀
  315.35 ▲
Cataplexy (idiopathic) — see Narcolepsy
Cataract (anterior cortical) (anterior polar)
  (black) (capsular) (central) (cortical) (hypermature) (immature) (incipient) (mature) 366.9
  anterior
    and posterior axial embryonal 743.33
    pyramidal 743.31
    subcapsular polar
      infantile, juvenile, or presenile 366.01
      senile 366.13
  associated with
    calcinosis 275.40 [366.42]
    craniofacial dysostosis 756.0 [366.44]
    galactosemia 271.1 [366.44]
    hypoparathyroidism 252.1 [366.42]
    myotonic disorders 359.21 [366.43]
    neovascularization 366.33
  blue dot 743.39
  cerulean 743.39
  complicated NEC 366.30
  congenital 743.30
    capsular or subcapsular 743.31
    cortical 743.32
    nuclear 743.33
    specified type NEC 743.39
    total or subtotal 743.34
    zonular 743.32
  coronary (congenital) 743.39
    acquired 366.12
  cupuliform 366.14
  diabetic 250.5 ☑ [366.41]
    due to secondary diabetes
      249.5 ☑ [366.41]
  drug-induced 366.45

Cataract — continued
  due to
    chalcosis 360.24 [366.34]
    chronic choroiditis (see also Choroiditis)
      363.20 [366.32]
    degenerative myopia 360.21 [366.34]
    glaucoma (see also Glaucoma)
      365.9 [366.31]
    infection, intraocular NEC 366.32
    inflammatory ocular disorder NEC 366.32
    iridocyclitis, chronic 364.10 [366.33]
    pigmentary retinal dystrophy
      362.74 [366.34]
    radiation 366.46
  electric 366.46
  glassblowers' 366.46
  heat ray 366.46
  heterochromic 366.33
  in eye disease NEC 366.30
  infantile (see also Cataract, juvenile) 366.00
  intumescent 366.12
  irradiational 366.46
  juvenile 366.00
    anterior subcapsular polar 366.01
    combined forms 366.09
    cortical 366.03
    lamellar 366.03
    nuclear 366.04
    posterior subcapsular polar 366.02
    specified NEC 366.09
    zonular 366.03
  lamellar 743.32
    infantile, juvenile, or presenile 366.03
  morgagnian 366.18
  myotonic 359.21 [366.43]
  myxedema 244.9 [366.44]
  nuclear 366.16
  posterior, polar (capsular) 743.31
    infantile, juvenile, or presenile 366.02
    senile 366.14
  presenile (see also Cataract, juvenile) 366.00
  punctate
    acquired 366.12
    congenital 743.39
  secondary (membrane) 366.50
    obscuring vision 366.53
    specified type, not obscuring vision
      366.52
  senile 366.10
    anterior subcapsular polar 366.13
    combined forms 366.19
    cortical 366.15
    hypermature 366.18
    immature 366.12
    incipient 366.12
    mature 366.17
    nuclear 366.16
    posterior subcapsular polar 366.14
    specified NEC 366.19
    total or subtotal 366.17
  snowflake 250.5 ☑ [366.41]
    due to secondary diabetes
      249.5 ☑ [366.41]
  specified NEC 366.8
  subtotal (senile) 366.17
    congenital 743.34
  sunflower 360.24 [366.34]
  tetanic NEC 252.1 [366.42]
  total (mature) (senile) 366.17
    congenital 743.34
    localized 366.21
    traumatic 366.22
  toxic 366.45
  traumatic 366.20
    partially resolved 366.23
    total 366.22
  zonular (perinuclear) 743.32
    infantile, juvenile, or presenile 366.03
Cataracta 366.10
  brunescens 366.16
  cerulea 743.39
  complicata 366.30
  congenita 743.30
  coralliformis 743.39
  coronaria (congenital) 743.39
    acquired 366.12

Cataracta — continued
  diabetic 250.5 ☑ [366.41]
    due to secondary diabetes
      249.5 ☑ [366.41]
  floriformis 360.24 [366.34]
  membranacea
    accreta 366.50
    congenita 743.39
  nigra 366.16
Catarrh, catarrhal (inflammation) — see also
  condition 460
  acute 460
  asthma, asthmatic (see also Asthma)
    493.9 ☑
  Bostock's (see also Fever, hay) 477.9
  bowel — see Enteritis
  bronchial 490
    acute 466.0
    chronic 491.0
    subacute 466.0
  cervix, cervical (canal) (uteri) — see Cervicitis
  chest (see also Bronchitis) 490
  chronic 472.0
  congestion 472.0
  conjunctivitis 372.03
  due to syphilis 095.9
    congenital 090.0
  enteric — see Enteritis
  epidemic ▶(see also Influenza)◀ 487.1
  Eustachian 381.50
  eye (acute) (vernal) 372.03
  fauces (see also Pharyngitis) 462
  febrile 460
  fibrinous acute 466.0
  gastroenteric — see Enteritis
  gastrointestinal — see Enteritis
  gingivitis 523.00
  hay (see also Fever, hay) 477.9
  infectious 460
  intestinal — see Enteritis
  larynx (see also Laryngitis, chronic) 476.0
  liver 070.1
    with hepatic coma 070.0
  lung (see also Bronchitis) 490
    acute 466.0
    chronic 491.0
  middle ear (chronic) — see Otitis media,
    chronic
  mouth 528.00
  nasal (chronic) (see also Rhinitis) 472.0
    acute 460
  nasobronchial 472.2
  nasopharyngeal (chronic) 472.2
    acute 460
  nose — see Catarrh, nasal
  ophthalmia 372.03
  pneumococcal, acute 466.0
  pulmonary (see also Bronchitis) 490
    acute 466.0
    chronic 491.0
  spring (eye) 372.13
  suffocating (see also Asthma) 493.9 ☑
  summer (hay) (see also Fever, hay) 477.9
  throat 472.1
  tracheitis 464.10
    with obstruction 464.11
  tubotympanal 381.4
    acute (see also Otitis media, acute, non-
      suppurative) 381.00
    chronic 381.10
  vasomotor (see also Fever, hay) 477.9
  vesical (bladder) — see Cystitis
Catarrhus aestivus — see also Fever, hay 477.9
Catastrophe, cerebral — see also Disease,
  cerebrovascular, acute 436
Catatonia, catatonic (acute) 781.99
  with
    affective psychosis — see Psychosis, af-
      fective
    agitation 295.2 ☑
    dementia (praecox) 295.2 ☑
    due to or associated with physical condition
      293.89
    excitation 295.2 ☑
    excited type 295.2 ☑
    in conditions classified elsewhere 293.89

Catatonia, catatonic — continued
  schizophrenia 295.2 ☑
  stupor 295.2 ☑
Cat's ear 744.29
Cat-scratch — see also Injury, superficial
  disease or fever 078.3
Cauda equina — see also condition
  syndrome 344.60
Cauliflower ear 738.7
Caul over face 768.9
Causalgia 355.9
  lower limb 355.71
  upper limb 354.4
Cause
  external, general effects NEC 994.9
  not stated 799.9
  unknown 799.9
Caustic burn — see also Burn, by site
  from swallowing caustic or corrosive sub-
    stance — see Burn, internal organs
Cavare's disease (familial periodic paralysis)
  359.3
Cave-in, injury
  crushing (severe) (see also Crush, by site)
    869.1
  suffocation 994.7
Cavernitis (penis) 607.2
  lymph vessel — see Lymphangioma
Cavernositis 607.2
Cavernous — see condition
Cavitation of lung — see also Tuberculosis
  011.2 ☑
  nontuberculous 518.89
  primary, progressive 010.8 ☑
Cavity
  lung — see Cavitation of lung
  optic papilla 743.57
  pulmonary — see Cavitation of lung
  teeth 521.00
  vitreous (humor) 379.21
Cavovarus foot, congenital 754.59
Cavus foot (congenital) 754.71
  acquired 736.73
Cazenave's
  disease (pemphigus) NEC 694.4
  lupus (erythematosus) 695.4
CDGS (carbohydrate-deficient glycoprotein
  syndrome) 271.8
Cecitis — see Appendicitis
Cecocele — see Hernia
Cecum — see condition
Celiac
  artery compression syndrome 447.4
  disease 579.0
  infantilism 579.0
Cell, cellular — see also condition
  anterior chamber (eye) (positive aqueous
    ray) 364.04
Cellulitis (diffuse) (with lymphangitis) — see
  also Abscess 682.9
  abdominal wall 682.2
  anaerobic (see also Gas gangrene) 040.0
  ankle 682.6
  anus 566
  areola 611.0
  arm (any part, above wrist) 682.3
  auditory canal (external) 380.10
  axilla 682.3
  back (any part) 682.2
  breast 611.0
    postpartum 675.1 ☑
  broad ligament (see also Disease, pelvis, in-
    flammatory) 614.4
    acute 614.3
  buttock 682.5
  cervical (neck region) 682.1
  cervix (uteri) (see also Cervicitis) 616.0
  cheek, external 682.0
    internal 528.3
  chest wall 682.2
  chronic NEC 682.9
  colostomy 569.61
  corpus cavernosum 607.2
  digit 681.9

☑ **Additional Digit Required** — Refer to the Tabular List for Digit Selection   ⓦ **Subterms under main terms may continue to next column or page**

44 — Volume 2 · October 2010   ▶◀ **Revised Text**   ● **New Line**   ▲ **Revised Code**   **2011 ICD-9-CM**

Index   Carrier — Cellulitis

Cellulitis — see also Abscess — continued
Douglas' cul-de-sac or pouch (chronic) (see also Disease, pelvis, inflammatory) 614.4
　acute 614.3
drainage site (following operation) 998.59
ear, external 380.10
enterostomy 569.61
erysipelar (see also Erysipelas) 035
esophagostomy 530.86
eyelid 373.13
face (any part, except eye) 682.0
finger (intrathecal) (periosteal) (subcutaneous) (subcuticular) 681.00
flank 682.2
foot (except toe) 682.7
forearm 682.3
gangrenous (see also Gangrene) 785.4
genital organ NEC
　female — see Abscess, genital organ, female
　male 608.4
glottis 478.71
gluteal (region) 682.5
gonococcal NEC 098.0
groin 682.2
hand (except finger or thumb) 682.4
head (except face) NEC 682.8
heel 682.7
hip 682.6
jaw (region) 682.0
knee 682.6
labium (majus) (minus) (see also Vulvitis) 616.10
larynx 478.71
leg, except foot 682.6
lip 528.5
mammary gland 611.0
mouth (floor) 528.3
multiple sites NEC 682.9
nasopharynx 478.21
navel 682.2
　newborn NEC 771.4
neck (region) 682.1
nipple 611.0
nose 478.19
　external 682.0
orbit, orbital 376.01
palate (soft) 528.3
pectoral (region) 682.2
pelvis, pelvic
　with
　　abortion — see Abortion, by type, with sepsis
　　ectopic pregnancy (see also categories 633.0–633.9) 639.0
　　molar pregnancy (see also categories 630–632) 639.0
　female (see also Disease, pelvis, inflammatory) 614.4
　　acute 614.3
　following
　　abortion 639.0
　　ectopic or molar pregnancy 639.0
　male 567.21
　puerperal, postpartum, childbirth 670.8 ☑
penis 607.2
perineal, perineum 682.2
perirectal 566
peritonsillar 475
periurethral 597.0
periuterine (see also Disease, pelvis, inflammatory) 614.4
　acute 614.3
pharynx 478.21
phlegmonous NEC 682.9
rectum 566
retromammary 611.0
retroperitoneal (see also Peritonitis) 567.2 ☑, 567.38
round ligament (see also Disease, pelvis, inflammatory) 614.4
　acute 614.3
scalp (any part) 682.8
　dissecting 704.8

Cellulitis — see also Abscess — continued
scrotum 608.4
seminal vesicle 608.0
septic NEC 682.9
shoulder 682.3
specified sites NEC 682.8
spermatic cord 608.4
submandibular (region) (space) (triangle) 682.0
　gland 527.3
submaxillary 528.3
　gland 527.3
submental (pyogenic) 682.0
　gland 527.3
suppurative NEC 682.9
testis 608.4
thigh 682.6
thumb (intrathecal) (periosteal) (subcutaneous) (subcuticular) 681.00
toe (intrathecal) (periosteal) (subcutaneous) (subcuticular) 681.10
tonsil 475
trunk 682.2
tuberculous (primary) (see also Tuberculosis) 017.0 ☑
tunica vaginalis 608.4
umbilical 682.2
　newborn NEC 771.4
vaccinal 999.39
vagina — see Vaginitis
vas deferens 608.4
vocal cords 478.5
vulva (see also Vulvitis) 616.10
wrist 682.4
Cementoblastoma, benign (M9273/0) 213.1
upper jaw (bone) 213.0
Cementoma (M9273/0) 213.1
gigantiform (M9276/0) 213.1
　upper jaw (bone) 213.0
upper jaw (bone) 213.0
Cementoperiostitis 523.40
acute 523.33
apical 523.40
Cephalgia, cephalagia — see also Headache 784.0
histamine 339.00
nonorganic origin 307.81
other trigeminal autonomic (TACS) 339.09
psychogenic 307.81
tension 307.81
Cephalhematocele, cephalematocele
due to birth injury 767.19
fetus or newborn 767.19
traumatic (see also Contusion, head) 920
Cephalhematoma, cephalematoma (calcified)
due to birth injury 767.19
fetus or newborn 767.19
traumatic (see also Contusion, head) 920
Cephalic — see condition
Cephalitis — see Encephalitis
Cephalocele 742.0
Cephaloma — see Neoplasm, by site, malignant
Cephalomenia 625.8
Cephalopelvic — see condition
Cercomoniasis 007.3
Cerebellitis — see Encephalitis
Cerebellum (cerebellar) — see condition
Cerebral — see condition
Cerebritis — see Encephalitis
Cerebrohepatorenal syndrome 759.89
Cerebromacular degeneration 330.1
Cerebromalacia — see also Softening, brain 348.89 ▲
　due to cerebrovascular accident 438.89 ●
Cerebrosidosis 272.7
Cerebrospasticity — see Palsy, cerebral
Cerebrospinal — see condition
Cerebrum — see condition
Ceroid storage disease 272.7
Cerumen (accumulation) (impacted) 380.4
Cervical — see also condition
auricle 744.43
high risk human papillomavirus (HPV) DNA test positive 795.05

Cervical — see also condition — continued
intraepithelial glandular neoplasia 233.1
low risk human papillomavirus (HPV) DNA test positive 795.09
rib 756.2
shortening — see Short, cervical
Cervicalgia 723.1
Cervicitis (acute) (chronic) (nonvenereal) (subacute) (with erosion or ectropion) 616.0
with
　abortion — see Abortion, by type, with sepsis
　ectopic pregnancy (see also categories 633.0–633.9) 639.0
　molar pregnancy (see also categories 630–632) 639.0
　ulceration 616.0
chlamydial 099.53
complicating pregnancy or puerperium 646.6 ☑
　affecting fetus or newborn 760.8
following
　abortion 639.0
　ectopic or molar pregnancy 639.0
gonococcal (acute) 098.15
　chronic or duration of 2 months or more 098.35
senile (atrophic) 616.0
syphilitic 095.8
trichomonal 131.09
tuberculous (see also Tuberculosis) 016.7 ☑
Cervicoaural fistula 744.49
Cervicocolpitis (emphysematosa) — see also Cervicitis 616.0
Cervix — see condition
Cesarean delivery, operation or section NEC 669.7 ☑
affecting fetus or newborn 763.4
post mortem, affecting fetus or newborn 761.6
previous, affecting management of pregnancy 654.2 ☑
Céstan-Chenais paralysis 344.89
Céstan-Raymond syndrome 433.8 ☑
Céstan's syndrome 344.89
Cestode infestation NEC 123.9
specified type NEC 123.8
Cestodiasis 123.9
CGF (congenital generalized fibromatosis) 759.89
Chabert's disease 022.9
Chacaleh 266.2
Chafing 709.8
Chagas' disease — see also Trypanosomiasis, American 086.2
with heart involvement 086.0
Chagres fever 084.0
Chalasia (cardiac sphincter) 530.81
Chalazion 373.2
Chalazoderma 757.39
Chalcosis 360.24
cornea 371.15
crystalline lens 360.24 [366.34]
retina 360.24
Chalicosis (occupational) (pulmonum) 502
Chancre (any genital site) (hard) (indurated) (infecting) (primary) (recurrent) 091.0
congenital 090.0
conjunctiva 091.2
Ducrey's 099.0
extragenital 091.2
eyelid 091.2
Hunterian 091.0
lip (syphilis) 091.2
mixed 099.8
nipple 091.2
Nisbet's 099.0
of
　carate 103.0
　pinta 103.0
　yaws 102.0
palate, soft 091.2
phagedenic 099.0
Ricord's 091.0
Rollet's (syphilitic) 091.0

Chancre — continued
seronegative 091.0
seropositive 091.0
simple 099.0
soft 099.0
　bubo 099.0
urethra 091.0
yaws 102.0
Chancriform syndrome 114.1
Chancroid 099.0
anus 099.0
penis (Ducrey's bacillus) 099.0
perineum 099.0
rectum 099.0
scrotum 099.0
urethra 099.0
vulva 099.0
Chandipura fever 066.8
Chandler's disease (osteochondritis dissecans, hip) 732.7
Change(s) (of) — see also Removal of
arteriosclerotic — see Arteriosclerosis
battery
　cardiac pacemaker V53.31
bone 733.90
　diabetic 250.8 ☑ [731.8]
　　due to secondary diabetes 249.8 ☑ [731.8]
　in disease, unknown cause 733.90
bowel habits 787.99
cardiorenal (vascular) (see also Hypertension, cardiorenal) 404.90
cardiovascular — see Disease, cardiovascular
circulatory 459.9
cognitive or personality change of other type, nonpsychotic 310.1
color, teeth, tooth
　during formation 520.8
　extrinsic 523.6
　intrinsic posteruptive 521.7
contraceptive device V25.42
cornea, corneal
　degenerative NEC 371.40
　membrane NEC 371.30
　senile 371.41
coronary (see also Ischemia, heart) 414.9
degenerative
　chamber angle (anterior) (iris) 364.56
　ciliary body 364.57
　spine or vertebra (see also Spondylosis) 721.90
dental pulp, regressive 522.2
drains V58.49
dressing
　wound V58.30
　　nonsurgical V58.30
　　surgical V58.31
fixation device V54.89
　external V54.89
　internal V54.01
heart (see also Disease, heart)
hip joint 718.95
hyperplastic larynx 478.79
hypertrophic
　nasal sinus (see also Sinusitis) 473.9
　turbinate, nasal 478.0
　upper respiratory tract 478.9
inflammatory — see Inflammation
joint (see also Derangement, joint) 718.90
　sacroiliac 724.6
Kirschner wire V54.89
knee 717.9
macular, congenital 743.55
malignant (M— —/3) (see also Neoplasm, by site, malignant)

> *Note — for malignant change occurring in a neoplasm, use the appropriate M code with behavior digit /3 e.g., malignant change in uterine fibroid — M8890/3. For malignant change occurring in a nonneoplastic condition (e.g., gastric ulcer) use the M code M8000/3.*

mental (status) NEC 780.97
　due to or associated with physical condition — see Syndrome, brain

☑ **Additional Digit Required** — Refer to the Tabular List for Digit Selection　　　　　　　　　　　▽ **Subterms under main terms may continue to next column or page**

2011 ICD-9-CM　　　▶◀ **Revised Text**　　　● **New Line**　　　▲ **Revised Code**　　　**October 2010 · Volume 2 — 45**

Cellulitis — Change(s)

Change(s) — see also Removal of — continued
  myocardium, myocardial — see Degeneration, myocardial
  of life (see also Menopause) 627.2
  pacemaker battery (cardiac) V53.31
  peripheral nerve 355.9
  personality (nonpsychotic) NEC 310.1
  plaster cast V54.89
  refractive, transient 367.81
  regressive, dental pulp 522.2
  retina 362.9
    myopic (degenerative) (malignant) 360.21
    vascular appearance 362.13
  sacroiliac joint 724.6
  scleral 379.19
    degenerative 379.16
  senile (see also Senility) 797
  sensory (see also Disturbance, sensation) 782.0
  skin texture 782.8
  spinal cord 336.9
  splint, external V54.89
  subdermal implantable contraceptive V25.5
  suture V58.32
  traction device V54.89
  trophic 355.9
    arm NEC 354.9
    leg NEC 355.8
    lower extremity NEC 355.8
    upper extremity NEC 354.9
  vascular 459.9
  vasomotor 443.9
  voice 784.49
    psychogenic 306.1
  wound packing V58.30
    nonsurgical V58.30
    surgical V58.31
Changing sleep-work schedule, affecting sleep 327.36
Changuinola fever 066.0
Chapping skin 709.8
Character
  depressive 301.12
Charcôt's
  arthropathy 094.0 [713.5]
  cirrhosis — see Cirrhosis, biliary
  disease 094.0
    spinal cord 094.0
  fever (biliary) (hepatic) (intermittent) — see Choledocholithiasis
  joint (disease) 094.0 [713.5]
    diabetic 250.6 ☑ [713.5]
      due to secondary diabetes 249.6 ☑ [713.5]
    syringomyelic 336.0 [713.5]
  syndrome (intermittent claudication) 443.9
    due to atherosclerosis 440.21
Charcôt-Marie-Tooth disease, paralysis, or syndrome 356.1
CHARGE association (syndrome) 759.89
Charleyhorse (quadriceps) 843.8
  muscle, except quadriceps — see Sprain, by site
Charlouis' disease — see also Yaws 102.9
Chauffeur's fracture — see Fracture, ulna, lower end
Cheadle (-Möller) (-Barlow) disease or syndrome (infantile scurvy) 267
Checking (of)
  contraceptive device (intrauterine) V25.42
  device
    fixation V54.89
      external V54.89
      internal V54.09
    traction V54.89
  Kirschner wire V54.89
  plaster cast V54.89
  splint, external V54.89
Checkup
  following treatment — see Examination
  health V70.0
  infant (over 28 days old) (not sick) V20.2
  newborn, routine
    8 to 28 days old V20.32

Checkup — continued
  newborn, routine — continued
    over 28 days old, routine V20.2
    under 8 days old V20.31
    weight V20.32
  pregnancy (normal) V22.1
    first V22.0
    high-risk pregnancy V23.9
    specified problem NEC V23.89
Chédiak-Higashi (-Steinbrinck) anomaly, disease, or syndrome (congenital gigantism of peroxidase granules) 288.2
Cheek — see also condition
  biting 528.9
Cheese itch 133.8
Cheese washers' lung 495.8
Cheilitis 528.5
  actinic (due to sun) 692.72
    chronic NEC 692.74
      due to radiation, except from sun 692.82
    due to radiation, except from sun 692.82
  acute 528.5
  angular 528.5
  catarrhal 528.5
  chronic 528.5
  exfoliative 528.5
  gangrenous 528.5
  glandularis apostematosa 528.5
  granulomatosa 351.8
  infectional 528.5
  membranous 528.5
  Miescher's 351.8
  suppurative 528.5
  ulcerative 528.5
  vesicular 528.5
Cheilodynia 528.5
Cheilopalatoschisis — see also Cleft, palate, with cleft lip 749.20
Cheilophagia 528.9
Cheiloschisis — see also Cleft, lip 749.10
Cheilosis 528.5
  with pellagra 265.2
  angular 528.5
  due to
    dietary deficiency 266.0
    vitamin deficiency 266.0
Cheiromegaly 729.89
Cheiropompholyx 705.81
Cheloid — see also Keloid 701.4
Chemical burn — see also Burn, by site
  from swallowing chemical — see Burn, internal organs
Chemodectoma (M8693/1) — see Paraganglioma, nonchromaffin
Chemoprophylaxis NEC V07.39
Chemosis, conjunctiva 372.73
Chemotherapy
  convalescence V66.2
  encounter (for) (oral) (intravenous) V58.11
  maintenance (oral) (intravenous) V58.11
  prophylactic NEC V07.39
    fluoride V07.31
Cherubism 526.89
Chest — see condition
Cheyne-Stokes respiration (periodic) 786.04
Chiari's
  disease or syndrome (hepatic vein thrombosis) 453.0
  malformation
    type I 348.4
    type II (see also Spina bifida) 741.0 ☑
    type III 742.0
    type IV 742.2
    network 746.89
Chiari-Frommel syndrome 676.6 ☑
Chicago disease (North American blastomycosis) 116.0
Chickenpox — see also Varicella 052.9
  exposure to V01.71
  vaccination and inoculation (prophylactic) V05.4
Chiclero ulcer 085.4
Chiggers 133.8
Chignon 111.2

Chignon — continued
  fetus or newborn (from vacuum extraction) 767.19
Chigoe disease 134.1
Chikungunya fever 066.3
Chilaiditi's syndrome (subphrenic displacement, colon) 751.4
Chilblains 991.5
  lupus 991.5
Child
  behavior causing concern V61.20
    adopted child V61.24
    biological child V61.23
    foster child V61.25
Childbed fever 670.8 ☑
Childbirth — see also Delivery
  puerperal complications — see Puerperal
Childhood, period of rapid growth V21.0
Chill(s) 780.64
  with fever 780.60
  without fever 780.64
  congestive 780.99
    in malarial regions 084.6
  septic — see Septicemia
  urethral 599.84
Chilomastigiasis 007.8
Chin — see condition
Chinese dysentery 004.9
Chiropractic dislocation — see also Lesion, nonallopathic, by site 739.9
Chitral fever 066.0
Chlamydia, chlamydial — see condition
Chloasma 709.09
  cachecticorum 709.09
  eyelid 374.52
    congenital 757.33
    hyperthyroid 242.0 ☑
  gravidarum 646.8 ☑
  idiopathic 709.09
  skin 709.09
  symptomatic 709.09
Chloroma (M9930/3) 205.3 ☑
Chlorosis 280.9
  Egyptian (see also Ancylostomiasis) 126.9
  miners' (see also Ancylostomiasis) 126.9
Chlorotic anemia 280.9
Chocolate cyst (ovary) 617.1
Choked
  disk or disc — see Papilledema
  on food, phlegm, or vomitus NEC (see also Asphyxia, food) 933.1
  phlegm 933.1
  while vomiting NEC (see also Asphyxia, food) 933.1
Chokes (resulting from bends) 993.3
Choking sensation 784.99
Cholangiectasis — see also Disease, gallbladder 575.8
Cholangiocarcinoma (M8160/3)
  and hepatocellular carcinoma, combined (M8180/3) 155.0
  liver 155.1
  specified site NEC — see Neoplasm, by site, malignant
  unspecified site 155.1
Cholangiohepatitis 575.8
  due to fluke infestation 121.1
Cholangiohepatoma (M8180/3) 155.0
Cholangiolitis (acute) (chronic) (extrahepatic) (gangrenous) 576.1
  intrahepatic 575.8
  paratyphoidal (see also Fever, paratyphoid) 002.9
  typhoidal 002.0
Cholangioma (M8160/0) 211.5
  malignant — see Cholangiocarcinoma
Cholangitis (acute) (ascending) (catarrhal) (chronic) (infective) (malignant) (primary) (recurrent) (sclerosing) (secondary) (stenosing) (suppurative) 576.1
  chronic nonsuppurative destructive 571.6
  nonsuppurative destructive (chronic) 571.6
Cholecystdocholithiasis — see Choledocholithiasis
Cholecystitis 575.10

Cholecystitis — continued
  with
    calculus, stones in
      bile duct (common) (hepatic) — see Choledocholithiasis
      gallbladder — see Cholelithiasis
  acute 575.0
  acute and chronic 575.12
  chronic 575.11
  emphysematous (acute) (see also Cholecystitis, acute) 575.0
  gangrenous (see also Cholecystitis, acute) 575.0
  paratyphoidal, current (see also Fever, paratyphoid) 002.9
  suppurative (see also Cholecystitis, acute) 575.0
  typhoidal 002.0
Choledochitis (suppurative) 576.1
Choledocholith — see Choledocholithiasis
Choledocholithiasis 574.5 ☑

Note — Use the following fifth-digit subclassification with category 574:

0   without mention of obstruction

1   with obstruction

  with
    cholecystitis 574.4 ☑
      acute 574.3 ☑
      chronic 574.4 ☑
    cholelithiasis 574.9 ☑
      with
        cholecystitis 574.7 ☑
          acute 574.6 ☑
          and chronic 574.8 ☑
          chronic 574.7 ☑
Cholelithiasis (impacted) (multiple) 574.2 ☑

Note — Use the following fifth-digit subclassification with category 574:

0   without mention of obstruction

1   with obstruction

  with
    cholecystitis 574.1 ☑
      acute 574.0 ☑
      chronic 574.1 ☑
    choledocholithiasis 574.9 ☑
      with
        cholecystitis 574.7 ☑
          acute 574.6 ☑
          and chronic 574.8 ☑
          chronic cholecystitis 574.7 ☑
Cholemia — see also Jaundice 782.4
  familial 277.4
  Gilbert's (familial nonhemolytic) 277.4
Cholemic gallstone — see Cholelithiasis
Choleperitoneum, choleperitonitis — see also Disease, gallbladder 567.81
Cholera (algid) (Asiatic) (asphyctic) (epidemic) (gravis) (Indian) (malignant) (morbus) (pestilential) (spasmodic) 001.9
  antimonial 985.4
  carrier (suspected) of V02.0
  classical 001.0
  contact V01.0
  due to
    Vibrio
      cholerae (Inaba, Ogawa, Hikojima serotypes) 001.0
      El Tor 001.1
  El Tor 001.1
  exposure to V01.0
  vaccination, prophylactic (against) V03.0
Cholerine — see also Cholera 001.9
Cholestasis 576.8
  due to total parenteral nutrition (TPN) 573.8
Cholesteatoma (ear) 385.30
  attic (primary) 385.31
  diffuse 385.35
  external ear (canal) 380.21
  marginal (middle ear) 385.32
    with involvement of mastoid cavity 385.33

☑ Additional Digit Required — Refer to the Tabular List for Digit Selection   ▽ Subterms under main terms may continue to next column or page

46 — Volume 2   ▶◀ Revised Text   ● New Line   ▲ Revised Code   2011 ICD-9-CM

Cholesteatoma — *continued*
  marginal — *continued*
      secondary (with middle ear involvement) 385.33
    mastoid cavity 385.30
    middle ear (secondary) 385.32
      with involvement of mastoid cavity 385.33
    postmastoidectomy cavity (recurrent) 383.32
    primary 385.31
    recurrent, postmastoidectomy cavity 383.32
    secondary (middle ear) 385.32
      with involvement of mastoid cavity 385.33
Cholesteatosis (middle ear) — *see also* Cholesteatoma 385.30
  diffuse 385.35
Cholesteremia 272.0
Cholesterin
  granuloma, middle ear 385.82
  in vitreous 379.22
Cholesterol
  deposit
    retina 362.82
    vitreous 379.22
  elevated (high) 272.0
    with elevated (high) triglycerides 272.2
  imbibition of gallbladder (*see also* Disease, gallbladder) 575.6
Cholesterolemia 272.0
  essential 272.0
  familial 272.0
  hereditary 272.0
Cholesterosis, cholesterolosis (gallbladder) 575.6
  with
    cholecystitis — *see* Cholecystitis
    cholelithiasis — *see* Cholelithiasis
  middle ear (*see also* Cholesteatoma) 385.30
Cholocolic fistula — *see also* Fistula, gallbladder 575.5
Choluria 791.4
Chondritis (purulent) 733.99
  auricle 380.03
  costal 733.6
    Tietze's 733.6
  patella, posttraumatic 717.7
  pinna 380.03
  posttraumatica patellae 717.7
  tuberculous (active) (*see also* Tuberculosis) 015.9 ☑
    intervertebral 015.0 ☑ [730.88]
Chondroangiopathia calcarea seu punctate 756.59
Chondroblastoma (M9230/0) — *see also* Neoplasm, bone, benign
  malignant (M9230/3) — *see* Neoplasm, bone, malignant
Chondrocalcinosis (articular) (crystal deposition) (dihydrate) — *see also* Arthritis, due to, crystals 275.49 [712.3] ☑
  due to
    calcium pyrophosphate 275.49 [712.2] ☑
    dicalcium phosphate crystals 275.49 [712.1] ☑
    pyrophosphate crystals 275.49 [712.2] ☑
Chondrodermatitis nodularis helicis 380.00
Chondrodysplasia 756.4
  angiomatose 756.4
  calcificans congenita 756.59
  epiphysialis punctata 756.59
  hereditary deforming 756.4
  rhizomelic punctata 277.86
Chondrodystrophia (fetalis) 756.4
  calcarea 756.4
  calcificans congenita 756.59
  fetalis hypoplastica 756.59
  hypoplastica calcinosa 756.59
  punctata 756.59
  tarda 277.5
Chondrodystrophy (familial) (hypoplastic) 756.4
  myotonic (congenital) 359.23
Chondroectodermal dysplasia 756.55

Chondrolysis 733.99
Chondroma (M9220/0) — *see also* Neoplasm, cartilage, benign
  juxtacortical (M9221/0) — *see* Neoplasm, bone, benign
  periosteal (M9221/0) — *see* Neoplasm, bone, benign
Chondromalacia 733.92
  epiglottis (congenital) 748.3
  generalized 733.92
  knee 717.7
  larynx (congenital) 748.3
  localized, except patella 733.92
  patella, patellae 717.7
  systemic 733.92
  tibial plateau 733.92
  trachea (congenital) 748.3
Chondromatosis (M9220/1) — *see* Neoplasm, cartilage, uncertain behavior
Chondromyxosarcoma (M9220/3) — *see* Neoplasm, cartilage, malignant
Chondro-osteodysplasia (Morquio-Brailsford type) 277.5
Chondro-osteodystrophy 277.5
Chondro-osteoma (M9210/0) — *see* Neoplasm, bone, benign
Chondropathia tuberosa 733.6
Chondrosarcoma (M9220/3) — *see also* Neoplasm, cartilage, malignant
  juxtacortical (M9221/3) — *see* Neoplasm, bone, malignant
  mesenchymal (M9240/3) — *see* Neoplasm, connective tissue, malignant
Chordae tendineae rupture (chronic) 429.5
Chordee (nonvenereal) 607.89
  congenital 752.63
  gonococcal 098.2
Chorditis (fibrinous) (nodosa) (tuberosa) 478.5
Chordoma (M9370/3) — *see* Neoplasm, by site, malignant
Chorea (gravis) (minor) (spasmodic) 333.5
  with
    heart involvement — *see* Chorea with rheumatic heart disease
    rheumatic heart disease (chronic, inactive, or quiescent) (conditions classifiable to 393–398) (*see* rheumatic heart condition involved)
      active or acute (conditions classifiable to 391) 392.0
  acute — *see* Chorea, Sydenham's
  apoplectic (*see also* Disease, cerebrovascular, acute) 436
  chronic 333.4
  electric 049.8
  gravidarum — *see* Eclampsia, pregnancy
  habit 307.22
  hereditary 333.4
  Huntington's 333.4
  posthemiplegic 344.89
  pregnancy — *see* Eclampsia, pregnancy
  progressive 333.4
    chronic 333.4
    hereditary 333.4
  rheumatic (chronic) 392.9
    with heart disease or involvement — *see* Chorea, with rheumatic heart disease
  senile 333.5
  Sydenham's 392.9
    with heart involvement — *see* Chorea, with rheumatic heart disease
    nonrheumatic 333.5
  variabilis 307.23
Choreoathetosis (paroxysmal) 333.5
Chorioadenoma (destruens) (M9100/1) 236.1
Chorioamnionitis 658.4 ☑
  affecting fetus or newborn 762.7
Chorioangioma (M9120/0) 219.8
Choriocarcinoma (M9100/3)
  combined with
    embryonal carcinoma (M9101/3) — *see* Neoplasm, by site, malignant
    teratoma (M9101/3) — *see* Neoplasm, by site, malignant

Choriocarcinoma — *continued*
  specified site — *see* Neoplasm, by site, malignant
  unspecified site
    female 181
    male 186.9
Chorioencephalitis, lymphocytic (acute) (serous) 049.0
Chorioepithelioma (M9100/3) — *see* Choriocarcinoma
Choriomeningitis (acute) (benign) (lymphocytic) (serous) 049.0
Chorionepithelioma (M9100/3) — *see* Choriocarcinoma
Chorionitis — *see also* Scleroderma 710.1
Chorioretinitis 363.20
  disseminated 363.10
    generalized 363.13
    in
      neurosyphilis 094.83
      secondary syphilis 091.51
    peripheral 363.12
    posterior pole 363.11
    tuberculous (*see also* Tuberculosis) 017.3 ☑ [363.13]
  due to
    histoplasmosis (*see also* Histoplasmosis) 115.92
    toxoplasmosis (acquired) 130.2
      congenital (active) 771.2
  focal 363.00
    juxtapapillary 363.01
    peripheral 363.04
    posterior pole NEC 363.03
  juxtapapillaris, juxtapapillary 363.01
  progressive myopia (degeneration) 360.21
  syphilitic (secondary) 091.51
    congenital (early) 090.0 [363.13]
    late 090.5 [363.13]
    late 095.8 [363.13]
  tuberculous (*see also* Tuberculosis) 017.3 ☑ [363.13]
Choristoma — *see* Neoplasm, by site, benign
Choroid — *see* condition
Choroideremia, choroidermia (initial stage) (late stage) (partial or total atrophy) 363.55
Choroiditis — *see also* Chorioretinitis 363.20
  leprous 030.9 [363.13]
  senile guttate 363.41
  sympathetic 360.11
  syphilitic (secondary) 091.51
    congenital (early) 090.0 [363.13]
    late 090.5 [363.13]
    late 095.8 [363.13]
  Tay's 363.41
  tuberculous (*see also* Tuberculosis) 017.3 ☑ [363.13]
Choroidopathy NEC 363.9
  degenerative (*see also* Degeneration, choroid) 363.40
  hereditary (*see also* Dystrophy, choroid) 363.50
  specified type NEC 363.8
Choroidoretinitis — *see* Chorioretinitis
Choroidosis, central serous 362.41
Choroidretinopathy, serous 362.41
Christian's syndrome (chronic histiocytosis X) 277.89
Christian-Weber disease (nodular nonsuppurative panniculitis) 729.30
Christmas disease 286.1
Chromaffinoma (M8700/0) — *see also* Neoplasm, by site, benign
  malignant (M8700/3) — *see* Neoplasm, by site, malignant
Chromatopsia 368.59
Chromhidrosis, chromidrosis 705.89
Chromoblastomycosis 117.2
Chromomycosis 117.2
Chromophytosis 111.0
Chromotrichomycosis 111.8
Chronic — *see* condition
Churg-Strauss syndrome 446.4
Chyle cyst, mesentery 457.8
Chylocele (nonfilarial) 457.8

Chylocele — *continued*
  filarial (*see also* Infestation, filarial) 125.9
  tunica vaginalis (nonfilarial) 608.84
    filarial (*see also* Infestation, filarial) 125.9
Chylomicronemia (fasting) (with hyperprebetalipoproteinemia) 272.3
Chylopericardium (acute) 420.90
Chylothorax (nonfilarial) 457.8
  filarial (*see also* Infestation, filarial) 125.9
Chylous
  ascites 457.8
  cyst of peritoneum 457.8
  hydrocele 603.9
  hydrothorax (nonfilarial) 457.8
    filarial (*see also* Infestation, filarial) 125.9
Chyluria 791.1
  bilharziasis 120.0
  due to
    Brugia (malayi) 125.1
    Wuchereria (bancrofti) 125.0
      malayi 125.1
  filarial (*see also* Infestation, filarial) 125.9
  filariasis (*see also* Infestation, filarial) 125.9
  nonfilarial 791.1
Cicatricial (deformity) — *see* Cicatrix
Cicatrix (adherent) (contracted) (painful) (vicious) 709.2
  adenoid 474.8
  alveolar process 525.8
  anus 569.49
  auricle 380.89
  bile duct (*see also* Disease, biliary) 576.8
  bladder 596.8
  bone 733.99
  brain 348.89
  cervix (postoperative) (postpartal) 622.3
    in pregnancy or childbirth 654.6 ☑
      causing obstructed labor 660.2 ☑
  chorioretinal 363.30
    disseminated 363.35
    macular 363.32
    peripheral 363.34
    posterior pole NEC 363.33
  choroid — *see* Cicatrix, chorioretinal
  common duct (*see also* Disease, biliary) 576.8
  congenital 757.39
  conjunctiva 372.64
  cornea 371.00
    tuberculous (*see also* Tuberculosis) 017.3 ☑ [371.05]
  duodenum (bulb) 537.3
  esophagus 530.3
  eyelid 374.46
    with
      ectropion — *see* Ectropion
      entropion — *see* Entropion
  hypopharynx 478.29
  knee, semilunar cartilage 717.5
  lacrimal
    canaliculi 375.53
    duct
      acquired 375.56
      neonatal 375.55
    punctum 375.52
    sac 375.54
  larynx 478.79
  limbus (cystoid) 372.64
  lung 518.89
  macular 363.32
    disseminated 363.35
    peripheral 363.34
  middle ear 385.89
  mouth 528.9
  muscle 728.89
  nasolacrimal duct
    acquired 375.56
    neonatal 375.55
  nasopharynx 478.29
  palate (soft) 528.9
  penis 607.89
  prostate 602.8
  rectum 569.49
  retina 363.30
    disseminated 363.35
    macular 363.32

☑ **Additional Digit Required — Refer to the Tabular List for Digit Selection**   ▽ **Subterms under main terms may continue to next column or page**

2011 ICD-9-CM   ▶◀ Revised Text   ● New Line   ▲ Revised Code   **Volume 2 — 47**

Index

Cicatrix — Closed bite

Cicatrix — *continued*
  retina — *continued*
    peripheral 363.34
    posterior pole NEC 363.33
  semilunar cartilage — *see* Derangement, meniscus
  seminal vesicle 608.89
  skin 709.2
    infected 686.8
    postinfectional 709.2
    tuberculous (*see also* Tuberculosis) 017.0 ☑
  specified site NEC 709.2
  throat 478.29
  tongue 529.8
  tonsil (and adenoid) 474.8
  trachea 478.9
  tuberculous NEC (*see also* Tuberculosis) 011.9 ☑
  ureter 593.89
  urethra 599.84
  uterus 621.8
  vagina 623.4
    in pregnancy or childbirth 654.7 ☑
      causing obstructed labor 660.2 ☑
  vocal cord 478.5
  wrist, constricting (annular) 709.2
CIDP (chronic inflammatory demyelinating polyneuropathy) 357.81
CIN I (cervical intraepithelial neoplasia I) 622.11
CIN II (cervical intraepithelial neoplasia II) 622.12
CIN III (cervical intraepithelial neoplasia III) 233.1
Cinchonism
  correct substance properly administered 386.9
  overdose or wrong substance given or taken 961.4
Circine herpes 110.5
Circle of Willis — *see* condition
Circular — *see also* condition
  hymen 752.49
Circulating, intrinsic anticoagulants causing hemorrhagic disorder 286.5
  following childbirth 666.3 ☑
  postpartum 666.3 ☑
Circulation
  collateral (venous), any site 459.89
  defective 459.9
    congenital 747.9
    lower extremity 459.89
  embryonic 747.9
  failure 799.89
    fetus or newborn 779.89
    peripheral 785.59
  fetal, persistent 747.83
  heart, incomplete 747.9
Circulatory system — *see* condition
Circulus senilis 371.41
Circumcision
  in absence of medical indication V50.2
  ritual V50.2
  routine V50.2
  status (post), female 629.20
Circumscribed — *see* condition
Circumvallata placenta — *see* Placenta, abnormal
Cirrhosis, cirrhotic 571.5
  with alcoholism 571.2
  alcoholic (liver) 571.2
  atrophic (of liver) — *see* Cirrhosis, portal
  Baumgarten-Cruveilhier 571.5
  biliary (cholangiolitic) (cholangitic) (cholestatic) (extrahepatic) (hypertrophic) (intrahepatic) (nonobstructive) (obstructive) (pericholangiolitic) (posthepatic) (primary) (secondary) (xanthomatous) 571.6
    due to
      clonorchiasis 121.1
      flukes 121.3
  brain 331.9
  capsular — *see* Cirrhosis, portal
  cardiac 571.5
    alcoholic 571.2

Cirrhosis, cirrhotic — *continued*
  central (liver) — *see* Cirrhosis, liver
  Charcôt's 571.6
  cholangiolitic — *see* Cirrhosis, biliary
  cholangitic — *see* Cirrhosis, biliary
  cholestatic — *see* Cirrhosis, biliary
  clitoris (hypertrophic) 624.2
  coarsely nodular 571.5
  congestive (liver) — *see* Cirrhosis, cardiac
  Cruveilhier-Baumgarten 571.5
  cryptogenic (of liver) 571.5
    alcoholic 571.2
  dietary (*see also* Cirrhosis, portal) 571.5
  due to
    bronzed diabetes 275.01 ▲
    congestive hepatomegaly — *see* Cirrhosis, cardiac
    cystic fibrosis 277.00
    hemochromatosis ▶(*see also* Hemochromatosis)◀ 275.03 ▲
    hepatolenticular degeneration 275.1
    passive congestion (chronic) — *see* Cirrhosis, cardiac
    Wilson's disease 275.1
    xanthomatosis 272.2
  extrahepatic (obstructive) — *see* Cirrhosis, biliary
  fatty 571.8
    alcoholic 571.0
  florid 571.2
  Glisson's — *see* Cirrhosis, portal
  Hanot's (hypertrophic) — *see* Cirrhosis, biliary
  hepatic — *see* Cirrhosis, liver
  hepatolienal — *see* Cirrhosis, liver
  hobnail — *see* Cirrhosis, portal
  hypertrophic (*see also* Cirrhosis, liver)
    biliary — *see* Cirrhosis, biliary
    Hanot's — *see* Cirrhosis, biliary
  infectious NEC — *see* Cirrhosis, portal
  insular — *see* Cirrhosis, portal
  intrahepatic (obstructive) (primary) (secondary) — *see* Cirrhosis, biliary
  juvenile (*see also* Cirrhosis, portal) 571.5
  kidney (*see also* Sclerosis, renal) 587
  Laennec's (of liver) 571.2
    nonalcoholic 571.5
  liver (chronic) (hepatolienal) (hypertrophic) (nodular) (splenomegalic) (unilobar) 571.5
    with alcoholism 571.2
    alcoholic 571.2
    congenital (due to failure of obliteration of umbilical vein) 777.8
    cryptogenic 571.5
      alcoholic 571.2
    fatty 571.8
      alcoholic 571.0
    macronodular 571.5
      alcoholic 571.2
    micronodular 571.5
      alcoholic 571.2
    nodular, diffuse 571.5
      alcoholic 571.2
    pigmentary 275.01 ▲
    portal 571.5
      alcoholic 571.2
    postnecrotic 571.5
      alcoholic 571.2
    syphilitic 095.3
  lung (chronic) (*see also* Fibrosis, lung) 515
  macronodular (of liver) 571.5
    alcoholic 571.2
  malarial 084.9
  metabolic NEC 571.5
  micronodular (of liver) 571.5
    alcoholic 571.2
  monolobular — *see* Cirrhosis, portal
  multilobular — *see* Cirrhosis, portal
  nephritis (*see also* Sclerosis, renal) 587
  nodular — *see* Cirrhosis, liver
  nutritional (fatty) 571.5
  obstructive (biliary) (extrahepatic) (intrahepatic) — *see* Cirrhosis, biliary
  ovarian 620.8

Cirrhosis, cirrhotic — *continued*
  paludal 084.9
  pancreas (duct) 577.8
  pericholangiolitic — *see* Cirrhosis, biliary
  periportal — *see* Cirrhosis, portal
  pigment, pigmentary (of liver) 275.01 ▲
  portal (of liver) 571.5
    alcoholic 571.2
  posthepatitic (*see also* Cirrhosis, postnecrotic) 571.5
  postnecrotic (of liver) 571.5
    alcoholic 571.2
  primary (intrahepatic) — *see* Cirrhosis, biliary
  pulmonary (*see also* Fibrosis, lung) 515
  renal (*see also* Sclerosis, renal) 587
  septal (*see also* Cirrhosis, postnecrotic) 571.5
  spleen 289.51
  splenomegalic (of liver) — *see* Cirrhosis, liver
  stasis (liver) — *see* Cirrhosis, liver
  stomach 535.4 ☑
  Todd's (*see also* Cirrhosis, biliary) 571.6
  toxic (nodular) — *see* Cirrhosis, postnecrotic
  trabecular — *see* Cirrhosis, postnecrotic
  unilobar — *see* Cirrhosis, liver
  vascular (of liver) — *see* Cirrhosis, liver
  xanthomatous (biliary) (*see also* Cirrhosis, biliary) 571.6
    due to xanthomatosis (familial) (metabolic) (primary) 272.2
Cistern, subarachnoid 793.0
Citrullinemia 270.6
Citrullinuria 270.6
Ciuffini-Pancoast tumor (M8010/3) (carcinoma, pulmonary apex) 162.3
Civatte's disease or poikiloderma 709.09
CJD (Creutzfeldt-Jakob disease) 046.19
  variant (vCJD) 046.11
Clam diggers' itch 120.3
Clap — *see* Gonorrhea
Clarke-Hadfield syndrome (pancreatic infantilism) 577.8
Clark's paralysis 343.9
Clastothrix 704.2
Claude Bernard-Horner syndrome — *see also* Neuropathy, peripheral, autonomic 337.9
Claude's syndrome 352.6
Claudication, intermittent 443.9
  cerebral (artery) (*see also* Ischemia, cerebral, transient) 435.9
  due to atherosclerosis 440.21
  spinal cord (arteriosclerotic) 435.1
    syphilitic 094.89
  spinalis 435.1
  venous (axillary) 453.89
Claudicatio venosa intermittens 453.89
Claustrophobia 300.29
Clavus (infected) 700
Clawfoot (congenital) 754.71
  acquired 736.74
Clawhand (acquired) 736.06
  congenital 755.59
Clawtoe (congenital) 754.71
  acquired 735.5
Clay eating 307.52
Clay shovelers' fracture — *see* Fracture, vertebra, cervical
Cleansing of artificial opening — *see also* Attention to artificial opening V55.9
Cleft (congenital) — *see also* Imperfect, closure
  alveolar process 525.8
  branchial (persistent) 744.41
    cyst 744.42
  clitoris 752.49
  cricoid cartilage, posterior 748.3
  facial (*see also* Cleft, lip) 749.10
  lip 749.10
    with cleft palate 749.20
      bilateral (lip and palate) 749.24
        with unilateral lip or palate 749.25
          complete 749.23
          incomplete 749.24
      unilateral (lip and palate) 749.22

Cleft — *see also* Imperfect, closure — *continued*
  lip — *continued*
    with cleft palate — *continued*
      unilateral — *continued*
        with bilateral lip or palate 749.25
          complete 749.21
          incomplete 749.22
      bilateral 749.14
        with cleft palate, unilateral 749.25
          complete 749.13
          incomplete 749.14
      unilateral 749.12
        with cleft palate, bilateral 749.25
          complete 749.11
          incomplete 749.12
  nose 748.1
  palate 749.00
    with cleft lip 749.20
      bilateral (lip and palate) 749.24
        with unilateral lip or palate 749.25
          complete 749.23
          incomplete 749.24
      unilateral (lip and palate) 749.22
        with bilateral lip or palate 749.25
          complete 749.21
          incomplete 749.22
    bilateral 749.04
      with cleft lip, unilateral 749.25
        complete 749.03
        incomplete 749.04
    unilateral 749.02
      with cleft lip, bilateral 749.25
        complete 749.01
        incomplete 749.02
  penis 752.69
  posterior, cricoid cartilage 748.3
  scrotum 752.89
  sternum (congenital) 756.3
  thyroid cartilage (congenital) 748.3
  tongue 750.13
  uvula 749.02
    with cleft lip (*see also* Cleft, lip, with cleft palate) 749.20
  water 366.12
Cleft hand (congenital) 755.58
Cleidocranial dysostosis 755.59
Cleidotomy, fetal 763.89
Cleptomania 312.32
Clérambault's syndrome 297.8
  erotomania 302.89
Clergyman's sore throat 784.49
Click, clicking
  systolic syndrome 785.2
Clifford's syndrome (postmaturity) 766.22
Climacteric — *see also* Menopause 627.2
  arthritis NEC (*see also* Arthritis, climacteric) 716.3 ☑
  depression (*see also* Psychosis, affective) 296.2 ☑
  disease 627.2
    recurrent episode 296.3 ☑
    single episode 296.2 ☑
  female (symptoms) 627.2
  male (symptoms) (syndrome) 608.89
  melancholia (*see also* Psychosis, affective) 296.2 ☑
    recurrent episode 296.3 ☑
    single episode 296.2 ☑
  paranoid state 297.2
  paraphrenia 297.2
  polyarthritis NEC 716.39
    male 608.89
  symptoms (female) 627.2
Clinical research investigation (control) (participant) V70.7
Clinodactyly 755.59
Clitoris — *see* condition
Cloaca, persistent 751.5
Clonorchiasis 121.1
Clonorchiosis 121.1
Clonorchis infection, liver 121.1
Clonus 781.0
Closed bite 524.20

Closed surgical procedure converted to open procedure
- arthroscopic V64.43
- laparoscopic V64.41
- thoracoscopic V64.42

Closure
- artificial opening (see also Attention to artificial opening) V55.9
- congenital, nose 748.0
- cranial sutures, premature 756.0
- defective or imperfect NEC — see Imperfect, closure
- fistula, delayed — see Fistula
- fontanelle, delayed 756.0
- foramen ovale, imperfect 745.5
- hymen 623.3
- interauricular septum, defective 745.5
- interventricular septum, defective 745.4
- lacrimal duct 375.56
  - congenital 743.65
  - neonatal 375.55
- nose (congenital) 748.0
  - acquired 738.0
- vagina 623.2
- valve — see Endocarditis
- vulva 624.8

Clot (blood)
- artery (obstruction) (occlusion) (see also Embolism) 444.9
- atrial appendage 429.89
- bladder 596.7
- brain (extradural or intradural) (see also Thrombosis, brain) 434.0 ☑
  - late effect — see Late effect(s) (of) cerebrovascular disease
- circulation 444.9
- heart (see also Infarct, myocardium) 410.9 ☑
  - without myocardial infarction 429.89
- vein (see also Thrombosis) 453.9

Clotting defect NEC — see also Defect, coagulation 286.9

Clouded state 780.09
- epileptic (see also Epilepsy) 345.9 ☑
- paroxysmal (idiopathic) (see also Epilepsy) 345.9 ☑

Clouding
- corneal graft 996.51

Cloudy
- antrum, antra 473.0
- dialysis effluent 792.5

Clouston's (hidrotic) ectodermal dysplasia 757.31

Clubbing of fingers 781.5

Clubfinger 736.29
- acquired 736.29
- congenital 754.89

Clubfoot (congenital) 754.70
- acquired 736.71
- equinovarus 754.51
- paralytic 736.71

Club hand (congenital) 754.89
- acquired 736.07

Clubnail (acquired) 703.8
- congenital 757.5

Clump kidney 753.3

Clumsiness 781.3
- syndrome 315.4

Cluttering ▶— see also Disorder, fluency◀ 315.35 ▲

Clutton's joints 090.5

Coagulation, intravascular (diffuse) (disseminated) — see also Fibrinolysis 286.6
- newborn 776.2

Coagulopathy — see also Defect, coagulation 286.9
- consumption 286.6
- intravascular (disseminated) NEC 286.6
  - newborn 776.2

Coalition
- calcaneoscaphoid 755.67
- calcaneus 755.67
- tarsal 755.67

Coal miners'
- elbow 727.2
- lung 500

Coal workers' lung or pneumoconiosis 500

Coarctation
- aorta (postductal) (preductal) 747.10
- pulmonary artery 747.3

Coated tongue 529.3

Coats' disease 362.12

Cocainism — see also Dependence 304.2 ☑

Coccidioidal granuloma 114.3

Coccidioidomycosis 114.9
- with pneumonia 114.0
- cutaneous (primary) 114.1
- disseminated 114.3
- extrapulmonary (primary) 114.1
- lung 114.5
  - acute 114.0
  - chronic 114.4
  - primary 114.0
- meninges 114.2
- primary (pulmonary) 114.0
  - acute 114.0
- prostate 114.3
- pulmonary 114.5
  - acute 114.0
  - chronic 114.4
  - primary 114.0
- specified site NEC 114.3

Coccidioidosis 114.9
- lung 114.5
  - acute 114.0
  - chronic 114.4
  - primary 114.0
- meninges 114.2

Coccidiosis (colitis) (diarrhea) (dysentery) 007.2

Cocciuria 791.9

Coccus in urine 791.9

Coccydynia 724.79

Coccygodynia 724.79

Coccyx — see condition

Cochin-China
- diarrhea 579.1
  - anguilluliasis 127.2
- ulcer 085.1

Cockayne's disease or syndrome (microcephaly and dwarfism) 759.89

Cockayne-Weber syndrome (epidermolysis bullosa) 757.39

Cocked-up toe 735.2

Cock's peculiar tumor 706.2

Codman's tumor (benign chondroblastoma) (M9230/0) — see Neoplasm, bone, benign

Coenurosis 123.8

Coffee workers' lung 495.8

Cogan's syndrome 370.52
- congenital oculomotor apraxia 379.51
- nonsyphilitic interstitial keratitis 370.52

Coiling, umbilical cord — see Complications, umbilical cord

Coitus, painful (female) 625.0
- male 608.89
- psychogenic 302.76

Cold 460
- with influenza, flu, or grippe ▶(see also Influenza)◀ 487.1
- abscess (see also Tuberculosis, abscess)
  - articular — see Tuberculosis, joint
- agglutinin
  - disease (chronic) or syndrome 283.0
  - hemoglobinuria 283.0
    - paroxysmal (cold) (nocturnal) 283.2
- allergic (see also Fever, hay) 477.9
- bronchus or chest — see Bronchitis
  - with grippe or influenza ▶(see also Influenza)◀ 487.1
- common (head) 460
  - vaccination, prophylactic (against) V04.7
- deep 464.10
- effects of 991.9
  - specified effect NEC 991.8
- excessive 991.9
  - specified effect NEC 991.8
- exhaustion from 991.8
- exposure to 991.9
  - specified effect NEC 991.8
- grippy ▶(see also Influenza)◀ 487.1
- head 460

Cold — continued
- injury syndrome (newborn) 778.2
- intolerance 780.99
- on lung — see Bronchitis
- rose 477.0
- sensitivity, autoimmune 283.0
- virus 460

Coldsore — see also Herpes, simplex 054.9

Colibacillosis 041.4
- generalized 038.42

Colibacilluria 791.9

Colic (recurrent) 789.7
- abdomen 789.7
  - psychogenic 307.89
- appendicular 543.9
- appendix 543.9
- bile duct — see Choledocholithiasis
- biliary — see Cholelithiasis
- bilious — see Cholelithiasis
- common duct — see Choledocholithiasis
- Devonshire NEC 984.9
  - specified type of lead — see Table of Drugs and Chemicals
- flatulent 787.3
- gallbladder or gallstone — see Cholelithiasis
- gastric 536.8
- hepatic (duct) — see Choledocholithiasis
- hysterical 300.11
- in
  - adult 789.0 ☑
  - child over 12 months old 789.0 ☑
  - infant 789.7
- infantile 789.7
- intestinal 789.7
- kidney 788.0
- lead NEC 984.9
  - specified type of lead — see Table of Drugs and Chemicals
- liver (duct) — see Choledocholithiasis
- mucous 564.9
  - psychogenic 316 [564.9]
- nephritic 788.0
- painter's NEC 984.9
- pancreas 577.8
- psychogenic 306.4
- renal 788.0
- saturnine NEC 984.9
  - specified type of lead — see Table of Drugs and Chemicals
- spasmodic 789.7
- ureter 788.0
- urethral 599.84
  - due to calculus 594.2
- uterus 625.8
  - menstrual 625.3
- vermicular 543.9
- virus 460
- worm NEC 128.9

Colicystitis — see also Cystitis 595.9

Colitis (acute) (catarrhal) (croupous) (cystica superficialis) (exudative) (hemorrhagic) (noninfectious) (phlegmonous) (presumed noninfectious) 558.9
- adaptive 564.9
- allergic 558.3
- amebic (see also Amebiasis) 006.9
  - nondysenteric 006.2
- anthrax 022.2
- bacillary (see also Infection, Shigella) 004.9
- balantidial 007.0
- chronic 558.9
  - ulcerative (see also Colitis, ulcerative) 556.9
- coccidial 007.2
- dietetic 558.9
- due to radiation 558.1
- eosinophilic 558.42
- functional 558.9
- gangrenous 009.0
- giardial 007.1
- granulomatous 555.1
- gravis (see also Colitis, ulcerative) 556.9
- infectious (see also Enteritis, due to, specific organism) 009.0
  - presumed 009.1
- ischemic 557.9

Colitis — continued
- ischemic — continued
  - acute 557.0
  - chronic 557.1
  - due to mesenteric artery insufficiency 557.1
- membranous 564.9
  - psychogenic 316 [564.9]
- mucous 564.9
  - psychogenic 316 [564.9]
- necrotic 009.0
- polyposa (see also Colitis, ulcerative) 556.9
- protozoal NEC 007.9
- pseudomembranous 008.45
- pseudomucinous 564.9
- regional 555.1
- segmental 555.1
- septic (see also Enteritis, due to, specific organism) 009.0
- spastic 564.9
  - psychogenic 316 [564.9]
- Staphylococcus 008.41
  - food 005.0
- thromboulcerative 557.0
- toxic 558.2
- transmural 555.1
- trichomonal 007.3
- tuberculous (ulcerative) 014.8 ☑
- ulcerative (chronic) (idiopathic) (nonspecific) 556.9
  - entero- 556.0
  - fulminant 557.0
  - ileo- 556.1
  - left-sided 556.5
  - procto- 556.2
  - proctosigmoid 556.3
  - psychogenic 316 [556] ☑
  - specified NEC 556.8
  - universal 556.6

Collagen disease NEC 710.9
- nonvascular 710.9
- vascular (allergic) (see also Angiitis, hypersensitivity) 446.20

Collagenosis — see also Collagen disease 710.9
- cardiovascular 425.4
- mediastinal 519.3

Collapse 780.2
- adrenal 255.8
- cardiorenal (see also Hypertension, cardiorenal) 404.90
- cardiorespiratory 785.51
  - fetus or newborn 779.85
- cardiovascular (see also Disease, heart) 785.51
  - fetus or newborn 779.85
- circulatory (peripheral) 785.59
  - with
    - abortion — see Abortion, by type, with shock
    - ectopic pregnancy (see also categories 633.0–633.9) 639.5
    - molar pregnancy (see also categories 630–632) 639.5
  - during or after labor and delivery 669.1 ☑
  - fetus or newborn 779.85
  - following
    - abortion 639.5
    - ectopic or molar pregnancy 639.5
  - during or after labor and delivery 669.1 ☑
  - fetus or newborn 779.89
- external ear canal 380.50
  - secondary to
    - inflammation 380.53
    - surgery 380.52
    - trauma 380.51
- general 780.2
- heart — see Disease, heart
- heat 992.1
- hysterical 300.11
- labyrinth, membranous (congenital) 744.05
- lung (massive) (see also Atelectasis) 518.0
  - pressure, during labor 668.0 ☑
- myocardial — see Disease, heart
- nervous (see also Disorder, mental, nonpsychotic) 300.9

☑ **Additional Digit Required** — Refer to the Tabular List for Digit Selection   ▽ **Subterms under main terms may continue to next column or page**

2011 ICD-9-CM   ▶◀ **Revised Text**   ● **New Line**   ▲ **Revised Code**   **October 2010 • Volume 2 — 49**

Complications — *continued*
  coronary bypass — *continued*
    occlusion NEC 996.72
    specified type NEC 996.72
    thrombus 996.72
  cystostomy 997.5
  delivery 669.9 ☑
    procedure (instrumental) (manual) (surgical) 669.4 ☑
    specified type NEC 669.8 ☑
  dialysis (hemodialysis) (peritoneal) (renal) NEC 999.9
    catheter NEC (*see also* Complications, due to (presence of) any device, implant, or graft classified to 996.0–996.5 NEC)
      infection or inflammation 996.62
        peritoneal 996.68
      mechanical 996.1
        peritoneal 996.56
  drug NEC 995.29
  due to (presence of) any device, implant, or graft classified to 996.0–996.5 NEC 996.70
    with infection or inflammation — *see* Complications, infection or inflammation, due to (presence of) any device, implant, or graft classified to 996.0–996.5 NEC
    arterial NEC 996.74
      coronary NEC 996.03
        atherosclerosis — *see* Arteriosclerosis, coronary
        embolism 996.72
        occlusion NEC 996.72
        specified type NEC 996.72
        thrombus 996.72
      renal dialysis 996.73
    arteriovenous fistula or shunt NEC 996.74
    bone growth stimulator 996.78
    breast NEC 996.79
    cardiac NEC 996.72
      defibrillator 996.72
      pacemaker 996.72
      valve prosthesis 996.71
    catheter NEC 996.79
      spinal 996.75
      urinary, indwelling 996.76
      vascular NEC 996.74
        renal dialysis 996.73
      ventricular shunt 996.75
    coronary (artery) bypass (graft) NEC 996.03
      atherosclerosis — *see* Arteriosclerosis, coronary
      embolism 996.72
      occlusion NEC 996.72
      thrombus 996.72
    electrodes
      brain 996.75
      heart 996.72
    esophagostomy 530.87
    gastrointestinal NEC 996.79
    genitourinary NEC 996.76
    heart valve prosthesis NEC 996.71
    infusion pump 996.74
    insulin pump 996.57
    internal
      joint prosthesis 996.77
      orthopedic NEC 996.78
      specified type NEC 996.79
    intrauterine contraceptive device NEC 996.76
    joint prosthesis, internal NEC 996.77
    mechanical — *see* Complications, mechanical
    nervous system NEC 996.75
    ocular lens NEC 996.79
    orbital NEC 996.79
    orthopedic NEC 996.78
      joint, internal 996.77
    renal dialysis 996.73
    specified type NEC 996.79
    urinary catheter, indwelling 996.76
    vascular NEC 996.74

Complications — *continued*
  due to any device, implant, or graft classified to 996.0–996.5 — *continued*
    ventricular shunt 996.75
  during dialysis NEC 999.9
  ectopic or molar pregnancy NEC 639.9
  electroshock therapy NEC 999.9
  enterostomy 569.60
    specified type NEC 569.69
  esophagostomy 530.87
    infection 530.86
    mechanical 530.87
  external (fixation) device with internal component(s) NEC 996.78
    infection or inflammation 996.67
    mechanical 996.49
  extracorporeal circulation NEC 999.9
  eye implant (prosthetic) NEC 996.79
    infection or inflammation 996.69
    mechanical
      ocular lens 996.53
      orbital globe 996.59
  fetal, from amniocentesis 679.1 ☑
  gastrointestinal, postoperative NEC (*see also* Complications, surgical procedures) 997.4
  gastrointestinal 536.40
    specified type NEC 536.49
  genitourinary device, implant or graft NEC 996.76
    infection or inflammation 996.65
      urinary catheter, indwelling 996.64
    mechanical (*see also* Complications, mechanical, by type) 996.30
      specified NEC 996.39
  graft (bypass) (patch) (*see also* Complications, due to (presence of) any device, implant, or graft classified to 996.0–996.5 NEC)
    bone marrow 996.85
    corneal NEC 996.79
      infection or inflammation 996.69
      rejection or reaction 996.51
      retroprosthetic membrane 996.51 ●
    mechanical — *see* Complications, mechanical, graft
    organ (immune or nonimmune cause) (partial) (total) 996.80
      bone marrow 996.85
      heart 996.83
      intestines 996.87
      kidney 996.81
      liver 996.82
      lung 996.84
      pancreas 996.86
      specified NEC 996.89
    skin NEC 996.79
      infection or inflammation 996.69
      rejection 996.52
        artificial 996.55
        decellularized allodermis 996.55
  heart (*see also* Disease, heart transplant (immune or nonimmune cause)) 996.83
  hematoma (intraoperative) (postoperative) 998.12
  hemorrhage (intraoperative) (postoperative) 998.11
  hyperalimentation therapy NEC 999.9
  immunization (procedure) — *see* Complications, vaccination
  implant (*see also* Complications, due to (presence of) any device, implant, or graft classified to 996.0–996.5 NEC)
    dental placement, hemorrhagic 525.71
    mechanical — *see* Complications, mechanical, implant
  infection and inflammation
    due to (presence of) any device, implant or graft classified to 996.0–996.5 NEC 996.60
      arterial NEC 996.62
        coronary 996.61
        renal dialysis 996.62
      arteriovenous fistula or shunt 996.62
      artificial heart 996.61

Complications — *continued*
  infection and inflammation — *continued*
    due to any device, implant or graft classified to 996.0–996.5 — *continued*
      bone growth stimulator 996.67
      breast 996.69
      cardiac 996.61
      catheter NEC 996.69
        central venous 999.31
        Hickman 999.31
        peripherally inserted central (PICC) 999.31
        peritoneal 996.68
        portacath (port-a-cath) 999.31
        spinal 996.63
        triple lumen 999.31
        umbilical venous 999.31
        urinary, indwelling 996.64
        vascular (arterial) (dialysis) (peripheral venous) NEC 996.62
        ventricular shunt 996.63
      central venous catheter 999.31
      coronary artery bypass 996.61
      electrodes
        brain 996.63
        heart 996.61
      gastrointestinal NEC 996.69
      genitourinary NEC 996.65
        indwelling urinary catheter 996.64
      heart assist device 996.61
      heart valve 996.61
      Hickman catheter 999.31
      infusion pump 996.62
      insulin pump 996.69
      intrauterine contraceptive device 996.65
      joint prosthesis, internal 996.66
      ocular lens 996.69
      orbital (implant) 996.69
      orthopedic NEC 996.67
        joint, internal 996.66
      peripherally inserted central catheter (PICC) 999.31
      portacath (port-a-cath) 999.31
      specified type NEC 996.69
      triple lumen catheter 999.31
      umbilical venous catheter 999.31
      urinary catheter, indwelling 996.64
      ventricular shunt 996.63
  infusion (procedure) 999.88
    blood — *see* Complications, transfusion
    infection NEC 999.39
    sepsis NEC 999.39
  inhalation therapy NEC 999.9
  injection (procedure) 999.9
    drug reaction (*see also* Reaction, drug) 995.27
    infection NEC 999.39
    sepsis NEC 999.39
    serum (prophylactic) (therapeutic) — *see* Complications, vaccination
    vaccine (any) — *see* Complications, vaccination
  inoculation (any) — *see* Complications, vaccination
  insulin pump 996.57
  internal device (catheter) (electronic) (fixation) (prosthetic) (*see also* Complications, due to (presence of) any device, implant, or graft classified to 996.0–996.5 NEC)
    mechanical — *see* Complications, mechanical
  intestinal pouch, specified NEC 569.79
  intestinal transplant (immune or nonimmune cause) 996.87
  intraoperative bleeding or hemorrhage 998.11
  intrauterine contraceptive device (*see also* Complications, contraceptive device) 996.76

Complications — *continued*
  intrauterine contraceptive device (*see also* Complications, contraceptive device) — *continued*
    with fetal damage affecting management of pregnancy 655.8 ☑
    infection or inflammation 996.65
  in utero procedure
    fetal 679.1 ☑
    maternal 679.0 ☑
  jejunostomy 569.60
  kidney transplant (immune or nonimmune cause) 996.81
  labor 669.9 ☑
    specified condition NEC 669.8 ☑
  liver transplant (immune or nonimmune cause) 996.82
  lumbar puncture 349.0
  mechanical
    anastomosis — *see* Complications, mechanical, graft
    artificial heart 996.09
    bypass — *see* Complications, mechanical, graft
    catheter NEC 996.59
      cardiac 996.09
      cystostomy 996.39
      dialysis (hemodialysis) 996.1
        peritoneal 996.56
      during a procedure 998.2
      urethral, indwelling 996.31
    colostomy 569.62
    device NEC 996.59
      balloon (counterpulsation), intra-aortic 996.1
      cardiac 996.00
        automatic implantable defibrillator 996.04
        long-term effect 429.4
        specified NEC 996.09
      contraceptive, intrauterine 996.32
      counterpulsation, intra-aortic 996.1
      fixation, external, with internal components 996.49
      fixation, internal (nail, rod, plate) 996.40
      genitourinary 996.30
        specified NEC 996.39
      insulin pump 996.57
      nervous system 996.2
      orthopedic, internal 996.40
        prosthetic joint (*see also* Complications, mechanical, device, orthopedic, prosthetic, joint) 996.47
      prosthetic NEC 996.59
        joint 996.47
          articular bearing surface wear 996.46
          aseptic loosening 996.41
          breakage 996.43
          dislocation 996.42
          failure 996.47
          fracture 996.43
            around prosthetic 996.44
            peri-prosthetic 996.44
          instability 996.42
          loosening 996.41
          peri-prosthetic osteolysis 996.45
          subluxation 996.42
          wear 996.46
      umbrella, vena cava 996.1
      vascular 996.1
    dorsal column stimulator 996.2
    electrode NEC 996.59
      brain 996.2
      cardiac 996.01
      spinal column 996.2
    enterostomy 569.62
    esophagostomy 530.87
    fistula, arteriovenous, surgically created 996.1
    gastrostomy 536.42
    graft NEC 996.52
      aortic (bifurcation) 996.1

☑ **Additional Digit Required** — Refer to the Tabular List for Digit Selection
▲▼ **Revised Text**   ● **New Line**   ▲ **Revised Code**
▽ **Subterms under main terms may continue to next column or page**
2011 ICD-9-CM   October 2010 • Volume 2 — 51

☑ **Additional Digit Required** — Refer to the Tabular List for Digit Selection   ▽ **Subterms under main terms may continue to next column or page**

Complications — *continued*
  transfusion (blood) (lymphocytes) (plasma) 999.80 ▲
    acute lung injury (TRALI) 518.7
    atrophy, liver, yellow, subacute (within 8 months of administration) — *see* Hepatitis, viral
    bone marrow 996.85
    embolism
      air 999.1
      thrombus 999.2
    febrile nonhemolytic reaction (FNHTR) ●
        780.66
    hemolysis NEC 999.89
      bone marrow 996.85
    hemolytic reaction, incompatibility ●
        unspecified 999.83 ●
        acute 999.84 ●
        delayed 999.85 ●
    hepatitis (serum) (type B) (within 8 months after administration) — *see* Hepatitis, viral
    incompatibility reaction
      ABO 999.60 ▲
        with hemolytic transfusion reac- ●
            tion (HTR) (not specified ●
            as acute or delayed) 999.61 ●
          acute 999.62 ●
          delayed 999.63 ●
        specified type NEC 999.69 ●
      minor blood group 999.89 ●
      non-ABO (minor antigens) (Duffy) ●
          (Kell) (Kidd) (Lewis) (M) (N) ●
          (P) (S) 999.75 ●
        with hemolytic transfusion reac- ●
            tion (HTR) (not specified ●
            as acute or delayed) 999.76 ●
          acute 999.77 ●
          delayed 999.78 ●
        specified type NEC 999.79 ●
      Rh ►antigen (C) (c) (D) (E) (e) (fac- ●
          tor)◄ 999.70 ●
        with hemolytic transfusion reac- ●
            tion (HTR) (not specified ●
            as acute or delayed) 999.71 ●
          acute 999.72 ●
          delayed 999.73 ●
        specified type NEC 999.74 ●
    infection 999.39
    jaundice (serum) (within 8 months after administration) — *see* Hepatitis, viral
    sepsis 999.39
    shock or reaction NEC 999.89
      bone marrow 996.85
    specified reaction NEC 999.89 ●
    subacute yellow atrophy of liver (within 8 months after administration) — *see* Hepatitis, viral
  thromboembolism 999.2
  transplant NEC (*see also* Complications, due to (presence of) any device, implant, or graft classified to 996.0–996.5 NEC)
    bone marrow 996.85
    organ (immune or nonimmune cause) (partial) (total) 996.80
      bone marrow 996.85
      heart 996.83
      intestines 996.87
      kidney 996.81
      liver 996.82
      lung 996.84
      pancreas 996.86
      specified NEC 996.89
  trauma NEC (early) 958.8
  ultrasound therapy NEC 999.9
  umbilical cord
    affecting fetus or newborn 762.6
    complicating delivery 663.9 ☑
      affecting fetus or newborn 762.6
      specified type NEC 663.8 ☑
  urethral catheter NEC 996.76

Complications — *continued*
  urethral catheter — *continued*
    infection or inflammation 996.64
    mechanical 996.31
  urinary, postoperative NEC 997.5
  vaccination 999.9
    anaphylaxis NEC 999.4
    cellulitis 999.39
    encephalitis or encephalomyelitis 323.51
    hepatitis (serum) (type B) (within 8 months after administration) — *see* Hepatitis, viral
    infection (general) (local) NEC 999.39
    jaundice (serum) (within 8 months after administration) — *see* Hepatitis, viral
    meningitis 997.09 *[321.8]*
    myelitis 323.52
    protein sickness 999.5
    reaction (allergic) 999.5
      Herxheimer's 995.0
      serum 999.5
    sepsis 999.39
    serum intoxication, sickness, rash, or other serum reaction NEC 999.5
    shock (allergic) (anaphylactic) 999.4
    subacute yellow atrophy of liver (within 8 months after administration) — *see* Hepatitis, viral
    vaccinia (generalized) 999.0
      localized 999.39
  vascular
    device, implant, or graft NEC 996.74
      infection or inflammation 996.62
      mechanical NEC 996.1
        cardiac (*see also* Complications, mechanical, by type) 996.00
    following infusion, perfusion, or transfusion 999.2
    postoperative NEC 997.2
      mesenteric artery 997.71
      other vessels 997.79
      peripheral vessels 997.2
      renal artery 997.72
  ventilation therapy NEC 999.9
  ventilator [respirator], mechanical V46.14
Compound presentation, complicating delivery 652.8 ☑
  causing obstructed labor 660.0 ☑
Compressed air disease 993.3
Compression
  with injury — *see* specific injury
  arm NEC 354.9
  artery 447.1
    celiac, syndrome 447.4
  brachial plexus 353.0
  brain (stem) 348.4
    due to
      contusion, brain — *see* Contusion, brain
      injury NEC (*see also* Hemorrhage, brain, traumatic)
        birth — *see* Birth, injury, brain
      laceration, brain — *see* Laceration, brain
    osteopathic 739.0
  bronchus 519.19
  by cicatrix — *see* Cicatrix
  cardiac 423.9
  cauda equina 344.60
    with neurogenic bladder 344.61
  celiac (artery) (axis) 447.4
  cerebral — *see* Compression, brain
  cervical plexus 353.2
  cord (umbilical) — *see* Compression, umbilical cord
  cranial nerve 352.9
    second 377.49
    third (partial) 378.51
      total 378.52
    fourth 378.53
    fifth 350.8
    sixth 378.54
    seventh 351.8
  divers' squeeze 993.3

Compression — *continued*
  duodenum (external) (*see also* Obstruction, duodenum) 537.3
  during birth 767.9
  esophagus 530.3
    congenital, external 750.3
  Eustachian tube 381.63
  facies (congenital) 754.0
  fracture — *see* Fracture, by site
  heart — *see* Disease, heart
  intestine (*see also* Obstruction, intestine) 560.9
    with hernia — *see* Hernia, by site, with obstruction
  laryngeal nerve, recurrent 478.79
  leg NEC 355.8
  lower extremity NEC 355.8
  lumbosacral plexus 353.1
  lung 518.89
  lymphatic vessel 457.1
  medulla — *see* Compression, brain
  nerve NEC (*see also* Disorder, nerve)
    arm NEC 354.9
    autonomic nervous system (*see also* Neuropathy, peripheral, autonomic) 337.9
    axillary 353.0
    cranial NEC 352.9
    due to displacement of intervertebral disc 722.2
      with myelopathy 722.70
      cervical 722.0
        with myelopathy 722.71
      lumbar, lumbosacral 722.10
        with myelopathy 722.73
      thoracic, thoracolumbar 722.11
        with myelopathy 722.72
    iliohypogastric 355.79
    ilioinguinal 355.79
    leg NEC 355.8
    lower extremity NEC 355.8
    median (in carpal tunnel) 354.0
    obturator 355.79
    optic 377.49
    plantar 355.6
    posterior tibial (in tarsal tunnel) 355.5
    root (by scar tissue) NEC 724.9
      cervical NEC 723.4
      lumbar NEC 724.4
      lumbosacral 724.4
      thoracic 724.4
    saphenous 355.79
    sciatic (acute) 355.0
    sympathetic 337.9
    traumatic — *see* Injury, nerve
    ulnar 354.2
    upper extremity NEC 354.9
  peripheral — *see* Compression, nerve
  spinal (cord) (old or nontraumatic) 336.9
    by displacement of intervertebral disc — *see* Displacement, intervertebral disc
    nerve
      root NEC 724.9
        postoperative 722.80
          cervical region 722.81
          lumbar region 722.83
          thoracic region 722.82
        traumatic — *see* Injury, nerve, spinal
      traumatic — *see* Injury, nerve, spinal
    spondylogenic 721.91
      cervical 721.1
      lumbar, lumbosacral 721.42
      thoracic 721.41
    traumatic (*see also* Injury, spinal, by site)
      with fracture, vertebra — *see* Fracture, vertebra, by site, with spinal cord injury
  spondylogenic — *see* Compression, spinal cord, spondylogenic
  subcostal nerve (syndrome) 354.8
  sympathetic nerve NEC 337.9
  syndrome 958.5
  thorax 512.8
    iatrogenic 512.1

Compression — *continued*
  thorax — *continued*
    postoperative 512.1
  trachea 519.19
    congenital 748.3
  ulnar nerve (by scar tissue) 354.2
  umbilical cord
    affecting fetus or newborn 762.5
      cord prolapsed 762.4
    complicating delivery 663.2 ☑
      cord around neck 663.1 ☑
      cord prolapsed 663.0 ☑
  upper extremity NEC 354.9
  ureter 593.3
  urethra — *see* Stricture, urethra
  vein 459.2
  vena cava (inferior) (superior) 459.2
  vertebral NEC — *see* Compression, spinal (cord)
Compulsion, compulsive
  eating 307.51
  neurosis (obsessive) 300.3
  personality 301.4
  states (mixed) 300.3
  swearing 300.3
    in Gilles de la Tourette's syndrome 307.23
  tics and spasms 307.22
  water drinking NEC (syndrome) 307.9
Concato's disease (pericardial polyserositis) 423.2
  peritoneal 568.82
  pleural — *see* Pleurisy
Concavity, chest wall 738.3
Concealed
  hemorrhage NEC 459.0
  penis 752.65
Concentric fading 368.12
Concern (normal) **about sick person in family** V61.49
Concrescence (teeth) 520.2
Concretio cordis 423.1
  rheumatic 393
Concretion — *see also* Calculus
  appendicular 543.9
  canaliculus 375.57
  clitoris 624.8
  conjunctiva 372.54
  eyelid 374.56
  intestine (impaction) (obstruction) 560.39
  lacrimal (passages) 375.57
  prepuce (male) 605
    female (clitoris) 624.8
  salivary gland (any) 527.5
  seminal vesicle 608.89
  stomach 537.89
  tonsil 474.8
Concussion (current) 850.9
  with
    loss of consciousness 850.5
      brief (less than one hour)
        30 minutes or less 850.11
        31-59 minutes 850.12
      moderate (1-24 hours) 850.2
      prolonged (more than 24 hours)
        (with complete recovery)
        (with return to pre-existing conscious level) 850.3
        without return to pre-existing conscious level 850.4
    mental confusion or disorientation (without loss of consciousness) 850.0
      with loss of consciousness — *see* Concussion, with, loss of consciousness
  without loss of consciousness 850.0
  blast (air) (hydraulic) (immersion) (underwater) 869.0
    with open wound into cavity 869.1
    abdomen or thorax — *see* Injury, internal, by site
    brain — *see* Concussion, brain
    ear (acoustic nerve trauma) 951.5

☑ **Additional Digit Required — Refer to the Tabular List for Digit Selection**   🔺 **Subterms under main terms may continue to next column or page**

2011 ICD-9-CM   ►◄ Revised Text   ● New Line   ▲ Revised Code   **October 2010 • Volume 2 — 53**

Concussion — continued
  blast — continued
    ear — continued
      with perforation, tympanic mem-
        brane — see Wound, open,
        ear drum
      thorax — see Injury, internal, intratho-
        racic organs NEC
  brain or cerebral (without skull fracture)
    850.9
    with
      loss of consciousness 850.5
        brief (less than one hour)
          30 minutes or less 850.11
          31-59 minutes 850.12
        moderate (1-24 hours) 850.2
        prolonged (more than 24 hours)
          (with complete recovery)
          (with return to pre-exist-
          ing conscious level) 850.3
          without return to pre-existing
          conscious level 850.4
      mental confusion or disorientation
        (without loss of conscious-
        ness) 850.0
      with loss of consciousness — see
        Concussion, brain, with,
        loss of consciousness
      skull fracture — see Fracture, skull,
        by site
      without loss of consciousness 850.0
  cauda equina 952.4
  cerebral — see Concussion, brain
  conus medullaris (spine) 952.4
  hydraulic — see Concussion, blast
  internal organs — see Injury, internal, by
    site
  labyrinth — see Injury, intracranial
  ocular 921.3
  osseous labyrinth — see Injury, intracranial
  spinal (cord) (see also Injury, spinal, by site)
    due to
      broken
        back — see Fracture, vertebra, by
          site, with spinal cord injury
        neck — see Fracture, vertebra,
          cervical, with spinal cord
          injury
      fracture, fracture dislocation, or
        compression fracture of spine
        or vertebra — see Fracture,
        vertebra, by site, with spinal
        cord injury
  syndrome 310.2
  underwater blast — see Concussion, blast
Condition — see also Disease
  fetal hematologic 678.0 ☑
  psychiatric 298.9
  respiratory NEC 519.9
    acute or subacute NEC 519.9
      due to
        external agent 508.9
          specified type NEC 508.8
        fumes or vapors (chemical) (in-
          halation) 506.3
        radiation 508.0
    chronic NEC 519.9
      due to
        external agent 508.9
          specified type NEC 508.8
        fumes or vapors (chemical) (in-
          halation) 506.4
        radiation 508.1
    due to
      external agent 508.9
        specified type NEC 508.8
      fumes or vapors (chemical) (inhala-
        tion) 506.9
Conduct disturbance — see also Disturbance,
    conduct 312.9
  adjustment reaction 309.3
  hyperkinetic 314.2
Condyloma NEC 078.11
  acuminatum 078.11
  gonorrheal 098.0
  latum 091.3

Condyloma — continued
  syphilitic 091.3
    congenital 090.0
  venereal, syphilitic 091.3
Confinement — see Delivery
Conflagration — see also Burn, by site
  asphyxia (by inhalation of smoke, gases,
    fumes, or vapors) 987.9
    specified agent — see Table of Drugs
      and Chemicals
Conflict
  family V61.9
    specified circumstance NEC V61.8
  interpersonal NEC V62.81
  marital V61.10
    involving
      divorce V61.03
      estrangement V61.09
  parent (guardian)-child V61.20
    adopted child V61.24
    biological child V61.23
    foster child V61.25
  partner V61.10
Confluent — see condition
Confusion, confused (mental) (state) — see
    also State, confusional 298.9
  acute 293.0
  epileptic 293.0
  postoperative 293.9
  psychogenic 298.2
  reactive (from emotional stress, psycholog-
    ical trauma) 298.2
  subacute 293.1
Congelation 991.9
Congenital — see also condition
  aortic septum 747.29
  generalized fibromatosis (CGF) 759.89
  intrinsic factor deficiency 281.0
  malformation — see Anomaly
Congestion, congestive
  asphyxia, newborn 768.9
  bladder 596.8
  bowel 569.89
  brain (see also Disease, cerebrovascular NEC)
    437.8
    malarial 084.9
  breast 611.79
  bronchi 519.19
  bronchial tube 519.19
  catarrhal 472.0
  cerebral — see Congestion, brain
  cerebrospinal — see Congestion, brain
  chest 786.9
  chill 786.9
    malarial (see also Malaria) 084.6
  circulatory NEC 459.9
  conjunctiva 372.71
  due to disturbance of circulation 459.9
  duodenum 537.3
  enteritis — see Enteritis
  eye 372.71
  fibrosis syndrome (pelvic) 625.5
  gastroenteritis — see Enteritis
  general 799.89
  glottis 476.0
  heart (see also Failure, heart) 428.0
  hepatic 573.0
  hypostatic (lung) 514
  intestine 569.89
  intracranial — see Congestion, brain
  kidney 593.89
  labyrinth 386.50
  larynx 476.0
  liver 573.0
  lung 786.9
    active or acute (see also Pneumonia) 486
      congenital 770.0
    chronic 514
    hypostatic 514
    idiopathic, acute 518.5
    passive 514
  malaria, malarial (brain) (fever) (see also
    Malaria) 084.6
  medulla — see Congestion, brain
  nasal 478.19

Congestion, congestive — continued
  nose 478.19
  orbit, orbital 376.33
    inflammatory (chronic) 376.10
    acute 376.00
  ovary 620.8
  pancreas 577.8
  pelvic, female 625.5
  pleural 511.0
  prostate (active) 602.1
  pulmonary — see Congestion, lung
  renal 593.89
  retina 362.89
  seminal vesicle 608.89
  spinal cord 336.1
  spleen 289.51
    chronic 289.51
  stomach 537.89
  trachea 464.11
  urethra 599.84
  uterus 625.5
    with subinvolution 621.1
  viscera 799.89
Congestive — see Congestion
Conical
  cervix 622.6
  cornea 371.60
  teeth 520.2
Conjoined twins 759.4
  causing disproportion (fetopelvic) 678.1 ☑
  fetal 678.1 ☑
Conjugal maladjustment V61.10
  involving
    divorce V61.03
    estrangement V61.09
Conjunctiva — see condition
Conjunctivitis (exposure) (infectious)
    (nondiphtheritic) (pneumococcal) (pus-
    tular) (staphylococcal) (streptococcal)
    NEC 372.30
  actinic 370.24
  acute 372.00
    atopic 372.05
    chemical 372.06
    contagious 372.03
    follicular 372.02
    hemorrhagic (viral) 077.4
    toxic 372.06
  adenoviral (acute) 077.3
  allergic (chronic) 372.14
    with hay fever 372.05
  anaphylactic 372.05
  angular 372.03
  Apollo (viral) 077.4
  atopic 372.05
  blennorrhagic (neonatorum) 098.40 ☑
  catarrhal 372.03
  chemical 372.06
    allergic 372.05
    meaning corrosion — see Burn, conjunc-
      tiva
  chlamydial 077.98
    due to
      Chlamydia trachomatis — see Tra-
        choma
      paratrachoma 077.0
  chronic 372.10
    allergic 372.14
    follicular 372.12
    simple 372.11
    specified type NEC 372.14
    vernal 372.13
  diphtheritic 032.81
  due to
    dust 372.05
    enterovirus type 70 077.4
    erythema multiforme 695.10 [372.33]
    filariasis (see also Filariasis) 125.9 [372.15]
    mucocutaneous
      disease NEC 372.33
      leishmaniasis 085.5 [372.15]
    Reiter's disease 099.3 [372.33]
    syphilis 095.8 [372.10]
    toxoplasmosis (acquired) 130.1
      congenital (active) 771.2
    trachoma — see Trachoma

Conjunctivitis — continued
  dust 372.05
  eczematous 370.31
  epidemic 077.1
    hemorrhagic 077.4
  follicular (acute) 372.02
    adenoviral (acute) 077.3
    chronic 372.12
  glare 370.24
  gonococcal (neonatorum) 098.40
  granular (trachomatous) 076.1
    late effect 139.1
  hemorrhagic (acute) (epidemic) 077.4
  herpetic (simplex) 054.43
    zoster 053.21
  inclusion 077.0
  infantile 771.6
  influenzal 372.03
  Koch-Weeks 372.03
  light 372.05
  medicamentosa 372.05
  membranous 372.04
  meningococcic 036.89
  Morax-Axenfeld 372.02
  mucopurulent NEC 372.03
  neonatal 771.6
    gonococcal 098.40
  Newcastle's 077.8
  nodosa 360.14
  of Beal 077.3
  parasitic 372.15
    filariasis (see also Filariasis) 125.9 [372.15]
    mucocutaneous leishmaniasis
      085.5 [372.15]
  Parinaud's 372.02
  petrificans 372.39
  phlyctenular 370.31
  pseudomembranous 372.04
    diphtheritic 032.81
  purulent 372.03
  Reiter's 099.3 [372.33]
  rosacea 695.3 [372.31]
  serous 372.01
    viral 077.99
  simple chronic 372.11
  specified NEC 372.39
  sunlamp 372.04
  swimming pool 077.0
  toxic 372.06
  trachomatous (follicular) 076.1
    acute 076.0
    late effect 139.1
  traumatic NEC 372.39
  tuberculous (see also Tuberculosis)
    017.3 ☑ [370.31]
  tularemic 021.3
  tularensis 021.3
  vernal 372.13
    limbar 372.13 [370.32]
  viral 077.99
    acute hemorrhagic 077.4
    specified NEC 077.8
Conjunctivochalasis 372.81
Conjunctoblepharitis — see Conjunctivitis
Connective tissue — see condition
Conn (-Louis) syndrome (primary aldostero-
    nism) 255.12
Conradi (-Hünermann) syndrome or disease
    (chondrodysplasia calcificans congenita)
    756.59
Consanguinity V19.7
Consecutive — see condition
Consolidated lung (base) — see Pneumonia,
    lobar
Constipation 564.00
  atonic 564.09
  drug induced
    correct substance properly administered
      564.09
    overdose or wrong substance given or
      taken 977.9
      specified drug — see Table of Drugs
        and Chemicals
  neurogenic 564.09
  other specified NEC 564.09
  outlet dysfunction 564.02

☑ **Additional Digit Required — Refer to the Tabular List for Digit Selection**   ▽ **Subterms under main terms may continue to next column or page**

Constipation — *continued*
  psychogenic 306.4
  simple 564.00
  slow transit 564.01
  spastic 564.09
Constitutional — *see also* condition
  arterial hypotension (*see also* Hypotension)
    458.9
  obesity 278.00
    morbid 278.01
  psychopathic state 301.9
  short stature in childhood 783.43
  state, developmental V21.9
    specified development NEC V21.8
  substandard 301.6
Constitutionally substandard 301.6
Constriction
  anomalous, meningeal bands or folds 742.8
  aortic arch (congenital) 747.10
  asphyxiation or suffocation by 994.7
  bronchus 519.19
  canal, ear (*see also* Stricture, ear canal, acquired) 380.50
  duodenum 537.3
  gallbladder (*see also* Obstruction, gallbladder) 575.2
    congenital 751.69
  intestine (*see also* Obstruction, intestine) 560.9
  larynx 478.74
    congenital 748.3
  meningeal bands or folds, anomalous 742.8
  organ or site, congenital NEC — *see* Atresia
  prepuce (congenital) 605
  pylorus 537.0
    adult hypertrophic 537.0
    congenital or infantile 750.5
    newborn 750.5
  ring (uterus) 661.4 ☑
    affecting fetus or newborn 763.7
  spastic (*see also* Spasm)
    ureter 593.3
    urethra — *see* Stricture, urethra
  stomach 537.89
  ureter 593.3
  urethra — *see* Stricture, urethra
  visual field (functional) (peripheral) 368.45
Constrictive — *see* condition
Consultation
  without complaint or sickness V65.9
    feared complaint unfounded V65.5
    specified reason NEC V65.8
  medical (*see also* Counseling, medical)
  specified reason NEC V65.8
Consumption — *see* Tuberculosis
Contact
  with
    AIDS virus V01.79
    anthrax V01.81
    asbestos V15.84
    cholera V01.0
    communicable disease V01.9
      specified type NEC V01.89
      viral NEC V01.79
    Escherichia coli (E. coli) V01.83
    German measles V01.4
    gonorrhea V01.6
    HIV V01.79
    human immunodeficiency virus V01.79
    lead V15.86
    meningococcus V01.84
    parasitic disease NEC V01.89
    poliomyelitis V01.2
    potentially hazardous body fluids V15.85
    rabies V01.5
    rubella V01.4
    SARS-associated coronavirus V01.82
    smallpox V01.3
    syphilis V01.6
    tuberculosis V01.1
    varicella V01.71
    venereal disease V01.6
    viral disease NEC V01.79
  dermatitis — *see* Dermatitis
Contamination, food — *see also* Poisoning, food 005.9

Contraception, contraceptive
  advice NEC V25.09
    family planning V25.09
    fitting of diaphragm V25.02
    prescribing or use of
      oral contraceptive agent V25.01
      specified agent NEC V25.02
  counseling NEC V25.09
    emergency V25.03
    family planning V25.09
    fitting of diaphragm V25.02
    prescribing or use of
      oral contraceptive agent V25.01
        emergency V25.03
        postcoital V25.03
      specified agent NEC V25.02
  device (in situ) V45.59
    causing menorrhagia 996.76
    checking V25.42
    complications 996.32
    insertion V25.11   ▲
    intrauterine V45.51
    reinsertion V25.13   ▲
    removal V25.12   ▲
      and reinsertion V25.13   ●
    replacement V25.13   ●
    subdermal V45.52
  fitting of diaphragm V25.02
  insertion
    intrauterine contraceptive device V25.11   ▲
    subdermal implantable V25.5
  maintenance V25.40
    examination V25.40
      oral contraceptive V25.41
      specified method NEC V25.49
      subdermal implantable V25.43
        intrauterine device V25.42
    intrauterine device V25.42
    oral contraceptive V25.41
    specified method NEC V25.49
    subdermal implantable V25.43
  management NEC V25.49
  prescription
    oral contraceptive agent V25.01
      emergency V25.03
      postcoital V25.03
      repeat V25.41
    specified agent NEC V25.02
      repeat V25.49
  sterilization V25.2
  surveillance V25.40
    intrauterine device V25.42
    oral contraceptive agent V25.41
      subdermal implantable V25.43
    specified method NEC V25.49
Contraction, contracture, contracted
  Achilles tendon (*see also* Short, tendon, Achilles) 727.81
  anus 564.89
  axilla 729.90
  bile duct (*see also* Disease, biliary) 576.8
  bladder 596.8
    neck or sphincter 596.0
  bowel (*see also* Obstruction, intestine) 560.9
  Braxton Hicks 644.1 ☑
  breast implant, capsular 611.83
  bronchus 519.19
  burn (old) — *see* Cicatrix
  capsular, of breast implant 611.83
  cecum (*see also* Obstruction, intestine) 560.9
  cervix (*see also* Stricture, cervix) 622.4
    congenital 752.49
  cicatricial — *see* Cicatrix
  colon (*see also* Obstruction, intestine) 560.9
  conjunctiva trachomatous, active 076.1
    late effect 139.1
  Dupuytren's 728.6
  eyelid 374.41
  eye socket (after enucleation) 372.64
  face 729.90
  fascia (lata) (postural) 728.89
    Dupuytren's 728.6
    palmar 728.6
    plantar 728.71
  finger NEC 736.29

Contraction, contracture, contracted — *continued*
  finger — *continued*
    congenital 755.59
    joint (*see also* Contraction, joint) 718.44
  flaccid, paralytic
    joint (*see also* Contraction, joint) 718.4 ☑
    muscle 728.85
      ocular 378.50
  gallbladder (*see also* Obstruction, gallbladder) 575.2
  hamstring 728.89
    tendon 727.81
  heart valve — *see* Endocarditis
  Hicks' 644.1 ☑
  hip (*see also* Contraction, joint) 718.4 ☑
  hourglass
    bladder 596.8
      congenital 753.8
    gallbladder (*see also* Obstruction, gallbladder) 575.2
      congenital 751.69
    stomach 536.8
      congenital 750.7
      psychogenic 306.4
    uterus 661.4 ☑
      affecting fetus or newborn 763.7
  hysterical 300.11
  infantile (*see also* Epilepsy) 345.6 ☑
  internal os (*see also* Stricture, cervix) 622.4
  intestine (*see also* Obstruction, intestine) 560.9
  joint (abduction) (acquired) (adduction) (flexion) (rotation) 718.40
    ankle 718.47
    congenital NEC 755.8
      generalized or multiple 754.89
        lower limb joints 754.89
      hip (*see also* Subluxation, congenital, hip) 754.32
      lower limb (including pelvic girdle) not involving hip 754.89
      upper limb (including shoulder girdle) 755.59
    elbow 718.42
    foot 718.47
    hand 718.44
    hip 718.45
    hysterical 300.11
    knee 718.46
    multiple sites 718.49
    pelvic region 718.45
    shoulder (region) 718.41
    specified site NEC 718.48
    wrist 718.43
  kidney (granular) (secondary) (*see also* Sclerosis, renal) 587
    congenital 753.3
    hydronephritic 591
    pyelonephritic (*see also* Pyelitis, chronic) 590.00
    tuberculous (*see also* Tuberculosis) 016.0 ☑
  ligament 728.89
    congenital 756.89
  liver — *see* Cirrhosis, liver
  muscle (postinfectional) (postural) NEC 728.85
    congenital 756.89
      sternocleidomastoid 754.1
    extraocular 378.60
    eye (extrinsic) (*see also* Strabismus) 378.9
      paralytic (*see also* Strabismus, paralytic) 378.50
    flaccid 728.85
    hysterical 300.11
    ischemic (Volkmann's) 958.6
    paralytic 728.85
    posttraumatic 958.6
    psychogenic 306.0
      specified as conversion reaction 300.11
  myotonic 728.85
  neck (*see also* Torticollis) 723.5
    congenital 754.1

Contraction, contracture, contracted — *continued*
  neck (*see also* Torticollis) — *continued*
    psychogenic 306.0
  ocular muscle (*see also* Strabismus) 378.9
    paralytic (*see also* Strabismus, paralytic) 378.50
  organ or site, congenital NEC — *see* Atresia
  outlet (pelvis) — *see* Contraction, pelvis
  palmar fascia 728.6
  paralytic
    joint (*see also* Contraction, joint) 718.4 ☑
    muscle 728.85
      ocular (*see also* Strabismus, paralytic) 378.50
  pelvis (acquired) (general) 738.6
    affecting fetus or newborn 763.1
    complicating delivery 653.1 ☑
      causing obstructed labor 660.1 ☑
      generally contracted 653.1 ☑
        causing obstructed labor 660.1 ☑
      inlet 653.2 ☑
        causing obstructed labor 660.1 ☑
      midpelvic 653.8 ☑
        causing obstructed labor 660.1 ☑
      midplane 653.8 ☑
        causing obstructed labor 660.1 ☑
      outlet 653.3 ☑
        causing obstructed labor 660.1 ☑
  plantar fascia 728.71
  premature
    atrial 427.61
    auricular 427.61
    auriculoventricular 427.61
    heart (junctional) (nodal) 427.60
    supraventricular 427.61
    ventricular 427.69
  prostate 602.8
  pylorus (*see also* Pylorospasm) 537.81
  rectosigmoid (*see also* Obstruction, intestine) 560.9
  rectum, rectal (sphincter) 564.89
    psychogenic 306.4
  ring (Bandl's) 661.4 ☑
    affecting fetus or newborn 763.7
  scar — *see* Cicatrix
  sigmoid (*see also* Obstruction, intestine) 560.9
  socket, eye 372.64
  spine (*see also* Curvature, spine) 737.9
  stomach 536.8
    hourglass 536.8
      congenital 750.7
    psychogenic 306.4
  tendon (sheath) (*see also* Short, tendon) 727.81
  toe 735.8
  ureterovesical orifice (postinfectional) 593.3
  urethra 599.84
  uterus 621.8
    abnormal 661.9 ☑
      affecting fetus or newborn 763.7
    clonic, hourglass or tetanic 661.4 ☑
      affecting fetus or newborn 763.7
    dyscoordinate 661.4 ☑
      affecting fetus or newborn 763.7
    hourglass 661.4 ☑
      affecting fetus or newborn 763.7
    hypotonic NEC 661.2 ☑
      affecting fetus or newborn 763.7
    incoordinate 661.4 ☑
      affecting fetus or newborn 763.7
    inefficient or poor 661.2 ☑
      affecting fetus or newborn 763.7
    irregular 661.2 ☑
      affecting fetus or newborn 763.7
    tetanic 661.4 ☑
      affecting fetus or newborn 763.7
  vagina (outlet) 623.2

☑ **Additional Digit Required** — **Refer to the Tabular List for Digit Selection**   ▽ **Subterms under main terms may continue to next column or page**

2011 ICD-9-CM   ▶◀ **Revised Text**   ● **New Line**   ▲ **Revised Code**   October 2010 • Volume 2 — 55

Contraction, contracture, contracted — *continued*
- *continued*
  - vesical 596.8
    - neck or urethral orifice 596.0
  - visual field, generalized 368.45
  - Volkmann's (ischemic) 958.6

Contusion (skin surface intact) 924.9
- with
  - crush injury — *see* Crush
  - dislocation — *see* Dislocation, by site
  - fracture — *see* Fracture, by site
  - internal injury (*see also* Injury, internal, by site)
    - heart — *see* Contusion, cardiac
    - kidney — *see* Contusion, kidney
    - liver — *see* Contusion, liver
    - lung — *see* Contusion, lung
    - spleen — *see* Contusion, spleen
  - intracranial injury — *see* Injury, intracranial
  - nerve injury — *see* Injury, nerve
  - open wound — *see* Wound, open, by site
- abdomen, abdominal (muscle) (wall) 922.2
  - organ(s) NEC 868.00
- adnexa, eye NEC 921.9
- ankle 924.21
  - with other parts of foot 924.20
- arm 923.9
  - lower (with elbow) 923.10
  - upper 923.03
    - with shoulder or axillary region 923.09
- auditory canal (external) (meatus) (and other part(s) of neck, scalp, or face, except eye) 920
- auricle, ear (and other part(s) of neck, scalp, or face except eye) 920
- axilla 923.02
  - with shoulder or upper arm 923.09
- back 922.31
- bone NEC 924.9
- brain (cerebral) (membrane) (with hemorrhage) 851.8 ☑

Note — Use the following fifth–digit subclassification with categories 851–854:

0   *unspecified state of consciousness*

1   *with no loss of consciousness*

2   *with brief [less than one hour] loss of consciousness*

3   *with moderate [1–24 hours] loss of consciousness*

4   *with prolonged [more than 24 hours] loss of consciousness and return to pre–existing conscious level*

5   *with prolonged [more than 24 hours] loss of consciousness, without return to pre–existing conscious level*

Use fifth–digit 5 to designate when a patient is unconscious and dies before regaining consciousness, regardless of the duration of the loss of consciousness

6   *with loss of consciousness of un-specified duration*

9   *with concussion, unspecified*

- with
  - open intracranial wound 851.9 ☑
  - skull fracture — *see* Fracture, skull, by site
- cerebellum 851.4 ☑
  - with open intracranial wound 851.5 ☑
- cortex 851.0 ☑
  - with open intracranial wound 851.1 ☑
- occipital lobe 851.4 ☑
  - with open intracranial wound 851.5 ☑

Contusion — *continued*
- brain — *continued*
  - stem 851.4 ☑
    - with open intracranial wound 851.5 ☑
- breast 922.0
- brow (and other part(s) of neck, scalp, or face, except eye) 920
- buttock 922.32
- canthus 921.1
- cardiac 861.01
  - with open wound into thorax 861.11
- cauda equina (spine) 952.4
- cerebellum — *see* Contusion, brain, cerebellum
- cerebral — *see* Contusion, brain
- cheek(s) (and other part(s) of neck, scalp, or face, except eye) 920
- chest (wall) 922.1
- chin (and other part(s) of neck, scalp, or face, except eye) 920
- clitoris 922.4
- conjunctiva 921.1
- conus medullaris (spine) 952.4
- cornea 921.3
- corpus cavernosum 922.4
- cortex (brain) (cerebral) — *see* Contusion, brain, cortex
- costal region 922.1
- ear (and other part(s) of neck, scalp, or face except eye) 920
- elbow 923.11
  - with forearm 923.10
- epididymis 922.4
- epigastric region 922.2
- eye NEC 921.9
- eyeball 921.3
- eyelid(s) (and periocular area) 921.1
- face (and neck, or scalp, any part, except eye) 920
- femoral triangle 922.2
- fetus or newborn 772.6
- finger(s) (nail) (subungual) 923.3
- flank 922.2
- foot (with ankle) (excluding toe(s)) 924.20
- forearm (and elbow) 923.10
- forehead (and other part(s) of neck, scalp, or face, except eye) 920
- genital organs, external 922.4
- globe (eye) 921.3
- groin 922.2
- gum(s) (and other part(s) of neck, scalp, or face, except eye) 920
- hand(s) (except fingers alone) 923.20
- head (any part, except eye) (and face) (and neck) 920
- heart — *see* Contusion, cardiac
- heel 924.20
- hip 924.01
  - with thigh 924.00
- iliac region 922.2
- inguinal region 922.2
- internal organs (abdomen, chest, or pelvis) NEC — *see* Injury, internal, by site
- interscapular region 922.33
- iris (eye) 921.3
- kidney 866.01
  - with open wound into cavity 866.11
- knee 924.11
  - with lower leg 924.10
- labium (majus) (minus) 922.4
- lacrimal apparatus, gland, or sac 921.1
- larynx (and other part(s) of neck, scalp, or face, except eye) 920
- late effect — *see* Late, effects (of), contusion
- leg 924.5
  - lower (with knee) 924.10
- lens 921.3
- lingual (and other part(s) of neck, scalp, or face, except eye) 920
- lip(s) (and other part(s) of neck, scalp, or face, except eye) 920
- liver 864.01
  - with
    - laceration — *see* Laceration, liver
    - open wound into cavity 864.11

Contusion — *continued*
- lower extremity 924.5
  - multiple sites 924.4
- lumbar region 922.31
- lung 861.21
  - with open wound into thorax 861.31
- malar region (and other part(s) of neck, scalp, or face, except eye) 920
- mandibular joint (and other part(s) of neck, scalp, or face, except eye) 920
- mastoid region (and other part(s) of neck, scalp, or face, except eye) 920
- membrane, brain — *see* Contusion, brain
- midthoracic region 922.1
- mouth (and other part(s) of neck, scalp, or face, except eye) 920
- multiple sites (not classifiable to same three-digit category) 924.8
  - lower limb 924.4
  - trunk 922.8
  - upper limb 923.8
- muscle NEC 924.9
- myocardium — *see* Contusion, cardiac
- nasal (septum) (and other part(s) of neck, scalp, or face, except eye) 920
- neck (and scalp or face, any part, except eye) 920
- nerve — *see* Injury, nerve, by site
- nose (and other part(s) of neck, scalp, or face, except eye) 920
- occipital region (scalp) (and neck or face, except eye) 920
  - lobe — *see* Contusion, brain, occipital lobe
- orbit (region) (tissues) 921.2
- palate (soft) (and other part(s) of neck, scalp, or face, except eye) 920
- parietal region (scalp) (and neck, or face, except eye) 920
  - lobe — *see* Contusion, brain
- penis 922.4
- pericardium — *see* Contusion, cardiac
- perineum 922.4
- periocular area 921.1
- pharynx (and other part(s) of neck, scalp, or face, except eye) 920
- popliteal space (*see also* Contusion, knee) 924.11
- prepuce 922.4
- pubic region 922.4
- pudenda 922.4
- pulmonary — *see* Contusion, lung
- quadriceps femoralis 924.00
- rib cage 922.1
- sacral region 922.32
- salivary ducts or glands (and other part(s) of neck, scalp, or face, except eye) 920
- scalp (and neck, or face any part, except eye) 920
- scapular region 923.01
  - with shoulder or upper arm 923.09
- sclera (eye) 921.3
- scrotum 922.4
- shoulder 923.00
  - with upper arm or axillar regions 923.09
- skin NEC 924.9
- skull 920
- spermatic cord 922.4
- spinal cord (*see also* Injury, spinal, by site)
  - cauda equina 952.4
  - conus medullaris 952.4
- spleen 865.01
  - with open wound into cavity 865.11
- sternal region 922.1
- stomach — *see* Injury, internal, stomach
- subconjunctival 921.1
- subcutaneous NEC 924.9
- submaxillary region (and other part(s) of neck, scalp, or face, except eye) 920
- submental region (and other part(s) of neck, scalp, or face, except eye) 920
- subperiosteal NEC 924.9
- supraclavicular fossa (and other part(s) of neck, scalp, or face, except eye) 920

Contusion — *continued*
- supraorbital (and other part(s) of neck, scalp, or face, except eye) 920
- temple (region) (and other part(s) of neck, scalp, or face, except eye) 920
- testis 924.00
- thigh (and hip) 924.00
- thorax 922.1
  - organ — *see* Injury, internal, intrathoracic
- throat (and other part(s) of neck, scalp, or face, except eye) 920
- thumb(s) (nail) (subungual) 923.3
- toe(s) (nail) (subungual) 924.3
- tongue (and other part(s) of neck, scalp, or face, except eye) 920
- trunk 922.9
  - multiple sites 922.8
  - specified site — *see* Contusion, by site
- tunica vaginalis 922.4
- tympanum (membrane) (and other part(s) of neck, scalp, or face, except eye) 920
- upper extremity 923.9
  - multiple sites 923.8
- uvula (and other part(s) of neck, scalp, or face, except eye) 920
- vagina 922.4
- vocal cord(s) (and other part(s) of neck, scalp, or face, except eye) 920
- vulva 922.4
- wrist 923.21
  - with hand(s), except finger(s) alone 923.20

Conus (any type) (congenital) 743.57
- acquired 371.60
- medullaris syndrome 336.8

Convalescence (following) V66.9
- chemotherapy V66.2
- medical NEC V66.5
- psychotherapy V66.3
- radiotherapy V66.1
- surgery NEC V66.0
- treatment (for) NEC V66.5
  - combined V66.6
  - fracture V66.4
  - mental disorder NEC V66.3
  - specified disorder NEC V66.5

Conversion
- closed surgical procedure to open procedure
  - arthroscopic V64.43
  - laparoscopic V64.41
  - thoracoscopic V64.42
- hysteria, hysterical, any type 300.11
- neurosis, any 300.11
- reaction, any 300.11

Converter, tuberculosis (test reaction) 795.5

Convulsions (idiopathic) 780.39
- apoplectiform (*see also* Disease, cerebrovascular, acute) 436
- brain 780.39
- cerebral 780.39
- cerebrospinal 780.39
- due to trauma NEC — *see* Injury, intracranial
- eclamptic (*see also* Eclampsia) 780.39
- epileptic (*see also* Epilepsy) 345.9 ☑
- epileptiform (*see also* Seizure, epileptiform) 780.39
- epileptoid (*see also* Seizure, epileptiform) 780.39
- ether
  - anesthetic
    - correct substance properly administered 780.39
    - overdose or wrong substance given 968.2
  - other specified type — *see* Table of Drugs and Chemicals
- febrile (simple) 780.31
  - complex 780.32
- generalized 780.39
- hysterical 300.11
- infantile 780.39
  - epilepsy — *see* Epilepsy
- internal 780.39

☑ **Additional Digit Required** — Refer to the Tabular List for Digit Selection   ▽ **Subterms under main terms may continue to next column or page**

56 — Volume 2   ▶◀ Revised Text   ● New Line   ▲ Revised Code   2011 ICD-9-CM

Convulsions — continued
  jacksonian (see also Epilepsy) 345.5 ☑
  myoclonic 333.2
  newborn 779.0
  paretic 094.1
  pregnancy (nephritic) (uremic) — see
    Eclampsia, pregnancy
  psychomotor (see also Epilepsy) 345.4 ☑
  puerperal, postpartum — see Eclampsia,
    pregnancy
  recurrent 780.39
    epileptic — see Epilepsy
  reflex 781.0
  repetitive 780.39
    epileptic — see Epilepsy
  salaam (see also Epilepsy) 345.6 ☑
  scarlatinal 034.1
  spasmodic 780.39
  tetanus, tetanic (see also Tetanus) 037
  thymic 254.8
  uncinate 780.39
  uremic 586
Convulsive — see also Convulsions
  disorder or state 780.39
    epileptic — see Epilepsy
  equivalent, abdominal (see also Epilepsy)
    345.5 ☑
Cooke-Apert-Gallais syndrome (adrenogenital) 255.2
Cooley's anemia (erythroblastic) 282.49
Coolie itch 126.9
Cooper's
  disease 610.1
  hernia — see Hernia, Cooper's
Coordination disturbance 781.3
Copper wire arteries, retina 362.13
Copra itch 133.8
Coprolith 560.39
Coprophilia 302.89
Coproporphyria, hereditary 277.1
Coprostasis 560.39
  with hernia (see also Hernia, by site, with
    obstruction)
    gangrenous — see Hernia, by site, with
      gangrene
Cor
  biloculare 745.7
  bovinum — see Hypertrophy, cardiac
  bovis (see also Hypertrophy, cardiac)
  pulmonale (chronic) 416.9
    acute 415.0
  triatriatum, triatrium 746.82
  triloculare 745.8
    biatriatum 745.3
    biventriculare 745.69
Corbus' disease 607.1
Cord — see also condition
  around neck (tightly) (with compression)
    affecting fetus or newborn 762.5
    complicating delivery 663.1 ☑
      without compression 663.3 ☑
        affecting fetus or newborn 762.6
  bladder NEC 344.61
    tabetic 094.0
  prolapse
    affecting fetus or newborn 762.4
    complicating delivery 663.0 ☑
Cord's angiopathy — see also Tuberculosis
  017.3 ☑ [362.18]
Cordis ectopia 746.87
Corditis (spermatic) 608.4
Corectopia 743.46
Cori type glycogen storage disease — see
  Disease, glycogen storage
Cork-handlers' disease or lung 495.3
Corkscrew esophagus 530.5
Corlett's pyosis (impetigo) 684
Corn (infected) 700
Cornea — see also condition
  donor V59.5
  guttata (dystrophy) 371.57
  plana 743.41
Cornelia de Lange's syndrome (Amsterdam dwarf, mental retardation, and brachycephaly) 759.89

Cornual gestation or pregnancy — see
  Pregnancy, cornual
Cornu cutaneum 702.8
Coronary (artery) — see also condition
  arising from aorta or pulmonary trunk
    746.85
Corpora — see also condition
  amylacea (prostate) 602.8
  cavernosa — see condition
Corpulence — see Obesity
Corpus — see condition
Corrigan's disease — see Insufficiency, aortic
Corrosive burn — see Burn, by site
Corsican fever — see Malaria 084.6
Cortical — see also condition
  blindness 377.75
  necrosis, kidney (bilateral) 583.6
Corticoadrenal — see condition
Corticosexual syndrome 255.2
Coryza (acute) 460
  with grippe or influenza ▶(see also Influenza)◀ 487.1
  syphilitic 095.8
    congenital (chronic) 090.0
Costen's syndrome or complex 524.60
Costiveness — see Constipation 564.00
Costochondritis 733.6
Cotard's syndrome (paranoia) 297.1
Cot death 798.0
Cotia virus 059.8
Cotungo's disease 724.3
Cough 786.2
  with hemorrhage (see also Hemoptysis)
    786.39 ▲
  affected 786.2
  bronchial 786.2
    with grippe or influenza ▶(see also Influenza)◀ 487.1
  chronic 786.2
  epidemic 786.2
  functional 306.1
  hemorrhagic 786.39 ▲
  hysterical 300.11
  laryngeal, spasmodic 786.2
  nervous 786.2
  psychogenic 306.1
  smokers' 491.0
  tea tasters' 112.89
Counseling NEC V65.40
  without complaint or sickness V65.49
  abuse victim NEC V62.89
    child V61.21
    partner V61.11
    spouse V61.11
  child abuse, maltreatment, or neglect
    V61.21
  contraceptive NEC V25.09
    device (intrauterine) V25.02
    maintenance V25.40
      intrauterine contraceptive device
        V25.42
      oral contraceptive (pill) V25.41
      specified type NEC V25.49
      subdermal implantable V25.43
    management NEC V25.9
    oral contraceptive (pill) V25.01
      emergency V25.03
      postcoital V25.03
    prescription NEC V25.02
      oral contraceptive (pill) V25.01
        emergency V25.03
        postcoital V25.03
        repeat prescription V25.41
      repeat prescription V25.40
    subdermal implantable V25.43
    surveillance NEC V25.40
  dietary V65.3
  exercise V65.41
  expectant parent(s)
    pediatric pre-adoption visit V65.11
    pediatric pre-birth visit V65.11
  explanation of
    investigation finding NEC V65.49
    medication NEC V65.49
  family planning V25.09

Counseling — continued
  family planning — continued
    natural
      procreative V26.41
      to avoid pregnancy V25.04
  for nonattending third party V65.19
  genetic V26.33
  gonorrhea V65.45
  health (advice) (education) (instruction) NEC
    V65.49
  HIV V65.44
  human immunodeficiency virus V65.44
  injury prevention V65.43
  insulin pump training V65.46
  marital V61.10
  medical (for) V65.9
    boarding school resident V60.6
    condition not demonstrated V65.5
    feared complaint and no disease found
      V65.5
    institutional resident V60.6
    on behalf of another V65.19
    person living alone V60.3
  natural family planning
    procreative V26.41
    to avoid pregnancy V25.04
  parent (guardian)-child conflict V61.20
    adopted child V61.24
    biological child V61.23
    foster child V61.25
    specified problem NEC V61.29
  partner abuse
    perpetrator V61.12
    victim V61.11
  pediatric
    pre-adoption visit for adoptive parent(s)
      V65.11
    pre-birth visit for expectant parents
      V65.11
  perpetrator of
    child abuse V62.83
      parental V61.22
    partner abuse V61.12
    spouse abuse V61.12
  procreative V65.49
  sex NEC V65.49
    transmitted disease NEC V65.45
      HIV V65.44
  specified reason NEC V65.49
  spousal abuse
    perpetrator V61.12
    victim V61.11
  substance use and abuse V65.42
  syphilis V65.45
  victim (of)
    abuse NEC V62.89
    child abuse V61.21
    partner abuse V61.11
    spousal abuse V61.11
Coupled rhythm 427.89
Couvelaire uterus (complicating delivery) —
  see Placenta, separation
Cowper's gland — see condition
Cowperitis — see also Urethritis 597.89
  gonorrheal (acute) 098.0
    chronic or duration of 2 months or over
      098.2
Cowpox (abortive) 051.01
  due to vaccination 999.0
  eyelid 051.01 [373.5]
    postvaccination 999.0 [373.5]
Coxa
  plana 732.1
  valga (acquired) 736.31
    congenital 755.61
    late effect of rickets 268.1
  vara (acquired) 736.32
    congenital 755.62
    late effect of rickets 268.1
Coxae malum senilis 715.25
Coxalgia (nontuberculous) 719.45
  tuberculous (see also Tuberculosis)
    015.1 ☑ [730.85]
Coxalgic pelvis 736.30
Coxitis 716.65
Coxsackie (infection) (virus) 079.2

Coxsackie — continued
  central nervous system NEC 048
  endocarditis 074.22
  enteritis 008.67
  meningitis (aseptic) 047.0
  myocarditis 074.23
  pericarditis 074.21
  pharyngitis 074.0
  pleurodynia 074.1
  specific disease NEC 074.8
Crabs, meaning pubic lice 132.2
Crack baby 760.75
Cracked
  nipple 611.2
    puerperal, postpartum 676.1 ☑
  tooth 521.81
Cradle cap 690.11
Craft neurosis 300.89
Craigiasis 007.8
Cramp(s) 729.82
  abdominal 789.0 ☑
  bathing 994.1
  colic 789.7
    infantile 789.7
    psychogenic 306.4
  due to immersion 994.1
  extremity (lower) (upper) NEC 729.82
  fireman 992.2
  heat 992.2
  hysterical 300.11
  immersion 994.1
  intestinal 789.0 ☑
    psychogenic 306.4
  linotypist's 300.89
    organic 333.84
  muscle (extremity) (general) 729.82
    due to immersion 994.1
    hysterical 300.11
  occupational (hand) 300.89
    organic 333.84
  psychogenic 307.89
  salt depletion 276.1
  sleep related leg 327.52
  stoker 992.2
  stomach 789.0 ☑
  telegraphers' 300.89
    organic 333.84
  typists' 300.89
    organic 333.84
  uterus 625.8
    menstrual 625.3
  writers' 333.84
    organic 333.84
    psychogenic 300.89
Cranial — see condition
Cranioclasis, fetal 763.89
Craniocleidodysostosis 755.59
Craniofenestria (skull) 756.0
Craniolacunia (skull) 756.0
Craniopagus 759.4
Craniopathy, metabolic 733.3
Craniopharyngeal — see condition
Craniopharyngioma (M9350/1) 237.0
Craniorachischisis (totalis) 740.1
Cranioschisis 756.0
Craniostenosis 756.0
Craniosynostosis 756.0
Craniotabes (cause unknown) 733.3
  rachitic 268.1
  syphilitic 090.5
Craniotomy, fetal 763.89
Cranium — see condition
Craw-craw 125.3
CRBSI (catheter-related bloodstream infection)
  999.31
Creaking joint 719.60
  ankle 719.67
  elbow 719.62
  foot 719.67
  hand 719.64
  hip 719.65
  knee 719.66
  multiple sites 719.69
  pelvic region 719.65
  shoulder (region) 719.61
  specified site NEC 719.68

☑ **Additional Digit Required** — Refer to the Tabular List for Digit Selection   ▽ **Subterms under main terms may continue to next column or page**

2011 ICD-9-CM   ▶◀ **Revised Text**   ● **New Line**   ▲ **Revised Code**   October 2010 • Volume 2 — 57

☑ **Additional Digit Required** — Refer to the Tabular List for Digit Selection
▽ **Subterms under main terms may continue to next column or page**

58 — Volume 2 ▶◀ Revised Text ● New Line ▲ Revised Code 2011 ICD-9-CM

Cutis — *see also* condition — *continued*
  marmorata 782.61
  osteosis 709.3
  pendula 756.83
    acquired 701.8
  rhomboidalis nuchae 701.8
  verticis gyrata 757.39
    acquired 701.8
Cyanopathy, newborn 770.83
Cyanosis 782.5
  autotoxic 289.7
  common atrioventricular canal 745.69
  congenital 770.83
  conjunctiva 372.71
  due to
    endocardial cushion defect 745.60
    nonclosure, foramen botalli 745.5
    patent foramen botalli 745.5
    persistent foramen ovale 745.5
  enterogenous 289.7
  fetus or newborn 770.83
  ostium primum defect 745.61
  paroxysmal digital 443.0
  retina, retinal 362.10
Cycle
  anovulatory 628.0
  menstrual, irregular 626.4
Cyclencephaly 759.89
Cyclical vomiting 536.2
  associated with migraine 346.2 ☑
  psychogenic 306.4
Cyclitic membrane 364.74
Cyclitis — *see also* Iridocyclitis 364.3
  acute 364.00
    primary 364.01
    recurrent 364.02
  chronic 364.10
    in
      sarcoidosis 135 *[364.11]*
      tuberculosis (*see also* Tuberculosis)
        017.3 ☑ *[364.11]*
  Fuchs' heterochromic 364.21
  granulomatous 364.10
  lens induced 364.23
  nongranulomatous 364.00
  posterior 363.21
  primary 364.01
  recurrent 364.02
  secondary (noninfectious) 364.04
    infectious 364.03
  subacute 364.00
    primary 364.01
    recurrent 364.02
Cyclokeratitis — *see* Keratitis
Cyclophoria 378.44
Cyclopia, cyclops 759.89
Cycloplegia 367.51
Cyclospasm 367.53
Cyclosporiasis 007.5
Cyclothymia 301.13
Cyclothymic personality 301.13
Cyclotropia 378.33
Cyesis — *see* Pregnancy
Cylindroma (M8200/3) — *see also* Neoplasm,
  by site, malignant
  eccrine dermal (M8200/0) — *see* Neoplasm,
    skin, benign
  skin (M8200/0) — *see* Neoplasm, skin, be-
    nign
Cylindruria 791.7
Cyllosoma 759.89
Cynanche
  diphtheritic 032.3
  tonsillaris 475
Cynorexia 783.6
Cyphosis — *see* Kyphosis
Cyprus fever — *see also* Brucellosis 023.9
Cyriax's syndrome (slipping rib) 733.99

Cyst (mucus) (retention) (serous) (simple)

Note — In general, cysts are not neoplastic and are classified to the appropriate category for disease of the specified anatomical site. This generalization does not apply to certain types of cysts which are neoplastic in nature, for example, dermoid, nor does it apply to cysts of certain structures, for example, branchial cleft, which are classified as developmental anomalies.

The following listing includes some of the most frequently reported sites of cysts as well as qualifiers which indicate the type of cyst. The latter qualifiers usually are not repeated under the anatomical sites. Since the code assignment for a given site may vary depending upon the type of cyst, the coder should refer to the listings under the specified type of cyst before consideration is given to the site.

  accessory, fallopian tube 752.11
  adenoid (infected) 474.8
  adrenal gland 255.8
    congenital 759.1
  air, lung 518.89
  allantoic 753.7
  alveolar process (jaw bone) 526.2
  amnion, amniotic 658.8 ☑
  anterior chamber (eye) 364.60
    exudative 364.62
    implantation (surgical) (traumatic)
      364.61
    parasitic 360.13
  anterior nasopalatine 526.1
  antrum 478.19
  anus 569.49
  apical (periodontal) (tooth) 522.8
  appendix 543.9
  arachnoid, brain 348.0
  arytenoid 478.79
  auricle 706.2
  Baker's (knee) 727.51
    tuberculous (*see also* Tuberculosis)
      015.2 ☑
  Bartholin's gland or duct 616.2
  bile duct (*see also* Disease, biliary) 576.8
  bladder (multiple) (trigone) 596.8
  Blessig's 362.62
  blood, endocardial (*see also* Endocarditis)
    424.90
  blue dome 610.0
  bone (local) 733.20
    aneurysmal 733.22
    jaw 526.2
      developmental (odontogenic) 526.0
      fissural 526.1
      latent 526.89
    solitary 733.21
    unicameral 733.21
  brain 348.0
    congenital 742.4
    hydatid (*see also* Echinococcus) 122.9
    third ventricle (colloid) 742.4
  branchial (cleft) 744.42
  branchiogenic 744.42
  breast (benign) (blue dome) (pedunculated)
    (solitary) (traumatic) 610.0
    involution 610.4
    sebaceous 610.8
  broad ligament (benign) 620.8
    embryonic 752.11
  bronchogenic (mediastinal) (sequestration)
    518.89
    congenital 748.4
  buccal 528.4
  bulbourethral gland (Cowper's) 599.89
  bursa, bursal 727.49
    pharyngeal 478.26
  calcifying odontogenic (M9301/0) 213.1
    upper jaw (bone) 213.0
  canal of Nuck (acquired) (serous) 629.1
    congenital 752.41
  canthus 372.75

Cyst — *continued*
  carcinomatous (M8010/3) — *see* Neoplasm,
    by site, malignant
  cartilage (joint) — *see* Derangement, joint
  cauda equina 336.8
  cavum septi pellucidi NEC 348.0
  celomic (pericardium) 746.89
  cerebellopontine (angle) — *see* Cyst, brain
  cerebellum — *see* Cyst, brain
  cerebral — *see* Cyst, brain
  cervical lateral 744.42
  cervix 622.8
    embryonal 752.41
    nabothian (gland) 616.0
  chamber, anterior (eye) 364.60
    exudative 364.62
    implantation (surgical) (traumatic)
      364.61
    parasitic 360.13
  chiasmal, optic NEC (*see also* Lesion, chiasmal) 377.54
  chocolate (ovary) 617.1
  choledochal (congenital) 751.69
    acquired 576.8
  choledochus 751.69
  chorion 658.8 ☑
  choroid plexus 348.0
  chyle, mesentery 457.8
  ciliary body 364.60
    exudative 364.64
    implantation 364.61
    primary 364.63
  clitoris 624.8
  coccyx (*see also* Cyst, bone) 733.20
  colloid
    third ventricle (brain) 742.4
    thyroid gland — *see* Goiter
  colon 569.89
  common (bile) duct (*see also* Disease, biliary)
    576.8
  congenital NEC 759.89
    adrenal glands 759.1
    epiglottis 748.3
    esophagus 750.4
    fallopian tube 752.11
    kidney 753.10
      multiple 753.19
      single 753.11
    larynx 748.3
    liver 751.62
    lung 748.4
    mediastinum 748.8
    ovary 752.0
    oviduct 752.11
    pancreas 751.7
    periurethral (tissue) 753.8
    prepuce NEC 752.69
      penis 752.69
    sublingual 750.26
    submaxillary gland 750.26
    thymus (gland) 759.2
    tongue 750.19
    ureterovesical orifice 753.4
    vulva 752.41
  conjunctiva 372.75
  cornea 371.23
  corpora quadrigemina 348.0
  corpus
    albicans (ovary) 620.2
    luteum (ruptured) 620.1
  Cowper's gland (benign) (infected) 599.89
  cranial meninges 348.0
  craniobuccal pouch 253.8
  craniopharyngeal pouch 253.8
  cystic duct (*see also* Disease, gallbladder)
    575.8
  Cysticercus (any site) 123.1
  Dandy-Walker 742.3
    with spina bifida (*see also* Spina bifida)
      741.0 ☑
  dental 522.8
    developmental 526.0
    eruption 526.0
    lateral periodontal 526.0
    primordial (keratocyst) 526.0
    root 522.8

Cyst — *continued*
  dentigerous 526.0
    mandible 526.0
    maxilla 526.0
  dermoid (M9084/0) (*see also* Neoplasm, by
    site, benign)
    with malignant transformation
      (M9084/3) 183.0
    implantation
      external area or site (skin) NEC 709.8
      iris 364.61
      skin 709.8
      vagina 623.8
      vulva 624.8
    mouth 528.4
    oral soft tissue 528.4
    sacrococcygeal 685.1
      with abscess 685.0
  developmental of ovary, ovarian 752.0
  dura (cerebral) 348.0
    spinal 349.2
  ear (external) 706.2
  echinococcal (*see also* Echinococcus) 122.9
  embryonal
    cervix uteri 752.41
    genitalia, female external 752.41
    uterus 752.39 ▲
    vagina 752.41
  endometrial 621.8
    ectopic 617.9
  endometrium (uterus) 621.8
    ectopic — *see* Endometriosis
  enteric 751.5
  enterogenous 751.5
  epidermal (inclusion) (*see also* Cyst, skin)
    706.2
  epidermoid (inclusion) (*see also* Cyst, skin)
    706.2
    mouth 528.4
    not of skin — *see* Cyst, by site
    oral soft tissue 528.4
  epididymis 608.89
  epiglottis 478.79
  epiphysis cerebri 259.8
  epithelial (inclusion) (*see also* Cyst, skin)
    706.2
  epoophoron 752.11
  eruption 526.0
  esophagus 530.89
  ethmoid sinus 478.19
  eye (retention) 379.8
    congenital 743.03
    posterior segment, congenital 743.54
  eyebrow 706.2
  eyelid (sebaceous) 374.84
    infected 373.13
    sweat glands or ducts 374.84
  falciform ligament (inflammatory) 573.8
  fallopian tube 620.8
    congenital 752.11
  female genital organs NEC 629.89
  fimbrial (congenital) 752.11
  fissural (oral region) 526.1
  follicle (atretic) (graafian) (ovarian) 620.0
    nabothian (gland) 616.0
  follicular (atretic) (ovarian) 620.0
    dentigerous 526.0
  frontal sinus 478.19
  gallbladder or duct 575.8
  ganglion 727.43
  Gartner's duct 752.41
  gas, of mesentery 568.89
  gingiva 523.8
  gland of moll 374.84
  globulomaxillary 526.1
  graafian follicle 620.0
  granulosal lutein 620.2
  hemangiomatous (M9121/0) (*see also* Hemangioma) 228.00
  hydatid (*see also* Echinococcus) 122.9
    fallopian tube (Morgagni) 752.11
    liver NEC 122.8
    lung NEC 122.9
    Morgagni 752.89
      fallopian tube 752.11
    specified site NEC 122.9

☑ **Additional Digit Required — Refer to the Tabular List for Digit Selection**   ◥ **Subterms under main terms may continue to next column or page**

2011 ICD-9-CM   ▶◀ Revised Text   ● New Line   ▲ Revised Code   October 2010 • Volume 2 — 59

Cutis — Cyst

Cyst — continued
  utriculus masculinus 599.89
  vagina, vaginal (squamous cell) (wall) 623.8
    embryonal 752.41
    implantation 623.8
    inclusion 623.8
  vallecula, vallecular 478.79
  ventricle, neuroepithelial 348.0
  verumontanum 599.89
  vesical (orifice) 596.8
  vitreous humor 379.29
  vulva (sweat glands) 624.8
    congenital 752.41
    implantation 624.8
    inclusion 624.8
    sebaceous gland 624.8
  vulvovaginal gland 624.8
  wolffian 752.89
Cystadenocarcinoma (M8440/3) — see also Neoplasm, by site, malignant
  bile duct type (M8161/3) 155.1
  endometrioid (M8380/3) — see Neoplasm, by site, malignant
  mucinous (M8470/3)
    papillary (M8471/3)
      specified site — see Neoplasm, by site, malignant
      unspecified site 183.0
    specified site — see Neoplasm, by site, malignant
    unspecified site 183.0
  papillary (M8450/3)
    mucinous (M8471/3)
      specified site — see Neoplasm, by site, malignant
      unspecified site 183.0
    pseudomucinous (M8471/3)
      specified site — see Neoplasm, by site, malignant
      unspecified site 183.0
    serous (M8460/3)
      specified site — see Neoplasm, by site, malignant
      unspecified site 183.0
    specified site — see Neoplasm, by site, malignant
    unspecified site 183.0
  pseudomucinous (M8470/3)
    papillary (M8471/3)
      specified site — see Neoplasm, by site, malignant
      unspecified site 183.0
    specified site — see Neoplasm, by site, malignant
    unspecified site 183.0
  serous (M8441/3)
    papillary (M8460/3)
      specified site — see Neoplasm, by site, malignant
      unspecified site 183.0
    specified site — see Neoplasm, by site, malignant
    unspecified site 183.0
Cystadenofibroma (M9013/0)
  clear cell (M8313/0) — see Neoplasm, by site, benign
  endometrioid (M8381/0) 220
    borderline malignancy (M8381/1) 236.2
    malignant (M8381/3) 183.0
  mucinous (M9015/0)
    specified site — see Neoplasm, by site, benign
    unspecified site 220
  serous (M9014/0)
    specified site — see Neoplasm, by site, benign
    unspecified site 220
  specified site — see Neoplasm, by site, benign
  unspecified site 220
Cystadenoma (M8440/0) — see also Neoplasm, by site, benign
  bile duct (M8161/0) 211.5
  endometrioid (M8380/0) (see also Neoplasm, by site, benign)

Cystadenoma — see also Neoplasm, by site, benign — continued
  endometrioid (see also Neoplasm, by site, benign) — continued
    borderline malignancy (M8380/1) — see Neoplasm, by site, uncertain behavior
    malignant (M8440/3) — see Neoplasm, by site, malignant
  mucinous (M8470/0)
    borderline malignancy (M8470/1)
      specified site — see Neoplasm, uncertain behavior
      unspecified site 236.2
    papillary (M8471/0)
      borderline malignancy (M8471/1)
        specified site — see Neoplasm, by site, uncertain behavior
        unspecified site 236.2
      specified site — see Neoplasm, by site, benign
      unspecified site 220
    specified site — see Neoplasm, by site, benign
    unspecified site 220
  papillary (M8450/0)
    borderline malignancy (M8450/1)
      specified site — see Neoplasm, by site, uncertain behavior
      unspecified site 236.2
    lymphomatosum (M8561/0) 210.2
    mucinous (M8471/0)
      borderline malignancy (M8471/1)
        specified site — see Neoplasm, by site, uncertain behavior
        unspecified site 236.2
      specified site — see Neoplasm, by site, benign
      unspecified site 220
    pseudomucinous (M8471/0)
      borderline malignancy (M8471/1)
        specified site — see Neoplasm, by site, uncertain behavior
        unspecified site 236.2
      specified site — see Neoplasm, by site, benign
      unspecified site 220
    serous (M8460/0)
      borderline malignancy (M8460/1)
        specified site — see Neoplasm, by site, uncertain behavior
        unspecified site 236.2
      specified site — see Neoplasm, by site, benign
      unspecified site 220
    specified site — see Neoplasm, by site, benign
    unspecified site 220
  pseudomucinous (M8470/0)
    borderline malignancy (M8470/1)
      specified site — see Neoplasm, by site, uncertain behavior
      unspecified site 236.2
    papillary (M8471/0)
      borderline malignancy (M8471/1)
        specified site — see Neoplasm, by site, uncertain behavior
        unspecified site 236.2
      specified site — see Neoplasm, by site, benign
      unspecified site 220
    specified site — see Neoplasm, by site, benign
    unspecified site 220
  serous (M8441/0)
    borderline malignancy (M8441/1)
      specified site — see Neoplasm, by site, uncertain behavior
      unspecified site 236.2
    papillary (M8460/0)
      borderline malignancy (M8460/1)
        specified site — see Neoplasm, by site, uncertain behavior
        unspecified site 236.2
      specified site — see Neoplasm, by site, benign

Cystadenoma — see also Neoplasm, by site, benign — continued
  serous — continued
    papillary — continued
      unspecified site 220
    specified site — see Neoplasm, by site, benign
    unspecified site 220
  thyroid 226
Cystathioninemia 270.4
Cystathioninuria 270.4
Cystic — see also condition
  breast, chronic 610.1
  corpora lutea 620.1
  degeneration, congenital
    brain 742.4
    kidney (see also Cystic, disease, kidney) 753.10
  disease
    breast, chronic 610.1
    kidney, congenital 753.10
      medullary 753.16
      multiple 753.19
      polycystic — see Polycystic, kidney
      single 753.11
      specified NEC 753.19
    liver, congenital 751.62
    lung 518.89
      congenital 748.4
    pancreas, congenital 751.7
    semilunar cartilage 717.5
  duct — see condition
  eyeball, congenital 743.03
  fibrosis (pancreas) 277.00
    with
      manifestations
        gastrointestinal 277.03
        pulmonary 277.02
        specified NEC 277.09
      meconium ileus 277.01
      pulmonary exacerbation 277.02
  hygroma (M9173/0) 228.1
  kidney, congenital 753.10
    medullary 753.16
    multiple 753.19
    polycystic — see Polycystic, kidney
    single 753.11
    specified NEC 753.19
  liver, congenital 751.62
  lung 518.89
    congenital 748.4
  mass — see Cyst
  mastitis, chronic 610.1
  ovary 620.2
  pancreas, congenital 751.7
Cysticerciasis 123.1
Cysticercosis (mammary) (subretinal) 123.1
Cysticercus 123.1
  cellulosae infestation 123.1
Cystinosis (malignant) 270.0
Cystinuria 270.0
Cystitis (bacillary) (colli) (diffuse) (exudative) (hemorrhagic) (purulent) (recurrent) (septic) (suppurative) (ulcerative) 595.9
  with
    abortion — see Abortion, by type, with urinary tract infection
    ectopic pregnancy (see also categories 633.0–633.9) 639.8
    fibrosis 595.1
    leukoplakia 595.1
    malakoplakia 595.1
    metaplasia 595.1
    molar pregnancy (see also categories 630–632) 639.8
  actinomycotic 039.8 [595.4]
  acute 595.0
    of trigone 595.3
  allergic 595.89
  amebic 006.8 [595.4]
  bilharzial 120.9 [595.4]
  blennorrhagic (acute) 098.11
    chronic or duration of 2 months or more 098.31
  bullous 595.89
  calculous 594.1

Cystitis — continued
  chlamydial 099.53
  chronic 595.2
    interstitial 595.1
    of trigone 595.3
  complicating pregnancy, childbirth, or puerperium 646.6 ☑
    affecting fetus or newborn 760.1
  cystic(a) 595.81
  diphtheritic 032.84
  echinococcal
    granulosus 122.3 [595.4]
    multilocularis 122.6 [595.4]
  emphysematous 595.89
  encysted 595.81
  follicular 595.3
  following
    abortion 639.8
    ectopic or molar pregnancy 639.8
  gangrenous 595.89
  glandularis 595.89
  gonococcal (acute) 098.11
    chronic or duration of 2 months or more 098.31
  incrusted 595.89
  interstitial 595.1
  irradiation 595.82
  irritation 595.89
  malignant 595.89
  monilial 112.2
  of trigone 595.3
  panmural 595.1
  polyposa 595.89
  prostatic 601.3
  radiation 595.82
  Reiter's (abacterial) 099.3
  specified NEC 595.89
  subacute 595.2
  submucous 595.1
  syphilitic 095.8
  trichomoniasis 131.09
  tuberculous (see also Tuberculosis) 016.1 ☑
  ulcerative 595.1
Cystocele
  female (without uterine prolapse) 618.01
    with uterine prolapse 618.4
      complete 618.3
      incomplete 618.2
    lateral 618.02
    midline 618.01
    paravaginal 618.02
  in pregnancy or childbirth 654.4 ☑
    affecting fetus or newborn 763.89
    causing obstructed labor 660.2 ☑
      affecting fetus or newborn 763.1
  male 596.8
Cystoid
  cicatrix limbus 372.64
  degeneration macula 362.53
Cystolithiasis 594.1
Cystoma (M8440/0) — see also Neoplasm, by site, benign
  endometrial, ovary 617.1
  mucinous (M8470/0)
    specified site — see Neoplasm, by site, benign
    unspecified site 220
  serous (M8441/0)
    specified site — see Neoplasm, by site, benign
    unspecified site 220
  simple (ovary) 620.2
Cystoplegia 596.53
Cystoptosis 596.8
Cystopyelitis — see also Pyelitis 590.80
Cystorrhagia 596.8
Cystosarcoma phyllodes (M9020/1) 238.3
  benign (M9020/0) 217
  malignant (M9020/3) — see Neoplasm, breast, malignant
Cystostomy status V44.50
  with complication 997.5
  appendico-vesicostomy V44.52
  cutaneous-vesicostomy V44.51
  specified type NEC V44.59
Cystourethritis — see also Urethritis 597.89

☑ **Additional Digit Required — Refer to the Tabular List for Digit Selection**   ⬛ **Subterms under main terms may continue to next column or page**

2011 ICD-9-CM   ▶◀ **Revised Text**   ● **New Line**   ▲ **Revised Code**   **Volume 2 — 61**

Cystourethrocele — *see also* Cystocele
    female (without uterine prolapse) 618.09
        with uterine prolapse 618.4
            complete 618.3
            incomplete 618.2
    male 596.8
Cytomegalic inclusion disease 078.5

Cytomegalic inclusion disease —
    continued
    congenital 771.1
Cytomycosis, reticuloendothelial — *see also*
    Histoplasmosis, American 115.00
Cytopenia 289.9

Cytopenia — *continued*
    refractory
        with
            multilineage dysplasia (RCMD)
                238.72
            and ringed sideroblasts (RCMD-
                RS) 238.72

☑ **Additional Digit Required — Refer to the Tabular List for Digit Selection**   ▽ **Subterms under main terms may continue to next column or page**

62 — Volume 2   ▶◀ **Revised Text**   ● **New Line**   ▲ **Revised Code**   **2011 ICD-9-CM**

D

Daae (-Finsen) disease (epidemic pleurodynia) 074.1
Dabney's grip 074.1
Da Costa's syndrome (neurocirculatory asthenia) 306.2
Dacryoadenitis, dacryadenitis 375.00
  acute 375.01
  chronic 375.02
Dacryocystitis 375.30
  acute 375.32
  chronic 375.42
  neonatal 771.6
  phlegmonous 375.33
  syphilitic 095.8
    congenital 090.0
  trachomatous, active 076.1
    late effect 139.1
  tuberculous (see also Tuberculosis) 017.3 ☑
Dacryocystoblenorrhea 375.42
Dacryocystocele 375.43
Dacryolith, dacryolithiasis 375.57
Dacryoma 375.43
Dacryopericystitis (acute) (subacute) 375.32
  chronic 375.42
Dacryops 375.11
Dacryosialadenopathy, atrophic 710.2
Dacryostenosis 375.56
  congenital 743.65
Dactylitis
  bone (see also Osteomyelitis) 730.2 ☑
  sickle-cell 282.62
    Hb-C 282.64
    Hb-SS 282.62
    specified NEC 282.69
  syphilitic 095.5
  tuberculous (see also Tuberculosis) 015.5 ☑
Dactylolysis spontanea 136.0
Dactylosymphysis — see also Syndactylism 755.10
Damage
  arteriosclerotic — see Arteriosclerosis
  brain 348.9
    anoxic, hypoxic 348.1
      during or resulting from a procedure 997.01
      ischemic, in newborn 768.70
        mild 768.71
        moderate 768.72
        severe 768.73
    child NEC 343.9
    due to birth injury 767.0
    minimal (child) (see also Hyperkinesia) 314.9
    newborn 767.0
  cardiac (see also Disease, heart)
  cardiorenal (vascular) (see also Hypertension, cardiorenal) 404.90
  central nervous system — see Damage, brain
  cerebral NEC — see Damage, brain
  coccyx, complicating delivery 665.6 ☑
  coronary (see also Ischemia, heart) 414.9
  eye, birth injury 767.8
  heart (see also Disease, heart)
    valve — see Endocarditis
  hypothalamus NEC 348.9
  liver 571.9
    alcoholic 571.3
  medication 995.20
  myocardium (see also Degeneration, myocardial) 429.1
  pelvic
    joint or ligament, during delivery 665.6 ☑
    organ NEC
      with
        abortion — see Abortion, by type, with damage to pelvic organs
        ectopic pregnancy (see also categories 633.0–633.9) 639.2
        molar pregnancy (see also categories 630–632) 639.2
      during delivery 665.5 ☑

Damage — continued
  pelvic — continued
    organ — continued
      following
        abortion 639.2
        ectopic or molar pregnancy 639.2
  renal (see also Disease, renal) 593.9
  skin, solar 692.79
    acute 692.72
    chronic 692.74
  subendocardium, subendocardial (see also Degeneration, myocardial) 429.1
  vascular 459.9
Dameshek's syndrome (erythroblastic anemia) 282.49
Dana-Putnam syndrome (subacute combined sclerosis with pernicious anemia) 281.0 [336.2]
Danbolt (-Closs) syndrome (acrodermatitis enteropathica) 686.8
Dandruff 690.18
Dandy fever 061
Dandy-Walker deformity or syndrome (atresia, foramen of Magendie) 742.3
  with spina bifida (see also Spina bifida) 741.0 ☑
Dangle foot 736.79
Danielssen's disease (anesthetic leprosy) 030.1
Danlos' syndrome 756.83
Darier's disease (congenital) (keratosis follicularis) 757.39
  due to vitamin A deficiency 264.8
  meaning erythema annulare centrifugum 695.0
Darier-Roussy sarcoid 135
Dark area on retina 239.81
Darling's
  disease (see also Histoplasmosis, American) 115.00
  histoplasmosis (see also Histoplasmosis, American) 115.00
Dartre 054.9
Darwin's tubercle 744.29
Davidson's anemia (refractory) 284.9
Davies-Colley syndrome (slipping rib) 733.99
Davies' disease 425.0
Dawson's encephalitis 046.2
Day blindness — see also Blindness, day 368.60
Dead
  fetus
    retained (in utero) 656.4 ☑
      early pregnancy (death before 22 completed weeks gestation) 632
      late (death after 22 completed weeks gestation) 656.4 ☑
    syndrome 641.3 ☑
  labyrinth 386.50
  ovum, retained 631
Deaf and dumb NEC 389.7
Deaf mutism (acquired) (congenital) NEC 389.7
  endemic 243
  hysterical 300.11
  syphilitic, congenital 090.0
Deafness (acquired) (complete) (congenital) (hereditary) (middle ear) (partial) 389.9
  with
    blindness V49.85
    blue sclera and fragility of bone 756.51
  auditory fatigue 389.9
  aviation 993.0
    nerve injury 951.5
  boilermakers' 951.5
  central 389.14
    with conductive hearing loss 389.20
      bilateral 389.22
      unilateral 389.21
  conductive (air) 389.00
    with sensorineural hearing loss 389.20
      bilateral 389.22
      unilateral 389.21
    bilateral 389.06
    combined types 389.08
    external ear 389.01

Deafness — continued
  conductive — continued
    inner ear 389.04
    middle ear 389.03
    multiple types 389.08
    tympanic membrane 389.02
    unilateral 389.05
  emotional (complete) 300.11
  functional (complete) 300.11
  high frequency 389.8
  hysterical (complete) 300.11
  injury 951.5
  low frequency 389.8
  mental 784.69
  mixed conductive and sensorineural 389.20
    bilateral 389.22
    unilateral 389.21
  nerve
    with conductive hearing loss 389.20
      bilateral 389.22
      unilateral 389.21
    bilateral 389.12
    unilateral 389.13
  neural
    with conductive hearing loss 389.20
      bilateral 389.22
      unilateral 389.21
    bilateral 389.12
    unilateral 389.13
  noise-induced 388.12
    nerve injury 951.5
  nonspeaking 389.7
  perceptive 389.10
    with conductive hearing loss 389.20
      bilateral 389.22
      unilateral 389.21
    central 389.14
    neural
      bilateral 389.12
      unilateral 389.13
    sensorineural 389.10
      asymmetrical 389.16
      bilateral 389.18
      unilateral 389.15
    sensory
      bilateral 389.11
      unilateral 389.17
  psychogenic (complete) 306.7
  sensorineural (see also Deafness, perceptive) 389.10
    asymmetrical 389.16
    bilateral 389.18
    unilateral 389.15
  sensory
    with conductive hearing loss 389.20
      bilateral 389.22
      unilateral 389.21
    bilateral 389.11
    unilateral 389.17
  specified type NEC 389.8
  sudden NEC 388.2
  syphilitic 094.89
  transient ischemic 388.02
  transmission — see Deafness, conductive
  traumatic 951.5
  word (secondary to organic lesion) 784.69
    developmental 315.31
Death
  after delivery (cause not stated) (sudden) 674.9 ☑
  anesthetic
    due to
      correct substance properly administered 995.4
      overdose or wrong substance given 968.4
      specified anesthetic — see Table of Drugs and Chemicals
    during delivery 668.9 ☑
  brain 348.89
  cardiac (sudden) (SCD) — code to underlying condition
    family history of V17.41
    personal history of, successfully resuscitated V12.53
  cause unknown 798.2

Death — continued
  cot (infant) 798.0
  crib (infant) 798.0
  fetus, fetal (cause not stated) (intrauterine) 779.9
    early, with retention (before 22 completed weeks gestation) 632
    from asphyxia or anoxia (before labor) 768.0
    during labor 768.1
    late, affecting management of pregnancy (after 22 completed weeks gestation) 656.4 ☑
  from pregnancy NEC 646.9 ☑
  instantaneous 798.1
  intrauterine (see also Death, fetus) 779.9
    complicating pregnancy 656.4 ☑
  maternal, affecting fetus or newborn 761.6
  neonatal NEC 779.9
  sudden (cause unknown) 798.1
    cardiac (SCD)
      family history of V17.41
      personal history of, successfully resuscitated V12.53
    during delivery 669.9 ☑
      under anesthesia NEC 668.9 ☑
    infant, syndrome (SIDS) 798.0
    puerperal, during puerperium 674.9 ☑
  unattended (cause unknown) 798.9
  under anesthesia NEC
    due to
      correct substance properly administered 995.4
      overdose or wrong substance given 968.4
      specified anesthetic — see Table of Drugs and Chemicals
    during delivery 668.9 ☑
  violent 798.1
de Beurmann-Gougerot disease (sporotrichosis) 117.1
Debility (general) (infantile) (postinfectional) 799.3
  with nutritional difficulty 269.9
  congenital or neonatal NEC 779.9
  nervous 300.5
  old age 797
  senile 797
Débove's disease (splenomegaly) 789.2
Decalcification
  bone (see also Osteoporosis) 733.00
  teeth 521.89
Decapitation 874.9
  fetal (to facilitate delivery) 763.89
Decapsulation, kidney 593.89
Decay
  dental 521.00
  senile 797
  tooth, teeth 521.00
Decensus, uterus — see Prolapse, uterus
Deciduitis (acute)
  with
    abortion — see Abortion, by type, with sepsis
    ectopic pregnancy (see also categories 633.0–633.9) 639.0
    molar pregnancy (see also categories 630–632) 639.0
  affecting fetus or newborn 760.8
  following
    abortion 639.0
    ectopic or molar pregnancy 639.0
  in pregnancy 646.6 ☑
  puerperal, postpartum 670.1 ☑
Deciduoma malignum (M9100/3) 181
Deciduous tooth (retained) 520.6
Decline (general) — see also Debility 799.3
Decompensation
  cardiac (acute) (chronic) (see also Disease, heart) 429.9
    failure — see Failure, heart
  cardiorenal (see also Hypertension, cardiorenal) 404.90
  cardiovascular (see also Disease, cardiovascular) 429.2
  heart (see also Disease, heart) 429.9

Decompensation — *continued*
  heart (*see also* Disease, heart) — *continued*
    failure — *see* Failure, heart
    hepatic 572.2
    myocardial (acute) (chronic) (*see also* Disease, heart) 429.9
    failure — *see* Failure, heart
    respiratory 519.9
Decompression sickness 993.3
Decrease, decreased
  blood
    platelets (*see also* Thrombocytopenia) 287.5
    pressure 796.3
      due to shock following
        injury 958.4
        operation 998.0
    white cell count 288.50
      specified NEC 288.59
  cardiac reserve — *see* Disease, heart
  estrogen 256.39
    postablative 256.2
  fetal movements 655.7 ☑
  fragility of erythrocytes 289.89
  function
    adrenal (cortex) 255.41
      medulla 255.5
    ovary in hypopituitarism 253.4
    parenchyma of pancreas 577.8
    pituitary (gland) (lobe) (anterior) 253.2
      posterior (lobe) 253.8
  functional activity 780.99
  glucose 790.29
  haptoglobin (serum) NEC 273.8
  leukocytes 288.50
  libido 799.81
  lymphocytes 288.51
  platelets (*see also* Thrombocytopenia) 287.5
  pulse pressure 785.9
  respiration due to shock following injury 958.4
  sexual desire 799.81
  tear secretion NEC 375.15
  tolerance
    fat 579.8
    salt and water 276.9
  vision NEC 369.9
  white blood cell count 288.50
Decubital gangrene — *see also* Ulcer, pressure 707.00 [785.4]
Decubiti — *see also* Ulcer, pressure 707.00
Decubitus (ulcer) — *see also* Ulcer, pressure 707.00
  with gangrene 707.00 [785.4]
  ankle 707.06
  back
    lower 707.03
    upper 707.02
  buttock 707.05
  coccyx 707.03
  elbow 707.01
  head 707.09
  heel 707.07
  hip 707.04
  other site 707.09
  sacrum 707.03
  shoulder blades 707.02
Deepening acetabulum 718.85
Defect, defective 759.9
  3-beta-hydroxysteroid dehydrogenase 255.2
  11-hydroxylase 255.2
  21-hydroxylase 255.2
  abdominal wall, congenital 756.70
  aorticopulmonary septum 745.0
  aortic septal 745.0
  atrial septal (ostium secundum type) 745.5
    acquired 429.71
    ostium primum type 745.61
    sinus venosus 745.8
  atrioventricular
    canal 745.69
    septum 745.4
      acquired 429.71
  atrium secundum 745.5
    acquired 429.71

Defect, defective — *continued*
  auricular septal 745.5
    acquired 429.71
  bilirubin excretion 277.4
  biosynthesis, testicular androgen 257.2
  bridge 525.60
  bulbar septum 745.0
  butanol-insoluble iodide 246.1
  chromosome — *see* Anomaly, chromosome
  circulation (acquired) 459.9
    congenital 747.9
    newborn 747.9
  clotting NEC (*see also* Defect, coagulation) 286.9
  coagulation (factor) (*see also* Deficiency, coagulation factor) 286.9
    with
      abortion — *see* Abortion, by type, with hemorrhage
      ectopic pregnancy (*see also* categories 634–638) 639.1
      molar pregnancy (*see also* categories 630–632) 639.1
    acquired (any) 286.7
    antepartum or intrapartum 641.3 ☑
      affecting fetus or newborn 762.1
    causing hemorrhage of pregnancy or delivery 641.3 ☑
    complicating pregnancy, childbirth, or puerperium 649.3 ☑
    due to
      liver disease 286.7
      vitamin K deficiency 286.7
    newborn, transient 776.3
    postpartum 666.3 ☑
    specified type NEC 286.9
  conduction (heart) 426.9
    bone (*see also* Deafness, conductive) 389.00
  congenital, organ or site NEC (*see also* Anomaly)
    circulation 747.9
    Descemet's membrane 743.9
      specified type NEC 743.49
    diaphragm 756.6
    ectodermal 757.9
    esophagus 750.9
    pulmonic cusps — *see* Anomaly, heart valve
    respiratory system 748.9
      specified type NEC 748.8
  crown 525.60
  cushion endocardial 745.60
  dental restoration 525.60
  dentin (hereditary) 520.5
  Descemet's membrane (congenital) 743.9
    acquired 371.30
    specific type NEC 743.49
  deutan 368.52
  developmental (*see also* Anomaly, by site)
    cauda equina 742.59
    left ventricle 746.9
      with atresia or hypoplasia of aortic orifice or valve, with hypoplasia of ascending aorta 746.7
      in hypoplastic left heart syndrome 746.7
    testis 752.9
    vessel 747.9
  diaphragm
    with elevation, eventration, or hernia — *see* Hernia, diaphragm
    congenital 756.6
      with elevation, eventration, or hernia 756.6
      gross (with elevation, eventration, or hernia) 756.6
  ectodermal, congenital 757.9
  Eisenmenger's (ventricular septal defect) 745.4
  endocardial cushion 745.60
    specified type NEC 745.69
  esophagus, congenital 750.9
  extensor retinaculum 728.9
  fibrin polymerization (*see also* Defect, coagulation) 286.3

Defect, defective — *continued*
  filling
    biliary tract 793.3
    bladder 793.5
    dental 525.60
    gallbladder 793.3
    kidney 793.5
    stomach 793.4
    ureter 793.5
  fossa ovalis 745.5
  gene, carrier (suspected) of V83.89
  Gerbode 745.4
  glaucomatous, without elevated tension 365.89
  Hageman (factor) (*see also* Defect, coagulation) 286.3
  hearing (*see also* Deafness) 389.9
  high grade 317
  homogentisic acid 270.2
  interatrial septal 745.5
    acquired 429.71
  interauricular septal 745.5
    acquired 429.71
  interventricular septal 745.4
    with pulmonary stenosis or atresia, dextraposition of aorta, and hypertrophy of right ventricle 745.2
    acquired 429.71
    in tetralogy of Fallot 745.2
  iodide trapping 246.1
  iodotyrosine dehalogenase 246.1
  kynureninase 270.2
  learning, specific 315.2
  major osseous 731.3
  mental (*see also* Retardation, mental) 319
  osseous, major 731.3
  osteochondral NEC 738.8
  ostium
    primum 745.61
    secundum 745.5
  pericardium 746.89
  peroxidase-binding 246.1
  placental blood supply — *see* Placenta, insufficiency
  platelet (qualitative) 287.1
    constitutional 286.4
  postural, spine 737.9
  protan 368.51
  pulmonic cusps, congenital 746.00
  renal pelvis 753.9
    obstructive 753.29
    specified type NEC 753.3
  respiratory system, congenital 748.9
    specified type NEC 748.8
  retina, retinal 361.30
    with detachment (*see also* Detachment, retina, with retinal defect) 361.00
    multiple 361.33
      with detachment 361.02
    nerve fiber bundle 362.85
    single 361.30
      with detachment 361.01
  septal (closure) (heart) NEC 745.9
    acquired 429.71
    atrial 745.5
    specified type NEC 745.8
  speech NEC 784.59
    developmental 315.39
    late effect of cerebrovascular disease — *see* Late effect(s) (of) cerebrovascular disease, speech and language deficit
    secondary to organic lesion 784.59
  Taussig-Bing (transposition, aorta and overriding pulmonary artery) 745.11
  teeth, wedge 521.20
  thyroid hormone synthesis 246.1
  tritan 368.53
  ureter 753.9
    obstructive 753.29
  vascular (acquired) (local) 459.9
    congenital (peripheral) NEC 747.60
      gastrointestinal 747.61
      lower limb 747.64
      renal 747.62
      specified NEC 747.69

Defect, defective — *continued*
  vascular — *continued*
    congenital — *continued*
      spinal 747.82
      upper limb 747.63
  ventricular septal 745.4
    with pulmonary stenosis or atresia, dextraposition of aorta, and hypertrophy of right ventricle 745.2
    acquired 429.71
    atrioventricular canal type 745.69
    between infundibulum and anterior portion 745.4
    in tetralogy of Fallot 745.2
    isolated anterior 745.4
  vision NEC 369.9
  visual field 368.40
    arcuate 368.43
    heteronymous, bilateral 368.47
    homonymous, bilateral 368.46
    localized NEC 368.44
    nasal step 368.44
    peripheral 368.44
    sector 368.43
  voice and resonance 784.40
  wedge, teeth (abrasion) 521.20
Defeminization syndrome 255.2
Deferentitis 608.4
  gonorrheal (acute) 098.14
    chronic or duration of 2 months or over 098.34
Defibrination syndrome — *see also* Fibrinolysis 286.6
Deficiency, deficient
  3-beta-hydroxysteroid dehydrogenase 255.2
  6-phosphogluconic dehydrogenase (anemia) 282.2
  11-beta-hydroxylase 255.2
  17-alpha-hydroxylase 255.2
  18-hydroxysteroid dehydrogenase 255.2
  20-alpha-hydroxylase 255.2
  21-hydroxylase 255.2
  AAT (alpha-1 antitrypsin) 273.4
  abdominal muscle syndrome 756.79
  accelerator globulin (Ac G) (blood) (*see also* Defect, coagulation) 286.3
  AC globulin (congenital) (*see also* Defect, coagulation) 286.3
    acquired 286.7
  activating factor (blood) (*see also* Defect, coagulation) 286.3
  adenohypophyseal 253.2
  adenosine deaminase 277.2
  aldolase (hereditary) 271.2
  alpha-1-antitrypsin 273.4
  alpha-1-trypsin inhibitor 273.4
  alpha-fucosidase 271.8
  alpha-lipoprotein 272.5
  alpha-mannosidase 271.8
  amino acid 270.9
  anemia — *see* Anemia, deficiency
  aneurin 265.1
    with beriberi 265.0
  antibody NEC 279.00
  antidiuretic hormone 253.5
  antihemophilic
    factor (A) 286.0
      B 286.1
      C 286.2
    globulin (AHG) NEC 286.0
  antithrombin III 289.81
  antitrypsin 273.4
  argininosuccinate synthetase or lyase 270.6
  ascorbic acid (with scurvy) 267
  autoprothrombin
    I (*see also* Defect, coagulation) 286.3
    II 286.1
    C (*see also* Defect, coagulation) 286.3
  bile salt 579.8
  biotin 266.2
  biotinidase 277.6
  bradykinase-1 277.6
  brancher enzyme (amylopectinosis) 271.0
  calciferol 268.9
    with
      osteomalacia 268.2

☑ Additional Digit Required — Refer to the Tabular List for Digit Selection   ▽ Subterms under main terms may continue to next column or page

64 — Volume 2   ▶◀ Revised Text   ● New Line   ▲ Revised Code   2011 ICD-9-CM

Deficiency, deficient — *continued*
  calciferol — *continued*
    with — *continued*
      rickets (*see also* Rickets) 268.0
  calcium 275.40
    dietary 269.3
  calorie, severe 261
  carbamyl phosphate synthetase 270.6
  cardiac (*see also* Insufficiency, myocardial)
    428.0
  carnitine 277.81
    due to
      hemodialysis 277.83
      inborn errors of metabolism 277.82
      valproic acid therapy 277.83
    iatrogenic 277.83
    palmitoyltransferase (CPT1, CPT2) 277.85
    palmityl transferase (CPT1, CPT2) 277.85
    primary 277.81
    secondary 277.84
  carotene 264.9
  Carr factor (*see also* Defect, coagulation)
    286.9
  central nervous system 349.9
  ceruloplasmin 275.1
  cevitamic acid (with scurvy) 267
  choline 266.2
  Christmas factor 286.1
  chromium 269.3
  citrin 269.1
  clotting (blood) (*see also* Defect, coagulation) 286.9
  coagulation factor NEC 286.9
    with
      abortion — *see* Abortion, by type,
        with hemorrhage
      ectopic pregnancy (*see also* categories 634–638) 639.1
      molar pregnancy (*see also* categories 630–632) 639.1
    acquired (any) 286.7
    antepartum or intrapartum 641.3 ☑
      affecting fetus or newborn 762.1
    complicating pregnancy, childbirth, or puerperium 649.3 ☑
    due to
      liver disease 286.7
      vitamin K deficiency 286.7
    newborn, transient 776.3
    postpartum 666.3 ☑
    specified type NEC 286.3
  color vision (congenital) 368.59
    acquired 368.55
  combined glucocorticoid and mineralocorticoid 255.41
  combined, two or more coagulation factors (*see also* Defect, coagulation) 286.9
  complement factor NEC 279.8
  contact factor (*see also* Defect, coagulation) 286.3
  copper NEC 275.1
  corticoadrenal 255.41
  craniofacial axis 756.0
  cyanocobalamin (vitamin B$_{12}$) 266.2
  debrancher enzyme (limit dextrinosis) 271.0
  desmolase 255.2
  diet 269.9
  dihydrofolate reductase 281.2
  dihydropteridine reductase 270.1
  dihydropyrimidine dehydrogenase (DPD) ●
    277.6
  disaccharidase (intestinal) 271.3
  disease NEC 269.9
  ear(s) V48.8
  edema 262
  endocrine 259.9
  enzymes, circulating NEC (*see also* Deficiency, by specific enzyme) 277.6
  ergosterol 268.9
    with
      osteomalacia 268.2
      rickets (*see also* Rickets) 268.0
  erythrocytic glutathione (anemia) 282.2
  eyelid(s) V48.8
  factor (*see also* Defect, coagulation) 286.9
    I (congenital) (fibrinogen) 286.3

Deficiency, deficient — *continued*
  factor (*see also* Defect, coagulation) — *continued*
    I — *continued*
      antepartum or intrapartum 641.3 ☑
        affecting fetus or newborn 762.1
      newborn, transient 776.3
      postpartum 666.3 ☑
    II (congenital) (prothrombin) 286.3
    V (congenital) (labile) 286.3
    VII (congenital) (stable) 286.3
    VIII (congenital) (functional) 286.0
      with
        functional defect 286.0
        vascular defect 286.4
    IX (Christmas) (congenital) (functional)
      286.1
    X (congenital) (Stuart-Prower) 286.3
    XI (congenital) (plasma thromboplastin antecedent) 286.2
    XII (congenital) (Hageman) 286.3
    XIII (congenital) (fibrin stabilizing) 286.3
    Hageman 286.3
    multiple (congenital) 286.9
      acquired 286.7
  fibrinase (*see also* Defect, coagulation) 286.3
  fibrinogen (congenital) (*see also* Defect, coagulation) 286.3
    acquired 286.6
  fibrin-stabilizing factor (congenital) (*see also* Defect, coagulation) 286.3
  finger — *see* Absence, finger
  fletcher factor (*see also* Defect, coagulation) 286.9
  fluorine 269.3
  folate, anemia 281.2
  folic acid (vitamin B$_c$) 266.2
    anemia 281.2
  follicle-stimulating hormone (FSH) 253.4
  fructokinase 271.2
  fructose-1, 6-diphosphate 271.2
  fructose-1-phosphate aldolase 271.2
  FSH (follicle-stimulating hormone) 253.4
  fucosidase 271.8
  galactokinase 271.1
  galactose-1-phosphate uridyl transferase
    271.1
  gamma globulin in blood 279.00
  glass factor (*see also* Defect, coagulation)
    286.3
  glucocorticoid 255.41
  glucose-6-phosphatase 271.0
  glucose-6-phosphate dehydrogenase anemia 282.2
  glucuronyl transferase 277.4
  glutathione-reductase (anemia) 282.2
  glycogen synthetase 271.0
  growth hormone 253.3
  Hageman factor (congenital) (*see also* Defect, coagulation) 286.3
  head V48.0
  hemoglobin (*see also* Anemia) 285.9
  hepatophosphorylase 271.0
  hexose monophosphate (HMP) shunt 282.2
  HGH (human growth hormone) 253.3
  HG-PRT 277.2
  homogentisic acid oxidase 270.2
  hormone (*see also* Deficiency, by specific hormone)
    anterior pituitary (isolated) (partial) NEC
      253.4
      growth (human) 253.3
    follicle-stimulating 253.4
    growth (human) (isolated) 253.3
    human growth 253.3
    interstitial cell-stimulating 253.4
    luteinizing 253.4
    melanocyte-stimulating 253.4
    testicular 257.2
  human growth hormone 253.3
  humoral 279.00
    with
      hyper-IgM 279.05
        autosomal recessive 279.05
        X-linked 279.05
      increased IgM 279.05

Deficiency, deficient — *continued*
  humoral — *continued*
    congenital hypogammaglobulinemia
      279.04
      non-sex-linked 279.06
    selective immunoglobulin NEC 279.03
      IgA 279.01
      IgG 279.03
      IgM 279.02
        increased 279.05
    specified NEC 279.09
  hydroxylase 255.2
  hypoxanthine-guanine phosphoribosyltransferase (HG-PRT) 277.2
  ICSH (interstitial cell-stimulating hormone)
    253.4
  immunity NEC 279.3
    cell-mediated 279.10
      with
        hyperimmunoglobulinemia 279.2
        thrombocytopenia and eczema
          279.12
      specified NEC 279.19
    combined (severe) 279.2
      syndrome 279.2
    common variable 279.06
    humoral NEC 279.00
      IgA (secretory) 279.01
      IgG 279.03
      IgM 279.02
    immunoglobulin, selective NEC 279.03
      IgA 279.01
      IgG 279.03
      IgM 279.02
  inositol (B complex) 266.2
  interferon 279.49
  internal organ V47.0
  interstitial cell-stimulating hormone (ICSH)
    253.4
  intrinsic factor (Castle's) (congenital) 281.0
  intrinsic (urethral) sphincter (ISD) 599.82
  invertase 271.3
  iodine 269.3
  iron, anemia 280.9
  labile factor (congenital) (*see also* Defect, coagulation) 286.3
    acquired 286.7
  lacrimal fluid (acquired) 375.15
    congenital 743.64
  lactase 271.3
  Laki-Lorand factor (*see also* Defect, coagulation) 286.3
  lecithin-cholesterol acyltranferase 272.5
  LH (luteinizing hormone) 253.4
  limb V49.0
    lower V49.0
      congenital (*see also* Deficiency, lower limb, congenital) 755.30
    upper V49.0
      congenital (*see also* Deficiency, upper limb, congenital) 755.20
  lipocaic 577.8
  lipoid (high-density) 272.5
  lipoprotein (familial) (high density) 272.5
  liver phosphorylase 271.0
  long chain 3-hydroxyacyl CoA dehydrogenase (LCHAD) 277.85
  long chain/very long chain acyl CoA dehydrogenase (LCAD, VLCAD) 277.85
  lower limb V49.0
    congenital 755.30
      with complete absence of distal elements 755.31
      longitudinal (complete) (partial) (with distal deficiencies, incomplete) 755.32
        with complete absence of distal elements 755.31
        combined femoral, tibial, fibular (incomplete) 755.33
        femoral 755.34
        fibular 755.37
        metatarsal(s) 755.38
        phalange(s) 755.39
          meaning all digits 755.31
        tarsal(s) 755.38

Deficiency, deficient — *continued*
  lower limb — *continued*
    congenital — *continued*
      longitudinal — *continued*
        tibia 755.36
        tibiofibular 755.35
        transverse 755.31
  luteinizing hormone (LH) 253.4
  lysosomal alpha-1, 4 glucosidase 271.0
  magnesium 275.2
  mannosidase 271.8
  medium chain acyl CoA dehydrogenase (MCAD) 277.85
  melanocyte-stimulating hormone (MSH)
    253.4
  menadione (vitamin K) 269.0
    newborn 776.0
  mental (familial) (hereditary) (*see also* Retardation, mental) 319
  methylenetetrahydrofolate reductase (MTHFR) 270.4
  mineral NEC 269.3
  mineralocorticoid 255.42
  molybdenum 269.3
  moral 301.7
  multiple, syndrome 260
  myocardial (*see also* Insufficiency, myocardial) 428.0
  myophosphorylase 271.0
  NADH-diaphorase or reductase (congenital)
    289.7
  NADH (DPNH)-methemoglobin-reductase (congenital) 289.7
  neck V48.1
  niacin (amide) (-tryptophan) 265.2
  nicotinamide 265.2
  nicotinic acid (amide) 265.2
  nose V48.8
  number of teeth (*see also* Anodontia) 520.0
  nutrition, nutritional 269.9
    specified NEC 269.8
  ornithine transcarbamylase 270.6
  ovarian 256.39
  oxygen (*see also* Anoxia) 799.02
  pantothenic acid 266.2
  parathyroid (gland) 252.1
  phenylalanine hydroxylase 270.1
  phosphoenolpyruvate carboxykinase 271.8
  phosphofructokinase 271.2
  phosphoglucomutase 271.0
  phosphohexosisomerase 271.8
  phosphomannomutase 271.8
  phosphomannose isomerase 271.8
  phosphomannosyl mutase 271.8
  phosphorylase kinase, liver 271.0
  pituitary (anterior) 253.2
    posterior 253.5
  placenta — *see* Placenta, insufficiency
  plasma
    cell 279.00
    protein (paraproteinemia) (pyroglobulinemia) 273.8
      gamma globulin 279.00
    thromboplastin
      antecedent (PTA) 286.2
      component (PTC) 286.1
  platelet NEC 287.1
    constitutional 286.4
  polyglandular 258.9
  potassium (K) 276.8
  proaccelerin (congenital) (*see also* Defect, congenital) 286.3
    acquired 286.7
  proconvertin factor (congenital) (*see also* Defect, coagulation) 286.3
    acquired 286.7
  prolactin 253.4
  protein 260
    anemia 281.4
    C 289.81
    plasma — *see* Deficiency, plasma, protein
    S 289.81
  prothrombin (congenital) (*see also* Defect, coagulation) 286.3
    acquired 286.7

☑ Additional Digit Required — Refer to the Tabular List for Digit Selection   ▿ Subterms under main terms may continue to next column or page

2011 ICD-9-CM   ▶◀ Revised Text   ● New Line   ▲ Revised Code   October 2010 • Volume 2 — 65

Deficiency, deficient — *continued*
  Prower factor (*see also* Defect, coagulation) 286.3
  PRT 277.2
  pseudocholinesterase 289.89
  psychobiological 301.6
  PTA 286.2
  PTC 286.1
  purine nucleoside phosphorylase 277.2
  pyracin (alpha) (beta) 266.1
  pyridoxal 266.1
  pyridoxamine 266.1
  pyridoxine (derivatives) 266.1
  pyruvate carboxylase 271.8
  pyruvate dehydrogenase 271.8
  pyruvate kinase (PK) 282.3
  riboflavin (vitamin B_2) 266.0
  saccadic eye movements 379.57
  salivation 527.7
  salt 276.1
  secretion
    ovary 256.39
    salivary gland (any) 527.7
    urine 788.5
  selenium 269.3
  serum
    antitrypsin, familial 273.4
    protein (congenital) 273.8
  short chain acyl CoA dehydrogenase (SCAD) 277.85
  short stature homeobox gene (SHOX)
    with
      dyschondrosteosis 756.89
      short stature (idiopathic) 783.43
      Turner's syndrome 758.6
  smooth pursuit movements (eye) 379.58
  sodium (Na) 276.1
  SPCA (*see also* Defect, coagulation) 286.3
  specified NEC 269.8
  stable factor (congenital) (*see also* Defect, coagulation) 286.3
    acquired 286.7
  Stuart (-Prower) factor (*see also* Defect, coagulation) 286.3
  sucrase 271.3
  sucrase-isomaltase 271.3
  sulfite oxidase 270.0
  syndrome, multiple 260
  thiamine, thiaminic (chloride) 265.1
  thrombokinase (*see also* Defect, coagulation) 286.3
    newborn 776.0
  thrombopoieten 287.39
  thymolymphatic 279.2
  thyroid (gland) 244.9
  tocopherol 269.1
  toe — *see* Absence, toe
  tooth bud (*see also* Anodontia) 520.0
  trunk V48.1
  UDPG-glycogen transferase 271.0
  upper limb V49.0
    congenital 755.20
      with complete absence of distal elements 755.21
      longitudinal (complete) (partial) (with distal deficiencies, incomplete) 755.22
        carpal(s) 755.28
        combined humeral, radial, ulnar (incomplete) 755.23
        humeral 755.24
        metacarpal(s) 755.28
        phalange(s) 755.29
          meaning all digits 755.21
        radial 755.26
        radioulnar 755.25
        ulnar 755.27
      transverse (complete) (partial) 755.21
  vascular 459.9
  vasopressin 253.5
  viosterol (*see also* Deficiency, calciferol) 268.9
  vitamin (multiple) NEC 269.2
    A 264.9
      with
        Bitôt's spot 264.1

Deficiency, deficient — *continued*
  vitamin — *continued*
    A — *continued*
      with — *continued*
        Bitôt's spot — *continued*
          corneal 264.2
            with corneal ulceration 264.3
        keratomalacia 264.4
        keratosis, follicular 264.8
        night blindness 264.5
        scar of cornea, xerophthalmic 264.6
        specified manifestation NEC 264.8
          ocular 264.7
        xeroderma 264.8
        xerophthalmia 264.7
        xerosis
          conjunctival 264.0
            with Bitôt's spot 264.1
          corneal 264.2
            with corneal ulceration 264.3
    B (complex) NEC 266.9
      with
        beriberi 265.0
        pellagra 265.2
      specified type NEC 266.2
    B_1 NEC 265.1
      beriberi 265.0
    B_2 266.0
    B_6 266.1
    B_{12} 266.2
    B_c (folic acid) 266.2
    C (ascorbic acid) (with scurvy) 267
    D (calciferol) (ergosterol) 268.9
      with
        osteomalacia 268.2
        rickets (*see also* Rickets) 268.0
    E 269.1
    folic acid 266.2
    G 266.0
    H 266.2
    K 269.0
      of newborn 776.0
    nicotinic acid 265.2
    P 269.1
    PP 265.2
    specified NEC 269.1
  zinc 269.3
Deficient — *see also* Deficiency
  blink reflex 374.45
  craniofacial axis 756.0
  number of teeth (*see also* Anodontia) 520.0
  secretion of urine 788.5
Deficit
  attention 799.51 ●
  cognitive communication 799.52 ●
  concentration 799.51 ●
  executive function 799.55 ●
  frontal lobe 799.55 ●
  neurologic NEC 781.99
    due to
      cerebrovascular lesion (*see also* Disease, cerebrovascular, acute) 436
        late effect — *see* Late effect(s) (of) cerebrovascular disease
      transient ischemic attack 435.9
    ischemic
      reversible (RIND) 434.91
        history of (personal) V12.54
      prolonged (PRIND) 434.91
        history of (personal) V12.54
  oxygen 799.02
  psychomotor 799.54 ●
  visuospatial 799.53 ●
Deflection
  radius 736.09
  septum (acquired) (nasal) (nose) 470
  spine — *see* Curvature, spine
  turbinate (nose) 470
Defluvium
  capillorum (*see also* Alopecia) 704.00
  cilium 374.55

Defluvium — *continued*
  unguium 703.8
Deformity 738.9
  abdomen, congenital 759.9
  abdominal wall
    acquired 738.8
    congenital 756.70
    muscle deficiency syndrome 756.79
  acquired (unspecified site) 738.9
    specified site NEC 738.8
  adrenal gland (congenital) 759.1
  alimentary tract, congenital 751.9
    lower 751.5
      specified type NEC 751.8
    upper (any part, except tongue) 750.9
      specified type NEC 750.8
      tongue 750.10
        specified type NEC 750.19
  ankle (joint) (acquired) 736.70
    abduction 718.47
    congenital 755.69
    contraction 718.47
    specified NEC 736.79
  anus (congenital) 751.5
    acquired 569.49
  aorta (congenital) 747.20
    acquired 447.8
    arch 747.21
      acquired 447.8
    coarctation 747.10
  aortic
    arch 747.21
      acquired 447.8
    cusp or valve (congenital) 746.9
      acquired (*see also* Endocarditis, aortic) 424.1
    ring 747.21
  appendix 751.5
  arm (acquired) 736.89
    congenital 755.50
  arteriovenous (congenital) (peripheral) NEC 747.60
    gastrointestinal 747.61
    lower limb 747.64
    renal 747.62
    specified NEC 747.69
    spinal 747.82
    upper limb 747.63
  artery (congenital) (peripheral) NEC (*see also* Deformity, vascular) 747.60
    acquired 447.8
    cerebral 747.81
    coronary (congenital) 746.85
      acquired (*see also* Ischemia, heart) 414.9
    retinal 743.9
    umbilical 747.5
  atrial septal (congenital) (heart) 745.5
  auditory canal (congenital) (external) (*see also* Deformity, ear) 744.3
    acquired 380.50
  auricle
    ear (congenital) (*see also* Deformity, ear) 744.3
      acquired 380.32
    heart (congenital) 746.9
  back (acquired) — *see* Deformity, spine
  Bartholin's duct (congenital) 750.9
  bile duct (congenital) 751.60
    acquired 576.8
      with calculus, choledocholithiasis, or stones — *see* Choledocholithiasis
  biliary duct or passage (congenital) 751.60
    acquired 576.8
      with calculus, choledocholithiasis, or stones — *see* Choledocholithiasis
  bladder (neck) (sphincter) (trigone) (acquired) 596.8
    congenital 753.9
  bone (acquired) NEC 738.9
    congenital 756.9
    turbinate 738.0
  boutonniere (finger) 736.21
  brain (congenital) 742.9

Deformity — *continued*
  brain — *continued*
    acquired 348.89
    multiple 742.4
    reduction 742.2
    vessel (congenital) 747.81
  breast (acquired) 611.89
    congenital 757.6
    reconstructed 612.0
  bronchus (congenital) 748.3
    acquired 519.19
  bursa, congenital 756.9
  canal of Nuck 752.9
  canthus (congenital) 743.9
    acquired 374.89
  capillary (acquired) 448.9
    congenital NEC (*see also* Deformity, vascular) 747.60
  cardiac — *see* Deformity, heart
  cardiovascular system (congenital) 746.9
  caruncle, lacrimal (congenital) 743.9
    acquired 375.69
  cascade, stomach 537.6
  cecum (congenital) 751.5
    acquired 569.89
  cerebral (congenital) 742.9
    acquired 348.89
  cervix (acquired) (uterus) 622.8
    congenital 752.40
  cheek (acquired) 738.19
    congenital 744.9
  chest (wall) (acquired) 738.3
    congenital 754.89
    late effect of rickets 268.1
  chin (acquired) 738.19
    congenital 744.9
  choroid (congenital) 743.9
    acquired 363.8
    plexus (congenital) 742.9
      acquired 349.2
  cicatricial — *see* Cicatrix
  cilia (congenital) 743.9
    acquired 374.89
  circulatory system (congenital) 747.9
  clavicle (acquired) 738.8
    congenital 755.51
  clitoris (congenital) 752.40
    acquired 624.8
  clubfoot — *see* Clubfoot
  coccyx (acquired) 738.6
    congenital 756.10
  colon (congenital) 751.5
    acquired 569.89
  concha (ear) (congenital) (*see also* Deformity, ear) 744.3
    acquired 380.32
  congenital, organ or site not listed (*see also* Anomaly) 759.9
  cornea (congenital) 743.9
    acquired 371.70
  coronary artery (congenital) 746.85
    acquired (*see also* Ischemia, heart) 414.9
  cranium (acquired) 738.19
    congenital (*see also* Deformity, skull, congenital) 756.0
  cricoid cartilage (congenital) 748.3
    acquired 478.79
  cystic duct (congenital) 751.60
    acquired 575.8
  Dandy-Walker 742.3
    with spina bifida (*see also* Spina bifida) 741.0 ☑
  diaphragm (congenital) 756.6
    acquired 738.8
  digestive organ(s) or system (congenital) NEC 751.9
    specified type NEC 751.8
  ductus arteriosus 747.0
  duodenal bulb 537.89
  duodenum (congenital) 751.5
    acquired 537.89
  dura (congenital) 742.9
    brain 742.4
      acquired 349.2
    spinal 742.59
      acquired 349.2

☑ **Additional Digit Required** — Refer to the Tabular List for Digit Selection   ▽ **Subterms under main terms may continue to next column or page**

Deformity — *continued*
ear (congenital) 744.3
  acquired 380.32
  auricle 744.3
    causing impairment of hearing 744.02
  causing impairment of hearing 744.00
  external 744.3
    causing impairment of hearing 744.02
  internal 744.05
  lobule 744.3
  middle 744.03
    ossicles 744.04
  ossicles 744.04
ectodermal (congenital) NEC 757.9
  specified type NEC 757.8
ejaculatory duct (congenital) 752.9
  acquired 608.89
elbow (joint) (acquired) 736.00
  congenital 755.50
  contraction 718.42
endocrine gland NEC 759.2
epididymis (congenital) 752.9
  acquired 608.89
  torsion 608.24
epiglottis (congenital) 748.3
  acquired 478.79
esophagus (congenital) 750.9
  acquired 530.89
Eustachian tube (congenital) NEC 744.3
  specified type NEC 744.24
extremity (acquired) 736.9
  congenital, except reduction deformity 755.9
    lower 755.60
    upper 755.50
  reduction — *see* Deformity, reduction
eye (congenital) 743.9
  acquired 379.8
  muscle 743.9
eyebrow (congenital) 744.89
eyelid (congenital) 743.9
  acquired 374.89
  specified type NEC 743.62
face (acquired) 738.19
  congenital (any part) 744.9
    due to intrauterine malposition and pressure 754.0
fallopian tube (congenital) 752.10
  acquired 620.8
femur (acquired) 736.89
  congenital 755.60
fetal
  with fetopelvic disproportion 653.7 ☑
    affecting fetus or newborn 763.1
  causing obstructed labor 660.1 ☑
    affecting fetus or newborn 763.1
  known or suspected, affecting management of pregnancy 655.9 ☑
finger (acquired) 736.20
  boutonniere type 736.21
  congenital 755.50
  flexion contracture 718.44
  swan neck 736.22
flexion (joint) (acquired) 736.9
  congenital NEC 755.9
  hip or thigh (acquired) 736.39
    congenital (*see also* Subluxation, congenital, hip) 754.32
foot (acquired) 736.70
  cavovarus 736.75
    congenital 754.59
  congenital NEC 754.70
    specified type NEC 754.79
  valgus (acquired) 736.79
    congenital 754.60
      specified type NEC 754.69
  varus (acquired) 736.79
    congenital 754.50
      specified type NEC 754.59
forearm (acquired) 736.00
  congenital 755.50
forehead (acquired) 738.19
  congenital (*see also* Deformity, skull, congenital) 756.0

Deformity — *continued*
frontal bone (acquired) 738.19
  congenital (*see also* Deformity, skull, congenital) 756.0
gallbladder (congenital) 751.60
  acquired 575.8
gastrointestinal tract (congenital) NEC 751.9
  acquired 569.89
  specified type NEC 751.8
genitalia, genital organ(s) or system NEC
  congenital 752.9
  female (congenital) 752.9
    acquired 629.89
    external 752.40
    internal 752.9
  male (congenital) 752.9
    acquired 608.89
globe (eye) (congenital) 743.9
  acquired 360.89
gum (congenital) 750.9
  acquired 523.9
gunstock 736.02
hand (acquired) 736.00
  claw 736.06
  congenital 755.50
  minus (and plus) (intrinsic) 736.09
  pill roller (intrinsic) 736.09
  plus (and minus) (intrinsic) 736.09
  swan neck (intrinsic) 736.09
head (acquired) 738.10
  congenital (*see also* Deformity, skull congenital) 756.0
  specified NEC 738.19
heart (congenital) 746.9
  auricle (congenital) 746.9
  septum 745.9
    auricular 745.5
    specified type NEC 745.8
    ventricular 745.4
  valve (congenital) NEC 746.9
    acquired — *see* Endocarditis
    pulmonary (congenital) 746.00
    specified type NEC 746.89
  ventricle (congenital) 746.9
heel (acquired) 736.76
  congenital 755.67
hepatic duct (congenital) 751.60
  acquired 576.8
    with calculus, choledocholithiasis, or stones — *see* Choledocholithiasis
hip (joint) (acquired) 736.30
  congenital NEC 755.63
  flexion 718.45
    congenital (*see also* Subluxation, congenital, hip) 754.32
hourglass — *see* Contraction, hourglass
humerus (acquired) 736.89
  congenital 755.50
hymen (congenital) 752.40
hypophyseal (congenital) 759.2
ileocecal (coil) (valve) (congenital) 751.5
  acquired 569.89
ileum (intestine) (congenital) 751.5
  acquired 569.89
ilium (acquired) 738.6
  congenital 755.60
integument (congenital) 757.9
intervertebral cartilage or disc (acquired) (*see also* Displacement, intervertebral disc)
  congenital 756.10
intestine (large) (small) (congenital) 751.5
  acquired 569.89
iris (acquired) 364.75
  congenital 743.9
  prolapse 364.89
ischium (acquired) 738.6
  congenital 755.60
jaw (acquired) (congenital) NEC 524.9
  due to intrauterine malposition and pressure 754.0
joint (acquired) NEC 738.8
  congenital 755.9

Deformity — *continued*
joint — *continued*
  contraction (abduction) (adduction) (extension) (flexion) — *see* Contraction, joint
kidney(s) (calyx) (pelvis) (congenital) 753.9
  acquired 593.89
  vessel 747.62
    acquired 459.9
Klippel-Feil (brevicollis) 756.16
knee (acquired) NEC 736.6
  congenital 755.64
labium (majus) (minus) (congenital) 752.40
  acquired 624.8
lacrimal apparatus or duct (congenital) 743.9
  acquired 375.69
larynx (muscle) (congenital) 748.3
  acquired 478.79
  web (glottic) (subglottic) 748.2
leg (lower) (upper) (acquired) NEC 736.89
  congenital 755.60
  reduction — *see* Deformity, reduction, lower limb
lens (congenital) 743.9
  acquired 379.39
lid (fold) (congenital) 743.9
  acquired 374.89
ligament (acquired) 728.9
  congenital 756.9
limb (acquired) 736.9
  congenital, except reduction deformity 755.9
  lower 755.60
    reduction (*see also* Deformity, reduction, lower limb) 755.30
  upper 755.50
    reduction (*see also* Deformity, reduction, upper limb) 755.20
  specified NEC 736.89
lip (congenital) NEC 750.9
  acquired 528.5
  specified type NEC 750.26
liver (congenital) 751.60
  acquired 573.8
  duct (congenital) 751.60
    acquired 576.8
      with calculus, choledocholithiasis, or stones — *see* Choledocholithi-asis
lower extremity — *see* Deformity, leg
lumbosacral (joint) (region) (congenital) 756.10
  acquired 738.5
lung (congenital) 748.60
  acquired 518.89
  specified type NEC 748.69
lymphatic system, congenital 759.9
Madelung's (radius) 755.54
maxilla (acquired) (congenital) 524.9
meninges or membrane (congenital) 742.9
  brain 742.4
    acquired 349.2
  spinal (cord) 742.59
    acquired 349.2
mesentery (congenital) 751.9
  acquired 568.89
metacarpus (acquired) 736.00
  congenital 755.50
metatarsus (acquired) 736.70
  congenital 754.70
middle ear, except ossicles (congenital) 744.03
  ossicles 744.04
mitral (leaflets) (valve) (congenital) 746.9
  acquired — *see* Endocarditis, mitral
  Ebstein's 746.89
  parachute 746.5
  specified type NEC 746.89
  stenosis, congenital 746.5
mouth (acquired) 528.9
  congenital NEC 750.9
    specified type NEC 750.26
multiple, congenital NEC 759.7

Deformity — *continued*
multiple, congenital — *continued*
  specified type NEC 759.89
muscle (acquired) 728.9
  congenital 756.9
    specified type NEC 756.89
  sternocleidomastoid (due to intrauterine malposition and pressure) 754.1
musculoskeletal system, congenital NEC 756.9
  specified type NEC 756.9
nail (acquired) 703.9
  congenital 757.9
nasal — *see* Deformity, nose
neck (acquired) NEC 738.2
  congenital (any part) 744.9
  sternocleidomastoid 754.1
nervous system (congenital) 742.9
nipple (congenital) 757.6
  acquired 611.89
nose, nasal (cartilage) (acquired) 738.0
  bone (turbinate) 738.0
  congenital 748.1
    bent 754.0
    squashed 754.0
  saddle 738.0
    syphilitic 090.5
  septum 470
    congenital 748.1
  sinus (wall) (congenital) 748.1
    acquired 738.0
  syphilitic (congenital) 090.5
    late 095.8
ocular muscle (congenital) 743.9
  acquired 378.60
opticociliary vessels (congenital) 743.9
orbit (congenital) (eye) 743.9
  acquired NEC 376.40
    associated with craniofacial deformities 376.44
    due to
      bone disease 376.43
      surgery 376.47
      trauma 376.47
organ of Corti (congenital) 744.05
ovary (congenital) 752.0
  acquired 620.8
oviduct (congenital) 752.10
  acquired 620.8
palate (congenital) 750.9
  acquired 526.89
  cleft (congenital) (*see also* Cleft, palate) 749.00
  hard, acquired 526.89
  soft, acquired 528.9
pancreas (congenital) 751.7
  acquired 577.8
parachute, mitral valve 746.5
parathyroid (gland) 759.2
parotid (gland) (congenital) 750.9
  acquired 527.8
patella (acquired) 736.6
  congenital 755.64
pelvis, pelvic (acquired) (bony) 738.6
  with disproportion (fetopelvic) 653.0 ☑
    affecting fetus or newborn 763.1
    causing obstructed labor 660.1 ☑
      affecting fetus or newborn 763.1
  congenital 755.60
  rachitic (late effect) 268.1
penis (glans) (congenital) 752.9
  acquired 607.89
pericardium (congenital) 746.9
  acquired — *see* Pericarditis
pharynx (congenital) 750.9
  acquired 478.29
Pierre Robin (congenital) 756.0
pinna (acquired) 380.32
  congenital 744.3
pituitary (congenital) 759.2
pleural folds (congenital) 748.8
portal vein (congenital) 747.40
posture — *see* Curvature, spine
prepuce (congenital) 752.9
  acquired 607.89

☑ **Additional Digit Required — Refer to the Tabular List for Digit Selection**   ▽ **Subterms under main terms may continue to next column or page**

2011 ICD-9-CM   ▶◀ Revised Text   ● New Line   ▲ Revised Code   **Volume 2 — 67**

Index

Deformity — Degeneration, degenerative

Deformity — *continued*
prostate (congenital) 752.9
  acquired 602.8
pulmonary valve — *see* Endocarditis, pulmonary
pupil (congenital) 743.9
  acquired 364.75
pylorus (congenital) 750.9
  acquired 537.89
rachitic (acquired), healed or old 268.1
radius (acquired) 736.00
  congenital 755.50
    reduction — *see* Deformity, reduction, upper limb
rectovaginal septum (congenital) 752.40
  acquired 623.8
rectum (congenital) 751.5
  acquired 569.49
reduction (extremity) (limb) 755.4
  brain 742.2
  lower limb 755.30
    with complete absence of distal elements 755.31
    longitudinal (complete) (partial) (with distal deficiencies, incomplete) 755.32
      with complete absence of distal elements 755.31
      combined femoral, tibial, fibular (incomplete) 755.33
      femoral 755.34
      fibular 755.37
      metatarsal(s) 755.38
      phalange(s) 755.39
        meaning all digits 755.31
      tarsal(s) 755.38
      tibia 755.36
      tibiofibular 755.35
    transverse 755.31
  upper limb 755.20
    with complete absence of distal elements 755.21
    longitudinal (complete) (partial) (with distal deficiencies, incomplete) 755.22
      with complete absence of distal elements 755.21
      carpal(s) 755.28
      combined humeral, radial, ulnar (incomplete) 755.23
      humeral 755.24
      metacarpal(s) 755.28
      phalange(s) 755.29
        meaning all digits 755.21
      radial 755.26
      radioulnar 755.25
      ulnar 755.27
    transverse (complete) (partial) 755.21
renal — *see* Deformity, kidney
respiratory system (congenital) 748.9
  specified type NEC 748.8
rib (acquired) 738.3
  congenital 756.3
    cervical 756.2
rotation (joint) (acquired) 736.9
  congenital 755.9
  hip or thigh 736.39
    congenital (*see also* Subluxation, congenital, hip) 754.32
sacroiliac joint (congenital) 755.69
  acquired 738.5
sacrum (acquired) 738.5
  congenital 756.10
saddle
  back 737.8
  nose 738.0
    syphilitic 090.5
salivary gland or duct (congenital) 750.9
  acquired 527.8
scapula (acquired) 736.89
  congenital 755.50
scrotum (congenital) 752.9
  acquired 608.89
sebaceous gland, acquired 706.8
seminal tract or duct (congenital) 752.9
  acquired 608.89

Deformity — *continued*
septum (nasal) (acquired) 470
  congenital 748.1
shoulder (joint) (acquired) 736.89
  congenital 755.50
    specified type NEC 755.59
  contraction 718.41
sigmoid (flexure) (congenital) 751.5
  acquired 569.89
sinus of Valsalva 747.29
skin (congenital) 757.9
  acquired NEC 709.8
skull (acquired) 738.19
  congenital 756.0
    with
      anencephalus 740.0
      encephalocele 742.0
      hydrocephalus 742.3
        with spina bifida (*see also* Spina bifida) 741.0 ☑
      microcephalus 742.1
    due to intrauterine malposition and pressure 754.0
soft parts, organs or tissues (of pelvis)
  in pregnancy or childbirth NEC 654.9 ☑
    affecting fetus or newborn 763.89
    causing obstructed labor 660.2 ☑
      affecting fetus or newborn 763.1
spermatic cord (congenital) 752.9
  acquired 608.89
    torsion 608.22
      extravaginal 608.21
      intravaginal 608.22
spinal
  column — *see* Deformity, spine
  cord (congenital) 742.9
    acquired 336.8
    vessel (congenital) 747.82
  nerve root (congenital) 742.9
    acquired 724.9
spine (acquired) NEC 738.5
  congenital 756.10
    due to intrauterine malposition and pressure 754.2
  kyphoscoliotic (*see also* Kyphoscoliosis) 737.30
  kyphotic (*see also* Kyphosis) 737.10
  lordotic (*see also* Lordosis) 737.20
  rachitic 268.1
  scoliotic (*see also* Scoliosis) 737.30
spleen
  acquired 289.59
  congenital 759.0
Sprengel's (congenital) 755.52
sternum (acquired) 738.3
  congenital 756.3
stomach (congenital) 750.9
  acquired 537.89
submaxillary gland (congenital) 750.9
  acquired 527.8
swan neck (acquired)
  finger 736.22
  hand 736.09
talipes — *see* Talipes
teeth, tooth NEC 520.9
testis (congenital) 752.9
  acquired 608.89
    torsion 608.20
thigh (acquired) 736.89
  congenital 755.60
thorax (acquired) (wall) 738.3
  congenital 754.89
  late effect of rickets 268.1
thumb (acquired) 736.20
  congenital 755.50
thymus (tissue) (congenital) 759.2
thyroid (gland) (congenital) 759.2
  cartilage 748.3
    acquired 478.79
tibia (acquired) 736.89
  congenital 755.60
  saber 090.5
toe (acquired) 735.9
  congenital 755.66
  specified NEC 735.8
tongue (congenital) 750.10

Deformity — *continued*
tongue — *continued*
  acquired 529.8
tooth, teeth NEC 520.9
trachea (rings) (congenital) 748.3
  acquired 519.19
transverse aortic arch (congenital) 747.21
tricuspid (leaflets) (valve) (congenital) 746.9
  acquired — *see* Endocarditis, tricuspid
  atresia or stenosis 746.1
  specified type NEC 746.89
trunk (acquired) 738.3
  congenital 759.9
ulna (acquired) 736.00
  congenital 755.50
upper extremity — *see* Deformity, arm
urachus (congenital) 753.7
ureter (opening) (congenital) 753.9
  acquired 593.89
urethra (valve) (congenital) 753.9
  acquired 599.84
urinary tract or system (congenital) 753.9
  urachus 753.7
uterus (congenital) 752.39 ▲
  acquired 621.8
uvula (congenital) 750.9
  acquired 528.9
vagina (congenital) 752.40
  acquired 623.8
valve, valvular (heart) (congenital) 746.9
  acquired — *see* Endocarditis
  pulmonary 746.00
  specified type NEC 746.89
vascular (congenital) (peripheral) NEC 747.60
  acquired 459.9
  gastrointestinal 747.61
  lower limb 747.64
  renal 747.62
  specified site NEC 747.69
  spinal 747.82
  upper limb 747.63
vas deferens (congenital) 752.9
  acquired 608.89
vein (congenital) NEC (*see also* Deformity, vascular) 747.60
  brain 747.81
  coronary 746.9
  great 747.40
vena cava (inferior) (superior) (congenital) 747.40
vertebra — *see* Deformity, spine
vesicourethral orifice (acquired) 596.8
  congenital NEC 753.9
    specified type NEC 753.8
vessels of optic papilla (congenital) 743.9
visual field (contraction) 368.45
vitreous humor (congenital) 743.9
  acquired 379.29
vulva (congenital) 752.40
  acquired 624.8
wrist (joint) (acquired) 736.00
  congenital 755.50
  contraction 718.43
  valgus 736.03
    congenital 755.59
  varus 736.04
    congenital 755.59

Degeneration, degenerative
adrenal (capsule) (gland) 255.8
  with hypofunction 255.41
  fatty 255.8
  hyaline 255.8
  infectional 255.8
  lardaceous 277.39
amyloid (any site) (general) 277.39
anterior cornua, spinal cord 336.8
anterior labral 840.8
aorta, aortic 440.0
  fatty 447.8
  valve (heart) (*see also* Endocarditis, aortic) 424.1
arteriovascular — *see* Arteriosclerosis
artery, arterial (atheromatous) (calcareous) (*see also* Arteriosclerosis)
  amyloid 277.39

Degeneration, degenerative — *continued*
artery, arterial (*see also* Arteriosclerosis) — *continued*
  lardaceous 277.39
  medial NEC (*see also* Arteriosclerosis, extremities) 440.20
articular cartilage NEC (*see also* Disorder, cartilage, articular) 718.0 ☑
  elbow 718.02
  knee 717.5
  patella 717.7
  shoulder 718.01
  spine (*see also* Spondylosis) 721.90
atheromatous — *see* Arteriosclerosis
bacony (any site) 277.39
basal nuclei or ganglia NEC 333.0
bone 733.90
brachial plexus 353.0
brain (cortical) (progressive) 331.9
  arteriosclerotic 437.0
  childhood 330.9
    specified type NEC 330.8
  congenital 742.4
  cystic 348.0
    congenital 742.4
  familial NEC 331.89
  grey matter 330.8
  heredofamilial NEC 331.89
  in
    alcoholism 303.9 ☑ [331.7]
    beriberi 265.0 [331.7]
    cerebrovascular disease 437.9 [331.7]
    congenital hydrocephalus 742.3 [331.7]
      with spina bifida (*see also* Spina bifida) 741.0 ☑ [331.7]
    Fabry's disease 272.7 [330.2]
    Gaucher's disease 272.7 [330.2]
    Hunter's disease or syndrome 277.5 [330.3]
    lipidosis
      cerebral 330.1
      generalized 272.7 [330.2]
    mucopolysaccharidosis 277.5 [330.3]
    myxedema (*see also* Myxedema) 244.9 [331.7]
    neoplastic disease NEC (M8000/1) 239.9 [331.7]
    Niemann-Pick disease 272.7 [330.2]
    sphingolipidosis 272.7 [330.2]
    vitamin B_{12} deficiency 266.2 [331.7]
  motor centers 331.89
  senile 331.2
  specified type NEC 331.89
breast — *see* Disease, breast
Bruch's membrane 363.40
bundle of His 426.50
  left 426.3
  right 426.4
calcareous NEC 275.49
capillaries 448.9
  amyloid 277.39
  fatty 448.9
  lardaceous 277.39
cardiac (brown) (calcareous) (fatty) (fibrous) (hyaline) (mural) (muscular) (pigmentary) (senile) (with arteriosclerosis) (*see also* Degeneration, myocardial) 429.1
  valve, valvular — *see* Endocarditis
cardiorenal (*see also* Hypertension, cardiorenal) 404.90
cardiovascular (*see also* Disease, cardiovascular) 429.2
  renal (*see also* Hypertension, cardiorenal) 404.90
cartilage (joint) — *see* Derangement, joint
cerebellar NEC 334.9
  primary (hereditary) (sporadic) 334.2
cerebral — *see* Degeneration, brain
cerebromacular 330.1
cerebrovascular 437.1
  due to hypertension 437.2
  late effect — *see* Late effect(s) (of) cerebrovascular disease
cervical plexus 353.2

☑ **Additional Digit Required — Refer to the Tabular List for Digit Selection**   ▽ **Subterms under main terms may continue to next column or page**

68 — Volume 2 · October 2010   ▶◀ **Revised Text**   ● **New Line**   ▲ **Revised Code**   **2011 ICD-9-CM**

Degeneration, degenerative — *continued*
cervix 622.8
   due to radiation (intended effect) 622.8
      adverse effect or misadventure 622.8
changes, spine or vertebra (*see also*
    Spondylosis) 721.90
chitinous 277.39
chorioretinal 363.40
   congenital 743.53
   hereditary 363.50
choroid (colloid) (drusen) 363.40
   hereditary 363.50
   senile 363.41
   diffuse secondary 363.42
cochlear 386.8
collateral ligament (knee) (medial) 717.82
   lateral 717.81
combined (spinal cord) (subacute)
   266.2 *[336.2]*
   with anemia (pernicious) 281.0 *[336.2]*
      due to dietary deficiency
         281.1 *[336.2]*
      due to vitamin B$_{12}$ deficiency anemia
         (dietary) 281.1 *[336.2]*
conjunctiva 372.50
   amyloid 277.39 *[372.50]*
cornea 371.40
   calcerous 371.44
   familial (hereditary) (*see also* Dystrophy,
      cornea) 371.50
      macular 371.55
      reticular 371.54
   hyaline (of old scars) 371.41
   marginal (Terrien's) 371.48
   mosaic (shagreen) 371.41
   nodular 371.46
   peripheral 371.48
   senile 371.41
cortical (cerebellar) (parenchymatous) 334.2
   alcoholic 303.9 ☑ *[334.4]*
   diffuse, due to arteriopathy 437.0
corticostriatal-spinal 334.8
cretinoid 243
cruciate ligament (knee) (posterior) 717.84
   anterior 717.83
cutis 709.3
   amyloid 277.39
dental pulp 522.2
disc disease — *see* Degeneration, interver-
    tebral disc
dorsolateral (spinal cord) — *see* Degenera-
    tion, combined
endocardial 424.90
extrapyramidal NEC 333.90
eye NEC 360.40
   macular (*see also* Degeneration, macula)
      362.50
      congenital 362.75
      hereditary 362.76
fatty (diffuse) (general) 272.8
   liver 571.8
      alcoholic 571.0
   localized site — *see* Degeneration, by
      site, fatty
   placenta — *see* Placenta, abnormal
globe (eye) NEC 360.40
   macular — *see* Degeneration, macula
grey matter 330.8
heart (brown) (calcareous) (fatty) (fibrous)
   (hyaline) (mural) (muscular) (pigmentary) (senile) (with arteriosclerosis)
   (*see also* Degeneration, myocardial)
   429.1
   amyloid 277.39 *[425.7]*
   atheromatous — *see* Arteriosclerosis,
      coronary
   gouty 274.82
   hypertensive (*see also* Hypertension,
      heart) 402.90
   ischemic 414.9
   valve, valvular — *see* Endocarditis
hepatolenticular (Wilson's) 275.1
hepatorenal 572.4
heredofamilial
   brain NEC 331.89
   spinal cord NEC 336.8

Degeneration, degenerative — *continued*
hyaline (diffuse) (generalized) 728.9
   localized (*see also* Degeneration, by site)
      cornea 371.41
      keratitis 371.41
hypertensive vascular — *see* Hypertension
infrapatellar fat pad 729.31
internal semilunar cartilage 717.3
intervertebral disc 722.6
   with myelopathy 722.70
   cervical, cervicothoracic 722.4
      with myelopathy 722.71
   lumbar, lumbosacral 722.52
      with myelopathy 722.73
   thoracic, thoracolumbar 722.51
      with myelopathy 722.72
intestine 569.89
   amyloid 277.39
   lardaceous 277.39
iris (generalized) (*see also* Atrophy, iris)
   364.59
   pigmentary 364.53
   pupillary margin 364.54
ischemic — *see* Ischemia
joint disease (*see also* Osteoarthrosis)
   715.9 ☑
   multiple sites 715.09
   spine (*see also* Spondylosis) 721.90
kidney (*see also* Sclerosis, renal) 587
   amyloid 277.39 *[583.81]*
   cyst, cystic (multiple) (solitary) 593.2
      congenital (*see also* Cystic, disease,
         kidney) 753.10
   fatty 593.89
   fibrocystic (congenital) 753.19
   lardaceous 277.39 *[583.81]*
   polycystic (congenital) 753.12
      adult type (APKD) 753.13
      autosomal dominant 753.13
      autosomal recessive 753.14
      childhood type (CPKD) 753.14
      infantile type 753.14
   waxy 277.39 *[583.81]*
Kuhnt-Junius (retina) 362.52
labyrinth, osseous 386.8
lacrimal passages, cystic 375.12
lardaceous (any site) 277.39
lateral column (posterior), spinal cord (*see
    also* Degeneration, combined)
   266.2 *[336.2]*
lattice 362.63
lens 366.9
   infantile, juvenile, or presenile 366.00
   senile 366.10
lenticular (familial) (progressive) (Wilson's)
   (with cirrhosis of liver) 275.1
   striate artery 437.0
lethal ball, prosthetic heart valve 996.02
ligament
   collateral (knee) (medial) 717.82
      lateral 717.81
   cruciate (knee) (posterior) 717.84
      anterior 717.83
liver (diffuse) 572.8
   amyloid 277.39
   congenital (cystic) 751.62
   cystic 572.8
      congenital 751.62
   fatty 571.8
      alcoholic 571.0
   hypertrophic 572.8
   lardaceous 277.39
   parenchymatous, acute or subacute (*see
      also* Necrosis, liver) 570
   pigmentary 572.8
   toxic (acute) 573.8
   waxy 277.39
lung 518.89
lymph gland 289.3
   hyaline 289.3
   lardaceous 277.39
macula (acquired) (senile) 362.50
   atrophic 362.51
   Best's 362.76
   congenital 362.75
   cystic 362.54

Degeneration, degenerative — *continued*
macula — *continued*
   cystoid 362.53
   disciform 362.52
   dry 362.51
   exudative 362.52
   familial pseudoinflammatory 362.77
   hereditary 362.76
   hole 362.54
   juvenile (Stargardt's) 362.75
   nonexudative 362.51
   pseudohole 362.54
   wet 362.52
medullary — *see* Degeneration, brain
membranous labyrinth, congenital (causing
    impairment of hearing) 744.05
meniscus — *see* Derangement, joint
microcystoid 362.62
mitral — *see* Insufficiency, mitral
Mönckeberg's (*see also* Arteriosclerosis, ex-
    tremities) 440.20
moral 301.7
motor centers, senile 331.2
mural (*see also* Degeneration, myocardial)
   429.1
   heart, cardiac (*see also* Degeneration,
      myocardial) 429.1
   myocardium, myocardial (*see also* Degen-
      eration, myocardial) 429.1
muscle 728.9
   fatty 728.9
   fibrous 728.9
   heart (*see also* Degeneration, myocar-
      dial) 429.1
   hyaline 728.9
muscular progressive 728.2
myelin, central nervous system NEC 341.9
myocardium, myocardial (brown) (calcareous) (fatty) (fibrous) (hyaline) (mural)
   (muscular) (pigmentary) (senile)
   (with arteriosclerosis) 429.1
   with rheumatic fever (conditions classifi-
      able to 390) 398.0
      active, acute, or subacute 391.2
         with chorea 392.0
      inactive or quiescent (with chorea)
         398.0
   amyloid 277.39 *[425.7]*
   congenital 746.89
   fetus or newborn 779.89
   gouty 274.82
   hypertensive (*see also* Hypertension,
      heart) 402.90
   ischemic 414.8
   rheumatic (*see also* Degeneration, my-
      ocardium, with rheumatic fever)
      398.0
   syphilitic 093.82
nasal sinus (mucosa) (*see also* Sinusitis)
   473.9
   frontal 473.1
   maxillary 473.0
nerve — *see* Disorder, nerve
nervous system 349.89
   amyloid 277.39 *[357.4]*
   autonomic (*see also* Neuropathy, periph-
      eral, autonomic) 337.9
   fatty 349.89
   peripheral autonomic NEC (*see also*
      Neuropathy, peripheral, autonom-
      ic) 337.9
nipple 611.9
nose 478.19
oculoacousticocerebral, congenital (progres-
    sive) 743.8
olivopontocerebellar (familial) (hereditary)
    333.0
osseous labyrinth 386.8
ovary 620.8
   cystic 620.2
   microcystic 620.2
pallidal, pigmentary (progressive) 333.0
pancreas 577.8
   tuberculous (*see also* Tuberculosis)
      017.9 ☑
papillary muscle 429.81

Degeneration, degenerative — *continued*
paving stone 362.61
penis 607.89
peritoneum 568.89
pigmentary (diffuse) (general)
   localized — *see* Degeneration, by site
   pallidal (progressive) 333.0
   secondary 362.65
pineal gland 259.8
pituitary (gland) 253.8
placenta (fatty) (fibrinoid) (fibroid) — *see*
    Placenta, abnormal
popliteal fat pad 729.31
posterolateral (spinal cord) (*see also* Degen-
    eration, combined) 266.2 *[336.2]*
pulmonary valve (heart) (*see also* Endocardi-
    tis, pulmonary) 424.3
pulp (tooth) 522.2
pupillary margin 364.54
renal (*see also* Sclerosis, renal) 587
   fibrocystic 753.19
   polycystic 753.12
      adult type (APKD) 753.13
      autosomal dominant 753.13
      autosomal recessive 753.14
      childhood type (CPKD) 753.14
      infantile type 753.14
reticuloendothelial system 289.89
retina (peripheral) 362.60
   with retinal defect (*see also* Detachment,
      retina, with retinal defect) 361.00
   cystic (senile) 362.50
   cystoid 362.53
   hereditary (*see also* Dystrophy, retina)
      362.70
      cerebroretinal 362.71
      congenital 362.75
      juvenile (Stargardt's) 362.75
      macula 362.76
   Kuhnt-Junius 362.52
   lattice 362.63
   macular (*see also* Degeneration, macula)
      362.50
   microcystoid 362.62
   palisade 362.63
   paving stone 362.61
   pigmentary (primary) 362.74
      secondary 362.65
   posterior pole (*see also* Degeneration,
      macula) 362.50
   secondary 362.66
   senile 362.60
      cystic 362.53
      reticular 362.64
saccule, congenital (causing impairment of
    hearing) 744.05
sacculocochlear 386.8
senile 797
   brain 331.2
   cardiac, heart, or myocardium (*see also*
      Degeneration, myocardial) 429.1
   motor centers 331.2
   reticule 362.64
   retina, cystic 362.50
   vascular — *see* Arteriosclerosis
silicone rubber poppet (prosthetic valve)
    996.02
sinus (cystic) (*see also* Sinusitis) 473.9
   polypoid 471.1
skin 709.3
   amyloid 277.39
   colloid 709.3
spinal (cord) 336.8
   amyloid 277.39
   column 733.90
   combined (subacute) (*see also* Degener-
      ation, combined) 266.2 *[336.2]*
      with anemia (pernicious)
         281.0 *[336.2]*
   dorsolateral (*see also* Degeneration,
      combined) 266.2 *[336.2]*
   familial NEC 336.8
   fatty 336.8
   funicular (*see also* Degeneration, com-
      bined) 266.2 *[336.2]*
   heredofamilial NEC 336.8

☑ **Additional Digit Required** — Refer to the Tabular List for Digit Selection   ✇ **Subterms under main terms may continue to next column or page**

2011 ICD-9-CM   ▶◀ **Revised Text**   ● **New Line**   ▲ **Revised Code**   **Volume 2 — 69**

Degeneration, degenerative — *continued*
 spinal — *continued*
  posterolateral (*see also* Degeneration, combined) 266.2 *[336.2]*
  subacute combined — *see* Degeneration, combined
  tuberculous (*see also* Tuberculosis) 013.8 ☑
 spine 733.90
 spleen 289.59
  amyloid 277.39
  lardaceous 277.39
 stomach 537.89
  lardaceous 277.39
 strionigral 333.0
 sudoriparous (cystic) 705.89
 suprarenal (capsule) (gland) 255.8
  with hypofunction 255.41
 sweat gland 705.89
 synovial membrane (pulpy) 727.9
 tapetoretinal 362.74
  adult or presenile form 362.50
 testis (postinfectional) 608.89
 thymus (gland) 254.8
  fatty 254.8
  lardaceous 277.39
 thyroid (gland) 246.8
 tricuspid (heart) (valve) — *see* Endocarditis, tricuspid
 tuberculous NEC (*see also* Tuberculosis) 011.9 ☑
 turbinate 733.90
 uterus 621.8
  cystic 621.8
 vascular (senile) (*see also* Arteriosclerosis)
  hypertensive — *see* Hypertension
 vitreoretinal (primary) 362.73
  secondary 362.66
 vitreous humor (with infiltration) 379.21
 wallerian NEC — *see* Disorder, nerve
 waxy (any site) 277.39
 Wilson's hepatolenticular 275.1
Deglutition
 paralysis 784.99
  hysterical 300.11
 pneumonia 507.0
Degos' disease or syndrome 447.8
Degradation disorder, branched-chain amino acid 270.3
Dehiscence
 anastomosis — *see* Complications, anastomosis
 cesarean wound 674.1 ☑
 closure of
  cornea 998.32
  fascia, superficial or muscular 998.31
  internal organ 998.31
  mucosa 998.32
  muscle or muscle flap 998.31
  ribs or rib cage 998.31
  skin 998.32
  skull or craniotomy 998.31
  sternum or sternotomy 998.31
  subcutaneous tissue 998.32
  tendon or ligament 998.31
  traumatic laceration (external) (internal) 998.33
 episiotomy 674.2 ☑
 operation wound 998.32
  deep 998.31
  external 998.32
  internal 998.31
  superficial 998.32
 perineal wound (postpartum) 674.2 ☑
 postoperative 998.32
  abdomen 998.32
   internal 998.31
  internal 998.31
 traumatic injury wound repair 998.33
 uterine wound 674.1 ☑
Dehydration (cachexia) 276.51
 with
  hypernatremia 276.0
  hyponatremia 276.1
 newborn 775.5
Deiters' nucleus syndrome 386.19

Déjérine's disease 356.0
Déjérine-Klumpke paralysis 767.6
Déjérine-Roussy syndrome 338.0
Déjérine-Sottas disease or neuropathy (hypertrophic) 356.0
Déjérine-Thomas atrophy or syndrome 333.0
de Lange's syndrome (Amsterdam dwarf, mental retardation, and brachycephaly) 759.89
Delay, delayed
 adaptation, cones or rods 368.63
 any plane in pelvis
  affecting fetus or newborn 763.1
  complicating delivery 660.1 ☑
 birth or delivery NEC 662.1 ☑
  affecting fetus or newborn 763.89
  second twin, triplet, or multiple mate 662.3 ☑
 closure (*see also* Fistula)
  cranial suture 756.0
  fontanel 756.0
 coagulation NEC 790.92
 conduction (cardiac) (ventricular) 426.9
 delivery NEC 662.1 ☑
  second twin, triplet, etc. 662.3 ☑
   affecting fetus or newborn 763.89
 development
  in childhood 783.40
   physiological 783.40
  intellectual NEC 315.9
  learning NEC 315.2
  reading 315.00
  sexual 259.0
  speech 315.39
   and language due to hearing loss 315.34
   associated with hyperkinesis 314.1
  spelling 315.09
 gastric emptying 536.8
 menarche 256.39
  due to pituitary hypofunction 253.4
 menstruation (cause unknown) 626.8
 milestone in childhood 783.42
 motility — *see* Hypomotility
 passage of meconium (newborn) 777.1
 primary respiration 768.9
 puberty 259.0
 separation of umbilical cord 779.83
 sexual maturation, female 259.0
 vaccination V64.00
Del Castillo's syndrome (germinal aplasia) 606.0
Déleage's disease 359.89
Deletion syndrome
 5p 758.31
 22q11.2 758.32
 autosomal NEC 758.39
 constitutional 5q deletion 758.39
Delhi (boil) (button) (sore) 085.1
Delinquency (juvenile) 312.9
 group (*see also* Disturbance, conduct) 312.2 ☑
 neurotic 312.4
Delirium, delirious 780.09
 acute 780.09 ▲
  due to conditions classified elsewhere ● 293.0 ●
 alcoholic 291.0
  acute 291.0
  chronic 291.1
 alcoholicum 291.0
 chronic (*see also* Psychosis) 293.89
  due to or associated with physical condition — *see* Psychosis, organic
 drug-induced 292.81
 due to conditions classified elsewhere 293.0
 eclamptic (*see also* Eclampsia) 780.39
 exhaustion (*see also* Reaction, stress, acute) 308.9
 hysterical 300.11
 in
  presenile dementia 290.11
  senile dementia 290.3
 induced by drug 292.81
 manic, maniacal (acute) (*see also* Psychosis, affective) 296.0 ☑

Delirium, delirious — *continued*
 manic, maniacal (*see also* Psychosis, affective) — *continued*
  recurrent episode 296.1 ☑
  single episode 296.0 ☑
 puerperal 293.9
 senile 290.3
 subacute (psychotic) 293.1
 thyroid (*see also* Thyrotoxicosis) 242.9 ☑
 traumatic (*see also* Injury, intracranial) with
   lesion, spinal cord — *see* Injury, spinal, by site
   shock, spinal — *see* Injury, spinal, by site
 tremens (impending) 291.0
 uremic — *see* Uremia
 withdrawal
  alcoholic (acute) 291.0
   chronic 291.1
  drug 292.0
Delivery

> Note — Use the following fifth-digit subclassification with categories 640–649, 651–676:
>
> 0   unspecified as to episode of care
>
> 1   delivered, with or without mention of antepartum condition
>
> 2   delivered, with mention of postpartum complication
>
> 3   antepartum condition or complication
>
> 4   postpartum condition or complication

 breech (assisted) (buttocks) (complete) (frank) (spontaneous) 652.2 ☑
  affecting fetus or newborn 763.0
  extraction NEC 669.6 ☑
 cesarean (for) 669.7 ☑
  abnormal
   cervix 654.6 ☑
   pelvic organs or tissues 654.9 ☑
   pelvis (bony) (major) NEC 653.0 ☑
   presentation or position 652.9 ☑
    in multiple gestation 652.6 ☑
   size, fetus 653.5 ☑
   soft parts (of pelvis) 654.9 ☑
   uterus, congenital 654.0 ☑
   vagina 654.7 ☑
   vulva 654.8 ☑
  abruptio placentae 641.2 ☑
  acromion presentation 652.8 ☑
  affecting fetus or newborn 763.4
  anteversion, cervix or uterus 654.4 ☑
  atony, uterus 661.2 ☑
   with hemorrhage 666.1 ☑
  bicornis or bicornuate uterus 654.0 ☑
  breech presentation (buttocks) (complete) (frank) 652.2 ☑
  brow presentation 652.4 ☑
  cephalopelvic disproportion (normally formed fetus) 653.4 ☑
  chin presentation 652.4 ☑
  cicatrix of cervix 654.6 ☑
  contracted pelvis (general) 653.1 ☑
   inlet 653.2 ☑
   outlet 653.3 ☑
  cord presentation or prolapse 663.0 ☑
  cystocele 654.4 ☑
  deformity (acquired) (congenital)
   pelvic organs or tissues NEC 654.9 ☑
   pelvis (bony) NEC 653.0 ☑
  displacement, uterus NEC 654.4 ☑
  disproportion NEC 653.9 ☑
  distress
   fetal 656.8 ☑
   maternal 669.0 ☑
  eclampsia 642.6 ☑
  face presentation 652.4 ☑
  failed
   forceps 660.7 ☑

Delivery — *continued*
 cesarean — *continued*
  failed — *continued*
   trial of labor NEC 660.6 ☑
   vacuum extraction 660.7 ☑
   ventouse 660.7 ☑
  fetal deformity 653.7 ☑
  fetal-maternal hemorrhage 656.0 ☑
  fetus, fetal
   distress 656.8 ☑
   prematurity 656.8 ☑
  fibroid (tumor) (uterus) 654.1 ☑
  footling 652.8 ☑
   with successful version 652.1 ☑
  hemorrhage (antepartum) (intrapartum) NEC 641.9 ☑
  hydrocephalic fetus 653.6 ☑
  incarceration of uterus 654.3 ☑
  incoordinate uterine action 661.4 ☑
  inertia, uterus 661.2 ☑
   primary 661.0 ☑
   secondary 661.1 ☑
  lateroversion, uterus or cervix 654.4 ☑
  mal lie 652.9 ☑
  malposition
   fetus 652.9 ☑
    in multiple gestation 652.6 ☑
   pelvic organs or tissues NEC 654.9 ☑
   uterus NEC or cervix 654.4 ☑
  malpresentation 652.9 ☑
   in multiple gestation 652.6 ☑
  maternal
   diabetes mellitus (conditions classifiable to 249 and 250) 648.0 ☑
   heart disease NEC 648.6 ☑
  meconium in liquor 656.8 ☑
   staining only 792.3
  oblique presentation 652.3 ☑
  oversize fetus 653.5 ☑
  pelvic tumor NEC 654.9 ☑
  placental insufficiency 656.5 ☑
  placenta previa 641.0 ☑
   with hemorrhage 641.1 ☑
  poor dilation, cervix 661.0 ☑
  pre-eclampsia 642.4 ☑
   severe 642.5 ☑
  previous
   cesarean delivery, section 654.2 ☑
   surgery (to)
    cervix 654.6 ☑
    gynecological NEC 654.9 ☑
    rectum 654.8 ☑
    uterus NEC 654.9 ☑
     previous cesarean delivery, section 654.2 ☑
    vagina 654.7 ☑
  prolapse
   arm or hand 652.7 ☑
   uterus 654.4 ☑
  prolonged labor 662.1 ☑
  rectocele 654.4 ☑
  retroversion, uterus or cervix 654.3 ☑
  rigid
   cervix 654.6 ☑
   pelvic floor 654.4 ☑
   perineum 654.8 ☑
   vagina 654.7 ☑
   vulva 654.8 ☑
  sacculation, pregnant uterus 654.4 ☑
  scar(s)
   cervix 654.6 ☑
   cesarean delivery, section 654.2 ☑
   uterus NEC 654.9 ☑
    due to previous cesarean delivery, section 654.2 ☑
  Shirodkar suture in situ 654.5 ☑
  shoulder presentation 652.8 ☑
  stenosis or stricture, cervix 654.6 ☑
  transverse presentation or lie 652.3 ☑
  tumor, pelvic organs or tissues NEC 654.4 ☑
  umbilical cord presentation or prolapse 663.0 ☑
 completely normal case — *see* category 650

☑ **Additional Digit Required** — **Refer to the Tabular List for Digit Selection**

▽ **Subterms under main terms may continue to next column or page**

▶◀ **Revised Text**   ● **New Line**   ▲ **Revised Code**

Index

Delivery — Delivery

Delivery — *continued*
complicated — *continued*
  separation
    placenta (premature) 641.2 ☑
    pubic bone 665.6 ☑
    symphysis pubis 665.6 ☑
  septate vagina 654.7 ☑
    causing obstructed labor 660.2 ☑
  shock (birth) (obstetric) (puerperal)
    669.1 ☑
  short cord syndrome 663.4 ☑
  shoulder
    girdle dystocia 660.4 ☑
    presentation 652.8 ☑
      causing obstructed labor
        660.0 ☑
  Siamese twins 678.1 ☑
  slow slope active phase 661.2 ☑
  spasm
    cervix 661.4 ☑
    uterus 661.4 ☑
  spondylolisthesis, pelvis 653.3 ☑
    causing obstructed labor 660.1 ☑
  spondylolysis (lumbosacral) 653.3 ☑
    causing obstructed labor 660.1 ☑
  spondylosis 653.0 ☑
    causing obstructed labor 660.1 ☑
  stenosis or stricture
    cervix 654.6 ☑
      causing obstructed labor
        660.2 ☑
    vagina 654.7 ☑
      causing obstructed labor
        660.2 ☑
  sudden death, unknown cause 669.9 ☑
  tear (pelvic organ) (*see also* Delivery,
    complicated, laceration) 664.9 ☑
    anal sphincter (healed) (old) 654.8 ☑
      not associated with third-degree
        perineal laceration
        664.6 ☑
  teratomas, sacral, fetal 653.7 ☑
    causing obstructed labor 660.1 ☑
  tetanic uterus 661.4 ☑
  tipping pelvis 653.0 ☑
    causing obstructed labor 660.1 ☑
  transverse
    arrest (deep) 660.3 ☑
    presentation or lie 652.3 ☑
      with successful version 652.1 ☑
      causing obstructed labor
        660.0 ☑
  trauma (obstetrical) NEC 665.9 ☑
    periurethral 664.8 ☑   ●
  tumor
    abdominal, fetal 653.7 ☑
      causing obstructed labor
        660.1 ☑
    pelvic organs or tissues NEC 654.9 ☑
      causing obstructed labor
        660.2 ☑
  umbilical cord (*see also* Delivery, compli-
    cated, cord) 663.9 ☑
    around neck tightly, or with compres-
      sion 663.1 ☑
    entanglement NEC 663.3 ☑
      with compression 663.2 ☑
    prolapse (complete) (occult) (partial)
      663.0 ☑
  unstable lie 652.0 ☑
    causing obstructed labor 660.0 ☑
  uterine
    inertia (*see also* Delivery, complicat-
      ed, inertia, uterus) 661.2 ☑
    spasm 661.4 ☑
  vasa previa 663.5 ☑
  velamentous insertion of cord 663.8 ☑
  young maternal age 659.8 ☑
delayed NEC 662.1 ☑
  following rupture of membranes (spon-
    taneous) 658.2 ☑
    artificial 658.3 ☑
  second twin, triplet, etc. 662.3 ☑
difficult NEC 669.9 ☑

Delivery — *continued*
difficult — *continued*
  previous, affecting management of
    pregnancy or childbirth V23.49
    specified type NEC 669.8 ☑
  early onset (spontaneous) 644.2 ☑
  footling 652.8 ☑
    with successful version 652.1 ☑
  forceps NEC 669.5 ☑
    affecting fetus or newborn 763.2
  missed (at or near term) 656.4 ☑
  multiple gestation NEC 651.9 ☑
    with fetal loss and retention of one or
      more fetus(es) 651.6 ☑
    following (elective) fetal reduction
      651.7 ☑
    specified type NEC 651.8 ☑
      with fetal loss and retention of one
        or more fetus(es) 651.6 ☑
      following (elective) fetal reduction
        651.7 ☑
  nonviable infant 656.4 ☑
  normal — *see* category 650
  precipitate 661.3 ☑
    affecting fetus or newborn 763.6
  premature NEC (before 37 completed weeks
    gestation) 644.2 ☑
    previous, affecting management of
      pregnancy V23.41
  quadruplet NEC 651.2 ☑
    with fetal loss and retention of one or
      more fetus(es) 651.5 ☑
    following (elective) fetal reduction
      651.7 ☑
  quintuplet NEC 651.8 ☑
    with fetal loss and retention of one or
      more fetus(es) 651.6 ☑
    following (elective) fetal reduction
      651.7 ☑
  sextuplet NEC 651.8 ☑
    with fetal loss and retention of one or
      more fetus(es) 651.6 ☑
    following (elective) fetal reduction
      651.7 ☑
  specified complication NEC 669.8 ☑
  stillbirth (near term) NEC 656.4 ☑
    early (before 22 completed weeks gesta-
      tion) 632
  term pregnancy (live birth) NEC — *see* cate-
    gory 650
    stillbirth NEC 656.4 ☑
  threatened premature 644.2 ☑
  triplets NEC 651.1 ☑
    with fetal loss and retention of one or
      more fetus(es) 651.4 ☑
    delayed delivery (one or more mates)
      662.3 ☑
    following (elective) fetal reduction
      651.7 ☑
    locked mates 660.5 ☑
  twins NEC 651.0 ☑
    with fetal loss and retention of one fetus
      651.3 ☑
    delayed delivery (one or more mates)
      662.3 ☑
    following (elective) fetal reduction
      locked mates 660.5 ☑
  uncomplicated — *see* category 650
  vacuum extractor NEC 669.5 ☑
    affecting fetus or newborn 763.3
  ventouse NEC 669.5 ☑
    affecting fetus or newborn 763.3
Dellen, cornea 371.41
Delusions (paranoid) 297.9
  grandiose 297.1
  parasitosis 300.29
  systematized 297.1
Dementia 294.8
  alcohol-induced persisting (*see also* Psy-
    chosis, alcoholic) 291.2
  Alzheimer's — *see* Alzheimer's, dementia
  arteriosclerotic (simple type) (uncomplicat-
    ed) 290.40
    with
      acute confusional state 290.41

Dementia — *continued*
arteriosclerotic — *continued*
  with — *continued*
    delirium 290.41
    delusions 290.42
    depressed mood 290.43
  depressed type 290.43
  paranoid type 290.42
Binswanger's 290.12
catatonic (acute) (*see also* Schizophrenia)
  295.2 ☑
congenital (*see also* Retardation, mental)
  319
degenerative 290.9
  presenile-onset — *see* Dementia, prese-
    nile
  senile-onset — *see* Dementia, senile
developmental (*see also* Schizophrenia)
  295.9 ☑
dialysis 294.8
  transient 293.9
drug-induced persisting (*see also* Psychosis,
  drug) 292.82
due to or associated with condition(s) classified elsewhere
  Alzheimer's
    with behavioral disturbance
      331.0 [294.11]
    without behavioral disturbance
      331.0 [294.10]
  cerebral lipidoses
    with behavioral disturbance
      330.1 [294.11]
    without behavioral disturbance
      330.1 [294.10]
  epilepsy
    with behavioral disturbance
      345.9 ☑ [294.11]
    without behavioral disturbance
      345.9 ☑ [294.10]
  hepatolenticular degeneration
    with behavioral disturbance
      275.1 [294.11]
    without behavioral disturbance
      275.1 [294.10]
  HIV
    with behavioral disturbance
      042 [294.11]
    without behavioral disturbance
      042 [294.10]
  Huntington's chorea
    with behavioral disturbance
      333.4 [294.11]
    without behavioral disturbance
      333.4 [294.10]
  Jakob-Creutzfeldt disease (CJD)
    with behavioral disturbance
      046.19 [294.11]
    without behavioral disturbance
      046.19 [294.10]
    variant (vCJD) 046.11
      with dementia
        with behavioral disturbance
          046.11 [294.11]
        without behavioral disbur-
          bance 046.11 [294.10]
  Lewy bodies
    with behavioral disturbance
      331.82 [294.11]
    without behavioral disturbance
      331.82 [294.10]
  multiple sclerosis
    with behavioral disturbance
      340 [294.11]
    without behavioral disturbance
      340 [294.10]
  neurosyphilis
    with behavioral disturbance
      094.9 [294.11]
    without behavioral disturbance
      094.9 [294.10]
  Parkinsonism
    with behavioral disturbance
      331.82 [294.11]
    without behavioral disturbance
      331.82 [294.10]

Dementia — *continued*
due to or associated with condition(s) classified elsewhere — *continued*
  Pelizaeus-Merzbacher disease
    with behavioral disturbance
      333.0 [294.11]
    without behavioral disturbance
      333.0 [294.10]
  Pick's disease
    with behavioral disturbance
      331.11 [294.11]
    without behavioral disturbance
      331.11 [294.10]
  polyarteritis nodosa
    with behavioral disturbance
      446.0 [294.11]
    without behavioral disturbance
      446.0 [294.10]
  syphilis
    with behavioral disturbance
      094.1 [294.11]
    without behavioral disturbance
      094.1 [294.10]
  Wilson's disease
    with behavioral disturbance
      275.1 [294.11]
    without behavioral disturbance
      275.1 [294.10]
frontal 331.19
  with behavioral disturbance
    331.19 [294.11]
  without behavioral disturbance
    331.19 [294.10]
frontotemporal 331.19
  with behavioral disturbance
    331.19 [294.11]
  without behavioral disturbance
    331.19 [294.10]
hebephrenic (acute) 295.1 ☑
Heller's (infantile psychosis) (*see also* Psychosis, childhood) 299.1 ☑
idiopathic 290.9
  presenile-onset — *see* Dementia, prese-
    nile
  senile-onset — *see* Dementia, senile
in
  arteriosclerotic brain disease 290.40
  senility 290.0
induced by drug 292.82
infantile, infantilia (*see also* Psychosis,
  childhood) 299.0 ☑
Lewy body 331.82
  with behavioral disturbance
    331.82 [294.11]
  without behavioral disturbance
    331.82 [294.10]
multi-infarct (cerebrovascular) (*see also* Dementia, arteriosclerotic) 290.40
old age 290.0
paralytica, paralytic 094.1
  juvenilis 090.40
  syphilitic 094.1
    congenital 090.40
  tabetic form 094.1
paranoid (*see also* Schizophrenia) 295.3 ☑
paraphrenic (*see also* Schizophrenia)
  295.3 ☑
paretic 094.1
praecox (*see also* Schizophrenia) 295.9 ☑
presenile 290.10
  with
    acute confusional state 290.11
    delirium 290.11
    delusional features 290.12
    depressive features 290.13
  depressed type 290.13
  paranoid type 290.12
  simple type 290.10
  uncomplicated 290.10
primary (acute) (*see also* Schizophrenia)
  295.0 ☑
progressive, syphilitic 094.1
puerperal — *see* Psychosis, puerperal
schizophrenic (*see also* Schizophrenia)
  295.9 ☑
senile 290.0

☑ Additional Digit Required — Refer to the Tabular List for Digit Selection   Subterms under main terms may continue to next column or page

2011 ICD-9-CM   ▶◀ Revised Text   ● New Line   ▲ Revised Code   October 2010 · Volume 2 — 73

Delivery — Dementia

Index

Dementia — Dependence

Dementia — *continued*
  senile — *continued*
    with
      acute confusional state 290.3
      delirium 290.3
      delusional features 290.20
      depressive features 290.21
    depressed type 290.21
    exhaustion 290.0
    paranoid type 290.20
    simple type (acute) (*see also* Schizophrenia) 295.0
    simplex (acute) (*see also* Schizophrenia) 295.0
    syphilitic 094.1
    uremic — *see* Uremia
  vascular 290.40
    with
      delirium 290.41
      delusions 290.42
      depressed mood 290.43
Demerol dependence — *see also* Dependence 304.0 ✓
Demineralization, ankle — *see also* Osteoporosis 733.00
Demodex folliculorum (infestation) 133.8
Demoralization 799.25
de Morgan's spots (senile angiomas) 448.1
Demyelinating
  polyneuritis, chronic inflammatory 357.81
Demyelination, demyelinization
  central nervous system 341.9
    specified NEC 341.8
  corpus callosum (central) 341.8
  global 340
Dengue (fever) 061
  sandfly 061
  vaccination, prophylactic (against) V05.1
  virus hemorrhagic fever 065.4
Dens
  evaginatus 520.2
  in dente 520.2
  invaginatus 520.2
Dense
  breast(s) — *omit code*
Density
  increased, bone (disseminated) (generalized) (spotted) 733.99
  lung (nodular) 518.89
Dental — *see also* condition
  examination only V72.2
Dentia praecox 520.6
Denticles (in pulp) 522.2
Dentigerous cyst 526.0
Dentin
  irregular (in pulp) 522.3
  opalescent 520.5
  secondary (in pulp) 522.3
  sensitive 521.89
Dentinogenesis imperfecta 520.5
Dentinoma (M9271/0) 213.1
  upper jaw (bone) 213.0
Dentition 520.7
  abnormal 520.6
  anomaly 520.6
  delayed 520.6
  difficult 520.7
  disorder of 520.6
  precocious 520.6
  retarded 520.6
Denture sore (mouth) 528.9
Dependence

> *Note* — Use the following fifth-digit subclassification with category 304:
> 0   unspecified
> 1   continuous
> 2   episodic
> 3   in remission

  with
    withdrawal symptoms
      alcohol 291.81
      drug 292.0
  14-hydroxy-dihydromorphinone 304.0 ✓
  absinthe 304.6 ✓

Dependence — *continued*
  acemorphan 304.0 ✓
  acetanilid(e) 304.6 ✓
  acetophenetidin 304.6 ✓
  acetorphine 304.0 ✓
  acetyldihydrocodeine 304.0 ✓
  acetyldihydrocodeinone 304.0 ✓
  Adalin 304.1 ✓
  Afghanistan black 304.3 ✓
  agrypnal 304.1 ✓
  alcohol, alcoholic (ethyl) (methyl) (wood) 303.9 ✓
    maternal, with suspected fetal damage affecting management of pregnancy 655.4 ✓
  allobarbitone 304.1 ✓
  allonal 304.1 ✓
  allylisopropylacetylurea 304.1 ✓
  alphaprodine (hydrochloride) 304.0 ✓
  Alurate 304.1 ✓
  Alvodine 304.0 ✓
  amethocaine 304.6 ✓
  amidone 304.0 ✓
  amidopyrine 304.6 ✓
  aminopyrine 304.6 ✓
  amobarbital 304.1 ✓
  amphetamine(s) (type) (drugs classifiable to 969.7) 304.4 ✓
  analgesic (drug) NEC 304.6 ✓
    synthetic with morphine-like effect 304.0 ✓
  anesthetic (agent) (drug) (gas) (general) (local) NEC 304.6 ✓
  Angel dust 304.6 ✓
  anileridine 304.0 ✓
  antipyrine 304.6 ✓
  anxiolytic 304.1 ✓
  aprobarbital 304.1 ✓
  aprobarbitone 304.1 ✓
  atropine 304.6 ✓
  Avertin (bromide) 304.6 ✓
  barbenyl 304.1 ✓
  barbital(s) 304.1 ✓
  barbitone 304.1 ✓
  barbiturate(s) (compounds) (drugs classifiable to 967.0) 304.1 ✓
  barbituric acid (and compounds) 304.1 ✓
  benzedrine 304.4 ✓
  benzylmorphine 304.0 ✓
  Beta-chlor 304.1 ✓
  bhang 304.3 ✓
  blue velvet 304.0 ✓
  Brevital 304.1 ✓
  bromal (hydrate) 304.1 ✓
  bromide(s) NEC 304.1 ✓
  bromine compounds NEC 304.1 ✓
  bromisovalum 304.1 ✓
  bromoform 304.1 ✓
  Bromo-seltzer 304.1 ✓
  bromural 304.1 ✓
  butabarbital (sodium) 304.1 ✓
  butabarpal 304.1 ✓
  butallylonal 304.1 ✓
  butethal 304.1 ✓
  buthalitone (sodium) 304.1 ✓
  Butisol 304.1 ✓
  butobarbitone 304.1 ✓
  butyl chloral (hydrate) 304.1 ✓
  caffeine 304.4 ✓
  cannabis (indica) (sativa) (resin) (derivatives) (type) 304.3 ✓
  carbamazepine 304.6 ✓
  Carbrital 304.1 ✓
  carbromal 304.1 ✓
  carisoprodol 304.6 ✓
  Catha (edulis) 304.4 ✓
  chloral (betaine) (hydrate) 304.1 ✓
  chloralamide 304.1 ✓
  chloralformamide 304.1 ✓

Dependence — *continued*
  chloralose 304.1 ✓
  chlordiazepoxide 304.1 ✓
  Chloretone 304.1 ✓
  chlorbutanol 304.1 ✓
  chlorodyne 304.1 ✓
  chloroform 304.6 ✓
  Cliradon 304.0 ✓
  coca (leaf) and derivatives 304.2 ✓
  cocaine 304.2 ✓
    hydrochloride 304.2 ✓
    salt (any) 304.2 ✓
  codeine 304.0 ✓
  combination of drugs (excluding morphine or opioid type drug) NEC 304.8 ✓
    morphine or opioid type drug with any other drug 304.7 ✓
  croton-chloral 304.1 ✓
  cyclobarbital 304.1 ✓
  cyclobarbitone 304.1 ✓
  dagga 304.3 ✓
  Delvinal 304.1 ✓
  Demerol 304.0 ✓
  desocodeine 304.0 ✓
  desomorphine 304.0 ✓
  desoxyephedrine 304.4 ✓
  DET 304.5 ✓
  dexamphetamine 304.4 ✓
  dexedrine 304.4 ✓
  dextromethorphan 304.0 ✓
  dextromoramide 304.0 ✓
  dextronorpseudoephedrine 304.4 ✓
  dextrorphan 304.0 ✓
  diacetylmorphine 304.0 ✓
  Dial 304.1 ✓
  diallylbarbituric acid 304.1 ✓
  diamorphine 304.0 ✓
  diazepam 304.1 ✓
  dibucaine 304.6 ✓
  dichloroethane 304.6 ✓
  diethyl barbituric acid 304.1 ✓
  diethylsulfone-diethylmethane 304.1 ✓
  difencloxazine 304.0 ✓
  dihydrocodeine 304.0 ✓
  dihydrocodeinone 304.0 ✓
  dihydrohydroxycodeinone 304.0 ✓
  dihydroisocodeine 304.0 ✓
  dihydromorphine 304.0 ✓
  dihydromorphinone 304.0 ✓
  dihydroxcodeinone 304.0 ✓
  Dilaudid 304.0 ✓
  dimenhydrinate 304.6 ✓
  dimethylmeperidine 304.0 ✓
  dimethyltriptamine 304.5 ✓
  Dionin 304.0 ✓
  diphenoxylate 304.6 ✓
  dipipanone 304.0 ✓
  d-lysergic acid diethylamide 304.5 ✓
  DMT 304.5 ✓
  Dolophine 304.0 ✓
  DOM 304.2 ✓
  Doriden 304.1 ✓
  dormiral 304.1 ✓
  Dormison 304.1 ✓
  Dromoran 304.0 ✓
  drug NEC 304.9 ✓
    analgesic NEC 304.6 ✓
    combination (excluding morphine or opioid type drug) NEC 304.8 ✓
      morphine or opioid type drug with any other drug 304.7 ✓
    complicating pregnancy, childbirth, or puerperium 648.3 ✓
      affecting fetus or newborn 779.5
    hallucinogenic 304.5 ✓
    hypnotic NEC 304.1 ✓
    narcotic NEC 304.9 ✓
    psychostimulant NEC 304.4 ✓
    sedative 304.1 ✓
    soporific NEC 304.1 ✓
    specified type NEC 304.6 ✓

Dependence — *continued*
  drug — *continued*
    suspected damage to fetus affecting management of pregnancy 655.5 ✓
    synthetic, with morphine-like effect 304.0 ✓
    tranquilizing 304.1 ✓
  duboisine 304.6 ✓
  ectylurea 304.1 ✓
  Endocaine 304.6 ✓
  Equanil 304.1 ✓
  Eskabarb 304.1 ✓
  ethchlorvynol 304.1 ✓
  ether (ethyl) (liquid) (vapor) (vinyl) 304.6 ✓
  ethidene 304.1 ✓
  ethinamate 304.1 ✓
  ethoheptazine 304.6 ✓
  ethyl
    alcohol 303.9 ✓
    bromide 304.6 ✓
    carbamate 304.6 ✓
    chloride 304.6 ✓
    morphine 304.0 ✓
  ethylene (gas) 304.6 ✓
    dichloride 304.6 ✓
  ethylidene chloride 304.6 ✓
  etilfen 304.1 ✓
  etorphine 304.0 ✓
  etoval 304.1 ✓
  eucodal 304.0 ✓
  euneryl 304.1 ✓
  Evipal 304.1 ✓
  Evipan 304.1 ✓
  fentanyl 304.0 ✓
  ganja 304.3 ✓
  gardenal 304.1 ✓
  gardenpanyl 304.1 ✓
  gelsemine 304.6 ✓
  Gelsemium 304.6 ✓
  Gemonil 304.1 ✓
  glucochloral 304.1 ✓
  glue (airplane) (sniffing) 304.6 ✓
  glutethimide 304.1 ✓
  hallucinogenics 304.5 ✓
  hashish 304.3 ✓
  headache powder NEC 304.6 ✓
  Heavenly Blue 304.5 ✓
  hedonal 304.1 ✓
  hemp 304.3 ✓
  heptabarbital 304.1 ✓
  Heptalgin 304.0 ✓
  heptobarbitone 304.1 ✓
  heroin 304.0 ✓
    salt (any) 304.0 ✓
  hexethal (sodium) 304.1 ✓
  hexobarbital 304.1 ✓
  Hycodan 304.0 ✓
  hydrocodone 304.0 ✓
  hydromorphinol 304.0 ✓
  hydromorphinone 304.0 ✓
  hydromorphone 304.0 ✓
  hydroxycodeine 304.0 ✓
  hypnotic NEC 304.1 ✓
  Indian hemp 304.3 ✓
  inhalant 304.6 ✓
  intranarcon 304.1 ✓
  Kemithal 304.1 ✓
  ketobemidone 304.0 ✓
  khat 304.4 ✓
  kif 304.3 ✓
  Lactuca (virosa) extract 304.1 ✓
  lactucarium 304.1 ✓
  laudanum 304.0 ✓
  Lebanese red 304.3 ✓
  Leritine 304.0 ✓
  lettuce opium 304.1 ✓
  Levanil 304.1 ✓
  Levo-Dromoran 304.0 ✓
  levo-iso-methadone 304.0 ✓
  levorphanol 304.0 ✓
  Librium 304.1 ✓
  Lomotil 304.6 ✓

☑ **Additional Digit Required — Refer to the Tabular List for Digit Selection**   ▼ **Subterms under main terms may continue to next column or page**

74 — Volume 2   ▶◀ Revised Text   ● New Line   ▲ Revised Code   **2011 ICD-9-CM**

Dependence — continued
Lotusate 304.1 ✓
LSD (-25) (and derivatives) 304.5 ✓
Luminal 304.1 ✓
lysergic acid 304.5 ✓
   amide 304.5 ✓
maconha 304.3 ✓
magic mushroom 304.5 ✓
marihuana 304.3 ✓
MDA (methylene dioxyamphetamine) 304.4 ✓
Mebaral 304.1 ✓
Medinal 304.1 ✓
Medomin 304.1 ✓
megahallucinogenics 304.5 ✓
meperidine 304.0 ✓
mephobarbital 304.1 ✓
meprobamate 304.1 ✓
mescaline 304.5 ✓
methadone 304.0 ✓
methamphetamine(s) 304.4 ✓
methaqualone 304.1 ✓
metharbital 304.1 ✓
methitural 304.1 ✓
methobarbitone 304.1 ✓
methohexital 304.1 ✓
methopholine 304.6 ✓
methyl
   alcohol 303.9 ✓
   bromide 304.6 ✓
   morphine 304.0 ✓
   sulfonal 304.1 ✓
methylaparafynol 304.1 ✓
methylated spirit 303.9 ✓
methylbutinol 304.6 ✓
methyldihydromorphinone 304.0 ✓
methylene
   chloride 304.6 ✓
   dichloride 304.6 ✓
   dioxyamphetamine (MDA) 304.4 ✓
methylphenidate 304.4 ✓
methyprylone 304.1 ✓
metopon 304.0 ✓
Miltown 304.1 ✓
morning glory seeds 304.5 ✓
morphinan(s) 304.0 ✓
morphine (sulfate) (sulfite) (type) (drugs classifiable to 965.00–965.09) 304.0 ✓
morphine or opioid type drug (drugs classifiable to 965.00–965.09) with any other drug 304.7 ✓
morphinol(s) 304.0 ✓
morphinon 304.0 ✓
morpholinylethylmorphine 304.0 ✓
mylomide 304.1 ✓
myristicin 304.5 ✓
narcotic (drug) NEC 304.9 ✓
nealbarbital 304.1 ✓
nealbarbitone 304.1 ✓
Nembutal 304.1 ✓
Neonal 304.1 ✓
Neraval 304.1 ✓
Neravan 304.1 ✓
neurobarb 304.1 ✓
nicotine 305.1
Nisentil 304.0 ✓
nitrous oxide 304.6 ✓
Noctec 304.1 ✓
Noludar 304.1 ✓
nonbarbiturate sedatives and tranquilizers with similar effect 304.1 ✓
noptil 304.1 ✓
normorphine 304.0 ✓
noscapine 304.0 ✓
Novocaine 304.6 ✓
Numorphan 304.0 ✓
nunol 304.1 ✓
Nupercaine 304.6 ✓
Oblivon 304.1 ✓
on
   aspirator V46.0
   hemodialysis V45.11

Dependence — continued
on — continued
   hyperbaric chamber V46.8
   iron lung V46.11
   machine (enabling) V46.9
     specified type NEC V46.8
   peritoneal dialysis V45.11
   Possum (Patient-Operated-Selector-Mechanism) V46.8
   renal dialysis machine V45.11
   respirator [ventilator] V46.11
     encounter
       during
         mechanical failure V46.14
         power failure V46.12
       for weaning V46.13
   supplemental oxygen V46.2
   wheelchair V46.3
opiate 304.0 ✓
opioids 304.0 ✓
opioid type drug 304.0 ✓
   with any other drug 304.7 ✓
opium (alkaloids) (derivatives) (tincture) 304.0 ✓
ortal 304.1 ✓
Oxazepam 304.1 ✓
oxycodone 304.0 ✓
oxymorphone 304.0 ✓
Palfium 304.0 ✓
Panadol 304.6 ✓
pantopium 304.0 ✓
pantopon 304.0 ✓
papaverine 304.0 ✓
paracetamol 304.6 ✓
paracodin 304.0 ✓
paraldehyde 304.1 ✓
paregoric 304.0 ✓
Parzone 304.0 ✓
PCP (phencyclidine) 304.6 ✓
Pearly Gates 304.5 ✓
pentazocine 304.0 ✓
pentobarbital 304.1 ✓
pentobarbitone (sodium) 304.1 ✓
Pentothal 304.1 ✓
Percaine 304.6 ✓
Percodan 304.0 ✓
Perichlor 304.1 ✓
Pernocton 304.1 ✓
Pernoston 304.1 ✓
peronine 304.0 ✓
pethidine (hydrochloride) 304.0 ✓
petrichloral 304.1 ✓
peyote 304.5 ✓
Phanodron 304.1 ✓
phenacetin 304.6 ✓
phenadoxone 304.0 ✓
phenaglycodol 304.1 ✓
phenazocine 304.0 ✓
phencyclidine 304.6 ✓
phenmetrazine 304.4 ✓
phenobal 304.1 ✓
phenobarbital 304.1 ✓
phenobarbitone 304.1 ✓
phenomorphan 304.0 ✓
phenonyl 304.1 ✓
phenoperidine 304.0 ✓
pholcodine 304.0 ✓
piminodine 304.0 ✓
Pipadone 304.0 ✓
Pitkin's solution 304.6 ✓
Placidyl 304.1 ✓
polysubstance 304.8 ✓
Pontocaine 304.6 ✓
pot 304.3 ✓
potassium bromide 304.1 ✓
Preludin 304.4 ✓
Prinadol 304.0 ✓
probarbital 304.1 ✓
procaine 304.6 ✓
propanal 304.1 ✓
propoxyphene 304.6 ✓
psilocibin 304.5 ✓
psilocin 304.5 ✓
psilocybin 304.5 ✓

Dependence — continued
psilocyline 304.5 ✓
psilocyn 304.5 ✓
psychedelic agents 304.5 ✓
psychostimulant NEC 304.4 ✓
psychotomimetic agents 304.5 ✓
pyrahexyl 304.3 ✓
Pyramidon 304.6 ✓
quinalbarbitone 304.1 ✓
racemoramide 304.0 ✓
racemorphan 304.0 ✓
Rela 304.6 ✓
scopolamine 304.6 ✓
secobarbital 304.1 ✓
Seconal 304.1 ✓
sedative NEC 304.1 ✓
   nonbarbiturate with barbiturate effect 304.1 ✓
Sedormid 304.1 ✓
sernyl 304.1 ✓
sodium bromide 304.1 ✓
Soma 304.6 ✓
Somnal 304.1 ✓
Somnos 304.1 ✓
Soneryl 304.1 ✓
soporific (drug) NEC 304.1 ✓
specified drug NEC 304.6 ✓
speed 304.4 ✓
spinocaine 304.6 ✓
Stovaine 304.6 ✓
STP 304.5 ✓
stramonium 304.6 ✓
Sulfonal 304.1 ✓
sulfonethylmethane 304.1 ✓
sulfonmethane 304.1 ✓
Surital 304.1 ✓
synthetic drug with morphine-like effect 304.0 ✓
talbutal 304.1 ✓
tetracaine 304.6 ✓
tetrahydrocannabinol 304.3 ✓
tetronal 304.1 ✓
THC 304.3 ✓
thebacon 304.0 ✓
thebaine 304.0 ✓
thiamil 304.1 ✓
thiamylal 304.1 ✓
thiopental 304.1 ✓
tobacco 305.1
toluene, toluol 304.6 ✓
tranquilizer NEC 304.1 ✓
   nonbarbiturate with barbiturate effect 304.1 ✓
tribromacetaldehyde 304.6 ✓
tribromethanol 304.6 ✓
tribromomethane 304.6 ✓
trichloroethanol 304.6 ✓
trichoroethyl phosphate 304.1 ✓
triclofos 304.1 ✓
Trional 304.1 ✓
Tuinal 304.1 ✓
Turkish Green 304.3 ✓
urethan(e) 304.6 ✓
Valium 304.1 ✓
Valmid 304.1 ✓
veganin 304.0 ✓
veramon 304.1 ✓
Veronal 304.1 ✓
versidyne 304.6 ✓
vinbarbital 304.1 ✓
vinbarbitone 304.1 ✓
vinyl bitone 304.1 ✓
vitamin B_6 266.1
wine 303.9 ✓
Zactane 304.6 ✓
Dependency
passive 301.6
reactions 301.6
Depersonalization (episode, in neurotic state) (neurotic) (syndrome) 300.6
Depletion
carbohydrates 271.9
complement factor 279.8

Depletion — continued
extracellular fluid 276.52
plasma 276.52
potassium 276.8
   nephropathy 588.89
salt or sodium 276.1
   causing heat exhaustion or prostration 992.4
   nephropathy 593.9
volume 276.50
   extracellular fluid 276.52
   plasma 276.52
Deployment (military)
personal history of V62.22
returned from V62.22
status V62.21
Deposit
argentous, cornea 371.16
bone, in Boeck's sarcoid 135
calcareous, calcium — see Calcification
cholesterol
   retina 362.82
   skin 709.3
   vitreous (humor) 379.22
conjunctival 372.56
cornea, corneal NEC 371.10
   argentous 371.16
   in
     cystinosis 270.0 [371.15]
     mucopolysaccharidosis 277.5 [371.15]
crystalline, vitreous (humor) 379.22
hemosiderin, in old scars of cornea 371.11
metallic, in lens 366.45
skin 709.3
teeth, tooth (betel) (black) (green) (materia alba) (orange) (soft) (tobacco) 523.6
urate, in kidney (see also Disease, renal) 593.9
Depraved appetite 307.52
Depression 311
acute (see also Psychosis, affective) 296.2 ✓
   recurrent episode 296.3 ✓
   single episode 296.2 ✓
agitated (see also Psychosis, affective) 296.2 ✓
   recurrent episode 296.3 ✓
   single episode 296.2 ✓
anaclitic 309.21
anxiety 300.4
arches 734
   congenital 754.61
autogenous (see also Psychosis, affective) 296.2 ✓
   recurrent episode 296.3 ✓
   single episode 296.2 ✓
basal metabolic rate (BMR) 794.7
bone marrow 289.9
central nervous system 799.1
   newborn 779.2
cerebral 331.9
   newborn 779.2
cerebrovascular 437.8
   newborn 779.2
chest wall 738.3
endogenous (see also Psychosis, affective) 296.2 ✓
   recurrent episode 296.3 ✓
   single episode 296.2 ✓
functional activity 780.99
hysterical 300.11
involutional, climacteric, or menopausal (see also Psychosis, affective) 296.2 ✓
   recurrent episode 296.3 ✓
   single episode 296.2 ✓
major 296.2 ✓   ●
   recurrent episode 296.3 ✓   ●
   single episode 296.2 ✓   ●
manic (see also Psychosis, affective) 296.80
medullary 348.89
   newborn 779.2
mental 300.4
metatarsal heads — see Depression, arches
metatarsus — see Depression, arches
monopolar (see also Psychosis, affective) 296.2 ✓

✓ **Additional Digit Required** — Refer to the Tabular List for Digit Selection   ⅶ **Subterms under main terms may continue to next column or page**

2011 ICD-9-CM   ▶◀ **Revised Text**   ● **New Line**   ▲ **Revised Code**   **October 2010 • Volume 2 — 75**

Depression — continued
  monopolar (see also Psychosis, affective) —
      continued
    recurrent episode 296.3 ☑
    single episode 296.2 ☑
  nervous 300.4
  neurotic 300.4
  nose 738.0
  postpartum 648.4 ☑
  psychogenic 300.4
    reactive 298.0
  psychoneurotic 300.4
  psychotic (see also Psychosis, affective)
      296.2 ☑
    reactive 298.0
    recurrent episode 296.3 ☑
    single episode 296.2 ☑
  reactive 300.4
    neurotic 300.4
    psychogenic 298.0
    psychoneurotic 300.4
    psychotic 298.0
  recurrent 296.3 ☑
  respiratory center 348.89
    newborn 770.89
  scapula 736.89
  senile 290.21
  situational (acute) (brief) 309.0
    prolonged 309.1
  skull 754.0
  sternum 738.3
  visual field 368.40

Depressive reaction — see also Reaction, de-
    pressive
  acute (transient) 309.0
    with anxiety 309.28
  prolonged 309.1
  situational (acute) 309.0
    prolonged 309.1

Deprivation
  cultural V62.4
  emotional V62.89
    affecting
      adult 995.82
      infant or child 995.51
  food 994.2
    specific substance NEC 269.8
  protein (familial) (kwashiorkor) 260
  sleep V69.4
  social V62.4
    affecting
      adult 995.82
      infant or child 995.51
  symptoms, syndrome
    alcohol 291.81
    drug 292.0
  vitamins (see also Deficiency, vitamin) 269.2
  water 994.3

de Quervain's
  disease (tendon sheath) 727.04
  syndrome 259.51
  thyroiditis (subacute granulomatous thy-
    roiditis) 245.1

Derangement
  ankle (internal) 718.97
    current injury (see also Dislocation, an-
      kle) 837.0
    recurrent 718.37
  cartilage (articular) NEC (see also Disorder,
    cartilage, articular) 718.0 ☑
    knee 717.9
      recurrent 718.36
    recurrent 718.3 ☑
  collateral ligament (knee) (medial) (tibial)
      717.82
    current injury 844.1
      lateral (fibular) 844.0
    lateral (fibular) 717.81
      current injury 844.0
  cruciate ligament (knee) (posterior) 717.84
    anterior 717.83
      current injury 844.2
    current injury 844.2
  elbow (internal) 718.92
    current injury (see also Dislocation, el-
      bow) 832.00

Derangement — continued
  elbow — continued
    recurrent 718.32
  gastrointestinal 536.9
  heart — see Disease, heart
  hip (joint) (internal) (old) 718.95
    current injury (see also Dislocation, hip)
      835.00
    recurrent 718.35
  intervertebral disc — see Displacement, in-
    tervertebral disc
  joint (internal) 718.90
    ankle 718.97
    current injury (see also Dislocation, by
      site)
      knee, meniscus or cartilage (see also
        Tear, meniscus) 836.2
    elbow 718.92
    foot 718.97
    hand 718.94
    hip 718.95
    knee 717.9
    multiple sites 718.99
    pelvic region 718.95
    recurrent 718.30
      ankle 718.37
      elbow 718.32
      foot 718.37
      hand 718.34
      hip 718.35
      knee 718.36
      multiple sites 718.39
      pelvic region 718.35
      shoulder (region) 718.31
      specified site NEC 718.38
      temporomandibular (old) 524.69
      wrist 718.33
    shoulder (region) 718.91
    specified site NEC 718.98
    spine NEC 724.9
    temporomandibular 524.69
    wrist 718.93
  knee (cartilage) (internal) 717.9
    current injury (see also Tear, meniscus)
      836.2
    ligament 717.89
      capsular 717.85
      collateral — see Derangement, collat-
        eral ligament
      cruciate — see Derangement, cruci-
        ate ligament
      specified NEC 717.85
    recurrent 718.36
  low back NEC 724.9
  meniscus NEC (knee) 717.5
    current injury (see also Tear, meniscus)
      836.2
    lateral 717.40
      anterior horn 717.42
      posterior horn 717.43
      specified NEC 717.49
    medial 717.3
      anterior horn 717.1
      posterior horn 717.2
    recurrent 718.3 ☑
    site other than knee — see Disorder,
      cartilage, articular
  mental (see also Psychosis) 298.9
  rotator cuff (recurrent) (tear) 726.10
    current 840.4
  sacroiliac (old) 724.6
    current — see Dislocation, sacroiliac
  semilunar cartilage (knee) 717.5
    current injury 836.2
      lateral 836.1
      medial 836.0
    recurrent 718.3 ☑
  shoulder (internal) 718.91
    current injury (see also Dislocation,
      shoulder) 831.00
    recurrent 718.31
  spine (recurrent) NEC 724.9
    current — see Dislocation, spine
  temporomandibular (internal) (joint) (old)
      524.69
    current — see Dislocation, jaw

Dercum's disease or syndrome (adiposis do-
    lorosa) 272.8
Derealization (neurotic) 300.6
Dermal — see condition
Dermaphytid — see Dermatophytosis
Dermatergosis — see Dermatitis
Dermatitis (allergic) (contact) (occupational)
    (venenata) 692.9
  ab igne 692.82
  acneiform 692.9
  actinic (due to sun) 692.70
    acute 692.72
    chronic NEC 692.74
    other than from sun NEC 692.82
  ambustionis
    due to
      burn or scald — see Burn, by site
      sunburn (see also Sunburn) 692.71
  amebic 006.6
  ammonia 691.0
  anaphylactoid NEC 692.9
  arsenical 692.4
  artefacta 698.4
    psychogenic 316 [698.4]
  asthmatic 691.8
  atopic (allergic) (intrinsic) 691.8
    psychogenic 316 [691.8]
  atrophicans 701.8
    diffusa 701.8
    maculosa 701.3
  autoimmune progesterone 279.49
  berlock, berloque 692.72
  blastomycetic 116.0
  blister beetle 692.89
  Brucella NEC 023.9
  bullosa 694.9
    striata pratensis 692.6
  bullous 694.9
    mucosynechial, atrophic 694.60
      with ocular involvement 694.61
    seasonal 694.8
  calorica
    due to
      burn or scald — see Burn, by site
      cold 692.89
      sunburn (see also Sunburn) 692.71
  caterpillar 692.89
  cercarial 120.3
  combustionis
    due to
      burn or scald — see Burn, by site
      sunburn (see also Sunburn) 692.71
  congelationis 991.5
  contusiformis 695.2
  diabetic 250.8 ☑
  diaper 691.0
  diphtheritica 032.85
  due to
    acetone 692.2
    acids 692.4
    adhesive plaster 692.4
    alcohol (skin contact) (substances classi-
      fiable to 980.0–980.9) 692.4
      taken internally 693.8
    alkalis 692.4
    allergy NEC 692.9
    ammonia (household) (liquid) 692.4
    animal
      dander (cat) (dog) 692.84
      hair (cat) (dog) 692.84
    arnica 692.3
    arsenic 692.4
      taken internally 693.8
    blister beetle 692.89
    cantharides 692.3
    carbon disulphide 692.2
    caterpillar 692.89
    caustics 692.4
    cereal (ingested) 693.1
      contact with skin 692.5
    chemical(s) NEC 692.4
      internal 693.8
      irritant NEC 692.4
        taken internally 693.8
    chlorocompounds 692.2
    coffee (ingested) 693.1

Dermatitis — continued
  due to — continued
    coffee — continued
      contact with skin 692.5
    cold weather 692.89
    cosmetics 692.81
    cyclohexanes 692.2
    dander, animal (cat) (dog) 692.84
    deodorant 692.81
    detergents 692.0
    dichromate 692.4
    drugs and medicinals (correct substance
      properly administered) (internal
      use) 693.0
      external (in contact with skin) 692.3
        wrong substance given or taken
          976.9
        specified substance — see
          Table of Drugs and
          Chemicals
      wrong substance given or taken
        977.9
        specified substance — see Table
          of Drugs and Chemicals
    dyes 692.89
      hair 692.89
    epidermophytosis — see Dermatophyto-
      sis
    esters 692.2
    external irritant NEC 692.9
      specified agent NEC 692.89
    eye shadow 692.81
    fish (ingested) 693.1
      contact with skin 692.5
    flour (ingested) 693.1
      contact with skin 692.5
    food (ingested) 693.1
      in contact with skin 692.5
    fruit (ingested) 693.1
      contact with skin 692.5
    fungicides 692.3
    furs 692.84
    glycols 692.2
    greases NEC 692.1
    hair, animal (cat) (dog) 692.84
    hair dyes 692.89
    hot
      objects and materials — see Burn, by
        site
      weather or places 692.89
    hydrocarbons 692.2
    infrared rays, except from sun 692.82
      solar NEC (see also Dermatitis, due to,
        sun) 692.70
    ingested substance 693.9
      drugs and medicinals (see also Der-
        matitis, due to, drugs and
        medicinals) 693.0
      food 693.1
      specified substance NEC 693.8
    ingestion or injection of chemical 693.8
      drug (correct substance properly ad-
        ministered) 693.0
      wrong substance given or taken
        977.9
        specified substance — see Table
          of Drugs and Chemicals
    insecticides 692.4
    internal agent 693.9
      drugs and medicinals (see also Der-
        matitis, due to, drugs and
        medicinals) 693.0
      food (ingested) 693.1
        in contact with skin 692.5
      specified agent NEC 693.8
    iodine 692.3
    iodoform 692.3
    irradiation 692.82
    jewelry 692.83
    keratolytics 692.3
    ketones 692.2
    lacquer tree (Rhus verniciflua) 692.6
    light (sun) NEC (see also Dermatitis, due
      to, sun) 692.70
      other 692.82
    low temperature 692.89

☑ Additional Digit Required — Refer to the Tabular List for Digit Selection　　　　　　🐃 Subterms under main terms may continue to next column or page

76 — Volume 2　　　　▶◀ Revised Text　　　● New Line　　▲ Revised Code　　　　2011 ICD-9-CM

Dermatitis — *continued*
  due to — *continued*
    mascara 692.81
    meat (ingested) 693.1
      contact with skin 692.5
    mercury, mercurials 692.3
    metals 692.83
    milk (ingested) 693.1
      contact with skin 692.5
    Neomycin 692.3
    nylon 692.4
    oils NEC 692.1
    paint solvent 692.2
    pediculocides 692.3
    petroleum products (substances classifiable to 981) 692.4
    phenol 692.3
    photosensitiveness, photosensitivity (sun) 692.72
      other light 692.82
    plants NEC 692.6
    plasters, medicated (any) 692.3
    plastic 692.4
    poison
      ivy (Rhus toxicodendron) 692.6
      oak (Rhus diversiloba) 692.6
      plant or vine 692.6
      sumac (Rhus venenata) 692.6
      vine (Rhus radicans) 692.6
    preservatives 692.89
    primrose (primula) 692.6
    primula 692.6
    radiation 692.82
      sun NEC (*see also* Dermatitis, due to, sun) 692.70
      tanning bed 692.82
    radioactive substance 692.82
    radium 692.82
    ragweed (Senecio jacobae) 692.6
    Rhus (diversiloba) (radicans) (toxicodendron) (venenata) (verniciflua) 692.6
    rubber 692.4
    scabicides 692.3
    Senecio jacobae 692.6
    solar radiation — *see* Dermatitis, due to, sun
    solvents (any) (substances classifiable to 982.0–982.8) 692.2
      chlorocompound group 692.2
      cyclohexane group 692.2
      ester group 692.2
      glycol group 692.2
      hydrocarbon group 692.2
      ketone group 692.2
      paint 692.2
    specified agent NEC 692.89
    sun 692.70
      acute 692.72
      chronic NEC 692.74
      specified NEC 692.79
    sunburn (*see also* Sunburn) 692.71
    sunshine NEC (*see also* Dermatitis, due to, sun) 692.70
    tanning bed 692.82
    tetrachlorethylene 692.2
    toluene 692.2
    topical medications 692.3
    turpentine 692.2
    ultraviolet rays, except from sun 692.82
      sun NEC (*see also* Dermatitis, due to, sun) 692.70
    vaccine or vaccination (correct substance properly administered) 693.0
      wrong substance given or taken
        bacterial vaccine 978.8
          specified — *see* Table of Drugs and Chemicals
        other vaccines NEC 979.9
          specified — *see* Table of Drugs and Chemicals
    varicose veins (*see also* Varicose, vein, inflamed or infected) 454.1
    x-rays 692.82
  dyshydrotic 705.81
  dysmenorrheica 625.8

Dermatitis — *continued*
  eczematoid NEC 692.9
    infectious 690.8
  eczematous NEC 692.9
  epidemica 695.89
  erysipelatosa 695.81
  escharotica — *see* Burn, by site
  exfoliativa, exfoliative 695.89
    generalized 695.89
    infantum 695.81
    neonatorum 695.81
  eyelid 373.31
    allergic 373.32
    contact 373.32
    eczematous 373.31
    herpes (zoster) 053.20
      simplex 054.41
    infective 373.5
      due to
        actinomycosis 039.3 *[373.5]*
        herpes
          simplex 054.41
          zoster 053.20
        impetigo 684 *[373.5]*
        leprosy (*see also* Leprosy) 030.0 *[373.4]*
        lupus vulgaris (tuberculous) (*see also* Tuberculosis) 017.0 ☑ *[373.4]*
        mycotic dermatitis (*see also* Dermatomycosis) 111.9 *[373.5]*
        vaccinia 051.02 *[373.5]*
          postvaccination 999.0 *[373.5]*
        yaws (*see also* Yaws) 102.9 *[373.4]*
  facta, factitia 698.4
    psychogenic 316 *[698.4]*
  ficta 698.4
    psychogenic 316 *[698.4]*
  flexural 691.8
  follicularis 704.8
  friction 709.8
  fungus 111.9
    specified type NEC 111.8
  gangrenosa, gangrenous (infantum) (*see also* Gangrene) 785.4
  gestationis 646.8 ☑
  gonococcal 098.89
  gouty 274.89
  harvest mite 133.8
  heat 692.89
  herpetiformis (bullous) (erythematous) (pustular) (vesicular) 694.0
    juvenile 694.2
    senile 694.5
  hiemalis 692.89
  hypostatic, hypostatica 454.1
    with ulcer 454.2
  impetiginous 684
  infantile (acute) (chronic) (intertriginous) (intrinsic) (seborrheic) 690.12
  infectiosa eczematoides 690.8
  infectious (staphylococcal) (streptococcal) 686.9
    eczematoid 690.8
  infective eczematoid 690.8
  Jacquet's (diaper dermatitis) 691.0
  leptus 133.8
  lichenified NEC 692.9
  lichenoid, chronic 701.0
  lichenoides purpurica pigmentosa 709.1
  meadow 692.6
  medicamentosa (correct substance properly administered) (internal use) (*see also* Dermatitis, due to, drugs or medicinals) 693.0
    due to contact with skin 692.3
  mite 133.8
  multiformis 694.0
    juvenile 694.2
    senile 694.5
  napkin 691.0
  neuro 698.3
  neurotica 694.0
  nummular NEC 692.9
  osteatosis, osteatotic 706.8

Dermatitis — *continued*
  papillaris capillitii 706.1
  pellagrous 265.2
  perioral 695.3
  perstans 696.1
  photosensitivity (sun) 692.72
    other light 692.82
  pigmented purpuric lichenoid 709.1
  polymorpha dolorosa 694.0
  primary irritant 692.9
  pruriginosa 694.0
  pruritic NEC 692.9
  psoriasiform nodularis 696.2
  psychogenic 316
  purulent 686.00
  pustular contagious 051.2
  pyococcal 686.00
  pyocyaneus 686.09
  pyogenica 686.00
  radiation 692.82
  repens 696.1
  Ritter's (exfoliativa) 695.81
  Schamberg's (progressive pigmentary dermatosis) 709.09
  schistosome 120.3
  seasonal bullous 694.8
  seborrheic 690.10
    infantile 690.12
  sensitization NEC 692.9
  septic (*see also* Septicemia) 686.00
    gonococcal 098.89
  solar, solare NEC (*see also* Dermatitis, due to, sun) 692.70
  stasis 454.1
    due to
      postphlebitic syndrome 459.12
        with ulcer 459.13
      varicose veins — *see* Varicose
    ulcerated or with ulcer (varicose) 454.2
  sunburn (*see also* Sunburn) 692.71
  suppurative 686.00
  traumatic NEC 709.8
  trophoneurotica 694.0
  ultraviolet, except from sun 692.82
    due to sun NEC (*see also* Dermatitis, due to, sun) 692.82
  varicose 454.1
    with ulcer 454.2
  vegetans 686.8
  verrucosa 117.2
  xerotic 706.8
Dermatoarthritis, lipoid 272.8 *[713.0]*
Dermatochalasia, dermatochalasis 374.87
Dermatofibroma (lenticulare) (M8832/0) — *see also* Neoplasm, skin, benign
  protuberans (M8832/1) — *see* Neoplasm, skin, uncertain behavior
Dermatofibrosarcoma (protuberans) (M8832/3) — *see* Neoplasm, skin, malignant
Dermatographia 708.3
Dermatolysis (congenital) (exfoliativa) 757.39
  acquired 701.8
  eyelids 374.34
  palpebrarum 374.34
  senile 701.8
Dermatomegaly NEC 701.8
Dermatomucomyositis 710.3
Dermatomycosis 111.9
  furfuracea 111.0
  specified type NEC 111.8
Dermatomyositis (acute) (chronic) 710.3
Dermatoneuritis of children 985.0
Dermatophiliasis 134.1
Dermatophytide — *see* Dermatophytosis
Dermatophytosis (Epidermophyton) (infection) (microsporum) (tinea) (Trichophyton) 110.9
  beard 110.0
  body 110.5
  deep seated 110.6
  fingernails 110.1
  foot 110.4
  groin 110.3
  hand 110.2
  nail 110.1

Dermatophytosis — *continued*
  perianal (area) 110.3
  scalp 110.0
  scrotal 110.8
  specified site NEC 110.8
  toenails 110.1
  vulva 110.8
Dermatopolyneuritis 985.0
Dermatorrhexis 756.83
  acquired 701.8
Dermatosclerosis — *see also* Scleroderma 710.1
  localized 701.0
Dermatosis 709.9
  Andrews' 686.8
  atopic 691.8
  Bowen's (M8081/2) — *see* Neoplasm, skin, in situ
  bullous 694.9
    specified type NEC 694.8
  erythematosquamous 690.8
  exfoliativa 695.89
  factitial 698.4
  gonococcal 098.89
  herpetiformis 694.0
    juvenile 694.2
    senile 694.5
  hysterical 300.11
  linear IgA 694.8
  menstrual NEC 709.8
  neutrophilic, acute febrile 695.89
  occupational (*see also* Dermatitis) 692.9
  papulosa nigra 709.8
  pigmentary NEC 709.00
    progressive 709.09
    Schamberg's 709.09
    Siemens-Bloch 757.33
  progressive pigmentary 709.09
  psychogenic 316
  pustular subcorneal 694.1
  Schamberg's (progressive pigmentary) 709.09
  senile NEC 709.3
  specified NEC 702.8
  Unna's (seborrheic dermatitis) 690.10
Dermographia 708.3
Dermographism 708.3
Dermoid (cyst) (M9084/0) — *see also* Neoplasm, by site, benign
  with malignant transformation (M9084/3) 183.0
Dermopathy
  infiltrative, with thyrotoxicosis 242.0 ☑
  nephrogenic fibrosing 701.8
  senile NEC 709.3
Dermophytosis — *see* Dermatophytosis
Descemet's membrane — *see* condition
Descemetocele 371.72
Descending — *see* condition
Descensus uteri (complete) (incomplete) (partial) (without vaginal wall prolapse) 618.1
  with mention of vaginal wall prolapse — *see* Prolapse, uterovaginal
Desensitization to allergens V07.1
Desert
  rheumatism 114.0
  sore (*see also* Ulcer, skin) 707.9
Desertion (child) (newborn) 995.52
  adult 995.84
Desmoid (extra-abdominal) (tumor) (M8821/1) — *see also* Neoplasm, connective tissue, uncertain behavior
  abdominal (M8822/1) — *see* Neoplasm, connective tissue, uncertain behavior
Despondency 300.4
Desquamative dermatitis NEC 695.89
Destruction
  articular facet (*see also* Derangement, joint) 718.9 ☑
    vertebra 724.9
  bone 733.90
    syphilitic 095.5
  joint (*see also* Derangement, joint) 718.9 ☑
    sacroiliac 724.6
  kidney 593.89

☑ **Additional Digit Required — Refer to the Tabular List for Digit Selection**   ⫧ **Subterms under main terms may continue to next column or page**

2011 ICD-9-CM   ▶◀ Revised Text   ● New Line   ▲ Revised Code   **Volume 2 — 77**

Destruction — *continued*
  live fetus to facilitate birth NEC 763.89
  ossicles (ear) 385.24
  rectal sphincter 569.49
  septum (nasal) 478.19
  tuberculous NEC (*see also* Tuberculosis)
      011.9 ☑
  tympanic membrane 384.82
  tympanum 385.89
  vertebral disc — *see* Degeneration, intervertebral disc
Destructiveness — *see also* Disturbance, conduct 312.9
  adjustment reaction 309.3
Detachment
  cartilage (*see also* Sprain, by site)
    knee — *see* Tear, meniscus
  cervix, annular 622.8
    complicating delivery 665.3 ☑
  choroid (old) (postinfectional) (simple)
      (spontaneous) 363.70
    hemorrhagic 363.72
    serous 363.71
  knee, medial meniscus (old) 717.3
    current injury 836.0
  ligament — *see* Sprain, by site
  placenta (premature) — *see* Placenta, separation
  retina (recent) 361.9
    with retinal defect (rhegmatogenous)
        361.00
      giant tear 361.03
      multiple 361.02
      partial
        with
            giant tear 361.03
            multiple defects 361.02
            retinal dialysis (juvenile)
                361.04
            single defect 361.01
        retinal dialysis (juvenile) 361.04
        single 361.01
        subtotal 361.05
        total 361.05
    delimited (old) (partial) 361.06
    old
      delimited 361.06
      partial 361.06
      total or subtotal 361.07
    pigment epithelium (RPE) (serous)
        362.42
      exudative 362.42
      hemorrhagic 362.43
    rhegmatogenous (*see also* Detachment,
        retina, with retinal defect) 361.00
    serous (without retinal defect) 361.2
    specified type NEC 361.89
    traction (with vitreoretinal organization)
        361.81
  vitreous humor 379.21
Detergent asthma 507.8
Deterioration
  epileptic
    with behavioral disturbance
        345.9 ☑ [294.11]
    without behavioral disturbance
        345.9 ☑ [294.10]
  heart, cardiac (*see also* Degeneration, myocardial) 429.1
  mental (*see also* Psychosis) 298.9
  myocardium, myocardial (*see also* Degeneration, myocardial) 429.1
  senile (simple) 797
  transplanted organ — *see* Complications,
      transplant, organ, by site
de Toni-Fanconi syndrome (cystinosis) 270.0
Deuteranomaly 368.52
Deuteranopia (anomalous trichromat) (complete) (incomplete) 368.52
Deutschländer's disease — *see* Fracture, foot
Development
  abnormal, bone 756.9
  arrested 783.40
    bone 733.91
    child 783.40

Development — *continued*
  arrested — *continued*
    due to malnutrition (protein-calorie)
        263.2
    fetus or newborn 764.9 ☑
    tracheal rings (congenital) 748.3
  defective, congenital (*see also* Anomaly)
    cauda equina 742.59
    left ventricle 746.9
      with atresia or hypoplasia of aortic
          orifice or valve with hypoplasia of ascending aorta 746.7
      in hypoplastic left heart syndrome
          746.7
  delayed (*see also* Delay, development)
      783.40
    arithmetical skills 315.1
    language (skills) 315.31
      and speech due to hearing loss
          315.34
      expressive 315.31
      mixed receptive-expressive 315.32
    learning skill, specified NEC 315.2
    mixed skills 315.5
    motor coordination 315.4
    reading 315.00
    specified
      learning skill NEC 315.2
      type NEC, except learning 315.8
    speech 315.39
      and language due to hearing loss
          315.34
      associated with hyperkinesia 314.1
      phonological 315.39
    spelling 315.09
    written expression 315.2
  imperfect, congenital (*see also* Anomaly)
    heart 746.9
    lungs 748.60
  improper (fetus or newborn) 764.9 ☑
  incomplete (fetus or newborn) 764.9 ☑
    affecting management of pregnancy
        656.5 ☑
    bronchial tree 748.3
    organ or site not listed — *see* Hypoplasia
    respiratory system 748.9
  sexual, precocious NEC 259.1
  tardy, mental (*see also* Retardation, mental)
      319
Developmental — *see* condition
Devergie's disease (pityriasis rubra pilaris)
    696.4
Deviation
  conjugate (eye) 378.87
    palsy 378.81
    spasm, spastic 378.82
  esophagus 530.89
  eye, skew 378.87
  mandible, opening and closing 524.53
  midline (jaw) (teeth) 524.29
    specified site NEC — *see* Malposition
  occlusal plane 524.76
  organ or site, congenital NEC — *see* Malposition, congenital
  septum (acquired) (nasal) 470
    congenital 754.0
  sexual 302.9
    bestiality 302.1
    coprophilia 302.89
    ego-dystonic
      homosexuality 302.0
      lesbianism 302.0
    erotomania 302.89
      Clérambault's 297.8
    exhibitionism (sexual) 302.4
    fetishism 302.81
      transvestic 302.3
    frotteurism 302.89
    homosexuality, ego-dystonic 302.0
      pedophilic 302.2
    lesbianism, ego-dystonic 302.0
    masochism 302.83
    narcissism 302.89
    necrophilia 302.89
    nymphomania 302.89
    pederosis 302.2

Deviation — *continued*
  sexual — *continued*
    pedophilia 302.2
    sadism 302.84
    sadomasochism 302.84
    satyriasis 302.89
    specified type NEC 302.89
    transvestic fetishism 302.3
    transvestism 302.3
    voyeurism 302.82
    zoophilia (erotica) 302.1
  teeth, midline 524.29
  trachea 519.19
  ureter (congenital) 753.4
Devic's disease 341.0
Device
  cerebral ventricle (communicating) in situ
      V45.2
  contraceptive — *see* Contraceptive, device
  drainage, cerebrospinal fluid V45.2
Devil's
  grip 074.1
  pinches (purpura simplex) 287.2
Devitalized tooth 522.9
Devonshire colic 984.9
  specified type of lead — *see* Table of Drugs
      and Chemicals
Dextraposition, aorta 747.21
  with ventricular septal defect, pulmonary
      stenosis or atresia, and hypertrophy
      of right ventricle 745.2
  in tetralogy of Fallot 745.2
Dextratransposition, aorta 745.11
Dextrinosis, limit (debrancher enzyme deficiency) 271.0
Dextrocardia (corrected) (false) (isolated)
    (secondary) (true) 746.87
  with
    complete transposition of viscera 759.3
    situs inversus 759.3
Dextroversion, kidney (left) 753.3
Dhobie itch 110.3
DHTR (delayed hemolytic transfusion reaction) — *see* Complications, transfusion ●
Diabetes, diabetic (brittle) (congenital) (familial) (mellitus) (severe) (slight) (without
    complication) 250.0 ☑

> *Note* — Use the following fifth-digit
> subclassification with category 250:
>
> 0   type II or unspecified type, not
>   stated as uncontrolled
>
> *Fifth-digit 0 is for use for type II patients, even if the patient requires insulin*
>
> 1   type I [juvenile type], not stated
>   as uncontrolled
>
> 2   type II or unspecified type, uncontrolled
>
> *Fifth-digit 2 is for use for type II patients, even if the patient requires insulin*
>
> 3   type I [juvenile type], uncontrolled

  with
    coma (with ketoacidosis) 250.3 ☑
      due to secondary diabetes 249.3 ☑
      hyperosmolar (nonketotic) 250.2 ☑
        due to secondary diabetes
            249.2 ☑
    complication NEC 250.9 ☑
      due to secondary diabetes 249.9 ☑
      specified NEC 250.8 ☑
        due to secondary diabetes
            249.8 ☑
    gangrene 250.7 ☑ [785.4]
      due to secondary diabetes
          249.7 ☑ [785.4]
    hyperglycemia — code to Diabetes, by
        type, with 5th digit for not stated
        as uncontrolled
    hyperosmolarity 250.2 ☑
      due to secondary diabetes 249.2 ☑
    ketosis, ketoacidosis 250.1 ☑
      due to secondary diabetes 249.1 ☑

Diabetes, diabetic — *continued*
  with — *continued*
    loss of protective sensation (LOPS) — ●
      see Diabetes, neuropathy   ●
    osteomyelitis 250.8 ☑ [731.8]
      due to secondary diabetes
          249.8 ☑ [731.8]
    specified manisfestations NEC 250.8 ☑
      due to secondary diabetes 249.8 ☑
  acetonemia 250.1 ☑
    due to secondary diabetes 249.1 ☑
  acidosis 250.1 ☑
    due to secondary diabetes 249.1 ☑
  amyotrophy 250.6 ☑ [353.5]
    due to secondary diabetes
        249.6 ☑ [353.5]
  angiopathy, peripheral 250.7 ☑ [443.81]
    due to secondary diabetes
        249.7 ☑ [443.81]
  asymptomatic 790.29
  autonomic neuropathy (peripheral)
      250.6 ☑ [337.1]
    due to secondary diabetes
        249.6 ☑ [337.1]
  bone change 250.8 ☑ [731.8]
    due to secondary diabetes
        249.8 ☑ [731.8]
  bronze, bronzed 275.01   ▲
  cataract 250.5 ☑ [366.41]
    due to secondary diabetes
        249.5 ☑ [366.41]
  chemical induced — *see* Diabetes, secondary
  complicating pregnancy, childbirth, or
      puerperium 648.0 ☑
  coma (with ketoacidosis) 250.3 ☑
    due to secondary diabetes 249.3 ☑
    hyperglycemic 250.3 ☑
      due to secondary diabetes 249.3 ☑
    hyperosmolar (nonketotic) 250.2 ☑
      due to secondary diabetes 249.2 ☑
    hypoglycemic 250.3 ☑
      due to secondary diabetes 249.3 ☑
    insulin 250.3 ☑
      due to secondary diabetes 249.3 ☑
  complicating pregnancy, childbirth, or
      puerperium (maternal) (conditions
      classifiable to 249 and 250) 648.0 ☑
    affecting fetus or newborn 775.0
  complication NEC 250.9 ☑
    due to secondary diabetes 249.9 ☑
    specified NEC 250.8 ☑
      due to secondary diabetes 249.8 ☑
  dorsal sclerosis 250.6 ☑ [340]
    due to secondary diabetes
        249.6 ☑ [340]
  drug-induced — *see also* Diabetes, secondary
    overdose or wrong substance given or
        taken — *see* Table of Drugs and
        Chemicals
  due to
    cystic fibrosis — *see* Diabetes, secondary
    infection — *see* Diabetes, secondary
  dwarfism-obesity syndrome 258.1
  gangrene 250.7 ☑ [785.4]
    due to secondary diabetes
        249.7 ☑ [785.4]
  gastroparesis 250.6 ☑ [536.3]
    due to secondary diabetes
        249.6 ☑ [536.3]
  gestational 648.8 ☑
    complicating pregnancy, childbirth, or
        puerperium 648.8 ☑
  glaucoma 250.5 ☑ [365.44]
    due to secondary diabetes
        249.5 ☑ [365.44]
  glomerulosclerosis (intercapillary)
      250.4 ☑ [581.81]
    due to secondary diabetes
        249.4 ☑ [581.81]
  glycogenosis, secondary 250.8 ☑ [259.8]
    due to secondary diabetes
        249.8 ☑ [259.8]

Diabetes, diabetic — *continued*
hemochromatosis ▶(*see also* Hemochromatosis)◀ 275.03 ▲
hyperosmolar coma 250.2 ☑
  due to secondary diabetes 249.2 ☑
hyperosmolarity 250.2 ☑
  due to secondary diabetes 249.2 ☑
hypertension-nephrosis syndrome 250.4 ☑ [581.81]
  due to secondary diabetes 249.4 ☑ [581.81]
hypoglycemia 250.8 ☑
  due to secondary diabetes 249.8 ☑
hypoglycemic shock 250.8 ☑
  due to secondary diabetes 249.8 ☑
inadequately controlled — code to Diabetes, by type, with 5th digit for not stated as uncontrolled
insipidus 253.5
  nephrogenic 588.1
  pituitary 253.5
  vasopressin-resistant 588.1
intercapillary glomerulosclerosis 250.4 ☑ [581.81]
  due to secondary diabetes 249.4 ☑ [581.81]
iritis 250.5 ☑ [364.42]
  due to secondary diabetes 249.5 ☑ [364.42]
ketosis, ketoacidosis 250.1 ☑
  due to secondary diabetes 249.1 ☑
Kimmelstiel (-Wilson) disease or syndrome (intercapillary glomerulosclerosis) 250.4 ☑ [581.81]
  due to secondary diabetes 249.4 ☑ [581.81]
Lancereaux's (diabetes mellitus with marked emaciation) 250.8 ☑ [261]
  due to secondary diabetes 249.8 ☑ [261]
latent (chemical) — *see* Diabetes, secondary
complicating pregnancy, childbirth, or puerperium 648.0 ☑
lipoidosis 250.8 ☑ [272.7]
  due to secondary diabetes 249.8 ☑ [272.7]
macular edema 250.5 ☑ [362.07]
  due to secondary diabetes 249.5 ☑ [362.07]
maternal
  with manifest disease in the infant 775.1
  affecting fetus or newborn 775.0
microaneurysms, retinal 250.5 ☑ [362.01]
  due to secondary diabetes 249.5 ☑ [362.01]
mononeuropathy 250.6 ☑ [355.9]
  due to secondary diabetes 249.6 ☑ [355.9]
neonatal, transient 775.1
nephropathy 250.4 ☑ [583.81]
  due to secondary diabetes 249.4 ☑ [583.81]
nephrosis (syndrome) 250.4 ☑ [581.81]
  due to secondary diabetes 249.4 ☑ [581.81]
neuralgia 250.6 ☑ [357.2]
  due to secondary diabetes 249.6 ☑ [357.2]
neuritis 250.6 ☑ [357.2]
  due to secondary diabetes 249.6 ☑ [357.2]
neurogenic arthropathy 250.6 ☑ [713.5]
  due to secondary diabetes 249.6 ☑ [713.5]
neuropathy 250.6 ☑ [357.2]
  autonomic (peripheral) 250.6 ☑ [337.1]
    due to secondary diabetes 249.6 ☑ [337.1]
  due to secondary diabetes 249.6 ☑ [357.2]
nonclinical 790.29
osteomyelitis 250.8 ☑ [731.8]
  due to secondary diabetes 249.8 ☑ [731.8]

Diabetes, diabetic — *continued*
out of control — code to Diabetes, by type, with 5th digit for uncontrolled
peripheral autonomic neuropathy 250.6 ☑ [337.1]
  due to secondary diabetes 249.6 ☑ [337.1]
phosphate 275.3
polyneuropathy 250.6 ☑ [357.2]
  due to secondary diabetes 249.6 ☑ [357.2]
poorly controlled — code to Diabetes, by type, with 5th digit for not stated as uncontrolled
renal (true) 271.4
retinal
  edema 250.5 ☑ [362.07]
    due to secondary diabetes 249.5 ☑ [362.07]
  hemorrhage 250.5 ☑ [362.01]
    due to secondary diabetes 249.5 ☑ [362.01]
  microaneurysms 250.5 ☑ [362.01]
    due to secondary diabetes 249.5 ☑ [362.01]
retinitis 250.5 ☑ [362.01]
  due to secondary diabetes 249.5 ☑ [362.01]
retinopathy 250.5 ☑ [362.01]
  background 250.5 ☑ [362.01]
    due to secondary diabetes 249.5 ☑ [362.01]
  due to secondary diabetes 249.5 ☑ [362.01]
  nonproliferative 250.5 ☑ [362.03]
    due to secondary diabetes 249.5 ☑ [362.03]
    mild 250.5 ☑ [362.04]
      due to secondary diabetes 249.5 ☑ [362.04]
    moderate 250.5 ☑ [362.05]
      due to secondary diabetes 249.5 ☑ [362.05]
    severe 250.5 ☑ [362.06]
      due to secondary diabetes 249.5 ☑ [362.06]
  proliferative 250.5 ☑ [362.02]
    due to secondary diabetes 249.5 ☑ [362.02]
secondary (chemical-induced) (due to chronic condition) (due to infection) (drug-induced) 249.0 ☑
  with
    coma (with ketoacidosis) 249.3 ☑
      hyperosmolar (nonketotic) 249.2 ☑
    complication NEC 249.9 ☑
      specified NEC 249.8 ☑
    gangrene 249.7 ☑ [785.4]
    hyperosmolarity 249.2 ☑
    ketosis, ketoacidosis 249.1 ☑
    osteomyelitis 249.8 ☑ [731.8]
    specified manifestations NEC 249.8 ☑
  acetonemia 249.1 ☑
  acidosis 249.1 ☑
  amyotrophy 249.6 ☑ [353.5]
  angiopathy, peripheral 249.7 ☑ [443.81]
  autonomic neuropathy (peripheral) 249.6 ☑ [337.1]
  bone change 249.8 ☑ [731.8]
  cataract 249.5 ☑ [366.41]
  coma (with ketoacidosis) 249.3 ☑
    hyperglycemic 249.3 ☑
    hyperosmolar (nonketotic) 249.2 ☑
    hypoglycemic 249.3 ☑
    insulin 249.3 ☑
  complicating pregnancy, childbirth, or puerperium (maternal) 648.0 ☑
    affecting fetus or newborn 775.0
  complication NEC 249.9 ☑
    specified NEC 249.8 ☑
  dorsal sclerosis 249.6 ☑ [340]

Diabetes, diabetic — *continued*
secondary — *continued*
  due to overdose or wrong substance given or taken — *see* Table of Drugs and Chemicals
  gangrene 249.7 ☑ [785.4]
  gastroparesis 249.6 ☑ [536.3]
  glaucoma 249.5 ☑ [365.44]
  glomerulosclerosis (intercapillary) 249.4 ☑ [581.81]
  glycogenosis, secondary 249.8 ☑ [259.8]
  hyperosmolar coma 249.2 ☑
  hyperosmolarity 249.2 ☑
  hypertension-nephrosis syndrome 249.4 ☑ [581.81]
  hypoglycemia 249.8 ☑
  hypoglycemic shock 249.8 ☑
  intercapillary glomerulosclerosis 249.4 ☑ [581.81]
  iritis 249.5 ☑ [364.42]
  ketosis, ketoacidosis 249.1 ☑
  Kimmelstiel (-Wilson) disease or syndrome (intercapillary glomerulosclerosis) 249.4 ☑ [581.81]
  Lancereaux's (diabetes mellitus with marked emaciation) 249.8 ☑ [261]
  lipoidosis 249.8 ☑ [272.7]
  macular edema 249.5 ☑ [362.07]
  maternal
    with manifest disease in the infant 775.1
    affecting fetus or newborn 775.0
  microaneurysms, retinal 249.5 ☑ [362.01]
  mononeuropathy 249.6 ☑ [355.9]
  nephropathy 249.4 ☑ [583.81]
  nephrosis (syndrome) 249.4 ☑ [581.81]
  neuralgia 249.6 ☑ [357.2]
  neuritis 249.6 ☑ [357.2]
  neurogenic arthropathy 249.6 ☑ [713.5]
  neuropathy 249.6 ☑ [357.2]
    autonomic (peripheral) 249.6 ☑ [337.1]
  osteomyelitis 249.8 ☑ [731.8]
  peripheral autonomic neuropathy 249.6 ☑ [337.1]
  polyneuropathy 249.6 ☑ [357.2]
  retinal
    edema 249.5 ☑ [362.07]
    hemorrhage 249.5 ☑ [362.01]
    microaneurysms 249.5 ☑ [362.01]
  retinitis 249.5 ☑ [362.01]
  retinopathy 249.5 ☑ [362.01]
    background 249.5 ☑ [362.01]
    nonproliferative 249.5 ☑ [362.03]
      mild 249.5 ☑ [362.04]
      moderate 249.5 ☑ [362.05]
      severe 249.5 ☑ [362.06]
    proliferative 249.5 ☑ [362.02]
  ulcer (skin) 249.8 ☑ [707.9]
    lower extemity 249.8 ☑ [707.10]
      ankle 249.8 ☑ [707.13]
      calf 249.8 ☑ [707.12]
      foot 249.8 ☑ [707.15]
      heel 249.8 ☑ [707.14]
      knee 249.8 ☑ [707.19]
      specified site NEC 249.8 ☑ [707.19]
      thigh 249.8 ☑ [707.11]
      toes 249.8 ☑ [707.15]
    specified site NEC 249.8 ☑ [707.8]
  xanthoma 249.8 ☑ [272.2]
  steroid induced — *see also* Diabetes, secondary
    overdose or wrong substance given or taken 962.0
stress 790.29
subclinical 790.29
subliminal 790.29
sugar 250.0 ☑
ulcer (skin) 250.8 ☑ [707.9]
  due to secondary diabetes 249.8 ☑ [707.9]

Diabetes, diabetic — *continued*
ulcer — *continued*
  lower extremity 250.8 ☑ [707.10]
    ankle 250.8 ☑ [707.13]
      due to secondary diabetes 249.8 ☑ [707.13]
    calf 250.8 ☑ [707.12]
      due to secondary diabetes 249.8 ☑ [707.12]
    foot 250.8 ☑ [707.15]
      due to secondary diabetes 249.8 ☑ [707.15]
    heel 250.8 ☑ [707.14]
      due to secondary diabetes 249.8 ☑ [707.14]
    knee 250.8 ☑ [707.19]
      due to secondary diabetes 249.8 ☑ [707.19]
    specified site NEC 250.8 ☑ [707.19]
      due to secondary diabetes 249.8 ☑ [707.19]
    thigh 250.8 ☑ [707.11]
      due to secondary diabetes 249.8 ☑ [707.11]
    toes 250.8 ☑ [707.15]
      due to secondary diabetes 249.8 ☑ [707.15]
  specified site NEC 250.8 ☑ [707.8]
    due to secondary diabetes 249.8 ☑ [707.8]
  xanthoma 250.8 ☑ [272.2]
    due to secondary diabetes 249.8 ☑ [272.2]
Diacyclothrombopathia 287.1
Diagnosis deferred 799.9
Dialysis (intermittent) (treatment)
anterior retinal (juvenile) (with detachment) 361.04
extracorporeal V56.0
hemodialysis V56.0
  status only V45.11
peritoneal V56.8
  status only V45.11
renal V56.0
  status only V45.11
specified type NEC V56.8
Diamond-Blackfan anemia or syndrome (congenital hypoplastic anemia) 284.01
Diamond-Gardener syndrome (autoerythrocyte sensitization) 287.2
Diaper rash 691.0
Diaphoresis (excessive) NEC — *see also* Hyperhidrosis) 780.8
Diaphragm — *see* condition
Diaphragmalgia 786.52
Diaphragmitis 519.4
Diaphyseal aclasis 756.4
Diaphysitis 733.99
Diarrhea, diarrheal (acute) (autumn) (bilious) (bloody) (catarrhal) (choleraic) (chronic) (gravis) (green) (infantile) (lienteric) (noninfectious) (presumed noninfectious) (putrefactive) (secondary) (sporadic) (summer) (symptomatic) (thermic) 787.91
achlorhydric 536.0
allergic 558.3
amebic (*see also* Amebiasis) 006.9
  with abscess — *see* Abscess, amebic
  acute 006.0
  chronic 006.1
  nondysenteric 006.2
bacillary — *see* Dysentery, bacillary
bacterial NEC 008.5
balantidial 007.0
bile salt-induced 579.8
cachectic NEC 787.91
chilomastix 007.8
choleriformis 001.1
coccidial 007.2
Cochin-China 579.1
  anguilluliasis 127.2
  psilosis 579.1
Dientamoeba 007.8

Index

Diarrhea, diarrheal — Diplegia

Diarrhea, diarrheal — *continued*
dietetic 787.91
due to
achylia gastrica 536.8
Aerobacter aerogenes 008.2
Bacillus coli — *see* Enteritis, E. coli
bacteria NEC 008.5
bile salts 579.8
Capillaria
hepatica 128.8
philippinensis 127.5
Clostridium perfringens (C) (F) 008.46
Enterobacter aerogenes 008.2
enterococci 008.49
Escherichia coli — *see* Enteritis, E. coli
Giardia lamblia 007.1
Heterophyes heterophyes 121.6
irritating foods 787.91
Metagonimus yokogawai 121.5
Necator americanus 126.1
Paracolobactrum arizonae 008.1
Paracolon bacillus NEC 008.47
Arizona 008.1
Proteus (bacillus) (mirabilis) (Morganii) 008.3
Pseudomonas aeruginosa 008.42
S. japonicum 120.2
specified organism NEC 008.8
bacterial 008.49
viral NEC 008.69
Staphylococcus 008.41
Streptococcus 008.49
anaerobic 008.46
Strongyloides stercoralis 127.2
Trichuris trichiuria 127.3
virus NEC (*see also* Enteritis, viral) 008.69
dysenteric 009.2
due to specified organism NEC 008.8
dyspeptic 787.91
endemic 009.3
due to specified organism NEC 008.8
epidemic 009.2
due to specified organism NEC 008.8
fermentative 787.91
flagellate 007.9
Flexner's (ulcerative) 004.1
functional 564.5
following gastrointestinal surgery 564.4
psychogenic 306.4
giardial 007.1
Giardia lamblia 007.1
hill 579.1
hyperperistalsis (nervous) 306.4
infectious 009.2
due to specified organism NEC 008.8
presumed 009.3
inflammatory 787.91
due to specified organism NEC 008.8
malarial (*see also* Malaria) 084.6
mite 133.8
mycotic 117.9
nervous 306.4
neurogenic 564.5
parenteral NEC 009.2
postgastrectomy 564.4
postvagotomy 564.4
prostaglandin induced 579.8
protozoal NEC 007.9
psychogenic 306.4
septic 009.2
due to specified organism NEC 008.8
specified organism NEC 008.8
bacterial 008.49
viral NEC 008.69
Staphylococcus 008.41
Streptococcus 008.49
anaerobic 008.46
toxic 558.2
travelers' 009.2
due to specified organism NEC 008.8
trichomonal 007.3
tropical 579.1
tuberculous 014.8 ☑
ulcerative (chronic) (*see also* Colitis, ulcerative) 556.9
viral (*see also* Enteritis, viral) 008.8

Diarrhea, diarrheal — *continued*
zymotic NEC 009.2
Diastasis
cranial bones 733.99
congenital 756.0
joint (traumatic) — *see* Dislocation, by site
muscle 728.84
congenital 756.89
recti (abdomen) 728.84
complicating delivery 665.8 ☑
congenital 756.79
Diastema, teeth, tooth 524.30
Diastematomyelia 742.51
Diataxia, cerebral, infantile 343.0
Diathesis
allergic V15.09
bleeding (familial) 287.9
cystine (familial) 270.0
gouty 274.9
hemorrhagic (familial) 287.9
newborn NEC 776.0
oxalic 271.8
scrofulous (*see also* Tuberculosis) 017.2 ☑
spasmophilic (*see also* Tetany) 781.7
ulcer 536.9
uric acid 274.9
Diaz's disease or osteochondrosis 732.5
Dibothriocephaliasis 123.4
larval 123.5
Dibothriocephalus (infection) (infestation) (latus) 123.4
larval 123.5
Dicephalus 759.4
Dichotomy, teeth 520.2
Dichromat, dichromata (congenital) 368.59
Dichromatopsia (congenital) 368.59
Dichuchwa 104.0
Dicrocoeliasis 121.8
Didelphys, didelphic — *see also* Double uterus 752.2
Didymitis — *see also* Epididymitis 604.90
Died — *see also* Death
without
medical attention (cause unknown) 798.9
sign of disease 798.2
Dientamoeba diarrhea 007.8
Dietary
inadequacy or deficiency 269.9
surveillance and counseling V65.3
Dietl's crisis 593.4
Dieulafoy lesion (hemorrhagic)
of
duodenum 537.84
esophagus 530.82
intestine 569.86
stomach 537.84
Difficult
birth, affecting fetus or newborn 763.9
delivery NEC 669.9 ☑
Difficulty
feeding 783.3
adult 783.3
breast 676.8 ☑
child 783.3
elderly 783.3
infant 783.3
newborn 779.31
nonorganic (infant) NEC 307.59
mechanical, gastroduodenal stoma 537.89
reading 315.00
specific, spelling 315.09
swallowing (*see also* Dysphagia) 787.20
walking 719.7
Diffuse — *see* condition
Diffused ganglion 727.42
Di George's syndrome (thymic hypoplasia) 279.11
Digestive — *see* condition
Di Guglielmo's disease or syndrome (M9841/3) 207.0 ☑
Dihydropyrimidine dehydrogenase disease (DPD) 277.6 ●
Diktyoma (M9051/3) — *see* Neoplasm, by site, malignant
Dilaceration, tooth 520.4

Dilatation
anus 564.89
venule — *see* Hemorrhoids
aorta (focal) (general) (*see also* ▶Ectasia, aortic)◀ 447.70 ▲
with aneurysm 441.9 ●
congenital 747.29
infectional 093.0
ruptured 441.5
syphilitic 093.0
appendix (cystic) 543.9
artery 447.8
bile duct (common) (cystic) (congenital) 751.69
acquired 576.8
bladder (sphincter) 596.8
congenital 753.8
in pregnancy or childbirth 654.4 ☑
causing obstructed labor 660.2 ☑
affecting fetus or newborn 763.1
blood vessel 459.89
bronchus, bronchi 494.0
with acute exacerbation 494.1
calyx (due to obstruction) 593.89
capillaries 448.9
cardiac (acute) (chronic) (*see also* Hypertrophy, cardiac) 429.3
congenital 746.89
valve NEC 746.89
pulmonary 746.09
hypertensive (*see also* Hypertension, heart) 402.90
cavum septi pellucidi 742.4
cecum 564.89
psychogenic 306.4
cervix (uteri) (*see also* Incompetency, cervix)
incomplete, poor, slow
affecting fetus or newborn 763.7
complicating delivery 661.0 ☑
affecting fetus or newborn 763.7
colon 564.7
congenital 751.3
due to mechanical obstruction 560.89
psychogenic 306.4
common bile duct (congenital) 751.69
acquired 576.8
with calculus, choledocholithiasis, or stones — *see* Choledocholithiasis
cystic duct 751.69
acquired (any bile duct) 575.8
duct, mammary 610.4
duodenum 564.89
esophagus 530.89
congenital 750.4
due to
achalasia 530.0
cardiospasm 530.0
Eustachian tube, congenital 744.24
fontanel 756.0
gallbladder 575.8
congenital 751.69
gastric 536.8
acute 536.1
psychogenic 306.4
heart (acute) (chronic) (*see also* Hypertrophy, cardiac) 429.3
congenital 746.89
hypertensive (*see also* Hypertension, heart) 402.90
valve (*see also* Endocarditis)
congenital 746.89
ileum 564.89
psychogenic 306.4
inguinal rings — *see* Hernia, inguinal
jejunum 564.89
psychogenic 306.4
kidney (calyx) (collecting structures) (cystic) (parenchyma) (pelvis) 593.89
lacrimal passages 375.69
lymphatic vessel 457.1
mammary duct 610.4
Meckel's diverticulum (congenital) 751.0
meningeal vessels, congenital 742.8
myocardium (acute) (chronic) (*see also* Hypertrophy, cardiac) 429.3

Dilatation — *continued*
organ or site, congenital NEC — *see* Distortion
pancreatic duct 577.8
pelvis, kidney 593.89
pericardium — *see* Pericarditis
pharynx 478.29
prostate 602.8
pulmonary
artery (idiopathic) 417.8
congenital 747.3
valve, congenital 746.09
pupil 379.43
rectum 564.89
renal 593.89
saccule vestibularis, congenital 744.05
salivary gland (duct) 527.8
sphincter ani 564.89
stomach 536.8
acute 536.1
psychogenic 306.4
submaxillary duct 527.8
trachea, congenital 748.3
ureter (idiopathic) 593.89
congenital 753.20
due to obstruction 593.5
urethra (acquired) 599.84
vasomotor 443.9
vein 459.89
ventricular, ventricle (acute) (chronic) (*see also* Hypertrophy, cardiac) 429.3
cerebral, congenital 742.4
hypertensive (*see also* Hypertension, heart) 402.90
venule 459.89
anus — *see* Hemorrhoids
vesical orifice 596.8
Dilated, dilation — *see* Dilatation
Diminished
hearing (acuity) (*see also* Deafness) 389.9
pulse pressure 785.9
vision NEC 369.9
vital capacity 794.2
Diminuta taenia 123.6
Diminution, sense or sensation (cold) (heat) (tactile) (vibratory) — *see also* Disturbance, sensation 782.0
Dimitri-Sturge-Weber disease (encephalocutaneous angiomatosis) 759.6
Dimple
parasacral 685.1
with abscess 685.0
pilonidal 685.1
with abscess 685.0
postanal 685.1
with abscess 685.0
Dioctophyma renale (infection) (infestation) 128.8
Dipetalonemiasis 125.4
Diphallus 752.69
Diphtheria, diphtheritic (gangrenous) (hemorrhagic) 032.9
carrier (suspected) of V02.4
cutaneous 032.85
cystitis 032.84
faucial 032.0
infection of wound 032.85
inoculation (anti) (not sick) V03.5
laryngeal 032.3
myocarditis 032.82
nasal anterior 032.2
nasopharyngeal 032.1
neurological complication 032.89
peritonitis 032.83
specified site NEC 032.89
Diphyllobothriasis (intestine) 123.4
larval 123.5
Diplacusis 388.41
Diplegia (upper limbs) 344.2
brain or cerebral 437.8
congenital 343.0
facial 351.0
congenital 352.6
infantile or congenital (cerebral) (spastic) (spinal) 343.0
lower limbs 344.1

☑ **Additional Digit Required** — Refer to the Tabular List for Digit Selection   ▽ **Subterms under main terms may continue to next column or page**

Diplegia — continued
　syphilitic, congenital 090.49
Diplococcus, diplococcal — see condition
Diplomyelia 742.59
Diplopia 368.2
　refractive 368.15
Dipsomania — see also Alcoholism 303.9 ☑
　with psychosis (see also Psychosis, alcoholic)
　　291.9
Dipylidiasis 123.8
　intestine 123.8
Direction, teeth, abnormal 524.30
Dirt-eating child 307.52
Disability
　heart — see Disease, heart
　learning NEC 315.2
　special spelling 315.09
Disarticulation — see also Derangement, joint
　718.9 ☑
　meaning
　　amputation
　　　status — see Absence, by site
　　　traumatic — see Amputation, trau-
　　　　matic
　　dislocation, traumatic or congenital —
　　　see Dislocation
Disaster, cerebrovascular — see also Disease,
　cerebrovascular, acute 436
Discharge
　anal NEC 787.99
　breast (female) (male) 611.79
　conjunctiva 372.89
　continued locomotor idiopathic (see also
　　Epilepsy) 345.5 ☑
　diencephalic autonomic idiopathic (see also
　　Epilepsy) 345.5 ☑
　ear 388.60
　　blood 388.69
　　cerebrospinal fluid 388.61
　excessive urine 788.42
　eye 379.93
　nasal 478.19
　nipple 611.79
　patterned motor idiopathic (see also
　　Epilepsy) 345.5 ☑
　penile 788.7
　postnasal — see Sinusitis
　sinus, from mediastinum 510.0
　umbilicus 789.9
　urethral 788.7
　　bloody 599.84
　vaginal 623.5
Discitis 722.90
　cervical, cervicothoracic 722.91
　lumbar, lumbosacral 722.93
　thoracic, thoracolumbar 722.92
Discogenic syndrome — see Displacement,
　intervertebral disc
Discoid
　kidney 753.3
　meniscus, congenital 717.5
　semilunar cartilage 717.5
Discoloration
　mouth 528.9
　nails 703.8
　teeth 521.7
　　due to
　　　drugs 521.7
　　　metals (copper) (silver) 521.7
　　　pulpal bleeding 521.7
　　during formation 520.8
　　extrinsic 523.6
　　intrinsic posteruptive 521.7
Discomfort
　chest 786.59
　visual 368.13
Discomycosis — see Actinomycosis
Discontinuity, ossicles, ossicular chain
　385.23
Discrepancy
　centric occlusion
　　maximum intercuspation 524.55
　　of teeth 524.55
　leg length (acquired) 736.81
　　congenital 755.30
　uterine size-date 649.6 ☑

Discrimination
　political V62.4
　racial V62.4
　religious V62.4
　sex V62.4
Disease, diseased — see also Syndrome
　Abrami's (acquired hemolytic jaundice)
　　283.9
　absorbent system 459.89
　accumulation — see Thesaurismosis
　acid-peptic 536.8
　Acosta's 993.2
　Adams-Stokes (-Morgagni) (syncope with
　　heart block) 426.9
　Addison's (bronze) (primary adrenal insuffi-
　　ciency) 255.41
　　anemia (pernicious) 281.0
　　tuberculous (see also Tuberculosis)
　　　017.6 ☑
　Addison-Gull — see Xanthoma
　adenoids (and tonsils) (chronic) 474.9
　adrenal (gland) (capsule) (cortex) 255.9
　　hyperfunction 255.3
　　hypofunction 255.41
　　specified type NEC 255.8
　ainhum (dactylolysis spontanea) 136.0
　akamushi (scrub typhus) 081.2
　Akureyri (epidemic neuromyasthenia) 049.8
　Albarrán's (colibacilluria) 791.9
　Albers-Schönberg's (marble bones) 756.52
　Albert's 726.71
　Albright (-Martin) (-Bantam) 275.49
　Alibert's (mycosis fungoides) (M9700/3)
　　202.1 ☑
　Alibert-Bazin (M9700/3) 202.1 ☑
　alimentary canal 569.9
　alligator skin (ichthyosis congenita) 757.1
　　acquired 701.1
　Almeida's (Brazilian blastomycosis) 116.1
　Alpers' 330.8
　alpine 993.2
　altitude 993.2
　alveoli, teeth 525.9
　Alzheimer's — see Alzheimer's
　amyloid (any site) 277.30
　anarthritic rheumatoid 446.5
　Anders' (adiposis tuberosa simplex) 272.8
　Andersen's (glycogenosis IV) 271.0
　Anderson's (angiokeratoma corporis dif-
　　fusum) 272.7
　Andes 993.2
　Andrews' (bacterid) 686.8
　angiospastic, angiospasmodic 443.9
　　cerebral 435.9
　　　with transient neurologic deficit
　　　　435.9
　　vein 459.89
　anterior
　　chamber 364.9
　　horn cell 335.9
　　　specified type NEC 335.8
　antral (chronic) 473.0
　　acute 461.0
　anus NEC 569.49
　aorta (nonsyphilitic) 447.9
　　syphilitic NEC 093.89
　aortic (heart) (valve) (see also Endocarditis,
　　aortic) 424.1
　apollo 077.4
　aponeurosis 726.90
　appendix 543.9
　aqueous (chamber) 364.9
　arc-welders' lung 503
　Armenian 277.31
　Arnold-Chiari (see also Spina bifida) 741.0 ☑
　arterial 447.9
　　occlusive (see also Occlusion, by site)
　　　444.22
　　　with embolus or thrombus — see
　　　　Occlusion, by site
　　　due to stricture or stenosis 447.1
　　　specified type NEC 447.8
　arteriocardiorenal (see also Hypertension,
　　cardiorenal) 404.90
　arteriolar (generalized) (obliterative) 447.9
　　specified type NEC 447.8

Disease, diseased — see also Syndrome —
　continued
　arteriorenal — see Hypertension, kidney
　arteriosclerotic (see also Arteriosclerosis)
　　cardiovascular 429.2
　　coronary — see Arteriosclerosis, coro-
　　　nary
　　heart — see Arteriosclerosis, coronary
　　vascular — see Arteriosclerosis
　artery 447.9
　　cerebral 437.9
　　coronary — see Arteriosclerosis, coro-
　　　nary
　　specified type NEC 447.8
　arthropod-borne NEC 088.9
　　specified type NEC 088.89
　Asboe-Hansen's (incontinentia pigmenti)
　　757.33
　atticoantral, chronic (with posterior or supe-
　　rior marginal perforation of ear
　　drum) 382.2
　auditory canal, ear 380.9
　Aujeszky's 078.89
　auricle, ear NEC 380.30
　Australian X 062.4
　autoimmune NEC 279.49
　　hemolytic (cold type) (warm type) 283.0
　　parathyroid 252.1
　　thyroid 245.2
　aviators' (see also Effect, adverse, high alti-
　　tude) 993.2
　ax(e)-grinders' 502
　Ayala's 756.89
　Ayerza's (pulmonary artery sclerosis with
　　pulmonary hypertension) 416.0
　Azorean (of the nervous system) 334.8
　Babington's (familial hemorrhagic telangiec-
　　tasia) 448.0
　back bone NEC 733.90
　bacterial NEC 040.89
　　zoonotic NEC 027.9
　　　specified type NEC 027.8
　Baehr-Schiffrin (thrombotic thrombocy-
　　topenic purpura) 446.6
　Baelz's (cheilitis glandularis apostematosa)
　　528.5
　Baerensprung's (eczema marginatum) 110.3
　Balfour's (chloroma) 205.3 ☑
　balloon (see also Effect, adverse, high alti-
　　tude) 993.2
　Baló's 341.1
　Bamberger (-Marie) (hypertrophic pul-
　　monary osteoarthropathy) 731.2
　Bang's (Brucella abortus) 023.1
　Bannister's 995.1
　Banti's (with cirrhosis) (with portal hyperten-
　　sion) — see Cirrhosis, liver
　Barcoo (see also Ulcer, skin) 707.9
　barium lung 503
　Barlow (-Möller) (infantile scurvy) 267
　barometer makers' 985.0
　Barraquer (-Simons) (progressive lipodystro-
　　phy) 272.6
　basal ganglia 333.90
　　degenerative NEC 333.0
　　specified NEC 333.89
　Basedow's (exophthalmic goiter) 242.0 ☑
　basement membrane NEC 583.89
　　with
　　　pulmonary hemorrhage (Goodpas-
　　　　ture's syndrome)
　　　　446.21 [583.81]
　Bateman's 078.0
　　purpura (senile) 287.2
　Batten's 330.1 [362.71]
　Batten-Mayou (retina) 330.1 [362.71]
　Batten-Steinert 359.21
　Battey 031.0
　Baumgarten-Cruveilhier (cirrhosis of liver)
　　571.5
　bauxite-workers' 503
　Bayle's (dementia paralytica) 094.1
　Bazin's (primary) (see also Tuberculosis)
　　017.1 ☑
　Beard's (neurasthenia) 300.5

Disease, diseased — see also Syndrome —
　continued
　Beau's (see also Degeneration, myocardial)
　　429.1
　Bechterew's (ankylosing spondylitis) 720.0
　Becker's
　　idiopathic mural endomyocardial dis-
　　　ease 425.2
　　myotonia congenita, recessive form
　　　359.22
　Begbie's (exophthalmic goiter) 242.0 ☑
　Behr's 362.50
　Beigel's (white piedra) 111.2
　Bekhterev's (ankylosing spondylitis) 720.0
　Bell's (see also Psychosis, affective) 296.0 ☑
　Bennett's (leukemia) 208.9 ☑
　Benson's 379.22
　Bergeron's (hysteroepilepsy) 300.11
　Berlin's 921.3
　Bernard-Soulier (thrombopathy) 287.1
　Bernhardt (-Roth) 355.1
　beryllium 503
　Besnier-Boeck (-Schaumann) (sarcoidosis)
　　135
　Best's 362.76
　Beurmann's (sporotrichosis) 117.1
　Bielschowsky (-Jansky) 330.1
　Biermer's (pernicious anemia) 281.0
　Biett's (discoid lupus erythematosus) 695.4
　bile duct (see also Disease, biliary) 576.9
　biliary (duct) (tract) 576.9
　　with calculus, choledocholithiasis, or
　　　stones — see Choledocholithiasis
　Billroth's (meningocele) (see also Spina bifi-
　　da) 741.9 ☑
　Binswanger's 290.12
　Bird's (oxaluria) 271.8
　bird fanciers' 495.2
　black lung 500
　bladder 596.9
　　specified NEC 596.8
　bleeder's 286.0
　Bloch-Sulzberger (incontinentia pigmenti)
　　757.33
　Blocq's (astasia-abasia) 307.9
　blood (-forming organs) 289.9
　　specified NEC 289.89
　　vessel 459.9
　Bloodgood's 610.1
　Blount's (tibia vara) 732.4
　blue 746.9
　Bodechtel-Guttmann (subacute sclerosing
　　panencephalitis) 046.2
　Boeck's (sarcoidosis) 135
　bone 733.90
　　fibrocystic NEC 733.29
　　　jaw 526.2
　　marrow 289.9
　　Paget's (osteitis deformans) 731.0
　　specified type NEC 733.99
　　von Recklinghausen's (osteitis fibrosa
　　　cystica) 252.01
　Bonfils' — see Disease, Hodgkin's
　Borna 062.9
　Bornholm (epidemic pleurodynia) 074.1
　Bostock's (see also Fever, hay) 477.9
　Bouchard's (myopathic dilatation of the
　　stomach) 536.1
　Bouillaud's (rheumatic heart disease) 391.9
　Bourneville (-Brissaud) (tuberous sclerosis)
　　759.5
　Bouveret (-Hoffmann) (paroxysmal tachycar-
　　dia) 427.2
　bowel 569.9
　　functional 564.9
　　　psychogenic 306.4
　Bowen's (M8081/2) — see Neoplasm, skin,
　　in situ
　Bozzolo's (multiple myeloma) (M9730/3)
　　203.0 ☑
　Bradley's (epidemic vomiting) 078.82
　Brailsford's 732.3
　　radius, head 732.3
　　tarsal, scaphoid 732.5
　Brailsford-Morquio (mucopolysaccharidosis
　　IV) 277.5

☑ **Additional Digit Required** — Refer to the Tabular List for Digit Selection　　　　　　☝ **Subterms under main terms may continue to next column or page**

2011 ICD-9-CM　　　　▶◀ **Revised Text**　　　● **New Line**　　　▲ **Revised Code**　　　**Volume 2 — 81**

Disease, diseased — Disease, diseased

Disease, diseased — *see also* Syndrome — *continued*

demyelinating, demyelinizating (brain stem) (central nervous system) 341.9
  multiple sclerosis 340
  specified NEC 341.8
de Quervain's (tendon sheath) 727.04
  thyroid (subacute granulomatous thyroiditis) 245.1
Dercum's (adiposis dolorosa) 272.8
Deutschländer's — *see* Fracture, foot
Devergie's (pityriasis rubra pilaris) 696.4
Devic's 341.0
diaphorase deficiency 289.7
diaphragm 519.4
diarrheal, infectious 009.2
diatomaceous earth 502
Diaz's (osteochondrosis astragalus) 732.5
digestive system 569.9
Di Guglielmo's (erythemic myelosis) (M9841/3) 207.0 ☑
Dimitri-Sturge-Weber (encephalocutaneous angiomatosis) 759.6
disc, degenerative — *see* Degeneration, intervertebral disc
discogenic (*see also* Disease, intervertebral disc) 722.90
diverticular — *see* Diverticula
Down's (mongolism) 758.0
Dubini's (electric chorea) 049.8
Dubois' (thymus gland) 090.5
Duchenne's 094.0
  locomotor ataxia 094.0
  muscular dystrophy 359.1
  paralysis 335.22
  pseudohypertrophy, muscles 359.1
Duchenne-Griesinger 359.1
ductless glands 259.9
Duhring's (dermatitis herpetiformis) 694.0
Dukes (-Filatov) 057.8
duodenum NEC 537.9
  specified NEC 537.89
Duplay's 726.2
Dupré's (meningism) 781.6
Dupuytren's (muscle contracture) 728.6
Durand-Nicolas-Favre (climatic bubo) 099.1
Duroziez's (congenital mitral stenosis) 746.5
Dutton's (trypanosomiasis) 086.9
Eales' 362.18
ear (chronic) (inner) NEC 388.9
  middle 385.9
    adhesive (*see also* Adhesions, middle ear) 385.10
    specified NEC 385.89
Eberth's (typhoid fever) 002.0
Ebstein's
  heart 746.2
  meaning diabetes 250.4 ☑ *[581.81]*
    due to secondary diabetes 249.4 ☑ *[581.81]*
Echinococcus (*see also* Echinococcus) 122.9
ECHO virus NEC 078.89
Economo's (encephalitis lethargica) 049.8
Eddowes' (brittle bones and blue sclera) 756.51
Edsall's 992.2
Eichstedt's (pityriasis versicolor) 111.0
Ellis-van Creveld (chondroectodermal dysplasia) 756.55
endocardium — *see* Endocarditis
endocrine glands or system NEC 259.9
  specified NEC 259.8
endomyocardial, idiopathic mural 425.2
Engelmann's (diaphyseal sclerosis) 756.59
Engel-von Recklinghausen (osteitis fibrosa cystica) 252.01
English (rickets) 268.0
Engman's (infectious eczematoid dermatitis) 690.8
enteroviral, enterovirus NEC 078.89
  central nervous system NEC 048
epidemic NEC 136.9
epididymis 608.9
epigastric, functional 536.9
  psychogenic 306.4
Erb (-Landouzy) 359.1

Disease, diseased — *see also* Syndrome — *continued*

Erb-Goldflam 358.00
Erdheim-Chester (ECD) 277.89
Erichsen's (railway spine) 300.16
esophagus 530.9
  functional 530.5
  psychogenic 306.4
Eulenburg's (congenital paramyotonia) 359.29
Eustachian tube 381.9
Evans' (thrombocytopenic purpura) 287.32
external auditory canal 380.9
extrapyramidal NEC 333.90
eye 379.90
  anterior chamber 364.9
  inflammatory NEC 364.3
  muscle 378.9
eyeball 360.9
eyelid 374.9
eyeworm of Africa 125.2
Fabry's (angiokeratoma corporis diffusum) 272.7
facial nerve (seventh) 351.9
  newborn 767.5
Fahr-Volhard (malignant nephrosclerosis) 403.00
fallopian tube, noninflammatory 620.9
  specified NEC 620.8
familial periodic 277.31
  paralysis 359.3
Fanconi's (congenital pancytopenia) 284.09
Farber's (disseminated lipogranulomatosis) 272.8
fascia 728.9
  inflammatory 728.9
Fauchard's (periodontitis) 523.40
Favre-Durand-Nicolas (climatic bubo) 099.1
Favre-Racouchot (elastoidosis cutanea nodularis) 701.8
Fede's 529.0
Feer's 985.0
Felix's (juvenile osteochondrosis, hip) 732.1
Fenwick's (gastric atrophy) 537.89
Fernels' (aortic aneurysm) 441.9
fibrocaseous, of lung (*see also* Tuberculosis, pulmonary) 011.9 ☑
fibrocystic (*see also* Fibrocystic, disease) newborn 277.01
Fiedler's (leptospiral jaundice) 100.0
fifth 057.0
Filatoff's (infectious mononucleosis) 075
Filatov's (infectious mononucleosis) 075
file-cutters' 984.9
  specified type of lead — *see* Table of Drugs and Chemicals
filterable virus NEC 078.89
fish skin 757.1
  acquired 701.1
Flajani (-Basedow) (exophthalmic goiter) 242.0 ☑
Flatau-Schilder 341.1
flax-dressers' 504
Fleischner's 732.3
flint 502
fluke — *see* Infestation, fluke
Følling's (phenylketonuria) 270.1
foot and mouth 078.4
foot process 581.3
Forbes' (glycogenosis III) 271.0
Fordyce's (ectopic sebaceous glands) (mouth) 750.26
Fordyce-Fox (apocrine miliaria) 705.82
Fothergill's
  meaning scarlatina anginosa 034.1
  neuralgia (*see also* Neuralgia, trigeminal) 350.1
Fournier's 608.83
fourth 057.8
Fox (-Fordyce) (apocrine miliaria) 705.82
Francis' (*see also* Tularemia) 021.9
Franklin's (heavy chain) 273.2
Frei's (climatic bubo) 099.1
Freiberg's (flattening metatarsal) 732.5
Friedländer's (endarteritis obliterans) — *see* Arteriosclerosis

Disease, diseased — *see also* Syndrome — *continued*

Friedreich's
  combined systemic or ataxia 334.0
  facial hemihypertrophy 756.0
  myoclonia 333.2
Fröhlich's (adiposogenital dystrophy) 253.8
Frommel's 676.6 ☑
frontal sinus (chronic) 473.1
  acute 461.1
Fuller's earth 502
fungus, fungous NEC 117.9
Gaisböck's (polycythemia hypertonica) 289.0
gallbladder 575.9
  congenital 751.60
Gamna's (siderotic splenomegaly) 289.51
Gamstorp's (adynamia episodica hereditaria) 359.3
Gandy-Nanta (siderotic splenomegaly) 289.51
Gannister (occupational) 502
Garré's (*see also* Osteomyelitis) 730.1 ☑
gastric (*see also* Disease, stomach) 537.9
gastroesophageal reflux (GERD) 530.81
gastrointestinal (tract) 569.9
  amyloid 277.39
  functional 536.9
    psychogenic 306.4
Gaucher's (adult) (cerebroside lipidosis) (infantile) 272.7
Gayet's (superior hemorrhagic polioencephalitis) 265.1
Gee (-Herter) (-Heubner) (-Thaysen) (nontropical sprue) 579.0
generalized neoplastic (M8000/6) 199.0
genital organs NEC
  female 629.9
    specified NEC 629.89
  male 608.9
Gerhardt's (erythromelalgia) 443.82
Gerlier's (epidemic vertigo) 078.81
Gibert's (pityriasis rosea) 696.3
Gibney's (perispondylitis) 720.9
Gierke's (glycogenosis I) 271.0
Gilbert's (familial nonhemolytic jaundice) 277.4
Gilchrist's (North American blastomycosis) 116.0
Gilford (-Hutchinson) (progeria) 259.8
Gilles de la Tourette's (motor-verbal tic) 307.23
Giovannini's 117.9
gland (lymph) 289.9
Glanzmann's (hereditary hemorrhagic thrombasthenia) 287.1
glassblowers' 527.1
Glénard's (enteroptosis) 569.89
Glisson's (*see also* Rickets) 268.0
glomerular
  membranous, idiopathic 581.1
  minimal change 581.3
glycogen storage (Andersen's) (Cori types 1-7) (Forbes') (McArdle-Schmid-Pearson') (Pompe's) (types I-VII) 271.0
  cardiac 271.0 *[425.7]*
  generalized 271.0
  glucose–6–phosphatase deficiency 271.0
  heart 271.0 *[425.7]*
  hepatorenal 271.0
  liver and kidneys 271.0
  myocardium 271.0 *[425.7]*
  von Gierke's (glycogenosis I) 271.0
Goldflam-Erb 358.00
Goldscheider's (epidermolysis bullosa) 757.39
Goldstein's (familial hemorrhagic telangiectasia) 448.0
gonococcal NEC 098.0
Goodall's (epidemic vomiting) 078.82
Gordon's (exudative enteropathy) 579.8
Gougerot's (trisymptomatic) 709.1
Gougerot-Carteaud (confluent reticulate papillomatosis) 701.8

Disease, diseased — *see also* Syndrome — *continued*

Gougerot-Hailey-Hailey (benign familial chronic pemphigus) 757.39
graft-versus-host 279.50
  acute 279.51
  on chronic 279.53
  chronic 279.52
grain-handlers' 495.8
Grancher's (splenopneumonia) — *see* Pneumonia
granulomatous (childhood) (chronic) 288.1
graphite lung 503
Graves' (exophthalmic goiter) 242.0 ☑
Greenfield's 330.0
green monkey 078.89
Griesinger's (*see also* Ancylostomiasis) 126.9
grinders' 502
Grisel's 723.5
Gruby's (tinea tonsurans) 110.0
Guertin's (electric chorea) 049.8
Guillain-Barré 357.0
Guinon's (motor-verbal tic) 307.23
Gull's (thyroid atrophy with myxedema) 244.8
Gull and Sutton's — *see* Hypertension, kidney
gum NEC 523.9
Günther's (congenital erythropoietic porphyria) 277.1
gynecological 629.9
  specified NEC 629.89
H 270.0
Haas' 732.3
Habermann's (acute parapsoriasis varioliformis) 696.2
Haff 985.1
Hageman (congenital factor XII deficiency) (*see also* Defect, congenital) 286.3
Haglund's (osteochondrosis os tibiale externum) 732.5
Hagner's (hypertrophic pulmonary osteoarthropathy) 731.2
Hailey-Hailey (benign familial chronic pemphigus) 757.39
hair (follicles) NEC 704.9
  specified type NEC 704.8
Hallervorden-Spatz 333.0
Hallopeau's (lichen sclerosus et atrophicus) 701.0
Hamman's (spontaneous mediastinal emphysema) 518.1
hand, foot, and mouth 074.3
Hand-Schüller-Christian (chronic histiocytosis X) 277.89
Hanot — *see* Cirrhosis, biliary
Hansen's (leprosy) 030.9
  benign form 030.1
  malignant form 030.0
Harada's 363.22
Harley's (intermittent hemoglobinuria) 283.2
Hartnup (pellagra-cerebellar ataxia-renal aminoaciduria) 270.0
Hart's (pellagra-cerebellar ataxia-renal aminoaciduria) 270.0
Hashimoto's (struma lymphomatosa) 245.2
Hb — *see* Disease, hemoglobin
heart (organic) 429.9
  with
    acute pulmonary edema (*see also* Failure, ventricular, left) 428.1
    hypertensive 402.91
      with renal failure 404.93
      benign 402.11
        with renal failure 404.13
      malignant 402.01
        with renal failure 404.03
    kidney disease — *see* Hypertension, cardiorenal
    rheumatic fever (conditions classifiable to 390)
      active 391.9
        with chorea 392.0
      inactive or quiescent (with chorea) 398.90

☑ **Additional Digit Required** — Refer to the Tabular List for Digit Selection   ▽ **Subterms under main terms may continue to next column or page**

2011 ICD-9-CM   ▶◀ Revised Text   ● New Line   ▲ Revised Code   Volume 2 — 83

Index

Disease, diseased — Disease, diseased

Disease, diseased — *see also* Syndrome — continued
heart — *continued*
  amyloid 277.39 *[425.7]*
  aortic (valve) (*see also* Endocarditis, aortic) 424.1
  arteriosclerotic or sclerotic (minimal) (senile) — *see* Arteriosclerosis, coronary
  artery, arterial — *see* Arteriosclerosis, coronary
  atherosclerotic — *see* Arteriosclerosis, coronary
  beer drinkers' 425.5
  beriberi 265.0 *[425.7]*
  black 416.0
  congenital NEC 746.9
    cyanotic 746.9
    maternal, affecting fetus or newborn 760.3
    specified type NEC 746.89
  congestive (*see also* Failure, heart) 428.0
  coronary 414.9
  cryptogenic 429.9
  due to
    amyloidosis 277.39 *[425.7]*
    beriberi 265.0 *[425.7]*
    cardiac glycogenosis 271.0 *[425.7]*
    Friedreich's ataxia 334.0 *[425.8]*
    gout 274.82
    mucopolysaccharidosis 277.5 *[425.7]*
    myotonia atrophica 359.21 *[425.8]*
    progressive muscular dystrophy 359.1 *[425.8]*
    sarcoidosis 135 *[425.8]*
  fetal 746.9
    inflammatory 746.89
  fibroid (*see also* Myocarditis) 429.0
  functional 427.9
    postoperative 997.1
    psychogenic 306.2
  glycogen storage 271.0 *[425.7]*
  gonococcal NEC 098.85
  gouty 274.82
  hypertensive (*see also* Hypertension, heart) 402.90
    benign 402.10
    malignant 402.00
  hyperthyroid (*see also* Hyperthyroidism) 242.9 ☑ *[425.7]*
  incompletely diagnosed — *see* Disease, heart
  ischemic (chronic) (*see also* Ischemia, heart) 414.9
    acute (*see also* Infarct, myocardium) 410.9 ☑
      without myocardial infarction 411.89
        with coronary (artery) occlusion 411.81
    asymptomatic 412
    diagnosed on ECG or other special investigation but currently presenting no symptoms 412
  kyphoscoliotic 416.1
  mitral (*see also* Endocarditis, mitral) 394.9
  muscular (*see also* Degeneration, myocardial) 429.1
  postpartum 674.8 ☑
  psychogenic (functional) 306.2
  pulmonary (chronic) 416.9
    acute 415.0
    specified NEC 416.8
  rheumatic (chronic) (inactive) (old) (quiescent) (with chorea) 398.90
    active or acute 391.9
      with chorea (active) (rheumatic) (Sydenham's) 392.0
      specified type NEC 391.8
    maternal, affecting fetus or newborn 760.3
  rheumatoid — *see* Arthritis, rheumatoid
  sclerotic — *see* Arteriosclerosis, coronary
  senile (*see also* Myocarditis) 429.0
  specified type NEC 429.89

Disease, diseased — *see also* Syndrome — continued
heart — *continued*
  syphilitic 093.89
    aortic 093.1
      aneurysm 093.0
    asymptomatic 093.89
    congenital 090.5
  thyroid (gland) (*see also* Hyper-thyroidism) 242.9 ☑ *[425.7]*
  thyrotoxic (*see also* Thyrotoxicosis) 242.9 ☑ *[425.7]*
  tuberculous (*see also* Tuberculosis) 017.9 ☑ *[425.8]*
  valve, valvular (obstructive) (regurgitant) (*see also* Endocarditis)
    congenital NEC (*see also* Anomaly, heart, valve) 746.9
    pulmonary 746.00
    specified type NEC 746.89
  vascular — *see* Disease, cardiovascular
heavy-chain (gamma G) 273.2
Heberden's 715.04
Hebra's
  dermatitis exfoliativa 695.89
  erythema multiforme exudativum 695.19
  pityriasis
    maculata et circinata 696.3
    rubra 695.89
    pilaris 696.4
  prurigo 698.2
Heerfordt's (uveoparotitis) 135
Heidenhain's 290.10
  with dementia 290.10
Heilmeyer-Schöner (M9842/3) 207.1 ☑
Heine-Medin (*see also* Poliomyelitis) 045.9 ☑
Heller's (*see also* Psychosis, childhood) 299.1 ☑
Heller-Döhle (syphilitic aortitis) 093.1
hematopoietic organs 289.9
hemoglobin (Hb) 282.7
  with thalassemia 282.49
  abnormal (mixed) NEC 282.7
    with thalassemia 282.49
  AS genotype 282.5
  Bart's 282.49
  C (Hb-C) 282.7
    with other abnormal hemoglobin NEC 282.7
    elliptocytosis 282.7
    Hb-S (without crisis) 282.63
      with
        crisis 282.64
          vaso-occlusive pain 282.64
    sickle-cell (without crisis) 282.63
      with
        crisis 282.64
          vaso-occlusive pain 282.64
    thalassemia 282.49
  constant spring 282.7
  D (Hb-D) 282.7
    with other abnormal hemoglobin NEC 282.7
    Hb-S (without crisis) 282.68
      with crisis 282.69
    sickle-cell (without crisis) 282.68
      with crisis 282.69
    thalassemia 282.49
  E (Hb-E) 282.7
    with other abnormal hemoglobin NEC 282.7
    Hb-S (without crisis) 282.68
      with crisis 282.69
    sickle-cell (without crisis) 282.68
      with crisis 282.69
    thalassemia 282.49
  elliptocytosis 282.7
  F (Hb-F) 282.7
  G (Hb-G) 282.7
  H (Hb-H) 282.49
  hereditary persistence, fetal (HPFH) ("Swiss variety") 282.7
  high fetal gene 282.7
  I thalassemia 282.49

Disease, diseased — *see also* Syndrome — continued
hemoglobin — *continued*
  M 289.7
  S (*see also* Disease, sickle-cell, Hb-S)
    thalassemia (without crisis) 282.41
      with
        crisis 282.42
          vaso-occlusive pain 282.42
    spherocytosis 282.7
    unstable, hemolytic 282.7
    Zurich (Hb-Zurich) 282.7
  hemolytic (fetus) (newborn) 773.2
    autoimmune (cold type) (warm type) 283.0
    due to or with incompatibility
      ABO (blood group) 773.1
      blood (group) (Duffy) (Kell) (Kidd) (Lewis) (M) (S) NEC 773.2
      Rh (blood group) (factor) 773.0
      Rh negative mother 773.0
    unstable hemoglobin 282.7
  hemorrhagic 287.9
    newborn 776.0
  Henoch (-Schönlein) (purpura nervosa) 287.0
  hepatic — *see* Disease, liver
  hepatolenticular 275.1
  heredodegenerative NEC
    brain 331.89
    spinal cord 336.8
  Hers' (glycogenosis VI) 271.0
  Herter (-Gee) (-Heubner) (nontropical sprue) 579.0
  Herxheimer's (diffuse idiopathic cutaneous atrophy) 701.8
  Heubner's 094.89
  Heubner-Herter (nontropical sprue) 579.0
  high fetal gene or hemoglobin thalassemia 282.49
  Hildenbrand's (typhus) 081.9
  hip (joint) NEC 719.95
    congenital 755.63
    suppurative 711.05
    tuberculous (*see also* Tuberculosis) 015.1 ☑ *[730.85]*
  Hippel's (retinocerebral angiomatosis) 759.6
  Hirschfeld's (acute diabetes mellitus) (*see also* Diabetes) 250.0 ☑
    due to secondary diabetes 249.0 ☑
  Hirschsprung's (congenital megacolon) 751.3
  His (-Werner) (trench fever) 083.1
  HIV 042
  Hodgkin's (M9650/3) 201.9 ☑

Note — Use the following fifth-digit subclassification with category 201:

0	*unspecified site*
1	*lymph nodes of head, face, and neck*
2	*intrathoracic lymph nodes*
3	*intra-abdominal lymph nodes*
4	*lymph nodes of axilla and upper limb*
5	*lymph nodes of inguinal region and lower limb*
6	*intrapelvic lymph nodes*
7	*spleen*
8	*lymph nodes of multiple sites*

  lymphocytic
    depletion (M9653/3) 201.7 ☑
      diffuse fibrosis (M9654/3) 201.7 ☑
      reticular type (M9655/3) 201.7 ☑
    predominance (M9651/3) 201.4 ☑
  lymphocytic-histiocytic predominance (M9651/3) 201.4 ☑
  mixed cellularity (M9652/3) 201.6 ☑
  nodular sclerosis (M9656/3) 201.5 ☑
    cellular phase (M9657/3) 201.5 ☑

Disease, diseased — *see also* Syndrome — continued
  Hodgson's 441.9
    ruptured 441.5
  Hoffa (-Kastert) (liposynovitis prepatellaris) 272.8
  Holla (*see also* Spherocytosis) 282.0
  homozygous-Hb-S 282.61
  hoof and mouth 078.4
  hookworm (*see also* Ancylostomiasis) 126.9
  Horton's (temporal arteritis) 446.5
  host-versus-graft (immune or nonimmune cause) 279.50
  HPFH (hereditary persistence of fetal hemoglobin) ("Swiss variety") 282.7
  Huchard's disease (continued arterial hypertension) 401.9
  Huguier's (uterine fibroma) 218.9
  human immunodeficiency (virus) 042
  hunger 251.1
  Hunt's
    dyssynergia cerebellaris myoclonica 334.2
    herpetic geniculate ganglionitis 053.11
  Huntington's 333.4
  Huppert's (multiple myeloma) (M9730/3) 203.0 ☑
  Hurler's (mucopolysaccharidosis I) 277.5
  Hutchinson-Boeck (sarcoidosis) 135
  Hutchinson-Gilford (progeria) 259.8
  Hutchinson's, meaning
    angioma serpiginosum 709.1
    cheiropompholyx 705.81
    prurigo estivalis 692.72
  hyaline (diffuse) (generalized) 728.9
    membrane (lung) (newborn) 769
  hydatid (*see also* Echinococcus) 122.9
  Hyde's (prurigo nodularis) 698.3
  hyperkinetic (*see also* Hyperkinesia) 314.9
    heart 429.82
  hypertensive (*see also* Hypertension) 401.9
  hypophysis 253.9
    hyperfunction 253.1
    hypofunction 253.2
  Iceland (epidemic neuromyasthenia) 049.8
  I cell 272.7
  ill-defined 799.89
  immunologic NEC 279.9
  immunoproliferative 203.8 ☑
  inclusion 078.5
    salivary gland 078.5
  infancy, early NEC 779.9
  infective NEC 136.9
  inguinal gland 289.9
  internal semilunar cartilage, cystic 717.5
  intervertebral disc 722.90
    with myelopathy 722.70
    cervical, cervicothoracic 722.91
      with myelopathy 722.71
    lumbar, lumbosacral 722.93
      with myelopathy 722.73
    thoracic, thoracolumbar 722.92
      with myelopathy 722.72
  intestine 569.9
    functional 564.9
      congenital 751.3
      psychogenic 306.4
    lardaceous 277.39
    organic 569.9
    protozoal NEC 007.9
  iris 364.9
    specified NEC 364.89
  iron
    metabolism ▶(*see also* Hemochromatosis)◀ 275.03 ▲
    storage ▶(*see also* Hemochromatosis)◀ 275.03 ▲
  Isambert's (*see also* Tuberculosis, larynx) 012.3 ☑
  Iselin's (osteochondrosis, fifth metatarsal) 732.5
  island (scrub typhus) 081.2
  itai-itai 985.5
  Jadassohn's (maculopapular erythroderma) 696.2
  Jadassohn-Pellizari's (anetoderma) 701.3

☑ **Additional Digit Required** — Refer to the Tabular List for Digit Selection   ▽ **Subterms under main terms may continue to next column or page**

84 — Volume 2 · October 2010   ▶◀ Revised Text   ● New Line   ▲ Revised Code   **2011 ICD-9-CM**

Disease, diseased — *see also* Syndrome — *continued*

Jakob-Creutzfeldt (CJD) 046.19
    with dementia
        with behavioral disturbance 046.19 [294.11]
        without behavioral disturbance 046.19 [294.10]
    familial 046.19
    iatrogenic 046.19
    specified NEC 046.19
    sporadic 046.19
    variant (vCJD) 046.11
        with dementia
            with behavioral disturbance 046.11 [294.11]
            without behavioral disturbance 046.11 [294.10]
Jaksch (-Luzet) (pseudoleukemia infantum) 285.8
Janet's 300.89
Jansky-Bielschowsky 330.1
jaw NEC 526.9
    fibrocystic 526.2
Jensen's 363.05
Jeune's (asphyxiating thoracic dystrophy) 756.4
jigger 134.1
Johnson-Stevens (erythema multiforme exudativum) 695.13
joint NEC 719.9 ☑
    ankle 719.97
    Charcôt 094.0 [713.5]
    degenerative (*see also* Osteoarthrosis) 715.9 ☑
        multiple 715.09
        spine (*see also* Spondylosis) 721.90
    elbow 719.92
    foot 719.97
    hand 719.94
    hip 719.95
    hypertrophic (chronic) (degenerative) (*see also* Osteoarthrosis) 715.9 ☑
        spine (*see also* Spondylosis) 721.90
    knee 719.96
    Luschka 721.90
    multiple sites 719.99
    pelvic region 719.95
    sacroiliac 724.6
    shoulder (region) 719.91
    specified site NEC 719.98
    spine NEC 724.9
        pseudarthrosis following fusion 733.82
        sacroiliac 724.6
    wrist 719.93
Jourdain's (acute gingivitis) 523.00
Jüngling's (sarcoidosis) 135
Kahler (-Bozzolo) (multiple myeloma) (M9730/3) 203.0 ☑
Kalischer's 759.6
Kaposi's 757.33
    lichen ruber 697.8
        acuminatus 696.4
        moniliformis 697.8
    xeroderma pigmentosum 757.33
Kaschin-Beck (endemic polyarthritis) 716.00
    ankle 716.07
    arm 716.02
        lower (and wrist) 716.03
        upper (and elbow) 716.02
    foot (and ankle) 716.07
    forearm (and wrist) 716.03
    hand 716.04
    leg 716.06
        lower 716.06
        upper 716.05
    multiple sites 716.09
    pelvic region (hip) (thigh) 716.05
    shoulder region 716.01
    specified site NEC 716.08
Katayama 120.2
Kawasaki 446.1
Kedani (scrub typhus) 081.2
kidney (functional) (pelvis) (*see also* Disease, renal) 593.9

Disease, diseased — *see also* Syndrome — *continued*

kidney (*see also* Disease, renal) — *continued*
    chronic 585.9
        requiring chronic dialysis 585.6
        stage
            I 585.1
            II (mild) 585.2
            III (moderate) 585.3
            IV (severe) 585.4
            V 585.5
    cystic (congenital) 753.10
        multiple 753.19
        single 753.11
        specified NEC 753.19
    fibrocystic (congenital) 753.19
    in gout 274.10
    polycystic (congenital) 753.12
        adult type (APKD) 753.13
        autosomal dominant 753.13
        autosomal recessive 753.14
        childhood type (CPKD) 753.14
        infantile type 753.14
Kienböck's (carpal lunate) (wrist) 732.3
Kimmelstiel (-Wilson) (intercapillary glomerulosclerosis) 250.4 ☑ [581.81]
    due to secondary diabetes 249.4 ☑ [581.81]
Kinnier Wilson's (hepatolenticular degeneration) 275.1
kissing 075
Kleb's (*see also* Nephritis) 583.9
Klinger's 446.4
Klippel's 723.8
Klippel-Feil (brevicollis) 756.16
knight's 911.1
Köbner's (epidermolysis bullosa) 757.39
Koenig-Wichmann (pemphigus) 694.4
Köhler's
    first (osteoarthrosis juvenilis) 732.5
    second (Freiberg's infraction, metatarsal head) 732.5
    patellar 732.4
    tarsal navicular (bone) (osteoarthrosis juvenilis) 732.5
Köhler-Freiberg (infraction, metatarsal head) 732.5
Köhler-Mouchet (osteoarthrosis juvenilis) 732.5
Köhler-Pellegrini-Stieda (calcification, knee joint) 726.62
Kok 759.89
König's (osteochondritis dissecans) 732.7
Korsakoff's (nonalcoholic) 294.0
    alcoholic 291.1
Kostmann's (infantile genetic agranulocytosis) 288.01
Krabbe's 330.0
Kraepelin-Morel (*see also* Schizophrenia) 295.9 ☑
Kraft-Weber-Dimitri 759.6
Kufs' 330.1
Kugelberg-Welander 335.11
Kuhnt-Junius 362.52
Kümmell's (-Verneuil) (spondylitis) 721.7
Kundrat's (lymphosarcoma) 200.1 ☑
kuru 046.0
Kussmaul (-Meier) (polyarteritis nodosa) 446.2
Kyasanur Forest 065.2
Kyrle's (hyperkeratosis follicularis in cutem penetrans) 701.1
labia
    inflammatory 616.10
    noninflammatory 624.9
        specified NEC 624.8
labyrinth, ear 386.8
lacrimal system (apparatus) (passages) 375.9
    gland 375.00
    specified NEC 375.89
Lafora's 333.2
Lagleyze-von Hippel (retinocerebral angiomatosis) 759.6
Lancereaux-Mathieu (leptospiral jaundice) 100.0

Disease, diseased — *see also* Syndrome — *continued*

Landry's 357.0
Lane's 569.89
lardaceous (any site) 277.39
Larrey-Weil (leptospiral jaundice) 100.0
Larsen (-Johansson) (juvenile osteopathia patellae) 732.4
larynx 478.70
Lasègue's (persecution mania) 297.9
Leber's 377.16
Lederer's (acquired infectious hemolytic anemia) 283.19
Legg's (capital femoral osteochondrosis) 732.1
Legg-Calvé-Perthes (capital femoral osteochondrosis) 732.1
Legg-Calvé-Waldenström (femoral capital osteochondrosis) 732.1
Legg-Perthes (femoral capital osteochrondosis) 732.1
Legionnaires' 482.84
Leigh's 330.8
Leiner's (exfoliative dermatitis) 695.89
Leloir's (lupus erythematosus) 695.4
Lenègre's 426.0
lens (eye) 379.39
Leriche's (osteoporosis, posttraumatic) 733.7
Letterer-Siwe (acute histiocytosis X) (M9722/3) 202.5 ☑
Lev's (acquired complete heart block) 426.0
Lewandowski's (*see also* Tuberculosis) 017.0 ☑
Lewandowski-Lutz (epidermodysplasia verruciformis) 078.19
Lewy body 331.82
    with dementia
        with behavioral disturbance 331.82 [294.11]
        without behavioral disturbance 331.82 [294.10]
Leyden's (periodic vomiting) 536.2
Libman-Sacks (verrucous endocarditis) 710.0 [424.91]
Lichtheim's (subacute combined sclerosis with pernicious anemia) 281.0 [336.2]
ligament 728.9
light chain 203.0 ☑
Lightwood's (renal tubular acidosis) 588.89
Lignac's (cystinosis) 270.0
Lindau's (retinocerebral angiomatosis) 759.6
Lindau-von Hippel (angiomatosis retinocerebellosa) 759.6
lip NEC 528.5
lipidosis 272.7
lipoid storage NEC 272.7
Lipschütz's 616.50
Little's — *see* Palsy, cerebral
liver 573.9
    alcoholic 571.3
        acute 571.1
        chronic 571.3
    chronic 571.9
        alcoholic 571.3
    cystic, congenital 751.62
    drug-induced 573.3
    due to
        chemicals 573.3
        fluorinated agents 573.3
        hypersensitivity drugs 573.3
        isoniazids 573.3
    end stage NEC 572.8
        due to hepatitis — *see* Hepatitis
    fibrocystic (congenital) 751.62
    glycogen storage 271.0
    organic 573.9
    polycystic (congenital) 751.62
Lobo's (keloid blastomycosis) 116.2
Lobstein's (brittle bones and blue sclera) 756.51
locomotor system 334.9
Lorain's (pituitary dwarfism) 253.3
Lou Gehrig's 335.20
Lucas-Championnière (fibrinous bronchitis) 466.0
Ludwig's (submaxillary cellulitis) 528.3

Disease, diseased — *see also* Syndrome — *continued*

luetic — *see* Syphilis
lumbosacral region 724.6
lung NEC 518.89
    black 500
    congenital 748.60
    cystic 518.89
        congenital 748.4
    fibroid (chronic) (*see also* Fibrosis, lung) 515
    fluke 121.2
        oriental 121.2
    in
        amyloidosis 277.39 [517.8]
        polymyositis 710.4 [517.8]
        sarcoidosis 135 [517.8]
        Sjögren's syndrome 710.2 [517.8]
        syphilis 095.1
        systemic lupus erythematosus 710.0 [517.8]
        systemic sclerosis 710.1 [517.2]
    interstitial (chronic) 515
        acute 136.3
    nonspecific, chronic 496
    obstructive (chronic) (COPD) 496
        with
            acute
                bronchitis 491.22
                    exacerbation NEC 491.21
            alveolitis, allergic (*see also* Alveolitis, allergic) 495.9
            asthma (chronic) (obstructive) 493.2 ☑
            bronchiectasis 494.0
                with acute exacerbation 494.1
            bronchitis (chronic) 491.20
                with
                    acute bronchitis 491.22
                    exacerbation (acute) 491.21
            decompensated 491.21
                with exacerbation 491.21
            emphysema NEC 492.8
        diffuse (with fibrosis) 496
    polycystic 518.89
        asthma (chronic) (obstructive) 493.2 ☑
        congenital 748.4
    purulent (cavitary) 513.0
    restrictive 518.89
    rheumatoid 714.81
        diffuse interstitial 714.81
    specified NEC 518.89
Lutembacher's (atrial septal defect with mitral stenosis) 745.5
Lutz-Miescher (elastosis perforans serpiginosa) 701.1
Lutz-Splendore-de Almeida (Brazilian blastomycosis) 116.1
Lyell's (toxic epidermal necrolysis) 695.15
    due to drug
        correct substance properly administered 695.15
        overdose or wrong substance given or taken 977.9
        specific drug — *see* Table of Drugs and Chemicals
Lyme 088.81
lymphatic (gland) (system) 289.9
    channel (noninfective) 457.9
    vessel (noninfective) 457.9
    specified NEC 457.8
lymphoproliferative (chronic) (M9970/1) 238.79
Machado-Joseph 334.8
Madelung's (lipomatosis) 272.8
Madura (actinomycotic) 039.9
    mycotic 117.4
Magitot's 526.4
Majocchi's (purpura annularis telangiectodes) 709.1
malarial (*see also* Malaria) 084.6
Malassez's (cystic) 608.89
Malibu 919.8
    infected 919.9

☑ **Additional Digit Required** — Refer to the Tabular List for Digit Selection   ▽ **Subterms under main terms may continue to next column or page**

2011 ICD-9-CM   ▶◀ Revised Text   ● New Line   ▲ Revised Code   Volume 2 — 85

Disease, diseased — *see also* Syndrome — *continued*

malignant (M8000/3) (*see also* Neoplasm, by site, malignant)
  previous, affecting management of pregnancy V23.89
Manson's 120.1
maple bark 495.6
maple syrup (urine) 270.3
Marburg (virus) 078.89
Marchiafava (-Bignami) 341.8
Marfan's 090.49
  congenital syphilis 090.49
  meaning Marfan's syndrome 759.82
Marie-Bamberger (hypertrophic pulmonary osteoarthropathy) (secondary) 731.2
  primary or idiopathic (acropachyderma) 757.39
  pulmonary (hypertrophic osteoarthropathy) 731.2
Marie-Strümpell (ankylosing spondylitis) 720.0
Marion's (bladder neck obstruction) 596.0
Marsh's (exophthalmic goiter) 242.0 ☑
Martin's 715.27
mast cell 757.33
  systemic (M9741/3) 202.6 ☑
mastoid (*see also* Mastoiditis) 383.9
  process 385.9
maternal, unrelated to pregnancy NEC, affecting fetus or newborn 760.9
Mathieu's (leptospiral jaundice) 100.0
Mauclaire's 732.3
Mauriac's (erythema nodosum syphiliticum) 091.3
Maxcy's 081.0
McArdle (-Schmid-Pearson) (glycogenosis V) 271.0
mediastinum NEC 519.3
Medin's (*see also* Poliomyelitis) 045.9 ☑
Mediterranean (with hemoglobinopathy) 282.49
medullary center (idiopathic) (respiratory) 348.89
Meige's (chronic hereditary edema) 757.0
Meleda 757.39
Ménétrier's (hypertrophic gastritis) 535.2 ☑
Ménière's (active) 386.00
  cochlear 386.02
  cochleovestibular 386.01
  inactive 386.04
  in remission 386.04
  vestibular 386.03
meningeal — *see* Meningitis
mental (*see also* Psychosis) 298.9
Merzbacher-Pelizaeus 330.0
mesenchymal 710.9
mesenteric embolic 557.0
metabolic NEC 277.9
metal polishers' 502
metastatic — *see* Metastasis
Mibelli's 757.39
microdrepanocytic 282.49
microvascular — code to condition
microvillus inclusion (MVD) 751.5 ●
Miescher's 709.3
Mikulicz's (dryness of mouth, absent or decreased lacrimation) 527.1
Milkman (-Looser) (osteomalacia with pseudofractures) 268.2
Miller's (osteomalacia) 268.2
Mills' 335.29
Milroy's (chronic hereditary edema) 757.0
Minamata 985.0
Minor's 336.1
Minot's (hemorrhagic disease, newborn) 776.0
Minot-von Willebrand-Jürgens (angiohemophilia) 286.4
Mitchell's (erythromelalgia) 443.82
mitral — *see* Endocarditis, mitral
Mljet (mal de Meleda) 757.39
Möbius', Moebius' 346.2 ☑
Moeller's 267
Möller (-Barlow) (infantile scurvy) 267

Mönckeberg's (*see also* Arteriosclerosis, extremities) 440.20
Mondor's (thrombophlebitis of breast) 451.89
Monge's 993.2
Morel-Kraepelin (*see also* Schizophrenia) 295.9 ☑
Morgagni's (syndrome) (hyperostosis frontalis interna) 733.3
Morgagni-Adams-Stokes (syncope with heart block) 426.9
Morquio (-Brailsford) (-Ullrich) (mucopolysaccharidosis IV) 277.5
Morton's (with metatarsalgia) 355.6
Morvan's 336.0
motor neuron (bulbar) (mixed type) 335.20
Mouchet's (juvenile osteochondrosis, foot) 732.5
mouth 528.9
Moyamoya 437.5
Mucha's (acute parapsoriasis varioliformis) 696.2
mu-chain 273.2
mucolipidosis (I) (II) (III) 272.7
Münchmeyer's (exostosis luxurians) 728.11
Murri's (intermittent hemoglobinuria) 283.2
muscle 359.9
  inflammatory 728.9
  ocular 378.9
musculoskeletal system 729.90
mushroom workers' 495.5
Myà's (congenital dilation, colon) 751.3
mycotic 117.9
myeloproliferative (chronic) (M9960/1) 238.79
myocardium, myocardial (*see also* Degeneration, myocardial) 429.1
  hypertensive (*see also* Hypertension, heart) 402.90
  primary (idiopathic) 425.4
myoneural 358.9
Naegeli's 287.1
nail 703.9
  specified type NEC 703.8
Nairobi sheep 066.1
nasal 478.19
  cavity NEC 478.19
  sinus (chronic) — *see* Sinusitis
navel (newborn) NEC 779.89
  delayed separation of umbilical cord 779.83
nemaline body 359.0
neoplastic, generalized (M8000/6) 199.0
nerve — *see* Disorder, nerve
nervous system (central) 349.9
  autonomic, peripheral (*see also* Neuropathy, peripheral, autonomic) 337.9
  congenital 742.9
  inflammatory — *see* Encephalitis
  parasympathetic (*see also* Neuropathy, peripheral, autonomic) 337.9
  peripheral NEC 355.9
  prion NEC 046.79
  specified NEC 349.89
  sympathetic (*see also* Neuropathy, peripheral, autonomic) 337.9
  vegetative (*see also* Neuropathy, peripheral, autonomic) 337.9
Nettleship's (urticaria pigmentosa) 757.33
Neumann's (pemphigus vegetans) 694.4
neurologic (central) NEC (*see also* Disease, nervous system) 349.9
  peripheral NEC 355.9
neuromuscular system NEC 358.9
Newcastle 077.8
Nicolas (-Durand) — Favre (climatic bubo) 099.1
Niemann-Pick (lipid histiocytosis) 272.7
nipple 611.9
  Paget's (M8540/3) 174.0
Nishimoto (-Takeuchi) 437.5
nonarthropod-borne NEC 078.89
  central nervous system NEC 049.9
  enterovirus NEC 078.89

nonautoimmune hemolytic NEC 283.10
Nonne-Milroy-Meige (chronic hereditary edema) 757.0
Norrie's (congenital progressive oculoacousticocerebral degeneration) 743.8
nose 478.19
nucleus pulposus — *see* Disease, intervertebral disc
nutritional 269.9
  maternal, affecting fetus or newborn 760.4
oasthouse, urine 270.2
obliterative vascular 447.1
Odelberg's (juvenile osteochondrosis) 732.1
Oguchi's (retina) 368.61
Ohara's (*see also* Tularemia) 021.9
Ollier's (chondrodysplasia) 756.4
Opitz's (congestive splenomegaly) 289.51
Oppenheim's 358.8
Oppenheim-Urbach (necrobiosis lipoidica diabeticorum) 250.8 ☑ [709.3]
  due to secondary diabetes 249.8 ☑ [709.3]
optic nerve NEC 377.49
orbit 376.9
  specified NEC 376.89
Oriental liver fluke 121.1
Oriental lung fluke 121.2
Ormond's 593.4
Osgood-Schlatter 732.4
Osgood's tibia (tubercle) 732.4
Osler (-Vaquez) (polycythemia vera) (M9950/1) 238.4
Osler-Rendu (familial hemorrhagic telangiectasia) 448.0
osteofibrocystic 252.01
Otto's 715.35
outer ear 380.9
ovary (noninflammatory) NEC 620.9
  cystic 620.2
  polycystic 256.4
  specified NEC 620.8
Owren's (congenital) (*see also* Defect, coagulation) 286.3
Paas' 756.59
Paget's (osteitis deformans) 731.0
  with infiltrating duct carcinoma of the breast (M8541/3) — *see* Neoplasm, breast, malignant
  bone 731.0
    osteosarcoma in (M9184/3) — *see* Neoplasm, bone, malignant
  breast (M8540/3) 174.0
  extramammary (M8542/3) (*see also* Neoplasm, skin, malignant)
    anus 154.3
    skin 173.5
  malignant (M8540/3)
    breast 174.0
    specified site NEC (M8542/3) — *see* Neoplasm, skin, malignant
    unspecified site 174.0
  mammary (M8540/3) 174.0
  nipple (M8540/3) 174.0
palate (soft) 528.9
Paltauf-Sternberg 201.9 ☑
pancreas 577.9
  cystic 577.2
    congenital 751.7
  fibrocystic 277.00
Panner's 732.3
  capitellum humeri 732.3
  head of humerus 732.3
  tarsal navicular (bone) (osteochondrosis) 732.5
panvalvular — *see* Endocarditis, mitral
parametrium 629.9
parasitic NEC 136.9
  cerebral NEC 123.9
  intestinal NEC 129
  mouth 112.0
  skin NEC 134.9
  specified type — *see* Infestation
  tongue 112.0

parathyroid (gland) 252.9
  specified NEC 252.8
Parkinson's 332.0
parodontal 523.9
Parrot's (syphilitic osteochondritis) 090.0
Parry's (exophthalmic goiter) 242.0 ☑
Parson's (exophthalmic goiter) 242.0 ☑
Pavy's 593.6
Paxton's (white piedra) 111.2
Payr's (splenic flexure syndrome) 569.89
pearl-workers' (chronic osteomyelitis) (*see also* Osteomyelitis) 730.1 ☑
Pel-Ebstein — *see* Disease, Hodgkin's
Pelizaeus-Merzbacher 330.0
  with dementia
    with behavioral disturbance 330.0 [294.11]
    without behavioral disturbance 330.0 [294.10]
Pellegrini-Stieda (calcification, knee joint) 726.62
pelvis, pelvic
  female NEC 629.9
    specified NEC 629.89
  gonococcal (acute) 098.19
    chronic or duration of 2 months or over 098.39
  infection (*see also* Disease, pelvis, inflammatory) 614.9
  inflammatory (female) (PID) 614.9
    with
      abortion — *see* Abortion, by type, with sepsis
      ectopic pregnancy (*see also* categories 633.0–633.9) 639.0
      molar pregnancy (*see also* categories 630–632) 639.0
    acute 614.3
    chronic 614.4
    complicating pregnancy 646.6 ☑
      affecting fetus or newborn 760.8
    following
      abortion 639.0
      ectopic or molar pregnancy 639.0
    peritonitis (acute) 614.5
      chronic NEC 614.7
    puerperal, postpartum, childbirth 670.8 ☑
    specified NEC 614.8
  organ, female NEC 629.9
    specified NEC 629.89
  peritoneum, female NEC 629.9
    specified NEC 629.89
penis 607.9
  inflammatory 607.2
peptic NEC 536.9
  acid 536.8
periapical tissues NEC 522.9
pericardium 423.9
  specified type NEC 423.8
perineum
  female
    inflammatory 616.9
      specified NEC 616.89
    noninflammatory 624.9
      specified NEC 624.8
  male (inflammatory) 682.2
periodic (familial) (Reimann's) NEC 277.31
  paralysis 359.3
periodontal NEC 523.9
  specified NEC 523.8
periosteum 733.90
peripheral
  arterial 443.9
  autonomic nervous system (*see also* Neuropathy, autonomic) 337.9
  nerve NEC (*see also* Neuropathy) 356.9
    multiple — *see* Polyneuropathy
  vascular 443.9
    specified type NEC 443.89
peritoneum 568.9
  pelvic, female 629.9
    specified NEC 629.89
Perrin-Ferraton (snapping hip) 719.65

Disease, diseased — *see also* Syndrome — *continued*

persistent mucosal (middle ear) (with posterior or superior marginal perforation of ear drum) 382.2

Perthes' (capital femoral osteochondrosis) 732.1

Petit's (*see also* Hernia, lumbar) 553.8

Peutz-Jeghers 759.6

Peyronie's 607.85

Pfeiffer's (infectious mononucleosis) 075

pharynx 478.20

Phocas' 610.1

photochromogenic (acid-fast bacilli) (pulmonary) 031.0

nonpulmonary 031.9

Pick's

brain 331.11

with dementia

with behavioral disturbance 331.11 [294.11]

without behavioral disturbance 331.11 [294.10]

cerebral atrophy 331.11

with dementia

with behavioral disturbance 331.11 [294.11]

without behavioral disturbance 331.11 [294.10]

lipid histiocytosis 272.7

liver (pericardial pseudocirrhosis of liver) 423.2

pericardium (pericardial pseudocirrhosis of liver) 423.2

polyserositis (pericardial pseudocirrhosis of liver) 423.2

Pierson's (osteochondrosis) 732.1

pigeon fanciers' or breeders' 495.2

pineal gland 259.8

pink 985.0

Pinkus' (lichen nitidus) 697.1

pinworm 127.4

pituitary (gland) 253.9

hyperfunction 253.1

hypofunction 253.2

pituitary snuff-takers' 495.8

placenta

affecting fetus or newborn 762.2

complicating pregnancy or childbirth 656.7 ☑

pleura (cavity) (*see also* Pleurisy) 511.0

Plummer's (toxic nodular goiter) 242.3 ☑

pneumatic

drill 994.9

hammer 994.9

policeman's 729.2

Pollitzer's (hidradenitis suppurativa) 705.83

polycystic (congenital) 759.89

congenital 748.4

kidney or renal 753.12

adult type (APKD) 753.13

autosomal dominant 753.13

autosomal recessive 753.14

childhood type (CPKD) 753.14

infantile type 753.14

liver or hepatic 751.62

lung or pulmonary 518.89

ovary, ovaries 256.4

spleen 759.0

Pompe's (glycogenosis II) 271.0

Poncet's (tuberculous rheumatism) (*see also* Tuberculosis) 015.9 ☑

Posada-Wernicke 114.9

Potain's (pulmonary edema) 514

Pott's (*see also* Tuberculosis) 015.0 ☑ [730.88]

osteomyelitis 015.0 ☑ [730.88]

paraplegia 015.0 ☑ [730.88]

spinal curvature 015.0 ☑ [737.43]

spondylitis 015.0 ☑ [720.81]

Potter's 753.0

Poulet's 714.2

pregnancy NEC (*see also* Pregnancy) 646.9 ☑

Preiser's (osteoporosis) 733.09

Pringle's (tuberous sclerosis) 759.5

Disease, diseased — *see also* Syndrome — *continued*

Profichet's 729.90

prostate 602.9

specified type NEC 602.8

protozoal NEC 136.8

intestine, intestinal NEC 007.9

pseudo-Hurler's (mucolipidosis III) 272.7

psychiatric (*see also* Psychosis) 298.9

psychotic (*see also* Psychosis) 298.9

Puente's (simple glandular cheilitis) 528.5

puerperal NEC (*see also* Puerperal) 674.9 ☑

pulmonary (*see also* Disease, lung)

amyloid 277.39 [517.8]

artery 417.9

circulation, circulatory 417.9

specified NEC 417.8

diffuse obstructive (chronic) 496

with

acute bronchitis 491.22

asthma (chronic) (obstructive) 493.2 ☑

exacerbation NEC (acute) 491.21

heart (chronic) 416.9

specified NEC 416.8

hypertensive (vascular) 416.0

cardiovascular 416.0

obstructive diffuse (chronic) 496

with

acute bronchitis 491.22

asthma (chronic) (obstructive) 493.2 ☑

bronchitis (chronic) 491.20

with

exacerbation (acute) 491.21

acute 491.22

exacerbation NEC (acute) 491.21

decompensated 491.21

with exacerbation 491.21

valve (*see also* Endocarditis, pulmonary) 424.3

pulp (dental) NEC 522.9

pulseless 446.7

Putnam's (subacute combined sclerosis with pernicious anemia) 281.0 [336.2]

Pyle (-Cohn) (craniometaphyseal dysplasia) 756.89

pyramidal tract 333.90

Quervain's

tendon sheath 727.04

thyroid (subacute granulomatous thyroiditis) 245.1

Quincke's — *see* Edema, angioneurotic

Quinquaud (acne decalvans) 704.09

rag sorters' 022.1

Raynaud's (paroxysmal digital cyanosis) 443.0

reactive airway — *see* Asthma

Recklinghausen's (M9540/1) 237.71

bone (osteitis fibrosa cystica) 252.01

Recklinghausen-Applebaum (hemochromatosis) ▶(*see also* Hemochromatosis)◀ 275.03 ▲

Reclus' (cystic) 610.1

rectum NEC 569.49

Refsum's (heredopathia atactica polyneuritiformis) 356.3

Reichmann's (gastrosuccorrhea) 536.8

Reimann's (periodic) 277.31

Reiter's 099.3

renal (functional) (pelvis) (*see also* Disease, kidney) 593.9

with

edema (*see also* Nephrosis) 581.9

exudative nephritis 583.89

lesion of interstitial nephritis 583.89

stated generalized cause — *see* Nephritis

acute 593.9

basement membrane NEC 583.89

with

pulmonary hemorrhage (Goodpasture's syndrome) 446.21 [583.81]

Disease, diseased — *see also* Syndrome — *continued*

renal (*see also* Disease, kidney) — *continued*

chronic (*see also* Disease, kidney, chronic) 585.9

complicating pregnancy or puerperium NEC 646.2 ☑

with hypertension — *see* Toxemia, of pregnancy

affecting fetus or newborn 760.1

cystic, congenital (*see also* Cystic, disease, kidney) 753.10

diabetic 250.4 ☑ [583.81]

due to secondary diabetes 249.4 ☑ [581.81]

due to

amyloidosis 277.39 [583.81]

diabetes mellitus 250.4 ☑ [583.81]

due to secondary diabetes 249.4 ☑ [581.81]

systemic lupus erythematosis 710.0 [583.81]

end-stage 585.6

exudative 583.89

fibrocystic (congenital) 753.19

gonococcal 098.19 [583.81]

gouty 274.10

hypertensive (*see also* Hypertension, kidney) 403.90

immune complex NEC 583.89

interstitial (diffuse) (focal) 583.89

lupus 710.0 [583.81]

maternal, affecting fetus or newborn 760.1

hypertensive 760.0

phosphate-losing (tubular) 588.0

polycystic (congenital) 753.12

adult type (APKD) 753.13

autosomal dominant 753.13

autosomal recessive 753.14

childhood type (CPKD) 753.14

infantile type 753.14

specified lesion or cause NEC (*see also* Glomerulonephritis) 583.89

subacute 581.9

syphilitic 095.4

tuberculous (*see also* Tuberculosis) 016.0 ☑ [583.81]

tubular (*see also* Nephrosis, tubular) 584.5

Rendu-Osler-Weber (familial hemorrhagic telangiectasia) 448.0

renovascular (arteriosclerotic) (*see also* Hypertension, kidney) 403.90

respiratory (tract) 519.9

acute or subacute (upper) NEC 465.9

due to fumes or vapors 506.3

multiple sites NEC 465.8

noninfectious 478.9

streptococcal 034.0

chronic 519.9

arising in the perinatal period 770.7

due to fumes or vapors 506.4

due to

aspiration of liquids or solids 508.9

external agents NEC 508.9

specified NEC 508.8

fumes or vapors 506.9

acute or subacute NEC 506.3

chronic 506.4

fetus or newborn NEC 770.9

obstructive 496

specified type NEC 519.8

upper (acute) (infectious) NEC 465.9

multiple sites NEC 465.8

noninfectious NEC 478.9

streptococcal 034.0

retina, retinal NEC 362.9

Batten's or Batten-Mayou 330.1 [362.71]

degeneration 362.89

vascular lesion 362.17

rheumatic (*see also* Arthritis) 716.8 ☑

heart — *see* Disease, heart, rheumatic

rheumatoid (heart) — *see* Arthritis, rheumatoid

Disease, diseased — *see also* Syndrome — *continued*

rickettsial NEC 083.9

specified type NEC 083.8

Riedel's (ligneous thyroiditis) 245.3

Riga (-Fede) (cachectic aphthae) 529.0

Riggs' (compound periodontitis) 523.40

Ritter's 695.81

Rivalta's (cervicofacial actinomycosis) 039.3

Robles' (onchocerciasis) 125.3 [360.13]

Roger's (congenital interventricular septal defect) 745.4

Rokitansky's (*see also* Necrosis, liver) 570

Romberg's 349.89

Rosenthal's (factor XI deficiency) 286.2

Rossbach's (hyperchlorhydria) 536.8

psychogenic 306.4

Roth (-Bernhardt) 355.1

Runeberg's (progressive pernicious anemia) 281.0

Rust's (tuberculous spondylitis) (*see also* Tuberculosis) 015.0 ☑ [720.81]

Rustitskii's (multiple myeloma) (M9730/3) 203.0 ☑

Ruysch's (Hirschsprung's disease) 751.3

Sachs (-Tay) 330.1

sacroiliac NEC 724.6

salivary gland or duct NEC 527.9

inclusion 078.5

streptococcal 034.0

virus 078.5

Sander's (paranoia) 297.1

Sandhoff's 330.1

sandworm 126.9

Savill's (epidemic exfoliative dermatitis) 695.89

Schamberg's (progressive pigmentary dermatosis) 709.09

Schaumann's (sarcoidosis) 135

Schenck's (sporotrichosis) 117.1

Scheuermann's (osteochondrosis) 732.0

Schilder (-Flatau) 341.1

Schimmelbusch's 610.1

Schlatter-Osgood 732.4

Schlatter's tibia (tubercle) 732.4

Schmorl's 722.30

cervical 722.39

lumbar, lumbosacral 722.32

specified region NEC 722.39

thoracic, thoracolumbar 722.31

Scholz's 330.0

Schönlein (-Henoch) (purpura rheumatica) 287.0

Schottmüller's (*see also* Fever, paratyphoid) 002.9

Schüller-Christian (chronic histiocytosis X) 277.89

Schultz's (agranulocytosis) 288.09

Schwalbe-Ziehen-Oppenheimer 333.6

Schwartz-Jampel 359.23

Schweninger-Buzzi (macular atrophy) 701.3

sclera 379.19

scrofulous (*see also* Tuberculosis) 017.2 ☑

scrotum 608.9

sebaceous glands NEC 706.9

Secretan's (posttraumatic edema) 782.3

semilunar cartilage, cystic 717.5

seminal vesicle 608.9

Senear-Usher (pemphigus erythematosus) 694.4

serum NEC 999.5

Sever's (osteochondrosis calcaneum) 732.5

sexually transmitted — *see* Disease, venereal

Sézary's (reticulosis) (M9701/3) 202.2 ☑

Shaver's (bauxite pneumoconiosis) 503

Sheehan's (postpartum pituitary necrosis) 253.2

shimamushi (scrub typhus) 081.2

shipyard 077.1

sickle cell 282.60

with

crisis 282.62

Hb-S disease 282.61

☑ **Additional Digit Required** — Refer to the Tabular List for Digit Selection

Ⓦ **Subterms under main terms may continue to next column or page**

Index

Disease, diseased — Disease, diseased

Disease, diseased — *see also* Syndrome — *continued*
sickle cell — *continued*
  with — *continued*
    other abnormal hemoglobin (Hb-D)
      (Hb-E) (Hb-G) (Hb-J) (Hb-K)
      (Hb-O) (Hb-P) (high fetal
      gene) (without crisis) 282.68
      with crisis 282.69
  elliptocytosis 282.60
  Hb-C (without crisis) 282.63
    with
      crisis 282.64
      vaso-occlusive pain 282.64
  Hb-S 282.61
    with
      crisis 282.62
      Hb-C (without crisis) 282.63
        with
          crisis 282.64
          vaso-occlusive pain 282.64
      other abnormal hemoglobin (Hb-
        D) (Hb-E) (Hb-G) (Hb-J)
        (Hb-K) (Hb-O) (Hb-P) (high
        fetal gene) (without crisis)
        282.68
        with crisis 282.69
  spherocytosis 282.60
  thalassemia (without crisis) 282.41
    with
      crisis 282.42
      vaso-occlusive pain 282.42
Siegal-Cattan-Mamou (periodic) 277.31
silo fillers' 506.9
Simian B 054.3
Simmonds' (pituitary cachexia) 253.2
Simons' (progressive lipodystrophy) 272.6
Sinding-Larsen (juvenile osteopathia patellae) 732.4
sinus (*see also* Sinusitis)
  brain 437.9
  specified NEC 478.19
Sirkari's 085.0
sixth (*see also* Exanthem subitum) 058.10
Sjögren (-Gougerot) 710.2
  with lung involvement 710.2 *[517.8]*
Skevas-Zerfus 989.5
skin NEC 709.9
  due to metabolic disorder 277.9
  specified type NEC 709.8
sleeping (*see also* Narcolepsy) 347.00
  meaning sleeping sickness (*see also* Trypanosomiasis) 086.5
small vessel 443.9
Smith-Strang (oasthouse urine) 270.2
Sneddon-Wilkinson (subcorneal pustular dermatosis) 694.1
South African creeping 133.8
Spencer's (epidemic vomiting) 078.82
Spielmeyer-Stock 330.1
Spielmeyer-Vogt 330.1
spine, spinal 733.90
  combined system (*see also* Degeneration, combined) 266.2 *[336.2]*
    with pernicious anemia 281.0 *[336.2]*
  cord NEC 336.9
    congenital 742.9
  demyelinating NEC 341.8
  joint (*see also* Disease, joint, spine) 724.9
  tuberculous 015.0 ☑ *[730.8]* ☑
spinocerebellar 334.9
  specified NEC 334.8
spleen (organic) (postinfectional) 289.50
  amyloid 277.39
  lardaceous 277.39
  polycystic 759.0
  specified NEC 289.59
sponge divers' 989.5
Stanton's (melioidosis) 025
Stargardt's 362.75
Startle 759.89
Steinert's 359.21
Sternberg's — *see* Disease, Hodgkin's
Stevens-Johnson (erythema multiforme exudativum) 695.13
Sticker's (erythema infectiosum) 057.0

Disease, diseased — *see also* Syndrome — *continued*
Stieda's (calcification, knee joint) 726.62
Still's (juvenile rheumatoid arthritis) 714.30
  adult onset 714.2
Stiller's (asthenia) 780.79
Stokes' (exophthalmic goiter) 242.0 ☑
Stokes-Adams (syncope with heart block) 426.9
Stokvis (-Talma) (enterogenous cyanosis) 289.7
stomach NEC (organic) 537.9
  functional 536.9
    psychogenic 306.4
  lardaceous 277.39
stonemasons' 502
storage
  glycogen (*see also* Disease, glycogen storage) 271.0
  lipid 272.7
  mucopolysaccharide 277.5
striatopallidal system 333.90
  specified NEC 333.89
Strümpell-Marie (ankylosing spondylitis) 720.0
Stuart's (congenital factor X deficiency) (*see also* Defect, coagulation) 286.3
Stuart-Prower (congenital factor X deficiency) (*see also* Defect, coagulation) 286.3
Sturge (-Weber) (-Dimitri) (encephalocutaneous angiomatosis) 759.6
Stuttgart 100.89
Sudeck's 733.7
supporting structures of teeth NEC 525.9
suprarenal (gland) (capsule) 255.9
  hyperfunction 255.3
  hypofunction 255.41
Sutton's 709.09
Sutton and Gull's — *see* Hypertension, kidney
sweat glands NEC 705.9
  specified type NEC 705.89
sweating 078.2
Sweeley-Klionsky 272.4
Swift (-Feer) 985.0
swimming pool (bacillus) 031.1
swineherd's 100.89
Sylvest's (epidemic pleurodynia) 074.1
Symmers (follicular lymphoma) (M9690/3) 202.0 ☑
sympathetic nervous system (*see also* Neuropathy, peripheral, autonomic) 337.9
synovium 727.9
syphilitic — *see* Syphilis
systemic tissue mast cell (M9741/3) 202.6 ☑
Taenzer's 757.4
Takayasu's (pulseless) 446.7
Talma's 728.85
Tangier (familial high-density lipoprotein deficiency) 272.5
Tarral-Besnier (pityriasis rubra pilaris) 696.4
Taylor's 701.8
Tay-Sachs 330.1
tear duct 375.69
teeth, tooth 525.9
  hard tissues 521.9
    specified NEC 521.89
  pulp NEC 522.9
tendon 727.9
  inflammatory NEC 727.9
terminal vessel 443.9
testis 608.9
Thaysen-Gee (nontropical sprue) 579.0
Thomsen's 359.22
Thomson's (congenital poikiloderma) 757.33
Thornwaldt's, Tornwaldt's (pharyngeal bursitis) 478.29
throat 478.20
  septic 034.0
thromboembolic (*see also* Embolism) 444.9
thymus (gland) 254.9
  specified NEC 254.8
thyroid (gland) NEC 246.9

Disease, diseased — *see also* Syndrome — *continued*
thyroid — *continued*
  heart (*see also* Hyperthyroidism) 242.9 ☑ *[425.7]*
  lardaceous 277.39
  specified NEC 246.8
Tietze's 733.6
Tommaselli's
  correct substance properly administered 599.70
  overdose or wrong substance given or taken 961.4
tongue 529.9
tonsils, tonsillar (and adenoids) (chronic) 474.9
  specified NEC 474.8
tooth, teeth 525.9
  hard tissues 521.9
    specified NEC 521.89
  pulp NEC 522.9
Tornwaldt's (pharyngeal bursitis) 478.29
Tourette's 307.23
trachea 519.19
tricuspid — *see* Endocarditis, tricuspid
triglyceride-storage, type I, II, III 272.7
triple vessel (coronary arteries) — *see* Arteriosclerosis, coronary
trisymptomatic, Gourgerot's 709.1
trophoblastic (*see also* Hydatidiform mole) 630
  previous, affecting management of pregnancy V23.1
tsutsugamushi (scrub typhus) 081.2
tube (fallopian), noninflammatory 620.9
  specified NEC 620.8
tuberculous NEC (*see also* Tuberculosis) 011.9 ☑
tubo-ovarian
  inflammatory (*see also* Salpingo-oophoritis) 614.2
  noninflammatory 620.9
    specified NEC 620.8
tubotympanic, chronic (with anterior perforation of ear drum) 382.1
tympanum 385.9
Uhl's 746.84
umbilicus (newborn) NEC 779.89
  delayed separation 779.83
Underwood's (sclerema neonatorum) 778.1
undiagnosed 799.9
Unna's (seborrheic dermatitis) 690.18
unstable hemoglobin hemolytic 282.7
Unverricht (-Lundborg) 345.1 ☑
Urbach-Oppenheim (necrobiosis lipoidica diabeticorum) 250.8 ☑ *[709.3]*
  due to secondary diabetes 249.8 ☑ *[709.3]*
Urbach-Wiethe (lipoid proteinosis) 272.8
ureter 593.9
urethra 599.9
  specified type NEC 599.84
urinary (tract) 599.9
  bladder 596.9
    specified NEC 596.8
  maternal, affecting fetus or newborn 760.1
Usher-Senear (pemphigus erythematosus) 694.4
uterus (organic) 621.9
  infective (*see also* Endometritis) 615.9
  inflammatory (*see also* Endometritis) 615.9
  noninflammatory 621.9
    specified type NEC 621.8
uveal tract
  anterior 364.9
  posterior 363.9
vagabonds' 132.1
vagina, vaginal
  inflammatory 616.10
  noninflammatory 623.9
    specified NEC 623.8
Valsuani's (progressive pernicious anemia, puerperal) 648.2 ☑

Disease, diseased — *see also* Syndrome — *continued*
Valsuani's — *continued*
  complicating pregnancy or puerperium 648.2 ☑
valve, valvular — *see also* Endocarditis
  congenital NEC (*see also* Anomaly, heart, valve) 746.9
    pulmonary 746.00
    specified type NEC 746.89
van Bogaert-Nijssen (-Peiffer) 330.0
van Creveld-von Gierke (glycogenosis I) 271.0
van den Bergh's (enterogenous cyanosis) 289.7
van Neck's (juvenile osteochondrosis) 732.1
Vaquez (-Osler) (polycythemia vera) (M9950/1) 238.4
vascular 459.9
  arteriosclerotic — *see* Arteriosclerosis
  hypertensive — *see* Hypertension
  obliterative 447.1
    peripheral 443.9
  occlusive 459.9
  peripheral (occlusive) 443.9
    in (due to) (with) diabetes mellitus 250.7 ☑ *[443.81]*
      in (due to) (with) secondary diabetes 249.7 ☑ *[443.81]*
    specified type NEC 443.89
vas deferens 608.9
vasomotor 443.9
vasospastic 443.9
vein 459.9
venereal 099.9
  chlamydial NEC 099.50
    anus 099.52
    bladder 099.53
    cervix 099.53
    epididymis 099.54
    genitourinary NEC 099.55
      lower 099.53
      specified NEC 099.54
    pelvic inflammatory disease 099.54
    perihepatic 099.56
    peritoneum 099.56
    pharynx 099.51
    rectum 099.52
    specified site NEC 099.59
    testis 099.54
    vagina 099.53
    vulva 099.53
  complicating pregnancy, childbirth, or puerperium 647.2 ☑
  fifth 099.1
  sixth 099.1
  specified nature or type NEC 099.8
    chlamydial — *see* Disease, venereal, chlamydial
Verneuil's (syphilitic bursitis) 095.7
Verse's (calcinosis intervertebralis) 275.49 *[722.90]*
vertebra, vertebral NEC 733.90
  disc — *see* Disease, Intervertebral disc
vibration NEC 994.9
Vidal's (lichen simplex chronicus) 698.3
Vincent's (trench mouth) 101
Virchow's 733.99
virus (filterable) NEC 078.89
  arbovirus NEC 066.9
  arthropod-borne NEC 066.9
  central nervous system NEC 049.9
    specified type NEC 049.8
  complicating pregnancy, childbirth, or puerperium 647.6 ☑
  contact (with) V01.79
    varicella V01.71
  exposure to V01.79
    varicella V01.71
  Marburg 078.89
  maternal
    with fetal damage affecting management of pregnancy 655.3 ☑
  nonarthropod-borne NEC 078.89
    central nervous system NEC 049.9
      specified NEC 049.8

☑ Additional Digit Required — Refer to the Tabular List for Digit Selection   Subterms under main terms may continue to next column or page

88 — Volume 2   ►◄ Revised Text   ● New Line   ▲ Revised Code   2011 ICD-9-CM

Disease, diseased — *see also* Syndrome — *continued*

virus — *continued*

vaccination, prophylactic (against) V04.89

vitreous 379.29

vocal cords NEC 478.5

Vogt's (Cecile) 333.71

Vogt-Spielmeyer 330.1

Volhard-Fahr (malignant nephrosclerosis) 403.00

Volkmann's

acquired 958.6

von Bechterew's (ankylosing spondylitis) 720.0

von Economo's (encephalitis lethargica) 049.8

von Eulenburg's (congenital paramyotonia) 359.29

von Gierke's (glycogenosis I) 271.0

von Graefe's 378.72

von Hippel's (retinocerebral angiomatosis) 759.6

von Hippel-Lindau (angiomatosis retinocerebellosa) 759.6

von Jaksch's (pseudoleukemia infantum) 285.8

von Recklinghausen's (M9540/1) 237.71

bone (osteitis fibrosa cystica) 252.01

von Recklinghausen-Applebaum (hemochromatosis) ▶*see also* Hemochromatosis*◄* 275.03 ▲

von Willebrand (-Jürgens) (angiohemophilia) 286.4

von Zambusch's (lichen sclerosus et atrophicus) 701.0

Voorhoeve's (dyschondroplasia) 756.4

Vrolik's (osteogenesis imperfecta) 756.51

vulva

inflammatory 616.10

noninflammatory 624.9

specified NEC 624.8

Wagner's (colloid milium) 709.3

Waldenström's (osteochondrosis capital femoral) 732.1

Wallgren's (obstruction of splenic vein with collateral circulation) 459.89

Wardrop's (with lymphangitis) 681.9

finger 681.02

toe 681.11

Wassilieff's (leptospiral jaundice) 100.0

wasting NEC 799.4

due to malnutrition 261

paralysis 335.21

Waterhouse-Friderichsen 036.3

waxy (any site) 277.39

Weber-Christian (nodular nonsuppurative panniculitis) 729.30

Wegner's (syphilitic osteochondritis) 090.0

Weil's (leptospiral jaundice) 100.0

of lung 100.0

Weir Mitchell's (erythromelalgia) 443.82

Werdnig-Hoffmann 335.0

Werlhof's (*see also* Purpura, thrombocytopenic) 287.39

Wermer's 258.01

Werner's (progeria adultorum) 259.8

Werner-His (trench fever) 083.1

Werner-Schultz (agranulocytosis) 288.09

Wernicke's (superior hemorrhagic polioencephalitis) 265.1

Wernicke-Posadas 114.9

Whipple's (intestinal lipodystrophy) 040.2

whipworm 127.3

White's (congenital) (keratosis follicularis) 757.39

white

blood cell 288.9

specified NEC 288.8

spot 701.0

Whitmore's (melioidosis) 025

Widal-Abrami (acquired hemolytic jaundice) 283.9

Wilkie's 557.1

Wilkinson-Sneddon (subcorneal pustular dermatosis) 694.1

Disease, diseased — *see also* Syndrome — *continued*

Willis' (diabetes mellitus) (*see also* Diabetes) 250.0 ☑

due to secondary diabetes 249.0 ☑

Wilson's (hepatolenticular degeneration) 275.1

Wilson-Brocq (dermatitis exfoliativa) 695.89

winter vomiting 078.82

Wise's 696.2

Wohlfart-Kugelberg-Welander 335.11

Woillez's (acute idiopathic pulmonary congestion) 518.5

Wolman's (primary familial xanthomatosis) 272.7

wool-sorters' 022.1

Zagari's (xerostomia) 527.7

Zahorsky's (exanthem subitum) 058.10

Ziehen-Oppenheim 333.6

zoonotic, bacterial NEC 027.9

specified type NEC 027.8

Disfigurement (due to scar) 709.2

head V48.6

limb V49.4

neck V48.7

trunk V48.7

Disgerminoma — *see* Dysgerminoma

Disinsertion, retina 361.04

Disintegration, complete, of the body 799.89

traumatic 869.1

Disk kidney 753.3

Dislocatable hip, congenital — *see also* Dislocation, hip, congenital 754.30

Dislocation (articulation) (closed) (displacement) (simple) (subluxation) 839.8

> *Note* — "Closed" includes simple, complete, partial, uncomplicated, and unspecified dislocation.
>
> "Open" includes dislocation specified as infected or compound and dislocation with foreign body.
>
> "Chronic," "habitual," "old," or "recurrent" dislocations should be coded as indicated under the entry "Dislocation, recurrent," and "pathological" as indicated under the entry "Dislocation, pathological."
>
> For late effect of dislocation see Late, effect, dislocation.

with fracture — *see* Fracture, by site

acromioclavicular (joint) (closed) 831.04

open 831.14

anatomical site (closed)

specified NEC 839.69

open 839.79

unspecified or ill-defined 839.8

open 839.9

ankle (scaphoid bone) (closed) 837.0

open 837.1

arm (closed) 839.8

open 839.9

astragalus (closed) 837.0

open 837.1

atlanto-axial (closed) 839.01

open 839.11

atlas (closed) 839.01

open 839.11

axis (closed) 839.02

open 839.12

back (closed) 839.8

open 839.9

Bell-Daly 723.8

breast bone (closed) 839.61

open 839.71

capsule, joint — *see* Dislocation, by site

carpal (bone) — *see* Dislocation, wrist

carpometacarpal (joint) (closed) 833.04

open 833.14

cartilage (joint) (*see also* Dislocation, by site)

knee — *see* Tear, meniscus

cervical, cervicodorsal, or cervicothoracic (spine) (vertebra) — *see* Dislocation, vertebra, cervical

---

Dislocation — *continued*

chiropractic (*see also* Lesion, nonallopathic) 739.9

chondrocostal — *see* Dislocation, costochondral

chronic — *see* Dislocation, recurrent

clavicle (closed) 831.04

open 831.14

coccyx (closed) 839.41

open 839.51

collar bone (closed) 831.04

open 831.14

compound (open) NEC 839.9

congenital NEC 755.8

hip (*see also* Dislocation, hip, congenital) 754.30

lens 743.37

rib 756.3

sacroiliac 755.69

spine NEC 756.19

vertebra 756.19

coracoid (closed) 831.09

open 831.19

costal cartilage (closed) 839.69

open 839.79

costochondral (closed) 839.69

open 839.79

cricoarytenoid articulation (closed) 839.69

open 839.79

cricothyroid (cartilage) articulation (closed) 839.69

open 839.79

dorsal vertebrae (closed) 839.21

open 839.31

ear ossicle 385.23

elbow (closed) 832.00

anterior (closed) 832.01

open 832.11

congenital 754.89

divergent (closed) 832.09

open 832.19

lateral (closed) 832.04

open 832.14

medial (closed) 832.03

open 832.13

open 832.10

posterior (closed) 832.02

open 832.12

recurrent 718.32

specified type NEC 832.09

open 832.19

eye 360.81

lateral 376.36

eyeball 360.81

lateral 376.36

femur

distal end (closed) 836.50

anterior 836.52

open 836.62

lateral 836.54

open 836.64

medial 836.53

open 836.63

open 836.60

posterior 836.51

open 836.61

proximal end (closed) 835.00

anterior (pubic) 835.03

open 835.13

obturator 835.02

open 835.12

open 835.10

posterior 835.01

open 835.11

fibula

distal end (closed) 837.0

open 837.1

proximal end (closed) 836.59

open 836.69

finger(s) (phalanx) (thumb) (closed) 834.00

interphalangeal (joint) 834.02

open 834.12

metacarpal (bone), distal end 834.01

open 834.11

metacarpophalangeal (joint) 834.01

open 834.11

Dislocation — *continued*

finger(s) — *continued*

open 834.10

recurrent 718.34

foot (closed) 838.00

open 838.10

recurrent 718.37

forearm (closed) 839.8

open 839.9

fracture — *see* Fracture, by site

glenoid (closed) 831.09

open 831.19

habitual — *see* Dislocation, recurrent

hand (closed) 839.8

open 839.9

hip (closed) 835.00

anterior 835.03

obturator 835.02

open 835.12

open 835.13

congenital (unilateral) 754.30

with subluxation of other hip 754.35

bilateral 754.31

developmental 718.75

open 835.10

posterior 835.01

open 835.11

recurrent 718.35

humerus (closed) 831.00

distal end (*see also* Dislocation, elbow) 832.00

open 831.10

proximal end (closed) 831.00

anterior (subclavicular) (subcoracoid) (subglenoid) (closed) 831.01

open 831.11

inferior (closed) 831.03

open 831.13

open 831.10

posterior (closed) 831.02

open 831.12

implant — *see* Complications, mechanical

incus 385.23

infracoracoid (closed) 831.01

open 831.11

innominate (pubic junction) (sacral junction) (closed) 839.69

acetabulum (*see also* Dislocation, hip) 835.00

open 839.79

interphalangeal (joint)

finger or hand (closed) 834.02

open 834.12

foot or toe (closed) 838.06

open 838.16

jaw (cartilage) (meniscus) (closed) 830.0

open 830.1

recurrent 524.69

joint NEC (closed) 839.8

developmental 718.7 ☑

open 839.9

pathological — *see* Dislocation, pathological

recurrent — *see* Dislocation, recurrent

knee (closed) 836.50

anterior 836.51

open 836.61

congenital (with genu recurvatum) 754.41

habitual 718.36

lateral 836.54

open 836.64

medial 836.53

open 836.63

old 718.36

open 836.60

posterior 836.52

open 836.62

recurrent 718.36

rotatory 836.59

open 836.69

lacrimal gland 375.16

leg (closed) 839.8

open 839.9

lens (crystalline) (complete) (partial) 379.32

anterior 379.33

Disease, diseased — Dislocation

☑ **Additional Digit Required** — Refer to the Tabular List for Digit Selection   ▼ **Subterms under main terms may continue to next column or page**

2011 ICD-9-CM   ▶◀ **Revised Text**   ● **New Line**   ▲ **Revised Code**   **October 2010 • Volume 2 — 89**

Dislocation — *continued*
lens — *continued*
  congenital 743.37
  ocular implant 996.53
  posterior 379.34
  traumatic 921.3
ligament — *see* Dislocation, by site
lumbar (vertebrae) (closed) 839.20
  open 839.30
lumbosacral (vertebrae) (closed) 839.20
  congenital 756.19
  open 839.30
mandible (closed) 830.0
  open 830.1
maxilla (inferior) (closed) 830.0
  open 830.1
meniscus (knee) (*see also* Tear, meniscus)
  other sites — *see* Dislocation, by site
metacarpal (bone)
  distal end (closed) 834.01
    open 834.11
  proximal end (closed) 833.05
    open 833.15
metacarpophalangeal (joint) (closed) 834.01
  open 834.11
metatarsal (bone) (closed) 838.04
  open 838.14
metatarsophalangeal (joint) (closed) 838.05
  open 838.15
midcarpal (joint) (closed) 833.03
  open 833.13
midtarsal (joint) (closed) 838.02
  open 838.12
Monteggia's — *see* Dislocation, hip
multiple locations (except fingers only or toes only) (closed) 839.8
  open 839.9
navicular (bone) foot (closed) 837.0
  open 837.1
neck (*see also* Dislocation, vertebra, cervical) 839.00
Nélaton's — *see* Dislocation, ankle
nontraumatic (joint) — *see* Dislocation, pathological
nose (closed) 839.69
  open 839.79
not recurrent, not current injury — *see* Dislocation, pathological
occiput from atlas (closed) 839.01
  open 839.11
old — *see* Dislocation, recurrent
open (compound) NEC 839.9
ossicle, ear 385.23
paralytic (flaccid) (spastic) — *see* Dislocation, pathological
patella (closed) 836.3
  congenital 755.64
  open 836.4
pathological NEC 718.20
  ankle 718.27
  elbow 718.22
  foot 718.27
  hand 718.24
  hip 718.25
  knee 718.26
  lumbosacral joint 724.6
  multiple sites 718.29
  pelvic region 718.25
  sacroiliac 724.6
  shoulder (region) 718.21
  specified site NEC 718.28
  spine 724.8
    sacroiliac 724.6
  wrist 718.23
pelvis (closed) 839.69
  acetabulum (*see also* Dislocation, hip) 835.00
  open 839.79
phalanx
  foot or toe (closed) 838.09
    open 838.19
  hand or finger (*see also* Dislocation, finger) 834.00
postpoliomyelitic — *see* Dislocation, pathological

Dislocation — *continued*
prosthesis, internal — *see* Complications, mechanical
radiocarpal (joint) (closed) 833.02
  open 833.12
radioulnar (joint)
  distal end (closed) 833.01
    open 833.11
  proximal end (*see also* Dislocation, elbow) 832.00
radius
  distal end (closed) 833.00
    open 833.10
  proximal end (closed) 832.01
    open 832.11
recurrent (*see also* Derangement, joint, recurrent) 718.3 ☑
  elbow 718.32
  hip 718.35
  joint NEC 718.38
  knee 718.36
  lumbosacral (joint) 724.6
  patella 718.36
  sacroiliac 724.6
  shoulder 718.31
  temporomandibular 524.69
rib (cartilage) (closed) 839.69
  congenital 756.3
  open 839.79
sacrococcygeal (closed) 839.42
  open 839.52
sacroiliac (joint) (ligament) (closed) 839.42
  congenital 755.69
  open 839.52
  recurrent 724.6
sacrum (closed) 839.42
  open 839.52
scaphoid (bone)
  ankle or foot (closed) 837.0
    open 837.1
  wrist (closed) (*see also* Dislocation, wrist) 833.00
    open 833.10
scapula (closed) 831.09
  open 831.19
semilunar cartilage, knee — *see* Tear, meniscus
septal cartilage (nose) (closed) 839.69
  open 839.79
septum (nasal) (old) 470
sesamoid bone — *see* Dislocation, by site
shoulder (blade) (ligament) (closed) 831.00
  anterior (subclavicular) (subcoracoid) (subglenoid) (closed) 831.01
    open 831.11
  chronic 718.31
  inferior 831.03
    open 831.13
    open 831.10
  posterior (closed) 831.02
    open 831.12
  recurrent 718.31
skull — *see* Injury, intracranial
Smith's — *see* Dislocation, foot
spine (articular process) (*see also* Dislocation, vertebra) (closed) 839.40
  atlanto-axial (closed) 839.01
    open 839.11
    recurrent 723.8
  cervical, cervicodorsal, cervicothoracic (closed) (*see also* Dislocation, vertebrae, cervical) 839.00
    open 839.10
    recurrent 723.8
  coccyx 839.41
    open 839.51
  congenital 756.19
  due to birth trauma 767.4
  open 839.50
  recurrent 724.9
  sacroiliac 839.42
    recurrent 724.6
  sacrum (sacrococcygeal) (sacroiliac) 839.42
    open 839.52

Dislocation — *continued*
spontaneous — *see* Dislocation, pathological
sternoclavicular (joint) (closed) 839.61
  open 839.71
sternum (closed) 839.61
  open 839.71
subastragalar — *see* Dislocation, foot
subglenoid (closed) 831.01
  open 831.11
symphysis
  jaw (closed) 830.0
    open 830.1
  mandibular (closed) 830.0
    open 830.1
  pubis (closed) 839.69
    open 839.79
tarsal (bone) (joint) 838.01
  open 838.11
tarsometatarsal (joint) 838.03
  open 838.13
temporomandibular (joint) (closed) 830.0
  open 830.1
  recurrent 524.69
thigh
  distal end (*see also* Dislocation, femur, distal end) 836.50
  proximal end (*see also* Dislocation, hip) 835.00
thoracic (vertebrae) (closed) 839.21
  open 839.31
thumb(s) (*see also* Dislocation, finger) 834.00
thyroid cartilage (closed) 839.69
  open 839.79
tibia
  distal end (closed) 837.0
    open 837.1
  proximal end (closed) 836.50
    anterior 836.51
      open 836.61
    lateral 836.54
      open 836.64
    medial 836.53
      open 836.63
      open 836.60
    posterior 836.52
      open 836.62
    rotatory 836.59
      open 836.69
tibiofibular
  distal (closed) 837.0
    open 837.1
  superior (closed) 836.59
    open 836.69
toe(s) (closed) 838.09
  open 838.19
trachea (closed) 839.69
  open 839.79
ulna
  distal end (closed) 833.09
    open 833.19
  proximal end — *see* Dislocation, elbow
vertebra (articular process) (body) (closed) (traumatic) 839.40
  cervical, cervicodorsal or cervicothoracic (closed) 839.00
    first (atlas) 839.01
      open 839.11
    second (axis) 839.02
      open 839.12
    third 839.03
      open 839.13
    fourth 839.04
      open 839.14
    fifth 839.05
      open 839.15
    sixth 839.06
      open 839.16
    seventh 839.07
      open 839.17
    congenital 756.19
    multiple sites 839.08
      open 839.18
      open 839.10
  congenital 756.19
  dorsal 839.21

Dislocation — *continued*
vertebra — *continued*
  dorsal — *continued*
    open 839.31
    recurrent 724.9
  lumbar, lumbosacral 839.20
    open 839.30
  non-traumatic — *see* Displacement, intervertebral disc
  open NEC 839.50
  recurrent 724.9
  specified region NEC 839.49
    open 839.59
  thoracic 839.21
    open 839.31
wrist (carpal bone) (scaphoid) (semilunar) (closed) 833.00
  carpometacarpal (joint) 833.04
    open 833.14
  metacarpal bone, proximal end 833.05
    open 833.15
  midcarpal (joint) 833.03
    open 833.13
  radiocarpal (joint) 833.02
    open 833.12
  radioulnar (joint) 833.01
    open 833.11
  recurrent 718.33
  specified site NEC 833.09
    open 833.19
  xiphoid cartilage (closed) 839.61
    open 839.71
Dislodgement
  artificial skin graft 996.55
  decellularized allodermis graft 996.55
Disobedience, hostile (covert) (overt) — *see also* Disturbance, conduct 312.0 ☑
Disorder — *see also* Disease
  academic underachievement, childhood and adolescence 313.83
  accommodation 367.51
    drug-induced 367.89
    toxic 367.89
  adjustment (*see also* Reaction, adjustment) 309.9
    with
      anxiety 309.24
      anxiety and depressed mood 309.28
      depressed mood 309.0
      disturbance of conduct 309.3
      disturbance of emotions and conduct 309.4
  adrenal (capsule) (cortex) (gland) 255.9
    specified type NEC 255.8
  adrenogenital 255.2
  affective (*see also* Psychosis, affective) 296.90
    atypical 296.81
  aggressive, unsocialized (*see also* Disturbance, conduct) 312.0 ☑
  alcohol, alcoholic (*see also* Alcohol) 291.9
  allergic — *see* Allergy
  amino acid (metabolic) (*see also* Disturbance, metabolism, amino acid) 270.9
    albinism 270.2
    alkaptonuria 270.2
    argininosuccinicaciduria 270.6
    beta-amino-isobutyricaciduria 277.2
    cystathioninuria 270.4
    cystinosis 270.0
    cystinuria 270.0
    glycinuria 270.0
    homocystinuria 270.4
    imidazole 270.5
    maple syrup (urine) disease 270.3
    neonatal, transitory 775.89
    oasthouse urine disease 270.2
    ochronosis 270.2
    phenylketonuria 270.1
    phenylpyruvic oligophrenia 270.1
    purine NEC 277.2
    pyrimidine NEC 277.2
    renal transport NEC 270.0
    specified type NEC 270.8

☑ **Additional Digit Required** — **Refer to the Tabular List for Digit Selection**   ▽ **Subterms under main terms may continue to next column or page**

90 — Volume 2   ▶◀ **Revised Text**   ● **New Line**   ▲ **Revised Code**   **2011 ICD-9-CM**

Disorder — *see also* Disease — *continued*
amino acid (*see also* Disturbance,
metabolism, amino acid) — *continued*
transport NEC 270.0
renal 270.0
xanthinuria 277.2
amnestic (*see also* Amnestic syndrome)
294.8
alcohol-induced persisting 291.1
drug-induced persisting 292.83
in conditions classified elsewhere 294.0
anaerobic glycolysis with anemia 282.3
anxiety (*see also* Anxiety) 300.00
due to or associated with physical condition 293.84
arteriole 447.9
specified type NEC 447.8
artery 447.9
specified type NEC 447.8
articulation — *see* Disorder, joint
Asperger's 299.8 ☑
attachment of infancy or early childhood
313.89
attention deficit 314.00
with hyperactivity 314.01
predominantly
combined hyperactive/inattentive
314.01
hyperactive/impulsive 314.01
inattentive 314.00
residual type 314.8
auditory processing disorder 388.45
acquired 388.45
developmental 315.32
autistic 299.0 ☑
autoimmune NEC 279.49
hemolytic (cold type) (warm type) 283.0
parathyroid 252.1
thyroid 245.2
avoidant, childhood or adolescence 313.21
balance
acid-base 276.9
mixed (with hypercapnia) 276.4
electrolyte 276.9
fluid 276.9
behavior NEC (*see also* Disturbance, conduct) 312.9
disruptive 312.9
bilirubin excretion 277.4
bipolar (affective) (alternating) 296.80

Note — Use the following fifth-digit
subclassification with categories
296.0–296.6:

0   unspecifed

1   mild

2   moderate

3   severe, without mention of psy-
    chotic behavior

4   severe, specified as with psychotic
    behavior

5   in partial or unspecified remission

6   in full remission

---

atypical 296.7
currently
depressed 296.5 ☑
hypomanic 296.4 ☑
manic 296.4 ☑
mixed 296.6 ☑
specified type NEC 296.89
type I 296.7
most recent episode (or current)
depressed 296.5 ☑
hypomanic 296.4 ☑
manic 296.4 ☑
mixed 296.6 ☑
unspecified 296.7
single manic episode 296.0 ☑
type II (recurrent major depressive
episodes with hypomania) 296.89
bladder 596.9
functional NEC 596.59

Disorder — *see also* Disease — *continued*
bladder — *continued*
specified NEC 596.8
bleeding 286.9
bone NEC 733.90
specified NEC 733.99
brachial plexus 353.0
branched-chain amino-acid degradation
270.3
breast 611.9
puerperal, postpartum 676.3 ☑
specified NEC 611.89
Briquet's 300.81
bursa 727.9
shoulder region 726.10
carbohydrate metabolism, congenital 271.9
cardiac, functional 427.9
postoperative 997.1
psychogenic 306.2
cardiovascular, psychogenic 306.2
cartilage NEC 733.90
articular 718.00
ankle 718.07
elbow 718.02
foot 718.07
hand 718.04
hip 718.05
knee 717.9
multiple sites 718.09
pelvic region 718.05
shoulder region 718.01
specified
site NEC 718.08
type NEC 733.99
wrist 718.03
catatonic — *see* Catatonia
central auditory processing 315.32
acquired 388.45
developmental 315.32
cervical region NEC 723.9
cervical root (nerve) NEC 353.2
character NEC (*see also* Disorder, personality) 301.9
ciliary body 364.9
specified NEC 364.89
coagulation (factor) (*see also* Defect, coagulation) 286.9
factor VIII (congenital) (functional) 286.0
factor IX (congenital) (functional) 286.1
neonatal, transitory 776.3
coccyx 724.70
specified NEC 724.79
cognitive 294.9
colon 569.9
functional 564.9
congenital 751.3
communication 307.9
conduct (*see also* Disturbance, conduct)
312.9
adjustment reaction 309.3
adolescent onset type 312.82
childhood onset type 312.81
compulsive 312.30
specified type NEC 312.39
hyperkinetic 314.2
onset unspecified 312.89
socialized (type) 312.20
aggressive 312.23
unaggressive 312.21
specified NEC 312.89
conduction, heart 426.9
specified NEC 426.89
conflict
sexual orientation 302.0
congenital
glycosylation (CDG) 271.8
convulsive (secondary) (*see also* Convulsions) 780.39
due to injury at birth 767.0
idiopathic 780.39
coordination 781.3
cornea NEC 371.89
due to contact lens 371.82
corticosteroid metabolism NEC 255.2
cranial nerve — *see* Disorder, nerve, cranial
cyclothymic 301.13

Disorder — *see also* Disease — *continued*
degradation, branched-chain amino acid
270.3
delusional 297.1
dentition 520.6
depersonalization 300.6
depressive NEC 311
atypical 296.82
major (*see also* Psychosis, affective)
296.2 ☑
recurrent episode 296.3 ☑
single episode 296.2 ☑
development, specific 315.9
associated with hyperkinesia 314.1
coordination 315.4
language 315.31
and speech due to hearing loss
315.34
learning 315.2
arithmetical 315.1
reading 315.00
mixed 315.5
motor coordination 315.4
specified type NEC 315.8
speech 315.39
and language due to hearing loss
315.34
diaphragm 519.4
digestive 536.9
fetus or newborn 777.9
specified NEC 777.8
psychogenic 306.4
disintegrative, childhood 299.1 ☑
dissociative 300.15
identity 300.14
nocturnal 307.47
drug-related 292.9
dysmorphic body 300.7
dysthymic 300.4
ear 388.9
degenerative NEC 388.00
external 380.9
specified 380.89
pinna 380.30
specified type NEC 388.8
vascular NEC 388.00
eating NEC 307.50
electrolyte NEC 276.9
with
abortion — *see* Abortion, by type,
with metabolic disorder
ectopic pregnancy (*see also* categories 633.0–633.9) 639.4
molar pregnancy (*see also* categories
630–632) 639.4
acidosis 276.2
metabolic 276.2
respiratory 276.2
alkalosis 276.3
metabolic 276.3
respiratory 276.3
following
abortion 639.4
ectopic or molar pregnancy 639.4
neonatal, transitory NEC 775.5
emancipation as adjustment reaction 309.22
emotional (*see also* Disorder, mental,
nonpsychotic) V40.9
endocrine 259.9
specified type NEC 259.8
esophagus 530.9
functional 530.5
psychogenic 306.4
explosive
intermittent 312.34
isolated 312.35
expressive language 315.31
eye 379.90
globe — *see* Disorder, globe
ill-defined NEC 379.99
limited duction NEC 378.63
specified NEC 379.8
eyelid 374.9
degenerative 374.50
sensory 374.44
specified type NEC 374.89

Disorder — *see also* Disease — *continued*
eyelid — *continued*
vascular 374.85
factitious (with combined psychological and
physical signs and symptoms) (with
predominantly physical signs and
symptoms) 300.19
with predominantly psychological signs
and symptoms 300.16
factor, coagulation (*see also* Defect, coagulation) 286.9
IX (congenital) (funcitonal) 286.1
VIII (congenital) (functional) 286.0
fascia 728.9
fatty acid oxidation 277.85
feeding — *see* Feeding
female sexual arousal 302.72
fluency 315.35 ●
adult onset 307.0 ●
childhood onset 315.35 ●
due to late effect of cerebrovascular ●
accident 438.14 ●
in conditions classified elsewhere ●
784.52 ●
fluid NEC 276.9
gastric (functional) 536.9
motility 536.8
psychogenic 306.4
secretion 536.8
gastrointestinal (functional) NEC 536.9
newborn (neonatal) 777.9
specified NEC 777.8
psychogenic 306.4
gender (child) 302.6
adult 302.85
gender identity (childhood) 302.6
adolescents 302.85
adults (-life) 302.85
genitourinary system, psychogenic 306.50
globe 360.9
degenerative 360.20
specified NEC 360.29
specified type NEC 360.89
hearing (*see also* Deafness)
conductive type (air) (*see also* Deafness,
conductive) 389.00
mixed conductive and sensorineural
389.20
bilateral 389.22
unilateral 389.21
nerve
bilateral 389.12
unilateral 389.13
perceptive (*see also* Deafness, perceptive) 389.10
sensorineural type NEC (*see also* Deafness, sensorineural 389.10
heart action 427.9
postoperative 997.1
hematological, transient neonatal 776.9
specified type NEC 776.8
hematopoietic organs 289.9
hemorrhagic NEC 287.9
due to intrinsic circulating anticoagulants 286.5
specified type NEC 287.8
hemostasis (*see also* Defect, coagulation)
286.9
homosexual conflict 302.0
hypomanic (chronic) 301.11
identity
childhood and adolescence 313.82
gender 302.6
immune mechanism (immunity) 279.9
single complement (C1-C9) 279.8
specified type NEC 279.8
impulse control (*see also* Disturbance, conduct, compulsive) 312.30
infant sialic acid storage 271.8
integument, fetus or newborn 778.9
specified type NEC 778.8
interactional psychotic (childhood) (*see also*
Psychosis, childhood) 299.1 ☑
intermittent explosive 312.34
intervertebral disc 722.90
cervical, cervicothoracic 722.91

Disorder — *see also* Disease — *continued*
intervertebral disc — *continued*
 lumbar, lumbosacral 722.93
 thoracic, thoracolumbar 722.92
intestinal 569.9
 functional NEC 564.9
  congenital 751.3
  postoperative 564.4
 psychogenic 306.4
introverted, of childhood and adolescence 313.22
involuntary emotional expression (IEED) 310.8
iris 364.9
 specified NEC 364.89
iron, metabolism 275.09   ▲
 specified type NEC 275.09   ●
isolated explosive 312.35
joint NEC 719.90
 ankle 719.97
 elbow 719.92
 foot 719.97
 hand 719.94
 hip 719.95
 knee 719.96
 multiple sites 719.99
 pelvic region 719.95
 psychogenic 306.0
 shoulder (region) 719.91
 specified site NEC 719.98
 temporomandibular 524.60
  sounds on opening or closing 524.64
  specified NEC 524.69
 wrist 719.93
kidney 593.9
 functional 588.9
  specified NEC 588.89
labyrinth, labyrinthine 386.9
 specified type NEC 386.8
lactation 676.9 ☑
language (developmental) (expressive) 315.31
 mixed receptive-expressive 315.32
learning 315.9
ligament 728.9
ligamentous attachments, peripheral (*see also* Enthesopathy)
 spine 720.1
limb NEC 729.90
 psychogenic 306.0
lipid
 metabolism, congenital 272.9
 storage 272.7
lipoprotein deficiency (familial) 272.5
low back NEC 724.9
 psychogenic 306.0
lumbosacral
 plexus 353.1
 root (nerve) NEC 353.4
lymphoproliferative (chronic) NEC (M9970/1) 238.79
 post-transplant (PTLD) 238.77
major depressive (*see also* Psychosis, affective) 296.2 ☑
 recurrent episode 296.3 ☑
 single episode 296.2 ☑
male erectile 607.84
 nonorganic origin 302.72
manic (*see also* Psychosis, affective) 296.0 ☑
 atypical 296.81
mathematics 315.1
meniscus NEC (*see also* Disorder, cartilage, articular) 718.0 ☑
menopausal 627.9
 specified NEC 627.8
menstrual 626.9
 psychogenic 306.52
 specified NEC 626.8
mental (nonpsychotic) 300.9
 affecting management of pregnancy, childbirth, or puerperium 648.4 ☑
 drug-induced 292.9
  hallucinogen persisting perception 292.89
  specified type NEC 292.89

Disorder — *see also* Disease — *continued*
mental — *continued*
 due to or associated with
  alcoholism 291.9
  drug consumption NEC 292.9
   specified type NEC 292.89
  physical condition NEC 293.9
 induced by drug 292.9
  specified type NEC 292.89
 neurotic (*see also* Neurosis) 300.9
 of infancy, childhood or adolescence 313.9
 persistent
  other
   due to conditions classified elsewhere 294.8
  unspecified
   due to conditions classified elsewhere 294.9
 presenile 310.1
  psychotic NEC 290.10
 previous, affecting management of pregnancy V23.89
 psychoneurotic (*see also* Neurosis) 300.9
 psychotic (*see also* Psychosis) 298.9
  brief 298.8
  senile 290.20
 specific, following organic brain damage 310.9
  cognitive or personality change of other type 310.1
  frontal lobe syndrome 310.0
  postconcussional syndrome 310.2
  specified type NEC 310.8
 transient
  in conditions classified elsewhere 293.9
metabolism NEC 277.9
 with
  abortion — *see* Abortion, by type, with metabolic disorder
  ectopic pregnancy (*see also* categories 633.0–633.9) 639.4
  molar pregnancy (*see also* categories 630–632) 639.4
 alkaptonuria 270.2
 amino acid (*see also* Disorder, amino acid) 270.9
  specified type NEC 270.8
 ammonia 270.6
 arginine 270.6
 argininosuccinic acid 270.6
 basal 794.7
 bilirubin 277.4
 calcium 275.40
 carbohydrate 271.9
  specified type NEC 271.8
 cholesterol 272.9
 citrulline 270.6
 copper 275.1
 corticosteroid 255.2
 cystine storage 270.0
 cystinuria 270.0
 fat 272.9
 fatty acid oxidation 277.85
 following
  abortion 639.4
  ectopic or molar pregnancy 639.4
 fructosemia 271.2
 fructosuria 271.2
 fucosidosis 271.8
 galactose-1-phosphate uridyl transferase 271.1
 glutamine 270.7
 glycine 270.7
 glycogen storage NEC 271.0
  hepatorenal 271.0
 hemochromatosis ►*(see also* Hemochromatosis)◄ 275.03   ▲
 in labor and delivery 669.0 ☑
 iron 275.09   ▲
 lactose 271.3
 lipid 272.9
  specified type NEC 272.8
  storage 272.7

Disorder — *see also* Disease — *continued*
metabolism — *continued*
 lipoprotein (*see also* Hyperlipemia deficiency (familial)) 272.5
 lysine 270.7
 magnesium 275.2
 mannosidosis 271.8
 mineral 275.9
  specified type NEC 275.8
 mitochondrial 277.87
 mucopolysaccharide 277.5
 nitrogen 270.9
 ornithine 270.6
 oxalosis 271.8
 pentosuria 271.8
 phenylketonuria 270.1
 phosphate 275.3
 phosphorous 275.3
 plasma protein 273.9
  specified type NEC 273.8
 porphyrin 277.1
 purine 277.2
 pyrimidine 277.2
 serine 270.7
 sodium 276.9
 specified type NEC 277.89
 steroid 255.2
 threonine 270.7
 urea cycle 270.6
 xylose 271.8
micturition NEC 788.69
 psychogenic 306.53
misery and unhappiness, of childhood and adolescence 313.1
mitochondrial metabolism 277.87
mitral valve 424.0
mood (*see also* Disorder, bipolar) 296.90
 episodic 296.90
  specified NEC 296.99
 in conditions classified elsewhere 293.83
motor tic 307.20
 chronic 307.22
 transient (childhood) 307.21
movement NEC 333.90
 hysterical 300.11
 medication-induced 333.90
 periodic limb 327.51
 sleep related, unspecified 780.58
  other organic 327.59
 specified type NEC 333.99
 stereotypic 307.3
mucopolysaccharide 277.5
muscle 728.9
 psychogenic 306.0
 specified type NEC 728.3
muscular attachments, peripheral (*see also* Enthesopathy)
 spine 720.1
musculoskeletal system NEC 729.90
 psychogenic 306.0
myeloproliferative (chronic) NEC (M9960/1) 238.79
myoneural 358.9
 due to lead 358.2
 specified type NEC 358.8
 toxic 358.2
myotonic 359.29
neck region NEC 723.9
nerve 349.9
 abducens NEC 378.54
 accessory 352.4
 acoustic 388.5
 auditory 388.5
 auriculotemporal 350.8
 axillary 353.0
 cerebral — *see* Disorder, nerve, cranial
 cranial 352.9
  first 352.0
  second 377.49
  third
   partial 378.51
   total 378.52
  fourth 378.53
  fifth 350.9
  sixth 378.54
  seventh NEC 351.9

Disorder — *see also* Disease — *continued*
nerve — *continued*
 cranial — *continued*
  eighth 388.5
  ninth 352.2
  tenth 352.3
  eleventh 352.4
  twelfth 352.5
  multiple 352.6
 entrapment — *see* Neuropathy, entrapment
 facial 351.9
  specified NEC 351.8
 femoral 355.2
 glossopharyngeal NEC 352.2
 hypoglossal 352.5
 iliohypogastric 355.79
 ilioinguinal 355.79
 intercostal 353.8
 lateral
  cutaneous of thigh 355.1
  popliteal 355.3
 lower limb NEC 355.8
 medial, popliteal 355.4
 median NEC 354.1
 obturator 355.79
 oculomotor
  partial 378.51
  total 378.52
 olfactory 352.0
 optic 377.49
  hypoplasia 377.43
  ischemic 377.41
  nutritional 377.33
  toxic 377.34
 peroneal 355.3
 phrenic 354.8
 plantar 355.6
 pneumogastric 352.3
 posterior tibial 355.5
 radial 354.3
 recurrent laryngeal 352.3
 root 353.9
  specified NEC 353.8
 saphenous 355.79
 sciatic NEC 355.0
 specified NEC 355.9
  lower limb 355.79
  upper limb 354.8
 spinal 355.9
 sympathetic NEC 337.9
 trigeminal 350.9
  specified NEC 350.8
 trochlear 378.53
 ulnar 354.2
 upper limb NEC 354.9
 vagus 352.3
nervous system NEC 349.9
 autonomic (peripheral) (*see also* Neuropathy, peripheral, autonomic) 337.9
 cranial 352.9
 parasympathetic (*see also* Neuropathy, peripheral, autonomic) 337.9
 specified type NEC 349.89
 sympathetic (*see also* Neuropathy, peripheral, autonomic) 337.9
 vegetative (*see also* Neuropathy, peripheral, autonomic) 337.9
neurohypophysis NEC 253.6
neurological NEC 781.99
 peripheral NEC 355.9
neuromuscular NEC 358.9
 hereditary NEC 359.1
 specified NEC 358.8
 toxic 358.2
neurotic 300.9
 specified type NEC 300.89
neutrophil, polymorphonuclear (functional) 288.1
nightmare 307.47
night terror 307.46
obsessive-compulsive 300.3
oppositional defiant, childhood and adolescence 313.81
optic
 chiasm 377.54

☑ Additional Digit Required — Refer to the Tabular List for Digit Selection   ▽ Subterms under main terms may continue to next column or page

92 — Volume 2 • October 2010   ►◄ Revised Text   ● New Line   ▲ Revised Code   2011 ICD-9-CM

Disorder — see also Disease — continued
 tendon 727.9
  shoulder region 726.10
 thoracic root (nerve) NEC 353.3
 thyrocalcitonin secretion 246.0
 thyroid (gland) NEC 246.9
  specified type NEC 246.8
 tic 307.20
  chronic (motor or vocal) 307.22
  motor-verbal 307.23
  organic origin 333.1
  transient (of childhood) 307.21
 tooth NEC 525.9
  development NEC 520.9
   specified type NEC 520.8
  eruption 520.6
  specified type NEC 525.8
 Tourette's 307.23
 transport, carbohydrate 271.9
  specified type NEC 271.8
 tubular, phosphate-losing 588.0
 tympanic membrane 384.9
 unaggressive, unsocialized (see also Disturbance, conduct) 312.1 ✓
 undersocialized, unsocialized (see also Disturbance, conduct)
  aggressive (type) 312.0 ✓
  unaggressive (type) 312.1 ✓
 vision, visual NEC 368.9
  binocular NEC 368.30
  cortex 377.73
   associated with
    inflammatory disorders 377.73
    neoplasms 377.71
    vascular disorders 377.72
  pathway NEC 377.63
   associated with
    inflammatory disorders 377.63
    neoplasms 377.61
    vascular disorders 377.62
 vocal tic
  chronic 307.22
 wakefulness (see also Hypersomnia) 780.54
  nonorganic origin (transient) 307.43
  persistent 307.44
 written expression 315.2
Disorganized globe 360.29
Displacement, displaced

> Note — For acquired displacement of bones, cartilage, joints, tendons, due to injury, see also Dislocation.
>
> Displacements at ages under one year should be considered congenital, provided there is no indication the condition was acquired after birth.

 acquired traumatic of bone, cartilage, joint, tendon NEC (without fracture) (see also Dislocation) 839.8
  with fracture — see Fracture, by site
 adrenal gland (congenital) 759.1
 alveolus and teeth, vertical 524.75
 appendix, retrocecal (congenital) 751.5
 auricle (congenital) 744.29
 bladder (acquired) 596.8
  congenital 753.8
 brachial plexus (congenital) 742.8
 brain stem, caudal 742.4
 canaliculus lacrimalis 743.65
 cardia, through esophageal hiatus 750.6
 cerebellum, caudal 742.4
 cervix — see Displacement, uterus
 colon (congenital) 751.4
 device, implant, or graft — see Complications, mechanical
 epithelium
  columnar of cervix 622.10
  cuboidal, beyond limits of external os (uterus) 752.49
 esophageal mucosa into cardia of stomach, congenital 750.4
 esophagus (acquired) 530.89
  congenital 750.4
 eyeball (acquired) (old) 376.36
  congenital 743.8
  current injury 871.3

Displacement, displaced — continued
 eyeball — continued
  lateral 376.36
 fallopian tube (acquired) 620.4
  congenital 752.19
  opening (congenital) 752.19
 gallbladder (congenital) 751.69
 gastric mucosa 750.7
  into
   duodenum 750.7
   esophagus 750.7
   Meckel's diverticulum, congenital 750.7
 globe (acquired) (lateral) (old) 376.36
  current injury 871.3
 graft
  artificial skin graft 996.55
  decellularized allodermis graft 996.55
 heart (congenital) 746.87
  acquired 429.89
 hymen (congenital) (upward) 752.49
 internal prosthesis NEC — see Complications, mechanical
 intervertebral disc (with neuritis, radiculitis, sciatica, or other pain) 722.2
  with myelopathy 722.70
  cervical, cervicodorsal, cervicothoracic 722.0
   with myelopathy 722.71
   due to major trauma — see Dislocation, vertebra, cervical
  due to trauma — see Dislocation, vertebra
  lumbar, lumbosacral 722.10
   with myelopathy 722.73
   due to major trauma — see Dislocation, vertebra, lumbar
  thoracic, thoracolumbar 722.11
   with myelopathy 722.72
   due to major trauma — see Dislocation, vertebra, thoracic
 intrauterine device 996.32
 kidney (acquired) 593.0
  congenital 753.3
 lacrimal apparatus or duct (congenital) 743.65
 macula (congenital) 743.55
 Meckel's diverticulum (congenital) 751.0
 nail (congenital) 757.5
  acquired 703.8
 opening of Wharton's duct in mouth 750.26
 organ or site, congenital NEC — see Malposition, congenital
 ovary (acquired) 620.4
  congenital 752.0
  free in peritoneal cavity (congenital) 752.0
  into hernial sac 620.4
 oviduct (acquired) 620.4
  congenital 752.19
 parathyroid (gland) 252.8
 parotid gland (congenital) 750.26
 punctum lacrimale (congenital) 743.65
 sacroiliac (congenital) (joint) 755.69
  current injury — see Dislocation, sacroiliac
  old 724.6
 spine (congenital) 756.19
 spleen, congenital 759.0
 stomach (congenital) 750.7
  acquired 537.89
 subglenoid (closed) 831.01
 sublingual duct (congenital) 750.26
 teeth, tooth 524.30
  horizontal 524.33
  vertical 524.34
 tongue (congenital) (downward) 750.19
 trachea (congenital) 748.3
 ureter or ureteric opening or orifice (congenital) 753.4
 uterine opening of oviducts or fallopian tubes 752.19
 uterus, uterine (see also Malposition, uterus) 621.6
  congenital 752.39   ▲
 ventricular septum 746.89

Displacement, displaced — continued
 ventricular septum — continued
  with rudimentary ventricle 746.89
  xyphoid bone (process) 738.3
Disproportion 653.9 ✓
 affecting fetus or newborn 763.1
 breast, reconstructed 612.1
  between native and reconstructed 612.1
 caused by
  conjoined twins 678.1 ✓
  contraction, pelvis (general) 653.1 ✓
   inlet 653.2 ✓
   midpelvic 653.8 ✓
   midplane 653.8 ✓
   outlet 653.3 ✓
  fetal
   ascites 653.7 ✓
   hydrocephalus 653.6 ✓
   hydrops 653.7 ✓
   meningomyelocele 653.7 ✓
   sacral teratoma 653.7 ✓
   tumor 653.7 ✓
  hydrocephalic fetus 653.6 ✓
  pelvis, pelvic, abnormality (bony) NEC 653.0 ✓
  unusually large fetus 653.5 ✓
 causing obstructed labor 660.1 ✓
 cephalopelvic, normally formed fetus 653.4 ✓
  causing obstructed labor 660.1 ✓
 fetal NEC 653.5 ✓
  causing obstructed labor 660.1 ✓
 fetopelvic, normally formed fetus 653.4 ✓
  causing obstructed labor 660.1 ✓
 mixed maternal and fetal origin, normally formed fetus 653.4 ✓
 pelvis, pelvic (bony) NEC 653.1 ✓
  causing obstructed labor 660.1 ✓
 specified type NEC 653.8 ✓
Disruption
 cesarean wound 674.1 ✓
 family V61.09
  due to
   child in
    care of non-parental family member V61.06
    foster care V61.06
    welfare custody V61.05
   death of family member V61.07
   divorce V61.03
   estrangement V61.09
    parent-child V61.04
   extended absence of family member NEC V61.08
   family member
    on military deployment V61.01
    return from military deployment V61.02
   legal separation V61.03
 gastrointestinal anastomosis 997.4
 ligament(s) (see also Sprain)
  knee
   current injury — see Dislocation, knee
   old 717.89
    capsular 717.85
    collateral (medial) 717.82
     lateral 717.81
    cruciate (posterior) 717.84
     anterior 717.83
    specified site NEC 717.85
 marital V61.10
  involving
   divorce V61.03
   estrangement V61.09
 operation wound (external) (see also Dehiscence) 998.32
  internal 998.31
 organ transplant, anastomosis site — see Complications, transplant, organ, by site
 ossicles, ossicular chain 385.23
  traumatic — see Fracture, skull, base

Disruption — continued
 parenchyma
  liver (hepatic) — see Laceration, liver, major
  spleen — see Laceration, spleen, parenchyma, massive
 phase-shift, of 24-hour sleep-wake cycle, unspecified 780.55
  nonorganic origin 307.45
 sleep-wake cycle (24-hour), unspecified 780.55
  circadian rhythm 327.33
  nonorganic origin 307.45
 suture line (external) (see also Dehiscence) 998.32
  internal 998.31
 wound 998.30
  cesarean operation 674.1 ✓
  episiotomy 674.2 ✓
  operation (surgical) 998.32
   cesarean 674.1 ✓
   internal 998.31
  perineal (obstetric) 674.2 ✓
  uterine 674.1 ✓
Disruptio uteri — see also Rupture, uterus
 complicating delivery — see Delivery, complicated, rupture, uterus
Dissatisfaction with
 employment V62.29
 school environment V62.3
Dissecting — see condition
Dissection
 aorta 441.00
  abdominal 441.02
  thoracic 441.01
  thoracoabdominal 441.03
 artery, arterial
  carotid 443.21
  coronary 414.12
  iliac 443.22
  renal 443.23
  specified NEC 443.29
  vertebral 443.24
 vascular 459.9
 wound — see Wound, open, by site
Disseminated — see condition
Dissociated personality NEC 300.15
Dissociation
 auriculoventricular or atrioventricular (any degree) (AV) 426.89
  with heart block 426.0
 interference 426.89
 isorhythmic 426.89
 rhythm
  atrioventricular (AV) 426.89
  interference 426.89
Dissociative
 identity disorder 300.14
 reaction NEC 300.15
Dissolution, vertebra — see also Osteoporosis 733.00
Distention
 abdomen (gaseous) 787.3
 bladder 596.8
 cecum 569.89
 colon 569.89
 gallbladder 575.8
 gaseous (abdomen) 787.3
 intestine 569.89
 kidney 593.89
 liver 573.9
 seminal vesicle 608.89
 stomach 536.8
  acute 536.1
  psychogenic 306.4
 ureter 593.5
 uterus 621.8
Distichia, distichiasis (eyelid) 743.63
Distoma hepaticum infestation 121.3
Distomiasis 121.9
 bile passages 121.3
  due to Clonorchis sinensis 121.1
 hemic 120.9
 hepatic (liver) 121.3
  due to Clonorchis sinensis (clonorchiasis) 121.1

☑ Additional Digit Required — Refer to the Tabular List for Digit Selection   🖑 Subterms under main terms may continue to next column or page

94 — Volume 2 • October 2010 ▶◀ Revised Text ● New Line ▲ Revised Code 2011 ICD-9-CM

Distomiasis — *continued*
  intestinal 121.4
  liver 121.3
    due to Clonorchis sinensis 121.1
  lung 121.2
  pulmonary 121.2
Distomolar (fourth molar) 520.1
  causing crowding 524.31
Disto-occlusion (division I) (division II) 524.22
Distortion (congenital)
  adrenal (gland) 759.1
  ankle (joint) 755.69
  anus 751.5
  aorta 747.29
  appendix 751.5
  arm 755.59
  artery (peripheral) NEC (*see also* Distortion,
      peripheral vascular system) 747.60
    cerebral 747.81
    coronary 746.85
    pulmonary 747.3
    retinal 743.58
    umbilical 747.5
  auditory canal 744.29
    causing impairment of hearing 744.02
  bile duct or passage 751.69
  bladder 753.8
  brain 742.4
  bronchus 748.3
  cecum 751.5
  cervix (uteri) 752.49
  chest (wall) 756.3
  clavicle 755.51
  clitoris 752.49
  coccyx 756.19
  colon 751.5
  common duct 751.69
  cornea 743.41
  cricoid cartilage 748.3
  cystic duct 751.69
  duodenum 751.5
  ear 744.29
    auricle 744.29
      causing impairment of hearing
          744.02
    causing impairment of hearing 744.09
    external 744.29
      causing impairment of hearing
          744.02
    inner 744.05
    middle, except ossicles 744.03
      ossicles 744.04
    ossicles 744.04
  endocrine (gland) NEC 759.2
  epiglottis 748.3
  Eustachian tube 744.24
  eye 743.8
    adnexa 743.69
  face bone(s) 756.0
  fallopian tube 752.19
  femur 755.69
  fibula 755.69
  finger(s) 755.59
  foot 755.67
  gallbladder 751.69
  genitalia, genital organ(s)
    female 752.89
      external 752.49
      internal NEC 752.89
    male 752.89
      penis 752.69
  glottis 748.3
  gyri 742.4
  hand bone(s) 755.59
  heart (auricle) (ventricle) 746.89
    valve (cusp) 746.89
  hepatic duct 751.69
  humerus 755.59
  hymen 752.49
  ileum 751.5
  intestine (large) (small) 751.5
    with anomalous adhesions, fixation or
        malrotation 751.4
  jaw NEC 524.89
  jejunum 751.5
  kidney 753.3

Distortion — *continued*
  knee (joint) 755.64
  labium (majus) (minus) 752.49
  larynx 748.3
  leg 755.69
  lens 743.36
  liver 751.69
  lumbar spine 756.19
    with disproportion (fetopelvic) 653.0 ☑
      affecting fetus or newborn 763.1
      causing obstructed labor 660.1 ☑
  lumbosacral (joint) (region) 756.19
  lung (fissures) (lobe) 748.69
  nerve 742.8
  nose 748.1
  organ
    of Corti 744.05
    of site not listed — *see* Anomaly, speci-
        fied type NEC
  ossicles, ear 744.04
  ovary 752.0
  oviduct 752.19
  pancreas 751.7
  parathyroid (gland) 759.2
  patella 755.64
  peripheral vascular system NEC 747.60
    gastrointestinal 747.61
    lower limb 747.64
    renal 747.62
    spinal 747.82
    upper limb 747.63
  pituitary (gland) 759.2
  radius 755.59
  rectum 751.5
  rib 756.3
  sacroiliac joint 755.69
  sacrum 756.19
  scapula 755.59
  shoulder girdle 755.59
  site not listed — *see* Anomaly, specified
      type NEC
  skull bone(s) 756.0
    with
      anencephalus 740.0
      encephalocele 742.0
      hydrocephalus 742.3
        with spina bifida (*see also* Spina
            bifida) 741.0 ☑
      microcephalus 742.1
  spinal cord 742.59
  spine 756.19
  spleen 759.0
  sternum 756.3
  thorax (wall) 756.3
  thymus (gland) 759.2
  thyroid (gland) 759.2
    cartilage 748.3
  tibia 755.69
  toe(s) 755.66
  tongue 750.19
  trachea (cartilage) 748.3
  ulna 755.59
  ureter 753.4
    causing obstruction 753.20
  urethra 753.8
    causing obstruction 753.6
  uterus 752.39   ▲
  vagina 752.49
  vein (peripheral) NEC (*see also* Distortion,
      peripheral vascular system) 747.60
    great 747.49
    portal 747.49
    pulmonary 747.49
  vena cava (inferior) (superior) 747.49
  vertebra 756.19
  visual NEC 368.15
    shape or size 368.14
  vulva 752.49
  wrist (bones) (joint) 755.59
Distress
  abdomen 789.0 ☑
  colon 564.9
  emotional V40.9
  epigastric 789.0 ☑
  fetal (syndrome) 768.4

Distress — *continued*
  fetal — *continued*
    affecting management of pregnancy or
        childbirth 656.8 ☑
    liveborn infant 768.4
      first noted
        before onset of labor 768.2
        during labor and delivery 768.3
    stillborn infant (death before onset of
        labor) 768.0
      death during labor 768.1
  gastrointestinal (functional) 536.9
    psychogenic 306.4
  intestinal (functional) NEC 564.9
    psychogenic 306.4
  intrauterine — *see* Distress, fetal
  leg 729.5
  maternal 669.0 ☑
  mental V40.9
  respiratory 786.09
    acute (adult) 518.82
    adult syndrome (following shock,
        surgery, or trauma) 518.5
      specified NEC 518.82
    fetus or newborn 770.89
    syndrome (idiopathic) (newborn) 769
  stomach 536.9
    psychogenic 306.4
Distribution vessel, atypical NEC 747.60
  coronary artery 746.85
  spinal 747.82
Districhiasis 704.2
Disturbance — *see also* Disease
  absorption NEC 579.9
    calcium 269.3
    carbohydrate 579.8
    fat 579.8
    protein 579.8
    specified type NEC 579.8
    vitamin (*see also* Deficiency, vitamin)
        269.2
  acid-base equilibrium 276.9
  activity and attention, simple, with hyperki-
      nesis 314.01
  amino acid (metabolic) (*see also* Disorder,
      amino acid) 270.9
    imidazole 270.5
    maple syrup (urine) disease 270.3
    transport 270.0
  assimilation, food 579.9
  attention, simple 314.00
    with hyperactivity 314.01
  auditory, nerve, except deafness 388.5
  behavior (*see also* Disturbance, conduct)
      312.9
  blood clotting (hypoproteinemia) (mecha-
      nism) (*see also* Defect, coagulation)
      286.9
  central nervous system NEC 349.9
  cerebral nerve NEC 352.9
  circulatory 459.9
  conduct 312.9

  *Note — Use the following fifth-digit
  subclassification with categories
  312.0–312.2:*

  0   unspecified
  1   mild
  2   moderate
  3   severe

    adjustment reaction 309.3
    adolescent onset type 312.82
    childhood onset type 312.81
    compulsive 312.30
      intermittent explosive disorder
          312.34
      isolated explosive disorder 312.35
      kleptomania 312.32
      pathological gambling 312.31
      pyromania 312.33
    hyperkinetic 314.2
    intermittent explosive 312.34
    isolated explosive 312.35
    mixed with emotions 312.4
    socialized (type) 312.20

Disturbance — *see also* Disease —
    continued
  conduct — *continued*
    socialized — *continued*
      aggressive 312.23
      unaggressive 312.21
    specified type NEC 312.89
    undersocialized, unsocialized
      aggressive (type) 312.0 ☑
      unaggressive (type) 312.1 ☑
  coordination 781.3
  cranial nerve NEC 352.9
  deep sensibility — *see* Disturbance, sensa-
      tion
  digestive 536.9
    psychogenic 306.4
  electrolyte — *see* Imbalance, electrolyte
  emotions specific to childhood or adoles-
      cence 313.9
    with
      academic underachievement 313.83
      anxiety and fearfulness 313.0
      elective mutism 313.23
      identity disorder 313.82
      jealousy 313.3
      misery and unhappiness 313.1
      oppositional defiant disorder 313.81
      overanxiousness 313.0
      sensitivity 313.21
      shyness 313.21
      social withdrawal 313.22
      withdrawal reaction 313.22
    involving relationship problems 313.3
    mixed 313.89
    specified type NEC 313.89
  endocrine (gland) 259.9
    neonatal, transitory 775.9
      specified NEC 775.89
  equilibrium 780.4
  feeding (elderly) (infant) 783.3
    newborn 779.31
      nonorganic origin NEC 307.59
      psychogenic NEC 307.59
  fructose metabolism 271.2
  gait 781.2
    hysterical 300.11
  gastric (functional) 536.9
    motility 536.8
    psychogenic 306.4
    secretion 536.8
  gastrointestinal (functional) 536.9
    psychogenic 306.4
  habit, child 307.9
  hearing, except deafness 388.40
  heart, functional (conditions classifiable to
      426, 427, 428)
    due to presence of (cardiac) prosthesis
        429.4
    postoperative (immediate) 997.1
      long-term effect of cardiac surgery
          429.4
    psychogenic 306.2
  hormone 259.9
  innervation uterus, sympathetic, parasym-
      pathetic 621.8
  keratinization NEC
    gingiva 523.10
    lip 528.5
    oral (mucosa) (soft tissue) 528.79
      residual ridge mucosa
        excessive 528.72
        minimal 528.71
    tongue 528.79
  labyrinth, labyrinthine (vestibule) 386.9
  learning, specific NEC 315.2
  memory (*see also* Amnesia) 780.93
    mild, following organic brain damage
        310.8
  mental (*see also* Disorder, mental) 300.9
    associated with diseases classified else-
        where 316
  metabolism (acquired) (congenital) (*see also*
      Disorder, metabolism) 277.9
    with
      abortion — *see* Abortion, by type,
          with metabolic disorder

☑ **Additional Digit Required** — Refer to the Tabular List for Digit Selection   🅥 **Subterms under main terms may continue to next column or page**

2011 ICD-9-CM   ▶◀ Revised Text   ● New Line   ▲ Revised Code   October 2010 • Volume 2 — 95

Disturbance — *see also* Disease — *continued*
  metabolism (*see also* Disorder, metabolism) — *continued*
    with — *continued*
      ectopic pregnancy (*see also* categories 633.0–633.9) 639.4
      molar pregnancy (*see also* categories 630–632) 639.4
    amino acid (*see also* Disorder, amino acid) 270.9
      aromatic NEC 270.2
      branched-chain 270.3
      specified type NEC 270.8
      straight-chain NEC 270.7
      sulfur-bearing 270.4
      transport 270.0
    ammonia 270.6
    arginine 270.6
    argininosuccinic acid 270.6
    carbohydrate NEC 271.9
    cholesterol 272.9
    citrulline 270.6
    cystathionine 270.4
    fat 272.9
    following
      abortion 639.4
      ectopic or molar pregnancy 639.4
    general 277.9
      carbohydrate 271.9
      iron 275.09   ▲
      phosphate 275.3
      sodium 276.9
    glutamine 270.7
    glycine 270.7
    histidine 270.5
    homocystine 270.4
    in labor or delivery 669.0 ☑
    iron 275.09   ▲
    isoleucine 270.3
    leucine 270.3
    lipoid 272.9
      specified type NEC 272.8
    lysine 270.7
    methionine 270.4
    neonatal, transitory 775.9
      specified type NEC 775.89
    nitrogen 788.99
    ornithine 270.6
    phosphate 275.3
    phosphatides 272.7
    serine 270.7
    sodium NEC 276.9
    threonine 270.7
    tryptophan 270.2
    tyrosine 270.2
    urea cycle 270.6
    valine 270.3
  motor 796.1
  nervous functional 799.21
  neuromuscular mechanism (eye) due to syphilis 094.84
  nutritional 269.9
    nail 703.8
  ocular motion 378.87
    psychogenic 306.7
  oculogyric 378.87
    psychogenic 306.7
  oculomotor NEC 378.87
    psychogenic 306.7
  olfactory nerve 781.1
  optic nerve NEC 377.49
  oral epithelium, including tongue 528.79
    residual ridge mucosa
      excessive 528.72
      minimal 528.71
  personality (pattern) (trait) (*see also* Disorder, personality) 301.9
    following organic brain damage 310.1
  polyglandular 258.9
  psychomotor 307.9
  pupillary 379.49
  reflex 796.1
  rhythm, heart 427.9
    postoperative (immediate) 997.1

Disturbance — *see also* Disease — *continued*
  rhythm, heart — *continued*
    postoperative — *continued*
      long-term effect of cardiac surgery 429.4
  psychogenic 306.2
  salivary secretion 527.7
  sensation (cold) (heat) (localization) (tactile discrimination localization) (texture) (vibratory) NEC 782.0
    hysterical 300.11
    skin 782.0
    smell 781.1
    taste 781.1
  sensory (*see also* Disturbance, sensation) 782.0
    innervation 782.0
  situational (transient) (*see also* Reaction, adjustment) 309.9
    acute 308.3
  sleep 780.50
    with apnea — *see* Apnea, sleep
    initiation or maintenance (*see also* Insomnia) 780.52
      nonorganic origin 307.41
    nonorganic origin 307.40
      specified type NEC 307.49
    specified NEC 780.59
      nonorganic origin 307.49
    wakefulness (*see also* Hypersomnia) 780.54
      nonorganic origin 307.43
  sociopathic 301.7
  speech NEC 784.59
    developmental 315.39
      associated with hyperkinesis 314.1
    secondary to organic lesion 784.59
  stomach (functional) (*see also* Disturbance, gastric) 536.9
  sympathetic (nerve) (*see also* Neuropathy, peripheral, autonomic) 337.9
  temperature sense 782.0
    hysterical 300.11
  tooth
    eruption 520.6
    formation 520.4
    structure, hereditary NEC 520.5
  touch (*see also* Disturbance, sensation) 782.0
  vascular 459.9
    arteriosclerotic — *see* Arteriosclerosis
  vasomotor 443.9
  vasospastic 443.9
  vestibular labyrinth 386.9
  vision, visual NEC 368.9
    psychophysical 368.16
    specified NEC 368.8
    subjective 368.10
  voice and resonance 784.40
  wakefulness (initiation or maintenance) (*see also* Hypersomnia) 780.54
    nonorganic origin 307.43
Disulfiduria, beta-mercaptolactate-cysteine 270.0
Disuse atrophy, bone 733.7
Ditthomska syndrome 307.81
Diuresis 788.42
Divers'
  palsy or paralysis 993.3
  squeeze 993.3
Diverticula, diverticulosis, diverticulum (acute) (multiple) (perforated) (ruptured) 562.10
  with diverticulitis 562.11
  aorta (Kommerell's) 747.21
  appendix (noninflammatory) 543.9
  bladder (acquired) (sphincter) 596.3
    congenital 753.8
  broad ligament 620.8
  bronchus (congenital) 748.3
    acquired 494.0
      with acute exacerbation 494.1
  calyx, calyceal (kidney) 593.89
  cardia (stomach) 537.1
  cecum 562.10

Diverticula, diverticulosis, diverticulum — *continued*
  cecum — *continued*
    with
      diverticulitis 562.11
        with hemorrhage 562.13
      hemorrhage 562.12
    congenital 751.5
  colon (acquired) 562.10
    with
      diverticulitis 562.11
        with hemorrhage 562.13
      hemorrhage 562.12
    congenital 751.5
  duodenum 562.00
    with
      diverticulitis 562.01
        with hemorrhage 562.03
      hemorrhage 562.02
    congenital 751.5
  epiphrenic (esophagus) 530.6
  esophagus (congenital) 750.4
    acquired 530.6
    epiphrenic 530.6
    pulsion 530.6
    traction 530.6
    Zenker's 530.6
  Eustachian tube 381.89
  fallopian tube 620.8
  gallbladder (congenital) 751.69
  gastric 537.1
  heart (congenital) 746.89
  ileum 562.00
    with
      diverticulitis 562.01
        with hemorrhage 562.03
      hemorrhage 562.02
  intestine (large) 562.10
    with
      diverticulitis 562.11
        with hemorrhage 562.13
      hemorrhage 562.12
    congenital 751.5
    small 562.00
      with
        diverticulitis 562.01
          with hemorrhage 562.03
        hemorrhage 562.02
      congenital 751.5
  jejunum 562.00
    with
      diverticulitis 562.01
        with hemorrhage 562.03
      hemorrhage 562.02
  kidney (calyx) (pelvis) 593.89
    with calculus 592.0
  Kommerell's 747.21
  laryngeal ventricle (congenital) 748.3
  Meckel's (displaced) (hypertrophic) 751.0
  midthoracic 530.6
  organ or site, congenital NEC — *see* Distortion
  pericardium (congenital) (cyst) 746.89
    acquired (true) 423.8
  pharyngoesophageal (pulsion) 530.6
  pharynx (congenital) 750.27
  pulsion (esophagus) 530.6
  rectosigmoid 562.10
    with
      diverticulitis 562.11
        with hemorrhage 562.13
      hemorrhage 562.12
    congenital 751.5
  rectum 562.10
    with
      diverticulitis 562.11
        with hemorrhage 562.13
      hemorrhage 562.12
  renal (calyces) (pelvis) 593.89
    with calculus 592.0
  Rokitansky's 530.6
  seminal vesicle 608.0
  sigmoid 562.10
    with
      diverticulitis 562.11
        with hemorrhage 562.13

Diverticula, diverticulosis, diverticulum — *continued*
  sigmoid — *continued*
    with — *continued*
      hemorrhage 562.12
    congenital 751.5
  small intestine 562.00
    with
      diverticulitis 562.01
        with hemorrhage 562.03
      hemorrhage 562.02
  stomach (cardia) (juxtacardia) (juxtapyloric) (acquired) 537.1
    congenital 750.7
  subdiaphragmatic 530.6
  trachea (congenital) 748.3
    acquired 519.19
  traction (esophagus) 530.6
  ureter (acquired) 593.89
    congenital 753.4
  ureterovesical orifice 593.89
  urethra (acquired) 599.2
    congenital 753.8
  ventricle, left (congenital) 746.89
  vesical (urinary) 596.3
    congenital 753.8
  Zenker's (esophagus) 530.6
Diverticulitis (acute) — *see also* Diverticula 562.11
  with hemorrhage 562.13
  bladder (urinary) 596.3
  cecum (perforated) 562.11
    with hemorrhage 562.13
  colon (perforated) 562.11
    with hemorrhage 562.13
  duodenum 562.01
    with hemorrhage 562.03
  esophagus 530.6
  ileum (perforated) 562.01
    with hemorrhage 562.03
  intestine (large) (perforated) 562.11
    with hemorrhage 562.13
    small 562.01
      with hemorrhage 562.03
  jejunum (perforated) 562.01
    with hemorrhage 562.03
  Meckel's (perforated) 751.0
  pharyngoesophageal 530.6
  rectosigmoid (perforated) 562.11
    with hemorrhage 562.13
  rectum 562.11
    with hemorrhage 562.13
  sigmoid (old) (perforated) 562.11
    with hemorrhage 562.13
  small intestine (perforated) 562.01
    with hemorrhage 562.03
  vesical (urinary) 596.3
Diverticulosis — *see* Diverticula
Division
  cervix uteri 622.8
    external os into two openings by frenum 752.44   ▲
    external (cervical) into two openings by frenum 752.44   ▲
  glans penis 752.69
  hymen 752.49
  labia minora (congenital) 752.49
  ligament (partial or complete) (current) (*see also* Sprain, by site)
    with open wound — *see* Wound, open, by site
  muscle (partial or complete) (current) (*see also* Sprain, by site)
    with open wound — *see* Wound, open, by site
  nerve — *see* Injury, nerve, by site
  penis glans 752.69
  spinal cord — *see* Injury, spinal, by site
  vein 459.9
    traumatic — *see* Injury, vascular, by site
Divorce V61.03
Dix-Hallpike neurolabyrinthitis 386.12
Dizziness 780.4
  hysterical 300.11
  psychogenic 306.9

☑ **Additional Digit Required — Refer to the Tabular List for Digit Selection**   ▽ **Subterms under main terms may continue to next column or page**

96 — Volume 2 • October 2010   ▶◀ **Revised Text**   ● **New Line**   ▲ **Revised Code**   **2011 ICD-9-CM**

Doan-Wiseman syndrome (primary splenic neutropenia) 289.53
Dog bite — *see* Wound, open, by site
Döhle body-panmyelopathic syndrome 288.2
Döhle-Heller aortitis 093.1
Dolichocephaly, dolichocephalus 754.0
Dolichocolon 751.5
Dolichostenomelia 759.82
Donohue's syndrome (leprechaunism) 259.8
Donor
　blood V59.01
　　other blood components V59.09
　　stem cells V59.02
　　whole blood V59.01
　bone V59.2
　　marrow V59.3
　cornea V59.5
　egg (oocyte) (ovum) V59.70
　　over age 35 V59.73
　　　anonymous recipient V59.73
　　　designated recipient V59.74
　　under age 35 V59.71
　　　anonymous recipient V59.71
　　　designated recipient V59.72
　heart V59.8
　kidney V59.4
　liver V59.6
　lung V59.8
　lymphocyte V59.8
　organ V59.9
　　specified NEC V59.8
　potential, examination of V70.8
　skin V59.1
　specified organ or tissue NEC V59.8
　sperm V59.8
　stem cells V59.02
　tissue V59.9
　　specified type NEC V59.8
Donovanosis (granuloma venereum) 099.2
DOPS (diffuse obstructive pulmonary syndrome) 496
Double
　albumin 273.8
　aortic arch 747.21
　auditory canal 744.29
　auricle (heart) 746.82
　bladder 753.8
　external (cervical) os 752.44 ▲
　kidney with double pelvis (renal) 753.3
　larynx 748.3
　meatus urinarius 753.8
　organ or site NEC — *see* Accessory
　orifice
　　heart valve NEC 746.89
　　　pulmonary 746.09
　outlet, right ventricle 745.11
　pelvis (renal) with double ureter 753.4
　penis 752.69
　tongue 750.13
　ureter (one or both sides) 753.4
　　with double pelvis (renal) 753.4
　urethra 753.8
　urinary meatus 753.8
　uterus (any degree) 752.2
　　with doubling of cervix and vagina 752.2
　　in pregnancy or childbirth 654.0 ☑
　　　affecting fetus or newborn 763.89
　vagina 752.47 ▲
　　with doubling of cervix and uterus 752.2
　vision 368.2
　vocal cords 748.3
　vulva 752.49
　whammy (syndrome) 360.81
Douglas' pouch, cul-de-sac — *see* condition
Down's disease or syndrome (mongolism) 758.0
Down-growth, epithelial (anterior chamber) 364.61
DPD (dihydropyrimidine dehydrogenase deficiency) 277.6 ●
Dracontiasis 125.7
Dracunculiasis 125.7
Dracunculosis 125.7
Drainage
　abscess (spontaneous) — *see* Abscess

Drainage — *continued*
　anomalous pulmonary veins to hepatic veins or right atrium 747.41
　stump (amputation) (surgical) 997.62
　suprapubic, bladder 596.8
Dream state, hysterical 300.13
Drepanocytic anemia — *see also* Disease, sickle cell 282.60
Dresbach's syndrome (elliptocytosis) 282.1
Dreschlera (infection) 118
　hawaiiensis 117.8
Dressler's syndrome (postmyocardial infarction) 411.0
Dribbling (post-void) 788.35
Drift, ulnar 736.09
Drinking (alcohol) — *see also* Alcoholism
　excessive, to excess NEC (*see also* Abuse, drugs, nondependent) 305.0 ☑
　　bouts, periodic 305.0 ☑
　　continual 303.9 ☑
　　episodic 305.0 ☑
　　habitual 303.9 ☑
　　periodic 305.0 ☑
Drip, postnasal (chronic) 784.91
　due to
　　allergic rhinitis — *see* Rhinitis, allergic
　　common cold 460
　　gastroesophageal reflux — *see* Reflux, gastroesophageal
　　nasopharyngitis — *see* Nasopharyngitis
　　other known condition — code to condition
　　sinusitis — *see* Sinusitis
Drivers' license examination V70.3
Droop
　Cooper's 611.81
　facial 781.94
Drop
　finger 736.29
　foot 736.79
　hematocrit (precipitous) 790.01
　hemoglobin 790.01
　toe 735.8
　wrist 736.05
Dropped
　dead 798.1
　heart beats 426.6
Dropsy, dropsical — *see also* Edema 782.3
　abdomen 789.59
　amnion (*see also* Hydramnios) 657.0 ☑
　brain — *see* Hydrocephalus
　cardiac (*see also* Failure, heart) 428.0
　cardiorenal (*see also* Hypertension, cardiorenal) 404.90
　chest 511.9
　fetus or newborn 778.0
　　due to isoimmunization 773.3
　gangrenous (*see also* Gangrene) 785.4
　heart (*see also* Failure, heart) 428.0
　hepatic — *see* Cirrhosis, liver
　infantile — *see* Hydrops, fetalis
　kidney (*see also* Nephrosis) 581.9
　liver — *see* Cirrhosis, liver
　lung 514
　malarial (*see also* Malaria) 084.9
　neonatorum — *see* Hydrops, fetalis
　nephritic 581.9
　newborn — *see* Hydrops, fetalis
　nutritional 269.9
　ovary 620.8
　pericardium (*see also* Pericarditis) 423.9
　renal (*see also* Nephrosis) 581.9
　uremic — *see* Uremia
Drowned, drowning (near) 994.1
　lung 518.5
Drowsiness 780.09
Drug — *see also* condition
　addiction (*see also* listing under Dependence) 304.9 ☑
　adverse effect, correct substance properly administered 995.20
　allergy 995.27
　dependence (*see also* listing under Dependence) 304.9 ☑
　habit (*see also* listing under Dependence) 304.9 ☑

Drug — *see also* condition — *continued*
　hypersensitivity 995.27
　induced
　　circadian rhythm sleep disorder 292.85
　　hypersomnia 292.85
　　insomnia 292.85
　　mental disorder 292.9
　　　anxiety 292.89
　　　mood 292.84
　　　sexual 292.89
　　　sleep 292.85
　　　specified type 292.89
　　parasomnia 292.85
　　persisting
　　　amnestic disorder 292.83
　　　dementia 292.82
　　psychotic disorder
　　　with
　　　　delusions 292.11
　　　　hallucinations 292.12
　　sleep disorder 292.85
　intoxication 292.89
　overdose — *see* Table of Drugs and Chemicals
　poisoning — *see* Table of Drugs and Chemicals
　therapy (maintenance) status NEC
　　chemotherapy, antineoplastic V58.11
　　immunotherapy, antineoplastic V58.12
　　long-term (current) ▶(prophylactic)◀ use V58.69
　　　antibiotics V58.62
　　　anticoagulants V58.61
　　　anti-inflammatories, non-steroidal (NSAID) V58.64
　　　antiplatelets V58.63
　　　antithrombotics V58.63
　　　aspirin V58.66
　　　high-risk medications NEC V58.69
　　　insulin V58.67
　　　methadone V58.69
　　　opiate analgesic V58.69
　　　steroids V58.65
　wrong substance given or taken in error — *see* Table of Drugs and Chemicals
Drunkenness — *see also* Abuse, drugs, nondependent 305.0 ☑
　acute in alcoholism (*see also* Alcoholism) 303.0 ☑
　chronic (*see also* Alcoholism) 303.9 ☑
　pathologic 291.4
　simple (acute) 305.0 ☑
　　in alcoholism 303.0 ☑
　sleep 307.47
Drusen
　optic disc or papilla 377.21
　retina (colloid) (hyaloid degeneration) 362.57
　　hereditary 362.77
Drusenfieber 075
Dry, dryness — *see also* condition
　eye 375.15
　　syndrome 375.15
　larynx 478.79
　mouth 527.7
　nose 478.19
　skin syndrome 701.1
　socket (teeth) 526.5
　throat 478.29
DSAP (disseminated superficial actinic porokeratosis) 692.75
DSTR (delayed serologic transfusion reaction) ●
　due to or resulting from ●
　　incompatibility ●
　　　ABO 999.69 ●
　　　non-ABO antigen (minor) (Duffy) ●
　　　　(Kell) (Kidd) (Lewis) (M) (N) ●
　　　　(P) (S) 999.79 ●
　　　Rh antigen (C) (c) (D) (E) (e) 999.74 ●
Duane's retraction syndrome 378.71
Duane-Stilling-Türk syndrome (ocular retraction syndrome) 378.71
Dubini's disease (electric chorea) 049.8
Dubin-Johnson disease or syndrome 277.4
Dubois' abscess or disease 090.5

Duchenne's
　disease 094.0
　　locomotor ataxia 094.0
　　muscular dystrophy 359.1
　　pseudohypertrophy, muscles 359.1
　paralysis 335.22
　syndrome 335.22
Duchenne-Aran myelopathic, muscular atrophy (nonprogressive) (progressive) 335.21
Duchenne-Griesinger disease 359.1
Ducrey's
　bacillus 099.0
　chancre 099.0
　disease (chancroid) 099.0
Duct, ductus — *see* condition
Duengero 061
Duhring's disease (dermatitis herpetiformis) 694.0
Dukes (-Filatov) disease 057.8
Dullness
　cardiac (decreased) (increased) 785.3
Dumb ague — *see also* Malaria 084.6
Dumbness — *see also* Aphasia 784.3
Dumdum fever 085.0
Dumping syndrome (postgastrectomy) 564.2
　nonsurgical 536.8
Duodenitis (nonspecific) (peptic) 535.60
　with hemorrhage 535.61
　due to
　　Strongyloides stercoralis 127.2
Duodenocholangitis 575.8
Duodenum, duodenal — *see* condition
Duplay's disease, periarthritis, or syndrome 726.2
Duplex — *see also* Accessory
　kidney 753.3
　placenta — *see* Placenta, abnormal
　uterus 752.2
Duplication — *see also* Accessory
　anus 751.5
　aortic arch 747.21
　appendix 751.5
　biliary duct (any) 751.69
　bladder 753.8
　cecum 751.5
　　and appendix 751.5
　cervical, cervix 752.44
　clitoris 752.49
　cystic duct 751.69
　digestive organs 751.8
　duodenum 751.5
　esophagus 750.4
　fallopian tube 752.19
　frontonasal process 756.0
　gallbladder 751.69
　ileum 751.5
　intestine (large) (small) 751.5
　jejunum 751.5
　kidney 753.3
　liver 751.69
　nose 748.1
　pancreas 751.7
　penis 752.69
　respiratory organs NEC 748.9
　salivary duct 750.22
　spinal cord (incomplete) 742.51
　stomach 750.7
　ureter 753.4
　vagina 752.47 ▲
　vas deferens 752.89
　vocal cords 748.3
Dupré's disease or syndrome (meningism) 781.6
Dupuytren's
　contraction 728.6
　disease (muscle contracture) 728.6
　fracture (closed) 824.4
　　ankle (closed) 824.4
　　　open 824.5
　　fibula (closed) 824.4
　　　open 824.5
　　open 824.5
　　radius (closed) 813.42
　　　open 813.52
　muscle contracture 728.6

☑ Additional Digit Required — Refer to the Tabular List for Digit Selection
🖝 Subterms under main terms may continue to next column or page
2011 ICD-9-CM　　▶◀ Revised Text　　● New Line　　▲ Revised Code
October 2010 · Volume 2 — 97

☑ **Additional Digit Required** — Refer to the Tabular List for Digit Selection   ▽ **Subterms under main terms may continue to next column or page**

Dysfunction — continued
  vestibular — continued
    specified type NEC 386.58
Dysgammaglobulinemia 279.06
Dysgenesis
  gonadal (due to chromosomal anomaly)
    758.6
    pure 752.7
  kidney(s) 753.0
  ovarian 758.6
  renal 753.0
  reticular 279.2
  seminiferous tubules 758.6
  tidal platelet 287.31
Dysgerminoma (M9060/3)
  specified site — see Neoplasm, by site, malignant
  unspecified site
    female 183.0
    male 186.9
Dysgeusia 781.1
Dysgraphia 781.3
Dyshidrosis 705.81
Dysidrosis 705.81
Dysinsulinism 251.8
Dyskaryotic cervical smear 795.09
Dyskeratosis — see also Keratosis 701.1
  bullosa hereditaria 757.39
  cervix 622.10
  congenital 757.39
  follicularis 757.39
    vitamin A deficiency 264.8
  gingiva 523.8
  oral soft tissue NEC 528.79
  tongue 528.79
  uterus NEC 621.8
Dyskinesia 781.3
  biliary 575.8
  esophagus 530.5
  hysterical 300.11
  intestinal 564.89
  neuroleptic-induced tardive 333.85
  nonorganic origin 307.9
  orofacial 333.82
    due to drugs 333.85
  psychogenic 307.9
  subacute, due to drugs 333.85
  tardive (oral) 333.85
Dyslalia 784.59
  developmental 315.39
Dyslexia 784.61
  developmental 315.02
  secondary to organic lesion 784.61
Dyslipidemia 272.4
Dysmaturity — see also Immaturity 765.1 ☑
  lung 770.4
  pulmonary 770.4
Dysmenorrhea (essential) (exfoliative) (functional) (intrinsic) (membranous) (primary) (secondary) 625.3
  psychogenic 306.52
Dysmetabolic syndrome X 277.7
Dysmetria 781.3
Dysmorodystrophia mesodermalis congenita 759.82
Dysnomia 784.3
Dysorexia 783.0
  hysterical 300.11
Dysostosis
  cleidocranial, cleidocranialis 755.59
  craniofacial 756.0
  Fairbank's (idiopathic familial generalized osteophytosis) 756.50
  mandibularis 756.0
  mandibulofacial, incomplete 756.0
  multiplex 277.5
  orodigitofacial 759.89
Dyspareunia (female) 625.0
  male 608.89
  psychogenic 302.76
Dyspepsia (allergic) (congenital) (fermentative) (flatulent) (functional) (gastric) (gastrointestinal) (neurogenic) (occupational) (reflex) 536.8
  acid 536.8
  atonic 536.3

Dyspepsia — continued
  atonic — continued
    psychogenic 306.4
  diarrhea 787.91
    psychogenic 306.4
  intestinal 564.89
    psychogenic 306.4
  nervous 306.4
  neurotic 306.4
  psychogenic 306.4
Dysphagia 787.20
  cervical 787.29
  functional 300.11
  hysterical 300.11
  nervous 300.11
  neurogenic 787.29
  oral phase 787.21
  oropharyngeal phase 787.22
  pharyngeal phase 787.23
  pharyngoesophageal phase 787.24
  psychogenic 306.4
  sideropenic 280.8
  spastica 530.5
  specified NEC 787.29
Dysphagocytosis, congenital 288.1
Dysphasia 784.59
Dysphonia 784.42
  clericorum 784.49
  functional 300.11
  hysterical 300.11
  psychogenic 306.1
  spastica 478.79
Dyspigmentation — see also Pigmentation
  eyelid (acquired) 374.52
Dyspituitarism 253.9
  hyperfunction 253.1
  hypofunction 253.2
  posterior lobe 253.6
Dysplasia — see also Anomaly
  anus 569.44
    intraepithelial neoplasia I (AIN I) (histologically confirmed) 569.44
    intraepithelial neoplasia II (AIN II) (histologically confirmed) 569.44
    intraepithelial neoplasia III (AIN III) 230.6
      anal canal 230.5
    mild (histologically confirmed) 569.44
    moderate (histologically confirmed) 569.44
    severe 230.6
      anal canal 230.5
  artery
    fibromuscular NEC 447.8
      carotid 447.8
      renal 447.3
  bladder 596.8
  bone (fibrous) NEC 733.29
    diaphyseal, progressive 756.59
    jaw 526.89
    monostotic 733.29
    polyostotic 756.54
    solitary 733.29
  brain 742.9
  bronchopulmonary, fetus or newborn 770.7
  cervix (uteri) 622.10
    cervical intraepithelial neoplasia I (CIN I) 622.11
    cervical intraepithelial neoplasia II (CIN II) 622.12
    cervical intraepithelial neoplasia III (CIN III) 233.1
    CIN I 622.11
    CIN II 622.12
    CIN III 233.1
    mild 622.11
    moderate 622.12
    severe 233.1
  chondroectodermal 756.55
  chondromatose 756.4
  colon 211.3
  craniocarpotarsal 759.89
  craniometaphyseal 756.89
  dentinal 520.5
  diaphyseal, progressive 756.59

Dysplasia — see also Anomaly — continued
  ectodermal (anhidrotic) (Bason) (Clouston's) (congenital) (Feinmesser) (hereditary) (hidrotic) (Marshall) (Robinson's) 757.31
  epiphysealis 756.9
    multiplex 756.56
    punctata 756.59
  epiphysis 756.9
    multiple 756.56
  epithelial
    epiglottis 478.79
    uterine cervix 622.10
  erythroid NEC 289.89
  eye (see also Microphthalmos) 743.10
  familial metaphyseal 756.89
  fibromuscular, artery NEC 447.8
    carotid 447.8
    renal 447.3
  fibrous
    bone NEC 733.29
    diaphyseal, progressive 756.59
    jaw 526.89
    monostotic 733.29
    polyostotic 756.54
    solitary 733.29
  high-grade, focal — see Neoplasm, by site, benign
  hip (congenital) 755.63
    with dislocation (see also Dislocation, hip, congenital) 754.30
  hypohidrotic ectodermal 757.31
  joint 755.8
  kidney 753.15
  leg 755.69
  linguofacialis 759.89
  lung 748.5
  macular 743.55
  mammary (benign) (gland) 610.9
    cystic 610.1
    specified type NEC 610.8
  metaphyseal 756.9
    familial 756.89
  monostotic fibrous 733.29
  muscle 756.89
  myeloid NEC 289.89
  nervous system (general) 742.9
  neuroectodermal 759.6
  oculoauriculovertebral 756.0
  oculodentodigital 759.89
  olfactogenital 253.4
  osteo-onycho-arthro (hereditary) 756.89
  periosteum 733.99
  polyostotic fibrous 756.54
  progressive diaphyseal 756.59
  prostate 602.3
    intraepithelial neoplasia I [PIN I] 602.3
    intraepithelial neoplasia II [PIN II] 602.3
    intraepithelial neoplasia III [PIN III] 233.4
  renal 753.15
  renofacialis 753.0
  retinal NEC 743.56
  retrolental (see also Retinopathy of prematurity) 362.21
  skin 709.8
  spinal cord 742.9
  thymic, with immunodeficiency 279.2
  vagina 623.0
    mild 623.0
    moderate 623.0
    severe 233.31
  vocal cord 478.5
  vulva 624.8
    intraepithelial neoplasia I (VIN I) 624.01
    intraepithelial neoplasia II (VIN II) 624.02
    intraepithelial neoplasia III (VIN III) 233.32
    mild 624.01
    moderate 624.02
    severe 233.32
    VIN I 624.01
    VIN II 624.02
    VIN III 233.32
Dyspnea (nocturnal) (paroxysmal) 786.09

Dyspnea — continued
  asthmatic (bronchial) (see also Asthma) 493.9 ☑
    with bronchitis (see also Asthma) 493.9 ☑
    chronic 493.2 ☑
  cardiac (see also Failure, ventricular, left) 428.1
  cardiac (see also Failure, ventricular, left) 428.1
  functional 300.11
  hyperventilation 786.01
  hysterical 300.11
  Monday morning 504
  newborn 770.89
  psychogenic 306.1
  uremic — see Uremia
Dyspraxia 781.3
  syndrome 315.4
Dysproteinemia 273.8
  transient with copper deficiency 281.4
Dysprothrombinemia (constitutional) — see also Defect, coagulation 286.3
Dysreflexia, autonomic 337.3
Dysrhythmia
  cardiac 427.9
    postoperative (immediate) 997.1
      long-term effect of cardiac surgery 429.4
    specified type NEC 427.89
  cerebral or cortical 348.30
Dyssecretosis, mucoserous 710.2
Dyssocial reaction, without manifest psychiatric disorder
  adolescent V71.02
  adult V71.01
  child V71.02
Dyssomnia NEC 780.56
  nonorganic origin 307.47
Dyssplenism 289.4
Dyssynergia
  biliary (see also Disease, biliary) 576.8
  cerebellaris myoclonica 334.2
  detrusor sphincter (bladder) 596.55
  ventricular 429.89
Dystasia, hereditary areflexic 334.3
Dysthymia 300.4
Dysthymic disorder 300.4
Dysthyroidism 246.9
Dystocia 660.9 ☑
  affecting fetus or newborn 763.1
  cervical 661.2 ☑
    affecting fetus or newborn 763.7
  contraction ring 661.4 ☑
    affecting fetus or newborn 763.7
  fetal 660.9 ☑
    abnormal size 653.5 ☑
      affecting fetus or newborn 763.1
    deformity 653.7 ☑
  maternal 660.9 ☑
    affecting fetus or newborn 763.1
  positional 660.0 ☑
    affecting fetus or newborn 763.1
  shoulder (girdle) 660.4 ☑
    affecting fetus or newborn 763.1
  uterine NEC 661.4 ☑
    affecting fetus or newborn 763.7
Dystonia
  acute
    due to drugs 333.72
      neuroleptic-induced acute 333.72
  deformans progressiva 333.6
  lenticularis 333.6
  musculorum deformans 333.6
  torsion (idiopathic) 333.6
    acquired 333.79
    fragments (of) 333.89
    genetic 333.6
    symptomatic 333.79
Dystonic
  movements 781.0
Dystopia kidney 753.3
Dystrophia myotonica 359.2 ☑
Dystrophy, dystrophia 783.9
  adiposogenital 253.8
  asphyxiating thoracic 756.4

☑ Additional Digit Required — Refer to the Tabular List for Digit Selection   ⬇ Subterms under main terms may continue to next column or page

2011 ICD-9-CM   ▶◀ Revised Text   ● New Line   ▲ Revised Code   Volume 2 — 99

Index

Dystrophy, dystrophia — Ectropion

Ectropion — continued
  uvea 364.54
Eczema (acute) (allergic) (chronic) (erythematous) (fissum) (occupational) (rubrum) (squamous) 692.9
  asteatotic 706.8
  atopic 691.8
  contact NEC 692.9
  dermatitis NEC 692.9
  due to specified cause — see Dermatitis, due to
  dyshidrotic 705.81
  external ear 380.22
  flexural 691.8
  gouty 274.89
  herpeticum 054.0
  hypertrophicum 701.8
  hypostatic — see Varicose, vein
  impetiginous 684
  infantile (acute) (chronic) (due to any substance) (intertriginous) (seborrheic) 690.12
  intertriginous NEC 692.9
    infantile 690.12
  intrinsic 691.8
  lichenified NEC 692.9
  marginatum 110.3
  nummular 692.9
  pustular 686.8
  seborrheic 690.18
    infantile 690.12
  solare 692.72
  stasis (lower extremity) 454.1
    ulcerated 454.2
  vaccination, vaccinatum 999.0
  varicose (lower extremity) — see Varicose, vein
  verrucosum callosum 698.3
Eczematoid, exudative 691.8
Eddowes' syndrome (brittle bones and blue sclera) 756.51
Edema, edematous 782.3
  with nephritis (see also Nephrosis) 581.9
  allergic 995.1
  angioneurotic (allergic) (any site) (with urticaria) 995.1
    hereditary 277.6
  angiospastic 443.9
  Berlin's (traumatic) 921.3
  brain ▶(cytotoxic) (vasogenic)◀ 348.5
    due to birth injury 767.8
    fetus or newborn 767.8
  cardiac (see also Failure, heart) 428.0
  cardiovascular (see also Failure, heart) 428.0
  cerebral — see Edema, brain
  cerebrospinal vessel — see Edema, brain
  cervix (acute) (uteri) 622.8
    puerperal, postpartum 674.8 ☑
  chronic hereditary 757.0
  circumscribed, acute 995.1
    hereditary 277.6
  complicating pregnancy (gestational) 646.1 ☑
    with hypertension — see Toxemia, of pregnancy
  conjunctiva 372.73
  connective tissue 782.3
  cornea 371.20
    due to contact lenses 371.24
    idiopathic 371.21
    secondary 371.22
  cystoid macular 362.53
  due to
    lymphatic obstruction — see Edema, lymphatic
    salt retention 276.0
  epiglottis — see Edema, glottis
  essential, acute 995.1
    hereditary 277.6
  extremities, lower — see Edema, legs
  eyelid NEC 374.82
  familial, hereditary (legs) 757.0
  famine 262
  fetus or newborn 778.5
  genital organs
    female 629.89

Edema, edematous — continued
  genital organs — continued
    male 608.86
  gestational 646.1 ☑
    with hypertension — see Toxemia, of pregnancy
  glottis, glottic, glottides (obstructive) (passive) 478.6
    allergic 995.1
      hereditary 277.6
    due to external agent — see Condition, respiratory, acute, due to specified agent
  heart (see also Failure, heart) 428.0
    newborn 779.89
  heat 992.7
  hereditary (legs) 757.0
  inanition 262
  infectious 782.3
  intracranial 348.5
    due to injury at birth 767.8
  iris 364.89
  joint (see also Effusion, joint) 719.0 ☑
  larynx (see also Edema, glottis) 478.6
  legs 782.3
    due to venous obstruction 459.2
    hereditary 757.0
  localized 782.3
    due to venous obstruction 459.2
      lower extremity 459.2
  lower extremities — see Edema, legs
  lung 514
    acute 518.4
      with heart disease or failure (see also Failure, ventricular, left) 428.1
        congestive 428.0
      chemical (due to fumes or vapors) 506.1
      due to
        external agent(s) NEC 508.9
          specified NEC 508.8
        fumes and vapors (chemical) (inhalation) 506.1
        radiation 508.0
    chemical (acute) 506.1
      chronic 506.4
    chronic 514
      chemical (due to fumes or vapors) 506.4
      due to
        external agent(s) NEC 508.9
          specified NEC 508.8
        fumes or vapors (chemical) (inhalation) 506.4
        radiation 508.1
    due to
      external agent 508.9
        specified NEC 508.8
      high altitude 993.2
      near drowning 994.1
    postoperative 518.4
    terminal 514
  lymphatic 457.1
    due to mastectomy operation 457.0
  macula 362.83
    cystoid 362.53
    diabetic 250.5 ☑ [362.07]
      due to secondary diabetes 249.5 ☑ [362.07]
  malignant (see also Gangrene, gas) 040.0
  Milroy's 757.0
  nasopharynx 478.25
  neonatorum 778.5
  nutritional (newborn) 262
    with dyspigmentation, skin and hair 260
  optic disc or nerve — see Papilledema
  orbit 376.33
    circulatory 459.89
  palate (soft) (hard) 528.9
  pancreas 577.8
  penis 607.83
  periodic 995.1
    hereditary 277.6
  pharynx 478.25
  pitting 782.3
  pulmonary — see Edema, lung

Edema, edematous — continued
  Quincke's 995.1
    hereditary 277.6
  renal (see also Nephrosis) 581.9
  retina (localized) (macular) (peripheral) 362.83
    cystoid 362.53
    diabetic 250.5 ☑ [362.07]
      due to secondary diabetes 249.5 ☑ [362.07]
  salt 276.0
  scrotum 608.86
  seminal vesicle 608.86
  spermatic cord 608.86
  spinal cord 336.1
  starvation 262
  stasis (see also Hypertension, venous) 459.30
  subconjunctival 372.73
  subglottic (see also Edema, glottis) 478.6
  supraglottic (see also Edema, glottis) 478.6
  testis 608.86
  toxic NEC 782.3
  traumatic NEC 782.3
  tunica vaginalis 608.86
  vas deferens 608.86
  vocal cord — see Edema, glottis
  vulva (acute) 624.8
Edentia (complete) (partial) — see also Absence, tooth 520.0
  acquired (see also Edentulism) 525.40
    due to
      caries 525.13
      extraction 525.10
      periodontal disease 525.12
      specified NEC 525.19
      trauma 525.11
  causing malocclusion 524.30
  congenital (deficiency of tooth buds) 520.0
Edentulism 525.40
  complete 525.40
    class I 525.41
    class II 525.42
    class III 525.43
    class IV 525.44
  partial 525.50
    class I 525.51
    class II 525.52
    class III 525.53
    class IV 525.54
Edsall's disease 992.2
Educational handicap V62.3
Edwards' syndrome 758.2
Effect, adverse NEC
  abnormal gravitational (G) forces or states 994.9
  air pressure — see Effect, adverse, atmospheric pressure
  altitude (high) — see Effect, adverse, high altitude
  anesthetic
    in labor and delivery NEC 668.9 ☑
      affecting fetus or newborn 763.5
  antitoxin — see Complications, vaccination
  atmospheric pressure 993.9
    due to explosion 993.4
    high 993.3
    low — see Effect, adverse, high altitude
    specified effect NEC 993.8
  biological, correct substance properly administered (see also Effect, adverse, drug) 995.20
  blood (derivatives) (serum) (transfusion) — see Complications, transfusion
  chemical substance NEC 989.9
    specified — see Table of Drugs and Chemicals
  cobalt, radioactive (see also Effect, adverse, radioactive substance) 990
  cold (temperature) (weather) 991.9
    chilblains 991.5
    frostbite — see Frostbite
    specified effect NEC 991.8
  drugs and medicinals 995.20
    correct substance properly administered 995.20

Effect, adverse — continued
  drugs and medicinals — continued
    overdose or wrong substance given or taken 977.9
      specified drug — see Table of Drugs and Chemicals
  electric current (shock) 994.8
    burn — see Burn, by site
  electricity (electrocution) (shock) 994.8
    burn — see Burn, by site
  exertion (excessive) 994.5
  exposure 994.9
    exhaustion 994.4
  external cause NEC 994.9
  fallout (radioactive) NEC 990
  fluoroscopy NEC 990
  foodstuffs
    allergic reaction (see also Allergy, food) 693.1
    anaphylactic shock due to food NEC 995.60
    noxious 988.9
      specified type NEC (see also Poisoning, by name of noxious foodstuff) 988.8
  gases, fumes, or vapors — see Table of Drugs and Chemicals
  glue (airplane) sniffing 304.6 ☑
  heat — see Heat
  high altitude NEC 993.2
    anoxia 993.2
    on
      ears 993.0
      sinuses 993.1
    polycythemia 289.0
  hot weather — see Heat
  hunger 994.2
  immersion, foot 991.4
  immunization — see Complications, vaccination
  immunological agents — see Complications, vaccination
  implantation (removable) of isotope or radium NEC 990
  infrared (radiation) (rays) NEC 990
    burn — see Burn, by site
    dermatitis or eczema 692.82
  infusion — see Complications, infusion
  ingestion or injection of isotope (therapeutic) NEC 990
  irradiation NEC (see also Effect, adverse, radiation) 990
  isotope (radioactive) NEC 990
  lack of care (child) (infant) (newborn) 995.52
    adult 995.84
  lightning 994.0
    burn — see Burn, by site
  Lirugin — see Complications, vaccination
  medicinal substance, correct, properly administered (see also Effect, adverse, drugs) 995.20
  mesothorium NEC 990
  motion 994.6
  noise, inner ear 388.10
  other drug, medicinal and biological substance 995.29
  overheated places — see Heat
  polonium NEC 990
  psychosocial, of work environment V62.1
  radiation (diagnostic) (fallout) (infrared) (natural source) (therapeutic) (tracer) (ultraviolet) (x-ray) NEC 990
    with pulmonary manifestations
      acute 508.0
      chronic 508.1
    dermatitis or eczema 692.82
      due to sun NEC (see also Dermatitis, due to, sun) 692.70
    fibrosis of lungs 508.1
    maternal with suspected damage to fetus affecting management of pregnancy 655.6 ☑
    pneumonitis 508.0
  radioactive substance NEC 990
    dermatitis or eczema 692.82
  radioactivity NEC 990

☑ **Additional Digit Required** — Refer to the Tabular List for Digit Selection   ▽ **Subterms under main terms may continue to next column or page**

2011 ICD-9-CM   ▶◀ Revised Text   ● New Line   ▲ Revised Code   October 2010 • Volume 2 — 101

Ectropion — Effect, adverse

Effect, adverse — continued
  radiotherapy NEC 990
    dermatitis or eczema 692.82
  radium NEC 990
  reduced temperature 991.9
    frostbite — see Frostbite
    immersion, foot (hand) 991.4
    specified effect NEC 991.8
  roentgenography NEC 990
  roentgenoscopy NEC 990
  roentgen rays NEC 990
  serum (prophylactic) (therapeutic) NEC
    999.5
  specified NEC 995.89
    external cause NEC 994.9
  strangulation 994.7
  submersion 994.1
  teletherapy NEC 990
  thirst 994.3
  transfusion — see Complications, transfu-
    sion
  ultraviolet (radiation) (rays) NEC 990
    burn (see also Burn, by site)
      from sun (see also Sunburn) 692.71
    dermatitis or eczema 692.82
      due to sun NEC (see also Dermatitis,
        due to, sun) 692.70
  uranium NEC 990
  vaccine (any) — see Complications, vaccina-
    tion
  weightlessness 994.9
  whole blood (see also Complications, trans-
    fusion)
    overdose or wrong substance given (see
      also Table of Drugs and Chemi-
      cals) 964.7
  working environment V62.1
  x-rays NEC 990
    dermatitis or eczema 692.82
Effect, remote
  of cancer — see condition
Effects, late — see Late, effect (of)
Effluvium, telogen 704.02
Effort
  intolerance 306.2
  syndrome (aviators) (psychogenic) 306.2
Effusion
  amniotic fluid (see also Rupture, mem-
    branes, premature) 658.1 ☑
  brain (serous) 348.5
  bronchial (see also Bronchitis) 490
  cerebral 348.5
  cerebrospinal (see also Meningitis) 322.9
    vessel 348.5
  chest — see Effusion, pleura
  intracranial 348.5
  joint 719.00
    ankle 719.07
    elbow 719.02
    foot 719.07
    hand 719.04
    hip 719.05
    knee 719.06
    multiple sites 719.09
    pelvic region 719.05
    shoulder (region) 719.01
    specified site NEC 719.08
    wrist 719.03
  meninges (see also Meningitis) 322.9
  pericardium, pericardial (see also Pericardi-
    tis) 423.9
    acute 420.90
  peritoneal (chronic) 568.82
  pleura, pleurisy, pleuritic, pleuropericardial
    511.9
    bacterial, nontuberculous 511.1
    fetus or newborn 511.9
    malignant 511.81
    nontuberculous 511.9
      bacterial 511.1
    pneumococcal 511.1
    staphylococcal 511.1
    streptococcal 511.1
    traumatic 862.29
      with open wound 862.39

Effusion — continued
  pleura, pleurisy, pleuritic, pleuropericardial
    — continued
    tuberculous (see also Tuberculosis,
      pleura) 012.0 ☑
      primary progressive 010.1 ☑
  pulmonary — see Effusion, pleura
  spinal (see also Meningitis) 322.9
  thorax, thoracic — see Effusion, pleura
Egg (oocyte) (ovum)
  donor V59.70
    over age 35 V59.73
      anonymous recipient V59.73
      designated recipient V59.74
    under age 35 V59.71
      anonymous recipient V59.71
      designated recipient V59.72
Eggshell nails 703.8
  congenital 757.5
Ego-dystonic
  homosexuality 302.0
  lesbianism 302.0
  sexual orientation 302.0
Egyptian splenomegaly 120.1
Ehlers-Danlos syndrome 756.83
Ehrlichiosis 082.40
  chaffeensis 082.41
  specified type NEC 082.49
Eichstedt's disease (pityriasis versicolor) 111.0
EIN (endometrial intraepithelial neoplasia)
  621.35
Eisenmenger's complex or syndrome (ventricular septal defect) 745.4
Ejaculation, semen
  painful 608.89
    psychogenic 306.59
  premature 302.75
  retrograde 608.87
Ekbom syndrome (restless legs) 333.94
Ekman's syndrome (brittle bones and blue
  sclera) 756.51
Elastic skin 756.83
  acquired 701.8
Elastofibroma (M8820/0) — see Neoplasm,
  connective tissue, benign
Elastoidosis
  cutanea nodularis 701.8
  cutis cystica et comedonica 701.8
Elastoma 757.39
  juvenile 757.39
  Miescher's (elastosis perforans serpiginosa)
    701.1
Elastomyofibrosis 425.3
Elastosis 701.8
  atrophicans 701.8
  perforans serpiginosa 701.1
  reactive perforating 701.1
  senilis 701.8
  solar (actinic) 692.74
Elbow — see condition
Electric
  current, electricity, effects (concussion) (fa-
    tal) (nonfatal) (shock) 994.8
    burn — see Burn, by site
  feet (foot) syndrome 266.2
  shock from electroshock gun (taser) 994.8
Electrocution 994.8
Electrolyte imbalance 276.9
  with
    abortion — see Abortion, by type, with
      metabolic disorder
    ectopic pregnancy (see also categories
      633.0–633.9) 639.4
    hyperemesis gravidarum (before 22
      completed weeks gestation)
      643.1 ☑
    molar pregnancy (see also categories
      630–632) 639.4
    following
      abortion 639.4
      ectopic or molar pregnancy 639.4
Elephantiasis (nonfilarial) 457.1
  arabicum (see also Infestation, filarial) 125.9
  congenita hereditaria 757.0
  congenital (any site) 757.0

Elephantiasis — continued
  due to
    Brugia (malayi) 125.1
    mastectomy operation 457.0
    Wuchereria (bancrofti) 125.0
      malayi 125.1
  eyelid 374.83
  filarial (see also Infestation, filarial) 125.9
  filariensis (see also Infestation, filarial) 125.9
  gingival 523.8
  glandular 457.1
  graecorum 030.9
  lymphangiectatic 457.1
  lymphatic vessel 457.1
    due to mastectomy operation 457.0
  neuromatosa 237.71
  postmastectomy 457.0
  scrotum 457.1
  streptococcal 457.1
  surgical 997.99
    postmastectomy 457.0
  telangiectodes 457.1
  vulva (nonfilarial) 624.8
Elephant man syndrome 237.71
Elevated — see Elevation
  findings on laboratory examination — see
    Findings, abnormal, without diagno-
    sis (examination) (laboratory test)
  GFR (glomerular filtration rate) — see Find-
    ings, abnormal, without diagnosis
    (examination) (laboratory test)
Elevation
  17-ketosteroids 791.9
  acid phosphatase 790.5
  alkaline phosphatase 790.5
  amylase 790.5
  antibody titers 795.79
  basal metabolic rate (BMR) 794.7
  blood pressure (see also Hypertension) 401.9
    reading (incidental) (isolated) (nonspe-
      cific), no diagnosis of hyperten-
      sion 796.2
  blood sugar 790.29
  body temperature (of unknown origin) (see
    also Pyrexia) 780.60
  cancer antigen 125 [CA 125] 795.82
  carcinoembryonic antigen [CEA] 795.81
  cholesterol 272.0
    with high triglycerides 272.2
  conjugate, eye 378.81
  C-reactive protein (CRP) 790.95
  CRP (C-reactive protein) 790.95
  diaphragm, congenital 756.6
  GFR (glomerular filtration rate) — see Find-
    ings, abnormal, without diagnosis
    (examination) (laboratory test)
  glucose
    fasting 790.21
    tolerance test 790.22
  immunoglobulin level 795.79
  indolacetic acid 791.9
  lactic acid dehydrogenase (LDH) level 790.4
  leukocytes 288.60
  lipase 790.5
  lipoprotein a level 272.8
  liver function test (LFT) 790.6
    alkaline phosphatase 790.5
    aminotransferase 790.4
    bilirubin 782.4
    hepatic enzyme NEC 790.5
    lactate dehydrogenase 790.4
  lymphocytes 288.61
  prostate specific antigen (PSA) 790.93
  renin 790.99
    in hypertension (see also Hypertension,
      renovascular) 405.91
  Rh titer ▶(see also Complications, transfu-
    sion)◀ 999.70 ▲
  scapula, congenital 755.52
  sedimentation rate 790.1
  SGOT 790.4
  SGPT 790.4
  transaminase 790.4
  triglycerides 272.1
    with high cholesterol 272.2
  vanillylmandelic acid 791.9

Elevation — continued
  venous pressure 459.89
  VMA 791.9
  white blood cell count 288.60
    specified NEC 288.69
Elliptocytosis (congenital) (hereditary) 282.1
  Hb-C (disease) 282.7
  hemoglobin disease 282.7
  sickle-cell (disease) 282.60
    trait 282.5
Ellison-Zollinger syndrome (gastric hypersecretion with pancreatic islet cell tumor) 251.5
Ellis-van Creveld disease or syndrome
  (chondroectodermal dysplasia) 756.55
Elongation, elongated (congenital) — see also
  Distortion
  bone 756.9
  cervix (uteri) 752.49
    acquired 622.6
    hypertrophic 622.6
  colon 751.5
  common bile duct 751.69
  cystic duct 751.69
  frenulum, penis 752.69
  labia minora, acquired 624.8
  ligamentum patellae 756.89
  petiolus (epiglottidis) 748.3
  styloid bone (process) 733.99
  tooth, teeth 520.2
  uvula 750.26
    acquired 528.9
Elschnig bodies or pearls 366.51
El Tor cholera 001.1
Emaciation (due to malnutrition) 261
Emancipation disorder 309.22
Embadomoniasis 007.8
Embarrassment heart, cardiac — see Disease,
  heart
Embedded
  fragment (status) — see Foreign body,   ●
    retained   ●
  splinter (status) — see Foreign body, re-   ●
    tained   ●
  tooth, teeth 520.6   ●
    root only 525.3
Embolic — see condition
Embolism 444.9
  with
    abortion — see Abortion, by type, with
      embolism
    ectopic pregnancy (see also categories
      633.0–633.9) 639.6
    molar pregnancy (see also categories
      630–632) 639.6
  air (any site) 958.0
    with
      abortion — see Abortion, by type,
        with embolism
      ectopic pregnancy (see also cate-
        gories 633.0–633.9) 639.6
      molar pregnancy (see also categories
        630–632) 639.6
    due to implanted device — see Compli-
      cations, due to (presence of) any
      device, implant, or graft classified
      to 996.0–996.5 NEC
    following
      abortion 639.6
      ectopic or molar pregnancy 639.6
      infusion, perfusion, or transfusion
        999.1
    in pregnancy, childbirth, or puerperium
      673.0 ☑
    traumatic 958.0
  amniotic fluid (pulmonary) 673.1 ☑
    with
      abortion — see Abortion, by type,
        with embolism
      ectopic pregnancy (see also cate-
        gories 633.0–633.9) 639.6
      molar pregnancy (see also categories
        630–632) 639.6
    following
      abortion 639.6
      ectopic or molar pregnancy 639.6

☑ Additional Digit Required — Refer to the Tabular List for Digit Selection   ▼ Subterms under main terms may continue to next column or page

102 — Volume 2 • October 2010   ▶◀ Revised Text   ● New Line   ▲ Revised Code   2011 ICD-9-CM

Embolism — *continued*
- aorta, aortic 444.1
  - abdominal 444.0
  - bifurcation 444.0
  - saddle 444.0
  - thoracic 444.1
- artery 444.9
  - auditory, internal 433.8 ☑
  - basilar (*see also* Occlusion, artery, basilar) 433.0 ☑
  - bladder 444.89
  - carotid (common) (internal) (*see also* Occlusion, artery, carotid) 433.1 ☑
  - cerebellar (anterior inferior) (posterior inferior) (superior) 433.8 ☑
  - cerebral (*see also* Embolism, brain) 434.1 ☑
  - choroidal (anterior) 433.8 ☑
  - communicating posterior 433.8 ☑
  - coronary (*see also* Infarct, myocardium) 410.9 ☑
    - without myocardial infarction 411.81
  - extremity 444.22
    - lower 444.22
    - upper 444.21
  - hypophyseal 433.8 ☑
  - mesenteric (with gangrene) 557.0
  - ophthalmic (*see also* Occlusion, retina) 362.30
  - peripheral 444.22
  - pontine 433.8 ☑
  - precerebral NEC — *see* Occlusion, artery, precerebral
  - pulmonary — *see* Embolism, pulmonary
  - pyemic 449
    - pulmonary 415.12
  - renal 593.81
  - retinal (*see also* Occlusion, retina) 362.30
  - septic 449
    - pulmonary 415.12
  - specified site NEC 444.89
  - vertebral (*see also* Occlusion, artery, vertebral) 433.2 ☑
- auditory, internal 433.8 ☑
- basilar (artery) (*see also* Occlusion, artery, basilar) 433.0 ☑
- birth, mother — *see* Embolism, obstetrical
- blood-clot
  - with
    - abortion — *see* Abortion, by type, with embolism
    - ectopic pregnancy (*see also* categories 633.0–633.9) 639.6
    - molar pregnancy (*see also* categories 630–632) 639.6
  - following
    - abortion 639.6
    - ectopic or molar pregnancy 639.6
  - in pregnancy, childbirth, or puerperium 673.2 ☑
- brain 434.1 ☑
  - with
    - abortion — *see* Abortion, by type, with embolism
    - ectopic pregnancy (*see also* categories 633.0–633.9) 639.6
    - molar pregnancy (*see also* categories 630–632) 639.6
  - following
    - abortion 639.6
    - ectopic or molar pregnancy 639.6
  - late effect — *see* Late effect(s) (of) cerebrovascular disease
  - puerperal, postpartum, childbirth 674.0 ☑
- capillary 448.9
- cardiac (*see also* Infarct, myocardium) 410.9 ☑
- carotid (artery) (common) (internal) (*see also* Occlusion, artery, carotid) 433.1 ☑
- cavernous sinus (venous) — *see* Embolism, intracranial venous sinus
- cerebral (*see also* Embolism, brain) 434.1 ☑
- cholesterol — *see* Atheroembolism
- choroidal (anterior) (artery) 433.8 ☑

Embolism — *continued*
- coronary (artery or vein) (systemic) (*see also* Infarct, myocardium) 410.9 ☑
  - without myocardial infarction 411.81
  - due to (presence of) any device, implant, or graft classifiable to 996.0–996.5 — *see* Complications, due to (presence of) any device, implant, or graft classified to 996.0–996.5 NEC
- encephalomalacia (*see also* Embolism, brain) 434.1 ☑
- extremities 444.22
  - lower 444.22
  - upper 444.21
- eye 362.30
- fat (cerebral) (pulmonary) (systemic) 958.1
  - with
    - abortion — *see* Abortion, by type, with embolism
    - ectopic pregnancy (*see also* categories 633.0–633.9) 639.6
    - molar pregnancy (*see also* categories 630–632) 639.6
  - complicating delivery or puerperium 673.8 ☑
  - following
    - abortion 639.6
    - ectopic or molar pregnancy 639.6
  - in pregnancy, childbirth, or the puerperium 673.8 ☑
- femoral (artery) 444.22
  - vein 453.6
    - deep 453.41
- following
  - abortion 639.6
  - ectopic or molar pregnancy 639.6
  - infusion, perfusion, or transfusion
    - air 999.1
    - thrombus 999.2
- heart (fatty) (*see also* Infarct, myocardium) 410.9 ☑
- hepatic (vein) 453.0
- iliac (artery) 444.81
- iliofemoral 444.81
- in pregnancy, childbirth, or puerperium (pulmonary) — *see* Embolism, obstetrical
- intestine (artery) (vein) (with gangrene) 557.0
- intracranial (*see also* Embolism, brain) 434.1 ☑
  - venous sinus (any) 325
    - late effect — *see* category 326
    - nonpyogenic 437.6
      - in pregnancy or puerperium 671.5 ☑
- kidney (artery) 593.81
- lateral sinus (venous) — *see* Embolism, intracranial venous sinus
- longitudinal sinus (venous) — *see* Embolism, intracranial venous sinus
- lower extremity 444.22
- lung (massive) — *see* Embolism, pulmonary
- meninges (*see also* Embolism, brain) 434.1 ☑
- mesenteric (artery) (with gangrene) 557.0
- multiple NEC 444.9
- obstetrical (pulmonary) 673.2 ☑
  - air 673.0 ☑
  - amniotic fluid (pulmonary) 673.1 ☑
  - blood-clot 673.2 ☑
  - cardiac 674.8 ☑
  - fat 673.8 ☑
  - heart 674.8 ☑
  - pyemic 673.3 ☑
  - septic 673.3 ☑
  - specified NEC 674.8 ☑
- ophthalmic (*see also* Occlusion, retina) 362.30
- paradoxical NEC 444.9
- penis 607.82
- peripheral arteries NEC 444.22
  - lower 444.22
  - upper 444.21
- pituitary 253.8
- popliteal (artery) 444.22

Embolism — *continued*
- portal (vein) 452
- postoperative NEC 997.2
  - cerebral 997.02
  - mesenteric artery 997.71
  - other vessels 997.79
  - peripheral vascular 997.2
  - pulmonary 415.11
    - septic 415.11
  - renal artery 997.72
- precerebral artery (*see also* Occlusion, artery, precerebral) 433.9 ☑
- puerperal — *see* Embolism, obstetrical
- pulmonary (acute) (artery) (vein) 415.19
  - with
    - abortion — *see* Abortion, by type, with embolism
    - ectopic pregnancy (*see also* categories 633.0–633.9) 639.6
    - molar pregnancy (*see also* categories 630–632) 639.6
  - chronic 416.2
  - following
    - abortion 639.6
    - ectopic or molar pregnancy 639.6
  - healed or old V12.51
  - iatrogenic 415.11
  - in pregnancy, childbirth, or puerperium — *see* Embolism, obstetrical
  - personal history of V12.51
  - postoperative 415.11
  - septic 415.12
- pyemic (multiple) (*see also* Septicemia) 415.12
  - with
    - abortion — *see* Abortion, by type, with embolism
    - ectopic pregnancy (*see also* categories 633.0–633.9) 639.6
    - molar pregnancy (*see also* categories 630–632) 639.6
  - Aerobacter aerogenes 415.12
  - enteric gram-negative bacilli 415.12
  - Enterobacter aerogenes 415.12
  - Escherichia coli 415.12
  - following
    - abortion 639.6
    - ectopic or molar pregnancy 639.6
  - Hemophilus influenzae 415.12
  - pneumococcal 415.12
  - Proteus vulgaris 415.12
  - Pseudomonas (aeruginosa) 415.12
  - puerperal, postpartum, childbirth (any organism) 673.3 ☑
  - Serratia 415.12
  - specified organism NEC 415.12
  - staphylococcal 415.12
    - aureus 415.12
    - specified organism NEC 415.12
  - streptococcal 415.12
- renal (artery) 593.81
  - vein 453.3
- retina, retinal (*see also* Occlusion, retina) 362.30
- saddle (aorta) 444.0
- septic 415.12
  - arterial 449
- septicemic — *see* Embolism, pyemic
- sinus — *see* Embolism, intracranial venous sinus
- soap
  - with
    - abortion — *see* Abortion, by type, with embolism
    - ectopic pregnancy (*see also* categories 633.0–633.9) 639.6
    - molar pregnancy (*see also* categories 630–632) 639.6
  - following
    - abortion 639.6
    - ectopic or molar pregnancy 639.6
- spinal cord (nonpyogenic) 336.1
  - in pregnancy or puerperium 671.5 ☑
  - pyogenic origin 324.1
    - late effect — *see* category 326
- spleen, splenic (artery) 444.89

Embolism — *continued*
- thrombus (thromboembolism) following infusion, perfusion, or transfusion 999.2
- upper extremity 444.21
- vein 453.9
  - with inflammation or phlebitis — *see* Thrombophlebitis
  - antecubital ►(acute)◄ 453.81
    - chronic 453.71
  - axillary ►(acute)◄ 453.84
    - chronic 453.74
  - basilic ►(acute)◄ 453.81
    - chronic 453.71
  - brachial ►(acute)◄ 453.82
    - chronic 453.72
  - brachiocephalic ►(acute)◄ (innominate) 453.87
    - chronic 453.77
  - cephalic ►(acute)◄ 453.81
    - chronic 453.71
  - cerebral (*see also* Embolism, brain) 434.1 ☑
  - coronary (*see also* Infarct, myocardium) 410.9 ☑
    - without myocardial infarction 411.81
  - hepatic 453.0
  - internal jugular ►(acute)◄ 453.86
    - chronic 453.76
  - lower extremity (superficial) 453.6
    - deep 453.40
      - acute 453.40
        - calf 453.42
        - distal (lower leg) 453.42
        - femoral 453.41
        - iliac 453.41
        - lower leg 453.42
        - peroneal 453.42
        - popliteal 453.42
        - proximal (upper leg) 453.41
        - thigh 453.41
        - tibial 453.42
      - chronic 453.50
        - calf 453.52
        - disal (lower leg) 453.52
        - femoral 453.51
        - iliac 453.51
        - lower leg 453.52
        - peroneal 453.52
        - popliteal 453.51
        - proximal (upper leg) 453.51
        - thigh 453.51
        - tibial 453.52
    - saphenous (greater) (lesser) 453.6
    - superficial 453.6
  - mesenteric (with gangrene) 557.0
  - portal 452
  - pulmonary — *see* Embolism, pulmonary
  - radial ►(acute)◄ 453.82
    - chronic 453.72
  - renal 453.3
  - saphenous (greater) (lesser) 453.6
  - specified NEC (acute) 453.89
    - with inflammation or phlebitis — *see* Thrombophlebitis
    - chronic 453.79
  - subclavian ►(acute)◄ 453.85
    - chronic 453.75
  - superior vena cava ►(acute)◄ 453.87
    - chronic 453.77
  - thoracic ►(acute)◄ 453.87
    - chronic 453.77
  - ulnar ►(acute)◄ 453.82
    - chronic 453.72
  - upper extremity 453.83
    - acute 453.83
      - deep 453.82
      - superficial 453.81
    - chronic 453.73
      - deep 453.72
      - superficial 453.71
- vena cava
  - inferior 453.2
  - superior ►(acute)◄ 453.87
    - chronic 453.77

☑ **Additional Digit Required** — Refer to the Tabular List for Digit Selection   ▽ **Subterms under main terms may continue to next column or page**

Embolism — *continued*
  vessels of brain (*see also* Embolism, brain) 434.1 ☑
Embolization — *see* **Embolism**
Embolus — *see* Embolism
Embryoma (M9080/1) — *see also* Neoplasm, by site, uncertain behavior
  benign (M9080/0) — *see* Neoplasm, by site, benign
    kidney (M8960/3) 189.0
    liver (M8970/3) 155.0
  malignant (M9080/3) (*see also* Neoplasm, by site, malignant)
    kidney (M8960/3) 189.0
    liver (M8970/3) 155.0
    testis (M9070/3) 186.9
      undescended 186.0
  testis (M9070/3) 186.9
    undescended 186.0
Embryonic
  circulation 747.9
  heart 747.9
  vas deferens 752.89
Embryopathia NEC 759.9
Embryotomy, fetal 763.89
Embryotoxon 743.43
  interfering with vision 743.42
Emesis — *see also* Vomiting
  bilious 787.04
  gravidarum — *see* Hyperemesis, gravidarum
Emissions, nocturnal (semen) 608.89
Emotional
  crisis — *see* Crisis, emotional
  disorder (*see also* Disorder, mental) 300.9
  instability (excessive) 301.3
  lability 799.24
  overlay — *see* Reaction, adjustment
  upset 300.9
Emotionality, pathological 301.3
Emotogenic disease — *see also* Disorder, psychogenic 306.9
Emphysema (atrophic) (centriacinar) (centrilobular) (chronic) (diffuse) (essential) (hypertrophic) (interlobular) (lung) (obstructive) (panlobular) (paracicatricial) (paracinar) (postural) (pulmonary) (senile) (subpleural) (traction) (unilateral) (unilobular) (vesicular) 492.8
  with bronchitis
    chronic 491.20
      with
        acute bronchitis 491.22
        exacerbation (acute) 491.21
  bullous (giant) 492.0
  cellular tissue 958.7
    surgical 998.81
  compensatory 518.2
  congenital 770.2
  conjunctiva 372.89
  connective tissue 958.7
    surgical 998.81
  due to fumes or vapors 506.4
  eye 376.89
  eyelid 374.85
    surgical 998.81
    traumatic 958.7
  fetus or newborn (interstitial) (mediastinal) (unilobular) 770.2
  heart 416.9
  interstitial 518.1
    congenital 770.2
    fetus or newborn 770.2
  laminated tissue 958.7
    surgical 998.81
  mediastinal 518.1
    fetus or newborn 770.2
  newborn (interstitial) (mediastinal) (unilobular) 770.2
  obstructive diffuse with fibrosis 492.8
  orbit 376.89
  subcutaneous 958.7
    due to trauma 958.7
    nontraumatic 518.1
    surgical 998.81
  surgical 998.81
  thymus (gland) (congenital) 254.8

Emphysema — *continued*
  traumatic 958.7
  tuberculous (*see also* Tuberculosis, pulmonary) 011.9 ☑
Employment examination (certification) V70.5
Empty sella (turcica) syndrome 253.8
Empyema (chest) (diaphragmatic) (double) (encapsulated) (general) (interlobar) (lung) (medial) (necessitatis) (perforating chest wall) (pleura) (pneumococcal) (residual) (sacculated) (streptococcal) (supradiaphragmatic) 510.9
  with fistula 510.0
  accessory sinus (chronic) (*see also* Sinusitis) 473.9
  acute 510.9
    with fistula 510.0
  antrum (acute) (*see also* Sinusitis, maxillary) 473.0
  brain (any part) (*see also* Abscess, brain) 324.0
  ethmoidal (sinus) (chronic) (*see also* Sinusitis, ethmoidal) 473.2
  extradural (*see also* Abscess, extradural) 324.9
  frontal (sinus) (chronic) (*see also* Sinusitis, frontal) 473.1
  gallbladder (*see also* Cholecystitis, acute) 575.0
  mastoid (process) (acute) (*see also* Mastoiditis, acute) 383.00
  maxilla, maxillary 526.4
    sinus (chronic) (*see also* Sinusitis, maxillary) 473.0
  nasal sinus (chronic) (*see also* Sinusitis) 473.9
  sinus (accessory) (nasal) (*see also* Sinusitis) 473.9
  sphenoidal (chronic) (sinus) (*see also* Sinusitis, sphenoidal) 473.3
  subarachnoid (*see also* Abscess, extradural) 324.9
  subdural (*see also* Abscess, extradural) 324.9
  tuberculous (*see also* Tuberculosis, pleura) 012.0 ☑
  ureter (*see also* Ureteritis) 593.89
  ventricular (*see also* Abscess, brain) 324.0
Enameloma 520.2
Encephalitis (bacterial) (chronic) (hemorrhagic) (idiopathic) (nonepidemic) (spurious) (subacute) 323.9
  acute (*see also* Encephalitis, viral)
    disseminated (postinfectious) NEC 136.9 *[323.61]*
      postimmunization or postvaccination 323.51
    inclusional 049.8
    inclusion body 049.8
    necrotizing 049.8
  arboviral, arbovirus NEC 064
  arthropod-borne (*see also* Encephalitis, viral, arthropod-borne) 064
  Australian X 062.4
  Bwamba fever 066.3
  California (virus) 062.5
  Central European 063.2
  Czechoslovakian 063.2
  Dawson's (inclusion body) 046.2
  diffuse sclerosing 046.2
  due to
    actinomycosis 039.8 *[323.41]*
    cat-scratch disease 078.3 *[323.01]*
    human herpesvirus NEC 058.29
    human herpesvirus 6 058.21
    human herpesvirus 7 058.29
    infection classified elsewhere 136.9 *[323.41]*
    infectious mononucleosis 075 *[323.01]*
    malaria (*see also* Malaria) 084.6 *[323.2]*
    Negishi virus 064
    ornithosis 073.7 *[323.01]*
    prophylactic inoculation against smallpox 323.51
    rickettsiosis (*see also* Rickettsiosis) 083.9 *[323.1]*
    rubella 056.01
    toxoplasmosis (acquired) 130.0

Encephalitis — *continued*
  due to — *continued*
    toxoplasmosis — *continued*
      congenital (active) 771.2 *[323.41]*
    typhus (fever) (*see also* Typhus) 081.9 *[323.1]*
    vaccination (smallpox) 323.51
  Eastern equine 062.2
  endemic 049.8
  epidemic 049.8
  equine (acute) (infectious) (viral) 062.9
    Eastern 062.2
    Venezuelan 066.2
    Western 062.1
  Far Eastern 063.0
  following vaccination or other immunization procedure 323.51
  herpes 054.3
  human herpesvirus NEC 058.29
  human herpesvirus 6 058.21
  human herpesvirus 7 058.29
  Ilheus (virus) 062.8
  inclusion body 046.2
  infectious (acute) (virus) NEC 049.8
  influenzal ▶(*see also* Influenza)◀ 487.8 *[323.41]*
  lethargic 049.8
  Japanese (B type) 062.0
  La Crosse 062.5
  Langat 063.8
  late effect — *see* Late, effect, encephalitis
  lead 984.9 *[323.71]*
  lethargic (acute) (infectious) (influenzal) 049.8
  lethargica 049.8
  louping ill 063.1
  lupus 710.0 *[323.81]*
  lymphatica 049.0
  Mengo 049.8
  meningococcal 036.1
  mumps 072.2
  Murray Valley 062.4
  myoclonic 049.8
  Negishi virus 064
  otitic NEC 382.4 *[323.41]*
  parasitic NEC 123.9 *[323.41]*
  periaxialis (concentrica) (diffusa) 341.1
  postchickenpox 052.0
  postexanthematous NEC 057.9 *[323.62]*
  postimmunization 323.51
  postinfectious NEC 136.9 *[323.62]*
  postmeasles 055.0
  posttraumatic 323.81
  postvaccinal (smallpox) 323.51
  postvaricella 052.0
  postviral NEC 079.99 *[323.62]*
    postexanthematous 057.9 *[323.62]*
    specified NEC 057.8 *[323.62]*
  Powassan 063.8
  progressive subcortical (Binswanger's) 290.12
  Rasmussen 323.81
  Rio Bravo 049.8
  rubella 056.01
  Russian
    autumnal 062.0
    spring-summer type (taiga) 063.0
  saturnine 984.9 *[323.71]*
  Semliki Forest 062.8
  serous 048
  slow-acting virus NEC 046.8
  specified cause NEC 323.81
  St. Louis type 062.3
  subacute sclerosing 046.2
  subcorticalis chronica 290.12
  summer 062.0
  suppurative 324.0
  syphilitic 094.81
    congenital 090.41
  tick-borne 063.9
  torula, torular 117.5 *[323.41]*
  toxic NEC 989.9 *[323.71]*
  toxoplasmic (acquired) 130.0
    congenital (active) 771.2 *[323.41]*
  trichinosis 124 *[323.41]*

Encephalitis — *continued*
  Trypanosomiasis (*see also* Trypanosomiasis) 086.9 *[323.2]*
  tuberculous (*see also* Tuberculosis) 013.6 ☑
  type B (Japanese) 062.0
  type C 062.3
  van Bogaert's 046.2
  Venezuelan 066.2
  Vienna type 049.8
  viral, virus 049.9
    arthropod-borne NEC 064
      mosquito-borne 062.9
        Australian X disease 062.4
        California virus 062.5
        Eastern equine 062.2
        Ilheus virus 062.8
        Japanese (B type) 062.0
        Murray Valley 062.4
        specified type NEC 062.8
        St. Louis 062.3
        type B 062.0
        type C 062.3
        Western equine 062.1
      tick-borne 063.9
        biundulant 063.2
        Central European 063.2
        Czechoslovakian 063.2
        diphasic meningoencephalitis 063.2
        Far Eastern 063.0
        Langat 063.8
        louping ill 063.1
        Powassan 063.8
        Russian spring-summer (taiga) 063.0
        specified type NEC 063.8
      vector unknown 064
      Western equine 062.1
    slow acting NEC 046.8
    specified type NEC 049.8
    vaccination, prophylactic (against) V05.0
  von Economo's 049.8
  Western equine 062.1
  West Nile type 066.41
Encephalocele 742.0
  orbit 376.81
Encephalocystocele 742.0
Encephalomalacia (brain) (cerebellar) (cerebral) (cerebrospinal) — *see also* Softening, brain 348.89 ▲
  due to
    hemorrhage (*see also* Hemorrhage, brain) 431
    recurrent spasm of artery 435.9
  embolic (cerebral) (*see also* Embolism, brain) 434.1 ☑
  subcorticalis chronicus arteriosclerotica 290.12
  thrombotic (*see also* Thrombosis, brain) 434.0 ☑
Encephalomeningitis — *see* Meningoencephalitis
Encephalomeningocele 742.0
Encephalomeningomyelitis — *see* Meningoencephalitis
Encephalomeningopathy — *see also* Meningoencephalitis 349.9
Encephalomyelitis (chronic) (granulomatous) (myalgic, benign) — *see also* Encephalitis 323.9
  abortive disseminated 049.8
  acute disseminated (ADEM) (postinfectious) 136.9 *[323.61]*
    infectious 136.9 *[323.61]*
    noninfectious 323.81
    postimmunization 323.51
  due to
    cat-scratch disease 078.3 *[323.01]*
    infectious mononucleosis 075 *[323.01]*
    ornithosis 073.7 *[323.01]*
    vaccination (any) 323.51
  equine (acute) (infectious) 062.9
    Eastern 062.2
    Venezuelan 066.2
    Western 062.1
  funicularis infectiosa 049.8

Encephalomyelitis — see also Encephalitis — continued
late effect — see Late, effect, encephalitis
Munch-Peterson's 049.8
postchickenpox 052.0
postimmunization 323.51
postmeasles 055.0
postvaccinal (smallpox) 323.51
rubella 056.01
specified cause NEC 323.81
syphilitic 094.81
West Nile 066.41
Encephalomyelocele 742.0
Encephalomyelomeningitis — see Meningoencephalitis
Encephalomyeloneuropathy 349.9
Encephalomyelopathy 349.9
subacute necrotizing (infantile) 330.8
Encephalomyeloradiculitis (acute) 357.0
Encephalomyeloradiculoneuritis (acute) 357.0
Encephalomyeloradiculopathy 349.9
Encephalomyocarditis 074.23
Encephalopathia hyperbilirubinemica, newborn 774.7
due to isoimmunization (conditions classifiable to 773.0–773.2) 773.4
Encephalopathy (acute) 348.30
alcoholic 291.2
anoxic — see Damage, brain, anoxic
arteriosclerotic 437.0
late effect — see Late effect(s) (of) cerebrovascular disease
bilirubin, newborn 774.7
due to isoimmunization 773.4
congenital 742.9
demyelinating (callosal) 341.8
due to
birth injury (intracranial) 767.8
dialysis 294.8
transient 293.9
drugs — (see also Table of Drugs and Chemicals) 348.39
hyperinsulinism — see Hyperinsulinism
influenza (virus) ▶(see also Influenza)◀ 487.8
identified ●
avian 488.09 ●
novel H1N1 488.19 ●
lack of vitamin (see also Deficiency, vitamin) 269.2
nicotinic acid deficiency 291.2
serum (nontherapeutic) (therapeutic) 999.5
syphilis 094.81
trauma (postconcussional) 310.2
current (see also Concussion, brain) 850.9
with skull fracture — see Fracture, skull, by site, with intracranial injury
vaccination 323.51
hepatic 572.2
hyperbilirubinemic, newborn 774.7
due to isoimmunization (conditions classifiable to 773.0–773.2) 773.4
hypertensive 437.2
hypoglycemic 251.2
hypoxic (see also Damage, brain, anoxic)
ischemic (HIE) 768.70
mild 768.71
moderate 768.72
severe 768.73
infantile cystic necrotizing (congenital) 341.8
lead 984.9 [323.71]
leukopolio 330.0
metabolic (see also Delirium) 348.31
toxic 349.82
necrotizing
hemorrhagic (acute) 323.61
subacute 330.8
other specified type NEC 348.39
pellagrous 265.2
portal-systemic 572.2
postcontusional 310.2

Encephalopathy — continued
posttraumatic 310.2
saturnine 984.9 [323.71]
septic 348.31
spongiform, subacute (viral) 046.19
subacute
necrotizing 330.8
spongiform 046.19
viral, spongiform 046.19
subcortical progressive (Schilder) 341.1
chronic (Binswanger's) 290.12
toxic 349.82
metabolic 349.82
traumatic (postconcussional) 310.2
current (see also Concussion, brain) 850.9
with skull fracture — see Fracture, skull, by site, with intracranial injury
vitamin B deficiency NEC 266.9
Wernicke's (superior hemorrhagic polioencephalitis) 265.1
Encephalorrhagia — see also Hemorrhage, brain 432.9
healed or old V12.54
late effect — see Late effect(s) (of) cerebrovascular disease
Encephalosis, posttraumatic 310.2
Enchondroma (M9220/0) — see also Neoplasm, bone, benign
multiple, congenital 756.4
Enchondromatosis (cartilaginous) (congenital) (multiple) 756.4
Enchondroses, multiple (cartilaginous) (congenital) 756.4
Encopresis — see also Incontinence, feces 787.60 ▲
nonorganic origin 307.7
Encounter for — see also Admission for
administrative purpose only V68.9
referral of patient without examination or treatment V68.81
specified purpose NEC V68.89
chemotherapy, (oral) (intravenous), antineoplastic V58.11
dialysis
extracorporeal (renal) V56.0
peritoneal V56.8
disability examination V68.01
end-of-life care V66.7
hospice care V66.7
immunizations (childhood) appropriate for age V20.2
immunotherapy, antineoplastic V58.12
palliative care V66.7
paternity testing V70.4
radiotherapy V58.0
respirator [ventilator] dependence during
mechanical failure V46.14
power failure V46.12
for weaning V46.13
routine infant and child vision and hearing testing V20.2
school examination V70.3
following surgery V67.09
screening mammogram NEC V76.12
for high-risk patient V76.11
terminal care V66.7
weaning from respirator [ventilator] V46.13
Encystment — see Cyst
Endamebiasis — see Amebiasis
Endamoeba — see Amebiasis
Endarteritis (bacterial, subacute) (infective) (septic) 447.6
brain, cerebral or cerebrospinal 437.4
late effect — see Late effect(s) (of) cerebrovascular disease
coronary (artery) — see Arteriosclerosis, coronary
deformans — see Arteriosclerosis
embolic (see also Embolism) 444.9
obliterans (see also Arteriosclerosis)
pulmonary 417.8
pulmonary 417.8
retina 362.18
senile — see Arteriosclerosis

Endarteritis — continued
syphilitic 093.89
brain or cerebral 094.89
congenital 090.5
spinal 094.89
tuberculous (see also Tuberculosis) 017.9 ☑
Endemic — see condition
Endocarditis (chronic) (indeterminate) (interstitial) (marantic) (nonbacterial thrombotic) (residual) (sclerotic) (sclerous) (senile) (valvular) 424.90
with
rheumatic fever (conditions classifiable to 390)
active — see Endocarditis, acute, rheumatic
inactive or quiescent (with chorea) 397.9
acute or subacute 421.9
rheumatic (aortic) (mitral) (pulmonary) (tricuspid) 391.1
with chorea (acute) (rheumatic) (Sydenham's) 392.0
aortic (heart) (nonrheumatic) (valve) 424.1
with
mitral (valve) disease 396.9
active or acute 391.1
with chorea (acute) (rheumatic) (Sydenham's) 392.0
bacterial 421.0
rheumatic fever (conditions classifiable to 390)
active — see Endocarditis, acute, rheumatic
inactive or quiescent (with chorea) 395.9
with mitral disease 396.9
acute or subacute 421.9
arteriosclerotic 424.1
congenital 746.89
hypertensive 424.1
rheumatic (chronic) (inactive) 395.9
with mitral (valve) disease 396.9
active or acute 391.1
with chorea (acute) (rheumatic) (Sydenham's) 392.0
active or acute 391.1
with chorea (acute) (rheumatic) (Sydenham's) 392.0
specified cause, except rheumatic 424.1
syphilitic 093.22
arteriosclerotic or due to arteriosclerosis 424.99
atypical verrucous (Libman-Sacks) 710.0 [424.91]
bacterial (acute) (any valve) (chronic) (subacute) 421.0
blastomycotic 116.0 [421.1]
candidal 112.81
congenital 425.3
constrictive 421.0
Coxsackie 074.22
due to
blastomycosis 116.0 [421.1]
candidiasis 112.81
Coxsackie (virus) 074.22
disseminated lupus erythematosus 710.0 [424.91]
histoplasmosis (see also Histoplasmosis) 115.94
hypertension (benign) 424.99
moniliasis 112.81
prosthetic cardiac valve 996.61
Q fever 083.0 [421.1]
serratia marcescens 421.0
typhoid (fever) 002.0 [421.1]
fetal 425.3
gonococcal 098.84
hypertensive 424.99
infectious or infective (acute) (any valve) (chronic) (subacute) 421.0
lenta (acute) (any valve) (chronic) (subacute) 421.0
Libman-Sacks 710.0 [424.91]

Endocarditis — continued
Loeffler's (parietal fibroplastic) 421.0
malignant (acute) (any valve) (chronic) (subacute) 421.0
meningococcal 036.42
mitral (chronic) (double) (fibroid) (heart) (inactive) (valve) (with chorea) 394.9
with
aortic (valve) disease 396.9
active or acute 391.1
with chorea (acute) (rheumatic) (Sydenham's) 392.0
rheumatic fever (conditions classifiable to 390)
active — see Endocarditis, acute, rheumatic
inactive or quiescent (with chorea) 394.9
with aortic valve disease 396.9
active or acute 391.1
with chorea (acute) (rheumatic) (Sydenham's) 392.0
bacterial 421.0
arteriosclerotic 424.0
congenital 746.09
hypertensive 424.0
nonrheumatic 424.0
acute or subacute 421.9
syphilitic 093.21
monilial 112.81
mycotic (acute) (any valve) (chronic) (subacute) 421.0
pneumococcic (acute) (any valve) (chronic) (subacute) 421.0
pulmonary (chronic) (heart) (valve) 424.3
with
rheumatic fever (conditions classifiable to 390)
active — see Endocarditis, acute, rheumatic
inactive or quiescent (with chorea) 397.1
acute or subacute 421.9
rheumatic 391.1
with chorea (acute) (rheumatic) (Sydenham's) 392.0
arteriosclerotic or due to arteriosclerosis 424.3
congenital 746.09
hypertensive or due to hypertension (benign) 424.3
rheumatic (chronic) (inactive) (with chorea) 397.1
active or acute 391.1
with chorea (acute) (rheumatic) (Sydenham's) 392.0
syphilitic 093.24
purulent (acute) (any valve) (chronic) (subacute) 421.0
rheumatic (chronic) (inactive) (with chorea) 397.9
active or acute (aortic) (mitral) (pulmonary) (tricuspid) 391.1
with chorea (acute) (rheumatic) (Sydenham's) 392.0
septic (acute) (any valve) (chronic) (subacute) 421.0
specified cause, except rheumatic 424.99
streptococcal (acute) (any valve) (chronic) (subacute) 421.0
subacute — see Endocarditis, acute
suppurative (any valve) (acute) (chronic) (subacute) 421.0
syphilitic NEC 093.20
toxic (see also Endocarditis, acute) 421.9
tricuspid (chronic) (heart) (inactive) (rheumatic) (valve) (with chorea) 397.0
with
rheumatic fever (conditions classifiable to 390)
active — see Endocarditis, acute, rheumatic
inactive or quiescent (with chorea) 397.0

☑ Additional Digit Required — Refer to the Tabular List for Digit Selection   ▽ Subterms under main terms may continue to next column or page

2011 ICD-9-CM   ▶◀ Revised Text   ● New Line   ▲ Revised Code   October 2010 • Volume 2 — 105

Endocarditis — continued
  tricuspid — continued
    active or acute 391.1
      with chorea (acute) (rheumatic)
        (Sydenham's) 392.0
    arteriosclerotic 424.2
    congenital 746.89
    hypertensive 424.2
    nonrheumatic 424.2
      acute or subacute 421.9
    specified cause, except rheumatic 424.2
    syphilitic 093.23
    tuberculous (see also Tuberculosis)
      017.9 ☑ [424.91]
    typhoid 002.0 [421.1]
    ulcerative (acute) (any valve) (chronic)
      (subacute) 421.0
    vegetative (acute) (any valve) (chronic)
      (subacute) 421.0
    verrucous (acute) (any valve) (chronic)
      (subacute) NEC 710.0 [424.91]
      nonbacterial 710.0 [424.91]
      nonrheumatic 710.0 [424.91]
Endocardium, endocardial — see also condition
  cushion defect 745.60
    specified type NEC 745.69
Endocervicitis — see also Cervicitis 616.0
  due to
    intrauterine (contraceptive) device
      996.65
  gonorrheal (acute) 098.15
    chronic or duration of 2 months or over
      098.35
  hyperplastic 616.0
  syphilitic 095.8
  trichomonal 131.09
  tuberculous (see also Tuberculosis) 016.7 ☑
Endocrine — see condition
Endocrinopathy, pluriglandular 258.9
Endodontitis 522.0
End-of-life care V66.7
Endomastoiditis — see also Mastoiditis 383.9
Endometrioma 617.9
Endometriosis 617.9
  appendix 617.5
  bladder 617.8
  bowel 617.5
  broad ligament 617.3
  cervix 617.0
  colon 617.5
  cul-de-sac (Douglas') 617.3
  exocervix 617.0
  fallopian tube 617.2
  female genital organ NEC 617.8
  gallbladder 617.8
  in scar of skin 617.6
  internal 617.0
  intestine 617.5
  lung 617.8
  myometrium 617.0
  ovary 617.1
  parametrium 617.3
  pelvic peritoneum 617.3
  peritoneal (pelvic) 617.3
  rectovaginal septum 617.4
  rectum 617.5
  round ligament 617.3
  skin 617.6
  specified site NEC 617.8
  stromal (M8931/1) 236.0
  umbilicus 617.8
  uterus 617.0
    internal 617.0
  vagina 617.4
  vulva 617.8
Endometritis (nonspecific) (purulent) (septic)
  (suppurative) 615.9
  with
    abortion — see Abortion, by type, with
      sepsis
    ectopic pregnancy (see also categories
      633.0–633.9) 639.0
    molar pregnancy (see also categories
      630–632) 639.0
  acute 615.0

Endometritis — continued
  blennorrhagic 098.16
    acute 098.16
    chronic or duration of 2 months or over
      098.36
  cervix, cervical (see also Cervicitis) 616.0
    hyperplastic 616.0
  chronic 615.1
  complicating pregnancy 670.1 ☑
    affecting fetus or newborn 760.8
    septic 670.2 ☑
  decidual 615.9
  following
    abortion 639.0
    ectopic or molar pregnancy 639.0
  gonorrheal (acute) 098.16
    chronic or duration of 2 months or over
      098.36
  hyperplastic (see also Hyperplasia, en-
    dometrium) 621.30
    cervix 616.0
  polypoid — see Endometritis, hyperplastic
  puerperal, postpartum, childbirth 670.1 ☑
    septic 670.2 ☑
  senile (atrophic) 615.9
  subacute 615.0
  tuberculous (see also Tuberculosis) 016.7 ☑
Endometrium — see condition
Endomyocardiopathy, South African 425.2
Endomyocarditis — see Endocarditis
Endomyofibrosis 425.0
Endomyometritis — see also Endometritis
  615.9
Endopericarditis — see Endocarditis
Endoperineuritis — see Disorder, nerve
Endophlebitis — see also Phlebitis 451.9
  leg 451.2
    deep (vessels) 451.19
    superficial (vessels) 451.0
  portal (vein) 572.1
  retina 362.18
  specified site NEC 451.89
  syphilitic 093.89
Endophthalmia — see also Endophthalmitis
  360.00
  gonorrheal 098.42
Endophthalmitis (globe) (infective)
  (metastatic) (purulent) (subacute) 360.00
  acute 360.01
  bleb associated 379.63
  chronic 360.03
  parasitic 360.13
  phacoanaphylactic 360.19
  specified type NEC 360.19
  sympathetic 360.11
Endosalpingioma (M9111/1) 236.2
Endosalpingiosis 629.89
Endosteitis — see Osteomyelitis
Endothelioma, bone (M9260/3) — see Neoplasm, bone, malignant
Endotheliosis 287.8
  hemorrhagic infectional 287.8
Endotoxemia — code to condition
Endotoxic shock 785.52
Endotrachelitis — see also Cervicitis 616.0
Enema rash 692.89
Engelmann's disease (diaphyseal sclerosis)
  756.9
**Engel-von Recklinghausen disease or syn-
  drome** (osteitis fibrosa cystica) 252.01
English disease — see also Rickets 268.0
Engman's disease (infectious eczematoid
  dermatitis) 690.8
Engorgement
  breast 611.79
    newborn 778.7
    puerperal, postpartum 676.2 ☑
  liver 573.9
  lung 514
  pulmonary 514
  retina, venous 362.37
  stomach 536.8
  venous, retina 362.37
Enlargement, enlarged — see also Hypertrophy
  abdomen 789.3 ☑

Enlargement, enlarged — see also
  Hypertrophy — continued
  adenoids 474.12
    and tonsils 474.10
  alveolar process or ridge 525.8
  apertures of diaphragm (congenital) 756.6
  blind spot, visual field 368.42
  gingival 523.8
  heart, cardiac (see also Hypertrophy, cardiac)
    429.3
  lacrimal gland, chronic 375.03
  liver (see also Hypertrophy, liver) 789.1
  lymph gland or node 785.6
  orbit 376.46
  organ or site, congenital NEC — see
    Anomaly, specified type NEC
  parathyroid (gland) 252.01
  pituitary fossa 793.0
  prostate (simple) (soft) 600.00
    with
      other lower urinary tract symptoms
        (LUTS) 600.01
      urinary
        obstruction 600.01
        retention 600.01
  sella turcica 793.0
  spleen (see also Splenomegaly) 789.2
    congenital 759.0
  thymus (congenital) (gland) 254.0
  thyroid (gland) (see also Goiter) 240.9
  tongue 529.8
  tonsils 474.11
    and adenoids 474.10
  uterus 621.2
Enophthalmos 376.50
  due to
    atrophy of orbital tissue 376.51
    surgery 376.52
    trauma 376.52
Enostosis 526.89
Entamebiasis — see Amebiasis
Entamebic — see Amebiasis
Entanglement, umbilical cord(s) 663.3 ☑
  with compression 663.2 ☑
  affecting fetus or newborn 762.5
  around neck with compression 663.1 ☑
  twins in monoamniotic sac 663.2 ☑
Enteralgia 789.0 ☑
Enteric — see condition
Enteritis (acute) (catarrhal) (choleraic) (chronic)
  (congestive) (diarrheal) (exudative) (follicular) (hemorrhagic) (infantile) (lienteric) (noninfectious) (perforative) (phlegmonous) (presumed noninfectious)
  (pseudomembranous) 558.9
  adaptive 564.9
  aertrycke infection 003.0
  allergic 558.3
  amebic (see also Amebiasis) 006.9
    with abscess — see Abscess, amebic
    acute 006.0
      with abscess — see Abscess, amebic
      nondysenteric 006.2
    chronic 006.1
      with abscess — see Abscess, amebic
      nondysenteric 006.2
    nondysenteric 006.2
  anaerobic (cocci) (gram-negative) (gram-
    positive) (mixed) NEC 008.46
  bacillary NEC 004.9
  bacterial NEC 008.5
    specified NEC 008.49
  Bacteroides (fragilis) (melaninogeniscus)
    (oralis) 008.46
  Butyrivibrio (fibriosolvens) 008.46
  Campylobacter 008.43
  Candida 112.85
  Chilomastix 007.8
  choleriformis 001.1
  chronic 558.9
    ulcerative (see also Colitis, ulcerative)
      556.9
  cicatrizing (chronic) 555.0
  Clostridium
    botulinum 005.1
    difficile 008.45

Enteritis — continued
  Clostridium — continued
    haemolyticum 008.46
    novyi 008.46
    perfringens (C) (F) 008.46
    specified type NEC 008.46
  coccidial 007.2
  dietetic 558.9
  due to
    achylia gastrica 536.8
    adenovirus 008.62
    Aerobacter aerogenes 008.2
    anaerobes (see also Enteritis, anaerobic)
      008.46
    Arizona (bacillus) 008.1
    astrovirus 008.66
    Bacillus coli — see Enteritis, E. coli
    bacteria NEC 008.5
      specified NEC 008.49
    Bacteroides (see also Enteritis, Bac-
      teroides) 008.46
    Butyrivibrio (fibriosolvens) 008.46
    calicivirus 008.65
    Camplyobacter 008.43
    Clostridium — see Enteritis, Clostridium
    Cockle agent 008.64
    Coxsackie (virus) 008.67
    Ditchling agent 008.64
    ECHO virus 008.67
    Enterobacter aerogenes 008.2
    enterococci 008.49
    enterovirus NEC 008.67
    Escherichia coli — see Enteritis, E. coli
    Eubacterium 008.46
    Fusobacterium (nucleatum) 008.46
    gram-negative bacteria NEC 008.47
      anaerobic NEC 008.46
    Hawaii agent 008.63
    irritating foods 558.9
    Klebsiella aerogenes 008.47
    Marin County agent 008.66
    Montgomery County agent 008.63
    norovirus 008.63
    Norwalk-like agent 008.63
    Norwalk virus 008.63
    Otofuke agent 008.63
    Paracolobactrum arizonae 008.1
    paracolon bacillus NEC 008.47
      Arizona 008.1
    Paramatta agent 008.64
    Peptococcus 008.46
    Peptostreptococcus 008.46
    Proprionibacterium 008.46
    Proteus (bacillus) (mirabilis) (morganii)
      008.3
    Pseudomonas aeruginosa 008.42
    Rotavirus 008.61
    Sapporo agent 008.63
    small round virus (SRV) NEC 008.64
      featureless NEC 008.63
      structured NEC 008.63
    Snow Mountain (SM) agent 008.63
    specified
      bacteria NEC 008.49
      organism, nonbacterial NEC 008.8
      virus NEC 008.69
    Staphylococcus 008.41
    Streptococcus 008.49
      anaerobic 008.46
    Taunton agent 008.63
    Torovirus 008.69
    Treponema 008.46
    Veillonella 008.46
    virus 008.8
      specified type NEC 008.69
    Wollan (W) agent 008.64
    Yersinia enterocolitica 008.44
  dysentery — see Dysentery
  E. coli 008.00
    enterohemorrhagic 008.04
    enteroinvasive 008.03
    enteropathogenic 008.01
    enterotoxigenic 008.02
    specified type NEC 008.09
  el tor 001.1
  embadomonial 007.8

☑ Additional Digit Required — Refer to the Tabular List for Digit Selection ▼ Subterms under main terms may continue to next column or page

106 — Volume 2 ▶◀ Revised Text ● New Line ▲ Revised Code 2011 ICD-9-CM

Enteritis — *continued*
eosinophilic 558.41
epidemic 009.0
Eubacterium 008.46
fermentative 558.9
fulminant 557.0
Fusobacterium (nucleatum) 008.46
gangrenous (*see also* Enteritis, due to, by organism) 009.0
giardial 007.1
gram-negative bacteria NEC 008.47
anaerobic NEC 008.46
infectious NEC (*see also* Enteritis, due to, by organism) 009.0
presumed 009.1
influenzal ▶(*see also* Influenza)◀ 487.8
ischemic 557.9
acute 557.0
chronic 557.1
due to mesenteric artery insufficiency 557.1
membranous 564.9
mucous 564.9
myxomembranous 564.9
necrotic (*see also* Enteritis, due to, by organism) 009.0
necroticans 005.2
necrotizing of fetus or newborn (*see also* Enterocolitis, necrotizing, newborn) 777.50
neurogenic 564.9
newborn 777.8
necrotizing (*see also* Enterocolitis, necrotizing, newborn) 777.50
parasitic NEC 129
paratyphoid (fever) (*see also* Fever, paratyphoid) 002.9
Peptococcus 008.46
Peptostreptococcus 008.46
Proprionibacterium 008.46
protozoal NEC 007.9
radiation 558.1
regional (of) 555.9
intestine
large (bowel, colon, or rectum) 555.1
with small intestine 555.2
small (duodenum, ileum, or jejunum) 555.0
with large intestine 555.2
Salmonella infection 003.0
salmonellosis 003.0
segmental (*see also* Enteritis, regional) 555.9
septic (*see also* Enteritis, due to, by organism) 009.0
Shigella 004.9
simple 558.9
spasmodic 564.9
spastic 564.9
staphylococcal 008.41
due to food 005.0
streptococcal 008.49
anaerobic 008.46
toxic 558.2
Treponema (denticola) (macrodentium) 008.46
trichomonal 007.3
tuberculous (*see also* Tuberculosis) 014.8 ☑
typhosa 002.0
ulcerative (chronic) (*see also* Colitis, ulcerative) 556.9
Veillonella 008.46
viral 008.8
adenovirus 008.62
enterovirus 008.67
specified virus NEC 008.69
Yersinia enterocolitica 008.44
zymotic 009.0
Enteroarticular syndrome 099.3
Enterobiasis 127.4
Enterobius vermicularis 127.4
Enterocele — *see also* Hernia 553.9
pelvis, pelvic (acquired) (congenital) 618.6
vagina, vaginal (acquired) (congenital) 618.6
Enterocolitis — *see also* Enteritis
fetus or newborn (*see also* Enterocolitis, necrotizing, newborn) 777.8

Enterocolitis — *see also* Enteritis — *continued*
fetus or newborn (*see also* Enterocolitis, necrotizing, newborn) — *continued*
necrotizing 777.50
fulminant 557.0
granulomatous 555.2
hemorrhagic (acute) 557.0
chronic 557.1
necrotizing (acute) (membranous) 557.0
newborn 777.50
with
perforation 777.53
pneumatosis and perforation 777.53
pneumatosis without perforation 777.52
without pneumatosis, without perforation 777.51
stage I 777.51
stage II 777.52
stage III 777.53
primary necrotizing (*see also* Enterocolitis, necrotizing, newborn) 777.50
pseudomembranous 008.45
newborn 008.45
radiation 558.1
newborn (*see also* Enterocolitis, necrotizing, newborn) 777.50
ulcerative 556.0
Enterocystoma 751.5
Enterogastritis — *see* Enteritis
Enterogenous cyanosis 289.7
Enterolith, enterolithiasis (impaction) 560.39
with hernia (*see also* Hernia, by site, with obstruction)
gangrenous — *see* Hernia, by site, with gangrene
Enteropathy 569.9
exudative (of Gordon) 579.8
gluten 579.0
hemorrhagic, terminal 557.0
protein-losing 579.8
Enteroperitonitis — *see also* Peritonitis 567.9
Enteroptosis 569.89
Enterorrhagia 578.9
Enterospasm 564.9
psychogenic 306.4
Enterostenosis — *see also* Obstruction, intestine 560.9
Enterostomy status V44.4
with complication 569.60
Enthesopathy 726.90
ankle and tarsus 726.70
elbow region 726.30
specified NEC 726.39
hip 726.5
knee 726.60
peripheral NEC 726.8
shoulder region 726.10
adhesive 726.0
spinal 720.1
wrist and carpus 726.4
Entrance, air into vein — *see* Embolism, air
Entrapment, nerve — *see* Neuropathy, entrapment
Entropion (eyelid) 374.00
cicatricial 374.04
congenital 743.62
late effect of trachoma (healed) 139.1
mechanical 374.02
paralytic 374.02
senile 374.01
spastic 374.03
Enucleation of eye (current) (traumatic) 871.3
Enuresis 788.30
habit disturbance 307.6
nocturnal 788.36
psychogenic 307.6
nonorganic origin 307.6
psychogenic 307.6
Enzymopathy 277.9
Eosinopenia 288.59
Eosinophilia 288.3
allergic 288.3

Eosinophilia — *continued*
hereditary 288.3
idiopathic 288.3
infiltrative 518.3
Loeffler's 518.3
myalgia syndrome 710.5
pulmonary (tropical) 518.3
secondary 288.3
tropical 518.3
Eosinophilic — *see also* condition
fasciitis 728.89
granuloma (bone) 277.89
infiltration lung 518.3
Ependymitis (acute) (cerebral) (chronic) (granular) — *see also* Meningitis 322.9
Ependymoblastoma (M9392/3)
specified site — *see* Neoplasm, by site, malignant
unspecified site 191.9
Ependymoma (epithelial) (malignant) (M9391/3)
anaplastic type (M9392/3)
specified site — *see* Neoplasm, by site, malignant
unspecified site 191.9
benign (M9391/0)
specified site — *see* Neoplasm, by site, benign
unspecified site 225.0
myxopapillary (M9394/1) 237.5
papillary (M9393/1) 237.5
specified site — *see* Neoplasm, by site, malignant
unspecified site 191.9
Ependymopathy 349.2
spinal cord 349.2
Ephelides, ephelis 709.09
Ephemeral fever — *see also* Pyrexia 780.60
Epiblepharon (congenital) 743.62
Epicanthus, epicanthic fold (congenital) (eyelid) 743.63
Epicondylitis (elbow) (lateral) 726.32
medial 726.31
Epicystitis — *see also* Cystitis 595.9
Epidemic — *see* condition
Epidermidalization, cervix — *see* condition
Epidermidization, cervix — *see* condition
Epidermis, epidermal — *see* condition
Epidermization, cervix — *see* condition
Epidermodysplasia verruciformis 078.19
Epidermoid
cholesteatoma — *see* Cholesteatoma
inclusion (*see also* Cyst, skin) 706.2
Epidermolysis
acuta (combustiformis) (toxica) 695.15
bullosa 757.39
necroticans combustiformis 695.15
due to drug
correct substance properly administered 695.15
overdose or wrong substance given or taken 977.9
specified drug — *see* Table of Drugs and Chemicals
Epidermophytid — *see* Dermatophytosis
Epidermophytosis (infected) — *see* Dermatophytosis
Epidermosis, ear (middle) — *see also* Cholesteatoma 385.30
Epididymis — *see* condition
Epididymitis (nonvenereal) 604.90
with abscess 604.0
acute 604.99
blennorrhagic (acute) 098.0
chronic or duration of 2 months or over 098.2
caseous (*see also* Tuberculosis) 016.4 ☑
chlamydial 099.54
diphtheritic 032.89 [604.91]
filarial 125.9 [604.91]
gonococcal (acute) 098.0
chronic or duration of 2 months or over 098.2
recurrent 604.99
residual 604.99
syphilitic 095.8 [604.91]

Epididymitis — *continued*
tuberculous (*see also* Tuberculosis) 016.4 ☑
Epididymo-orchitis — *see also* Epididymitis 604.90
with abscess 604.0
chlamydial 099.54
gonococcal (acute) 098.13
chronic or duration of 2 months or over 098.33
Epidural — *see* condition
Epigastritis — *see also* Gastritis 535.5 ☑
Epigastrium, epigastric — *see* condition
Epigastrocele — *see also* Hernia, epigastric 553.29
Epiglottiditis (acute) 464.30
with obstruction 464.31
chronic 476.1
viral 464.30
with obstruction 464.31
Epiglottis — *see* condition
Epiglottitis (acute) 464.30
with obstruction 464.31
chronic 476.1
viral 464.30
with obstruction 464.31
Epignathus 759.4
Epilepsia
partialis continua (*see also* Epilepsy) 345.7 ☑
procursiva (*see also* Epilepsy) 345.8 ☑
Epilepsy, epileptic (idiopathic) 345.9 ☑

Note — use the following fifth-digit subclassification with categories 345.0, 345.1, 345.4–345.9:

0   without mention of intractable epilepsy

1   with intractable epilepsy

  pharmacoresistant (pharmacologically resistant)

  poorly controlled

  refractory (medically)

  treatment resistant

abdominal 345.5 ☑
absence (attack) 345.0 ☑
akinetic 345.0 ☑
psychomotor 345.4 ☑
automatism 345.4 ☑
autonomic diencephalic 345.5 ☑
brain 345.9 ☑
Bravais-Jacksonian 345.5 ☑
cerebral 345.9 ☑
climacteric 345.9 ☑
clonic 345.1 ☑
clouded state 345.9 ☑
coma 345.3
communicating 345.4 ☑
complicating pregnancy, childbirth, or the puerperium 649.4 ☑
congenital 345.9 ☑
convulsions 345.9 ☑
cortical (focal) (motor) 345.5 ☑
cursive (running) 345.8 ☑
cysticercosis 123.1
deterioration
with behavioral disturbance 345.9 ☑ [294.11]
without behavioral disturbance 345.9 ☑ [294.10]
due to syphilis 094.89
equivalent 345.5 ☑
fit 345.9 ☑
focal (motor) 345.5 ☑
gelastic 345.8 ☑
generalized 345.9 ☑
convulsive 345.1 ☑
flexion 345.1 ☑
nonconvulsive 345.0 ☑
grand mal (idiopathic) 345.1 ☑
Jacksonian (motor) (sensory) 345.5 ☑
Kojevnikoff's, Kojevnikov's, Kojewnikoff's 345.7 ☑

☑ **Additional Digit Required** — Refer to the Tabular List for Digit Selection   ▽ **Subterms under main terms may continue to next column or page**

2011 ICD-9-CM   ▶◀ Revised Text   ● New Line   ▲ Revised Code   October 2010 · Volume 2 — 107

Epilepsy, epileptic — *continued*
laryngeal 786.2
limbic system 345.4 ☑
localization related (focal) (partial) and
    epileptic syndromes
    with
        complex partial seizures 345.4 ☑
        simple partial seizures 345.5 ☑
major (motor) 345.1 ☑
minor 345.0 ☑
mixed (type) 345.9 ☑
motor partial 345.5 ☑
musicogenic 345.1 ☑
myoclonus, myoclonic 345.1 ☑
    progressive (familial) 345.1 ☑
nonconvulsive, generalized 345.0 ☑
parasitic NEC 123.9
partial (focalized) 345.5 ☑
    with
        impairment of consciousness
            345.4 ☑
        memory and ideational disturbances
            345.4 ☑
    without impairment of consciousness
        345.5 ☑
    abdominal type 345.5 ☑
    motor type 345.5 ☑
    psychomotor type 345.4 ☑
    psychosensory type 345.4 ☑
    secondarily generalized 345.4 ☑
    sensory type 345.5 ☑
    somatomotor type 345.5 ☑
    somatosensory type 345.5 ☑
    temporal lobe type 345.4 ☑
    visceral type 345.5 ☑
    visual type 345.5 ☑
peripheral 345.9 ☑
petit mal 345.0 ☑
photokinetic 345.8 ☑
progressive myoclonic (familial) 345.1 ☑
psychic equivalent 345.5 ☑
psychomotor 345.4 ☑
psychosensory 345.4 ☑
reflex 345.1 ☑
seizure 345.9 ☑
senile 345.9 ☑
sensory-induced 345.5 ☑
sleep (*see also* Narcolepsy) 347.00
somatomotor type 345.5 ☑
somatosensory 345.5 ☑
specified type NEC 345.8 ☑
status (grand mal) 345.3
    focal motor 345.7 ☑
    petit mal 345.2
    psychomotor 345.7 ☑
    temporal lobe 345.7 ☑
symptomatic 345.9 ☑
temporal lobe 345.4 ☑
tonic (-clonic) 345.1 ☑
traumatic (injury unspecified) 907.0
    injury specified — *see* Late, effect (of)
        specified injury
twilight 293.0
uncinate (gyrus) 345.4 ☑
Unverricht (-Lundborg) (familial myoclonic)
    345.1 ☑
visceral 345.5 ☑
visual 345.5 ☑
Epileptiform
convulsions 780.39
seizure 780.39
Epiloia 759.5
Epimenorrhea 626.2
Epipharyngitis — *see also* Nasopharyngitis
    460
Epiphora 375.20
due to
    excess lacrimation 375.21
    insufficient drainage 375.22
Epiphyseal arrest 733.91
femoral head 732.2
Epiphyseolysis, epiphysiolysis — *see also*
    Osteochondrosis 732.9
Epiphysitis — *see also* Osteochondrosis 732.9

Epiphysitis — *see also* Osteochondrosis —
    continued
juvenile 732.6
marginal (Scheuermann's) 732.0
os calcis 732.5
syphilitic (congenital) 090.0
vertebral (Scheuermann's) 732.0
Epiplocele — *see also* Hernia 553.9
Epiploitis — *see also* Peritonitis 567.9
Epiplosarcomphalocele — *see also* Hernia,
    umbilicus 553.1
Episcleritis 379.00
gouty 274.89 [379.09]
nodular 379.02
periodica fugax 379.01
    angioneurotic — *see* Edema, angioneu-
        rotic
specified NEC 379.09
staphylococcal 379.00
suppurative 379.00
syphilitic 095.0
tuberculous (*see also* Tuberculosis)
    017.3 ☑ [379.09]
Episode
brain (*see also* Disease, cerebrovascular,
    acute) 436
cerebral (*see also* Disease, cerebrovascular,
    acute) 436
depersonalization (in neurotic state) 300.6
hyporesponsive 780.09
psychotic (*see also* Psychosis) 298.9
    organic, transient 293.9
schizophrenic (acute) NEC (*see also*
    Schizophrenia) 295.4 ☑
Epispadias
female 753.8
male 752.62
Episplenitis 289.59
Epistaxis (multiple) 784.7
hereditary 448.0
vicarious menstruation 625.8
Epithelioma (malignant) (M8011/3) — *see also*
    Neoplasm, by site, malignant
adenoides cysticum (M8100/0) — *see* Neo-
    plasm, skin, benign
basal cell (M8090/3) — *see* Neoplasm, skin,
    malignant
benign (M8011/0) — *see* Neoplasm, by site,
    benign
Bowen's (M8081/2) — *see* Neoplasm, skin,
    in situ
calcifying (benign) (Malherbe's) (M8110/0)
    — *see* Neoplasm, skin, benign
external site — *see* Neoplasm, skin, malig-
    nant
intraepidermal, Jadassohn (M8096/0) — *see*
    Neoplasm, skin, benign
squamous cell (M8070/3) — *see* Neoplasm,
    by site, malignant
Epitheliopathy
pigment, retina 363.15
posterior multifocal placoid (acute) 363.15
Epithelium, epithelial — *see* condition
Epituberculosis (allergic) (with atelectasis) —
    see also Tuberculosis 010.8 ☑
Eponychia 757.5
Epstein's
nephrosis or syndrome (*see also* Nephrosis)
    581.9
pearl (mouth) 528.4
Epstein-Barr infection (viral) 075
chronic 780.79 [139.8]
Epulis (giant cell) (gingiva) 523.8
Equinia 024
Equinovarus (congenital) 754.51
acquired 736.71
Equivalent
angina 413.9
convulsive (abdominal) (*see also* Epilepsy)
    345.5 ☑
epileptic (psychic) (*see also* Epilepsy)
    345.5 ☑
Erb's
disease 359.1
palsy, paralysis (birth) (brachial) (newborn)
    767.6

Erb's — *continued*
palsy, paralysis — *continued*
    spinal (spastic) syphilitic 094.89
pseudohypertrophic muscular dystrophy
    359.1
Erb-Goldflam disease or syndrome 358.00
Erb (-Duchenne) paralysis (birth injury)
    (newborn) 767.6
Erdheim-Chester disease (ECD) 277.89
Erdheim's syndrome (acromegalic
    macrospondylitis) 253.0
Erection, painful (persistent) 607.3
Ergosterol deficiency (vitamin D) 268.9
with
    osteomalacia 268.2
    rickets (*see also* Rickets) 268.0
Ergotism (ergotized grain) 988.2
from ergot used as drug (migraine therapy)
    correct substance properly administered
        349.82
    overdose or wrong substance given or
        taken 975.0
Erichsen's disease (railway spine) 300.16
Erlacher-Blount syndrome (tibia vara) 732.4
Erosio interdigitalis blastomycetica 112.3
Erosion
arteriosclerotic plaque — *see* Arteriosclero-
    sis, by site
artery NEC 447.2
    without rupture 447.8
bone 733.99
bronchus 519.19
cartilage (joint) 733.99
cervix (uteri) (acquired) (chronic) (congeni-
    tal) 622.0
    with mention of cervicitis 616.0
cornea (recurrent) (*see also* Keratitis) 371.42
    traumatic 918.1
dental (idiopathic) (occupational) 521.30
    extending into
        dentine 521.32
        pulp 521.33
    generalized 521.35
    limited to enamel 521.31
    localized 521.34
duodenum, postpyloric — *see* Ulcer, duode-
    num
esophagus 530.89
gastric 535.4 ☑
intestine 569.89
lymphatic vessel 457.8
pylorus, pyloric (ulcer) 535.4 ☑
sclera 379.16
spine, aneurysmal 094.89
spleen 289.59
stomach 535.4 ☑
teeth (idiopathic) (occupational) (*see also*
    Erosion, dental) 521.30
    due to
        medicine 521.30
        persistent vomiting 521.30
urethra 599.84
uterus 621.8
vertebra 733.99
Erotomania 302.89
Clérambault's 297.8
Error
in diet 269.9
refractive 367.9
    astigmatism (*see also* Astigmatism)
        367.20
    drug-induced 367.89
    hypermetropia 367.0
    hyperopia 367.0
    myopia 367.1
    presbyopia 367.4
    toxic 367.89
Eructation 787.3
nervous 306.4
psychogenic 306.4
Eruption
creeping 126.9
drug — *see* Dermatitis, due to, drug
Hutchinson, summer 692.72
Kaposi's varicelliform 054.0
napkin (psoriasiform) 691.0

Eruption — *continued*
polymorphous
    light (sun) 692.72
        other source 692.82
psoriasiform, napkin 691.0
recalcitrant pustular 694.8
ringed 695.89
skin (*see also* Dermatitis) 782.1
    creeping (meaning hookworm) 126.9
    due to
        chemical(s) NEC 692.4
            internal use 693.8
        drug — *see* Dermatitis, due to, drug
        prophylactic inoculation or vaccina-
            tion against disease — *see*
            Dermatitis, due to, vaccine
        smallpox vaccination NEC — *see*
            Dermatitis, due to, vaccine
    erysipeloid 027.1
    feigned 698.4
    Hutchinson, summer 692.72
    Kaposi's, varicelliform 054.0
        vaccinia 999.0
    lichenoid, axilla 698.3
    polymorphous, due to light 692.72
    toxic NEC 695.0
    vesicular 709.8
teeth, tooth
    accelerated 520.6
    delayed 520.6
    difficult 520.6
    disturbance of 520.6
    in abnormal sequence 520.6
    incomplete 520.6
    late 520.6
    natal 520.6
    neonatal 520.6
    obstructed 520.6
    partial 520.6
    persistent primary 520.6
    premature 520.6
    prenatal 520.6
vesicular 709.8
Erysipelas (gangrenous) (infantile) (newborn)
    (phlegmonous) (suppurative) 035
external ear 035 [380.13]
puerperal, postpartum, childbirth 670.8 ☑
Erysipelatoid (Rosenbach's) 027.1
Erysipeloid (Rosenbach's) 027.1
Erythema, erythematous (generalized) 695.9
ab igne — *see* Burn, by site, first degree
annulare (centrifugum) (rheumaticum)
    695.0
arthriticum epidemicum 026.1
brucellum (*see also* Brucellosis) 023.9
bullosum 695.19
caloricum — *see* Burn, by site, first degree
chronicum migrans 088.81
circinatum 695.19
diaper 691.0
due to
    chemical (contact) NEC 692.4
        internal 693.8
    drug (internal use) 693.0
        contact 692.3
elevatum diutinum 695.89
endemic 265.2
epidemic, arthritic 026.1
figuratum perstans 695.0
gluteal 691.0
gyratum (perstans) (repens) 695.19
heat — *see* Burn, by site, first degree
ichthyosiforme congenitum 757.1
induratum (primary) (scrofulosorum) (*see*
    also Tuberculosis) 017.1 ☑
    nontuberculous 695.2
infantum febrile 057.8
infectional NEC 695.9
infectiosum 057.0
inflammation NEC 695.9
intertrigo 695.89
iris 695.10
lupus (discoid) (localized) (*see also* Lupus,
    erythematosus) 695.4
marginatum 695.0
    rheumaticum — *see* Fever, rheumatic

Erythema, erythematous — *continued*
  medicamentosum — *see* Dermatitis, due to, drug
  migrans 529.1
    chronicum 088.81
  multiforme 695.10
    bullosum 695.19
    conjunctiva 695.19
    exudativum (Hebra) 695.19
    major 695.12
    minor 695.11
    pemphigoides 694.5
  napkin 691.0
  neonatorum 778.8
  nodosum 695.2
    tuberculous (*see also* Tuberculosis) 017.1 ☑
  nummular, nummulare 695.19
  palmar 695.0
  palmaris hereditarium 695.0
  pernio 991.5
  perstans solare 692.72
  rash, newborn 778.8
  scarlatiniform (exfoliative) (recurrent) 695.0
  simplex marginatum 057.8
  solare (*see also* Sunburn) 692.71
  streptogenes 696.5
  toxic, toxicum NEC 695.0
    newborn 778.8
  tuberculous (primary) (*see also* Tuberculosis) 017.0 ☑
  venenatum 695.0
Erythematosus — *see* condition
Erythematous — *see* condition
Erythermalgia (primary) 443.82
Erythralgia 443.82
Erythrasma 039.0
Erythredema 985.0
  polyneuritica 985.0
  polyneuropathy 985.0
Erythremia (acute) (M9841/3) 207.0 ☑
  chronic (M9842/3) 207.1 ☑
  secondary 289.0
Erythroblastopenia (acquired) 284.89
  congenital 284.01
Erythroblastophthisis 284.01
Erythroblastosis (fetalis) (newborn) 773.2
  due to
    ABO
      antibodies 773.1
      incompatibility, maternal/fetal 773.1
      isoimmunization 773.1
    Rh
      antibodies 773.0
      incompatibility, maternal/fetal 773.0
      isoimmunization 773.0
Erythrocyanosis (crurum) 443.89
Erythrocythemia — *see* Erythremia
Erythrocytopenia 285.9
Erythrocytosis (megalosplenic)
  familial 289.6
  oval, hereditary (*see also* Elliptocytosis) 282.1
  secondary 289.0
  stress 289.0
Erythroderma — *see also* Erythema 695.9
  desquamativa (in infants) 695.89
  exfoliative 695.89
  ichthyosiform, congenital 757.1
  infantum 695.89
  maculopapular 696.2
  neonatorum 778.8
  psoriaticum 696.1
  secondary 695.9
Erythrodysesthesia, palmar plantar (PPE) 693.0
Erythrogenesis imperfecta 284.09
Erythroleukemia (M9840/3) 207.0 ☑
Erythromelalgia 443.82
Erythromelia 701.8
Erythropenia 285.9
Erythrophagocytosis 289.9
Erythrophobia 300.23
Erythroplakia
  oral mucosa 528.79
  tongue 528.79

Erythroplasia (Queyrat) (M8080/2)
  specified site — *see* Neoplasm, skin, in situ
  unspecified site 233.5
Erythropoiesis, idiopathic ineffective 285.0
Escaped beats, heart 427.60
  postoperative 997.1
Esoenteritis — *see* Enteritis
Esophagalgia 530.89
Esophagectasis 530.89
  due to cardiospasm 530.0
Esophagismus 530.5
Esophagitis (alkaline) (chemical) (chronic) (infectional) (necrotic) (peptic) (postoperative) (regurgitant) 530.10
  acute 530.12
  candidal 112.84
  eosinophilic 530.13
  reflux 530.11
  specified NEC 530.19
  tuberculous (*see also* Tuberculosis) 017.8 ☑
  ulcerative 530.19
Esophagocele 530.6
Esophagodynia 530.89
Esophagomalacia 530.89
Esophagoptosis 530.89
Esophagospasm 530.5
Esophagostenosis 530.3
Esophagostomiasis 127.7
Esophagostomy
  complication 530.87
    infection 530.86
    malfunctioning 530.87
    mechanical 530.87
Esophagotracheal — *see* condition
Esophagus — *see* condition
Esophoria 378.41
  convergence, excess 378.84
  divergence, insufficiency 378.85
Esotropia (nonaccommodative) 378.00
  accommodative 378.35
  alternating 378.05
    with
      A pattern 378.06
      specified noncomitancy NEC 378.08
      V pattern 378.07
      X pattern 378.08
      Y pattern 378.08
    intermittent 378.22
  intermittent 378.20
    alternating 378.22
    monocular 378.21
  monocular 378.01
    with
      A pattern 378.02
      specified noncomitancy NEC 378.04
      V pattern 378.03
      X pattern 378.04
      Y pattern 378.04
    intermittent 378.21
Espundia 085.5
Essential — *see* condition
Esterapenia 289.89
Esthesioneuroblastoma (M9522/3) 160.0
Esthesioneurocytoma (M9521/3) 160.0
Esthesioneuroepithelioma (M9523/3) 160.0
Esthiomene 099.1
Estivo-autumnal
  fever 084.0
  malaria 084.0
Estrangement V61.09
Estriasis 134.0
Ethanolaminuria 270.8
Ethanolism — *see also* Alcoholism 303.9 ☑
Ether dependence, dependency — *see also* Dependence 304.6 ☑
Etherism — *see also* Dependence 304.6 ☑
Ethmoid, ethmoidal — *see* condition
Ethmoiditis (chronic) (nonpurulent) (purulent) — *see also* Sinusitis, ethmoidal 473.2
  influenzal ▶(*see also* Influenza)◀ 487.1
  Woakes' 471.1
Ethylism — *see also* Alcoholism 303.9 ☑
Eulenburg's disease (congenital paramyotonia) 359.29
Eunuchism 257.2
Eunuchoidism 257.2

Eunuchoidism — *continued*
  hypogonadotropic 257.2
European blastomycosis 117.5
Eustachian — *see* condition
Euthyroidism 244.9
Euthyroid sick syndrome 790.94
Evaluation
  fetal lung maturity 659.8 ☑
  for suspected condition (*see also* Observation) V71.9
    abuse V71.81
    exposure
      anthrax V71.82
      biologic agent NEC V71.83
      SARS V71.83
    neglect V71.81
    newborn — *see* Observation, suspected, condition, newborn
    specified condition NEC V71.89
  mental health V70.2
    requested by authority V70.1
  nursing care V63.8
  social service V63.8
Evans' syndrome (thrombocytopenic purpura) 287.32
Event, apparent life threatening in newborn and infant (ALTE) 799.82
Eventration
  colon into chest — *see* Hernia, diaphragm
  diaphragm (congenital) 756.6
Eversion
  bladder 596.8
  cervix (uteri) 622.0
    with mention of cervicitis 616.0
  foot NEC 736.79
    congenital 755.67
  lacrimal punctum 375.51
  punctum lacrimale (postinfectional) (senile) 375.51
  ureter (meatus) 593.89
  urethra (meatus) 599.84
  uterus 618.1
    complicating delivery 665.2 ☑
      affecting fetus or newborn 763.89
    puerperal, postpartum 674.8 ☑
Evidence
  of malignancy
    cytologic
      without histologic confirmation
        anus 796.76
        cervix 795.06
        vagina 795.16
Evisceration
  birth injury 767.8
  bowel (congenital) — *see* Hernia, ventral
  congenital (*see also* Hernia, ventral) 553.29
  operative wound 998.32
  traumatic NEC 869.1
    eye 871.3
Evulsion — *see* Avulsion
Ewing's
  angioendothelioma (M9260/3) — *see* Neoplasm, bone, malignant
  sarcoma (M9260/3) — *see* Neoplasm, bone, malignant
  tumor (M9260/3) — *see* Neoplasm, bone, malignant
Exaggerated lumbosacral angle (with impinging spine) 756.12
Examination (general) (routine) (of) (for) V70.9
  allergy V72.7
  annual V70.0
  cardiovascular preoperative V72.81
  cervical Papanicolaou smear V76.2
    as a part of routine gynecological examination V72.31
    to confirm findings of recent normal smear following initial abnormal smear V72.32
  child care (routine) V20.2
  clinical research investigation (normal control patient) (participant) V70.7
  dental V72.2
  developmental testing (child) (infant) V20.2
  donor (potential) V70.8
  ear V72.19

Examination — *continued*
  eye V72.0
  following
    accident (motor vehicle) V71.4
    alleged rape or seduction (victim or culprit) V71.5
    inflicted injury (victim or culprit) NEC V71.6
    rape or seduction, alleged (victim or culprit) V71.5
    treatment (for) V67.9
      combined V67.6
      fracture V67.4
      involving high-risk medication NEC V67.51
      mental disorder V67.3
      specified condition NEC V67.59
  follow-up (routine) (following) V67.9
    cancer chemotherapy V67.2
    chemotherapy V67.2
    disease NEC V67.59
    high-risk medication NEC V67.51
    injury NEC V67.59
    population survey V70.6
    postpartum V24.2
    psychiatric V67.3
    psychotherapy V67.3
    radiotherapy V67.1
    specified surgery NEC V67.09
    surgery V67.00
    vaginal pap smear V67.01
  gynecological V72.31
    for contraceptive maintenance V25.40
      intrauterine device V25.42
      pill V25.41
      specified method NEC V25.49
  health (of)
    armed forces personnel V70.5
    checkup V70.0
    child, routine V20.2
    defined subpopulation NEC V70.5
    inhabitants of institutions V70.5
    occupational V70.5
    pre-employment screening V70.5
    preschool children V70.5
      for admission to school V70.3
    prisoners V70.5
      for entrance into prison V70.3
    prostitutes V70.5
    refugees V70.5
    school children V70.5
    students V70.5
  hearing V72.19
    following failed hearing screening V72.11
  infant
    8 to 28 days old V20.32
    over 28 days old, routine V20.2
    under 8 days old V20.31
  laboratory V72.60
    ordered as part of a routine general medical examination V72.62
    pre-operative V72.63
    pre-procedural V72.63
    specified NEC V72.69
  lactating mother V24.1
  medical (for) (of) V70.9
    administrative purpose NEC V70.3
    admission to
      old age home V70.3
      prison V70.3
      school V70.3
    adoption V70.3
    armed forces personnel V70.5
    at health care facility V70.0
    camp V70.3
    child, routine V20.2
    clinical research (control) (normal comparison) (participant) V70.7
    defined subpopulation NEC V70.5
    donor (potential) V70.8
    driving license V70.3
    general V70.9
      routine V70.0
      specified reason NEC V70.8
    immigration V70.3

☑ **Additional Digit Required** — Refer to the Tabular List for Digit Selection   ⁿᵉᵂ **Subterms under main terms may continue to next column or page**

Examination — *continued*
 medical — *continued*
  inhabitants of institutions V70.5
  insurance certification V70.3
  marriage V70.3
  medicolegal reasons V70.4
  naturalization V70.3
  occupational V70.5
  population survey V70.6
  pre-employment V70.5
  preschool children V70.5
   for admission to school V70.3
  prison V70.3
  prisoners V70.5
   for entrance into prison V70.3
  prostitutes V70.5
  refugees V70.5
  school children V70.5
  specified reason NEC V70.8
  sport competition V70.3
  students V70.5
 medicolegal reason V70.4
 pelvic (annual) (periodic) V72.31
 periodic (annual) (routine) V70.0
 postpartum
  immediately after delivery V24.0
  routine follow-up V24.2
 pregnancy (unconfirmed) (possible) V72.40
  negative result V72.41
  positive result V72.42
 prenatal V22.1
  first pregnancy V22.0
  high-risk pregnancy V23.9
   specified problem NEC V23.89
 preoperative V72.84
  cardiovascular V72.81
  respiratory V72.82
  specified NEC V72.83
 preprocedural V72.84
  cardiovascular V72.81
  general physical V72.83
  respiratory V72.82
  specified NEC V72.83
 prior to chemotherapy V72.83
 psychiatric V70.2
  follow-up not needing further care V67.3
  requested by authority V70.1
 radiological NEC V72.5
 respiratory preoperative V72.82
 screening — *see* Screening
 sensitization V72.7
 skin V72.7
  hypersensitivity V72.7
 special V72.9
 specified type or reason NEC V72.85
  preoperative V72.83
   specified NEC V72.83
 teeth V72.2
 vaginal Papanicolaou smear V76.47
  following hysterectomy for malignant condition V67.01
 victim or culprit following
  alleged rape or seduction V71.5
  inflicted injury NEC V71.6
 vision V72.0
 well baby V20.2
Exanthem, exanthema — *see also* Rash 782.1
 Boston 048
 epidemic, with meningitis 048
 lichenoid psoriasiform 696.2
 subitum 058.10
  due to
   human herpesvirus 6 058.11
   human herpesvirus 7 058.12
 viral, virus NEC 057.9
  specified type NEC 057.8
Excess, excessive, excessively
 alcohol level in blood 790.3
 carbohydrate tissue, localized 278.1
 carotene (dietary) 278.3
 cold 991.9
  specified effect NEC 991.8
 convergence 378.84
 crying 780.95
  of
   adolescent 780.95

Excess, excessive, excessively — *continued*
 crying — *continued*
  of — *continued*
   adult 780.95
   baby 780.92
   child 780.95
   infant (baby) 780.92
   newborn 780.92
 development, breast 611.1
 diaphoresis (*see also* Hyperhidrosis) 780.8
 distance, interarch 524.28
 divergence 378.85
 drinking (alcohol) NEC (*see also* Abuse, drugs, nondependent) 305.0 ☑
  continual (*see also* Alcoholism) 303.9 ☑
  habitual (*see also* Alcoholism) 303.9 ☑
 eating 783.6
 eyelid fold (congenital) 743.62
 fat 278.02
  in heart (*see also* Degeneration, myocardial) 429.1
  tissue, localized 278.1
 foreskin 605
 gas 787.3
 gastrin 251.5
 glucagon 251.4
 heat (*see also* Heat) 992.9
 horizontal
  overjet 524.26
  overlap 524.26
 interarch distance 524.28
 intermaxillary vertical dimension 524.37
 interocclusal distance of teeth 524.37
 large
  colon 564.7
   congenital 751.3
  fetus or infant 766.0
   with obstructed labor 660.1 ☑
    affecting management of pregnancy 656.6 ☑
   causing disproportion 653.5 ☑
  newborn (weight of 4500 grams or more) 766.0
  organ or site, congenital NEC — *see* Anomaly, specified type NEC
 lid fold (congenital) 743.62
 long
  colon 751.5
  organ or site, congenital NEC — *see* Anomaly, specified type NEC
  umbilical cord (entangled)
   affecting fetus or newborn 762.5
   in pregnancy or childbirth 663.3 ☑
    with compression 663.2 ☑
 menstruation 626.2
 number of teeth 520.1
  causing crowding 524.31
 nutrients (dietary) NEC 783.6
 potassium (K) 276.7
 salivation (*see also* Ptyalism) 527.7
 secretion (*see also* Hypersecretion)
  milk 676.6 ☑
  sputum 786.4
  sweat (*see also* Hyperhidrosis) 780.8
 short
  organ or site, congenital NEC — *see* Anomaly, specified type NEC
  umbilical cord
   affecting fetus or newborn 762.6
   in pregnancy or childbirth 663.4 ☑
 skin NEC 701.9
  eyelid 743.62
   acquired 374.30
 sodium (Na) 276.0
 spacing of teeth 524.32
 sputum 786.4
 sweating (*see also* Hyperhidrosis) 780.8
 tearing (ducts) (eye) (*see also* Epiphora) 375.20
 thirst 783.5
  due to deprivation of water 994.3
 tissue in reconstructed breast 612.0
 tuberosity 524.07
 vitamin
  A (dietary) 278.2

Excess, excessive, excessively — *continued*
 vitamin — *continued*
  A — *continued*
   administered as drug (chronic) (prolonged excessive intake) 278.2
    reaction to sudden overdose 963.5
  D (dietary) 278.4
   administered as drug (chronic) (prolonged excessive intake) 278.4
    reaction to sudden overdose 963.5
 weight 278.02
  gain 783.1
   of pregnancy 646.1 ☑
  loss 783.21
Excitability, abnormal, under minor stress 309.29
Excitation
 catatonic (*see also* Schizophrenia) 295.2 ☑
 psychogenic 298.0
 reactive (from emotional stress, psychological trauma) 298.1
Excitement
 manic (*see also* Psychosis, affective) 296.0 ☑
  recurrent episode 296.1 ☑
  single episode 296.0 ☑
 mental, reactive (from emotional stress, psychological trauma) 298.1
 state, reactive (from emotional stress, psychological trauma) 298.1
Excluded pupils 364.76
Excoriation (traumatic) — *see also* Injury, superficial, by site 919.8
 neurotic 698.4
Excyclophoria 378.44
Excyclotropia 378.33
Exencephalus, exencephaly 742.0
Exercise
 breathing V57.0
 remedial NEC V57.1
 therapeutic NEC V57.1
Exfoliation
 skin
  due to erythematous condition 695.50
   involving (percent of body surface)
    less than 10 percent 695.50
    10-19 percent 695.51
    20-29 percent 695.52
    30-39 percent 695.53
    40-49 percent 695.54
    50-59 percent 695.55
    60-69 percent 695.56
    70-79 percent 695.57
    80-89 percent 695.58
    90 percent or more 695.59
 teeth
  due to systemic causes 525.0
Exfoliative — *see also* condition
 dermatitis 695.89
Exhaustion, exhaustive (physical NEC) 780.79
 battle (*see also* Reaction, stress, acute) 308.9
 cardiac (*see also* Failure, heart) 428.9
 delirium (*see also* Reaction, stress, acute) 308.9
 due to
  cold 991.8
  excessive exertion 994.5
  exposure 994.4
  overexertion 994.5
 fetus or newborn 779.89
 heart (*see also* Failure, heart) 428.9
 heat 992.5
  due to
   salt depletion 992.4
   water depletion 992.3
 manic (*see also* Psychosis, affective) 296.0 ☑
  recurrent episode 296.1 ☑
  single episode 296.0 ☑
 maternal, complicating delivery 669.8 ☑
  affecting fetus or newborn 763.89
 mental 300.5
 myocardium, myocardial (*see also* Failure, heart) 428.9
 nervous 300.5

Exhaustion, exhaustive — *continued*
 old age 797
 postinfectional NEC 780.79
 psychogenic 300.5
 psychosis (*see also* Reaction, stress, acute) 308.9
 senile 797
  dementia 290.0
Exhibitionism (sexual) 302.4
Exomphalos 756.72
Exophoria 378.42
 convergence, insufficiency 378.83
 divergence, excess 378.85
Exophthalmic
 cachexia 242.0 ☑
 goiter 242.0 ☑
 ophthalmoplegia 242.0 ☑ *[376.22]*
Exophthalmos 376.30
 congenital 743.66
 constant 376.31
 endocrine NEC 259.9 *[376.22]*
 hyperthyroidism 242.0 ☑ *[376.21]*
 intermittent NEC 376.34
 malignant 242.0 ☑ *[376.21]*
 pulsating 376.35
  endocrine NEC 259.9 *[376.22]*
 thyrotoxic 242.0 ☑ *[376.21]*
Exostosis 726.91
 cartilaginous (M9210/0) — *see* Neoplasm, bone, benign
 congenital 756.4
 ear canal, external 380.81
 gonococcal 098.89
 hip 726.5
 intracranial 733.3
 jaw (bone) 526.81
 luxurians 728.11
 multiple (cancellous) (congenital) (hereditary) 756.4
 nasal bones 726.91
 orbit, orbital 376.42
 osteocartilaginous (M9210/0) — *see* Neoplasm, bone, benign
 spine 721.8
  with spondylosis — *see* Spondylosis
 syphilitic 095.5
 wrist 726.4
Exotropia 378.10
 alternating 378.15
  with
   A pattern 378.16
    specified noncomitancy NEC 378.18
   V pattern 378.17
   X pattern 378.18
   Y pattern 378.18
  intermittent 378.24
 intermittent 378.20
  alternating 378.24
  monocular 378.23
 monocular 378.11
  with
   A pattern 378.12
    specified noncomitancy NEC 378.14
   V pattern 378.13
   X pattern 378.14
   Y pattern 378.14
  intermittent 378.23
Explanation of
 investigation finding V65.4 ☑
 medication V65.4 ☑
Exposure (suspected) 994.9
 algae bloom V87.32
 cold 991.9
  specified effect NEC 991.8
 effects of 994.9
 exhaustion due to 994.4
 to
  AIDS virus V01.79
  anthrax V01.81
  aromatic
   amines V87.11
   dyes V87.19
  arsenic V87.01
  asbestos V15.84
  benzene V87.12
  body fluids (hazardous) V15.85

Exposure — *continued*
to — *continued*
cholera V01.0
chromium compounds V87.09
communicable disease V01.9
specified type NEC V01.89
dyes V87.2
aromatic V87.19
Escherichia coli (E. coli) V01.83
German measles V01.4
gonorrhea V01.6
hazardous
aromatic compounds NEC V87.19
body fluids V15.85
chemicals NEC V87.2
metals V87.09
substances V87.39
HIV V01.79
human immunodeficiency virus V01.79
lead V15.86
meningococcus V01.84
mold V87.31
nickel dust V87.09
parasitic disease V01.89
poliomyelitis V01.2
polycyclic aromatic hydrocarbons V87.19
potentially hazardous body fluids V15.85
rabies V01.5
rubella V01.4
SARS-associated coronavirus V01.82
smallpox V01.3
syphilis V01.6
tuberculosis V01.1
varicella V01.71
venereal disease V01.6
viral disease NEC V01.79
varicella V01.71
Exsanguination, fetal 772.0
Exstrophy
abdominal content 751.8
bladder (urinary) 753.5
Extensive — *see* condition
Extra — *see also* Accessory
rib 756.3
cervical 756.2
Extraction
with hook 763.89
breech NEC 669.6 ☑
affecting fetus or newborn 763.0
cataract postsurgical V45.61
manual NEC 669.8 ☑
affecting fetus or newborn 763.89
Extrasystole 427.60
atrial 427.61
postoperative 997.1
ventricular 427.69
Extrauterine gestation or pregnancy — *see* Pregnancy, ectopic
Extravasation
blood 459.0
lower extremity 459.0
chemotherapy, vesicant 999.81
chyle into mesentery 457.8
pelvicalyceal 593.4
pyelosinus 593.4
urine 788.8
from ureter 788.8
vesicant
agent NEC 999.82
chemotherapy 999.81
Extremity — *see* condition
Extrophy — *see* Exstrophy
Extroversion
bladder 753.5
uterus 618.1
complicating delivery 665.2 ☑
affecting fetus or newborn 763.89
postpartal (old) 618.1
Extruded tooth 524.34
Extrusion
alveolus and teeth 524.75
breast implant (prosthetic) 996.54
device, implant, or graft — *see* Complications, mechanical
eye implant (ball) (globe) 996.59

Extrusion — *continued*
intervertebral disc — *see* Displacement, intervertebral disc
lacrimal gland 375.43
mesh (reinforcing) 996.59
ocular lens implant 996.53
prosthetic device NEC — *see* Complications, mechanical
vitreous 379.26
Exudate, pleura — *see* Effusion, pleura
Exudates, retina 362.82
Exudative — *see* condition
Eye, eyeball, eyelid — *see* condition
Eyestrain 368.13
Eyeworm disease of Africa 125.2

F

Faber's anemia or syndrome (achlorhydric anemia) 280.9
Fabry's disease (angiokeratoma corporis diffusum) 272.7
Face, facial — *see* condition
Facet of cornea 371.44
Faciocephalalgia, autonomic — *see also* Neuropathy, peripheral, autonomic 337.9
Facioscapulohumeral myopathy 359.1
Factitious disorder, illness — *see* Illness, factitious
Factor
deficiency — *see* Deficiency, factor
psychic, associated with diseases classified elsewhere 316
risk — *see* Problem
Fahr-Volhard disease (malignant nephrosclerosis) 403.00
Failure, failed
adenohypophyseal 253.2
attempted abortion (legal) (*see also* Abortion, failed) 638.9
bone marrow (anemia) 284.9
acquired (secondary) 284.89
congenital 284.09
idiopathic 284.9
cardiac (*see also* Failure, heart) 428.9
newborn 779.89
cardiorenal (chronic) 428.9
hypertensive (*see also* Hypertension, cardiorenal) 404.93
cardiorespiratory 799.1
specified during or due to a procedure 997.1
long-term effect of cardiac surgery 429.4
cardiovascular (chronic) 428.9
cerebrovascular 437.8
cervical dilatation in labor 661.0 ☑
affecting fetus or newborn 763.7
circulation, circulatory 799.89
fetus or newborn 779.89
peripheral 785.50
compensation — *see* Disease, heart
congestive (*see also* Failure, heart) 428.0
conscious sedation, during procedure 995.24
coronary (*see also* Insufficiency, coronary) 411.89
dental implant 525.79
due to
infection 525.71
lack of attached gingiva 525.72
occlusal trauma (caused by poor prosthetic design) 525.72
parafunctional habits 525.72
periodontal infection (peri-implantitis) 525.72
poor oral hygiene 525.72
unintentional loading 525.71
endosseous NEC 525.79
mechanical 525.73
osseointegration 525.71
due to
complications of systemic disease 525.71
poor bone quality 525.71
premature loading 525.71

Failure, failed — *continued*
dental implant — *continued*
osseointegration — *continued*
iatrogenic 525.71
prior to intentional prosthetic loading 525.71
post-osseointegration
biological 525.72
iatrogenic 525.72
due to complications of systemic disease 525.72
mechanical 525.73
pre-integration 525.71
pre-osseointegration 525.71
dental prosthesis causing loss of dental implant 525.73
dental restoration
marginal integrity 525.61
periodontal anatomical integrity 525.65
descent of head (at term) 652.5 ☑
affecting fetus or newborn 763.1
in labor 660.0 ☑
affecting fetus or newborn 763.1
device, implant, or graft — *see* Complications, mechanical
engagement of head NEC 652.5 ☑
in labor 660.0 ☑
affecting fetus or newborn 763.1
extrarenal 788.99
fetal head to enter pelvic brim 652.5 ☑
affecting fetus or newborn 763.1
in labor 660.0 ☑
affecting fetus or newborn 763.1
forceps NEC 660.7 ☑
affecting fetus or newborn 763.1
fusion (joint) (spinal) 996.49
growth in childhood 783.43
heart (acute) (sudden) 428.9
with
abortion — *see* Abortion, by type, with specified complication NEC
acute pulmonary edema (*see also* Failure, ventricular, left) 428.1
with congestion (*see also* Failure, heart) 428.0
decompensation (*see also* Failure, heart) 428.0
dilation — *see* Disease, heart
ectopic pregnancy (*see also* categories 633.0–633.9) 639.8
molar pregnancy (*see also* categories 630–632) 639.8
arteriosclerotic 440.9
combined left-right sided 428.0
combined systolic and diastolic 428.40
acute 428.41
acute on chronic 428.43
chronic 428.42
compensated (*see also* Failure, heart) 428.0
complicating
abortion — *see* Abortion, by type, with specified complication NEC
delivery (cesarean) (instrumental) 669.4 ☑
ectopic pregnancy (*see also* categories 633.0–633.9) 639.8
molar pregnancy (*see also* categories 630–632) 639.8
obstetric anesthesia or sedation 668.1 ☑
surgery 997.1
congestive (compensated) (decompensated) (*see also* Failure, heart) 428.0
with rheumatic fever (conditions classifiable to 390)
active 391.8
inactive or quiescent (with chorea) 398.91
fetus or newborn 779.89
hypertensive (*see also* Hypertension, heart) 402.91

Failure, failed — *continued*
heart — *continued*
congestive (*see also* Failure, heart) — *continued*
hypertensive (*see also* Hypertension, heart) — *continued*
with renal disease (*see also* Hypertension, cardiorenal) 404.91
with renal failure 404.93
benign 402.11
malignant 402.01
rheumatic (chronic) (inactive) (with chorea) 398.91
active or acute 391.8
with chorea (Sydenham's) 392.0
decompensated (*see also* Failure, heart) 428.0
degenerative (*see also* Degeneration, myocardial) 429.1
diastolic 428.30
acute 428.31
acute on chronic 428.33
chronic 428.32
due to presence of (cardiac) prosthesis 429.4
fetus or newborn 779.89
following
abortion 639.8
cardiac surgery 429.4
ectopic or molar pregnancy 639.8
high output NEC 428.9
hypertensive (*see also* Hypertension, heart) 402.91
with renal disease (*see also* Hypertension, cardiorenal) 404.91
with renal failure 404.93
benign 402.11
malignant 402.01
left (ventricular) (*see also* Failure, ventricular, left) 428.1
with right-sided failure (*see also* Failure, heart) 428.0
low output (syndrome) NEC 428.9
organic — *see* Disease, heart
postoperative (immediate) 997.1
long term effect of cardiac surgery 429.4
rheumatic (chronic) (congestive) (inactive) 398.91
right (secondary to left heart failure, conditions classifiable to 428.1) (ventricular) (*see also* Failure, heart) 428.0
senile 797
specified during or due to a procedure 997.1
long-term effect of cardiac surgery 429.4
systolic 428.20
acute 428.21
acute on chronic 428.23
chronic 428.22
thyrotoxic (*see also* Thyrotoxicosis) 242.9 ☑ [425.7]
valvular — *see* Endocarditis
hepatic 572.8
acute 570
due to a procedure 997.4
hepatorenal 572.4
hypertensive heart (*see also* Hypertension, heart) 402.91
benign 402.11
malignant 402.01
induction (of labor) 659.1 ☑
abortion (legal) (*see also* Abortion, failed) 638.9
affecting fetus or newborn 763.89
by oxytocic drugs 659.1 ☑
instrumental 659.0 ☑
mechanical 659.0 ☑
medical 659.1 ☑
surgical 659.0 ☑
initial alveolar expansion, newborn 770.4
involution, thymus (gland) 254.8

☑ Additional Digit Required — Refer to the Tabular List for Digit Selection   ҉ Subterms under main terms may continue to next column or page

2011 ICD-9-CM   ▶◀ Revised Text   ● New Line   ▲ Revised Code   Volume 2 — 111

Failure, failed — continued
kidney — see Failure, renal
lactation 676.4 ☑
Leydig's cell, adult 257.2
liver 572.8
   acute 570
medullary 799.89
mitral — see Endocarditis, mitral
moderate sedation, during procedure 995.24
myocardium, myocardial (see also Failure, heart) 428.9
   chronic (see also Failure, heart) 428.0
   congestive (see also Failure, heart) 428.0
ovarian (primary) 256.39
   iatrogenic 256.2
   postablative 256.2
   postirradiation 256.2
   postsurgical 256.2
ovulation 628.0
prerenal 788.99
renal (kidney) 586
   with
      abortion — see Abortion, by type, with renal failure
      ectopic pregnancy (see also categories 633.0–633.9) 639.3
      edema (see also Nephrosis) 581.9
      hypertension (see also Hypertension, kidney) 403.91
      hypertensive heart disease (conditions classifiable to 402) 404.92
         with heart failure 404.93
         benign 404.12
            with heart failure 404.13
         malignant 404.02
            with heart failure 404.03
      molar pregnancy (see also categories 630–632) 639.3
      tubular necrosis (acute) 584.5
   acute 584.9
      with lesion of
         necrosis
            cortical (renal) 584.6
            medullary (renal) (papillary) 584.7
            tubular 584.5
         specified pathology NEC 584.8
   chronic 585.9
      hypertensive or with hypertension (see also Hypertension, kidney) 403.91
   due to a procedure 997.5
   following
      abortion 639.3
      crushing 958.5
      ectopic or molar pregnancy 639.3
      labor and delivery (acute) 669.3 ☑
   hypertensive (see also Hypertension, kidney) 403.91
   puerperal, postpartum 669.3 ☑
respiration, respiratory 518.81
   acute 518.81
   acute and chronic 518.84
   center 348.89
      newborn 770.84
   chronic 518.83
   due to trauma, surgery or shock 518.5
   newborn 770.84
rotation
   cecum 751.4
   colon 751.4
   intestine 751.4
   kidney 753.3
sedation, during procedure
   conscious 995.24
   moderate 995.24
segmentation (see also Fusion)
   fingers (see also Syndactylism, fingers) 755.11
   toes (see also Syndactylism, toes) 755.13
seminiferous tubule, adult 257.2
senile (general) 797
   with psychosis 290.20
testis, primary (seminal) 257.2

Failure, failed — continued
to progress 661.2 ☑
to thrive
   adult 783.7
   child 783.41
   newborn 779.34
transplant 996.80
   bone marrow 996.85
   organ (immune or nonimmune cause) 996.80
      bone marrow 996.85
      heart 996.83
      intestines 996.87
      kidney 996.81
      liver 996.82
      lung 996.84
      pancreas 996.86
      specified NEC 996.89
   skin 996.52
      artificial 996.55
      decellularized allodermis 996.55
      temporary allograft or pigskin graft — omit code
trial of labor NEC 660.6 ☑
   affecting fetus or newborn 763.1
tubal ligation 998.89
urinary 586
vacuum extraction
   abortion — see Abortion, failed
   delivery NEC 660.7 ☑
      affecting fetus or newborn 763.1
vasectomy 998.89
ventouse NEC 660.7 ☑
   affecting fetus or newborn 763.1
ventricular (see also Failure, heart) 428.9
   left 428.1
      with rheumatic fever (conditions classifiable to 390)
         active 391.8
            with chorea 392.0
         inactive or quiescent (with chorea) 398.91
      hypertensive (see also Hypertension, heart) 402.91
         benign 402.11
         malignant 402.01
      rheumatic (chronic) (inactive) (with chorea) 398.91
         active or acute 391.8
            with chorea 392.0
   right (see also Failure, heart) 428.0
vital centers, fetus or newborn 779.89
weight gain in childhood 783.41
Fainting (fit) (spell) 780.2
Falciform hymen 752.49
Fallen arches 734
Falling, any organ or part — see Prolapse
Fall, maternal, affecting fetus or newborn 760.5
Fallopian
   insufflation
      fertility testing V26.21
      following sterilization reversal V26.22
   tube — see condition
Fallot's
   pentalogy 745.2
   tetrad or tetralogy 745.2
   triad or trilogy 746.09
Fallout, radioactive (adverse effect) NEC 990
False — see also condition
   bundle branch block 426.50
   bursa 727.89
   croup 478.75
   joint 733.82
   labor (pains) 644.1 ☑
   opening, urinary, male 752.69
   passage, urethra (prostatic) 599.4
   positive
      serological test for syphilis 795.6
      Wassermann reaction 795.6
   pregnancy 300.11
Family, familial — see also condition
   affected by
      family member
         currently on deployment (military) V61.01

Family, familial — see also condition — continued
   affected by — continued
      family member — continued
         returned from deployment (military) (current or past conflict) V61.02
   disruption (see also Disruption, family) V61.09
   estrangement V61.09
   hemophagocytic
      lymphohistiocytosis 288.4
      reticulosis 288.4
   Li-Fraumeni (syndrome) V84.01
   planning advice V25.09
      natural
         procreative V26.41
         to avoid pregnancy V25.04
      problem V61.9
         specified circumstance NEC V61.8
   retinoblastoma (syndrome) 190.5
Famine 994.2
   edema 262
Fanconi's anemia (congenital pancytopenia) 284.09
Fanconi (-de Toni) (-Debré) syndrome (cystinosis) 270.0
Farber (-Uzman) syndrome or disease (disseminated lipogranulomatosis) 272.8
Farcin 024
Farcy 024
Farmers'
   lung 495.0
   skin 692.74
Farsightedness 367.0
Fascia — see condition
Fasciculation 781.0
Fasciculitis optica 377.32
Fasciitis 729.4
   eosinophilic 728.89
   necrotizing 728.86
   nodular 728.79
   perirenal 593.4
   plantar 728.71
   pseudosarcomatous 728.79
   traumatic (old) NEC 728.79
      current — see Sprain, by site
Fasciola hepatica infestation 121.3
Fascioliasis 121.3
Fasciolopsiasis (small intestine) 121.4
Fasciolopsis (small intestine) 121.4
Fast pulse 785.0
Fat
   embolism (cerebral) (pulmonary) (systemic) 958.1
      with
         abortion — see Abortion, by type, with embolism
         ectopic pregnancy (see also categories 633.0–633.9) 639.6
         molar pregnancy (see also categories 630–632) 639.6
      complicating delivery or puerperium 673.8 ☑
      following
         abortion 639.6
         ectopic or molar pregnancy 639.6
      in pregnancy, childbirth, or the puerperium 673.8 ☑
   excessive 278.02
      in heart (see also Degeneration, myocardial) 429.1
   general 278.02
   hernia, herniation 729.30
      eyelid 374.34
      knee 729.31
      orbit 374.34
      retro-orbital 374.34
      retropatellar 729.31
      specified site NEC 729.39
   indigestion 579.8
   in stool 792.1
   localized (pad) 278.1
      heart (see also Degeneration, myocardial) 429.1
      knee 729.31

Fat — continued
   localized — continued
      retropatellar 729.31
   necrosis (see also Fatty, degeneration)
      breast (aseptic) (segmental) 611.3
      mesentery 567.82
      omentum 567.82
      peritoneum 567.82
   pad 278.1
Fatal familial insomnia (FFI) 046.72
Fatal syncope 798.1
Fatigue 780.79
   auditory deafness (see also Deafness) 389.9
   chronic, syndrome 780.71
   combat (see also Reaction, stress, acute) 308.9
   during pregnancy 646.8 ☑
   general 780.79
      psychogenic 300.5
   heat (transient) 992.6
   muscle 729.89
   myocardium (see also Failure, heart) 428.9
   nervous 300.5
   neurosis 300.5
   operational 300.89
   postural 729.89
   posture 729.89
   psychogenic (general) 300.5
   senile 797
   syndrome NEC 300.5
      chronic 780.71
   undue 780.79
   voice 784.49
Fatness 278.02
Fatty — see also condition
   apron 278.1
   degeneration (diffuse) (general) NEC 272.8
      localized — see Degeneration, by site, fatty
      placenta — see Placenta, abnormal
   heart (enlarged) (see also Degeneration, myocardial) 429.1
   infiltration (diffuse) (general) (see also Degeneration, by site, fatty) 272.8
      heart (enlarged) (see also Degeneration, myocardial) 429.1
   liver 571.8
      alcoholic 571.0
   necrosis — see Degeneration, fatty
   phanerosis 272.8
Fauces — see condition
Fauchard's disease (periodontitis) 523.40
Faucitis 478.29
Faulty — see also condition
   position of teeth 524.30
Favism (anemia) 282.2
Favre-Racouchot disease (elastoidosis cutanea nodularis) 701.8
Favus 110.9
   beard 110.0
   capitis 110.0
   corporis 110.5
   eyelid 110.8
   foot 110.4
   hand 110.4
   scalp 110.0
   specified site NEC 110.8
Feared complaint unfounded V65.5
Fear, fearfulness (complex) (reaction) 300.20
   child 313.0
   of
      animals 300.29
      closed spaces 300.29
      crowds 300.29
      eating in public 300.23
      heights 300.29
      open spaces 300.22
         with panic attacks 300.21
      public speaking 300.23
      streets 300.22
         with panic attacks 300.21
      travel 300.22
         with panic attacks 300.21
      washing in public 300.23
   transient 308.0

☑ **Additional Digit Required** — Refer to the Tabular List for Digit Selection   � **Subterms under main terms may continue to next column or page**

112 — Volume 2   ▶◀ Revised Text   ● New Line   ▲ Revised Code   2011 ICD-9-CM

Index

Failure, failed — Fear, fearfulness

Febricula (continued) (simple) — *see also*
    Pyrexia 780.60
Febrile — *see also* Pyrexia 780.60
    convulsion (simple) 780.31
        complex 780.32
    nonhemolytic transfusion reaction (FN-
        HTR) 780.66 ●
    seizure (simple) 780.31
        atypical 780.32
        complex 780.32
        complicated 780.32
Febris — *see also* Fever 780.60
    aestiva (*see also* Fever, hay) 477.9
    flava (*see also* Fever, yellow) 060.9
    melitensis 023.0
    pestis (*see also* Plague) 020.9
    puerperalis 672.0 ☑
    recurrens (*see also* Fever, relapsing) 087.9
        pediculo vestimenti 087.0
    rubra 034.1
    typhoidea 002.0
    typhosa 002.0
Fecal — *see* condition
Fecalith (impaction) 560.32 ▲
    with hernia (*see also* Hernia, by site, with
        obstruction)
        gangrenous — *see* Hernia, by site, with
            gangrene
    appendix 543.9
    congenital 777.1
Fede's disease 529.0
Feeble-minded 317
Feeble rapid pulse due to shock following
    injury 958.4
Feeding
    faulty (elderly) (infant) 783.3
        newborn 779.31
    formula check V20.2
    improper (elderly) (infant) 783.3
        newborn 779.31
    problem (elderly) (infant) 783.3
        newborn 779.31
        nonorganic origin 307.59
Feeling of foreign body in throat 784.99
Feer's disease 985.0
Feet — *see* condition
Feigned illness V65.2
Feil-Klippel syndrome (brevicollis) 756.16
Feinmesser's (hidrotic) **ectodermal dysplasia**
    757.31
Felix's disease (juvenile osteochondrosis, hip)
    732.1
Felon (any digit) (with lymphangitis) 681.01
    herpetic 054.6
Felty's syndrome (rheumatoid arthritis with
    splenomegaly and leukopenia) 714.1
Feminism in boys 302.6
Feminization, testicular 259.51
    with pseudohermaphroditism, male 259.51
Femoral hernia — *see* Hernia, femoral
Femora vara 736.32
Femur, femoral — *see* condition
Fenestrata placenta — *see* Placenta, abnormal
Fenestration, fenestrated — *see also* Imper-
    fect, closure
    aorta-pulmonary 745.0
    aorticopulmonary 745.0
    aortopulmonary 745.0
    cusps, heart valve NEC 746.89
        pulmonary 746.09
    hymen 752.49
    pulmonic cusps 746.09
Fenwick's disease 537.89
Fermentation (gastric) (gastrointestinal)
    (stomach) 536.8
    intestine 564.89
        psychogenic 306.4
    psychogenic 306.4
Fernell's disease (aortic aneurysm) 441.9
Fertile eunuch syndrome 257.2
Fertility, meaning multiparity — *see* Multi-
    parity
Fetal
    alcohol syndrome 760.71
    anemia 678.0 ☑
    thrombocytopenia 678.0 ☑

Fetal — *continued*
    twin to twin transfusion 678.0 ☑
Fetalis uterus 752.39   ▲
Fetid
    breath 784.99
    sweat 705.89
Fetishism 302.81
    transvestic 302.3
Fetomaternal hemorrhage
    affecting management of pregnancy
        656.0 ☑
    fetus or newborn 772.0
Fetus, fetal — *see also* condition
    papyraceous 779.89
    type lung tissue 770.4
Fever 780.60
    with chills 780.60
        in malarial regions (*see also* Malaria)
            084.6
    abortus NEC 023.9
    aden 061
    African tick-borne 087.1
    American
        mountain tick 066.1
        spotted 082.0
    and ague (*see also* Malaria) 084.6
    aphthous 078.4
    arbovirus hemorrhagic 065.9
    Assam 085.0
    Australian A or Q 083.0
    Bangkok hemorrhagic 065.4
    biliary, Charcôt's intermittent — *see* Chole-
        docholithiasis
    bilious, hemoglobinuric 084.8
    blackwater 084.8
    blister 054.9
    Bonvale Dam 780.79
    boutonneuse 082.1
    brain 323.9
        late effect — *see* category 326
    breakbone 061
    Bullis 082.8
    Bunyamwera 066.3
    Burdwan 085.0
    Bwamba (encephalitis) 066.3
    Cameroon (*see also* Malaria) 084.6
    Canton 081.9
    catarrhal (acute) 460
        chronic 472.0
    cat-scratch 078.3
    cerebral 323.9
        late effect — *see* category 326
    cerebrospinal (meningococcal) (*see also*
        Meningitis, cerebrospinal) 036.0
    Chagres 084.0
    Chandipura 066.8
    changuinola 066.0
    Charcôt's (biliary) (hepatic) (intermittent)
        — *see* Choledocholithiasis
    Chikungunya (viral) 066.3
        hemorrhagic 065.4
    childbed 670.8 ☑
    Chitral 066.0
    Colombo (*see also* Fever, paratyphoid) 002.9
    Colorado tick (virus) 066.1
    congestive
        malarial (*see also* Malaria) 084.6
        remittent (*see also* Malaria) 084.6
    Congo virus 065.0
    continued 780.60
        malarial 084.0
    Corsican (*see also* Malaria) 084.6
    Crimean hemorrhagic 065.0
    Cyprus (*see also* Brucellosis) 023.9
    dandy 061
    deer fly (*see also* Tularemia) 021.9
    dehydration, newborn 778.4
    dengue (virus) 061
        hemorrhagic 065.4
    desert 114.0
    due to heat 992.0
    Dumdum 085.0
    enteric 002.0
    ephemeral (of unknown origin) (*see also*
        Pyrexia) 780.60
    epidemic, hemorrhagic of the Far East 065.0

Fever — *continued*
    erysipelatous (*see also* Erysipelas) 035
    estivo-autumnal (malarial) 084.0
    etiocholanolone 277.31
    famine (*see also* Fever, relapsing)
        meaning typhus — *see* Typhus
    Far Eastern hemorrhagic 065.0
    five day 083.1
    Fort Bragg 100.89
    gastroenteric 002.0
    gastromalarial (*see also* Malaria) 084.6
    Gibraltar (*see also* Brucellosis) 023.9
    glandular 075
    Guama (viral) 066.3
    Haverhill 026.1
    hay (allergic) (with rhinitis) 477.9
        with
            asthma (bronchial) (*see also* Asthma)
                493.0 ☑
        due to
            dander, animal (cat) (dog) 477.2
            dust 477.8
            fowl 477.8
            hair, animal (cat) (dog) 477.2
            pollen, any plant or tree 477.0
            specified allergen other than pollen
                477.8
    heat (effects) 992.0
    hematuric, bilious 084.8
    hemoglobinuric (malarial) 084.8
        bilious 084.8
    hemorrhagic (arthropod-borne) NEC 065.9
        with renal syndrome 078.6
        arenaviral 078.7
        Argentine 078.7
        Bangkok 065.4
        Bolivian 078.7
        Central Asian 065.0
        chikungunya 065.4
        Crimean 065.0
        dengue (virus) 065.4
        Ebola 065.8
        epidemic 078.6
            of Far East 065.0
        Far Eastern 065.0
        Junin virus 078.7
        Korean 078.6
        Kyasanur forest 065.2
        Machupo virus 078.7
        mite-borne NEC 065.8
        mosquito-borne 065.4
        Omsk 065.1
        Philippine 065.4
        Russian (Yaroslav) 078.6
        Singapore 065.4
        Southeast Asia 065.4
        Thailand 065.4
        tick-borne NEC 065.3
    hepatic (*see also* Cholecystitis) 575.8
        intermittent (Charcôt's) — *see* Choledo-
            cholithiasis
    herpetic (*see also* Herpes) 054.9
    Hyalomma tick 065.0
    icterohemorrhagic 100.0
    inanition 780.60
        newborn 778.4
    in conditions classified elsewhere 780.61
    infective NEC 136.9
    intermittent (bilious) (*see also* Malaria) 084.6
        hepatic (Charcôt) — *see* Choledocholithi-
            asis
        of unknown origin (*see also* Pyrexia)
            780.60
        pernicious 084.0
    iodide
        correct substance properly administered
            780.60
        overdose or wrong substance given or
            taken 975.5
    Japanese river 081.2
    jungle yellow 060.0
    Junin virus, hemorrhagic 078.7
    Katayama 120.2
    Kedani 081.2
    Kenya 082.1
    Korean hemorrhagic 078.6

Fever — *continued*
    Lassa 078.89
    Lone Star 082.8
    lung — *see* Pneumonia
    Machupo virus, hemorrhagic 078.7
    malaria, malarial (*see also* Malaria) 084.6
    Malta (*see also* Brucellosis) 023.9
    Marseilles 082.1
    marsh (*see also* Malaria) 084.6
    Mayaro (viral) 066.3
    Mediterranean (*see also* Brucellosis) 023.9
        familial 277.31
        tick 082.1
    meningeal — *see* Meningitis
    metal fumes NEC 985.8
    Meuse 083.1
    Mexican — *see* Typhus, Mexican
    Mianeh 087.1
    miasmatic (*see also* Malaria) 084.6
    miliary 078.2
    milk, female 672.0 ☑
    mill 504
    mite-borne hemorrhagic 065.8
    Monday 504
    mosquito-borne NEC 066.3
        hemorrhagic NEC 065.4
    mountain 066.1
        meaning
            Rocky Mountain spotted 082.0
            undulant fever (*see also* Brucellosis)
                023.9
        tick (American) 066.1
    Mucambo (viral) 066.3
    mud 100.89
    Neapolitan (*see also* Brucellosis) 023.9
    neutropenic 288.00
    newborn (environmentally-induced) 778.4
    nine-mile 083.0
    nonexanthematous tick 066.1
    North Asian tick-borne typhus 082.2
    Omsk hemorrhagic 065.1
    O'nyong-nyong (viral) 066.3
    Oropouche (viral) 066.3
    Oroya 088.0
    paludal (*see also* Malaria) 084.6
    Panama 084.0
    pappataci 066.0
    paratyphoid 002.9
        A 002.1
        B (Schottmüller's) 002.2
        C (Hirschfeld) 002.3
    parrot 073.9
    periodic 277.31
    pernicious, acute 084.0
    persistent (of unknown origin) (*see also*
        Pyrexia) 780.60
    petechial 036.0
    pharyngoconjunctival 077.2
        adenoviral type 3 077.2
    Philippine hemorrhagic 065.4
    phlebotomus 066.0
    Piry 066.8
    Pixuna (viral) 066.3
    Plasmodium ovale 084.3
    pleural (*see also* Pleurisy) 511.0
    pneumonic — *see* Pneumonia
    polymer fume 987.8
    postimmunization 780.63
    postoperative 780.62
        due to infection 998.59
    posttransfusion 780.66   ●
    postvaccination 780.63
    pretibial 100.89
    puerperal, postpartum 672.0 ☑
    putrid — *see* Septicemia
    pyemic — *see* Septicemia
    Q 083.0
        with pneumonia 083.0 [484.8]
    quadrilateral 083.0
    quartan (malaria) 084.2
    Queensland (coastal) 083.0
        seven-day 100.89
    Quintan (A) 083.1
    quotidian 084.0
    rabbit (*see also* Tularemia) 021.9
    rat-bite 026.9

☑ **Additional Digit Required** — Refer to the Tabular List for Digit Selection   ▽ **Subterms under main terms may continue to next column or page**

Fibro-osteoma (M9262/0) — *see* Neoplasm, bone, benign
Fibroplasia, retrolental (*see also* Retinopathy of prematurity) 362.21
Fibropurulent — *see* condition
Fibrosarcoma (M8810/3) — *see also* Neoplasm, connective tissue, malignant
  ameloblastic (M9330/3) 170.1
    upper jaw (bone) 170.0
  congenital (M8814/3) — *see* Neoplasm, connective tissue, malignant
  fascial (M8813/3) — *see* Neoplasm, connective tissue, malignant
  infantile (M8814/3) — *see* Neoplasm, connective tissue, malignant
  odontogenic (M9330/3) 170.1
    upper jaw (bone) 170.0
  periosteal (M8812/3) — *see* Neoplasm, bone, malignant
Fibrosclerosis
  breast 610.3
  corpora cavernosa (penis) 607.89
  familial multifocal NEC 710.8
  multifocal (idiopathic) NEC 710.8
  penis (corpora cavernosa) 607.89
Fibrosis, fibrotic
  adrenal (gland) 255.8
  alveolar (diffuse) 516.3
  amnion 658.8 ☑
  anal papillae 569.49
  anus 569.49
  appendix, appendiceal, noninflammatory 543.9
  arteriocapillary — *see* Arteriosclerosis
  bauxite (of lung) 503
  biliary 576.8
    due to Clonorchis sinensis 121.1
  bladder 596.8
    interstitial 595.1
    localized submucosal 595.1
    panmural 595.1
  bone, diffuse 756.59
  breast 610.3
  capillary (*see also* Arteriosclerosis)
    lung (chronic) (*see also* Fibrosis, lung) 515
  cardiac (*see also* Myocarditis) 429.0
  cervix 622.8
  chorion 658.8 ☑
  corpus cavernosum 607.89
  cystic (of pancreas) 277.00
    with
      manifestations
        gastrointestinal 277.03
        pulmonary 277.02
        specified NEC 277.09
      meconium ileus 277.01
      pulmonary exacerbation 277.02
  due to (presence of) any device, implant, or graft — *see* Complications, due to (presence of) any device, implant, or graft classified to 996.0–996.5 NEC
  ejaculatory duct 608.89
  endocardium (*see also* Endocarditis) 424.90
  endomyocardial (African) 425.0
  epididymis 608.89
  eye muscle 378.62
  graphite (of lung) 503
  heart (*see also* Myocarditis) 429.0
  hepatic (*see also* Cirrhosis, liver)
    due to Clonorchis sinensis 121.1
  hepatolienal — *see* Cirrhosis, liver
  hepatosplenic — *see* Cirrhosis, liver
  infrapatellar fat pad 729.31
  interstitial pulmonary, newborn 770.7
  intrascrotal 608.89
  kidney (*see also* Sclerosis, renal) 587
  liver — *see* Cirrhosis, liver
  lung (atrophic) (capillary) (chronic) (confluent) (massive) (perialveolar) (peribronchial) 515
    with
      anthracosilicosis (occupational) 500
      anthracosis (occupational) 500
      asbestosis (occupational) 501
      bagassosis (occupational) 495.1

Fibrosis, fibrotic — *continued*
  lung — *continued*
    with — *continued*
      bauxite 503
      berylliosis (occupational) 503
      byssinosis (occupational) 504
      calcicosis (occupational) 502
      chalicosis (occupational) 502
      dust reticulation (occupational) 504
      farmers' lung 495.0
      gannister disease (occupational) 502
      graphite 503
      pneumoconiosis (occupational) 505
      pneumosiderosis (occupational) 503
      siderosis (occupational) 503
      silicosis (occupational) 502
      tuberculosis (*see also* Tuberculosis) 011.4 ☑
    diffuse (idiopathic) (interstitial) 516.3
    due to
      bauxite 503
      fumes or vapors (chemical) (inhalation) 506.4
      graphite 503
    following radiation 508.1
    postinflammatory 515
    silicotic (massive) (occupational) 502
    tuberculous (*see also* Tuberculosis) 011.4 ☑
  lymphatic gland 289.3
  median bar 600.90
    with
      other lower urinary tract symptoms (LUTS) 600.91
      urinary
        obstruction 600.91
        retention 600.91
  mediastinum (idiopathic) 519.3
  meninges 349.2
  muscle NEC 728.2
    iatrogenic (from injection) 999.9
  myocardium, myocardial (*see also* Myocarditis) 429.0
  oral submucous 528.8
  ovary 620.8
  oviduct 620.8
  pancreas 577.8
    cystic 277.00
      with
        manifestations
          gastrointestinal 277.03
          pulmonary 277.02
          specified NEC 277.09
        meconium ileus 277.01
        pulmonary exacerbation 277.02
  penis 607.89
  periappendiceal 543.9
  periarticular (*see also* Ankylosis) 718.5 ☑
  pericardium 423.1
  perineum, in pregnancy or childbirth 654.8 ☑
    affecting fetus or newborn 763.89
    causing obstructed labor 660.2 ☑
      affecting fetus or newborn 763.1
  perineural NEC 355.9
    foot 355.6
  periureteral 593.89
  placenta — *see* Placenta, abnormal
  pleura 511.0
  popliteal fat pad 729.31
  preretinal 362.56
  prostate (chronic) 600.90
    with
      other lower urinary tract symptoms (LUTS) 600.91
      urinary
        obstruction 600.91
        retention 600.91
  pulmonary (chronic) (*see also* Fibrosis, lung) 515
    alveolar capillary block 516.3
    interstitial
      diffuse (idiopathic) 516.3
      newborn 770.7
  radiation — *see* Effect, adverse, radiation

Fibrosis, fibrotic — *continued*
  rectal sphincter 569.49
  retroperitoneal, idiopathic 593.4
  sclerosing mesenteric (idiopathic) 567.82
  scrotum 608.89
  seminal vesicle 608.89
  senile 797
  skin NEC 709.2
  spermatic cord 608.89
  spleen 289.59
    bilharzial (*see also* Schistosomiasis) 120.9
  subepidermal nodular (M8832/0) — *see* Neoplasm, skin, benign
  submucous NEC 709.2
    oral 528.8
    tongue 528.8
  syncytium — *see* Placenta, abnormal
  testis 608.89
    chronic, due to syphilis 095.8
  thymus (gland) 254.8
  tunica vaginalis 608.89
  ureter 593.89
  urethra 599.84
  uterus (nonneoplastic) 621.8
    bilharzial (*see also* Schistosomiasis) 120.9
    neoplastic (*see also* Leiomyoma, uterus) 218.9
  vagina 623.8
  valve, heart (*see also* Endocarditis) 424.90
  vas deferens 608.89
  vein 459.89
    lower extremities 459.89
  vesical 595.1
Fibrositis (periarticular) (rheumatoid) 729.0
  humeroscapular region 726.2
  nodular, chronic
    Jaccoud's 714.4
    rheumatoid 714.4
  ossificans 728.11
  scapulohumeral 726.2
Fibrothorax 511.0
Fibrotic — *see* Fibrosis
Fibrous — *see* condition
Fibroxanthoma (M8831/0) — *see also* Neoplasm, connective tissue, benign
  atypical (M8831/1) — *see* Neoplasm, connective tissue, uncertain behavior
  malignant (M8831/3) — *see* Neoplasm, connective tissue, malignant
Fibroxanthosarcoma (M8831/3) — *see* Neoplasm, connective tissue, malignant
Fiedler's
  disease (leptospiral jaundice) 100.0
  myocarditis or syndrome (acute isolated myocarditis) 422.91
Fiessinger-Leroy (-Reiter) syndrome 099.3
Fiessinger-Rendu syndrome (erythema muliforme exudativum) 695.19
Fifth disease (eruptive) 057.0
  venereal 099.1
Filaria, filarial — *see* Infestation, filarial
Filariasis — *see also* Infestation, filarial 125.9
  bancroftian 125.0
  Brug's 125.1
  due to
    bancrofti 125.0
    Brugia (Wuchereria) (malayi) 125.1
    Loa loa 125.2
    malayi 125.1
    organism NEC 125.6
    Wuchereria (bancrofti) 125.0
      malayi 125.1
  Malayan 125.1
  ozzardi 125.5
  specified type NEC 125.6
Filatoff's, Filatov's, Filatow's disease (infectious mononucleosis) 075
File-cutters' disease 984.9
  specified type of lead — *see* Table of Drugs and Chemicals
Filling defect
  biliary tract 793.3
  bladder 793.5
  duodenum 793.4
  gallbladder 793.3
  gastrointestinal tract 793.4

Filling defect — *continued*
  intestine 793.4
  kidney 793.5
  stomach 793.4
  ureter 793.5
Filtering bleb, eye (postglaucoma) (status) V45.69
  with complication or rupture 997.99
  postcataract extraction (complication) 997.99
Fimbrial cyst (congenital) 752.11
Fimbriated hymen 752.49
Financial problem affecting care V60.2
Findings, (abnormal), without diagnosis (examination) (laboratory test) 796.4
  17-ketosteroids, elevated 791.9
  acetonuria 791.6
  acid phosphatase 790.5
  albumin-globulin ratio 790.99
  albuminuria 791.0
  alcohol in blood 790.3
  alkaline phosphatase 790.5
  amniotic fluid 792.3
  amylase 790.5
  anisocytosis 790.09
  antenatal screening 796.5
  anthrax, positive 795.31
  antibody titers, elevated 795.79
  anticardiolipin antibody 795.79
  antigen-antibody reaction 795.79
  antiphospholipid antibody 795.79
  bacteriuria 791.9
  ballistocardiogram 794.39
  bicarbonate 276.9
  bile in urine 791.4
  bilirubin 277.4
  bleeding time (prolonged) 790.92
  blood culture, positive 790.7
  blood gas level (arterial) 790.91
  blood sugar level 790.29
    high 790.29
      fasting glucose 790.21
      glucose tolerance test 790.22
    low 251.2
  calcium 275.40
  cancer antigen 125 [CA 125] 795.82
  carbonate 276.9
  carcinoembryonic antigen [CEA] 795.81
  casts, urine 791.7
  catecholamines 791.9
  cells, urine 791.7
  cerebrospinal fluid (color) (content) (pressure) 792.0
  cervical
    high risk human papillomavirus (HPV) DNA test positive 795.05
    low risk human papillomavirus (HPV) DNA test positive 795.09
    non-atypical endometrial cells 795.09 ●
  chloride 276.9
  cholesterol 272.9
    high 272.0
      with high triglycerides 272.2
  chromosome analysis 795.2
  chyluria 791.1
  circulation time 794.39
  cloudy dialysis effluent 792.5
  cloudy urine 791.9
  coagulation study 790.92
  cobalt, blood 790.6
  color of urine (unusual) NEC 791.9
  copper, blood 790.6
  C-reactive protein (CRP) 790.95
  creatinine clearance 794.4
  crystals, urine 791.9
  culture, positive NEC 795.39
    blood 790.7
    HIV V08
    human immunodeficiency virus V08
    nose 795.39
      Staphylococcus — *see* Carrier (suspected) of, Staphylococcus
    skin lesion NEC 795.39
    spinal fluid 792.0
    sputum 795.39
    stool 792.1

Fish
hook stomach 537.89
meal workers' lung 495.8

Fisher's syndrome 357.0

Fissure, fissured
abdominal wall (congenital) 756.79
anus, anal 565.0
  congenital 751.5
buccal cavity 528.9
clitoris (congenital) 752.49
ear, lobule (congenital) 744.29
epiglottis (congenital) 748.3
larynx 478.79
  congenital 748.3
lip 528.5
  congenital (see also Cleft, lip) 749.10
nipple 611.2
  puerperal, postpartum 676.1 ☑
palate (congenital) (see also Cleft, palate) 749.00
postanal 565.0
rectum 565.0
skin 709.8
  streptococcal 686.9
spine (congenital) (see also Spina bifida) 741.9 ☑
sternum (congenital) 756.3
tongue (acquired) 529.5
  congenital 750.13

Fistula (sinus) 686.9
abdomen (wall) 569.81
  bladder 596.2
  intestine 569.81
  ureter 593.82
  uterus 619.2
abdominorectal 569.81
abdominosigmoidal 569.81
abdominothoracic 510.0
abdominouterine 619.2
  congenital 752.39 ▲
abdominovesical 596.2
accessory sinuses (see also Sinusitis) 473.9
actinomycotic — see Actinomycosis
alveolar
  antrum (see also Sinusitis, maxillary) 473.0
  process 522.7
anorectal 565.1
antrobuccal (see also Sinusitis, maxillary) 473.0
antrum (see also Sinusitis, maxillary) 473.0
anus, anal (infectional) (recurrent) 565.1
  congenital 751.5
  tuberculous (see also Tuberculosis) 014.8 ☑
aortic sinus 747.29
aortoduodenal 447.2
appendix, appendicular 543.9
arteriovenous (acquired) 447.0
  brain 437.3
    congenital 747.81
      ruptured (see also Hemorrhage, subarachnoid) 430
    ruptured (see also Hemorrhage, subarachnoid) 430
  cerebral 437.3
    congenital 747.81
  congenital (peripheral) 747.60
    brain — see Fistula, arteriovenous, brain, congenital
    coronary 746.85
    gastrointestinal 747.61
    lower limb 747.64
    pulmonary 747.3
    renal 747.62
    specified site NEC 747.69
    upper limb 747.63
  coronary 414.19
    congenital 746.85
  heart 414.19
  pulmonary (vessels) 417.0
    congenital 747.3
  surgically created (for dialysis) V45.11
    complication NEC 996.73
      atherosclerosis — see Arteriosclerosis, extremities

Fistula — continued
arteriovenous — continued
  surgically created — continued
    complication — continued
      embolism 996.74
      infection or inflammation 996.62
      mechanical 996.1
      occlusion NEC 996.74
      thrombus 996.74
  traumatic — see Injury, blood vessel, by site
artery 447.2
aural 383.81
  congenital 744.49
auricle 383.81
  congenital 744.49
Bartholin's gland 619.8
bile duct (see also Fistula, biliary) 576.4
biliary (duct) (tract) 576.4
  congenital 751.69
bladder (neck) (sphincter) 596.2
  into seminal vesicle 596.2
bone 733.99
brain 348.89
  arteriovenous — see Fistula, arteriovenous, brain
branchial (cleft) 744.41
branchiogenous 744.41
breast 611.0
  puerperal, postpartum 675.1 ☑
bronchial 510.0
bronchocutaneous, bronchomediastinal, bronchopleural, bronchopleuromediastinal (infective) 510.0
  tuberculous (see also Tuberculosis) 011.3 ☑
bronchoesophageal 530.89
  congenital 750.3
buccal cavity (infective) 528.3
canal, ear 380.89
carotid-cavernous
  congenital 747.81
    with hemorrhage 430
  traumatic 900.82
    with hemorrhage (see also Hemorrhage, brain, traumatic) 853.0 ☑
    late effect 908.3
cecosigmoidal 569.81
cecum 569.81
cerebrospinal (fluid) 349.81
cervical, lateral (congenital) 744.41
cervicoaural (congenital) 744.49
cervicosigmoidal 619.1
cervicovesical 619.0
cervix 619.8
chest (wall) 510.0
cholecystocolic (see also Fistula, gallbladder) 575.5
cholecystocolonic (see also Fistula, gallbladder) 575.5
cholecystoduodenal (see also Fistula, gallbladder) 575.5
cholecystoenteric (see also Fistula, gallbladder) 575.5
cholecystogastric (see also Fistula, gallbladder) 575.5
cholecystointestinal (see also Fistula, gallbladder) 575.5
choledochoduodenal 576.4
cholocolic (see also Fistula, gallbladder) 575.5
coccyx 685.1
  with abscess 685.0
colon 569.81
colostomy 569.69
colovaginal (acquired) 619.1
common duct (bile duct) 576.4
congenital, NEC — see Anomaly, specified type NEC
cornea, causing hypotony 360.32
coronary, arteriovenous 414.19
  congenital 746.85
costal region 510.0
cul-de-sac, Douglas' 619.8
cutaneous 686.9

Fistula — continued
cystic duct (see also Fistula, gallbladder) 575.5
  congenital 751.69
dental 522.7
diaphragm 510.0
  bronchovisceral 510.0
  pleuroperitoneal 510.0
  pulmonoperitoneal 510.0
duodenum 537.4
ear (canal) (external) 380.89
enterocolic 569.81
enterocutaneous 569.81
enteroenteric 569.81
entero-uterine 619.1
  congenital 752.39 ▲
enterovaginal 619.1
  congenital 752.49
enterovesical 596.1
epididymis 608.89
  tuberculous (see also Tuberculosis) 016.4 ☑
esophagobronchial 530.89
  congenital 750.3
esophagocutaneous 530.89
esophagopleurocutaneous 530.89
esophagotracheal 530.84
  congenital 750.3
esophagus 530.89
  congenital 750.4
ethmoid (see also Sinusitis, ethmoidal) 473.2
eyeball (cornea) (sclera) 360.32
eyelid 373.11
fallopian tube (external) 619.2
fecal 569.81
  congenital 751.5
from periapical lesion 522.7
frontal sinus (see also Sinusitis, frontal) 473.1
gallbladder 575.5
  with calculus, cholelithiasis, stones (see also Cholelithiasis) 574.2 ☑
  congenital 751.69
gastric 537.4
gastrocolic 537.4
  congenital 750.7
  tuberculous (see also Tuberculosis) 014.8 ☑
gastroenterocolic 537.4
gastroesophageal 537.4
gastrojejunal 537.4
gastrojejunocolic 537.4
genital
  organs
    female 619.9
      specified site NEC 619.8
    male 608.89
  tract-skin (female) 619.2
hepatopleural 510.0
hepatopulmonary 510.0
horseshoe 565.1
ileorectal 569.81
ileosigmoidal 569.81
ileostomy 569.69
ileovesical 596.1
ileum 569.81
in ano 565.1
  tuberculous (see also Tuberculosis) 014.8 ☑
inner ear (see also Fistula, labyrinth) 386.40
intestine 569.81
intestinocolonic (abdominal) 569.81
intestinoureteral 593.82
intestinouterine 619.1
intestinovaginal 619.1
  congenital 752.49
intestinovesical 596.1
involving female genital tract 619.9
  digestive-genital 619.1
  genital tract-skin 619.2
  specified site NEC 619.8
  urinary-genital 619.0
ischiorectal (fossa) 566
jejunostomy 569.69
jejunum 569.81
joint 719.80
  ankle 719.87

Fistula — continued
joint — continued
  elbow 719.82
  foot 719.87
  hand 719.84
  hip 719.85
  knee 719.86
  multiple sites 719.89
  pelvic region 719.85
  shoulder (region) 719.81
  specified site NEC 719.88
  tuberculous — see Tuberculosis, joint
  wrist 719.83
kidney 593.89
labium (majus) (minus) 619.8
labyrinth, labyrinthine NEC 386.40
  combined sites 386.48
  multiple sites 386.48
  oval window 386.42
  round window 386.41
  semicircular canal 386.43
lacrimal, lachrymal (duct) (gland) (sac) 375.61
lacrimonasal duct 375.61
laryngotracheal 748.3
larynx 478.79
lip 528.5
  congenital 750.25
lumbar, tuberculous (see also Tuberculosis) 015.0 ☑ [730.8] ☑
lung 510.0
lymphatic (node) (vessel) 457.8
mamillary 611.0
mammary (gland) 611.0
  puerperal, postpartum 675.1 ☑
mastoid (process) (region) 383.1
maxillary (see also Sinusitis, maxillary) 473.0
mediastinal 510.0
mediastinobronchial 510.0
mediastinocutaneous 510.0
middle ear 385.89
mouth 528.3
nasal 478.19
  sinus (see also Sinusitis) 473.9
nasopharynx 478.29
nipple — see Fistula, breast
nose 478.19
oral (cutaneous) 528.3
  maxillary (see also Sinusitis, maxillary) 473.0
  nasal (with cleft palate) (see also Cleft, palate) 749.00
orbit, orbital 376.10
oro-antral (see also Sinusitis, maxillary) 473.0
oval window (internal ear) 386.42
oviduct (external) 619.2
palate (hard) 526.89
  soft 528.9
pancreatic 577.8
pancreaticoduodenal 577.8
parotid (gland) 527.4
  region 528.3
pelvoabdominointestinal 569.81
penis 607.89
perianal 565.1
pericardium (pleura) (sac) (see also Pericarditis) 423.8
pericecal 569.81
perineal — see Fistula, perineum
perineorectal 569.81
perineosigmoidal 569.81
perineo-urethroscrotal 608.89
perineum, perineal (with urethral involvement) NEC 599.1
  tuberculous (see also Tuberculosis) 017.9 ☑
  ureter 593.82
perirectal 565.1
  tuberculous (see also Tuberculosis) 014.8 ☑
peritoneum (see also Peritonitis) 567.22
periurethral 599.1
pharyngo-esophageal 478.29
pharynx 478.29
  branchial cleft (congenital) 744.41
pilonidal (infected) (rectum) 685.1

☑ Additional Digit Required — Refer to the Tabular List for Digit Selection
2011 ICD-9-CM ▶◄ Revised Text ● New Line ▲ Revised Code
Subterms under main terms may continue to next column or page
October 2010 • Volume 2 — 117

Index

Fish — Fistula

Index

Fistula — Flexion

Fistula — *continued*
pilonidal — *continued*
  with abscess 685.0
pleura, pleural, pleurocutaneous, pleuroperitoneal 510.0
  stomach 510.0
  tuberculous (*see also* Tuberculosis)
    012.0 ☑
pleuropericardial 423.8
postauricular 383.81
postoperative, persistent 998.6
preauricular (congenital) 744.46
prostate 602.8
pulmonary 510.0
  arteriovenous 417.0
    congenital 747.3
  tuberculous (*see also* Tuberculosis, pulmonary) 011.9 ☑
pulmonoperitoneal 510.0
rectolabial 619.1
rectosigmoid (intercommunicating) 569.81
rectoureteral 593.82
rectourethral 599.1
  congenital 753.8
rectouterine 619.1
  congenital 752.39 ▲
rectovaginal 619.1
  congenital 752.49
  old, postpartal 619.1
  tuberculous (*see also* Tuberculosis)
    014.8 ☑
rectovesical 596.1
  congenital 753.8
rectovesicovaginal 619.1
rectovulvar 619.1
  congenital 752.49
rectum (to skin) 565.1
  tuberculous (*see also* Tuberculosis)
    014.8 ☑
renal 593.89
retroauricular 383.81
round window (internal ear) 386.41
salivary duct or gland 527.4
  congenital 750.24
sclera 360.32
scrotum (urinary) 608.89
  tuberculous (*see also* Tuberculosis)
    016.5 ☑
semicircular canals (internal ear) 386.43
sigmoid 569.81
  vesicoabdominal 596.1
sigmoidovaginal 619.1
  congenital 752.49
skin 686.9
  ureter 593.82
  vagina 619.2
sphenoidal sinus (*see also* Sinusitis, sphenoidal) 473.3
splenocolic 289.59
stercoral 569.81
stomach 537.4
sublingual gland 527.4
  congenital 750.24
submaxillary
  gland 527.4
    congenital 750.24
  region 528.3
thoracic 510.0
  duct 457.8
thoracicoabdominal 510.0
thoracicogastric 510.0
thoracicointestinal 510.0
thoracoabdominal 510.0
thoracogastric 510.0
thorax 510.0
thyroglossal duct 759.2
thyroid 246.8
trachea (congenital) (external) (internal) 748.3
tracheoesophageal 530.84
  congenital 750.3
  following tracheostomy 519.09
traumatic
  arteriovenous (*see also* Injury, blood vessel, by site) 904.9
  brain — *see* Injury, intracranial

Fistula — *continued*
tuberculous — *see* Tuberculosis, by site
typhoid 002.0
umbilical 759.89
umbilico-urinary 753.8
urachal, urachus 753.7
ureter (persistent) 593.82
ureteroabdominal 593.82
ureterocervical 593.82
ureterorectal 593.82
ureterosigmoido-abdominal 593.82
ureterovaginal 619.0
ureterovesical 596.2
urethra 599.1
  congenital 753.8
  tuberculous (*see also* Tuberculosis)
    016.3 ☑
urethroperineal 599.1
urethroperineovesical 596.2
urethrorectal 599.1
  congenital 753.8
urethroscrotal 608.89
urethrovaginal 619.0
urethrovesical 596.2
urethrovesicovaginal 619.0
urinary (persistent) (recurrent) 599.1
uteroabdominal (anterior wall) 619.2
  congenital 752.39 ▲
uteroenteric 619.1
uterofecal 619.1
uterointestinal 619.1
  congenital 752.39 ▲
uterorectal 619.1
  congenital 752.39 ▲
uteroureteric 619.0
uterovaginal 619.8
uterovesical 619.0
  congenital 752.39 ▲
uterus 619.8
vagina (wall) 619.8
  postpartal, old 619.8
vaginocutaneous (postpartal) 619.2
vaginoileal (acquired) 619.1
vaginoperineal 619.2
vesical NEC 596.2
vesicoabdominal 596.2
vesicocervicovaginal 619.0
vesicocolic 596.1
vesicocutaneous 596.2
vesicoenteric 596.1
vesicointestinal 596.1
vesicometrorectal 619.1
vesicoperineal 596.2
vesicorectal 596.1
  congenital 753.8
vesicosigmoidal 596.1
vesicosigmoidovaginal 619.1
vesicoureteral 596.2
vesicoureterovaginal 619.0
vesicourethral 596.2
vesicourethrorectal 596.1
vesicouterine 619.0
  congenital 752.39 ▲
vesicovaginal 619.0
vulvorectal 619.1
  congenital 752.49

Fit 780.39
apoplectic (*see also* Disease, cerebrovascular, acute) 436
  late effect — *see* Late effect(s) (of) cerebrovascular disease
epileptic (*see also* Epilepsy) 345.9 ☑
fainting 780.2
hysterical 300.11
newborn 779.0

Fitting (of)
artificial
  arm (complete) (partial) V52.0
  breast V52.4
    implant exchange (different material) (different size) V52.4
  eye(s) V52.2
  leg(s) (complete) (partial) V52.1
brain neuropacemaker V53.02
cardiac pacemaker V53.31
carotid sinus pacemaker V53.39

Fitting — *continued*
cerebral ventricle (communicating) shunt V53.01
colostomy belt V53.5 ☑
contact lenses V53.1
cystostomy device V53.6
defibrillator, automatic implantable cardiac
  ▶(with synchronous cardiac pacemaker)◀ V53.32
dentures V52.3
device, unspecified type V53.90
  abdominal V53.59
  cardiac
    defibrillator, automatic implantable
    ▶(with synchronous cardiac pacemaker)◀ V53.32
    pacemaker V53.31
    specified NEC V53.39
  cerebral ventricle (communicating)
    shunt V53.01
  gastrointestinal NEC V53.59
  insulin pump V53.91
  intestinal V53.50
  intrauterine contraceptive
    insertion V25.11 ●
    removal V25.12 ●
      and reinsertion V25.13 ●
    replacement V25.13 ●
  nervous system V53.09
  orthodontic V53.4
  orthoptic V53.1
  other device V53.99
  prosthetic V52.9
    breast V52.4
    dental V52.3
    eye V52.2
    specified type NEC V52.8
  special senses V53.09
  substitution
    auditory V53.09
    nervous system V53.09
    visual V53.09
  urinary V53.6
diaphragm (contraceptive) V25.02
gastric lap band V53.51
gastrointestinal appliance and device NEC V53.59
glasses (reading) V53.1
growth rod V54.02
hearing aid V53.2
ileostomy device V53.5 ☑
intestinal appliance and device V53.50
intestinal appliance or device NEC V53.5 ☑
intrauterine contraceptive device
  insertion V25.11 ●
  removal V25.12 ●
    and reinsertion V25.13 ●
  replacement V25.13 ●
neuropacemaker (brain) (peripheral nerve) (spinal cord) V53.02
orthodontic device V53.4
orthopedic (device) V53.7
  brace V53.7
  cast V53.7
  corset V53.7
  shoes V53.7
pacemaker (cardiac) V53.31
  brain V53.02
  carotid sinus V53.39
  peripheral nerve V53.02
  spinal cord V53.02
prosthesis V52.9
  arm (complete) (partial) V52.0
  breast V52.4
    implant exchange (different material) (different size) V52.4
  dental V52.3
  eye V52.2
  leg (complete) (partial) V52.1
  specified type NEC V52.8
spectacles V53.1
wheelchair V53.8

Fitz-Hugh and Curtis syndrome 098.86
due to
  Chlamydia trachomatis 099.56

Fitz-Hugh and Curtis syndrome — *continued*
due to — *continued*
  Neisseria gonorrhoeae (gonococcal peritonitis) 098.86
Fitz's syndrome (acute hemorrhagic pancreatitis) 577.0
Fixation
joint — *see* Ankylosis
larynx 478.79
pupil 364.76
stapes 385.22
  deafness (*see also* Deafness, conductive) 389.04
uterus (acquired) — *see* Malposition, uterus
vocal cord 478.5
Flaccid — *see also* condition
foot 736.79
forearm 736.09
palate, congenital 750.26
Flail
chest 807.4
  newborn 767.3
joint (paralytic) 718.80
  ankle 718.87
  elbow 718.82
  foot 718.87
  hand 718.84
  hip 718.85
  knee 718.86
  multiple sites 718.89
  pelvic region 718.85
  shoulder (region) 718.81
  specified site NEC 718.88
  wrist 718.83
Flajani (-Basedow) syndrome or disease (exophthalmic goiter) 242.0 ☑
Flap, liver 572.8
Flare, anterior chamber (aqueous) (eye) 364.04
Flashback phenomena (drug) (hallucinogenic) 292.89
Flat
chamber (anterior) (eye) 360.34
chest, congenital 754.89
electroencephalogram (EEG) 348.89
foot (acquired) (fixed type) (painful) (postural) (spastic) 734
  congenital 754.61
    rocker bottom 754.61
    vertical talus 754.61
  rachitic 268.1
  rocker bottom (congenital) 754.61
  vertical talus, congenital 754.61
organ or site, congenital NEC — *see* Anomaly, specified type NEC
pelvis 738.6
  with disproportion (fetopelvic) 653.2 ☑
    affecting fetus or newborn 763.1
    causing obstructed labor 660.1 ☑
      affecting fetus or newborn 763.1
  congenital 755.69
Flatau-Schilder disease 341.1
Flattening
head, femur 736.39
hip 736.39
lip (congenital) 744.89
nose (congenital) 754.0
  acquired 738.0
Flatulence 787.3
Flatus 787.3
vaginalis 629.89
Flax dressers' disease 504
Flea bite — *see* Injury, superficial, by site
Fleischer (-Kayser) ring (corneal pigmentation) 275.1 [371.14]
Fleischner's disease 732.3
Fleshy mole 631
Flexibilitas cerea — *see also* Catalepsy 300.11
Flexion
cervix — *see* Flexion, uterus
contracture, joint (*see also* Contraction, joint) 718.4 ☑
deformity, joint (*see also* Contraction, joint) 736.9

☑ **Additional Digit Required — Refer to the Tabular List for Digit Selection**   ▽ **Subterms under main terms may continue to next column or page**

☑ Additional Digit Required — Refer to the Tabular List for Digit Selection   ⑊ Subterms under main terms may continue to next column or page

2011 ICD-9-CM   ▶◀ Revised Text   ● New Line   ▲ Revised Code   October 2010 • Volume 2 — 119

Foreign body — *continued*
  old or residual — *continued*
    soft tissue 729.6
      with granuloma 709.4
    subcutaneous tissue 729.6
      with granuloma 709.4
  operation wound, left accidentally 998.4
  orbit 870.4
    retained or old 376.6
  posterior wall, eye 871.6
    magnetic 871.5
      retained or old 360.55
    retained or old 360.65
  respiratory tree 934.9
    specified site NEC 934.8
  retained (old) (nonmagnetic) (in)
    V90.9 ▲
    anterior chamber (eye) 360.61
      magnetic 360.51
    ciliary body 360.62
      magnetic 360.52
    eyelid 374.86
    fragment(s)
      acrylics V90.2
      animal quills V90.31
      animal spines V90.31
      cement V90.83
      concrete V90.83
      crystalline V90.83
      depleted
        isotope V90.09
        uranium V90.01
      diethylhexylphthalates V90.2
      glass V90.81
      isocyanate V90.2
      metal V90.10
        magnetic V90.11
        nonmagnetic V90.12
      organic NEC V90.39
      plastic V90.2
      radioactive
        nontherapeutic V90.09
        specified NEC V90.09
      stone V90.83
      tooth V90.32
      wood V90.33
    globe 360.60
      magnetic 360.50
    intraocular 360.60
      magnetic 360.50
      specified site NEC 360.69
        magnetic 360.59
    iris 360.62
      magnetic 360.52
    lens 360.63
      magnetic 360.53
    muscle 729.6
    orbit 376.6
    posterior wall of globe 360.65
      magnetic 360.55
    retina 360.65
      magnetic 360.55
    retrobulbar 376.6
    skin 729.6
      with granuloma 709.4
    soft tissue 729.6
      with granuloma 709.4
    specified NEC V90.89
    subcutaneous tissue 729.6
      with granuloma 709.4
    vitreous 360.64
      magnetic 360.54
  retina 871.6
    magnetic 871.5
      retained or old 360.55
    retained or old 360.65
  superficial, without major open wound (*see also* Injury, superficial, by site) 919.6
  swallowed NEC 938
  throat, feeling of 784.99
  vitreous (humor) 871.6
    magnetic 871.5
      retained or old 360.54
    retained or old 360.64
Forking, aqueduct of Sylvius 742.3

Forking, aqueduct of Sylvius — *continued*
  with spina bifida (*see also* Spina bifida)
    741.0 ☑
Formation
  bone in scar tissue (skin) 709.3
  connective tissue in vitreous 379.25
  Elschnig pearls (postcataract extraction)
    366.51
  hyaline in cornea 371.49
  sequestrum in bone (due to infection) (*see also* Osteomyelitis) 730.1 ☑
  valve
    colon, congenital 751.5
    ureter (congenital) 753.29
Formication 782.0
Fort Bragg fever 100.89
Fossa — *see also* condition
  pyriform — *see* condition
Foster care (status) V60.81
Foster-Kennedy syndrome 377.04
Fothergill's
  disease, meaning scarlatina anginosa 034.1
  neuralgia (*see also* Neuralgia, trigeminal) 350.1
Foul breath 784.99
Found dead (cause unknown) 798.9
Foundling V20.0
Fournier's disease (idiopathic gangrene) 608.83
Fourth
  cranial nerve — *see* condition
  disease 057.8
  molar 520.1
Foville's syndrome 344.89
Fox's
  disease (apocrine miliaria) 705.82
  impetigo (contagiosa) 684
Fox-Fordyce disease (apocrine miliaria) 705.82
Fracture (abduction) (adduction) (avulsion) (compression) (crush) (dislocation) (oblique) (separation) (closed) 829.0

> *Note* — For fracture of any of the following sites with fracture of other bones — *see* Fracture, multiple.
>
> *"Closed" includes the following descriptions of fractures, with or without delayed healing, unless they are specified as open or compound:*
>
> | | |
> |---|---|
> | comminuted | linear |
> | depressed | simple |
> | elevated | slipped epiphysis |
> | fissured | spiral |
> | greenstick | unspecified |
> | impacted | |
>
> *"Open" includes the following descriptions of fractures, with or without delayed healing:*
>
> | | |
> |---|---|
> | compound | puncture |
> | infected | with foreign body |
> | missile | |
>
> *For late effect of fracture, see Late, effect, fracture, by site.*

  with
    internal injuries in same region (conditions classifiable to 860–869) (*see also* Injury, internal, by site)
    pelvic region — *see* Fracture, pelvis
  acetabulum (with visceral injury) (closed) 808.0
    open 808.1
  acromion (process) (closed) 811.01
    open 811.11
  alveolus (closed) 802.8
    open 802.9
  ankle (malleolus) (closed) 824.8
    bimalleolar (Dupuytren's) (Pott's) 824.4
      open 824.5
    bone 825.21
      open 825.31

Fracture — *continued*
  ankle — *continued*
    lateral malleolus only (fibular) 824.2
      open 824.3
    medial malleolus only (tibial) 824.0
      open 824.1
    open 824.9
    pathologic 733.16
    talus 825.21
      open 825.31
    trimalleolar 824.6
      open 824.7
  antrum — *see* Fracture, skull, base
  arm (closed) 818.0
    and leg(s) (any bones) 828.0
      open 828.1
    both (any bones) (with rib(s)) (with sternum) 819.0
      open 819.1
    lower 813.80
      open 813.90
    open 818.1
    upper — *see* Fracture, humerus
  astragalus (closed) 825.21
    open 825.31
  atlas — *see* Fracture, vertebra, cervical, first
  axis — *see* Fracture, vertebra, cervical, second
  back — *see* Fracture, vertebra, by site
  Barton's — *see* Fracture, radius, lower end
  basal (skull) — *see* Fracture, skull, base
  Bennett's (closed) 815.01
    open 815.11
  bimalleolar (closed) 824.4
    open 824.5
  bone (closed) NEC 829.0
    birth injury NEC 767.3
    open 829.1
    pathologic NEC (*see also* Fracture, pathologic) 733.10
    stress NEC (*see also* Fracture, stress) 733.95
  boot top — *see* Fracture, fibula
  boxers' — *see* Fracture, metacarpal bone(s)
  breast bone — *see* Fracture, sternum
  bucket handle (semilunar cartilage) — *see* Tear, meniscus
  buckle — *see* Fracture, torus
  burst — *see* Fracture, traumatic, by site
  bursting — *see* Fracture, phalanx, hand, distal
  calcaneus (closed) 825.0
    open 825.1
  capitate (bone) (closed) 814.07
    open 814.17
  capitellum (humerus) (closed) 812.49
    open 812.59
  carpal bone(s) (wrist NEC) (closed) 814.00
    open 814.10
    specified site NEC 814.09
      open 814.19
  cartilage, knee (semilunar) — *see* Tear, meniscus
  cervical — *see* Fracture, vertebra, cervical
  chauffeur's — *see* Fracture, ulna, lower end
  chisel — *see* Fracture, radius, upper end
  chronic — *see* Fracture, pathologic
  clavicle (interligamentous part) (closed) 810.00
    acromial end 810.03
      open 810.13
    due to birth trauma 767.2
    open 810.10
    shaft (middle third) 810.02
      open 810.12
    sternal end 810.01
      open 810.11
  clayshovelers' — *see* Fracture, vertebra, cervical
  coccyx (*see also* Fracture, vertebra, coccyx)
    complicating delivery 665.6 ☑
  collar bone — *see* Fracture, clavicle
  Colles' (reversed) (closed) 813.41
    open 813.51
  comminuted — *see* Fracture, by site
  compression (*see also* Fracture, by site)

Fracture — *continued*
  compression (*see also* Fracture, by site) — *continued*
    nontraumatic — *see* Fracture, pathologic
  congenital 756.9
  coracoid process (closed) 811.02
    open 811.12
  coronoid process (ulna) (closed) 813.02
    mandible (closed) 802.23
      open 802.33
    open 813.12
  corpus cavernosum penis 959.13
  costochondral junction — *see* Fracture, rib
  costosternal junction — *see* Fracture, rib
  cranium — *see* Fracture, skull, by site
  cricoid cartilage (closed) 807.5
    open 807.6
  cuboid (ankle) (closed) 825.23
    open 825.33
  cuneiform
    foot (closed) 825.24
      open 825.34
    wrist (closed) 814.03
      open 814.13
  dental implant 525.73
  dental restorative material
    with loss of material 525.64
    without loss of material 525.63
  due to
    birth injury — *see* Birth injury, fracture
    gunshot — *see* Fracture, by site, open
    neoplasm — *see* Fracture, pathologic
    osteoporosis — *see* Fracture, pathologic
  Dupuytren's (ankle) (fibula) (closed) 824.4
    open 824.5
    radius 813.42
      open 813.52
  Duverney's — *see* Fracture, ilium
  elbow (*see also* Fracture, humerus, lower end)
    olecranon (process) (closed) 813.01
      open 813.11
    supracondylar (closed) 812.41
      open 812.51
  ethmoid (bone) (sinus) — *see* Fracture, skull, base
  face bone(s) (closed) NEC 802.8
    with
      other bone(s) — *see* Fracture, multiple, skull
      skull (*see also* Fracture, skull)
        involving other bones — *see* Fracture, multiple, skull
    open 802.9
  fatigue — *see* Fracture, march
  femur, femoral (closed) 821.00
    cervicotrochanteric 820.03
      open 820.13
    condyles, epicondyles 821.21
      open 821.31
    distal end — *see* Fracture, femur, lower end
    epiphysis (separation)
      capital 820.01
        open 820.11
      head 820.01
        open 820.11
      lower 821.22
        open 821.32
      trochanteric 820.01
        open 820.11
      upper 820.01
        open 820.11
    head 820.09
      open 820.19
    lower end or extremity (distal end) (closed) 821.20
      condyles, epicondyles 821.21
        open 821.31
      epiphysis (separation) 821.22
        open 821.32
      multiple sites 821.29
        open 821.39
      open 821.30
      specified site NEC 821.29
        open 821.39

☑ **Additional Digit Required** — Refer to the Tabular List for Digit Selection   ▽ **Subterms under main terms may continue to next column or page**

120 — Volume 2 · October 2010   ▶◀ **Revised Text**   ● **New Line**   ▲ **Revised Code**   **2011 ICD-9-CM**

Fracture — *continued*
femur, femoral — *continued*
  lower end or extremity — *continued*
    supracondylar 821.23
      open 821.33
    T-shaped 821.21
      open 821.31
    neck (closed) 820.8
      base (cervicotrochanteric) 820.03
        open 820.13
      extracapsular 820.20
        open 820.30
      intertrochanteric (section) 820.21
        open 820.31
      intracapsular 820.00
        open 820.10
      intratrochanteric 820.21
        open 820.31
      midcervical 820.02
        open 820.12
      open 820.9
      pathologic 733.14
        specified part NEC 733.15
      specified site NEC 820.09
        open 820.19
      transcervical 820.02
        open 820.12
      transtrochanteric 820.20
        open 820.30
    open 821.10
    pathologic 733.14
      specified part NEC 733.15
    peritrochanteric (section) 820.20
      open 820.30
    shaft (lower third) (middle third) (upper third) 821.01
      open 821.11
    subcapital 820.09
      open 820.19
    subtrochanteric (region) (section) 820.22
      open 820.32
    supracondylar 821.23
      open 821.33
    transepiphyseal 820.01
      open 820.11
    trochanter (greater) (lesser) (*see also* Fracture, femur, neck, by site) 820.20
      open 820.30
    T-shaped, into knee joint 821.21
      open 821.31
    upper end 820.8
      open 820.9
fibula (closed) 823.81
  with tibia 823.82
    open 823.92
  distal end 824.8
    open 824.9
  epiphysis
    lower 824.8
      open 824.9
    upper — *see* Fracture, fibula, upper end
  head — *see* Fracture, fibula, upper end
  involving ankle 824.2
    open 824.3
  lower end or extremity 824.8
    open 824.9
  malleolus (external) (lateral) 824.2
    open 824.3
  open NEC 823.91
  pathologic 733.16
  proximal end — *see* Fracture, fibula, upper end
  shaft 823.21
    with tibia 823.22
      open 823.32
    open 823.31
  stress 733.93
  torus 823.41
    with tibia 823.42
  upper end or extremity (epiphysis) (head) (proximal end) (styloid) 823.01
    with tibia 823.02
      open 823.12

Fracture — *continued*
fibula — *continued*
  upper end or extremity — *continued*
    open 823.11
finger(s), of one hand (closed) (*see also* Fracture, phalanx, hand) 816.00
  with
    metacarpal bone(s), of same hand 817.0
      open 817.1
    thumb of same hand 816.03
      open 816.13
  open 816.10
foot, except toe(s) alone (closed) 825.20
  open 825.30
forearm (closed) NEC 813.80
  lower end (distal end) (lower epiphysis) 813.40
    open 813.50
    open 813.90
  shaft 813.20
    open 813.30
  upper end (proximal end) (upper epiphysis) 813.00
    open 813.10
fossa, anterior, middle, or posterior — *see* Fracture, skull, base
Fracture (abduction) (adduction) (avulsion) (compression) (crush) (dislocation) (oblique) (separation) (closed) 829.0
frontal (bone) (*see also* Fracture, skull, vault)
  sinus — *see* Fracture, skull, base
Galeazzi's — *see* Fracture, radius, lower end
glenoid (cavity) (fossa) (scapula) (closed) 811.03
  open 811.13
Gosselin's — *see* Fracture, ankle
greenstick — *see* Fracture, by site
grenade-throwers' — *see* Fracture, humerus, shaft
gutter — *see* Fracture, skull, vault
hamate (closed) 814.08
  open 814.18
hand, one (closed) 815.00
  carpals 814.00
    open 814.10
    specified site NEC 814.09
      open 814.19
  metacarpals 815.00
    open 815.10
  multiple, bones of one hand 817.0
    open 817.1
  open 815.10
  phalanges (*see also* Fracture, phalanx, hand) 816.00
    open 816.10
healing
  aftercare (*see also* Aftercare, fracture) V54.89
  change of cast V54.89
  complications — *see* condition
  convalescence V66.4
  removal of
    cast V54.89
    fixation device
      external V54.89
      internal V54.01
heel bone (closed) 825.0
  open 825.1
Hill-Sachs 812.09
hip (closed) (*see also* Fracture, femur, neck) 820.8
  open 820.9
  pathologic 733.14
humerus (closed) 812.20
  anatomical neck 812.02
    open 812.12
  articular process (*see also* Fracture humerus, condyle(s)) 812.44
    open 812.54
  capitellum 812.49
    open 812.59
  condyle(s) 812.44
    lateral (external) 812.42
      open 812.52
    medial (internal epicondyle) 812.43

Fracture — *continued*
humerus — *continued*
  condyle(s) — *continued*
    medial — *continued*
      open 812.53
      open 812.54
    distal end — *see* Fracture, humerus, lower end
  epiphysis
    lower (*see also* Fracture, humerus, condyle(s)) 812.44
      open 812.54
    upper 812.09
      open 812.19
  external condyle 812.42
    open 812.52
  great tuberosity 812.03
    open 812.13
  head 812.09
    open 812.19
  internal epicondyle 812.43
    open 812.53
  lesser tuberosity 812.09
    open 812.19
  lower end or extremity (distal end) (*see also* Fracture, humerus, by site) 812.40
    multiple sites NEC 812.49
      open 812.59
    open 812.50
    specified site NEC 812.49
      open 812.59
  neck 812.01
    open 812.11
  open 812.30
  pathologic 733.11
  proximal end — *see* Fracture, humerus, upper end
  shaft 812.21
    open 812.31
  supracondylar 812.41
    open 812.51
  surgical neck 812.01
    open 812.11
  trochlea 812.49
    open 812.59
  T-shaped 812.44
    open 812.54
  tuberosity — *see* Fracture, humerus, upper end
  upper end or extremity (proximal end) (*see also* Fracture, humerus, by site) 812.00
    open 812.10
    specified site NEC 812.09
      open 812.19
hyoid bone (closed) 807.5
  open 807.6
hyperextension — *see* Fracture, radius, lower end
ilium (with visceral injury) (closed) 808.41
  open 808.51
impaction, impacted — *see* Fracture, by site
incus — *see* Fracture, skull, base
innominate bone (with visceral injury) (closed) 808.49
  open 808.59
instep, of one foot (closed) 825.20
  with toe(s) of same foot 827.0
    open 827.1
  open 825.30
insufficiency — *see* Fracture, pathologic, by site
internal
  ear — *see* Fracture, skull, base
  semilunar cartilage, knee — *see* Tear, meniscus, medial
intertrochanteric — *see* Fracture, femur, neck, intertrochanteric
ischium (with visceral injury) (closed) 808.42
  open 808.52
jaw (bone) (lower) (closed) (*see also* Fracture, mandible) 802.20
  angle 802.25
    open 802.35
  open 802.30

Fracture — *continued*
jaw (*see also* Fracture, mandible) — *continued*
  upper — *see* Fracture, maxilla
knee
  cap (closed) 822.0
    open 822.1
  cartilage (semilunar) — *see* Tear, meniscus
labyrinth (osseous) — *see* Fracture, skull, base
larynx (closed) 807.5
  open 807.6
late effect — *see* Late, effects (of), fracture
Le Fort's — *see* Fracture, maxilla
leg (closed) 827.0
  with rib(s) or sternum 828.0
    open 828.1
  both (any bones) 828.0
    open 828.1
  lower — *see* Fracture, tibia
  open 827.1
  upper — *see* Fracture, femur
limb
  lower (multiple) (closed) NEC 827.0
    open 827.1
  upper (multiple) (closed) NEC 818.0
    open 818.1
long bones, due to birth trauma — *see* Birth injury, fracture
lower end or extremity (anterior lip) (posterior) 824.8
  open 824.9
lumbar — *see* Fracture, vertebra, lumbar
lunate bone (closed) 814.02
  open 814.12
malar bone (closed) 802.4
  open 802.5
Malgaigne's (closed) 808.43
  open 808.53
malleolus (closed) 824.8
  bimalleolar 824.4
    open 824.5
  lateral 824.2
    and medial (*see also* Fracture, malleolus, bimalleolar)
      with lip of tibia — *see* Fracture, malleolus, trimalleolar
    open 824.3
  medial (closed) 824.0
    and lateral (*see also* Fracture, malleolus, bimalleolar)
      with lip of tibia — *see* Fracture, malleolus, trimalleolar
    open 824.1
  open 824.9
  trimalleolar (closed) 824.6
    open 824.7
malleus — *see* Fracture, skull, base
malunion 733.81
mandible (closed) 802.20
  angle 802.25
    open 802.35
  body 802.28
    alveolar border 802.27
      open 802.37
    open 802.38
    symphysis 802.26
      open 802.36
  condylar process 802.21
    open 802.31
  coronoid process 802.23
    open 802.33
  multiple sites 802.29
    open 802.39
  open 802.30
  ramus NEC 802.24
    open 802.34
  subcondylar 802.22
    open 802.32
manubrium — *see* Fracture, sternum
march 733.95
  fibula 733.93
  metatarsals 733.94
  tibia 733.93

☑ Additional Digit Required — Refer to the Tabular List for Digit Selection   🔄 Subterms under main terms may continue to next column or page

2011 ICD-9-CM   ▶◀ Revised Text   ● New Line   ▲ Revised Code   Volume 2 — 121

Index

Fracture — Fracture

Fracture — *continued*

maxilla, maxillary (superior) (upper jaw) (closed) 802.4
  inferior — *see* Fracture, mandible
  open 802.5
meniscus, knee — *see* Tear, meniscus
metacarpus, metacarpal (bone(s)), of one hand (closed) 815.00
  with phalanx, phalanges, hand (finger(s)) (thumb) of same hand 817.0
    open 817.1
  base 815.02
    first metacarpal 815.01
      open 815.11
    open 815.12
    thumb 815.01
      open 815.11
  multiple sites 815.09
    open 815.19
  neck 815.04
    open 815.14
  open 815.10
  shaft 815.03
    open 815.13
metatarsus, metatarsal (bone(s)), of one foot (closed) 825.25
  with tarsal bone(s) 825.29
    open 825.39
  open 825.35
Monteggia's (closed) 813.03
  open 813.13
Moore's — *see* Fracture, radius, lower end
multangular bone (closed)
  larger 814.05
    open 814.15
  smaller 814.06
    open 814.16
multiple (closed) 829.0

Note — *Multiple fractures of sites classifiable to the same three- or four-digit category are coded to that category, except for sites classifiable to 810–818 or 820–827 in different limbs.*

Multiple fractures of sites classifiable to different fourth-digit subdivisions within the same three–digit category should be dealt with according to coding rules.

Multiple fractures of sites classifiable to different three–digit categories (identifiable from the listing under "Fracture"), and of sites classifiable to 810–818 or 820–827 in different limbs should be coded according to the following list, which should be referred to in the following priority order: skull or face bones, pelvis or vertebral column, legs, arms.

  arm (multiple bones in same arm except in hand alone) (sites classifiable to 810–817 with sites classifiable to a different three–digit category in 810–817 in same arm) (closed) 818.0
    open 818.1
  arms, both or arm(s) with rib(s) or sternum (sites classifiable to 810–818 with sites classifiable to same range of categories in other limb or to 807) (closed) 819.0
    open 819.1
  bones of trunk NEC (closed) 809.0
    open 809.1
  hand, metacarpal bone(s) with phalanx or phalanges of same hand (sites classifiable to 815 with sites classifiable to 816 in same hand) (closed) 817.0
    open 817.1
  leg (multiple bones in same leg) (sites classifiable to 820–826 with sites classifiable to a different three–digit category in that range in same leg) (closed) 827.0
    open 827.1

Fracture — *continued*

multiple — *continued*
  legs, both or leg(s) with arm(s), rib(s), or sternum (sites classifiable to 820–827 with sites classifiable to same range of categories in other leg or to 807 or 810–819) (closed) 828.0
    open 828.1
  open 829.1
  pelvis with other bones except skull or face bones (sites classifiable to 808 with sites classifiable to 805–807 or 810–829) (closed) 809.0
    open 809.1
  skull, specified or unspecified bones, or face bone(s) with any other bone(s) (sites classifiable to 800–803 with sites classifiable to 805–829) (closed) 804.0 ☑

Note — *Use the following fifth-digit subclassification with categories 800, 801, 803, and 804:*

0 *unspecified state of consciousness*

1 *with no loss of consciousness*

2 *with brief [less than one hour] loss of consciousness*

3 *with moderate [1–24 hours] loss of consciousness*

4 *with prolonged [more than 24 hours] loss of consciousness and return to pre–existing conscious level*

5 *with prolonged [more than 24 hours] loss of consciousness, without return to pre–existing conscious level*

Use fifth-digit 5 to designate when a patient is unconscious and dies before regaining consciousness, regardless of the duration of the loss of consciousness

6 *with loss of consciousness of unspecified duration*

9 *with concussion, unspecified*

  with
    contusion, cerebral 804.1 ☑
    epidural hemorrhage 804.2 ☑
    extradural hemorrhage 804.2 ☑
    hemorrhage (intracranial) NEC 804.3 ☑
    intracranial injury NEC 804.4 ☑
    laceration, cerebral 804.1 ☑
    subarachnoid hemorrhage 804.2 ☑
    subdural hemorrhage 804.2 ☑
  open 804.5 ☑
    with
      contusion, cerebral 804.6 ☑
      epidural hemorrhage 804.7 ☑
      extradural hemorrhage 804.7 ☑
      hemorrhage (intracranial) NEC 804.8 ☑
      intracranial injury NEC 804.9 ☑
      laceration, cerebral 804.6 ☑
      subarachnoid hemorrhage 804.7 ☑
      subdural hemorrhage 804.7 ☑
  vertebral column with other bones, except skull or face bones (sites classifiable to 805 or 806 with sites classifiable to 807–808 or 810–829) (closed) 809.0
    open 809.1
nasal (bone(s)) (closed) 802.0
  open 802.1
  sinus — *see* Fracture, skull, base

Fracture — *continued*

navicular
  carpal (wrist) (closed) 814.01
    open 814.11
  tarsal (ankle) (closed) 825.22
    open 825.32
neck — *see* Fracture, vertebra, cervical
neural arch — *see* Fracture, vertebra, by site
nonunion 733.82
nose, nasal, (bone) (septum) (closed) 802.0
  open 802.1
occiput — *see* Fracture, skull, base
odontoid process — *see* Fracture, vertebra, cervical
olecranon (process) (ulna) (closed) 813.01
  open 813.11
open 829.1
orbit, orbital (bone) (region) (closed) 802.8
  floor (blow-out) 802.6
    open 802.7
  open 802.9
  roof — *see* Fracture, skull, base
  specified part NEC 802.8
    open 802.9
os
  calcis (closed) 825.0
    open 825.1
  magnum (closed) 814.07
    open 814.17
  pubis (with visceral injury) (closed) 808.2
    open 808.3
  triquetrum (closed) 814.03
    open 814.13
osseous
  auditory meatus — *see* Fracture, skull, base
  labyrinth — *see* Fracture, skull, base
ossicles, auditory (incus) (malleus) (stapes) — *see* Fracture, skull, base
osteoporotic — *see* Fracture, pathologic
palate (closed) 802.8
  open 802.9
paratrooper — *see* Fracture, tibia, lower end
parietal bone — *see* Fracture, skull, vault
parry — *see* Fracture, Monteggia's
patella (closed) 822.0
  open 822.1
pathologic (cause unknown) 733.10
  ankle 733.16
  femur (neck) 733.14
    specified NEC 733.15
  fibula 733.16
  hip 733.14
  humerus 733.11
  radius (distal) 733.12
  specified site NEC 733.19
  tibia 733.16
  ulna 733.12
  vertebrae (collapse) 733.13
  wrist 733.12
pedicle (of vertebral arch) — *see* Fracture, vertebra, by site
pelvis, pelvic (bone(s)) (with visceral injury) (closed) 808.8
  multiple ▶with disruption of pelvic circle◀ 808.43
    open 808.53
  open 808.9
  rim (closed) 808.49
    open 808.59
peritrochanteric (closed) 820.20
  open 820.30
phalanx, phalanges, of one
  foot (closed) 826.0
    with bone(s) of same lower limb 827.0
      open 827.1
    open 826.1
  hand (closed) 816.00
    with metacarpal bone(s) of same hand 817.0
      open 817.1
    distal 816.02
      open 816.12
    middle 816.01
      open 816.11

Fracture — *continued*

phalanx, phalanges, of one — *continued*
  hand — *continued*
    multiple sites NEC 816.03
      open 816.13
    open 816.10
    proximal 816.01
      open 816.11
pisiform (closed) 814.04
  open 814.14
pond — *see* Fracture, skull, vault
Pott's (closed) 824.4
  open 824.5
prosthetic device, internal — *see* Complications, mechanical
pubis (with visceral injury) (closed) 808.2
  open 808.3
Quervain's (closed) 814.01
  open 814.11
radius (alone) (closed) 813.81
  with ulna NEC 813.83
    open 813.93
  distal end — *see* Fracture, radius, lower end
  epiphysis
    lower — *see* Fracture, radius, lower end
    upper — *see* Fracture, radius, upper end
  head — *see* Fracture, radius, upper end
  lower end or extremity (distal end) (lower epiphysis) 813.42
    with ulna (lower end) 813.44
      open 813.54
    open 813.52
    torus 813.45
      with ulna 813.47
  neck — *see* Fracture, radius, upper end
  open NEC 813.91
  pathologic 733.12
  proximal end — *see* Fracture, radius, upper end
  shaft (closed) 813.21
    with ulna (shaft) 813.23
      open 813.33
    open 813.31
  upper end 813.07
    with ulna (upper end) 813.08
      open 813.18
    epiphysis 813.05
      open 813.15
    head 813.05
      open 813.15
    multiple sites 813.07
      open 813.17
    neck 813.06
      open 813.16
    open 813.17
    specified site NEC 813.07
      open 813.17
ramus
  inferior or superior (with visceral injury) (closed) 808.2
    open 808.3
  ischium — *see* Fracture, ischium
  mandible 802.24
    open 802.34

☑ **Additional Digit Required** — **Refer to the Tabular List for Digit Selection**

▽ **Subterms under main terms may continue to next column or page**

Fracture — *continued*
  rib(s) (closed) 807.0 ☑

> *Note* — *Use the following fifth-digit subclassification with categories 807.0–807.1:*
>
> 0 *rib(s), unspecified*
>
> 1 *one rib*
>
> 2 *two ribs*
>
> 3 *three ribs*
>
> 4 *four ribs*
>
> 5 *five ribs*
>
> 6 *six ribs*
>
> 7 *seven ribs*
>
> 8 *eight or more ribs*
>
> 9 *multiple ribs, unspecified*

      with flail chest (open) 807.4
      open 807.1 ☑
  root, tooth 873.63
      complicated 873.73
  sacrum — *see* Fracture, vertebra, sacrum
  scaphoid
      ankle (closed) 825.22
        open 825.32
      wrist (closed) 814.01
        open 814.11
  scapula (closed) 811.00
      acromial, acromion (process) 811.01
        open 811.11
      body 811.09
        open 811.19
      coracoid process 811.02
        open 811.12
      glenoid (cavity) (fossa) 811.03
        open 811.13
      neck 811.03
        open 811.13
        open 811.10
  semilunar
      bone, wrist (closed) 814.02
        open 814.12
      cartilage (interior) (knee) — *see* Tear, meniscus
  sesamoid bone — *see* Fracture, by site
  Shepherd's (closed) 825.21
      open 825.31
  shoulder (*see also* Fracture, humerus, upper end)
      blade — *see* Fracture, scapula
  silverfork — *see* Fracture, radius, lower end
  sinus (ethmoid) (frontal) (maxillary) (nasal) (sphenoidal) — *see* Fracture, skull, base
  Skillern's — *see* Fracture, radius, shaft

Fracture — *continued*
  skull (multiple NEC) (with face bones) (closed) 803.0 ☑

> *Note* — *Use the following fifth-digit subclassification with categories 800, 801, 803, and 804:*
>
> 0 *unspecified state of consciousness*
>
> 1 *with no loss of consciousness*
>
> 2 *with brief [less than one hour] loss of consciousness*
>
> 3 *with moderate [1-24 hours] loss of consciousness*
>
> 4 *with prolonged [more than 24 hours] loss of consciousness and return to pre-existing conscious level*
>
> 5 *with prolonged [more than 24 hours] loss of consciousness, without return to pre-existing conscious level*
>
> *Use fifth-digit 5 to designate when a patient is unconscious and dies before regaining consciousness, regardless of the duration of the loss of consciousness*
>
> 6 *with loss of consciousness of unspecified duration*
>
> 9 *with concussion, unspecified*

      with
        contusion, cerebral 803.1 ☑
        epidural hemorrhage 803.2 ☑
        extradural hemorrhage 803.2 ☑
        hemorrhage (intracranial) NEC 803.3 ☑
        intracranial injury NEC 803.4 ☑
        laceration, cerebral 803.1 ☑
        other bones — *see* Fracture, multiple, skull
        subarachnoid hemorrhage 803.2 ☑
        subdural hemorrhage 803.2 ☑
      base (antrum) (ethmoid bone) (fossa) (internal ear) (nasal sinus) (occiput) (sphenoid) (temporal bone) (closed) 801.0 ☑
        with
          contusion, cerebral 801.1 ☑
          epidural hemorrhage 801.2 ☑
          extradural hemorrhage 801.2 ☑
          hemorrhage (intracranial) NEC 801.3 ☑
          intracranial injury NEC 801.4 ☑
          laceration, cerebral 801.1 ☑
          subarachnoid hemorrhage 801.2 ☑
          subdural hemorrhage 801.2 ☑
        open 801.5 ☑
          with
            contusion, cerebral 801.6 ☑
            epidural hemorrhage 801.7 ☑
            extradural hemorrhage 801.7 ☑
            hemorrhage (intracranial) NEC 801.8 ☑
            intracranial injury NEC 801.9 ☑
            laceration, cerebral 801.6 ☑
            subarachnoid hemorrhage 801.7 ☑
            subdural hemorrhage 801.7 ☑
      birth injury 767.3
      face bones — *see* Fracture, face bones
      open 803.5 ☑

Fracture — *continued*
  skull — *continued*
      open — *continued*
        with
          contusion, cerebral 803.6 ☑
          epidural hemorrhage 803.7 ☑
          extradural hemorrhage 803.7 ☑
          hemorrhage (intracranial) NEC 803.8 ☑
          intracranial injury NEC 803.9 ☑
          laceration, cerebral 803.6 ☑
          subarachnoid hemorrhage 803.7 ☑
          subdural hemorrhage 803.7 ☑
      vault (frontal bone) (parietal bone) (vertex) (closed) 800.0 ☑
        with
          contusion, cerebral 800.1 ☑
          epidural hemorrhage 800.2 ☑
          extradural hemorrhage 800.2 ☑
          hemorrhage (intracranial) NEC 800.3 ☑
          intracranial injury NEC 800.4 ☑
          laceration, cerebral 800.1 ☑
          subarachnoid hemorrhage 800.2 ☑
          subdural hemorrhage 800.2 ☑
        open 800.5 ☑
          with
            contusion, cerebral 800.6 ☑
            epidural hemorrhage 800.7 ☑
            extradural hemorrhage 800.7 ☑
            hemorrhage (intracranial) NEC 800.8 ☑
            intracranial injury NEC 800.9 ☑
            laceration, cerebral 800.6 ☑
            subarachnoid hemorrhage 800.7 ☑
            subdural hemorrhage 800.7 ☑
  Smith's 813.41
      open 813.51
  sphenoid (bone) (sinus) — *see* Fracture, skull, base
  spine (*see also* Fracture, vertebra, by site due to birth trauma) 767.4
  spinous process — *see* Fracture, vertebra, by site
  spontaneous — *see* Fracture, pathologic
  sprinters' — *see* Fracture, ilium
  stapes — *see* Fracture, skull, base
  stave (*see also* Fracture, metacarpus, metacarpal bone(s))
      spine — *see* Fracture, tibia, upper end
  sternum (closed) 807.2
      with flail chest (open) 807.4
      open 807.3
  Stieda's — *see* Fracture, femur, lower end
  stress 733.95
      fibula 733.93
      metatarsals 733.94
      specified site NEC 733.95
      tibia 733.93
  styloid process
      metacarpal (closed) 815.02
        open 815.12
      radius — *see* Fracture, radius, lower end
      temporal bone — *see* Fracture, skull, base
      ulna — *see* Fracture, ulna, lower end
  supracondylar, elbow 812.41
      open 812.51

Fracture — *continued*
  symphysis pubis (with visceral injury) (closed) 808.2
      open 808.3
  talus (ankle bone) (closed) 825.21
      open 825.31
  tarsus, tarsal bone(s) (with metatarsus) of one foot (closed) NEC 825.29
      open 825.39
  temporal bone (styloid) — *see* Fracture, skull, base
  tendon — *see* Sprain, by site
  thigh — *see* Fracture, femur, shaft
  thumb (and finger(s)) of one hand (closed) (*see also* Fracture, phalanx, hand) 816.00
      with metacarpal bone(s) of same hand 817.0
        open 817.1
      metacarpal(s) — *see* Fracture, metacarpus
      open 816.10
  thyroid cartilage (closed) 807.5
      open 807.6
  tibia (closed) 823.80
      with fibula 823.82
        open 823.92
      condyles — *see* Fracture, tibia, upper end
      distal end 824.8
        open 824.9
      epiphysis
        lower 824.8
          open 824.9
        upper — *see* Fracture, tibia, upper end
      head (involving knee joint) — *see* Fracture, tibia, upper end
      intercondyloid eminence — *see* Fracture, tibia, upper end
      involving ankle 824.0
        open 824.9
      lower end or extremity (anterior lip) (posterior lip) 824.8
        open 824.9
      malleolus (internal) (medial) 824.0
        open 824.1
      open NEC 823.90
      pathologic 733.16
      proximal end — *see* Fracture, tibia, upper end
      shaft 823.20
        with fibula 823.22
          open 823.32
        open 823.30
      spine — *see* Fracture, tibia, upper end
      stress 733.93
      torus 823.40
        with fibula 823.42
      tuberosity — *see* Fracture, tibia, upper end
      upper end or extremity (condyle) (epiphysis) (head) (spine) (proximal end) (tuberosity) 823.00
        with fibula 823.02
          open 823.12
        open 823.10
  toe(s), of one foot (closed) 826.0
      with bone(s) of same lower limb 827.0
        open 827.1
      open 826.1
  tooth (root) 873.63
      complicated 873.73
  torus
      fibula 823.41
        with tibia 823.42
      humerus 812.49
      radius (alone) 813.45
        with ulna 813.47
      tibia 823.40
        with fibula 823.42
      ulna (alone) 813.46
        with radius 813.47
  trachea (closed) 807.5
      open 807.6

☑ Additional Digit Required — Refer to the Tabular List for Digit Selection   ▽ Subterms under main terms may continue to next column or page

2011 ICD-9-CM   ▶◀ Revised Text   ● New Line   ▲ Revised Code   Volume 2 — 123

Fracture — *continued*
- transverse process — *see* Fracture, vertebra, by site
- trapezium (closed) 814.05
  - open 814.15
- trapezoid bone (closed) 814.06
  - open 814.16
- trimalleolar (closed) 824.6
  - open 824.7
- triquetral (bone) (closed) 814.03
  - open 814.13
- trochanter (greater) (lesser) (closed) (*see also* Fracture, femur, neck, by site) 820.20
  - open 820.30
- trunk (bones) (closed) 809.0
  - open 809.1
- tuberosity (external) — *see* Fracture, by site
- ulna (alone) (closed) 813.82
  - with radius NEC 813.83
    - open 813.93
  - coronoid process (closed) 813.02
    - open 813.12
  - distal end — *see* Fracture, ulna, lower end
  - epiphysis
    - lower — *see* Fracture, ulna, lower end
    - upper — *see* Fracture, ulna, upper end
  - head — *see* Fracture, ulna, lower end
  - lower end (distal end) (head) (lower epiphysis) (styloid process) 813.43
    - with radius (lower end) 813.44
      - open 813.54
    - open 813.53
  - olecranon process (closed) 813.01
    - open 813.11
  - open NEC 813.92
  - pathologic 733.12
  - proximal end — *see* Fracture, ulna, upper end
  - shaft 813.22
    - with radius (shaft) 813.23
      - open 813.33
    - open 813.32
  - styloid process — *see* Fracture, ulna, lower end
  - torus 813.46
    - with radius 813.47
  - transverse — *see* Fracture, ulna, by site
  - upper end (epiphysis) 813.04
    - with radius (upper end) 813.08
      - open 813.18
    - multiple sites 813.04
      - open 813.14
    - open 813.14
    - specified site NEC 813.04
      - open 813.14
- unciform (closed) 814.08
  - open 814.18
- vertebra, vertebral (back) (body) (column) (neural arch) (pedicle) (spine) (spinous process) (transverse process) (closed) 805.8
  - with
    - hematomyelia — *see* Fracture, vertebra, by site, with spinal cord injury
    - injury to
      - cauda equina — *see* Fracture, vertebra, sacrum, with spinal cord injury
      - nerve — *see* Fracture, vertebra, by site, with spinal cord injury
    - paralysis — *see* Fracture, vertebra, by site, with spinal cord injury
    - paraplegia — *see* Fracture, vertebra, by site, with spinal cord injury
    - quadriplegia — *see* Fracture, vertebra, by site, with spinal cord injury
    - spinal concussion — *see* Fracture, vertebra, by site, with spinal cord injury

Fracture — *continued*
- vertebra, vertebral — *continued*
  - with — *continued*
    - spinal cord injury (closed) NEC 806.8

Note — *Use the following fifth-digit subclassification with categories 806.0–806.3:*

C_1–C_4 *or unspecified level and* D_1–D_6 (T_1–T_6) *or unspecified level with*

- 0 *unspecified spinal cord injury*
- 1 *complete lesion of cord*
- 2 *anterior cord syndrome*
- 3 *central cord syndrome*
- 4 *specified injury NEC*

C_5–C_7 *level and* D_7–D_{12} *level with:*

- 5 *unspecified spinal cord injury*
- 6 *complete lesion of cord*
- 7 *anterior cord syndrome*
- 8 *central cord syndrome*
- 9 *specified injury NEC*

  - cervical 806.0 ☑
    - open 806.1 ☑
  - dorsal, dorsolumbar 806.2 ☑
    - open 806.3 ☑
  - open 806.9
  - thoracic, thoracolumbar 806.2 ☑
    - open 806.3 ☑
- atlanto-axial — *see* Fracture, vertebra, cervical
- cervical (hangman) (teardrop) (closed) 805.00
  - with spinal cord injury — *see* Fracture, vertebra, with spinal cord injury, cervical
  - first (atlas) 805.01
    - open 805.11
  - second (axis) 805.02
    - open 805.12
  - third 805.03
    - open 805.13
  - fourth 805.04
    - open 805.14
  - fifth 805.05
    - open 805.15
  - sixth 805.06
    - open 805.16
  - seventh 805.07
    - open 805.17
  - multiple sites 805.08
    - open 805.18
  - open 805.10
- chronic 733.13
- coccyx (closed) 805.6
  - with spinal cord injury (closed) 806.60
    - cauda equina injury 806.62
      - complete lesion 806.61
        - open 806.71
      - open 806.72
    - open 806.70
    - specified type NEC 806.69
      - open 806.79
  - open 805.7
- collapsed 733.13
- compression, not due to trauma 733.13
- dorsal (closed) 805.2
  - with spinal cord injury — *see* Fracture, vertebra, with spinal cord injury, dorsal
  - open 805.3
- dorsolumbar (closed) 805.2
  - with spinal cord injury — *see* Fracture, vertebra, with spinal cord injury, dorsal
  - open 805.3
- due to osteoporosis 733.13
- fetus or newborn 767.4
- lumbar (closed) 805.4
  - with spinal cord injury (closed) 806.4

Fracture — *continued*
- vertebra, vertebral — *continued*
  - lumbar — *continued*
    - with spinal cord injury — *continued*
      - open 806.5
    - open 805.5
  - nontraumatic 733.13
  - open NEC 805.9
  - pathologic (any site) 733.13
  - sacrum (closed) 805.6
    - with spinal cord injury 806.60
      - cauda equina injury 806.62
        - complete lesion 806.61
          - open 806.71
        - open 806.72
      - open 806.70
      - specified type NEC 806.69
        - open 806.79
    - open 805.7
  - site unspecified (closed) 805.8
    - with spinal cord injury (closed) 806.8
      - open 806.9
    - open 805.9
  - stress (any site) 733.95
  - thoracic (closed) 805.2
    - with spinal cord injury — *see* Fracture, vertebra, with spinal cord injury, thoracic
    - open 805.3
  - vertex — *see* Fracture, skull, vault
  - vomer (bone) 802.0
    - open 802.1
- Wagstaffe's — *see* Fracture, ankle
- wrist (closed) 814.00
  - open 814.10
  - pathologic 733.12
- xiphoid (process) — *see* Fracture, sternum
- zygoma (zygomatic arch) (closed) 802.4
  - open 802.5

Fragile X syndrome 759.83

Fragilitas
- crinium 704.2
- hair 704.2
- ossium 756.51
  - with blue sclera 756.51
- unguium 703.8
  - congenital 757.5

Fragility
- bone 756.51
  - with deafness and blue sclera 756.51
- capillary (hereditary) 287.8
- hair 704.2
- nails 703.8

Fragmentation — *see* Fracture, by site

Frailty 797

Frambesia, frambesial (tropica) — *see also* Yaws 102.9
- initial lesion or ulcer 102.0
- primary 102.0

Frambeside
- gummatous 102.4
- of early yaws 102.2

Frambesioma 102.1

Franceschetti's syndrome (mandibulofacial dysostosis) 756.0

Francis' disease — *see also* Tularemia 021.9

Franklin's disease (heavy chain) 273.2

Frank's essential thrombocytopenia — *see also* Purpura, thrombocytopenic 287.39

Fraser's syndrome 759.89

Freckle 709.09
- malignant melanoma in (M8742/3) — *see* Melanoma
- melanotic (of Hutchinson) (M8742/2) — *see* Neoplasm, skin, in situ
- retinal 239.81

Freeman-Sheldon syndrome 759.89

Freezing 991.9
- specified effect NEC 991.8

Freiberg's
- disease (osteochondrosis, second metatarsal) 732.5
- infraction of metatarsal head 732.5
- osteochondrosis 732.5

Frei's disease (climatic bubo) 099.1

Fremitus, friction, cardiac 785.3

Frenulum linguae 750.0

Frenum
- external os 752.44 ▲
- tongue 750.0

Frequency (urinary) NEC 788.41
- micturition 788.41
- nocturnal 788.43
- polyuria 788.42
- psychogenic 306.53

Frey's syndrome (auriculotemporal syndrome) 705.22

Friction
- burn (*see also* Injury, superficial, by site) 919.0
- fremitus, cardiac 785.3
- precordial 785.3
- sounds, chest 786.7

Friderichsen-Waterhouse syndrome or disease 036.3

Friedländer's
- B (bacillus) NEC (*see also* condition) 041.3
  - sepsis or septicemia 038.49
- disease (endarteritis obliterans) — *see* Arteriosclerosis

Friedreich's
- ataxia 334.0
- combined systemic disease 334.0
- disease 333.2
  - combined systemic 334.0
- myoclonia 333.2
- sclerosis (spinal cord) 334.0

Friedrich-Erb-Arnold syndrome (acropachyderma) 757.39

Frigidity 302.72
- psychic or psychogenic 302.72

Fröhlich's disease or syndrome (adiposogenital dystrophy) 253.8

Froin's syndrome 336.8

Frommel-Chiari syndrome 676.6 ☑

Frommel's disease 676.6 ☑

Frontal — *see also* condition
- lobe syndrome 310.0

Frostbite 991.3
- face 991.0
- foot 991.2
- hand 991.1
- specified site NEC 991.3

Frotteurism 302.89

Frozen 991.9
- pelvis 620.8
- shoulder 726.0

Fructosemia 271.2

Fructosuria (benign) (essential) 271.2

Fuchs'
- black spot (myopic) 360.21
- corneal dystrophy (endothelial) 371.57
- heterochromic cyclitis 364.21

Fucosidosis 271.8

Fugue 780.99
- dissociative 300.13
- hysterical (dissociative) 300.13
- reaction to exceptional stress (transient) 308.1

Fukuhara syndrome 277.87

Fuller Albright's syndrome (osteitis fibrosa disseminata) 756.59

Fuller's earth disease 502

Fulminant, fulminating — *see* condition

Functional — *see* condition

Functioning
- borderline intellectual V62.89

Fundus — *see also* condition
- flavimaculatus 362.76

Fungemia 117.9

Fungus, fungous
- cerebral 348.89
- disease NEC 117.9
- infection — *see* Infection, fungus
- testis (*see also* Tuberculosis) 016.5 ☑ [608.81]

Funiculitis (acute) 608.4
- chronic 608.4
- endemic 608.4
- gonococcal (acute) 098.14

Funiculitis — *continued*
  gonococcal — *continued*
    chronic or duration of 2 months or over
      098.34
  tuberculous (*see also* Tuberculosis) 016.5 ☑
Funnel
  breast (acquired) 738.3
    congenital 754.81
    late effect of rickets 268.1
  chest (acquired) 738.3
    congenital 754.81
    late effect of rickets 268.1
  pelvis (acquired) 738.6
    with disproportion (fetopelvic) 653.3 ☑
      affecting fetus or newborn 763.1
      causing obstructed labor 660.1 ☑
        affecting fetus or newborn 763.1
    congenital 755.69
    tuberculous (*see also* Tuberculosis)
      016.9 ☑
FUO — *see also* Pyrexia 780.60
Furfur 690.18
  microsporon 111.0
Furor, paroxysmal (idiopathic) — *see also*
  Epilepsy 345.8 ☑
Furriers' lung 495.8
Furrowed tongue 529.5
  congenital 750.13
Furrowing nail(s) (transverse) 703.8
  congenital 757.5
Furuncle 680.9
  abdominal wall 680.2
  ankle 680.6
  anus 680.5
  arm (any part, above wrist) 680.3
  auditory canal, external 680.0
  axilla 680.3
  back (any part) 680.2
  breast 680.2
  buttock 680.5
  chest wall 680.2
  corpus cavernosum 607.2

Furuncle — *continued*
  ear (any part) 680.0
  eyelid 373.13
  face (any part, except eye) 680.0
  finger (any) 680.4
  flank 680.2
  foot (any part) 680.7
  forearm 680.3
  gluteal (region) 680.5
  groin 680.2
  hand (any part) 680.4
  head (any part, except face) 680.8
  heel 680.7
  hip 680.6
  kidney (*see also* Abscess, kidney) 590.2
  knee 680.6
  labium (majus) (minus) 616.4
  lacrimal
    gland (*see also* Dacryoadenitis) 375.00
    passages (duct) (sac) (*see also* Dacryocys-
      titis) 375.30
  leg, any part except foot 680.6
  malignant 022.0
  multiple sites 680.9
  neck 680.1
  nose (external) (septum) 680.0
  orbit 376.01
  partes posteriores 680.5
  pectoral region 680.2
  penis 607.2
  perineum 680.2
  pinna 680.0
  scalp (any part) 680.8
  scrotum 608.4
  seminal vesicle 608.0
  shoulder 680.3
  skin NEC 680.9
  specified site NEC 680.8
  spermatic cord 608.4
  temple (region) 680.0
  testis 604.90
  thigh 680.6

Furuncle — *continued*
  thumb 680.4
  toe (any) 680.7
  trunk 680.2
  tunica vaginalis 608.4
  umbilicus 680.2
  upper arm 680.3
  vas deferens 608.4
  vulva 616.4
  wrist 680.4
Furunculosis — *see also* Furuncle 680.9
  external auditory meatus 680.0 *[380.13]*
Fusarium (infection) 118
Fusion, fused (congenital)
  anal (with urogenital canal) 751.5
  aorta and pulmonary artery 745.0
  astragaloscaphoid 755.67
  atria 745.5
  atrium and ventricle 745.69
  auditory canal 744.02
  auricles, heart 745.5
  binocular, with defective stereopsis 368.33
  bone 756.9
  cervical spine — *see* Fusion, spine
  choanal 748.0
  commissure, mitral valve 746.5
  cranial sutures, premature 756.0
  cusps, heart valve NEC 746.89
    mitral 746.5
    tricuspid 746.89
  ear ossicles 744.04
  fingers (*see also* Syndactylism, fingers)
    755.11
  hymen 752.42
  hymeno-urethral 599.89
    causing obstructed labor 660.1 ☑
      affecting fetus or newborn 763.1
  joint (acquired) (*see also* Ankylosis)
    congenital 755.8
  kidneys (incomplete) 753.3
  labium (majus) (minus) 752.49
  larynx and trachea 748.3

Fusion, fused — *continued*
  limb 755.8
    lower 755.69
    upper 755.59
  lobe, lung 748.5
  lumbosacral (acquired) 724.6
    congenital 756.15
    surgical V45.4
  nares (anterior) (posterior) 748.0
  nose, nasal 748.0
  nostril(s) 748.0
  organ or site NEC — *see* Anomaly, specified
    type NEC
  ossicles 756.9
    auditory 744.04
  pulmonary valve segment 746.02
  pulmonic cusps 746.02
  ribs 756.3
  sacroiliac (acquired) (joint) 724.6
    congenital 755.69
    surgical V45.4
  skull, imperfect 756.0
  spine (acquired) 724.9
    arthrodesis status V45.4
    congenital (vertebra) 756.15
    postoperative status V45.4
  sublingual duct with submaxillary duct at
    opening in mouth 750.26
  talonavicular (bar) 755.67
  teeth, tooth 520.2
  testes 752.89
  toes (*see also* Syndactylism, toes) 755.13
  trachea and esophagus 750.3
  twins 759.4
  urethral-hymenal 599.89
  vagina 752.49
  valve cusps — *see* Fusion, cusps, heart valve
  ventricles, heart 745.4
  vertebra (arch) — *see* Fusion, spine
  vulva 752.49
Fusospirillosis (mouth) (tongue) (tonsil) 101
Fussy infant (baby) 780.91

☑ **Additional Digit Required** — Refer to the Tabular List for Digit Selection   ⁿᵉʷ **Subterms under main terms may continue to next column or page**

2011 ICD-9-CM   ▶◀ Revised Text   ● New Line   ▲ Revised Code   Volume 2 — 125

G

Gafsa boil 085.1
Gain, weight (abnormal) (excessive) — *see also* Weight, gain 783.1
Gaisböck's disease or syndrome (polycythemia hypertonica) 289.0
Gait
  abnormality 781.2
    hysterical 300.11
  ataxic 781.2
    hysterical 300.11
  disturbance 781.2
    hysterical 300.11
  paralytic 781.2
  scissor 781.2
  spastic 781.2
  staggering 781.2
    hysterical 300.11
Galactocele (breast) (infected) 611.5
  puerperal, postpartum 676.8 ☑
Galactophoritis 611.0
  puerperal, postpartum 675.2 ☑
Galactorrhea 676.6 ☑
  not associated with childbirth 611.6
Galactosemia (classic) (congenital) 271.1
Galactosuria 271.1
Galacturia 791.1
  bilharziasis 120.0
Galen's vein — *see* condition
Gallbladder — *see also* condition
  acute (*see also* Disease, gallbladder) 575.0
Gall duct — *see* condition
Gallop rhythm 427.89
Gallstone (cholemic) (colic) (impacted) — *see also* Cholelithiasis
  causing intestinal obstruction 560.31
Gambling, pathological 312.31
Gammaloidosis 277.39
Gammopathy 273.9
  macroglobulinemia 273.3
  monoclonal (benign) (essential) (idiopathic) (with lymphoplasmacytic dyscrasia) 273.1
Gamna's disease (sideriotic splenomegaly) 289.51
Gampsodactylia (congenital) 754.71
Gamstorp's disease (adynamia episodica hereditaria) 359.3
Gandy-Nanta disease (sideriotic splenomegaly) 289.51
Gang activity, without manifest psychiatric disorder V71.09
  adolescent V71.02
  adult V71.01
  child V71.02
Gangliocytoma (M9490/0) — *see* Neoplasm, connective tissue, benign
Ganglioglioma (M9505/1) — *see* Neoplasm, by site, uncertain behavior
Ganglion 727.43
  joint 727.41
  of yaws (early) (late) 102.6
  periosteal (*see also* Periostitis) 730.3 ☑
  tendon sheath (compound) (diffuse) 727.42
  tuberculous (*see also* Tuberculosis) 015.9 ☑
Ganglioneuroblastoma (M9490/3) — *see* Neoplasm, connective tissue, malignant
Ganglioneuroma (M9490/0) — *see also* Neoplasm, connective tissue, benign
  malignant (M9490/3) — *see* Neoplasm, connective tissue, malignant
Ganglioneuromatosis (M9491/0) — *see* Neoplasm, connective tissue, benign
Ganglionitis
  fifth nerve (*see also* Neuralgia, trigeminal) 350.1
  gasserian 350.1
  geniculate 351.1
    herpetic 053.11
    newborn 767.5
  herpes zoster 053.11
  herpetic geniculate (Hunt's syndrome) 053.11
Gangliosidosis 330.1
Gangosa 102.5

Gangrene, gangrenous (anemia) (artery) (cellulitis) (dermatitis) (dry) (infective) (moist) (pemphigus) (septic) (skin) (stasis) (ulcer) 785.4
  with
    arteriosclerosis (native artery) 440.24
      bypass graft 440.30
        autologous vein 440.31
        nonautologous biological 440.32
    diabetes (mellitus) 250.7 ☑ [785.4]
      due to secondary diabetes 249.7 ☑ [785.4]
  abdomen (wall) 785.4
  adenitis 683
  alveolar 526.5
  angina 462
    diphtheritic 032.0
  anus 569.49
  appendices epiploicae — *see* Gangrene, mesentery
  appendix — *see* Appendicitis, acute
  arteriosclerotic — *see* Arteriosclerosis, with, gangrene
  auricle 785.4
  Bacillus welchii (*see also* Gangrene, gas) 040.0
  bile duct (*see also* Cholangitis) 576.8
  bladder 595.89
  bowel — *see* Gangrene, intestine
  cecum — *see* Gangrene, intestine
  Clostridium perfringens or welchii (*see also* Gangrene, gas) 040.0
  colon — *see* Gangrene, intestine
  connective tissue 785.4
  cornea 371.40
  corpora cavernosa (infective) 607.2
    noninfective 607.89
  cutaneous, spreading 785.4
  decubital (*see also* Ulcer, pressure) 707.00 [785.4]
  diabetic (any site) 250.7 ☑ [785.4]
    due to secondary diabetes 249.7 ☑ [785.4]
  dropsical 785.4
  emphysematous (*see also* Gangrene, gas) 040.0
  epidemic (ergotized grain) 988.2
  epididymis (infectional) (*see also* Epididymitis) 604.99
  erysipelas (*see also* Erysipelas) 035
  extremity (lower) (upper) 785.4
  gallbladder or duct (*see also* Cholecystitis, acute) 575.0
  gas (bacillus) 040.0
    with
      abortion — *see* Abortion, by type, with sepsis
      ectopic pregnancy (*see also* categories 633.0–633.9) 639.0
      molar pregnancy (*see also* categories 630–632) 639.0
    following
      abortion 639.0
      ectopic or molar pregnancy 639.0
    puerperal, postpartum, childbirth 670.8 ☑
  glossitis 529.0
  gum 523.8
  hernia — *see* Hernia, by site, with gangrene
  hospital noma 528.1
  intestine, intestinal (acute) (hemorrhagic) (massive) 557.0
    with
      hernia — *see* Hernia, by site, with gangrene
      mesenteric embolism or infarction 557.0
      obstruction (*see also* Obstruction, intestine) 560.9
  laryngitis 464.00
    with obstruction 464.01
  liver 573.8
  lung 513.0
    spirochetal 104.8
  lymphangitis 457.2
  Meleney's (cutaneous) 686.09

Gangrene, gangrenous — *continued*
  mesentery 557.0
    with
      embolism or infarction 557.0
      intestinal obstruction (*see also* Obstruction, intestine) 560.9
  mouth 528.1
  noma 528.1
  orchitis 604.90
  ovary (*see also* Salpingo-oophoritis) 614.2
  pancreas 577.0
  penis (infectional) 607.2
    noninfective 607.89
  perineum 785.4
  pharynx 462
  pneumonia 513.0
  Pott's 440.24
  presenile 443.1
  pulmonary 513.0
  pulp, tooth 522.1
  quinsy 475
  Raynaud's (symmetric gangrene) 443.0 [785.4]
  rectum 569.49
  retropharyngeal 478.24
  rupture — *see* Hernia, by site, with gangrene
  scrotum 608.4
    noninfective 608.83
  senile 440.24
  septic 034.0
  septic 034.0
  sore throat 462
  spermatic cord 608.4
    noninfective 608.89
  spine 785.4
  spirochetal NEC 104.8
  spreading cutaneous 785.4
  stomach 537.89
  stomatitis 528.1
  symmetrical 443.0 [785.4]
  testis (infectional) (*see also* Orchitis) 604.99
    noninfective 608.89
  throat 462
    diphtheritic 032.0
  thyroid (gland) 246.8
  tonsillitis (acute) 463
  tooth (pulp) 522.1
  tuberculous NEC (*see also* Tuberculosis) 011.9 ☑
  tunica vaginalis 608.4
    noninfective 608.89
  umbilicus 785.4
  uterus (*see also* Endometritis) 615.9
  uvulitis 528.3
  vas deferens 608.4
    noninfective 608.89
  vulva (*see also* Vulvitis) 616.10
Gannister disease (occupational) 502
  with tuberculosis — *see* Tuberculosis, pulmonary
Ganser's syndrome, hysterical 300.16
Gardner-Diamond syndrome (autoerythrocyte sensitization) 287.2
Gargoylism 277.5
Garré's
  disease (*see also* Osteomyelitis) 730.1 ☑
  osteitis (sclerosing) (*see also* Osteomyelitis) 730.1 ☑
  osteomyelitis (*see also* Osteomyelitis) 730.1 ☑
Garrod's pads, knuckle 728.79
Gartner's duct
  cyst 752.41
  persistent 752.41
Gas 787.3
  asphyxia, asphyxiation, inhalation, poisoning, suffocation NEC 987.9
    specified gas — *see* Table of Drugs and Chemicals
  bacillus gangrene or infection — *see* Gas, gangrene
  cyst, mesentery 568.89
  excessive 787.3
  gangrene 040.0

Gas — *continued*
  gangrene — *continued*
    with
      abortion — *see* Abortion, by type, with sepsis
      ectopic pregnancy (*see also* categories 633.0–633.9) 639.0
      molar pregnancy (*see also* categories 630–632) 639.0
    following
      abortion 639.0
      ectopic or molar pregnancy 639.0
    puerperal, postpartum, childbirth 670.8 ☑
  on stomach 787.3
  pains 787.3
Gastradenitis 535.0 ☑
Gastralgia 536.8
  psychogenic 307.89
Gastrectasis, gastrectasia 536.1
  psychogenic 306.4
Gastric — *see* condition
Gastrinoma (M8153/1)
  malignant (M8153/3)
    pancreas 157.4
    specified site NEC — *see* Neoplasm, by site, malignant
    unspecified site 157.4
  specified site — *see* Neoplasm, by site, uncertain behavior
  unspecified site 235.5
Gastritis 535.5 ☑

Note — Use the following fifth-digit subclassification for category 535:

0   without mention of hemorrhage

1   with hemorrhage

  acute 535.0 ☑
  alcoholic 535.3 ☑
  allergic 535.4 ☑
  antral 535.4 ☑
  atrophic 535.1 ☑
  atrophic-hyperplastic 535.1 ☑
  bile-induced 535.4 ☑
  catarrhal 535.0 ☑
  chronic (atrophic) 535.1 ☑
  cirrhotic 535.4 ☑
  corrosive (acute) 535.4 ☑
  dietetic 535.4 ☑
  due to diet deficiency 269.9 [535.4] ☑
  eosinophilic 535.7 ☑
  erosive 535.4 ☑
  follicular 535.4 ☑
    chronic 535.1 ☑
  giant hypertrophic 535.2 ☑
  glandular 535.4 ☑
    chronic 535.1 ☑
  hypertrophic (mucosa) 535.2 ☑
    chronic giant 211.1
  irritant 535.4 ☑
  nervous 306.4
  phlegmonous 535.0 ☑
  psychogenic 306.4
  sclerotic 535.4 ☑
  spastic 536.8
  subacute 535.0 ☑
  superficial 535.4 ☑
  suppurative 535.0 ☑
  toxic 535.4 ☑
  tuberculous (*see also* Tuberculosis) 017.9 ☑
Gastrocarcinoma (M8010/3) 151.9
Gastrocolic — *see* condition
Gastrocolitis — *see* Enteritis
Gastrodisciasis 121.8
Gastroduodenitis — *see also* Gastritis 535.5 ☑
  catarrhal 535.0 ☑
  infectional 535.0 ☑
  virus, viral 008.8
    specified type NEC 008.69
Gastrodynia 536.8
Gastroenteritis (acute) (catarrhal) (congestive) (hemorrhagic) (noninfectious) — *see also* Enteritis 558.9
  aertrycke infection 003.0

☑ Additional Digit Required — Refer to the Tabular List for Digit Selection   ▽ Subterms under main terms may continue to next column or page

2011 ICD-9-CM   ▶◀ Revised Text   ● New Line   ▲ Revised Code   Volume 2 — 127

Gastroenteritis — see also Enteritis — continued
  allergic 558.3
  chronic 558.9
    ulcerative (see also Colitis, ulcerative) 556.9
  dietetic 558.9
  due to
    antineoplastic chemotherapy 558.9
    food poisoning (see also Poisoning, food) 005.9
    radiation 558.1
  eosinophilic 558.41
  epidemic 009.0
  functional 558.9
  infectious (see also Enteritis, due to, by organism) 009.0
    presumed 009.1
  salmonella 003.0
  septic (see also Enteritis, due to, by organism) 009.0
  toxic 558.2
  tuberculous (see also Tuberculosis) 014.8 ☑
  ulcerative (see also Colitis, ulcerative) 556.9
  viral NEC 008.8
    specified type NEC 008.69
  zymotic 009.0
Gastroenterocolitis — see Enteritis
Gastroenteropathy, protein-losing 579.8
Gastroenteroptosis 569.89
Gastroesophageal laceration-hemorrhage syndrome 530.7
Gastroesophagitis 530.19
Gastrohepatitis — see also Gastritis 535.5 ☑
Gastrointestinal — see condition
Gastrojejunal — see condition
Gastrojejunitis — see also Gastritis 535.5 ☑
Gastrojejunocolic — see condition
Gastroliths 537.89
Gastromalacia 537.89
Gastroparalysis 536.3
  diabetic 250.6 ☑ [536.3]
    due to secondary diabetes 249.6 ☑ [536.3]
Gastroparesis 536.3
  diabetic 250.6 ☑ [536.3]
    due to secondary diabetes 249.6 ☑ [536.3]
Gastropathy 537.9
  congestive portal 537.89
  erythematous 535.5 ☑
  exudative 579.8
  portal hypertensive 537.89
Gastroptosis 537.5
Gastrorrhagia 578.0
Gastrorrhea 536.8
  psychogenic 306.4
Gastroschisis (congenital) 756.73
  acquired 569.89
Gastrospasm (neurogenic) (reflex) 536.8
  neurotic 306.4
  psychogenic 306.4
Gastrostaxis 578.0
Gastrostenosis 537.89
Gastrostomy
  attention to V55.1
  complication 536.40
    specified type 536.49
  infection 536.41
  malfunctioning 536.42
  status V44.1
Gastrosuccorrhea (continuous) (intermittent) 536.8
  neurotic 306.4
  psychogenic 306.4
Gaucher's
  disease (adult) (cerebroside lipidosis) (infantile) 272.7
  hepatomegaly 272.7
  splenomegaly (cerebroside lipidosis) 272.7
GAVE (gastric antral vascular ectasia) 537.82
  with hemorrhage 537.83
  without hemorrhage 537.82
Gayet's disease (superior hemorrhagic polioencephalitis) 265.1

Gayet-Wernicke's syndrome (superior hemorrhagic polioencephalitis) 265.1
Gee (-Herter) (-Heubner) (-Thaysen) disease or syndrome (nontropical sprue) 579.0
Gélineau's syndrome — see also Narcolepsy 347.00
Gemination, teeth 520.2
Gemistocytoma (M9411/3)
  specified site — see Neoplasm, by site, malignant
  unspecified site 191.9
General, generalized — see condition
Genetic
  susceptibility to
    MEN (multiple endocrine neoplasia) V84.81
    neoplasia
      multiple endocrine (MEN) V84.81
    neoplasm
      malignant, of
        breast V84.01
        endometrium V84.04
        other V84.09
        ovary V84.02
        prostate V84.03
    specified disease NEC V84.89
Genital — see condition
  warts 078.11
Genito-anorectal syndrome 099.1
Genitourinary system — see condition
Genu
  congenital 755.64
  extrorsum (acquired) 736.42
    congenital 755.64
    late effects of rickets 268.1
  introrsum (acquired) 736.41
    congenital 755.64
    late effects of rickets 268.1
  rachitic (old) 268.1
  recurvatum (acquired) 736.5
    congenital 754.40
      with dislocation of knee 754.41
    late effects of rickets 268.1
  valgum (acquired) (knock-knee) 736.41
    congenital 755.64
    late effects of rickets 268.1
  varum (acquired) (bowleg) 736.42
    congenital 755.64
    late effect of rickets 268.1
Geographic tongue 529.1
Geophagia 307.52
Geotrichosis 117.9
  intestine 117.9
  lung 117.9
  mouth 117.9
Gephyrophobia 300.29
Gerbode defect 745.4
GERD (gastroesophageal reflux disease) 530.81
Gerhardt's
  disease (erythromelalgia) 443.82
  syndrome (vocal cord paralysis) 478.30
Gerlier's disease (epidemic vertigo) 078.81
German measles 056.9
  exposure to V01.4
Germinoblastoma (diffuse) (M9614/3) 202.8 ☑
  follicular (M9692/3) 202.0 ☑
Germinoma (M9064/3) — see Neoplasm, by site, malignant
Gerontoxon 371.41
Gerstmann-Sträussler-Scheinker syndrome (GSS) 046.71
Gerstmann's syndrome (finger agnosia) 784.69
Gestation (period) — see also Pregnancy
  ectopic NEC (see also Pregnancy, ectopic) 633.90
    with intrauterine pregnancy 633.91
  multiple ●
    placenta status ●
      quadruplet ●
        two or more monoamniotic fetuses V91.22 ●
        two or more monochorionic fetuses V91.21 ●

Gestation — see also Pregnancy — continued
  multiple — continued
    placenta status — continued
      quadruplet — continued
        unable to determine number of ●
          placenta and number of ●
          amniotic sacs V91.29 ●
        unspecified number of placenta ●
          and unspecified number ●
          of amniotic sacs V91.20 ●
      specified (greater than quadruplets) NEC ●
        two or more monoamniotic fetuses V91.92 ●
        two or more monochorionic fetuses V91.91 ●
        unable to determine number of ●
          placenta and number of ●
          amniotic sacs V91.99 ●
        unspecified number of placenta ●
          and unspecified number ●
          of amniotic sacs V91.90 ●
      triplet ●
        two or more monoamniotic fetuses V91.12 ●
        two or more monochorionic fetuses V91.11 ●
        unable to determine number of ●
          placenta and number of ●
          amniotic sacs V91.19 ●
        unspecified number of placenta, unspecified number ●
          of amniotic sacs V91.10 ●
      twin ●
        dichorionic/diamniotic (two ●
          placentae, two amniotic ●
          sacs) V91.03 ●
        monochorionic/diamniotic (one ●
          placenta, two amniotic ●
          sacs) V91.02 ●
        monochorionic/monoamniotic ●
          (one placenta, one amni- ●
          otic sac) V91.01 ●
        unable to determine number of ●
          placenta and number of ●
          amniotic sacs V91.09 ●
        unspecified number of placen- ●
          ta, unspecified number ●
          of amniotic sacs V91.00 ●
Gestational proteinuria 646.2 ☑
  with hypertension — see Toxemia, of pregnancy
Ghon tubercle primary infection — see also Tuberculosis 010.0 ☑
Ghost
  teeth 520.4
  vessels, cornea 370.64
Ghoul hand 102.3
Gianotti Crosti syndrome 057.8
  due to known virus — see Infection, virus
  due to unknown virus 057.8
Giant
  cell
    epulis 523.8
    peripheral (gingiva) 523.8
    tumor, tendon sheath 727.02
  colon (congenital) 751.3
  esophagus (congenital) 750.4
  kidney 753.3
  urticaria 995.1
    hereditary 277.6
Giardia lamblia infestation 007.1
Giardiasis 007.1
Gibert's disease (pityriasis rosea) 696.3
Gibraltar fever — see Brucellosis
Giddiness 780.4
  hysterical 300.11
  psychogenic 306.9
Gierke's disease (glycogenosis I) 271.0
Gigantism (cerebral) (hypophyseal) (pituitary) 253.0
Gilbert's disease or cholemia (familial nonhemolytic jaundice) 277.4
Gilchrist's disease (North American blastomycosis) 116.0

Gilford (-Hutchinson) disease or syndrome (progeria) 259.8
Gilles de la Tourette's disease (motor-verbal tic) 307.23
Gillespie's syndrome (dysplasia oculodentodigitalis) 759.89
Gingivitis 523.10
  acute 523.00
    necrotizing 101
    non-plaque induced 523.01
    plaque induced 523.00
  catarrhal 523.00
  chronic 523.10
    non-plaque induced 523.11
  desquamative 523.10
  expulsiva 523.40
  hyperplastic 523.10
  marginal, simple 523.10
  necrotizing, acute 101
  non-plaque induced 523.11
  pellagrous 265.2
  plaque induced 523.10
  ulcerative 523.10
    acute necrotizing 101
    Vincent's 101
Gingivoglossitis 529.0
Gingivopericementitis 523.40
Gingivosis 523.10
Gingivostomatitis 523.10
  herpetic 054.2
Giovannini's disease 117.9
GISA (glycopeptide intermediate staphylococcus aureus) V09.8 ☑
Glanders 024
Gland, glandular — see condition
Glanzmann (-Naegeli) disease or thrombasthenia 287.1
Glassblowers' disease 527.1
Glaucoma (capsular) (inflammatory) (noninflammatory) (primary) 365.9
  with increased episcleral venous pressure 365.82
  absolute 360.42
  acute 365.22
    narrow angle 365.22
    secondary 365.60
  angle closure 365.20
    acute 365.22
    chronic 365.23
    intermittent 365.21
    interval 365.21
    residual stage 365.24
    subacute 365.21
  borderline 365.00
  chronic 365.11
    noncongestive 365.11
    open angle 365.11
    simple 365.11
  closed angle — see Glaucoma, angle closure
  congenital 743.20
    associated with other eye anomalies 743.22
    simple 743.21
  congestive — see Glaucoma, narrow angle
  corticosteroid-induced (glaucomatous stage) 365.31
    residual stage 365.32
  hemorrhagic 365.60
  hypersecretion 365.81
  infantile 365.14
    congenital 743.20
      associated with other eye anomalies 743.22
      simple 743.21
  in or with
    aniridia 365.42
    Axenfeld's anomaly 365.41
    congenital syndromes NEC 759.89 [365.44]
    disorder of lens NEC 365.59
    inflammation, ocular 365.62
    iris
      anomalies NEC 365.42
      atrophy, essential 365.42
      bombé 365.61
    microcornea 365.43

☑ **Additional Digit Required** — Refer to the Tabular List for Digit Selection   ▽ **Subterms under main terms may continue to next column or page**

128 — Volume 2 · October 2010   ▶◀ Revised Text   ● New Line   ▲ Revised Code   **2011 ICD-9-CM**

Glaucoma — *continued*
in or with — *continued*
  neurofibromatosis 237.71 *[365.44]*
  ocular
    cysts NEC 365.64
    disorders NEC 365.60
    trauma 365.65
    tumors NEC 365.64
  pupillary block or seclusion 365.61
  Rieger's anomaly or syndrome 365.41
  seclusion of pupil 365.61
  Sturge-Weber (-Dimitri) syndrome
    759.6 *[365.44]*
  systemic syndrome NEC 365.44
  tumor of globe 365.64
  vascular disorders NEC 365.63
juvenile 365.14
low tension 365.12
malignant 365.83
narrow angle (primary) 365.20
  acute 365.22
  chronic 365.23
  intermittent 365.21
  interval 365.21
  residual stage 365.24
  subacute 365.21
newborn 743.20
  associated with other eye anomalies
    743.22
  simple 743.21
noncongestive (chronic) 365.11
nonobstructive (chronic) 365.11
obstructive 365.60
  due to lens changes 365.59
open angle 365.10
  with
    borderline intraocular pressure
      365.01
    cupping of optic discs 365.01
  primary 365.11
  residual stage 365.15
phacolytic 365.51
pigmentary 365.13
postinfectious 365.60
pseudoexfoliation 365.52
secondary NEC 365.60
simple (chronic) 365.11
simplex 365.11
steroid responders 365.03
suspect 365.00
syphilitic 095.8
traumatic NEC 365.65
  newborn 767.8
wide angle (*see also* Glaucoma, open angle)
  365.10
Glaucomatous flecks (subcapsular) 366.31
Glazed tongue 529.4
Gleet 098.2
Glénard's disease or syndrome (enteroptosis)
  569.89
Glinski-Simmonds syndrome (pituitary
  cachexia) 253.2
Glioblastoma (multiforme) (M9440/3)
with sarcomatous component (M9442/3)
  specified site — *see* Neoplasm, by site,
    malignant
  unspecified site 191.9
giant cell (M9441/3)
  specified site — *see* Neoplasm, by site,
    malignant
  unspecified site 191.9
specified site — *see* Neoplasm, by site, malignant
unspecified site 191.9
Glioma (malignant) (M9380/3)
astrocytic (M9400/3)
  specified site — *see* Neoplasm, by site,
    malignant
  unspecified site 191.9
mixed (M9382/3)
  specified site — *see* Neoplasm, by site,
    malignant
  unspecified site 191.9
nose 748.1
specified site NEC — *see* Neoplasm, by site,
  malignant

Glioma — *continued*
subependymal (M9383/1) 237.5
unspecified site 191.9
Gliomatosis cerebri (M9381/3) 191.0
Glioneuroma (M9505/1) — *see* Neoplasm, by
  site, uncertain behavior
Gliosarcoma (M9380/3)
specified site — *see* Neoplasm, by site, malignant
unspecified site 191.9
Gliosis (cerebral) 349.89
spinal 336.0
Glisson's
cirrhosis — *see* Cirrhosis, portal
disease (*see also* Rickets) 268.0
Glissonitis 573.3
Globinuria 791.2
Globus 306.4
hystericus 300.11
Glomangioma (M8712/0) — *see also* Hemangioma 228.00
Glomangiosarcoma (M8710/3) — *see* Neoplasm, connective tissue, malignant
Glomerular nephritis — *see also* Nephritis
  583.9
Glomerulitis — *see also* Nephritis 583.9
Glomerulonephritis — *see also* Nephritis 583.9
with
  edema (*see also* Nephrosis) 581.9
  lesion of
    exudative nephritis 583.89
    interstitial nephritis (diffuse) (focal)
      583.89
    necrotizing glomerulitis 583.4
      acute 580.4
      chronic 582.4
    renal necrosis 583.9
      cortical 583.6
      medullary 583.7
    specified pathology NEC 583.89
      acute 580.89
      chronic 582.89
  necrosis, renal 583.9
    cortical 583.6
    medullary (papillary) 583.7
  specified pathology or lesion NEC 583.89
acute 580.9
  with
    exudative nephritis 580.89
    interstitial nephritis (diffuse) (focal)
      580.89
    necrotizing glomerulitis 580.4
    extracapillary with epithelial crescents
      580.4
  poststreptococcal 580.0
  proliferative (diffuse) 580.0
  rapidly progressive 580.4
  specified pathology NEC 580.89
arteriolar (*see also* Hypertension, kidney)
  403.90
arteriosclerotic (*see also* Hypertension, kidney) 403.90
ascending (*see also* Pyelitis) 590.80
basement membrane NEC 583.89
  with
    pulmonary hemorrhage (Goodpas-
      ture's syndrome)
      446.21 *[583.81]*
chronic 582.9
  with
    exudative nephritis 582.89
    interstitial nephritis (diffuse) (focal)
      582.89
    necrotizing glomerulitis 582.4
    specified pathology or lesion NEC
      582.89
  endothelial 582.2
  extracapillary with epithelial crescents
    582.4
  hypocomplementemic persistent 582.2
  lobular 582.2
  membranoproliferative 582.2
  membranous 582.1
    and proliferative (mixed) 582.2
    sclerosing 582.1
  mesangiocapillary 582.2

Glomerulonephritis — *see also* Nephritis —
continued
chronic — *continued*
  mixed membranous and proliferative
    582.2
  proliferative (diffuse) 582.0
  rapidly progressive 582.4
  sclerosing 582.1
cirrhotic — *see* Sclerosis, renal
desquamative — *see* Nephrosis
due to or associated with
  amyloidosis 277.39 *[583.81]*
    with nephrotic syndrome
      277.39 *[581.81]*
    chronic 277.39 *[582.81]*
  diabetes mellitus 250.4 ☑ *[583.81]*
    with nephrotic syndrome
      250.4 ☑ *[581.81]*
    due to secondary diabetes
      249.4 ☑ *[581.81]*
    due to secondary diabetes
      249.4 ☑ *[581.81]*
  diphtheria 032.89 *[580.81]*
  gonococcal infection (acute)
    098.19 *[583.81]*
    chronic or duration of 2 months or
      over 098.39 *[583.81]*
  infectious hepatitis 070.9 *[580.81]*
  malaria (with nephrotic syndrome)
    084.9 *[581.81]*
  mumps 072.79 *[580.81]*
  polyarteritis (nodosa) (with nephrotic
    syndrome) 446.0 *[581.81]*
  specified pathology NEC 583.89
    acute 580.89
    chronic 582.89
  streptotrichosis 039.8 *[583.81]*
  subacute bacterial endocarditis
    421.0 *[580.81]*
  syphilis (late) 095.4
    congenital 090.5 *[583.81]*
    early 091.69 *[583.81]*
  systemic lupus erythematosus
    710.0 *[583.81]*
    with nephrotic syndrome
      710.0 *[581.81]*
    chronic 710.0 *[582.81]*
  tuberculosis (*see also* Tuberculosis)
    016.0 ☑ *[583.81]*
  typhoid fever 002.0 *[580.81]*
extracapillary with epithelial crescents 583.4
  acute 580.4
  chronic 582.4
exudative 583.89
  acute 580.89
  chronic 582.89
focal (*see also* Nephritis) 583.9
  embolic 580.4
granular 582.89
granulomatous 582.89
hydremic (*see also* Nephrosis) 581.9
hypocomplementemic persistent 583.2
  with nephrotic syndrome 581.2
  chronic 582.2
immune complex NEC 583.89
infective (*see also* Pyelitis) 590.80
interstitial (diffuse) (focal) 583.89
  with nephrotic syndrome 581.89
  acute 580.89
  chronic 582.89
latent or quiescent 582.9
lobular 583.2
  with nephrotic syndrome 581.2
  chronic 582.2
membranoproliferative 583.2
  with nephrotic syndrome 581.2
  chronic 582.2
membranous 583.1
  with nephrotic syndrome 581.1
  and proliferative (mixed) 583.2
    with nephrotic syndrome 581.2
    chronic 582.2
  chronic 582.1
  sclerosing 582.1
    with nephrotic syndrome 581.1
mesangiocapillary 583.2

Glomerulonephritis — *see also* Nephritis —
continued
mesangiocapillary — *continued*
  with nephrotic syndrome 581.2
  chronic 582.2
minimal change 581.3
mixed membranous and proliferative 583.2
  with nephrotic syndrome 581.2
  chronic 582.2
necrotizing 583.4
  acute 580.4
  chronic 582.4
nephrotic (*see also* Nephrosis) 581.9
old — *see* Glomerulonephritis, chronic
parenchymatous 581.89
poststreptococcal 580.0
proliferative (diffuse) 583.0
  with nephrotic syndrome 581.0
  acute 580.0
  chronic 582.0
purulent (*see also* Pyelitis) 590.80
quiescent — *see* Nephritis, chronic
rapidly progressive 583.4
  acute 580.4
  chronic 582.4
sclerosing membranous (chronic) 582.1
  with nephrotic syndrome 581.1
septic (*see also* Pyelitis) 590.80
specified pathology or lesion NEC 583.89
  with nephrotic syndrome 581.89
  acute 580.89
  chronic 582.89
suppurative (acute) (disseminated) (*see also*
  Pyelitis) 590.80
toxic — *see* Nephritis, acute
tubal, tubular — *see* Nephrosis, tubular
type II (Ellis) — *see* Nephrosis
vascular — *see* Hypertension, kidney
Glomerulosclerosis — *see also* Sclerosis, renal
  587
focal 582.1
  with nephrotic syndrome 581.1
intercapillary (nodular) (with diabetes)
  250.4 ☑ *[581.81]*
  due to secondary diabetes
    249.4 ☑ *[581.81]*
Glossagra 529.6
Glossalgia 529.6
Glossitis 529.0
areata exfoliativa 529.1
atrophic 529.4
benign migratory 529.1
gangrenous 529.0
Hunter's 529.4
median rhomboid 529.2
Moeller's 529.4
pellagrous 265.2
Glossocele 529.8
Glossodynia 529.6
exfoliativa 529.4
Glossoncus 529.8
Glossophytia 529.3
Glossoplegia 529.8
Glossoptosis 529.8
Glossopyrosis 529.6
Glossotrichia 529.3
Glossy skin 701.9
Glottis — *see* condition
Glottitis — *see* Glossitis
Glucagonoma (M8152/0)
malignant (M8152/3)
  pancreas 157.4
  specified site NEC — *see* Neoplasm, by
    site, malignant
  unspecified site 157.4
pancreas 211.7
specified site NEC — *see* Neoplasm, by site,
  benign
unspecified site 211.7
Glucoglycinuria 270.7
Glue ear syndrome 381.20
Glue sniffing (airplane glue) — *see also* Depen-
  dence 304.6 ☑
Glycemia (with methylmalonic acidemia)
  270.7
Glycinuria (renal) (with ketosis) 270.0

Glaucoma — Glycinuria

☑ **Additional Digit Required** — Refer to the Tabular List for Digit Selection   ⓦ **Subterms under main terms may continue to next column or page**

2011 ICD-9-CM   ▶◀ **Revised Text**   ● **New Line**   ▲ **Revised Code**   **Volume 2 — 129**

Glycogen
  infiltration (see also Disease, glycogen storage) 271.0
  storage disease (see also Disease, glycogen storage) 271.0
Glycogenosis — see also Disease, glycogen storage 271.0
  cardiac 271.0 [425.7]
  Cori, types I-VII 271.0
  diabetic, secondary 250.8 ☑ [259.8]
    due to secondary diabetes 249.8 ☑ [259.8]
  diffuse (with hepatic cirrhosis) 271.0
  generalized 271.0
  glucose-6-phosphatase deficiency 271.0
  hepatophosphorylase deficiency 271.0
  hepatorenal 271.0
  myophosphorylase deficiency 271.0
Glycopenia 251.2
Glycopeptide
  intermediate staphylococcus aureus (GISA) V09.8 ☑
  resistant
    enterococcus V09.8 ☑
    staphylococcus aureus (GRSA) V09.8 ☑
Glycoprolinuria 270.8
Glycosuria 791.5
  renal 271.4
Gnathostoma (spinigerum) (infection) (infestation) 128.1
  wandering swellings from 128.1
Gnathostomiasis 128.1
Goiter (adolescent) (colloid) (diffuse) (dipping) (due to iodine deficiency) (endemic) (euthyroid) (heart) (hyperplastic) (internal) (intrathoracic) (juvenile) (mixed type) (nonendemic) (parenchymatous) (plunging) (sporadic) (subclavicular) (substernal) 240.9
  with
    hyperthyroidism (recurrent) (see also Goiter, toxic) 242.0 ☑
    thyrotoxicosis (see also Goiter, toxic) 242.0 ☑
  adenomatous (see also Goiter, nodular) 241.9
  cancerous (M8000/3) 193
  complicating pregnancy, childbirth, or puerperium 648.1 ☑
  congenital 246.1
  cystic (see also Goiter, nodular) 241.9
  due to enzyme defect in synthesis of thyroid hormone (butane-insoluble iodine) (coupling) (deiodinase) (iodide trapping or organification) (iodotyrosine dehalogenase) (peroxidase) 246.1
  dyshormonogenic 246.1
  exophthalmic (see also Goiter, toxic) 242.0 ☑
  familial (with deaf-mutism) 243
  fibrous 245.3
  lingual 759.2
  lymphadenoid 245.2
  malignant (M8000/3) 193
  multinodular (nontoxic) 241.1
    toxic or with hyperthyroidism (see also Goiter, toxic) 242.2 ☑
  nodular (nontoxic) 241.9
    with
      hyperthyroidism (see also Goiter, toxic) 242.3 ☑
      thyrotoxicosis (see also Goiter, toxic) 242.3 ☑
    endemic 241.9
    exophthalmic (diffuse) (see also Goiter, toxic) 242.0 ☑
    multinodular (nontoxic) 241.1
    sporadic 241.9
    toxic (see also Goiter, toxic) 242.3 ☑
    uninodular (nontoxic) 241.0
  nontoxic (nodular) 241.9
    multinodular 241.1
    uninodular 241.0
  pulsating (see also Goiter, toxic) 242.0 ☑
  simple 240.0

Goiter — continued
  toxic 242.0 ☑

Note — Use the following fifth-digit subclassification with category 242:

0   without mention of thyrotoxic crisis or storm

1   with mention of thyrotoxic crisis or storm

    adenomatous 242.3 ☑
      multinodular 242.2 ☑
      uninodular 242.1 ☑
    multinodular 242.2 ☑
    nodular 242.3 ☑
      multinodular 242.2 ☑
      uninodular 242.1 ☑
    uninodular 242.1 ☑
  uninodular (nontoxic) 241.0
  toxic or with hyperthyroidism (see also Goiter, toxic) 242.1 ☑
Goldberg (-Maxwell) (-Morris) syndrome (testicular feminization) 259.51
Goldblatt's
  hypertension 440.1
  kidney 440.1
Goldenhar's syndrome (oculoauriculovertebral dysplasia) 756.0
Goldflam-Erb disease or syndrome 358.00
Goldscheider's disease (epidermolysis bullosa) 757.39
Goldstein's disease (familial hemorrhagic telangiectasia) 448.0
Golfer's elbow 726.32
Goltz-Gorlin syndrome (dermal hypoplasia) 757.39
Gonadoblastoma (M9073/1)
  specified site — see Neoplasm, by site uncertain behavior
  unspecified site
    female 236.2
    male 236.4
Gonecystitis — see also Vesiculitis 608.0
Gongylonemiasis 125.6
  mouth 125.6
Goniosynechiae 364.73
Gonococcemia 098.89
Gonococcus, gonococcal (disease) (infection) — see also condition 098.0
  anus 098.7
  bursa 098.52
  chronic NEC 098.2
  complicating pregnancy, childbirth, or puerperium 647.1 ☑
    affecting fetus or newborn 760.2
  conjunctiva, conjunctivitis (neonatorum) 098.40
  dermatosis 098.89
  endocardium 098.84
  epididymo-orchitis 098.13
    chronic or duration of 2 months or over 098.33
  eye (newborn) 098.40
  fallopian tube (chronic) 098.37
    acute 098.17
  genitourinary (acute) (organ) (system) (tract) (see also Gonorrhea) 098.0
    lower 098.0
      chronic 098.2
    upper 098.10
      chronic 098.30
  heart NEC 098.85
  joint 098.50
  keratoderma 098.81
  keratosis (blennorrhagica) 098.81
  lymphatic (gland) (node) 098.89
  meninges 098.82
  orchitis (acute) 098.13
    chronic or duration of 2 months or over 098.33
  pelvis (acute) 098.19
    chronic or duration of 2 months or over 098.39
  pericarditis 098.83
  peritonitis 098.86
  pharyngitis 098.6

Gonococcus, gonococcal — see also condition — continued
  pharynx 098.6
  proctitis 098.7
  pyosalpinx (chronic) 098.37
    acute 098.17
  rectum 098.7
  septicemia 098.89
  skin 098.89
  specified site NEC 098.89
  synovitis 098.51
  tendon sheath 098.51
  throat 098.6
  urethra (acute) 098.0
    chronic or duration of 2 months or over 098.2
  vulva (acute) 098.0
    chronic or duration of 2 months or over 098.2
Gonocytoma (M9073/1)
  specified site — see Neoplasm, by site, uncertain behavior
  unspecified site
    female 236.2
    male 236.4
Gonorrhea 098.0
  acute 098.0
  Bartholin's gland (acute) 098.0
    chronic or duration of 2 months or over 098.2
  bladder (acute) 098.11
    chronic or duration of 2 months or over 098.31
  carrier (suspected of) V02.7
  cervix (acute) 098.15
    chronic or duration of 2 months or over 098.35
  chronic 098.2
  complicating pregnancy, childbirth, or puerperium 647.1 ☑
    affecting fetus or newborn 760.2
  conjunctiva, conjunctivitis (neonatorum) 098.40
  contact V01.6
  Cowper's gland (acute) 098.0
    chronic or duration of 2 months or over 098.2
  duration of two months or over 098.2
  exposure to V01.6
  fallopian tube (chronic) 098.37
    acute 098.17
  genitourinary (acute) (organ) (system) (tract) 098.0
    chronic 098.2
    duration of two months or over 098.2
  kidney (acute) 098.19
    chronic or duration of 2 months or over 098.39
  ovary (acute) 098.19
    chronic or duration of 2 months or over 098.39
  pelvis (acute) 098.19
    chronic or duration of 2 months or over 098.39
  penis (acute) 098.0
    chronic or duration of 2 months or over 098.2
  prostate (acute) 098.12
    chronic or duration of 2 months or over 098.32
  seminal vesicle (acute) 098.14
    chronic or duration of 2 months or over 098.34
  specified site NEC — see Gonococcus
  spermatic cord (acute) 098.14
    chronic or duration of 2 months or over 098.34
  urethra (acute) 098.0
    chronic or duration of 2 months or over 098.2
  vagina (acute) 098.0
    chronic or duration of 2 months or over 098.2
  vas deferens (acute) 098.14
    chronic or duration of 2 months or over 098.34

Gonorrhea — continued
  vulva (acute) 098.0
    chronic or duration of 2 months or over 098.2
Goodpasture's syndrome (pneumorenal) 446.21
Good's syndrome 279.06
Gopalan's syndrome (burning feet) 266.2
Gordon's disease (exudative enteropathy) 579.8
Gorlin-Chaudhry-Moss syndrome 759.89
Gougerot-Blum syndrome (pigmented purpuric lichenoid dermatitis) 709.1
Gougerot-Carteaud disease or syndrome (confluent reticulate papillomatosis) 701.8
Gougerot-Hailey-Hailey disease (benign familial chronic pemphigus) 757.39
Gougerot (-Houwer) -Sjögren syndrome (keratoconjunctivitis sicca) 710.2
Gougerot's syndrome (trisymptomatic) 709.1
Gouley's syndrome (constrictive pericarditis) 423.2
Goundou 102.6
Gout, gouty 274.9
  with
    specified manifestations NEC 274.89
    tophi (tophus) 274.03
  acute 274.01
  arthritis 274.00
    acute 274.01
  arthropathy 274.00
    acute 274.01
    chronic (without mention of tophus (tophi)) 274.02
      with tophus (tophi) 274.03
  attack 274.01
  chronic 274.02
    tophaceous 274.03
  degeneration, heart 274.82
  diathesis 274.9
  eczema 274.89
  episcleritis 274.89 [379.09]
  external ear (tophus) 274.81
  flare 274.01
  glomerulonephritis 274.10
  iritis 274.89 [364.11]
  joint 274.00
  kidney 274.10
  lead 984.9
    specified type of lead — see Table of Drugs and Chemicals
  nephritis 274.10
  neuritis 274.89 [357.4]
  phlebitis 274.89 [451.9]
  rheumatic 714.0
  saturnine 984.9
    specified type of lead — see Table of Drugs and Chemicals
  spondylitis 274.00
  synovitis 274.00
  syphilitic 095.8
  tophi 274.03
    ear 274.81
    heart 274.82
    specified site NEC 274.82
Gowers'
  muscular dystrophy 359.1
  syndrome (vasovagal attack) 780.2
Gowers-Paton-Kennedy syndrome 377.04
Gradenigo's syndrome 383.02
Graft-versus-host disease 279.50
  due to organ transplant NEC — see Complications, transplant, organ
Graham Steell's murmur (pulmonic regurgitation) — see also Endocarditis, pulmonary 424.3
Grain-handlers' disease or lung 495.8
Grain mite (itch) 133.8
Grand
  mal (idiopathic) (see also Epilepsy) 345.1 ☑
    hysteria of Charcôt 300.11
    nonrecurrent or isolated 780.39
  multipara
    affecting management of labor and delivery 659.4 ☑

☑ **Additional Digit Required** — Refer to the Tabular List for Digit Selection   ▽ **Subterms under main terms may continue to next column or page**

Grand — *continued*
  multipara — *continued*
    status only (not pregnant) V61.5
Granite workers' lung 502
Granular — *see also* condition
  inflammation, pharynx 472.1
  kidney (contracting) (*see also* Sclerosis, renal) 587
  liver — *see* Cirrhosis, liver
  nephritis — *see* Nephritis
Granulation tissue, abnormal — *see also* Granuloma
  abnormal or excessive 701.5
  postmastoidectomy cavity 383.33
  postoperative 701.5
  skin 701.5
Granulocytopenia, granulocytopenic (primary) 288.00
  malignant 288.09
Granuloma NEC 686.1
  abdomen (wall) 568.89
    skin (pyogenicum) 686.1
      from residual foreign body 709.4
  annulare 695.89
  anus 569.49
  apical 522.6
  appendix 543.9
  aural 380.23
  beryllium (skin) 709.4
    lung 503
  bone (*see also* Osteomyelitis) 730.1 ☑
    eosinophilic 277.89
    from residual foreign body 733.99
  canaliculus lacrimalis 375.81
  cerebral 348.89
  cholesterin, middle ear 385.82
  coccidioidal (progressive) 114.3
    lung 114.4
    meninges 114.2
    primary (lung) 114.0
  colon 569.89
  conjunctiva 372.61
  dental 522.6
  ear, middle (cholesterin) 385.82
    with otitis media — *see* Otitis media
  eosinophilic 277.89
    bone 277.89
    lung 277.89
    oral mucosa 528.9
  exuberant 701.5
  eyelid 374.89
  facial
    lethal midline 446.3
    malignant 446.3
  faciale 701.8
  fissuratum (gum) 523.8
  foot NEC 686.1
  foreign body (in soft tissue) NEC 728.82
    bone 733.99
    in operative wound 998.4
    muscle 728.82
    skin 709.4
    subcutaneous tissue 709.4
  fungoides 202.1 ☑
  gangraenescens 446.3
  giant cell (central) (jaw) (reparative) 526.3
    gingiva 523.8
    peripheral (gingiva) 523.8
  gland (lymph) 289.3
  Hodgkin's (M9661/3) 201.1 ☑
  ileum 569.89
  infectious NEC 136.9
  inguinale (Donovan) 099.2
    venereal 099.2
  intestine 569.89
  iridocyclitis 364.10
  jaw (bone) 526.3
    reparative giant cell 526.3
  kidney (*see also* Infection, kidney) 590.9
  lacrimal sac 375.81
  larynx 478.79
  lethal midline 446.3
  lipid 277.89
  lipoid 277.89
  liver 572.8
  lung (infectious) (*see also* Fibrosis, lung) 515

Granuloma — *continued*
  lung (*see also* Fibrosis, lung) — *continued*
    coccidioidal 114.4
    eosinophilic 277.89
  lymph gland 289.3
  Majocchi's 110.6
  malignant, face 446.3
  mandible 526.3
  mediastinum 519.3
  midline 446.3
  monilial 112.3
  muscle 728.82
    from residual foreign body 728.82
  nasal sinus (*see also* Sinusitis) 473.9
  operation wound 998.59
    foreign body 998.4
    stitch (external) 998.89
      internal wound 998.89
    talc 998.7
  oral mucosa, eosinophilic or pyogenic 528.9
  orbit, orbital 376.11
  paracoccidioidal 116.1
  penis, venereal 099.2
  periapical 522.6
  peritoneum 568.89
    due to ova of helminths NEC (*see also* Helminthiasis) 128.9
  postmastoidectomy cavity 383.33
  postoperative — *see* Granuloma, operation wound
  prostate 601.8
  pudendi (ulcerating) 099.2
  pudendorum (ulcerative) 099.2
  pulp, internal (tooth) 521.49
  pyogenic, pyogenicum (skin) 686.1
    maxillary alveolar ridge 522.6
    oral mucosa 528.9
  rectum 569.49
  reticulohistiocytic 277.89
  rubrum nasi 705.89
  sarcoid 135
  Schistosoma 120.9
  septic (skin) 686.1
  silica (skin) 709.4
  sinus (accessory) (infectional) (nasal) (*see also* Sinusitis) 473.9
  skin (pyogenicum) 686.1
    from foreign body or material 709.4
  sperm 608.89
  spine
    syphilitic (epidural) 094.89
    tuberculous (*see also* Tuberculosis) 015.0 ☑ *[730.88]*
  stitch (postoperative) 998.89
    internal wound 998.89
  suppurative (skin) 686.1
  suture (postoperative) 998.89
    internal wound 998.89
  swimming pool 031.1
  talc 728.82
    in operation wound 998.7
  telangiectaticum (skin) 686.1
  tracheostomy 519.09
  trichophyticum 110.6
  tropicum 102.4
  umbilicus 686.1
    newborn 771.4
  urethra 599.84
  uveitis 364.10
  vagina 099.2
  venereum 099.2
  vocal cords 478.5
  Wegener's (necrotizing respiratory granulomatosis) 446.4
Granulomatosis NEC 686.1
  disciformis chronica et progressiva 709.3
  infantiseptica 771.2
  lipoid 277.89
  lipophagic, intestinal 040.2
  miliary 027.0
  necrotizing, respiratory 446.4
  progressive, septic 288.1
  Wegener's (necrotizing respiratory) 446.4
Granulomatous tissue — *see* Granuloma
Granulosis rubra nasi 705.89

Graphite fibrosis (of lung) 503
Graphospasm 300.89
  organic 333.84
Grating scapula 733.99
Gravel (urinary) — *see also* Calculus 592.9
Graves' disease (exophthalmic goiter) — *see also* Goiter, toxic 242.0 ☑
Gravis — *see* condition
Grawitz's tumor (hypernephroma) (M8312/3) 189.0
Grayness, hair (premature) 704.3
  congenital 757.4
Gray or grey syndrome (chloramphenicol) (newborn) 779.4
Greenfield's disease 330.0
Green sickness 280.9
Greenstick fracture — *see* Fracture, by site
Greig's syndrome (hypertelorism) 756.0
Grief 309.0
Griesinger's disease — *see also* Ancylostomiasis 126.9
Grinders'
  asthma 502
  lung 502
  phthisis (*see also* Tuberculosis) 011.4 ☑
Grinding, teeth 306.8
Grip
  Dabney's 074.1
  devil's 074.1
Grippe, grippal — *see also* Influenza
  Balkan 083.0
  intestinal ▶(*see also* Influenza)◀ 487.8
  summer 074.8
Grippy cold ▶— *see also* Influenza◀ 487.1
Grisel's disease 723.5
Groin — *see* condition
Grooved
  nails (transverse) 703.8
  tongue 529.5
    congenital 750.13
Ground itch 126.9
Growing pains, children 781.99
Growth (fungoid) (neoplastic) (new) (M8000/1) — *see also* Neoplasm, by site, unspecified nature
  adenoid (vegetative) 474.12
  benign (M8000/0) — *see* Neoplasm, by site, benign
  fetal, poor 764.9 ☑
    affecting management of pregnancy 656.5 ☑
  malignant (M8000/3) — *see* Neoplasm, by site, malignant
  rapid, childhood V21.0
  secondary (M8000/6) — *see* Neoplasm, by site, malignant, secondary
GRSA (glycopeptide resistant staphylococcus aureus) V09.8 ☑
Gruber's hernia — *see* Hernia, Gruber's
Gruby's disease (tinea tonsurans) 110.0
GSS (Gerstmann-Sträussler-Scheinker syndrome) 046.71
G-trisomy 758.0
Guama fever 066.3
Gubler (-Millard) paralysis or syndrome 344.89
Guérin-Stern syndrome (arthrogryposis multiplex congenita) 754.89
Guertin's disease (electric chorea) 049.8
Guillain-Barré disease or syndrome 357.0
Guinea worms (infection) (infestation) 125.7
Guinon's disease (motor-verbal tic) 307.23
Gull and Sutton's disease — *see* Hypertension, kidney
Gull's disease (thyroid atrophy with myxedema) 244.8
Gum — *see* condition
Gumboil 522.7
Gumma (syphilitic) 095.9
  artery 093.89
    cerebral or spinal 094.89
  bone 095.5
    of yaws (late) 102.6
  brain 094.89
  cauda equina 094.89
  central nervous system NEC 094.9

Gumma — *continued*
  ciliary body 095.8 *[364.11]*
  congenital 090.5
    testis 090.5
  eyelid 095.8 *[373.5]*
  heart 093.89
  intracranial 094.89
  iris 095.8 *[364.11]*
  kidney 095.4
  larynx 095.8
  leptomeninges 094.2
  liver 095.3
  meninges 094.2
  myocardium 093.82
  nasopharynx 095.8
  neurosyphilitic 094.9
  nose 095.8
  orbit 095.8
  palate (soft) 095.8
  penis 095.8
  pericardium 093.81
  pharynx 095.8
  pituitary 095.8
  scrofulous (*see also* Tuberculosis) 017.0 ☑
  skin 095.8
  specified site NEC 095.8
  spinal cord 094.89
  tongue 095.8
  tonsil 095.8
  trachea 095.8
  tuberculous (*see also* Tuberculosis) 017.0 ☑
  ulcerative due to yaws 102.4
  ureter 095.8
  yaws 102.4
    bone 102.6
Gunn's syndrome (jaw-winking syndrome) 742.8
Gunshot wound — *see also* Wound, open, by site
  fracture — *see* Fracture, by site, open
  internal organs (abdomen, chest, or pelvis) — *see* Injury, internal, by site, with open wound
  intracranial — *see* Laceration, brain, with open intracranial wound
Günther's disease or syndrome (congenital erythropoietic porphyria) 277.1
Gustatory hallucination 780.1
Gynandrism 752.7
Gynandroblastoma (M8632/1)
  specified site — *see* Neoplasm, by site, uncertain behavior
  unspecified site
    female 236.2
    male 236.4
Gynandromorphism 752.7
Gynatresia (congenital) 752.49
Gynecoid pelvis, male 738.6
Gynecological examination V72.31
  for contraceptive maintenance V25.40
Gynecomastia 611.1
Gynephobia 300.29
Gyrate scalp 757.39

H

Haas' disease (osteochondrosis head of humerus) 732.3
Habermann's disease (acute parapsoriasis varioliformis) 696.2
Habit, habituation
  chorea 307.22
  disturbance, child 307.9
  drug (*see also* Dependence) 304.9 ☑
  laxative (*see also* Abuse, drugs, nondependent) 305.9 ☑
  spasm 307.20
    chronic 307.22
    transient (of childhood) 307.21
  tic 307.20
    chronic 307.22
    transient (of childhood) 307.21
  use of
    nonprescribed drugs (*see also* Abuse, drugs, nondependent) 305.9 ☑
    patent medicines (*see also* Abuse, drugs, nondependent) 305.9 ☑

☑ **Additional Digit Required — Refer to the Tabular List for Digit Selection**
▽ **Subterms under main terms may continue to next column or page**

Habit, habituation — *continued*
vomiting 536.2
Hadfield-Clarke syndrome (pancreatic infantilism) 577.8
Haff disease 985.1
Hageman factor defect, deficiency, or disease — *see also* Defect, coagulation 286.3
Haglund's disease (osteochondrosis os tibiale externum) 732.5
Haglund-Läwen-Fründ syndrome 717.89
Hagner's disease (hypertrophic pulmonary osteoarthropathy) 731.2
Hag teeth, tooth 524.39
Hailey-Hailey disease (benign familial chronic pemphigus) 757.39
Hair — *see also* condition
plucking 307.9
Hairball in stomach 935.2
Hairy black tongue 529.3
Half vertebra 756.14
Halitosis 784.99
Hallermann-Streiff syndrome 756.0
Hallervorden-Spatz disease or syndrome 333.0
Hallopeau's
acrodermatitis (continua) 696.1
disease (lichen sclerosis et atrophicus) 701.0
Hallucination (auditory) (gustatory) (olfactory) (tactile) 780.1
alcohol-induced 291.3
drug-induced 292.12
visual 368.16
Hallucinosis 298.9
alcohol-induced (acute) 291.3
drug-induced 292.12
Hallus — *see* Hallux
Hallux 735.9
limitus 735.8
malleus (acquired) 735.3
rigidus (acquired) 735.2
congenital 755.66
late effects of rickets 268.1
valgus (acquired) 735.0
congenital 755.66
varus (acquired) 735.1
congenital 755.66
Halo, visual 368.15
Hamartoblastoma 759.6
Hamartoma 759.6
epithelial (gingival), odontogenic, central, or peripheral (M9321/0) 213.1
upper jaw (bone) 213.0
vascular 757.32
Hamartosis, hamartoses NEC 759.6
Hamman's disease or syndrome (spontaneous mediastinal emphysema) 518.1
Hamman-Rich syndrome (diffuse interstitial pulmonary fibrosis) 516.3
Hammer toe (acquired) 735.4
congenital 755.66
late effects of rickets 268.1
Hand — *see* condition
Hand-foot syndrome 693.0
Hand-Schüller-Christian disease or syndrome (chronic histiocytosis x) 277.89
Hanging (asphyxia) (strangulation) (suffocation) 994.7
Hangnail (finger) (with lymphangitis) 681.02
Hangover (alcohol) — *see also* Abuse, drugs, nondependent 305.0 ☑
Hanot-Chauffard (-Troisier) syndrome (bronze diabetes) 275.01 ▲
Hanot's cirrhosis or disease — *see* Cirrhosis, biliary
Hansen's disease (leprosy) 030.9
benign form 030.1
malignant form 030.0
Harada's disease or syndrome 363.22
Hard chancre 091.0
Hardening
artery — *see* Arteriosclerosis
brain 348.89
liver 571.8
Hard firm prostate 600.10

Hard firm prostate — *continued*
with
urinary
obstruction 600.11
retention 600.11
Harelip — *see also* Cleft, lip 749.10
Hare's syndrome (M8010/3) (carcinoma, pulmonary apex) 162.3
Harkavy's syndrome 446.0
Harlequin (fetus) 757.1
color change syndrome 779.89
Harley's disease (intermittent hemoglobinuria) 283.2
Harris'
lines 733.91
syndrome (organic hyperinsulinism) 251.1
Hart's disease or syndrome (pellagra-cerebellar ataxia-renal aminoaciduria) 270.0
Hartmann's pouch (abnormal sacculation of gallbladder neck) 575.8
of intestine V44.3
attention to V55.3
Hartnup disease (pellagra-cerebellar ataxia-renal aminoaciduria) 270.0
Harvester lung 495.0
Hashimoto's disease or struma (struma lymphomatosa) 245.2
Hassall-Henle bodies (corneal warts) 371.41
Haut mal — *see also* Epilepsy 345.1 ☑
Haverhill fever 026.1
Hawaiian wood rose dependence 304.5 ☑
Hawkins' keloid 701.4
Hay
asthma (*see also* Asthma) 493.0 ☑
fever (allergic) (with rhinitis) 477.9
with asthma (bronchial) (*see also* Asthma) 493.0 ☑
allergic, due to grass, pollen, ragweed, or tree 477.0
conjunctivitis 372.05
due to
dander, animal (cat) (dog) 477.2
dust 477.8
fowl 477.8
hair, animal (cat) (dog) 477.2
pollen 477.0
specified allergen other than pollen 477.8
Hayem-Faber syndrome (achlorhydric anemia) 280.9
Hayem-Widal syndrome (acquired hemolytic jaundice) 283.9
Haygarth's nodosities 715.04
Hazard-Crile tumor (M8350/3) 193
Hb (abnormal)
disease — *see* Disease, hemoglobin
trait — *see* Trait
H disease 270.0
Head — *see also* condition
banging 307.3
Headache 784.0
allergic 339.00
associated with sexual activity 339.82
cluster 339.00
chronic 339.02
episodic 339.01
daily
chronic 784.0
new persistent (NPDH) 339.42
drug induced 339.3
due to
loss, spinal fluid 349.0
lumbar puncture 349.0
saddle block 349.0
emotional 307.81
histamine 339.00
hypnic 339.81
lumbar puncture 349.0
medication overuse 339.3
menopausal 627.2
menstrual 346.4 ☑
migraine 346.9 ☑
nasal septum 784.0
nonorganic origin 307.81
orgasmic 339.82
postspinal 349.0

Headache — *continued*
post-traumatic 339.20
acute 339.21
chronic 339.22
premenstrual 346.4 ☑
preorgasmic 339.82
primary
cough 339.83
exertional 339.84
stabbing 339.85
thunderclap 339.43
psychogenic 307.81
psychophysiologic 307.81
rebound 339.3
short lasting unilateral neuralgiform with conjunctival injection and tearing (SUNCT) 339.05
sick 346.9 ☑
spinal 349.0
complicating labor and delivery 668.8 ☑
postpartum 668.8 ☑
spinal fluid loss 349.0
syndrome
cluster 339.00
complicated NEC 339.44
periodic in child or adolescent 346.2 ☑
specified NEC 339.89
tension 307.81
type 339.10
chronic 339.12
episodic 339.11
vascular 784.0
migraine type 346.9 ☑
vasomotor 346.9 ☑
Health
advice V65.4 ☑
audit V70.0
checkup V70.0
education V65.4 ☑
hazard (*see also* History of) V15.9
falling V15.88
specified cause NEC V15.89
instruction V65.4 ☑
services provided because of (of)
boarding school residence V60.6
holiday relief for person providing home care V60.5
inadequate
housing V60.1
resources V60.2
lack of housing V60.0
no care available in home V60.4
person living alone V60.3
poverty V60.3
residence in institution V60.6
specified cause NEC V60.89
vacation relief for person providing home care V60.5
Healthy
donor (*see also* Donor) V59.9
infant or child
accompanying sick mother V65.0
receiving care V20.1
person
accompanying sick relative V65.0
admitted for sterilization V25.2
receiving prophylactic inoculation or vaccination (*see also* Vaccination, prophylactic) V05.9
Hearing
conservation and treatment V72.12
examination V72.19
following failed hearing screening V72.11
Heart — *see* condition
Heartburn 787.1
psychogenic 306.4
Heat (effects) 992.9
apoplexy 992.0
burn (*see also* Burn, by site)
from sun (*see also* Sunburn) 692.71
collapse 992.1
cramps 992.2
dermatitis or eczema 692.89
edema 992.7
erythema — *see* Burn, by site

Heat — *continued*
excessive 992.9
specified effect NEC 992.8
exhaustion 992.5
anhydrotic 992.3
due to
salt (and water) depletion 992.4
water depletion 992.3
fatigue (transient) 992.6
fever 992.0
hyperpyrexia 992.0
prickly 705.1
prostration — *see* Heat, exhaustion
pyrexia 992.0
rash 705.1
specified effect NEC 992.8
stroke 992.0
sunburn (*see also* Sunburn) 692.71
syncope 992.1
Heavy-chain disease 273.2
Heavy-for-dates (fetus or infant) 766.1
4500 grams or more 766.0
exceptionally 766.0
Hebephrenia, hebephrenic (acute) — *see also* Schizophrenia 295.1 ☑
dementia (praecox) (*see also* Schizophrenia) 295.1 ☑
schizophrenia (*see also* Schizophrenia) 295.1 ☑
Heberden's
disease or nodes 715.04
syndrome (angina pectoris) 413.9
Hebra's disease
dermatitis exfoliativa 695.89
erythema multiforme exudativum 695.19
pityriasis 695.89
maculata et circinata 696.3
rubra 695.89
pilaris 696.4
prurigo 698.2
Hebra, nose 040.1
Hedinger's syndrome (malignant carcinoid) 259.2
Heel — *see* condition
Heerfordt's disease or syndrome (uveoparotitis) 135
Hegglin's anomaly or syndrome 288.2
Heidenhain's disease 290.10
with dementia 290.10
Heilmeyer-Schöner disease (M9842/3) 207.1 ☑
Heine-Medin disease — *see also* Poliomyelitis 045.9 ☑
Heinz-body anemia, congenital 282.7
Heller's disease or syndrome (infantile psychosis) — *see also* Psychosis, childhood 299.1 ☑
H.E.L.L.P 642.5 ☑
Helminthiasis — *see also* Infestation, by specific parasite 128.9
Ancylostoma (*see also* Ancylostoma) 126.9
intestinal 127.9
mixed types (types classifiable to more than one of the categories 120.0–127.7) 127.8
specified type 127.7
mixed types (intestinal) (types classifiable to more than one of the categories 120.0–127.7) 127.8
Necator americanus 126.1
specified type NEC 128.8
Trichinella 124
Heloma 700
Hemangioblastoma (M9161/1) — *see also* Neoplasm, connective tissue, uncertain behavior
malignant (M9161/3) — *see* Neoplasm, connective tissue, malignant
Hemangioblastomatosis, cerebelloretinal 759.6
Hemangioendothelioma (M9130/1) — *see also* Neoplasm, by site, uncertain behavior
benign (M9130/0) 228.00
bone (diffuse) (M9130/3) — *see* Neoplasm, bone, malignant

Hemangioendothelioma — *see also*
  Neoplasm, by site, uncertain behavior —
   continued
  malignant (M9130/3) — *see* Neoplasm,
   connective tissue, malignant
  nervous system (M9130/0) 228.09
Hemangioendotheliosarcoma (M9130/3) —
  see Neoplasm, connective tissue, malignant
Hemangiofibroma (M9160/0) — *see* Neoplasm, by site, benign
Hemangiolipoma (M8861/0) — *see* Lipoma
Hemangioma (M9120/0) 228.00
  arteriovenous (M9123/0) — *see* Hemangioma, by site
  brain 228.02
  capillary (M9131/0) — *see* Hemangioma, by
   site
  cavernous (M9121/0) — *see* Hemangioma,
   by site
  central nervous system NEC 228.09
  choroid 228.09
  heart 228.09
  infantile (M9131/0) — *see* Hemangioma, by
   site
  intra-abdominal structures 228.04
  intracranial structures 228.02
  intramuscular (M9132/0) — *see* Hemangioma, by site
  iris 228.09
  juvenile (M9131/0) — *see* Hemangioma, by
   site
  malignant (M9120/3) — *see* Neoplasm,
   connective tissue, malignant
  meninges 228.09
   brain 228.02
   spinal cord 228.09
  peritoneum 228.04
  placenta — *see* Placenta, abnormal
  plexiform (M9131/0) — *see* Hemangioma,
   by site
  racemose (M9123/0) — *see* Hemangioma,
   by site
  retina 228.03
  retroperitoneal tissue 228.04
  sclerosing (M8832/0) — *see* Neoplasm, skin,
   benign
  simplex (M9131/0) — *see* Hemangioma, by
   site
  skin and subcutaneous tissue 228.01
  specified site NEC 228.09
  spinal cord 228.09
  venous (M9122/0) — *see* Hemangioma, by
   site
  verrucous keratotic (M9142/0) — *see* Hemangioma, by site
Hemangiomatosis (systemic) 757.32
  involving single site — *see* Hemangioma
Hemangiopericytoma (M9150/1) — *see also*
  Neoplasm, connective tissue, uncertain
  behavior
  benign (M9150/0) — *see* Neoplasm, connective tissue, benign
  malignant (M9150/3) — *see* Neoplasm,
   connective tissue, malignant
Hemangiosarcoma (M9120/3) — *see* Neoplasm, connective tissue, malignant
Hemarthrosis (nontraumatic) 719.10
  ankle 719.17
  elbow 719.12
  foot 719.17
  hand 719.14
  hip 719.15
  knee 719.16
  multiple sites 719.19
  pelvic region 719.15
  shoulder (region) 719.11
  specified site NEC 719.18
  traumatic — *see* Sprain, by site
  wrist 719.13
Hematemesis 578.0
  with ulcer — *see* Ulcer, by site, with hemorrhage
  due to S. japonicum 120.2
  Goldstein's (familial hemorrhagic telangiectasia) 448.0

Hematemesis — *continued*
  newborn 772.4
   due to swallowed maternal blood 777.3
Hematidrosis 705.89
Hematinuria — *see also* Hemoglobinuria 791.2
  malarial 084.8
  paroxysmal 283.2
Hematite miners' lung 503
Hematobilia 576.8
Hematocele (congenital) (diffuse) (idiopathic)
  608.83
  broad ligament 620.7
  canal of Nuck 629.0
  cord, male 608.83
  fallopian tube 620.8
  female NEC 629.0
  ischiorectal 569.89
  male NEC 608.83
  ovary 629.0
  pelvis, pelvic
   female 629.0
    with ectopic pregnancy (*see also*
     Pregnancy, ectopic) 633.90
    with intrauterine pregnancy
     633.91
   male 608.83
  periuterine 629.0
  retrouterine 629.0
  scrotum 608.83
  spermatic cord (diffuse) 608.83
  testis 608.84
  traumatic — *see* Injury, internal, pelvis
  tunica vaginalis 608.83
  uterine ligament 629.0
  uterus 621.4
  vagina 623.6
  vulva 624.5
Hematocephalus 742.4
Hematochezia — *see also* Melena 578.1
Hematochyluria — *see also* Infestation, filarial
  125.9
Hematocolpos 626.8
Hematocornea 371.12
Hematogenous — *see* condition
Hematoma (skin surface intact) (traumatic) —
  see also Contusion

*Note — Hematomas are coded accord-
ing to origin and the nature and site
of the hematoma or the accompanying
injury. Hematomas of unspecified origin
are coded as injuries of the sites involved, except:*

*(a) hematomas of genital organs
which are coded as diseases of
the organ involved unless they
complicate pregnancy or delivery*

*(b) hematomas of the eye which are
coded as diseases of the eye.*

*For late effect of hematoma classifiable
to 920–924 see Late, effect, contusion*

  with
   crush injury — *see* Crush
   fracture — *see* Fracture, by site
   injury of internal organs (*see also* Injury,
    internal, by site)
    kidney — *see* Hematoma, kidney
     traumatic
    liver — *see* Hematoma, liver, traumat-
     ic
    spleen — *see* Hematoma, spleen
   nerve injury — *see* Injury, nerve
   open wound — *see* Wound, open, by
    site
   skin surface intact — *see* Contusion
  abdomen (wall) — *see* Contusion, abdomen
  amnion 658.8 ☑
  aorta, dissecting 441.00
   abdominal 441.02
   thoracic 441.01
   thoracoabdominal 441.03
  arterial (complicating trauma) 904.9
   specified site — *see* Injury, blood vessel,
    by site
  auricle (ear) 380.31

Hematoma — *see also* Contusion —
  continued
  birth injury 767.8
   skull 767.19
  brain (traumatic) 853.0 ☑

*Note — Use the following fifth-digit
subclassification with categories
851–854:*

0 unspecified state of consciousness

1 with no loss of consciousness

*2 with brief [less than one hour]
   loss of consciousness*

*3 with moderate [1–24 hours] loss
   of consciousness*

*4 with prolonged [more than 24
   hours] loss of consciousness and
   return to pre–existing conscious
   level*

*5 with prolonged [more than 24
   hours] loss of consciousness,
   without return to pre–existing
   conscious level*

*Use fifth-digit 5 to designate when a
patient is unconscious and dies before
regaining consciousness, regardless of
the duration of the loss of consciousness*

*6 with loss of consciousness of un-
   specified duration*

9 with concussion, unspecified

  with
   cerebral
    contusion — *see* Contusion, brain
    laceration — *see* Laceration, brain
   open intracranial wound 853.1 ☑
   skull fracture — *see* Fracture, skull,
    by site
  extradural or epidural 852.4 ☑
   with open intracranial wound
    852.5 ☑
   fetus or newborn 767.0
   nontraumatic 432.0
  fetus or newborn NEC 767.0
  nontraumatic (*see also* Hemorrhage,
   brain) 431
   epidural or extradural 432.0
   newborn NEC 772.8
   subarachnoid, arachnoid, or
    meningeal (*see also* Hemor-
    rhage, subarachnoid) 430
   subdural (*see also* Hemorrhage, sub-
    dural) 432.1
  subarachnoid, arachnoid, or meningeal
   852.0 ☑
   with open intracranial wound
    852.1 ☑
   fetus or newborn 772.2
   nontraumatic (*see also* Hemorrhage,
    subarachnoid) 430
  subdural 852.2 ☑
   with open intracranial wound
    852.3 ☑
   fetus or newborn (localized) 767.0
   nontraumatic (*see also* Hemorrhage,
    subdural) 432.1
  breast (nontraumatic) 611.89
  broad ligament (nontraumatic) 620.7
   complicating delivery 665.7 ☑
   traumatic — *see* Injury, internal, broad
    ligament
  calcified NEC 959.9
  capitis 920
   due to birth injury 767.19
   newborn 767.19
  cerebral — *see* Hematoma, brain
  cesarean section wound 674.3 ☑
  chorion — *see* Placenta, abnormal
  complicating delivery (perineum) (vulva)
   664.5 ☑
   pelvic 665.7 ☑
   vagina 665.7 ☑

Hematoma — *see also* Contusion —
  continued
  corpus
   cavernosum (nontraumatic) 607.82
   luteum (nontraumatic) (ruptured) 620.1
  dura (mater) — *see* Hematoma, brain, subdural
  epididymis (nontraumatic) 608.83
  epidural (traumatic) (*see also* Hematoma,
   brain, extradural)
   spinal — *see* Injury, spinal, by site
  episiotomy 674.3 ☑
  external ear 380.31
  extradural (*see also* Hematoma, brain, extradural)
   fetus or newborn 767.0
   nontraumatic 432.0
    fetus or newborn 767.0
  fallopian tube 620.8
  genital organ (nontraumatic)
   female NEC 629.89
   male NEC 608.83
   traumatic (external site) 922.4
    internal — *see* Injury, internal, geni-
     tal organ
  graafian follicle (ruptured) 620.0
  internal organs (abdomen, chest, or pelvis)
   (*see also* Injury, internal, by site)
   kidney — *see* Hematoma, kidney, trau-
    matic
   liver — *see* Hematoma, liver, traumatic
   spleen — *see* Hematoma, spleen
  intracranial — *see* Hematoma, brain
  kidney, cystic 593.81
   traumatic 866.01
    with open wound into cavity 866.11
  labia (nontraumatic) 624.5
  lingual (and other parts of neck, scalp, or
   face, except eye) 920
  liver (subcapsular) 573.8
   birth injury 767.8
   fetus or newborn 767.8
   traumatic NEC 864.01
    with
     laceration — *see* Laceration, liver
     open wound into cavity 864.11
  mediastinum — *see* Injury, internal, mediastinum
  meninges, meningeal (brain) (*see also*
   Hematoma, brain, subarachnoid)
   spinal — *see* Injury, spinal, by site
  mesosalpinx (nontraumatic) 620.8
   traumatic — *see* Injury, internal, pelvis
  muscle (traumatic) — *see* Contusion, by site
   nontraumatic 729.92
  nasal (septum) (and other part(s) of neck,
   scalp, or face, except eye) 920
  obstetrical surgical wound 674.3 ☑
  orbit, orbital (nontraumatic) 376.32
   traumatic 921.2
  ovary (corpus luteum) (nontraumatic) 620.1
   traumatic — *see* Injury, internal, ovary
  pelvis (female) (nontraumatic) 629.89
   complicating delivery 665.7 ☑
   male 608.93
   traumatic (*see also* Injury, internal, pelvis)
    specified organ NEC (*see also* Injury,
     internal, pelvis) 867.6
  penis (nontraumatic) 607.82
  pericranial (and neck, or face any part, except eye) 920
   due to injury at birth 767.19
  perineal wound (obstetrical) 674.3 ☑
   complicating delivery 664.5 ☑
  perirenal, cystic 593.81
  pinna 380.31
  placenta — *see* Placenta, abnormal
  postoperative 998.12
  retroperitoneal (nontraumatic) 568.81
   traumatic — *see* Injury, internal,
    retroperitoneum
  retropubic, male 568.81
  scalp (and neck, or face any part, except eye)
   920
   fetus or newborn 767.19
  scrotum (nontraumatic) 608.83

☑ **Additional Digit Required** — Refer to the Tabular List for Digit Selection   ▽ **Subterms under main terms may continue to next column or page**

2011 ICD-9-CM   ▶◀ **Revised Text**   ● **New Line**   ▲ **Revised Code**   **Volume 2 — 133**

Index

Hematoma — Hemophilus influenzae

Hematoma — *see also* Contusion — *continued*
  scrotum — *continued*
    traumatic 922.4
  seminal vesicle (nontraumatic) 608.83
    traumatic — *see* Injury, internal, seminal, vesicle
  soft tissue 729.92
  spermatic cord (*see also* Injury, internal, spermatic cord)
    nontraumatic 608.83
  spinal (cord) (meninges) (*see also* Injury, spinal, by site)
    fetus or newborn 767.4
    nontraumatic 336.1
  spleen 865.01
    with
      laceration — *see* Laceration, spleen
      open wound into cavity 865.11
  sternocleidomastoid, birth injury 767.8
  sternomastoid, birth injury 767.8
  subarachnoid (*see also* Hematoma, brain, subarachnoid)
    fetus or newborn 772.2
    nontraumatic (*see also* Hemorrhage, subarachnoid) 430
      newborn 772.2
  subdural (*see also* Hematoma, brain, subdural)
    fetus or newborn (localized) 767.0
    nontraumatic (*see also* Hemorrhage, subdural) 432.1
  subperiosteal (syndrome) 267
    traumatic — *see* Hematoma, by site
  superficial, fetus or newborn 772.6
  syncytium — *see* Placenta, abnormal
  testis (nontraumatic) 608.83
    birth injury 767.8
    traumatic 922.4
  tunica vaginalis (nontraumatic) 608.83
  umbilical cord 663.6 ☑
    affecting fetus or newborn 762.6
  uterine ligament (nontraumatic) 620.7
    traumatic — *see* Injury, internal, pelvis
  uterus 621.4
    traumatic — *see* Injury, internal, pelvis
  vagina (nontraumatic) (ruptured) 623.6
    complicating delivery 665.7 ☑
    traumatic 922.4
  vas deferens (nontraumatic) 608.83
    traumatic — *see* Injury, internal, vas deferens
  vitreous 379.23
  vocal cord 920
  vulva (nontraumatic) 624.5
    complicating delivery 664.5 ☑
    fetus or newborn 767.8
    traumatic 922.4
Hematometra 621.4
Hematomyelia 336.1
  with fracture of vertebra (*see also* Fracture, vertebra, by site, with spinal cord injury) 806.8
  fetus or newborn 767.4
Hematomyelitis 323.9
  late effect — *see* category 326
Hematoperitoneum — *see also* Hemoperitoneum 568.81
Hematopneumothorax — *see also* Hemothorax 511.89
Hematopoiesis, cyclic 288.02
Hematoporphyria (acquired) (congenital) 277.1
Hematoporphyrinuria (acquired) (congenital) 277.1
Hematorachis, hematorrhachis 336.1
  fetus or newborn 767.4
Hematosalpinx 620.8
  with
    ectopic pregnancy (*see also* categories 633.0–633.9) 639.2
    infectional (*see also* Salpingo-oophoritis) 614.2
    molar pregnancy (*see also* categories 630–632) 639.2
Hematospermia 608.82

Hematothorax — *see also* Hemothorax 511.89
Hematotympanum 381.03
Hematuria (benign) (essential) (idiopathic) 599.70
  due to S. hematobium 120.0
  endemic 120.0
  gross 599.71
  intermittent 599.70
  malarial 084.8
  microscopic 599.72
  paroxysmal 599.70
  sulfonamide
    correct substance properly administered 599.70
    overdose or wrong substance given or taken 961.0
  tropical (bilharziasis) 120.0
  tuberculous (*see also* Tuberculosis) 016.9 ☑
Hematuric bilious fever 084.8
Hemeralopia 368.10
Hemiabiotrophy 799.89
Hemi-akinesia 781.8
Hemianalgesia — *see also* Disturbance, sensation 782.0
Hemianencephaly 740.0
Hemianesthesia — *see also* Disturbance, sensation 782.0
Hemianopia, hemianopsia (altitudinal) (homonymous) 368.46
  binasal 368.47
  bitemporal 368.47
  heteronymous 368.47
  syphilitic 095.8
Hemiasomatognosia 307.9
Hemiathetosis 781.0
Hemiatrophy 799.89
  cerebellar 334.8
  face 349.89
    progressive 349.89
  fascia 728.9
  leg 728.2
  tongue 529.8
Hemiballism (us) 333.5
Hemiblock (cardiac) (heart) (left) 426.2
Hemicardia 746.89
Hemicephalus, hemicephaly 740.0
Hemichorea 333.5
Hemicrania 346.9 ☑
  congenital malformation 740.0
  continua 339.41
  paroxysmal 339.03
    chronic 339.04
    episodic 339.03
Hemidystrophy — *see* Hemiatrophy
Hemiectromelia 755.4
Hemihypalgesia — *see also* Disturbance, sensation 782.0
Hemihypertrophy (congenital) 759.89
  cranial 756.0
Hemihypesthesia — *see also* Disturbance, sensation 782.0
Hemi-inattention 781.8
Hemimelia 755.4
  lower limb 755.30
    paraxial (complete) (incomplete) (intercalary) (terminal) 755.32
      fibula 755.37
      tibia 755.36
    transverse (complete) (partial) 755.31
  upper limb 755.20
    paraxial (complete) (incomplete) (intercalary) (terminal) 755.22
      radial 755.26
      ulnar 755.27
    transverse (complete) (partial) 755.21
Hemiparalysis — *see also* Hemiplegia 342.9 ☑
Hemiparesis — *see also* Hemiplegia 342.9 ☑
Hemiparesthesia — *see also* Disturbance, sensation 782.0
Hemiplegia 342.9 ☑
  acute (*see also* Disease, cerebrovascular, acute) 436
  alternans facialis 344.89
  apoplectic (*see also* Disease, cerebrovascular, acute) 436

Hemiplegia — *continued*
  apoplectic (*see also* Disease, cerebrovascular, acute) — *continued*
    late effect or residual
      affecting
        dominant side 438.21
        nondominant side 438.22
        unspecified side 438.20
  arteriosclerotic 437.0
    late effect or residual
      affecting
        dominant side 438.21
        nondominant side 438.22
        unspecified side 438.20
  ascending (spinal) NEC 344.89
  attack (*see also* Disease, cerebrovascular, acute) 436
  brain, cerebral (current episode) 437.8
    congenital 343.1
  cerebral — *see* Hemiplegia, brain
  congenital (cerebral) (spastic) (spinal) 343.1
  conversion neurosis (hysterical) 300.11
  cortical — *see* Hemiplegia, brain
  due to
    arteriosclerosis 437.0
      late effect or residual
        affecting
          dominant side 438.21
          nondominant side 438.22
          unspecified side 438.20
    cerebrovascular lesion (*see also* Disease, cerebrovascular, acute) 436
      late effect
        affecting
          dominant side 438.21
          nondominant side 438.22
          unspecified side 438.20
  embolic (current) (*see also* Embolism, brain) 434.1 ☑
    late effect
      affecting
        dominant side 438.21
        nondominant side 438.22
        unspecified side 438.20
  flaccid 342.0 ☑
  hypertensive (current episode) 437.8
  infantile (postnatal) 343.4
  late effect
    birth injury, intracranial or spinal 343.4
    cerebrovascular lesion — *see* Late effect(s) (of) cerebrovascular disease
    viral encephalitis 139.0
  middle alternating NEC 344.89
  newborn NEC 767.0
  seizure (current episode) (*see also* Disease, cerebrovascular, acute) 436
  spastic 342.1 ☑
    congenital or infantile 343.1
  specified NEC 342.8 ☑
  thrombotic (current) (*see also* Thrombosis, brain) 434.0 ☑
    late effect — *see* Late effect(s) (of) cerebrovascular disease
Hemisection, spinal cord — *see* Fracture, vertebra, by site, with spinal cord injury
Hemispasm 781.0
  facial 781.0
Hemispatial neglect 781.8
Hemisporosis 117.9
Hemitremor 781.0
Hemivertebra 756.14
Hemobilia 576.8
Hemocholecyst 575.8
Hemochromatosis (acquired) (liver) (myocardium) (secondary) 275.03 ▲
  with refractory anemia 238.72
  diabetic 275.01 ●
  due to repeated red blood cell transfusions 275.02 ●
  hereditary 275.01 ●
  primary idiopathic 275.01 ●
  specified NEC 275.03 ●
  transfusion associated (red blood cell) 275.02 ●
Hemodialysis V56.0

Hemoglobin — *see also* condition
  abnormal (disease) — *see* Disease, hemoglobin
  AS genotype 282.5
  fetal, hereditary persistence 282.7
  high-oxygen-affinity 289.0
  low NEC 285.9
  S (Hb-S), heterozygous 282.5
Hemoglobinemia 283.2
  due to blood transfusion NEC 999.89
    bone marrow 996.85
  paroxysmal 283.2
Hemoglobinopathy (mixed) — *see also* Disease, hemoglobin 282.7
  with thalassemia 282.49
  sickle-cell 282.60
    with thalassemia (without crisis) 282.41
      with
        crisis 282.42
        vaso-occlusive pain 282.42
Hemoglobinuria, hemoglobinuric 791.2
  with anemia, hemolytic, acquired (chronic) NEC 283.2
  cold (agglutinin) (paroxysmal) (with Raynaud's syndrome) 283.2
  due to
    exertion 283.2
    hemolysis (from external causes) NEC 283.2
  exercise 283.2
  fever (malaria) 084.8
  infantile 791.2
  intermittent 283.2
  malarial 084.8
  march 283.2
  nocturnal (paroxysmal) 283.2
  paroxysmal (cold) (nocturnal) 283.2
Hemolymphangioma (M9175/0) 228.1
Hemolysis
  fetal — *see* Jaundice, fetus or newborn
  intravascular (disseminated) NEC 286.6
    with
      abortion — *see* Abortion, by type, with hemorrhage, delayed or excessive
      ectopic pregnancy (*see also* categories 633.0–633.9) 639.1
      hemorrhage of pregnancy 641.3 ☑
        affecting fetus or newborn 762.1
      molar pregnancy (*see also* categories 630–632) 639.1
    acute 283.2
    following
      abortion 639.1
      ectopic or molar pregnancy 639.1
  neonatal — *see* Jaundice, fetus or newborn
  transfusion NEC 999.89
    bone marrow 996.85
Hemolytic — *see also* condition
  anemia — *see* Anemia, hemolytic
  uremic syndrome 283.11
Hemometra 621.4
Hemopericardium (with effusion) 423.0
  newborn 772.8
  traumatic (*see also* Hemothorax, traumatic) 860.2
    with open wound into thorax 860.3
Hemoperitoneum 568.81
  infectional (*see also* Peritonitis) 567.29
  traumatic — *see* Injury, internal, peritoneum
Hemophagocytic syndrome 288.4
  infection-associated 288.4
Hemophilia (familial) (hereditary) 286.0
  A 286.0
    carrier (asymptomatic) V83.01
      symptomatic V83.02
  acquired 286.5
  B (Leyden) 286.1
  C 286.2
  calcipriva (*see also* Fibrinolysis) 286.7
  classical 286.0
  nonfamilial 286.7
  secondary 286.5
  vascular 286.4
Hemophilus influenzae NEC 041.5
  arachnoiditis (basic) (brain) (spinal) 320.0

☑ **Additional Digit Required** — **Refer to the Tabular List for Digit Selection**   ▽ **Subterms under main terms may continue to next column or page**

Hemophilus influenzae — *continued*
  arachnoiditis — *continued*
    late effect — *see* category 326
  bronchopneumonia 482.2
  cerebral ventriculitis 320.0
    late effect — *see* category 326
  cerebrospinal inflammation 320.0
    late effect — *see* category 326
  infection NEC 041.5
  leptomeningitis 320.0
    late effect — *see* category 326
  meningitis (cerebral) (cerebrospinal) (spinal) 320.0
    late effect — *see* category 326
  meningomyelitis 320.0
    late effect — *see* category 326
  pachymeningitis (adhesive) (fibrous) (hemorrhagic) (hypertrophic) (spinal) 320.0
    late effect — *see* category 326
  pneumonia (broncho-) 482.2
Hemophthalmos 360.43
Hemopneumothorax — *see also* Hemothorax 511.89
  traumatic 860.4
    with open wound into thorax 860.5
Hemoptysis 786.30 ▲
  due to Paragonimus (westermani) 121.2
  newborn 770.3
  specified NEC 786.39 ●
  tuberculous (*see also* Tuberculosis, pulmonary) 011.9 ☑
Hemorrhage, hemorrhagic (nontraumatic) 459.0
  abdomen 459.0
  accidental (antepartum) 641.2 ☑
    affecting fetus or newborn 762.1
  adenoid 474.8
  adrenal (capsule) (gland) (medulla) 255.41
    newborn 772.5
  after labor — *see* Hemorrhage, postpartum
  alveolar
    lung, newborn 770.3
    process 525.8
  alveolus 525.8
  amputation stump (surgical) 998.11
    secondary, delayed 997.69
  anemia (chronic) 280.0
    acute 285.1
  antepartum — *see* Hemorrhage, pregnancy
  anus (sphincter) 569.3
  apoplexy (stroke) 432.9
  arachnoid — *see* Hemorrhage, subarachnoid
  artery NEC 459.0
    brain (*see also* Hemorrhage, brain) 431
    middle meningeal — *see* Hemorrhage, subarachnoid
  basilar (ganglion) (*see also* Hemorrhage, brain) 431
  bladder 596.8
  blood dyscrasia 289.9
  bowel 578.9
    newborn 772.4
  brain (miliary) (nontraumatic) 431
    with
      birth injury 767.0
      arachnoid — *see* Hemorrhage, subarachnoid
      due to
        birth injury 767.0
        rupture of aneurysm (congenital) (*see also* Hemorrhage, subarachnoid) 430
          mycotic 431
        syphilis 094.89
    epidural or extradural — *see* Hemorrhage, extradural
    fetus or newborn (anoxic) (hypoxic) (due to birth trauma) (nontraumatic) 767.0
      intraventricular 772.10
        grade I 772.11
        grade II 772.12
        grade III 772.13
        grade IV 772.14

Hemorrhage, hemorrhagic — *continued*
  brain — *continued*
    iatrogenic 997.02
    postoperative 997.02
    puerperal, postpartum, childbirth 674.0 ☑
    stem 431
    subarachnoid, arachnoid, or meningeal — *see* Hemorrhage, subarachnoid
    subdural — *see* Hemorrhage, subdural
    traumatic NEC 853.0 ☑

> *Note* — Use the following fifth-digit subclassification with categories 851–854:
>
> 0   unspecified state of consciousness
>
> 1   with no loss of consciousness
>
> 2   with brief [less than one hour] loss of consciousness
>
> 3   with moderate [1–24 hours] loss of consciousness
>
> 4   with prolonged [more than 24 hours] loss of consciousness and return to pre–existing conscious level
>
> 5   with prolonged [more than 24 hours] loss of consciousness, without return to pre–existing conscious level
>
> Use fifth-digit 5 to designate when a patient is unconscious and dies before regaining consciousness, regardless of the duration of the loss of consciousness
>
> 6   with loss of consciousness of unspecified duration
>
> 9   with concussion, unspecified

    with
      cerebral
        contusion — *see* Contusion, brain
        laceration — *see* Laceration, brain
      open intracranial wound 853.1 ☑
      skull fracture — *see* Fracture, skull, by site
    extradural or epidural 852.4 ☑
      with open intracranial wound 852.5 ☑
    subarachnoid 852.0 ☑
      with open intracranial wound 852.1 ☑
    subdural 852.2 ☑
      with open intracranial wound 852.3 ☑
  breast 611.79
  bronchial tube — *see* Hemorrhage, lung
  bronchopulmonary — *see* Hemorrhage, lung
  bronchus (cause unknown) (*see also* Hemorrhage, lung) 786.30 ▲
  bulbar (*see also* Hemorrhage, brain) 431
  bursa 727.89
  capillary 448.9
    primary 287.8
  capsular — *see* Hemorrhage, brain
  cardiovascular 429.89
  cecum 578.9
  cephalic (*see also* Hemorrhage, brain) 431
  cerebellar (*see also* Hemorrhage, brain) 431
  cerebellum (*see also* Hemorrhage, brain) 431
  cerebral (*see also* Hemorrhage, brain) 431
    fetus or newborn (anoxic) (traumatic) 767.0
  cerebromeningeal (*see also* Hemorrhage, brain) 431
  cerebrospinal (*see also* Hemorrhage, brain) 431
  cerebrovascular accident — *see* Hemorrhage, brain
  cerebrum (*see also* Hemorrhage, brain) 431
  cervix (stump) (uteri) 622.8

Hemorrhage, hemorrhagic — *continued*
  cesarean section wound 674.3 ☑
  chamber, anterior (eye) 364.41
  childbirth — *see* Hemorrhage, complicating, delivery
  choroid 363.61
    expulsive 363.62
  ciliary body 364.41
  cochlea 386.8
  colon — *see* Hemorrhage, intestine
  complicating
    delivery 641.9 ☑
      affecting fetus or newborn 762.1
      associated with
        afibrinogenemia 641.3 ☑
          affecting fetus or newborn 763.89
        coagulation defect 641.3 ☑
          affecting fetus or newborn 763.89
        hyperfibrinolysis 641.3 ☑
          affecting fetus or newborn 763.89
        hypofibrinogenemia 641.3 ☑
          affecting fetus or newborn 763.89
      due to
        low-lying placenta 641.1 ☑
          affecting fetus or newborn 762.0
        placenta previa 641.1 ☑
          affecting fetus or newborn 762.0
        premature separation of placenta 641.2 ☑
          affecting fetus or newborn 762.1
      retained
        placenta 666.0 ☑
        secundines 666.2 ☑
      trauma 641.8 ☑
        affecting fetus or newborn 763.89
      uterine leiomyoma 641.8 ☑
        affecting fetus or newborn 763.89
    surgical procedure 998.11
  complication(s)
    of dental implant placement 525.71
  concealed NEC 459.0
  congenital 772.9
  conjunctiva 372.72
    newborn 772.8
  cord, newborn 772.0
    slipped ligature 772.3
    stump 772.3
  corpus luteum (ruptured) 620.1
  cortical (*see also* Hemorrhage, brain) 431
  cranial 432.9
  cutaneous 782.7
    newborn 772.6
  cystitis — *see* Cystitis
  cyst, pancreas 577.2
  delayed
    with
      abortion — *see* Abortion, by type, with hemorrhage, delayed or excessive
      ectopic pregnancy (*see also* categories 633.0–633.9) 639.1
      molar pregnancy (*see also* categories 630–632) 639.1
    following
      abortion 639.1
      ectopic or molar pregnancy 639.1
    postpartum 666.2 ☑
  diathesis (familial) 287.9
    newborn 776.0
  disease 287.9
    newborn 776.0
    specified type NEC 287.8
  disorder 287.9
    due to intrinsic circulating anticoagulants 286.5
    specified type NEC 287.8

Hemorrhage, hemorrhagic — *continued*
  due to
    any device, implant or graft (presence of) classifiable to 996.0–996.5 — *see* Complications, due to (presence of) any device, implant, or graft classified to 996.0–996.5NEC
    intrinsic circulating anticoagulant 286.5
  duodenum, duodenal 537.89
    ulcer — *see* Ulcer, duodenum, with hemorrhage
  dura mater — *see* Hemorrhage, subdural
  endotracheal — *see* Hemorrhage, lung
  epicranial subaponeurotic (massive) 767.11
  epidural — *see* Hemorrhage, extradural
  episiotomy 674.3 ☑
  esophagus 530.82
    varix (*see also* Varix, esophagus, bleeding) 456.0
  excessive
    with
      abortion — *see* Abortion, by type, with hemorrhage, delayed or excessive
      ectopic pregnancy (*see also* categories 633.0–633.9) 639.1
      molar pregnancy (*see also* categories 630–632) 639.1
    following
      abortion 639.1
      ectopic or molar pregnancy 639.1
  external 459.0
  extradural (traumatic) (*see also* Hemorrhage, brain, traumatic, extradural)
    birth injury 767.0
    fetus or newborn (anoxic) (traumatic) 767.0
    nontraumatic 432.0
  eye 360.43
    chamber (anterior) (aqueous) 364.41
    fundus 362.81
  eyelid 374.81
  fallopian tube 620.8
  fetomaternal 772.0
    affecting management of pregnancy or puerperium 656.0 ☑
  fetus, fetal, affecting newborn 772.0
    from
      cut end of co-twin's cord 772.0
      placenta 772.0
      ruptured cord 772.0
      vasa previa 772.0
    into
      co-twin 772.0
      mother's circulation 772.0
        affecting management of pregnancy or puerperium 656.0 ☑
  fever (*see also* Fever, hemorrhagic) 065.9
    with renal syndrome 078.6
    arthropod-borne NEC 065.9
    Bangkok 065.4
    Crimean 065.0
    dengue virus 065.4
    epidemic 078.6
    Junin virus 078.7
    Korean 078.6
    Machupo virus 078.7
    mite-borne 065.8
    mosquito-borne 065.4
    Philippine 065.4
    Russian (Yaroslav) 078.6
    Singapore 065.4
    southeast Asia 065.4
    Thailand 065.4
    tick-borne NEC 065.3
  fibrinogenolysis (*see also* Fibrinolysis) 286.6
  fibrinolytic (acquired) (*see also* Fibrinolysis) 286.6
  fontanel 767.19
  from tracheostomy stoma 519.09
  fundus, eye 362.81
  funis
    affecting fetus or newborn 772.0
    complicating delivery 663.8 ☑

☑ **Additional Digit Required** — Refer to the Tabular List for Digit Selection

ⓦ **Subterms under main terms may continue to next column or page**

Hemorrhage, hemorrhagic — *continued*
gastric (*see also* Hemorrhage, stomach)
578.9
gastroenteric 578.9
newborn 772.4
gastrointestinal (tract) 578.9
newborn 772.4
genitourinary (tract) NEC 599.89
gingiva 523.8
globe 360.43
gravidarum — *see* Hemorrhage, pregnancy
gum 523.8
heart 429.89
hypopharyngeal (throat) 784.8
intermenstrual 626.6
irregular 626.6
regular 626.5
internal (organs) 459.0
capsule (*see also* Hemorrhage, brain) 431
ear 386.8
newborn 772.8
intestine 578.9
congenital 772.4
newborn 772.4
into
bladder wall 596.7
bursa 727.89
corpus luysii (*see also* Hemorrhage,
brain) 431
intra-abdominal 459.0
during or following surgery 998.11
intra-alveolar, newborn (lung) 770.3
intracerebral (*see also* Hemorrhage, brain)
431
intracranial NEC 432.9
puerperal, postpartum, childbirth
674.0 ☑
traumatic — *see* Hemorrhage, brain,
traumatic
intramedullary NEC 336.1
intraocular 360.43
intraoperative 998.11
intrapartum — *see* Hemorrhage, complicating, delivery
intrapelvic
female 629.89
male 459.0
intraperitoneal 459.0
intrapontine (*see also* Hemorrhage, brain)
431
intrauterine 621.4
complicating delivery — *see* Hemorrhage, complicating, delivery
in pregnancy or childbirth — *see* Hemorrhage, pregnancy
postpartum (*see also* Hemorrhage,
postpartum) 666.1 ☑
intraventricular (*see also* Hemorrhage, brain)
431
fetus or newborn (anoxic) (traumatic)
772.10
grade I 772.11
grade II 772.12
grade III 772.13
grade IV 772.14
intravesical 596.7
iris (postinfectional) (postinflammatory)
(toxic) 364.41
joint (nontraumatic) 719.10
ankle 719.17
elbow 719.12
foot 719.17
forearm 719.13
hand 719.14
hip 719.15
knee 719.16
lower leg 719.16
multiple sites 719.19
pelvic region 719.15
shoulder (region) 719.11
specified site NEC 719.18
thigh 719.15
upper arm 719.12
wrist 719.13
kidney 593.81
knee (joint) 719.16

Hemorrhage, hemorrhagic — *continued*
labyrinth 386.8
leg NEC 459.0
lenticular striate artery (*see also* Hemorrhage, brain) 431
ligature, vessel 998.11
liver 573.8
lower extremity NEC 459.0
lung 786.30 ▲
newborn 770.3
tuberculous (*see also* Tuberculosis, pulmonary) 011.9 ☑
malaria 084.8
marginal sinus 641.2 ☑
massive subaponeurotic, birth injury 767.11
maternal, affecting fetus or newborn 762.1
mediastinum 786.30 ▲
medulla (*see also* Hemorrhage, brain) 431
membrane (brain) (*see also* Hemorrhage,
subarachnoid) 430
spinal cord — *see* Hemorrhage, spinal
cord
meninges, meningeal (brain) (middle) (*see
also* Hemorrhage, subarachnoid) 430
spinal cord — *see* Hemorrhage, spinal
cord
mesentery 568.81
metritis 626.8
midbrain (*see also* Hemorrhage, brain) 431
mole 631
mouth 528.9
mucous membrane NEC 459.0
newborn 772.8
muscle 728.89
nail (subungual) 703.8
nasal turbinate 784.7
newborn 772.8
nasopharynx 478.29
navel, newborn 772.3
newborn 772.9
adrenal 772.5
alveolar (lung) 770.3
brain (anoxic) (hypoxic) (due to birth
trauma) 767.0
cerebral (anoxic) (hypoxic) (due to birth
trauma) 767.0
conjunctiva 772.8
cutaneous 772.6
diathesis 776.0
due to vitamin K deficiency 776.0
epicranial subaponeurotic (massive)
767.11
gastrointestinal 772.4
internal (organs) 772.8
intestines 772.4
intra-alveolar (lung) 770.3
intracranial (from any perinatal cause)
767.0
intraventricular (from any perinatal
cause) 772.10
grade I 772.11
grade II 772.12
grade III 772.13
grade IV 772.14
lung 770.3
pulmonary (massive) 770.3
spinal cord, traumatic 767.4
stomach 772.4
subaponeurotic (massive) 767.11
subarachnoid (from any perinatal cause)
772.2
subconjunctival 772.8
subgaleal 767.11
umbilicus 772.0
slipped ligature 772.3
vasa previa 772.0
nipple 611.79
nose 784.7
newborn 772.8
obstetrical surgical wound 674.3 ☑
omentum 568.89
newborn 772.4
optic nerve (sheath) 377.42
orbit 376.32
ovary 620.1
oviduct 620.8

Hemorrhage, hemorrhagic — *continued*
pancreas 577.8
parathyroid (gland) (spontaneous) 252.8
parturition — *see* Hemorrhage, complicating, delivery
penis 607.82
pericardium, pericarditis 423.0
perineal wound (obstetrical) 674.3 ☑
peritoneum, peritoneal 459.0
peritonsillar tissue 474.8
after operation on tonsils 998.11
due to infection 475
petechial 782.7
pituitary (gland) 253.8
placenta NEC 641.9 ☑
affecting fetus or newborn 762.1
from surgical or instrumental damage
641.8 ☑
affecting fetus or newborn 762.1
previa 641.1 ☑
affecting fetus or newborn 762.0
pleura — *see* Hemorrhage, lung
polioencephalitis, superior 265.1
polymyositis — *see* Polymyositis
pons (*see also* Hemorrhage, brain) 431
pontine (*see also* Hemorrhage, brain) 431
popliteal 459.0
postcoital 626.7
postextraction (dental) 998.11
postmenopausal 627.1
postnasal 784.7
postoperative 998.11
postpartum (atonic) (following delivery of
placenta) 666.1 ☑
delayed or secondary (after 24 hours)
666.2 ☑
retained placenta 666.0 ☑
third stage 666.0 ☑
pregnancy (concealed) 641.9 ☑
accidental 641.2 ☑
affecting fetus or newborn 762.1
affecting fetus or newborn 762.1
before 22 completed weeks gestation
640.9 ☑
affecting fetus or newborn 762.1
due to
abruptio placenta 641.2 ☑
affecting fetus or newborn 762.1
afibrinogenemia or other coagulation defect (conditions classifiable to 286.0–286.9) 641.3 ☑
affecting fetus or newborn 762.1
coagulation defect 641.3 ☑
affecting fetus or newborn 762.1
hyperfibrinolysis 641.3 ☑
affecting fetus or newborn 762.1
hypofibrinogenemia 641.3 ☑
affecting fetus or newborn 762.1
leiomyoma, uterus 641.8 ☑
affecting fetus or newborn 762.1
low-lying placenta 641.1 ☑
affecting fetus or newborn 762.1
marginal sinus (rupture) 641.2 ☑
affecting fetus or newborn 762.1
placenta previa 641.1 ☑
affecting fetus or newborn 762.0
premature separation of placenta
(normally implanted) 641.2 ☑
affecting fetus or newborn 762.1
threatened abortion 640.0 ☑
affecting fetus or newborn 762.1
trauma 641.8 ☑
affecting fetus or newborn 762.1
early (before 22 completed weeks gestation) 640.9 ☑
affecting fetus or newborn 762.1
previous, affecting management of
pregnancy or childbirth V23.49
unavoidable — *see* Hemorrhage, pregnancy, due to placenta previa
prepartum (mother) — *see* Hemorrhage,
pregnancy
preretinal, cause unspecified 362.81
prostate 602.1

Hemorrhage, hemorrhagic — *continued*
puerperal (*see also* Hemorrhage, postpartum) 666.1 ☑
pulmonary (*see also* Hemorrhage, lung)
786.30 ▲
acute idiopathic in infants (AIPHI) (over ●
28 days old) 786.31 ●
newborn (massive) 770.3
renal syndrome 446.21
purpura (primary) (*see also* Purpura, thrombocytopenic) 287.39
rectum (sphincter) 569.3
recurring, following initial hemorrhage at
time of injury 958.2
renal 593.81
pulmonary syndrome 446.21
respiratory tract (*see also* Hemorrhage, lung)
786.30 ▲
retina, retinal (deep) (superficial) (vessels)
362.81
diabetic 250.5 ☑ [362.01]
due to secondary diabetes
249.5 ☑ [362.01]
due to birth injury 772.8
retrobulbar 376.89
retroperitoneal 459.0
retroplacental (*see also* Placenta, separation)
641.2 ☑
scalp 459.0
due to injury at birth 767.19
scrotum 608.83
secondary (nontraumatic) 459.0
following initial hemorrhage at time of
injury 958.2
seminal vesicle 608.83
skin 782.7
newborn 772.6
spermatic cord 608.83
spinal (cord) 336.1
aneurysm (ruptured) 336.1
syphilitic 094.89
due to birth injury 767.4
fetus or newborn 767.4
spleen 289.59
spontaneous NEC 459.0
petechial 782.7
stomach 578.9
newborn 772.4
ulcer — *see* Ulcer, stomach, with hemorrhage
subaponeurotic, newborn 767.11
massive (birth injury) 767.11
subarachnoid (nontraumatic) 430
fetus or newborn (anoxic) (traumatic)
772.2
puerperal, postpartum, childbirth
674.0 ☑
traumatic — *see* Hemorrhage, brain,
traumatic, subarachnoid
subconjunctival 372.72
due to birth injury 772.8
newborn 772.8
subcortical (*see also* Hemorrhage, brain) 431
subcutaneous 782.7
subdiaphragmatic 459.0
subdural (nontraumatic) 432.1
due to birth injury 767.0
fetus or newborn (anoxic) (hypoxic) (due
to birth trauma) 767.0
puerperal, postpartum, childbirth
674.0 ☑
spinal 336.1
traumatic — *see* Hemorrhage, brain,
traumatic, subdural
subgaleal 767.11
subhyaloid 362.81
subperiosteal 733.99
subretinal 362.81
subtentorial (*see also* Hemorrhage, subdural) 432.1
subungual 703.8
due to blood dyscrasia 287.8
suprarenal (capsule) (gland) 255.41
fetus or newborn 772.2
tentorium (traumatic) (*see also* Hemorrhage,
brain, traumatic)

☑ Additional Digit Required — Refer to the Tabular List for Digit Selection

▽ Subterms under main terms may continue to next column or page

Hemorrhage, hemorrhagic — *continued*
tentorium (*see also* Hemorrhage, brain,
   traumatic) — *continued*
   fetus or newborn 767.0
   nontraumatic — *see* Hemorrhage, sub-
    dural
testis 608.83
thigh 459.0
third stage 666.0 ☑
thorax — *see* Hemorrhage, lung
throat 784.8
thrombocythemia 238.71
thymus (gland) 254.8
thyroid (gland) 246.3
   cyst 246.3
tongue 529.8
tonsil 474.8
   postoperative 998.11
tooth socket (postextraction) 998.11
trachea — *see* Hemorrhage, lung
traumatic (*see also* nature of injury)
   brain — *see* Hemorrhage, brain, traumat-
    ic
   recurring or secondary (following initial
    hemorrhage at time of injury)
    958.2
tuberculous NEC (*see also* Tuberculosis,
   pulmonary) 011.9 ☑
tunica vaginalis 608.83
ulcer — *see* Ulcer, by site, with hemorrhage
umbilicus, umbilical cord 772.0
   after birth, newborn 772.3
   complicating delivery 663.8 ☑
    affecting fetus or newborn 772.0
   slipped ligature 772.3
   stump 772.3
unavoidable (due to placenta previa)
   641.1 ☑
   affecting fetus or newborn 762.0
upper extremity 459.0
urethra (idiopathic) 599.84
uterus, uterine (abnormal) 626.9
   climacteric 627.0
   complicating delivery — *see* Hemor-
    rhage, complicating, delivery
   due to
    intrauterine contraceptive device
     996.76
     perforating uterus 996.32
   functional or dysfunctional 626.8
   in pregnancy — *see* Hemorrhage, preg-
    nancy
   intermenstrual 626.6
    irregular 626.6
    regular 626.5
   postmenopausal 627.1
   postpartum (*see also* Hemorrhage,
    postpartum) 666.1 ☑
   prepubertal 626.8
   pubertal 626.3
   puerperal (immediate) 666.1 ☑
vagina 623.8
vasa previa 663.5 ☑
   affecting fetus or newborn 772.0
vas deferens 608.83
ventricular (*see also* Hemorrhage, brain) 431
vesical 596.8
viscera 459.0
   newborn 772.8
vitreous (humor) (intraocular) 379.23
vocal cord 478.5
vulva 624.8
Hemorrhoids (anus) (rectum) (without complication) 455.6
bleeding, prolapsed, strangulated, or ulcerated NEC 455.8
   external 455.5
   internal 455.2
complicated NEC 455.8
complicating pregnancy and puerperium
   671.8 ☑
external 455.3
   with complication NEC 455.5
   bleeding, prolapsed, strangulated, or
    ulcerated 455.5
   thrombosed 455.4

Hemorrhoids — *continued*
internal 455.0
   with complication NEC 455.2
   bleeding, prolapsed, strangulated, or
    ulcerated 455.2
   thrombosed 455.1
residual skin tag 455.9
sentinel pile 455.9
thrombosed NEC 455.7
   external 455.4
   internal 455.1
Hemosalpinx 620.8
Hemosiderosis 275.09   ▲
dietary 275.09   ▲
pulmonary (idiopathic) 275.09 [516.1]   ▲
transfusion NEC 275.02   ▲
   bone marrow 996.85
Hemospermia 608.82
Hemothorax 511.89
bacterial, nontuberculous 511.1
newborn 772.8
nontuberculous 511.89
   bacterial 511.1
pneumococcal 511.1
postoperative 998.11
staphylococcal 511.1
streptococcal 511.1
traumatic 860.2
   with
    open wound into thorax 860.3
    pneumothorax 860.4
     with open wound into thorax
     860.5
tuberculous (*see also* Tuberculosis, pleura)
   012.0 ☑
Hemotympanum 385.89
Hench-Rosenberg syndrome (palindromic
   arthritis) — *see also* Rheumatism, palindromic 719.3 ☑
Henle's warts 371.41
Henoch (-Schönlein)
disease or syndrome (allergic purpura) 287.0
purpura (allergic) 287.0
Henpue, henpuye 102.6
Heparin-induced thrombocytopenia (HIT)
   289.84
Heparitinuria 277.5
Hepar lobatum 095.3
Hepatalgia 573.8
Hepatic — *see also* condition
flexure syndrome 569.89
Hepatitis 573.3
acute (*see also* Necrosis, liver) 570
   alcoholic 571.1
   infective 070.1
    with hepatic coma 070.0
alcoholic 571.1
amebic — *see* Abscess, liver, amebic
anicteric (acute) — *see* Hepatitis, viral
antigen-associated (HAA) — *see* Hepatitis,
   viral, type B
Australian antigen (positive) — *see* Hepatitis, viral, type B
autoimmune 571.42
catarrhal (acute) 070.1
   with hepatic coma 070.0
   chronic 571.40
   newborn 070.1
    with hepatic coma 070.0
chemical 573.3
cholangiolitic 573.8
cholestatic 573.8
chronic 571.40
   active 571.49
    viral — *see* Hepatitis, viral
   aggressive 571.49
   persistent 571.41
   viral — *see* Hepatitis, viral
cytomegalic inclusion virus 078.5 [573.1]
diffuse 573.3
"dirty needle" — *see* Hepatitis, viral
drug-induced 573.3
due to
   Coxsackie 074.8 [573.1]
   cytomegalic inclusion virus 078.5 [573.1]
   infectious mononucleosis 075 [573.1]

Hepatitis — *continued*
due to — *continued*
   malaria 084.9 [573.2]
   mumps 072.71
   secondary syphilis 091.62
   toxoplasmosis (acquired) 130.5
    congenital (active) 771.2
epidemic — *see* Hepatitis, viral, type A
fetus or newborn 774.4
fibrous (chronic) 571.49
   acute 570
from injection, inoculation, or transfusion
   (blood) (other substance) (plasma)
   (serum) (onset within 8 months after
   administration) — *see* Hepatitis, viral
fulminant (viral) (*see also* Hepatitis, viral)
   070.9
   with hepatic coma 070.6
   type A 070.1
    with hepatic coma 070.0
   type B — *see* Hepatitis, viral, type B
giant cell (neonatal) 774.4
hemorrhagic 573.8
history of
   B V12.09
   C V12.09
homologous serum — *see* Hepatitis, viral
hypertrophic (chronic) 571.49
   acute 570
infectious, infective (acute) (chronic) (subacute) 070.1
   with hepatic coma 070.0
inoculation — *see* Hepatitis, viral
interstitial (chronic) 571.49
   acute 570
lupoid 571.49
malarial 084.9 [573.2]
malignant (*see also* Necrosis, liver) 570
neonatal (toxic) 774.4
newborn 774.4
parenchymatous (acute) (*see also* Necrosis,
   liver) 570
peliosis 573.3
persistent, chronic 571.41
plasma cell 571.49
postimmunization — *see* Hepatitis, viral
postnecrotic 571.49
posttransfusion — *see* Hepatitis, viral
recurrent 571.49
septic 573.3
serum — *see* Hepatitis, viral
   carrier (suspected of) V02.61
subacute (*see also* Necrosis, liver) 570
suppurative (diffuse) 572.0
syphilitic (late) 095.3
   congenital (early) 090.0 [573.2]
    late 090.5 [573.2]
   secondary 091.62
toxic (noninfectious) 573.3
   fetus or newborn 774.4
tuberculous (*see also* Tuberculosis) 017.9 ☑
viral (acute) (anicteric) (cholangiolitic)
   (cholestatic) (chronic) (subacute)
   070.9
   with hepatic coma 070.6
   AU-SI I type virus — *see* Hepatitis, viral,
    type B
   Australian antigen — *see* Hepatitis, viral,
    type B
   B-antigen — *see* Hepatitis, viral, type B
   Coxsackie 074.8 [573.1]
   cytomegalic inclusion 078.5 [573.1]
   IH (virus) — *see* Hepatitis, viral, type A
   infectious hepatitis virus — *see* Hepati-
    tis, viral, type A
   serum hepatitis virus — *see* Hepatitis,
    viral, type B
   SH — *see* Hepatitis, viral, type B
   specified type NEC 070.59
    with hepatic coma 070.49
   type A 070.1
    with hepatic coma 070.0
   type B (acute) 070.30
    with
     hepatic coma 070.20
      with hepatitis delta 070.21

Hepatitis — *continued*
viral — *continued*
   type B — *continued*
    with — *continued*
     hepatitis delta 070.31
      with hepatic coma 070.21
    carrier status V02.61
    chronic 070.32
     with
      hepatic coma 070.22
       with hepatitis delta 070.23
      hepatitis delta 070.33
       with hepatic coma 070.23
   type C
    acute 070.51
     with hepatic coma 070.41
    carrier status V02.62
    chronic 070.54
     with hepatic coma 070.44
    in remission 070.54
    unspecified 070.70
     with hepatic coma 070.71
   type delta (with hepatitis B carrier state)
    070.52
    with
     active hepatitis B disease — *see*
      Hepatitis, viral, type B
     hepatic coma 070.42
   type E 070.53
    with hepatic coma 070.43
   vaccination and inoculation (prophylac-
    tic) V05.3
   Waldenström's (lupoid hepatitis) 571.49
Hepatization, lung (acute) — *see also* Pneu-
   monia, lobar
chronic (*see also* Fibrosis, lung) 515
Hepatoblastoma (M8970/3) 155.0
Hepatocarcinoma (M8170/3) 155.0
Hepatocholangiocarcinoma (M8180/3) 155.0
Hepatocholangioma, benign (M8180/0) 211.5
Hepatocholangitis 573.8
Hepatocystitis — *see also* Cholecystitis 575.10
Hepatodystrophy 570
Hepatolenticular degeneration 275.1
Hepatolithiasis — *see* Choledocholithiasis
Hepatoma (malignant) (M8170/3) 155.0
benign (M8170/0) 211.5
congenital (M8970/3) 155.0
embryonal (M8970/3) 155.0
Hepatomegalia glycogenica diffusa 271.0
Hepatomegaly — *see also* Hypertrophy, liver
   789.1
congenital 751.69
   syphilitic 090.0
due to Clonorchis sinensis 121.1
Gaucher's 272.7
syphilitic (congenital) 090.0
Hepatoptosis 573.8
Hepatorrhexis 573.8
Hepatosis, toxic 573.8
Hepatosplenomegaly 571.8
due to S. japonicum 120.2
hyperlipemic (Bürger-Grutz type) 272.3
Herald patch 696.3
Hereditary — *see* condition
Heredodegeneration 330.9
macular 362.70
Heredopathia atactica polyneuritiformis
   356.3
Heredosyphilis — *see also* Syphilis, congenital
   090.9
Hermaphroditism (true) 752.7
with specified chromosomal anomaly —
   see Anomaly, chromosomes, sex
Hernia, hernial (acquired) (recurrent) 553.9
with
   gangrene (obstructed) NEC 551.9
   obstruction NEC 552.9
    and gangrene 551.9
abdomen (wall) — *see* Hernia, ventral
abdominal, specified site NEC 553.8
   with
    gangrene (obstructed) 551.8
    obstruction 552.8
     and gangrene 551.8
appendix 553.8

Index

Hemorrhage, hemorrhagic — Hernia, hernial

☑ **Additional Digit Required** — Refer to the Tabular List for Digit Selection   Ⓦ **Subterms under main terms may continue to next column or page**

2011 ICD-9-CM   ▶◀ Revised Text   ● New Line   ▲ Revised Code   October 2010 • Volume 2 — 137

Hernia, hernial — *continued*
  appendix — *continued*
    with
      gangrene (obstructed) 551.8
      obstruction 552.8
        and gangrene 551.8
  bilateral (inguinal) — *see* Hernia, inguinal
  bladder (sphincter)
    congenital (female) (male) 756.71
    female (*see also* Cystocele, female)
      618.01
    male 596.8
  brain 348.4
    congenital 742.0
  broad ligament 553.8
  cartilage, vertebral — *see* Displacement,
    intervertebral disc
  cerebral 348.4
    congenital 742.0
    endaural 742.0
  ciliary body 364.89
    traumatic 871.1
  colic 553.9
    with
      gangrene (obstructed) 551.9
      obstruction 552.9
        and gangrene 551.9
  colon 553.9
    with
      gangrene (obstructed) 551.9
      obstruction 552.9
        and gangrene 551.9
  colostomy (stoma) 569.69
  Cooper's (retroperitoneal) 553.8
    with
      gangrene (obstructed) 551.8
      obstruction 552.8
        and gangrene 551.8
  crural — *see* Hernia, femoral
  diaphragm, diaphragmatic 553.3
    with
      gangrene (obstructed) 551.3
      obstruction 552.3
        and gangrene 551.3
    congenital 756.6
    due to gross defect of diaphragm 756.6
    traumatic 862.0
      with open wound into cavity 862.1
  direct (inguinal) — *see* Hernia, inguinal
  disc, intervertebral — *see* Displacement,
    intervertebral disc
  diverticulum, intestine 553.9
    with
      gangrene (obstructed) 551.9
      obstruction 552.9
        and gangrene 551.9
  double (inguinal) — *see* Hernia, inguinal
  due to adhesion with obstruction
    552.9   ▲
  duodenojejunal 553.8
    with
      gangrene (obstructed) 551.8
      obstruction 552.8
        and gangrene 551.8
  en glissade — *see* Hernia, inguinal
  enterostomy (stoma) 569.69
  epigastric 553.29
    with
      gangrene (obstruction) 551.29
      obstruction 552.29
        and gangrene 551.29
    recurrent 553.21
      with
        gangrene (obstructed) 551.21
        obstruction 552.21
          and gangrene 551.21
  esophageal hiatus (sliding) 553.3
    with
      gangrene (obstructed) 551.3
      obstruction 552.3
        and gangrene 551.3
    congenital 750.6
  external (inguinal) — *see* Hernia, inguinal
  fallopian tube 620.4
  fascia 728.89
  fat 729.30

Hernia, hernial — *continued*
  fat — *continued*
    eyelid 374.34
    orbital 374.34
    pad 729.30
      eye, eyelid 374.34
      knee 729.31
      orbit 374.34
      popliteal (space) 729.31
      specified site NEC 729.39
  femoral (unilateral) 553.00
    with
      gangrene (obstructed) 551.00
      obstruction 552.00
        with gangrene 551.00
    bilateral 553.02
      gangrenous (obstructed) 551.02
      obstructed 552.02
        with gangrene 551.02
      recurrent 553.03
        gangrenous (obstructed) 551.03
        obstructed 552.03
          with gangrene 551.03
    recurrent (unilateral) 553.01
      bilateral 553.03
        gangrenous (obstructed) 551.03
        obstructed 552.03
          with gangrene 551.01
      gangrenous (obstructed) 551.01
      obstructed 552.01
        with gangrene 551.01
  foramen
    Bochdalek 553.3
      with
        gangrene (obstructed) 551.3
        obstruction 552.3
          and gangrene 551.3
      congenital 756.6
    magnum 348.4
    Morgagni, Morgagnian 553.3
      with
        gangrene 551.3
        obstruction 552.3
          and gangrene 551.3
      congenital 756.6
  funicular (umbilical) 553.1
    with
      gangrene (obstructed) 551.1
      obstruction 552.1
        and gangrene 551.1
    spermatic cord — *see* Hernia, inguinal
  gangrenous — *see* Hernia, by site, with
    gangrene
  gastrointestinal tract 553.9
    with
      gangrene (obstructed) 551.9
      obstruction 552.9
        and gangrene 551.9
  gluteal — *see* Hernia, femoral
  Gruber's (internal mesogastric) 553.8
    with
      gangrene (obstructed) 551.8
      obstruction 552.8
        and gangrene 551.8
  Hesselbach's 553.8
    with
      gangrene (obstructed) 551.8
      obstruction 552.8
        and gangrene 551.8
  hiatal (esophageal) (sliding) 553.3
    with
      gangrene (obstructed) 551.3
      obstruction 552.3
        and gangrene 551.3
    congenital 750.6
  incarcerated (*see also* Hernia, by site, with
    obstruction) 552.9
  gangrenous (*see also* Hernia, by site, with
    gangrene) 551.9
  incisional 553.21
    with
      gangrene (obstructed) 551.21
      obstruction 552.21
        and gangrene 551.21
    lumbar — *see* Hernia, lumbar
    recurrent 553.21

Hernia, hernial — *continued*
  incisional — *continued*
    recurrent — *continued*
      with
        gangrene (obstructed) 551.21
        obstruction 552.21
          and gangrene 551.21
  indirect (inguinal) — *see* Hernia, inguinal
  infantile — *see* Hernia, inguinal
  infrapatellar fat pad 729.31
  inguinal (direct) (double) (encysted) (exter-
    nal) (funicular) (indirect) (infantile)
    (internal) (interstitial) (oblique)
    (scrotal) (sliding) 550.9 ☑

Note — Use the following fifth-digit
subclassification with category 550:

0 *unilateral or unspecified (not*
   specified as recurrent)

1 *unilateral or unspecified, recurrent*

2 *bilateral (not specified as recur-*
   rent)

3 *bilateral, recurrent*

---

      with
        gangrene (obstructed) 550.0 ☑
        obstruction 550.1 ☑
          and gangrene 550.0 ☑
  internal 553.8
    with
      gangrene (obstructed) 551.8
      obstruction 552.8
        and gangrene 551.8
    inguinal — *see* Hernia, inguinal
  interstitial 553.9
    with
      gangrene (obstructed) 551.9
      obstruction 552.9
        and gangrene 551.9
    inguinal — *see* Hernia, inguinal
  intervertebral cartilage or disc — *see* Dis-
    placement, intervertebral disc
  intestine, intestinal 553.9
    with
      gangrene (obstructed) 551.9
      obstruction 552.9
        and gangrene 551.9
  intra-abdominal 553.9
    with
      gangrene (obstructed) 551.9
      obstruction 552.9
        and gangrene 551.9
  intraparietal 553.9
    with
      gangrene (obstructed) 551.9
      obstruction 552.9
        and gangrene 551.9
  iris 364.89
    traumatic 871.1
  irreducible (*see also* Hernia, by site, with
    obstruction) 552.9
    gangrenous (with obstruction) (*see also*
      Hernia, by site, with gangrene)
      551.9
  ischiatic 553.8
    with
      gangrene (obstructed) 551.8
      obstruction 552.8
        and gangrene 551.8
  ischiorectal 553.8
    with
      gangrene (obstructed) 551.8
      obstruction 552.8
        and gangrene 551.8
  lens 379.32
    traumatic 871.1
  linea
    alba — *see* Hernia, epigastric
    semilunaris — *see* Hernia, spigelian
  Littre's (diverticular) 553.9
    with
      gangrene (obstructed) 551.9
      obstruction 552.9
        and gangrene 551.9
  lumbar 553.8

Hernia, hernial — *continued*
  lumbar — *continued*
    with
      gangrene (obstructed) 551.8
      obstruction 552.8
        and gangrene 551.8
    intervertebral disc 722.10
  lung (subcutaneous) 518.89
    congenital 748.69
  mediastinum 519.3
  mesenteric (internal) 553.8
    with
      gangrene (obstructed) 551.8
      obstruction 552.8
        and gangrene 551.8
  mesocolon 553.8
    with
      gangrene (obstructed) 551.8
      obstruction 552.8
        and gangrene 551.8
  muscle (sheath) 728.89
  nucleus pulposus — *see* Displacement, in-
    tervertebral disc
  oblique (inguinal) — *see* Hernia, inguinal
  obstructive (*see also* Hernia, by site, with
    obstruction) 552.9
    gangrenous (with obstruction) (*see also*
      Hernia, by site, with gangrene)
      551.9
  obturator 553.8
    with
      gangrene (obstructed) 551.8
      obstruction 552.8
        and gangrene 551.8
  omental 553.8
    with
      gangrene (obstructed) 551.8
      obstruction 552.8
        and gangrene 551.8
  orbital fat (pad) 374.34
  ovary 620.4
  oviduct 620.4
  paracolostomy (stoma) 569.69
  paraduodenal 553.8
    with
      gangrene (obstructed) 551.8
      obstruction 552.8
        and gangrene 551.8
  paraesophageal 553.3
    with
      gangrene (obstructed) 551.3
      obstruction 552.3
        and gangrene 551.3
    congenital 750.6
  parahiatal 553.3
    with
      gangrene (obstructed) 551.3
      obstruction 552.3
        and gangrene 551.3
  paraumbilical 553.1
    with
      gangrene (obstructed) 551.1
      obstruction 552.1
        and gangrene 551.1
  parietal 553.9
    with
      gangrene (obstructed) 551.9
      obstruction 552.9
        and gangrene 551.9
  perineal 553.8
    with
      gangrene (obstructed) 551.8
      obstruction 552.8
        and gangrene 551.8
  peritoneal sac, lesser 553.8
    with
      gangrene (obstructed) 551.8
      obstruction 552.8
        and gangrene 551.8
  popliteal fat pad 729.31
  postoperative 553.21
    with
      gangrene (obstructed) 551.21
      obstruction 552.21
        and gangrene 551.21
  pregnant uterus 654.4 ☑

☑ **Additional Digit Required** — **Refer to the Tabular List for Digit Selection**

▽ **Subterms under main terms may continue to next column or page**

▶◀ **Revised Text**   ● **New Line**   ▲ **Revised Code**

Hernia, hernial — *continued*
  prevesical 596.8
  properitoneal 553.8
    with
      gangrene (obstructed) 551.8
      obstruction 552.8
        and gangrene 551.8
  pudendal 553.8
    with
      gangrene (obstructed) 551.8
      obstruction 552.8
        and gangrene 551.8
  rectovaginal 618.6
  retroperitoneal 553.8
    with
      gangrene (obstructed) 551.8
      obstruction 552.8
        and gangrene 551.8
  Richter's (parietal) 553.9
    with
      gangrene (obstructed) 551.9
      obstruction 552.9
        and gangrene 551.9
  Rieux's, Riex's (retrocecal) 553.8
    with
      gangrene (obstructed) 551.8
      obstruction 552.8
        and gangrene 551.8
  sciatic 553.8
    with
      gangrene (obstructed) 551.8
      obstruction 552.8
        and gangrene 551.8
  scrotum, scrotal — *see* Hernia, inguinal
  sliding (inguinal) (*see also* Hernia, inguinal)
    hiatus — *see* Hernia, hiatal
  spigelian 553.29
    with
      gangrene (obstructed) 551.29
      obstruction 552.29
        and gangrene 551.29
  spinal (*see also* Spina bifida) 741.9 ☑
    with hydrocephalus 741.0 ☑
  strangulated (*see also* Hernia, by site, with obstruction) 552.9
    gangrenous (with obstruction) (*see also* Hernia, by site, with gangrene) 551.9
  supraumbilicus (linea alba) — *see* Hernia, epigastric
  tendon 727.9
  testis (nontraumatic) 550.9 ☑
    meaning
      scrotal hernia 550.9 ☑
      symptomatic late syphilis 095.8
  Treitz's (fossa) 553.8
    with
      gangrene (obstructed) 551.8
      obstruction 552.8
        and gangrene 551.8
  tunica
    albuginea 608.89
    vaginalis 752.89
  umbilicus, umbilical 553.1
    with
      gangrene (obstructed) 551.1
      obstruction 552.1
        and gangrene 551.1
  ureter 593.89
    with obstruction 593.4
  uterus 621.8
    pregnant 654.4 ☑
  vaginal (posterior) 618.6
  Velpeau's (femoral) (*see also* Hernia, femoral) 553.00
  ventral 553.20
    with
      gangrene (obstructed) 551.20
      obstruction 552.20
        and gangrene 551.20
    incisional 553.21
    recurrent 553.21
      with
        gangrene (obstructed) 551.21
        obstruction 552.21
          and gangrene 551.21

Hernia, hernial — *continued*
  vesical
    congenital (female) (male) 756.71
    female (*see also* Cystocele, female) 618.01
    male 596.8
  vitreous (into anterior chamber) 379.21
    traumatic 871.1
Herniation — *see also* Hernia
  brain (stem) 348.4
  cerebral 348.4
  gastric mucosa (into duodenal bulb) 537.89
  mediastinum 519.3
  nucleus pulposus — *see* Displacement, intervertebral disc
Herpangina 074.0
Herpes, herpetic 054.9
  auricularis (zoster) 053.71
    simplex 054.73
  blepharitis (zoster) 053.20
    simplex 054.41
  circinate 110.5
  circinatus 110.5
    bullous 694.5
  conjunctiva (simplex) 054.43
    zoster 053.21
  cornea (simplex) 054.43
    disciform (simplex) 054.43
    zoster 053.21
  encephalitis 054.3
  eye (zoster) 053.29
    simplex 054.40
  eyelid (zoster) 053.20
    simplex 054.41
  febrilis 054.9
  fever 054.9
  geniculate ganglionitis 053.11
  genital, genitalis 054.10
    specified site NEC 054.19
  gestationis 646.8 ☑
  gingivostomatitis 054.2
  iridocyclitis (simplex) 054.44
    zoster 053.22
  iris (any site) 695.10
  iritis (simplex) 054.44
  keratitis (simplex) 054.43
    dendritic 054.42
    disciform 054.43
    interstitial 054.43
      zoster 053.21
  keratoconjunctivitis (simplex) 054.43
    zoster 053.21
  labialis 054.9
    meningococcal 036.89
  lip 054.9
  meningitis (simplex) 054.72
    zoster 053.0
  ophthalmicus (zoster) 053.20
    simplex 054.40
  otitis externa (zoster) 053.71
    simplex 054.73
  penis 054.13
  perianal 054.10
  pharyngitis 054.79
  progenitalis 054.10
  scrotum 054.19
  septicemia 054.5
  simplex 054.9
    complicated 054.8
      ophthalmic 054.40
        specified NEC 054.49
      specified NEC 054.79
    congenital 771.2
    external ear 054.73
    keratitis 054.43
      dendritic 054.42
    meningitis 054.72
    myelitis 054.74
    neuritis 054.79
    specified complication NEC 054.79
      ophthalmic 054.49
    visceral 054.71
  stomatitis 054.2
  tonsurans 110.0
    maculosus (of Hebra) 696.3
  visceral 054.71

Herpes, herpetic — *continued*
  vulva 054.12
  vulvovaginitis 054.11
  whitlow 054.6
  zoster 053.9
    auricularis 053.71
    complicated 053.8
      specified NEC 053.79
    conjunctiva 053.21
    cornea 053.21
    ear 053.71
    eye 053.29
    geniculate 053.11
    keratitis 053.21
      interstitial 053.21
    myelitis 053.14
    neuritis 053.10
    ophthalmicus(a) 053.20
    oticus 053.71
    otitis externa 053.71
    specified complication NEC 053.79
    specified site NEC 053.9
  zosteriform, intermediate type 053.9
Herrick's
  anemia (hemoglobin S disease) 282.61
  syndrome (hemoglobin S disease) 282.61
Hers' disease (glycogenosis VI) 271.0
Herter (-Gee) disease or syndrome (nontropical sprue) 579.0
Herter's infantilism (nontropical sprue) 579.0
Herxheimer's disease (diffuse idiopathic cutaneous atrophy) 701.8
Herxheimer's reaction 995.0
Hesitancy, urinary 788.64
Hesselbach's hernia — *see* Hernia, Hesselbach's
Heterochromia (congenital) 743.46
  acquired 364.53
  cataract 366.33
  cyclitis 364.21
  hair 704.3
  iritis 364.21
  retained metallic foreign body 360.62
    magnetic 360.52
  uveitis 364.21
Heterophoria 378.40
  alternating 378.45
  vertical 378.43
Heterophyes, small intestine 121.6
Heterophyiasis 121.6
Heteropsia 368.8
Heterotopia, heterotopic — *see also* Malposition, congenital
  cerebralis 742.4
  pancreas, pancreatic 751.7
  spinalis 742.59
Heterotropia 378.30
  intermittent 378.20
    vertical 378.31
  vertical (constant) (intermittent) 378.31
Heubner's disease 094.89
Heubner-Herter disease or syndrome (nontropical sprue) 579.0
Hexadactylism 755.0 ☑
Heyd's syndrome (hepatorenal) 572.4
HGSIL (high grade squamous intraepithelial lesion) (cytologic finding) (Pap smear finding)
  anus 796.74
  cervix 795.04
    biopsy finding — code to CIN II or CIN III
  vagina 795.14
Hibernoma (M8880/0) — *see* Lipoma
Hiccough 786.8
  epidemic 078.89
  psychogenic 306.1
Hiccup — *see also* Hiccough 786.8
Hicks (-Braxton) contractures 644.1 ☑
Hidden penis 752.65
Hidradenitis (axillaris) (suppurative) 705.83
Hidradenoma (nodular) (M8400/0) — *see also* Neoplasm, skin, benign
  clear cell (M8402/0) — *see* Neoplasm, skin, benign

Hidradenoma — *see also* Neoplasm, skin, benign — *continued*
  papillary (M8405/0) — *see* Neoplasm, skin, benign
Hidrocystoma (M8404/0) — *see* Neoplasm, skin, benign
HIE (hypoxic-ischemic encephalopathy) 768.70
  mild 768.71
  moderate 768.72
  severe 768.73
High
  A₂ anemia 282.49
  altitude effects 993.2
    anoxia 993.2
    on
      ears 993.0
      sinuses 993.1
    polycythemia 289.0
  arch
    foot 755.67
    palate 750.26
  artery (arterial) tension (*see also* Hypertension) 401.9
    without diagnosis of hypertension 796.2
  basal metabolic rate (BMR) 794.7
  blood pressure (*see also* Hypertension) 401.9
    incidental reading (isolated) (nonspecific), no diagnosis of hypertension 796.2
  cholesterol 272.0
    with high triglycerides 272.2
  compliance bladder 596.4
  diaphragm (congenital) 756.6
  frequency deafness (congenital) (regional) 389.8
  head at term 652.5 ☑
    affecting fetus or newborn 763.1
  output failure (cardiac) (*see also* Failure, heart) 428.9
  oxygen-affinity hemoglobin 289.0
  palate 750.26
  risk
    behavior — *see* Problem
    family situation V61.9
      specified circumstance NEC V61.8
    human papillomavirus (HPV) DNA test positive
      anal 796.75
      cervical 795.05
      vaginal 795.15
    individual NEC V62.89
    infant NEC V20.1
    patient taking drugs (prescribed) V67.51
      nonprescribed (*see also* Abuse, drugs, nondependent) 305.9 ☑
    pregnancy V23.9
      inadequate prenatal care V23.7
      specified problem NEC V23.89
  temperature (of unknown origin) (*see also* Pyrexia) 780.60
  thoracic rib 756.3
  triglycerides 272.1
    with high cholesterol 272.2
Hildenbrand's disease (typhus) 081.9
Hilger's syndrome 337.09
Hill diarrhea 579.1
Hilliard's lupus — *see also* Tuberculosis 017.0 ☑
Hilum — *see* condition
Hip — *see* condition
Hippel's disease (retinocerebral angiomatosis) 759.6
Hippus 379.49
Hirschfeld's disease (acute diabetes mellitus) — *see also* Diabetes 250.0 ☑
  due to secondary diabetes 249.0 ☑
Hirschsprung's disease or megacolon (congenital) 751.3
Hirsuties — *see also* Hypertrichosis 704.1
Hirsutism — *see also* Hypertrichosis 704.1
Hirudiniasis (external) (internal) 134.2
Hiss-Russell dysentery 004.1
Histamine cephalgia 339.00
Histidinemia 270.5
Histidinuria 270.5
Histiocytic syndromes 288.4

☑ Additional Digit Required — Refer to the Tabular List for Digit Selection   ▽ Subterms under main terms may continue to next column or page

2011 ICD-9-CM   ▶◀ Revised Text   ● New Line   ▲ Revised Code   Volume 2 — 139

Histiocytoma (M8832/0) — *see also* Neoplasm, skin, benign
  fibrous (M8830/0) (*see also* Neoplasm, skin, benign)
    atypical (M8830/1) — *see* Neoplasm, connective tissue, uncertain behavior
    malignant (M8830/3) — *see* Neoplasm, connective tissue, malignant
Histiocytosis (acute) (chronic) (subacute) 277.89
  acute differentiated progressive (M9722/3) 202.5 ☑
  cholesterol 277.89
  essential 277.89
  lipid, lipoid (essential) 272.7
  lipochrome (familial) 288.1 ☑
  malignant (M9720/3) 202.3 ☑
  non-Langerhans cell 277.89
  polyostotic sclerosing 277.89
  X (chronic) 277.89
    acute (progressive) (M9722/3) 202.5 ☑
Histoplasmosis 115.90
  with
    endocarditis 115.94
    meningitis 115.91
    pericarditis 115.93
    pneumonia 115.95
    retinitis 115.92
    specified manifestation NEC 115.99
  African (due to Histoplasma duboisii) 115.10
    with
      endocarditis 115.14
      meningitis 115.11
      pericarditis 115.13
      pneumonia 115.15
      retinitis 115.12
      specified manifestation NEC 115.19
  American (due to Histoplasma capsulatum) 115.00
    with
      endocarditis 115.04
      meningitis 115.01
      pericarditis 115.03
      pneumonia 115.05
      retinitis 115.02
      specified manifestation NEC 115.09
  Darling's — *see* Histoplasmosis, American
  large form (*see also* Histoplasmosis, African) 115.10
  lung 115.05
  small form (*see also* Histoplasmosis, American) 115.00
History (personal) of
  abuse
    emotional V15.42
    neglect V15.42
    physical V15.41
    sexual V15.41
  affective psychosis V11.1
  alcoholism V11.3
    specified as drinking problem (*see also* Abuse, drugs, nondependent) 305.0 ☑
  allergy ▶to◀ V15.09   ▲
    analgesic agent NEC V14.6
    anesthetic NEC V14.4
    antibiotic agent NEC V14.1
      penicillin V14.0
    anti-infective agent NEC V14.3
    arachnid bite V15.06
    diathesis V15.09
    drug V14.9
      specified type NEC V14.8
    eggs V15.03
    food additives V15.05
    insect bite V15.06
    latex V15.07
    medicinal agents V14.9
      specified type NEC V14.8
    milk products V15.02
    narcotic agent NEC V14.5
    nuts V15.05
      peanuts V15.01
    penicillin V14.0
    radiographic dye V15.08

History of — *continued*
  allergy ▶to◀ — *continued*
    seafood V15.04
    serum V14.7
    specified food NEC V15.05
    specified nonmedicinal agents NEC V15.09
    spider bite V15.06
    sulfa V14.2
    sulfonamides V14.2
    therapeutic agent NEC V15.09
    vaccine V14.7
  anaphylactic shock V15.09   ●
  anemia V12.3
  arrest, sudden cardiac V12.53
  arthritis V13.4
  attack, transient ischemic (TIA) V12.54
  benign neoplasm of brain V12.41
  blood disease V12.3
  calculi, urinary V13.01
  cardiovascular disease V12.50
    myocardial infarction 412
  chemotherapy, antineoplastic V87.41
  child abuse V15.41
  cigarette smoking V15.82
  circulatory system disease V12.50
    myocardial infarction 412
  cleft lip and palate, corrected V13.64   ●
  combat and operational stress reaction   ●
    V11.4   ●
  congenital malformation ▶(corrected)◀
    circulatory system V13.65   ●
    digestive system V13.67   ●
    ear V13.64   ●
    eye V13.64   ●
    face V13.64   ●
    genitourinary system V13.62   ●
    heart V13.65   ●
    integument V13.68   ●
    limbs V13.68   ●
    musculoskeletal V13.68   ●
    neck V13.64   ●
    nervous system V13.63   ●
    respiratory system V13.66   ●
    specified type NEC V13.69   ●
  contraception V15.7
  death, sudden, successfully resuscitated V12.53
  deficit
    prolonged reversible ischemic neurologic (PRIND) V12.54
    reversible ischemic neurologic (RIND) V12.54
  diathesis, allergic V15.09
  digestive system disease V12.70
    peptic ulcer V12.71
    polyps, colonic V12.72
    specified NEC V12.79
  disease (of) V13.9
    blood V12.3
    blood-forming organs V12.3
    cardiovascular system V12.50
    circulatory system V12.50
      specified NEC V12.59
    digestive system V12.70
      peptic ulcer V12.71
      polyps, colonic V12.72
      specified NEC V12.79
    infectious V12.00
      malaria V12.03
      methicillin resistant Staphylococcus aureus (MRSA) V12.04
      MRSA (methicillin resistant Staphylococcus aureus) V12.04
      poliomyelitis V12.02
      specified NEC V12.09
      tuberculosis V12.01
    parasitic V12.00
      specified NEC V12.09
    respiratory system V12.60
      pneumonia V12.61
      specified NEC V12.69
    skin V13.3
    specified site NEC V13.8
    subcutaneous tissue V13.3
    trophoblastic V13.1

History of — *continued*
  disease — *continued*
    trophoblastic — *continued*
      affecting management of pregnancy V23.1
  disorder (of) V13.9
    endocrine V12.2
    genital system V13.29
    hematological V12.3
    immunity V12.2
    mental V11.9
      affective type V11.1
      manic-depressive V11.1
      neurosis V11.2
      schizophrenia V11.0
      specified type NEC V11.8
    metabolic V12.2
    musculoskeletal NEC V13.59
    nervous system V12.40
      specified type NEC V12.49
    obstetric V13.29
      affecting management of current pregnancy V23.49
        pre-term labor V23.41
      pre-term labor V13.21
    sense organs V12.40
      specified type NEC V12.49
    specified site NEC V13.8
    urinary system V13.00
      calculi V13.01
      infection V13.02
      nephrotic syndrome V13.03
      specified NEC V13.09
  drug use
    nonprescribed (*see also* Abuse, drugs, nondependent) 305.9 ☑
    patent (*see also* Abuse, drugs, non-dependent) 305.9 ☑
  dysplasia
    cervical (conditions classifiable to 622.10-622.12) V13.22
    vaginal (conditions classifiable to 623.0) V13.23   ●
    vulvar (conditions classifiable to 624.01-624.02) V13.24   ●
  effect NEC of external cause V15.89
  embolism (pulmonary) V12.51
  emotional abuse V15.42
  encephalitis V12.42
  endocrine disorder V12.2
  estrogen therapy V87.43
  extracorporeal membrane oxygenation (ECMO) V15.87
  failed
    conscious sedation V15.80
    moderate sedation V15.80
  falling V15.88
  family
    allergy V19.6
    anemia V18.2
    arteriosclerosis V17.49
    arthritis V17.7
    asthma V17.5
    blindness V19.0
    blood disorder NEC V18.3
    cardiovascular disease V17.49
    carrier, genetic disease V18.9
    cerebrovascular disease V17.1
    chronic respiratory condition NEC V17.6
    colonic polyps V18.51
    congenital anomalies V19.5
    consanguinity V19.7
    coronary artery disease V17.3
    cystic fibrosis V18.19
    deafness V19.2
    diabetes mellitus V18.0
    digestive disorders V18.59
    disease or disorder (of)
      allergic V19.6
      blood NEC V18.3
      cardiovascular NEC V17.49
      cerebrovascular V17.1
      colonic polyps V18.51
      coronary artery V17.3
      death, sudden cardiac (SCD) V17.41
      digestive V18.59

History of — *continued*
  family — *continued*
    disease or disorder — *continued*
      ear NEC V19.3
      endocrine V18.19
        multiple neoplasia (MEN) syndrome V18.11
      eye NEC V19.1
      genitourinary NEC V18.7
      hypertensive V17.49
      infectious V18.8
      ischemic heart V17.3
      kidney V18.69
        polycystic V18.61
      mental V17.0
      metabolic V18.19
      musculoskeletal NEC V17.89
        osteoporosis V17.81
      neurological NEC V17.2
      parasitic V18.8
      psychiatric condition V17.0
      skin condition V19.4
    ear disorder NEC V19.3
    endocrine disease V18.19
      multiple neoplasia (MEN) syndrome V18.11
    epilepsy V17.2
    eye disorder NEC V19.1
    genetic disease carrier V18.9
    genitourinary disease NEC V18.7
    glomerulonephritis V18.69
    gout V18.19
    hay fever V17.6
    hearing loss V19.2
    hematopoietic neoplasia V16.7
    Hodgkin's disease V16.7
    Huntington's chorea V17.2
    hydrocephalus V19.5
    hypertension V17.49
    infarction, myocardial V17.3
    infectious disease V18.8
    ischemic heart disease V17.3
    kidney disease V18.69
      polycystic V18.61
    leukemia V16.6
    lymphatic malignant neoplasia NEC V16.7
    malignant neoplasm (of) NEC V16.9
      anorectal V16.0
      anus V16.0
      appendix V16.0
      bladder V16.52
      bone V16.8
      brain V16.8
      breast V16.3
        male V16.8
      bronchus V16.1
      cecum V16.0
      cervix V16.49
      colon V16.0
      duodenum V16.0
      esophagus V16.0
      eye V16.8
      gallbladder V16.0
      gastrointestinal tract V16.0
      genital organs V16.40
      hemopoietic NEC V16.7
      ileum V16.0
      ilium V16.8
      intestine V16.0
      intrathoracic organs NEC V16.2
      kidney V16.51
      larynx V16.2
      liver V16.0
      lung V16.1
      lymphatic NEC V16.7
      ovary V16.41
      oviduct V16.41
      pancreas V16.0
      penis V16.49
      prostate V16.42
      rectum V16.0
      respiratory organs NEC V16.2
      skin V16.8
      specified site NEC V16.8
      stomach V16.0

☑ **Additional Digit Required** — Refer to the Tabular List for Digit Selection   ▽ **Subterms under main terms may continue to next column or page**

140 — Volume 2 · October 2010   ▶◀ Revised Text   ● New Line   ▲ Revised Code   2011 ICD-9-CM

History of — *continued*
  family — *continued*
    malignant neoplasm — *continued*
      testis V16.43
      trachea V16.1
      ureter V16.59
      urethra V16.59
      urinary organs V16.59
      uterus V16.49
      vagina V16.49
      vulva V16.49
    MEN (multiple endocrine neoplasia syndrome) V18.11
    mental retardation V18.4
    metabolic disease NEC V18.19
    mongolism V19.5
    multiple
      endocrine neoplasia (MEN) syndrome V18.11
      myeloma V16.7
    musculoskeletal disease NEC V17.89
      osteoporosis V17.81
    myocardial infarction V17.3
    nephritis V18.69
    nephrosis V18.69
    osteoporosis V17.81
    parasitic disease V18.8
    polycystic kidney disease V18.61
    psychiatric disorder V17.0
    psychosis V17.0
    retardation, mental V18.4
    retinitis pigmentosa V19.1
    schizophrenia V17.0
    skin conditions V19.4
    specified condition NEC V19.8
    stroke (cerebrovascular) V17.1
    sudden cardiac death (SCD) V17.41
    visual loss V19.0
  foreign body fully removed V15.53 ●
  fracture, healed
    pathologic V13.51
    stress V13.52
    traumatic V15.51
  genital system disorder V13.29
    pre-term labor V13.21
  health hazard V15.9
    falling V15.88
    specified cause NEC V15.89
  hepatitis
    B V12.09
    C V12.09
  Hodgkin's disease V10.72
  hypospadias ▶(corrected)◀ V13.61
  immunity disorder V12.2
  immunosuppression therapy V87.46
  infarction, cerebral, without residual deficits V12.54
  infection
    central nervous system V12.42
    urinary (tract) V13.02
  infectious disease V12.00
    malaria V12.03
    methicillin resistant Staphylococcus aureus (MRSA) V12.04
    MRSA (methicillin resistant Staphylococcus aureus) V12.04
    poliomyelitis V12.02
    specified NEC V12.09
    tuberculosis V12.01
  injury NEC V15.59
    traumatic brain V15.52
  insufficient prenatal care V23.7
  in utero procedure
    during pregnancy V15.21
    while a fetus V15.22
  irradiation V15.3
  leukemia V10.60
    lymphoid V10.61
    monocytic V10.63
    myeloid V10.62
    specified type NEC V10.69
  little or no prenatal care V23.7
  low birth weight (*see also* Status, low birth weight) V21.30
  lymphosarcoma V10.71
  malaria V12.03

History of — *continued*
  malignant carcinoid tumor V10.91
  malignant neoplasm (of) V10.90
    accessory sinus V10.22
    adrenal V10.88
    anus V10.06
    bile duct V10.09
    bladder V10.51
    bone V10.81
    brain V10.85
    breast V10.3
    bronchus V10.11
    cervix uteri V10.41
    colon V10.05
    connective tissue NEC V10.89
    corpus uteri V10.42
    digestive system V10.00
      specified part NEC V10.09
    duodenum V10.09
    endocrine gland NEC V10.88
    epididymis V10.48
    esophagus V10.03
    eye V10.84
    fallopian tube V10.44
    female genital organ V10.40
      specified site NEC V10.44
    gallbladder V10.09
    gastrointestinal tract V10.00
    gum V10.02
    hematopoietic NEC V10.79
    hypopharynx V10.02
    ileum V10.09
    intrathoracic organs NEC V10.20
    jejunum V10.09
    kidney V10.52
    large intestine V10.05
    larynx V10.21
    lip V10.02
    liver V10.07
    lung V10.11
    lymphatic NEC V10.79
    lymph glands or nodes NEC V10.79
    male genital organ V10.45
      specified site NEC V10.49
    mediastinum V10.29
    melanoma (of skin) V10.82
    middle ear V10.22
    mouth V10.02
      specified part NEC V10.02
    nasal cavities V10.22
    nasopharynx V10.02
    nervous system NEC V10.86
    nose V10.22
    oropharynx V10.02
    ovary V10.43
    pancreas V10.09
    parathyroid V10.88
    penis V10.49
    pharynx V10.02
    pineal V10.88
    pituitary V10.88
    placenta V10.44
    pleura V10.29
    prostate V10.46
    rectosigmoid junction V10.06
    rectum V10.06
    renal pelvis V10.53
    respiratory organs NEC V10.20
    salivary gland V10.02
    skin V10.83
      melanoma V10.82
    small intestine NEC V10.09
    soft tissue NEC V10.89
    specified site NEC V10.89
    stomach V10.04
    testis V10.47
    thymus V10.29
    thyroid V10.87
    tongue V10.01
    trachea V10.12
    ureter V10.59
    urethra V10.59
    urinary organ V10.50
    uterine adnexa V10.44
    uterus V10.42
    vagina V10.44

History of — *continued*
  malignant neoplasm — *continued*
    vulva V10.44
  malignant neuroendocrine tumor V10.91
  manic-depressive psychosis V11.1
  meningitis V12.42
  mental disorder V11.9
    affective type V11.1
    manic-depressive V11.1
    neurosis V11.2
    schizophrenia V11.0
    specified type NEC V11.8
  Merkel cell carcinoma V10.91
  metabolic disorder V12.2
  methicillin resistant Staphylococcus aureus (MRSA) V12.04
  MRSA (methicillin resistant Staphylococcus aureus) V12.04
  musculoskeletal disorder NEC V13.59
  myocardial infarction 412
  neglect (emotional) V15.42
  nephrotic syndrome V13.03
  nervous system disorder V12.40
    specified type NEC V12.49
  neurosis V11.2
  noncompliance with medical treatment V15.81
  nutritional deficiency V12.1
  obstetric disorder V13.29
    affecting management of current pregnancy V23.49
      pre-term labor V23.41
    pre-term labor V13.21
  parasitic disease V12.00
    specified NEC V12.09
  perinatal problems V13.7
    low birth weight (*see also* Status, low birth weight) V21.30
  physical abuse V15.41
  poisoning V15.6
  poliomyelitis V12.02
  polyps, colonic V12.72
  poor obstetric V13.29
    affecting management of current pregnancy V23.49
      pre-term labor V23.41
    pre-term labor V13.21
  prolonged reversible ischemic neurologic deficit (PRIND) V12.54
  psychiatric disorder V11.9
    affective type V11.1
    manic-depressive V11.1
    neurosis V11.2
    schizophrenia V11.0
    specified type NEC V11.8
  psychological trauma V15.49
    emotional abuse V15.42
    neglect V15.42
    physical abuse V15.41
    rape V15.41
  psychoneurosis V11.2
  radiation therapy V15.3
  rape V15.41
  respiratory system disease V12.60
    pneumonia V12.61
    specified NEC V12.69
  reticulosarcoma V10.71
  return from military deployment V62.22
  reversible ischemic neurologic deficit (RIND) V12.54
  schizophrenia V11.0
  skin disease V13.3
  smoking (tobacco) V15.82
  steroid therapy V87.45
    inhaled V87.44
    systemic V87.45
  stroke without residual deficits V12.54
  subcutaneous tissue disease V13.3
  sudden
    cardiac
      arrest V12.53
      death (successfully resuscitated) V12.53
  surgery to
    great vessels V15.1
    heart V15.1

History of — *continued*
  surgery to — *continued*
    in utero
      during pregnancy V15.21
      while a fetus V15.22
    organs NEC V15.29
  syndrome, nephrotic V13.03
  therapy
    antineoplastic drug V87.41
    drug NEC V87.49
    estrogen V87.43
    immunosuppression V87.46
    monoclonal drug V87.42
    steroid V87.45
      inhaled V87.44
      systemic V87.45
  thrombophlebitis V12.52
  thrombosis V12.51
  tobacco use V15.82
  trophoblastic disease V13.1
    affecting management of pregnancy V23.1
  tuberculosis V12.01
  ulcer, peptic V12.71
  urinary system disorder V13.00
    calculi V13.01
    infection V13.02
    nephrotic syndrome V13.03
    specified NEC V13.09
His-Werner disease (trench fever) 083.1
HIT (heparin-induced thrombocytopenia) 289.84
Hives (bold) — *see also* Urticaria 708.9
HIV infection (disease) (illness) — *see* Human immunodeficiency virus (disease) (illness) (infection)
Hoarseness 784.42
Hobnail liver — *see* Cirrhosis, portal
Hobo, hoboism V60.0
Hodgkin's
  disease (M9650/3) 201.9 ☑
    lymphocytic
      depletion (M9653/3) 201.7 ☑
        diffuse fibrosis (M9654/3) 201.7 ☑
        reticular type (M9655/3) 201.7 ☑
      predominance (M9651/3) 201.4 ☑
    lymphocytic-histiocytic predominance (M9651/3) 201.4 ☑
    mixed cellularity (M9652/3) 201.6 ☑
    nodular sclerosis (M9656/3) 201.5 ☑
      cellular phase (M9657/3) 201.5 ☑
  granuloma (M9661/3) 201.1 ☑
  lymphogranulomatosis (M9650/3) 201.9 ☑
  lymphoma (M9650/3) 201.9 ☑
  lymphosarcoma (M9650/3) 201.9 ☑
  paragranuloma (M9660/3) 201.0 ☑
  sarcoma (M9662/3) 201.2 ☑
Hodgson's disease (aneurysmal dilatation of aorta) 441.9
  ruptured 441.5
Hodi-potsy 111.0
Hoffa (-Kastert) disease or syndrome (liposynovitis prepatellaris) 272.8
Hoffmann-Bouveret syndrome (paroxysmal tachycardia) 427.2
Hoffman's syndrome 244.9 *[359.5]*
Hole
  macula 362.54
  optic disc, crater-like 377.22
  retina (macula) 362.54
    round 361.31
      with detachment 361.01
Holla disease — *see also* Spherocytosis 282.0
Holländer-Simons syndrome (progressive lipodystrophy) 272.6
Hollow foot (congenital) 754.71
  acquired 736.73
Holmes' syndrome (visual disorientation) 368.16
Holoprosencephaly 742.2
  due to
    trisomy 13 758.1
    trisomy 18 758.2
Holthouse's hernia — *see* Hernia, in
Homesickness 309.89

☑ **Additional Digit Required — Refer to the Tabular List for Digit Selection**   ▽ **Subterms under main terms may continue to next colu**

2011 ICD-9-CM   ▶◀ **Revised Text**   ● **New Line**   ▲ **Revised Code**   **October 2010 • Volum**

Homicidal ideation V62.85 ●
Homocystinemia 270.4
Homocystinuria 270.4
Homologous serum jaundice (prophylactic)
   (therapeutic) — see Hepatitis, viral
Homosexuality — omit code
   ego-dystonic 302.0
   pedophilic 302.2
   problems with 302.0
Homozygous Hb-S disease 282.61
Honeycomb lung 518.89
   congenital 748.4
Hong Kong ear 117.3
HOOD (hereditary osteo-onychodysplasia)
   756.89
Hooded
   clitoris 752.49
   penis 752.69
Hookworm (anemia) (disease) (infestation) —
   see Ancylostomiasis
Hoppe-Goldflam syndrome 358.00
Hordeolum (external) (eyelid) 373.11
   internal 373.12
Horn
   cutaneous 702.8
      cheek 702.8
      eyelid 702.8
      penis 702.8
   iliac 756.89
   nail 703.8
      congenital 757.5
   papillary 700
Horner's
   syndrome (see also Neuropathy, peripheral,
      autonomic) 337.9
   traumatic 954.0
   teeth 520.4
Horseshoe kidney (congenital) 753.3
Horton's
   disease (temporal arteritis) 446.5
   headache or neuralgia 339.00
Hospice care V66.7
Hospitalism (in children) NEC 309.83
Hourglass contraction, contracture
   bladder 596.8
   gallbladder 575.2
      congenital 751.69
   stomach 536.8
      congenital 750.7
      psychogenic 306.4
   uterus 661.4 ☑
      affecting fetus or newborn 763.7
Household circumstance affecting care V60.9
   specified type NEC V60.89
Housemaid's knee 727.2
Housing circumstance affecting care V60.9
   specified type NEC V60.89
HTLV-I infection 079.51
HTLV-II infection 079.52
HTLV-III/LAV (disease) (illness) (infection) —
   see Human immunodeficiency virus
   (disease) (illness) (infection)
HTLV-III (disease) (illness) (infection) — see
   Human immunodeficiency virus (dis-
   ease) (illness) (infection)
HTR (hemolytic transfusion reaction) ●
   due to or resulting from ●
      incompatibility ●
         ABO 999.61 ●
            acute 999.62 ●
            delayed 999.63 ●
         non-ABO antigen (minor) (Duffy) ●
            (Kell) (Kidd) (Lewis) (M) (N) ●
            (P) (S) 999.76 ●
            acute 999.77 ●
            delayed 999.78 ●
         Rh antigen (C) (c) (D) (E) (e) 999.71 ●
            acute 999.72 ●
            delayed 999.73 ●
Huchard's disease (continued arterial hypertension) 401.9
Hudson-Stähli lines 371.11
Huguier's disease (uterine fibroma) 218.9
Human bite (open wound) — see also Wound,
   open, by site
   intact skin surface — see Contusion

Human immunodeficiency virus (disease)
   (illness) 042
   infection V08
      with symptoms, symptomatic 042
Human immunodeficiency virus-2 infection
   079.53
Human immunovirus (disease) (illness) (infection) — see Human immunodeficiency
   virus (disease) (illness) (infection)
Human papillomavirus 079.4
   high risk, DNA test positive
      anal 796.75
      cervical 795.05
      vaginal 795.15
   low risk, DNA test positive
      anal 796.79
      cervical 795.09
      vaginal 795.19
Human parvovirus 079.83
**Human T-cell lymphotrophic virus-I infec-
   tion** 079.51
**Human T-cell lymphotrophic virus-II infec-
   tion** 079.52
Human T-cell lymphotrophic virus-III (disease) (illness) (infection) — see Human
   immunodeficiency virus (disease) (ill-
   ness) (infection)
Humpback (acquired) 737.9
   congenital 756.19
Hum, venous — omit code
Hunchback (acquired) 737.9
   congenital 756.19
Hunger 994.2
   air, psychogenic 306.1
   disease 251.1
Hungry bone syndrome 275.5
Hunner's ulcer — see also Cystitis 595.1
Hunt's
   neuralgia 053.11
   syndrome (herpetic geniculate ganglionitis)
      053.11
      dyssynergia cerebellaris myoclonica
         334.2
Hunter's glossitis 529.4
Hunterian chancre 091.0
Hunter (-Hurler) syndrome (mucopolysaccharidosis II) 277.5
Huntington's
   chorea 333.4
   disease 333.4
Huppert's disease (multiple myeloma)
   (M9730/3) 203.0 ☑
Hurler (-Hunter) disease or syndrome (mucopolysaccharidosis II) 277.5
Hürthle cell
   adenocarcinoma (M8290/3) 193
   adenoma (M8290/0) 226
   carcinoma (M8290/3) 193
   tumor (M8290/0) 226
Hutchinson's
   disease meaning
      angioma serpiginosum 709.1
      cheiropompholyx 705.81
      prurigo estivalis 692.72
      summer eruption, or summer prurigo
         692.72
   incisors 090.5
   melanotic freckle (M8742/2) (see also Neo-
      plasm, skin, in situ)
      malignant melanoma in (M8742/3) —
         see Melanoma
   teeth or incisors (congenital syphilis) 090.5
Hutchinson-Boeck disease or syndrome
   (sarcoidosis) 135
Hutchinson-Gilford disease or syndrome
   (progeria) 259.8
Hyaline
   degeneration (diffuse) (generalized) 728.9
      localized — see Degeneration, by site
   membrane (disease) (lung) (newborn) 769
Hyalinosis cutis et mucosae 272.8
Hyalin plaque, sclera, senile 379.16
Hyalitis (asteroid) 379.22
   syphilitic 095.8
Hydatid
   cyst or tumor (see also Echinococcus) —

Hydatid — continued
   cyst or tumor (see also Echinococcus) —
      continued
      fallopian tube 752.11
   mole — see Hydatidiform mole
   Morgagni (congenital) 752.89
      fallopian tube 752.11
Hydatidiform mole (benign) (complicating
   pregnancy) (delivered) (undelivered) 630
   invasive (M9100/1) 236.1
   malignant (M9100/1) 236.1
   previous, affecting management of pregnan-
      cy V23.1
Hydatidosis — see Echinococcus
Hyde's disease (prurigo nodularis) 698.3
Hydradenitis 705.83
Hydradenoma (M8400/0) — see Hidradenoma
Hydralazine lupus or syndrome
   correct substance properly administered
      695.4
   overdose or wrong substance given or taken
      972.6
Hydramnios 657.0 ☑
   affecting fetus or newborn 761.3
Hydrancephaly 742.3
   with spina bifida (see also Spina bifida)
      741.0 ☑
Hydranencephaly 742.3
   with spina bifida (see also Spina bifida)
      741.0 ☑
Hydrargyrism NEC 985.0
Hydrarthrosis — see also Effusion, joint
   719.0 ☑
   gonococcal 098.50
   intermittent (see also Rheumatism, palin-
      dromic) 719.3 ☑
   of yaws (early) (late) 102.6
   syphilitic 095.8
      congenital 090.5
Hydremia 285.9
Hydrencephalocele (congenital) 742.0
Hydrencephalomeningocele (congenital)
   742.0
Hydroa 694.0
   aestivale 692.72
   gestationis 646.8 ☑
   herpetiformis 694.0
   pruriginosa 694.0
   vacciniforme 692.72
Hydroadenitis 705.83
Hydrocalycosis — see also Hydronephrosis 591
   congenital 753.29
Hydrocalyx — see also Hydronephrosis 591
Hydrocele (calcified) (chylous) (idiopathic)
   (infantile) (inguinal canal) (recurrent)
   (senile) (spermatic cord) (testis) (tunica
   vaginalis) 603.9
   canal of Nuck (female) 629.1
      male 603.9
   congenital 778.6
   encysted 603.0
      congenital 778.6
   female NEC 629.89
   infected 603.1
   round ligament 629.89
   specified type NEC 603.8
      congenital 778.6
   spinalis (see also Spina bifida) 741.9 ☑
   vulva 624.8
Hydrocephalic fetus
   affecting management or pregnancy
      655.0 ☑
   causing disproportion 653.6 ☑
      with obstructed labor 660.1 ☑
         affecting fetus or newborn 763.1
Hydrocephalus (acquired) (external) (internal)
   (malignant) (noncommunicating) (obstructive) (recurrent) 331.4
   aqueduct of Sylvius stricture 742.3
      with spina bifida (see also Spina bifida)
         741.0 ☑
   chronic 742.3
      with spina bifida (see also Spina bifida)
         741.0 ☑
   communicating 331.3
   congenital (external) (internal) 742.3

Hydrocephalus — continued
   congenital — continued
      with spina bifida (see also Spina bifida)
         741.0 ☑
   due to
      stricture of aqueduct of Sylvius 742.3
         with spina bifida (see also Spina bifi-
            da) 741.0 ☑
      toxoplasmosis (congenital) 771.2
   fetal affecting management of pregnancy
      655.0 ☑
   foramen Magendie block (acquired) 331.3
      congenital 742.3
         with spina bifida (see also Spina bifi-
            da) 741.0 ☑
   newborn 742.3
      with spina bifida (see also Spina bifida)
         741.0 ☑
   normal pressure 331.5
      idiopathic (INPH) 331.5
      secondary 331.3
   otitic 348.2
   syphilitic, congenital 090.49
   tuberculous (see also Tuberculosis) 013.8 ☑
Hydrocolpos (congenital) 623.8
Hydrocystoma (M8404/0) — see Neoplasm,
   skin, benign
Hydroencephalocele (congenital) 742.0
Hydroencephalomeningocele (congenital)
   742.0
Hydrohematopneumothorax — see also
   Hemothorax 511.89
Hydromeningitis — see also Meningitis
Hydromeningocele (spinal) — see also Spina
   bifida 741.9 ☑
   cranial 742.0
Hydrometra 621.8
Hydrometrocolpos 623.8
Hydromicrocephaly 742.1
Hydromphalus (congenital) (since birth)
   757.39
Hydromyelia 742.53
Hydromyelocele — see also Spina bifida
   741.9 ☑
Hydronephrosis 591
   atrophic 591
   congenital 753.29
   due to S. hematobium 120.0
   early 591
   functionless (infected) 591
   infected 591
   intermittent 591
   primary 591
   secondary 591
   tuberculous (see also Tuberculosis) 016.0 ☑
Hydropericarditis — see also Pericarditis 423.9
Hydropericardium — see also Pericarditis
   423.9
Hydroperitoneum 789.59
Hydrophobia 071
Hydrophthalmos — see also Buphthalmia
   743.20
Hydropneumohemothorax — see also
   Hemothorax 511.89
Hydropneumopericarditis — see also Pericarditis 423.9
Hydropneumopericardium — see also Pericarditis 423.9
Hydropneumothorax 511.89
   nontuberculous 511.89
      bacterial 511.1
      pneumococcal 511.1
      staphylococcal 511.1
      streptococcal 511.1
   traumatic 860.0
      with open wound into thorax 860.1
   tuberculous (see also Tuberculosis, pleura)
      012.0 ☑
Hydrops 782.3
   abdominis 789.59
   amnii (complicating pregnancy) (see also
      Hydramnios) 657.0 ☑
   articulorum intermittens (see also Rheuma-
      tism, palindromic) 719.3 ☑
   cardiac (see also Failure, heart) 428.0
   congenital — see Hydrops, fetalis

☑ **Additional Digit Required** — Refer to the Tabular List for Digit Selection   ▽ **Subterms under main terms may continue to next column or page**

— **Volume 2 • October 2010**   ▶◀ **Revised Text**   ● **New Line**   ▲ **Revised Code**   **2011 ICD-9-CM**

Hydrops — continued
  endolymphatic (see also Disease, Ménière's)
    386.00
  fetal(is) or newborn 778.0
    due to isoimmunization 773.3
    not due to isoimmunization 778.0
  gallbladder 575.3
  idiopathic (fetus or newborn) 778.0
  joint (see also Effusion, joint) 719.0 ☑
  labyrinth (see also Disease, Ménière's) 386.00
  meningeal NEC 331.4
  nutritional 262
  pericardium — see Pericarditis
  pleura (see also Hydrothorax) 511.89
  renal (see also Nephrosis) 581.9
  spermatic cord (see also Hydrocele) 603.9
Hydropyonephrosis — see also Pyelitis 590.80
  chronic 590.00
Hydrorachis 742.53
Hydrorrhea (nasal) 478.19
  gravidarum 658.1 ☑
  pregnancy 658.1 ☑
Hydrosadenitis 705.83
Hydrosalpinx (fallopian tube) (follicularis)
  614.1
Hydrothorax (double) (pleural) 511.89
  chylous (nonfilarial) 457.8
    filaria (see also Infestation, filarial) 125.9
  nontuberculous 511.89
    bacterial 511.1
    pneumococcal 511.1
    staphylococcal 511.1
    streptococcal 511.1
  traumatic 862.29
    with open wound into thorax 862.39
  tuberculous (see also Tuberculosis, pleura)
    012.0 ☑
Hydroureter 593.5
  congenital 753.22
Hydroureteronephrosis — see also Hydronephrosis 591
Hydrourethra 599.84
Hydroxykynureninuria 270.2
Hydroxyprolinemia 270.8
Hydroxyprolinuria 270.8
Hygroma (congenital) (cystic) (M9173/0) 228.1
  prepatellar 727.3
  subdural — see Hematoma, subdural
Hymen — see condition
Hymenolepiasis (diminuta) (infection) (infestation) (nana) 123.6
Hymenolepsis (diminuta) (infection) (infestation) (nana) 123.6
Hypalgesia — see also Disturbance, sensation 782.0
Hyperabduction syndrome 447.8
Hyperacidity, gastric 536.8
  psychogenic 306.4
Hyperactive, hyperactivity 314.01
  basal cell, uterine cervix 622.10
  bladder 596.51
  bowel (syndrome) 564.9
    sounds 787.5
  cervix epithelial (basal) 622.10
  child 314.01
  colon 564.9
  gastrointestinal 536.8
    psychogenic 306.4
  intestine 564.9
  labyrinth (unilateral) 386.51
    with loss of labyrinthine reactivity 386.58
    bilateral 386.52
  nasal mucous membrane 478.19
  stomach 536.8
  thyroid (gland) (see also Thyrotoxicosis)
    242.9 ☑
Hyperacusis 388.42
Hyperadrenalism (cortical) 255.3
  medullary 255.6
Hyperadrenocorticism 255.3
  congenital 255.2
  iatrogenic
    correct substance properly administered 255.3
    overdose or wrong substance given or taken 962.0

Hyperaffectivity 301.11
Hyperaldosteronism (atypical) (hyperplastic) (normoaldosteronal) (normotensive) (primary) 255.10
  secondary 255.14
Hyperalgesia — see also Disturbance, sensation 782.0
Hyperalimentation 783.6
  carotene 278.3
  specified NEC 278.8
  vitamin A 278.2
  vitamin D 278.4
Hyperaminoaciduria 270.9
  arginine 270.6
  citrulline 270.6
  cystine 270.0
  glycine 270.0
  lysine 270.7
  ornithine 270.6
  renal (types I, II, III) 270.0
Hyperammonemia (congenital) 270.6
Hyperamnesia 780.99
Hyperamylasemia 790.5
Hyperaphia 782.0
Hyperazotemia 791.9
Hyperbetalipoproteinemia (acquired) (essential) (familial) (hereditary) (primary) (secondary) 272.0
  with prebetalipoproteinemia 272.2
Hyperbilirubinemia 782.4
  congenital 277.4
  constitutional 277.4
  neonatal (transient) (see also Jaundice, fetus or newborn) 774.6
  of prematurity 774.2
Hyperbilirubinemia encephalopathia, newborn 774.7
  due to isoimmunization 773.4
Hypercalcemia, hypercalcemic (idiopathic) 275.42
  nephropathy 588.89
Hypercalcinuria 275.40
Hypercapnia 786.09
  with mixed acid-based disorder 276.4
  fetal, affecting newborn 770.89
Hypercarotinemia 278.3
Hypercementosis 521.5
Hyperchloremia 276.9
Hyperchlorhydria 536.8
  neurotic 306.4
  psychogenic 306.4
Hypercholesterinemia — see Hypercholesterolemia
Hypercholesterolemia 272.0
  with hyperglyceridemia, endogenous 272.2
  essential 272.0
  familial 272.0
  hereditary 272.0
  primary 272.0
  pure 272.0
Hypercholesterolosis 272.0
Hyperchylia gastrica 536.8
  psychogenic 306.4
Hyperchylomicronemia (familial) (with hyperbetalipoproteinemia) 272.3
Hypercoagulation syndrome (primary) 289.81
  secondary 289.82
Hypercorticosteronism
  correct substance properly administered 255.3
  overdose or wrong substance given or taken 962.0
Hypercortisonism
  correct substance properly administered 255.3
  overdose or wrong substance given or taken 962.0
Hyperdynamic beta-adrenergic state or syndrome (circulatory) 429.82
Hyperekplexia 759.89
Hyperelectrolytemia 276.9
Hyperemesis 536.2
  arising during pregnancy — see Hyperemesis, gravidarum
  gravidarum (mild) (before 22 completed weeks gestation) 643.0 ☑

Hyperemesis — continued
  gravidarum — continued
    with
      carbohydrate depletion 643.1 ☑
      dehydration 643.1 ☑
      electrolyte imbalance 643.1 ☑
      metabolic disturbance 643.1 ☑
    affecting fetus or newborn 761.8
    severe (with metabolic disturbance) 643.1 ☑
  psychogenic 306.4
Hyperemia (acute) 780.99
  anal mucosa 569.49
  bladder 596.7
  cerebral 437.8
  conjunctiva 372.71
  ear, internal, acute 386.30
  enteric 564.89
  eye 372.71
  eyelid (active) (passive) 374.82
  intestine 564.89
  iris 364.41
  kidney 593.81
  labyrinth 386.30
  liver (active) (passive) 573.8
  lung 514
  ovary 620.8
  passive 780.99
  pulmonary 514
  renal 593.81
  retina 362.89
  spleen 289.59
  stomach 537.89
Hyperesthesia (body surface) — see also Disturbance, sensation 782.0
  larynx (reflex) 478.79
    hysterical 300.11
  pharynx (reflex) 478.29
Hyperestrinism 256.0
Hyperestrogenism 256.0
Hyperestrogenosis 256.0
Hyperexplexia 759.89
Hyperextension, joint 718.80
  ankle 718.87
  elbow 718.82
  foot 718.87
  hand 718.84
  hip 718.85
  knee 718.86
  multiple sites 718.89
  pelvic region 718.85
  shoulder (region) 718.81
  specified site NEC 718.88
  wrist 718.83
Hyperfibrinolysis — see Fibrinolysis
Hyperfolliculinism 256.0
Hyperfructosemia 271.2
Hyperfunction
  adrenal (cortex) 255.3
    androgenic, acquired benign 255.3
    medulla 255.6
    virilism 255.2
  corticoadrenal NEC 255.3
  labyrinth — see Hyperactive, labyrinth
  medulloadrenal 255.6
  ovary 256.1
    estrogen 256.0
  pancreas 577.8
  parathyroid (gland) 252.00
  pituitary (anterior) (gland) (lobe) 253.1
  testicular 257.0
Hypergammaglobulinemia 289.89
  monoclonal, benign (BMH) 273.1
  polyclonal 273.0
  Waldenström's 273.0
Hyperglobulinemia 273.8
Hyperglycemia 790.29
  maternal
    affecting fetus or newborn 775.0
    manifest diabetes in infant 775.1
  postpancreatectomy (complete) (partial) 251.3
Hyperglyceridemia 272.1
  endogenous 272.1
  essential 272.1
  familial 272.1

Hyperglyceridemia — continued
  hereditary 272.1
  mixed 272.3
  pure 272.1
Hyperglycinemia 270.7
Hypergonadism
  ovarian 256.1
  testicular (infantile) (primary) 257.0
Hyperheparinemia — see also Circulating anticoagulants 286.5
Hyperhidrosis, hyperidrosis 705.21
  axilla 705.21
  face 705.21
  focal (localized) 705.21
    primary 705.21
      axilla 705.21
      face 705.21
      palms 705.21
      soles 705.21
    secondary 705.22
      axilla 705.22
      face 705.22
      palms 705.22
      soles 705.22
  generalized 780.8
  palms 705.21
  psychogenic 306.3
  secondary 780.8
  soles 705.21
Hyperhistidinemia 270.5
Hyperinsulinism (ectopic) (functional) (organic) NEC 251.1
  iatrogenic 251.0
  reactive 251.2
  spontaneous 251.2
  therapeutic misadventure (from administration of insulin) 962.3
Hyperiodemia 276.9
Hyperirritability (cerebral), in newborn 779.1
Hyperkalemia 276.7
Hyperkeratosis — see also Keratosis 701.1
  cervix 622.2
  congenital 757.39
  cornea 371.89
  due to yaws (early) (late) (palmar or plantar) 102.3
  eccentrica 757.39
  figurata centrifuga atrophica 757.39
  follicularis 757.39
    in cutem penetrans 701.1
  limbic (cornea) 371.89
  palmoplantaris climacterica 701.1
  pinta (carate) 103.1
  senile (with pruritus) 702.0
  tongue 528.79
  universalis congenita 757.1
  vagina 623.1
  vocal cord 478.5
  vulva 624.09
Hyperkinesia, hyperkinetic (disease) (reaction) (syndrome) 314.9
  with
    attention deficit — see Disorder, attention deficit
    conduct disorder 314.2
    developmental delay 314.1
    simple disturbance of activity and attention 314.01
    specified manifestation NEC 314.8
  heart (disease) 429.82
  of childhood or adolescence NEC 314.9
Hyperlacrimation — see also Epiphora 375.20
Hyperlipemia — see also Hyperlipidemia 272.4
Hyperlipidemia 272.4
  carbohydrate-induced 272.1
  combined 272.2
  endogenous 272.1
  exogenous 272.3
  fat-induced 272.3
  group
    A 272.0
    B 272.1
    C 272.2
    D 272.3
  mixed 272.2
  specified type NEC 272.4

☑ Additional Digit Required — Refer to the Tabular List for Digit Selection   Subterms under main terms may continue to next column or page

2011 ICD-9-CM   ►◄ Revised Text   ● New Line   ▲ Revised Code   Volume 2 — 143

Hyperlipidosis 272.7
  hereditary 272.7
Hyperlipoproteinemia (acquired) (essential) (familial) (hereditary) (primary) (secondary) 272.4
  Fredrickson type
    I 272.3
    IIa 272.0
    IIb 272.2
    III 272.2
    IV 272.1
    V 272.3
  low-density-lipoid-type (LDL) 272.0
  very-low-density-lipoid-type (VLDL) 272.1
Hyperlucent lung, unilateral 492.8
Hyperluteinization 256.1
Hyperlysinemia 270.7
Hypermagnesemia 275.2
  neonatal 775.5
Hypermaturity (fetus or newborn)
  post-term infant 766.21
  prolonged gestation infant 766.22
Hypermenorrhea 626.2
Hypermetabolism 794.7
Hypermethioninemia 270.4
Hypermetropia (congenital) 367.0
Hypermobility
  cecum 564.9
  coccyx 724.71
  colon 564.9
    psychogenic 306.4
  ileum 564.89
  joint (acquired) 718.80
    ankle 718.87
    elbow 718.82
    foot 718.87
    hand 718.84
    hip 718.85
    knee 718.86
    multiple sites 718.89
    pelvic region 718.85
    shoulder (region) 718.81
    specified site NEC 718.88
    wrist 718.83
  kidney, congenital 753.3
  meniscus (knee) 717.5
  scapula 718.81
  stomach 536.8
    psychogenic 306.4
  syndrome 728.5
  testis, congenital 752.52
  urethral 599.81
Hypermotility
  gastrointestinal 536.8
  intestine 564.9
    psychogenic 306.4
  stomach 536.8
Hypernasality 784.43
Hypernatremia 276.0
  with water depletion 276.0
Hypernephroma (M8312/3) 189.0
Hyperopia 367.0
Hyperorexia 783.6
Hyperornithinemia 270.6
Hyperosmia — see also Disturbance, sensation 781.1
Hyperosmolality 276.0
Hyperosteogenesis 733.99
Hyperostosis 733.99
  calvarial 733.3
  cortical 733.3
    infantile 756.59
  frontal, internal of skull 733.3
  interna frontalis 733.3
  monomelic 733.99
  skull 733.3
    congenital 756.0
  vertebral 721.8
    with spondylosis — see Spondylosis
    ankylosing 721.6
Hyperovarianism 256.1
Hyperovarism, hyperovaria 256.1
Hyperoxaluria (primary) 271.8
Hyperoxia 987.8
Hyperparathyroidism 252.00
  ectopic 259.3

Hyperparathyroidism — continued
  other 252.08
  primary 252.01
  secondary (of renal origin) 588.81
    non-renal 252.02
  tertiary 252.08
Hyperpathia — see also Disturbance, sensation 782.0
  psychogenic 307.80
Hyperperistalsis 787.4
  psychogenic 306.4
Hyperpermeability, capillary 448.9
Hyperphagia 783.6
Hyperphenylalaninemia 270.1
Hyperphoria 378.40
  alternating 378.45
Hyperphosphatemia 275.3
Hyperpiesia — see also Hypertension 401.9
Hyperpiesis — see also Hypertension 401.9
Hyperpigmentation — see Pigmentation
Hyperpinealism 259.8
Hyperpipecolatemia 270.7
Hyperpituitarism 253.1
Hyperplasia, hyperplastic
  adenoids (lymphoid tissue) 474.12
    and tonsils 474.10
  adrenal (capsule) (cortex) (gland) 255.8
    with
      sexual precocity (male) 255.2
      virilism, adrenal 255.2
      virilization (female) 255.2
    congenital 255.2
    due to excess ACTH (ectopic) (pituitary) 255.0
    medulla 255.8
  alpha cells (pancreatic)
    with
      gastrin excess 251.5
      glucagon excess 251.4
  appendix (lymphoid) 543.0
  artery, fibromuscular NEC 447.8
    carotid 447.8
    renal 447.3
  bone 733.99
    marrow 289.9
  breast (see also Hypertrophy, breast) 611.1
    ductal 610.8
      atypical 610.8
  carotid artery 447.8
  cementation, cementum (teeth) (tooth) 521.5
  cervical gland 785.6
  cervix (uteri) 622.10
    basal cell 622.10
    congenital 752.49
    endometrium 622.10
    polypoid 622.10
  chin 524.05
  clitoris, congenital 752.49
  dentin 521.5
  endocervicitis 616.0
  endometrium, endometrial (adenomatous) (atypical) (cystic) (glandular) (polypoid) (uterus) 621.30
    with atypia 621.33
    without atypia
      complex 621.32
      simple 621.31
    benign 621.34
    cervix 622.10
  epithelial 709.8
    focal, oral, including tongue 528.79
    mouth (focal) 528.79
    nipple 611.89
    skin 709.8
    tongue (focal) 528.79
    vaginal wall 623.0
  erythroid 289.9
  fascialis ossificans (progressiva) 728.11
  fibromuscular, artery NEC 447.8
    carotid 447.8
    renal 447.3
  genital
    female 629.89
    male 608.89
  gingiva 523.8

Hyperplasia, hyperplastic — continued
  glandularis
    cystica uteri 621.30
    endometrium (uterus) 621.30
    interstitialis uteri 621.30
  granulocytic 288.69
  gum 523.8
  hymen, congenital 752.49
  islands of Langerhans 251.1
  islet cell (pancreatic) 251.9
    alpha cells
      with excess
        gastrin 251.5
        glucagon 251.4
    beta cells 251.1
  juxtaglomerular (complex) (kidney) 593.89
  kidney (congenital) 753.3
  liver (congenital) 751.69
  lymph node (gland) 785.6
  lymphoid (diffuse) (nodular) 785.6
    appendix 543.0
    intestine 569.89
  mandibular 524.02
    alveolar 524.72
    unilateral condylar 526.89
  Marchand multiple nodular (liver) — see Cirrhosis, postnecrotic
  maxillary 524.01
    alveolar 524.71
  medulla, adrenal 255.8
  myometrium, myometrial 621.2
  nose (lymphoid) (polypoid) 478.19
  oral soft tissue (inflammatory) (irritative) (mucosa) NEC 528.9
    gingiva 523.8
    tongue 529.8
  organ or site, congenital NEC — see Anomaly, specified type NEC
  ovary 620.8
  palate, papillary 528.9
  pancreatic islet cells 251.9
    alpha
      with excess
        gastrin 251.5
        glucagon 251.4
    beta 251.1
  parathyroid (gland) 252.01
  persistent, vitreous (primary) 743.51
  pharynx (lymphoid) 478.29
  prostate 600.90
    with
      other lower urinary tract symptoms (LUTS) 600.91
    urinary
      obstruction 600.91
      retention 600.91
    adenofibromatous 600.20
      with
        other lower urinary tract symptoms (LUTS) 600.21
      urinary
        obstruction 600.21
        retention 600.21
    nodular 600.10
      with
        urinary
          obstruction 600.11
          retention 600.11
  renal artery (fibromuscular) 447.3
  reticuloendothelial (cell) 289.9
  salivary gland (any) 527.1
  Schimmelbusch's 610.1
  suprarenal (capsule) (gland) 255.8
  thymus (gland) (persistent) 254.0
  thyroid (see also Goiter) 240.9
    primary 242.0 ☑
    secondary 242.2 ☑
  tonsil (lymphoid tissue) 474.11
    and adenoids 474.10
  urethrovaginal 599.89
  uterus, uterine (myometrium) 621.2
    endometrium (see also Hyperplasia, endometrium) 621.30
  vitreous (humor), primary persistent 743.51
  vulva 624.3
  zygoma 738.11

Hyperpnea — see also Hyperventilation 786.01
Hyperpotassemia 276.7
Hyperprebetalipoproteinemia 272.1
  with chylomicronemia 272.3
  familial 272.1
Hyperprolactinemia 253.1
Hyperprolinemia 270.8
Hyperproteinemia 273.8
Hyperprothrombinemia 289.89
Hyperpselaphesia 782.0
Hyperpyrexia 780.60
  heat (effects of) 992.0
  malarial (see also Malaria) 084.6
  malignant, due to anesthetic 995.86
  rheumatic — see Fever, rheumatic
  unknown origin (see also Pyrexia) 780.60
Hyperreactor, vascular 780.2
Hyperreflexia 796.1
  bladder, autonomic 596.54
    with cauda equina 344.61
  detrusor 344.61
Hypersalivation — see also Ptyalism 527.7
Hypersarcosinemia 270.8
Hypersecretion
  ACTH 255.3
  androgens (ovarian) 256.1
  calcitonin 246.0
  corticoadrenal 255.3
  cortisol 255.0
  estrogen 256.0
  gastric 536.8
    psychogenic 306.4
  gastrin 251.5
  glucagon 251.4
  hormone
    ACTH 255.3
    anterior pituitary 253.1
    growth NEC 253.0
    ovarian androgen 256.1
    testicular 257.0
    thyroid stimulating 242.8 ☑
  insulin — see Hyperinsulinism
  lacrimal glands (see also Epiphora) 375.20
  medulloadrenal 255.6
  milk 676.6 ☑
  ovarian androgens 256.1
  pituitary (anterior) 253.1
  salivary gland (any) 527.7
  testicular hormones 257.0
  thyrocalcitonin 246.0
  upper respiratory 478.9
Hypersegmentation, hereditary 288.2
  eosinophils 288.2
  neutrophil nuclei 288.2
Hypersensitive, hypersensitiveness, hypersensitivity — see also Allergy
  angiitis 446.20
    specified NEC 446.29
  carotid sinus 337.01
  colon 564.9
    psychogenic 306.4
  DNA (deoxyribonucleic acid) NEC 287.2
  drug (see also Allergy, drug) 995.27
    due to correct medical substance properly administered 995.27
  esophagus 530.89
  insect bites — see Injury, superficial, by site
  labyrinth 386.58
  pain (see also Disturbance, sensation) 782.0
  pneumonitis NEC 495.9
  reaction (see also Allergy) 995.3
    upper respiratory tract NEC 478.8
  stomach (allergic) (nonallergic) 536.8
    psychogenic 306.4
Hypersomatotropism (classic) 253.0
Hypersomnia, unspecified 780.54
  with sleep apnea, unspecified 780.53
  alcohol induced 291.82
  drug induced 292.85
  due to
    medical condition classified elsewhere 327.14
    mental disorder 327.15
  idiopathic
    with long sleep time 327.11
    without long sleep time 327.12

☑ **Additional Digit Required** — Refer to the Tabular List for Digit Selection   ▽ **Subterms under main terms may continue to next column or page**

Hypersomnia, unspecified — *continued*
   menstrual related 327.13
   nonorganic origin 307.43
      persistent (primary) 307.44
      transient 307.43

Hypersomnia, unspecified — *continued*
   organic 327.10
      other 327.19
   primary 307.44
   recurrent 327.13

Hypersplenia 289.4
Hypersplenism 289.4
Hypersteatosis 706.3
Hyperstimulation, ovarian 256.1
Hypersuprarenalism 255.3

Hypersusceptibility — *see* Allergy
Hyper-TBG-nemia 246.8
Hypertelorism 756.0
   orbit, orbital 376.41

☑ Additional Digit Required — Refer to the Tabular List for Digit Selection   ▽ Subterms under main terms may continue to next column or page

2011 ICD-9-CM   ▶◀ Revised Text   ● New Line   ▲ Revised Code   Volume 2 — 145

	Malignant	Benign	Unspecified
Hypertension, hypertensive (arterial) (arteriolar) (crisis) (degeneration) (disease) (essential) (fluctuating) (idiopathic) (intermittent) (labile) (low renin) (orthostatic) (paroxysmal) (primary) (systemic) (uncontrolled) (vascular)	401.0	401.1	401.9
with			
chronic kidney disease			
stage I through stage IV, or unspecified	403.00	403.10	403.90
stage V or end stage renal disese	403.01	403.11	403.91
heart involvement (conditions classifiable to 429.0–429.3, 429.8, 429.9 due to hypertension) (*see also* Hypertension, heart)	402.00	402.10	402.90
with kidney involvement — *see* Hypertension, cardiorenal			
renal (kidney) involvement (only conditions classifiable to 585, ▶587◀ (excludes conditions classifiable to 584) (*see also* Hypertension, kidney)	403.00	403.10	403.90
with heart involvement — *see* Hypertension, cardiorenal			
failure (and sclerosis) (*see also* Hypertension, kidney)	403.01	403.11	403.91
sclerosis without failure (*see also* Hypertension, kidney)	403.00	403.10	403.90
accelerated (*see also* Hypertension, by type, malignant)	401.0	—	—
antepartum — *see* Hypertension, complicating pregnancy, childbirth, or the puerperium			
cardiorenal (disease)	404.00	404.10	404.90
with			
chronic kidney disease			
stage I through stage IV, or unspecified	404.00	404.10	404.90
and heart failure	404.01	404.11	404.91
stage V or end stage renal disease	404.02	404.12	404.92
and heart failure	404.03	404.13	404.93
heart failure	404.01	404.11	404.91
and chronic kidney disease	404.01	404.11	404.91
stage I through stage IV or unspecified	404.01	404.11	404.91
stave V or end stage renal disease	404.03	404.13	404.93
cardiovascular disease (arteriosclerotic) (sclerotic)	402.00	402.10	402.90
with			
heart failure	402.01	402.11	402.91
renal involvement (conditions classifiable to 403) (*see also* Hypertension, cardiorenal)	404.00	404.10	404.90
cardiovascular renal (disease) (sclerosis) (*see also* Hypertension, cardiorenal)	404.00	404.10	404.90
cerebrovascular disease NEC	437.2	437.2	437.2
complicating pregnancy, childbirth, or the puerperium	642.2 ☑	642.0 ☑	642.9 ☑
with			
albuminuria (and edema) (mild)	—	—	642.4 ☑
severe	—	—	642.5 ☑
chronic kidney diseae	642.2 ☑	642.2 ☑	642.2 ☑
and heart disease	642.2 ☑	642.2 ☑	642.2 ☑
edema (mild)	—	—	642.4 ☑
severe	—	—	642.5 ☑
heart disease	642.2 ☑	642.2 ☑	642.2 ☑
and chronic kidney disease	642.2 ☑	642.2 ☑	642.2 ☑
renal disease	642.2 ☑	642.2 ☑	642.2 ☑
and heart disease	642.2 ☑	642.2 ☑	642.2 ☑
chronic	642.2 ☑	642.0 ☑	642.0 ☑
with pre-eclampsia or eclampsia	642.7 ☑	642.7 ☑	642.7 ☑
fetus or newborn	760.0	760.0	760.0
essential	—	642.0 ☑	642.0 ☑
with pre-eclampsia or eclampsia	—	642.7 ☑	642.7 ☑
fetus or newborn	760.0	760.0	760.0
fetus or newborn	760.0	760.0	760.0
gestational	—	—	642.3 ☑
pre-existing	642.2 ☑	642.0 ☑	642.0 ☑
with pre-eclampsia or eclampsia	642.7 ☑	642.7 ☑	642.7 ☑
fetus or newborn	760.0	760.0	760.0
secondary to renal disease	642.1 ☑	642.1 ☑	642.1 ☑
with pre-eclampsia or eclampsia	642.7 ☑	642.7 ☑	642.7 ☑
fetus or newborn	760.0	760.0	760.0
transient	—	—	642.3 ☑
due to			
aldosteronism, primary	405.09	405.19	405.99
brain tumor	405.09	405.19	405.99
bulbar poliomyelitis	405.09	405.19	405.99
calculus			
kidney	405.09	405.19	405.99

	Malignant	Benign	Unspecified
Hypertension, hypertensive — *continued*			
due to — *continued*			
calculus — *continued*			
ureter	405.09	405.19	405.99
coarctation, aorta	405.09	405.19	405.99
Cushing's disease	405.09	405.19	405.99
glomerulosclerosis (*see also* Hypertension, kidney)	403.00	403.10	403.90
periarteritis nodosa	405.09	405.19	405.99
pheochromocytoma	405.09	405.19	405.99
polycystic kidney(s)	405.09	405.19	405.99
polycythemia	405.09	405.19	405.99
porphyria	405.09	405.19	405.99
pyelonephritis	405.09	405.19	405.99
renal (artery)			
aneurysm	405.01	405.11	405.91
anomaly	405.01	405.11	405.91
embolism	405.01	405.11	405.91
fibromuscular hyperplasia	405.01	405.11	405.91
occlusion	405.01	405.11	405.91
stenosis	405.01	405.11	405.91
thrombosis	405.01	405.11	405.91
encephalopathy	437.2	437.2	437.2
gestational (transient) NEC	—	—	642.3 ☑
Goldblatt's	440.1	440.1	440.1
heart (disease) (conditions classifiable to 429.0–429.3, 429.8, 429.9 due to hypertension)	402.00	402.10	402.90
with heart failure	402.01	402.11	402.91
hypertensive kidney disease (conditions classifiable to 403) (*see also* Hypertension, cardiorenal)	404.00	404.10	404.90
renal sclerosis (*see also* Hypertension, cardiorenal)	404.00	404.10	404.90
intracranial, benign	—	348.2	—
intraocular	—	—	365.04
kidney	403.00	403.10	403.90
with			
chronic kidney disease			
stage I through stage IV, or unspecified	403.00	403.10	403.90
stage V or end stage renal disese	403.01	403.11	403.91
heart involvement (conditions classifiable to 429.0–429.3, 429.8, 429.9 due to hypertension) (*see also* Hypertension, cardiorenal)	404.00	404.10	404.90
hypertensive heart (disease) (conditions classifiable to 402) (*see also* Hypertension, cardiorenal)	404.00	404.10	404.90
lesser circulation	—	—	416.0
necrotizing	401.0	—	—
ocular	—	—	365.04
pancreatic duct — code to underlying condition			
with			
chronic pancreatitis	—	—	577.1
portal (due to chronic liver disease)	—	—	572.3
postoperative	—	—	997.91
psychogenic	—	—	306.2
puerperal, postpartum — *see* Hypertension, complicating pregnancy, childbirth, or the puerperium			
pulmonary (artery) ▶(secondary)◀	—	—	416.8
with cor pulmonale (chronic)	—	—	416.8
acute	—	—	415.0
idiopathic	—	—	416.0
primary	—	—	416.0
of newborn	—	—	747.83
secondary	—	—	416.8
renal (disease) (*see also* Hypertension, kidney)	403.00	403.10	403.90
renovascular NEC	405.01	405.11	405.91
secondary NEC	405.09	405.19	405.99
due to			
aldosteronism, primary	405.09	405.19	405.99
brain tumor	405.09	405.19	405.99
bulbar poliomyelitis	405.09	405.19	405.99
calculus			
kidney	405.09	405.19	405.99
ureter	405.09	405.19	405.99
coarctation, aorta	405.09	405.19	405.99
Cushing's disease	405.09	405.19	405.99
glomerulosclerosis (*see also* Hypertension, kidney)	403.00	403.10	403.90
periarteritis nodosa	405.09	405.19	405.99
pheochromocytoma	405.09	405.19	405.99
polycystic kidney(s)	405.09	405.19	405.99

☑ **Additional Digit Required** — Refer to the Tabular List for Digit Selection   ᵛᵉᵇˢ **Subterms under main terms may continue to next column or page**

	Malignant	Benign	Unspecified
Hypertension, hypertensive — *continued*			
secondary — *continued*			
due to — *continued*			
polycythemia	405.09	405.19	405.99
porphyria	405.09	405.19	405.99
pyelonephritis	405.09	405.19	405.99
renal (artery)			
aneurysm	405.01	405.11	405.91
anomaly	405.01	405.11	405.91
embolism	405.01	405.11	405.91
fibromuscular hyperplasia	405.01	405.11	405.91
occlusion	405.01	405.11	405.91
stenosis	405.01	405.11	405.91
thrombosis	405.01	405.11	405.91
transient	—	—	796.2
of pregnancy	—	—	642.3 ☑
vascular degeneration	401.0	401.1	401.9
venous, chronic (asymptomatic) (idiopathic)	—	—	459.30
with			
complication, NEC	—	—	459.39
inflammation	—	—	459.32
with ulcer	—	—	459.33
ulcer	—	—	459.31
with inflammation	—	—	459.33
due to			
deep vein thrombosis (*see also* Syndrome, postphlebetic)	—	—	459.10

Hypertensive urgency — see Hypertension ●
Hyperthecosis, ovary 256.8
Hyperthermia (of unknown origin) — see also
    Pyrexia 780.60
    malignant (due to anesthesia) 995.86
    newborn 778.4
Hyperthymergasia — see also Psychosis, affec-
    tive 296.0 ☑
    reactive (from emotional stress, psycholog-
      ical trauma) 298.1
    recurrent episode 296.1 ☑
    single episode 296.0 ☑
Hyperthymism 254.8
Hyperthyroid (recurrent) — see Hyperthy-
    roidism
Hyperthyroidism (latent) (preadult) (recurrent)
    (without goiter) 242.9 ☑

> Note — Use the following fifth-digit
> subclassification with category 242:
> 0 without mention of thyrotoxic
>   crisis or storm
> 1 with mention of thyrotoxic crisis
>   or storm

    with
      goiter (diffuse) 242.0 ☑
        adenomatous 242.3 ☑
          multinodular 242.2 ☑
          uninodular 242.1 ☑
        nodular 242.3 ☑
          multinodular 242.2 ☑
          uninodular 242.1 ☑
      thyroid nodule 242.1 ☑
      complicating pregnancy, childbirth, or
        puerperium 648.1 ☑
      neonatal (transient) 775.3
Hypertonia — see Hypertonicity
Hypertonicity
    bladder 596.51
    fetus or newborn 779.89
    gastrointestinal (tract) 536.8
    infancy 779.89
      due to electrolyte imbalance 779.89
    muscle 728.85
    stomach 536.8
      psychogenic 306.4
    uterus, uterine (contractions) 661.4 ☑
      affecting fetus or newborn 763.7
Hypertony — see Hypertonicity
Hypertransaminemia 790.4
Hypertrichosis 704.1
    congenital 757.4
    eyelid 374.54
    lanuginosa 757.4
      acquired 704.1
Hypertriglyceridemia, essential 272.1
Hypertrophy, hypertrophic
    adenoids (infectional) 474.12
      and tonsils (faucial) (infective) (lingual)
        (lymphoid) 474.10
    adrenal 255.8
    alveolar process or ridge 525.8
    anal papillae 569.49
    apocrine gland 705.82
    artery NEC 447.8
      carotid 447.8
      congenital (peripheral) NEC 747.60
        gastrointestinal 747.61
        lower limb 747.64
        renal 747.62
        specified NEC 747.69
        spinal 747.82
        upper limb 747.63
      renal 447.3
    arthritis (chronic) (see also Osteoarthrosis)
      715.9 ☑
      spine (see also Spondylosis) 721.90
    arytenoid 478.79
    asymmetrical (heart) 429.9
    auricular — see Hypertrophy, cardiac
    Bartholin's gland 624.8
    bile duct 576.8
    bladder (sphincter) (trigone) 596.8
    blind spot, visual field 368.42
    bone 733.99

Hypertrophy, hypertrophic — continued
    brain 348.89
    breast 611.1
      cystic 610.1
      fetus or newborn 778.7
      fibrocystic 610.1
      massive pubertal 611.1
      puerperal, postpartum 676.3 ☑
      senile (parenchymatous) 611.1
    cardiac (chronic) (idiopathic) 429.3
      with
        rheumatic fever (conditions classifi-
          able to 390)
          active 391.8
            with chorea 392.0
          inactive or quiescent (with
            chorea) 398.99
      congenital NEC 746.89
      fatty (see also Degeneration, myocardial)
        429.1
      hypertensive (see also Hypertension,
        heart) 402.90
      rheumatic (with chorea) 398.99
        active or acute 391.8
          with chorea 392.0
      valve (see also Endocarditis) 424.90
        congenital NEC 746.89
    cartilage 733.99
    cecum 569.89
    cervix (uteri) 622.6
      congenital 752.49
      elongation 622.6
    clitoris (cirrhotic) 624.2
      congenital 752.49
    colon 569.89
      congenital 751.3
    conjunctiva, lymphoid 372.73
    cornea 371.89
    corpora cavernosa 607.89
    duodenum 537.89
    endometrium (uterus) (see also Hyperplasia,
      endometrium) 621.30
      cervix 622.6
    epididymis 608.89
    esophageal hiatus (congenital) 756.6
      with hernia — see Hernia, diaphragm
    eyelid 374.30
    falx, skull 733.99
    fat pad 729.30
      infrapatellar 729.31
      knee 729.31
      orbital 374.34
      popliteal 729.31
      prepatellar 729.31
      retropatellar 729.31
      specified site NEC 729.39
    foot (congenital) 755.67
    frenum, frenulum (tongue) 529.8
      linguae 529.8
      lip 528.5
    gallbladder or cystic duct 575.8
    gastric mucosa 535.2 ☑
    gingiva 523.8
    gland, glandular (general) NEC 785.6
    gum (mucous membrane) 523.8
    heart (idiopathic) (see also Hypertrophy,
      cardiac)
      valve (see also Endocarditis)
        congenital NEC 746.89
    hemifacial 754.0
    hepatic — see Hypertrophy, liver
    hiatus (esophageal) 756.6
    hilus gland 785.6
    hymen, congenital 752.49
    ileum 569.89
    infrapatellar fat pad 729.31
    intestine 569.89
    jejunum 569.89
    kidney (compensatory) 593.1
      congenital 753.3
    labial frenulum 528.5
    labium (majus) (minus) 624.3
    lacrimal gland, chronic 375.03
    ligament 728.9
      spinal 724.8
    linguae frenulum 529.8

Hypertrophy, hypertrophic — continued
    lingual tonsil (infectional) 474.11
    lip (frenum) 528.5
      congenital 744.81
    liver 789.1
      acute 573.8
      cirrhotic — see Cirrhosis, liver
      congenital 751.69
      fatty — see Fatty, liver
    lymph gland 785.6
      tuberculous — see Tuberculosis, lymph
        gland
    mammary gland — see Hypertrophy, breast
    maxillary frenulum 528.5
    Meckel's diverticulum (congenital) 751.0
    medial meniscus, acquired 717.3
    median bar 600.90
      with
        other lower urinary tract symptoms
          (LUTS) 600.91
        urinary
          obstruction 600.91
          retention 600.91
    mediastinum 519.3
    meibomian gland 373.2
    meniscus, knee, congenital 755.64
    metatarsal head 733.99
    metatarsus 733.99
    mouth 528.9
    mucous membrane
      alveolar process 523.8
      nose 478.19
      turbinate (nasal) 478.0
    muscle 728.9
    muscular coat, artery NEC 447.8
      carotid 447.8
      renal 447.3
    myocardium (see also Hypertrophy, cardiac)
      429.3
      idiopathic 425.4
    myometrium 621.2
    nail 703.8
      congenital 757.5
    nasal 478.19
      alae 478.19
      bone 738.0
      cartilage 478.19
      mucous membrane (septum) 478.19
      sinus (see also Sinusitis) 473.9
      turbinate 478.0
    nasopharynx, lymphoid (infectional) (tissue)
      (wall) 478.29
    neck, uterus 622.6
    nipple 611.1
    normal aperture diaphragm (congenital)
      756.6
    nose (see also Hypertrophy, nasal) 478.19
    orbit 376.46
    organ or site, congenital NEC — see
      Anomaly, specified type NEC
    osteoarthropathy (pulmonary) 731.2
    ovary 620.8
    palate (hard) 526.89
      soft 528.9
    pancreas (congenital) 751.7
    papillae
      anal 569.49
      tongue 529.3
    parathyroid (gland) 252.01
    parotid gland 527.1
    penis 607.89
    phallus 607.89
      female (clitoris) 624.2
    pharyngeal tonsil 474.12
    pharyngitis 472.1
    pharynx 478.29
      lymphoid (infectional) (tissue) (wall)
        478.29
    pituitary (fossa) (gland) 253.8
    popliteal fat pad 729.31
    preauricular (lymph) gland (Hampstead)
      785.6
    prepuce (congenital) 605
      female 624.2
    prostate (asymptomatic) (early) (recurrent)
      600.90

Hypertrophy, hypertrophic — continued
    prostate — continued
      with
        other lower urinary tract symptoms
          (LUTS) 600.91
        urinary
          obstruction 600.91
          retention 600.91
      adenofibromatous 600.20
        with
          other lower urinary tract symp-
            toms (LUTS) 600.21
          urinary
            obstruction 600.21
            retention 600.21
      benign 600.00
        with
          other lower urinary tract symp-
            toms (LUTS) 600.01
          urinary
            obstruction 600.01
            retention 600.01
      congenital 752.89
    pseudoedematous hypodermal 757.0
    pseudomuscular 359.1
    pylorus (muscle) (sphincter) 537.0
      congenital 750.5
      infantile 750.5
    rectal sphincter 569.49
    rectum 569.49
    renal 593.1
    rhinitis (turbinate) 472.0
    salivary duct or gland 527.1
      congenital 750.26
    scaphoid (tarsal) 733.99
    scar 701.4
    scrotum 608.89
    sella turcica 253.8
    seminal vesicle 608.89
    sigmoid 569.89
    skin condition NEC 701.9
    spermatic cord 608.89
    spinal ligament 724.8
    spleen — see Splenomegaly
    spondylitis (spine) (see also Spondylosis)
      721.90
    stomach 537.89
    subaortic stenosis (idiopathic) 425.1
    sublingual gland 527.1
      congenital 750.26
    submaxillary gland 527.1
    suprarenal (gland) 255.8
    tendon 727.9
    testis 608.89
      congenital 752.89
    thymic, thymus (congenital) (gland) 254.0
    thyroid (gland) (see also Goiter) 240.9
      primary 242.0 ☑
      secondary 242.2 ☑
    toe (congenital) 755.65
      acquired 735.8
    tongue 529.8
      congenital 750.15
      frenum 529.8
      papillae (foliate) 529.3
    tonsil (faucial) (infective) (lingual) (lym-
      phoid) 474.11
      with
        adenoiditis 474.01
        tonsillitis 474.00
          and adenoiditis 474.02
      and adenoids 474.10
    tunica vaginalis 608.89
    turbinate (mucous membrane) 478.0
    ureter 593.89
    urethra 599.84
    uterus 621.2
      puerperal, postpartum 674.8 ☑
    uvula 528.9
    vagina 623.8
    vas deferens 608.89
    vein 459.89
    ventricle, ventricular (heart) (left) (right) (see
      also Hypertrophy, cardiac)
      congenital 746.89

☑ Additional Digit Required — Refer to the Tabular List for Digit Selection   ▽ Subterms under main terms may continue to next column or page

148 — Volume 2 · October 2010   ▶◀ Revised Text   ● New Line   ▲ Revised Code   2011 ICD-9-CM

Hypertrophy, hypertrophic — *continued*
  ventricle, ventricular (*see also* Hypertrophy, cardiac) — *continued*
    due to hypertension (left) (right) (*see also* Hypertension, heart) 402.90
      benign 402.10
      malignant 402.00
    right with ventricular septal defect, pulmonary stenosis or atresia, and dextraposition of aorta 745.2
  verumontanum 599.89
  vesical 596.8
  vocal cord 478.5
  vulva 624.3
    stasis (nonfilarial) 624.3
Hypertropia (intermittent) (periodic) 378.31
Hypertyrosinemia 270.2
Hyperuricemia 790.6
Hypervalinemia 270.3
Hyperventilation (tetany) 786.01
  hysterical 300.11
  psychogenic 306.1
  syndrome 306.1
Hyperviscidosis 277.00
Hyperviscosity (of serum) (syndrome) NEC 273.3
  polycythemic 289.0
  sclerocythemic 282.8
Hypervitaminosis (dietary) NEC 278.8
  A (dietary) 278.2
  D (dietary) 278.4
  from excessive administration or use of vitamin preparations (chronic) 278.8
    reaction to sudden overdose 963.5
    vitamin A 278.2
      reaction to sudden overdose 963.5
    vitamin D 278.4
      reaction to sudden overdose 963.5
    vitamin K
      correct substance properly administered 278.8
      overdose or wrong substance given or taken 964.3
Hypervolemia 276.69 ▲
Hypesthesia — *see also* Disturbance, sensation 782.0
  cornea 371.81
Hyphema (anterior chamber) (ciliary body) (iris) 364.41
  traumatic 921.3
Hyphemia — *see* Hyphema
Hypoacidity, gastric 536.8
  psychogenic 306.4
Hypoactive labyrinth (function) — *see* Hypofunction, labyrinth
Hypoadrenalism 255.41
  tuberculous (*see also* Tuberculosis) 017.6 ☑
Hypoadrenocorticism 255.41
  pituitary 253.4
Hypoalbuminemia 273.8
Hypoaldosteronism 255.42
Hypoalphalipoproteinemia 272.5
Hypobarism 993.2
Hypobaropathy 993.2
Hypobetalipoproteinemia (familial) 272.5
Hypocalcemia 275.41
  cow's milk 775.4
  dietary 269.3
  neonatal 775.4
  phosphate-loading 775.4
Hypocalcification, teeth 520.4
Hypochloremia 276.9
Hypochlorhydria 536.8
  neurotic 306.4
  psychogenic 306.4
Hypocholesteremia 272.5
Hypochondria (reaction) 300.7
Hypochondriac 300.7
Hypochondriasis 300.7
Hypochromasia blood cells 280.9
Hypochromic anemia 280.9
  due to blood loss (chronic) 280.0
    acute 285.1
  microcytic 280.9
Hypocoagulability — *see also* Defect, coagulation 286.9

Hypocomplementemia 279.8
Hypocythemia (progressive) 284.9
Hypodontia — *see also* Anodontia 520.0
Hypoeosinophilia 288.59
Hypoesthesia — *see also* Disturbance, sensation 782.0
  cornea 371.81
  tactile 782.0
Hypoestrinism 256.39
Hypoestrogenism 256.39
Hypoferremia 280.9
  due to blood loss (chronic) 280.0
Hypofertility
  female 628.9
  male 606.1
Hypofibrinogenemia 286.3
  acquired 286.6
  congenital 286.3
Hypofunction
  adrenal (gland) 255.41
    cortex 255.41
    medulla 255.5
    specified NEC 255.5
  cerebral 331.9
  corticoadrenal NEC 255.41
  intestinal 564.89
  labyrinth (unilateral) 386.53
    with loss of labyrinthine reactivity 386.55
    bilateral 386.54
      with loss of labyrinthine reactivity 386.56
  Leydig cell 257.2
  ovary 256.39
    postablative 256.2
  pituitary (anterior) (gland) (lobe) 253.2
    posterior 253.5
  testicular 257.2
    iatrogenic 257.1
    postablative 257.1
    postirradiation 257.1
    postsurgical 257.1
Hypogammaglobulinemia 279.00
  acquired primary 279.06
  non-sex-linked, congenital 279.06
  sporadic 279.06
  transient of infancy 279.09
Hypogenitalism (congenital) (female) (male) 752.89
  penis 752.69
Hypoglycemia (spontaneous) 251.2
  coma 251.0
    diabetic 250.3 ☑
      due to secondary diabetes 249.3 ☑
  diabetic 250.8 ☑
    due to secondary diabetes 249.8 ☑
  due to insulin 251.0
    therapeutic misadventure 962.3
  familial (idiopathic) 251.2
  following gastrointestinal surgery 579.3
  infantile (idiopathic) 251.2
  in infant of diabetic mother 775.0
  leucine-induced 270.3
  neonatal 775.6
  reactive 251.2
  specified NEC 251.1
Hypoglycemic shock 251.0
  diabetic 250.8 ☑
    due to secondary diabetes 249.8 ☑
  due to insulin 251.0
  functional (syndrome) 251.1
Hypogonadism
  female 256.39
  gonadotrophic (isolated) 253.4
  hypogonadotropic (isolated) (with anosmia) 253.4
  isolated 253.4
  male 257.2
    hereditary familial (Reifenstein's syndrome) 259.52
  ovarian (primary) 256.39
  pituitary (secondary) 253.4
  testicular (primary) (secondary) 257.2
Hypohidrosis 705.0
Hypohidrotic ectodermal dysplasia 757.31
Hypoidrosis 705.0
Hypoinsulinemia, postsurgical 251.3

Hypoinsulinemia, postsurgical — *continued*
  postpancreatectomy (complete) (partial) 251.3
Hypokalemia 276.8
Hypokinesia 780.99
Hypoleukia splenica 289.4
Hypoleukocytosis 288.50
Hypolipidemia 272.5
Hypolipoproteinemia 272.5
Hypomagnesemia 275.2
  neonatal 775.4
Hypomania, hypomanic reaction — *see also* Psychosis, affective 296.0 ☑
  recurrent episode 296.1 ☑
  single episode 296.0 ☑
Hypomastia (congenital) 611.82
Hypomenorrhea 626.1
Hypometabolism 783.9
Hypomotility
  gastrointestinal tract 536.8
    psychogenic 306.4
  intestine 564.89
    psychogenic 306.4
  stomach 536.8
    psychogenic 306.4
Hyponasality 784.44
Hyponatremia 276.1
Hypo-ovarianism 256.39
Hypo-ovarism 256.39
Hypoparathyroidism (idiopathic) (surgically induced) 252.1
  neonatal 775.4
Hypoperfusion (in) ●
  newborn 779.89 ●
Hypopharyngitis 462
Hypophoria 378.40
Hypophosphatasia 275.3
Hypophosphatemia (acquired) (congenital) (familial) 275.3
  renal 275.3
Hypophyseal, hypophysis — *see also* condition
  dwarfism 253.3
  gigantism 253.0
  syndrome 253.8
Hypophyseothalamic syndrome 253.8
Hypopiesis — *see* Hypotension
Hypopigmentation 709.00
  eyelid 374.53
Hypopinealism 259.8
Hypopituitarism (juvenile) (syndrome) 253.2
  due to
    hormone therapy 253.7
    hypophysectomy 253.7
    radiotherapy 253.7
  postablative 253.7
  postpartum hemorrhage 253.2
Hypoplasia, hypoplasis 759.89
  adrenal (gland) 759.1
  alimentary tract 751.8
    lower 751.2
    upper 750.8
  anus, anal (canal) 751.2
  aorta 747.22
  aortic
    arch (tubular) 747.10
    orifice or valve with hypoplasia of ascending aorta and defective development of left ventricle (with mitral valve atresia) 746.7
  appendix 751.2
  areola 757.6
  arm (*see also* Absence, arm, congenital) 755.20
  artery (congenital) (peripheral) 747.60
    brain 747.81
    cerebral 747.81
    coronary 746.85
    gastrointestinal 747.61
    lower limb 747.64
    pulmonary 747.3
    renal 747.62
    retinal 743.58
    specified NEC 747.69
    spinal 747.82

Hypoplasia, hypoplasis — *continued*
  artery — *continued*
    umbilical 747.5
    upper limb 747.63
  auditory canal 744.29
    causing impairment of hearing 744.02
  biliary duct (common) or passage 751.61
  bladder 753.8
  bone NEC 756.9
    face 756.0
    malar 756.0
    mandible 524.04
      alveolar 524.74
    marrow 284.9
      acquired (secondary) 284.89
      congenital 284.09
      idiopathic 284.9
    maxilla 524.03
      alveolar 524.73
    skull (*see also* Hypoplasia, skull) 756.0
  brain 742.1
    gyri 742.2
    specified part 742.2
  breast (areola) 611.82
  bronchus (tree) 748.3
  cardiac 746.89
    valve — *see* Hypoplasia, heart, valve
    vein 746.89
  carpus (*see also* Absence, carpal, congenital) 755.28
  cartilaginous 756.9
  cecum 751.2
  cementum 520.4
    hereditary 520.5
  cephalic 742.1
  cerebellum 742.2
  cervix (uteri) 752.43 ▲
  chin 524.06
  clavicle 755.51
  coccyx 756.19
  colon 751.2
  corpus callosum 742.2
  cricoid cartilage 748.3
  dermal, focal (Goltz) 757.39
  digestive organ(s) or tract NEC 751.8
    lower 751.2
    upper 750.8
  ear 744.29
    auricle 744.23
    lobe 744.29
    middle, except ossicles 744.03
      ossicles 744.04
    ossicles 744.04
  enamel of teeth (neonatal) (postnatal) (prenatal) 520.4
    hereditary 520.5
  endocrine (gland) NEC 759.2
  endometrium 621.8
  epididymis 752.89
  epiglottis 748.3
  erythroid, congenital 284.01
  erythropoietic, chronic acquired 284.81
  esophagus 750.3
  Eustachian tube 744.24
  eye (*see also* Microphthalmos) 743.10
    lid 743.62
  face 744.89
    bone(s) 756.0
  fallopian tube 752.19
  femur (*see also* Absence, femur, congenital) 755.34
  fibula (*see also* Absence, fibula, congenital) 755.37
  finger (*see also* Absence, finger, congenital) 755.29
  focal dermal 757.39
  foot 755.31
  gallbladder 751.69
  genitalia, genital organ(s)
    female 752.89
      external 752.49
      internal NEC 752.89
    in adiposogenital dystrophy 253.8
    male 752.89
      penis 752.69
  glottis 748.3

Hypoplasia, hypoplasis — *continued*
hair 757.4
hand 755.21
heart 746.89
   left (complex) (syndrome) 746.7
   valve NEC 746.89
      pulmonary 746.01
humerus (*see also* Absence, humerus, congenital) 755.24
hymen 752.49
intestine (small) 751.1
   large 751.2
iris 743.46
jaw 524.09
kidney(s) 753.0
labium (majus) (minus) 752.49
labyrinth, membranous 744.05
lacrimal duct (apparatus) 743.65
larynx 748.3
leg (*see also* Absence, limb, congenital,
   lower) 755.30
limb 755.4
   lower (*see also* Absence, limb, congeni-
      tal, lower) 755.30
   upper (*see also* Absence, limb, congeni-
      tal, upper) 755.20
liver 751.69
lung (lobe) 748.5
mammary (areolar) 611.82
mandibular 524.04
   alveolar 524.74
   unilateral condylar 526.89
maxillary 524.03
   alveolar 524.73
medullary 284.9
megakaryocytic 287.30
metacarpus (*see also* Absence, metacarpal,
   congenital) 755.28
metatarsus (*see also* Absence, metatarsal,
   congenital) 755.38
muscle 756.89
   eye 743.69
myocardium (congenital) (Uhl's anomaly)
   746.84
nail(s) 757.5
nasolacrimal duct 743.65
nervous system NEC 742.8
neural 742.8
nose, nasal 748.1
ophthalmic (*see also* Microphthalmos)
   743.10
optic nerve 377.43
organ
   of Corti 744.05
   or site NEC — *see* Anomaly, by site
osseous meatus (ear) 744.03
ovary 752.0
oviduct 752.19
pancreas 751.7
parathyroid (gland) 759.2
parotid gland 750.26
patella 755.64
pelvis, pelvic girdle 755.69
penis 752.69
peripheral vascular system (congenital) NEC
   747.60
   gastrointestinal 747.61
   lower limb 747.64
   renal 747.62
   specified NEC 747.69
   spinal 747.82
   upper limb 747.63
pituitary (gland) 759.2
pulmonary 748.5
   arteriovenous 747.3
   artery 747.3
   valve 746.01

Hypoplasia, hypoplasis — *continued*
punctum lacrimale 743.65
radioulnar (*see also* Absence, radius, congenital, with ulna) 755.25
radius (*see also* Absence, radius, congenital)
   755.26
rectum 751.2
respiratory system NEC 748.9
rib 756.3
sacrum 756.19
scapula 755.59
shoulder girdle 755.59
skin 757.39
skull (bone) 756.0
   with
      anencephalus 740.0
      encephalocele 742.0
      hydrocephalus 742.3
         with spina bifida (*see also* Spina
            bifida) 741.0 ☑
      microcephalus 742.1
spinal (cord) (ventral horn cell) 742.59
   vessel 747.82
spine 756.19
spleen 759.0
sternum 756.3
tarsus (*see also* Absence, tarsal, congenital)
   755.38
testis, testicle 752.89
thymus (gland) 279.11
thyroid (gland) 243
   cartilage 748.3
tibiofibular (*see also* Absence, tibia, congenital, with fibula) 755.35
toe (*see also* Absence, toe, congenital)
   755.39
tongue 750.16
trachea (cartilage) (rings) 748.3
Turner's (tooth) 520.4
ulna (*see also* Absence, ulna, congenital)
   755.27
umbilical artery 747.5
ureter 753.29
uterus 752.32 ▲
vagina 752.45 ▲
vascular (peripheral) NEC (*see also* Hypoplasia, peripheral vascular system)
   747.60
   brain 747.81
vein(s) (peripheral) NEC (*see also* Hypoplasia,
   peripheral vascular system) 747.60
   brain 747.81
   cardiac 746.89
   great 747.49
   portal 747.49
   pulmonary 747.49
vena cava (inferior) (superior) 747.49
vertebra 756.19
vulva 752.49
zonule (ciliary) 743.39
zygoma 738.12
Hypopotassemia 276.8
Hypoproaccelerinemia — *see also* Defect,
   coagulation 286.3
Hypoproconvertinemia (congenital) — *see*
   also Defect, coagulation 286.3
Hypoproteinemia (essential) (hypermetabolic)
   (idiopathic) 273.8
Hypoproteinosis 260
Hypoprothrombinemia (congenital) (hereditary) (idiopathic) — *see also* Defect, coagulation 286.3
   acquired 286.7
   newborn 776.3
Hypopselaphesia 782.0
Hypopyon (anterior chamber) (eye) 364.05
   iritis 364.05

Hypopyon — *continued*
   ulcer (cornea) 370.04
Hypopyrexia 780.99
Hyporeflex 796.1
Hyporeninemia, extreme 790.99
   in primary aldosteronism 255.10
Hyporesponsive episode 780.09
Hyposecretion
   ACTH 253.4
   ovary 256.39
      postablative 256.2
   salivary gland (any) 527.7
Hyposegmentation of neutrophils, heredi-
   tary 288.2
Hyposiderinemia 280.9
Hyposmolality 276.1
   syndrome 276.1
Hyposomatotropism 253.3
Hyposomnia, unspecified — *see also* Insom-
   nia 780.52
   with sleep apnea, unspecified 780.51
Hypospadias (male) 752.61
   female 753.8
Hypospermatogenesis 606.1
Hyposphagma 372.72
Hyposplenism 289.59
Hypostasis, pulmonary 514
Hypostatic — *see* condition
Hyposthenuria 593.89
Hyposuprarenalism 255.41
Hypo-TBG-nemia 246.8
Hypotension (arterial) (constitutional) 458.9
   chronic 458.1
   iatrogenic 458.29
   maternal, syndrome (following labor and
      delivery) 669.2 ☑
   of hemodialysis 458.21
   orthostatic (chronic) 458.0
      dysautonomic-dyskinetic syndrome
         333.0
   permanent idiopathic 458.1
   postoperative 458.29
   postural 458.0
   specified type NEC 458.8
   transient 796.3
Hypothermia (accidental) 991.6
   anesthetic 995.89
   associated with low environmental temper-
      ature 991.6
   newborn NEC 778.3
   not associated with low environmental
      temperature 780.65
Hypothymergasia — *see also* Psychosis, affective 296.2 ☑
   recurrent episode 296.3 ☑
   single episode 296.2 ☑
Hypothyroidism (acquired) 244.9
   complicating pregnancy, childbirth, or
      puerperium 648.1 ☑
   congenital 243
   due to
      ablation 244.1
         radioactive iodine 244.1
         surgical 244.0
      iodine (administration) (ingestion) 244.2
         radioactive 244.1
      irradiation therapy 244.1
      p-aminosalicylic acid (PAS) 244.3
      phenylbutazone 244.3
      resorcinol 244.3
      specified cause NEC 244.8
      surgery 244.0
   goitrous (sporadic) 246.1
   iatrogenic NEC 244.3
   iodine 244.2
   pituitary 244.8
   postablative NEC 244.1

Hypothyroidism — *continued*
   postsurgical 244.0
   primary 244.9
   secondary NEC 244.8
   specified cause NEC 244.8
   sporadic goitrous 246.1
Hypotonia, hypotonicity, hypotony 781.3
   benign congenital 358.8
   bladder 596.4
   congenital 779.89
      benign 358.8
   eye 360.30
      due to
         fistula 360.32
         ocular disorder NEC 360.33
      following loss of aqueous or vitreous
         360.33
      primary 360.31
   infantile muscular (benign) 359.0
   muscle 728.9
   uterus, uterine (contractions) — *see* Inertia,
      uterus
Hypotrichosis 704.09
   congenital 757.4
   lid (congenital) 757.4
      acquired 374.55
   postinfectional NEC 704.09
Hypotropia 378.32
Hypoventilation 786.09
   congenital central alveolar syndrome 327.25
   idiopathic sleep related nonobstructive
      alveolar 327.24
   obesity 278.03   ●
   sleep related, in conditions classifiable
      elsewhere 327.26
Hypovitaminosis — *see also* Deficiency, vitamin 269.2
Hypovolemia 276.52
   surgical shock 998.0
   traumatic (shock) 958.4
Hypoxemia — *see also* Anoxia 799.02
   sleep related, in conditions classifiable
      elsewhere 327.26
Hypoxia — *see also* Anoxia 799.02
   cerebral 348.1
      during or resulting from a procedure
         997.01
      newborn 770.88
         mild or moderate 768.6
         severe 768.5
   fetal, affecting newborn 770.88
   intrauterine — *see* Distress, fetal
   myocardial (*see also* Insufficiency, coronary)
      411.89
      arteriosclerotic — *see* Arteriosclerosis,
         coronary
   newborn 770.88
   sleep related 327.24
Hypoxic-ischemic encephalopathy (HIE)
   768.70
   mild 768.71
   moderate 768.72
   severe 768.73
Hypsarrhythmia — *see also* Epilepsy 345.6 ☑
Hysteralgia, pregnant uterus 646.8 ☑
Hysteria, hysterical 300.10
   anxiety 300.20
   Charcôt's gland 300.11
   conversion (any manifestation) 300.11
   dissociative type NEC 300.15
   psychosis, acute 298.1
Hysteroepilepsy 300.11
Hysterotomy, affecting fetus or newborn
   763.89

☑ **Additional Digit Required — Refer to the Tabular List for Digit Selection**   Ⓦ **Subterms under main terms may continue to next column or page**

150 — Volume 2 · October 2010   ▶◀ **Revised Text**   ● **New Line**   ▲ **Revised Code**   **2011 ICD-9-CM**

I

Iatrogenic syndrome of excess cortisol 255.0
IBM (inclusion body myositis) 359.71
Iceland disease (epidemic neuromyasthenia) 049.8
Ichthyosis (congenita) 757.1
  acquired 701.1
  fetalis gravior 757.1
  follicularis 757.1
  hystrix 757.39
  lamellar 757.1
  lingual 528.6
  palmaris and plantaris 757.39
  simplex 757.1
  vera 757.1
  vulgaris 757.1
Ichthyotoxism 988.0
  bacterial (*see also* Poisoning, food) 005.9
Icteroanemia, hemolytic (acquired) 283.9
  congenital (*see also* Spherocytosis) 282.0
Icterus — *see also* Jaundice 782.4
  catarrhal — *see* Icterus, infectious
  conjunctiva 782.4
    newborn 774.6
  epidemic — *see* Icterus, infectious
  febrilis — *see* Icterus, infectious
  fetus or newborn — *see* Jaundice, fetus or newborn
  gravis (*see also* Necrosis, liver) 570
    complicating pregnancy 646.7 ☑
      affecting fetus or newborn 760.8
    fetus or newborn NEC 773.0
    obstetrical 646.7 ☑
      affecting fetus or newborn 760.8
  hematogenous (acquired) 283.9
  hemolytic (acquired) 283.9
    congenital (*see also* Spherocytosis) 282.0
  hemorrhagic (acute) 100.0
    leptospiral 100.0
    newborn 776.0
    spirochetal 100.0
  infectious 070.1
    with hepatic coma 070.0
    leptospiral 100.0
    spirochetal 100.0
  intermittens juvenilis 277.4
  malignant (*see also* Necrosis, liver) 570
  neonatorum (*see also* Jaundice, fetus or newborn) 774.6
  pernicious (*see also* Necrosis, liver) 570
  spirochetal 100.0
Ictus solaris, solis 992.0
Ideation
  homicidal V62.85   ●
  suicidal V62.84
Identity disorder 313.82
  dissociative 300.14
  gender role (child) 302.6
    adult 302.85
  psychosexual (child) 302.6
    adult 302.85
Idioglossia 307.9
Idiopathic — *see* condition
Idiosyncrasy — *see also* Allergy 995.3
  drug, medicinal substance, and biological — *see* Allergy, drug
Idiot, idiocy (congenital) 318.2
  amaurotic (Bielschowsky) (-Jansky) (family) (infantile) (late) (juvenile) (late) (Vogt-Spielmeyer) 330.1
  microcephalic 742.1
  Mongolian 758.0
  oxycephalic 756.0
Id reaction (due to bacteria) 692.89
IEED (involuntary emotional expression disorder) 310.8
IFIS (intraoperative floppy iris syndrome) 364.81
IgE asthma 493.0 ☑
Ileitis (chronic) — *see also* Enteritis 558.9
  infectious 009.0
  noninfectious 558.9
  regional (ulcerative) 555.0
    with large intestine 555.2
  segmental 555.0

Ileitis — *see also* Enteritis — *continued*
  segmental — *continued*
    with large intestine 555.2
  terminal (ulcerative) 555.0
    with large intestine 555.2
Ileocolitis — *see also* Enteritis 558.9
  infectious 009.0
  regional 555.2
  ulcerative 556.1
Ileostomy status V44.2
  with complication 569.60
Ileotyphus 002.0
Ileum — *see* condition
Ileus (adynamic) (bowel) (colon) (inhibitory) (intestine) (neurogenic) (paralytic) 560.1
  arteriomesenteric duodenal 537.2
  due to gallstone (in intestine) 560.31
  duodenal, chronic 537.2
  following gastrointestinal surgery 997.4
  gallstone 560.31
  mechanical (*see also* Obstruction, intestine) 560.9
  meconium 777.1
    due to cystic fibrosis 277.01
  myxedema 564.89
  postoperative 997.4
  transitory, newborn 777.4
Iliac — *see* condition
Iliotibial band friction syndrome 728.89
Illegitimacy V61.6
Ill, louping 063.1
Illness — *see also* Disease
  factitious 300.19
    with
      combined psychological and physical signs and symptoms 300.19
      predominantly
        physical signs and symptoms 300.19
        psychological symptoms 300.16
    chronic (with physical symptoms) 301.51
  heart — *see* Disease, heart
  manic-depressive (*see also* Psychosis, affective) 296.80
  mental (*see also* Disorder, mental) 300.9
Imbalance 781.2
  autonomic (*see also* Neuropathy, peripheral, autonomic) 337.9
  electrolyte 276.9
    with
      abortion — *see* Abortion, by type, with metabolic disorder
      ectopic pregnancy (*see also* categories 633.0–633.9) 639.4
      hyperemesis gravidarum (before 22 completed weeks gestation) 643.1 ☑
      molar pregnancy (*see also* categories 630–632) 639.4
    following
      abortion 639.4
      ectopic or molar pregnancy 639.4
    neonatal, transitory NEC 775.5
  endocrine 259.9
  eye muscle NEC 378.9
    heterophoria — *see* Heterophoria
  glomerulotubular NEC 593.89
  hormone 259.9
  hysterical (*see also* Hysteria) 300.10
  labyrinth NEC 386.50
  posture 729.90
  sympathetic (*see also* Neuropathy, peripheral, autonomic) 337.9
Imbecile, imbecility 318.0
  moral 301.7
  old age 290.9
  senile 290.9
  specified IQ — *see* IQ
  unspecified IQ 318.0
Imbedding, intrauterine device 996.32
Imbibition, cholesterol (gallbladder) 575.6
Imerslund (-Gräsbeck) syndrome (anemia due to familial selective vitamin B_{12} malabsorption) 281.1
Iminoacidopathy 270.8
Iminoglycinuria, familial 270.8

Immature — *see also* Immaturity
  personality 301.89
Immaturity 765.1 ☑
  extreme 765.0 ☑
  fetus or infant light-for-dates — *see* Light-for-dates
  lung, fetus or newborn 770.4
  organ or site NEC — *see* Hypoplasia
  pulmonary, fetus or newborn 770.4
  reaction 301.89
  sexual (female) (male) 259.0
Immersion 994.1
  foot 991.4
  hand 991.4
Immobile, immobility
  complete
    due to severe physical disability or frailty 780.72
  intestine 564.89
  joint — *see* Ankylosis
  syndrome (paraplegic) 728.3
Immunization
  ABO
    affecting management of pregnancy 656.2 ☑
      fetus or newborn 773.1
  complication — *see* Complications, vaccination
  Rh factor
    affecting management of pregnancy 656.1 ☑
      fetus or newborn 773.0
    from transfusion ▶(*see also* Complications, transfusion)◀ 999.70 ▲
Immunodeficiency 279.3
  with
    adenosine-deaminase deficiency 279.2
    defect, predominant
      B-cell 279.00
      T-cell 279.10
    hyperimmunoglobulinemia 279.2
    lymphopenia, hereditary 279.2
    thrombocytopenia and eczema 279.12
    thymic
      aplasia 279.2
      dysplasia 279.2
  autosomal recessive, Swiss-type 279.2
  common variable 279.06
  severe combined (SCID) 279.2
  to Rh factor
    affecting management of pregnancy 656.1 ☑
      fetus or newborn 773.0
  X-linked, with increased IgM 279.05
Immunotherapy, prophylactic V07.2
  antineoplastic V58.12
Impaction, impacted
  bowel, colon, rectum 560.30
    with hernia (*see also* Hernia, by site, with obstruction)
      gangrenous — *see* Hernia, by site, with gangrene
    by
      calculus 560.39
      gallstone 560.31
      fecal 560.32   ▲
      specified type NEC 560.39
  calculus — *see* Calculus
  cerumen (ear) (external) 380.4
  cuspid 520.6
  dental 520.6
  fecal, feces 560.32   ▲
    with hernia (*see also* Hernia, by site, with obstruction)
      gangrenous — *see* Hernia, by site, with gangrene
  fracture — *see* Fracture, by site
  gallbladder — *see* Cholelithiasis
  gallstone(s) — *see* Cholelithiasis
    in intestine (any part) 560.31
  intestine(s) 560.30
    with hernia (*see also* Hernia, by site, with obstruction)
      gangrenous — *see* Hernia, by site, with gangrene

Impaction, impacted — *continued*
  intestine(s) — *continued*
    by
      calculus 560.39
      gallstone 560.31
      fecal 560.32   ▲
      specified type NEC 560.39
  intrauterine device (IUD) 996.32
  molar 520.6
  shoulder 660.4 ☑
    affecting fetus or newborn 763.1
  tooth, teeth 520.6
  turbinate 733.99
Impaired, impairment (function)
  arm V49.1
    movement, involving
      musculoskeletal system V49.1
      nervous system V49.2
  auditory discrimination 388.43
  back V48.3
  body (entire) V49.89
  cognitive, mild, so stated 331.83
  combined visual hearing V49.85
  dual sensory V49.85
  glucose
    fasting 790.21
    tolerance test (oral) 790.22
  hearing (*see also* Deafness) 389.9
    combined with visual impairment V49.85
  heart — *see* Disease, heart
  kidney (*see also* Disease, renal) 593.9
    disorder resulting from 588.9
      specified NEC 588.89
  leg V49.1
    movement, involving
      musculoskeletal system V49.1
      nervous system V49.2
  limb V49.1
    movement, involving
      musculoskeletal system V49.1
      nervous system V49.2
  liver 573.8
  mastication 524.9
  mild cognitive, so stated 331.83
  mobility
    ear ossicles NEC 385.22
    incostapedial joint 385.22
    malleus 385.21
  myocardium, myocardial (*see also* Insufficiency, myocardial) 428.0
  neuromusculoskeletal NEC V49.89
    back V48.3
    head V48.2
    limb V49.2
    neck V48.3
    spine V48.3
    trunk V48.3
  rectal sphincter 787.99
  renal (*see also* Disease, renal) 593.9
    disorder resulting from 588.9
      specified NEC 588.89
  spine V48.3
  vision NEC 369.9
    both eyes NEC 369.3
      combined with hearing impairment V49.85
      moderate 369.74
        both eyes 369.25
          with impairment of lesser eye (specified as)
            blind, not further specified 369.15
            low vision, not further specified 369.23
            near-total 369.17
            profound 369.18
            severe 369.24
            total 369.16
        one eye 369.74
          with vision of other eye (specified as)
            near-normal 369.75
            normal 369.76
      near-total 369.64
        both eyes 369.04

☑ **Additional Digit Required** — Refer to the Tabular List for Digit Selection   ⒩ **Subterms under main terms may continue to next column or page**

2011 ICD-9-CM   ▶◀ **Revised Text**   ● **New Line**   ▲ **Revised Code**   October 2010 • Volume 2 — 151

Impaired, impairment — *continued*
  vision — *continued*
    near-total — *continued*
      both eyes — *continued*
        with impairment of lesser eye (specified as)
          blind, not further specified 369.02
            total 369.03
      one eye 369.64
        with vision of other eye (specified as)
          near normal 369.65
          normal 369.66
    one eye 369.60
      with low vision of other eye 369.10
    profound 369.67
      both eyes 369.08
        with impairment of lesser eye (specified as)
          blind, not further specified 369.05
          near-total 369.07
          total 369.06
      one eye 369.67
        with vision of other eye (specified as)
          near-normal 369.68
          normal 369.69
    severe 369.71
      both eyes 369.22
        with impairment of lesser eye (specified as)
          blind, not further specified 369.11
          low vision, not further specified 369.21
          near-total 369.13
          profound 369.14
          total 369.12
      one eye 369.71
        with vision of other eye (specified as)
          near-normal 369.72
          normal 369.73
    total
      both eyes 369.01
      one eye 369.61
        with vision of other eye (specified as)
          near-normal 369.62
          normal 369.63
Impaludism — *see* Malaria
Impediment, speech NEC 784.59
  psychogenic 307.9
  secondary to organic lesion 784.59
Impending
  cerebrovascular accident or attack 435.9
  coronary syndrome 411.1
  delirium tremens 291.0
  myocardial infarction 411.1
Imperception, auditory (acquired) (congenital) 389.9
Imperfect
  aeration, lung (newborn) 770.5
  closure (congenital)
    alimentary tract NEC 751.8
      lower 751.5
      upper 750.8
    atrioventricular ostium 745.69
    atrium (secundum) 745.5
      primum 745.61
    branchial cleft or sinus 744.41
    choroid 743.59
    cricoid cartilage 748.3
    cusps, heart valve NEC 746.89
      pulmonary 746.09
    ductus
      arteriosus 747.0
      Botalli 747.0
    ear drum 744.29
      causing impairment of hearing 744.03
    endocardial cushion 745.60
    epiglottis 748.3

Imperfect — *continued*
  closure — *continued*
    esophagus with communication to bronchus or trachea 750.3
    Eustachian valve 746.89
    eyelid 743.62
    face, facial (*see also* Cleft, lip) 749.10
    foramen
      Botalli 745.5
      ovale 745.5
    genitalia, genital organ(s) or system
      female 752.89
        external 752.49
        internal NEC 752.89
        uterus 752.39 ▲
      male 752.89
        penis 752.69
    glottis 748.3
    heart valve (cusps) NEC 746.89
    interatrial ostium or septum 745.5
    interauricular ostium or septum 745.5
    interventricular ostium or septum 745.4
    iris 743.46
    kidney 753.3
    larynx 748.3
    lens 743.36
    lip (*see also* Cleft, lip) 749.10
    nasal septum or sinus 748.1
    nose 748.1
    omphalomesenteric duct 751.0
    optic nerve entry 743.57
    organ or site NEC — *see* Anomaly, specified type, by site
    ostium
      interatrial 745.5
      interauricular 745.5
      interventricular 745.4
    palate (*see also* Cleft, palate) 749.00
    preauricular sinus 744.46
    retina 743.56
    roof of orbit 742.0
    sclera 743.47
    septum
      aortic 745.0
      aorticopulmonary 745.0
      atrial (secundum) 745.5
        primum 745.61
      between aorta and pulmonary artery 745.0
      heart 745.9
      interatrial (secundum) 745.5
        primum 745.61
      interauricular (secundum) 745.5
        primum 745.61
      interventricular 745.4
        with pulmonary stenosis or atresia, dextraposition of aorta, and hypertrophy of right ventricle 745.2
          in tetralogy of Fallot 745.2
      nasal 748.1
      ventricular 745.4
        with pulmonary stenosis or atresia, dextraposition of aorta, and hypertrophy of right ventricle 745.2
          in tetralogy of Fallot 745.2
    skull 756.0
      with
        anencephalus 740.0
        encephalocele 742.0
        hydrocephalus 742.3
          with spina bifida (*see also* Spina bifida) 741.0 ☑
        microcephalus 742.1
      spine (with meningocele) (*see also* Spina bifida) 741.90
    thyroid cartilage 748.3
    trachea 748.3
    tympanic membrane 744.29
      causing impairment of hearing 744.03
    uterus (with communication to bladder, intestine, or rectum) 752.39 ▲
    uvula 749.02

Imperfect — *continued*
  closure — *continued*
    uvula — *continued*
      with cleft lip (*see also* Cleft, palate, with cleft lip) 749.20
      vitelline duct 751.0
    development — *see* Anomaly, by site
    erection 607.84
    fusion — *see* Imperfect, closure
    inflation lung (newborn) 770.5
    intestinal canal 751.5
    poise 729.90
    rotation — *see* Malrotation
    septum, ventricular 745.4
Imperfectly descended testis 752.51
Imperforate (congenital) — *see also* Atresia
  anus 751.2
  bile duct 751.61
  cervix (uteri) 752.49
  esophagus 750.3
  hymen 752.42
  intestine (small) 751.1
    large 751.2
  jejunum 751.1
  pharynx 750.29
  rectum 751.2
  salivary duct 750.23
  urethra 753.6
  urinary meatus 753.6
  vagina 752.49
Impervious (congenital) — *see also* Atresia
  anus 751.2
  bile duct 751.61
  esophagus 750.3
  intestine (small) 751.1
    large 751.2
  rectum 751.2
  urethra 753.6
Impetiginization of other dermatoses 684
Impetigo (any organism) (any site) (bullous) (circinate) (contagiosa) (neonatorum) (simplex) 684
  Bockhart's (superficial folliculitis) 704.8
  external ear 684 [380.13]
  eyelid 684 [373.5]
  Fox's (contagiosa) 684
  furfuracea 696.5
  herpetiformis 694.3
    nonobstetrical 694.3
  staphylococcal infection 684
  ulcerative 686.8
  vulgaris 684
Impingement, soft tissue between teeth 524.89
  anterior 524.81
  posterior 524.82
Implantation
  anomalous (*see also* Anomaly, specified type, by site)
    ureter 753.4
  cyst
    external area or site (skin) NEC 709.8
    iris 364.61
    vagina 623.8
    vulva 624.8
  dermoid (cyst)
    external area or site (skin) NEC 709.8
    iris 364.61
    vagina 623.8
    vulva 624.8
  placenta, low or marginal — *see* Placenta previa
Implant, endometrial 617.9
Impotence (sexual) 607.84
  organic origin NEC 607.84
  psychogenic 302.72
Impoverished blood 285.9
Impression, basilar 756.0
Imprisonment V62.5
Improper
  development, infant 764.9 ☑
Improperly tied umbilical cord (causing hemorrhage) 772.3
Impulses, obsessional 300.3
Impulsive 799.23
  neurosis 300.3

Impulsiveness 799.23
Inaction, kidney — *see also* Disease, renal 593.9
Inactive — *see* condition
Inadequate, inadequacy
  aesthetics of dental restoration 525.67
  biologic 301.6
  cardiac and renal — *see* Hypertension, cardiorenal
  constitutional 301.6
  development
    child 783.40
    fetus 764.9 ☑
      affecting management of pregnancy 656.5 ☑
    genitalia
      after puberty NEC 259.0
      congenital — *see* Hypoplasia, genitalia
    lungs 748.5
    organ or site NEC — *see* Hypoplasia, by site
  dietary 269.9
  distance, interarch 524.28
  education V62.3
  environment
    economic problem V60.2
    household condition NEC V60.1
    poverty V60.2
    unemployment V62.0
  functional 301.6
  household care, due to
    family member
      handicapped or ill V60.4
        temporarily away from home V60.4
          on vacation V60.5
      technical defects in home V60.1
    temporary absence from home of person rendering care V60.4
  housing (heating) (space) V60.1
  interarch distance 524.28
  material resources V60.2
  mental (*see also* Retardation, mental) 319
  nervous system 799.29
  personality 301.6
  prenatal care in current pregnancy V23.7
  pulmonary
    function 786.09
      newborn 770.89
    ventilation, newborn 770.89
  respiration 786.09
    newborn 770.89
  sample
    cytology
      anal 796.78
      cervical 795.08
      vaginal 795.18
  social 301.6
Inanition 263.9
  with edema 262
  due to
    deprivation of food 994.2
    malnutrition 263.9
  fever 780.60
Inappropriate secretion
  ACTH 255.0
  antidiuretic hormone (ADH) (excessive) 253.6
    deficiency 253.5
  ectopic hormone NEC 259.3
  pituitary (posterior) 253.6
Inattention after or at birth 995.52
Inborn errors of metabolism — *see* Disorder, metabolism
Incarceration, incarcerated
  bubonocele (*see also* Hernia, inguinal, with obstruction)
    gangrenous — *see* Hernia, inguinal, with gangrene
  colon (by hernia) (*see also* Hernia, by site with obstruction)
    gangrenous — *see* Hernia, by site, with gangrene
  enterocele 552.9
    gangrenous 551.9
  epigastrocele 552.29

☑ **Additional Digit Required** — Refer to the Tabular List for Digit Selection   ⫸ **Subterms under main terms may continue to next column or page**

Incarceration, incarcerated — *continued*
  epigastrocele — *continued*
    gangrenous 551.29
  epiplocele 552.9
    gangrenous 551.9
  exomphalos 552.1
    gangrenous 551.1
  fallopian tube 620.8
  hernia (see also Hernia, by site, with obstruction)
    gangrenous — see Hernia, by site, with gangrene
  iris, in wound 871.1
  lens, in wound 871.1
  merocele (see also Hernia, femoral, with obstruction) 552.00
  omentum (by hernia) (see also Hernia, by site, with obstruction)
    gangrenous — see Hernia, by site, with gangrene
  omphalocele 756.72
  rupture (meaning hernia) (see also Hernia, by site, with obstruction) 552.9
    gangrenous (see also Hernia, by site, with gangrene) 551.9
  sarcoepiplocele 552.9
    gangrenous 551.9
  sarcoepiplomphalocele 552.1
    with gangrene 551.1
  uterus 621.8
    gravid 654.3 ☑
      causing obstructed labor 660.2 ☑
        affecting fetus or newborn 763.1
Incident, cerebrovascular — see also Disease, cerebrovascular, acute 436
Incineration (entire body) (from fire, conflagration, electricity, or lightning) — see Burn, multiple, specified sites
Incised wound
  external — see Wound, open, by site
  internal organs (abdomen, chest, or pelvis) — see Injury, internal, by site, with open wound
Incision, incisional
  hernia — see Hernia, incisional
  surgical, complication — see Complications, surgical procedures
  traumatic
    external — see Wound, open, by site
    internal organs (abdomen, chest, or pelvis) — see Injury, Internal, by site, with open wound
Inclusion
  azurophilic leukocytic 288.2
  blennorrhea (neonatal) (newborn) 771.6
  cyst — see Cyst, skin
  gallbladder in liver (congenital) 751.69
Incompatibility
  ABO
    affecting management of pregnancy 656.2 ☑
    fetus or newborn 773.1
    infusion or transfusion reaction ▶(see also Complications, transfusion)◀ 999.60 ▲
  blood (group) (Duffy) (E) (K(ell)) (Kidd) (Lewis) (M) (N) (P) (S) NEC
    affecting management of pregnancy 656.2 ☑
    fetus or newborn 773.2
    infusion or transfusion reaction ▶(see also Complications, transfusion)◀ 999.75 ▲
  contour of existing restoration of tooth with oral health 525.65
  marital V61.10
    involving
      divorce V61.03
      estrangement V61.09
  non-ABO (see also Complications, transfusion) 999.75 ●
  Rh ▶(antigen) (C) (c) (D) (E) (e)◀ (blood group) (factor)
    affecting management of pregnancy 656.1 ☑
    fetus or newborn 773.0

Incompatibility — *continued*
  Rh — *continued*
    infusion or transfusion reaction ▶(see also Complications, transfusion)◀ 999.70 ▲
  Rhesus — see Incompatibility, Rh
Incompetency, incompetence, incompetent
  annular
    aortic (valve) (see also Insufficiency, aortic) 424.1
    mitral (valve) (see also Insufficiency, mitral) 424.0
    pulmonary valve (heart) (see also Endocarditis, pulmonary) 424.3
  aortic (valve) (see also Insufficiency, aortic) 424.1
    syphilitic 093.22
  cardiac (orifice) 530.0
    valve — see Endocarditis
  cervix, cervical (os) 622.5
    in pregnancy 654.5 ☑
      affecting fetus or newborn 761.0
  chronotropic 426.89
    with
      autonomic dysfunction 337.9
      ischemic heart disease 414.9
      left ventricular dysfunction 429.89
      sinus node dysfunction 427.81
  esophagogastric (junction) (sphincter) 530.0
  heart valve, congenital 746.89
  mitral (valve) — see Insufficiency, mitral
  papillary muscle (heart) 429.81
  pelvic fundus
    pubocervical tissue 618.81
    rectovaginal tissue 618.82
  pulmonary valve (heart) (see also Endocarditis, pulmonary) 424.3
    congenital 746.09
  tricuspid (annular) (rheumatic) (valve) (see also Endocarditis, tricuspid) 397.0
  valvular — see Endocarditis
  vein, venous (saphenous) (varicose) (see also Varicose, vein) 454.9
  velopharyngeal (closure)
    acquired 528.9
    congenital 750.29
Incomplete — see also condition
  bladder emptying 788.21
  defecation 787.61 ●
  expansion lungs (newborn) 770.5
  gestation (liveborn) — see Immaturity
  rotation — see Malrotation
Inconclusive
  image test due to excess body fat 793.91
  mammogram, mammography 793.82
    due to dense breasts 793.82
Incontinence 788.30
  without sensory awareness 788.34
  anal sphincter 787.60 ▲
  continuous leakage 788.37
  feces, ▶fecal◀ 787.60 ▲
    due to hysteria 300.11
    nonorganic origin 307.7
  hysterical 300.11
  mixed (male) (female) (urge and stress) 788.33
  overflow 788.38
  paradoxical 788.39
  rectal 787.60 ▲
  specified NEC 788.39
  stress (female) 625.6
    male NEC 788.32
  urethral sphincter 599.84
  urge 788.31
    and stress (male) (female) 788.33
  urine 788.30
    active 788.30
    due to
      cognitive impairment 788.91
      immobility 788.91
      severe physical disability 788.91
    functional 788.91
    male 788.30
      stress 788.32
        and urge 788.33
    neurogenic 788.39

Incontinence — *continued*
  urine — *continued*
    nonorganic origin 307.6
    stress (female) 625.6
      male NEC 788.32
    urge 788.31
      and stress 788.33
Incontinentia pigmenti 757.33
Incoordinate
  uterus (action) (contractions) 661.4 ☑
    affecting fetus or newborn 763.7
Incoordination
  esophageal-pharyngeal (newborn) 787.24
  muscular 781.3
  papillary muscle 429.81
Increase, increased
  abnormal, in development 783.9
  androgens (ovarian) 256.1
  anticoagulants (antithrombin) (anti-VIIIa) (anti-IXa) (anti-Xa) (anti-XIa) 286.5
    postpartum 666.3 ☑
  cold sense (see also Disturbance, sensation) 782.0
  estrogen 256.0
  function
    adrenal (cortex) 255.3
      medulla 255.6
    pituitary (anterior) (gland) (lobe) 253.1
      posterior 253.6
  heat sense (see also Disturbance, sensation) 782.0
  intracranial pressure 781.99
    injury at birth 767.8
  light reflex of retina 362.13
  permeability, capillary 448.9
  pressure
    intracranial 781.99
      injury at birth 767.8
    intraocular 365.00
  pulsations 785.9
  pulse pressure 785.9
  sphericity, lens 743.36
  splenic activity 289.4
  venous pressure 459.89
    portal 572.3
Incrustation, cornea, lead or zinc 930.0
Incyclophoria 378.44
Incyclotropia 378.33
Indeterminate sex 752.7
India rubber skin 756.83
Indicanuria 270.2
Indigestion (bilious) (functional) 536.8
  acid 536.8
  catarrhal 536.8
  due to decomposed food NEC 005.9
  fat 579.8
  nervous 306.4
  psychogenic 306.4
Indirect — see condition
Indolent bubo NEC 099.8
Induced
  abortion — see Abortion, induced
  birth, affecting fetus or newborn 763.89
  delivery — see Delivery
  labor — see Delivery
Induration, Indurated
  brain 348.89
  breast (fibrous) 611.79
    puerperal, postpartum 676.3 ☑
  broad ligament 620.8
  chancre 091.0
    anus 091.1
    congenital 090.0
    extragenital NEC 091.2
  corpora cavernosa (penis) (plastic) 607.89
  liver (chronic) 573.8
    acute 573.8
  lung (black) (brown) (chronic) (fibroid) (see also Fibrosis, lung) 515
    essential brown 275.09 [516.1] ▲
  penile 607.89
  phlebitic — see Phlebitis
  skin 782.8
  stomach 537.89
Induratio penis plastica 607.89
Industrial — see condition

Inebriety — see also Abuse, drugs, nondependent 305.0 ☑
Inefficiency
  kidney (see also Disease, renal) 593.9
  thyroid (acquired) (gland) 244.9
Inelasticity, skin 782.8
Inequality, leg (acquired) (length) 736.81
  congenital 755.30
Inertia
  bladder 596.4
    neurogenic 596.54
      with cauda equina syndrome 344.61
  stomach 536.8
    psychogenic 306.4
  uterus, uterine 661.2 ☑
    affecting fetus or newborn 763.7
    primary 661.0 ☑
    secondary 661.1 ☑
  vesical 596.4
    neurogenic 596.54
      with cauda equina 344.61
Infant — see also condition
  excessive crying of 780.92
  fussy (baby) 780.91
  held for adoption V68.89
  newborn — see Newborn
  post-term (gestation period over 40 completed weeks to 42 completed weeks) 766.21
  prolonged gestation of (period over 42 completed weeks) 766.22
  syndrome of diabetic mother 775.0
"Infant Hercules" syndrome 255.2
Infantile — see also condition
  genitalia, genitals 259.0
    in pregnancy or childbirth NEC 654.4 ☑
      affecting fetus or newborn 763.89
      causing obstructed labor 660.2 ☑
        affecting fetus or newborn 763.1
  heart 746.9
  kidney 753.3
  lack of care 995.52
  macula degeneration 362.75
  melanodontia 521.05
  os, uterus (see also Infantile, genitalia) 259.0
  pelvis 738.6
    with disproportion (fetopelvic) 653.1 ☑
      affecting fetus or newborn 763.1
      causing obstructed labor 660.1 ☑
        affecting fetus or newborn 763.1
  penis 259.0
  testis 257.2
  uterus (see also Infantile, genitalia) 259.0
  vulva 752.49
Infantilism 259.9
  with dwarfism (hypophyseal) 253.3
  Brissaud's (infantile myxedema) 244.9
  celiac 579.0
  Herter's (nontropical sprue) 579.0
  hypophyseal 253.3
  hypothalamic (with obesity) 253.8
  idiopathic 259.9
  intestinal 579.0
  pancreatic 577.8
  pituitary 253.3
  renal 588.0
  sexual (with obesity) 259.0
Infants, healthy liveborn — see Newborn
Infarct, infarction
  adrenal (capsule) (gland) 255.41
  amnion 658.8 ☑
  anterior (with contiguous portion of intraventricular septum) NEC (see also Infarct, myocardium) 410.1 ☑
  appendices epiploicae 557.0
  bowel 557.0
  brain (stem) 434.91
    embolic (see also Embolism, brain) 434.11
    healed or old without residuals V12.54
    iatrogenic 997.02
    lacunar 434.91
    late effect — see Late effect(s) (of) cerebrovascular disease
    postoperative 997.02

☑ Additional Digit Required — Refer to the Tabular List for Digit Selection   ▽ Subterms under main terms may continue to next column or page

2011 ICD-9-CM   ▶◀ Revised Text   ● New Line   ▲ Revised Code   October 2010 · Volume 2 — 153

Index

Infarct, infarction — Infection, infected, infective

Infarct, infarction — *continued*
brain — *continued*
    puerperal, postpartum, childbirth 674.0 ☑
    thrombotic (*see also* Thrombosis, brain) 434.01
breast 611.89
Brewer's (kidney) 593.81
cardiac (*see also* Infarct, myocardium) 410.9 ☑
cerebellar (*see also* Infarct, brain) 434.91
    embolic (*see also* Embolism, brain) 434.11
cerebral (*see also* Infarct, brain) 434.91
    aborted 434.91
    embolic (*see also* Embolism, brain) 434.11
    thrombotic (*see also* Infarct, brain) 434.01
chorion 658.8 ☑
colon (acute) (agnogenic) (embolic) (hemorrhagic) (nonocclusive) (nonthrombotic) (occlusive) (segmental) (thrombotic) (with gangrene) 557.0
coronary artery (*see also* Infarct, myocardium) 410.9 ☑
cortical 434.91
embolic (*see also* Embolism) 444.9
fallopian tube 620.8
gallbladder 575.8
heart (*see also* Infarct, myocardium) 410.9 ☑
hepatic 573.4
hypophysis (anterior lobe) 253.8
impending (myocardium) 411.1
intestine (acute) (agnogenic) (embolic) (hemorrhagic) (nonocclusive) (nonthrombotic) (occlusive) (thrombotic) (with gangrene) 557.0
kidney 593.81
lacunar 434.91
liver 573.4
lung (embolic) (thrombotic) 415.19
    with
        abortion — *see* Abortion, by type, with, embolism
        ectopic pregnancy (*see also* categories 633.0–633.9) 639.6
        molar pregnancy (*see also* categories 630–632) 639.6
    following
        abortion 639.6
        ectopic or molar pregnancy 639.6
    iatrogenic 415.11
    in pregnancy, childbirth, or puerperium — *see* Embolism, obstetrical
    postoperative 415.11
    septic 415.12
lymph node or vessel 457.8
medullary (brain) — *see* Infarct, brain
meibomian gland (eyelid) 374.85
mesentery, mesenteric (embolic) (thrombotic) (with gangrene) 557.0
midbrain — *see* Infarct, brain
myocardium, myocardial (acute or with a stated duration of 8 weeks or less) (with hypertension) 410.9 ☑

Note — Use the following fifth-digit subclassification with category 410:
0   episode unspecified
1   initial episode
2   subsequent episode without recurrence

    with symptoms after 8 weeks from date of infarction 414.8
    anterior (wall) (with contiguous portion of intraventricular septum) NEC 410.1 ☑
    anteroapical (with contiguous portion of intraventricular septum) 410.1 ☑
    anterolateral (wall) 410.0 ☑

Infarct, infarction — *continued*
myocardium, myocardial — *continued*
    anteroseptal (with contiguous portion of intraventricular septum) 410.1 ☑
    apical-lateral 410.5 ☑
    atrial 410.8 ☑
    basal-lateral 410.5 ☑
    chronic (with symptoms after 8 weeks from date of infarction) 414.8
    diagnosed on ECG, but presenting no symptoms 412
    diaphragmatic wall (with contiguous portion of intraventricular septum) 410.4 ☑
    healed or old, currently presenting no symptoms 412
    high lateral 410.5 ☑
    impending 411.1
    inferior (wall) (with contiguous portion of intraventricular septum) 410.4 ☑
    inferolateral (wall) 410.2 ☑
    inferoposterior wall 410.3 ☑
    intraoperative 997.1
    lateral wall 410.5 ☑
    non-Q wave 410.7 ☑
    non-ST elevation (NSTEMI)
    nontransmural 410.7 ☑
    papillary muscle 410.8 ☑
    past (diagnosed on ECG or other special investigation, but currently presenting no symptoms) 412
        with symptoms NEC 414.8
    posterior (strictly) (true) (wall) 410.6 ☑
    posterobasal 410.6 ☑
    posteroinferior 410.3 ☑
    posterolateral 410.5 ☑
    postprocedural 997.1
    previous, currently presenting no symptoms 412
    Q wave (*see also* Infarct, myo-cardium, by site) 410.9 ☑
    septal 410.8 ☑
    specified site NEC 410.8 ☑
    ST elevation (STEMI) 410.9 ☑
        anterior (wall) 410.1 ☑
        anterolateral (wall) 410.0 ☑
        inferior (wall) 410.4 ☑
        inferolateral (wall) 410.2 ☑
        inferoposterior wall 410.3 ☑
        lateral wall 410.5 ☑
        posterior (strictly) (true) (wall) 410.6 ☑
        specified site NEC 410.8 ☑
        subendocardial 410.7 ☑
    syphilitic 093.82
    non-ST elevation myocardial infarction (NSTEMI) 410.7 ☑
    nontransmural 410.7 ☑
omentum 557.0
ovary 620.8
pancreas 577.8
papillary muscle (*see also* Infarct, myocardium) 410.8 ☑
parathyroid gland 252.8
pituitary (gland) 253.8
placenta (complicating pregnancy) 656.7 ☑
    affecting fetus or newborn 762.2
pontine — *see* Infarct, brain
posterior NEC (*see also* Infarct, myocardium) 410.6 ☑
prostate 602.8
pulmonary (artery) (hemorrhagic) (vein) 415.19
    with
        abortion — *see* Abortion, by type, with embolism
        ectopic pregnancy (*see also* categories 633.0–633.9) 639.6
        molar pregnancy (*see also* categories 630–632) 639.6
    following
        abortion 639.6
        ectopic or molar pregnancy 639.6

Infarct, infarction — *continued*
pulmonary — *continued*
    iatrogenic 415.11
    in pregnancy, childbirth, or puerperium — *see* Embolism, obstetrical
    postoperative 415.11
    septic 415.12
renal 593.81
    embolic or thrombotic 593.81
retina, retinal 362.84
    with occlusion — *see* Occlusion, retina
spinal (acute) (cord) (embolic) (nonembolic) 336.1
spleen 289.59
    embolic or thrombotic 444.89
subchorionic — *see* Infarct, placenta
subendocardial (*see also* Infarct, myocardium) 410.7 ☑
suprarenal (capsule) (gland) 255.41
syncytium — *see* Infarct, placenta
testis 608.83
thrombotic (*see also* Thrombosis) 453.9
    artery, arterial — *see* Embolism
thyroid (gland) 246.3
ventricle (heart) (*see also* Infarct, myocardium) 410.9 ☑
Infecting — *see* condition
Infection, infected, infective (opportunistic) 136.9
with lymphangitis — *see* Lymphangitis
abortion — *see* Abortion, by type, with, sepsis
abscess (skin) — *see* Abscess, by site
Absidia 117.7
acanthamoeba 136.21
Acanthocheilonema (perstans) 125.4
    streptocerca 125.6
accessory sinus (chronic) (*see also* Sinusitis) 473.9
Achorion — *see* Dermatophytosis
Acremonium falciforme 117.4
acromioclavicular (joint) 711.91
actinobacillus
    lignieresii 027.8
    mallei 024
    muris 026.1
actinomadura — *see* Actinomycosis
Actinomyces (israelii) (*see also* Actinomycosis)
    muris-ratti 026.1
Actinomycetales (actinomadura) (Actinomyces) (Nocardia) (Streptomyces) — *see* Actinomycosis
actinomycotic NEC (*see also* Actinomycosis) 039.9
adenoid (chronic) 474.01
    acute 463
    and tonsil (chronic) 474.02
        acute or subacute 463
adenovirus NEC 079.0
    in diseases classified elsewhere — *see* category 079
    unspecified nature or site 079.0
Aerobacter aerogenes NEC 041.85
    enteritis 008.2
aerogenes capsulatus (*see also* Gangrene, gas) 040.0
aertrycke (*see also* Infection, Salmonella) 003.9
ajellomyces dermatitidis 116.0
alimentary canal NEC (*see also* Enteritis, due to, by organism) 009.0
Allescheria boydii 117.6
Alternaria 118
alveolus, alveolar (process) (pulpal origin) 522.4
ameba, amebic (histolytica) (*see also* Amebiasis) 006.9
    acute 006.0
    chronic 006.1
    free-living 136.29
    hartmanni 007.8
    specified
        site NEC 006.8
        type NEC 007.8
amniotic fluid or cavity 658.4 ☑

Infection, infected, infective — *continued*
amniotic fluid or cavity — *continued*
    affecting fetus or newborn 762.7
anaerobes (cocci) (gram-negative) (gram-positive) (mixed) NEC 041.84
anal canal 569.49
Ancylostoma braziliense 126.2
Angiostrongylus cantonensis 128.8
anisakiasis 127.1
Anisakis larva 127.1
anthrax (*see also* Anthrax) 022.9
antrum (chronic) (*see also* Sinusitis, maxillary) 473.0
anus (papillae) (sphincter) 569.49
arbor virus NEC 066.9
arbovirus NEC 066.9
argentophil-rod 027.0
Ascaris lumbricoides 127.0
ascomycetes 117.4
Aspergillus (flavus) (fumigatus) (terreus) 117.3
atypical
    acid-fast (bacilli) (*see also* Mycobacterium, atypical) 031.9
    mycobacteria (*see also* Mycobacterium, atypical) 031.9
auditory meatus (circumscribed) (diffuse) (external) (*see also* Otitis, externa) 380.10
auricle (ear) (*see also* Otitis, externa) 380.10
axillary gland 683
Babesiasis 088.82
Babesiosis 088.82
Bacillus NEC 041.89
    abortus 023.1
    anthracis (*see also* Anthrax) 022.9
    cereus (food poisoning) 005.89
    coli — *see* Infection, Escherichia coli
    coliform NEC 041.85
    Ducrey's (any location) 099.0
    Flexner's 004.1
    Friedländer's NEC 041.3
    fusiformis 101
    gas (gangrene) (*see also* Gangrene, gas) 040.0
    mallei 024
    melitensis 023.0
    paratyphoid, paratyphosus 002.9
        A 002.1
        B 002.2
        C 002.3
    Schmorl's 040.3
    Shiga 004.0
    suipestifer (*see also* Infection, Salmonella) 003.9
    swimming pool 031.1
    typhosa 002.0
    welchii (*see also* Gangrene, gas) 040.0
    Whitmore's 025
bacterial NEC 041.9
    specified NEC 041.89
        anaerobic NEC 041.84
        gram-negative NEC 041.85
            anaerobic NEC 041.84
Bacterium
    paratyphosum 002.9
        A 002.1
        B 002.2
        C 002.3
    typhosum 002.0
Bacteroides (fragilis) (melaninogenicus) (oralis) NEC 041.82
balantidium coli 007.0
Bartholin's gland 616.89
Basidiobolus 117.7
Bedsonia 079.98
    specified NEC 079.88
bile duct 576.1
bladder (*see also* Cystitis) 595.9
Blastomyces, blastomycotic 116.0
    brasiliensis 116.1
    dermatitidis 116.0
    European 117.5
    loboi 116.2
    North American 116.0
    South American 116.1

Infection, infected, infective — *continued*
bleb
  postprocedural 379.60
    stage 1 379.61
    stage 2 379.62
    stage 3 379.63
blood stream — *see also* Septicemia
  catheter-related (CRBSI) 999.31
bone 730.9 ☑
  specified — *see* Osteomyelitis
Bordetella 033.9
  bronchiseptica 033.8
  parapertussis 033.1
  pertussis 033.0
Borrelia
  bergdorfi 088.81
  vincentii (mouth) (pharynx) (tonsil) 101
bovine stomatitis 059.11
brain (*see also* Encephalitis) 323.9
  late effect — *see* category 326
  membranes (*see also* Meningitis) 322.9
  septic 324.0
    late effect — *see* category 326
  meninges (*see also* Meningitis) 320.9
branchial cyst 744.42
breast 611.0
  puerperal, postpartum 675.2 ☑
    with nipple 675.9 ☑
      specified type NEC 675.8 ☑
    nonpurulent 675.2 ☑
    purulent 675.1 ☑
bronchus (*see also* Bronchitis) 490
  fungus NEC 117.9
Brucella 023.9
  abortus 023.1
  canis 023.3
  melitensis 023.0
  mixed 023.8
  suis 023.2
Brugia (Wuchereria) malayi 125.1
bursa — *see* Bursitis
buttocks (skin) 686.9
Candida (albicans) (tropicalis) (*see also* Candidiasis) 112.9
  congenital 771.7
Candiru 136.8
Capillaria
  hepatica 128.8
  philippinensis 127.5
cartilage 733.99
catheter-related bloodstream (CRBSI) 999.31
cat liver fluke 121.0
cellulitis — *see* Cellulitis, by site
Cephalosporum falciforme 117.4
Cercomonas hominis (intestinal) 007.3
cerebrospinal (*see also* Meningitis) 322.9
  late effect — *see* category 326
cervical gland 683
cervix (*see also* Cervicitis) 616.0
cesarean section wound 674.3 ☑
Chilomastix (intestinal) 007.8
Chlamydia 079.98
  specified NEC 079.88
cholera (*see also* Cholera) 001.9
chorionic plate 658.8 ☑
Cladosporium
  bantianum 117.8
  carrionii 117.2
  mansoni 111.1
  trichoides 117.8
  wernecki 111.1
Clonorchis (sinensis) (liver) 121.1
Clostridium (haemolyticum) (novyi) NEC 041.84
  botulinum 005.1
  histolyticum (*see also* Gangrene, gas) 040.0
  oedematiens (*see also* Gangrene, gas) 040.0
  perfringens 041.83
    due to food 005.2
  septicum (*see also* Gangrene, gas) 040.0
  sordellii (*see also* Gangrene, gas) 040.0
  welchii (*see also* Gangrene, gas) 040.0
    due to food 005.2

Infection, infected, infective — *continued*
Coccidioides (immitis) (*see also* Coccidioidomycosis) 114.9
coccus NEC 041.89
colon (*see also* Enteritis, due to, by organism) 009.0
  bacillus — *see* Infection, Escherichia coli
colostomy or enterostomy 569.61
common duct 576.1
complicating pregnancy, childbirth, or puerperium NEC 647.9 ☑
  affecting fetus or newborn 760.2
Condiobolus 117.7
congenital NEC 771.89
  Candida albicans 771.7
  chronic 771.2
  cytomegalovirus 771.1
  hepatitis, viral 771.2
  herpes simplex 771.2
  listeriosis 771.2
  malaria 771.2
  poliomyelitis 771.2
  rubella 771.0
  toxoplasmosis 771.2
  tuberculosis 771.2
  urinary (tract) 771.82
  vaccinia 771.2
coronavirus 079.89
  SARS-associated 079.82
corpus luteum (*see also* Salpingo-oophoritis) 614.2
Corynebacterium diphtheriae — *see* Diphtheria
cotia virus 059.8
Coxsackie (*see also* Coxsackie) 079.2
  endocardium 074.22
  heart NEC 074.20
  in diseases classified elsewhere — *see* category 079 ☑
  meninges 047.0
  myocardium 074.23
  pericardium 074.21
  pharynx 074.0
  specified disease NEC 074.8
  unspecified nature or site 079.2
Cryptococcus neoformans 117.5
Cryptosporidia 007.4
Cunninghamella 117.7
cyst — *see* Cyst
Cysticercus cellulosae 123.1
cytomegalovirus 078.5
  congenital 771.1
dental (pulpal origin) 522.4
deuteromycetes 117.4
Dicrocoelium dendriticum 121.8
Dipetalonema (perstans) 125.4
  streptocerca 125.6
diphtherial — *see* Diphtheria
Diphyllobothrium (adult) (latum) (pacificum) 123.4
  larval 123.5
Diplogonoporus (grandis) 123.8
Dipylidium (caninum) 123.8
Dirofilaria 125.6
dog tapeworm 123.8
Dracunculus medinensis 125.7
Dreschlera 118
  hawaiiensis 117.8
Ducrey's bacillus (any site) 099.0
due to or resulting from
  central venous catheter 999.31
  device, implant, or graft (any) (presence of) — *see* Complications, infection and inflammation, due to (presence of) any device, implant, or graft classified to 996.0–996.5 NEC
  injection, inoculation, infusion, transfusion, or vaccination (prophylactic) (therapeutic) 999.39
  injury NEC — *see* Wound, open, by site, complicated
  surgery 998.59
duodenum 535.6 ☑
ear (*see also* Otitis)
  external (*see also* Otitis, externa) 380.10

Infection, infected, infective — *continued*
ear (*see also* Otitis) — *continued*
  inner (*see also* Labyrinthitis) 386.30
  middle — *see* Otitis, media
Eaton's agent NEC 041.81
Eberthella typhosa 002.0
Ebola 078.89
echinococcosis 122.9
Echinococcus (*see also* Echinococcus) 122.9
Echinostoma 121.8
ECHO virus 079.1
  in diseases classified elsewhere — *see* category 079 ☑
  unspecified nature or site 079.1
Ehrlichiosis 082.40
  chaffeensis 082.41
  specified type NEC 082.49
Endamoeba — *see* Infection, ameba
endocardium (*see also* Endocarditis) 421.0
endocervix (*see also* Cervicitis) 616.0
Entamoeba — *see* Infection, ameba
enteric (*see also* Enteritis, due to, by organism) 009.0
Enterobacter aerogenes NEC 041.85
Enterobacter sakazakii 041.85
Enterobius vermicularis 127.4
enterococcus NEC 041.04
enterovirus NEC 079.89
  central nervous system NEC 048
  enteritis 008.67
  meningitis 047.9
Entomophthora 117.7
Epidermophyton — *see* Dermatophytosis
epidermophytosis — *see* Dermatophytosis
episiotomy 674.3 ☑
Epstein-Barr virus 075
  chronic 780.79 [139.8]
erysipeloid 027.1
Erysipelothrix (insidiosa) (rhusiopathiae) 027.1
erythema infectiosum 057.0
Escherichia coli NEC 041.4
  enteritis — *see* Enteritis, E. coli
  generalized 038.42
  intestinal — *see* Enteritis, E. coli
esophagostomy 530.86
ethmoidal (chronic) (sinus) (*see also* Sinusitis, ethmoidal) 473.2
Eubacterium 041.84
Eustachian tube (ear) 381.50
  acute 381.51
  chronic 381.52
exanthema subitum (*see also* Exanthem subitum) 058.10
external auditory canal (meatus) (*see also* Otitis, externa) 380.10
eye NEC 360.00
eyelid 373.9
  specified NEC 373.8
fallopian tube (*see also* Salpingo-oophoritis) 614.2
fascia 728.89
Fasciola
  gigantica 121.3
  hepatica 121.3
Fasciolopsis (buski) 121.4
fetus (intra-amniotic) — *see* Infection, congenital
filarial — *see* Infestation, filarial
finger (skin) 686.9
  abscess (with lymphangitis) 681.00
    pulp 681.01
  cellulitis (with lymphangitis) 681.00
  distal closed space (with lymphangitis) 681.00
  nail 681.02
    fungus 110.1
fish tapeworm 123.4
  larval 123.5
flagellate, intestinal 007.9
fluke — *see* Infestation, fluke
focal
  teeth (pulpal origin) 522.4
  tonsils 474.00
    and adenoids 474.02

Infection, infected, infective — *continued*
Fonsecaea
  compactum 117.2
  pedrosoi 117.2
food (*see also* Poisoning, food) 005.9
foot (skin) 686.9
  fungus 110.4
Francisella tularensis (*see also* Tularemia) 021.9
frontal sinus (chronic) (*see also* Sinusitis, frontal) 473.1
fungus NEC 117.9
  beard 110.0
  body 110.5
  dermatiacious NEC 117.8
  foot 110.4
  groin 110.3
  hand 110.2
  nail 110.1
  pathogenic to compromised host only 118
  perianal (area) 110.3
  scalp 110.0
  scrotum 110.8
  skin 111.9
    foot 110.4
    hand 110.2
  toenails 110.1
  trachea 117.9
Fusarium 118
Fusobacterium 041.84
gallbladder (*see also* Cholecystitis, acute) 575.0
Gardnerella vaginalis 041.89
gas bacillus (*see also* Gas, gangrene) 040.0
gastric (*see also* Gastritis) 535.5 ☑
Gastrodiscoides hominis 121.8
gastroenteric (*see also* Enteritis, due to, by organism) 009.0
gastrointestinal (*see also* Enteritis, due to, by organism) 009.0
gastrostomy 536.41
generalized NEC (*see also* Septicemia) 038.9
genital organ or tract NEC
  female 614.9
    with
      abortion — *see* Abortion, by type, with sepsis
      ectopic pregnancy (*see also* categories 633.0–633.9) 639.0
      molar pregnancy (*see also* categories 630–632) 639.0
    complicating pregnancy 646.6 ☑
      affecting fetus or newborn 760.8
    following
      abortion 639.0
      ectopic or molar pregnancy 639.0
    puerperal, postpartum, childbirth 670.8 ☑
      minor or localized 646.6 ☑
        affecting fetus or newborn 760.8
  male 608.4
genitourinary tract NEC 599.0
Ghon tubercle, primary (*see also* Tuberculosis) 010.0 ☑
Giardia lamblia 007.1
gingival (chronic) 523.10
  acute 523.00
  Vincent's 101
glanders 024
Glenosporopsis amazonica 116.2
Gnathostoma spinigerum 128.1
Gongylonema 125.6
gonococcal NEC (*see also* Gonococcus) 098.0
gram-negative bacilli NEC 041.85
  anaerobic 041.84
guinea worm 125.7
gum (*see also* Infection, gingival) 523.10
Hantavirus 079.81
heart 429.89
Helicobacter pylori [H. pylori] 041.86
helminths NEC 128.9
  intestinal 127.9

☑ **Additional Digit Required** — Refer to the Tabular List for Digit Selection   ꙮ **Subterms under main terms may continue to next column or page**

2011 ICD-9-CM   ▶◀ **Revised Text**   ● **New Line**   ▲ **Revised Code**   **Volume 2 — 155**

Infection, infected, infective — *continued*
helminths — *continued*
  intestinal — *continued*
    mixed (types classifiable to more
      than one category in
      120.0–127.7) 127.8
    specified type NEC 127.7
    specified type NEC 128.8
Hemophilus influenzae NEC 041.5
  generalized 038.41
herpes (simplex) (*see also* Herpes, simplex)
  054.9
  congenital 771.2
  zoster (*see also* Herpes, zoster) 053.9
    eye NEC 053.29
Heterophyes heterophyes 121.6
Histoplasma (*see also* Histoplasmosis) 115.90
  capsulatum (*see also* Histoplasmosis,
    American) 115.00
  duboisii (*see also* Histoplasmosis, African)
    115.10
HIV V08
  with symptoms, symptomatic 042
hookworm (*see also* Ancylostomiasis) 126.9
human herpesvirus NEC 058.89
human herpesvirus 6 058.81
human herpesvirus 7 058.82
human herpesvirus 8 058.89
human immunodeficiency virus V08
  with symptoms, symptomatic 042
human papillomavirus 079.4
hydrocele 603.1
hydronephrosis 591
Hymenolepis 123.6
hypopharynx 478.29
inguinal glands 683
  due to soft chancre 099.0
intestine, intestinal (*see also* Enteritis, due
  to, by organism) 009.0
intrauterine (*see also* Endometritis) 615.9
  complicating delivery 646.6 ☑
isospora belli or hominis 007.2
Japanese B encephalitis 062.0
jaw (bone) (acute) (chronic) (lower) (subacute) (upper) 526.4
joint — *see* Arthritis, infectious or infective
Kaposi's sarcoma-associated herpesvirus
  058.89
kidney (cortex) (hematogenous) 590.9
  with
    abortion — *see* Abortion, by type,
      with urinary tract infection
    calculus 592.0
    ectopic pregnancy (*see also* cate-
      gories 633.0–633.9) 639.8
    molar pregnancy (*see also* categories
      630–632) 639.8
  complicating pregnancy or puerperium
    646.6 ☑
    affecting fetus or newborn 760.1
  following
    abortion 639.8
    ectopic or molar pregnancy 639.8
  pelvis and ureter 590.3
Klebsiella pneumoniae NEC 041.3
knee (skin) NEC 686.9
  joint — *see* Arthritis, infectious
Koch's (*see also* Tuberculosis, pulmonary)
  011.9 ☑
labia (majora) (minora) (*see also* Vulvitis)
  616.10
lacrimal
  gland (*see also* Dacryoadenitis) 375.00
  passages (duct) (sac) (*see also* Dacryocys-
    titis) 375.30
larynx NEC 478.79
leg (skin) NEC 686.9
Leishmania (*see also* Leishmaniasis) 085.9
  braziliensis 085.5
  donovani 085.0
  ethiopica 085.3
  furunculosa 085.1
  infantum 085.0
  mexicana 085.4
  tropica (minor) 085.1
    major 085.2

Infection, infected, infective — *continued*
Leptosphaeria senegalensis 117.4
leptospira (*See also* Leptospirosis) 100.9
  Australis 100.89
  Bataviae 100.89
  pyrogenes 100.89
  specified type NEC 100.89
leptospirochetal NEC (*see also* Leptospirosis)
  100.9
Leptothrix — *see* Actinomycosis
Listeria monocytogenes (listeriosis) 027.0
  congenital 771.2
liver fluke — *see* Infestation, fluke, liver
Loa loa 125.2
  eyelid 125.2 [373.6]
Loboa loboi 116.2
local, skin (staphylococcal) (streptococcal)
  NEC 686.9
  abscess — *see* Abscess, by site
  cellulitis — *see* Cellulitis, by site
  ulcer (*see also* Ulcer, skin) 707.9
Loefflerella
  mallei 024
  whitmori 025
lung 518.89
  atypical Mycobacterium 031.0
    tuberculous (*see also* Tuberculosis,
      pulmonary) 011.9 ☑
  basilar 518.89
  chronic 518.89
  fungus NEC 117.9
  spirochetal 104.8
  virus — *see* Pneumonia, virus
lymph gland (axillary) (cervical) (inguinal)
  683
  mesenteric 289.2
lymphoid tissue, base of tongue or posterior
  pharynx, NEC 474.00
madurella
  grisea 117.4
  mycetomii 117.4
major
  with
    abortion — *see* Abortion, by type,
      with sepsis
    ectopic pregnancy (*see also* cate-
      gories 633.0–633.9) 639.0
    molar pregnancy (*see also* categories
      630–632) 639.0
  following
    abortion 639.0
    ectopic or molar pregnancy 639.0
  puerperal, postpartum, childbirth
    670.0 ☑
Malassezia furfur 111.0
Malleomyces
  mallei 024
  pseudomallei 025
mammary gland 611.0
  puerperal, postpartum 675.2 ☑
Mansonella (ozzardi) 125.5
mastoid (suppurative) — *see* Mastoiditis
maxilla, maxillary 526.4
  sinus (chronic) (*see also* Sinusitis, maxil-
    lary) 473.0
mediastinum 519.2
medina 125.7
meibomian
  cyst 373.12
  gland 373.12
melioidosis 025
meninges (*see also* Meningitis) 320.9
meningococcal (*see also* condition) 036.9
  brain 036.1
  cerebrospinal 036.0
  endocardium 036.42
  generalized 036.2
  meninges 036.0
  meningococcemia 036.2
  specified site NEC 036.89
mesenteric lymph nodes or glands NEC
  289.2
Metagonimus 121.5
metatarsophalangeal 711.97

Infection, infected, infective — *continued*
methicillin
  resistant Staphylococcus aureus (MRSA)
    041.12
  susceptible Staphylococcus aureus
    (MSSA) 041.11
microorganism resistant to drugs — *see*
  Resistance (to), drugs by microorganisms
Microsporidia 136.8
microsporum, microsporic — *see* Dermatophytosis
Mima polymorpha NEC 041.85
mixed flora NEC 041.89
Monilia (*see also* Candidiasis) 112.9
  neonatal 771.7
monkeypox 059.01
Monosporium apiospermum 117.6
mouth (focus) NEC 528.9
  parasitic 136.9
MRSA (methicillin resistant Staphylococcus
  aureus) 041.12
MSSA (methicillin susceptible Staphylococcus aureus) 041.11
Mucor 117.7
muscle NEC 728.89
mycelium NEC 117.9
mycetoma
  actinomycotic NEC (*see also* Actinomyco-
    sis) 039.9
  mycotic NEC 117.4
Mycobacterium, mycobacterial (*see also*
  Mycobacterium) 031.9
Mycoplasma NEC 041.81
mycotic NEC 117.9
  pathogenic to compromised host only
    118
  skin NEC 111.9
  systemic 117.9
myocardium NEC 422.90
nail (chronic) (with lymphangitis) 681.9
  finger 681.02
    fungus 110.1
  ingrowing 703.0
  toe 681.11
    fungus 110.1
nasal sinus (chronic) (*see also* Sinusitis) 473.9
nasopharynx (chronic) 478.29
  acute 460
navel 686.9
  newborn 771.4
Neisserian — *see* Gonococcus
Neotestudina rosatii 117.4
newborn, generalized 771.89
nipple 611.0
  puerperal, postpartum 675.0 ☑
    with breast 675.9 ☑
      specified type NEC 675.8 ☑
Nocardia — *see* Actinomycosis
nose 478.19
nostril 478.19
obstetrical surgical wound 674.3 ☑
Oesophagostomum (apiostomum) 127.7
Oestrus ovis 134.0
Oidium albicans (*see also* Candidiasis) 112.9
Onchocerca (volvulus) 125.3
  eye 125.3 [360.13]
  eyelid 125.3 [373.6]
operation wound 998.59
Opisthorchis (felineus) (tenuicollis) (viverrini) 121.0
orbit 376.00
  chronic 376.10
orthopoxvirus 059.00
  specified NEC 059.09
ovary (*see also* Salpingo-oophoritis) 614.2
Oxyuris vermicularis 127.4
pancreas 577.0
Paracoccidioides brasiliensis 116.1
Paragonimus (westermani) 121.2
parainfluenza virus 079.89
parameningococcus NEC 036.9
  with meningitis 036.0
parapoxvirus 059.10
  specified NEC 059.19
parasitic NEC 136.9

Infection, infected, infective — *continued*
paratyphoid 002.9
  type A 002.1
  type B 002.2
  type C 002.3
paraurethral ducts 597.89
parotid gland 527.2
Pasteurella NEC 027.2
  multocida (cat-bite) (dog-bite) 027.2
  pestis (*see also* Plague) 020.9
  pseudotuberculosis 027.2
  septica (cat-bite) (dog-bite) 027.2
  tularensis (*see also* Tularemia) 021.9
pelvic, female (*see also* Disease, pelvis, inflammatory) 614.9
penis (glans) (retention) NEC 607.2
  herpetic 054.13
Peptococcus 041.84
Peptostreptococcus 041.84
periapical (pulpal origin) 522.4
peridental 523.30
perineal wound (obstetrical) 674.3 ☑
periodontal 523.31
periorbital 376.00
  chronic 376.10
perirectal 569.49
perirenal (*see also* Infection, kidney) 590.9
peritoneal (*see also* Peritonitis) 567.9
periureteral 593.89
periurethral 597.89
Petriellidium boydii 117.6
pharynx 478.29
  Coxsackie virus 074.0
  phlegmonous 462
  posterior, lymphoid 474.00
Phialophora
  gougerotii 117.8
  jeanselmei 117.8
  verrucosa 117.2
Piedraia hortai 111.3
pinna, acute 380.11
pinta 103.9
  intermediate 103.1
  late 103.2
  mixed 103.3
  primary 103.0
pinworm 127.4
pityrosporum furfur 111.0
pleuropneumonia-like organisms NEC (PP-
  LO) 041.81
pneumococcal NEC 041.2
  generalized (purulent) 038.2
Pneumococcus NEC 041.2
postoperative wound 998.59
posttraumatic NEC 958.3
postvaccinal 999.39
poxvirus 059.9
  specified NEC 059.8
prepuce NEC 607.1
Proprionibacterium 041.84
prostate (capsule) (*see also* Prostatitis) 601.9
Proteus (mirabilis) (morganii) (vulgaris) NEC
  041.6
  enteritis 008.3
protozoal NEC 136.8
  intestinal NEC 007.9
Pseudomonas NEC 041.7
  mallei 024
  pneumonia 482.1
  pseudomallei 025
psittacosis 073.9
puerperal, postpartum (major) 670.0 ☑
  minor 646.6 ☑
pulmonary — *see* Infection, lung
purulent — *see* Abscess
putrid, generalized — *see* Septicemia
pyemic — *see* Septicemia
Pyrenochaeta romeroi 117.4
Q fever 083.0
rabies 071
rectum (sphincter) 569.49
renal (*see also* Infection, kidney) 590.9
  pelvis and ureter 590.3
resistant to drugs — *see* Resistance (to),
  drugs by microorganisms
respiratory 519.8

☑ **Additional Digit Required** — Refer to the Tabular List for Digit Selection
           Subterms under main terms may continue to next column or page

Infection, infected, infective — *continued*
respiratory — *continued*
  chronic 519.8
  influenzal (acute) (upper) ▶(*see also* Influenza)◀ 487.1
  lung 518.89
  rhinovirus 460
  syncytial virus 079.6
  upper (acute) (infectious) NEC 465.9
    with flu, grippe, or influenza ▶(*see also* Influenza)◀ 487.1
    influenzal ▶(*see also* Influenza)◀ 487.1
    multiple sites NEC 465.8
    streptococcal 034.0
    viral NEC 465.9
respiratory syncytial virus (RSV) 079.6
resulting from presence of shunt or other internal prosthetic device — *see* Complications, infection and inflammation, due to (presence of) any device, implant, or graft classified to 996.0–996.5 NEC
retroperitoneal 567.39
retrovirus 079.50
  human immunodeficiency virus type 2 (HIV2) 079.53
  human T-cell lymphotrophic virus type I (HTLV-I) 079.51
  human T-cell lymphotrophic virus type II (HTLV-II) 079.52
  specified NEC 079.59
Rhinocladium 117.1
Rhinosporidium — *see* beri 117.0
rhinovirus
  in diseases classified elsewhere — *see* category 079 ☑
  unspecified nature or site 079.3
Rhizopus 117.7
rickettsial 083.9
rickettsialpox 083.2
rubella (*see also* Rubella) 056.9
  congenital 771.0
Saccharomyces (*see also* Candidiasis) 112.9
Saksenaea 117.7
salivary duct or gland (any) 527.2
Salmonella (aertrycke) (callinarum) (choleraesuis) (enteritidis) (suipestifer) (typhimurium) 003.9
  with
    arthritis 003.23
    gastroenteritis 003.0
    localized infection 003.20
      specified type NEC 003.29
    meningitis 003.21
    osteomyelitis 003.24
    pneumonia 003.22
    septicemia 003.1
    specified manifestation NEC 003.8
  due to food (poisoning) (any serotype) (*see also* Poisoning, food, due to, Salmonella)
  hirschfeldii 002.3
  localized 003.20
    specified type NEC 003.29
  paratyphi 002.9
    A 002.1
    B 002.2
    C 002.3
  schottmuelleri 002.2
  specified type NEC 003.8
  typhi 002.0
  typhosa 002.0
saprophytic 136.8
Sarcocystis, lindemanni 136.5
SARS-associated coronavirus 079.82
scabies 133.0
Schistosoma — *see* Infestation, Schistosoma
Schmorl's bacillus 040.3
scratch or other superficial injury — *see* Injury, superficial, by site
scrotum (acute) NEC 608.4
sealpox 059.12
secondary, burn or open wound (dislocation) (fracture) 958.3
seminal vesicle (*see also* Vesiculitis) 608.0

Infection, infected, infective — *continued*
septic
  generalized — *see* Septicemia
  localized, skin (*see also* Abscess) 682.9
septicemic — *see* Septicemia
seroma 998.51
Serratia (marcescens) 041.85
  generalized 038.44
sheep liver fluke 121.3
Shigella 004.9
  boydii 004.2
  dysenteriae 004.0
  flexneri 004.1
  group
    A 004.0
    B 004.1
    C 004.2
    D 004.3
  Schmitz (-Stutzer) 004.0
  schmitzii 004.0
  Shiga 004.0
  sonnei 004.3
  specified type NEC 004.8
Sin Nombre virus 079.81
sinus (*see also* Sinusitis) 473.9
  pilonidal 685.1
    with abscess 685.0
  skin NEC 686.9
Skene's duct or gland (*see also* Urethritis) 597.89
skin (local) (staphylococcal) (streptococcal) NEC 686.9
  abscess — *see* Abscess, by site
  cellulitis — *see* Cellulitis, by site
  due to fungus 111.9
    specified type NEC 111.8
  mycotic 111.9
    specified type NEC 111.8
  ulcer (*see also* Ulcer, skin) 707.9
slow virus 046.9
  specified condition NEC 046.8
Sparganum (mansoni) (proliferum) 123.5
spermatic cord NEC 608.4
sphenoidal (chronic) (sinus) (*see also* Sinusitis, sphenoidal) 473.3
Spherophorus necrophorus 040.3
spinal cord NEC (*see also* Encephalitis) 323.9
  abscess 324.1
    late effect — *see* category 326
  late effect — *see* category 326
  meninges — *see* Meningitis
  streptococcal 320.2
Spirillum
  minus or minor 026.0
  morsus muris 026.0
  obermeieri 087.0
spirochetal NEC 104.9
  lung 104.8
  specified nature or site NEC 104.8
spleen 289.59
Sporothrix schenckii 117.1
Sporotrichum (schenckii) 117.1
Sporozoa 136.8
staphylococcal NEC 041.10
  aureus 041.11
    methicillin
      resistant (MRSA) 041.12
      susceptible (MSSA) 041.11
  food poisoning 005.0
  generalized (purulent) 038.10
    aureus 038.11
      methicillin
        resistant 038.12
        susceptible 038.11
    specified organism NEC 038.19
  pneumonia 482.40
    aureus 482.41
      methicillin
        resistant (MRSA) 482.42
        susceptible (MSSA) 482.41
    MRSA (methicillin resistant Staphylococcus aureus) 482.42
    MSSA (methicillin susceptible Staphylococcus aureus) 482.41
    specified type NEC 482.49

Infection, infected, infective — *continued*
staphylococcal — *continued*
  septicemia 038.10
    aureus 038.11
      methicillin
        resistant (MRSA) 038.12
        susceptible (MSSA) 038.11
    MRSA (methicillin resistant Staphylococcus aureus) 038.12
    MSSA (methicillin susceptible Staphylococcus aureus) 038.11
    specified organism NEC 038.19
  specified NEC 041.19
steatoma 706.2
Stellantchasmus falcatus 121.6
Streptobacillus moniliformis 026.1
streptococcal NEC 041.00
  generalized (purulent) 038.0
  Group
    A 041.01
    B 041.02
    C 041.03
    D [enterococcus] 041.04
    G 041.05
  pneumonia — *see* Pneumonia, streptococcal
  septicemia 038.0
  sore throat 034.0
  specified NEC 041.09
Streptomyces — *see* Actinomycosis
streptotrichosis — *see* Actinomycosis
Strongyloides (stercoralis) 127.2
stump (amputation) (posttraumatic) (surgical) 997.62
  traumatic — *see* Amputation, traumatic, by site, complicated
subcutaneous tissue, local NEC 686.9
submaxillary region 528.9
suipestifer (*see also* Infection, Salmonella) 003.9
swimming pool bacillus 031.1
syphilitic — *see* Syphilis
systemic — *see* Septicemia
Taenia — *see* Infestation, Taenia
Taeniarhynchus saginatus 123.2
tanapox 059.21
tapeworm — *see* Infestation, tapeworm
tendon (sheath) 727.89
Ternidens diminutus 127.7
testis (*see also* Orchitis) 604.90
thigh (skin) 686.9
threadworm 127.4
throat 478.29
  pneumococcal 462
  staphylococcal 462
  streptococcal 034.0
  viral NEC (*see also* Pharyngitis) 462
thumb (skin) 686.9
  abscess (with lymphangitis) 681.00
    pulp 681.01
  cellulitis (with lymphangitis) 681.00
  nail 681.02
thyroglossal duct 529.8
toe (skin) 686.9
  abscess (with lymphangitis) 681.10
  cellulitis (with lymphangitis) 681.10
  nail 681.11
    fungus 110.1
tongue NEC 529.0
  parasitic 112.0
tonsil (faucial) (lingual) (pharyngeal) 474.00
  acute or subacute 463
  and adenoid 474.02
  tag 474.00
tooth, teeth 522.4
  periapical (pulpal origin) 522.4
  peridental 523.30
  periodontal 523.31
  pulp 522.0
  socket 526.5
TORCH — *see* Infection, congenital NEC
  without active infection 760.2
Torula histolytica 117.5
Toxocara (cani) (cati) (felis) 128.0

Infection, infected, infective — *continued*
Toxoplasma gondii (*see also* Toxoplasmosis) 130.9
trachea, chronic 491.8
  fungus 117.9
traumatic NEC 958.3
trematode NEC 121.9
trench fever 083.1
Treponema
  denticola 041.84
  macrodenticum 041.84
  pallidum (*see also* Syphilis) 097.9
Trichinella (spiralis) 124
Trichomonas 131.9
  bladder 131.09
  cervix 131.09
  hominis 007.3
  intestine 007.3
  prostate 131.03
  specified site NEC 131.8
  urethra 131.02
  urogenitalis 131.00
  vagina 131.01
  vulva 131.01
Trichophyton, trichophytid — *see* Dermatophytosis
Trichosporon (beigelii) cutaneum 111.2
Trichostrongylus 127.6
Trichuris (trichiuria) 127.3
Trombicula (irritans) 133.8
Trypanosoma (*see also* Trypanosomiasis) 086.9
  cruzi 086.2
tubal (*see also* Salpingo-oophoritis) 614.2
tuberculous NEC (*see also* Tuberculosis) 011.9 ☑
tubo-ovarian (*see also* Salpingo-oophoritis) 614.2
tunica vaginalis 608.4
tympanic membrane — *see* Myringitis
typhoid (abortive) (ambulant) (bacillus) 002.0
typhus 081.9
  flea-borne (endemic) 081.0
  louse-borne (epidemic) 080
  mite-borne 081.2
  recrudescent 081.1
  tick-borne 082.9
    African 082.1
    North Asian 082.2
umbilicus (septic) 686.9
  newborn NEC 771.4
ureter 593.89
urethra (*see also* Urethritis) 597.80
urinary (tract) NEC 599.0
  with
    abortion — *see* Abortion, by type, with urinary tract infection
    ectopic pregnancy (*see also* categories 633.0–633.9) 639.8
    molar pregnancy (*see also* categories 630–632) 639.8
  candidal 112.2
  complicating pregnancy, childbirth, or puerperium 646.6 ☑
    affecting fetus or newborn 760.1
    asymptomatic 646.5 ☑
      affecting fetus or newborn 760.1
  diplococcal (acute) 098.0
    chronic 098.2
  due to Trichomonas (vaginalis) 131.00
  following
    abortion 639.8
    ectopic or molar pregnancy 639.8
  gonococcal (acute) 098.0
    chronic or duration of 2 months or over 098.2
  newborn 771.82
  trichomonal 131.00
  tuberculous (*see also* Tuberculosis) 016.3 ☑
  uterus, uterine (*see also* Endometritis) 615.9
  utriculus masculinus NEC 597.89
vaccination 999.39

Infection, infected, infective — *continued*
urinary — *continued*
  vagina (granulation tissue) (wall) (*see also* Vaginitis) 616.10
  varicella 052.9
  varicose veins — *see* Varicose, veins
  variola 050.9
    major 050.0
    minor 050.1
  vas deferens NEC 608.4
  Veillonella 041.84
  verumontanum 597.89
  vesical (*see also* Cystitis) 595.9
  Vibrio
    cholerae 001.0
      El Tor 001.1
    parahaemolyticus (food poisoning) 005.4
    vulnificus 041.85
  Vincent's (gums) (mouth) (tonsil) 101
  vaccination 999.39
  virus, viral 079.99
    adenovirus
      in diseases classified elsewhere — *see* category 079 ☑
      unspecified nature or site 079.0
    central nervous system NEC 049.9
      enterovirus 048
        meningitis 047.9
          specified type NEC 047.8
      slow virus 046.9
      specified condition NEC 046.8
    chest 519.8
    conjunctivitis 077.99
      specified type NEC 077.8
    coronavirus 079.89
      SARS-associated 079.82
    Coxsackie (*see also* Infection, Coxsackie) 079.2
    Ebola 065.8
    ECHO
      in diseases classified elsewhere — *see* category 079 ☑
      unspecified nature or site 079.1
    encephalitis 049.9
      arthropod-borne NEC 064
      tick-borne 063.9
        specified type NEC 063.8
    enteritis NEC (*see also* Enteritis, viral) 008.8
    exanthem NEC 057.9
    Hantavirus 079.81
    human papilloma 079.4
    in diseases classified elsewhere — *see* category 079 ☑
    intestine (*see also* Enteritis, viral) 008.8
    lung — *see* Pneumonia, viral
    respiratory syncytial (RSV) 079.6
    retrovirus 079.50
    rhinovirus
      in diseases classified elsewhere — *see* category 079 ☑
      unspecified nature or site 079.3
    salivary gland disease 078.5
    slow 046.9
      specified condition NEC 046.8
    specified type NEC 079.89
      in diseases classified elsewhere — *see* category 079 ☑
      unspecified nature or site 079.99
    warts 078.10
      specified NEC 078.19
    yaba monkey tumor 059.22
  vulva (*see also* Vulvitis) 616.10
  whipworm 127.3
  Whitmore's bacillus 025
  wound (local) (posttraumatic) NEC 958.3
    with
      dislocation — *see* Dislocation, by site, open
      fracture — *see* Fracture, by site, open
      open wound — *see* Wound, open, by site, complicated
    postoperative 998.59
    surgical 998.59
  Wuchereria 125.0

Infection, infected, infective — *continued*
Wuchereria — *continued*
  bancrofti 125.0
  malayi 125.1
yaba monkey tumor virus 059.22
yatapoxvirus 059.20
yaws — *see* Yaws
yeast (*see also* Candidiasis) 112.9
yellow fever (*see also* Fever, yellow) 060.9
Yersinia pestis (*see also* Plague) 020.9
Zeis' gland 373.12
zoonotic bacterial NEC 027.9
Zopfia senegalensis 117.4
Infective, infectious — *see* condition
Inferiority complex 301.9
  constitutional psychopathic 301.9
Infertility
female 628.9
  age related 628.8
  associated with
    adhesions, peritubal 614.6 *[628.2]*
    anomaly
      cervical mucus 628.4
      congenital
        cervix 628.4
        fallopian tube 628.2
        uterus 628.3
        vagina 628.4
    anovulation 628.0
    dysmucorrhea 628.4
    endometritis, tuberculous (*see also* Tuberculosis) 016.7 ☑ *[628.3]*
    Stein-Leventhal syndrome 256.4 *[628.0]*
  due to
    adiposogenital dystrophy 253.8 *[628.1]*
    anterior pituitary disorder NEC 253.4 *[628.1]*
      hyperfunction 253.1 *[628.1]*
    cervical anomaly 628.4
    fallopian tube anomaly 628.2
    ovarian failure 256.39 *[628.0]*
    Stein-Leventhal syndrome 256.4 *[628.0]*
    uterine anomaly 628.3
    vaginal anomaly 628.4
  nonimplantation 628.3
  origin
    cervical 628.4
    pituitary-hypothalamus NEC 253.8 *[628.1]*
      anterior pituitary NEC 253.4 *[628.1]*
        hyperfunction NEC 253.1 *[628.1]*
      dwarfism 253.3 *[628.1]*
      panhypopituitarism 253.2 *[628.1]*
    specified NEC 628.8
    tubal (block) (occlusion) (stenosis) 628.2
      adhesions 614.6 *[628.2]*
    uterine 628.3
    vaginal 628.4
  previous, requiring supervision of pregnancy V23.0
male 606.9
  absolute 606.0
  due to
    azoospermia 606.0
    drug therapy 606.8
    extratesticular cause NEC 606.8
    germinal cell
      aplasia 606.0
      desquamation 606.1
    hypospermatogenesis 606.1
    infection 606.8
    obstruction, afferent ducts 606.8
    oligospermia 606.1
    radiation 606.8
    spermatogenic arrest (complete) 606.0
      incomplete 606.1
    systemic disease 606.8
Infestation 134.9
  Acanthocheilonema (perstans) 125.4

Infestation — *continued*
Acanthocheilonema — *continued*
  streptocerca 125.6
Acariasis 133.9
  demodex folliculorum 133.8
  Sarcoptes scabiei 133.0
  trombiculae 133.8
Agamofilaria streptocerca 125.6
Ancylostoma, Ankylostoma 126.9
  americanum 126.1
  braziliense 126.2
  canium 126.8
  ceylanicum 126.3
  duodenale 126.0
  new world 126.1
  old world 126.0
Angiostrongylus cantonensis 128.8
anisakiasis 127.1
Anisakis larva 127.1
arthropod NEC 134.1
Ascaris lumbricoides 127.0
Bacillus fusiformis 101
Balantidium coli 007.0
beef tapeworm 123.2
Bothriocephalus (latus) 123.4
  larval 123.5
broad tapeworm 123.4
  larval 123.5
Brugia malayi 125.1
Candiru 136.8
Capillaria
  hepatica 128.8
  philippinensis 127.5
cat liver fluke 121.0
Cercomonas hominis (intestinal) 007.3
cestodes 123.9
  specified type NEC 123.8
chigger 133.8
chigoe 134.1
Chilomastix 007.8
Clonorchis (sinensis) (liver) 121.1
coccidia 007.2
complicating pregnancy, childbirth, or puerperium 647.9 ☑
  affecting fetus or newborn 760.8
Cysticercus cellulosae 123.1
Demodex folliculorum 133.8
Dermatobia (hominis) 134.0
Dibothriocephalus (latus) 123.4
  larval 123.5
Dicrocoelium dendriticum 121.8
Diphyllobothrium (adult) (intestinal) (latum) (pacificum) 123.4
  larval 123.5
Diplogonoporus (grandis) 123.8
Dipylidium (caninum) 123.8
Distoma hepaticum 121.3
dog tapeworm 123.8
Dracunculus medinensis 125.7
dragon worm 125.7
dwarf tapeworm 123.6
Echinococcus (*see also* Echinococcus) 122.9
Echinostoma ilocanum 121.8
Embadomonas 007.8
Endamoeba (histolytica) — *see* Infection, ameba
Entamoeba (histolytica) — *see* Infection, ameba
Enterobius vermicularis 127.4
Epidermophyton — *see* Dermatophytosis
eyeworm 125.2
Fasciola
  gigantica 121.3
  hepatica 121.3
Fasciolopsis (buski) (small intestine) 121.4
  blood NEC (*see also* Schistosomiasis) 120.9
  cat liver 121.0
  filarial 125.9
  due to
    Acanthocheilonema (perstans) 125.4
    streptocerca 125.6
    Brugia (Wuchereria) malayi 125.1
    Dracunculus medinensis 125.7
    guinea worms 125.7

Infestation — *continued*
Fasciolopsis — *continued*
  filarial — *continued*
    due to — *continued*
      Mansonella (ozzardi) 125.5
      Onchocerca volvulus 125.3
        eye 125.3 *[360.13]*
        eyelid 125.3 *[373.6]*
      Wuchereria (bancrofti) 125.0
        malayi 125.1
    specified type NEC 125.6
fish tapeworm 123.4
  larval 123.5
fluke 121.9
intestinal (giant) 121.4
liver (sheep) 121.3
  cat 121.0
  Chinese 121.1
  clonorchiasis 121.1
  fascioliasis 121.3
  Oriental 121.1
lung (oriental) 121.2
sheep liver 121.3
fly larva 134.0
Gasterophilus (intestinalis) 134.0
Gastrodiscoides hominis 121.8
Giardia lamblia 007.1
Gnathostoma (spinigerum) 128.1
Gongylonema 125.6
guinea worm 125.7
helminth NEC 128.9
  intestinal 127.9
    mixed (types classifiable to more than one category in 120.0–127.7) 127.8
    specified type NEC 127.7
  specified type NEC 128.8
Heterophyes heterophyes (small intestine) 121.6
hookworm (*see also* Infestation, ancylostoma) 126.9
Hymenolepis (diminuta) (nana) 123.6
intestinal NEC 129
leeches (aquatic) (land) 134.2
Leishmania — *see* Leishmaniasis
lice (*see also* Infestation, pediculus) 132.9
Linguatulidae, linguatula (pentastoma) (serrata) 134.1
Loa loa 125.2
  eyelid 125.2 *[373.6]*
louse (*see also* Infestation, pediculus) 132.9
  body 132.1
  head 132.0
  pubic 132.2
maggots 134.0
Mansonella (ozzardi) 125.5
medina 125.7
Metagonimus yokogawai (small intestine) 121.5
Microfilaria streptocerca 125.3
  eye 125.3 *[360.13]*
  eyelid 125.3 *[373.6]*
Microsporon furfur 111.0
microsporum — *see* Dermatophytosis
mites 133.9
  scabic 133.0
  specified type NEC 133.8
monilia (albicans) (*see also* Candidiasis) 112.9
  vagina 112.1
  vulva 112.1
mouth 112.0
Necator americanus 126.1
nematode (intestinal) 127.9
  Ancylostoma (*see also* Ancylostoma) 126.9
  Ascaris lumbricoides 127.0
  conjunctiva NEC 128.9
  Dioctophyma 128.8
  Enterobius vermicularis 127.4
  Gnathostoma spinigerum 128.1
  Oesophagostomum (apiostomum) 127.7
  Physaloptera 127.4
  specified type NEC 127.7
  Strongyloides stercoralis 127.2
  Ternidens diminutus 127.7

☑ **Additional Digit Required** — Refer to the Tabular List for Digit Selection   ▽ **Subterms under main terms may continue to next column or page**

158 — Volume 2   ▶◀ Revised Text   ● New Line   ▲ Revised Code   2011 ICD-9-CM

Infestation — *continued*
  nematode — *continued*
    Trichinella spiralis 124
    Trichostrongylus 127.6
    Trichuris (trichiuria) 127.3
  Oesophagostomum (apiostomum) 127.7
  Oestrus ovis 134.0
  Onchocerca (volvulus) 125.3
    eye 125.3 [360.13]
    eyelid 125.3 [373.6]
  Opisthorchis (felineus) (tenuicollis) (viverrini) 121.0
  Oxyuris vermicularis 127.4
  Paragonimus (westermani) 121.2
  parasite, parasitic NEC 136.9
    eyelid 134.9 [373.6]
    intestinal 129
    mouth 112.0
    orbit 376.13
    skin 134.9
    tongue 112.0
  pediculus 132.9
    capitis (humanus) (any site) 132.0
    corporis (humanus) (any site) 132.1
    eyelid 132.0 [373.6]
    mixed (classifiable to more than one category in 132.0–132.2) 132.3
    pubis (any site) 132.2
  phthirus (pubis) (any site) 132.2
    with any infestation classifiable to 132.0, 132.1 and 132.3
  pinworm 127.4
  pork tapeworm (adult) 123.0
  protozoal NEC 136.8
  pubic louse 132.2
  rat tapeworm 123.6
  red bug 133.8
  roundworm (large) NEC 127.0
  sand flea 134.1
  saprophytic NEC 136.8
  Sarcoptes scabiei 133.0
  scabies 133.0
  Schistosoma 120.9
    bovis 120.8
    cercariae 120.3
    hematobium 120.0
    intercalatum 120.8
    japonicum 120.2
    mansoni 120.1
    mattheii 120.8
    specified
      site — *see* Schistosomiasis
      type NEC 120.8
    spindale 120.8
  screw worms 134.0
  skin NEC 134.9
  Sparganum (mansoni) (proliferum) 123.5
    larval 123.5
  specified type NEC 134.8
  Spirometra larvae 123.5
  Sporozoa NEC 136.8
  Stellantchasmus falcatus 121.6
  Strongyloides 127.2
  Strongylus (gibsoni) 127.7
  Taenia 123.3
    diminuta 123.6
    Echinococcus (*see also* Echinococcus) 122.9
    mediocanellata 123.2
    nana 123.6
    saginata (mediocanellata) 123.2
    solium (intestinal form) 123.0
      larval form 123.1
  Taeniarhynchus saginatus 123.2
  tapeworm 123.9
    beef 123.2
    broad 123.4
      larval 123.5
    dog 123.8
    dwarf 123.6
    fish 123.4
      larval 123.5
    pork 123.0
    rat 123.6
  Ternidens diminutus 127.7
  Tetranychus molestissimus 133.8

Infestation — *continued*
  threadworm 127.4
  tongue 112.0
  Toxocara (cani) (cati) (felis) 128.0
  trematode(s) NEC 121.9
  Trichina spiralis 124
  Trichinella spiralis 124
  Trichocephalus 127.3
  Trichomonas 131.9
    bladder 131.09
    cervix 131.09
    intestine 007.3
    prostate 131.03
    specified site NEC 131.8
    urethra (female) (male) 131.02
    urogenital 131.00
    vagina 131.01
    vulva 131.01
  Trichophyton — *see* Dermatophytosis
  Trichostrongylus instabilis 127.6
  Trichuris (trichiuria) 127.3
  Trombicula (irritans) 133.8
  Trypanosoma — *see* Trypanosomiasis
  Tunga penetrans 134.1
  Uncinaria americana 126.1
  whipworm 127.3
  worms NEC 128.9
    intestinal 127.9
  Wuchereria 125.0
    bancrofti 125.0
    malayi 125.1

Infiltrate, infiltration
  with an iron compound 275.09 ▲
  amyloid (any site) (generalized) 277.39
  calcareous (muscle) NEC 275.49
    localized — *see* Degeneration, by site
  calcium salt (muscle) 275.49
  chemotherapy, vesicant 999.81
  corneal (*see also* Edema, cornea) 371.20
  eyelid 373.9
  fatty (diffuse) (generalized) 272.8
    localized — *see* Degeneration, by site, fatty
  glycogen, glycogenic (*see also* Disease, glycogen storage) 271.0
  heart, cardiac
    fatty (*see also* Degeneration, myocardial) 429.1
    glycogenic 271.0 [425.7]
  inflammatory in vitreous 379.29
  kidney (*see also* Disease, renal) 593.9
  leukemic (M9800/3) — *see* Leukemia
  liver 573.8
    fatty — *see* Fatty, liver
    glycogen (*see also* Disease, glycogen storage) 271.0
  lung (*see also* Infiltrate, pulmonary) 518.3
    eosinophilic 518.3
    x-ray finding only 793.1
  lymphatic (*see also* Leukemia, lymphatic) 204.9 ☑
    gland, pigmentary 289.3
  muscle, fatty 728.9
  myelogenous (*see also* Leukemia, myeloid) 205.9 ☑
  myocardium, myocardial
    fatty (*see also* Degeneration, myocardial) 429.1
    glycogenic 271.0 [425.7]
  pulmonary 518.3
    with
      eosinophilia 518.3
      pneumonia — *see* Pneumonia, by type
    x-ray finding only 793.1
  Ranke's primary (*see also* Tuberculosis) 010.0 ☑
  skin, lymphocytic (benign) 709.8
  thymus (gland) (fatty) 254.8
  urine 788.8
  vesicant
    agent NEC 999.82
    chemotherapy 999.81
  vitreous humor 379.29
Infirmity 799.89
  senile 797

Inflammation, inflamed, inflammatory (with exudation)
  abducens (nerve) 378.54
  accessory sinus (chronic) (*see also* Sinusitis) 473.9
  adrenal (gland) 255.8
  alimentary canal — *see* Enteritis
  alveoli (teeth) 526.5
    scorbutic 267
  amnion — *see* Amnionitis
  anal canal 569.49
  antrum (chronic) (*see also* Sinusitis, maxillary) 473.0
  anus 569.49
  appendix (*see also* Appendicitis) 541
  arachnoid — *see* Meningitis
  areola 611.0
    puerperal, postpartum 675.0 ☑
  areolar tissue NEC 686.9
  artery — *see* Arteritis
  auditory meatus (external) (*see also* Otitis, externa) 380.10
  Bartholin's gland 616.89
  bile duct or passage 576.1
  bladder (*see also* Cystitis) 595.9
  bleb
    postprocedural 379.60
      stage 1 379.61
      stage 2 379.62
      stage 3 379.63
  bone — *see* Osteomyelitis
  bowel (*see also* Enteritis) 558.9
  brain (*see also* Encephalitis) 323.9
    late effect — *see* category 326
    membrane — *see* Meningitis
  breast 611.0
    puerperal, postpartum 675.2 ☑
  broad ligament (*see also* Disease, pelvis, inflammatory) 614.4
    acute 614.3
  bronchus — *see* Bronchitis
  bursa — *see* Bursitis
  capsule
    liver 573.3
    spleen 289.59
  catarrhal (*see also* Catarrh) 460
    vagina 616.10
  cecum (*see also* Appendicitis) 541
  cerebral (*see also* Encephalitis) 323.9
    late effect — *see* category 326
    membrane — *see* Meningitis
  cerebrospinal (*see also* Meningitis) 322.9
    late effect — *see* category 326
    meningococcal 036.0
    tuberculous (*see also* Tuberculosis) 013.6 ☑
  cervix (uteri) (*see also* Cervicitis) 616.0
  chest 519.9
  choroid NEC (*see also* Choroiditis) 363.20
  cicatrix (tissue) — *see* Cicatrix
  colon (*see also* Enteritis) 558.9
    granulomatous 555.1
    newborn 558.9
  connective tissue (diffuse) NEC 728.9
  cornea (*see also* Keratitis) 370.9
    with ulcer (*see also* Ulcer, cornea) 370.00
  corpora cavernosa (penis) 607.2
  cranial nerve — *see* Disorder, nerve, cranial
  diarrhea — *see* Diarrhea
  disc (intervertebral) (space) 722.90
    cervical, cervicothoracic 722.91
    lumbar, lumbosacral 722.93
    thoracic, thoracolumbar 722.92
  Douglas' cul-de-sac or pouch (chronic) (*see also* Disease, pelvis, inflammatory) 614.4
    acute 614.3
  due to (presence of) any device, implant, or graft classifiable to 996.0–996.5 — *see* Complications, infection and inflammation, due to (presence of) any device, implant, or graft classified to 996.0–996.5 NEC
  duodenum 535.6 ☑
  dura mater — *see* Meningitis
  ear (*see also* Otitis)

Inflammation, inflamed, inflammatory — *continued*
  ear (*see also* Otitis) — *continued*
    external (*see also* Otitis, externa) 380.10
    inner (*see also* Labyrinthitis) 386.30
    middle — *see* Otitis media
  esophagus 530.10
  ethmoidal (chronic) (sinus) (*see also* Sinusitis, ethmoidal) 473.2
  Eustachian tube (catarrhal) 381.50
    acute 381.51
    chronic 381.52
  extrarectal 569.49
  eye 379.99
  eyelid 373.9
    specified NEC 373.8
  fallopian tube (*see also* Salpingo-oophoritis) 614.2
  fascia 728.9
  fetal membranes (acute) 658.4 ☑
    affecting fetus or newborn 762.7
  follicular, pharynx 472.1
  frontal (chronic) (sinus) (*see also* Sinusitis, frontal) 473.1
  gallbladder (*see also* Cholecystitis, acute) 575.0
  gall duct (*see also* Cholecystitis) 575.10
  gastrointestinal (*see also* Enteritis) 558.9
  genital organ (diffuse) (internal)
    female 614.9
      with
        abortion — *see* Abortion, by type, with sepsis
        ectopic pregnancy (*see also* categories 633.0–633.9) 639.0
        molar pregnancy (*see also* categories 630–632) 639.0
      complicating pregnancy, childbirth, or puerperium 646.6 ☑
        affecting fetus or newborn 760.8
      following
        abortion 639.0
        ectopic or molar pregnancy 639.0
    male 608.4
  gland (lymph) (*see also* Lymphadenitis) 289.3
  glottis (*see also* Laryngitis) 464.00
    with obstruction 464.01
  granular, pharynx 472.1
  gum 523.10
  heart (*see also* Carditis) 429.89
  hepatic duct 576.8
  hernial sac — *see* Hernia, by site
  ileum (*see also* Enteritis) 558.9
    terminal or regional 555.0
      with large intestine 555.2
  intervertebral disc 722.90
    cervical, cervicothoracic 722.91
    lumbar, lumbosacral 722.93
    thoracic, thoracolumbar 722.92
  intestine (*see also* Enteritis) 558.9
  jaw (acute) (bone) (chronic) (lower) (suppurative) (upper) 526.4
  jejunum — *see* Enteritis
  joint NEC (*see also* Arthritis) 716.9 ☑
    sacroiliac 720.2
  kidney (*see also* Nephritis) 583.9
  knee (joint) 716.66
    tuberculous (active) (*see also* Tuberculosis) 015.2 ☑
  labium (majus) (minus) (*see also* Vulvitis) 616.10
  lacrimal
    gland (*see also* Dacryoadenitis) 375.00
    passages (duct) (sac) (*see also* Dacryocystitis) 375.30
  larynx (*see also* Laryngitis) 464.00
    with obstruction 464.01
    diphtheritic 032.3
  leg NEC 686.9
  lip 528.5
  liver (capsule) (*see also* Hepatitis) 573.3
    acute 570
    chronic 571.40
    suppurative 572.0
  lung (acute) (*see also* Pneumonia) 486

☑ **Additional Digit Required** — Refer to the Tabular List for Digit Selection   ▽ **Subterms under main terms may continue to next column or page**

2011 ICD-9-CM   ▶◀ Revised Text   ● New Line   ▲ Revised Code   October 2010 • Volume 2 — 159

Infestation — Inflammation, inflamed, inflammatory

☑ **Additional Digit Required — Refer to the Tabular List for Digit Selection**   ▽ **Subterms under main terms may continue to next column or page**

160 — Volume 2 · October 2010   ▶◀ **Revised Text**   ● **New Line**   ▲ **Revised Code**   2011 ICD-9-CM

Injury — *continued*
blood vessel — *continued*
abdomen 902.9
multiple 902.87
specified NEC 902.89
aorta (thoracic) 901.0
abdominal 902.0
arm NEC 903.9
axillary 903.00
artery 903.01
vein 903.02
azygos vein 901.89
basilic vein 903.1
brachial (artery) (vein) 903.1
bronchial 901.89
carotid artery 900.00
common 900.01
external 900.02
internal 900.03
celiac artery 902.20
specified branch NEC 902.24
cephalic vein (arm) 903.1
colica dextra 902.26
cystic
artery 902.24
vein 902.39
deep plantar 904.6
digital (artery) (vein) 903.5
due to accidental puncture or laceration
during procedure 998.2
extremity
lower 904.8
multiple 904.7
specified NEC 904.7
upper 903.9
multiple 903.8
specified NEC 903.8
femoral
artery (superficial) 904.1
above profunda origin 904.0
common 904.0
vein 904.2
gastric
artery 902.21
vein 902.39
head 900.9
intracranial — *see* Injury, intracranial
multiple 900.82
specified NEC 900.89
hemiazygos vein 901.89
hepatic
artery 902.22
vein 902.11
hypogastric 902.59
artery 902.51
vein 902.52
ileocolic
artery 902.26
vein 902.31
iliac 902.50
artery 902.53
specified branch NEC 902.59
vein 902.54
innominate
artery 901.1
vein 901.3
intercostal (artery) (vein) 901.81
jugular vein (external) 900.81
internal 900.1
leg NEC 904.8
mammary (artery) (vein) 901.82
mesenteric
artery 902.20
inferior 902.27
specified branch NEC 902.29
superior (trunk) 902.25
branches, primary 902.26
vein 902.39
inferior 902.32
superior (and primary subdivisions) 902.31
neck 900.9
multiple 900.82
specified NEC 900.89
ovarian 902.89
artery 902.81

Injury — *continued*
blood vessel — *continued*
ovarian — *continued*
vein 902.82
palmar artery 903.4
pelvis 902.9
multiple 902.87
specified NEC 902.89
plantar (deep) (artery) (vein) 904.6
popliteal 904.40
artery 904.41
vein 904.42
portal 902.33
pulmonary 901.40
artery 901.41
vein 901.42
radial (artery) (vein) 903.2
renal 902.40
artery 902.41
specified NEC 902.49
vein 902.42
saphenous
artery 904.7
vein (greater) (lesser) 904.3
splenic
artery 902.23
vein 902.34
subclavian
artery 901.1
vein 901.3
suprarenal 902.49
thoracic 901.9
multiple 901.83
specified NEC 901.89
tibial 904.50
artery 904.50
anterior 904.51
posterior 904.53
vein 904.50
anterior 904.52
posterior 904.54
ulnar (artery) (vein) 903.3
uterine 902.59
artery 902.55
vein 902.56
vena cava
inferior 902.10
specified branches NEC 902.19
superior 901.2
brachial plexus 953.4
newborn 767.6
brain (traumatic) NEC (*see also* Injury, intracranial) 854.0 ☑
due to fracture of skull — *see* Fracture, skull, by site
breast 959.19
broad ligament — *see* Injury, internal, broad ligament
bronchus, bronchi — *see* Injury, internal, bronchus
brow 959.09
buttock 959.19
canthus, eye 921.1
cathode ray 990
cauda equina 952.4
with fracture, vertebra — *see* Fracture, vertebra, sacrum
cavernous sinus (*see also* Injury, intracranial) 854.0 ☑
cecum — *see* Injury, internal, cecum
celiac ganglion or plexus 954.1
cerebellum (*see also* Injury, intracranial) 854.0 ☑
cervix (uteri) — *see* Injury, internal, cervix
cheek 959.09
chest (*see also* Injury, internal, chest) wall 959.11
childbirth (*see also* Birth, injury)
maternal NEC 665.9 ☑
chin 959.09
choroid (eye) 921.3
clitoris 959.14
coccyx 959.19
complicating delivery 665.6 ☑
colon — *see* Injury, internal, colon

Injury — *continued*
common duct — *see* Injury, internal, common duct
conjunctiva 921.1
superficial 918.2
cord
spermatic — *see* Injury, internal, spermatic cord
spinal — *see* Injury, spinal, by site
cornea 921.3
abrasion 918.1
due to contact lens 371.82
penetrating — *see* Injury, eyeball, penetrating
superficial 918.1
due to contact lens 371.82
cortex (cerebral) (*see also* Injury, intracranial) 854.0 ☑
visual 950.3
costal region 959.11
costochondral 959.11
cranial
bones — *see* Fracture, skull, by site
cavity (*see also* Injury, intracranial) 854.0 ☑
nerve — *see* Injury, nerve, cranial
crushing — *see* Crush
cutaneous sensory nerve
lower limb 956.4
upper limb 955.5
deep tissue — *see* Contusion, by site
meaning pressure ulcer 707.25
delivery (*see also* Birth, injury)
maternal NEC 665.9 ☑
Descemet's membrane — *see* Injury, eyeball, penetrating
diaphragm — *see* Injury, internal, diaphragm
diffuse axonal — *see* Injury, intracranial
duodenum — *see* Injury, internal, duodenum
ear (auricle) (canal) (drum) (external) 959.09
elbow (and forearm) (and wrist) 959.3
epididymis 959.14
epigastric region 959.12
epiglottis 959.09
epiphyseal, current — *see* Fracture, by site
esophagus — *see* Injury, internal, esophagus
Eustachian tube 959.09
extremity (lower) (upper) NEC 959.8
eye 921.9
penetrating eyeball — *see* Injury, eyeball, penetrating
superficial 918.9
eyeball 921.3
penetrating 871.7
with
partial loss (of intraocular tissue) 871.2
prolapse or exposure (of intraocular tissue) 871.1
without prolapse 871.0
foreign body (nonmagnetic) 871.6
magnetic 871.5
superficial 918.9
eyebrow 959.09
eyelid(s) 921.1
laceration — *see* Laceration, eyelid
superficial 918.0
face (and neck) 959.09
fallopian tube — *see* Injury, internal, fallopian tube
finger(s) (nail) 959.5
flank 959.19
foot (and ankle) (and knee) (and leg, except thigh) 959.7
forceps NEC 767.9
scalp 767.19
forearm (and elbow) (and wrist) 959.3
forehead 959.09
gallbladder — *see* Injury, internal, gallbladder
gasserian ganglion 951.2
gastrointestinal tract — *see* Injury, internal, gastrointestinal tract

Injury — *continued*
genital organ(s)
with
abortion — *see* Abortion, by type, with, damage to pelvic organs
ectopic pregnancy (*see also* categories 633.0–633.9) 639.2
molar pregnancy (*see also* categories 630–632) 639.2
external 959.14
fracture of corpus cavernosum penis 959.13
following
abortion 639.2
ectopic or molar pregnancy 639.2
internal — *see* Injury, internal, genital organs
obstetrical trauma NEC 665.9 ☑
affecting fetus or newborn 763.89
gland
lacrimal 921.1
laceration 870.8
parathyroid 959.09
salivary 959.09
thyroid 959.09
globe (eye) (*see also* Injury, eyeball) 921.3
grease gun — *see* Wound, open, by site, complicated
groin 959.19
gum 959.09
hand(s) (except fingers) 959.4
head NEC 959.01
with
loss of consciousness 850.5
skull fracture — *see* Fracture, skull, by site
heart — *see* Injury, internal, heart
heel 959.7
hip (and thigh) 959.6
hymen 959.14
hyperextension (cervical) (vertebra) 847.0
ileum — *see* Injury, internal, ileum
iliac region 959.19
infrared rays NEC 990
instrumental (during surgery) 998.2
birth injury — *see* Birth, injury
nonsurgical (*see also* Injury, by site) 959.9
obstetrical 665.9 ☑
affecting fetus or newborn 763.89
bladder 665.5 ☑
cervix 665.3 ☑
high vaginal 665.4 ☑
perineal NEC 664.9 ☑
urethra 665.5 ☑
uterus 665.5 ☑
internal 869.0

Note — For injury of internal organ(s) by foreign body entering through a natural orifice (e.g., inhaled, ingested, or swallowed) — see Foreign body, entering through orifice.

For internal injury of any of the following sites with internal injury of any other of the sites — see Injury, internal, multiple.

with
fracture
pelvis — *see* Fracture, pelvis
specified site, except pelvis — *see* Injury, internal, by site
open wound into cavity 869.1
abdomen, abdominal (viscera) NEC 868.00
with
fracture, pelvis — *see* Fracture, pelvis
open wound into cavity 868.10
specified site NEC 868.09
with open wound into cavity 868.19
adrenal (gland) 868.01
with open wound into cavity 868.11
aorta (thoracic) 901.0
abdominal 902.0

Index

Injury — Injury

Injury — continued
  internal — continued
    appendix 863.85
      with open wound into cavity 863.95
    bile duct 868.02
      with open wound into cavity 868.12
    bladder (sphincter) 867.0
      with
        abortion — see Abortion, by type,
          with damage to pelvic or-
          gans
        ectopic pregnancy (see also cate-
          gories 633.0–633.9) 639.2
        molar pregnancy (see also cate-
          gories 630–632) 639.2
        open wound into cavity 867.1
      following
        abortion 639.2
        ectopic or molar pregnancy 639.2
      obstetrical trauma 665.5 ☑
        affecting fetus or newborn 763.89
    blood vessel — see Injury, blood vessel,
      by site
    broad ligament 867.6
      with open wound into cavity 867.7
    bronchus, bronchi 862.21
      with open wound into cavity 862.31
    cecum 863.89
      with open wound into cavity 863.99
    cervix (uteri) 867.4
      with
        abortion — see Abortion, by type,
          with damage to pelvic or-
          gans
        ectopic pregnancy (see also cate-
          gories 633.0–633.9) 639.2
        molar pregnancy (see also cate-
          gories 630–632) 639.2
        open wound into cavity 867.5
      following
        abortion 639.2
        ectopic or molar pregnancy 639.2
      obstetrical trauma 665.3 ☑
        affecting fetus or newborn 763.89
    chest (see also Injury, internal, intratho-
      racic organs) 862.8
      with open wound into cavity 862.9
    colon 863.40
      with
        open wound into cavity 863.50
        rectum 863.46
          with open wound into cavity
            863.56
      ascending (right) 863.41
        with open wound into cavity
          863.51
      descending (left) 863.43
        with open wound into cavity
          863.53
      multiple sites 863.46
        with open wound into cavity
          863.56
      sigmoid 863.44
        with open wound into cavity
          863.54
      specified site NEC 863.49
        with open wound into cavity
          863.59
      transverse 863.42
        with open wound into cavity
          863.52
    common duct 868.02
      with open wound into cavity 868.12
    complicating delivery 665.9 ☑
      affecting fetus or newborn 763.89
    diaphragm 862.0
      with open wound into cavity 862.1
    duodenum 863.21
      with open wound into cavity 863.31
    esophagus (intrathoracic) 862.22
      with open wound into cavity 862.32
      cervical region 874.4
        complicated 874.5
    fallopian tube 867.6
      with open wound into cavity 867.7
    gallbladder 868.02

Injury — continued
  internal — continued
    gallbladder — continued
      with open wound into cavity 868.12
    gastrointestinal tract NEC 863.80
      with open wound into cavity 863.90
    genital organ NEC 867.6
      with open wound into cavity 867.7
    heart 861.00
      with open wound into thorax 861.10
    ileum 863.29
      with open wound into cavity 863.39
    intestine NEC 863.89
      with open wound into cavity 863.99
      large NEC 863.40
        with open wound into cavity
          863.50
      small NEC 863.20
        with open wound into cavity
          863.30
    intra-abdominal (organ) 868.00
      with open wound into cavity 868.10
      multiple sites 868.09
        with open wound into cavity
          868.19
      specified site NEC 868.09
        with open wound into cavity
          868.19
    intrathoracic organs (multiple) 862.8
      with open wound into cavity 862.9
      diaphragm (only) — see Injury, inter-
        nal, diaphragm
      heart (only) — see Injury, internal,
        heart
      lung (only) — see Injury, internal,
        lung
      specified site NEC 862.29
        with open wound into cavity
          862.39
    intrauterine (see also Injury, internal,
      uterus) 867.4
      with open wound into cavity 867.5
    jejunum 863.29
      with open wound into cavity 863.39
    kidney (subcapsular) 866.00
      with
        disruption of parenchyma (com-
          plete) 866.03
          with open wound into cavity
            866.13
        hematoma (without rupture of
          capsule) 866.01
          with open wound into cavity
            866.11
        laceration 866.02
          with open wound into cavity
            866.12
        open wound into cavity 866.10
    liver 864.00
      with
        contusion 864.01
          with open wound into cavity
            864.11
        hematoma 864.01
          with open wound into cavity
            864.11
        laceration 864.05
          with open wound into cavity
            864.15
        major (disruption of hepatic
          parenchyma) 864.04
          with open wound into
            cavity 864.14
        minor (capsule only) 864.02
          with open wound into
            cavity 864.12
        moderate (involving
          parenchyma) 864.03
          with open wound into
            cavity 864.13
        multiple 864.04
        stellate 864.04
          with open wound into
            cavity 864.14
      open wound into cavity 864.10
    lung 861.20

Injury — continued
  internal — continued
    lung — continued
      with open wound into thorax 861.30
      hemopneumothorax — see Hemop-
        neumothorax, traumatic
      hemothorax — see Hemothorax,
        traumatic
      pneumohemothorax — see Pneumo-
        hemothorax, traumatic
      pneumothorax — see Pneumotho-
        rax, traumatic
      transfusion related, acute (TRALI)
        518.7
    mediastinum 862.29
      with open wound into cavity 862.39
    mesentery 863.89
      with open wound into cavity 863.99
    mesosalpinx 867.6
      with open wound into cavity 867.7
    multiple 869.0

> Note — Multiple internal injuries of sites
> classifiable to the same three- or four-
> digit category should be classified to
> that category.
>
> Multiple injuries classifiable to different
> fourth-digit subdivisions of 861 (heart
> and lung injuries) should be dealt with
> according to coding rules.

      internal
        with open wound into cavity
          869.1
      intra-abdominal organ (sites classifi-
        able to 863–868)
        with
          intrathoracic organ(s) (sites
            classifiable to 861–862)
            869.0
            with open wound into
              cavity 869.1
          other intra-abdominal or-
            gan(s) (sites classifiable
            to 863–868, except
            where classifiable to
            the same three-digit
            category) 868.09
            with open wound into
              cavity 868.19
      intrathoracic organ (sites classifiable
        to 861–862)
        with
          intra-abdominal organ(s)
            (sites classifiable to
            863–868) 869.0
            with open wound into
              cavity 869.1
          other intrathoracic organ(s)
            (sites classifiable to
            861–862, except where
            classifiable to the same
            three-digit category)
            862.8
            with open wound into
              cavity 862.9
    myocardium — see Injury, internal, heart
    ovary 867.6
      with open wound into cavity 867.7
    pancreas (multiple sites) 863.84
      with open wound into cavity 863.94
      body 863.82
        with open wound into cavity
          863.92
      head 863.81
        with open wound into cavity
          863.91
      tail 863.83
        with open wound into cavity
          863.93
    pelvis, pelvic (organs) (viscera) 867.8
      with
        fracture, pelvis — see Fracture,
          pelvis
        open wound into cavity 867.9
      specified site NEC 867.6

Injury — continued
  internal — continued
    pelvis, pelvic — continued
      specified site — continued
        with open wound into cavity
          867.7
    peritoneum 868.03
      with open wound into cavity 868.13
    pleura 862.29
      with open wound into cavity 862.39
    prostate 867.6
      with open wound into cavity 867.7
    rectum 863.45
      with
        colon 863.46
          with open wound into cavity
            863.56
        open wound into cavity 863.55
    retroperitoneum 868.04
      with open wound into cavity 868.14
    round ligament 867.6
      with open wound into cavity 867.7
    seminal vesicle 867.6
      with open wound into cavity 867.7
    spermatic cord 867.6
      with open wound into cavity 867.7
    scrotal — see Wound, open, spermat-
      ic cord
    spleen 865.00
      with
        disruption of parenchyma (mas-
          sive) 865.04
          with open wound into cavity
            865.14
        hematoma (without rupture of
          capsule) 865.01
          with open wound into cavity
            865.11
        open wound into cavity 865.10
        tear, capsular 865.02
          with open wound into cavity
            865.12
          extending into parenchyma
            865.03
            with open wound into
              cavity 865.13
    stomach 863.0
      with open wound into cavity 863.1
    suprarenal gland (multiple) 868.01
      with open wound into cavity 868.11
    thorax, thoracic (cavity) (organs) (multi-
      ple) (see also Injury, internal, in-
      trathoracic organs) 862.8
      with open wound into cavity 862.9
    thymus (gland) 862.29
      with open wound into cavity 862.39
    trachea (intrathoracic) 862.29
      with open wound into cavity 862.39
      cervical region (see also Wound,
        open, trachea) 874.02
    ureter 867.2
      with open wound into cavity 867.3
    urethra (sphincter) 867.0
      with
        abortion — see Abortion, by type,
          with damage to pelvic or-
          gans
        ectopic pregnancy (see also cate-
          gories 633.0–633.9) 639.2
        molar pregnancy (see also cate-
          gories 630–632) 639.2
        open wound into cavity 867.1
      following
        abortion 639.2
        ectopic or molar pregnancy 639.2
      obstetrical trauma 665.5 ☑
        affecting fetus or newborn 763.89
    uterus 867.4
      with
        abortion — see Abortion, by type,
          with damage to pelvic or-
          gans
        ectopic pregnancy (see also cate-
          gories 633.0–633.9) 639.2
        molar pregnancy (see also cate-
          gories 630–632) 639.2

Injury — *continued*
  internal — *continued*
    uterus — *continued*
      with — *continued*
        open wound into cavity 867.5
      following
        abortion 639.2
        ectopic or molar pregnancy 639.2
      obstetrical trauma NEC 665.5 ☑
        affecting fetus or newborn 763.89
    vas deferens 867.6
      with open wound into cavity 867.7
    vesical (sphincter) 867.0
      with open wound into cavity 867.1
    viscera (abdominal) (*see also* Injury, internal, multiple) 868.00
      with
        fracture, pelvis — *see* Fracture, pelvis
        open wound into cavity 868.10
      thoracic NEC (*see also* Injury, internal, intrathoracic organs) 862.8
        with open wound into cavity 862.9
  interscapular region 959.19
  intervertebral disc 959.19
  intestine — *see* Injury, internal, intestine
  intra-abdominal (organs) NEC — *see* Injury, internal, intra-abdominal
  intracranial (traumatic) 854.0 ☑

Note — *Use the following fifth-digit subclassification with categories 851–854:*

0 *unspecified state of consciousness*

1 *with no loss of consciousness*

2 *with brief [less than one hour] loss of consciousness*

3 *with moderate [1–24 hours] loss of consciousness*

4 *with prolonged [more than 24 hours] loss of consciousness and return to pre-existing conscious level*

5 *with prolonged [more than 24 hours] loss of consciousness, without return to pre-existing conscious level*

Use fifth-digit 5 to designate when a patient is unconscious and dies before regaining consciousness, regardless of the duration of the loss of consciousness

6 *with loss of consciousness of unspecified duration*

9 *with concussion, unspecified*

    with
      open intracranial wound 854.1 ☑
      skull fracture — *see* Fracture, skull, by site
    contusion 851.8 ☑
      with open intracranial wound 851.9 ☑
      brain stem 851.4 ☑
        with open intracranial wound 851.5 ☑
      cerebellum 851.4 ☑
        with open intracranial wound 851.5 ☑
      cortex (cerebral) 851.0 ☑
        with open intracranial wound 851.2 ☑
    hematoma — *see* Injury, intracranial, hemorrhage
    hemorrhage 853.0 ☑
      with
        laceration — *see* Injury, intracranial, laceration
        open intracranial wound 853.1 ☑
      extradural 852.4 ☑
        with open intracranial wound 852.5 ☑
      subarachnoid 852.0 ☑

Injury — *continued*
  intracranial — *continued*
    hemorrhage — *continued*
      subarachnoid — *continued*
        with open intracranial wound 852.1 ☑
      subdural 852.2 ☑
        with open intracranial wound 852.3 ☑
    laceration 851.8 ☑
      with open intracranial wound 851.9 ☑
      brain stem 851.6 ☑
        with open intracranial wound 851.7 ☑
      cerebellum 851.6 ☑
        with open intracranial wound 851.7 ☑
      cortex (cerebral) 851.2 ☑
        with open intracranial wound 851.3 ☑
  intraocular — *see* Injury, eyeball, penetrating
  intrathoracic organs (multiple) — *see* Injury, internal, intrathoracic organs
  intrauterine — *see* Injury, internal, intrauterine
  iris 921.3
    penetrating — *see* Injury, eyeball, penetrating
  jaw 959.09
  jejunum — *see* Injury, internal, jejunum
  joint NEC 959.9
    old or residual 718.80
      ankle 718.87
      elbow 718.82
      foot 718.87
      hand 718.84
      hip 718.85
      knee 718.86
      multiple sites 718.89
      pelvic region 718.85
      shoulder (region) 718.81
      specified site NEC 718.88
      wrist 718.83
  kidney — *see* Injury, internal, kidney
    acute (nontraumatic) 584.9
  knee (and ankle) (and foot) (and leg, except thigh) 959.7
  labium (majus) (minus) 959.14
  labyrinth, ear 959.09
  lacrimal apparatus, gland, or sac 921.1
    laceration 870.8
  larynx 959.09
  late effect — *see* Late, effects (of), injury
  leg, except thigh (and ankle) (and foot) (and knee) 959.7
    upper or thigh 959.6
  lens, eye 921.3
    penetrating — *see* Injury, eyeball, penetrating
  lid, eye — *see* Injury, eyelid
  lip 959.09
  liver — *see* Injury, internal, liver
  lobe, parietal — *see* Injury, intracranial
  lumbar (region) 959.19
    plexus 953.5
  lumbosacral (region) 959.19
    plexus 953.5
  lung — *see* Injury, internal, lung
  malar region 959.09
  mastoid region 959.09
  maternal, during pregnancy, affecting fetus or newborn 760.5
  maxilla 959.09
  mediastinum — *see* Injury, internal, mediastinum
  membrane
    brain (*see also* Injury, intracranial) 854.0 ☑
    tympanic 959.09
  meningeal artery — *see* Hemorrhage, brain, traumatic, subarachnoid
  meninges (cerebral) — *see* Injury, intracranial

Injury — *continued*
  mesenteric
    artery — *see* Injury, blood vessel, mesenteric, artery
    plexus, inferior 954.1
    vein — *see* Injury, blood vessel, mesenteric, vein
  mesentery — *see* Injury, internal, mesentery
  mesosalpinx — *see* Injury, internal, mesosalpinx
  middle ear 959.09
  midthoracic region 959.11
  mouth 959.09
  multiple (sites not classifiable to the same four-digit category in 959.0–959.7) 959.8
    internal 869.0
      with open wound into cavity 869.1
  musculocutaneous nerve 955.4
  nail
    finger 959.5
    toe 959.7
  nasal (septum) (sinus) 959.09
  nasopharynx 959.09
  neck (and face) 959.09
  nerve 957.9
    abducens 951.3
    abducent 951.3
    accessory 951.6
    acoustic 951.5
    ankle and foot 956.9
    anterior crural, femoral 956.1
    arm (*see also* Injury, nerve, upper limb) 955.9
    auditory 951.5
    axillary 955.0
    brachial plexus 953.4
    cervical sympathetic 954.0
    cranial 951.9
      first or olfactory 951.8
      second or optic 950.0
      third or oculomotor 951.0
      fourth or trochlear 951.1
      fifth or trigeminal 951.2
      sixth or abducens 951.3
      seventh or facial 951.4
      eighth, acoustic, or auditory 951.5
      ninth or glossopharyngeal 951.8
      tenth, pneumogastric, or vagus 951.8
      eleventh or accessory 951.6
      twelfth or hypoglossal 951.7
      newborn 767.7
    cutaneous sensory
      lower limb 956.4
      upper limb 955.5
    digital (finger) 955.6
      toe 956.5
    facial 951.4
      newborn 767.5
    femoral 956.1
    finger 955.9
    foot and ankle 956.9
    forearm 955.9
    glossopharyngeal 951.8
    hand and wrist 955.9
    head and neck, superficial 957.0
    hypoglossal 951.7
    involving several parts of body 957.8
    leg (*see also* Injury, nerve, lower limb) 956.9
    lower limb 956.9
      multiple 956.8
      specified site NEC 956.5
    lumbar plexus 953.5
    lumbosacral plexus 953.5
    median 955.1
      forearm 955.1
      wrist and hand 955.1
    multiple (in several parts of body) (sites not classifiable to the same three-digit category) 957.8
    musculocutaneous 955.4
    musculospiral 955.3
      upper arm 955.3
    oculomotor 951.0
    olfactory 951.8

Injury — *continued*
  nerve — *continued*
    optic 950.0
    pelvic girdle 956.9
      multiple sites 956.8
      specified site NEC 956.5
    peripheral 957.9
      multiple (in several regions) (sites not classifiable to the same three-digit category) 957.8
      specified site NEC 957.1
    peroneal 956.3
      ankle and foot 956.3
      lower leg 956.3
    plantar 956.5
    plexus 957.9
      celiac 954.1
      mesenteric, inferior 954.1
      spinal 953.9
        brachial 953.4
        lumbosacral 953.5
        multiple sites 953.8
      sympathetic NEC 954.1
    pneumogastric 951.8
    radial 955.3
      wrist and hand 955.3
    sacral plexus 953.5
    sciatic 956.0
      thigh 956.0
    shoulder girdle 955.9
      multiple 955.8
      specified site NEC 955.7
    specified site NEC 957.1
    spinal 953.9
      plexus — *see* Injury, nerve, plexus, spinal
      root 953.9
        cervical 953.0
        dorsal 953.1
        lumbar 953.2
        multiple sites 953.8
        sacral 953.3
    splanchnic 954.1
    sympathetic NEC 954.1
      cervical 954.0
    thigh 956.9
    tibial 956.5
      ankle and foot 956.2
      lower leg 956.5
      posterior 956.2
    toe 956.9
    trigeminal 951.2
    trochlear 951.1
    trunk, excluding shoulder and pelvic girdles 954.9
      specified site NEC 954.8
      sympathetic NEC 954.1
    ulnar 955.2
      forearm 955.2
      wrist (and hand) 955.2
    upper limb 955.9
      multiple 955.8
      specified site NEC 955.7
    vagus 951.8
    wrist and hand 955.9
  nervous system, diffuse 957.8
  nose (septum) 959.09
  obstetrical NEC 665.9 ☑
    affecting fetus or newborn 763.89
  occipital (region) (scalp) 959.09
    lobe (*see also* Injury, intracranial) 854.0 ☑
  optic 950.9
    chiasm 950.1
    cortex 950.3
    nerve 950.0
    pathways 950.2
  orbit, orbital (region) 921.2
    penetrating 870.3
      with foreign body 870.4
  ovary — *see* Injury, internal, ovary
  paint-gun — *see* Wound, open, by site, complicated
  palate (soft) 959.09
  pancreas — *see* Injury, internal, pancreas
  parathyroid (gland) 959.09

☑ Additional Digit Required — Refer to the Tabular List for Digit Selection   ▽ Subterms under main terms may continue to next column or page

2011 ICD-9-CM   ▶◀ Revised Text   ● New Line   ▲ Revised Code   Volume 2 — 163

Injury — *continued*

parietal (region) (scalp) 959.09
  lobe — *see* Injury, intracranial
pelvic
  floor 959.19
    complicating delivery 664.1 ☑
      affecting fetus or newborn 763.89
  joint or ligament, complicating delivery 665.6 ☑
    affecting fetus or newborn 763.89
  organs (*see also* Injury, internal, pelvis)
    with
      abortion — *see* Abortion, by type, with damage to pelvic organs
      ectopic pregnancy (*see also* categories 633.0–633.9) 639.2
      molar pregnancy (*see also* categories 633.0–633.9) 639.2
    following
      abortion 639.2
      ectopic or molar pregnancy 639.2
    obstetrical trauma 665.5 ☑
      affecting fetus or newborn 763.89
pelvis 959.19
penis 959.14
  fracture of corpus cavernosum 959.13
perineum 959.14
peritoneum — *see* Injury, internal, peritoneum
periurethral tissue
  with
    abortion — *see* Abortion, by type, with damage to pelvic organs
    ectopic pregnancy (*see also* categories 633.0–633.9) 639.2
    molar pregnancy (*see also* categories 630–632) 639.2
  complicating delivery 664.8 ☑ ▲
    affecting fetus or newborn 763.89
  following
    abortion 639.2
    ectopic or molar pregnancy 639.2
phalanges
  foot 959.7
  hand 959.5
pharynx 959.09
pleura — *see* Injury, internal, pleura
popliteal space 959.7
post-cardiac surgery (syndrome) 429.4
prepuce 959.14
prostate — *see* Injury, internal, prostate
pubic region 959.19
pudenda 959.14
radiation NEC 990
radioactive substance or radium NEC 990
rectovaginal septum 959.14
rectum — *see* Injury, internal, rectum
retina 921.3
  penetrating — *see* Injury, eyeball, penetrating
retroperitoneal — *see* Injury, internal, retroperitoneum
roentgen rays NEC 990
round ligament — *see* Injury, internal, round ligament
sacral (region) 959.19
  plexus 953.5
sacroiliac ligament NEC 959.19
sacrum 959.19
salivary ducts or glands 959.09
scalp 959.09
  due to birth trauma 767.19
  fetus or newborn 767.19
scapular region 959.2
sclera 921.3
  penetrating — *see* Injury, eyeball, penetrating
  superficial 918.2
scrotum 959.14
seminal vesicle — *see* Injury, internal, seminal vesicle
shoulder (and upper arm) 959.2
sinus
  cavernous (*see also* Injury, intracranial) 854.0 ☑

Injury — *continued*

sinus — *continued*
  nasal 959.09
skeleton NEC, birth injury 767.3
skin NEC 959.9
skull — *see* Fracture, skull, by site
soft tissue (of external sites) (severe) — *see* Wound, open, by site
specified site NEC 959.8
spermatic cord — *see* Injury, internal, spermatic cord
spinal (cord) 952.9
  with fracture, vertebra — *see* Fracture, vertebra, by site, with spinal cord injury
  cervical (C₁-C₄) 952.00
    with
      anterior cord syndrome 952.02
      central cord syndrome 952.03
      complete lesion of cord 952.01
      incomplete lesion NEC 952.04
      posterior cord syndrome 952.04
    C₅-C₇ level 952.05
      with
        anterior cord syndrome 952.07
        central cord syndrome 952.08
        complete lesion of cord 952.06
        incomplete lesion NEC 952.09
        posterior cord syndrome 952.09
    specified type NEC 952.09
    specified type NEC 952.04
  dorsal (D₁-D₆) (T₁-T₆) (thoracic) 952.10
    with
      anterior cord syndrome 952.12
      central cord syndrome 952.13
      complete lesion of cord 952.11
      incomplete lesion NEC 952.14
      posterior cord syndrome 952.14
    D₇-D₁₂ level (T₇-T₁₂) 952.15
      with
        anterior cord syndrome 952.17
        central cord syndrome 952.18
        complete lesion of cord 952.16
        incomplete lesion NEC 952.19
        posterior cord syndrome 952.19
      specified type NEC 952.19
    specified type NEC 952.14
  lumbar 952.2
  multiple sites 952.8
  nerve (root) NEC — *see* Injury, nerve, spinal, root
  plexus 953.9
    brachial 953.4
    lumbosacral 953.5
    multiple sites 953.8
  sacral 952.3
  thoracic (*see also* Injury, spinal, dorsal) 952.10
spleen — *see* Injury, internal, spleen
stellate ganglion 954.1
sternal region 959.11
stomach — *see* Injury, internal, stomach
subconjunctival 921.1
subcutaneous 959.9
subdural — *see* Injury, intracranial
submaxillary region 959.09
submental region 959.09
subungual
  fingers 959.5
  toes 959.7

Injury — *continued*

superficial 919 ☑

> Note — Use the following fourth-digit subdivisions with categories 910–919:
>
> 0   Abrasion or friction burn without mention of infection
> 1   Abrasion or friction burn, infected
> 2   Blister without mention of infection
> 3   Blister, infected
> 4   Insect bite, nonvenomous, without mention of infection
> 5   Insect bite, nonvenomous, infected
> 6   Superficial foreign body (splinter) without major open wound and without mention of infection
> 7   Superficial foreign body (splinter) without major open wound, infected
> 8   Other and unspecified superficial injury without mention of infection
> 9   Other and unspecified superficial injury, infected
>
> For late effects of superficial injury, see category 906.2.

  abdomen, abdominal (muscle) (wall) (and other part(s) of trunk) 911 ☑
  ankle (and hip, knee, leg, or thigh) 916 ☑
  anus (and other part(s) of trunk) 911 ☑
  arm 913 ☑
    upper (and shoulder) 912 ☑
  auditory canal (external) (meatus) (and other part(s) of face, neck, or scalp, except eye) 910 ☑
  axilla (and upper arm) 912 ☑
  back (and other part(s) of trunk) 911 ☑
  breast (and other part(s) of trunk) 911 ☑
  brow (and other part(s) of face, neck, or scalp, except eye) 910 ☑
  buttock (and other part(s) of trunk) 911 ☑
  canthus, eye 918.0
  cheek(s) (and other part(s) of face, neck, or scalp, except eye) 910 ☑
  chest wall (and other part(s) of trunk) 911 ☑
  chin (and other part(s) of face, neck, or scalp, except eye) 910 ☑
  clitoris (and other part(s) of trunk) 911 ☑
  conjunctiva 918.2
  cornea 918.1
    due to contact lens 371.82
  costal region (and other part(s) of trunk) 911 ☑
  ear(s) (auricle) (canal) (drum) (external) (and other part(s) of face, neck, or scalp, except eye) 910 ☑
  elbow (and forearm) (and wrist) 913 ☑
  epididymis (and other part(s) of trunk) 911 ☑
  epigastric region (and other part(s) of trunk) 911 ☑
  epiglottis (and other part(s) of face, neck, or scalp, except eye) 910 ☑
  eye(s) (and adnexa) NEC 918.9
  eyelid(s) (and periocular area) 918.0
  face (any part(s), except eye) (and neck or scalp) 910 ☑
  finger(s) (nail) (any) 915 ☑
  flank (and other part(s) of trunk) 911 ☑
  foot (phalanges) (and toe(s)) 917 ☑
  forearm (and elbow) (and wrist) 913 ☑
  forehead (and other part(s) of face, neck, or scalp, except eye) 910 ☑
  globe (eye) 918.9

Injury — *continued*

superficial — *continued*
  groin (and other part(s) of trunk) 911 ☑
  gum(s) (and other part(s) of face, neck, or scalp, except eye) 910 ☑
  hand(s) (except fingers alone) 914 ☑
  head (and other part(s) of face, neck, or scalp, except eye) 910 ☑
  heel (and foot or toe) 917 ☑
  hip (and ankle, knee, leg, or thigh) 916 ☑
  iliac region (and other part(s) of trunk) 911 ☑
  interscapular region (and other part(s) of trunk) 911 ☑
  iris 918.9
  knee (and ankle, hip, leg, or thigh) 916 ☑
  labium (majus) (minus) (and other part(s) of trunk) 911 ☑
  lacrimal (apparatus) (gland) (sac) 918.0
  leg (lower) (upper) (and ankle, hip, knee, or thigh) 916 ☑
  lip(s) (and other part(s) of face, neck, or scalp, except eye) 910 ☑
  lower extremity (except foot) 916 ☑
  lumbar region (and other part(s) of trunk) 911 ☑
  malar region (and other part(s) of face, neck, or scalp, except eye) 910 ☑
  mastoid region (and other part(s) of face, neck, or scalp, except eye) 910 ☑
  midthoracic region (and other part(s) of trunk) 911 ☑
  mouth (and other part(s) of face, neck, or scalp, except eye) 910 ☑
  multiple sites (not classifiable to the same three-digit category) 919 ☑
  nasal (septum) (and other part(s) of face, neck, or scalp, except eye) 910 ☑
  neck (and face or scalp, any part(s), except eye) 910 ☑
  nose (septum) (and other part(s) of face, neck, or scalp, except eye) 910 ☑
  occipital region (and other part(s) of face, neck, or scalp, except eye) 910 ☑
  orbital region 918.0
  palate (soft) (and other part(s) of face, neck, or scalp, except eye) 910 ☑
  parietal region (and other part(s) of face, neck, or scalp, except eye) 910 ☑
  penis (and other part(s) of trunk) 911 ☑
  perineum (and other part(s) of trunk) 911 ☑
  periocular area 918.0
  pharynx (and other part(s) of face, neck, or scalp, except eye) 910 ☑
  popliteal space (and ankle, hip, leg, or thigh) 916 ☑
  prepuce (and other part(s) of trunk) 911 ☑
  pubic region (and other part(s) of trunk) 911 ☑
  pudenda (and other part(s) of trunk) 911 ☑
  sacral region (and other part(s) of trunk) 911 ☑
  salivary (ducts) (glands) (and other part(s) of face, neck, or scalp, except eye) 910 ☑
  scalp (and other part(s) of face or neck, except eye) 910 ☑
  scapular region (and upper arm) 912 ☑
  sclera 918.2
  scrotum (and other part(s) of trunk) 911 ☑
  shoulder (and upper arm) 912 ☑
  skin NEC 919 ☑
  specified site(s) NEC 919 ☑
  sternal region (and other part(s) of trunk) 911 ☑
  subconjunctival 918.2
  subcutaneous NEC 919 ☑

☑ Additional Digit Required — Refer to the Tabular List for Digit Selection   ✅ Subterms under main terms may continue to next column or page

Injury — continued
superficial — continued
submaxillary region (and other part(s) of face, neck, or scalp, except eye) 910 ☑
submental region (and other part(s) of face, neck, or scalp, except eye) 910 ☑
supraclavicular fossa (and other part(s) of face, neck, or scalp, except eye) 910 ☑
supraorbital 918.0
temple (and other part(s) of face, neck, or scalp, except eye) 910 ☑
temporal region (and other part(s) of face, neck, or scalp, except eye) 910 ☑
testis (and other part(s) of trunk) 911 ☑
thigh (and ankle, hip, knee, or leg) 916 ☑
thorax, thoracic (external) (and other part(s) of trunk) 911 ☑
throat (and other part(s) of face, neck, or scalp, except eye) 910 ☑
thumb(s) (nail) 915 ☑
toe(s) (nail) (subungual) (and foot) 917 ☑
tongue (and other part(s) of face, neck, or scalp, except eye) 910 ☑
tooth, teeth (see also Abrasion, dental) 521.20
trunk (any part(s)) 911 ☑
tunica vaginalis 959.14
tympanum, tympanic membrane (and other part(s) of face, neck, or scalp, except eye) 910 ☑
upper extremity NEC 913 ☑
uvula (and other part(s) of face, neck, or scalp, except eye) 910 ☑
vagina (and other part(s) of trunk) 911 ☑
vulva (and other part(s) of trunk) 911 ☑
wrist (and elbow) (and forearm) 913 ☑
supraclavicular fossa 959.19
supraorbital 959.09
surgical complication (external or internal site) 998.2
symphysis pubis 959.19
complicating delivery 665.6 ☑
affecting fetus or newborn 763.89
temple 959.09
temporal region 959.09
testis 959.14
thigh (and hip) 959.6
thorax, thoracic (external) 959.11
cavity — see Injury, internal, thorax
internal — see Injury, internal, intrathoracic organs
throat 959.09
thumb(s) (nail) 959.5
thymus — see Injury, internal, thymus
thyroid (gland) 959.09
toe (nail) (any) 959.7
tongue 959.09
tonsil 959.09
tooth NEC 873.63
complicated 873.73
trachea — see Injury, internal, trachea
trunk 959.19
tunica vaginalis 959.14
tympanum, tympanic membrane 959.09
ultraviolet rays NEC 990
ureter — see Injury, internal, ureter
urethra (sphincter) — see Injury, internal, urethra
uterus — see Injury, internal, uterus
uvula 959.09
vagina 959.14
vascular — see Injury, blood vessel
vas deferens — see Injury, internal, vas deferens
vein (see also Injury, blood vessel, by site) 904.9
vena cava
inferior 902.10
superior 901.2

Injury — continued
vesical (sphincter) — see Injury, internal, vesical
viscera (abdominal) — see Injury, internal, viscera
with fracture, pelvis — see Fracture, pelvis
visual 950.9
cortex 950.3
vitreous (humor) 871.2
vulva 959.14
whiplash (cervical spine) 847.0
wringer — see Crush, by site
wrist (and elbow) (and forearm) 959.3
x-ray NEC 990
Inoculation — see also Vaccination
complication or reaction — see Complication, vaccination
INPH (idiopathic normal pressure hydrocephalus) 331.5
Insanity, insane — see also Psychosis 298.9
adolescent (see also Schizophrenia) 295.9 ☑
alternating (see also Psychosis, affective, circular) 296.7
confusional 298.9
acute 293.0
subacute 293.1
delusional 298.9
paralysis, general 094.1
progressive 094.1
paresis, general 094.1
senile 290.20
Insect
bite — see Injury, superficial, by site
venomous, poisoning by 989.5
Insemination, artificial V26.1
Insensitivity
adrenocorticotropin hormone (ACTH) 255.41
androgen 259.50
complete 259.51
partial 259.52
Insertion
cord (umbilical) lateral or velamentous 663.8 ☑
affecting fetus or newborn 762.6
intrauterine contraceptive device V25.11 ▲
placenta, vicious — see Placenta, previa
subdermal implantable contraceptive V25.5
velamentous, umbilical cord 663.8 ☑
affecting fetus or newborn 762.6
Insolation 992.0
meaning sunstroke 992.0
Insomnia, unspecified 780.52
with sleep apnea, unspecified 780.51
adjustment 307.41
alcohol induced 291.82
behavioral, of childhood V69.5
drug induced 292.85
due to
medical condition classified elsewhere 327.01
mental disorder 327.02
fatal familial (FFI) 046.72
idiopathic 307.42
nonorganic origin 307.41
persistent (primary) 307.42
transient 307.41
organic 327.00
other 327.09
paradoxical 307.42
primary 307.42
psychophysiological 307.42
subjective complaint 307.49
Inspiration
food or foreign body (see also Asphyxia, food or foreign body) 933.1
mucus (see also Asphyxia, mucus) 933.1
Inspissated bile syndrome, newborn 774.4
Instability
detrusor 596.59
emotional (excessive) 301.3
joint (posttraumatic) 718.80
ankle 718.87
elbow 718.82

Instability — continued
joint — continued
foot 718.87
hand 718.84
hip 718.85
knee 718.86
lumbosacral 724.6
multiple sites 718.89
pelvic region 718.85
sacroiliac 724.6
shoulder (region) 718.81
specified site NEC 718.88
wrist 718.83
lumbosacral 724.6
nervous 301.89
personality (emotional) 301.59
thyroid, paroxysmal 242.9 ☑
urethral 599.83
vasomotor 780.2
Insufficiency, insufficient
accommodation 367.4
adrenal (gland) (acute) (chronic) 255.41
medulla 255.5
primary 255.41
specified site NEC 255.5
adrenocortical 255.41
anterior (occlusal) guidance 524.54
anus 569.49
aortic (valve) 424.1
with
mitral (valve) disease 396.1
insufficiency, incompetence, or regurgitation 396.3
stenosis or obstruction 396.1
stenosis or obstruction 424.1
with mitral (valve) disease 396.8
congenital 746.4
rheumatic 395.1
with
mitral (valve) disease 396.1
insufficiency, incompetence, or regurgitation 396.3
stenosis or obstruction 396.1
stenosis or obstruction 395.2
with mitral (valve) disease 396.8
specified cause NEC 424.1
syphilitic 093.22
arterial 447.1
basilar artery 435.0
carotid artery 435.8
cerebral 437.1
coronary (acute or subacute) 411.89
mesenteric 557.1
peripheral 443.9
precerebral 435.9
vertebral artery 435.1
vertebrobasilar 435.3
arteriovenous 459.9
basilar artery 435.0
biliary 575.8
cardiac (see also Insufficiency, myocardial) 428.0
complicating surgery 997.1
due to presence of (cardiac) prosthesis 429.4
postoperative 997.1
long-term effect of cardiac surgery 429.4
specified during or due to a procedure 997.1
long-term effect of cardiac surgery 429.4
cardiorenal (see also Hypertension, cardiorenal) 404.90
cardiovascular (see also Disease, cardiovascular) 429.2
renal (see also Hypertension, cardiorenal) 404.90
carotid artery 435.8
cerebral (vascular) 437.9
cerebrovascular 437.9
with transient focal neurological signs and symptoms 435.9
acute 437.1

Insufficiency, insufficient — continued
cerebrovascular — continued
acute — continued
with transient focal neurological signs and symptoms 435.9
circulatory NEC 459.9
fetus or newborn 779.89
convergence 378.83
coronary (acute or subacute) 411.89
chronic or with a stated duration of over 8 weeks 414.8
corticoadrenal 255.41
dietary 269.9
divergence 378.85
food 994.2
gastroesophageal 530.89
gonadal
ovary 256.39
testis 257.2
gonadotropic hormone secretion 253.4
heart (see also Insufficiency, myocardial)
fetus or newborn 779.89
valve (see also Endocarditis) 424.90
congenital NEC 746.89
hepatic 573.8
idiopathic autonomic 333.0
interocclusal distance of teeth (ridge) 524.36
kidney
acute 593.9
chronic 585.9
labyrinth, labyrinthine (function) 386.53
bilateral 386.54
unilateral 386.53
lacrimal 375.15
liver 573.8
lung (acute) (see also Insufficiency, pulmonary) 518.82
following trauma, surgery, or shock 518.5
newborn 770.89
mental (congenital) (see also Retardation, mental) 319
mesenteric 557.1
mitral (valve) 424.0
with
aortic (valve) disease 396.3
insufficiency, incompetence, or regurgitation 396.3
stenosis or obstruction 396.2
obstruction or stenosis 394.2
with aortic valve disease 396.8
congenital 746.6
rheumatic 394.1
with
aortic (valve) disease 396.3
insufficiency, incompetence, or regurgitation 396.3
stenosis or obstruction 396.2
obstruction or stenosis 394.2
with aortic valve disease 396.8
active or acute 391.1
with chorea, rheumatic (Sydenham's) 392.0
specified cause, except rheumatic 424.0
muscle
heart — see Insufficiency, myocardial
ocular (see also Strabismus) 378.9
myocardial, myocardium (with arteriosclerosis) 428.0
with rheumatic fever (conditions classifiable to 390)
active, acute, or subacute 391.2
with chorea 392.0
inactive or quiescent (with chorea) 398.0
congenital 746.89
due to presence of (cardiac) prosthesis 429.4
fetus or newborn 779.89
following cardiac surgery 429.4
hypertensive (see also Hypertension, heart) 402.91
benign 402.11
malignant 402.01
postoperative 997.1

☑ Additional Digit Required — Refer to the Tabular List for Digit Selection ⓦ Subterms under main terms may continue to next column or page

2011 ICD-9-CM ►◄ Revised Text ● New Line ▲ Revised Code October 2010 • Volume 2 — 165

Index

Insufficiency, insufficient — Inversion

Insufficiency, insufficient — *continued*
  myocardial, myocardium — *continued*
    postoperative — *continued*
      long-term effect of cardiac surgery 429.4
      rheumatic 398.0
        active, acute, or subacute 391.2
          with chorea (Sydenham's) 392.0
    syphilitic 093.82
  nourishment 994.2
  organic 799.89
  ovary 256.39
    postablative 256.2
  pancreatic 577.8
  parathyroid (gland) 252.1
  peripheral vascular (arterial) 443.9
  pituitary (anterior) 253.2
    posterior 253.5
  placental — *see* Placenta, insufficiency
  platelets 287.5
  prenatal care in current pregnancy V23.7
  progressive pluriglandular 258.9
  pseudocholinesterase 289.89
  pulmonary (acute) 518.82
    following
      shock 518.5
      surgery 518.5
      trauma 518.5
    newborn 770.89
    valve (*see also* Endocarditis, pulmonary) 424.3
      congenital 746.09
  pyloric 537.0
  renal 593.9
    acute 593.9
    chronic 585.9
    due to a procedure 997.5
  respiratory 786.09
    acute 518.82
      following shock, surgery, or trauma 518.5
    newborn 770.89
  rotation — *see* Malrotation
  suprarenal 255.41
    medulla 255.5
  tarso-orbital fascia, congenital 743.66
  tear film 375.15
  testis 257.2
  thyroid (gland) (acquired) (*see also* Hypothyroidism)
    congenital 243
  tricuspid (*see also* Endocarditis, tricuspid) 397.0
    congenital 746.89
    syphilitic 093.23
  urethral sphincter 599.84
  valve, valvular (heart) (*see also* Endocarditis) 424.90
  vascular 459.9
    intestine NEC 557.9
    mesenteric 557.1
    peripheral 443.9
    renal (*see also* Hypertension, kidney) 403.90
  velopharyngeal
    acquired 528.9
    congenital 750.29
  venous (peripheral) 459.81
  ventricular — *see* Insufficiency, myocardial
  vertebral artery 435.1
  vertebrobasilar artery 435.3
  weight gain during pregnancy 646.8 ☑
  zinc 269.3
Insufflation
  fallopian
    fertility testing V26.21
    following sterilization reversal V26.22
  meconium 770.11
    with respiratory symptoms 770.12
Insular — *see* condition
Insulinoma (M8151/0)
  malignant (M8151/3)
    pancreas 157.4
    specified site — *see* Neoplasm, by site, malignant
    unspecified site 157.4

Insulinoma — *continued*
  pancreas 211.7
  specified site — *see* Neoplasm, by site, benign
  unspecified site 211.7
Insuloma — *see* Insulinoma
Insult
  brain 437.9
    acute 436
    cerebral 437.9
      acute 436
    cerebrovascular 437.9
      acute 436
    vascular NEC 437.9
      acute 436
Insurance examination (certification) V70.3
Intemperance — *see also* Alcoholism 303.9 ☑
Interception of pregnancy (menstrual extraction) V25.3
Interference
  balancing side 524.56
  non-working side 524.56
Intermenstrual
  bleeding 626.6
    irregular 626.6
    regular 626.5
  hemorrhage 626.6
    irregular 626.6
    regular 626.5
  pain(s) 625.2
Intermittent — *see* condition
Internal — *see* condition
Interproximal wear 521.10
Interruption
  aortic arch 747.11
  bundle of His 426.50
  fallopian tube (for sterilization) V25.2
  phase-shift, sleep cycle 307.45
  repeated REM-sleep 307.48
  sleep
    due to perceived environmental disturbances 307.48
    phase-shift, of 24-hour sleep-wake cycle 307.45
    repeated REM-sleep type 307.48
  vas deferens (for sterilization) V25.2
Intersexuality 752.7
Interstitial — *see* condition
Intertrigo 695.89
  labialis 528.5
Intervertebral disc — *see* condition
Intestine, intestinal — *see also* condition
  flu 487.8
Intolerance
  carbohydrate NEC 579.8
  cardiovascular exercise, with pain (at rest) (with less than ordinary activity) (with ordinary activity) V47.2
  cold 780.99
  dissacharide (hereditary) 271.3
  drug
    correct substance properly administered 995.27
    wrong substance given or taken in error 977.9
      specified drug — *see* Table of Drugs and Chemicals
  effort 306.2
  fat NEC 579.8
  foods NEC 579.8
  fructose (hereditary) 271.2
  glucose (-galactose) (congenital) 271.3
  gluten 579.0
  lactose (hereditary) (infantile) 271.3
  lysine (congenital) 270.7
  milk NEC 579.8
  protein (familial) 270.7
  starch NEC 579.8
  sucrose (-isomaltose) (congenital) 271.3
Intoxicated NEC — *see also* Alcoholism 305.0 ☑
Intoxication
  acid 276.2
  acute
    alcoholic 305.0 ☑
      with alcoholism 303.0 ☑

Intoxication — *continued*
  acute — *continued*
    alcoholic — *continued*
      hangover effects 305.0 ☑
      caffeine 305.9 ☑
      hallucinogenic (*see also* Abuse, drugs, nondependent) 305.3 ☑
    alcohol (acute) 305.0 ☑
      with alcoholism 303.0 ☑
      hangover effects 305.0 ☑
      idiosyncratic 291.4
      pathological 291.4
    alimentary canal 558.2
    ammonia (hepatic) 572.2
    caffeine 305.9 ☑
    chemical (*see also* Table of Drugs and Chemicals)
      via placenta or breast milk 760.70
        alcohol 760.71
        anticonvulsants
        antifungals
        anti-infective agents 760.74
        antimetabolics
        cocaine 760.75
        "crack" 760.75
        hallucinogenic agents NEC 760.73
        medicinal agents NEC 760.79
        narcotics 760.72
        obstetric anesthetic or analgesic drug 763.5
        specified agent NEC 760.79
        suspected, affecting management of pregnancy 655.5 ☑
    cocaine, through placenta or breast milk 760.75
    delirium
      alcohol 291.0
      drug 292.81
    drug 292.89
      with delirium 292.81
      correct substance properly administered (*see also* Allergy, drug) 995.27
      newborn 779.4
      obstetric anesthetic or sedation 668.9 ☑
        affecting fetus or newborn 763.5
      overdose or wrong substance given or taken — *see* Table of Drugs and Chemicals
      pathologic 292.2
      specific to newborn 779.4
      via placenta or breast milk 760.70
        alcohol 760.71
        anticonvulsants 760.77
        antifungals 760.74
        anti-infective agents 760.74
        antimetabolics 760.78
        cocaine 760.75
        "crack" 760.75
        hallucinogenic agents 760.73
        medicinal agents NEC 760.79
        narcotics 760.72
        obstetric anesthetic or analgesic drug 763.5
        specified agent NEC 760.79
        suspected, affecting management of pregnancy 655.5 ☑
    enteric — *see* Intoxication, intestinal
    fetus or newborn, via placenta or breast milk 760.70
      alcohol 760.71
      anticonvulsants 760.77
      antifungals 760.74
      anti-infective agents 760.74
      antimetabolics 760.78
      cocaine 760.75
      "crack" 760.75
      hallucinogenic agents 760.73
      medicinal agents NEC 760.79
      narcotics 760.72
      obstetric anesthetic or analgesic drug 763.5
      specified agent NEC 760.79
      suspected, affecting management of pregnancy 655.5 ☑
    food — *see* Poisoning, food
    gastrointestinal 558.2

Intoxication — *continued*
  hallucinogenic (acute) 305.3 ☑
  hepatocerebral 572.2
  idiosyncratic alcohol 291.4
  intestinal 569.89
    due to putrefaction of food 005.9
  methyl alcohol (*see also* Alcoholism) 305.0 ☑
    with alcoholism 303.0 ☑
  non-foodborne due to toxins of Clostridium botulinum [C. botulinum] — *see* Botulism
  pathologic 291.4
    drug 292.2
  potassium (K) 276.7
  septic
    with
      abortion — *see* Abortion, by type, with sepsis
      ectopic pregnancy (*see also* categories 633.0–633.9) 639.0
      molar pregnancy (*see also* categories 630–632) 639.0
    during labor 659.3 ☑
    following
      abortion 639.0
      ectopic or molar pregnancy 639.0
    generalized — *see* Septicemia
    puerperal, postpartum, childbirth 670.2 ☑
  serum (prophylactic) (therapeutic) 999.5
  uremic — *see* Uremia
  water 276.69   ▲
Intracranial — *see* condition
Intrahepatic gallbladder 751.69
Intraligamentous — *see also* condition
  pregnancy — *see* Pregnancy, cornual
Intraocular — *see also* condition
  sepsis 360.00
Intrathoracic — *see also* condition
  kidney 753.3
  stomach — *see* Hernia, diaphragm
Intrauterine contraceptive device
  checking V25.42
  insertion V25.11   ▲
  in situ V45.51
  management V25.42
  prescription V25.02
    repeat V25.42
  reinsertion V25.13   ▲
  removal V25.12   ▲
    and reinsertion V25.13   ●
  replacement V25.13   ●
Intraventricular — *see* condition
Intrinsic deformity — *see* Deformity
Intruded tooth 524.34
Intrusion, repetitive, of sleep (due to environmental disturbances) (with atypical polysomnographic features) 307.48
Intumescent, lens (eye) NEC 366.9
  senile 366.12
Intussusception (colon) (enteric) (intestine) (rectum) 560.0
  appendix 543.9
  congenital 751.5
  fallopian tube 620.8
  ileocecal 560.0
  ileocolic 560.0
  ureter (with obstruction) 593.4
Invagination
  basilar 756.0
  colon or intestine 560.0
Invalid (since birth) 799.89
Invalidism (chronic) 799.89
Inversion
  albumin-globulin (A-G) ratio 273.8
  bladder 596.8
  cecum (*see also* Intussusception) 560.0
  cervix 622.8
  nipple 611.79
    congenital 757.6
    puerperal, postpartum 676.3 ☑
  optic papilla 743.57
  organ or site, congenital NEC — *see* Anomaly, specified type NEC
  sleep rhythm 327.39

Inversion — *continued*
  sleep rhythm — *continued*
    nonorganic origin 307.45
  testis (congenital) 752.51
  uterus (postinfectional) (postpartal, old)
    621.7
    chronic 621.7
    complicating delivery 665.2 ☑
      affecting fetus or newborn 763.89
  vagina — *see* Prolapse, vagina
Investigation
  allergens V72.7
  clinical research (control) (normal comparison) (participant) V70.7
Inviability — *see* Immaturity
Involuntary movement, abnormal 781.0
Involution, involutional — *see also* condition
  breast, cystic or fibrocystic 610.1
  depression (*see also* Psychosis, affective)
    296.2 ☑
    recurrent episode 296.3 ☑
    single episode 296.2 ☑
  melancholia (*see also* Psychosis, affective)
    296.2 ☑
    recurrent episode 296.3 ☑
    single episode 296.2 ☑
  ovary, senile 620.3
  paranoid state (reaction) 297.2
  paraphrenia (climacteric) (menopause)
    297.2
  psychosis 298.8
  thymus failure 254.8
IQ
  under 20 318.2
  20-34 318.1
  35-49 318.0
  50-70 317
IRDS 769
Irideremia 743.45
Iridis rubeosis 364.42
  diabetic 250.5 ☑ *[364.42]*
    due to secondary diabetes
      249.5 ☑ *[364.42]*
Iridochoroiditis (panuveitis) 360.12
Iridocyclitis NEC 364.3
  acute 364.00
    primary 364.01
    recurrent 364.02
  chronic 364.10
    in
      lepromatous leprosy 030.0 *[364.11]*
      sarcoidosis 135 *[364.11]*
      tuberculosis (*see also* Tuberculosis)
        017.3 ☑ *[364.11]*
  due to allergy 364.04
  endogenous 364.01
  gonococcal 098.41
  granulomatous 364.10
  herpetic (simplex) 054.44
    zoster 053.22
  hypopyon 364.05
  lens induced 364.23
  nongranulomatous 364.00
  primary 364.01
  recurrent 364.02
  rheumatic 364.10
  secondary 364.04
    infectious 364.03
    noninfectious 364.04
  subacute 364.00
    primary 364.01
    recurrent 364.02
  sympathetic 360.11
  syphilitic (secondary) 091.52
  tuberculous (chronic) (*see also* Tuberculosis)
    017.3 ☑ *[364.11]*
Iridocyclochoroiditis (panuveitis) 360.12
Iridodialysis 364.76
Iridodonesis 364.89
Iridoplegia (complete) (partial) (reflex) 379.49
Iridoschisis 364.52
Iris — *see* condition
Iritis 364.3
  acute 364.00
    primary 364.01
    recurrent 364.02

Iritis — *continued*
  chronic 364.10
    in
      sarcoidosis 135 *[364.11]*
      tuberculosis (*see also* Tuberculosis)
        017.3 ☑ *[364.11]*
  diabetic 250.5 ☑ *[364.42]*
    due to secondary diabetes
      249.5 ☑ *[364.42]*
  due to
    allergy 364.04
    herpes simplex 054.44
    leprosy 030.0 *[364.11]*
  endogenous 364.01
  gonococcal 098.41
  gouty 274.89 *[364.11]*
  granulomatous 364.10
  hypopyon 364.05
  lens induced 364.23
  nongranulomatous 364.00
  papulosa 095.8 *[364.11]*
  primary 364.01
  recurrent 364.02
  rheumatic 364.10
  secondary 364.04
    infectious 364.03
    noninfectious 364.04
  subacute 364.00
    primary 364.01
    recurrent 364.02
  sympathetic 360.11
  syphilitic (secondary) 091.52
    congenital 090.0 *[364.11]*
    late 095.8 *[364.11]*
  tuberculous (*see also* Tuberculosis)
    017.3 ☑ *[364.11]*
  uratic 274.89 *[364.11]*
Iron
  deficiency anemia 280.9
  metabolism disease 275.09 ▲
  storage disease 275.09 ▲
Iron-miners' lung 503
Irradiated enamel (tooth, teeth) 521.89
Irradiation
  burn — *see* Burn, by site
  effects, adverse 990
Irreducible, irreducibility — *see* condition
Irregular, irregularity
  action, heart 427.9
  alveolar process 525.8
  bleeding NEC 626.4
  breathing 786.09
  colon 569.89
  contour
    acquired 371.70
    of cornea 743.41
      acquired 371.70
    reconstructed breast 612.0
  dentin in pulp 522.3
  eye movements NEC 379.59
  menstruation (cause unknown) 626.4
  periods 626.4
  prostate 602.9
  pupil 364.75
  respiratory 786.09
  septum (nasal) 470
  shape, organ or site, congenital NEC — *see* Distortion
  sleep-wake rhythm (non-24-hour) 327.39
    nonorganic origin 307.45
  vertebra 733.99
Irritability 799.22
  bladder 596.8
    neurogenic 596.54
      with cauda equina syndrome 344.61
  bowel (syndrome) 564.1
  bronchial (*see also* Bronchitis) 490
  cerebral, newborn 779.1
  colon 564.1
    psychogenic 306.4
  duodenum 564.89
  heart (psychogenic) 306.2
  ileum 564.89
  jejunum 564.89
  myocardium 306.2
  nervousness 799.21

Irritability — *continued*
  rectum 564.89
  stomach 536.9
    psychogenic 306.4
  sympathetic (nervous system) (*see also* Neuropathy, peripheral, autonomic) 337.9
  urethra 599.84
  ventricular (heart) (psychogenic) 306.2
Irritable — *see also* Irritability 799.22
Irritation
  anus 569.49
  axillary nerve 353.0
  bladder 596.8
  brachial plexus 353.0
  brain (traumatic) (*see also* Injury, intracranial) 854.0 ☑
    nontraumatic — *see* Encephalitis
  bronchial (*see also* Bronchitis) 490
  cerebral (traumatic) (*see also* Injury, intracranial) 854.0 ☑
    nontraumatic — *see* Encephalitis
  cervical plexus 353.2
  cervix (*see also* Cervicitis) 616.0
  choroid, sympathetic 360.11
  cranial nerve — *see* Disorder, nerve, cranial
  digestive tract 536.9
    psychogenic 306.4
  gastric 536.9
    psychogenic 306.4
  gastrointestinal (tract) 536.9
    functional 536.9
    psychogenic 306.4
  globe, sympathetic 360.11
  intestinal (bowel) 564.9
  labyrinth 386.50
  lumbosacral plexus 353.1
  meninges (traumatic) (*see also* Injury, intracranial) 854.0 ☑
    nontraumatic — *see* Meningitis
  myocardium 306.2
  nerve — *see* Disorder, nerve
  nervous 799.21
  nose 478.19
  penis 607.89
  perineum 709.9
  peripheral
    autonomic nervous system (*see also* Neuropathy, peripheral, autonomic) 337.9
    nerve — *see* Disorder, nerve
  peritoneum (*see also* Peritonitis) 567.9
  pharynx 478.29
  plantar nerve 355.6
  spinal (cord) (traumatic) (*see also* Injury, spinal, by site)
    nerve — *see* Disorder, nerve
      root NEC 724.9
      traumatic — *see* Injury, nerve, spinal
    nontraumatic — *see* Myelitis
  stomach 536.9
    psychogenic 306.4
  sympathetic nerve NEC (*see also* Neuropathy, peripheral, autonomic) 337.9
  ulnar nerve 354.2
  vagina 623.9
Isambert's disease 012.3 ☑
Ischemia, ischemic 459.9
  basilar artery (with transient neurologic deficit) 435.0
  bone NEC 733.40
  bowel (transient) 557.9
    acute 557.0
    chronic 557.1
    due to mesenteric artery insufficiency 557.1
  brain (*see also* Ischemia, cerebral)
    recurrent focal 435.9
  cardiac (*see also* Ischemia, heart) 414.9
  cardiomyopathy 414.8
  carotid artery (with transient neurologic deficit) 435.8
  cerebral (chronic) (generalized) 437.1
    arteriosclerotic 437.0
    intermittent (with transient neurologic deficit) 435.9

Ischemia, ischemic — *continued*
  cerebral — *continued*
    newborn 779.2
    puerperal, postpartum, childbirth 674.0 ☑
    recurrent focal (with transient neurologic deficit) 435.9
    transient (with transient neurologic deficit) 435.9
  colon 557.9
    acute 557.0
    chronic 557.1
    due to mesenteric artery insufficiency 557.1
  coronary (chronic) (*see also* Ischemia, heart) 414.9
  demand 411.89 •
  heart (chronic or with a stated duration of over 8 weeks) 414.9
    acute or with a stated duration of 8 weeks or less (*see also* Infarct, myocardium) 410.9 ☑
    without myocardial infarction 411.89
      with coronary (artery) occlusion 411.81
    subacute 411.89
  intestine (transient) 557.9
    acute 557.0
    chronic 557.1
    due to mesenteric artery insufficiency 557.1
  kidney 593.81
  labyrinth 386.50
  muscles, leg 728.89
  myocardium, myocardial (chronic or with a stated duration of over 8 weeks) 414.8
    acute (*see also* Infarct, myocardium) 410.9 ☑
    without myocardial infarction 411.89
      with coronary (artery) occlusion 411.81
  renal 593.81
  retina, retinal 362.84
  small bowel 557.9
    acute 557.0
    chronic 557.1
    due to mesenteric artery insufficiency 557.1
  spinal cord 336.1
  subendocardial (*see also* Insufficiency, coronary) 411.89
  supply (*see also* Angina) 414.9 •
  vertebral artery (with transient neurologic deficit) 435.1
Ischialgia — *see also* Sciatica 724.3
Ischiopagus 759.4
Ischium, ischial — *see* condition
Ischomenia 626.8
Ischuria 788.5
Iselin's disease or osteochondrosis 732.5
Islands of
  parotid tissue in
    lymph nodes 750.26
    neck structures 750.26
  submaxillary glands in
    fascia 750.26
    lymph nodes 750.26
    neck muscles 750.26
Islet cell tumor, pancreas (M8150/0) 211.7
Isoimmunization NEC — *see also* Incompatibility 656.2 ☑
  anti-E 656.2 ☑
  fetus or newborn 773.2
    ABO blood groups 773.1
    Rhesus (Rh) factor 773.0
Isolation V07.0
  social V62.4
Isosporosis 007.2
Issue
  medical certificate NEC V68.09
    cause of death V68.09
    disability examination V68.01
    fitness V68.09
    incapacity V68.09
  repeat prescription NEC V68.1

☑ **Additional Digit Required** — Refer to the Tabular List for Digit Selection

▽ **Subterms under main terms may continue to next column or page**

Issue — *continued*
  repeat prescription — *continued*
    appliance V68.1
    contraceptive V25.40
      device NEC V25.49
        intrauterine V25.42
        specified type NEC V25.49
      pill V25.41
    glasses V68.1
    medicinal substance V68.1
Itch — *see also* Pruritus 698.9
  bakers' 692.89
  barbers' 110.0
  bricklayers' 692.89

Itch — *see also* Pruritus — *continued*
  cheese 133.8
  clam diggers' 120.3
  coolie 126.9
  copra 133.8
  Cuban 050.1
  dew 126.9
  dhobie 110.3
  eye 379.99
  filarial (*see also* Infestation, filarial) 125.9
  grain 133.8
  grocers' 133.8
  ground 126.9
  harvest 133.8

Itch — *see also* Pruritus — *continued*
  jock 110.3
  Malabar 110.9
    beard 110.0
    foot 110.4
    scalp 110.0
  meaning scabies 133.0
  Norwegian 133.0
  perianal 698.0
  poultrymen's 133.8
  sarcoptic 133.0
  scrub 134.1
  seven year V61.10
    meaning scabies 133.0

Itch — *see also* Pruritus — *continued*
  straw 133.8
  swimmers' 120.3
  washerwoman's 692.4
  water 120.3
  winter 698.8
Itsenko-Cushing syndrome (pituitary basophilism) 255.0
Ivemark's syndrome (asplenia with congenital heart disease) 759.0
Ivory bones 756.52
Ixodes 134.8
Ixodiasis 134.8

☑ **Additional Digit Required — Refer to the Tabular List for Digit Selection**
▽ **Subterms under main terms may continue to next column or page**

168 — Volume 2   ▶◀ **Revised Text**   ● **New Line**   ▲ **Revised Code**   **2011 ICD-9-CM**

J

Jaccoud's nodular fibrositis, chronic (Jaccoud's syndrome) 714.4
Jackson's
membrane 751.4
paralysis or syndrome 344.89
veil 751.4
Jacksonian
epilepsy (see also Epilepsy) 345.5 ☑
seizures (focal) (see also Epilepsy) 345.5 ☑
Jacob's ulcer (M8090/3) — see Neoplasm, skin, malignant, by site
Jacquet's dermatitis (diaper dermatitis) 691.0
Jadassohn's
blue nevus (M8780/0) — see Neoplasm, skin, benign
disease (maculopapular erythroderma) 696.2
intraepidermal epithelioma (M8096/0) — see Neoplasm, skin, benign
Jadassohn-Lewandowski syndrome (pachyonychia congenita) 757.5
Jadassohn-Pellizari's disease (anetoderma) 701.3
Jadassohn-Tièche nevus (M8780/0) — see Neoplasm, skin, benign
Jaffe-Lichtenstein (-Uehlinger) syndrome 252.01
Jahnke's syndrome (encephalocutaneous angiomatosis) 759.6
Jakob-Creutzfeldt disease (CJD) (syndrome) 046.19
with dementia
with behavioral disturbance 046.19 [294.11]
without behavioral disturbance 046.19 [294.10]
familial 046.19
iatrogenic 046.19
specified NEC 046.19
sporadic 046.19
variant (vCJD) 046.11
with dementia
with behavioral disturbance 046.11 [294.11]
without behavioral disturbance 046.11 [294.10]
Jaksch (-Luzet) disease or syndrome (pseudoleukemia infantum) 285.8
Jamaican
neuropathy 349.82
paraplegic tropical ataxic-spastic syndrome 349.82
Janet's disease (psychasthenia) 300.89
Janiceps 759.4
Jansky-Bielschowsky amaurotic familial idiocy 330.1
Japanese
B type encephalitis 062.0
river fever 081.2
seven-day fever 100.89
Jaundice (yellow) 782.4
acholuric (familial) (splenomegalic) (see also Spherocytosis) 282.0
acquired 283.9
breast milk 774.39
catarrhal (acute) 070.1
with hepatic coma 070.0
chronic 571.9
epidemic — see Jaundice, epidemic
cholestatic (benign) 782.4
chronic idiopathic 277.4
epidemic (catarrhal) 070.1
with hepatic coma 070.0
leptospiral 100.0
spirochetal 100.0
febrile (acute) 070.1
with hepatic coma 070.0
leptospiral 100.0
spirochetal 100.0
fetus or newborn 774.6
due to or associated with
ABO
absence or deficiency of enzyme system for bilirubin conjugation (congenital) 774.39

Jaundice — continued
fetus or newborn — continued
due to or associated with — continued
antibodies 773.1
blood group incompatibility NEC 773.2
breast milk inhibitors to conjugation 774.39
associated with preterm delivery 774.2
bruising 774.1
Crigler-Najjar syndrome 277.4 [774.31]
delayed conjugation 774.30
associated with preterm delivery 774.2
development 774.39
drugs or toxins transmitted from mother 774.1
G-6-PD deficiency 282.2 [774.0]
galactosemia 271.1 [774.5]
Gilbert's syndrome 277.4 [774.31]
hepatocellular damage 774.4
hereditary hemolytic anemia (see also Anemia, hemolytic) 282.9 [774.0]
hypothyroidism, congenital 243 [774.31]
incompatibility, maternal/fetal NEC 773.2
incompatibility, maternal/fetal 773.1
infection 774.1
inspissated bile syndrome 774.4
isoimmunization NEC 773.2
isoimmunization 773.1
mucoviscidosis 277.01 [774.5]
obliteration of bile duct, congenital 751.61 [774.5]
polycythemia 774.1
preterm delivery 774.2
red cell defect 282.9 [774.0]
Rh
antibodies 773.0
incompatibility, maternal/fetal 773.0
isoimmunization 773.0
spherocytosis (congenital) 282.0 [774.0]
swallowed maternal blood 774.1
physiological NEC 774.6
from injection, inoculation, infusion, or transfusion (blood) (plasma) (serum) (other substance) (onset within 8 months after administration) — see Hepatitis, viral
Gilbert's (familial nonhemolytic) 277.4
hematogenous 283.9
hemolytic (acquired) 283.9
congenital (see also Spherocytosis) 282.0
hemorrhagic (acute) 100.0
leptospiral 100.0
newborn 776.0
spirochetal 100.0
hepatocellular 573.8
homologous (serum) — see Hepatitis, viral
idiopathic, chronic 277.4
infectious (acute) (subacute) 070.1
with hepatic coma 070.0
leptospiral 100.0
spirochetal 100.0
leptospiral 100.0
malignant (see also Necrosis, liver) 570
newborn (physiological) (see also Jaundice, fetus or newborn) 774.6
nonhemolytic, congenital familial (Gilbert's) 277.4
nuclear, newborn (see also Kernicterus of newborn) 774.7
obstructive NEC (see also Obstruction, biliary) 576.8
postimmunization — see Hepatitis, viral
posttransfusion — see Hepatitis, viral
regurgitation (see also Obstruction, biliary) 576.8

Jaundice — continued
serum (homologous) (prophylactic) (therapeutic) — see Hepatitis, viral
spirochetal (hemorrhagic) 100.0
symptomatic 782.4
newborn 774.6
Jaw — see condition
Jaw-blinking 374.43
congenital 742.8
Jaw-winking phenomenon or syndrome 742.8
Jealousy
alcoholic 291.5
childhood 313.3
sibling 313.3
Jejunitis — see also Enteritis 558.9
Jejunostomy status V44.4
Jejunum, jejunal — see condition
Jensen's disease 363.05
Jericho boil 085.1
Jerks, myoclonic 333.2
Jervell-Lange-Nielsen syndrome 426.82
Jeune's disease or syndrome (asphyxiating thoracic dystrophy) 756.4
Jigger disease 134.1
Job's syndrome (chronic granulomatous disease) 288.1
Jod-Basedow phenomenon 242.8 ☑
Johnson-Stevens disease (erythema multiforme exudativum) 695.13
Joint — see also condition
Charcôt's 094.0 [713.5]
false 733.82
flail — see Flail, joint
mice — see Loose, body, joint, by site
sinus to bone 730.9 ☑
von Gies' 095.8
Jordan's anomaly or syndrome 288.2
Josephs-Diamond-Blackfan anemia (congenital hypoplastic) 284.01
Joubert syndrome 759.89
Jumpers' knee 727.2
Jungle yellow fever 060.0
Jüngling's disease (sarcoidosis) 135
Junin virus hemorrhagic fever 078.7
Juvenile — see also condition
delinquent 312.9
group (see also Disturbance, conduct) 312.2 ☑
neurotic 312.4

K

Kabuki syndrome 759.89
Kahler (-Bozzolo) disease (multiple myeloma) (M9730/3) 203.0 ☑
Kakergasia 300.9
Kakke 265.0
Kala-azar (Indian) (infantile) (Mediterranean) (Sudanese) 085.0
Kalischer's syndrome (encephalocutaneous angiomatosis) 759.6
Kallmann's syndrome (hypogonadotropic hypogonadism with anosmia) 253.4
Kanner's syndrome (autism) — see also Psychosis, childhood 299.0 ☑
Kaolinosis 502
Kaposi's
disease 757.33
lichen ruber 696.4
acuminatus 696.4
moniliformis 697.8
xeroderma pigmentosum 757.33
sarcoma (M9140/3) 176.9
adipose tissue 176.1
aponeurosis 176.1
artery 176.1
associated herpesvirus infection 058.89
blood vessel 176.1
bursa 176.1
connective tissue 176.1
external genitalia 176.8
fascia 176.1
fatty tissue 176.1
fibrous tissue 176.1
gastrointestinal tract NEC 176.3
ligament 176.1

Kaposi's — continued
sarcoma — continued
lung 176.4
lymph
gland(s) 176.5
node(s) 176.5
lymphatic(s) NEC 176.1
muscle (skeletal) 176.1
oral cavity NEC 176.8
palate 176.2
scrotum 176.8
skin 176.0
soft tissue 176.1
specified site NEC 176.8
subcutaneous tissue 176.1
synovia 176.1
tendon (sheath) 176.1
vein 176.1
vessel 176.1
viscera NEC 176.9
vulva 176.8
varicelliform eruption 054.0
vaccinia 999.0
Kartagener's syndrome or triad (sinusitis, bronchiectasis, situs inversus) 759.3
Kasabach-Merritt syndrome (capillary hemangioma associated with thrombocytopenic purpura) 287.39
Kaschin-Beck disease (endemic polyarthritis) — see Disease, Kaschin-Beck
Kast's syndrome (dyschondroplasia with hemangiomas) 756.4
Katatonia — see Catatonia
Katayama disease or fever 120.2
Kathisophobia 781.0
Kawasaki disease 446.1
Kayser-Fleischer ring (cornea) (pseudosclerosis) 275.1 [371.14]
Kaznelson's syndrome (congenital hypoplastic anemia) 284.01
Kearns-Sayre syndrome 277.87
Kedani fever 081.2
Kelis 701.4
Kelly (-Patterson) syndrome (sideropenic dysphagia) 280.8
Keloid, cheloid 701.4
Addison's (morphea) 701.0
cornea 371.00
Hawkins' 701.4
scar 701.4
Keloma 701.4
Kenya fever 082.1
Keratectasia 371.71
congenital 743.41
Keratinization NEC
alveolar ridge mucosa
excessive 528.72
minimal 528.71
Keratitis (nodular) (nonulcerative) (simple) (zonular) NEC 370.9
with ulceration (see also Ulcer, cornea) 370.00
actinic 370.24
arborescens 054.42
areolar 370.22
bullosa 370.8
deep — see Keratitis, interstitial
dendritic(a) 054.42
desiccation 370.34
diffuse interstitial 370.52
disciform(is) 054.43
varicella 052.7 [370.44]
epithelialis vernalis 372.13 [370.32]
exposure 370.34
filamentary 370.23
gonococcal (congenital) (prenatal) 098.43
herpes, herpetic (simplex) NEC 054.43
zoster 053.21
hypopyon 370.04
in
chickenpox 052.7 [370.44]
exanthema (see also Exanthem) 057.9 [370.44]
paravaccinia (see also Paravaccinia) 051.9 [370.44]

☑ Additional Digit Required — Refer to the Tabular List for Digit Selection   ▽ Subterms under main terms may continue to next column or page

2011 ICD-9-CM   ▶◀ Revised Text   ● New Line   ▲ Revised Code   Volume 2 — 169

Keratitis — continued

in — continued

smallpox (see also Smallpox)
050.9 [370.44]

vernal conjunctivitis 372.13 [370.32]

interstitial (nonsyphilitic) 370.50

with ulcer (see also Ulcer, cornea) 370.00

diffuse 370.52

herpes, herpetic (simplex) 054.43

zoster 053.21

syphilitic (congenital) (hereditary) 090.3

tuberculous (see also Tuberculosis)
017.3 [370.59]

lagophthalmic 370.34

macular 370.22

neuroparalytic 370.35

neurotrophic 370.35

nummular 370.22

oyster-shuckers' 370.8

parenchymatous — see Keratitis, interstitial

petrificans 370.8

phlyctenular 370.31

postmeasles 055.71

punctata, punctate 370.21

leprosa 030.0 [370.21]

profunda 090.3

superficial (Thygeson's) 370.21

purulent 370.8

pustuliformis profunda 090.3

rosacea 695.3 [370.49]

sclerosing 370.54

specified type NEC 370.8

stellate 370.22

striate 370.22

superficial 370.20

with conjunctivitis (see also Keratoconjunctivitis) 370.40

punctate (Thygeson's) 370.21

suppurative 370.8

syphilitic (congenital) (prenatal) 090.3

trachomatous 076.1

late effect 139.1

tuberculous (phlyctenular) (see also Tuberculosis) 017.3 ☑ [370.31]

ulcerated (see also Ulcer, cornea) 370.00

vesicular 370.8

welders' 370.24

xerotic (see also Keratomalacia) 371.45

vitamin A deficiency 264.4

Keratoacanthoma 238.2

Keratocele 371.72

Keratoconjunctivitis — see also Keratitis 370.40

adenovirus type 8 077.1

epidemic 077.1

exposure 370.34

gonococcal 098.43

herpetic (simplex) 054.43

zoster 053.21

in

chickenpox 052.7 [370.44]

exanthema (see also Exanthem) 057.9 [370.44]

paravaccinia (see also Paravaccinia) 051.9 [370.44]

smallpox (see also Smallpox) 050.9 [370.44]

infectious 077.1

neurotrophic 370.35

phlyctenular 370.31

postmeasles 055.71

shipyard 077.1

sicca (Sjögren's syndrome) 710.2

not in Sjögren's syndrome 370.33

specified type NEC 370.49

tuberculous (phlyctenular) (see also Tuberculosis) 017.3 ☑ [370.31]

Keratoconus 371.60

acute hydrops 371.62

congenital 743.41

stable 371.61

Keratocyst (dental) 526.0

Keratoderma, keratodermia (congenital) (palmaris et plantaris) (symmetrical) 757.39

acquired 701.1

Keratoderma, keratodermia — continued

blennorrhagica 701.1

gonococcal 098.81

climacterium 701.1

eccentrica 757.39

gonorrheal 098.81

punctata 701.1

tylodes, progressive 701.1

Keratodermatocele 371.72

Keratoglobus 371.70

congenital 743.41

associated with buphthalmos 743.22

Keratohemia 371.12

Keratoiritis — see also Iridocyclitis 364.3

syphilitic 090.3

tuberculous (see also Tuberculosis) 017.3 [364.11]

Keratolysis exfoliativa (congenital) 757.39

acquired 695.89

neonatorum 757.39

Keratoma 701.1

congenital 757.39

malignum congenitale 757.1

palmaris et plantaris hereditarium 757.39

senile 702.0

Keratomalacia 371.45

vitamin A deficiency 264.4

Keratomegaly 743.41

Keratomycosis 111.1

nigricans (palmaris) 111.1

Keratopathy 371.40

band (see also Keratitis) 371.43

bullous (see also Keratitis) 371.23

degenerative (see also Degeneration, cornea) 371.40

hereditary (see also Dystrophy, cornea) 371.50

discrete colliquative 371.49

Keratoscleritis, tuberculous — see also Tuberculosis 017.3 ☑ [370.31]

Keratosis 701.1

actinic 702.0

arsenical 692.4

blennorrhagica 701.1

gonococcal 098.81

congenital (any type) 757.39

ear (middle) (see also Cholesteatoma) 385.30

female genital (external) 629.89

follicularis 757.39

acquired 701.1

congenital (acneiformis) (Siemens') 757.39

spinulosa (decalvans) 757.39

vitamin A deficiency 264.8

follicular, vitamin A deficiency 264.8

gonococcal 098.81

larynx, laryngeal 478.79

male genital (external) 608.89

middle ear (see also Cholesteatoma) 385.30

nigricans 701.2

congenital 757.39

obturans 380.21

oral epithelium

residual ridge mucosa

excessive 528.72

minimal 528.71

palmaris et plantaris (symmetrical) 757.39

penile 607.89

pharyngeus 478.29

pilaris 757.39

acquired 701.1

punctata (palmaris et plantaris) 701.1

scrotal 608.89

seborrheic 702.19

inflamed 702.11

senilis 702.0

solar 702.0

suprafollicularis 757.39

tonsillaris 478.29

vagina 623.1

vegetans 757.39

vitamin A deficiency 264.8

Kerato-uveitis — see also Iridocyclitis 364.3

Keraunoparalysis 994.0

Kerion (celsi) 110.0

Kernicterus of newborn (not due to isoimmunization) 774.7

due to isoimmunization (conditions classifiable to 773.0–773.2) 773.4

Ketoacidosis 276.2

diabetic 250.1 ☑

due to secondary diabetes 249.1 ☑

Ketonuria 791.6

branched-chain, intermittent 270.3

Ketosis 276.2

diabetic 250.1 ☑

due to secondary diabetes 249.1 ☑

Kidney — see condition

Kienböck's

disease 732.3

adult 732.8

osteochondrosis 732.3

Kimmelstiel (-Wilson) disease or syndrome (intercapillary glomerulosclerosis) 250.4 ☑ [581.81]

due to secondary diabetes 249.4 ☑ [581.81]

Kink, kinking

appendix 543.9

artery 447.1

cystic duct, congenital 751.61

hair (acquired) 704.2

ileum or intestine (see also Obstruction, intestine) 560.9

Lane's (see also Obstruction, intestine) 560.9

organ or site, congenital NEC — see Anomaly, specified type NEC, by site

ureter (pelvic junction) 593.3

congenital 753.20

vein(s) 459.2

caval 459.2

peripheral 459.2

Kinnier Wilson's disease (hepatolenticular degeneration) 275.1

Kissing

osteophytes 721.5

spine 721.5

vertebra 721.5

Klauder's syndrome (erythema multiforme, exudativum) 695.19

Klebs' disease — see also Nephritis 583.9

Kleine-Levin syndrome 327.13

Klein-Waardenburg syndrome (ptosisepicanthus) 270.2

Kleptomania 312.32

Klinefelter's syndrome 758.7

Klinger's disease 446.4

Klippel's disease 723.8

Klippel-Feil disease or syndrome (brevicollis) 756.16

Klippel-Trenaunay syndrome 759.89

Klumpke (-Déjérine) palsy, paralysis (birth) (newborn) 767.6

Klüver-Bucy (-Terzian) syndrome 310.0

Knee — see condition

Knifegrinders' rot — see also Tuberculosis 011.4 ☑

Knock-knee (acquired) 736.41

congenital 755.64

Knot

intestinal, syndrome (volvulus) 560.2

umbilical cord (true) 663.2 ☑

affecting fetus or newborn 762.5

Knots, surfer 919.8

infected 919.9

Knotting (of)

hair 704.2

intestine 560.2

Knuckle pads (Garrod's) 728.79

Köbner's disease (epidermolysis bullosa) 757.39

Koch's

infection (see also Tuberculosis, pulmonary) 011.9 ☑

relapsing fever 087.9

Koch-Weeks conjunctivitis 372.03

Koenig-Wichman disease (pemphigus) 694.4

Köhler's disease (osteochondrosis) 732.5

first (osteochondrosis juvenilis) 732.5

second (Freiburg's infarction, metatarsal head) 732.5

patellar 732.4

Köhler's disease — continued

tarsal navicular (bone) (osteoarthrosis juvenilis) 732.5

Köhler-Mouchet disease (osteoarthrosis juvenilis) 732.5

Köhler-Pellegrini-Stieda disease or syndrome (calcification, knee joint) 726.62

Koilonychia 703.8

congenital 757.5

Kojevnikov's, Kojewnikoff's epilepsy — see also Epilepsy 345.7 ☑

König's

disease (osteochondritis dissecans) 732.7

syndrome 564.89

Koniophthisis — see also Tuberculosis 011.4 ☑

Koplik's spots 055.9

Kopp's asthma 254.8

Korean hemorrhagic fever 078.6

Korsakoff (-Wernicke) disease, psychosis, or syndrome (nonalcoholic) 294.0

alcoholic 291.1

Korsakov's disease — see Korsakoff's disease

Korsakow's disease — see Korsakoff's disease

Kostmann's disease or syndrome (infantile genetic agranulocytosis) 288.01

Krabbe's

disease (leukodystrophy) 330.0

syndrome

congenital muscle hypoplasia 756.89

cutaneocerebral angioma 759.6

Kraepelin-Morel disease — see also Schizophrenia 295.9 ☑

Kraft-Weber-Dimitri disease 759.6

Kraurosis

ani 569.49

penis 607.0

vagina 623.8

vulva 624.09

Kreotoxism 005.9

Krukenberg's

spindle 371.13

tumor (M8490/6) 198.6

Kufs' disease 330.1

Kugelberg-Welander disease 335.11

Kuhnt-Junius degeneration or disease 362.52

Kulchitsky's cell carcinoma (carcinoid tumor of intestine) 259.2

Kümmell's disease or spondylitis 721.7

Kundrat's disease (lymphosarcoma) 200.1 ☑

Kunekune — see Dermatophytosis

Kunkel syndrome (lupoid hepatitis) 571.49

Kupffer cell sarcoma (M9124/3) 155.0

Kuru 046.0

Kussmaul's

coma (diabetic) 250.3 ☑

due to secondary diabetes 249.3 ☑

disease (polyarteritis nodosa) 446.0

respiration (air hunger) 786.09

Kwashiorkor (marasmus type) 260

Kyasanur Forest disease 065.2

Kyphoscoliosis, kyphoscoliotic (acquired) — see also Scoliosis 737.30

congenital 756.19

due to radiation 737.33

heart (disease) 416.1

idiopathic 737.30

infantile

progressive 737.32

resolving 737.31

late effect of rickets 268.1 [737.43]

specified NEC 737.39

thoracogenic 737.34

tuberculous (see also Tuberculosis) 015.0 ☑ [737.43]

Kyphosis, kyphotic (acquired) (postural) 737.10

adolescent postural 737.0

congenital 756.19

dorsalis juvenilis 732.0

due to or associated with

Charcôt-Marie-Tooth disease 356.1 [737.41]

mucopolysaccharidosis 277.5 [737.41]

neurofibromatosis 237.71 [737.41]

☑ **Additional Digit Required** — Refer to the Tabular List for Digit Selection   ▽ **Subterms under main terms may continue to next column or page**

170 — Volume 2   ▶◀ Revised Text   ● New Line   ▲ Revised Code   **2011 ICD-9-CM**

Kyphosis, kyphotic — *continued*
  due to or associated with — *continued*
    osteitis
      deformans 731.0 *[737.41]*
      fibrosa cystica 252.01 *[737.41]*
    osteoporosis (*see also* Osteoporosis)
        733.0 *[737.41]*
    poliomyelitis (*see also* Poliomyelitis)
        138 *[737.41]*
    radiation 737.11
    tuberculosis (*see also* Tuberculosis)
        015.0 ☑ *[737.41]*
  Kümmell's 721.7
  late effect of rickets 268.1 *[737.41]*
  Morquio-Brailsford type (spinal)
      277.5 *[737.41]*
  pelvis 738.6
  postlaminectomy 737.12
  specified cause NEC 737.19
  syphilitic, congenital 090.5 *[737.41]*
  tuberculous (*see also* Tuberculosis)
      015.0 ☑ *[737.41]*
Kyrle's disease (hyperkeratosis follicularis in cutem penetrans) 701.1

L

Labia, labium — *see* condition
Labiated hymen 752.49
Labile
  blood pressure 796.2
  emotions, emotionality 301.3
  vasomotor system 443.9
Lability, emotional 799.24
Labioglossal paralysis 335.22
Labium leporinum — *see also* Cleft, lip 749.10
Labor — *see also* Delivery
  with complications — *see* Delivery, complicated
  abnormal NEC 661.9 ☑
    affecting fetus or newborn 763.7
  arrested active phase 661.1 ☑
    affecting fetus or newborn 763.7
  desultory 661.2 ☑
    affecting fetus or newborn 763.7
  dyscoordinate 661.4 ☑
    affecting fetus or newborn 763.7
  early onset (22-36 weeks gestation)
      644.2 ☑
  failed
    induction 659.1 ☑
      mechanical 659.0 ☑
      medical 659.1 ☑
      surgical 659.0 ☑
    trial (vaginal delivery) 660.6 ☑
  false 644.1 ☑
  forced or induced, affecting fetus or newborn 763.89
  hypertonic 661.4 ☑
    affecting fetus or newborn 763.7
  hypotonic 661.2 ☑
    affecting fetus or newborn 763.7
    primary 661.0 ☑
      affecting fetus or newborn 763.7
    secondary 661.1 ☑
      affecting fetus or newborn 763.7
  incoordinate 661.4 ☑
    affecting fetus or newborn 763.7
  irregular 661.2 ☑
    affecting fetus or newborn 763.7
  long — *see* Labor, prolonged
  missed (at or near term) 656.4 ☑
  obstructed NEC 660.9 ☑
    affecting fetus or newborn 763.1
    due to female genital mutilation
        660.8 ☑
    specified cause NEC 660.8 ☑
      affecting fetus or newborn 763.1
  pains, spurious 644.1 ☑
  precipitate 661.3 ☑
    affecting fetus or newborn 763.6
  premature 644.2 ☑
    threatened 644.0 ☑
  prolonged or protracted 662.1 ☑
    first stage 662.0 ☑
      affecting fetus or newborn 763.89

Labor — *see also* Delivery — *continued*
  prolonged or protracted — *continued*
    second stage 662.2 ☑
      affecting fetus or newborn 763.89
      affecting fetus or newborn 763.89
    threatened NEC 644.1 ☑
    undelivered 644.1 ☑
Labored breathing — *see also* Hyperventilation 786.09
Labyrinthitis (inner ear) (destructive) (latent)
    386.30
  circumscribed 386.32
  diffuse 386.31
  focal 386.32
  purulent 386.33
  serous 386.31
  suppurative 386.33
  syphilitic 095.8
  toxic 386.34
  viral 386.35
Laceration — *see also* Wound, open, by site
  accidental, complicating surgery 998.2
  Achilles tendon 845.09
    with open wound 892.2
  anus (sphincter) 879.6
    with
      abortion — *see* Abortion, by type, with damage to pelvic organs
      ectopic pregnancy (*see also* categories 633.0–633.9) 639.2
      molar pregnancy (*see also* categories 630–632) 639.2
    complicated 879.7
    complicating delivery (healed) (old) 654.8 ☑
      with laceration of anal or rectal mucosa 664.3 ☑
      not associated with third-degree perineal laceration 664.6 ☑
    following
      abortion 639.2
      ectopic or molar pregnancy 639.2
    nontraumatic, nonpuerperal (healed) (old) 569.43
  bladder (urinary)
    with
      abortion — *see* Abortion, by type, with damage to pelvic organs
      ectopic pregnancy (*see also* categories 633.0–633.9) 639.2
      molar pregnancy (*see also* categories 630–632) 639.2
    following
      abortion 639.2
      ectopic or molar pregnancy 639.2
    obstetrical trauma 665.5 ☑
  blood vessel — *see* Injury, blood vessel, by site
  bowel
    with
      abortion — *see* Abortion, by type, with damage to pelvic organs
      ectopic pregnancy (*see also* categories 633.0–633.9) 639.2
      molar pregnancy (*see also* categories 630–632) 639.2
    following
      abortion 639.2
      ectopic or molar pregnancy 639.2
    obstetrical trauma 665.5 ☑

Laceration — *see also* Wound, open, by site — *continued*
  brain (cerebral) (membrane) (with hemorrhage) 851.8 ☑

> *Note* — Use the following fifth-digit subclassification with categories 851–854:
>
> 0 unspecified state of consciousness
>
> 1 with no loss of consciousness
>
> 2 with brief [less than one hour] loss of consciousness
>
> 3 with moderate [1–24 hours] loss of consciousness
>
> 4 with prolonged [more than 24 hours] loss of consciousness and return to pre–existing conscious level
>
> 5 with prolonged [more than 24 hours] loss of consciousness, without return to pre–existing conscious level
>
> Use fifth-digit 5 to designate when a patient is unconscious and dies before regaining consciousness, regardless of the duration of the loss of consciousness
>
> 6 with loss of consciousness of unspecified duration
>
> 9 with concussion, unspecified

    with
      open intracranial wound 851.9 ☑
      skull fracture — *see* Fracture, skull, by site
    cerebellum 851.6 ☑
      with open intracranial wound 851.7 ☑
    cortex 851.2 ☑
      with open intracranial wound 851.3 ☑
    during birth 767.0
    stem 851.6 ☑
      with open intracranial wound 851.7 ☑
  broad ligament
    with
      abortion — *see* Abortion, by type, with damage to pelvic organs
      ectopic pregnancy (*see also* categories 633.0–633.9) 639.2
      molar pregnancy (*see also* categories 630–632) 639.2
    following
      abortion 639.2
      ectopic or molar pregnancy 639.2
    nontraumatic 620.6
    obstetrical trauma 665.6 ☑
    syndrome (nontraumatic) 620.6
  capsule, joint — *see* Sprain, by site
  cardiac — *see* Laceration, heart
  causing eversion of cervix uteri (old) 622.0
  central, complicating delivery 664.4 ☑
  cerebellum — *see* Laceration, brain, cerebellum
  cerebral (*see also* Laceration, brain)
    during birth 767.0
  cervix (uteri)
    with
      abortion — *see* Abortion, by type, with damage to pelvic organs
      ectopic pregnancy (*see also* categories 633.0–633.9) 639.2
      molar pregnancy (*see also* categories 630–632) 639.2
    following
      abortion 639.2
      ectopic or molar pregnancy 639.2
    nonpuerperal, nontraumatic 622.3
    obstetrical trauma (current) 665.3 ☑
    old (postpartal) 622.3
    traumatic — *see* Injury, internal, cervix
  chordae heart 429.5
  complicated 879.9

Laceration — *see also* Wound, open, by site — *continued*
  cornea — *see* Laceration, eyeball
    superficial 918.1
  cortex (cerebral) — *see* Laceration, brain, cortex
  esophagus 530.89
  eye(s) — *see* Laceration, ocular
  eyeball NEC 871.4
    with prolapse or exposure of intraocular tissue 871.1
    penetrating — *see* Penetrating wound, eyeball
    specified as without prolapse of intraocular tissue 871.0
  eyelid NEC 870.8
    full thickness 870.1
      involving lacrimal passages 870.2
    skin (and periocular area) 870.0
      penetrating — *see* Penetrating wound, orbit
  fourchette
    with
      abortion — *see* Abortion, by type, with damage to pelvic organs
      ectopic pregnancy (*see also* categories 633.0–633.9) 639.2
      molar pregnancy (*see also* categories 630–632) 639.2
    complicating delivery 664.0 ☑
    following
      abortion 639.2
      ectopic or molar pregnancy 639.2
  heart (without penetration of heart chambers) 861.02
    with
      open wound into thorax 861.12
      penetration of heart chambers 861.03
        with open wound into thorax 861.13
  hernial sac — *see* Hernia, by site
  internal organ (abdomen) (chest) (pelvis)
      NEC — *see* Injury, internal, by site
      NEC — *see* Injury, internal, by site
  kidney (parenchyma) 866.02
    with
      complete disruption of parenchyma (rupture) 866.03
        with open wound into cavity 866.13
      open wound into cavity 866.12
  labia
    complicating delivery 664.0 ☑
  ligament (*see also* Sprain, by site)
    with open wound — *see* Wound, open, by site
  liver 864.05
    with open wound into cavity 864.15
    major (disruption of hepatic parenchyma) 864.04
      with open wound into cavity 864.14
    minor (capsule only) 864.02
      with open wound into cavity 864.12
    moderate (involving parenchyma without major disruption) 864.03
      with open wound into cavity 864.13
    multiple 864.04
      with open wound into cavity 864.14
    stellate 864.04
      with open wound into cavity 864.14
  lung 861.22
    with open wound into thorax 861.32
  meninges — *see* Laceration, brain
  meniscus (knee) (*see also* Tear, meniscus) 836.2
    old 717.5
    site other than knee (*see also* Sprain, by site)
      old NEC (*see also* Disorder, cartilage, articular) 718.0 ☑
  muscle (*see also* Sprain, by site)
    with open wound — *see* Wound, open, by site
  myocardium — *see* Laceration, heart

☑ **Additional Digit Required — Refer to the Tabular List for Digit Selection**

⩗ **Subterms under main terms may continue to next column or page**

Laceration — *see also* Wound, open, by site — *continued*
nerve — *see* Injury, nerve, by site
ocular NEC (*see also* Laceration, eyeball) 871.4
  adnexa NEC 870.8
    penetrating 870.3
      with foreign body 870.4
orbit (eye) 870.8
  penetrating 870.3
    with foreign body 870.4
pelvic
  floor (muscles)
    with
      abortion — *see* Abortion, by type, with damage to pelvic organs
      ectopic pregnancy (*see also* categories 633.0–633.9) 639.2
      molar pregnancy (*see also* categories 630–632) 639.2
    complicating delivery 664.1 ☑
    following
      abortion 639.2
      ectopic or molar pregnancy 639.2
    nonpuerperal 618.7
    old (postpartal) 618.7
  organ NEC
    with
      abortion — *see* Abortion, by type, with damage to pelvic organs
      ectopic pregnancy (*see also* categories 633.0–633.9) 639.2
      molar pregnancy (*see also* categories 630–632) 639.2
    complicating delivery 665.5 ☑
      affecting fetus or newborn 763.89
    following
      abortion 639.2
      ectopic or molar pregnancy 639.2
    obstetrical trauma 665.5 ☑
perineum, perineal (old) (postpartal) 618.7
  with
    abortion — *see* Abortion, by type, with damage to pelvic floor
    ectopic pregnancy (*see also* categories 633.0–633.9) 639.2
    molar pregnancy (*see also* categories 630–632) 639.2
  complicating delivery 664.4 ☑
    first degree 664.0 ☑
    second degree 664.1 ☑
    third degree 664.2 ☑
    fourth degree 664.3 ☑
    anal sphincter (healed) (old) 654.8 ☑
      not associated with third-degree perineal laceration 664.6 ☑
    sphincter (anal) (healed) (old) 654.8 ☑
      not associated with third-degree perineal laceration 664.6 ☑
    central 664.4 ☑
    involving
      anal sphincter 664.2 ☑
      fourchette 664.0 ☑
      hymen 664.0 ☑
      labia 664.0 ☑
      pelvic floor 664.1 ☑
      perineal muscles 664.1 ☑
      rectovaginal septum 664.2 ☑
        with anal mucosa 664.3 ☑
      skin 664.0 ☑
      sphincter (anal) 664.2 ☑
        with anal mucosa 664.3 ☑
      vagina 664.0 ☑
      vaginal muscles 664.1 ☑
      vulva 664.0 ☑
    secondary 674.2 ☑
  following
    abortion 639.2
    ectopic or molar pregnancy 639.2
  male 879.6

Laceration — *see also* Wound, open, by site — *continued*
perineum, perineal — *continued*
  male — *continued*
    complicated 879.7
    muscles, complicating delivery 664.1 ☑
    nonpuerperal, current injury 879.6
      complicated 879.7
  secondary (postpartal) 674.2 ☑
peritoneum
  with
    abortion — *see* Abortion, by type, with damage to pelvic organs
    ectopic pregnancy (*see also* categories 633.0–633.9) 639.2
    molar pregnancy (*see also* categories 630–632) 639.2
  following
    abortion 639.2
    ectopic or molar pregnancy 639.2
  obstetrical trauma 665.5 ☑
periurethral tissue
  with
    abortion — *see* Abortion, by type, with damage to pelvic organs
    ectopic pregnancy (*see also* categories 633.0–633.9) 639.2
    molar pregnancy (*see also* categories 630–632) 639.2
  following
    abortion 639.2
    ectopic or molar pregnancy 639.2
  obstetrical trauma 664.8 ☑ ▲
rectovaginal (septum)
  with
    abortion — *see* Abortion, by type, with damage to pelvic organs
    ectopic pregnancy (*see also* categories 633.0–633.9) 639.2
    molar pregnancy (*see also* categories 630–632) 639.2
  complicating delivery 665.4 ☑
    with perineum 664.2 ☑
      involving anal or rectal mucosa 664.3 ☑
  following
    abortion 639.2
    ectopic or molar pregnancy 639.2
  nonpuerperal 623.4
  old (postpartal) 623.4
spinal cord (meninges) (*see also* Injury, spinal, by site)
  due to injury at birth 767.4
  fetus or newborn 767.4
spleen 865.09
  with
    disruption of parenchyma (massive) 865.04
      with open wound into cavity 865.14
    open wound into cavity 865.19
  capsule (without disruption of parenchyma) 865.02
    with open wound into cavity 865.12
  parenchyma 865.03
    with open wound into cavity 865.13
    massive disruption (rupture) 865.04
      with open wound into cavity 865.14
tendon 848.9
  with open wound — *see* Wound, open, by site
  Achilles 845.09
    with open wound 892.2
  lower limb NEC 844.9
    with open wound NEC 894.2
  upper limb NEC 840.9
    with open wound NEC 884.2
tentorium cerebelli — *see* Laceration, brain, cerebellum
tongue 873.64
  complicated 873.74
urethra
  with
    abortion — *see* Abortion, by type, with damage to pelvic organs

Laceration — *see also* Wound, open, by site — *continued*
urethra — *continued*
  with — *continued*
    ectopic pregnancy (*see also* categories 633.0–633.9) 639.2
    molar pregnancy (*see also* categories 630–632) 639.2
  following
    abortion 639.2
    ectopic or molar pregnancy 639.2
  nonpuerperal, nontraumatic 599.84
  obstetrical trauma 665.5 ☑
uterus
  with
    abortion — *see* Abortion, by type, with damage to pelvic organs
    ectopic pregnancy (*see also* categories 633.0–633.9) 639.2
    molar pregnancy (*see also* categories 630–632) 639.2
  following
    abortion 639.2
    ectopic or molar pregnancy 639.2
  nonpuerperal, nontraumatic 621.8
  obstetrical trauma NEC 665.5 ☑
  old (postpartal) 621.8
vagina
  with
    abortion — *see* Abortion, by type, with damage to pelvic organs
    ectopic pregnancy (*see also* categories 633.0–633.9) 639.2
    molar pregnancy (*see also* categories 630–632) 639.2
    perineal involvement, complicating delivery 664.0 ☑
  complicating delivery 665.4 ☑
    first degree 664.0 ☑
    second degree 664.1 ☑
    third degree 664.2 ☑
    fourth degree 664.3 ☑
    high 665.4 ☑
    muscles 664.1 ☑
    sulcus 665.4 ☑
    wall 665.4 ☑
  following
    abortion 639.2
    ectopic or molar pregnancy 639.2
  nonpuerperal, nontraumatic 623.4
  old (postpartal) 623.4
valve, heart — *see* Endocarditis
vulva
  with
    abortion — *see* Abortion, by type, with damage to pelvic organs
    ectopic pregnancy (*see also* categories 633.0–633.9) 639.2
    molar pregnancy (*see also* categories 630–632) 639.2
  complicating delivery 664.0 ☑
  following
    abortion 639.2
    ectopic or molar pregnancy 639.2
  nonpuerperal, nontraumatic 624.4
  old (postpartal) 624.4
Lachrymal — *see* condition
Lachrymonasal duct — *see* condition
Lack of
adequate intermaxillary vertical dimension 524.36
appetite (*see also* Anorexia) 783.0
care
  in home V60.4
  of adult 995.84
  of infant (at or after birth) 995.52
coordination 781.3
development (*see also* Hypoplasia)
  physiological in childhood 783.40
education V62.3
energy 780.79
financial resources V60.2
food 994.2
  in environment V60.89
growth in childhood 783.43
heating V60.1

Lack of — *continued*
housing (permanent) (temporary) V60.0
  adequate V60.1
material resources V60.2
medical attention 799.89
memory (*see also* Amnesia) 780.93
  mild, following organic brain damage 310.8
ovulation 628.0
person able to render necessary care V60.4
physical exercise V69.0
physiologic development in childhood 783.40
posterior occlusal support 524.57
prenatal care in current pregnancy V23.7
shelter V60.0
sleep V69.4
water 994.3
Lacrimal — *see* condition
Lacrimation, abnormal — *see also* Epiphora 375.20
Lacrimonasal duct — *see* condition
Lactation, lactating (breast) (puerperal) (postpartum)
defective 676.4 ☑
disorder 676.9 ☑
  specified type NEC 676.8 ☑
excessive 676.6 ☑
failed 676.4 ☑
mastitis NEC 675.2 ☑
mother (care and/or examination) V24.1
nonpuerperal 611.6
suppressed 676.5 ☑
Lacticemia 271.3
excessive 276.2
Lactosuria 271.3
Lacunar skull 756.0
Laennec's cirrhosis (alcoholic) 571.2
nonalcoholic 571.5
Lafora's disease 333.2
Lagleyze-von Hippel disease (retinocerebral angiomatosis) 759.6
Lag, lid (nervous) 374.41
Lagophthalmos (eyelid) (nervous) 374.20
cicatricial 374.23
keratitis (*see also* Keratitis) 370.34
mechanical 374.22
paralytic 374.21
La grippe — *see* Influenza
Lahore sore 085.1
Lakes, venous (cerebral) 437.8
Laki-Lorand factor deficiency — *see also* Defect, coagulation 286.3
Lalling 307.9
Lambliasis 007.1
Lame back 724.5
Lancereaux's diabetes (diabetes mellitus with marked emaciation) 250.8 ☑ [261]
due to secondary diabetes 249.8 ☑ [261]
Landau-Kleffner syndrome 345.8 ☑
Landouzy-Déjérine dystrophy (fascioscapulohumeral atrophy) 359.1
Landry's disease or paralysis 357.0
Landry-Guillain-Barré syndrome 357.0
Lane's
band 751.4
disease 569.89
kink (*see also* Obstruction, intestine) 560.9
Langdon Down's syndrome (mongolism) 758.0
Language abolition 784.69
Lanugo (persistent) 757.4
Laparoscopic surgical procedure converted to open procedure V64.41
Lardaceous
degeneration (any site) 277.39
disease 277.39
kidney 277.39 [583.81]
liver 277.39
Large
baby (regardless of gestational age) 766.1
  exceptionally (weight of 4500 grams or more) 766.0
  of diabetic mother 775.0
ear 744.22
fetus (*see also* Oversize, fetus)

☑ Additional Digit Required — Refer to the Tabular List for Digit Selection   ▽ Subterms under main terms may continue to next column or page

172 — Volume 2 · October 2010   ▶◀ Revised Text   ● New Line   ▲ Revised Code   2011 ICD-9-CM

Large — *continued*
  fetus (*see also* Oversize, fetus) — *continued*
    causing disproportion 653.5 ☑
      with obstructed labor 660.1 ☑
    for dates
      fetus or newborn (regardless of gestational age) 766.1
        affecting management of pregnancy 656.6 ☑
      exceptionally (weight of 4500 grams or more) 766.0
    physiological cup 743.57
    stature 783.9
    waxy liver 277.39
    white kidney — *see* Nephrosis
Larsen-Johansson disease (juvenile osteopathia patellae) 732.4
Larsen's syndrome (flattened facies and multiple congenital dislocations) 755.8
Larva migrans
  cutaneous NEC 126.9
    ancylostoma 126.9
  of Diptera in vitreous 128.0
  visceral NEC 128.0
Laryngeal — *see also* condition 786.2
  syncope 786.2
Laryngismus (acute) (infectious) (stridulous) 478.75
  congenital 748.3
  diphtheritic 032.3
Laryngitis (acute) (edematous) (fibrinous) (gangrenous) (infective) (infiltrative) (malignant) (membranous) (phlegmonous) (pneumococcal) (pseudomembranous) (septic) (subglottic) (suppurative) (ulcerative) (viral) 464.00
  with
    influenza, flu, or grippe ▶(*see also* Influenza)◀ 487.1
    obstruction 464.01
    tracheitis (*see also* Laryngotracheitis) 464.20
      with obstruction 464.21
      acute 464.20
        with obstruction 464.21
      chronic 476.1
  atrophic 476.0
  Borrelia vincentii 101
  catarrhal 476.0
  chronic 476.0
    with tracheitis (chronic) 476.1
    due to external agent — *see* Condition, respiratory, chronic, due to
  diphtheritic (membranous) 032.3
  due to external agent — *see* Inflammation, respiratory, upper, due to
  Hemophilus influenzae 464.00
    with obstruction 464.01
  H. influenzae 464.00
    with obstruction 464.01
  hypertrophic 476.0
  influenzal ▶(*see also* Influenza)◀ 487.1
  pachydermic 478.79
  sicca 476.0
  spasmodic 478.75
    acute 464.00
      with obstruction 464.01
  streptococcal 034.0
  stridulous 478.75
  syphilitic 095.8
    congenital 090.5
  tuberculous (*see also* Tuberculosis, larynx) 012.3 ☑
  Vincent's 101
Laryngocele (congenital) (ventricular) 748.3
Laryngofissure 478.79
  congenital 748.3
Laryngomalacia (congenital) 748.3
Laryngopharyngitis (acute) 465.0
  chronic 478.9
    due to external agent — *see* Condition, respiratory, chronic, due to
  due to external agent — *see* Inflammation, respiratory, upper, due to
  septic 034.0

Laryngoplegia — *see also* Paralysis, vocal cord 478.30
Laryngoptosis 478.79
Laryngospasm 478.75
  due to external agent — *see* Condition, respiratory, acute, due to
Laryngostenosis 478.74
  congenital 748.3
Laryngotracheitis (acute) (infectional) (viral) — *see also* Laryngitis 464.20
  with obstruction 464.21
  atrophic 476.1
  Borrelia vincenti 101
  catarrhal 476.1
  chronic 476.1
    due to external agent — *see* Condition, respiratory, chronic, due to
  diphtheritic (membranous) 032.3
  due to external agent — *see* Inflammation, respiratory, upper, due to
  H. influenzae 464.20
    with obstruction 464.21
  hypertrophic 476.1
  influenzal ▶(*see also* Influenza)◀ 487.1
  pachydermic 478.75
  sicca 476.1
  spasmodic 478.75
    acute 464.20
      with obstruction 464.21
  streptococcal 034.0
  stridulous 478.75
  syphilitic 095.8
    congenital 090.5
  tuberculous (*see also* Tuberculosis, larynx) 012.3 ☑
  Vincent's 101
Laryngotracheobronchitis — *see also* Bronchitis 490
  acute 466.0
  chronic 491.8
  viral 466.0
Laryngotracheobronchopneumonitis — *see* Pneumonia, broncho-
Larynx, laryngeal — *see* condition
Lasègue's disease (persecution mania) 297.9
Lassa fever 078.89
Lassitude — *see also* Weakness 780.79
Late — *see also* condition
  effect(s) (of) (*see also* condition)
    abscess
      intracranial or intraspinal (conditions classifiable to 324) — *see* category 326
    adverse effect of drug, medicinal or biological substance 909.5
    allergic reaction 909.9
    amputation
      postoperative (late) 997.60
      traumatic (injury classifiable to 885–887 and 895–897) 905.9
    burn (injury classifiable to 948–949) 906.9
      extremities NEC (injury classifiable to 943 or 945) 906.7
      hand or wrist (injury classifiable to 944) 906.6
      eye (injury classifiable to 940) 906.5
      face, head, and neck (injury classifiable to 941) 906.5
      specified site NEC (injury classifiable to 942 and 946–947) 906.8
    cerebrovascular disease (conditions classifiable to 430–437) 438.9
      with
        alterations of sensations 438.6
        aphasia 438.11
        apraxia 438.81
        ataxia 438.84
        cognitive deficits 438.0
        disturbances of vision 438.7
        dysarthria 438.13
        dysphagia 438.82
        dysphasia 438.12
        facial droop 438.83
        facial weakness 438.83
        fluency disorder 438.14

Late — *see also* condition — *continued*
  effect(s) (*see also* condition) — *continued*
    cerebrovascular disease — *continued*
      with — *continued*
        hemiplegia/hemiparesis
          affecting
            dominant side 438.21
            nondominant side 438.22
            unspecified side 438.20
        monoplegia of lower limb
          affecting
            dominant side 438.41
            nondominant side 438.42
            unspecified side 438.40
        monoplegia of upper limb
          affecting
            dominant side 438.31
            nondominant side 438.32
            unspecified side 438.30
        paralytic syndrome NEC
          affecting
            bilateral 438.53
            dominant side 438.51
            nondominant side 438.52
            unspecified side 438.50
        speech and language deficit 438.10
          specified type NEC 438.19
        stuttering 438.14
        vertigo 438.85
      specified type NEC 438.89
    childbirth complication(s) 677
    complication(s) of
      childbirth 677
      delivery 677
      pregnancy 677
      puerperium 677
      surgical and medical care (conditions classifiable to 996–999) 909.3
      trauma (conditions classifiable to 958) 908.6
    contusion (injury classifiable to 920–924) 906.3
    crushing (injury classifiable to 925–929) 906.4
    delivery complication(s) 677
    dislocation (injury classifiable to 830–839) 905.6
    encephalitis or encephalomyelitis (conditions classifiable to 323) — *see* category 326
      in infectious diseases 139.8
        viral (conditions classifiable to 049.8, 049.9, 062–064) 139.0
    external cause NEC (conditions classifiable to 995) 909.9
      certain conditions classifiable to categories 991–994 909.4
    foreign body in orifice (injury classifiable to 930–939) 908.5
    fracture (multiple) (injury classifiable to 828–829) 905.5
      extremity
        lower (injury classifiable to 821–827) 905.4
          neck of femur (injury classifiable to 820) 905.3
        upper (injury classifiable to 810–819) 905.2
      face and skull (injury classifiable to 800–804) 905.0
      skull and face (injury classifiable to 800–804) 905.0
      spine and trunk (injury classifiable to 805 and 807–809) 905.1
        with spinal cord lesion (injury classifiable to 806) 907.2
    infection
      pyogenic, intracranial — *see* category 326
    infectious diseases (conditions classifiable to 001–136) NEC 139.8
    injury (injury classifiable to 959) 908.9

Late — *see also* condition — *continued*
  effect(s) (*see also* condition) — *continued*
    injury — *continued*
      blood vessel 908.3
        abdomen and pelvis (injury classifiable to 902) 908.4
        extremity (injury classifiable to 903–904) 908.3
        head and neck (injury classifiable to 900) 908.3
        intracranial (injury classifiable to 850–854) 907.0
          with skull fracture 905.0
        thorax (injury classifiable to 901) 908.4
      internal organ NEC (injury classifiable to 867 and 869) 908.2
        abdomen (injury classifiable to 863–866 and 868) 908.1
        thorax (injury classifiable to 860–862) 908.0
      intracranial (injury classifiable to 850–854) 907.0
        with skull fracture (injury classifiable to 800–801 and 803–804) 905.0
      nerve NEC (injury classifiable to 957) 907.9
        cranial (injury classifiable to 950–951) 907.1
        peripheral NEC (injury classifiable to 957) 907.9
          lower limb and pelvic girdle (injury classifiable to 956) 907.5
          upper limb and shoulder girdle (injury classifiable to 955) 907.4
        roots and plexus(es), spinal (injury classifiable to 953) 907.3
        trunk (injury classifiable to 954) 907.3
      spinal
        cord (injury classifiable to 806 and 952) 907.2
        nerve root(s) and plexus(es) (injury classifiable to 953) 907.3
      superficial (injury classifiable to 910–919) 906.2
      tendon (tendon injury classifiable to 840–848, 880–884 with .2, and 890–894 with .2) 905.8
    meningitis
      bacterial (conditions classifiable to 320) — *see* category 326
      unspecified cause (conditions classifiable to 322) — *see* category 326
    myelitis (*see also* Late, effect(s) (of), encephalitis) — *see* category 326
    parasitic diseases (conditions classifiable to 001–136 NEC) 139.8
    phlebitis or thrombophlebitis of intracranial venous sinuses (conditions classifiable to 325) — *see* category 326
    poisoning due to drug, medicinal or biological substance (conditions classifiable to 960–979) 909.0
    poliomyelitis, acute (conditions classifiable to 045) 138
    pregnancy complication(s) 677
    puerperal complication(s) 677
    radiation (conditions classifiable to 990) 909.2
    rickets 268.1
    sprain and strain without mention of tendon injury (injury classifiable to 840–848, except tendon injury) 905.7
      tendon involvement 905.8

Large — Late

Late — see also condition — continued
  effect(s) (see also condition) — continued
    toxic effect of
      drug, medicinal or biological substance (conditions classifiable to 960–979) 909.0
      nonmedical substance (conditions classifiable to 980–989) 909.1
    trachoma (conditions classifiable to 076) 139.1
    tuberculosis 137.0
      bones and joints (conditions classifiable to 015) 137.3
      central nervous system (conditions classifiable to 013) 137.1
      genitourinary (conditions classifiable to 016) 137.2
      pulmonary (conditions classifiable to 010–012) 137.0
      specified organs NEC (conditions classifiable to 014, 017–018) 137.4
    viral encephalitis (conditions classifiable to 049.8, 049.9, 062–064) 139.0
    wound, open
      extremity (injury classifiable to 880–884 and 890–894, except .2) 906.1
        tendon (injury classifiable to 880–884 with .2 and 890–894 with .2) 905.8
      head, neck, and trunk (injury classifiable to 870–879) 906.0
  infant
    post-term (gestation period over 40 completed weeks to 42 completed weeks) 766.21
    prolonged gestation (period over 42 completed weeks) 766.22
Latent — see condition
Lateral — see condition
Laterocession — see Lateroversion
Lateroflexion — see Lateroversion
Lateroversion
  cervix — see Lateroversion, uterus
  uterus, uterine (cervix) (postinfectional) (postpartal, old) 621.6
    congenital 752.39 ▲
    in pregnancy or childbirth 654.4 ☑
      affecting fetus or newborn 763.89
Lathyrism 988.2
Launois-Bensaude's lipomatosis 272.8
Launois-Cléret syndrome (adiposogenital dystrophy) 253.8
Launois' syndrome (pituitary gigantism) 253.0
Laurence-Moon-Biedl syndrome (obesity, polydactyly, and mental retardation) 759.89
LAV (disease) (illness) (infection) — see Human immunodeficiency virus (disease) (illness) (infection)
LAV/HTLV-III (disease) (illness) (infection) — see Human immunodeficiency virus (disease) (illness) (infection)
Lawford's syndrome (encephalocutaneous angiomatosis) 759.6
Laxative habit — see also Abuse, drugs, non-dependent 305.9 ☑
Lax, laxity — see also Relaxation
  ligament 728.4
  skin (acquired) 701.8
    congenital 756.83
Lazy leukocyte syndrome 288.09
LCAD (long chain/very long chain acyl CoA dehydrogenase deficiency, VLCAD) 277.85
LCHAD (long chain 3-hydroxyacyl CoA dehydrogenase deficiency) 277.85
Lead — see also condition
  exposure (suspected) to V15.86
  incrustation of cornea 371.15
  poisoning 984.9
    specified type of lead — see Table of Drugs and Chemicals
Lead miners' lung 503

Leakage
  amniotic fluid 658.1 ☑
    with delayed delivery 658.2 ☑
      affecting fetus or newborn 761.1
  bile from drainage tube (T tube) 997.4
  blood (microscopic), fetal, into maternal circulation 656.0 ☑
    affecting management of pregnancy or puerperium 656.0 ☑
  device, implant, or graft — see Complications, mechanical
  spinal fluid at lumbar puncture site 997.09
  urine, continuous 788.37
Leaky heart — see Endocarditis
Learning defect, specific NEC (strephosymbolia) 315.2
Leather bottle stomach (M8142/3) 151.9
Leber's
  congenital amaurosis 362.76
  optic atrophy (hereditary) 377.16
Lederer's anemia or disease (acquired infectious hemolytic anemia) 283.19
Lederer-Brill syndrome (acquired infectious hemolytic anemia) 283.19
Leeches (aquatic) (land) 134.2
Left-sided neglect 781.8
Leg — see condition
Legal investigation V62.5
Legg (-Calvé) -Perthes disease or syndrome (osteochondrosis, femoral capital) 732.1
Legionnaires' disease 482.84
Leigh's disease 330.8
Leiner's disease (exfoliative dermatitis) 695.89
Leiofibromyoma (M8890/0) — see also Leiomyoma
  uterus (cervix) (corpus) (see also Leiomyoma, uterus) 218.9
Leiomyoblastoma (M8891/1) — see Neoplasm, connective tissue, uncertain behavior
Leiomyofibroma (M8890/0) — see also Neoplasm, connective tissue, benign
  uterus (cervix) (corpus) (see also Leiomyoma, uterus) 218.9
Leiomyoma (M8890/0) — see also Neoplasm, connective tissue, benign
  bizarre (M8893/0) — see Neoplasm, connective tissue, benign
  cellular (M8892/1) — see Neoplasm, connective tissue, uncertain behavior
  epithelioid (M8891/1) — see Neoplasm, connective tissue, uncertain behavior
  prostate (polypoid) 600.20
    with
      other lower urinary tract symptoms (LUTS) 600.21
      urinary
        obstruction 600.21
        retention 600.21
  uterus (cervix) (corpus) 218.9
    interstitial 218.1
    intramural 218.1
    submucous 218.0
    subperitoneal 218.2
    subserous 218.2
  vascular (M8894/0) — see Neoplasm, connective tissue, benign
Leiomyomatosis (intravascular) (M8890/1) — see Neoplasm, connective tissue, uncertain behavior
Leiomyosarcoma (M8890/3) — see also Neoplasm, connective tissue, malignant
  epithelioid (M8891/3) — see Neoplasm, connective tissue, malignant
Leishmaniasis 085.9
  American 085.5
    cutaneous 085.4
      mucocutaneous 085.5
  Asian desert 085.2
  Brazilian 085.5
  cutaneous 085.9
    acute necrotizing 085.2
    American 085.4
    Asian desert 085.2
    diffuse 085.3
    dry form 085.1

Leishmaniasis — continued
  cutaneous — continued
    Ethiopian 085.3
    eyelid 085.5 [373.6]
    late 085.1
    lepromatous 085.3
    recurrent 085.1
    rural 085.2
    ulcerating 085.1
    urban 085.1
    wet form 085.2
    zoonotic form 085.2
  dermal (see also Leishmaniasis, cutaneous)
    post kala-azar 085.0
  eyelid 085.5 [373.6]
  infantile 085.0
  Mediterranean 085.0
  mucocutaneous (American) 085.5
  naso-oral 085.5
  nasopharyngeal 085.5
  Old World 085.1
  tegumentaria diffusa 085.4
  vaccination, prophylactic (against) V05.2
  visceral (Indian) 085.0
Leishmanoid, dermal — see also Leishmaniasis, cutaneous
  post kala-azar 085.0
Leloir's disease 695.4
Lemiere syndrome 451.89
Lenegre's disease 426.0
Lengthening, leg 736.81
Lennox-Gastaut syndrome 345.0 ☑
  with tonic seizures 345.1 ☑
Lennox's syndrome — see also Epilepsy 345.0 ☑
Lens — see condition
Lenticonus (anterior) (posterior) (congenital) 743.36
Lenticular degeneration, progressive 275.1
Lentiglobus (posterior) (congenital) 743.36
Lentigo (congenital) 709.09
  juvenile 709.09
  Maligna (M8742/2) (see also Neoplasm, skin, in situ)
    melanoma (M8742/3) — see Melanoma
  senile 709.09
Leonine leprosy 030.0
Leontiasis
  ossium 733.3
  syphilitic 095.8
    congenital 090.5
Léopold-Lévi's syndrome (paroxysmal thyroid instability) 242.9 ☑
Lepore hemoglobin syndrome 282.49
Lepothrix 039.0
Lepra 030.9
  Willan's 696.1
Leprechaunism 259.8
Lepromatous leprosy 030.0
Leprosy 030.9
  anesthetic 030.1
  beriberi 030.1
  borderline (group B) (infiltrated) (neuritic) 030.3
  cornea (see also Leprosy, by type) 030.9 [371.89]
  dimorphous (group B) (infiltrated) (lepromatous) (neuritic) (tuberculoid) 030.3
  eyelid 030.0 [373.4]
  indeterminate (group I) (macular) (neuritic) (uncharacteristic) 030.2
  leonine 030.0
  lepromatous (diffuse) (infiltrated) (macular) (neuritic) (nodular) (type L) 030.0
  macular (early) (neuritic) (simple) 030.2
  maculoanesthetic 030.1
  mixed 030.0
  neuro 030.1
  nodular 030.0
  primary neuritic 030.3
  specified type or group NEC 030.8
  tubercular 030.1
  tuberculoid (macular) (maculoanesthetic) (major) (minor) (neuritic) (type T) 030.1
Leptocytosis, hereditary 282.49

Leptomeningitis (chronic) (circumscribed) (hemorrhagic) (nonsuppurative) — see also Meningitis 322.9
  aseptic 047.9
    adenovirus 049.1
    Coxsackie virus 047.0
    ECHO virus 047.1
    enterovirus 047.9
    lymphocytic choriomeningitis 049.0
  epidemic 036.0
  late effect — see category 326
  meningococcal 036.0
  pneumococcal 320.1
  syphilitic 094.2
  tuberculous (see also Tuberculosis, meninges) 013.0 ☑
Leptomeningopathy — see also Meningitis 322.9
Leptospiral — see condition
Leptospirochetal — see condition
Leptospirosis 100.9
  autumnalis 100.89
  canicula 100.89
  grippotyphosa 100.89
  hebdomidis 100.89
  icterohemorrhagica 100.0
  nanukayami 100.89
  pomona 100.89
  Weil's disease 100.0
Leptothricosis — see Actinomycosis
Leptothrix infestation — see Actinomycosis
Leptotricosis — see Actinomycosis
Leptus dermatitis 133.8
Leriche's syndrome (aortic bifurcation occlusion) 444.0
Léris pleonosteosis 756.89
Léri-Weill syndrome 756.59
Lermoyez's syndrome — see also Disease, Ménière's 386.00
Lesbianism — omit code
  ego-dystonic 302.0
  problems with 302.0
Lesch-Nyhan syndrome (hypoxanthineguanine-phosphoribosyltransferase deficiency) 277.2
Lesion(s)
  abducens nerve 378.54
  alveolar process 525.8
  anorectal 569.49
  aortic (valve) — see Endocarditis, aortic
  auditory nerve 388.5
  basal ganglion 333.90
  bile duct (see also Disease, biliary) 576.8
  bladder 596.9
  bone 733.90
  brachial plexus 353.0
  brain 348.89
    congenital 742.9
    vascular (see also Lesion, cerebrovascular) 437.9
      degenerative 437.1
      healed or old without residuals V12.54
      hypertensive 437.2
      late effect — see Late effect(s) (of) cerebrovascular disease
  buccal 528.9
  calcified — see Calcification
  canthus 373.9
  carate — see Pinta, lesions
  cardia 537.89
  cardiac — see also Disease, heart
    congenital 746.9
    valvular — see Endocarditis
  cauda equina 344.60
    with neurogenic bladder 344.61
  cecum 569.89
  cerebral — see Lesion, brain
  cerebrovascular (see also Disease, cerebrovascular NEC) 437.9
    degenerative 437.1
      healed or old without residuals V12.54
    hypertensive 437.2
    specified type NEC 437.8
  cervical root (nerve) NEC 353.2

☑ Additional Digit Required — Refer to the Tabular List for Digit Selection   Subterms under main terms may continue to next column or page

174 — Volume 2 · October 2010   ►◄ Revised Text   ● New Line   ▲ Revised Code   2011 ICD-9-CM

Lesion(s) — *continued*
  chiasmal 377.54
    associated with
      inflammatory disorders 377.54
      neoplasm NEC 377.52
        pituitary 377.51
      pituitary disorders 377.51
      vascular disorders 377.53
  chorda tympani 351.8
  coin, lung 793.1
  colon 569.89
  congenital — *see* Anomaly
  conjunctiva 372.9
  coronary artery (*see also* Ischemia, heart) 414.9
  cranial nerve 352.9
    first 352.0
    second 377.49
    third
      partial 378.51
      total 378.52
    fourth 378.53
    fifth 350.9
    sixth 378.54
    seventh 351.9
    eighth 388.5
    ninth 352.2
    tenth 352.3
    eleventh 352.4
    twelfth 352.5
  cystic — *see* Cyst
  degenerative — *see* Degeneration
  dermal (skin) 709.9
  Dieulafoy (hemorrhagic)
    of
      duodenum 537.84
      intestine 569.86
      stomach 537.84
  duodenum 537.89
    with obstruction 537.3
  eyelid 373.9
  gasserian ganglion 350.8
  gastric 537.89
  gastroduodenal 537.89
  gastrointestinal 569.89
  glossopharyngeal nerve 352.2
  heart (organic) (*see also* Disease, heart)
    vascular — *see* Disease, cardiovascular
  helix (ear) 709.9
  high grade myelodysplastic syndrome 238.73
  hyperchromic, due to pinta (carate) 103.1
  hyperkeratotic (*see also* Hyperkeratosis) 701.1
  hypoglossal nerve 352.5
  hypopharynx 478.29
  hypothalamic 253.9
  ileocecal coil 569.89
  ileum 569.89
  iliohypogastric nerve 355.79
  ilioinguinal nerve 355.79
  in continuity — *see* Injury, nerve, by site
  inflammatory — *see* Inflammation
  intestine 569.89
  intracerebral — *see* Lesion, brain
  intrachiasmal (optic) (*see also* Lesion, chiasmal) 377.54
  intracranial, space-occupying NEC 784.2
  joint 719.90
    ankle 719.97
    elbow 719.92
    foot 719.97
    hand 719.94
    hip 719.95
    knee 719.96
    multiple sites 719.99
    pelvic region 719.95
    sacroiliac (old) 724.6
    shoulder (region) 719.91
    specified site NEC 719.98
    wrist 719.93
  keratotic (*see also* Keratosis) 701.1
  kidney (*see also* Disease, renal) 593.9
  laryngeal nerve (recurrent) 352.3
  leonine 030.0
  lip 528.5

Lesion(s) — *continued*
  liver 573.8
  low grade myelodysplastic syndrome 238.72
  lumbosacral
    plexus 353.1
    root (nerve) NEC 353.4
  lung 518.89
    coin 793.1
  maxillary sinus 473.0
  mitral — *see* Endocarditis, mitral
  Morel Lavallée — *see* Hematoma, by site
  motor cortex 348.89
  nerve (*see also* Disorder, nerve) 355.9
  nervous system 349.9
    congenital 742.9
  nonallopathic NEC 739.9
    in region (of)
      abdomen 739.9
      acromioclavicular 739.7
      cervical, cervicothoracic 739.1
      costochondral 739.8
      costovertebral 739.8
      extremity
        lower 739.6
        upper 739.7
      head 739.0
      hip 739.5
      lower extremity 739.6
      lumbar, lumbosacral 739.3
      occipitocervical 739.0
      pelvic 739.5
      pubic 739.5
      rib cage 739.8
      sacral, sacrococcygeal, sacroiliac 739.4
      sternochondral 739.8
      sternoclavicular 739.7
      thoracic, thoracolumbar 739.2
      upper extremity 739.7
  nose (internal) 478.19
  obstructive — *see* Obstruction
  obturator nerve 355.79
  occlusive
    artery — *see* Embolism, artery
  organ or site NEC — *see* Disease, by site
  osteolytic 733.90
  paramacular, of retina 363.32
  peptic 537.89
  periodontal, due to traumatic occlusion 523.8
  perirectal 569.49
  peritoneum (granulomatous) 568.89
  pigmented (skin) 709.00
  pinta — *see* Pinta, lesions
  polypoid — *see* Polyp
  prechiasmal (optic) (*see also* Lesion, chiasmal) 377.54
  primary (*see also* Syphilis, primary)
    carate 103.0
    pinta 103.0
    yaws 102.0
  pulmonary 518.89
    valve (*see also* Endocarditis, pulmonary) 424.3
  pylorus 537.89
  radiation NEC 990
  radium NEC 990
  rectosigmoid 569.89
  retina, retinal (*see also* Retinopathy)
    vascular 362.17
  retroperitoneal 568.89
  romanus 720.1
  sacroiliac (joint) 724.6
  salivary gland 527.8
    benign lymphoepithelial 527.8
  saphenous nerve 355.79
  secondary — *see* Syphilis, secondary
  sigmoid 569.89
  sinus (accessory) (nasal) (*see also* Sinusitis) 473.9
  skin 709.9
    suppurative 686.00
  SLAP (superior glenoid labrum) 840.7
  space-occupying, intracranial NEC 784.2
  spinal cord 336.9
    congenital 742.9

Lesion(s) — *continued*
  spinal cord — *continued*
    traumatic (complete) (incomplete) (transverse) (*see also* Injury, spinal, by site)
      with
        broken
          back — *see* Fracture, vertebra, by site, with spinal cord injury
          neck — *see* Fracture, vertebra, cervical, with spinal cord injury
        fracture, vertebra — *see* Fracture, vertebra, by site, with spinal cord injury
  spleen 289.50
  stomach 537.89
  superior glenoid labrum (SLAP) 840.7
  syphilitic — *see* Syphilis
  tertiary — *see* Syphilis, tertiary
  thoracic root (nerve) 353.3
  tonsillar fossa 474.9
  tooth, teeth 525.8
    white spot 521.01
  traumatic NEC (*see also* nature and site of injury) 959.9
  tricuspid (valve) — *see* Endocarditis, tricuspid
  trigeminal nerve 350.9
  ulcerated or ulcerative — *see* Ulcer
  uterus NEC 621.9
  vagina 623.8
  vagus nerve 352.3
  valvular — *see* Endocarditis
  vascular 459.9
    affecting central nervous system (*see also* Lesion, cerebrovascular) 437.9
    following trauma (*see also* Injury, blood vessel, by site) 904.9
    retina 362.17
    traumatic — *see* Injury, blood vessel, by site
    umbilical cord 663.6 ☑
      affecting fetus or newborn 762.6
  visual
    cortex NEC (*see also* Disorder, visual, cortex) 377.73
    pathway NEC (*see also* Disorder, visual, pathway) 377.63
  warty — *see* Verruca
  white spot, on teeth 521.01
  x-ray NEC 990
Lethargic — *see* condition
Lethargy 780.79
Letterer-Siwe disease (acute histiocytosis X) (M9722/3) 202.5 ☑
Leucinosis 270.3
Leucocoria 360.44
Leucosarcoma (M9850/3) 207.8 ☑
Leukasmus 270.2
Leukemia, leukemic (congenital) (M9800/3) 208.9 ☑

> *Note* – Use the following fifth-digit subclassification for categories 203–208:
>
> 0 *without mention of having achieved remission*
>
>   *failed remission*
>
> 1 *with remission*
>
> 2 *in relapse*

  acute NEC (M9801/3) 208.0 ☑
  aleukemic NEC (M9804/3) 208.8 ☑
    granulocytic (M9864/3) 205.8 ☑
  basophilic (M9870/3) 205.1 ☑
  blast (cell) (M9801/3) 208.0 ☑
  blastic (M9801/3) 208.0 ☑
    granulocytic (M9861/3) 205.0 ☑
  chronic NEC (M9803/3) 208.1 ☑
  compound (M9810/3) 207.8 ☑
  eosinophilic (M9880/3) 205.1 ☑
  giant cell (M9910/3) 207.2 ☑
  granulocytic (M9860/3) 205.9 ☑
    acute (M9861/3) 205.0 ☑

Leukemia, leukemic — *continued*
  granulocytic — *continued*
    aleukemic (M9864/3) 205.8 ☑
    blastic (M9861/3) 205.0 ☑
    chronic (M9863/3) 205.1 ☑
    subacute (M9862/3) 205.2 ☑
    subleukemic (M9864/3) 205.8 ☑
  hairy cell (M9940/3) 202.4 ☑
  hemoblastic (M9801/3) 208.0 ☑
  histiocytic (M9890/3) 206.9 ☑
  lymphatic (M9820/3) 204.9 ☑
    acute (M9821/3) 204.0 ☑
    aleukemic (M9824/3) 204.8 ☑
    chronic (M9823/3) 204.1 ☑
    subacute (M9822/3) 204.2 ☑
    subleukemic (M9824/3) 204.8 ☑
  lymphoblastic (M9821/3) 204.0 ☑
  lymphocytic (M9820/3) 204.9 ☑
    acute (M9821/3) 204.0 ☑
    aleukemic (M9824/3) 204.8 ☑
    chronic (M9823/3) 204.1 ☑
    granular
      large T-cell 204.8 ☑
    subacute (M9822/3) 204.2 ☑
    subleukemic (M9824/3) 204.8 ☑
  lymphogenous (M9820/3) — *see* Leukemia, lymphoid
  lymphoid (M9820/3) 204.9 ☑
    acute (M9821/3) 204.0 ☑
    aleukemic (M9824/3) 204.8 ☑
    blastic (M9821/3) 204.0 ☑
    chronic (M9823/3) 204.1 ☑
    subacute (M9822/3) 204.2 ☑
    subleukemic (M9824/3) 204.8 ☑
  lymphosarcoma cell (M9850/3) 207.8 ☑
  mast cell (M9900/3) 207.8 ☑
  megakaryocytic (M9910/3) 207.2 ☑
  megakaryocytoid (M9910/3) 207.2 ☑
  mixed (cell) (M9810/3) 207.8 ☑
  monoblastic (M9891/3) 206.0 ☑
  monocytic (Schilling-type) (M9890/3) 206.9 ☑
    acute (M9891/3) 206.0 ☑
    aleukemic (M9894/3) 206.8 ☑
    chronic (M9893/3) 206.1 ☑
    Naegeli-type (M9863/3) 205.1 ☑
    subacute (M9892/3) 206.2 ☑
    subleukemic (M9894/3) 206.8 ☑
  monocytoid (M9890/3) 206.9 ☑
    acute (M9891/3) 206.0 ☑
    aleukemic (M9894/3) 206.8 ☑
    chronic (M9893/3) 206.1 ☑
    myelogenous (M9863/3) 205.1 ☑
    subacute (M9892/3) 206.2 ☑
    subleukemic (M9894/3) 206.8 ☑
  monomyelocytic (M9860/3) — *see* Leukemia, myelomonocytic
  myeloblastic (M9861/3) 205.0 ☑
  myelocytic (M9863/3) 205.1 ☑
    acute (M9861/3) 205.0 ☑
  myelogenous (M9860/3) 205.9 ☑
    acute (M9861/3) 205.0 ☑
    aleukemic (M9864/3) 205.8 ☑
    chronic (M9863/3) 205.1 ☑
    monocytoid (M9863/3) 205.1 ☑
    subacute (M9862/3) 205.2 ☑
    subleukemic (M9864) 205.8 ☑
  myeloid (M9860/3) 205.9 ☑
    acute (M9861/3) 205.0 ☑
    aleukemic (M9864/3) 205.8 ☑
    chronic (M9863/3) 205.1 ☑
    subacute (M9862/3) 205.2 ☑
    subleukemic (M9864/3) 205.8 ☑
  myelomonocytic (M9860/3) 205.9 ☑
    acute (M9861/3) 205.0 ☑
    chronic (M9863/3) 205.1 ☑
  Naegeli-type monocytic (M9863/3) 205.1 ☑
  neutrophilic (M9865/3) 205.1 ☑
  plasma cell (M9830/3) 203.1 ☑
  plasmacytic (M9830/3) 203.1 ☑
  prolymphocytic (M9825/3) — *see* Leukemia, lymphoid
  promyelocytic, acute (M9866/3) 205.0 ☑

☑ Additional Digit Required — Refer to the Tabular List for Digit Selection   ⚐ Subterms under main terms may continue to next column or page

2011 ICD-9-CM   ▶◀ Revised Text   ● New Line   ▲ Revised Code   Volume 2 — 175

Leukemia, leukemic — *continued*
Schilling-type monocytic (M9890/3) — *see*
Leukemia, monocytic
stem cell (M9801/3) 208.0 ☑
subacute NEC (M9802/3) 208.2 ☑
subleukemic NEC (M9804/3) 208.8 ☑
thrombocytic (M9910/3) 207.2 ☑
undifferentiated (M9801/3) 208.0 ☑
Leukemoid reaction (basophilic) (lymphocytic)
(monocytic) (myelocytic) (neutrophilic)
288.62
Leukoaraiosis (hypertensive) 437.1
Leukoariosis — *see* Leukoaraiosis
Leukoclastic vasculitis 446.29
Leukocoria 360.44
Leukocythemia — *see* Leukemia
Leukocytopenia 288.50
Leukocytosis 288.60
basophilic 288.8
eosinophilic 288.3
lymphocytic 288.8
monocytic 288.8
neutrophilic 288.8
Leukoderma 709.09
syphilitic 091.3
late 095.8
Leukodermia — *see also* Leukoderma 709.09
Leukodystrophy (cerebral) (globoid cell)
(metachromatic) (progressive) (sudanophilic) 330.0
Leukoedema, mouth or tongue 528.79
Leukoencephalitis
acute hemorrhagic (postinfectious) NEC
136.9 [323.61]
postimmunization or postvaccinal
323.51
subacute sclerosing 046.2
van Bogaert's 046.2
van Bogaert's (sclerosing) 046.2
Leukoencephalopathy — *see also* Encephalitis
323.9
acute necrotizing hemorrhagic (postinfectious) 136.9 [323.61]
postimmunization or postvaccinal
323.51
Binswanger's 290.12
metachromatic 330.0
multifocal (progressive) 046.3
progressive multifocal 046.3
reversible, posterior 348.5
Leukoerythroblastosis 289.9
Leukoerythrosis 289.0
Leukokeratosis — *see also* Leukoplakia 702.8
mouth 528.6
nicotina palati 528.79
tongue 528.6
Leukokoria 360.44
Leukokraurosis vulva, vulvae 624.09
Leukolymphosarcoma (M9850/3) 207.8 ☑
Leukoma (cornea) (interfering with central vision) 371.03
adherent 371.04
Leukomalacia, periventricular 779.7
Leukomelanopathy, hereditary 288.2
Leukonychia (punctata) (striata) 703.8
congenital 757.5
Leukopathia
unguium 703.8
congenital 757.5
Leukopenia 288.50
basophilic 288.59
cyclic 288.02
eosinophilic 288.59
familial 288.59
malignant (*see also* Agranulocytosis) 288.09
periodic 288.02
transitory neonatal 776.7
Leukopenic — *see* condition
Leukoplakia 702.8
anus 569.49
bladder (postinfectional) 596.8
buccal 528.6
cervix (uteri) 622.2
esophagus 530.83
gingiva 528.6
kidney (pelvis) 593.89

Leukoplakia — *continued*
larynx 478.79
lip 528.6
mouth 528.6
oral soft tissue (including tongue) (mucosa)
528.6
palate 528.6
pelvis (kidney) 593.89
penis (infectional) 607.0
rectum 569.49
syphilitic 095.8
tongue 528.6
tonsil 478.29
ureter (postinfectional) 593.89
urethra (postinfectional) 599.84
uterus 621.8
vagina 623.1
vesical 596.8
vocal cords 478.5
vulva 624.09
Leukopolioencephalopathy 330.0
Leukorrhea (vagina) 623.5
due to trichomonas (vaginalis) 131.00
trichomonal (Trichomonas vaginalis) 131.00
Leukosarcoma (M9850/3) 207.8 ☑
Leukosis (M9800/3) — *see* Leukemia
Lev's disease or syndrome (acquired complete heart block) 426.0
Levi's syndrome (pituitary dwarfism) 253.3
Levocardia (isolated) 746.87
with situs inversus 759.3
Levulosuria 271.2
Lewandowski's disease (primary) — *see also*
Tuberculosis 017.0 ☑
Lewandowski-Lutz disease (epidermodysplasia verruciformis) 078.19
Lewy body dementia 331.82
Lewy body disease 331.82
Leyden's disease (periodic vomiting) 536.2
Leyden-Möbius dystrophy 359.1
Leydig cell
carcinoma (M8650/3)
specified site — *see* Neoplasm, by site,
malignant
unspecified site
female 183.0
male 186.9
tumor (M8650/1)
benign (M8650/0)
specified site — *see* Neoplasm, by
site, benign
unspecified site
female 220
male 222.0
malignant (M8650/3)
specified site — *see* Neoplasm, by
site, malignant
unspecified site
female 183.0
male 186.9
specified site — *see* Neoplasm, by site,
uncertain behavior
unspecified site
female 236.2
male 236.4
Leydig-Sertoli cell tumor (M8631/0)
specified site — *see* Neoplasm, by site, benign
unspecified site
female 220
male 222.0
LGSIL (low grade squamous intraepithelial lesion)
anus 796.73
cervix 795.03
vagina 795.13
Liar, pathologic 301.7
Libman-Sacks disease or syndrome
710.0 [424.91]
Lice (infestation) 132.9
body (pediculus corporis) 132.1
crab 132.2
head (pediculus capitis) 132.0
mixed (classifiable to more than one of the
categories 132.0–132.2) 132.3
pubic (pediculus pubis) 132.2

Lichen 697.9
albus 701.0
annularis 695.89
atrophicus 701.0
corneus obtusus 698.3
myxedematous 701.8
nitidus 697.1
pilaris 757.39
acquired 701.1
planopilaris 697.0
planus (acute) (chronicus) (hypertrophic)
(verrucous) 697.0
morphoeicus 701.0
sclerosus (et atrophicus) 701.0
ruber 696.4
acuminatus 696.4
moniliformis 697.8
obtusus corneus 698.3
of Wilson 697.0
planus 697.0
sclerosus (et atrophicus) 701.0
scrofulosus (primary) (*see also* Tuberculosis)
017.0 ☑
simplex (Vidal's) 698.3
chronicus 698.3
circumscriptus 698.3
spinulosus 757.39
mycotic 117.9
striata 697.8
urticatus 698.2
Lichenification 698.3
nodular 698.3
Lichenoides tuberculosis (primary) — *see also*
Tuberculosis 017.0 ☑
Lichtheim's disease or syndrome (subacute
combined sclerosis with pernicious anemia) 281.0 [336.2]
Lien migrans 289.59
Lientery — *see also* Diarrhea 787.91
infectious 009.2
Life circumstance problem NEC V62.89
Li-Fraumeni cancer syndrome V84.01
Ligament — *see* condition
Light-for-dates (infant) 764.0 ☑
with signs of fetal malnutrition 764.1 ☑
affecting management of pregnancy
656.5 ☑
Light-headedness 780.4
Lightning (effects) (shock) (stroke) (struck by)
994.0
burn — *see* Burn, by site
foot 266.2
Lightwood's disease or syndrome (renal
tubular acidosis) 588.89
Lignac's disease (cystinosis) 270.0
Lignac (-Fanconi) syndrome (cystinosis) 270.0
**Lignac (-de Toni) (-Fanconi) (-Debré) syn-
drome** (cystinosis) 270.0
Ligneous thyroiditis 245.3
Likoff's syndrome (angina in menopausal
women) 413.9
Limb — *see* condition
Limitation of joint motion — *see also* Stiff-
ness, joint 719.5 ☑
sacroiliac 724.6
Limit dextrinosis 271.0
Limited
cardiac reserve — *see* Disease, heart
duction, eye NEC 378.63
mandibular range of motion 524.52
Lindau (-von Hippel) disease (angiomatosis
retinocerebellosa) 759.6
Lindau's disease (retinocerebral angiomatosis)
759.6
Linea corneae senilis 371.41
Lines
Beau's (transverse furrows on fingernails)
703.8
Harris' 733.91
Hudson-Stähli 371.11
Stähli's 371.11
Lingua
geographical 529.1
nigra (villosa) 529.3
plicata 529.5
congenital 750.13

Lingua — *continued*
tylosis 528.6
Lingual (tongue) — *see also* condition
thyroid 759.2
Linitis (gastric) 535.4 ☑
plastica (M8142/3) 151.9
Lioderma essentialis (cum melanosis et
telangiectasia) 757.33
Lip — *see also* condition
biting 528.9
Lipalgia 272.8
Lipedema — *see* Edema
Lipemia — *see also* Hyperlipidemia 272.4
retina, retinalis 272.3
Lipidosis 272.7
cephalin 272.7
cerebral (infantile) (juvenile) (late) 330.1
cerebroretinal 330.1 [362.71]
cerebroside 272.7
cerebrospinal 272.7
chemically-induced 272.7
cholesterol 272.7
diabetic 250.8 ☑ [272.7]
due to secondary diabetes
249.8 ☑ [272.7]
dystopic (hereditary) 272.7
glycolipid 272.7
hepatosplenomegalic 272.3
hereditary, dystopic 272.7
sulfatide 330.0
Lipoadenoma (M8324/0) — *see* Neoplasm, by
site, benign
Lipoblastoma (M8881/0) — *see* Lipoma, by
site
Lipoblastomatosis (M8881/0) — *see* Lipoma,
by site
Lipochondrodystrophy 277.5
Lipochrome histiocytosis (familial) 288.1
Lipodystrophia progressiva 272.6
Lipodystrophy (progressive) 272.6
insulin 272.6
intestinal 040.2
mesenteric 567.82
Lipofibroma (M8851/0) — *see* Lipoma, by site
Lipoglycoproteinosis 272.8
Lipogranuloma, sclerosing 709.8
Lipogranulomatosis (disseminated) 272.8
kidney 272.8
Lipoid — *see also* condition
histiocytosis 272.7
essential 272.7
nephrosis (*see also* Nephrosis) 581.3
proteinosis of Urbach 272.8
Lipoidemia — *see also* Hyperlipidemia 272.4
Lipoidosis — *see also* Lipidosis 272.7
Lipoma (M8850/0) 214.9
breast (skin) 214.1
face 214.0
fetal (M8881/0) (*see also* Lipoma, by site)
fat cell (M8880/0) — *see* Lipoma, by site
infiltrating (M8856/0) — *see* Lipoma, by site
intra-abdominal 214.3
intramuscular (M8856/0) — *see* Lipoma, by
site
intrathoracic 214.2
kidney 214.3
mediastinum 214.2
muscle 214.8
peritoneum 214.3
retroperitoneum 214.3
skin 214.1
face 214.0
spermatic cord 214.4
spindle cell (M8857/0) — *see* Lipoma, by
site
stomach 214.3
subcutaneous tissue 214.1
face 214.0
thymus 214.2
thyroid gland 214.2
Lipomatosis (dolorosa) 272.8
epidural 214.8
fetal (M8881/0) — *see* Lipoma, by site
Launois-Bensaude's 272.8

Lipomyohemangioma (M8860/0)
  specified site — *see* Neoplasm, connective tissue, benign
  unspecified site 223.0
Lipomyoma (M8860/0)
  specified site — *see* Neoplasm, connective tissue, benign
  unspecified site 223.0
Lipomyxoma (M8852/0) — *see* Lipoma, by site
Lipomyxosarcoma (M8852/3) — *see* Neoplasm, connective tissue, malignant
Lipophagocytosis 289.89
Lipoproteinemia (alpha) 272.4
  broad-beta 272.2
  floating-beta 272.2
  hyper-pre-beta 272.1
Lipoproteinosis (Rössle-Urbach-Wiethe) 272.8
Liposarcoma (M8850/3) — *see also* Neoplasm, connective tissue, malignant
  differentiated type (M8851/3) — *see* Neoplasm, connective tissue, malignant
  embryonal (M8852/3) — *see* Neoplasm, connective tissue, malignant
  mixed type (M8855/3) — *see* Neoplasm, connective tissue, malignant
  myxoid (M8852/3) — *see* Neoplasm, connective tissue, malignant
  pleomorphic (M8854/3) — *see* Neoplasm, connective tissue, malignant
  round cell (M8853/3) — *see* Neoplasm, connective tissue, malignant
  well differentiated type (M8851/3) — *see* Neoplasm, connective tissue, malignant
Liposynovitis prepatellaris 272.8
Lipping
  cervix 622.0
  spine (*see also* Spondylosis) 721.90
  vertebra (*see also* Spondylosis) 721.90
Lip pits (mucus), congenital 750.25
Lipschütz disease or ulcer 616.50
Lipuria 791.1
  bilharziasis 120.0
Liquefaction, vitreous humor 379.21
Lisping 307.9
Lissauer's paralysis 094.1
Lissencephalia, lissencephaly 742.2
Listerellose 027.0
Listeriose 027.0
Listeriosis 027.0
  congenital 771.2
  fetal 771.2
  suspected fetal damage affecting management of pregnancy 655.4 ☑
Listlessness 780.79
Lithemia 790.6
Lithiasis — *see also* Calculus
  hepatic (duct) — *see* Choledocholithiasis
  urinary 592.9
Lithopedion 779.9
  affecting management of pregnancy 656.8 ☑
Lithosis (occupational) 502
  with tuberculosis — *see* Tuberculosis, pulmonary
Lithuria 791.9
Litigation V62.5
Little
  league elbow 718.82
  stroke syndrome 435.9
Little's disease — *see* Palsy, cerebral
Littre's
  gland — *see* condition
  hernia — *see* Hernia, Littre's
Littritis — *see also* Urethritis 597.89
Livedo 782.61
  annularis 782.61
  racemose 782.61
  reticularis 782.61
Live flesh 781.0
Liver — *see also* condition
  donor V59.6
Livida, asphyxia
  newborn 768.6
Living
  alone V60.3

Living — *continued*
  alone — *continued*
    with handicapped person V60.4
Lloyd's syndrome 258.1
Loa loa 125.2
Loasis 125.2
Lobe, lobar — *see* condition
Lobo's disease or blastomycosis 116.2
Lobomycosis 116.2
Lobotomy syndrome 310.0
Lobstein's disease (brittle bones and blue sclera) 756.51
Lobster-claw hand 755.58
Lobulation (congenital) — *see also* Anomaly, specified type NEC, by site
  kidney, fetal 753.3
  liver, abnormal 751.69
  spleen 759.0
Lobule, lobular — *see* condition
Local, localized — *see* condition
Locked bowel or intestine — *see also* Obstruction, intestine 560.9
Locked-in state 344.81
Locked twins 660.5 ☑
  affecting fetus or newborn 763.1
Locking
  joint (*see also* Derangement, joint) 718.90
  knee 717.9
Lockjaw — *see also* Tetanus 037
Locomotor ataxia (progressive) 094.0
Löffler's
  endocarditis 421.0
  eosinophilia or syndrome 518.3
  pneumonia 518.3
  syndrome (eosinophilic pneumonitis) 518.3
Löfgren's syndrome (sarcoidosis) 135
Loiasis 125.2
  eyelid 125.2 [373.6]
Loneliness V62.89
Lone star fever 082.8
Longitudinal stripes or grooves, nails 703.8
  congenital 757.5
Long labor 662.1 ☑
  affecting fetus or newborn 763.89
  first stage 662.0 ☑
  second stage 662.2 ☑
Long-term (current) ▶(prophylactic)◀ **drug use** V58.69
  antibiotics V58.62
  anticoagulants V58.61
  anti-inflammatories, non-steroidal (NSAID) V58.64
  antiplatelets/antithrombotics V58.63
  aspirin V58.66
  high-risk medications NEC V58.69
  insulin V58.67
  methadone V58.69
  opiate analgesic V58.69
  pain killers V58.69
    anti-inflammatories, non-steroidal (NSAID) V58.64
    aspirin V58.66
  steroids V58.65
  tamoxifen V07.51
Loop
  intestine (*see also* Volvulus) 560.2
  intrascleral nerve 379.29
  vascular on papilla (optic) 743.57
Loose — *see also* condition
  body
    in tendon sheath 727.82
    joint 718.10
      ankle 718.17
      elbow 718.12
      foot 718.17
      hand 718.14
      hip 718.15
      knee 717.6
      multiple sites 718.19
      pelvic region 718.15
      prosthetic implant — *see* Complications, mechanical
      shoulder (region) 718.11
      specified site NEC 718.18
      wrist 718.13

Loose — *see also* condition — *continued*
  cartilage (joint) (*see also* Loose, body, joint) 718.1 ☑
    knee 717.6
  facet (vertebral) 724.9
  prosthetic implant — *see* Complications, mechanical
  sesamoid, joint (*see also* Loose, body, joint) 718.1 ☑
  tooth, teeth 525.8
Loosening epiphysis 732.9
Looser (-Debray)-Milkman syndrome (osteomalacia with pseudofractures) 268.2
Lop ear (deformity) 744.29
Lorain's disease or syndrome (pituitary dwarfism) 253.3
Lorain-Levi syndrome (pituitary dwarfism) 253.3
Lordosis (acquired) (postural) 737.20
  congenital 754.2
  due to or associated with
    Charcôt-Marie-Tooth disease 356.1 [737.42]
    mucopolysaccharidosis 277.5 [737.42]
    neurofibromatosis 237.71 [737.42]
    osteitis
      deformans 731.0 [737.42]
      fibrosa cystica 252.01 [737.42]
    osteoporosis (*see also* Osteoporosis) 733.00 [737.42]
    poliomyelitis (*see also* Poliomyelitis) 138 [737.42]
    tuberculosis (*see also* Tuberculosis) 015.0 ☑ [737.42]
  late effect of rickets 268.1 [737.42]
  postlaminectomy 737.21
  postsurgical NEC 737.22
  rachitic 268.1 [737.42]
  specified NEC 737.29
  tuberculous (*see also* Tuberculosis) 015.0 ☑ [737.42]
Loss
  appetite 783.0
    hysterical 300.11
    nonorganic origin 307.59
    psychogenic 307.59
  blood — *see* Hemorrhage
  central vision 368.41
  consciousness 780.09
    transient 780.2
  control, sphincter, rectum 787.60 ▲
    nonorganic origin 307.7
  ear ossicle, partial 385.24
  elasticity, skin 782.8
  extremity or member, traumatic, current — *see* Amputation, traumatic
  fluid (acute) 276.50
    with
      hypernatremia 276.0
      hyponatremia 276.1
    fetus or newborn 775.5
  hair 704.00
  hearing (*see also* Deafness)
    central 389.14
    conductive (air) 389.00
      with sensorineural hearing loss 389.20
        bilateral 389.22
        unilateral 389.21
      bilateral 389.06
      combined types 389.08
      external ear 389.01
      inner ear 389.04
      middle ear 389.03
      multiple types 389.08
      tympanic membrane 389.02
      unilateral 389.05
    mixed conductive and sensorineural 389.20
      bilateral 389.22
      unilateral 389.21
    mixed type 389.20
      bilateral 389.22
      unilateral 389.21
    nerve
      bilateral 389.12

Loss — *continued*
  hearing (*see also* Deafness) — *continued*
    nerve — *continued*
      unilateral 389.13
    neural
      bilateral 389.12
      unilateral 389.13
    noise-induced 388.12
    perceptive NEC (*see also* Loss, hearing, sensorineural) 389.10
    sensorineural 389.10
      with conductive hearing loss 389.20
        bilateral 389.22
        unilateral 389.21
      asymmetrical 389.16
      bilateral 389.18
      central 389.14
      neural 389.12
        bilateral 389.12
        unilateral 389.13
      sensory
        bilateral 389.11
        unilateral 389.17
      unilateral 389.15
    sensory
      bilateral 389.11
      unilateral 389.17
    specified type NEC 389.8
    sudden NEC 388.2
  height 781.91
  labyrinthine reactivity (unilateral) 386.55
    bilateral 386.56
  memory (*see also* Amnesia) 780.93
    mild, following organic brain damage 310.8
  mind (*see also* Psychosis) 298.9
  occlusal vertical dimension 524.37
  organ or part — *see* Absence, by site, acquired
  recurrent pregnancy — *see* Pregnancy, ●
    management affected by, abortion, ●
    habitual ●
  sensation 782.0
  sense of
    smell (*see also* Disturbance, sensation) 781.1
    taste (*see also* Disturbance, sensation) 781.1
    touch (*see also* Disturbance, sensation) 781.1
  sight (acquired) (complete) (congenital) — *see* Blindness
  spinal fluid
    headache 349.0
  substance of
    bone (*see also* Osteoporosis) 733.00
    cartilage 733.99
      ear 380.32
    vitreous (humor) 379.26
  tooth, teeth
    acquired 525.10
      due to
        caries 525.13
        extraction 525.10
        periodontal disease 525.12
        specified NEC 525.19
        trauma 525.11
  vision, visual (*see also* Blindness) 369.9
    both eyes (*see also* Blindness, both eyes) 369.3
    complete (*see also* Blindness, both eyes) 369.00
    one eye 369.8
    sudden 368.11
    transient 368.12
  vitreous 379.26
  voice (*see also* Aphonia) 784.41
  weight (cause unknown) 783.21
Lou Gehrig's disease 335.20
Louis-Bar syndrome (ataxia-telangiectasia) 334.8
Louping ill 063.1
Lousiness — *see* Lice
Low
  back syndrome 724.2
  basal metabolic rate (BMR) 794.7

☑ **Additional Digit Required — Refer to the Tabular List for Digit Selection**   ℳ **Subterms under main terms may continue to next column or page**

2011 ICD-9-CM   ▶◀ **Revised Text**   ● **New Line**   ▲ **Revised Code**   **October 2010 • Volume 2 — 177**

Low — continued
- birthweight 765.1 ☑
  - extreme (less than 1000 grams) 765.0 ☑
  - for gestational age 764.0 ☑
  - status (see also Status, low birth weight) V21.30
- bladder compliance 596.52
- blood pressure (see also Hypotension) 458.9
  - reading (incidental) (isolated) (nonspecific) 796.3
- cardiac reserve — see Disease, heart
- compliance bladder 596.52
- frequency deafness — see Disorder, hearing
- function (see also Hypofunction)
  - kidney (see also Disease, renal) 593.9
  - liver 573.9
- hemoglobin 285.9
- implantation, placenta — see Placenta, previa
- insertion, placenta — see Placenta, previa
- lying
  - kidney 593.0
  - organ or site, congenital — see Malposition, congenital
  - placenta — see Placenta, previa
- output syndrome (cardiac) (see also Failure, heart) 428.9
- platelets (blood) (see also Thrombocytopenia) 287.5
- reserve, kidney (see also Disease, renal) 593.9
- risk
  - human papillomavirus (HPA) DNA test positive
    - anal 796.79
    - cervical 795.09
    - vaginal 795.19
- salt syndrome 593.9
- tension glaucoma 365.12
- vision 369.9
  - both eyes 369.20
  - one eye 369.70

Lower extremity — see condition
Lowe (-Terrey-MacLachlan) syndrome (oculocerebrorenal dystrophy) 270.8
Lown (-Ganong) -Levine syndrome (short P-R interval, normal QRS complex, and paroxysmal supraventricular tachycardia) 426.81
LSD reaction — see also Abuse, drugs, nondependent 305.3 ☑
L-shaped kidney 753.3
Lucas-Championnière disease (fibrinous bronchitis) 466.0
Lucey-Driscoll syndrome (jaundice due to delayed conjugation) 774.30
Ludwig's
- angina 528.3
- disease (submaxillary cellulitis) 528.3
Lues (venerea), **luetic** — see Syphilis
Luetscher's syndrome (dehydration) 276.51
Lumbago 724.2
- due to displacement, intervertebral disc 722.10
Lumbalgia 724.2
- due to displacement, intervertebral disc 722.10
Lumbar — see condition
Lumbarization, vertebra 756.15
Lumbermen's itch 133.8
Lump — see also Mass
- abdominal 789.3 ☑
- breast 611.72
- chest 786.6
- epigastric 789.3 ☑
- head 784.2
- kidney 753.3
- liver 789.1
- lung 786.6
- mediastinal 786.6
- neck 784.2
- nose or sinus 784.2
- pelvic 789.3 ☑
- skin 782.2
- substernal 786.6
- throat 784.2

Lump — see also Mass — continued
- umbilicus 789.3 ☑
Lunacy — see also Psychosis 298.9
Lunatomalacia 732.3
Lung — see also condition
- donor V59.8
- drug addict's 417.8
- mainliners' 417.8
- vanishing 492.0
Lupoid (miliary) **of Boeck** 135
Lupus 710.0
- anticoagulant 289.81
- Cazenave's (erythematosus) 695.4
- discoid (local) 695.4
- disseminated 710.0
- erythematodes (discoid) (local) 695.4
- erythematosus (discoid) (local) 695.4
  - disseminated 710.0
  - eyelid 373.34
  - systemic 710.0
    - with
      - encephalitis 710.0 [323.81]
      - lung involvement 710.0 [517.8]
    - inhibitor (presence of) 286.5
- exedens 017.0 ☑
- eyelid (see also Tuberculosis)
  - 017.0 ☑ [373.4]
- Hilliard's 017.0 ☑
- hydralazine
  - correct substance properly administered 695.4
  - overdose or wrong substance given or taken 972.6
- miliaris disseminatus faciei 017.0 ☑
- nephritis 710.0 [583.81]
  - acute 710.0 [580.81]
  - chronic 710.0 [582.81]
- nontuberculous, not disseminated 695.4
- pernio (Besnier) 135
- tuberculous (see also Tuberculosis) 017.0 ☑
  - eyelid (see also Tuberculosis)
    - 017.0 ☑ [373.4]
- vulgaris 017.0 ☑
Luschka's joint disease 721.90
Luteinoma (M8610/0) 220
Lutembacher's disease or syndrome (atrial septal defect with mitral stenosis) 745.5
Luteoma (M8610/0) 220
Lutz-Miescher disease (elastosis perforans serpiginosa) 701.1
Lutz-Splendore-de Almeida disease (Brazilian blastomycosis) 116.1
Luxatio
- bulbi due to birth injury 767.8
- coxae congenita (see also Dislocation, hip, congenital) 754.30
- erecta — see Dislocation, shoulder
- imperfecta — see Sprain, by site
- perinealis — see Dislocation, hip
Luxation — see also Dislocation, by site
- eyeball 360.81
  - due to birth injury 767.8
  - lateral 376.36
- genital organs (external) NEC — see Wound, open, genital organs
- globe (eye) 360.81
  - lateral 376.36
- lacrimal gland (postinfectional) 375.16
- lens (old) (partial) 379.32
  - congenital 743.37
    - syphilitic 090.49 [379.32]
  - Marfan's disease 090.49
  - spontaneous 379.32
- penis — see Wound, open, penis
- scrotum — see Wound, open, scrotum
- testis — see Wound, open, testis
L-xyloketosuria 271.8
Lycanthropy — see also Psychosis 298.9
Lyell's disease or syndrome (toxic epidermal necrolysis) 695.15
- due to drug
  - correct substance properly administered 695.15
  - overdose or wrong substance given or taken 977.9

Lyell's disease or syndrome — continued
- due to drug — continued
  - overdose or wrong substance given or taken — continued
    - specified drug — see Table of Drugs and Chemicals
Lyme disease 088.81
Lymph
- gland or node — see condition
- scrotum (see also Infestation, filarial) 125.9
Lymphadenitis 289.3
- with
  - abortion — see Abortion, by type, with sepsis
  - ectopic pregnancy (see also categories 633.0–633.9) 639.0
  - molar pregnancy (see also categories 630–632) 639.0
- acute 683
  - mesenteric 289.2
- any site, except mesenteric 289.3
  - acute 683
  - chronic 289.1
  - mesenteric (acute) (chronic) (nonspecific) (subacute) 289.2
  - subacute 289.1
    - mesenteric 289.2
- breast, puerperal, postpartum 675.2 ☑
- chancroidal (congenital) 099.0
- chronic 289.1
  - mesenteric 289.2
- dermatopathic 695.89
- due to
  - anthracosis (occupational) 500
  - Brugia (Wuchereria) malayi 125.1
  - diphtheria (toxin) 032.89
  - lymphogranuloma venereum 099.1
  - Wuchereria bancrofti 125.0
- following
  - abortion 639.0
  - ectopic or molar pregnancy 639.0
- generalized 289.3
- gonorrheal 098.89
- granulomatous 289.1
- infectional 683
- mesenteric (acute) (chronic) (nonspecific) (subacute) 289.2
  - due to Bacillus typhi 002.0
  - tuberculous (see also Tuberculosis) 014.8 ☑
- mycobacterial 031.8
- purulent 683
- pyogenic 683
- regional 078.3
- septic 683
- streptococcal 683
- subacute, unspecified site 289.1
- suppurative 683
- syphilitic (early) (secondary) 091.4
  - late 095.8
- tuberculous — see Tuberculosis, lymph gland
- venereal 099.1
Lymphadenoid goiter 245.2
Lymphadenopathy (general) 785.6
- due to toxoplasmosis (acquired) 130.7
  - congenital (active) 771.2
Lymphadenopathy-associated virus (disease) (illness) (infection) — see Human immunodeficiency virus (disease) (illness) (infection)
Lymphadenosis 785.6
- acute 075
Lymphangiectasis 457.1
- conjunctiva 372.89
- postinfectional 457.1
- scrotum 457.1
Lymphangiectatic elephantiasis, nonfilarial 457.1
Lymphangioendothelioma (M9170/0) 228.1
- malignant (M9170/3) — see Neoplasm, connective tissue, malignant
Lymphangioma (M9170/0) 228.1
- capillary (M9171/0) 228.1
- cavernous (M9172/0) 228.1
- cystic (M9173/0) 228.1

Lymphangioma — continued
- malignant (M9170/3) — see Neoplasm, connective tissue, malignant
Lymphangiomyoma (M9174/0) 228.1
Lymphangiomyomatosis (M9174/1) — see Neoplasm, connective tissue, uncertain behavior
Lymphangiosarcoma (M9170/3) — see Neoplasm, connective tissue, malignant
Lymphangitis 457.2
- with
  - abortion — see Abortion, by type, with sepsis
  - abscess — see Abscess, by site
  - cellulitis — see Abscess, by site
  - ectopic pregnancy (see also categories 633.0–633.9) 639.0
  - molar pregnancy (see also categories 630–632) 639.0
- acute (with abscess or cellulitis) 682.9
  - specified site — see Abscess, by site
- breast, puerperal, postpartum 675.2 ☑
- chancroidal 099.0
- chronic (any site) 457.2
- due to
  - Brugia (Wuchereria) malayi 125.1
  - Wuchereria bancrofti 125.0
- following
  - abortion 639.0
  - ectopic or molar pregnancy 639.0
- gangrenous 457.2
- penis
  - acute 607.2
  - gonococcal (acute) 098.0
    - chronic or duration of 2 months or more 098.2
- puerperal, postpartum, childbirth 670.8 ☑
- strumous, tuberculous (see also Tuberculosis) 017.2 ☑
- subacute (any site) 457.2
- tuberculous — see Tuberculosis, lymph gland
Lymphatic (vessel) — see condition
Lymphatism 254.8
- scrofulous (see also Tuberculosis) 017.2 ☑
Lymphectasia 457.1
Lymphedema — see also Elephantiasis 457.1
- acquired (chronic) 457.1
- chronic hereditary 757.0
- congenital 757.0
- idiopathic hereditary 757.0
- praecox 457.1
- secondary 457.1
- surgical NEC 997.99
  - postmastectomy (syndrome) 457.0
Lymph-hemangioma (M9120/0) — see Hemangioma, by site
Lymphoblastic — see condition
Lymphoblastoma (diffuse) (M9630/3) 200.1 ☑
- giant follicular (M9690/3) 202.0 ☑
- macrofollicular (M9690/3) 202.0 ☑
Lymphoblastosis, acute benign 075
Lymphocele 457.8
Lymphocythemia 288.51
Lymphocytic — see condition
- chorioencephalitis (acute) (serous) 049.0
- choriomeningitis (acute) (serous) 049.0
Lymphocytoma (diffuse) (malignant) (M9620/3) 200.1 ☑
Lymphocytomatosis (M9620/3) 200.1 ☑
Lymphocytopenia 288.51
Lymphocytosis (symptomatic) 288.61
- infectious (acute) 078.89
Lymphoepithelioma (M8082/3) — see Neoplasm, by site, malignant
Lymphogranuloma (malignant) (M9650/3) 201.9 ☑
- inguinale 099.1
- venereal (any site) 099.1
  - with stricture of rectum 099.1
- venereum 099.1
Lymphogranulomatosis (malignant) (M9650/3) 201.9 ☑
- benign (Boeck's sarcoid) (Schaumann's) 135
- Hodgkin's (M9650/3) 201.9 ☑

☑ Additional Digit Required — Refer to the Tabular List for Digit Selection   ▽ Subterms under main terms may continue to next column or page

Lymphohistiocytosis, familial hemophagocytic 288.4
Lymphoid — see condition
Lympholeukoblastoma (M9850/3) 207.8 ☑
Lympholeukosarcoma (M9850/3) 207.8 ☑
Lymphoma (malignant) (M9590/3) 202.8 ☑

Note — Use the following fifth-digit subclassification with categories 200–202:

0 unspecified site, extranodal and solid organ sites

1 lymph nodes of head, face, and neck

2 intrathoracic lymph nodes

3 intra–abdominal lymph nodes

4 lymph nodes of axilla and upper limb

5 lymph nodes of inguinal region and lower limb

6 intrapelvic lymph nodes

7 spleen

8 lymph nodes of multiple sites

benign (M9590/0) — see Neoplasm, by site, benign
Burkitt's type (lymphoblastic) (undifferentiated) (M9750/3) 200.2 ☑
Castleman's (mediastinal lymph node hyperplasia) 785.6
centroblastic-centrocytic
diffuse (M9614/3) 202.8 ☑
follicular (M9692/3) 202.0 ☑
centroblastic type (diffuse) (M9632/3) 202.8 ☑
follicular (M9697/3) 202.0 ☑
centrocytic (M9622/3) 202.8 ☑
compound (M9613/3) 200.8 ☑
convoluted cell type (lymphoblastic) (M9602/3) 202.8 ☑
diffuse NEC (M9590/3) 202.8 ☑
large B cell 202.8 ☑
follicular (giant) (M9690/3) 202.0 ☑
center cell (diffuse) (M9615/3) 202.8 ☑
cleaved (diffuse) (M9623/3) 202.8 ☑
follicular (M9695/3) 202.0 ☑
non-cleaved (diffuse) (M9633/3) 202.8 ☑
follicular (M9698/3) 202.0 ☑
centroblastic-centrocytic (M9692/3) 202.0 ☑
centroblastic type (M9697/3) 202.0 ☑
large cell 202.0 ☑
lymphocytic
intermediate differentiation (M9694/3) 202.0 ☑
poorly differentiated (M9696/3) 202.0 ☑
mixed (cell type) (lymphocytic-histiocytic) (small cell and large cell) (M9691/3) 202.0 ☑
germinocytic (M9622/3) 202.8 ☑
giant, follicular or follicle (M9690/3) 202.0 ☑
histiocytic (diffuse) (M9640/3) 200.0 ☑
nodular (M9642/3) 200.0 ☑
pleomorphic cell type (M9641/3) 200.0 ☑
Hodgkin's (M9650/3) (see also Disease, Hodgkin's) 201.9 ☑
immunoblastic (type) (M9612/3) 200.8 ☑
large cell (M9640/3) 200.7 ☑
anaplastic 200.6 ☑
nodular (M9642/3) 202.0 ☑
pleomorphic cell type (M9641/3) 200.0 ☑
lymphoblastic (diffuse) (M9630/3) 200.1 ☑
Burkitt's type (M9750/3) 200.2 ☑
convoluted cell type (M9602/3) 202.8 ☑
lymphocytic (cell type) (diffuse) (M9620/3) 200.1 ☑

Lymphoma — continued
lymphocytic — continued
with plasmacytoid differentiation, diffuse (M9611/3) 200.8 ☑
intermediate differentiation (diffuse) (M9621/3) 200.1 ☑
follicular (M9694/3) 202.0 ☑
nodular (M9694/3) 202.0 ☑
nodular (M9690/3) 202.0 ☑
poorly differentiated (diffuse) (M9630/3) 200.1 ☑
follicular (M9696/3) 202.0 ☑
nodular (M9696/3) 202.0 ☑
well differentiated (diffuse) (M9620/3) 200.1 ☑
follicular (M9693/3) 202.0 ☑
nodular (M9693/3) 202.0 ☑
lymphocytic-histiocytic, mixed (diffuse) (M9613/3) 200.8 ☑
follicular (M9691/3) 202.0 ☑
nodular (M9691/3) 202.0 ☑
lymphoplasmacytoid type (M9611/3) 200.8 ☑
lymphosarcoma type (M9610/3) 200.1 ☑
macrofollicular (M9690/3) 202.0 ☑
mantle cell 200.4 ☑
marginal zone 200.3 ☑
extranodal B-cell 200.3 ☑
nodal B-cell 200.3 ☑
splenic B-cell 200.3 ☑
mixed cell type (diffuse) (M9613/3) 200.8 ☑
follicular (M9691/3) 202.0 ☑
nodular (M9691/3) 202.0 ☑
nodular (M9690/3) 202.0 ☑
histiocytic (M9642/3) 200.0 ☑
lymphocytic (M9690/3) 202.0 ☑
intermediate differentiation (M9694/3) 202.0 ☑
poorly differentiated (M9696/3) 202.0 ☑
mixed (cell type) (lymphocytic-histiocytic) (small cell and large cell) (M9691/3) 202.0 ☑
non-Hodgkin's type NEC (M9591/3) 202.8 ☑
peripheral T-cell 202.7 ☑
primary central nervous system 200.5 ☑
reticulum cell (type) (M9640/3) 200.0 ☑
small cell and large cell, mixed (diffuse) (M9613/3) 200.8 ☑
follicular (M9691/3) 202.0 ☑
nodular (9691/3) 202.0 ☑
stem cell (type) (M9601/3) 202.8 ☑
T-cell 202.1 ☑
peripheral 202.7 ☑
undifferentiated (cell type) (non-Burkitt's) (M9600/3) 202.8 ☑
Burkitt's type (M9750/3) 200.2 ☑
Lymphomatosis (M9590/3) — see also Lymphoma
granulomatous 099.1
Lymphopathia
venereum 099.1
veneris 099.1
Lymphopenia 288.51
familial 279.2
Lymphoreticulosis, benign (of inoculation) 078.3
Lymphorrhea 457.8
Lymphosarcoma (M9610/3) 200.1 ☑
diffuse (M9610/3) 200.1 ☑
with plasmacytoid differentiation (M9611/3) 200.8 ☑
lymphoplasmacytic (M9611/3) 200.8 ☑
follicular (giant) (M9690/3) 202.0 ☑
lymphoblastic (M9696/3) 202.0 ☑
lymphocytic, intermediate differentiation (M9694/3) 202.0 ☑
mixed cell type (M9691/3) 202.0 ☑
giant follicular (M9690/3) 202.0 ☑
Hodgkin's (M9650/3) 201.9 ☑
immunoblastic (M9612/3) 200.8 ☑
lymphoblastic (diffuse) (M9630/3) 200.1 ☑
follicular (M9696/3) 202.0 ☑
nodular (M9696/3) 202.0 ☑

Lymphosarcoma — continued
lymphocytic (diffuse) (M9620/3) 200.1 ☑
intermediate differentiation (diffuse) (M9621/3) 200.1 ☑
follicular (M9694/3) 202.0 ☑
nodular (M9694/3) 202.0 ☑
mixed cell type (diffuse) (M9613/3) 200.8 ☑
follicular (M9691/3) 202.0 ☑
nodular (M9691/3) 202.0 ☑
nodular (M9690/3) 202.0 ☑
lymphoblastic (M9696/3) 202.0 ☑
lymphocytic, intermediate differentiation (M9694/3) 202.0 ☑
mixed cell type (M9691/3) 202.0 ☑
prolymphocytic (M9631/3) 200.1 ☑
reticulum cell (M9640/3) 200.0 ☑
Lymphostasis 457.8
Lypemania — see also Melancholia 296.2 ☑
Lyssa 071

M

Macacus ear 744.29
Maceration
fetus (cause not stated) 779.9
wet feet, tropical (syndrome) 991.4
Machado-Joseph disease 334.8
Machupo virus hemorrhagic fever 078.7
Macleod's syndrome (abnormal transradiancy, one lung) 492.8
Macrocephalia, macrocephaly 756.0
Macrocheilia (congenital) 744.81
Macrochilia (congenital) 744.81
Macrocolon (congenital) 751.3
Macrocornea 743.41
associated with buphthalmos 743.22
Macrocytic — see condition
Macrocytosis 289.89
Macrodactylia, macrodactylism (fingers) (thumbs) 755.57
toes 755.65
Macrodontia 520.2
Macroencephaly 742.4
Macrogenia 524.05
Macrogenitosomia (female) (male) (praecox) 255.2
Macrogingivae 523.8
Macroglobulinemia (essential) (idiopathic) (monoclonal) (primary) (syndrome) (Waldenström's) 273.3
Macroglossia (congenital) 750.15
acquired 529.8
Macrognathia, macrognathism (congenital) 524.00
mandibular 524.02
alveolar 524.72
maxillary 524.01
alveolar 524.71
Macrogyria (congenital) 742.4
Macrohydrocephalus — see also Hydrocephalus 331.4
Macromastia — see also Hypertrophy, breast 611.1
Macropsia 368.14
Macrosigmoid 564.7
congenital 751.3
Macrospondylitis, acromegalic 253.0
Macrostomia (congenital) 744.83
Macrotia (external ear) (congenital) 744.22
Macula
cornea, corneal
congenital 743.43
interfering with vision 743.42
interfering with central vision 371.03
not interfering with central vision 371.02
degeneration (see also Degeneration, macula) 362.50
hereditary (see also Dystrophy, retina) 362.70
edema, cystoid 362.53
Maculae ceruleae 132.1
Macules and papules 709.8
Maculopathy, toxic 362.55
Madarosis 374.55

Madelung's
deformity (radius) 755.54
disease (lipomatosis) 272.8
lipomatosis 272.8
Madness — see also Psychosis 298.9
myxedema (acute) 293.0
subacute 293.1
Madura
disease (actinomycotic) 039.9
mycotic 117.4
foot (actinomycotic) 039.4
mycotic 117.4
Maduromycosis (actinomycotic) 039.9
mycotic 117.4
Maffucci's syndrome (dyschondroplasia with hemangiomas) 756.4
Magenblase syndrome 306.4
Main en griffe (acquired) 736.06
congenital 755.59
Maintenance
chemotherapy regimen or treatment V58.11
dialysis regimen or treatment
extracorporeal (renal) V56.0
peritoneal V56.8
renal V56.0
drug therapy or regimen
chemotherapy, antineoplastic V58.11
immunotherapy, antineoplastic V58.12
external fixation NEC V54.89
radiotherapy V58.0
traction NEC V54.89
Majocchi's
disease (purpura annularis telangiectodes) 709.1
granuloma 110.6
Major — see condition
Mal
cerebral (idiopathic) (see also Epilepsy) 345.9 ☑
comital (see also Epilepsy) 345.9 ☑
de los pintos (see also Pinta) 103.9
de Meleda 757.39
de mer 994.6
lie — see Presentation, fetal
perforant (see also Ulcer, lower extremity) 707.15
Malabar itch 110.9
beard 110.0
foot 110.4
scalp 110.0
Malabsorption 579.9
calcium 579.8
carbohydrate 579.8
disaccharide 271.3
drug-induced 579.8
due to bacterial overgrowth 579.8
fat 579.8
folate, congenital 281.2
galactose 271.1
glucose-galactose (congenital) 271.3
intestinal 579.9
isomaltose 271.3
lactose (hereditary) 271.3
methionine 270.4
monosaccharide 271.8
postgastrectomy 579.3
postsurgical 579.3
protein 579.8
sucrose (-isomaltose) (congenital) 271.3
syndrome 579.9
postgastrectomy 579.3
postsurgical 579.3
Malacia, bone 268.2
juvenile (see also Rickets) 268.0
Kienböck's (juvenile) (lunate) (wrist) 732.3
adult 732.8
Malacoplakia
bladder 596.8
colon 569.89
pelvis (kidney) 593.89
ureter 593.89
urethra 599.84
Malacosteon 268.2
juvenile (see also Rickets) 268.0
Maladaptation — see Maladjustment
Maladie de Roger 745.4

☑ Additional Digit Required — Refer to the Tabular List for Digit Selection ⏷ Subterms under main terms may continue to next column or page

2011 ICD-9-CM ▶◀ Revised Text ● New Line ▲ Revised Code Volume 2 — 179

Index

Maladjustment — Malposition

Maladjustment
  conjugal V61.10
    involving
      divorce V61.03
      estrangement V61.09
  educational V62.3
  family V61.9
    specified circumstance NEC V61.8
  marital V61.10
    involving
      divorce V61.03
      estrangement V61.09
  occupational V62.29
    current military deployment status V62.21
  simple, adult (see also Reaction, adjustment) 309.9
  situational acute (see also Reaction, adjustment) 309.9
  social V62.4
Malaise 780.79
Malakoplakia — see Malacoplakia
Malaria, malarial (fever) 084.6
  algid 084.9
  any type, with
    algid malaria 084.9
    blackwater fever 084.8
    fever
      blackwater 084.8
      hemoglobinuric (bilious) 084.8
    hemoglobinuria, malarial 084.8
    hepatitis 084.9 [573.2]
    nephrosis 084.9 [581.81]
    pernicious complication NEC 084.9
      cardiac 084.9
      cerebral 084.9
  cardiac 084.9
  carrier (suspected) of V02.9
  cerebral 084.9
  complicating pregnancy, childbirth, or puerperium 647.4 ☑
  congenital 771.2
  congestion, congestive 084.6
    brain 084.9
  continued 084.0
  estivo-autumnal 084.0
  falciparum (malignant tertian) 084.0
  hematinuria 084.8
  hematuria 084.8
  hemoglobinuria 084.8
  hemorrhagic 084.6
  induced (therapeutically) 084.7
    accidental — see Malaria, by type
  liver 084.9 [573.2]
  malariae (quartan) 084.2
  malignant (tertian) 084.0
  mixed infections 084.5
  monkey 084.4
  ovale 084.3
  pernicious, acute 084.0
  Plasmodium, P.
    falciparum 084.0
    malariae 084.2
    ovale 084.3
    vivax 084.1
  quartan 084.2
  quotidian 084.0
  recurrent 084.6
    induced (therapeutically) 084.7
      accidental — see Malaria, by type
  remittent 084.6
  specified types NEC 084.4
  spleen 084.6
  subtertian 084.0
  tertian (benign) 084.1
    malignant 084.0
  tropical 084.0
  typhoid 084.6
  vivax (benign tertian) 084.1
Malassez's disease (testicular cyst) 608.89
Malassimilation 579.9
Maldescent, testis 752.51
Maldevelopment — see also Anomaly, by site
  brain 742.9
  colon 751.5
  hip (joint) 755.63

Maldevelopment — see also Anomaly, by site — continued
  hip — continued
    congenital dislocation (see also Dislocation, hip, congenital) 754.30
  mastoid process 756.0
  middle ear, except ossicles 744.03
    ossicles 744.04
  newborn (not malformation) 764.9 ☑
  ossicles, ear 744.04
  spine 756.10
  toe 755.66
Male type pelvis 755.69
  with disproportion (fetopelvic) 653.2 ☑
    affecting fetus or newborn 763.1
    causing obstructed labor 660.1 ☑
      affecting fetus or newborn 763.1
Malformation (congenital) — see also Anomaly
  bone 756.9
  bursa 756.9
  Chiari
    type I 348.4
    type II (see also Spina bifida) 741.0 ☑
    type III 742.0
    type IV 742.2
  circulatory system NEC 747.9
    specified type NEC 747.89
  cochlea 744.05
  digestive system NEC 751.9
    lower 751.5
    specified type NEC 751.8
    upper 750.9
  eye 743.9
  gum 750.9
  heart NEC 746.9
    specified type NEC 746.89
    valve 746.9
  internal ear 744.05
  joint NEC 755.9
    specified type NEC 755.8
  Mondini's (congenital) (malformation, cochlea) 744.05
  muscle 756.9
  nervous system (central) 742.9
  pelvic organs or tissues
    in pregnancy or childbirth 654.9 ☑
      affecting fetus or newborn 763.89
      causing obstructed labor 660.2 ☑
        affecting fetus or newborn 763.1
  placenta (see also Placenta, abnormal) 656.7 ☑
  respiratory organs 748.9
    specified type NEC 748.8
  Rieger's 743.44
  sense organs NEC 742.9
    specified type NEC 742.8
  skin 757.9
    specified type NEC 757.8
  spinal cord 742.9
  teeth, tooth NEC 520.9
  tendon 756.9
  throat 750.9
  umbilical cord (complicating delivery) 663.9 ☑
    affecting fetus or newborn 762.6
  umbilicus 759.9
  urinary system NEC 753.9
    specified type NEC 753.8
  venous — see Anomaly, vein
Malfunction — see also Dysfunction
  arterial graft 996.1
  cardiac pacemaker 996.01
  catheter device — see Complications, mechanical, catheter
  colostomy 569.62
    valve 569.62
  cystostomy 997.5
  device, implant, or graft NEC — see Complications, mechanical
  enteric stoma 569.62
  enterostomy 569.62
  esophagostomy 530.87
  gastroenteric 536.8
  gastrostomy 536.42

Malfunction — see also Dysfunction — continued
  ileostomy
    valve 569.62
  nephrostomy 997.5
  pacemaker — see Complications, mechanical, pacemaker
  prosthetic device, internal — see Complications, mechanical
  tracheostomy 519.02
  valve
    colostomy 569.62
    ileostomy 569.62
  vascular graft or shunt 996.1
Malgaigne's fracture (closed) 808.43
  open 808.53
Malherbe's
  calcifying epithelioma (M8110/0) — see Neoplasm, skin, benign
  tumor (M8110/0) — see Neoplasm, skin, benign
Malibu disease 919.8
  infected 919.9
Malignancy (M8000/3) — see Neoplasm, by site, malignant
Malignant — see condition
Malingerer, malingering V65.2
Mallet, finger (acquired) 736.1
  congenital 755.59
  late effect of rickets 268.1
Malleus 024
Mallory's bodies 034.1
Mallory-Weiss syndrome 530.7
Malnutrition (calorie) 263.9
  complicating pregnancy 648.9 ☑
  degree
    first 263.1
    second 263.0
    third 262
    mild ▶(protein)◀ 263.1
    moderate ▶(protein)◀ 263.0
    severe 261
      protein-calorie 262
  fetus 764.2 ☑
    "light-for-dates" 764.1 ☑
  following gastrointestinal surgery 579.3
  intrauterine or fetal 764.2 ☑
    fetus or infant "light-for-dates" 764.1 ☑
  lack of care, or neglect (child) (infant) 995.52
    adult 995.84
  malignant 260
  mild ▶(protein)◀ 263.1
  moderate ▶(protein)◀ 263.0
  protein 260
  protein-calorie 263.9
    mild 263.1   ●
    moderate 263.0   ●
    severe 262
    specified type NEC 263.8
  severe 261
    protein-calorie NEC 262
Malocclusion (teeth) 524.4
  angle's class I 524.21
  angle's class II 524.22
  angle's class III 524.23
  due to
    abnormal swallowing 524.59
    accessory teeth (causing crowding) 524.31
    dentofacial abnormality NEC 524.89
    impacted teeth (causing crowding) 520.6
    missing teeth 524.30
    mouth breathing 524.59
    sleep postures 524.59
    supernumerary teeth (causing crowding) 524.31
    thumb sucking 524.59
    tongue, lip, or finger habits 524.59
  temporomandibular (joint) 524.69
Malposition
  cardiac apex (congenital) 746.87
  cervix — see Malposition, uterus
  congenital
    adrenal (gland) 759.1
    alimentary tract 751.8
      lower 751.5

Malposition — continued
  congenital — continued
    alimentary tract — continued
      upper 750.8
    aorta 747.21
    appendix 751.5
    arterial trunk 747.29
    artery (peripheral) NEC (see also Malposition, congenital, peripheral vascular system) 747.60
      coronary 746.85
      pulmonary 747.3
    auditory canal 744.29
      causing impairment of hearing 744.02
    auricle (ear) 744.29
      causing impairment of hearing 744.02
      cervical 744.43
    biliary duct or passage 751.69
    bladder (mucosa) 753.8
      exteriorized or extroverted 753.5
    brachial plexus 742.8
    brain tissue 742.4
    breast 757.6
    bronchus 748.3
    cardiac apex 746.87
    cecum 751.5
    clavicle 755.51
    colon 751.5
    digestive organ or tract NEC 751.8
      lower 751.5
      upper 750.8
    ear (auricle) (external) 744.29
      ossicles 744.04
    endocrine (gland) NEC 759.2
    epiglottis 748.3
    Eustachian tube 744.24
    eye 743.8
    facial features 744.89
    fallopian tube 752.19
    finger(s) 755.59
      supernumerary 755.01
    foot 755.67
    gallbladder 751.69
    gastrointestinal tract 751.8
    genitalia, genital organ(s) or tract
      female 752.89
        external 752.49
        internal NEC 752.89
      male 752.89
        penis 752.69
        scrotal transposition 752.81
    glottis 748.3
    hand 755.59
    heart 746.87
      dextrocardia 746.87
        with complete transposition of viscera 759.3
    hepatic duct 751.69
    hip (joint) (see also Dislocation, hip, congenital) 754.30
    intestine (large) (small) 751.5
      with anomalous adhesions, fixation, or malrotation 751.4
    joint NEC 755.8
    kidney 753.3
    larynx 748.3
    limb 755.8
      lower 755.69
      upper 755.59
    liver 751.69
    lung (lobe) 748.69
    nail(s) 757.5
    nerve 742.8
    nervous system NEC 742.8
    nose, nasal (septum) 748.1
    organ or site NEC — see Anomaly, specified type NEC, by site
    ovary 752.0
    pancreas 751.7
    parathyroid (gland) 759.2
    patella 755.64
    peripheral vascular system 747.60
      gastrointestinal 747.61
      lower limb 747.64

☑ Additional Digit Required — Refer to the Tabular List for Digit Selection   ▽ **Subterms under main terms may continue to next column or page**

180 — Volume 2 · October 2010   ▶◀ Revised Text   ● New Line   ▲ Revised Code   **2011 ICD-9-CM**

Malposition — *continued*
  congenital — *continued*
    peripheral vascular system — *continued*
      renal 747.62
      specified NEC 747.69
      spinal 747.82
      upper limb 747.63
    pituitary (gland) 759.2
    respiratory organ or system NEC 748.9
    rib (cage) 756.3
      supernumerary in cervical region 756.2
    scapula 755.59
    shoulder 755.59
    spinal cord 742.59
    spine 756.19
    spleen 759.0
    sternum 756.3
    stomach 750.7
    symphysis pubis 755.69
    testis (undescended) 752.51
    thymus (gland) 759.2
    thyroid (gland) (tissue) 759.2
      cartilage 748.3
    toe(s) 755.66
      supernumerary 755.02
    tongue 750.19
    trachea 748.3
    uterus 752.39 ▲
    vein(s) (peripheral) NEC (*see also* Malposition, congenital, peripheral vascular system) 747.60
      great 747.49
      portal 747.49
      pulmonary 747.49
    vena cava (inferior) (superior) 747.49
  device, implant, or graft — *see* Complications, mechanical
  fetus NEC (*see also* Presentation, fetal) 652.9 ☑
    with successful version 652.1 ☑
    affecting fetus or newborn 763.1
    before labor, affecting fetus or newborn 761.7
    causing obstructed labor 660.0 ☑
    in multiple gestation (one fetus or more) 652.6 ☑
      with locking 660.5 ☑
      causing obstructed labor 660.0 ☑
  gallbladder (*see also* Disease, gallbladder) 575.8
  gastrointestinal tract 569.89
    congenital 751.8
  heart (*see also* Malposition, congenital, heart) 746.87
  intestine 569.89
    congenital 751.5
  pelvic organs or tissues
    in pregnancy or childbirth 654.4 ☑
      affecting fetus or newborn 763.89
      causing obstructed labor 660.2 ☑
        affecting fetus or newborn 763.1
  placenta — *see* Placenta, previa
  stomach 537.89
    congenital 750.7
  tooth, teeth 524.30
    with impaction 520.6
  uterus (acquired) (acute) (adherent) (any degree) (asymptomatic) (postinfectional) (postpartal, old) 621.6
    anteflexion or anteversion (*see also* Anteversion, uterus) 621.6
      congenital 752.39 ▲
    flexion 621.6
      lateral (*see also* Lateroversion, uterus) 621.6
    in pregnancy or childbirth 654.4 ☑
      affecting fetus or newborn 763.89
      causing obstructed labor 660.2 ☑
        affecting fetus or newborn 763.1
    inversion 621.6
    lateral (flexion) (version) (*see also* Lateroversion, uterus) 621.6
    lateroflexion (*see also* Lateroversion, uterus) 621.6

Malposition — *continued*
  uterus — *continued*
    lateroversion (*see also* Lateroversion, uterus) 621.6
    retroflexion or retroversion (*see also* Retroversion, uterus) 621.6
Malposture 729.90
Malpresentation, fetus — *see also* Presentation, fetal 652.9 ☑
Malrotation
  cecum 751.4
  colon 751.4
  intestine 751.4
  kidney 753.3
MALT (mucosa associated lymphoid tissue) 200.3 ☑
Malta fever — *see also* Brucellosis 023.9
Maltosuria 271.3
Maltreatment (of)
  adult 995.80
    emotional 995.82
    multiple forms 995.85
    neglect (nutritional) 995.84
    physical 995.81
    psychological 995.82
    sexual 995.83
  child 995.50
    emotional 995.51
    multiple forms 995.59
    neglect (nutritional) 995.52
    physical 995.54
      shaken infant syndrome 995.55
    psychological 995.51
    sexual 995.53
  spouse (*see also* Maltreatment, adult) 995.80
Malt workers' lung 495.4
Malum coxae senilis 715.25
Malunion, fracture 733.81
Mammillitis — *see also* Mastitis 611.0
  puerperal, postpartum 675.2 ☑
Mammitis — *see also* Mastitis 611.0
  puerperal, postpartum 675.2 ☑
Mammographic
  calcification 793.89
  calculus 793.89
  microcalcification 793.81
Mammoplasia 611.1
Management
  contraceptive V25.9
    specified type NEC V25.8
  procreative V26.9
    specified type NEC V26.89
Mangled NEC — *see also* nature and site of injury 959.9
Mania (monopolar) — *see also* Psychosis, affective 296.0 ☑
  alcoholic (acute) (chronic) 291.9
  Bell's — *see* Mania, chronic
  chronic 296.0 ☑
    recurrent episode 296.1 ☑
    single episode 296.0 ☑
  compulsive 300.3
  delirious (acute) 296.0 ☑
    recurrent episode 296.1 ☑
    single episode 296.0 ☑
  epileptic (*see also* Epilepsy) 345.4 ☑
  hysterical 300.10
  inhibited 296.89
  puerperal (after delivery) 296.0 ☑
    recurrent episode 296.1 ☑
    single episode 296.0 ☑
  recurrent episode 296.1 ☑
  senile 290.8
  single episode 296.0 ☑
  stupor 296.89
  stuporous 296.89
  unproductive 296.89
Manic-depressive insanity, psychosis, reaction, or syndrome — *see also* Psychosis, affective 296.80
  circular (alternating) 296.7
    currently
      depressed 296.5 ☑
      episode unspecified 296.7
      hypomanic, previously depressed 296.4 ☑

Manic-depressive insanity, psychosis, reaction, or syndrome — *see also* Psychosis, affective — *continued*
  circular — *continued*
    currently — *continued*
      manic 296.4 ☑
      mixed 296.6 ☑
    depressed (type), depressive 296.2 ☑
      atypical 296.82
      recurrent episode 296.3 ☑
      single episode 296.2 ☑
    hypomanic 296.0 ☑
      recurrent episode 296.1 ☑
      single episode 296.0 ☑
    manic 296.0 ☑
      atypical 296.81
      recurrent episode 296.1 ☑
      single episode 296.0 ☑
    mixed NEC 296.89
    perplexed 296.89
    stuporous 296.89
Manifestations, rheumatoid
  lungs 714.81
  pannus — *see* Arthritis, rheumatoid
  subcutaneous nodules — *see* Arthritis, rheumatoid
Mankowsky's syndrome (familial dysplastic osteopathy) 731.2
Mannoheptulosuria 271.8
Mannosidosis 271.8
Manson's
  disease (schistosomiasis) 120.1
  pyosis (pemphigus contagiosus) 684
  schistosomiasis 120.1
Mansonellosis 125.5
Manual — *see* condition
Maple bark disease 495.6
Maple bark-strippers' lung 495.6
Maple syrup (urine) disease or syndrome 270.3
Marable's syndrome (celiac artery compression) 447.4
Marasmus 261
  brain 331.9
  due to malnutrition 261
  intestinal 569.89
  nutritional 261
  senile 797
  tuberculous NEC (*see also* Tuberculosis) 011.9 ☑
Marble
  bones 756.52
  skin 782.61
Marburg disease (virus) 078.89
March
  foot 733.94
  hemoglobinuria 283.2
Marchand multiple nodular hyperplasia (liver) 571.5
Marchesani (-Weill) syndrome (brachymorphism and ectopia lentis) 759.89
Marchiafava (-Bignami) disease or syndrome 341.8
Marchiafava-Micheli syndrome (paroxysmal nocturnal hemoglobinuria) 283.2
Marcus Gunn's syndrome (jaw-winking syndrome) 742.8
Marfan's
  congenital syphilis 090.49
  disease 090.49
  syndrome (arachnodactyly) 759.82
    meaning congenital syphilis 090.49
    with luxation of lens 090.49 [379.32]
Marginal
  implantation, placenta — *see* Placenta, previa
  placenta — *see* Placenta, previa
  sinus (hemorrhage) (rupture) 641.2 ☑
    affecting fetus or newborn 762.1
Marie's
  cerebellar ataxia 334.2
  syndrome (acromegaly) 253.0
Marie-Bamberger disease or syndrome (hypertrophic) (pulmonary) (secondary) 731.2
  idiopathic (acropachyderma) 757.39

Marie-Bamberger disease or syndrome — *continued*
  primary (acropachyderma) 757.39
Marie-Charcôt-Tooth neuropathic atrophy, muscle 356.1
Marie-Strümpell arthritis or disease (ankylosing spondylitis) 720.0
Marihuana, marijuana
  abuse (*see also* Abuse, drugs, nondependent) 305.2 ☑
  dependence (*see also* Dependence) 304.3 ☑
Marion's disease (bladder neck obstruction) 596.0
Marital conflict V61.10
Mark
  port wine 757.32
  raspberry 757.32
  strawberry 757.32
  stretch 701.3
  tattoo 709.09
Maroteaux-Lamy syndrome (mucopolysaccharidosis VI) 277.5
Marriage license examination V70.3
Marrow (bone)
  arrest 284.9
  megakaryocytic 287.30
  poor function 289.9
Marseilles fever 082.1
Marshall's (hidrotic) **ectodermal dysplasia** 757.31
Marsh's disease (exophthalmic goiter) 242.0 ☑
Marsh fever — *see also* Malaria 084.6
Martin-Albright syndrome (pseudohypoparathyroidism) 275.49
Martin's disease 715.27
Martorell-Fabre syndrome (pulseless disease) 446.7
Masculinization, female, with adrenal hyperplasia 255.2
Masculinovoblastoma (M8670/0) 220
Masochism 302.83
Masons' lung 502
Mass
  abdominal 789.3 ☑
  anus 787.99
  bone 733.90
  breast 611.72
  cheek 784.2
  chest 786.6
  cystic — *see* Cyst
  ear 388.8
  epigastric 789.3 ☑
  eye 379.92
  female genital organ 625.8
  gum 784.2
  head 784.2
  intracranial 784.2
  joint 719.60
    ankle 719.67
    elbow 719.62
    foot 719.67
    hand 719.64
    hip 719.65
    knee 719.66
    multiple sites 719.69
    pelvic region 719.65
    shoulder (region) 719.61
    specified site NEC 719.68
    wrist 719.63
  kidney (*see also* Disease, kidney) 593.9
  lung 786.6
  lymph node 785.6
  malignant (M8000/3) — *see* Neoplasm, by site, malignant
  mediastinal 786.6
  mouth 784.2
  muscle (limb) 729.89
  neck 784.2
  nose or sinus 784.2
  palate 784.2
  pelvis, pelvic 789.3 ☑
  penis 607.89
  perineum 625.8
  rectum 787.99
  scrotum 608.89

☑ Additional Digit Required — Refer to the Tabular List for Digit Selection   ⌐ Subterms under main terms may continue to next column or page

2011 ICD-9-CM   ▶◀ Revised Text   ● New Line   ▲ Revised Code   October 2010 · Volume 2 — 181

Mass — continued
skin 782.2
specified organ NEC — see Disease of specified organ or site
splenic 789.2
substernal 786.6
thyroid (see also Goiter) 240.9
superficial (localized) 782.2
testes 608.89
throat 784.2
tongue 784.2
umbilicus 789.3 ☑
uterus 625.8
vagina 625.8
vulva 625.8
Massive — see condition
Mastalgia 611.71
psychogenic 307.89
Mast cell
disease 757.33
systemic (M9741/3) 202.6 ☑
leukemia (M9900/3) 207.8 ☑
sarcoma (M9742/3) 202.6 ☑
tumor (M9740/1) 238.5
malignant (M9740/3) 202.6 ☑
Masters-Allen syndrome 620.6
Mastitis (acute) (adolescent) (diffuse) (interstitial) (lobular) (nonpuerperal) (nonsuppurative) (parenchymatous) (phlegmonous) (simple) (subacute) (suppurative) 611.0
chronic (cystic) (fibrocystic) 610.1
cystic 610.1
Schimmelbusch's type 610.1
fibrocystic 610.1
infective 611.0
lactational 675.2 ☑
lymphangitis 611.0
neonatal (noninfective) 778.7
infective 771.5
periductal 610.4
plasma cell 610.4
puerperalis 675.2 ☑
puerperal, postpartum, (interstitial) (nonpurulent) (parenchymatous) 675.2 ☑
purulent 675.1 ☑
stagnation 676.2 ☑
retromammary 611.0
puerperal, postpartum 675.1 ☑
submammary 611.0
puerperal, postpartum 675.1 ☑
Mastocytoma (M9740/1) 238.5
malignant (M9740/3) 202.6 ☑
Mastocytosis 757.33
malignant (M9741/3) 202.6 ☑
systemic (M9741/3) 202.6 ☑
Mastodynia 611.71
psychogenic 307.89
Mastoid — see condition
Mastoidalgia — see also Otalgia 388.70
Mastoiditis (coalescent) (hemorrhagic) (pneumococcal) (streptococcal) (suppurative) 383.9
acute or subacute 383.00
with
Gradenigo's syndrome 383.02
petrositis 383.02
specified complication NEC 383.02
subperiosteal abscess 383.01
chronic (necrotic) (recurrent) 383.1
tuberculous (see also Tuberculosis) 015.6 ☑
Mastopathy, mastopathia 611.9
chronica cystica 610.1
diffuse cystic 610.1
estrogenic 611.89
ovarian origin 611.89
Mastoplasia 611.1
Masturbation 307.9
Maternal condition, affecting fetus or newborn
acute yellow atrophy of liver 760.8
albuminuria 760.1
anesthesia or analgesia 763.5
blood loss 762.1
chorioamnionitis 762.7

Maternal condition, affecting fetus or newborn — continued
circulatory disease, chronic (conditions classifiable to 390–459, 745–747) 760.3
congenital heart disease (conditions classifiable to 745–746) 760.3
cortical necrosis of kidney 760.1
death 761.6
diabetes mellitus 775.0
manifest diabetes in the infant 775.1
disease NEC 760.9
circulatory system, chronic (conditions classifiable to 390–459, 745–747) 760.3
genitourinary system (conditions classifiable to 580–599) 760.1
respiratory (conditions classifiable to 490–519, 748) 760.3
eclampsia 760.0
hemorrhage NEC 762.1
hepatitis acute, malignant, or subacute 760.8
hyperemesis (gravidarum) 761.8
hypertension (arising during pregnancy) (conditions classifiable to 642) 760.0
infection
disease classifiable to 001-136 ☑, 760.2
genital tract NEC 760.8
urinary tract 760.1
influenza 760.2
manifest influenza in the infant 771.2
injury (conditions classifiable to 800–996) 760.5
malaria 760.2
manifest malaria in infant or fetus 771.2
malnutrition 760.4
necrosis of liver 760.8
nephritis (conditions classifiable to 580–583) 760.1
nephrosis (conditions classifiable to 581) 760.1
noxious substance transmitted via breast milk or placenta 760.70
alcohol 760.71
anticonvulsants 760.77
antifungals 760.74
anti-infective agents 760.74
antimetabolics 760.78
cocaine 760.75
"crack" 760.75
diethylstilbestrol [DES] 760.76
hallucinogenic agents 760.73
medicinal agents NEC 760.79
narcotics 760.72
obstetric anesthetic or analgesic drug 760.72
specified agent NEC 760.79
nutritional disorder (conditions classifiable to 260–269) 760.4
operation unrelated to current delivery (see also Newborn, affected by) 760.64
pre-eclampsia 760.0
pyelitis or pyelonephritis, arising during pregnancy (conditions classifiable to 590) 760.1
renal disease or failure 760.1
respiratory disease, chronic (conditions classifiable to 490–519, 748) 760.3
rheumatic heart disease (chronic) (conditions classifiable to 393–398) 760.3
rubella (conditions classifiable to 056) 760.2
manifest rubella in the infant or fetus 771.0
surgery unrelated to current delivery (see also Newborn, affected by) 760.64
to uterus or pelvic organs 760.64
syphilis (conditions classifiable to 090–097) 760.2
manifest syphilis in the infant or fetus 090.0
thrombophlebitis 760.3
toxemia (of pregnancy) 760.0
pre-eclamptic 760.0
toxoplasmosis (conditions classifiable to 130) 760.2

Maternal condition, affecting fetus or newborn — continued
toxoplasmosis — continued
manifest toxoplasmosis in the infant or fetus 771.2
transmission of chemical substance through the placenta 760.70
alcohol 760.71
anticonvulsants 760.77
antifungals 760.74
anti-infective 760.74
antimetabolics 760.78
cocaine 760.75
"crack" 760.75
diethylstilbestrol [DES] 760.76
hallucinogenic agents 760.73
narcotics 760.72
specified substance NEC 760.79
uremia 760.1
urinary tract conditions (conditions classifiable to 580–599) 760.1
vomiting (pernicious) (persistent) (vicious) 761.8
Maternity — see Delivery
Matheiu's disease (leptospiral jaundice) 100.0
Mauclaire's disease or osteochondrosis 732.3
Maxcy's disease 081.0
Maxilla, maxillary — see condition
May (-Hegglin) anomaly or syndrome 288.2
Mayaro fever 066.3
Mazoplasia 610.8
MBD (minimal brain dysfunction), child — see also Hyperkinesia 314.9
MCAD (medium chain acyl CoA dehydrogenase deficiency) 277.85
McArdle (-Schmid-Pearson) disease or syndrome (glycogenosis V) 271.0
McCune-Albright syndrome (osteitis fibrosa disseminata) 756.59
MCLS (mucocutaneous lymph node syndrome) 446.1
McQuarrie's syndrome (idiopathic familial hypoglycemia) 251.2
Measles (black) (hemorrhagic) (suppressed) 055.9
with
encephalitis 055.0
keratitis 055.71
keratoconjunctivitis 055.71
otitis media 055.2
pneumonia 055.1
complication 055.8
specified type NEC 055.79
encephalitis 055.0
French 056.9
German 056.9
keratitis 055.71
keratoconjunctivitis 055.71
liberty 056.9
otitis media 055.2
pneumonia 055.1
specified complications NEC 055.79
vaccination, prophylactic (against) V04.2
Meatitis, urethral — see also Urethritis 597.89
Meat poisoning — see Poisoning, food
Meatus, meatal — see condition
Meat-wrappers' asthma 506.9
Meckel's
diverticulitis 751.0
diverticulum (displaced) (hypertrophic) 751.0
Meconium
aspiration 770.11
with
pneumonia 770.12
pneumonitis 770.12
respiratory symptoms 770.12
below vocal cords 770.11
with respiratory symptoms 770.12
syndrome 770.12
delayed passage in newborn 777.1
ileus 777.1
due to cystic fibrosis 277.01
in liquor 792.3
noted during delivery 656.8 ☑
insufflation 770.11

Meconium — continued
insufflation — continued
with respiratory symptoms 770.12
obstruction
fetus or newborn 777.1
in mucoviscidosis 277.01
passage of 792.3
noted during delivery 763.84
peritonitis 777.6
plug syndrome (newborn) NEC 777.1
staining 779.84
Median — see also condition
arcuate ligament syndrome 447.4
bar (prostate) 600.90
with
other lower urinary tract symptoms (LUTS) 600.91
urinary
obstruction 600.91
retention 600.91
rhomboid glossitis 529.2
vesical orifice 600.90
with
other lower urinary tract symptoms (LUTS) 600.91
urinary
obstruction 600.91
retention 600.91
Mediastinal shift 793.2
Mediastinitis (acute) (chronic) 519.2
actinomycotic 039.8
syphilitic 095.8
tuberculous (see also Tuberculosis) 012.8 ☑
Mediastinopericarditis — see also Pericarditis 423.9
acute 420.90
chronic 423.8
rheumatic 393
rheumatic, chronic 393
Mediastinum, mediastinal — see condition
Medical services provided for — see Health, services provided because (of)
Medicine poisoning (by overdose) (wrong substance given or taken in error) 977.9
specified drug or substance — see Table of Drugs and Chemicals
Medin's disease (poliomyelitis) 045.9 ☑
Mediterranean
anemia (with other hemoglobinopathy) 282.49
disease or syndrome (hemipathic) 282.49
fever (see also Brucellosis) 023.9
familial 277.31
kala-azar 085.0
leishmaniasis 085.0
tick fever 082.1
Medulla — see condition
Medullary
cystic kidney 753.16
sponge kidney 753.17
Medullated fibers
optic (nerve) 743.57
retina 362.85
Medulloblastoma (M9470/3)
desmoplastic (M9471/3) 191.6
specified site — see Neoplasm, by site, malignant
unspecified site 191.6
Medulloepithelioma (M9501/3) — see also Neoplasm, by site, malignant
teratoid (M9502/3) — see Neoplasm, by site, malignant
Medullomyoblastoma (M9472/3)
specified site — see Neoplasm, by site, malignant
unspecified site 191.6
Meekeren-Ehlers-Danlos syndrome 756.83
Megacaryocytic — see condition
Megacolon (acquired) (functional) (not Hirschsprung's disease) 564.7
aganglionic 751.3
congenital, congenitum 751.3
Hirschsprung's (disease) 751.3
psychogenic 306.4
toxic (see also Colitis, ulcerative) 556.9
Megaduodenum 537.3

☑ Additional Digit Required — Refer to the Tabular List for Digit Selection ▽ Subterms under main terms may continue to next column or page

2011 ICD-9-CM ▶◀ Revised Text ● New Line ▲ Revised Code October 2010 · Volume 2 — 183

Megaesophagus — Meningioma

Meningioma — see also Neoplasm, meninges, benign — continued
  malignant (M9530/3) — see Neoplasm, meninges, malignant
  meningiothelial (M9531/0) — see Neoplasm, meninges, benign
  meningotheliomatous (M9531/0) — see Neoplasm, meninges, benign
  mixed (M9537/0) — see Neoplasm, meninges, benign
  multiple (M9530/1) 237.6
  papillary (M9538/1) 237.6
  psammomatous (M9533/0) — see Neoplasm, meninges, benign
  syncytial (M9531/0) — see Neoplasm, meninges, benign
  transitional (M9537/0) — see Neoplasm, meninges, benign
Meningiomatosis (diffuse) (M9530/1) 237.6
Meningism — see also Meningismus 781.6
Meningismus (infectional) (pneumococcal) 781.6
  due to serum or vaccine 997.09 [321.8]
  influenzal NEC ▶(see also Influenza)◀ 487.8
Meningitis (basal) (basic) (basilar) (brain) (cerebral) (cervical) (congestive) (diffuse) (hemorrhagic) (infantile) (membranous) (metastatic) (nonspecific) (pontine) (progressive) (simple) (spinal) (subacute) (sympathetica) (toxic) 322.9
  abacterial NEC (see also Meningitis, aseptic) 047.9
  actinomycotic 039.8 [320.7]
  adenoviral 049.1
  Aerobacter aerogenes 320.82
    anaerobes (cocci) (gram-negative) (gram-positive) (mixed) (NEC) 320.81
  arbovirus NEC 066.9 [321.2]
    specified type NEC 066.8 [321.2]
  aseptic (acute) NEC 047.9
    adenovirus 049.1
    Coxsackie virus 047.0
    due to
      adenovirus 049.1
      Coxsackie virus 047.0
      ECHO virus 047.1
      enterovirus 047.9
      mumps 072.1
      poliovirus (see also Poliomyelitis) 045.2 ☑ [321.2]
    ECHO virus 047.1
    herpes (simplex) virus 054.72
      zoster 053.0
    leptospiral 100.81
    lymphocytic choriomeningitis 049.0
    noninfective 322.0
  Bacillus pyocyaneus 320.89
  bacterial NEC 320.9
    anaerobic 320.81
    gram-negative 320.82
      anaerobic 320.81
  Bacteroides (fragilis) (oralis) (melaninogenicus) 320.81
  cancerous (M8000/6) 198.4
  candidal 112.83
  carcinomatous (M8010/6) 198.4
  caseous (see also Tuberculosis, meninges) 013.0 ☑
  cerebrospinal (acute) (chronic) (diplococcal) (endemic) (epidemic) (fulminant) (infectious) (malignant) (meningococcal) (sporadic) 036.0
    carrier (suspected) of V02.59
  chronic NEC 322.2
  clear cerebrospinal fluid NEC 322.0
  Clostridium (haemolyticum) (novyi) NEC 320.81
  coccidioidomycosis 114.2
  Coxsackie virus 047.0
  cryptococcal 117.5 [321.0]
  diplococcal 036.0
    gram-negative 036.0
    gram-positive 320.1
  Diplococcus pneumoniae 320.1

Meningitis — continued
  due to
    actinomycosis 039.8 [320.7]
    adenovirus 049.1
    coccidiomycosis 114.2
    enterovirus 047.9
      specified NEC 047.8
    histoplasmosis (see also Histoplasmosis) 115.91
    Listerosis 027.0 [320.7]
    Lyme disease 088.81 [320.7]
    moniliasis 112.83
    mumps 072.1
    neurosyphilis 094.2
    nonbacterial organisms NEC 321.8
    oidiomycosis 112.83
    poliovirus (see also Poliomyelitis) 045.2 ☑ [321.2]
    preventive immunization, inoculation, or vaccination 997.09 [321.8]
    sarcoidosis 135 [321.4]
    sporotrichosis 117.1 [321.1]
    syphilis 094.2
      acute 091.81
      congenital 090.42
      secondary 091.81
    trypanosomiasis (see also Trypanosomiasis) 086.9 [321.3]
    whooping cough 033.9 [320.7]
  ECHO virus 047.1
  E. coli 320.82
  endothelial-leukocytic, benign, recurrent 047.9
  Enterobacter aerogenes 320.82
  enteroviral 047.9
    specified type NEC 047.8
  enterovirus 047.9
    specified NEC 047.8
  eosinophilic 322.1
  epidemic NEC 036.0
  Escherichia coli (E. coli) 320.82
  Eubacterium 320.81
  fibrinopurulent NEC 320.9
    specified type NEC 320.89
  Friedländer (bacillus) 320.82
  fungal NEC 117.9 [321.1]
  Fusobacterium 320.81
  gonococcal 098.82
  gram-negative bacteria NEC 320.82
    anaerobic 320.81
    cocci 036.0
      specified NEC 320.82
  gram-negative cocci NEC 036.0
    specified NEC 320.82
  gram-positive cocci NEC 320.9
  herpes (simplex) virus 054.72
    zoster 053.0
  H. influenzae 320.0
  infectious NEC 320.9
  influenzal 320.0
  Klebsiella pneumoniae 320.82
  late effect — see Late, effect, meningitis
  leptospiral (aseptic) 100.81
  Listerella (monocytogenes) 027.0 [320.7]
  Listeria monocytogenes 027.0 [320.7]
  lymphocytic (acute) (benign) (serous) 049.0
    choriomeningitis virus 049.0
  meningococcal (chronic) 036.0
  Mima polymorpha 320.82
  Mollaret's 047.9
  monilial 112.83
  mumps (virus) 072.1
  mycotic NEC 117.9 [321.1]
  Neisseria 036.0
  neurosyphilis 094.2
  nonbacterial NEC (see also Meningitis, aseptic) 047.9
  nonpyogenic NEC 322.0
  oidiomycosis 112.83
  ossificans 349.2
  Peptococcus 320.81
  Peptostreptococcus 320.81
  pneumococcal 320.1
  poliovirus (see also Poliomyelitis) 045.2 ☑ [321.2]
  Proprionibacterium 320.81

Meningitis — continued
  Proteus morganii 320.82
  Pseudomonas (aeruginosa) (pyocyaneus) 320.82
  purulent NEC 320.9
    specified organism NEC 320.89
  pyogenic NEC 320.9
    specified organism NEC 320.89
  Salmonella 003.21
  septic NEC 320.9
    specified organism NEC 320.89
  serosa circumscripta NEC 322.0
  serous NEC (see also Meningitis, aseptic) 047.9
    lymphocytic 049.0
    syndrome 348.2
  Serratia (marcescens) 320.82
  specified organism NEC 320.89
  sporadic cerebrospinal 036.0
  sporotrichosis 117.1 [321.1]
  staphylococcal 320.3
  sterile 997.09
  streptococcal (acute) 320.2
  suppurative 320.9
    specified organism NEC 320.89
  syphilitic 094.2
    acute 091.81
    congenital 090.42
    secondary 091.81
  torula 117.5 [321.0]
  traumatic (complication of injury) 958.8
  Treponema (denticola) (macrodenticum) 320.81
  trypanosomiasis 086.1 [321.3]
  tuberculous (see also Tuberculosis, meninges) 013.0 ☑
  typhoid 002.0 [320.7]
  Veillonella 320.81
  Vibrio vulnificus 320.82
  viral, virus NEC (see also Meningitis, aseptic) 047.9
  Wallgren's (see also Meningitis, aseptic) 047.9
Meningocele (congenital) (spinal) — see also Spina bifida 741.9 ☑
  acquired (traumatic) 349.2
  cerebral 742.0
  cranial 742.0
Meningocerebritis — see Meningoencephalitis
Meningococcemia (acute) (chronic) 036.2
Meningococcus, meningococcal — see also condition
  adrenalitis, hemorrhagic 036.3
  carditis 036.40
  carrier (suspected) of V02.59
  cerebrospinal fever 036.0
  encephalitis 036.1
  endocarditis 036.42
  exposure to V01.84
  infection NEC 036.9
  meningitis (cerebrospinal) 036.0
  myocarditis 036.43
  optic neuritis 036.81
  pericarditis 036.41
  septicemia (chronic) 036.2
Meningoencephalitis — see also Encephalitis 323.9
  acute NEC 048
  bacterial, purulent, pyogenic, or septic — see Meningitis
  chronic NEC 094.1
  diffuse NEC 094.1
  diphasic 063.2
  due to
    actinomycosis 039.8 [320.7]
    blastomycosis NEC (see also Blastomycosis) 116.0 [323.41]
    free-living amebae 136.29
    Listeria monocytogenes 027.0 [320.7]
    Lyme disease 088.81 [320.7]
    mumps 072.2
    Naegleria (amebae) (gruberi) (organisms) 136.29
    rubella 056.01
    sporotrichosis 117.1 [321.1]

Meningoencephalitis — see also Encephalitis — continued
  due to — continued
    toxoplasmosis (acquired) 130.0
      congenital (active) 771.2 [323.41]
    Trypanosoma 086.1 [323.2]
  epidemic 036.0
  herpes 054.3
  herpetic 054.3
  H. influenzae 320.0
  infectious (acute) 048
  influenzal 320.0
  late effect — see category 326
  Listeria monocytogenes 027.0 [320.7]
  lymphocytic (serous) 049.0
  mumps 072.2
  parasitic NEC 123.9 [323.41]
  pneumococcal 320.1
  primary amebic 136.29
  rubella 056.01
  serous 048
    lymphocytic 049.0
  specific 094.2
  staphylococcal 320.3
  streptococcal 320.2
  syphilitic 094.2
  toxic NEC 989.9 [323.71]
    due to
      carbon tetrachloride (vapor) 987.8 [323.71]
      hydroxyquinoline derivatives poisoning 961.3 [323.71]
      lead 984.9 [323.71]
      mercury 985.0 [323.71]
      thallium 985.8 [323.71]
  toxoplasmosis (acquired) 130.0
  trypanosomic 086.1 [323.2]
  tuberculous (see also Tuberculosis, meninges) 013.0 ☑
  virus NEC 048
Meningoencephalocele 742.0
  syphilitic 094.89
  congenital 090.49
Meningoencephalomyelitis — see also Meningoencephalitis 323.9
  acute NEC 048
    disseminated (postinfectious) 136.9 [323.61]
    postimmunization or postvaccination 323.51
  due to
    actinomycosis 039.8 [320.7]
    torula 117.5 [323.41]
    toxoplasma or toxoplasmosis (acquired) 130.0
      congenital (active) 771.2 [323.41]
  late effect — see category 326
Meningoencephalomyelopathy — see also Meningoencephalomyelitis 349.9
Meningoencephalopathy — see also Meningoencephalitis 348.39
Meningoencephalopoliomyelitis — see also Poliomyelitis, bulbar 045.0 ☑
  late effect 138
Meningomyelitis — see also Meningoencephalitis 323.9
  blastomycotic NEC (see also Blastomycosis) 116.0 [323.41]
  due to
    actinomycosis 039.8 [320.7]
    blastomycosis (see also Blastomycosis) 116.0 [323.41]
    Meningococcus 036.0
    sporotrichosis 117.1 [323.41]
    torula 117.5 [323.41]
  late effect — see category 326
  lethargic 049.8
  meningococcal 036.0
  syphilitic 094.2
  tuberculous (see also Tuberculosis, meninges) 013.0 ☑
Meningomyelocele — see also Spina bifida 741.9 ☑
  syphilitic 094.89
Meningomyeloneuritis — see Meningoencephalitis

☑ **Additional Digit Required** — Refer to the Tabular List for Digit Selection

🔻 **Subterms under main terms may continue to next column or page**

184 — Volume 2 · October 2010
  ▶◀ **Revised Text**
  ● **New Line**
  ▲ **Revised Code**
  2011 ICD-9-CM

Meningoradiculitis — *see* Meningitis
Meningovascular — *see* condition
Meniscocytosis 282.60
Menkes' syndrome — *see* Syndrome, Menkes'
Menolipsis 626.0
Menometrorrhagia 626.2
Menopause, menopausal (symptoms) (syndrome) 627.2
  arthritis (any site) NEC 716.3 ☑
  artificial 627.4
  bleeding 627.0
  crisis 627.2
  depression (*see also* Psychosis, affective) 296.2 ☑
    agitated 296.2 ☑
      recurrent episode 296.3 ☑
      single episode 296.2 ☑
    psychotic 296.2 ☑
      recurrent episode 296.3 ☑
      single episode 296.2 ☑
    recurrent episode 296.3 ☑
    single episode 296.2 ☑
  melancholia (*see also* Psychosis, affective) 296.2 ☑
    recurrent episode 296.3 ☑
    single episode 296.2 ☑
  paranoid state 297.2
  paraphrenia 297.2
  postsurgical 627.4
  premature 256.31
    postirradiation 256.2
    postsurgical 256.2
  psychoneurosis 627.2
  psychosis NEC 298.8
  surgical 627.4
  toxic polyarthritis NEC 716.39
Menorrhagia (primary) 626.2
  climacteric 627.0
  menopausal 627.0
  postclimacteric 627.1
  postmenopausal 627.1
  preclimacteric 627.0
  premenopausal 627.0
  puberty (menses retained) 626.3
Menorrhalgia 625.3
Menoschesis 626.8
Menostaxis 626.2
Menses, retention 626.8
Menstrual — *see also* Menstruation
  cycle, irregular 626.4
  disorders NEC 626.9
  extraction V25.3
  fluid, retained 626.8
  molimen 625.4
  period, normal V65.5
  regulation V25.3
Menstruation
  absent 626.0
  anovulatory 628.0
  delayed 626.8
  difficult 625.3
  disorder 626.9
    psychogenic 306.52
    specified NEC 626.8
  during pregnancy 640.8 ☑
  excessive 626.2
  frequent 626.2
  infrequent 626.1
  irregular 626.4
  latent 626.8
  membranous 626.8
  painful (primary) (secondary) 625.3
    psychogenic 306.52
  passage of clots 626.2
  precocious 259.1
  protracted 626.8
  retained 626.8
  retrograde 626.8
  scanty 626.1
  suppression 626.8
  vicarious (nasal) 625.8
Mentagra — *see also* Sycosis 704.8
Mental — *see also* condition
  deficiency (*see also* Retardation, mental) 319
  deterioration (*see also* Psychosis) 298.9
  disorder (*see also* Disorder, mental) 300.9

Mental — *see also* condition — *continued*
  exhaustion 300.5
  insufficiency (congenital) (*see also* Retardation, mental) 319
  observation without need for further medical care NEC V71.09
  retardation (*see also* Retardation, mental) 319
  subnormality (*see also* Retardation, mental) 319
    mild 317
    moderate 318.0
    profound 318.2
    severe 318.1
  upset (*see also* Disorder, mental) 300.9
Meralgia paresthetica 355.1
Mercurial — *see* condition
Mercurialism NEC 985.0
Merergasia 300.9
Merkel cell tumor — *see* Carcinoma, Merkel cell
Merocele — *see also* Hernia, femoral 553.00
Meromelia 755.4
  lower limb 755.30
    intercalary 755.32
      femur 755.34
        tibiofibular (complete) (incomplete) 755.33
      fibula 755.37
      metatarsal(s) 755.38
      tarsal(s) 755.38
      tibia 755.36
      tibiofibular 755.35
    terminal (complete) (partial) (transverse) 755.31
      longitudinal 755.32
        metatarsal(s) 755.38
        phalange(s) 755.39
        tarsal(s) 755.38
      transverse 755.31
  upper limb 755.20
    intercalary 755.22
      carpal(s) 755.28
      humeral 755.24
        radioulnar (complete) (incomplete) 755.23
      metacarpal(s) 755.28
      phalange(s) 755.29
      radial 755.26
      radioulnar 755.25
      ulnar 755.27
    terminal (complete) (partial) (transverse) 755.21
      longitudinal 755.22
        carpal(s) 755.28
        metacarpal(s) 755.28
        phalange(s) 755.29
      transverse 755.21
Merosmia 781.1
MERRF syndrome (myoclonus with epilepsy and with ragged red fibers) 277.87
Merycism — *see also* Vomiting
  psychogenic 307.53
Merzbacher-Pelizaeus disease 330.0
Mesaortitis — *see* Aortitis
Mesarteritis — *see* Arteritis
Mesencephalitis — *see also* Encephalitis 323.9
  late effect — *see* category 326
Mesenchymoma (M8990/1) — *see also* Neoplasm, connective tissue, uncertain behavior
  benign (M8990/0) — *see* Neoplasm, connective tissue, benign
  malignant (M8990/3) — *see* Neoplasm, connective tissue, malignant
Mesenteritis
  retractile 567.82
  sclerosing 567.82
Mesentery, mesenteric — *see* condition
Mesiodens, mesiodentes 520.1
  causing crowding 524.31
Mesio-occlusion 524.23
Mesocardia (with asplenia) 746.87
Mesocolon — *see* condition
Mesonephroma (malignant) (M9110/3) — *see also* Neoplasm, by site, malignant

Mesonephroma — *see also* Neoplasm, by site, malignant — *continued*
  benign (M9110/0) — *see* Neoplasm, by site, benign
Mesophlebitis — *see* Phlebitis
Mesostromal dysgenesis 743.51
Mesothelioma (malignant) (M9050/3) — *see also* Neoplasm, by site, malignant
  benign (M9050/0) — *see* Neoplasm, by site, benign
  biphasic type (M9053/3) (*see also* Neoplasm, by site, malignant)
    benign (M9053/0) — *see* Neoplasm, by site, benign
  epithelioid (M9052/3) (*see also* Neoplasm, by site, malignant)
    benign (M9052/0) — *see* Neoplasm, by site, benign
  fibrous (M9051/3) (*see also* Neoplasm, by site, malignant)
    benign (M9051/0) — *see* Neoplasm, by site, benign
Metabolic syndrome 277.7
Metabolism disorder 277.9
  specified type NEC 277.89
Metagonimiasis 121.5
Metagonimus infestation (small intestine) 121.5
Metal
  pigmentation (skin) 709.00
  polishers' disease 502
Metalliferous miners' lung 503
Metamorphopsia 368.14
Metaplasia
  bone, in skin 709.3
  breast 611.89
  cervix — *omit code*
  endometrium (squamous) 621.8
  esophagus 530.85
  intestinal, of gastric mucosa 537.89
  kidney (pelvis) (squamous) (*see also* Disease, renal) 593.89
  myelogenous 289.89
  myeloid 289.89
    agnogenic 238.76
    megakaryocytic 238.76
  spleen 289.59
  squamous cell
    amnion 658.8 ☑
    bladder 596.8
    cervix — *see* condition
    trachea 519.19
    tracheobronchial tree 519.19
    uterus 621.8
      cervix — *see* condition
Metastasis, metastatic
  abscess — *see* Abscess
  calcification 275.40
  cancer, neoplasm, or disease
    from specified site (M8000/3) — *see* Neoplasm, by site, malignant
    to specified site (M8000/6) — *see* Neoplasm, by site, secondary
  deposits (in) (M8000/6) — *see* Neoplasm, by site, secondary
  mesentery of neuroendocrine tumor 209.71
  pneumonia 038.8 [484.8]
  spread (to) (M8000/6) — *see* Neoplasm, by site, secondary
Metatarsalgia 726.70
  anterior 355.6
  due to Freiberg's disease 732.5
  Morton's 355.6
Metatarsus, metatarsal — *see also* condition
  abductus valgus (congenital) 754.60
  adductus varus (congenital) 754.53
    primus varus 754.52
  valgus (adductus) (congenital) 754.60
  varus (abductus) (congenital) 754.53
    primus 754.52
Methadone use 304.00
Methemoglobinemia 289.7
  acquired (with sulfhemoglobinemia) 289.7
  congenital 289.7
  enzymatic 289.7
  Hb-M disease 289.7

Methemoglobinemia — *continued*
  hereditary 289.7
  toxic 289.7
Methemoglobinuria — *see also* Hemoglobinuria 791.2
Methicillin
  resistant staphyloccocus aureus (MRSA) 041.12
    colonization V02.54
    personal history of V12.04
  susceptible staphylococcus aureus (MSSA) 041.11
    colonization V02.53
Methioninemia 270.4
Metritis (catarrhal) (septic) (suppurative) — *see also* Endometritis 615.9
  blennorrhagic 098.16
    chronic or duration of 2 months or over 098.36
  cervical (*see also* Cervicitis) 616.0
  gonococcal 098.16
    chronic or duration of 2 months or over 098.36
  hemorrhagic 626.8
  puerperal, postpartum, childbirth 670.1 ☑
    septic 670.2 ☑
  tuberculous (*see also* Tuberculosis) 016.7 ☑
Metropathia hemorrhagica 626.8
Metroperitonitis — *see also* Peritonitis, pelvic, female 614.5
Metrorrhagia 626.6
  arising during pregnancy — *see* Hemorrhage, pregnancy
  postpartum NEC 666.2 ☑
  primary 626.6
  psychogenic 306.59
  puerperal 666.2 ☑
Metrorrhexis — *see* Rupture, uterus
Metrosalpingitis — *see also* Salpingo-oophoritis 614.2
Metrostaxis 626.6
Metrovaginitis — *see also* Endometritis 615.9
  gonococcal (acute) 098.16
    chronic or duration of 2 months or over 098.36
Mexican fever — *see* Typhus, Mexican
Meyenburg-Altherr-Uehlinger syndrome 733.99
Meyer-Schwickerath and Weyers syndrome (dysplasia oculodentodigitalis) 759.89
Meynert's amentia (nonalcoholic) 294.0
  alcoholic 291.1
Mibelli's disease 757.39
Mice, joint — *see also* Loose, body, joint 718.1 ☑
  knee 717.6
Micheli-Rietti syndrome (thalassemia minor) 282.49
Michotte's syndrome 721.5
Micrencephalon, micrencephaly 742.1
Microalbuminuria 791.0
Microaneurysm, retina 362.14
  diabetic 250.5 ☑ [362.01]
    due to secondary diabetes 249.5 ☑ [362.01]
Microangiopathy 443.9
  diabetic (peripheral) 250.7 ☑ [443.81]
    due to secondary diabetes 249.7 ☑ [443.81]
    retinal 250.5 ☑ [362.01]
      due to secondary diabetes 249.5 ☑ [362.01]
  peripheral 443.9
    diabetic 250.7 ☑ [443.81]
      due to secondary diabetes 249.7 ☑ [443.81]
  retinal 362.18
    diabetic 250.5 ☑ [362.01]
      due to secondary diabetes 249.5 ☑ [362.01]
  thrombotic 446.6
    Moschcowitz's (thrombotic thrombocytopenic purpura) 446.6
Microcalcification, mammographic 793.81
Microcephalus, microcephalic, microcephaly 742.1

☑ **Additional Digit Required** — Refer to the Tabular List for Digit Selection   ▽ **Subterms under main terms may continue to next column or page**

2011 ICD-9-CM   ▶◀ Revised Text   ● New Line   ▲ Revised Code   October 2010 · Volume 2 — 185

Microcephalus, microcephalic, microcephaly — *continued*
  due to toxoplasmosis (congenital) 771.2
Microcheilia 744.82
Microcolon (congenital) 751.5
Microcornea (congenital) 743.41
Microcytic — *see* condition
Microdeletions NEC 758.33
Microdontia 520.2
Microdrepanocytosis (thalassemia-Hb-S disease) 282.49
Microembolism
  atherothrombotic — *see* Atheroembolism
  retina 362.33
Microencephalon 742.1
Microfilaria streptocerca infestation 125.3
Microgastria (congenital) 750.7
Microgenia 524.06
Microgenitalia (congenital) 752.89
  penis 752.64
Microglioma (M9710/3)
  specified site — *see* Neoplasm, by site, malignant
  unspecified site 191.9
Microglossia (congenital) 750.16
Micrognathia, micrognathism (congenital) 524.00
  mandibular 524.04
    alveolar 524.74
  maxillary 524.03
    alveolar 524.73
Microgyria (congenital) 742.2
Microinfarct, heart — *see also* Insufficiency, coronary 411.89
Microlithiasis, alveolar, pulmonary 516.2
Micromastia 611.82
Micromyelia (congenital) 742.59
Micropenis 752.64
Microphakia (congenital) 743.36
Microphthalmia (congenital) — *see also* Microphthalmos 743.10
Microphthalmos (congenital) 743.10
  associated with eye and adnexal anomalies NEC 743.12
  due to toxoplasmosis (congenital) 771.2
  isolated 743.11
  simple 743.11
  syndrome 759.89
Micropsia 368.14
Microsporidiosis 136.8
Microsporon furfur infestation 111.0
Microsporosis — *see also* Dermatophytosis 110.9
  nigra 111.1
Microstomia (congenital) 744.84
Microthelia 757.6
Microthromboembolism — *see* Embolism
Microtia (congenital) (external ear) 744.23
Microtropia 378.34
Microvillus inclusion disease (MVD) 751.5 ●
Micturition
  disorder NEC 788.69
    psychogenic 306.53
  frequency 788.41
    psychogenic 306.53
  nocturnal 788.43
  painful 788.1
    psychogenic 306.53
Middle
  ear — *see* condition
  lobe (right) syndrome 518.0
Midplane — *see* condition
Miescher's disease 709.3
  cheilitis 351.8
  granulomatosis disciformis 709.3
Miescher-Leder syndrome or granulomatosis 709.3
Mieten's syndrome 759.89

Migraine (idiopathic) 346.9 ☑

Note — The following fifth digit subclassification is for use with category 346:

0   *without mention of intractable migraine without mention of status migrainosus*

1   *with intractable migraine, so stated, without mention of status migrainosus*

2   *without mention of intractable migraine with status migrainosus*

3   *with intractable migraine, so stated, with status migrainosus*

  with aura (acute-onset) (without headache) (prolonged) (typical) 346.0 ☑
  without aura 346.1 ☑
    chronic 346.7 ☑
    transformed 346.7 ☑
  abdominal (syndrome) 346.2 ☑
  allergic (histamine) 346.2 ☑
  atypical 346.8 ☑
  basilar 346.0 ☑
  chronic without aura 346.7 ☑
  classic(al) 346.0 ☑
  common 346.1 ☑
  hemiplegic 346.3 ☑
    familial 346.3 ☑
    sporadic 346.3 ☑
  lower-half 339.00
  menstrual 346.4 ☑
  menstrually related 346.4 ☑
  ophthalmic 346.8 ☑
  ophthalmoplegic 346.2 ☑
  premenstrual 346.4 ☑
  pure menstrual 346.4 ☑
  retinal 346.0 ☑
  specified form NEC 346.8 ☑
  transformed without aura 346.7 ☑
  variant 346.2 ☑
Migrant, social V60.0
Migratory, migrating — *see also* condition
  person V60.0
  testis, congenital 752.52
Mikulicz's disease or syndrome (dryness of mouth, absent or decreased lacrimation) 527.1
Milian atrophia blanche 701.3
Miliaria (crystallina) (rubra) (tropicalis) 705.1
  apocrine 705.82
Miliary — *see* condition
Milium — *see also* Cyst, sebaceous 706.2
  colloid 709.3
  eyelid 374.84
Milk
  crust 690.11
  excess secretion 676.6 ☑
  fever, female 672.0 ☑
  poisoning 988.8
  retention 676.2 ☑
  sickness 988.8
  spots 423.1
Milkers' nodes 051.1
Milk-leg (deep vessels) 671.4 ☑
  complicating pregnancy 671.3 ☑
  nonpuerperal 451.19
  puerperal, postpartum, childbirth 671.4 ☑
Milkman (-Looser) disease or syndrome (osteomalacia with pseudofractures) 268.2
Milky urine — *see also* Chyluria 791.1
Millar's asthma (laryngismus stridulus) 478.75
Millard-Gubler-Foville paralysis 344.89
Millard-Gubler paralysis or syndrome 344.89
Miller-Dieker syndrome 758.33
Miller's disease (osteomalacia) 268.2
Miller Fisher's syndrome 357.0
Milles' syndrome (encephalocutaneous angiomatosis) 759.6
Mills' disease 335.29
Millstone makers' asthma or lung 502
Milroy's disease (chronic hereditary edema) 757.0
Miners' — *see also* condition

Miners' — *see also* condition — *continued*
  asthma 500
  elbow 727.2
  knee 727.2
  lung 500
  nystagmus 300.89
  phthisis (*see also* Tuberculosis) 011.4 ☑
  tuberculosis (see also Tuberculosis) 011.4 ☑
Minkowski-Chauffard syndrome — *see also* Spherocytosis 282.0
Minor — *see* condition
Minor's disease 336.1
Minot's disease (hemorrhagic disease, newborn) 776.0
Minot-von Willebrand (-Jürgens) disease or syndrome (angiohemophilia) 286.4
Minus (and plus) hand (intrinsic) 736.09
Miosis (persistent) (pupil) 379.42
Mirizzi's syndrome (hepatic duct stenosis) — *see also* Obstruction, biliary 576.2
  with calculus, cholelithiasis, or stones — *see* Choledocholithiasis
Mirror writing 315.09
  secondary to organic lesion 784.69
Misadventure (prophylactic) (therapeutic) — *see also* Complications 999.9
  administration of insulin 962.3
  infusion — *see* Complications, infusion
  local applications (of fomentations, plasters, etc.) 999.9
    burn or scald — *see* Burn, by site
  medical care (early) (late) NEC 999.9
    adverse effect of drugs or chemicals — *see* Table of Drugs and Chemicals
    burn or scald — *see* Burn, by site
  radiation NEC 990
  radiotherapy NEC 990
  surgical procedure (early) (late) — *see* Complications, surgical procedure
  transfusion — *see* Complications, transfusion
  vaccination or other immunological procedure — *see* Complications, vaccination
Misanthropy 301.7
Miscarriage — *see* Abortion, spontaneous
Mischief, malicious, child — *see also* Disturbance, conduct 312.0 ☑
Misdirection
  aqueous 365.83
Mismanagement, feeding 783.3
Misplaced, misplacement
  kidney (*see also* Disease, renal) 593.0
    congenital 753.3
  organ or site, congenital NEC — *see* Malposition, congenital
Missed
  abortion 632
  delivery (at or near term) 656.4 ☑
  labor (at or near term) 656.4 ☑
Misshapen reconstructed breast 612.0
Missing — *see also* Absence
  teeth (acquired) 525.10
    congenital (see also Anodontia) 520.0
    due to
      caries 525.13
      extraction 525.10
      periodontal disease 525.12
      specified NEC 525.19
      trauma 525.11
  vertebrae (congenital) 756.13
Misuse of drugs NEC — *see also* Abuse, drug, nondependent 305.9 ☑
Mitchell's disease (erythromelalgia) 443.82
Mite(s)
  diarrhea 133.8
  grain (itch) 133.8
  hair follicle (itch) 133.8
  in sputum 133.8
Mitochondrial encephalopathy, lactic acidosis and stroke-like episodes (MELAS syndrome) 277.87
Mitochondrial neurogastrointestinal encephalopathy syndrome (MNGIE) 277.87
Mitral — *see* condition
Mittelschmerz 625.2

Mixed — *see* condition
Mljet disease (mal de Meleda) 757.39
Mobile, mobility
  cecum 751.4
  coccyx 733.99
  excessive — *see* Hypermobility
  gallbladder 751.69
  kidney 593.0
    congenital 753.3
  organ or site, congenital NEC — *see* Malposition, congenital
  spleen 289.59
Mobitz heart block (atrioventricular) 426.10
  type I (Wenckebach's) 426.13
  type II 426.12
Möbius'
  disease 346.2 ☑
  syndrome
    congenital oculofacial paralysis 352.6
    ophthalmoplegic migraine 346.2 ☑
Moeller(-Barlow) disease (infantile scurvy) 267
  glossitis 529.4
Mohr's syndrome (types I and II) 759.89
Mola destruens (M9100/1) 236.1
Molarization, premolars 520.2
Molar pregnancy 631
  hydatidiform (delivered) (undelivered) 630
Molding, head (during birth) — *omit code*
Mold(s) in vitreous 117.9
Mole (pigmented) (M8720/0) — *see also* Neoplasm, skin, benign
  blood 631
  Breus' 631
  cancerous (M8720/3) — *see* Melanoma
  carneous 631
  destructive (M9100/1) 236.1
  ectopic — *see* Pregnancy, ectopic
  fleshy 631
  hemorrhagic 631
  hydatid, hydatidiform (benign) (complicating pregnancy) (delivered) (undelivered) (*see also* Hydatidiform mole) 630
    invasive (M9100/1) 236.1
    malignant (M9100/1) 236.1
    previous, affecting management of pregnancy V23.1
  invasive (hydatidiform) (M9100/1) 236.1
  malignant
    meaning
      malignant hydatidiform mole (9100/1) 236.1
      melanoma (M8720/3) — *see* Melanoma
  nonpigmented (M8730/0) — *see* Neoplasm, skin, benign
  pregnancy NEC 631
  skin (M8720/0) — *see* Neoplasm, skin, benign
  tubal — *see* Pregnancy, tubal
  vesicular (*see also* Hydatidiform mole) 630
Molimen, molimina (menstrual) 625.4
Mollaret's meningitis 047.9
Mollities (cerebellar) (cerebral) 437.8
  ossium 268.2
Molluscum
  contagiosum 078.0
  epitheliale 078.0
  fibrosum (M8851/0) — *see* Lipoma, by site
  pendulum (M8851/0) — *see* Lipoma, by site
Mönckeberg's arteriosclerosis, degeneration, disease, or sclerosis — *see also* Arteriosclerosis, extremities 440.20
Monday fever 504
Monday morning dyspnea or asthma 504
Mondini's malformation (cochlea) 744.05
Mondor's disease (thrombophlebitis of breast) 451.89
Mongolian, mongolianism, mongolism, mongoloid 758.0
  spot 757.33
Monilethrix (congenital) 757.4
Monilia infestation — *see* Candidiasis
Moniliasis — *see also* Candidiasis
  neonatal 771.7

☑ **Additional Digit Required** — Refer to the Tabular List for Digit Selection   ▽ **Subterms under main terms may continue to next column or page**

186 — Volume 2 · October 2010   ►◄ Revised Text   ● New Line   ▲ Revised Code   2011 ICD-9-CM

Moniliasis — see also Candidiasis — continued
  vulvovaginitis 112.1
Monkeypox 059.01
Monoarthritis 716.60
  ankle 716.67
  arm 716.62
    lower (and wrist) 716.63
    upper (and elbow) 716.62
  foot (and ankle) 716.67
  forearm (and wrist) 716.63
  hand 716.64
  leg 716.66
    lower 716.66
    upper 716.65
  pelvic region (hip) (thigh) 716.65
  shoulder (region) 716.61
  specified site NEC 716.68
Monoblastic — see condition
Monochromatism (cone) (rod) 368.54
Monocytic — see condition
Monocytopenia 288.59
Monocytosis (symptomatic) 288.63
Monofixation syndrome 378.34
Monomania — see also Psychosis 298.9
Mononeuritis 355.9
  cranial nerve — see Disorder, nerve, cranial
  femoral nerve 355.2
  lateral
    cutaneous nerve of thigh 355.1
    popliteal nerve 355.3
  lower limb 355.8
    specified nerve NEC 355.79
  medial popliteal nerve 355.4
  median nerve 354.1
  multiplex 354.5
  plantar nerve 355.6
  posterior tibial nerve 355.5
  radial nerve 354.3
  sciatic nerve 355.0
  ulnar nerve 354.2
  upper limb 354.9
    specified nerve NEC 354.8
  vestibular 388.5
Mononeuropathy — see also Mononeuritis 355.9
  diabetic NEC 250.6 ☑ [355.9]
    due to secondary diabetes 249.6 ☑ [355.9]
    lower limb 250.6 ☑ [355.8]
      due to secondary diabetes 249.6 ☑ [355.8]
    upper limb 250.6 ☑ [354.9]
      due to secondary diabetes 249.6 ☑ [354.9]
  iliohypogastric nerve 355.79
  ilioinguinal nerve 355.79
  obturator nerve 355.79
  saphenous nerve 355.79
Mononucleosis, infectious 075
  with hepatitis 075 [573.1]
Monoplegia 344.5
  brain (current episode) (see also Paralysis, brain) 437.8
    fetus or newborn 767.8
  cerebral (current episode) (see also Paralysis, brain) 437.8
  congenital or infantile (cerebral) (spastic) (spinal) 343.3
  embolic (current) (see also Embolism, brain) 434.1 ☑
    late effect — see Late effect(s) (of) cerebrovascular disease
  infantile (cerebral) (spastic) (spinal) 343.3
  lower limb 344.30
    affecting
      dominant side 344.31
      nondominant side 344.32
    due to late effect of cerebrovascular accident — see Late effect(s) (of) cerebrovascular accident
  newborn 767.8
  psychogenic 306.0
    specified as conversion reaction 300.11
  thrombotic (current) (see also Thrombosis, brain) 434.0 ☑

Monoplegia — continued
  thrombotic (see also Thrombosis, brain) — continued
    late effect — see Late effect(s) (of) cerebrovascular disease
  transient 781.4
  upper limb 344.40
    affecting
      dominant side 344.41
      nondominant side 344.42
    due to late effect of cerebrovascular accident — see Late effect(s) (of) cerebrovascular accident
Monorchism, monorchidism 752.89
Monteggia's fracture (closed) 813.03
  open 813.13
Mood swings
  brief compensatory 296.99
  rebound 296.99
Mooren's ulcer (cornea) 370.07
Moore's syndrome — see also Epilepsy 345.5 ☑
Mooser bodies 081.0
Mooser-Neill reaction 081.0
Moral
  deficiency 301.7
  imbecility 301.7
Morax-Axenfeld conjunctivitis 372.03
Morbilli — see also Measles 055.9
Morbus
  anglicus, anglorum 268.0
  Beigel 111.2
  caducus (see also Epilepsy) 345.9 ☑
  caeruleus 746.89
  celiacus 579.0
  comitialis (see also Epilepsy) 345.9 ☑
  cordis (see also Disease, heart)
    valvulorum — see Endocarditis
  coxae 719.95
    tuberculous (see also Tuberculosis) 015.1 ☑
  hemorrhagicus neonatorum 776.0
  maculosus neonatorum 772.6
  renum 593.2
  senilis (see also Osteoarthrosis) 715.9 ☑
Morel-Kraepelin disease — see also Schizophrenia 295.9 ☑
Morel-Moore syndrome (hyperostosis frontalis interna) 733.3
Morel-Morgagni syndrome (hyperostosis frontalis interna) 733.3
Morgagni
  cyst, organ, hydatid, or appendage 752.89
    fallopian tube 752.11
  disease or syndrome (hyperostosis frontalis interna) 733.3
Morgagni-Adams-Stokes syndrome (syncope with heart block) 426.9
Morgagni-Stewart-Morel syndrome (hyperostosis frontalis interna) 733.3
Moria — see also Psychosis 298.9
Morning sickness 643.0 ☑
Moron 317
Morphea (guttate) (linear) 701.0
Morphine dependence — see also Dependence 304.0 ☑
Morphinism — see also Dependence 304.0 ☑
Morphinomania — see also Dependence 304.0 ☑
Morphoea 701.0
Morquio (-Brailsford) (-Ullrich) disease or syndrome (mucopolysaccharidosis IV) 277.5
  kyphosis 277.5
Morris syndrome (testicular feminization) 259.51
Morsus humanus (open wound) — see also Wound, open, by site
  skin surface intact — see Contusion
Mortification (dry) (moist) — see also Gangrene 785.4
Morton's
  disease 355.6
  foot 355.6
  metatarsalgia (syndrome) 355.6
  neuralgia 355.6

Morton's — continued
  neuroma 355.6
  syndrome (metatarsalgia) (neuralgia) 355.6
  toe 355.6
Morvan's disease 336.0
Mosaicism, mosaic (chromosomal) 758.9
  autosomal 758.5
  sex 758.81
Moschcowitz's syndrome (thrombotic thrombocytopenic purpura) 446.6
Mother yaw 102.0
Motion sickness (from travel, any vehicle) (from roundabouts or swings) 994.6
Mottled teeth (enamel) (endemic) (nonendemic) 520.3
Mottling enamel (endemic) (nonendemic) (teeth) 520.3
Mouchet's disease 732.5
Mould(s) (in vitreous) 117.9
Moulders'
  bronchitis 502
  tuberculosis (see also Tuberculosis) 011.4 ☑
Mounier-Kuhn syndrome 748.3
  with
    acute exacerbation 494.1
    bronchiectasis 494.0
      with (acute) exacerbation 494.1
  acquired 519.19
    with bronchiectasis 494.0
      with (acute) exacerbation 494.1
Mountain
  fever — see Fever, mountain
  sickness 993.2
    with polycythemia, acquired 289.0
    acute 289.0
  tick fever 066.1
Mouse, joint — see also Loose, body, joint 718.1 ☑
  knee 717.6
Mouth — see condition
Movable
  coccyx 724.71
  kidney (see also Disease, renal) 593.0
    congenital 753.3
  organ or site, congenital NEC — see Malposition, congenital
  spleen 289.59
Movement
  abnormal (dystonic) (involuntary) 781.0
  decreased fetal 655.7 ☑
  paradoxical facial 374.43
Moya Moya disease 437.5
Mozart's ear 744.29
MRSA (methicillin-resistant staphylococcus aureus) 041.12
  colonization V02.54
  personal history of V12.04
MSSA (methicillin susceptible staphylococcus aureus) 041.11
  colonization V02.53
Mucha's disease (acute parapsoriasis varioliformis) 696.2
Mucha-Haberman syndrome (acute parapsoriasis varioliformis) 696.2
Mu-chain disease 273.2
Mucinosis (cutaneous) (papular) 701.8
Mucocele
  appendix 543.9
  buccal cavity 528.9
  gallbladder (see also Disease, gallbladder) 575.3
  lacrimal sac 375.43
  orbit (eye) 376.81
  salivary gland (any) 527.6
  sinus (accessory) (nasal) 478.19
  turbinate (bone) (middle) (nasal) 478.19
  uterus 621.8
Mucocutaneous lymph node syndrome (acute) (febrile) (infantile) 446.1
Mucoenteritis 564.9
Mucolipidosis I, II, III 272.7
Mucopolysaccharidosis (types 1-6) 277.5
  cardiopathy 277.5 [425.7]
Mucormycosis (lung) 117.7
Mucosa associated lymphoid tissue (MALT) 200.3 ☑

Mucositis — see also Inflammation, by site 528.00
  cervix (ulcerative) 616.81
  due to
    antineoplastic therapy (ulcerative) 528.01
    other drugs (ulcerative) 528.02
    specified NEC 528.09
  gastrointestinal (ulcerative) 538
  nasal (ulcerative) 478.11
  necroticans agranulocytica (see also Agranulocytosis) 288.09
  ulcerative 528.00
  vagina (ulcerative) 616.81
  vulva (ulcerative) 616.81
Mucous — see also condition
  patches (syphilitic) 091.3
    congenital 090.0
Mucoviscidosis 277.00
  with meconium obstruction 277.01
Mucus
  asphyxia or suffocation (see also Asphyxia, mucus) 933.1
    newborn 770.18
  in stool 792.1
  plug (see also Asphyxia, mucus) 933.1
    aspiration, of newborn 770.17
    tracheobronchial 519.19
      newborn 770.18
Muguet 112.0
Mulberry molars 090.5
Müllerian mixed tumor (M8950/3) — see Neoplasm, by site, malignant
Multicystic kidney 753.19
Multilobed placenta — see Placenta, abnormal
Multinodular prostate 600.10
  with
    urinary
      obstruction 600.11
      retention 600.11
Multiparity V61.5
  affecting
    fetus or newborn 763.89
    management of
      labor and delivery 659.4 ☑
      pregnancy V23.3
  requiring contraceptive management (see also Contraception) V25.9
Multipartita placenta — see Placenta, abnormal
Multiple, multiplex — see also condition
  birth
    affecting fetus or newborn 761.5
    healthy liveborn — see Newborn, multiple
  digits (congenital) 755.00
    fingers 755.01
    toes 755.02
  organ or site NEC — see Accessory
  personality 300.14
  renal arteries 747.62
Mumps 072.9
  with complication 072.8
    specified type NEC 072.79
  encephalitis 072.2
  hepatitis 072.71
  meningitis (aseptic) 072.1
  meningoencephalitis 072.2
  oophoritis 072.79
  orchitis 072.0
  pancreatitis 072.3
  polyneuropathy 072.72
  vaccination, prophylactic (against) V04.6
Mumu — see also Infestation, filarial 125.9
Münchausen syndrome 301.51
Münchmeyer's disease or syndrome (exostosis luxurians) 728.11
Mural — see condition
Murmur (cardiac) (heart) (nonorganic) (organic) 785.2
  abdominal 787.5
  aortic (valve) (see also Endocarditis, aortic) 424.1
  benign — omit code
  cardiorespiratory 785.2

Murmur — continued
  diastolic — see condition
  Flint (see also Endocarditis, aortic) 424.1
  functional — omit code
  Graham Steell (pulmonic regurgitation) (see also Endocarditis, pulmonary) 424.3
  innocent — omit code
  insignificant — omit code
  midsystolic 785.2
  mitral (valve) — see Stenosis, mitral
  physiologic — see condition
  presystolic, mitral — see Insufficiency, mitral
  pulmonic (valve) (see also Endocarditis, pulmonary) 424.3
  Still's (vibratory) — omit code
  systolic (valvular) — see condition
  tricuspid (valve) — see Endocarditis, tricuspid
  undiagnosed 785.2
  valvular — see condition
  vibratory — omit code
Murri's disease (intermittent hemoglobinuria) 283.2
Muscae volitantes 379.24
Muscle, muscular — see condition
Musculoneuralgia 729.1
Mushrooming hip 718.95
Mushroom workers' (pickers') lung 495.5
Mutation
  factor V leiden 289.81
  prothrombin gene 289.81
Mutism — see also Aphasia 784.3
  akinetic 784.3
  deaf (acquired) (congenital) 389.7
  hysterical 300.11
  selective (elective) 313.23
    adjustment reaction 309.83
MVD (microvillus inclusion disease) 751.5 ●
Myà's disease (congenital dilation, colon) 751.3
Myalgia (intercostal) 729.1
  eosinophilia syndrome 710.5
  epidemic 074.1
    cervical 078.89
  psychogenic 307.89
  traumatic NEC 959.9
Myasthenia 358.00
  cordis — see Failure, heart
  gravis 358.00
    with exacerbation (acute) 358.01
    in crisis 358.01
    neonatal 775.2
    pseudoparalytica 358.00
  stomach 536.8
    psychogenic 306.4
  syndrome
    in
      botulism 005.1 [358.1]
      diabetes mellitus 250.6 ☑ [358.1]
        due to secondary diabetes 249.6 ☑ [358.1]
      hypothyroidism (see also Hypothyroidism) 244.9 [358.1]
      malignant neoplasm NEC 199.1 [358.1]
      pernicious anemia 281.0 [358.1]
      thyrotoxicosis (see also Thyrotoxicosis) 242.9 ☑ [358.1]
Myasthenic 728.87
Mycelium infection NEC 117.9
Mycetismus 988.1
Mycetoma (actinomycotic) 039.9
  bone 039.8
    mycotic 117.4
  foot 039.4
    mycotic 117.4
  madurae 039.9
    mycotic 117.4
  maduromycotic 039.9
    mycotic 117.4
  mycotic 117.4
  nocardial 039.9
Mycobacteriosis — see Mycobacterium
Mycobacterium, mycobacterial (infection) 031.9
  acid-fast (bacilli) 031.9

Mycobacterium, mycobacterial — continued
  anonymous (see also Mycobacterium, atypical) 031.9
  atypical (acid-fast bacilli) 031.9
    cutaneous 031.1
    pulmonary 031.0
      tuberculous (see also Tuberculosis, pulmonary) 011.9 ☑
    specified site NEC 031.8
  avium 031.0
    intracellulare complex bacteremia (MAC) 031.2
  balnei 031.1
  Battey 031.0
  cutaneous 031.1
  disseminated 031.2
    avium-intracellulare complex (DMAC) 031.2
  fortuitum 031.0
  intracellulare (battey bacillus) 031.0
  kakerifu 031.8
  kansasii 031.0
  kasongo 031.8
  leprae — see Leprosy
  luciflavum 031.0
  marinum 031.1
  pulmonary 031.0
    tuberculous (see also Tuberculosis, pulmonary) 011.9 ☑
  scrofulaceum 031.1
  tuberculosis (human, bovine) (see also Tuberculosis)
    avian type 031.0
  ulcerans 031.1
  xenopi 031.0
Mycosis, mycotic 117.9
  cutaneous NEC 111.9
  ear 111.8 [380.15]
  fungoides (M9700/3) 202.1 ☑
  mouth 112.0
  pharynx 117.9
  skin NEC 111.9
  stomatitis 112.0
  systemic NEC 117.9
  tonsil 117.9
  vagina, vaginitis 112.1
Mydriasis (persistent) (pupil) 379.43
Myelatelia 742.59
Myelinoclasis, perivascular, acute (postinfectious) NEC 136.9 [323.61]
  postimmunization or postvaccinal 323.51
Myelinosis, central pontine 341.8
Myelitis (ascending) (cerebellar) (childhood) (chronic) (descending) (diffuse) (disseminated) (pressure) (progressive) (spinal cord) (subacute) — see also Encephalitis 323.9
  acute (transverse) 341.20
    idiopathic 341.22
    in conditions classified elsewhere 341.21
  due to
    infection classified elsewhere 136.9 [323.42]
    specified cause NEC 323.82
    vaccination (any) 323.52
    viral diseases classified elsewhere 323.02
  herpes simplex 054.74
  herpes zoster 053.14
  late effect — see category 326
  optic neuritis in 341.0
  postchickenpox 052.2
  postimmunization 323.52
  postinfectious 136.9 [323.63]
  postvaccinal 323.52
  postvaricella 052.2
  syphilitic (transverse) 094.89
  toxic 989.9 [323.72]
  transverse 323.82
    acute 341.20
      idiopathic 341.22
      in conditions classified elsewhere 341.21
    idiopathic 341.22
  tuberculous (see also Tuberculosis) 013.6 ☑
  virus 049.9

Myeloblastic — see condition
Myelocele — see also Spina bifida 741.9 ☑
  with hydrocephalus 741.0 ☑
Myelocystocele — see also Spina bifida 741.9 ☑
Myelocytic — see condition
Myelocytoma 205.1 ☑
Myelodysplasia (spinal cord) 742.59
  meaning myelodysplastic syndrome — see Syndrome, myelodysplastic
Myeloencephalitis — see Encephalitis
Myelofibrosis 289.83
  with myeloid metaplasia 238.76
  idiopathic (chronic) 238.76
  megakaryocytic 238.79
  primary 238.76
  secondary 289.83
Myelogenous — see condition
Myeloid — see condition
Myelokathexis 288.09
Myeloleukodystrophy 330.0
Myelolipoma (M8870/0) — see Neoplasm, by site, benign
Myeloma (multiple) (plasma cell) (plasmacytic) (M9730/3) 203.0 ☑
  monostotic (M9731/1) 238.6
  solitary (M9731/1) 238.6
Myelomalacia 336.8
Myelomata, multiple (M9730/3) 203.0 ☑
Myelomatosis (M9730/3) 203.0 ☑
Myelomeningitis — see Meningoencephalitis
Myelomeningocele (spinal cord) — see also Spina bifida 741.9 ☑
  fetal, causing fetopelvic disproportion 653.7 ☑
Myelo-osteo-musculodysplasia hereditaria 756.89
Myelopathic — see condition
Myelopathy (spinal cord) 336.9
  cervical 721.1
  diabetic 250.6 ☑ [336.3]
    due to secondary diabetes 249.6 ☑ [336.3]
  drug-induced 336.8
  due to or with
    carbon tetrachloride 987.8 [323.72]
    degeneration or displacement, intervertebral disc 722.70
      cervical, cervicothoracic 722.71
      lumbar, lumbosacral 722.73
      thoracic, thoracolumbar 722.72
    hydroxyquinoline derivatives 961.3 [323.72]
    infection — see Encephalitis
    intervertebral disc disorder 722.70
      cervical, cervicothoracic 722.71
      lumbar, lumbosacral 722.73
      thoracic, thoracolumbar 722.72
    lead 984.9 [323.72]
    mercury 985.0 [323.72]
    neoplastic disease (see also Neoplasm, by site) 239.9 [336.3]
    pernicious anemia 281.0 [336.3]
    spondylosis 721.91
      cervical 721.1
      lumbar, lumbosacral 721.42
      thoracic 721.41
    thallium 985.8 [323.72]
  lumbar, lumbosacral 721.42
  necrotic (subacute) 336.1
  radiation-induced 336.8
  spondylogenic NEC 721.91
    cervical 721.1
    lumbar, lumbosacral 721.42
    thoracic 721.41
  thoracic 721.41
  toxic NEC 989.9 [323.72]
  transverse (see also Myelitis) 323.82
  vascular 336.1
Myelophthisis 284.2
Myeloproliferative disease (M9960/1) 238.79
Myeloradiculitis — see also Polyneuropathy 357.0
Myeloradiculodysplasia (spinal) 742.59
Myelosarcoma (M9930/3) 205.3 ☑
Myelosclerosis 289.89

Myelosclerosis — continued
  with myeloid metaplasia (M9961/1) 238.76
  disseminated, of nervous system 340
  megakaryocytic (M9961/1) 238.79
Myelosis (M9860/3) — see also Leukemia, myeloid 205.9 ☑
  acute (M9861/3) 205.0 ☑
  aleukemic (M9864/3) 205.8 ☑
  chronic (M9863/3) 205.1 ☑
  erythremic (M9840/3) 207.0 ☑
    acute (M9841/3) 207.0 ☑
  megakaryocytic (M9920/3) 207.2 ☑
  nonleukemic (chronic) 288.8
  subacute (M9862/3) 205.2 ☑
Myesthenia — see Myasthenia
Myiasis (cavernous) 134.0
  orbit 134.0 [376.13]
Myoadenoma, prostate 600.20
  with
    other lower urinary tract symptoms (LUTS) 600.21
    urinary
      obstruction 600.21
      retention 600.21
Myoblastoma
  granular cell (M9580/0) (see also Neoplasm, connective tissue, benign)
    malignant (M9580/3) — see Neoplasm, connective tissue, malignant
    tongue (M9580/0) 210.1
Myocardial — see condition
Myocardiopathy (congestive) (constrictive) (familial) (hypertrophic nonobstructive) (idiopathic) (infiltrative) (obstructive) (primary) (restrictive) (sporadic) 425.4
  alcoholic 425.5
  amyloid 277.39 [425.7]
  beriberi 265.0 [425.7]
  cobalt-beer 425.5
  due to
    amyloidosis 277.39 [425.7]
    beriberi 265.0 [425.7]
    cardiac glycogenosis 271.0 [425.7]
    Chagas' disease 086.0
    Friedreich's ataxia 334.0 [425.8]
    influenza ▶(see also Influenza)◀ 487.8 [425.8]
    mucopolysaccharidosis 277.5 [425.7]
    myotonia atrophica 359.21 [425.8]
    progressive muscular dystrophy 359.1 [425.8]
    sarcoidosis 135 [425.8]
  glycogen storage 271.0 [425.7]
  hypertrophic obstructive 425.1
  metabolic NEC 277.9 [425.7]
  nutritional 269.9 [425.7]
  obscure (African) 425.2
  peripartum 674.5 ☑
  postpartum 674.5 ☑
  secondary 425.9
  thyrotoxic (see also Thyrotoxicosis) 242.9 ☑ [425.7]
  toxic NEC 425.9
Myocarditis (fibroid) (interstitial) (old) (progressive) (senile) (with arteriosclerosis) 429.0
  with
    rheumatic fever (conditions classifiable to 390) 398.0
      active (see also Myocarditis, acute, rheumatic) 391.2
      inactive or quiescent (with chorea) 398.0
  active (nonrheumatic) 422.90
    rheumatic 391.2
      with chorea (acute) (rheumatic) (Sydenham's) 392.0
  acute or subacute (interstitial) 422.90
    due to Streptococcus (beta-hemolytic) 391.2
    idiopathic 422.91
    rheumatic 391.2
      with chorea (acute) (rheumatic) (Sydenham's) 392.0
    specified type NEC 422.99
  aseptic of newborn 074.23
  bacterial (acute) 422.92

☑ **Additional Digit Required** — Refer to the Tabular List for Digit Selection   ▽ **Subterms under main terms may continue to next column or page**

188 — Volume 2 · October 2010   ▶◀ Revised Text   ● New Line   ▲ Revised Code   2011 ICD-9-CM

Myocarditis — continued
  chagasic 086.0
  chronic (interstitial) 429.0
  congenital 746.89
  constrictive 425.4
  Coxsackie (virus) 074.23
  diphtheritic 032.82
  due to or in
    Coxsackie (virus) 074.23
    diphtheria 032.82
    epidemic louse-borne typhus 080 *[422.0]*
    influenza ▶(see also Influenza)◀
      487.8 *[422.0]*
    Lyme disease 088.81 *[422.0]*
    scarlet fever 034.1 *[422.0]*
    toxoplasmosis (acquired) 130.3
    tuberculosis (see also Tuberculosis)
      017.9 ☑ *[422.0]*
    typhoid 002.0 *[422.0]*
    typhus NEC 081.9 *[422.0]*
  eosinophilic 422.91
  epidemic of newborn 074.23
  Fiedler's (acute) (isolated) (subacute) 422.91
  giant cell (acute) (subacute) 422.91
  gonococcal 098.85
  granulomatous (idiopathic) (isolated) (non-
    specific) 422.91
  hypertensive (see also Hypertension, heart)
    402.90
  idiopathic 422.91
    granulomatous 422.91
  infective 422.92
  influenzal ▶(see also Influenza)◀
    487.8 *[422.0]*
  isolated (diffuse) (granulomatous) 422.91
  malignant 422.99
  meningococcal 036.43
  nonrheumatic, active 422.90
  parenchymatous 422.90
  pneumococcal (acute) (subacute) 422.92
  rheumatic (chronic) (inactive) (with chorea)
    398.0
    active or acute 391.2
      with chorea (acute) (rheumatic)
        (Sydenham's) 392.0
  septic 422.92
  specific (giant cell) (productive) 422.91
  staphylococcal (acute) (subacute) 422.92
  suppurative 422.92
  syphilitic (chronic) 093.82
  toxic 422.93
    rheumatic (see also Myocarditis, acute
      rheumatic) 391.2
  tuberculous (see also Tuberculosis)
    017.9 ☑ *[422.0]*
  typhoid 002.0 *[422.0]*
  valvular — see Endocarditis
  viral, except Coxsackie 422.91
    Coxsackie 074.23
    of newborn (Coxsackie) 074.23
Myocardium, myocardial — see condition
Myocardosis — see also Cardiomyopathy 425.4
Myoclonia (essential) 333.2
  epileptica 345.1 ☑
  Friedrich's 333.2
  massive 333.2
Myoclonic
  epilepsy, familial (progressive) 345.1 ☑
  jerks 333.2
Myoclonus (familial essential) (multifocal)
  (simplex) 333.2
  with epilepsy and with ragged red fibers
    (MERRF syndrome) 277.87
  facial 351.8
  massive (infantile) 333.2
  palatal 333.2
  pharyngeal 333.2
Myocytolysis 429.1
Myodiastasis 728.84
Myoendocarditis — see also Endocarditis
  acute or subacute 421.9
Myoepithelioma (M8982/0) — see Neoplasm,
  by site, benign
Myofascitis (acute) 729.1
  low back 724.2

Myofibroma (M8890/0) — see also Neoplasm,
  connective tissue, benign
  uterus (cervix) (corpus) (also Leiomy-
    oma) 218.9
Myofibromatosis
  infantile 759.89
Myofibrosis 728.2
  heart (see also Myocarditis) 429.0
  humeroscapular region 726.2
  scapulohumeral 726.2
Myofibrositis — see also Myositis 729.1
  scapulohumeral 726.2
Myogelosis (occupational) 728.89
Myoglobinuria 791.3
Myoglobulinuria, primary 791.3
Myokymia — see also Myoclonus
  facial 351.8
Myolipoma (M8860/0)
  specified site — see Neoplasm, connective
    tissue, benign
  unspecified site 223.0
Myoma (M8895/0) — see also Neoplasm, connective tissue, benign
  cervix (stump) (uterus) (see also Leiomyoma)
    218.9
  malignant (M8895/3) — see Neoplasm,
    connective tissue, malignant
  prostate 600.20
    with
      other lower urinary tract symptoms
        (LUTS) 600.21
      urinary
        obstruction 600.21
        retention 600.21
  uterus (cervix) (corpus) (see also Leiomy-
    oma) 218.9
    in pregnancy or childbirth 654.1 ☑
      affecting fetus or newborn 763.89
      causing obstructed labor 660.2 ☑
        affecting fetus or newborn 763.1
Myomalacia 728.9
  cordis, heart (see also Degeneration, myocar-
    dial) 429.1
Myometritis — see also Endometritis 615.9
Myometrium — see condition
Myonecrosis, clostridial 040.0
Myopathy 359.9
  alcoholic 359.4
  amyloid 277.39 *[359.6]*
  benign, congenital 359.0
  central core 359.0
  centronuclear 359.0
  congenital (benign) 359.0
  critical illness 359.81
  distal 359.1
  due to drugs 359.4
  endocrine 259.9 *[359.5]*
    specified type NEC 259.8 *[359.5]*
  extraocular muscles 376.82
  facioscapulohumeral 359.1
  in
    Addison's disease 255.41 *[359.5]*
    amyloidosis 277.39 *[359.6]*
    cretinism 243 *[359.5]*
    Cushing's syndrome 255.0 *[359.5]*
    disseminated lupus erythematosus
      710.0 *[359.6]*
    giant cell arteritis 446.5 *[359.6]*
    hyperadrenocorticism NEC 255.3 *[359.5]*
    hyperparathyroidism 252.01 *[359.5]*
    hypopituitarism 253.2 *[359.5]*
    hypothyroidism (see also Hypothy-
      roidism) 244.9 *[359.5]*
    malignant neoplasm NEC (M8000/3)
      199.1 *[359.6]*
    myxedema (see also Myxedema)
      244.9 *[359.5]*
    polyarteritis nodosa 446.0 *[359.6]*
    rheumatoid arthritis 714.0 *[359.6]*
    sarcoidosis 135 *[359.6]*
    scleroderma 710.1 *[359.6]*
    Sjögren's disease 710.2 *[359.5]*
    thyrotoxicosis (see also Thyrotoxicosis)
      242.9 ☑ *[359.5]*
  inflammatory 359.79
    immune NEC 359.79

Myopathy — continued
  inflammatory — continued
    specified NEC 359.79
  intensive care (ICU) 359.81
  limb-girdle 359.1
  myotubular 359.0
  necrotizing, acute 359.81
  nemaline 359.0
  ocular 359.1
  oculopharyngeal 359.1
  of critical illness 359.81
  primary 359.89
  progressive NEC 359.89
  proximal myotonic (PROMM) 359.21
  quadriplegic, acute 359.81
  rod body 359.0
  scapulohumeral 359.1
  specified type NEC 359.89
  toxic 359.4
Myopericarditis — see also Pericarditis 423.9
Myopia (axial) (congenital) (increased curvature
  or refraction, nucleus of lens) 367.1
  degenerative, malignant 360.21
  malignant 360.21
  progressive high (degenerative) 360.21
Myosarcoma (M8895/3) — see Neoplasm,
  connective tissue, malignant
Myosis (persistent) 379.42
  stromal (endolymphatic) (M8931/1) 236.0
Myositis 729.1
  clostridial 040.0
  due to posture 729.1
  epidemic 074.1
  fibrosa or fibrous (chronic) 728.2
    Volkmann's (complicating trauma) 958.6
  inclusion body (IBM) 359.71
  infective 728.0
  interstitial 728.81
  multiple — see Polymyositis
  occupational 729.1
  orbital, chronic 376.12
  ossificans 728.12
    circumscribed 728.12
    progressive 728.11
    traumatic 728.12
  progressive fibrosing 728.11
  purulent 728.0
  rheumatic 729.1
  rheumatoid 729.1
  suppurative 728.0
  syphilitic 095.6
  traumatic (old) 729.1
Myospasia impulsiva 307.23
Myotonia (acquisita) (intermittens) 728.85
  atrophica 359.21
  congenita 359.22
    acetazolamide responsive 359.22
    dominant form 359.22
    recessive form 359.22
  drug-induced 359.24
  dystrophica 359.21
  fluctuans 359.29
  levior 359.22
  permanens 359.29
Myotonic pupil 379.46
Myriapodiasis 134.1
Myringitis
  with otitis media — see Otitis media
  acute 384.00
    specified type NEC 384.09
  bullosa hemorrhagica 384.01
  bullous 384.01
  chronic 384.1
Mysophobia 300.29
Mytilotoxism 988.0
Myxadenitis labialis 528.5
Myxedema (adult) (idiocy) (infantile) (juvenile)
  (thyroid gland) — see also Hypothyroidism 244.9
  circumscribed 242.9 ☑
  congenital 243
  cutis 701.8
  localized (pretibial) 242.9 ☑
  madness (acute) 293.0
    subacute 293.1
  papular 701.8

Myxedema — see also Hypothyroidism —
  continued
  pituitary 244.8
  postpartum 674.8 ☑
  pretibial 242.9 ☑
  primary 244.9
Myxochondrosarcoma (M9220/3) — see
  Neoplasm, cartilage, malignant
Myxofibroma (M8811/0) — see also Neoplasm,
  connective tissue, benign
  odontogenic (M9320/0) 213.1
    upper jaw (bone) 213.0
Myxofibrosarcoma (M8811/3) — see Neoplasm, connective tissue, malignant
Myxolipoma (M8852/0) — see also Lipoma, by
  site 214.9
Myxoliposarcoma (M8852/3) — see Neoplasm,
  connective tissue, malignant
Myxoma (M8840/0) — see also Neoplasm,
  connective tissue, benign
  odontogenic (M9320/0) 213.1
    upper jaw (bone) 213.0
Myxosarcoma (M8840/3) — see Neoplasm,
  connective tissue, malignant

N

Naegeli's
  disease (hereditary hemorrhagic thrombas-
    thenia) 287.1
  leukemia, monocytic (M9863/3) 205.1 ☑
  syndrome (incontinentia pigmenti) 757.33
Naffziger's syndrome 353.0
Naga sore — see also Ulcer, skin 707.9
Nägele's pelvis 738.6
  with disproportion (fetopelvic) 653.0 ☑
    affecting fetus or newborn 763.1
    causing obstructed labor 660.1 ☑
      affecting fetus or newborn 763.1
Nager-de Reynier syndrome (dysostosis
  mandibularis) 756.0
Nail — see also condition
  biting 307.9
  patella syndrome (hereditary osteoony-
    chodysplasia) 756.89
Nanism, nanosomia — see also Dwarfism
  259.4
  hypophyseal 253.3
  pituitary 253.3
  renis, renalis 588.0
Nanukayami 100.89
Napkin rash 691.0
Narcissism 301.81
Narcolepsy 347.00
  with cataplexy 347.01
  in conditions classified elsewhere 347.10
    with cataplexy 347.11
Narcosis
  carbon dioxide (respiratory) 786.09
  due to drug
    correct substance properly administered
      780.09
    overdose or wrong substance given or
      taken 977.9
      specified drug — see Table of Drugs
        and Chemicals
Narcotism (chronic) — see also Dependence
  304.9 ☑
  acute
    correct substance properly administered
      349.82
    overdose or wrong substance given or
      taken 967.8
      specified drug — see Table of Drugs
        and Chemicals
NARP (ataxia and retinitis pigmentosa) 277.87
Narrow
  anterior chamber angle 365.02
  pelvis (inlet) (outlet) — see Contraction,
    pelvis
Narrowing
  artery NEC 447.1
    auditory, internal 433.8 ☑
    basilar 433.0 ☑
      with other precerebral artery
        433.3 ☑

☑ **Additional Digit Required — Refer to the Tabular List for Digit Selection**   **Subterms under main terms may continue to next column or page**

2011 ICD-9-CM   ▶◀ Revised Text   ● New Line   ▲ Revised Code   **October 2010 · Volume 2 — 189**

Narrowing — continued
artery — continued
basilar — continued
bilateral 433.3 ☑
carotid 433.1 ☑
with other precerebral artery 433.3 ☑
bilateral 433.3 ☑
cerebellar 433.8 ☑
choroidal 433.8 ☑
communicating posterior 433.8 ☑
coronary (see also Arteriosclerosis, coronary)
congenital 746.85
due to syphilis 090.5
hypophyseal 433.8 ☑
pontine 433.8 ☑
precerebral NEC 433.9 ☑
multiple or bilateral 433.3 ☑
specified NEC 433.8 ☑
vertebral 433.2 ☑
with other precerebral artery 433.3 ☑
bilateral 433.3 ☑
auditory canal (external) (see also Stricture, ear canal, acquired) 380.50
cerebral arteries 437.0
cicatricial — see Cicatrix
congenital — see Anomaly, congenital
coronary artery — see Narrowing, artery, coronary
ear, middle 385.22
Eustachian tube (see also Obstruction, Eustachian tube) 381.60
eyelid 374.46
congenital 743.62
intervertebral disc or space NEC — see Degeneration, intervertebral disc
joint space, hip 719.85
larynx 478.74
lids 374.46
congenital 743.62
mesenteric artery (with gangrene) 557.0
palate 524.89
palpebral fissure 374.46
retinal artery 362.13
ureter 593.3
urethra (see also Stricture, urethra) 598.9
Narrowness, abnormal, eyelid 743.62
Nasal — see condition
Nasolacrimal — see condition
Nasopharyngeal — see also condition
bursa 478.29
pituitary gland 759.2
torticollis 723.5
Nasopharyngitis (acute) (infective) (subacute) 460
chronic 472.2
due to external agent — see Condition, respiratory, chronic, due to
due to external agent — see Condition, respiratory, due to
septic 034.0
streptococcal 034.0
suppurative (chronic) 472.2
ulcerative (chronic) 472.2
Nasopharynx, nasopharyngeal — see condition
Natal tooth, teeth 520.6
Nausea — see also Vomiting 787.02
with vomiting 787.01
epidemic 078.82
gravidarum — see Hyperemesis, gravidarum
marina 994.6
Navel — see condition
Neapolitan fever — see also Brucellosis 023.9
Near drowning 994.1
Nearsightedness 367.1
Near-syncope 780.2
Nebécourt's syndrome 253.3
Nebula, cornea (eye) 371.01
congenital 743.43
interfering with vision 743.42
Necator americanus infestation 126.1
Necatoriasis 126.1
Neck — see condition

Necrencephalus — see also Softening, brain 437.8
Necrobacillosis 040.3
Necrobiosis 799.89
brain or cerebral (see also Softening, brain) 437.8
lipoidica 709.3
diabeticorum 250.8 ☑ [709.3]
due to secondary diabetes 249.8 ☑ [709.3]
Necrodermolysis 695.15
Necrolysis, toxic epidermal 695.15
due to drug
correct substance properly administered 695.15
overdose or wrong substance given or taken 977.9
specified drug — see Table of Drugs and Chemicals
Stevens-Johnson syndrome overlap (SJS-TEN overlap syndrome) 695.14
Necrophilia 302.89
Necrosis, necrotic
adrenal (capsule) (gland) 255.8
antrum, nasal sinus 478.19
aorta (hyaline) (see also Aneurysm, aorta) 441.9
cystic medial 441.00
abdominal 441.02
thoracic 441.01
thoracoabdominal 441.03
ruptured 441.5
arteritis 446.0
artery 447.5
aseptic, bone 733.40
femur (head) (neck) 733.42
medial condyle 733.43
humoral head 733.41
jaw 733.45
medial femoral condyle 733.43
specific site NEC 733.49
talus 733.44
avascular, bone NEC (see also Necrosis, aseptic, bone) 733.40
bladder (aseptic) (sphincter) 596.8
bone (see also Osteomyelitis) 730.1 ☑
acute 730.0 ☑
aseptic or avascular 733.40
femur (head) (neck) 733.42
medial condyle 733.43
humoral head 733.41
jaw 733.45
medial femoral condyle 733.43
specified site NEC 733.49
talus 733.44
ethmoid 478.19
ischemic 733.40
jaw 526.4
asceptic 733.45
marrow 289.89
Paget's (osteitis deformans) 731.0
tuberculous — see Tuberculosis, bone
brain (softening) (see also Softening, brain) 437.8
breast (aseptic) (fat) (segmental) 611.3
bronchus, bronchi 519.19
central nervous system NEC (see also Softening, brain) 437.8
cerebellar (see also Softening, brain) 437.8
cerebral (softening) (see also Softening, brain) 437.8
cerebrospinal (softening) (see also Softening, brain) 437.8
colon 557.0
cornea (see also Keratitis) 371.40
cortical, kidney 583.6
cystic medial (aorta) 441.00
abdominal 441.02
thoracic 441.01
thoracoabdominal 441.03
dental 521.09
pulp 522.1
due to swallowing corrosive substance — see Burn, by site
ear (ossicle) 385.24
esophagus 530.89

Necrosis, necrotic — continued
ethmoid (bone) 478.19
eyelid 374.50
fat, fatty (generalized) (see also Degeneration, fatty) 272.8
abdominal wall 567.82
breast (aseptic) (segmental) 611.3
intestine 569.89
localized — see Degeneration, by site, fatty
mesentery 567.82
omentum 567.82
pancreas 577.8
peritoneum 567.82
skin (subcutaneous) 709.3
newborn 778.1
femur (aseptic) (avascular) 733.42
head 733.42
medial condyle 733.43
neck 733.42
gallbladder (see also Cholecystitis, acute) 575.0
gangrenous 785.4
gastric 537.89
glottis 478.79
heart (myocardium) — see Infarct, myocardium
hepatic (see also Necrosis, liver) 570
hip (aseptic) (avascular) 733.42
intestine (acute) (hemorrhagic) (massive) 557.0
ischemic 785.4
jaw 526.4
asceptic 733.45
kidney (bilateral) 583.9
acute 584.9
cortical 583.6
acute 584.6
with
abortion — see Abortion, by type, with renal failure
ectopic pregnancy (see also categories 633.0–633.9) 639.3
molar pregnancy (see also categories 630–632) 639.3
complicating pregnancy 646.2 ☑
affecting fetus or newborn 760.1
following labor and delivery 669.3 ☑
medullary (papillary) (see also Pyelitis) 590.80
in
acute renal failure 584.7
nephritis, nephropathy 583.7
papillary (see also Pyelitis) 590.80
in
acute renal failure 584.7
nephritis, nephropathy 583.7
tubular 584.5
with
abortion — see Abortion, by type, with renal failure
ectopic pregnancy (see also categories 633.0–633.9) 639.3
molar pregnancy (see also categories 630–632) 639.3
complicating
abortion 639.3
ectopic or molar pregnancy 639.3
pregnancy 646.2 ☑
affecting fetus or newborn 760.1
following labor and delivery 669.3 ☑
traumatic 958.5
larynx 478.79
liver (acute) (congenital) (diffuse) (massive) (subacute) 570
with
abortion — see Abortion, by type, with specified complication NEC
ectopic pregnancy (see also categories 633.0–633.9) 639.8

Necrosis, necrotic — continued
liver — continued
with — continued
molar pregnancy (see also categories 630–632) 639.8
complicating pregnancy 646.7 ☑
affecting fetus or newborn 760.8
following
abortion 639.8
ectopic or molar pregnancy 639.8
obstetrical 646.7 ☑
postabortal 639.8
puerperal, postpartum 674.8 ☑
toxic 573.3
lung 513.0
lymphatic gland 683
mammary gland 611.3
mastoid (chronic) 383.1
mesentery 557.0
fat 567.82
mitral valve — see Insufficiency, mitral
myocardium, myocardial — see Infarct, myocardium
nose (septum) 478.19
omentum 557.0
with mesenteric infarction 557.0
fat 567.82
orbit, orbital 376.10
ossicles, ear (aseptic) 385.24
ovary (see also Salpingo-oophoritis) 614.2
pancreas (aseptic) (duct) (fat) 577.8
acute 577.0
infective 577.0
papillary, kidney (see also Pyelitis) 590.80
perineum 624.8
peritoneum 567.82
with mesenteric infarction 557.0
fat 567.82
pharynx 462
in granulocytopenia 288.09
phosphorus 983.9
pituitary (gland) (postpartum) (Sheehan) 253.2
placenta (see also Placenta, abnormal) 656.7 ☑
pneumonia 513.0
pulmonary 513.0
pulp (dental) 522.1
pylorus 537.89
radiation — see Necrosis, by site
radium — see Necrosis, by site
renal — see Necrosis, kidney
sclera 379.19
scrotum 608.89
skin or subcutaneous tissue 709.8
due to burn — see Burn, by site
gangrenous 785.4
spine, spinal (column) 730.18
acute 730.18
cord 336.1
spleen 289.59
stomach 537.89
stomatitis 528.1
subcutaneous fat 709.3
fetus or newborn 778.1
subendocardial — see Infarct, myocardium
suprarenal (capsule) (gland) 255.8
teeth, tooth 521.09
testis 608.89
thymus (gland) 254.8
tonsil 474.8
trachea 519.19
tuberculous NEC — see Tuberculosis
tubular (acute) (anoxic) (toxic) 584.5
due to a procedure 997.5
umbilical cord, affecting fetus or newborn 762.6
vagina 623.8
vertebra (lumbar) 730.18
acute 730.18
tuberculous (see also Tuberculosis) 015.0 ☑ [730.8]
vesical (aseptic) (bladder) 596.8
vulva 624.8
x-ray — see Necrosis, by site
Necrospermia 606.0

☑ **Additional Digit Required** — Refer to the Tabular List for Digit Selection   ▽ **Subterms under main terms may continue to next column or page**

190 — Volume 2   ▶◀ Revised Text   ● New Line   ▲ Revised Code   2011 ICD-9-CM

Necrotizing angiitis 446.0
Negativism 301.7
Neglect (child) (newborn) NEC 995.52
   adult 995.84
   after or at birth 995.52
   hemispatial 781.8
   left-sided 781.8
   sensory 781.8
   visuospatial 781.8
Negri bodies 071
Neill-Dingwall syndrome (microcephaly and dwarfism) 759.89

Neisserian infection NEC — *see* Gonococcus
Nematodiasis NEC — *see also* Infestation, Nematode 127.9
   ancylostoma (*see also* Ancylostomiasis) 126.9
Neoformans cryptococcus infection 117.5
Neonatal — *see also* condition
   abstinence syndrome 779.5
   adrenoleukodystrophy 277.86
   teeth, tooth 520.6
Neonatorum — *see* condition

Neoplasia
   anal intraepithelial I (AIN I) (histologically confirmed) 569.44
   anal intraepithelial II (AIN II) (histologically confirmed) 569.44
   anal intraepithelial III (AIN III) 230.6
      anal canal 230.5
   endometrial intraepithelial (EIN) 621.35
   multiple endocrine (MEN)
      type I 258.01
      type IIA 258.02
      type IIB 258.03

Neoplasia — *continued*
   vaginal intraepithelial I (VAIN I) 623.0
   vaginal intraepithelial II (VAIN II) 623.0
   vaginal intraepithelial III (VAIN III) 233.31
   vulvular intraepithelial I (VIN I) 624.01
   vulvular intraepithelial II (VIN II) 624.02
   vulvular intraepithelial III (VIN III) 233.32

☑ Additional Digit Required — Refer to the Tabular List for Digit Selection   ▽ Subterms under main terms may continue to next column or page

2011 ICD-9-CM   ►◄ Revised Text   ● New Line   ▲ Revised Code   Volume 2 — 191

	Malignant					
	Primary	Secondary	Ca in situ	Benign	Uncertain Behavior	Unspecified
Neoplasm, neoplastic	199.1	199.1	234.9	229.9	238.9	239.9

Notes — 1. The list below gives the code numbers for neoplasms by anatomical site. For each site there are six possible code numbers according to whether the neoplasm in question is malignant, benign, in situ, of uncertain behavior, or of unspecified nature. The description of the neoplasm will often indicate which of the six columns is appropriate; e.g., malignant melanoma of skin, benign fibroadenoma of breast, carcinoma in situ of cervix uteri.

Where such descriptors are not present, the remainder of the Index should be consulted where guidance is given to the appropriate column for each morphological (histological) variety listed; e.g., Mesonephroma — see Neoplasm, malignant; Embryoma — see also Neoplasm, uncertain behavior; Disease, Bowen's — see Neoplasm, skin, in situ. However, the guidance in the Index can be overridden if one of the descriptors mentioned above is present; e.g., malignant adenoma of colon is coded to 153.9 and not to 211.3 as the adjective "malignant" overrides the Index entry "Adenoma — see also Neoplasm, benign."

2. Sites marked with the sign * (e.g., face NEC*) should be classified to malignant neoplasm of skin of these sites if the variety of neoplasm is a squamous cell carcinoma or an epidermoid carcinoma, and to benign neoplasm of skin of these sites if the variety of neoplasm is a papilloma (any type).

	Primary	Secondary	Ca in situ	Benign	Uncertain Behavior	Unspecified
abdomen, abdominal	195.2	198.89	234.8	229.8	238.8	239.89
cavity	195.2	198.89	234.8	229.8	238.8	239.89
organ	195.2	198.89	234.8	229.8	238.8	239.89
viscera	195.2	198.89	234.8	229.8	238.8	239.89
wall	173.5	198.2	232.5	216.5	238.2	239.2
connective tissue	171.5	198.89	—	215.5	238.1	239.2
abdominopelvic	195.8	198.89	234.8	229.8	238.8	239.89
accessory sinus — see Neoplasm, sinus						
acoustic nerve	192.0	198.4	—	225.1	237.9	239.7
acromion (process)	170.4	198.5	—	213.4	238.0	239.2
adenoid (pharynx) (tissue)	147.1	198.89	230.0	210.7	235.1	239.0
adipose tissue (see also Neoplasm, connective tissue)	171.9	198.89	—	215.9	238.1	239.2
adnexa (uterine)	183.9	198.82	233.39	221.8	236.3	239.5
adrenal (cortex) (gland) (medulla)	194.0	198.7	234.8	227.0	237.2	239.7
ala nasi (external)	173.3	198.2	232.3	216.3	238.2	239.2
alimentary canal or tract NEC	159.9	197.8	230.9	211.9	235.5	239.0
alveolar	143.9	198.89	230.0	210.4	235.1	239.0
mucosa	143.9	198.89	230.0	210.4	235.1	239.0
lower	143.1	198.89	230.0	210.4	235.1	239.0
upper	143.0	198.89	230.0	210.4	235.1	239.0
ridge or process	170.1	198.5	—	213.1	238.0	239.2
carcinoma	143.9	—	—	—	—	—
lower	143.1	—	—	—	—	—
upper	143.0	—	—	—	—	—
lower	170.1	198.5	—	213.1	238.0	239.2
mucosa	143.9	198.89	230.0	210.4	235.1	239.0
lower	143.1	198.89	230.0	210.4	235.1	239.0
upper	143.0	198.89	230.0	210.4	235.1	239.0
upper	170.0	198.5	—	213.0	238.0	239.2
sulcus	145.1	198.89	230.0	210.4	235.1	239.0
alveolus	143.9	198.89	230.0	210.4	235.1	239.0
lower	143.1	198.89	230.0	210.4	235.1	239.0
upper	143.0	198.89	230.0	210.4	235.1	239.0
ampulla of Vater	156.2	197.8	230.8	211.5	235.3	239.0
ankle NEC*	195.5	198.89	232.7	229.8	238.8	239.89
anorectum, anorectal (junction)	154.8	197.5	230.7	211.4	235.2	239.0
antecubital fossa or space*	195.4	198.89	232.6	229.8	238.8	239.89
antrum (Highmore) (maxillary)	160.2	197.3	231.8	212.0	235.9	239.1
pyloric	151.2	197.8	230.2	211.1	235.2	239.0
tympanicum	160.1	197.3	231.8	212.0	235.9	239.1
anus, anal	154.3	197.5	230.6	211.4	235.5	239.0
canal	154.2	197.5	230.5	211.4	235.5	239.0

	Primary	Secondary	Ca in situ	Benign	Uncertain Behavior	Unspecified
Neoplasm, neoplastic — continued						
anus, anal — continued						
contiguous sites with rectosigmoid junction or rectum	154.8	—	—	—	—	—
margin	173.5	198.2	232.5	216.5	238.2	239.2
skin	173.5	198.2	232.5	216.5	238.2	239.2
sphincter	154.2	197.5	230.5	211.4	235.5	239.0
aorta (thoracic)	171.4	198.89	—	215.4	238.1	239.2
abdominal	171.5	198.89	—	215.5	238.1	239.2
aortic body	194.6	198.89	—	227.6	237.3	239.7
aponeurosis	171.9	198.89	—	215.9	238.1	239.2
palmar	171.2	198.89	—	215.2	238.1	239.2
plantar	171.3	198.89	—	215.3	238.1	239.2
appendix	153.5	197.5	230.3	211.3	235.2	239.0
arachnold (cerebral)	192.1	198.4	—	225.2	237.6	239.7
spinal	192.3	198.4	—	225.4	237.6	239.7
areola (female)	174.0	198.81	233.0	217	238.3	239.3
male	175.0	198.81	233.0	217	238.3	239.3
arm NEC*	195.4	198.89	232.6	229.8	238.8	239.89
artery — see Neoplasm, connective tissue						
aryepiglottic fold	148.2	198.89	230.0	210.8	235.1	239.0
hypopharyngeal aspect	148.2	198.89	230.0	210.8	235.1	239.0
laryngeal aspect	161.1	197.3	231.0	212.1	235.6	239.1
marginal zone	148.2	198.89	230.0	210.8	235.1	239.0
arytenoid (cartilage)	161.3	197.3	231.0	212.1	235.6	239.1
fold — see Neoplasm, aryepiglottic						
associated with transplanted organ	199.2	—	—	—	—	—
atlas	170.2	198.5	—	213.2	238.0	239.2
atrium, cardiac	164.1	198.89	—	212.7	238.8	239.89
auditory canal (external) (skin)	173.2	198.2	232.2	216.2	238.2	239.2
internal	160.1	197.3	231.8	212.0	235.9	239.1
nerve	192.0	198.4	—	225.1	237.9	239.7
tube	160.1	197.3	231.8	212.0	235.9	239.1
Eustachian	160.1	197.3	231.8	212.0	235.9	239.1
opening	147.2	198.89	230.0	210.7	235.1	239.0
auricle, ear	173.2	198.2	232.2	216.2	238.2	239.2
cartilage	171.0	198.89	—	215.0	238.1	239.2
auricular canal (external)	173.2	198.2	232.2	216.2	238.2	239.2
internal	160.1	197.3	231.8	212.0	235.9	239.1
autonomic nerve or nervous system NEC	171.9	198.89	—	215.9	238.1	239.2
axilla, axillary	195.1	198.89	234.8	229.8	238.8	239.89
fold	173.5	198.2	232.5	216.5	238.2	239.2
back NEC*	195.8	198.89	232.5	229.8	238.8	239.89
Bartholin's gland	184.1	198.82	233.32	221.2	236.3	239.5
basal ganglia	191.0	198.3	—	225.0	237.5	239.6
basis pedunculi	191.7	198.3	—	225.0	237.5	239.6
bile or biliary (tract)	156.9	197.8	230.8	211.5	235.3	239.0
canaliculi (biliferi) (intrahepatic)	155.1	197.8	230.8	211.5	235.3	239.0
canals, interlobular	155.1	197.8	230.8	211.5	235.3	239.0
contiguous sites	156.8	—	—	—	—	—
duct or passage (common) (cystic) (extrahepatic)	156.1	197.8	230.8	211.5	235.3	239.0
contiguous sites with gallbladder	156.8	—	—	—	—	—
interlobular	155.1	197.8	230.8	211.5	235.3	239.0
intrahepatic	155.1	197.8	230.8	211.5	235.3	239.0

☑ **Additional Digit Required — Refer to the Tabular List for Digit Selection**

▽ **Subterms under main terms may continue to next column or page**

Neoplasm, neoplastic — continued
bile or biliary — continued
duct or passage — continued
intrahepatic — continued

	Malignant					
	Primary	Secondary	Ca in situ	Benign	Uncertain Behavior	Unspecified
and extrahepatic	156.9	197.8	230.8	211.5	235.3	239.0
bladder (urinary)	188.9	198.1	233.7	223.3	236.7	239.4
contiguous sites	188.8	—	—	—	—	—
dome	188.1	198.1	233.7	223.3	236.7	239.4
neck	188.5	198.1	233.7	223.3	236.7	239.4
orifice	188.9	198.1	233.7	223.3	236.7	239.4
ureteric	188.6	198.1	233.7	223.3	236.7	239.4
urethral	188.5	198.1	233.7	223.3	236.7	239.4
sphincter	188.8	198.1	233.7	223.3	236.7	239.4
trigone	188.0	198.1	233.7	223.3	236.7	239.4
urachus	188.7	—	233.7	223.3	236.7	239.4
wall	188.9	198.1	233.7	223.3	236.7	239.4
anterior	188.3	198.1	233.7	223.3	236.7	239.4
lateral	188.2	198.1	233.7	223.3	236.7	239.4
posterior	188.4	198.1	233.7	223.3	236.7	239.4

blood vessel — *see* Neoplasm, connective tissue

	Primary	Secondary	Ca in situ	Benign	Uncertain Behavior	Unspecified
bone (periosteum)	170.9	198.5	—	213.9	238.0	239.2

Note — Carcinomas and adenocarcinomas, of any type other than intraosseous or odontogenic, of the sites listed under "Neoplasm, bone" should be considered as constituting metastatic spread from an unspecified primary site and coded to 198.5 for morbidity coding.

	Primary	Secondary	Ca in situ	Benign	Uncertain Behavior	Unspecified
acetabulum	170.6	198.5	—	213.6	238.0	239.2
acromion (process)	170.4	198.5	—	213.4	238.0	239.2
ankle	170.8	198.5	—	213.8	238.0	239.2
arm NEC	170.4	198.5	—	213.4	238.0	239.2
astragalus	170.8	198.5	—	213.8	238.0	239.2
atlas	170.2	198.5	—	213.2	238.0	239.2
axis	170.2	198.5	—	213.2	238.0	239.2
back NEC	170.2	198.5	—	213.2	238.0	239.2
calcaneus	170.8	198.5	—	213.8	238.0	239.2
calvarium	170.0	198.5	—	213.0	238.0	239.2
carpus (any)	170.5	198.5	—	213.5	238.0	239.2
cartilage NEC	170.9	198.5	—	213.9	238.0	239.2
clavicle	170.3	198.5	—	213.3	238.0	239.2
clivus	170.0	198.5	—	213.0	238.0	239.2
coccygeal vertebra	170.6	198.5	—	213.6	238.0	239.2
coccyx	170.6	198.5	—	213.6	238.0	239.2
costal cartilage	170.3	198.5	—	213.3	238.0	239.2
costovertebral joint	170.3	198.5	—	213.3	238.0	239.2
cranial	170.0	198.5	—	213.0	238.0	239.2
cuboid	170.8	198.5	—	213.8	238.0	239.2
cuneiform	170.9	198.5	—	213.9	238.0	239.2
ankle	170.8	198.5	—	213.8	238.0	239.2
wrist	170.5	198.5	—	213.5	238.0	239.2
digital	170.9	198.5	—	213.9	238.0	239.2
finger	170.5	198.5	—	213.5	238.0	239.2
toe	170.8	198.5	—	213.8	238.0	239.2
elbow	170.4	198.5	—	213.4	238.0	239.2
ethmoid (labyrinth)	170.0	198.5	—	213.0	238.0	239.2
face	170.0	198.5	—	213.0	238.0	239.2
lower jaw	170.1	198.5	—	213.1	238.0	239.2
femur (any part)	170.7	198.5	—	213.7	238.0	239.2
fibula (any part)	170.7	198.5	—	213.7	238.0	239.2
finger (any)	170.5	198.5	—	213.5	238.0	239.2
foot	170.8	198.5	—	213.8	238.0	239.2
forearm	170.4	198.5	—	213.4	238.0	239.2
frontal	170.0	198.5	—	213.0	238.0	239.2
hand	170.5	198.5	—	213.5	238.0	239.2
heel	170.8	198.5	—	213.8	238.0	239.2
hip	170.6	198.5	—	213.6	238.0	239.2

Neoplasm, neoplastic — continued
bone — continued

	Malignant					
	Primary	Secondary	Ca in situ	Benign	Uncertain Behavior	Unspecified
humerus (any part)	170.4	198.5	—	213.4	238.0	239.2
hyoid	170.0	198.5	—	213.0	238.0	239.2
ilium	170.6	198.5	—	213.6	238.0	239.2
innominate	170.6	198.5	—	213.6	238.0	239.2
intervertebral cartilage or disc	170.2	198.5	—	213.2	238.0	239.2
ischium	170.6	198.5	—	213.6	238.0	239.2
jaw (lower)	170.1	198.5	—	213.1	238.0	239.2
upper	170.0	198.5	—	213.0	238.0	239.2
knee	170.7	198.5	—	213.7	238.0	239.2
leg NEC	170.7	198.5	—	213.7	238.0	239.2
limb NEC	170.9	198.5	—	213.9	238.0	239.2
lower (long bones)	170.7	198.5	—	213.7	238.0	239.2
short bones	170.8	198.5	—	213.8	238.0	239.2
upper (long bones)	170.4	198.5	—	213.4	238.0	239.2
short bones	170.5	198.5	—	213.5	238.0	239.2
long	170.9	198.5	—	213.9	238.0	239.2
lower limbs NEC	170.7	198.5	—	213.7	238.0	239.2
upper limbs NEC	170.4	198.5	—	213.4	238.0	239.2
malar	170.0	198.5	—	213.0	238.0	239.2
mandible	170.1	198.5	—	213.1	238.0	239.2
marrow NEC	202.9 ☑	198.5	—	—	—	238.79
mastoid	170.0	198.5	—	213.0	238.0	239.2
maxilla, maxillary (superior)	170.0	198.5	—	213.0	238.0	239.2
inferior	170.1	198.5	—	213.1	238.0	239.2
metacarpus (any)	170.5	198.5	—	213.5	238.0	239.2
metatarsus (any)	170.8	198.5	—	213.8	238.0	239.2
navicular (ankle)	170.8	198.5	—	213.8	238.0	239.2
hand	170.5	198.5	—	213.5	238.0	239.2
nose, nasal	170.0	198.5	—	213.0	238.0	239.2
occipital	170.0	198.5	—	213.0	238.0	239.2
orbit	170.0	198.5	—	213.0	238.0	239.2
parietal	170.0	198.5	—	213.0	238.0	239.2
patella	170.8	198.5	—	213.8	238.0	239.2
pelvic	170.6	198.5	—	213.6	238.0	239.2
phalanges	170.9	198.5	—	213.9	238.0	239.2
foot	170.8	198.5	—	213.8	238.0	239.2
hand	170.5	198.5	—	213.5	238.0	239.2
pubic	170.6	198.5	—	213.6	238.0	239.2
radius (any part)	170.4	198.5	—	213.4	238.0	239.2
rib	170.3	198.5	—	213.3	238.0	239.2
sacral vertebra	170.6	198.5	—	213.6	238.0	239.2
sacrum	170.6	198.5	—	213.6	238.0	239.2
scaphoid (of hand)	170.5	198.5	—	213.5	238.0	239.2
of ankle	170.8	198.5	—	213.8	238.0	239.2
scapula (any part)	170.4	198.5	—	213.4	238.0	239.2
sella turcica	170.0	198.5	—	213.0	238.0	239.2
short	170.9	198.5	—	213.9	238.0	239.2
lower limb	170.8	198.5	—	213.8	238.0	239.2
upper limb	170.5	198.5	—	213.5	238.0	239.2
shoulder	170.4	198.5	—	213.4	238.0	239.2
skeleton, skeletal NEC	170.9	198.5	—	213.9	238.0	239.2
skull	170.0	198.5	—	213.0	238.0	239.2
sphenoid	170.0	198.5	—	213.0	238.0	239.2
spine, spinal (column)	170.2	198.5	—	213.2	238.0	239.2
coccyx	170.6	198.5	—	213.6	238.0	239.2
sacrum	170.6	198.5	—	213.6	238.0	239.2
sternum	170.3	198.5	—	213.3	238.0	239.2
tarsus (any)	170.8	198.5	—	213.8	238.0	239.2
temporal	170.0	198.5	—	213.0	238.0	239.2
thumb	170.5	198.5	—	213.5	238.0	239.2

☑ **Additional Digit Required — Refer to the Tabular List for Digit Selection**

▽ **Subterms under main terms may continue to next column or page**

	Malignant					
	Primary	Secondary	Ca in situ	Benign	Uncertain Behavior	Unspecified
Neoplasm, neoplastic — *continued*						
bone — *continued*						
tibia (any part)	170.7	198.5	—	213.7	238.0	239.2
toe (any)	170.8	198.5	—	213.8	238.0	239.2
trapezium	170.5	198.5	—	213.5	238.0	239.2
trapezoid	170.5	198.5	—	213.5	238.0	239.2
turbinate	170.0	198.5	—	213.0	238.0	239.2
ulna (any part)	170.4	198.5	—	213.4	238.0	239.2
unciform	170.5	198.5	—	213.5	238.0	239.2
vertebra (column)	170.2	198.5	—	213.2	238.0	239.2
coccyx	170.6	198.5	—	213.6	238.0	239.2
sacrum	170.6	198.5	—	213.6	238.0	239.2
vomer	170.0	198.5	—	213.0	238.0	239.2
wrist	170.5	198.5	—	213.5	238.0	239.2
xiphoid process	170.3	198.5	—	213.3	238.0	239.2
zygomatic	170.0	198.5	—	213.0	238.0	239.2
book-leaf (mouth)	145.8	198.89	230.0	210.4	235.1	239.0
bowel — *see* Neoplasm, intestine						
brachial plexus	171.2	198.89	—	215.2	238.1	239.2
brain NEC	191.9	198.3	—	225.0	237.5	239.6
basal ganglia	191.0	198.3	—	225.0	237.5	239.6
cerebellopontine angle	191.6	198.3	—	225.0	237.5	239.6
cerebellum NOS	191.6	198.3	—	225.0	237.5	239.6
cerebrum	191.0	198.3	—	225.0	237.5	239.6
choroid plexus	191.5	198.3	—	225.0	237.5	239.6
contiguous sites	191.8	—	—	—	—	—
corpus callosum	191.8	198.3	—	225.0	237.5	239.6
corpus striatum	191.0	198.3	—	225.0	237.5	239.6
cortex (cerebral)	191.0	198.3	—	225.0	237.5	239.6
frontal lobe	191.1	198.3	—	225.0	237.5	239.6
globus pallidus	191.0	198.3	—	225.0	237.5	239.6
hippocampus	191.2	198.3	—	225.0	237.5	239.6
hypothalamus	191.0	198.3	—	225.0	237.5	239.6
internal capsule	191.0	198.3	—	225.0	237.5	239.6
medulla oblongata	191.7	198.3	—	225.0	237.5	239.6
meninges	192.1	198.4	—	225.2	237.6	239.7
midbrain	191.7	198.3	—	225.0	237.5	239.6
occipital lobe	191.4	198.3	—	225.0	237.5	239.6
parietal lobe	191.3	198.3	—	225.0	237.5	239.6
peduncle	191.7	198.3	—	225.0	237.5	239.6
pons	191.7	198.3	—	225.0	237.5	239.6
stem	191.7	198.3	—	225.0	237.5	239.6
tapetum	191.8	198.3	—	225.0	237.5	239.6
temporal lobe	191.2	198.3	—	225.0	237.5	239.6
thalamus	191.0	198.3	—	225.0	237.5	239.6
uncus	191.2	198.3	—	225.0	237.5	239.6
ventricle (floor)	191.5	198.3	—	225.0	237.5	239.6
branchial (cleft) (vestiges)	146.8	198.89	230.0	210.6	235.1	239.0
breast (connective tissue) (female) (glandular tissue) (soft parts)	174.9	198.81	233.0	217	238.3	239.3
areola	174.0	198.81	233.0	217	238.3	239.3
male	175.0	198.81	233.0	217	238.3	239.3
axillary tail	174.6	198.81	233.0	217	238.3	239.3
central portion	174.1	198.81	233.0	217	238.3	239.3
contiguous sites	174.8	—	—	—	—	—
ectopic sites	174.8	198.81	233.0	217	238.3	239.3
inner	174.8	198.81	233.0	217	238.3	239.3
lower	174.8	198.81	233.0	217	238.3	239.3
lower-inner quadrant	174.3	198.81	233.0	217	238.3	239.3
lower-outer quadrant	174.5	198.81	233.0	217	238.3	239.3
male	175.9	198.81	233.0	217	238.3	239.3
areola	175.0	198.81	233.0	217	238.3	239.3
ectopic tissue	175.9	198.81	233.0	217	238.3	239.3
nipple	175.0	198.81	233.0	217	238.3	239.3
mastectomy site (skin)	173.5	198.2	—	—	—	—

	Malignant					
	Primary	Secondary	Ca in situ	Benign	Uncertain Behavior	Unspecified
Neoplasm, neoplastic — *continued*						
breast — *continued*						
mastectomy site — *continued*						
specified as breast tissue	174.8	198.81	—	—	—	—
midline	174.8	198.81	233.0	217	238.3	239.3
nipple	174.0	198.81	233.0	217	238.3	239.3
male	175.0	198.81	233.0	217	238.3	239.3
outer	174.8	198.81	233.0	217	238.3	239.3
skin	173.5	198.2	232.5	216.5	238.2	239.2
tail (axillary)	174.6	198.81	233.0	217	238.3	239.3
upper	174.8	198.81	233.0	217	238.3	239.3
upper-inner quadrant	174.2	198.81	233.0	217	238.3	239.3
upper-outer quadrant	174.4	198.81	233.0	217	238.3	239.3
broad ligament	183.3	198.82	233.39	221.0	236.3	239.5
bronchiogenic, bronchogenic (lung)	162.9	197.0	231.2	212.3	235.7	239.1
bronchiole	162.9	197.0	231.2	212.3	235.7	239.1
bronchus	162.9	197.0	231.2	212.3	235.7	239.1
carina	162.2	197.0	231.2	212.3	235.7	239.1
contiguous sites with lung or trachea	162.8	—	—	—	—	—
lower lobe of lung	162.5	197.0	231.2	212.3	235.7	239.1
main	162.2	197.0	231.2	212.3	235.7	239.1
middle lobe of lung	162.4	197.0	231.2	212.3	235.7	239.1
upper lobe of lung	162.3	197.0	231.2	212.3	235.7	239.1
brow	173.3	198.2	232.3	216.3	238.2	239.2
buccal (cavity)	145.9	198.89	230.0	210.4	235.1	239.0
commissure	145.0	198.89	230.0	210.4	235.1	239.0
groove (lower) (upper)	145.1	198.89	230.0	210.4	235.1	239.0
mucosa	145.0	198.89	230.0	210.4	235.1	239.0
sulcus (lower) (upper)	145.1	198.89	230.0	210.4	235.1	239.0
bulbourethral gland	189.3	198.1	233.9	223.81	236.99	239.5
bursa — *see* Neoplasm, connective tissue						
buttock NEC*	195.3	198.89	232.5	229.8	238.8	239.89
calf*	195.5	198.89	232.7	229.8	238.8	239.89
calvarium	170.0	198.5	—	213.0	238.0	239.2
calyx, renal	189.1	198.0	233.9	223.1	236.91	239.5
canal						
anal	154.2	197.5	230.5	211.4	235.5	239.0
auditory (external)	173.2	198.2	232.2	216.2	238.2	239.2
auricular (external)	173.2	198.2	232.2	216.2	238.2	239.2
canaliculi, biliary (biliferi) (intrahepatic)	155.1	197.8	230.8	211.5	235.3	239.0
canthus (eye) (inner) (outer)	173.1	198.2	232.1	216.1	238.2	239.2
capillary — *see* Neoplasm, connective tissue						
caput coli	153.4	197.5	230.3	211.3	235.2	239.0
cardia (gastric)	151.0	197.8	230.2	211.1	235.2	239.0
cardiac orifice (stomach)	151.0	197.8	230.2	211.1	235.2	239.0
cardio-esophageal junction	151.0	197.8	230.2	211.1	235.2	239.0
cardio-esophagus	151.0	197.8	230.2	211.1	235.2	239.0
carina (bronchus)	162.2	197.0	231.2	212.3	235.7	239.1
carotid (artery)	171.0	198.89	—	215.0	238.1	239.2
body	194.5	198.89	—	227.5	237.3	239.7
carpus (any bone)	170.5	198.5	—	213.5	238.0	239.2
cartilage (articular) (joint) NEC (*see also*	170.9	198.5	—	213.9	238.0	239.2

☑ **Additional Digit Required** — Refer to the Tabular List for Digit Selection　　　　　　　Ⓝᴱᶜ **Subterms under main terms may continue to next column or page**

2011 ICD-9-CM　　　　▶◀ Revised Text　　　　● New Line　　　▲ Revised Code　　　　**Volume 2 — 195**

Index

Neoplasm, cartilage — Neoplasm, connective tissue

Neoplasm, neoplastic—	Malignant Primary	Malignant Secondary	Malignant Ca in situ	Benign	Uncertain Behavior	Unspecified
continued						
cartilage (*see also* Neoplasm, bone)— *continued* Neoplasm, bone)						
arytenoid	161.3	197.3	231.0	212.1	235.6	239.1
auricular	171.0	198.89	—	215.0	238.1	239.2
bronchi	162.2	197.3	—	212.3	235.7	239.1
connective tissue — *see* Neoplasm, connective tissue						
costal	170.3	198.5	—	213.3	238.0	239.2
cricoid	161.3	197.3	231.0	212.1	235.6	239.1
cuneiform	161.3	197.3	231.0	212.1	235.6	239.1
ear (external)	171.0	198.89	—	215.0	238.1	239.2
ensiform	170.3	198.5	—	213.3	238.0	239.2
epiglottis	161.1	197.3	231.0	212.1	235.6	239.1
anterior surface	146.4	198.89	230.0	210.6	235.1	239.0
eyelid	171.0	198.89	—	215.0	238.1	239.2
intervertebral	170.2	198.5	—	213.2	238.0	239.2
larynx, laryngeal	161.3	197.3	231.0	212.1	235.6	239.1
nose, nasal	160.0	197.3	231.8	212.0	235.9	239.1
pinna	171.0	198.89	—	215.0	238.1	239.2
rib	170.3	198.5	—	213.3	238.0	239.2
semilunar (knee)	170.7	198.5	—	213.7	238.0	239.2
thyroid	161.3	197.3	231.0	212.1	235.6	239.1
trachea	162.0	197.3	231.1	212.2	235.7	239.1
cauda equina	192.2	198.3	—	225.3	237.5	239.7
cavity						
buccal	145.9	198.89	230.0	210.4	235.1	239.0
nasal	160.0	197.3	231.8	212.0	235.9	239.1
oral	145.9	198.89	230.0	210.4	235.1	239.0
peritoneal	158.9	197.6	—	211.8	235.4	239.0
tympanic	160.1	197.3	231.8	212.0	235.9	239.1
cecum	153.4	197.5	230.3	211.3	235.2	239.0
central nervous system — *see* Neoplasm, nervous system						
white matter	191.0	198.3	—	225.0	237.5	239.6
cerebellopontine (angle)	191.6	198.3	—	225.0	237.5	239.6
cerebellum, cerebellar	191.6	198.3	—	225.0	237.5	239.6
cerebrum, cerebral (cortex) (hemisphere) (white matter)	191.0	198.3	—	225.0	237.5	239.6
meninges	192.1	198.4	—	225.2	237.6	239.7
peduncle	191.7	198.3	—	225.0	237.5	239.6
ventricle (any)	191.5	198.3	—	225.0	237.5	239.6
cervical region	195.0	198.89	234.8	229.8	238.8	239.89
cervix (cervical) (uteri) (uterus)	180.9	198.82	233.1	219.0	236.0	239.5
canal	180.0	198.82	233.1	219.0	236.0	239.5
contiguous sites	180.8	—	—	—	—	—
endocervix (canal) (gland)	180.0	198.82	233.1	219.0	236.0	239.5
exocervix	180.1	198.82	233.1	219.0	236.0	239.5
external os	180.1	198.82	233.1	219.0	236.0	239.5
internal os	180.0	198.82	233.1	219.0	236.0	239.5
nabothian gland	180.0	198.82	233.1	219.0	236.0	239.5
squamocolumnar junction	180.8	198.82	233.1	219.0	236.0	239.5
stump	180.8	198.82	233.1	219.0	236.0	239.5
cheek	195.0	198.89	234.8	229.8	238.8	239.89
external	173.3	198.2	232.3	216.3	238.2	239.2
inner aspect	145.0	198.89	230.0	210.4	235.1	239.0
internal	145.0	198.89	230.0	210.4	235.1	239.0
mucosa	145.0	198.89	230.0	210.4	235.1	239.0
chest (wall) NEC	195.1	198.89	234.8	229.8	238.8	239.89
chiasma opticum	192.0	198.4	—	225.1	237.9	239.7
chin	173.3	198.2	232.3	216.3	238.2	239.2
choana	147.3	198.89	230.0	210.7	235.1	239.0

Neoplasm, neoplastic—	Malignant Primary	Malignant Secondary	Malignant Ca in situ	Benign	Uncertain Behavior	Unspecified
continued						
cholangiole	155.1	197.8	230.8	211.5	235.3	239.0
choledochal duct	156.1	197.8	230.8	211.5	235.3	239.0
choroid	190.6	198.4	234.0	224.6	238.8	239.81
plexus	191.5	198.3	—	225.0	237.5	239.6
ciliary body	190.0	198.4	234.0	224.0	238.8	239.89
clavicle	170.3	198.5	—	213.3	238.0	239.2
clitoris	184.3	198.82	233.32	221.2	236.3	239.5
clivus	170.0	198.5	—	213.0	238.0	239.2
cloacogenic zone	154.8	197.5	230.7	211.4	235.5	239.0
coccygeal body or glomus	194.6	198.89	—	227.6	237.3	239.7
vertebra	170.6	198.5	—	213.6	238.0	239.2
coccyx	170.6	198.5	—	213.6	238.0	239.2
colon — *see also* Neoplasm, intestine, large ●	153.9	197.5	230.3	211.3	235.2	239.0
with rectum ●	154.0	197.5	230.4	211.4	235.2	239.0
columnella	173.3	198.2	232.3	216.3	238.2	239.2
column, spinal — *see* Neoplasm, spine						
commissure labial, lip	140.6	198.89	230.0	210.4	235.1	239.0
laryngeal	161.0	197.3	231.0	212.1	235.6	239.1
common (bile) duct	156.1	197.8	230.8	211.5	235.3	239.0
concha	173.2	198.2	232.2	216.2	238.2	239.2
nose	160.0	197.3	231.8	212.0	235.9	239.1
conjunctiva	190.3	198.4	234.0	224.3	238.8	239.89
connective tissue NEC	171.9	198.89	—	215.9	238.1	239.2

Note — For neoplasms of connective tissue (blood vessel, bursa, fascia, ligament, muscle, peripheral nerves, sympathetic and parasympathetic nerves and ganglia, synovia, tendon, etc.) or of morphological types that indicate connective tissue, code according to the list under "Neoplasm, connective tissue"; for sites that do not appear in this list, code to neoplasm of that site; e.g.,

liposarcoma, shoulder 171.2

leiomyosarcoma, stomach 151.9

neurofibroma, chest wall 215.4

Morphological types that indicate connective tissue appear in the proper place in the alphabetic index with the instruction "see Neoplasm, connective tissue…"

	Primary	Secondary	Ca in situ	Benign	Uncertain Behavior	Unspecified
abdomen	171.5	198.89	—	215.5	238.1	239.2
abdominal wall	171.5	198.89	—	215.5	238.1	239.2
ankle	171.3	198.89	—	215.3	238.1	239.2
antecubital fossa or space	171.2	198.89	—	215.2	238.1	239.2
arm	171.2	198.89	—	215.2	238.1	239.2
auricle (ear)	171.0	198.89	—	215.0	238.1	239.2
axilla	171.4	198.89	—	215.4	238.1	239.2
back	171.7	198.89	—	215.7	238.1	239.2
breast (female) (*see also* Neoplasm, breast)	174.9	198.81	233.0	217	238.3	239.3
male	175.9	198.81	233.0	217	238.3	239.3
buttock	171.6	198.89	—	215.6	238.1	239.2
calf	171.3	198.89	—	215.3	238.1	239.2
cervical region	171.0	198.89	—	215.0	238.1	239.2
cheek	171.0	198.89	—	215.0	238.1	239.2
chest (wall)	171.4	198.89	—	215.4	238.1	239.2
chin	171.0	198.89	—	215.0	238.1	239.2
contiguous sites	171.8	—	—	—	—	—
diaphragm	171.4	198.89	—	215.4	238.1	239.2
ear (external)	171.0	198.89	—	215.0	238.1	239.2
elbow	171.2	198.89	—	215.2	238.1	239.2
extrarectal	171.6	198.89	—	215.6	238.1	239.2
extremity	171.8	198.89	—	215.8	238.1	239.2
lower	171.3	198.89	—	215.3	238.1	239.2
upper	171.2	198.89	—	215.2	238.1	239.2
eyelid	171.0	198.89	—	215.0	238.1	239.2
face	171.0	198.89	—	215.0	238.1	239.2
finger	171.2	198.89	—	215.2	238.1	239.2
flank	171.7	198.89	—	215.7	238.1	239.2

☑ **Additional Digit Required** — Refer to the Tabular List for Digit Selection   ▽ **Subterms under main terms may continue to next column or page**

Neoplasm, neoplastic—	Malignant			Benign	Uncertain Behavior	Unspecified
	Primary	Secondary	Ca in situ			
continued						
connective tissue —						
continued						
foot	171.3	198.89	—	215.3	238.1	239.2
forearm	171.2	198.89	—	215.2	238.1	239.2
forehead	171.0	198.89	—	215.0	238.1	239.2
gastric	171.5	198.89	—	215.5	238.1	—
gastrointestinal	171.5	198.89	—	215.5	238.1	—
gluteal region	171.6	198.89	—	215.6	238.1	239.2
great vessels						
NEC	171.4	198.89	—	215.4	238.1	239.2
groin	171.6	198.89	—	215.6	238.1	239.2
hand	171.2	198.89	—	215.2	238.1	239.2
head	171.0	198.89	—	215.0	238.1	239.2
heel	171.3	198.89	—	215.3	238.1	239.2
hip	171.3	198.89	—	215.3	238.1	239.2
hypochondrium	171.5	198.89	—	215.5	238.1	239.2
iliopsoas muscle	171.6	198.89	—	215.5	238.1	239.2
infraclavicular						
region	171.4	198.89	—	215.4	238.1	239.2
inguinal (canal)						
(region)	171.6	198.89	—	215.6	238.1	239.2
intestine	171.5	198.89	—	215.5	238.1	—
intrathoracic	171.4	198.89	—	215.4	238.1	239.2
ischorectal fossa	171.6	198.89	—	215.6	238.1	239.2
jaw	143.9	198.89	230.0	210.4	235.1	239.0
knee	171.3	198.89	—	215.3	238.1	239.2
leg	171.3	198.89	—	215.3	238.1	239.2
limb NEC	171.9	198.89	—	215.8	238.1	239.2
lower	171.3	198.89	—	215.3	238.1	239.2
upper	171.2	198.89	—	215.2	238.1	239.2
nates	171.6	198.89	—	215.6	238.1	239.2
neck	171.0	198.89	—	215.0	238.1	239.2
orbit	190.1	198.4	234.0	224.1	238.8	239.89
pararectal	171.6	198.89	—	215.6	238.1	239.2
para-urethral	171.6	198.89	—	215.6	238.1	239.2
paravaginal	171.6	198.89	—	215.6	238.1	239.2
pelvis (floor)	171.6	198.89	—	215.6	238.1	239.2
pelvo-abdominal	171.8	198.89	—	215.8	238.1	239.2
perineum	171.6	198.89	—	215.6	238.1	239.2
perirectal (tissue)	171.6	198.89	—	215.6	238.1	239.2
periurethral						
(tissue)	171.6	198.89	—	215.6	238.1	239.2
popliteal fossa or						
space	171.3	198.89	—	215.3	238.1	239.2
presacral	171.6	198.89	—	215.6	238.1	239.2
psoas muscle	171.5	198.89	—	215.5	238.1	239.2
pterygoid fossa	171.0	198.89	—	215.0	238.1	239.2
rectovaginal septum						
or wall	171.6	198.89	—	215.6	238.1	239.2
rectovesical	171.6	198.89	—	215.6	238.1	239.2
retroperitoneum	158.0	197.6	—	211.8	235.4	239.0
sacrococcygeal						
region	171.6	198.89	—	215.6	238.1	239.2
scalp	171.0	198.89	—	215.0	238.1	239.2
scapular region	171.4	198.89	—	215.4	238.1	239.2
shoulder	171.2	198.89	—	215.2	238.1	239.2
skin (dermis)						
NEC	173.9	198.2	232.9	216.9	238.2	239.2
stomach	171.5	198.89	—	215.5	238.1	—
submental	171.0	198.89	—	215.0	238.1	239.2
supraclavicular						
region	171.0	198.89	—	215.0	238.1	239.2
temple	171.0	198.89	—	215.0	238.1	239.2
temporal region	171.0	198.89	—	215.0	238.1	239.2
thigh	171.3	198.89	—	215.3	238.1	239.2
thoracic (duct)						
(wall)	171.4	198.89	—	215.4	238.1	239.2
thorax	171.4	198.89	—	215.4	238.1	239.2
thumb	171.2	198.89	—	215.2	238.1	239.2
toe	171.3	198.89	—	215.3	238.1	239.2
trunk	171.7	198.89	—	215.7	238.1	239.2
umbilicus	171.5	198.89	—	215.5	238.1	239.2
vesicorectal	171.6	198.89	—	215.6	238.1	239.2
wrist	171.2	198.89	—	215.2	238.1	239.2

Neoplasm, neoplastic—	Malignant			Benign	Uncertain Behavior	Unspecified
	Primary	Secondary	Ca in situ			
continued						
conus medullaris	192.2	198.3	—	225.3	237.5	239.7
cord (true) (vocal)	161.0	197.3	231.0	212.1	235.6	239.1
false	161.1	197.3	231.0	212.1	235.6	239.1
spermatic	187.6	198.82	233.6	222.8	236.6	239.5
spinal (cervical)						
(lumbar)						
(thoracic)	192.2	198.3	—	225.3	237.5	239.7
cornea (limbus)	190.4	198.4	234.0	224.4	238.8	239.89
corpus						
albicans	183.0	198.6	233.39	220	236.2	239.5
callosum, brain	191.8	198.3	—	225.0	237.5	239.6
cavernosum	187.3	198.82	233.5	222.1	236.6	239.5
gastric	151.4	197.8	230.2	211.1	235.2	239.0
penis	187.3	198.82	233.5	222.1	236.6	239.5
striatum,						
cerebrum	191.0	198.3	—	225.0	237.5	239.6
uteri	182.0	198.82	233.2	219.1	236.0	239.5
isthmus	182.1	198.82	233.2	219.1	236.0	239.5
cortex						
adrenal	194.0	198.7	234.8	227.0	237.2	239.7
cerebral	191.0	198.3	—	225.0	237.5	239.6
costal cartilage	170.3	198.5	—	213.3	238.0	239.2
costovertebral						
joint	170.3	198.5	—	213.3	238.0	239.2
Cowper's gland	189.3	198.1	233.9	223.81	236.99	239.5
cranial (fossa, any)	191.9	198.3	—	225.0	237.5	239.6
meninges	192.1	198.4	—	225.2	237.6	239.7
nerve (any)	192.0	198.4	—	225.1	237.9	239.7
craniobuccal						
pouch	194.3	198.89	234.8	227.3	237.0	239.7
craniopharyngeal (duct)						
(pouch)	194.3	198.89	234.8	227.3	237.0	239.7
cricoid	148.0	198.89	230.0	210.8	235.1	239.0
cartilage	161.3	197.3	231.0	212.1	235.6	239.1
cricopharynx	148.0	198.89	230.0	210.8	235.1	239.0
crypt of Morgagni	154.8	197.5	230.7	211.4	235.2	239.0
crystalline lens	190.0	198.4	234.0	224.0	238.8	239.89
cul-de-sac						
(Douglas')	158.8	197.6	—	211.8	235.4	239.0
cuneiform						
cartilage	161.3	197.3	231.0	212.1	235.6	239.1
cutaneous — *see*						
Neoplasm, skin						
cutis — *see* Neoplasm,						
skin						
cystic (bile) duct						
(common)	156.1	197.8	230.8	211.5	235.3	239.0
dermis — *see*						
Neoplasm, skin						
diaphragm	171.4	198.89	—	215.4	238.1	239.2
digestive organs,						
system, tube, or						
tract NEC	159.9	197.8	230.9	211.9	235.5	239.0
contiguous sites with						
peritoneum	159.8	—	—	—	—	—
disc, intervertebral	170.2	198.5	—	213.2	238.0	239.2
disease,						
generalized	199.0	199.0	234.9	229.9	238.9	199.0
disseminated	199.0	199.0	234.9	229.9	238.9	199.0
Douglas' cul-de-sac or						
pouch	158.8	197.6	—	211.8	235.4	239.0
duodenojejunal						
junction	152.8	197.4	230.7	211.2	235.2	239.0
duodenum	152.0	197.4	230.7	211.2	235.2	239.0
dura (cranial)						
(mater)	192.1	198.4	—	225.2	237.6	239.7
cerebral	192.1	198.4	—	225.2	237.6	239.7
spinal	192.3	198.4	—	225.4	237.6	239.7
ear (external)	173.2	198.2	232.2	216.2	238.2	239.2
auricle or auris	173.2	198.2	232.2	216.2	238.2	239.2
canal, external	173.2	198.2	232.2	216.2	238.2	239.2
cartilage	171.0	198.89	—	215.0	238.1	239.2
external meatus	173.2	198.2	232.2	216.2	238.2	239.2
inner	160.1	197.3	231.8	212.0	235.9	239.89
lobule	173.2	198.2	232.2	216.2	238.2	239.2

☑ Additional Digit Required — Refer to the Tabular List for Digit Selection
▽ Subterms under main terms may continue to next column or page

2011 ICD-9-CM ▶◀ Revised Text ● New Line ▲ Revised Code Volume 2 — 197

Index

Neoplasm, ear — Neoplasm, ganglia

	Malignant					
	Primary	Secondary	Ca in situ	Benign	Uncertain Behavior	Unspecified
Neoplasm, neoplastic— *continued*						
ear — *continued*						
middle	160.1	197.3	231.8	212.0	235.9	239.89
contiguous sites with accessory sinuses or nasal cavities	160.8	—	—	—	—	—
skin	173.2	198.2	232.2	216.2	238.2	239.2
earlobe	173.2	198.2	232.2	216.2	238.2	239.2
ejaculatory duct ...	187.8	198.82	233.6	222.8	236.6	239.5
elbow NEC*	195.4	198.89	232.6	229.8	238.8	239.89
endocardium	164.1	198.89	—	212.7	238.8	239.89
endocervix (canal) (gland)	180.0	198.82	233.1	219.0	236.0	239.5
endocrine gland NEC	194.9	198.89	—	227.9	237.4	239.7
pluriglandular NEC	194.8	198.89	234.8	227.8	237.4	239.7
endometrium (gland) (stroma)	182.0	198.82	233.2	219.1	236.0	239.5
ensiform cartilage	170.3	198.5	—	213.3	238.0	239.2
enteric — *see* Neoplasm, intestine						
ependyma (brain)	191.5	198.3	—	225.0	237.5	239.6
epicardium	164.1	198.89	—	212.7	238.8	239.89
epididymis	187.5	198.82	233.6	222.3	236.6	239.5
epidural	192.9	198.4	—	225.9	237.9	239.7
epiglottis	161.1	197.3	231.0	212.1	235.6	239.1
anterior aspect or surface	146.4	198.89	230.0	210.6	235.1	239.0
cartilage	161.3	197.3	231.0	212.1	235.6	239.1
free border (margin)	146.4	198.89	230.0	210.6	235.1	239.0
junctional region	146.5	198.89	230.0	210.6	235.1	239.0
posterior (laryngeal) surface	161.1	197.3	231.0	212.1	235.6	239.1
suprahyoid portion	161.1	197.3	231.0	212.1	235.6	239.1
esophagogastric junction	151.0	197.8	230.2	211.1	235.2	239.0
esophagus	150.9	197.8	230.1	211.0	235.5	239.0
abdominal	150.2	197.8	230.1	211.0	235.5	239.0
cervical	150.0	197.8	230.1	211.0	235.5	239.0
contiguous sites	150.8	—	—	—	—	—
distal (third)	150.5	197.8	230.1	211.0	235.5	239.0
lower (third)	150.5	197.8	230.1	211.0	235.5	239.0
middle (third)	150.4	197.8	230.1	211.0	235.5	239.0
proximal (third)	150.3	197.8	230.1	211.0	235.5	239.0
specified part NEC	150.8	197.8	230.1	211.0	235.5	239.0
thoracic	150.1	197.8	230.1	211.0	235.5	239.0
upper (third)	150.3	197.8	230.1	211.0	235.5	239.0
ethmoid (sinus)	160.3	197.3	231.8	212.0	235.9	239.1
bone or labyrinth	170.0	198.5	—	213.0	238.0	239.2
Eustachian tube	160.1	197.3	231.8	212.0	235.9	239.1
exocervix	180.1	198.82	233.1	219.0	236.0	239.5
external meatus (ear)	173.2	198.2	232.2	216.2	238.2	239.2
os, cervix uteri	180.1	198.82	233.1	219.0	236.0	239.5
extradural	192.9	198.4	—	225.9	237.9	239.7
extrahepatic (bile) duct	156.1	197.8	230.8	211.5	235.3	239.0
contiguous sites with gallbladder	156.8	—	—	—	—	—
extraocular muscle	190.1	198.4	234.0	224.1	238.8	239.89
extrarectal	195.3	198.89	234.8	229.8	238.8	239.89
extremity*	195.8	198.89	232.8	229.8	238.8	239.89
lower*	195.5	198.89	232.7	229.8	238.8	239.89
upper*	195.4	198.89	232.6	229.8	238.8	239.89
eye NEC	190.9	198.4	234.0	224.9	238.8	239.89
contiguous sites	190.8	—	—	—	—	—
specified sites NEC	190.8	198.4	234.0	224.8	238.8	239.89
Neoplasm, neoplastic— *continued*						
eyeball	190.0	198.4	234.0	224.0	238.8	239.89
eyebrow	173.3	198.2	232.3	216.3	238.2	239.2
eyelid (lower) (skin) (upper)	173.1	198.2	232.1	216.1	238.2	239.2
cartilage	171.0	198.89	—	215.0	238.1	239.2
face NEC*	195.0	198.89	232.3	229.8	238.8	239.89
fallopian tube (accessory)	183.2	198.82	233.39	221.0	236.3	239.5
falx (cerebelli) (cerebri)	192.1	198.4		225.2	237.6	239.7
fascia (*see also* Neoplasm, connective tissue)						
palmar	171.2	198.89	—	215.2	238.1	239.2
plantar	171.3	198.89	—	215.3	238.1	239.2
fatty tissue — *see* Neoplasm, connective tissue						
fauces, faucial NEC	146.9	198.89	230.0	210.6	235.1	239.0
pillars	146.2	198.89	230.0	210.6	235.1	239.0
tonsil	146.0	198.89	230.0	210.5	235.1	239.0
femur (any part)	170.7	198.5	—	213.7	238.0	239.2
fetal membrane	181	198.82	233.2	219.8	236.1	239.5
fibrous tissue — *see* Neoplasm, connective tissue						
fibula (any part)	170.7	198.5	—	213.7	238.0	239.2
filum terminale	192.2	198.3	—	225.3	237.5	239.7
finger NEC*	195.4	198.89	232.6	229.8	238.8	239.89
flank NEC*	195.8	198.89	232.5	229.8	238.8	239.89
follicle, nabothian	180.0	198.82	233.1	219.0	236.0	239.5
foot NEC*	195.5	198.89	232.7	229.8	238.8	239.89
forearm NEC*	195.4	198.89	232.6	229.8	238.8	239.89
forehead (skin)	173.3	198.2	232.3	216.3	238.2	239.2
foreskin	187.1	198.82	233.5	222.1	236.6	239.5
fornix pharyngeal	147.3	198.89	230.0	210.7	235.1	239.0
vagina	184.0	198.82	233.31	221.1	236.3	239.5
fossa (of) anterior (cranial)	191.9	198.3	—	225.0	237.5	239.6
cranial	191.9	198.3	—	225.0	237.5	239.6
ischiorectal	195.3	198.89	234.8	229.8	238.8	239.89
middle (cranial)	191.9	198.3	—	225.0	237.5	239.6
pituitary	194.3	198.89	234.8	227.3	237.0	239.7
posterior (cranial)	191.9	198.3	—	225.0	237.5	239.6
pterygoid	171.0	198.89	—	215.0	238.1	239.2
pyriform	148.1	198.89	230.0	210.8	235.1	239.0
Rosenmüller	147.2	198.89	230.0	210.7	235.1	239.0
tonsillar	146.1	198.89	230.0	210.6	235.1	239.0
fourchette	184.4	198.82	233.32	221.2	236.3	239.5
frenulum labii — *see* Neoplasm, lip, internal						
linguae	141.3	198.89	230.0	210.1	235.1	239.0
frontal bone	170.0	198.5	—	213.0	238.0	239.2
lobe, brain	191.1	198.3	—	225.0	237.5	239.6
meninges	192.1	198.4	—	225.2	237.6	239.7
pole	191.1	198.3	—	225.0	237.5	239.6
sinus	160.4	197.3	231.8	212.0	235.9	239.1
fundus stomach	151.3	197.8	230.2	211.1	235.2	239.0
uterus	182.0	198.82	233.2	219.1	236.0	239.5
gallbladder	156.0	197.8	230.8	211.5	235.3	239.0
contiguous sites with extrahepatic bile ducts	156.8	—	—	—	—	—
gall duct (extrahepatic)	156.1	197.8	230.8	211.5	235.3	239.0
intrahepatic	155.1	197.8	230.8	211.5	235.3	239.0
ganglia (*see also* Neoplasm, connective tissue)	171.9	198.89	—	215.9	238.1	239.2

☑ **Additional Digit Required — Refer to the Tabular List for Digit Selection**   ▽ **Subterms under main terms may continue to next column or page**

198 — Volume 2   ▶◀ Revised Text   ● New Line   ▲ Revised Code   2011 ICD-9-CM

	Malignant					
	Primary	Secondary	Ca in situ	Benign	Uncertain Behavior	Unspecified
Neoplasm, neoplastic — *continued*						
ganglia (*see also* Neoplasm, connective tissue) — *continued*						
basal	191.0	198.3	—	225.0	237.5	239.6
ganglion (*see also* Neoplasm, connective tissue)	171.9	198.89	—	215.9	238.1	239.2
cranial nerve	192.0	198.4	—	225.1	237.9	239.7
Gartner's duct	184.0	198.82	233.31	221.1	236.3	239.5
gastric — *see* Neoplasm, stomach						
gastrocolic	159.8	197.8	230.9	211.9	235.5	239.0
gastroesophageal junction	151.0	197.8	230.2	211.1	235.2	239.0
gastrointestinal (tract) NEC	159.9	197.8	230.9	211.9	235.5	239.0
generalized	199.0	199.0	234.9	229.9	238.9	199.0
genital organ or tract						
female NEC	184.9	198.82	233.39	221.9	236.3	239.5
contiguous sites	184.8	—	—	—	—	—
specified site NEC	184.8	198.82	233.39	221.8	236.3	239.5
male NEC	187.9	198.82	233.6	222.9	236.6	239.5
contiguous sites	187.8	—	—	—	—	—
specified site NEC	187.8	198.82	233.6	222.8	236.6	239.5
genitourinary tract						
female	184.9	198.82	233.39	221.9	236.3	239.5
male	187.9	198.82	233.6	222.9	236.6	239.5
gingiva (alveolar) (marginal)	143.9	198.89	230.0	210.4	235.1	239.0
lower	143.1	198.89	230.0	210.4	235.1	239.0
mandibular	143.1	198.89	230.0	210.4	235.1	239.0
maxillary	143.0	198.89	230.0	210.4	235.1	239.0
upper	143.0	198.89	230.0	210.4	235.1	239.0
gland, glandular (lymphatic) (system) (*see also* Neoplasm, lymph gland)						
endocrine NEC	194.9	198.89	—	227.9	237.4	239.7
salivary — *see* Neoplasm, salivary, gland						
glans penis	187.2	198.82	233.5	222.1	236.6	239.5
globus pallidus	191.0	198.3	—	225.0	237.5	239.6
glomus						
coccygeal	194.6	198.89	—	227.6	237.3	239.7
jugularis	194.6	198.89	—	227.6	237.3	239.7
glosso-epiglottic fold(s)	146.4	198.89	230.0	210.6	235.1	239.0
glossopalatine fold	146.2	198.89	230.0	210.6	235.1	239.0
glossopharyngeal sulcus	146.1	198.89	230.0	210.6	235.1	239.0
glottis	161.0	197.3	231.0	212.1	235.6	239.1
gluteal region*	195.3	198.89	232.5	229.8	238.8	239.89
great vessels NEC	171.4	198.89	—	215.4	238.1	239.2
groin NEC	195.3	198.89	232.5	229.8	238.8	239.89
gum	143.9	198.89	230.0	210.4	235.1	239.0
contiguous sites	143.8	—	—	—	—	—
lower	143.1	198.89	230.0	210.4	235.1	239.0
upper	143.0	198.89	230.0	210.4	235.1	239.0
hand NEC*	195.4	198.89	232.6	229.8	238.8	239.89
head NEC*	195.0	198.89	232.4	229.8	238.8	239.89
heart	164.1	198.89	—	212.7	238.8	239.89
contiguous sites with mediastinum or thymus	164.8	—	—	—	—	—
heel NEC*	195.5	198.89	232.7	229.8	238.8	239.89
helix	173.2	198.2	232.2	216.2	238.2	239.2

	Malignant					
	Primary	Secondary	Ca in situ	Benign	Uncertain Behavior	Unspecified
Neoplasm, neoplastic — *continued*						
hematopoietic, hemopoietic tissue NEC	202.8 ☑	198.89	—	—	—	238.79
hemisphere, cerebral	191.0	198.3	—	225.0	237.5	239.6
hemorrhoidal zone	154.2	197.5	230.5	211.4	235.5	239.0
hepatic	155.2	197.7	230.8	211.5	235.3	239.0
duct (bile)	156.1	197.8	230.8	211.5	235.3	239.0
flexure (colon)	153.0	197.5	230.3	211.3	235.2	239.0
primary	155.0	—	—	—	—	—
hilus of lung	162.2	197.0	231.2	212.3	235.7	239.1
hip NEC*	195.5	198.89	232.7	229.8	238.8	239.89
hippocampus, brain	191.2	198.3	—	225.0	237.5	239.6
humerus (any part)	170.4	198.5	—	213.4	238.0	239.2
hymen	184.0	198.82	233.31	221.1	236.3	239.5
hypopharynx, hypopharyngeal NEC	148.9	198.89	230.0	210.8	235.1	239.0
contiguous sites	148.8	—	—	—	—	—
postcricoid region	148.0	198.89	230.0	210.8	235.1	239.0
posterior wall	148.3	198.89	230.0	210.8	235.1	239.0
pyriform fossa (sinus)	148.1	198.89	230.0	210.8	235.1	239.0
specified site NEC	148.8	198.89	230.0	210.8	235.1	239.0
wall	148.9	198.89	230.0	210.8	235.1	239.0
posterior	148.3	198.89	230.0	210.8	235.1	239.0
hypophysis	194.3	198.89	234.8	227.3	237.0	239.7
hypothalamus	191.0	198.3	—	225.0	237.5	239.6
ileocecum, ileocecal (coil) (junction) (valve)	153.4	197.5	230.3	211.3	235.2	239.0
ileum	152.2	197.4	230.7	211.2	235.2	239.0
ilium	170.6	198.5	—	213.6	238.0	239.2
immunoproliferative NEC	203.8 ☑	—	—	—	—	—
infraclavicular (region)*	195.1	198.89	232.5	229.8	238.8	239.89
inguinal (region)*	195.3	198.89	232.5	229.8	238.8	239.89
insula	191.0	198.3	—	225.0	237.5	239.6
insular tissue (pancreas)	157.4	197.8	230.9	211.7	235.5	239.0
brain	191.0	198.3	—	225.0	237.5	239.6
interarytenoid fold	148.2	198.89	230.0	210.8	235.1	239.0
hypopharyngeal aspect	148.2	198.89	230.0	210.8	235.1	239.0
laryngeal aspect	161.1	197.3	231.0	212.1	235.6	239.1
marginal zone	148.2	198.89	230.0	210.8	235.1	239.0
interdental papillae	143.9	198.89	230.0	210.4	235.1	239.0
lower	143.1	198.89	230.0	210.4	235.1	239.0
upper	143.0	198.89	230.0	210.4	235.1	239.0
internal capsule	191.0	198.3	—	225.0	237.5	239.6
os (cervix)	180.0	198.82	233.1	219.0	236.0	239.5
intervertebral cartilage or disc	170.2	198.5	—	213.2	238.0	239.2
intestine, intestinal	159.0	197.8	230.7	211.9	235.2	239.0
large	153.9	197.5	230.3	211.3	235.2	239.0
appendix	153.5	197.5	230.3	211.3	235.2	239.0
caput coli	153.4	197.5	230.3	211.3	235.2	239.0
cecum	153.4	197.5	230.3	211.3	235.2	239.0
colon	153.9	197.5	230.3	211.3	235.2	239.0
and rectum	154.0	197.5	230.4	211.4	235.2	239.0
ascending	153.6	197.5	230.3	211.3	235.2	239.0
caput	153.4	197.5	230.3	211.3	235.2	239.0
contiguous sites	153.8	—	—	—	—	—
descending	153.2	197.5	230.3	211.3	235.2	239.0
distal	153.2	197.5	230.3	211.3	235.2	239.0
left	153.2	197.5	230.3	211.3	235.2	239.0
pelvic	153.3	197.5	230.3	211.3	235.2	239.0
right	153.6	197.5	230.3	211.3	235.2	239.0

☑ Additional Digit Required — Refer to the Tabular List for Digit Selection   ⬮ Subterms under main terms may continue to next column or page

2011 ICD-9-CM   ▶◀ Revised Text   ● New Line   ▲ Revised Code   Volume 2 — 199

Neoplasm, ganglia — Neoplasm, intestine, intestinal

Neoplasm, neoplastic— continued	Malignant			Benign	Uncertain Behavior	Unspecified
	Primary	Secondary	Ca in situ			
intestine, intestinal — continued						
large — continued						
colon — continued						
sigmoid (flexure)	153.3	197.5	230.3	211.3	235.2	239.0
transverse	153.1	197.5	230.3	211.3	235.2	239.0
contiguous sites	153.8	—	—	—	—	—
hepatic flexure	153.0	197.5	230.3	211.3	235.2	239.0
ileocecum, ileocecal (coil) (valve)	153.4	197.5	230.3	211.3	235.2	239.0
sigmoid flexure (lower) (upper)	153.3	197.5	230.3	211.3	235.2	239.0
splenic flexure	153.7	197.5	230.3	211.3	235.2	239.0
small	152.9	197.4	230.7	211.2	235.2	239.0
contiguous sites	152.8	—	—	—	—	—
duodenum	152.0	197.4	230.7	211.2	235.2	239.0
ileum	152.2	197.4	230.7	211.2	235.2	239.0
jejunum	152.1	197.4	230.7	211.2	235.2	239.0
tract NEC	159.0	197.8	230.7	211.9	235.2	239.0
intra-abdominal	195.2	198.89	234.8	229.8	238.8	239.89
intracranial NEC	191.9	198.3	—	225.0	237.5	239.6
intrahepatic (bile) duct	155.1	197.8	230.8	211.5	235.3	239.0
intraocular	190.0	198.4	234.0	224.0	238.8	239.89
intraorbital	190.1	198.4	234.0	224.1	238.8	239.89
intrasellar	194.3	198.89	234.8	227.3	237.0	239.7
intrathoracic (cavity) (organs NEC)	195.1	198.89	234.8	229.8	238.8	239.89
contiguous sites with respiratory organs	165.8	—	—	—	—	—
iris	190.0	198.4	234.0	224.0	238.8	239.89
ischiorectal (fossa)	195.3	198.89	234.8	229.8	238.8	239.89
ischium	170.6	198.5	—	213.6	238.0	239.2
island of Reil	191.0	198.3	—	225.0	237.5	239.6
islands or islets of Langerhans	157.4	197.8	230.9	211.7	235.5	239.0
isthmus uteri	182.1	198.82	233.2	219.1	236.0	239.5
jaw	195.0	198.89	234.8	229.8	238.8	239.89
bone	170.1	198.5	—	213.1	238.0	239.2
carcinoma	143.9	—	—	—	—	—
lower	143.1	—	—	—	—	—
upper	143.0	—	—	—	—	—
lower	170.1	198.5	—	213.1	238.0	239.2
upper	170.0	198.5	—	213.0	238.0	239.2
carcinoma (any type) (lower)						
(upper)	195.0	—	—	—	—	—
skin	173.3	198.2	232.3	216.3	238.2	239.2
soft tissues	143.9	198.89	230.0	210.4	235.1	239.0
lower	143.1	198.89	230.0	210.4	235.1	239.0
upper	143.0	198.89	230.0	210.4	235.1	239.0
jejunum	152.1	197.4	230.7	211.2	235.2	239.0
joint NEC (see also Neoplasm, bone)	170.9	198.5	—	213.9	238.0	239.2
acromioclavicular	170.4	198.5	—	213.4	238.0	239.2
bursa or synovial membrane — see Neoplasm, connective tissue						
costovertebral	170.3	198.5	—	213.3	238.0	239.2
sternocostal	170.3	198.5	—	213.3	238.0	239.2
temporomandibular	170.1	198.5	—	213.1	238.0	239.2
junction						
anorectal	154.8	197.5	230.7	211.4	235.5	239.0
cardioesophageal	151.0	197.8	230.2	211.1	235.2	239.0
esophagogastric	151.0	197.8	230.2	211.1	235.2	239.0
gastroesophageal	151.0	197.8	230.2	211.1	235.2	239.0

Neoplasm, neoplastic— continued	Malignant			Benign	Uncertain Behavior	Unspecified
	Primary	Secondary	Ca in situ			
junction — continued						
hard and soft palate	145.5	198.89	230.0	210.4	235.1	239.0
ileocecal	153.4	197.5	230.3	211.3	235.2	239.0
pelvirectal	154.0	197.5	230.4	211.4	235.2	239.0
pelviureteric	189.1	198.0	233.9	223.1	236.91	239.5
rectosigmoid	154.0	197.5	230.4	211.4	235.2	239.0
squamocolumnar, of cervix	180.8	198.82	233.1	219.0	236.0	239.5
kidney (parenchyma)	189.0	198.0	233.9	223.0	236.91	239.5
calyx	189.1	198.0	233.9	223.1	236.91	239.5
hilus	189.1	198.0	233.9	223.1	236.91	239.5
pelvis	189.1	198.0	233.9	223.1	236.91	239.5
knee NEC*	195.5	198.89	232.7	229.8	238.8	239.89
labia (skin)	184.4	198.82	233.32	221.2	236.3	239.5
majora	184.1	198.82	233.32	221.2	236.3	239.5
minora	184.2	198.82	233.32	221.2	236.3	239.5
labial (see also Neoplasm, lip) sulcus (lower) (upper)	145.1	198.89	230.0	210.4	235.1	239.0
labium (skin)	184.4	198.82	233.32	221.2	236.3	239.5
majus	184.1	198.82	233.32	221.2	236.3	239.5
minus	184.2	198.82	233.32	221.2	236.3	239.5
lacrimal						
canaliculi	190.7	198.4	234.0	224.7	238.8	239.89
duct (nasal)	190.7	198.4	234.0	224.7	238.8	239.89
gland	190.2	198.4	234.0	224.2	238.8	239.89
punctum	190.7	198.4	234.0	224.7	238.8	239.89
sac	190.7	198.4	234.0	224.7	238.8	239.89
Langerhans, islands or islets	157.4	197.8	230.9	211.7	235.5	239.0
laryngopharynx	148.9	198.89	230.0	210.8	235.1	239.0
larynx, laryngeal NEC	161.9	197.3	231.0	212.1	235.6	239.1
aryepiglottic fold	161.1	197.3	231.0	212.1	235.6	239.1
cartilage (arytenoid) (cricoid) (cuneiform) (thyroid)	161.3	197.3	231.0	212.1	235.6	239.1
commissure (anterior) (posterior)	161.0	197.3	231.0	212.1	235.6	239.1
contiguous sites	161.8	—	—	—	—	—
extrinsic NEC	161.1	197.3	231.0	212.1	235.6	239.1
meaning hypopharynx	148.9	198.89	230.0	210.8	235.1	239.0
interarytenoid fold	161.1	197.3	231.0	212.1	235.6	239.1
intrinsic	161.0	197.3	231.0	212.1	235.6	239.1
ventricular band	161.1	197.3	231.0	212.1	235.6	239.1
leg NEC*	195.5	198.89	232.7	229.8	238.8	239.89
lens, crystalline	190.0	198.4	234.0	224.0	238.8	239.89
lid (lower) (upper)	173.1	198.2	232.1	216.1	238.2	239.2
ligament (see also Neoplasm, connective tissue)						
broad	183.3	198.82	233.39	221.0	236.3	239.5
Mackenrodt's	183.8	198.82	233.39	221.8	236.3	239.5
non-uterine — see Neoplasm, connective tissue						
round	183.5	198.82	—	221.0	236.3	239.5
sacro-uterine	183.4	198.82	—	221.0	236.3	239.5
uterine	183.4	198.82	—	221.0	236.3	239.5
utero-ovarian	183.8	198.82	233.39	221.8	236.3	239.5
uterosacral	183.4	198.82	—	221.0	236.3	239.5
limb*	195.8	198.89	232.8	229.8	238.8	239.89
lower*	195.5	198.89	232.7	229.8	238.8	239.89
upper*	195.4	198.89	232.6	229.8	238.8	239.89
limbus of cornea	190.4	198.4	234.0	224.4	238.8	239.89
lingual NEC (see also Neoplasm, tongue)	141.9	198.89	230.0	210.1	235.1	239.0
lingula, lung	162.3	197.0	231.2	212.3	235.7	239.1

☑ Additional Digit Required — Refer to the Tabular List for Digit Selection   ▽ Subterms under main terms may continue to next column or page

Neoplasm, lip — Neoplasm, lymph, lymphatic

Neoplasm, neoplastic—	Malignant					
continued	Primary	Secondary	Ca in situ	Benign	Uncertain Behavior	Unspecified
lip (external) (lipstick area) (vermillion border)	140.9	198.89	230.0	210.0	235.1	239.0
buccal aspect — *see* Neoplasm, lip, internal						
commissure	140.6	198.89	230.0	210.4	235.1	239.0
contiguous sites	140.8	—	—	—	—	—
with oral cavity or pharynx	149.8	—	—	—	—	—
frenulum — *see* Neoplasm, lip, internal						
inner aspect — *see* Neoplasm, lip, internal						
internal (buccal) (frenulum) (mucosa) (oral)	140.5	198.89	230.0	210.0	235.1	239.0
lower	140.4	198.89	230.0	210.0	235.1	239.0
upper	140.3	198.89	230.0	210.0	235.1	239.0
lower	140.1	198.89	230.0	210.0	235.1	239.0
internal (buccal) (frenulum) (mucosa) (oral)	140.4	198.89	230.0	210.0	235.1	239.0
mucosa — *see* Neoplasm, lip, internal						
oral aspect — *see* Neoplasm, lip, internal						
skin (commissure) (lower) (upper)	173.0	198.2	232.0	216.0	238.2	239.2
upper	140.0	198.89	230.0	210.0	235.1	239.0
internal (buccal) (frenulum) (mucosa) (oral)	140.3	198.89	230.0	210.0	235.1	239.0
liver	155.2	197.7	230.8	211.5	235.3	239.0
primary	155.0	—	—	—	—	—
lobe						
azygos	162.3	197.0	231.2	212.3	235.7	239.1
frontal	191.1	198.3	—	225.0	237.5	239.6
lower	162.5	197.0	231.2	212.3	235.7	239.1
middle	162.4	197.0	231.2	212.3	235.7	239.1
occipital	191.4	198.3	—	225.0	237.5	239.6
parietal	191.3	198.3	—	225.0	237.5	239.6
temporal	191.2	198.3	—	225.0	237.5	239.6
upper	162.3	197.0	231.2	212.3	235.7	239.1
lumbosacral plexus	171.6	198.4	—	215.6	238.1	239.2
lung	162.9	197.0	231.2	212.3	235.7	239.1
azygos lobe	162.3	197.0	231.2	212.3	235.7	239.1
carina	162.2	197.0	231.2	212.3	235.7	239.1
contiguous sites with bronchus or trachea	162.8	—	—	—	—	—
hilus	162.2	197.0	231.2	212.3	235.7	239.1
lingula	162.3	197.0	231.2	212.3	235.7	239.1
lobe NEC	162.9	197.0	231.2	212.3	235.7	239.1
lower lobe	162.5	197.0	231.2	212.3	235.7	239.1
main bronchus	162.2	197.0	231.2	212.3	235.7	239.1
middle lobe	162.4	197.0	231.2	212.3	235.7	239.1
upper lobe	162.3	197.0	231.2	212.3	235.7	239.1
lymph, lymphatic channel NEC (*see also* Neoplasm, connective tissue)	171.9	198.89	—	215.9	238.1	239.2
gland (secondary)	—	196.9	—	229.0	238.8	239.89
abdominal	—	196.2	—	229.0	238.8	239.89
aortic	—	196.2	—	229.0	238.8	239.89
arm	—	196.3	—	229.0	238.8	239.89

Neoplasm, neoplastic—	Malignant					
continued	Primary	Secondary	Ca in situ	Benign	Uncertain Behavior	Unspecified
lymph, lymphatic — *continued*						
gland — *continued*						
auricular (anterior) (posterior)	—	196.0	—	229.0	238.8	239.89
axilla, axillary	—	196.3	—	229.0	238.8	239.89
brachial	—	196.3	—	229.0	238.8	239.89
bronchial	—	196.1	—	229.0	238.8	239.89
bronchopulmonary	—	196.1	—	229.0	238.8	239.89
celiac	—	196.2	—	229.0	238.8	239.89
cervical	—	196.0	—	229.0	238.8	239.89
cervicofacial	—	196.0	—	229.0	238.8	239.89
Cloquet	—	196.5	—	229.0	238.8	239.89
colic	—	196.2	—	229.0	238.8	239.89
common duct	—	196.2	—	229.0	238.8	239.89
cubital	—	196.3	—	229.0	238.8	239.89
diaphragmatic	—	196.1	—	229.0	238.8	239.89
epigastric, inferior	—	196.6	—	229.0	238.8	239.89
epitrochlear	—	196.3	—	229.0	238.8	239.89
esophageal	—	196.1	—	229.0	238.8	239.89
face	—	196.0	—	229.0	238.8	239.89
femoral	—	196.5	—	229.0	238.8	239.89
gastric	—	196.2	—	229.0	238.8	239.89
groin	—	196.5	—	229.0	238.8	239.89
head	—	196.0	—	229.0	238.8	239.89
hepatic	—	196.2	—	229.0	238.8	239.89
hilar (pulmonary)	—	196.1	—	229.0	238.8	239.89
splenic	—	196.2	—	229.0	238.8	239.89
hypogastric	—	196.6	—	229.0	238.8	239.89
ileocolic	—	196.2	—	229.0	238.8	239.89
iliac	—	196.6	—	229.0	238.8	239.89
infraclavicular	—	196.3	—	229.0	238.8	239.89
inguina, inguinal	—	196.5	—	229.0	238.8	239.89
innominate	—	196.1	—	229.0	238.8	239.89
intercostal	—	196.1	—	229.0	238.8	239.89
intestinal	—	196.2	—	229.0	238.8	239.89
intra-abdominal	—	196.2	—	229.0	238.8	239.89
intrapelvic	—	196.6	—	229.0	238.8	239.89
intrathoracic	—	196.1	—	229.0	238.8	239.9
jugular	—	196.0	—	229.0	238.8	239.89
leg	—	196.5	—	229.0	238.8	239.89
limb lower	—	196.5	—	229.0	238.8	239.9 ▲
upper	—	196.3	—	229.0	238.8	239.89
lower limb	—	196.5	—	229.0	238.8	239.9 ▲
lumbar	—	196.2	—	229.0	238.8	239.89
mandibular	—	196.0	—	229.0	238.8	239.89
mediastinal	—	196.1	—	229.0	238.8	239.89
mesenteric (inferior) (superior)	—	196.2	—	229.0	238.8	239.89
midcolic	—	196.2	—	229.0	238.8	239.89
multiple sites in categories 196.0–196.6	—	196.8	—	229.0	238.8	239.89
neck	—	196.0	—	229.0	238.8	239.89
obturator	—	196.6	—	229.0	238.8	239.89
occipital	—	196.0	—	229.0	238.8	239.89
pancreatic	—	196.2	—	229.0	238.8	239.89
para-aortic	—	196.2	—	229.0	238.8	239.89
paracervical	—	196.6	—	229.0	238.8	239.89
parametrial	—	196.6	—	229.0	238.8	239.89
parasternal	—	196.1	—	229.0	238.8	239.89
parotid	—	196.0	—	229.0	238.8	239.89
pectoral	—	196.3	—	229.0	238.8	239.89
pelvic	—	196.6	—	229.0	238.8	239.89
peri-aortic	—	196.2	—	229.0	238.8	239.89
peripancreatic	—	196.2	—	229.0	238.8	239.89
popliteal	—	196.5	—	229.0	238.8	239.89
porta hepatis	—	196.2	—	229.0	238.8	239.89
portal	—	196.2	—	229.0	238.8	239.89
preauricular	—	196.0	—	229.0	238.8	239.89

Index

Neoplasm, lymph, lymphatic — Neoplasm, mucosa

	Malignant			Benign	Uncertain Behavior	Unspecified
	Primary	Secondary	Ca in situ			
Neoplasm, neoplastic — *continued*						
lymph, lymphatic — *continued*						
gland — *continued*						
prelaryngeal	—	196.0	—	229.0	238.8	239.89
presymphysial	—	196.6	—	229.0	238.8	239.89
pretracheal	—	196.0	—	229.0	238.8	239.89
primary (any site) NEC	202.9 ☑	—	—	—	—	—
pulmonary (hiler)	—	196.1	—	229.0	238.8	239.89
pyloric	—	196.2	—	229.0	238.8	239.89
retroperitoneal	—	196.2	—	229.0	238.8	239.89
retropharyngeal	—	196.0	—	229.0	238.8	239.89
Rosenmüller's	—	196.5	—	229.0	238.8	239.89
sacral	—	196.6	—	229.0	238.8	239.89
scalene	—	196.0	—	229.0	238.8	239.89
site NEC	—	196.9	—	229.0	238.8	239.89
splenic (hilar)	—	196.2	—	229.0	238.8	239.89
subclavicular	—	196.3	—	229.0	238.8	239.89
subinguinal	—	196.5	—	229.0	238.8	239.89
sublingual	—	196.0	—	229.0	238.8	239.89
submandibular	—	196.0	—	229.0	238.8	239.89
submaxillary	—	196.0	—	229.0	238.8	239.89
submental	—	196.0	—	229.0	238.8	239.89
subscapular	—	196.3	—	229.0	238.8	239.89
supraclavicular	—	196.0	—	229.0	238.8	239.89
thoracic	—	196.1	—	229.0	238.8	239.89
tibial	—	196.5	—	229.0	238.8	239.89
tracheal	—	196.1	—	229.0	238.8	239.89
tracheobronchial	—	196.1	—	229.0	238.8	239.89
upper limb	—	196.3	—	229.0	238.8	239.89
Virchow's	—	196.0	—	229.0	238.8	239.89
node (see also Neoplasm, lymph gland)						
primary NEC	202.9 ☑	—	—	—	—	—
vessel (see also Neoplasm, connective tissue)	171.9	198.89	—	215.9	238.1	239.2
Mackenrodt's ligament	183.8	198.82	233.39	221.8	236.3	239.5
malar	170.0	198.5	—	213.0	238.0	239.2
region — *see* Neoplasm, cheek						
mammary gland — *see* Neoplasm, breast						
mandible	170.1	198.5	—	213.1	238.0	239.2
alveolar						
mucosa	143.1	198.89	230.0	210.4	235.1	239.0
mucose	143.1	198.89	230.0	210.4	235.1	239.0
ridge or process	170.1	198.5	—	213.1	238.0	239.2
carcinoma	143.1	—	—	—	—	—
carcinoma	143.1	—	—	—	—	—
marrow (bone) NEC	202.9 ☑	198.5	—	—	—	238.79
mastectomy site (skin)	173.5	198.2	—	—	—	—
specified as breast tissue	174.8	198.81	—	—	—	—
mastoid (air cells) (antrum) (cavity)	160.1	197.3	231.8	212.0	235.9	239.1
bone or process	170.0	198.5	—	213.0	238.0	239.2
maxilla, maxillary (superior)	170.0	198.5	—	213.0	238.0	239.2
alveolar						
mucosa	143.0	198.89	230.0	210.4	235.1	239.0
ridge or process	170.0	198.5	—	213.0	238.0	239.2
carcinoma	143.0	—	—	—	—	—
antrum	160.2	197.3	231.8	212.0	235.9	239.1
carcinoma	143.0	—	—	—	—	—

	Malignant			Benign	Uncertain Behavior	Unspecified
	Primary	Secondary	Ca in situ			
Neoplasm, neoplastic — *continued*						
maxilla, maxillary — *continued*						
inferior — *see* Neoplasm, mandible						
sinus	160.2	197.3	231.8	212.0	235.9	239.1
meatus						
external (ear)	173.2	198.2	232.2	216.2	238.2	239.2
Meckel's diverticulum	152.3	197.4	230.7	211.2	235.2	239.0
mediastinum, mediastinal	164.9	197.1	—	212.5	235.8	239.89
anterior	164.2	197.1	—	212.5	235.8	239.89
contiguous sites with heart and thymus	164.8	—	—	—	—	—
posterior	164.3	197.1	—	212.5	235.8	239.89
medulla						
adrenal	194.0	198.7	234.8	227.0	237.2	239.7
oblongata	191.7	198.3	—	225.0	237.5	239.6
meibomian gland	173.1	198.2	232.1	216.1	238.2	239.2
meninges (brain) (cerebral) (cranial) (intracranial)	192.1	198.4	—	225.2	237.6	239.7
spinal (cord)	192.3	198.4	—	225.4	237.6	239.7
meniscus, knee joint (lateral) (medial)	170.7	198.5	—	213.7	238.0	239.2
mesentery, mesenteric	158.8	197.6	—	211.8	235.4	239.0
mesoappendix	158.8	197.6	—	211.8	235.4	239.0
mesocolon	158.8	197.6	—	211.8	235.4	239.0
mesopharynx — *see* Neoplasm, oropharynx						
mesosalpinx	183.3	198.82	233.39	221.0	236.3	239.5
mesovarium	183.3	198.82	233.39	221.0	236.3	239.5
metacarpus (any bone)	170.5	198.5	—	213.5	238.0	239.2
metastatic NEC (see also Neoplasm, by site, secondary)	—	199.1	—	—	—	—
metatarsus (any bone)	170.8	198.5	—	213.8	238.0	239.2
midbrain	191.7	198.3	—	225.0	237.5	239.6
milk duct — *see* Neoplasm, breast						
mons						
pubis	184.4	198.82	233.32	221.2	236.3	239.5
veneris	184.4	198.82	233.32	221.2	236.3	239.5
motor tract	192.9	198.4	—	225.9	237.9	239.7
brain	191.9	198.3	—	225.0	237.5	239.6
spinal	192.2	198.3	—	225.3	237.5	239.7
mouth	145.9	198.89	230.0	210.4	235.1	239.0
contiguous sites	145.8	—	—	—	—	—
floor	144.9	198.89	230.0	210.3	235.1	239.0
anterior portion	144.0	198.89	230.0	210.3	235.1	239.0
contiguous sites	144.8	—	—	—	—	—
lateral portion	144.1	198.89	230.0	210.3	235.1	239.0
roof	145.5	198.89	230.0	210.4	235.1	239.0
specified part NEC	145.8	198.89	230.0	210.4	235.1	239.0
vestibule	145.1	198.89	230.0	210.4	235.1	239.0
mucosa						
alveolar (ridge or process)	143.9	198.89	230.0	210.4	235.1	239.0
lower	143.1	198.89	230.0	210.4	235.1	239.0
upper	143.0	198.89	230.0	210.4	235.1	239.0
buccal	145.0	198.89	230.0	210.4	235.1	239.0
cheek	145.0	198.89	230.0	210.4	235.1	239.0
lip — *see* Neoplasm, lip, internal						
nasal	160.0	197.3	231.8	212.0	235.9	239.1
oral	145.0	198.89	230.0	210.4	235.1	239.0

☑ **Additional Digit Required — Refer to the Tabular List for Digit Selection**   ▽ **Subterms under main terms may continue to next column or page**

Neoplasm, neoplastic—	Malignant Primary	Secondary	Ca in situ	Benign	Uncertain Behavior	Unspecified
continued						
Müllerian duct						
female	184.8	198.82	233.39	221.8	236.3	239.5
male	187.8	198.82	233.6	222.8	236.6	239.5
multiple sites NEC	199.0	199.0	234.9	229.9	238.9	199.0
muscle (*see also* Neoplasm, connective tissue)						
extraocular	190.1	198.4	234.0	224.1	238.8	239.89
myocardium	164.1	198.89	—	212.7	238.8	239.89
myometrium	182.0	198.82	233.2	219.1	236.0	239.5
myopericardium	164.1	198.89	—	212.7	238.8	239.89
nabothian gland (follicle)	180.0	198.82	233.1	219.0	236.0	239.5
nail	173.9	198.2	232.9	216.9	238.2	239.2
finger	173.6	198.2	232.6	216.6	238.2	239.2
toe	173.7	198.2	232.7	216.7	238.2	239.2
nares, naris (anterior) (posterior)	160.0	197.3	231.8	212.0	235.9	239.1
nasal — *see* Neoplasm, nose						
nasolabial groove	173.3	198.2	232.3	216.3	238.2	239.2
nasolacrimal duct	190.7	198.4	234.0	224.7	238.8	239.89
nasopharynx, nasopharyngeal	147.9	198.89	230.0	210.7	235.1	239.0
contiguous sites	147.8	—	—	—	—	—
floor	147.3	198.89	230.0	210.7	235.1	239.0
roof	147.0	198.89	230.0	210.7	235.1	239.0
specified site NEC	147.8	198.89	230.0	210.7	235.1	239.0
wall	147.9	198.89	230.0	210.7	235.1	239.0
anterior	147.3	198.89	230.0	210.7	235.1	239.0
lateral	147.2	198.89	230.0	210.7	235.1	239.0
posterior	147.1	198.89	230.0	210.7	235.1	239.0
superior	147.0	198.89	230.0	210.7	235.1	239.0
nates	173.5	198.2	232.5	216.5	238.2	239.2
neck NEC*	195.0	198.89	234.8	229.8	238.8	239.89
nerve (autonomic) (ganglion) (parasympathetic) (peripheral) (sympathetic) (*see also* Neoplasm, connective tissue)						
abducens	192.0	198.4	—	225.1	237.9	239.7
accessory (spinal)	192.0	198.4	—	225.1	237.9	239.7
acoustic	192.0	198.4	—	225.1	237.9	239.7
auditory	192.0	198.4	—	225.1	237.9	239.7
brachial	171.2	198.89	—	215.2	238.1	239.2
cranial (any)	192.0	198.4	—	225.1	237.9	239.7
facial	192.0	198.4	—	225.1	237.9	239.7
femoral	171.3	198.89	—	215.3	238.1	239.2
glossopharyngeal	192.0	198.4	—	225.1	237.9	239.7
hypoglossal	192.0	198.4	—	225.1	237.9	239.7
intercostal	171.4	198.89	—	215.4	238.1	239.2
lumbar	171.7	198.89	—	215.7	238.1	239.2
median	171.2	198.89	—	215.2	238.1	239.2
obturator	171.3	198.89	—	215.3	238.1	239.2
oculomotor	192.0	198.4	—	225.1	237.9	239.7
olfactory	192.0	198.4	—	225.1	237.9	239.7
optic	192.0	198.4	—	225.1	237.9	239.7
peripheral NEC	171.9	198.89	—	215.9	238.1	239.2
radial	171.2	198.89	—	215.2	238.1	239.2
sacral	171.6	198.89	—	215.6	238.1	239.2
sciatic	171.3	198.89	—	215.3	238.1	239.2
spinal NEC	171.9	198.89	—	215.9	238.1	239.2
trigeminal	192.0	198.4	—	225.1	237.9	239.7
trochlear	192.0	198.4	—	225.1	237.9	239.7
ulnar	171.2	198.89	—	215.2	238.1	239.2
vagus	192.0	198.4	—	225.1	237.9	239.7
nervous system (central) NEC	192.9	198.4	—	225.9	237.9	239.7
autonomic NEC	171.9	198.89	—	215.9	238.1	239.2

Neoplasm, neoplastic—	Malignant Primary	Secondary	Ca in situ	Benign	Uncertain Behavior	Unspecified
continued						
nervous system — *continued*						
brain (*see also* Neoplasm, brain)						
membrane or meninges	192.1	198.4	—	225.2	237.6	239.7
contiguous sites	192.8	—	—	—	—	—
parasympathetic NEC	171.9	198.89	—	215.9	238.1	239.2
sympathetic NEC	171.9	198.89	—	215.9	238.1	239.2
nipple (female)	174.0	198.81	233.0	217	238.3	239.3
male	175.0	198.81	233.0	217	238.3	239.3
nose, nasal	195.0	198.89	234.8	229.8	238.8	239.89
ala (external)	173.3	198.2	232.3	216.3	238.2	239.2
bone	170.0	198.5	—	213.0	238.0	239.2
cartilage	160.0	197.3	231.8	212.0	235.9	239.1
cavity	160.0	197.3	231.8	212.0	235.9	239.1
contiguous sites with accessory sinuses or middle ear	160.8	—	—	—	—	—
choana	147.3	198.89	230.0	210.7	235.1	239.0
external (skin)	173.3	198.2	232.3	216.3	238.2	239.2
fossa	160.0	197.3	231.8	212.0	235.9	239.1
internal	160.0	197.3	231.8	212.0	235.9	239.1
mucosa	160.0	197.3	231.8	212.0	235.9	239.1
septum	160.0	197.3	231.8	212.0	235.9	239.1
posterior margin	147.3	198.89	230.0	210.7	235.1	239.0
sinus — *see* Neoplasm, sinus						
skin	173.3	198.2	232.3	216.3	238.2	239.2
turbinate (mucosa)	160.0	197.3	231.8	212.0	235.9	239.1
bone	170.0	198.5	—	213.0	238.0	239.2
vestibule	160.0	197.3	231.8	212.0	235.9	239.1
nostril	160.0	197.3	231.8	212.0	235.9	239.1
nucleus pulposus	170.2	198.5	—	213.2	238.0	239.2
occipital bone	170.0	198.5	—	213.0	238.0	239.2
lobe or pole, brain	191.4	198.3	—	225.0	237.5	239.6
odontogenic — *see* Neoplasm, jaw bone						
oesophagus — *see* Neoplasm, esophagus						
olfactory nerve or bulb	192.0	198.4	—	225.1	237.9	239.7
olive (brain)	191.7	198.3	—	225.0	237.5	239.6
omentum	158.8	197.6	—	211.8	235.4	239.0
operculum (brain)	191.0	198.3	—	225.0	237.5	239.6
optic nerve, chiasm, or tract	192.0	198.4	—	225.1	237.9	239.7
oral (cavity)	145.9	198.89	230.0	210.4	235.1	239.0
contiguous sites with lip or pharynx	149.8	—	—	—	—	—
ill-defined	149.9	198.89	230.0	210.4	235.1	239.0
mucosa	145.9	198.89	230.0	210.4	235.1	239.0
orbit	190.1	198.4	234.0	224.1	238.8	239.89
bone	170.0	198.5	—	213.0	238.0	239.2
eye	190.1	198.4	234.0	224.1	238.8	239.89
soft parts	190.1	198.4	234.0	224.1	238.8	239.89
organ of Zuckerkandl	194.6	198.89	—	227.6	237.3	239.7
oropharynx	146.9	198.89	230.0	210.6	235.1	239.0
branchial cleft (vestige)	146.8	198.89	230.0	210.6	235.1	239.0
contiguous sites	146.8	—	—	—	—	—
junctional region	146.5	198.89	230.0	210.6	235.1	239.0
lateral wall	146.6	198.89	230.0	210.6	235.1	239.0
pillars of fauces	146.2	198.89	230.0	210.6	235.1	239.0
posterior wall	146.7	198.89	230.0	210.6	235.1	239.0

☑ Additional Digit Required — Refer to the Tabular List for Digit Selection ▽ Subterms under main terms may continue to next column or page

2011 ICD-9-CM   ▶◀ Revised Text   ● New Line   ▲ Revised Code   Volume 2 — 203

Neoplasm, Müllerian duct — Neoplasm, oropharynx

Left column table:

| | Malignant | | | | | |
	Primary	Secondary	Ca in situ	Benign	Uncertain Behavior	Unspecified
Neoplasm, neoplastic — *continued*						
oropharynx — *continued*						
specified part						
NEC	146.8	198.89	230.0	210.6	235.1	239.0
vallecula	146.3	198.89	230.0	210.6	235.1	239.0
os						
external	180.1	198.82	233.1	219.0	236.0	239.5
internal	180.0	198.82	233.1	219.0	236.0	239.5
ovary	183.0	198.6	233.39	220	236.2	239.5
oviduct	183.2	198.82	233.39	221.0	236.3	239.5
palate	145.5	198.89	230.0	210.4	235.1	239.0
hard	145.2	198.89	230.0	210.4	235.1	239.0
junction of hard and soft palate	145.5	198.89	230.0	210.4	235.1	239.0
soft	145.3	198.89	230.0	210.4	235.1	239.0
nasopharyngeal surface	147.3	198.89	230.0	210.7	235.1	239.0
posterior surface	147.3	198.89	230.0	210.7	235.1	239.0
superior surface	147.3	198.89	230.0	210.7	235.1	239.0
palatoglossal arch	146.2	198.89	230.0	210.6	235.1	239.0
palatopharyngeal arch	146.2	198.89	230.0	210.6	235.1	239.0
pallium	191.0	198.3	—	225.0	237.5	239.6
palpebra	173.1	198.2	232.1	216.1	238.2	239.2
pancreas	157.9	197.8	230.9	211.6	235.5	239.0
body	157.1	197.8	230.9	211.6	235.5	239.0
contiguous sites	157.8	—	—	—	—	—
duct (of Santorini) (of Wirsung)	157.3	197.8	230.9	211.6	235.5	239.0
ectopic tissue	157.8	197.8	230.9	211.6	235.5	239.0
head	157.0	197.8	230.9	211.6	235.5	239.0
islet cells	157.4	197.8	230.9	211.7	235.5	239.0
neck	157.8	197.8	230.9	211.6	235.5	239.0
tail	157.2	197.8	230.9	211.6	235.5	239.0
para-aortic body	194.6	198.89	—	227.6	237.3	239.7
paraganglion NEC	194.6	198.89	—	227.6	237.3	239.7
parametrium	183.4	198.82	—	221.0	236.3	239.5
paranephric	158.0	197.6	—	211.8	235.4	239.0
pararectal	195.3	198.89	—	229.8	238.8	239.89
parasagittal (region)	195.0	198.89	234.8	229.8	238.8	239.89
parasellar	192.9	198.4	—	225.9	237.9	239.7
parathyroid (gland)	194.1	198.89	234.8	227.1	237.4	239.7
paraurethral	195.3	198.89	—	229.8	238.8	239.89
gland	189.4	198.1	233.9	223.89	236.99	239.5
paravaginal	195.3	198.89	—	229.8	238.8	239.89
parenchyma, kidney	189.0	198.0	233.9	223.0	236.91	239.5
parietal						
bone	170.0	198.5	—	213.0	238.0	239.2
lobe, brain	191.3	198.3	—	225.0	237.5	239.6
paroophoron	183.3	198.82	233.39	221.0	236.3	239.5
parotid (duct) (gland)	142.0	198.89	230.0	210.2	235.0	239.0
parovarium	183.3	198.82	233.39	221.0	236.3	239.5
patella	170.8	198.5	—	213.8	238.0	239.2
peduncle, cerebral	191.7	198.3	—	225.0	237.5	239.6
pelvirectal junction	154.0	197.5	230.4	211.4	235.2	239.0
pelvis, pelvic	195.3	198.89	234.8	229.8	238.8	239.89
bone	170.6	198.5	—	213.6	238.0	239.2
floor	195.3	198.89	234.8	229.8	238.8	239.89
renal	189.1	198.0	233.9	223.1	236.91	239.5
viscera	195.3	198.89	234.8	229.8	238.8	239.89
wall	195.3	198.89	234.8	229.8	238.8	239.89
pelvo-abdominal	195.8	198.89	234.8	229.8	238.8	239.89
penis	187.4	198.82	233.5	222.1	236.6	239.5
body	187.3	198.82	233.5	222.1	236.6	239.5
corpus (cavernosum)	187.3	198.82	233.5	222.1	236.6	239.5
glans	187.2	198.82	233.5	222.1	236.6	239.5
skin NEC	187.4	198.82	233.5	222.1	236.6	239.5
periadrenal (tissue)	158.0	197.6	—	211.8	235.4	239.0

Right column table:

| | Malignant | | | | | |
	Primary	Secondary	Ca in situ	Benign	Uncertain Behavior	Unspecified
Neoplasm, neoplastic — *continued*						
perianal (skin)	173.5	198.2	232.5	216.5	238.2	239.2
pericardium	164.1	198.89	—	212.7	238.8	239.89
perinephric	158.0	197.6	—	211.8	235.4	239.0
perineum	195.3	198.89	234.8	229.8	238.8	239.89
periodontal tissue NEC	143.9	198.89	230.0	210.4	235.1	239.0
periosteum — *see* Neoplasm, bone						
peripancreatic	158.0	197.6	—	211.8	235.4	239.0
peripheral nerve NEC	171.9	198.89	—	215.9	238.1	239.2
perirectal (tissue)	195.3	198.89	—	229.8	238.8	239.89
perirenal (tissue)	158.0	197.6	—	211.8	235.4	239.0
peritoneum, peritoneal (cavity)	158.9	197.6	—	211.8	235.4	239.0
contiguous sites	158.8	—	—	—	—	—
with digestive organs	159.8	—	—	—	—	—
parietal	158.8	197.6	—	211.8	235.4	239.0
pelvic	158.8	197.6	—	211.8	235.4	239.0
specified part NEC	158.8	197.6	—	211.8	235.4	239.0
peritonsillar (tissue)	195.0	198.89	234.8	229.8	238.8	239.89
periurethral tissue	195.3	198.89	—	229.8	238.8	239.89
phalanges	170.9	198.5	—	213.9	238.0	239.2
foot	170.8	198.5	—	213.8	238.0	239.2
hand	170.5	198.5	—	213.5	238.0	239.2
pharynx, pharyngeal	149.0	198.89	230.0	210.9	235.1	239.0
bursa	147.1	198.89	230.0	210.7	235.1	239.0
fornix	147.3	198.89	230.0	210.7	235.1	239.0
recess	147.2	198.89	230.0	210.7	235.1	239.0
region	149.0	198.89	230.0	210.9	235.1	239.0
tonsil	147.1	198.89	230.0	210.7	235.1	239.0
wall (lateral) (posterior)	149.0	198.89	230.0	210.9	235.1	239.0
pia mater (cerebral) (cranial)	192.1	198.4	—	225.2	237.6	239.7
spinal	192.3	198.4	—	225.4	237.6	239.7
pillars of fauces	146.2	198.89	230.0	210.6	235.1	239.0
pineal (body) (gland)	194.4	198.89	234.8	227.4	237.1	239.7
pinna (ear) NEC	173.2	198.2	232.2	216.2	238.2	239.2
cartilage	171.0	198.89	—	215.0	238.1	239.2
piriform fossa or sinus	148.1	198.89	230.0	210.8	235.1	239.0
pituitary (body) (fossa) (gland) (lobe)	194.3	198.89	234.8	227.3	237.0	239.7
placenta	181	198.82	233.2	219.8	236.1	239.5
pleura, pleural (cavity)	163.9	197.2	—	212.4	235.8	239.1
contiguous sites	163.8	—	—	—	—	—
parietal	163.0	197.2	—	212.4	235.8	239.1
visceral	163.1	197.2	—	212.4	235.8	239.1
plexus						
brachial	171.2	198.89	—	215.2	238.1	239.2
cervical	171.0	198.89	—	215.0	238.1	239.2
choroid	191.5	198.3	—	225.0	237.5	239.6
lumbosacral	171.6	198.89	—	215.6	238.1	239.2
sacral	171.6	198.89	—	215.6	238.1	239.2
pluri-endocrine	194.8	198.89	234.8	227.8	237.4	239.7
pole						
frontal	191.1	198.3	—	225.0	237.5	239.6
occipital	191.4	198.3	—	225.0	237.5	239.6
pons (varolii)	191.7	198.3	—	225.0	237.5	239.6
popliteal fossa or space*	195.5	198.89	234.8	229.8	238.8	239.89
postcricoid (region)	148.0	198.89	230.0	210.8	235.1	239.0
posterior fossa (cranial)	191.9	198.3	—	225.0	237.5	239.6
postnasal space	147.9	198.89	230.0	210.7	235.1	239.0
prepuce	187.1	198.82	233.5	222.1	236.6	239.5
prepylorus	151.1	197.8	230.2	211.1	235.2	239.0

☑ Additional Digit Required — Refer to the Tabular List for Digit Selection   ▽ Subterms under main terms may continue to next column or page

Neoplasm, neoplastic— continued	Malignant Primary	Malignant Secondary	Malignant Ca in situ	Benign	Uncertain Behavior	Unspecified
presacral (region)	195.3	198.89	—	229.8	238.8	239.89
prostate (gland)	185	198.82	233.4	222.2	236.5	239.5
utricle	189.3	198.1	233.9	223.81	236.99	239.5
pterygoid fossa	171.0	198.89	—	215.0	238.1	239.2
pubic bone	170.6	198.5	—	213.6	238.0	239.2
pudenda, pudendum (female)	184.4	198.82	233.32	221.2	236.3	239.5
pulmonary	162.9	197.0	231.2	212.3	235.7	239.1
putamen	191.0	198.3	—	225.0	237.5	239.6
pyloric antrum	151.2	197.8	230.2	211.1	235.2	239.0
canal	151.1	197.8	230.2	211.1	235.2	239.0
pylorus	151.1	197.8	230.2	211.1	235.2	239.0
pyramid (brain)	191.7	198.3	—	225.0	237.5	239.6
pyriform fossa or sinus	148.1	198.89	230.0	210.8	235.1	239.0
radius (any part)	170.4	198.5	—	213.4	238.0	239.2
Rathke's pouch	194.3	198.89	234.8	227.3	237.0	239.7
rectosigmoid (colon) (junction)	154.0	197.5	230.4	211.4	235.2	239.0
contiguous sites with anus or rectum	154.8	—	—	—	—	—
rectouterine pouch	158.8	197.6	—	211.8	235.4	239.0
rectovaginal septum or wall	195.3	198.89	234.8	229.8	238.8	239.89
rectovesical septum	195.3	198.89	234.8	229.8	238.8	239.89
rectum (ampulla)	154.1	197.5	230.4	211.4	235.2	239.0
and colon	154.0	197.5	230.4	211.4	235.2	239.0
contiguous sites with anus or rectosigmoid junction	154.8	—	—	—	—	—
renal	189.0	198.0	233.9	223.0	236.91	239.5
calyx	189.1	198.0	233.9	223.1	236.91	239.5
hilus	189.1	198.0	233.9	223.1	236.91	239.5
parenchyma	189.0	198.0	233.9	223.0	236.91	239.5
pelvis	189.1	198.0	233.9	223.1	236.91	239.5
respiratory organs or system NEC	165.9	197.3	231.9	212.9	235.9	239.1
contiguous sites with intrathoracic organs	165.8	—	—	—	—	—
specified sites NEC	165.8	197.3	231.8	212.8	235.9	239.1
tract NEC	165.9	197.3	231.9	212.9	235.9	239.1
upper	165.0	197.3	231.9	212.5	235.9	239.1
retina	190.5	198.4	234.0	224.5	238.8	239.81
retrobulbar	190.1	198.4	—	224.1	238.8	239.89
retrocecal	158.0	197.6	—	211.8	235.4	239.0
retromolar (area) (triangle) (trigone)	145.6	198.89	230.0	210.4	235.1	239.0
retro-orbital	195.0	198.89	234.8	229.8	238.8	239.89
retroperitoneal (space) (tissue)	158.0	197.6	—	211.8	235.4	239.0
contiguous sites	158.8	—	—	—	—	—
retroperitoneum	158.0	197.6	—	211.8	235.4	239.0
contiguous sites	158.8	—	—	—	—	—
retropharyngeal	149.0	198.89	230.0	210.9	235.1	239.0
retrovesical (septum)	195.3	198.89	234.8	229.8	238.8	239.89
rhinencephalon	191.0	198.3	—	225.0	237.5	239.6
rib	170.3	198.5	—	213.3	238.0	239.2
Rosenmüller's fossa	147.2	198.89	230.0	210.7	235.1	239.0
round ligament	183.5	198.82	—	221.0	236.3	239.5
sacrococcyx, sacrococcygeal	170.6	198.5	—	213.6	238.0	239.2
region	195.3	198.89	234.8	229.8	238.8	239.89
sacrouterine ligament	183.4	198.82	—	221.0	236.3	239.5
sacrum, sacral (vertebra)	170.6	198.5	—	213.6	238.0	239.2
salivary gland or duct (major)	142.9	198.89	230.0	210.2	235.0	239.0
contiguous sites	142.8	—	—	—	—	—
minor NEC	145.9	198.89	230.0	210.4	235.1	239.0
parotid	142.0	198.89	230.0	210.2	235.0	239.0
pluriglandular	142.8	198.89	—	210.2	235.0	239.0
sublingual	142.2	198.89	230.0	210.2	235.0	239.0
submandibular	142.1	198.89	230.0	210.2	235.0	239.0
submaxillary	142.1	198.89	230.0	210.2	235.0	239.0
salpinx (uterine)	183.2	198.82	233.39	221.0	236.3	239.5
Santorini's duct	157.3	197.8	230.9	211.6	235.5	239.0
scalp	173.4	198.2	232.4	216.4	238.2	239.2
scapula (any part)	170.4	198.5	—	213.4	238.0	239.2
scapular region	195.1	198.89	234.8	229.8	238.8	239.89
scar NEC (see also Neoplasm, skin)	173.9	198.2	232.9	216.9	238.2	239.2
sciatic nerve	171.3	198.89	—	215.3	238.1	239.2
sclera	190.0	198.4	234.0	224.0	238.8	239.89
scrotum (skin)	187.7	198.82	—	222.4	236.6	239.5
sebaceous gland — see Neoplasm, skin						
sella turcica	194.3	198.89	234.8	227.3	237.0	239.7
bone	170.0	198.5	—	213.0	238.0	239.2
semilunar cartilage (knee)	170.7	198.5	—	213.7	238.0	239.2
seminal vesicle	187.8	198.82	233.6	222.8	236.6	239.5
septum nasal	160.0	197.3	231.8	212.0	235.9	239.1
posterior margin	147.3	198.89	230.0	210.7	235.1	239.0
rectovaginal	195.3	198.89	234.8	229.8	238.8	239.89
rectovesical	195.3	198.89	234.8	229.8	238.8	239.89
urethrovaginal	184.9	198.82	233.39	221.9	236.3	239.5
vesicovaginal	184.9	198.82	233.39	221.9	236.3	239.5
shoulder NEC*	195.4	198.89	232.6	229.8	238.8	239.89
sigmoid flexure (lower) (upper)	153.3	197.5	230.3	211.3	235.2	239.0
sinus (accessory)	160.9	197.3	231.8	212.0	235.9	239.1
bone (any)	170.0	198.5	—	213.0	238.0	239.2
contiguous sites with middle ear or nasal cavities	160.8	—	—	—	—	—
ethmoidal	160.3	197.3	231.8	212.0	235.9	239.1
frontal	160.4	197.3	231.8	212.0	235.9	239.1
maxillary	160.2	197.3	231.8	212.0	235.9	239.1
nasal, paranasal NEC	160.9	197.3	231.8	212.0	235.9	239.1
pyriform	148.1	198.89	230.0	210.8	235.1	239.0
sphenoidal	160.5	197.3	231.8	212.0	235.9	239.1
skeleton, skeletal NEC	170.9	198.5	—	213.9	238.0	239.2
Skene's gland	189.4	198.1	233.9	223.89	236.99	239.5
skin NEC	173.9	198.2	232.9	216.9	238.2	239.2
abdominal wall	173.5	198.2	232.5	216.5	238.2	239.2
ala nasi	173.3	198.2	232.3	216.3	238.2	239.2
ankle	173.7	198.2	232.7	216.7	238.2	239.2
antecubital space	173.6	198.2	232.6	216.6	238.2	239.2
anus	173.5	198.2	232.5	216.5	238.2	239.2
arm	173.6	198.2	232.6	216.6	238.2	239.2
auditory canal (external)	173.2	198.2	232.2	216.2	238.2	239.2
auricle (ear)	173.2	198.2	232.2	216.2	238.2	239.2
auricular canal (external)	173.2	198.2	232.2	216.2	238.2	239.2
axilla, axillary fold	173.5	198.2	232.5	216.5	238.2	239.2
back	173.5	198.2	232.5	216.5	238.2	239.2
breast	173.5	198.2	232.5	216.5	238.2	239.2
brow	173.3	198.2	232.3	216.3	238.2	239.2
buttock	173.5	198.2	232.5	216.5	238.2	239.2
calf	173.7	198.2	232.7	216.7	238.2	239.2

☑ Additional Digit Required — Refer to the Tabular List for Digit Selection   ▽ Subterms under main terms may continue to next column or page

2011 ICD-9-CM   ▶◀ Revised Text   ● New Line   ▲ Revised Code   Volume 2 — 205

Neoplasm, presacral — Neoplasm, skin

	Malignant							Malignant					
	Primary	Secondary	Ca in situ	Benign	Uncertain Behavior	Unspecified		Primary	Secondary	Ca in situ	Benign	Uncertain Behavior	Unspecified
Neoplasm, neoplastic— *continued*							**Neoplasm, neoplastic**— *continued*						
skin — *continued*							skin — *continued*						
canthus (eye) (inner)							popliteal fossa or						
(outer)	173.1	198.2	232.1	216.1	238.2	239.2	space	173.7	198.2	232.7	216.7	238.2	239.2
cervical region	173.4	198.2	232.4	216.4	238.2	239.2	prepuce	187.1	198.82	233.5	222.1	236.6	239.5
cheek (external)	173.3	198.2	232.3	216.3	238.2	239.2	pubes	173.5	198.2	232.5	216.5	238.2	239.2
chest (wall)	173.5	198.2	232.5	216.5	238.2	239.2	sacrococcygeal						
chin	173.3	198.2	232.3	216.3	238.2	239.2	region	173.5	198.2	232.5	216.5	238.2	239.2
clavicular area	173.5	198.2	232.5	216.5	238.2	239.2	scalp	173.4	198.2	232.4	216.4	238.2	239.2
clitoris	184.3	198.82	233.32	221.2	236.3	239.5	scapular region	173.5	198.2	232.5	216.5	238.2	239.2
columnella	173.3	198.2	232.3	216.3	238.2	239.2	scrotum	187.7	198.82	233.6	222.4	236.6	239.5
concha	173.2	198.2	232.2	216.2	238.2	239.2	shoulder	173.6	198.2	232.6	216.6	238.2	239.2
contiguous sites	173.8	—	—	—	—	—	sole (foot)	173.7	198.2	232.7	216.7	238.2	239.2
ear (external)	173.2	198.2	232.2	216.2	238.2	239.2	specified sites						
elbow	173.6	198.2	232.6	216.6	238.2	239.2	NEC	173.8	198.2	232.8	216.8	232.8	239.2
eyebrow	173.3	198.2	232.3	216.3	238.2	239.2	submammary						
eyelid	173.1	198.2	232.1	—	238.2	239.2	fold	173.5	198.2	232.5	216.5	238.2	239.2
face NEC	173.3	198.2	232.3	216.3	238.2	239.2	supraclavicular						
female genital organs							region	173.4	198.2	232.4	216.4	238.2	239.2
(external)	184.4	198.82	233.30	221.2	236.3	239.5	temple	173.3	198.2	232.3	216.3	238.2	239.2
clitoris	184.3	198.82	233.32	221.2	236.3	239.5	thigh	173.7	198.2	232.7	216.7	238.2	239.2
labium NEC	184.4	198.82	233.32	221.2	236.3	239.5	thoracic wall	173.5	198.2	232.5	216.5	238.2	239.2
majus	184.1	198.82	233.32	221.2	236.3	239.5	thumb	173.6	198.2	232.6	216.6	238.2	239.2
minus	184.2	198.82	233.32	221.2	236.3	239.5	toe	173.7	198.2	232.7	216.7	238.2	239.2
pudendum	184.4	198.82	233.32	221.2	236.3	239.5	tragus	173.2	198.2	232.2	216.2	238.2	239.2
vulva	184.4	198.82	233.32	221.2	236.3	239.5	trunk	173.5	198.2	232.5	216.5	238.2	239.2
finger	173.6	198.2	232.6	216.6	238.2	239.2	umbilicus	173.5	198.2	232.5	216.5	238.2	239.2
flank	173.5	198.2	232.5	216.5	238.2	239.2	vulva	184.4	198.82	233.32	221.2	236.3	239.5
foot	173.7	198.2	232.7	216.7	238.2	239.2	wrist	173.6	198.2	232.6	216.6	238.2	239.2
forearm	173.6	198.2	232.6	216.6	238.2	239.2	skull	170.0	198.5	—	213.0	238.0	239.2
forehead	173.3	198.2	232.3	216.3	238.2	239.2	soft parts or tissues — *see* Neoplasm, connective tissue						
glabella	173.3	198.2	232.3	216.3	238.2	239.2	specified site NEC	195.8	198.89	234.8	229.8	238.8	239.89
gluteal region	173.5	198.2	232.5	216.5	238.2	239.2	specified site — *see* Neoplasm, skin						
groin	173.5	198.2	232.5	216.5	238.2	239.2	spermatic cord	187.6	198.82	233.6	222.8	236.6	239.5
hand	173.6	198.2	232.6	216.6	238.2	239.2	sphenoid	160.5	197.3	231.8	212.0	235.9	239.1
head NEC	173.4	198.2	232.4	216.4	238.2	239.2	bone	170.0	198.5	—	213.0	238.0	239.2
heel	173.7	198.2	232.7	216.7	238.2	239.2	sinus	160.5	197.3	231.8	212.0	235.9	239.1
helix	173.2	198.2	—	216.2	238.2	239.2	sphincter						
hip	173.7	198.2	232.7	216.7	238.2	239.2	anal	154.2	197.5	230.5	211.4	235.5	239.0
infraclavicular							of Oddi	156.1	197.8	230.8	211.5	235.3	239.0
region	173.5	198.2	232.5	216.5	238.2	239.2	spine, spinal						
inguinal region	173.5	198.2	232.5	216.5	238.2	239.2	(column)	170.2	198.5	—	213.2	238.0	239.2
jaw	173.3	198.2	232.3	216.3	238.2	239.2	bulb	191.7	198.3	—	225.0	237.5	239.6
knee	173.7	198.2	232.7	216.7	238.2	239.2	coccyx	170.6	198.5	—	213.6	238.0	239.2
labia							cord (cervical) (lumbar) (sacral) (thoracic)	192.2	198.3	—	225.3	237.5	239.7
majora	184.1	198.82	233.32	221.2	236.3	239.5	dura mater	192.3	198.4	—	225.4	237.6	239.7
minora	184.2	198.82	233.32	221.2	236.3	239.5	lumbosacral	170.2	198.5	—	213.2	238.0	239.2
leg	173.7	198.2	232.7	216.7	238.2	239.2	membrane	192.3	198.4	—	225.4	237.6	239.7
lid (lower)							meninges	192.3	198.4	—	225.4	237.6	239.7
(upper)	—	198.2	232.1	216.1	238.2	239.2	nerve (root)	171.9	198.89	—	215.9	238.1	239.2
limb NEC	173.9	198.2	232.9	216.9	238.2	239.5	pia mater	192.3	198.4	—	225.4	237.6	239.7
lower	173.7	198.2	232.7	216.7	238.2	239.2	root	171.9	198.89	—	215.9	238.1	239.2
upper	173.6	198.2	232.6	216.6	238.2	239.2	sacrum	170.6	198.5	—	213.6	238.0	239.2
lip (lower)							spleen, splenic						
(upper)	173.0	198.2	232.0	216.0	238.2	239.2	NEC	159.1	197.8	230.9	211.9	235.5	239.0
male genital							flexure (colon)	153.7	197.5	230.3	211.3	235.2	239.0
organs	187.9	198.82	233.6	222.9	236.6	239.5	stem, brain	191.7	198.3	—	225.0	237.5	239.6
penis	187.4	198.82	233.5	222.1	236.6	239.5	Stensen's duct	142.0	198.89	230.0	210.2	235.0	239.0
prepuce	187.1	198.82	233.5	222.1	236.6	239.5	sternum	170.3	198.5	—	213.3	238.0	239.2
scrotum	187.7	198.82	233.6	222.4	236.6	239.5	stomach	151.9	197.8	230.2	211.1	235.2	239.0
mastectomy site	173.5	198.2	—	—	—	—	antrum (pyloric)	151.2	197.8	230.2	211.1	235.2	239.0
specified as breast tissue	174.8	198.81	—	—	—	—	body	151.4	197.8	230.2	211.1	235.2	239.0
meatus, acoustic							cardia	151.0	197.8	230.2	211.1	235.2	239.0
(external)	173.2	198.2	232.2	216.2	238.2	239.2	cardiac orifice	151.0	197.8	230.2	211.1	235.2	239.0
nates	173.5	198.2	232.5	216.5	238.2	239.0	contiguous sites	151.8	—	—	—	—	—
neck	173.4	198.2	232.4	216.4	238.2	239.2	corpus	151.4	197.8	230.2	211.1	235.2	239.0
nose (external)	173.3	198.2	232.3	216.3	238.2	239.2	fundus	151.3	197.8	230.2	211.1	235.2	239.0
palm	173.6	198.2	232.6	216.6	238.2	239.2	greater curvature						
palpebra	173.1	198.2	232.1	216.1	238.2	239.2	NEC	151.6	197.8	230.2	211.1	235.2	239.0
penis NEC	187.4	198.82	233.5	222.1	236.6	239.5	lesser curvature						
perianal	173.5	198.2	232.5	216.5	238.2	239.2	NEC	151.5	197.8	230.2	211.1	235.2	239.0
perineum	173.5	198.2	232.5	216.5	238.2	239.2							
pinna	173.2	198.2	232.2	216.2	238.2	239.2							
plantar	173.7	198.2	232.7	216.7	238.2	239.2							

☑ **Additional Digit Required** — Refer to the Tabular List for Digit Selection   ▽ **Subterms under main terms may continue to next column or page**

Neoplasm, neoplastic—continued	Malignant Primary	Malignant Secondary	Malignant Ca in situ	Benign	Uncertain Behavior	Unspecified
stomach — *continued*						
prepylorus	151.1	197.8	230.2	211.1	235.2	239.0
pylorus	151.1	197.8	230.2	211.1	235.2	239.0
wall NEC	151.9	197.8	230.2	211.1	235.2	239.0
anterior NEC	151.8	197.8	230.2	211.1	235.2	239.0
posterior NEC	151.8	197.8	230.2	211.1	235.2	239.0
stroma, endometrial	182.0	198.82	233.2	219.1	236.0	239.5
stump, cervical	180.8	198.82	233.1	219.0	236.0	239.5
subcutaneous (nodule) (tissue) NEC — *see* Neoplasm, connective tissue						
subdural	192.1	198.4	—	225.2	237.6	239.7
subglottis, subglottic	161.2	197.3	231.0	212.1	235.6	239.1
sublingual	144.9	198.89	230.0	210.3	235.1	239.0
gland or duct	142.2	198.89	230.0	210.2	235.0	239.0
submandibular gland	142.1	198.89	230.0	210.2	235.0	239.0
submaxillary gland or duct	142.1	198.89	230.0	210.2	235.0	239.0
submental	195.0	198.89	234.8	229.8	238.8	239.89
subpleural	162.9	197.0	—	212.3	235.7	239.1
substernal	164.2	197.1	—	212.5	235.8	239.89
sudoriferous, sudoriparous gland, site unspecified	173.9	198.2	232.9	216.9	238.2	239.2
specified site — *see* Neoplasm, skin						
supraclavicular region	195.0	198.89	234.8	229.8	238.8	239.89
supraglottis	161.1	197.3	231.0	212.1	235.6	239.1
suprarenal (capsule) (cortex) (gland) (medulla)	194.0	198.7	234.8	227.0	237.2	239.7
suprasellar (region)	191.9	198.3	—	225.0	237.5	239.6
sweat gland (apocrine) (eccrine), site unspecified	173.9	198.2	232.9	216.9	238.2	239.2
sympathetic nerve or nervous system NEC	171.9	198.89	—	215.9	238.1	239.2
symphysis pubis	170.6	198.5	—	213.6	238.0	239.2
synovial membrane — *see* Neoplasm, connective tissue						
tapetum, brain	191.8	198.3	—	225.0	237.5	239.6
tarsus (any bone)	170.8	198.5	—	213.8	238.0	239.2
temple (skin)	173.3	198.2	232.3	216.3	238.2	239.2
temporal bone	170.0	198.5	—	213.0	238.0	239.2
lobe or pole	191.2	198.3	—	225.0	237.5	239.6
region	195.0	198.89	234.8	229.8	238.8	239.89
skin	173.3	198.2	232.3	216.3	238.2	239.2
tendon (sheath) — *see* Neoplasm, connective tissue						
tentorium (cerebelli)	192.1	198.4	—	225.2	237.6	239.7
testis, testes (descended) (scrotal)	186.9	198.82	233.6	222.0	236.4	239.5
ectopic	186.0	198.82	233.6	222.0	236.4	239.5
retained	186.0	198.82	233.6	222.0	236.4	239.5
undescended	186.0	198.82	233.6	222.0	236.4	239.5
thalamus	191.0	198.3	—	225.0	237.5	239.6
thigh NEC*	195.5	198.89	234.8	229.8	238.8	239.89
thorax, thoracic (cavity) (organs NEC)	195.1	198.89	234.8	229.8	238.8	239.89
duct	171.4	198.89	—	215.4	238.1	239.2
wall NEC	195.1	198.89	234.8	229.8	238.8	239.89
throat	149.0	198.89	230.0	210.9	235.1	239.0
thumb NEC*	195.4	198.89	232.6	229.8	238.8	239.89

Neoplasm, neoplastic—continued	Malignant Primary	Malignant Secondary	Malignant Ca in situ	Benign	Uncertain Behavior	Unspecified
thymus (gland)	164.0	198.89	—	212.6	235.8	239.89
contiguous sites with heart and mediastinum	164.8	—	—	—	—	—
thyroglossal duct	193	198.89	234.8	226	237.4	239.7
thyroid (gland)	193	198.89	234.8	226	237.4	239.7
cartilage	161.3	197.3	231.0	212.1	235.6	239.1
tibia (any part)	170.7	198.5	—	213.7	238.0	239.2
toe NEC*	195.5	198.89	232.7	229.8	238.8	239.89
tongue	141.9	198.89	230.0	210.1	235.1	239.0
anterior (two-thirds) NEC	141.4	198.89	230.0	210.1	235.1	239.0
dorsal surface	141.1	198.89	230.0	210.1	235.1	239.0
ventral surface	141.3	198.89	230.0	210.1	235.1	239.0
base (dorsal surface)	141.0	198.89	230.0	210.1	235.1	239.0
border (lateral)	141.2	198.89	230.0	210.1	235.1	239.0
contiguous sites	141.8	—	—	—	—	—
dorsal surface NEC	141.1	198.89	230.0	210.1	235.1	239.0
fixed part NEC	141.0	198.89	230.0	210.1	235.1	239.0
foreamen cecum	141.1	198.89	230.0	210.1	235.1	239.0
frenulum linguae	141.3	198.89	230.0	210.1	235.1	239.0
junctional zone	141.5	198.89	230.0	210.1	235.1	239.0
margin (lateral)	141.2	198.89	230.0	210.1	235.1	239.0
midline NEC	141.1	198.89	230.0	210.1	235.1	239.0
mobile part NEC	141.4	198.89	230.0	210.1	235.1	239.0
posterior (third)	141.0	198.89	230.0	210.1	235.1	239.0
root	141.0	198.89	230.0	210.1	235.1	239.0
surface (dorsal)	141.1	198.89	230.0	210.1	235.1	239.0
base	141.0	198.89	230.0	210.1	235.1	239.0
ventral	141.3	198.89	230.0	210.1	235.1	239.0
tip	141.2	198.89	230.0	210.1	235.1	239.0
tonsil	141.6	198.89	230.0	210.1	235.1	239.0
tonsil	146.0	198.89	230.0	210.5	235.1	239.0
fauces, faucial	146.0	198.89	230.0	210.5	235.1	239.0
lingual	141.6	198.89	230.0	210.1	235.1	239.0
palatine	146.0	198.89	230.0	210.5	235.1	239.0
pharyngeal	147.1	198.89	230.0	210.7	235.1	239.0
pillar (anterior) (posterior)	146.2	198.89	230.0	210.6	235.1	239.0
tonsillar fossa	146.1	198.89	230.0	210.6	235.1	239.0
tooth socket NEC	143.9	198.89	230.0	210.4	235.1	239.0
trachea (cartilage) (mucosa)	162.0	197.3	231.1	212.2	235.7	239.1
contiguous sites with bronchus or lung	162.8	—	—	—	—	—
tracheobronchial	162.8	197.3	231.1	212.2	235.7	239.1
contiguous sites with lung	162.8	—	—	—	—	—
tragus	173.2	198.2	232.2	216.2	238.2	239.2
trunk NEC*	195.8	198.89	232.5	229.8	238.8	239.89
tubo-ovarian	183.8	198.82	233.39	221.8	236.3	239.5
tunica vaginalis	187.8	198.82	233.6	222.8	236.6	239.5
turbinate (bone)	170.0	198.5	—	213.0	238.0	239.2
nasal	160.0	197.3	231.8	212.0	235.9	239.1
tympanic cavity	160.1	197.3	231.8	212.0	235.9	239.1
ulna (any part)	170.4	198.5	—	213.4	238.0	239.2
umbilicus, umbilical	173.5	198.2	232.5	216.5	238.2	239.2
uncus, brain	191.2	198.3	—	225.0	237.5	239.6
unknown site or unspecified	199.1	199.1	234.9	229.9	238.9	239.9
urachus	188.7	198.1	233.7	223.3	236.7	239.4
ureter-bladder (junction)	188.6	198.1	233.7	223.3	236.7	239.4
ureter, ureteral	189.2	198.1	233.9	223.2	236.91	239.5
orifice (bladder)*	188.6	198.1	233.7	223.3	236.7	239.4
urethra, urethral (gland)	189.3	198.1	233.9	223.81	236.99	239.5
orifice, internal	188.5	198.1	233.7	223.3	236.7	239.4
urethrovaginal (septum)	184.9	198.82	233.39	221.9	236.3	239.5

☑ **Additional Digit Required** — Refer to the Tabular List for Digit Selection   ▽ **Subterms under main terms may continue to next column or page**

Neoplasm, neoplastic—	Malignant					
	Primary	Secondary	Ca in situ	Benign	Uncertain Behavior	Unspecified
continued						
urinary organ or system						
NEC	189.9	198.1	233.9	223.9	236.99	239.5
bladder — *see* Neoplasm, bladder						
contiguous sites	189.8	—	—	—	—	—
specified sites NEC	189.8	198.1	233.9	223.89	236.99	239.5
utero-ovarian	183.8	198.82	233.39	221.8	236.3	239.5
ligament	183.3	198.82		221.0	236.3	239.5
uterosacral ligament	183.4	198.82	—	221.0	236.3	239.5
uterus, uteri, uterine	179	198.82	233.2	219.9	236.0	239.5
adnexa NEC	183.9	198.82	233.39	221.8	236.3	239.5
contiguous sites	183.8	—	—	—	—	—
body	182.0	198.82	233.2	219.1	236.0	239.5
contiguous sites	182.8	—	—	—	—	—
cervix	180.9	198.82	233.1	219.0	236.0	239.5
cornu	182.0	198.82	233.2	219.1	236.0	239.5
corpus	182.0	198.82	233.2	219.1	236.0	239.5
endocervix (canal) (gland)	180.0	198.82	233.1	219.0	236.0	239.5
endometrium	182.0	198.82	233.2	219.1	236.0	239.5
exocervix	180.1	198.82	233.1	219.0	236.0	239.5
external os	180.1	198.82	233.1	219.0	236.0	239.5
fundus	182.0	198.82	233.2	219.1	236.0	239.5
internal os	180.0	198.82	233.1	219.0	236.0	239.5
isthmus	182.1	198.82	233.2	219.1	236.0	239.5
ligament	183.4	198.82	—	221.0	236.3	239.5
broad	183.3	198.82	233.39	221.0	236.3	239.5
round	183.5	198.82	—	221.0	236.3	239.5
lower segment	182.1	198.82	233.2	219.1	236.0	239.5
myometrium	182.0	198.82	233.2	219.1	236.0	239.5
squamocolumnar junction	180.8	198.82	233.1	219.0	236.0	239.5
tube	183.2	198.82	233.39	221.0	236.3	239.5
utricle, prostatic	189.3	198.1	233.9	223.81	236.99	239.5
uveal tract	190.0	198.4	234.0	224.0	238.8	239.89
uvula	145.4	198.89	230.0	210.4	235.1	239.0
vagina, vaginal (fornix) (vault) (wall)	184.0	198.82	233.31	221.1	236.3	239.5
vaginovesical	184.9	198.82	233.39	221.9	236.3	239.5
septum	184.9	198.82	233.39	221.9	236.3	239.5
vallecula (epiglottis)	146.3	198.89	230.0	210.6	235.1	239.0
vascular — *see* Neoplasm, connective tissue						
vas deferens	187.6	198.82	233.6	222.8	236.6	239.5
Vater's ampulla	156.2	197.8	230.8	211.5	235.3	239.0
vein, venous — *see* Neoplasm, connective tissue						
vena cava (abdominal) (inferior)	171.5	198.89	—	215.5	238.1	239.2
superior	171.4	198.89	—	215.4	238.1	239.2
ventricle (cerebral) (floor) (fourth) (lateral) (third)	191.5	198.3	—	225.0	237.5	239.6
cardiac (left) (right)	164.1	198.89		212.7	238.8	239.89
ventricular band of larynx	161.1	197.3	231.0	212.1	235.6	239.1
ventriculus — *see* Neoplasm, stomach						
vermillion border — *see* Neoplasm, lip						
vermis, cerebellum	191.6	198.3	—	225.0	237.5	239.6
vertebra (column)	170.2	198.5	—	213.2	238.0	239.2
coccyx	170.6	198.5	—	213.6	238.0	239.2
sacrum	170.6	198.5	—	213.6	238.0	239.2

Neoplasm, neoplastic—	Malignant					
	Primary	Secondary	Ca in situ	Benign	Uncertain Behavior	Unspecified
continued						
vesical — *see* Neoplasm, bladder						
vesicle, seminal	187.8	198.82	233.6	222.8	236.6	239.5
vesicocervical tissue	184.9	198.82	233.39	221.9	236.3	239.5
vesicorectal	195.3	198.89	234.8	229.8	238.8	239.89
vesicovaginal	184.9	198.82	233.39	221.9	236.3	239.5
septum	184.9	198.82	233.39	221.9	236.3	239.5
vessel (blood) — *see* Neoplasm, connective tissue						
vestibular gland, greater	184.1	198.82	233.32	221.2	236.3	239.5
vestibule						
mouth	145.1	198.89	230.0	210.4	235.1	239.0
nose	160.0	197.3	231.8	212.0	235.9	239.1
Virchow's gland	—	196.0	—	229.0	238.8	239.89
viscera NEC	195.8	198.89	234.8	229.8	238.8	239.89
vocal cords (true)	161.0	197.3	231.0	212.1	235.6	239.1
false	161.1	197.3	231.0	212.1	235.6	239.1
vomer	170.0	198.5	—	213.0	238.0	239.2
vulva	184.4	198.82	233.32	221.2	236.3	239.5
vulvovaginal gland	184.4	198.82	233.32	221.2	236.3	239.5
Waldeyer's ring	149.1	198.89	230.0	210.9	235.1	239.0
Wharton's duct	142.1	198.89	230.0	210.2	235.0	239.0
white matter (central) (cerebral)	191.0	198.3	—	225.0	237.5	239.6
windpipe	162.0	197.3	231.1	212.2	235.7	239.1
Wirsung's duct	157.3	197.8	230.9	211.6	235.5	239.0
wolffian (body) (duct) female	184.8	198.82	233.39	221.8	236.3	239.5
male	187.8	198.82	233.6	222.8	236.6	239.5
womb — *see* Neoplasm, uterus						
wrist NEC*	195.4	198.89	232.6	229.8	238.8	239.89
xiphoid process	170.3	198.5	—	213.3	238.0	239.2
Zuckerkandl's organ	194.6	198.89	—	227.6	237.3	239.7

☑ **Additional Digit Required — Refer to the Tabular List for Digit Selection**

▽ **Subterms under main terms may continue to next column or page**

Neovascularization
 choroid 362.16
 ciliary body 364.42
 cornea 370.60
  deep 370.63
  localized 370.61
 iris 364.42
 retina 362.16
 subretinal 362.16
Nephralgia 788.0
Nephritis, nephritic (albuminuric) (azotemic)
  (congenital) (degenerative) (diffuse)
  (disseminated) (epithelial) (familial) (focal) (granulomatous) (hemorrhagic) (infantile) (nonsuppurative, excretory)
  (uremic) 583.9
 with
  edema — see Nephrosis
  lesion of
   glomerulonephritis
    hypocomplementemic persistent
     583.2
     with nephrotic syndrome
      581.2
      chronic 582.2
    lobular 583.2
     with nephrotic syndrome
      581.2
      chronic 582.2
    membranoproliferative 583.2
     with nephrotic syndrome
      581.2
      chronic 582.2
    membranous 583.1
     with nephrotic syndrome
      581.1
      chronic 582.1
    mesangiocapillary 583.2
     with nephrotic syndrome
      581.2
      chronic 582.2
    mixed membranous and prolifer-
     ative 583.2
     with nephrotic syndrome
      581.2
      chronic 582.2
    proliferative (diffuse) 583.0
     with nephrotic syndrome
      581.0
     acute 580.0
     chronic 582.0
    rapidly progressive 583.4
     acute 580.4
     chronic 582.4
   interstitial nephritis (diffuse) (focal)
    583.89
    with nephrotic syndrome 581.89
    acute 580.89
    chronic 582.89
   necrotizing glomerulitis 583.4
    acute 580.4
    chronic 582.4
   renal necrosis 583.9
    cortical 583.6
    medullary 583.7
   specified pathology NEC 583.89
    with nephrotic syndrome 581.89
    acute 580.89
    chronic 582.89
  necrosis, renal 583.9
   cortical 583.6
   medullary (papillary) 583.7
  nephrotic syndrome (see also Nephrosis)
   581.9
  papillary necrosis 583.7
  specified pathology NEC 583.89
 acute 580.9
  extracapillary with epithelial crescents
   580.4
  hypertensive (see also Hypertension,
   kidney) 403.90
  necrotizing 580.4
  poststreptococcal 580.0
  proliferative (diffuse) 580.0
  rapidly progressive 580.4
  specified pathology NEC 580.89

Nephritis, nephritic — continued
 amyloid 277.39 [583.81]
  chronic 277.39 [582.81]
 arteriolar (see also Hypertension, kidney)
  403.90
 arteriosclerotic (see also Hypertension, kidney) 403.90
 ascending (see also Pyelitis) 590.80
 atrophic 582.9
 basement membrane NEC 583.89
  with
   pulmonary hemorrhage (Goodpas-
    ture's syndrome)
    446.21 [583.81]
 calculous, calculus 592.0
 cardiac (see also Hypertension, kidney)
  403.90
 cardiovascular (see also Hypertension, kidney) 403.90
 chronic 582.9
  arteriosclerotic (see also Hypertension,
   kidney) 403.90
  hypertensive (see also Hypertension,
   kidney) 403.90
 cirrhotic (see also Sclerosis, renal) 587
 complicating pregnancy, childbirth, or
  puerperium 646.2 ☑
  with hypertension 642.1 ☑
   affecting fetus or newborn 760.0
  affecting fetus or newborn 760.1
 croupous 580.9
 desquamative — see Nephrosis
 due to
  amyloidosis 277.39 [583.81]
   chronic 277.39 [582.81]
  arteriosclerosis (see also Hypertension,
   kidney) 403.90
  diabetes mellitus 250.4 ☑ [583.81]
   with nephrotic syndrome
    250.4 ☑ [581.81]
    due to secondary diabetes
     249.4 ☑ [583.81]
   due to secondary diabetes
    249.4 ☑ [583.81]
  diphtheria 032.89 [580.81]
  gonococcal infection (acute)
   098.19 [583.81]
   chronic or duration of 2 months or
    over 098.39 [583.81]
  gout 274.10
  infectious hepatitis 070.9 [580.81]
  mumps 072.79 [580.81]
  specified kidney pathology NEC 583.89
   acute 580.89
   chronic 582.89
  streptotrichosis 039.8 [583.81]
  subacute bacterial endocarditis
   421.0 [580.81]
  systemic lupus erythematosus
   710.0 [583.81]
   chronic 710.0 [582.81]
  typhoid fever 002.0 [580.81]
 endothelial 582.2
 end stage (chronic) (terminal) NEC 585.6
 epimembranous 581.1
 exudative 583.89
  with nephrotic syndrome 581.89
  acute 580.89
  chronic 582.89
 gonococcal (acute) 098.19 [583.81]
  chronic or duration of 2 months or over
   098.39 [583.81]
 gouty 274.10
 hereditary (Alport's syndrome) 759.89
 hydremic — see Nephrosis
 hypertensive (see also Hypertension, kidney)
  403.90
 hypocomplementemic persistent 583.2
  with nephrotic syndrome 581.2
  chronic 582.2
 immune complex NEC 583.89
 infective (see also Pyelitis) 590.80
 interstitial (diffuse) (focal) 583.89
  with nephrotic syndrome 581.89
  acute 580.89
  chronic 582.89

Nephritis, nephritic — continued
 latent or quiescent — see Nephritis, chronic
 lead 984.9
  specified type of lead — see Table of
   Drugs and Chemicals
 lobular 583.2
  with nephrotic syndrome 581.2
  chronic 582.2
 lupus 710.0 [583.81]
  acute 710.0 [580.81]
  chronic 710.0 [582.81]
 membranoproliferative 583.2
  with nephrotic syndrome 581.2
  chronic 582.2
 membranous 583.1
  with nephrotic syndrome 581.1
  chronic 582.1
 mesangiocapillary 583.2
  with nephrotic syndrome 581.2
  chronic 582.2
 minimal change 581.3
 mixed membranous and proliferative 583.2
  with nephrotic syndrome 581.2
  chronic 582.2
 necrotic, necrotizing 583.4
  acute 580.4
  chronic 582.4
 nephrotic — see Nephrosis
 old — see Nephritis, chronic
 parenchymatous 581.89
 polycystic 753.12
  adult type (APKD) 753.13
  autosomal dominant 753.13
  autosomal recessive 753.14
  childhood type (CPKD) 753.14
  infantile type 753.14
 poststreptococcal 580.0
 pregnancy — see Nephritis, complicating
  pregnancy
 proliferative 583.0
  with nephrotic syndrome 581.0
  acute 580.0
  chronic 582.0
 purulent (see also Pyelitis) 590.80
 rapidly progressive 583.4
  acute 580.4
  chronic 582.4
 salt-losing or salt-wasting (see also Disease,
  renal) 593.9
 saturnine 984.9
  specified type of lead — see Table of
   Drugs and Chemicals
 septic (see also Pyelitis) 590.80
 specified pathology NEC 583.89
  acute 580.89
  chronic 582.89
 staphylococcal (see also Pyelitis) 590.80
 streptotrichosis 039.8 [583.81]
 subacute (see also Nephrosis) 581.9
 suppurative (see also Pyelitis) 590.80
 syphilitic (late) 095.4
  congenital 090.5 [583.81]
  early 091.69 [583.81]
 terminal (chronic) (end-stage) NEC 585.6
 toxic — see Nephritis, acute
 tubal, tubular — see Nephrosis, tubular
 tuberculous (see also Tuberculosis)
  016.0 ☑ [583.81]
 type II (Ellis) — see Nephrosis
 vascular — see Hypertension, kidney
 war 580.9
Nephroblastoma (M8960/3) 189.0
 epithelial (M8961/3) 189.0
 mesenchymal (M8962/3) 189.0
Nephrocalcinosis 275.49
Nephrocystitis, pustular — see also Pyelitis
 590.80
Nephrolithiasis (congenital) (pelvis) (recurrent)
 592.0
 uric acid 274.11
Nephroma (M8960/3) 189.0
 mesoblastic (M8960/1) 236.9 ☑
Nephronephritis — see also Nephrosis 581.9
Nephronopthisis 753.16
Nephropathy — see also Nephritis 583.9

Nephropathy — see also Nephritis —
  continued
 with
  exudative nephritis 583.89
  interstitial nephritis (diffuse) (focal)
   583.89
  medullary necrosis 583.7
  necrosis 583.9
   cortical 583.6
   medullary or papillary 583.7
  papillary necrosis 583.7
  specified lesion or cause NEC 583.89
 analgesic 583.89
  with medullary necrosis, acute 584.7
 arteriolar (see also Hypertension, kidney)
  403.90
 arteriosclerotic (see also Hypertension, kidney) 403.90
 complicating pregnancy 646.2 ☑
 diabetic 250.4 ☑ [583.81]
  due to secondary diabetes
   249.4 ☑ [583.81]
 gouty 274.10
  specified type NEC 274.19
 hereditary amyloid 277.31
 hypercalcemic 588.89
 hypertensive (see also Hypertension, kidney)
  403.90
 hypokalemic (vacuolar) 588.89
 IgA 583.9
 obstructive 593.89
  congenital 753.20
 phenacetin 584.7
 phosphate-losing 588.0
 potassium depletion 588.89
 proliferative (see also Nephritis, proliferative)
  583.0
 protein-losing 588.89
 salt-losing or salt-wasting (see also Disease,
  renal) 593.9
 sickle-cell (see also Disease, sickle-cell)
  282.60 [583.81]
 toxic 584.5
 vasomotor 584.5
 water-losing 588.89
Nephroptosis — see also Disease, renal 593.0
 congenital (displaced) 753.3
Nephropyosis — see also Abscess, kidney
 590.2
Nephrorrhagia 593.81
Nephrosclerosis (arteriolar) (arteriosclerotic)
 (chronic) (hyaline) — see also Hypertension, kidney 403.90
 gouty 274.10
 hyperplastic (arteriolar) (see also Hypertension, kidney) 403.90
 senile (see also Sclerosis, renal) 587
Nephrosis, nephrotic (Epstein's) (syndrome)
 581.9
 with
  lesion of
   focal glomerulosclerosis 581.1
   glomerulonephritis
    endothelial 581.2
    hypocomplementemic persistent
     581.2
    lobular 581.2
    membranoproliferative 581.2
    membranous 581.1
    mesangiocapillary 581.2
    minimal change 581.3
    mixed membranous and prolifer-
     ative 581.2
    proliferative 581.0
   segmental hyalinosis 581.1
   specified pathology NEC 581.89
 acute — see Nephrosis, tubular
 anoxic — see Nephrosis, tubular
 arteriosclerotic (see also Hypertension, kidney) 403.90
 chemical — see Nephrosis, tubular
 cholemic 572.4
 complicating pregnancy, childbirth, or
  puerperium — see Nephritis, complicating pregnancy
 diabetic 250.4 ☑ [581.81]

☑ Additional Digit Required — Refer to the Tabular List for Digit Selection
▽ Subterms under main terms may continue to next column or page
2011 ICD-9-CM
▶◀ Revised Text
● New Line
▲ Revised Code
Volume 2 — 209

Nephrosis, nephrotic — *continued*
  diabetic — *continued*
    due to secondary diabetes
      249.4 ☑ *[581.81]*
  Finnish type (congenital) 759.89
  hemoglobinuric — *see* Nephrosis, tubular
  in
    amyloidosis 277.39 *[581.81]*
    diabetes mellitus 250.4 ☑ *[581.81]*
      due to secondary diabetes
        249.4 ☑ *[581.81]*
    epidemic hemorrhagic fever 078.6
    malaria 084.9 *[581.81]*
    polyarteritis 446.0 *[581.81]*
    systemic lupus erythematosus
      710.0 *[581.81]*
  ischemic — *see* Nephrosis, tubular
  lipoid 581.3
  lower nephron — *see* Nephrosis, tubular
  lupoid 710.0 *[581.81]*
  lupus 710.0 *[581.81]*
  malarial 084.9 *[581.81]*
  minimal change 581.3
  necrotizing — *see* Nephrosis, tubular
  osmotic (sucrose) 588.89
  polyarteritic 446.0 *[581.81]*
  radiation 581.9
  specified lesion or cause NEC 581.89
  syphilitic 095.4
  toxic — *see* Nephrosis, tubular
  tubular (acute) 584.5
    due to a procedure 997.5
    radiation 581.9
Nephrosonephritis hemorrhagic (endemic)
  078.6
Nephrostomy status V44.6
  with complication 997.5
Nerve — *see* condition
Nerves 799.21
Nervous — *see also* condition 799.21
  breakdown 300.9
  heart 306.2
  stomach 306.4
  tension 799.21
Nervousness 799.21
Nesidioblastoma (M8150/0)
  pancreas 211.7
  specified site NEC — *see* Neoplasm, by site,
    benign
  unspecified site 211.7
Netherton's syndrome (ichthyosiform erythroderma) 757.1
Nettle rash 708.8
Nettleship's disease (urticaria pigmentosa)
  757.33
Neumann's disease (pemphigus vegetans)
  694.4
Neuralgia, neuralgic (acute) — *see also* Neuritis 729.2
  accessory (nerve) 352.4
  acoustic (nerve) 388.5
  ankle 355.8
  anterior crural 355.8
  anus 787.99
  arm 723.4
  auditory (nerve) 388.5
  axilla 353.0
  bladder 788.1
  brachial 723.4
  brain — *see* Disorder, nerve, cranial
  broad ligament 625.9
  cerebral — *see* Disorder, nerve, cranial
  ciliary 339.00
  cranial nerve (*see also* Disorder, nerve, cra-
    nial)
      fifth or trigeminal (*see also* Neuralgia,
        trigeminal) 350.1
  ear 388.71
    middle 352.1
  facial 351.8
  finger 354.9
  flank 355.8
  foot 355.8
  forearm 354.9
  Fothergill's (*see also* Neuralgia, trigeminal)
    350.1

Neuralgia, neuralgic — *see also* Neuritis —
  continued
  Fothergill's (*see also* Neuralgia, trigeminal)
    — *continued*
      postherpetic 053.12
  glossopharyngeal (nerve) 352.1
  groin 355.8
  hand 354.9
  heel 355.8
  Horton's 339.00
  Hunt's 053.11
  hypoglossal (nerve) 352.5
  iliac region 355.8
  infraorbital (*see also* Neuralgia, trigeminal)
    350.1
  inguinal 355.8
  intercostal (nerve) 353.8
    postherpetic 053.19
  jaw 352.1
  kidney 788.0
  knee 355.8
  loin 355.8
  malarial (*see also* Malaria) 084.6
  mastoid 385.89
  maxilla 352.1
  median thenar 354.1
  metatarsal 355.6
  middle ear 352.1
  migrainous 339.00
  Morton's 355.6
  nerve, cranial — *see* Disorder, nerve, cranial
  nose 352.0
  occipital 723.8
  olfactory (nerve) 352.0
  ophthalmic 377.30
    postherpetic 053.19
  optic (nerve) 377.30
  penis 607.9
  perineum 355.8
  pleura 511.0
  postherpetic NEC 053.19
    geniculate ganglion 053.11
    ophthalmic 053.19
    trifacial 053.12
    trigeminal 053.12
  pubic region 355.8
  radial (nerve) 723.4
  rectum 787.99
  sacroiliac joint 724.3
  sciatic (nerve) 724.3
  scrotum 608.9
  seminal vesicle 608.9
  shoulder 354.9
  Sluder's 337.09
  specified nerve NEC — *see* Disorder, nerve
  spermatic cord 608.9
  sphenopalatine (ganglion) 337.09
  subscapular (nerve) 723.4
  suprascapular (nerve) 723.4
  testis 608.89
  thenar (median) 354.1
  thigh 355.8
  tongue 352.5
  trifacial (nerve) (*see also* Neuralgia, trigemi-
    nal) 350.1
  trigeminal (nerve) 350.1
    postherpetic 053.12
  tympanic plexus 388.71
  ulnar (nerve) 723.4
  vagus (nerve) 352.3
  wrist 354.9
  writers' 300.89
    organic 333.84
Neurapraxia — *see* Injury, nerve, by site
Neurasthenia 300.5
  cardiac 306.2
  gastric 306.4
  heart 306.2
  postfebrile 780.79
  postviral 780.79
Neurilemmoma (M9560/0) — *see also* Neoplasm, connective tissue, benign
  acoustic (nerve) 225.1
  malignant (M9560/3) (*see also* Neoplasm,
    connective tissue, malignant)
      acoustic (nerve) 192.0

Neurilemmosarcoma (M9560/3) — *see* Neoplasm, connective tissue, malignant
Neurilemoma — *see* Neurilemmoma
Neurinoma (M9560/0) — *see* Neurilemmoma
Neurinomatosis (M9560/1) — *see also* Neoplasm, connective tissue, uncertain behavior
  centralis 759.5
Neuritis — *see also* Neuralgia 729.2
  abducens (nerve) 378.54
  accessory (nerve) 352.4
  acoustic (nerve) 388.5
    syphilitic 094.86
  alcoholic 357.5
    with psychosis 291.1
  amyloid, any site 277.39 *[357.4]*
  anterior crural 355.8
  arising during pregnancy 646.4 ☑
  arm 723.4
  ascending 355.2
  auditory (nerve) 388.5
  brachial (nerve) NEC 723.4
    due to displacement, intervertebral disc
      722.0
  cervical 723.4
  chest (wall) 353.8
  costal region 353.8
  cranial nerve (*see also* Disorder, nerve, cra-
    nial)
      first or olfactory 352.0
      second or optic 377.30
      third or oculomotor 378.52
      fourth or trochlear 378.53
      fifth or trigeminal (*see also* Neuralgia,
        trigeminal) 350.1
      sixth or abducens 378.54
      seventh or facial 351.8
        newborn 767.5
      eighth or acoustic 388.5
      ninth or glossopharyngeal 352.1
      tenth or vagus 352.3
      eleventh or accessory 352.4
      twelfth or hypoglossal 352.5
  Déjérine-Sottas 356.0
  diabetic 250.6 ☑ *[357.2]*
    due to secondary diabetes
      249.6 ☑ *[357.2]*
  diphtheritic 032.89 *[357.4]*
  due to
    beriberi 265.0 *[357.4]*
    displacement, prolapse, protrusion, or
      rupture of intervertebral disc
      722.2
        cervical 722.0
        lumbar, lumbosacral 722.10
        thoracic, thoracolumbar 722.11
    herniation, nucleus pulposus 722.2
        cervical 722.0
        lumbar, lumbosacral 722.10
        thoracic, thoracolumbar 722.11
  endemic 265.0 *[357.4]*
  facial (nerve) 351.8
    newborn 767.5
  general — *see* Polyneuropathy
  geniculate ganglion 351.1
    due to herpes 053.11
  glossopharyngeal (nerve) 352.1
  gouty 274.89 *[357.4]*
  hypoglossal (nerve) 352.5
  ilioinguinal (nerve) 355.8
  in diseases classified elsewhere — *see*
      Polyneuropathy, in
  infectious (multiple) 357.0
  intercostal (nerve) 353.8
  interstitial hypertrophic progressive NEC
      356.9
  leg 355.8
  lumbosacral NEC 724.4
  median (nerve) 354.1
    thenar 354.1
  multiple (acute) (infective) 356.9
    endemic 265.0 *[357.4]*
  multiplex endemica 265.0 *[357.4]*
  nerve root (*see also* Radiculitis) 729.2
  oculomotor (nerve) 378.52
  olfactory (nerve) 352.0

Neuritis — *see also* Neuralgia — *continued*
  optic (nerve) 377.30
    in myelitis 341.0
    meningococcal 036.81
  pelvic 355.8
  peripheral (nerve) (*see also* Neuropathy,
    peripheral)
      complicating pregnancy or puerperium
        646.4 ☑
      specified nerve NEC — *see* Mononeuritis
  pneumogastric (nerve) 352.3
  postchickenpox 052.7
  postherpetic 053.19
  progressive hypertrophic interstitial NEC
      356.9
  puerperal, postpartum 646.4 ☑
  radial (nerve) 723.4
  retrobulbar 377.32
    syphilitic 094.85
  rheumatic (chronic) 729.2
  sacral region 355.8
  sciatic (nerve) 724.3
    due to displacement of intervertebral
      disc 722.10
  serum 999.5
  specified nerve NEC — *see* Disorder, nerve
  spinal 355.9
    root (*see also* Radiculitis) 729.2
  subscapular (nerve) 723.4
  suprascapular (nerve) 723.4
  syphilitic 095.8
  thenar (median) 354.1
  thoracic NEC 724.4
  toxic NEC 357.7
  trochlear (nerve) 378.53
  ulnar (nerve) 723.4
  vagus (nerve) 352.3
Neuroangiomatosis, encephalofacial 759.6
Neuroastrocytoma (M9505/1) — *see* Neoplasm, by site, uncertain behavior
Neuro-avitaminosis 269.2
Neuroblastoma (M9500/3)
  olfactory (M9522/3) 160.0
  specified site — *see* Neoplasm, by site, ma-
    lignant
  unspecified site 194.0
Neurochorioretinitis — *see also* Chorioretinitis
  363.20
Neurocirculatory asthenia 306.2
Neurocytoma (M9506/0) — *see* Neoplasm, by
  site, benign
Neurodermatitis (circumscribed) (circumscripta) (local) 698.3
  atopic 691.8
  diffuse (Brocq) 691.8
  disseminated 691.8
  nodulosa 698.3
Neuroencephalomyelopathy, optic 341.0
Neuroendocrine tumor — *see* Tumor, neuroendocrine
Neuroepithelioma (M9503/3) — *see also*
  Neoplasm, by site, malignant
  olfactory (M9521/3) 160.0
Neurofibroma (M9540/0) — *see also* Neoplasm, connective tissue, benign
  melanotic (M9541/0) — *see* Neoplasm,
    connective tissue, benign
  multiple (M9540/1) 237.70
    type 1 237.71
    type 2 237.72
  plexiform (M9550/0) — *see* Neoplasm,
    connective tissue, benign
Neurofibromatosis (multiple) (M9540/1)
  237.70
  acoustic 237.72
  malignant (M9540/3) — *see* Neoplasm,
    connective tissue, malignant
  Schwannomatosis 237.73   ●
  specified type NEC 237.79   ●
  type 1 237.71
  type 2 237.72
  von Recklinghausen's 237.71
Neurofibrosarcoma (M9540/3) — *see* Neoplasm, connective tissue, malignant
Neurogenic — *see also* condition

☑ **Additional Digit Required** — Refer to the Tabular List for Digit Selection   ▽ **Subterms under main terms may continue to next column or page**

210 — Volume 2 · October 2010   ►◄ Revised Text   ● New Line   ▲ Revised Code   **2011 ICD-9-CM**

Neurogenic — *see also* condition —
continued
  bladder (atonic) (automatic) (autonomic)
    (flaccid) (hypertonic) (hypotonic)
    (inertia) (infranuclear) (irritable)
    (motor) (nonreflex) (nuclear) (paraly-
    sis) (reflex) (sensory) (spastic)
    (supranuclear) (uninhibited) 596.54
    with cauda equina syndrome 344.61
  bowel 564.81
  heart 306.2
Neuroglioma (M9505/1) — *see* Neoplasm,
  by site, uncertain behavior
Neurolabyrinthitis (of Dix and Hallpike) 386.12
Neurolathyrism 988.2
Neuroleprosy 030.1
Neuroleptic malignant syndrome 333.92
Neurolipomatosis 272.8
Neuroma (M9570/0) — *see also* Neoplasm,
  connective tissue, benign
  acoustic (nerve) (M9560/0) 225.1
  amputation (traumatic) (*see also* Injury,
    nerve, by site)
    surgical complication (late) 997.61
  appendix 211.3
  auditory nerve 225.1
  digital 355.6
    toe 355.6
  interdigital (toe) 355.6
  intermetatarsal 355.6
  Morton's 355.6
  multiple 237.70
    type 1 237.71
    type 2 237.72
  nonneoplastic 355.9
    arm NEC 354.9
    leg NEC 355.8
    lower extremity NEC 355.8
    specified site NEC — *see* Mononeuritis,
      by site
    upper extremity NEC 354.9
  optic (nerve) 225.1
  plantar 355.6
  plexiform (M9550/0) — *see* Neoplasm,
    connective tissue, benign
  surgical (nonneoplastic) 355.9
    arm NEC 354.9
    leg NEC 355.8
    lower extremity NEC 355.8
    upper extremity NEC 354.9
  traumatic (*see also* Injury, nerve, by site)
    old — *see* Neuroma, nonneoplastic
Neuromyalgia 729.1
Neuromyasthenia (epidemic) 049.8
Neuromyelitis 341.8
  ascending 357.0
  optica 341.0
Neuromyopathy NEC 358.9
Neuromyositis 729.1
Neuronevus (M8725/0) — *see* Neoplasm, skin,
  benign
Neuronitis 357.0
  ascending (acute) 355.2
  vestibular 386.12
Neuroparalytic — *see* condition
Neuropathy, neuropathic — *see also* Disorder,
  nerve 355.9
  acute motor 357.82
  alcoholic 357.5
    with psychosis 291.1
  arm NEC 354.9
  ataxia and retinitis pigmentosa (NARP syn-
    drome) 277.87
  autonomic (peripheral) — *see* Neuropathy,
    peripheral, autonomic
  axillary nerve 353.0
  brachial plexus 353.0
  cervical plexus 353.2
  chronic
    progressive segmentally demyelinating
      357.89
    relapsing demyelinating 357.89
  congenital sensory 356.2
  Déjérine-Sottas 356.0
  diabetic 250.6 ☑ *[357.2]*
    autonomic (peripheral) 250.6 ☑ *[337.1]*

Neuropathy, neuropathic — *see also* Disorder,
  nerve — *continued*
  diabetic — *continued*
    due to secondary diabetes
      249.6 ☑ *[357.2]*
      autonomic (peripheral)
        249.6 ☑ *[337.1]*
  entrapment 355.9
    iliohypogastric nerve 355.79
    ilioinguinal nerve 355.79
    lateral cutaneous nerve of thigh 355.1
    median nerve 354.0
    obturator nerve 355.79
    peroneal nerve 355.3
    posterior tibial nerve 355.5
    saphenous nerve 355.79
    ulnar nerve 354.2
  facial nerve 351.9
  hereditary 356.9
    peripheral 356.0
    sensory (radicular) 356.2
  hypertrophic
    Charcôt-Marie-Tooth 356.1
    Déjérine-Sottas 356.0
    interstitial 356.9
    Refsum 356.3
  intercostal nerve 354.8
  ischemic — *see* Disorder, nerve
  Jamaican (ginger) 357.7
  leg NEC 355.8
  lower extremity NEC 355.8
  lumbar plexus 353.1
  median nerve 354.1
  motor
    acute 357.82
  multiple (acute) (chronic) (*see also*
    Polyneuropathy) 356.9
  optic 377.39
    ischemic 377.41
    nutritional 377.33
    toxic 377.34
  peripheral (nerve) (*see also* Polyneuropathy)
    356.9
    arm NEC 354.9
    autonomic 337.9
      amyloid 277.39 *[337.1]*
      idiopathic 337.00
      in
        amyloidosis 277.39 *[337.1]*
        diabetes (mellitus)
          250.6 ☑ *[337.1]*
          due to secondary diabetes
            249.6 ☑ *[337.1]*
        diseases classified elsewhere
          337.1
        gout 274.89 *[337.1]*
        hyperthyroidism 242.9 ☑ *[337.1]*
    due to
      antitetanus serum 357.6
      arsenic 357.7
      drugs 357.6
      lead 357.7
      organophosphate compounds 357.7
      toxic agent NEC 357.7
    hereditary 356.0
    idiopathic 356.9
      progressive 356.4
      specified type NEC 356.8
    in diseases classified elsewhere — *see*
      Polyneuropathy, in
    leg NEC 355.8
    lower extremity NEC 355.8
    upper extremity NEC 354.9
  plantar nerves 355.6
  progressive
    hypertrophic interstitial 356.9
    inflammatory 357.89
  radicular NEC 729.2
    brachial 723.4
    cervical NEC 723.4
    hereditary sensory 356.2
    lumbar 724.4
    lumbosacral 724.4
    thoracic NEC 724.4
  sacral plexus 353.1
  sciatic 355.0

Neuropathy, neuropathic — *see also* Disorder,
  nerve — *continued*
  spinal nerve NEC 355.9
    root (*see also* Radiculitis) 729.2
  toxic 357.7
  trigeminal sensory 350.8
  ulnar nerve 354.2
  upper extremity NEC 354.9
  uremic 585.9 *[357.4]*
  vitamin B$_{12}$ 266.2 *[357.4]*
    with anemia (pernicious) 281.0 *[357.4]*
    due to dietary deficiency
      281.1 *[357.4]*
Neurophthisis — *see also* Disorder, nerve
  diabetic 250.6 ☑ *[357.2]*
    due to secondary diabetes
      249.6 ☑ *[357.2]*
  peripheral 356.9
Neuropraxia — *see* Injury, nerve
Neuroretinitis 363.05
  syphilitic 094.85
Neurosarcoma (M9540/3) — *see* Neoplasm,
  connective tissue, malignant
Neurosclerosis — *see* Disorder, nerve
Neurosis, neurotic 300.9
  accident 300.16
  anancastic, anankastic 300.3
  anxiety (state) 300.00
    generalized 300.02
    panic type 300.01
  asthenic 300.5
  bladder 306.53
  cardiac (reflex) 306.2
  cardiovascular 306.2
  climacteric, unspecified type 627.2
  colon 306.4
  compensation 300.16
  compulsive, compulsion 300.3
  conversion 300.11
  craft 300.89
  cutaneous 306.3
  depersonalization 300.6
  depressive (reaction) (type) 300.4
  endocrine 306.6
  environmental 300.89
  fatigue 300.5
  functional (*see also* Disorder, psychosomat-
    ic) 306.9
  gastric 306.4
  gastrointestinal 306.4
  genitourinary 306.50
  heart 306.2
  hypochondriacal 300.7
  hysterical 300.10
    conversion type 300.11
    dissociative type 300.15
  impulsive 300.3
  incoordination 306.0
    larynx 306.1
    vocal cord 306.1
  intestine 306.4
  larynx 306.1
    hysterical 300.11
    sensory 306.1
  menopause, unspecified type 627.2
  mixed NEC 300.89
  musculoskeletal 306.0
  obsessional 300.3
    phobia 300.3
  obsessive-compulsive 300.3
  occupational 300.89
  ocular 306.7
  oral ▶(*see also* Disorder, fluency)◀
    315.35 ▲
  organ (*see also* Disorder, psychosomatic)
    306.9
  pharynx 306.1
  phobic 300.20
  posttraumatic (acute) (situational) 309.81
    chronic 309.81
  psychasthenic (type) 300.89
  railroad 300.16
  rectum 306.4
  respiratory 306.1
  rumination 306.4
  senile 300.89

Neurosis, neurotic — *continued*
  sexual 302.70
  situational 300.89
  specified type NEC 300.89
  state 300.9
    with depersonalization episode 300.6
  stomach 306.4
  vasomotor 306.2
  visceral 306.4
  war 300.16
Neurospongioblastosis diffusa 759.5
Neurosyphilis (arrested) (early) (inactive) (late)
  (latent) (recurrent) 094.9
  with ataxia (cerebellar) (locomotor) (spastic)
    (spinal) 094.0
  acute meningitis 094.2
  aneurysm 094.89
  arachnoid (adhesive) 094.2
  arteritis (any artery) 094.89
  asymptomatic 094.3
  congenital 090.40
  dura (mater) 094.89
  general paresis 094.1
  gumma 094.9
  hemorrhagic 094.9
  juvenile (asymptomatic) (meningeal) 090.40
  leptomeninges (aseptic) 094.2
  meningeal 094.2
  meninges (adhesive) 094.2
  meningovascular (diffuse) 094.2
  optic atrophy 094.84
  parenchymatous (degenerative) 094.1
  paresis (*see also* Paresis, general) 094.1
  paretic (*see also* Paresis, general) 094.1
  relapse 094.9
  remission in (sustained) 094.9
  serological 094.3
  specified nature or site NEC 094.89
  tabes (dorsalis) 094.0
    juvenile 090.40
  tabetic 094.0
    juvenile 090.40
  taboparesis 094.1
    juvenile 090.40
  thrombosis 094.89
  vascular 094.89
Neurotic — *see also* Neurosis 300.9
  excoriation 698.4
    psychogenic 306.3
Neurotmesis — *see* Injury, nerve, by site
Neurotoxemia — *see* Toxemia
Neutro-occlusion 524.21
Neutropenia, neutropenic (idiopathic) (pernicious) (primary) 288.00
  chronic 288.09
    hypoplastic 288.09
  congenital (nontransient) 288.01
  cyclic 288.02
  drug induced 288.03
  due to infection 288.04
  fever 288.00
  genetic 288.01
  immune 288.09
  infantile 288.01
  malignant 288.09
  neonatal, transitory (isoimmune) (maternal
    transfer) 776.7
  periodic 288.02
  splenic 289.53
  splenomegaly 289.53
  toxic 288.09
Neutrophilia, hereditary giant 288.2
Nevocarcinoma (M8720/3) — *see* Melanoma
Nevus (M8720/0) — *see also* Neoplasm, skin,
  benign

> *Note* — Except where otherwise indicat-
> ed, varieties of nevus in the list below
> that are followed by a morphology code
> number (M----/0) should be coded by
> site as for "Neoplasm, skin, benign."

  acanthotic 702.8
  achromic (M8730/0)
  amelanotic (M8730/0)
  anemic, anemicus 709.09
  angiomatous (M9120/0) (*see also* Heman-
    gioma) 228.00

☑ Additional Digit Required — Refer to the Tabular List for Digit Selection   ▽ Subterms under main terms may continue to next column or page

2011 ICD-9-CM   ▶◀ Revised Text   ● New Line   ▲ Revised Code   October 2010 • Volume 2 — 211

Nevus — *see also* Neoplasm, skin, benign —
  continued
  araneus 448.1
  avasculosus 709.09
  balloon cell (M8722/0)
  bathing trunk (M8761/1) 238.2
  blue (M8780/0)
    cellular (M8790/0)
    giant (M8790/0)
    Jadassohn's (M8780/0)
    malignant (M8780/3) — *see* Melanoma
  capillary (M9131/0) (*see also* Hemangioma)
    228.00
  cavernous (M9121/0) (*see also* Heman-
    gioma) 228.00
  cellular (M8720/0)
    blue (M8790/0)
  comedonicus 757.33
  compound (M8760/0)
  conjunctiva (M8720/0) 224.3
  dermal (M8750/0)
    and epidermal (M8760/0)
  epithelioid cell (and spindle cell) (M8770/0)
  flammeus 757.32
    osteohypertrophic 759.89
  hairy (M8720/0)
  halo (M8723/0)
  hemangiomatous (M9120/0) (*see also* He-
    mangioma) 228.00
  intradermal (M8750/0)
  intraepidermal (M8740/0)
  involuting (M8724/0)
  Jadassohn's (blue) (M8780/0)
  junction, junctional (M8740/0)
    malignant melanoma in (M8740/3) —
      see Melanoma
  juvenile (M8770/0)
  lymphatic (M9170/0) 228.1
  magnocellular (M8726/0)
    specified site — *see* Neoplasm, by site,
      benign
    unspecified site 224.0
  malignant (M8720/3) — *see* Melanoma
  meaning hemangioma (M9120/0) (*see also*
    Hemangioma) 228.00
  melanotic (pigmented) (M8720/0)
  multiplex 759.5
  nonneoplastic 448.1
  nonpigmented (M8730/0)
  nonvascular (M8720/0)
  oral mucosa, white sponge 750.26
  osteohypertrophic, flammeus 759.89
  papillaris (M8720/0)
  papillomatosus (M8720/0)
  pigmented (M8720/0)
    giant (M8761/1) (*see also* Neoplasm, skin,
      uncertain behavior)
      malignant melanoma in (M8761/3)
        — *see* Melanoma
    systematicus 757.33
  pilosus (M8720/0)
  port wine 757.32
  sanguineous 757.32
  sebaceous (senile) 702.8
  senile 448.1
  spider 448.1
  spindle cell (and epithelioid cell) (M8770/0)
  stellar 448.1
  strawberry 757.32
  syringocystadenomatous papilliferous
    (M8406/0)
  unius lateris 757.33
  Unna's 757.32
  vascular 757.32
  verrucous 757.33
  white sponge (oral mucosa) 750.26

Newborn (infant) (liveborn)
  abstinence syndrome 779.5
  affected by
    amniocentesis 760.61
    maternal abuse of drugs (gestational)
      (via placenta) (via breast milk)
      (*see also* Noxious, substances
      transmitted through placenta or
      breast milk (affecting fetus or
      newborn)) 760.70

Newborn — *continued*
  affected by — *continued*
    maternal abuse of drugs (*see also* Nox-
      ious, substances transmitted
      through placenta or breast milk)
      — *continued*
      methamphetamine(s) 760.72
    procedure
      amniocentesis 760.61
      in utero NEC 760.62
      surgical on mother
        during pregnancy NEC 760.63
        previous not associated with
          pregnancy 760.64
  apnea 770.81
    obstructive 770.82
    specified NEC 770.82
  breast buds 779.89
  cardiomyopathy 425.4
    congenital 425.3
  convulsion 779.0
  electrolyte imbalance NEC (transitory) 775.5
  fever (environmentally-induced) 778.4
  gestation
    24 completed weeks 765.22
    25-26 completed weeks 765.23
    27-28 completed weeks 765.24
    29-30 completed weeks 765.25
    31-32 completed weeks 765.26
    33-34 completed weeks 765.27
    35-36 completed weeks 765.28
    37 or more completed weeks 765.29
    less than 24 completed weeks 765.21
    unspecified completed weeks 765.20
  infection 771.89
    candida 771.7
    mastitis 771.5
    specified NEC 771.89
    urinary tract 771.82
  mastitis 771.5
  multiple NEC
    born in hospital (without mention of
      cesarean delivery or section)
      V37.00
      with cesarean delivery or section
        V37.01
    born outside hospital
      hospitalized V37.1
      not hospitalized V37.2
    mates all liveborn
      born in hospital (without mention of
        cesarean delivery or section)
        V34.00
        with cesarean delivery or section
          V34.01
      born outside hospital
        hospitalized V34.1
        not hospitalized V34.2
    mates all stillborn
      born in hospital (without mention of
        cesarean delivery or section)
        V35.00
        with cesarean delivery or section
          V35.01
      born outside hospital
        hospitalized V35.1
        not hospitalized V35.2
    mates liveborn and stillborn
      born in hospital (without mention of
        cesarean delivery or section)
        V36.00
        with cesarean delivery or section
          V36.01
      born outside hospital
        hospitalized V36.1
        not hospitalized V36.2
  omphalitis 771.4
  seizure 779.0
  sepsis 771.81
  single
    born in hospital (without mention of
      cesarean delivery or section)
      V30.00
      with cesarean delivery or section
        V30.01

Newborn — *continued*
  single — *continued*
    born outside hospital
      hospitalized V30.1
      not hospitalized V30.2
    specified condition NEC 779.89
    twin NEC
      born in hospital (without mention of
        cesarean delivery or section)
        V33.00
        with cesarean delivery or section
          V33.01
      born outside hospital
        hospitalized V33.1
        not hospitalized V33.2
      mate liveborn
        born in hospital V31.0 ☑
        born outside hospital
          hospitalized V31.1
          not hospitalized V31.2
      mate stillborn
        born in hospital V32.0 ☑
        born outside hospital
          hospitalized V32.1
          not hospitalized V32.2
    unspecified as to single or multiple birth
      born in hospital (without mention of
        cesarean delivery or section)
        V39.00
        with cesarean delivery or section
          V39.01
      born outside hospital
        hospitalized V39.1
        not hospitalized V39.2
  weight check V20.32

Newcastle's conjunctivitis or disease 077.8
Nezelof's syndrome (pure alymphocytosis)
  279.13
Niacin (amide) **deficiency** 265.2
Nicolas-Durand-Favre disease (climatic bubo)
  099.1
Nicolas-Favre disease (climatic bubo) 099.1
Nicotinic acid (amide) **deficiency** 265.2
Niemann-Pick disease (lipid histiocytosis)
  (splenomegaly) 272.7
Night
  blindness (*see also* Blindness, night) 368.60
    congenital 368.61
    vitamin A deficiency 264.5
  cramps 729.82
  sweats 780.8
  terrors, child 307.46
Nightmare 307.47
  REM-sleep type 307.47
Nipple — *see* condition
Nisbet's chancre 099.0
Nishimoto (-Takeuchi) disease 437.5
Nitritoid crisis or reaction — *see* Crisis, nitritoid
Nitrogen retention, extrarenal 788.99
Nitrosohemoglobinemia 289.89
Njovera 104.0
No
  diagnosis 799.9
  disease (found) V71.9
  room at the inn V65.0
Nocardiasis — *see* Nocardiosis
Nocardiosis 039.9
  with pneumonia 039.1
  lung 039.1
  specified type NEC 039.8
Nocturia 788.43
  psychogenic 306.53
Nocturnal — *see also* condition
  dyspnea (paroxysmal) 786.09
  emissions 608.89
  enuresis 788.36
    psychogenic 307.6
  frequency (micturition) 788.43
    psychogenic 306.53
Nodal rhythm disorder 427.89
Nodding of head 781.0
Node(s) — *see also* Nodule(s)
  Heberden's 715.04
  larynx 478.79
  lymph — *see* condition

Node(s) — *see also* Nodule(s) — *continued*
  milkers' 051.1
  Osler's 421.0
  rheumatic 729.89
  Schmorl's 722.30
    lumbar, lumbosacral 722.32
    specified region NEC 722.39
    thoracic, thoracolumbar 722.31
  singers' 478.5
  skin NEC 782.2
  tuberculous — *see* Tuberculosis, lymph
    gland
  vocal cords 478.5
Nodosities, Haygarth's 715.04
Nodule(s), nodular
  actinomycotic (*see also* Actinomycosis) 039.9
  arthritic — *see* Arthritis, nodosa
  breast 793.89
  cutaneous 782.2
  Haygarth's 715.04
  inflammatory — *see* Inflammation
  juxta-articular 102.7
    syphilitic 095.7
    yaws 102.7
  larynx 478.79
  lung, solitary 518.89
    emphysematous 492.8
  milkers' 051.1
  prostate 600.10
    with
      urinary
        obstruction 600.11
        retention 600.11
  retrocardiac 785.9
  rheumatic 729.89
  rheumatoid — *see* Arthritis, rheumatoid
  scrotum (inflammatory) 608.4
  singers' 478.5
  skin NEC 782.2
  solitary, lung 518.89
    emphysematous 492.8
  subcutaneous 782.2
  thyroid (gland) (nontoxic) (uninodular)
    241.0
    with
      hyperthyroidism 242.1 ☑
      thyrotoxicosis 242.1 ☑
    toxic or with hyperthyroidism 242.1 ☑
  vocal cords 478.5
Noma (gangrenous) (hospital) (infective) 528.1
  auricle (*see also* Gangrene) 785.4
  mouth 528.1
  pudendi (*see also* Vulvitis) 616.10
  vulvae (*see also* Vulvitis) 616.10
Nomadism V60.0
Non-adherence
  artificial skin graft 996.55
  decellularized allodermis graft 996.55
Non-autoimmune hemolytic anemia NEC
  283.10
Nonclosure — *see also* Imperfect, closure
  ductus
    arteriosus 747.0
    Botalli 747.0
  Eustachian valve 746.89
  foramen
    Botalli 745.5
    ovale 745.5
Noncompliance with medical treatment
  V15.81
  renal dialysis V45.12
Nondescent (congenital) — *see also* Malposition, congenital
  cecum 751.4
  colon 751.4
  testis 752.51
Nondevelopment
  brain 742.1
    specified part 742.2
  heart 746.89
  organ or site, congenital NEC — *see* Hypopla-
    sia
Nonengagement
  head NEC 652.5 ☑
    in labor 660.1 ☑
      affecting fetus or newborn 763.1

☑ Additional Digit Required — Refer to the Tabular List for Digit Selection   ▽ Subterms under main terms may continue to next column or page

Nonexanthematous tick fever 066.1
Nonexpansion, lung (newborn) NEC 770.4
Nonfunctioning
    cystic duct (*see also* Disease, gallbladder) 575.8
    gallbladder (*see also* Disease, gallbladder) 575.8
    kidney (*see also* Disease, renal) 593.9
    labyrinth 386.58
Nonhealing
    stump (surgical) 997.69
    wound, surgical 998.83
Nonimplantation of ovum, causing infertility 628.3
Noninsufflation, fallopian tube 628.2
Nonne-Milroy-Meige syndrome (chronic hereditary edema) 757.0
Nonovulation 628.0
Nonpatent fallopian tube 628.2
Nonpneumatization, lung NEC 770.4
Nonreflex bladder 596.54
    with cauda equina 344.61
Nonretention of food — *see* Vomiting
Nonrotation — *see* Malrotation
Nonsecretion, urine — *see also* Anuria 788.5
    newborn 753.3
Nonunion
    fracture 733.82
    organ or site, congenital NEC — *see* Imperfect, closure
    symphysis pubis, congenital 755.69
    top sacrum, congenital 756.19
Nonviability 765.0 ☑
Nonvisualization, gallbladder 793.3
Nonvitalized tooth 522.9
Non-working side interference 524.56
Normal
    delivery — *see* category 650
    menses V65.5
    state (feared complaint unfounded) V65.5
Normoblastosis 289.89

Normocytic anemia (infectional) 285.9
    due to blood loss (chronic) 280.0
        acute 285.1
Norrie's disease (congenital) (progressive oculoacousticocerebral degeneration) 743.8
North American blastomycosis 116.0
Norwegian itch 133.0
Nosebleed 784.7
Nose, nasal — *see* condition
Nosomania 298.9
Nosophobia 300.29
Nostalgia 309.89
Notched lip, congenital — *see also* Cleft, lip 749.10
Notching nose, congenital (tip) 748.1
Notch of iris 743.46
Nothnagel's
    syndrome 378.52
    vasomotor acroparesthesia 443.89
Novy's relapsing fever (American) 087.1
Noxious
    foodstuffs, poisoning by
        fish 988.0
        fungi 988.1
        mushrooms 988.1
        plants (food) 988.2
        shellfish 988.0
        specified type NEC 988.8
        toadstool 988.1
    substances transmitted through placenta or breast milk (affecting fetus or newborn) 760.70
        acetretin 760.78
        alcohol 760.71
        aminopterin 760.78
        antiandrogens 760.79
        anticonvulsant 760.77
        antifungal 760.74
        anti-infective agents 760.74
        antimetabolic 760.78

Noxious — *continued*
    substances transmitted through placenta or breast milk — *continued*
        atorvastatin 760.78
        carbamazepine 760.77
        cocaine 760.75
        "crack" 760.75
        diethylstilbestrol (DES) 760.76
        divalproex sodium 760.77
        endocrine disrupting chemicals 760.79
        estrogens 760.79
        etretinate 760.78
        fluconazole 760.74
        fluvastatin 760.78
        hallucinogenic agents NEC 760.73
        hormones 760.79
        lithium 760.79
        lovastatin 760.78
        medicinal agents NEC 760.79
        methotrexate 760.78
        misoprostil 760.79
        narcotics 760.72
        obstetric anesthetic or analgesic 763.5
        phenobarbital 760.77
        phenytoin 760.77
        pravastatin 760.78
        progestins 760.79
        retinoic acid 760.78
        simvastatin 760.78
        solvents 760.79
        specified agent NEC 760.79
        statins 760.78
        suspected, affecting management of pregnancy 655.5 ☑
        tetracycline 760.74
        thalidomide 760.79
        trimethadione 760.77
        valproate 760.77
        valproic acid 760.77
        vitamin A 760.78
NPDH (new persistent daily headache) 339.42

Nuchal hitch (arm) 652.8 ☑
Nucleus pulposus — *see* condition
Numbness 782.0
Nuns' knee 727.2
Nursemaid's
    elbow 832.2
    shoulder 831.0 ☑
Nutmeg liver 573.8
Nutrition, deficient or insufficient (particular kind of food) 269.9
    due to
        insufficient food 994.2
        lack of
            care (child) (infant) 995.52
                adult 995.84
            food 994.2
Nyctalopia — *see also* Blindness, night 368.60
    vitamin A deficiency 264.5
Nycturia 788.43
    psychogenic 306.53
Nymphomania 302.89
Nystagmus 379.50
    associated with vestibular system disorders 379.54
    benign paroxysmal positional 386.11
    central positional 386.2
    congenital 379.51
    deprivation 379.53
    dissociated 379.55
    latent 379.52
    miners' 300.89
    positional
        benign paroxysmal 386.11
        central 386.2
    specified NEC 379.56
    vestibular 379.54
    visual deprivation 379.53

☑ **Additional Digit Required** — Refer to the Tabular List for Digit Selection   ▽ **Subterms under main terms may continue to next column or page**

O

Oasthouse urine disease 270.2
Obermeyer's relapsing fever (European) 087.0
Obesity (constitutional) (exogenous) (familial) (nutritional) (simple) 278.00
  adrenal 255.8
  complicating pregnancy, childbirth, or puerperium 649.1 ☑
  due to hyperalimentation 278.00
  endocrine NEC 259.9
  endogenous 259.9
  Fröhlich's (adiposogenital dystrophy) 253.8
  glandular NEC 259.9
  hypothyroid (see also Hypothyroidism) 244.9
  hypoventilation syndrome 278.03 ●
  morbid 278.01
  of pregnancy 649.1 ☑
  pituitary 253.8
  severe 278.01
  thyroid (see also Hypothyroidism) 244.9
Oblique — see also condition
  lie before labor, affecting fetus or newborn 761.7
Obliquity, pelvis 738.6
Obliteration
  abdominal aorta 446.7
  appendix (lumen) 543.9
  artery 447.1
  ascending aorta 446.7
  bile ducts 576.8
    with calculus, choledocholithiasis, or stones — see Choledocholithiasis
    congenital 751.61
      jaundice from 751.61 [774.5]
  common duct 576.8
    with calculus, choledocholithiasis, or stones — see Choledocholithiasis
    congenital 751.61
  cystic duct 575.8
    with calculus, choledocholithiasis, or stones — see Choledocholithiasis
    congenital 751.61
  disease, arteriolar 447.1
  endometrium 621.8
  eye, anterior chamber 360.34
  fallopian tube 628.2
  lymphatic vessel 457.1
    postmastectomy 457.0
  organ or site, congenital NEC — see Atresia
  placental blood vessels — see Placenta, abnormal
  supra-aortic branches 446.7
  ureter 593.89
  urethra 599.84
  vein 459.9
  vestibule (oral) 525.8
Observation (for) V71.9
  without need for further medical care V71.9
  accident NEC V71.4
    at work V71.3
  criminal assault V71.6
  deleterious agent ingestion V71.89
  disease V71.9
    cardiovascular V71.7
    heart V71.7
    mental V71.09
    specified condition NEC V71.89
  foreign body ingestion V71.89
  growth and development variations V21.8
  injuries (accidental) V71.4
    inflicted NEC V71.6
      during alleged rape or seduction V71.5
  malignant neoplasm, suspected V71.1
  postpartum
    immediately after delivery V24.0
    routine follow-up V24.2
  pregnancy
    high-risk V23.9
      specified problem NEC V23.89
    normal (without complication) V22.1
      with nonobstetric complication V22.2
      first V22.0
  rape or seduction, alleged V71.5
    injury during V71.5
  suicide attempt, alleged V71.89

Observation — continued
  suspected (undiagnosed) (unproven)
    abuse V71.81
    cardiovascular disease V71.7
    child or wife battering victim V71.6
    concussion (cerebral) V71.6
    condition NEC V71.89
      infant — see Observation, suspected, condition, newborn
      maternal and fetal
        amniotic cavity and membrane problem V89.01
        cervical shortening V89.05
        fetal anomaly V89.03
        fetal growth problem V89.04
        oligohydramnios V89.01
        other specified problem NEC V89.09
        placental problem V89.02
        polyhydramnios V89.01
      newborn V29.9
        cardiovascular disease V29.8
        congenital anomaly V29.8
        genetic V29.3
        infectious V29.0
        ingestion foreign object V29.8
        injury V29.8
        metabolic V29.3
        neoplasm V29.8
        neurological V29.1
        poison, poisoning V29.8
        respiratory V29.2
        specified NEC V29.8
    exposure
      anthrax V71.82
      biologic agent NEC V71.83
      SARS V71.83
    infectious disease not requiring isolation V71.89
    malignant neoplasm V71.1
    mental disorder V71.09
    neglect V71.81
    neoplasm
      benign V71.89
      malignant V71.1
    specified condition NEC V71.89
    tuberculosis V71.2
  tuberculosis, suspected V71.2
Obsession, obsessional 300.3
  ideas and mental images 300.3
  impulses 300.3
  neurosis 300.3
  phobia 300.3
  psychasthenia 300.3
  ruminations 300.3
  state 300.3
  syndrome 300.3
Obsessive-compulsive 300.3
  neurosis 300.3
  personality 301.4
  reaction 300.3
Obstetrical trauma NEC (complicating delivery) 665.9 ☑
  with
    abortion — see Abortion, by type, with damage to pelvic organs
    ectopic pregnancy (see also categories 633.0–633.9) 639.2
    molar pregnancy (see also categories 630–632) 639.2
  affecting fetus or newborn 763.89
  following
    abortion 639.2
    ectopic or molar pregnancy 639.2
Obstipation — see also Constipation 564.00
  psychogenic 306.4
Obstruction, obstructed, obstructive
  airway NEC 519.8
    with
      allergic alveolitis NEC 495.9
      asthma NEC (see also Asthma) 493.9 ☑
      bronchiectasis 494.0
        with acute exacerbation 494.1
      bronchitis (chronic) (see also Bronchitis, with, obstruction) 491.20

Obstruction, obstructed, obstructive — continued
  airway — continued
    with — continued
      emphysema NEC 492.8
      chronic 496
        with
          allergic alveolitis NEC 495.5
          asthma NEC (see also Asthma) 493.2 ☑
          bronchiectasis 494.0
            with acute exacerbation 494.1
          bronchitis (chronic) (see also Bronchitis, with, obstruction) 491.20
          emphysema NEC 492.8
      due to
        bronchospasm 519.11
        foreign body 934.9
        inhalation of fumes or vapors 506.9
        laryngospasm 478.75
  alimentary canal (see also Obstruction, intestine) 560.9
  ampulla of Vater 576.2
    with calculus, cholelithiasis, or stones — see Choledocholithiasis
  aortic (heart) (valve) (see also Stenosis, aortic) 424.1
    rheumatic (see also Stenosis, aortic, rheumatic) 395.0
  aortoiliac 444.0
  aqueduct of Sylvius 331.4
    congenital 742.3
      with spina bifida (see also Spina bifida) 741.0 ☑
  Arnold-Chiari (see also Spina bifida) 741.0 ☑
  artery (see also Embolism, artery) 444.9
    basilar (complete) (partial) (see also Occlusion, artery, basilar) 433.0 ☑
    carotid (complete) (partial) (see also Occlusion, artery, carotid) 433.1 ☑
    precerebral — see Occlusion, artery, precerebral NEC
    retinal (central) (see also Occlusion, retina) 362.30
    vertebral (complete) (partial) (see also Occlusion, artery, vertebral) 433.2 ☑
  asthma (chronic) (with obstructive pulmonary disease) 493.2 ☑
  band (intestinal) 560.81
  bile duct or passage (see also Obstruction, biliary) 576.2
    congenital 751.61
      jaundice from 751.61 [774.5]
  biliary (duct) (tract) 576.2
    with calculus 574.51
      with cholecystitis (chronic) 574.41
        acute 574.31
    congenital 751.61
      jaundice from 751.61 [774.5]
    gallbladder 575.2
      with calculus 574.21
        with cholecystitis (chronic) 574.11
          acute 574.01
  bladder neck (acquired) 596.0
    congenital 753.6
  bowel (see also Obstruction, intestine) 560.9
  bronchus 519.19
  canal, ear (see also Stricture, ear canal, acquired) 380.50
  cardia 537.89
  caval veins (inferior) (superior) 459.2
  cecum (see also Obstruction, intestine) 560.9
  circulatory 459.9
  colon (see also Obstruction, intestine) 560.9
    sympathicotonic 560.89
  common duct (see also Obstruction, biliary) 576.2
    congenital 751.61
  coronary (artery) (heart) (see also Arteriosclerosis, coronary)
    acute (see also Infarct, myocardium) 410.9 ☑
      without myocardial infarction 411.81

Obstruction, obstructed, obstructive — continued
  cystic duct (see also Obstruction, gallbladder) 575.2
    congenital 751.61
  device, implant, or graft — see Complications, due to (presence of) any device, implant, or graft classified to 996.0–996.5 NEC
  due to foreign body accidentally left in operation wound 998.4
  duodenum 537.3
    congenital 751.1
    due to
      compression NEC 537.3
      cyst 537.3
      intrinsic lesion or disease NEC 537.3
      scarring 537.3
      torsion 537.3
      ulcer 532.91
      volvulus 537.3
  ejaculatory duct 608.89
  endocardium 424.90
    arteriosclerotic 424.99
    specified cause, except rheumatic 424.99
  esophagus 530.3
  eustachian tube (complete) (partial) 381.60
    cartilaginous
      extrinsic 381.63
      intrinsic 381.62
    due to
      cholesteatoma 381.61
      osseous lesion NEC 381.61
      polyp 381.61
    osseous 381.61
  fallopian tube (bilateral) 628.2
  fecal 560.32 ▲
    with hernia (see also Hernia, by site, with obstruction)
      gangrenous — see Hernia, by site, with gangrene
  foramen of Monro (congenital) 742.3
    with spina bifida (see also Spina bifida) 741.0 ☑
  foreign body — see Foreign body
  gallbladder 575.2
    with calculus, cholelithiasis, or stones 574.21
      with cholecystitis (chronic) 574.11
        acute 574.01
    congenital 751.69
      jaundice from 751.69 [774.5]
  gastric outlet 537.0
  gastrointestinal (see also Obstruction, intestine) 560.9
  glottis 478.79
  hepatic 573.8
    duct (see also Obstruction, biliary) 576.2
      congenital 751.61
  icterus (see also Obstruction, biliary) 576.8
    congenital 751.61
  ileocecal coil (see also Obstruction, intestine) 560.9
  ileum (see also Obstruction, intestine) 560.9
  iliofemoral (artery) 444.81
  internal anastomosis — see Complications, mechanical, graft
  intestine (mechanical) (neurogenic) (paroxysmal) (postinfectional) (reflex) 560.9
    with
      adhesions (intestinal) (peritoneal) 560.81
      hernia (see also Hernia, by site, with obstruction)
        gangrenous — see Hernia, by site, with gangrene
    adynamic (see also Ileus) 560.1
    by gallstone 560.31
    congenital or infantile (small) 751.1
      large 751.2
    due to
      Ascaris lumbricoides 127.0
      mural thickening 560.89
      procedure 997.4
        involving urinary tract 997.5
    impaction 560.39

☑ Additional Digit Required — Refer to the Tabular List for Digit Selection   ▽ Subterms under main terms may continue to next column or page

2011 ICD-9-CM   ▶◀ Revised Text   ● New Line   ▲ Revised Code   October 2010 · Volume 2 — 215

Obstruction, obstructed, obstructive — *continued*
- intestine — *continued*
  - infantile — *see* Obstruction, intestine, congenital
  - newborn
    - due to
      - fecaliths 777.1
      - inspissated milk 777.2
      - meconium (plug) 777.1
        - in mucoviscidosis 277.01
      - transitory 777.4
    - specified cause NEC 560.89
    - transitory, newborn 777.4
    - volvulus 560.2
  - intracardiac ball valve prosthesis 996.02
  - jaundice (*see also* Obstruction, biliary) 576.8
    - congenital 751.61
  - jejunum (*see also* Obstruction, intestine) 560.9
  - kidney 593.89
  - labor 660.9 ☑
    - affecting fetus or newborn 763.1
    - by
      - bony pelvis (conditions classifiable to 653.0–653.9) 660.1 ☑
      - deep transverse arrest 660.3 ☑
      - impacted shoulder 660.4 ☑
      - locked twins 660.5 ☑
      - malposition (fetus) (conditions classifiable to 652.0–652.9) 660.0 ☑
        - head during labor 660.3 ☑
        - persistent occipitoposterior position 660.3 ☑
      - soft tissue, pelvic (conditions classifiable to 654.0–654.9) 660.2 ☑
  - lacrimal
    - canaliculi 375.53
    - congenital 743.65
    - punctum 375.52
    - sac 375.54
  - lacrimonasal duct 375.56
    - congenital 743.65
    - neonatal 375.55
  - lacteal, with steatorrhea 579.2
  - laryngitis (*see also* Laryngitis) 464.01
  - larynx 478.79
    - congenital 748.3
  - liver 573.8
    - cirrhotic (*see also* Cirrhosis, liver) 571.5
  - lung 518.89
    - with
      - asthma — *see* Asthma
      - bronchitis (chronic) 491.20
      - emphysema NEC 492.8
    - airway, chronic 496
    - chronic NEC 496
      - with
        - asthma (chronic) (obstructive) 493.2 ☑
    - disease, chronic 496
      - with
        - asthma (chronic) (obstructive) 493.2 ☑
    - emphysematous 492.8
  - lymphatic 457.1
  - meconium
    - fetus or newborn 777.1
      - in mucoviscidosis 277.01
    - newborn due to fecaliths 777.1
  - mediastinum 519.3
  - mitral (rheumatic) — *see* Stenosis, mitral
  - nasal 478.19
    - duct 375.56
      - neonatal 375.55
    - sinus — *see* Sinusitis
  - nasolacrimal duct 375.56
    - congenital 743.65
    - neonatal 375.55
  - nasopharynx 478.29
  - nose 478.19
  - organ or site, congenital NEC — *see* Atresia
  - pancreatic duct 577.8
  - parotid gland 527.8

Obstruction, obstructed, obstructive — *continued*
- pelviureteral junction (*see also* Obstruction, ureter) 593.4
- pharynx 478.29
- portal (circulation) (vein) 452
- prostate 600.90
  - with
    - other lower urinary tract symptoms (LUTS) 600.91
    - urinary
      - obstruction 600.91
      - retention 600.91
  - valve (urinary) 596.0
- pulmonary
  - valve (heart) (*see also* Endocarditis, pulmonary) 424.3
  - vein, isolated 747.49
- pyemic — *see* Septicemia
- pylorus (acquired) 537.0
  - congenital 750.5
  - infantile 750.5
- rectosigmoid (*see also* Obstruction, intestine) 560.9
- rectum 569.49
- renal 593.89
- respiratory 519.8
  - chronic 496
- retinal (artery) (vein) (central) (*see also* Occlusion, retina) 362.30
- salivary duct (any) 527.8
  - with calculus 527.5
- sigmoid (*see also* Obstruction, intestine) 560.9
- sinus (accessory) (nasal) (*see also* Sinusitis) 473.9
- Stensen's duct 527.8
- stomach 537.89
  - acute 536.1
  - congenital 750.7
- submaxillary gland 527.8
  - with calculus 527.5
- thoracic duct 457.1
- thrombotic — *see* Thrombosis
- tooth eruption 520.6
- trachea 519.19
- tracheostomy airway 519.09
- tricuspid — *see* Endocarditis, tricuspid
- upper respiratory, congenital 748.8
- ureter (functional) 593.4
  - congenital 753.20
  - due to calculus 592.1
- ureteropelvic junction, congenital 753.21
- ureterovesical junction, congenital 753.22
- urethra 599.60
  - congenital 753.6
- urinary (moderate) 599.60
  - organ or tract (lower) 599.60
    - due to
      - benign prostatic hypertrophy (BPH) - see category 600
    - specified NEC 599.69
      - due to
        - benign prostatic hypertrophy (BPH) — see category 600
  - prostatic valve 596.0
- uropathy 599.60
- uterus 621.8
- vagina 623.2
- valvular — *see* Endocarditis
- vascular graft or shunt 996.1
  - atherosclerosis — *see* Arteriosclerosis, coronary
  - embolism 996.74
  - occlusion NEC 996.74
  - thrombus 996.74
- vein, venous 459.2
  - caval (inferior) (superior) 459.2
  - thrombotic — *see* Thrombosis
- vena cava (inferior) (superior) 459.2
- ventricular shunt 996.2
- vesical 596.0
- vesicourethral orifice 596.0
- vessel NEC 459.9

Obturator — *see* condition

Occlusal
- plane deviation 524.76
- wear, teeth 521.10

Occlusion
- anus 569.49
  - congenital 751.2
  - infantile 751.2
- aortoiliac (chronic) 444.0
- aqueduct of Sylvius 331.4
  - congenital 742.3
    - with spina bifida (*see also* Spina bifida) 741.0 ☑
- arteries of extremities, lower 444.22
  - without thrombus or embolus (*see also* Arteriosclerosis, extremities) 440.20
  - due to stricture or stenosis 447.1
  - upper 444.21
    - without thrombus or embolus (*see also* Arteriosclerosis, extremities) 440.20
    - due to stricture or stenosis 447.1
- artery NEC (*see also* Embolism, artery) 444.9
  - auditory, internal 433.8 ☑
  - basilar 433.0 ☑
    - with other precerebral artery 433.3 ☑
    - bilateral 433.3 ☑
  - brain or cerebral (*see also* Infarct, brain) 434.9 ☑
  - carotid 433.1 ☑
    - with other precerebral artery 433.3 ☑
    - bilateral 433.3 ☑
  - cerebellar (anterior inferior) (posterior inferior) (superior) 433.8 ☑
  - cerebral (*see also* Infarct, brain) 434.9 ☑
  - choroidal (anterior) 433.8 ☑
  - chronic total
    - coronary 414.2
    - extremity(ies) 440.4
  - communicating posterior 433.8 ☑
  - complete
    - coronary 414.2
    - extremity(ies) 440.4
  - coronary (thrombotic) (*see also* Infarct, myocardium) 410.9 ☑
    - acute 410.9 ☑
      - without myocardial infarction 411.81
    - chronic total 414.2
    - complete 414.2
    - healed or old 412
    - total 414.2
  - extremity(ies)
    - chronic total 440.4
    - complete 440.4
    - total 440.4
  - hypophyseal 433.8 ☑
  - iliac (artery) 444.81
  - mesenteric (embolic) (thrombotic) (with gangrene) 557.0
  - pontine 433.8 ☑
  - precerebral NEC 433.9 ☑
    - late effect — *see* Late effect(s) (of) cerebrovascular disease
    - multiple or bilateral 433.3 ☑
    - puerperal, postpartum, childbirth 674.0 ☑
    - specified NEC 433.8 ☑
  - renal 593.81
  - retinal — *see* Occlusion, retina, artery
  - spinal 433.8 ☑
  - vertebral 433.2 ☑
    - with other precerebral artery 433.3 ☑
    - bilateral 433.3 ☑
- basilar (artery) — *see* Occlusion, artery, basilar
- bile duct (any) (*see also* Obstruction, biliary) 576.2
- bowel (*see also* Obstruction, intestine) 560.9
- brain (artery) (vascular) (*see also* Infarct, brain) 434.9 ☑
- breast (duct) 611.89

Occlusion — *continued*
- carotid (artery) (common) (internal) — *see* Occlusion, artery, carotid
- cerebellar (anterior inferior) (artery) (posterior inferior) (superior) 433.8 ☑
- cerebral (artery) (*see also* Infarct, brain) 434.9 ☑
- cerebrovascular (*see also* Infarct, brain) 434.9 ☑
  - diffuse 437.0
- cervical canal (*see also* Stricture, cervix) 622.4
  - by falciparum malaria 084.0
- cervix (uteri) (*see also* Stricture, cervix) 622.4
- choanal 748.0
- choroidal (artery) 433.8 ☑
- colon (*see also* Obstruction, intestine) 560.9
- communicating posterior artery 433.8 ☑
- coronary (artery) (thrombotic) (*see also* Infarct, myocardium) 410.9 ☑
  - without myocardial infarction 411.81
  - acute 410.9 ☑
    - without myocardial infarction 411.81
  - healed or old 412
- cystic duct (*see also* Obstruction, gallbladder) 575.2
  - congenital 751.69
- disto
  - division I 524.22
  - division II 524.22
- embolic — *see* Embolism
- fallopian tube 628.2
  - congenital 752.19
- gallbladder (*see also* Obstruction, gallbladder) 575.2
  - congenital 751.69
    - jaundice from 751.69 [774.5]
- gingiva, traumatic 523.8
- hymen 623.3
  - congenital 752.42
- hypophyseal (artery) 433.8 ☑
- iliac artery 444.81
- intestine (*see also* Obstruction, intestine) 560.9
- kidney 593.89
- lacrimal apparatus — *see* Stenosis, lacrimal
- lung 518.89
- lymph or lymphatic channel 457.1
- mammary duct 611.89
- mesenteric artery (embolic) (thrombotic) (with gangrene) 557.0
- nose 478.1 ☑
  - congenital 748.0
- organ or site, congenital NEC — *see* Atresia
- oviduct 628.2
  - congenital 752.19
- periodontal, traumatic 523.8
- peripheral arteries (lower extremity) 444.22
  - without thrombus or embolus (*see also* Arteriosclerosis, extremities) 440.20
  - due to stricture or stenosis 447.1
  - upper extremity 444.21
    - without thrombus or embolus (*see also* Arteriosclerosis, extremities) 440.20
    - due to stricture or stenosis 447.1
- pontine (artery) 433.8 ☑
- posterior lingual, of mandibular teeth 524.29
- precerebral artery — *see* Occlusion, artery, precerebral NEC
- puncta lacrimalia 375.52
- pupil 364.74
- pylorus (*see also* Stricture, pylorus) 537.0
- renal artery 593.81
- retina, retinal (vascular) 362.30
  - artery, arterial 362.30
    - branch 362.32
    - central (total) 362.31
    - partial 362.33
    - transient 362.34
    - tributary 362.32
  - vein 362.30
    - branch 362.36
    - central (total) 362.35

☑ **Additional Digit Required** — Refer to the Tabular List for Digit Selection　　　　　　　▽ **Subterms under main terms may continue to next column or page**

216 — Volume 2　　　　　　▶◀ Revised Text　　　　● New Line　　　▲ Revised Code　　　　　　　**2011 ICD-9-CM**

Occlusion — *continued*
  retina, retinal — *continued*
    vein — *continued*
      incipient 362.37
      partial 362.37
      tributary 362.36
  spinal artery 433.8 ☑
  stent
    coronary 996.72
  teeth (mandibular) (posterior lingual) 524.29
  thoracic duct 457.1
  tubal 628.2
  ureter (complete) (partial) 593.4
    congenital 753.29
  urethra (*see also* Stricture, urethra) 598.9
    congenital 753.6
  uterus 621.8
  vagina 623.2
  vascular NEC 459.9
  vein — *see* Thrombosis
  vena cava
    inferior 453.2
    superior ▶(acute)◀ 453.87   ▲
      chronic 453.77
  ventricle (brain) NEC 331.4
  vertebral (artery) — *see* Occlusion, artery, vertebral
  vessel (blood) NEC 459.9
  vulva 624.8
Occlusio pupillae 364.74
Occupational
  problems NEC V62.29
  therapy V57.21
Ochlophobia 300.29
Ochronosis (alkaptonuric) (congenital) (endogenous) 270.2
  with chloasma of eyelid 270.2
Ocular muscle — *see also* condition
  myopathy 359.1
  torticollis 781.93
Oculoauriculovertebral dysplasia 756.0
Oculogyric
  crisis or disturbance 378.87
    psychogenic 306.7
Oculomotor syndrome 378.81
Oddi's sphincter spasm 576.5
Odelberg's disease (juvenile osteochondrosis) 732.1
Odontalgia 525.9
Odontoameloblastoma (M9311/0) 213.1
  upper jaw (bone) 213.0
Odontoclasia 521.05
Odontoclasis 873.63
  complicated 873.73
Odontodysplasia, regional 520.4
Odontogenesis imperfecta 520.5
Odontoma (M9280/0) 213.1
  ameloblastic (M9311/0) 213.1
    upper jaw (bone) 213.0
  calcified (M9280/0) 213.1
    upper jaw (bone) 213.0
  complex (M9282/0) 213.1
    upper jaw (bone) 213.0
  compound (M9281/0) 213.1
    upper jaw (bone) 213.0
  fibroameloblastic (M9290/0) 213.1
    upper jaw (bone) 213.0
  follicular 526.0
    upper jaw (bone) 213.0
Odontomyelitis (closed) (open) 522.0
Odontonecrosis 521.09
Odontorrhagia 525.8
Odontosarcoma, ameloblastic (M9290/3) 170.1
  upper jaw (bone) 170.0
Odynophagia 787.20
Oesophagostomiasis 127.7
Oesophagostomum infestation 127.7
Oestriasis 134.0
Ogilvie's syndrome (sympathicotonic colon obstruction) 560.89
Oguchi's disease (retina) 368.61
Ohara's disease — *see also* Tularemia 021.9
Oidiomycosis — *see also* Candidiasis 112.9
Oidiomycotic meningitis 112.83

Oidium albicans infection — *see also* Candidiasis 112.9
Old age 797
  dementia (of) 290.0
Olfactory — *see* condition
Oligemia 285.9
Oligergasia — *see also* Retardation, mental 319
Oligoamnios 658.0 ☑
  affecting fetus or newborn 761.2
Oligoastrocytoma, mixed (M9382/3)
  specified site — *see* Neoplasm, by site, malignant
  unspecified site 191.9
Oligocythemia 285.9
Oligodendroblastoma (M9460/3)
  specified site — *see* Neoplasm, by site, malignant
  unspecified site 191.9
Oligodendroglioma (M9450/3)
  anaplastic type (M9451/3)
    specified site — *see* Neoplasm, by site, malignant
    unspecified site 191.9
  specified site — *see* Neoplasm, by site, malignant
  unspecified site 191.9
Oligodendroma — *see* Oligodendroglioma
Oligodontia — *see also* Anodontia 520.0
Oligoencephalon 742.1
Oligohydramnios 658.0 ☑
  affecting fetus or newborn 761.2
  due to premature rupture of membranes 658.1 ☑
    affecting fetus or newborn 761.2
Oligohydrosis 705.0
Oligomenorrhea 626.1
Oligophrenia — *see also* Retardation, mental 319
  phenylpyruvic 270.1
Oligospermia 606.1
Oligotrichia 704.09
  congenita 757.4
Oliguria 788.5
  with
    abortion — *see* Abortion, by type, with renal failure
    ectopic pregnancy (*see also* categories 633–633.9) 639.3
    molar pregnancy (*see also* categories 630–632) 639.3
  complicating
    abortion 639.3
    ectopic or molar pregnancy 639.3
    pregnancy 646.2 ☑
      with hypertension — *see* Toxemia, of pregnancy
  due to a procedure 997.5
  following labor and delivery 669.3 ☑
  heart or cardiac — *see* Failure, heart
  puerperal, postpartum 669.3 ☑
  specified due to a procedure 997.5
Ollier's disease (chondrodysplasia) 756.4
Omentitis — *see also* Peritonitis 567.9
Omentocele — *see also* Hernia, omental 553.8
Omentum, omental — *see* condition
Omphalitis (congenital) (newborn) 771.4
  not of newborn 686.9
  tetanus 771.3
Omphalocele 756.72
Omphalomesenteric duct, persistent 751.0
Omphalorrhagia, newborn 772.3
Omsk hemorrhagic fever 065.1
Onanism 307.9
Onchocerciasis 125.3
  eye 125.3 *[360.13]*
Onchocercosis 125.3
Oncocytoma (M8290/0) — *see* Neoplasm, by site, benign
Ondine's curse 348.89
Oneirophrenia — *see also* Schizophrenia 295.4 ☑
Onychauxis 703.8
  congenital 757.5
Onychia (with lymphangitis) 681.9
  dermatophytic 110.1

Onychia — *continued*
  finger 681.02
  toe 681.11
Onychitis (with lymphangitis) 681.9
  finger 681.02
  toe 681.11
Onychocryptosis 703.0
Onychodystrophy 703.8
  congenital 757.5
Onychogryphosis 703.8
Onychogryposis 703.8
Onycholysis 703.8
Onychomadesis 703.8
Onychomalacia 703.8
Onychomycosis 110.1
  finger 110.1
  toe 110.1
Onycho-osteodysplasia 756.89
Onychophagy 307.9
Onychoptosis 703.8
Onychorrhexis 703.8
  congenital 757.5
Onychoschizia 703.8
Onychotrophia — *see also* Atrophy, nail 703.8
O'nyong-nyong fever 066.3
Onyxis (finger) (toe) 703.0
Onyxitis (with lymphangitis) 681.9
  finger 681.02
  toe 681.11
Oocyte (egg) (ovum)
  donor V59.70
    over age 35 V59.73
      anonymous recipient V59.73
      designated recipient V59.74
    under age 35 V59.71
      anonymous recipient V59.71
      designated recipient V59.72
Oophoritis (cystic) (infectional) (interstitial) — *see also* Salpingo-oophoritis 614.2
  complicating pregnancy 646.6 ☑
  fetal (acute) 752.0
  gonococcal (acute) 098.19
    chronic or duration of 2 months or over 098.39
  tuberculous (*see also* Tuberculosis) 016.6 ☑
Opacity, opacities
  cornea 371.00
    central 371.03
    congenital 743.43
      interfering with vision 743.42
    degenerative (*see also* Degeneration, cornea) 371.40
    hereditary (*see also* Dystrophy, cornea) 371.50
    inflammatory (*see also* Keratitis) 370.9
    late effect of trachoma (healed) 139.1
    minor 371.01
    peripheral 371.02
  enamel (fluoride) (nonfluoride) (teeth) 520.3
  lens (*see also* Cataract) 366.9
  snowball 379.22
  vitreous (humor) 379.24
    congenital 743.51
Opalescent dentin (hereditary) 520.5
Open, opening
  abnormal, organ or site, congenital — *see* Imperfect, closure
  angle with
    borderline intraocular pressure 365.01
    cupping of discs 365.01
  bite
    anterior 524.24
    posterior 524.25
  false — *see* Imperfect, closure
  margin on tooth restoration 525.61
  restoration margins 525.61
  wound — *see* Wound, open, by site
Operation
  causing mutilation of fetus 763.89
  destructive, on live fetus, to facilitate birth 763.89
  for delivery, fetus or newborn 763.89
  maternal, unrelated to current delivery, affecting fetus or newborn (*see also* Newborn, affected by) 760.64
Operational fatigue 300.89

Operative — *see* condition
Operculitis (chronic) 523.40
  acute 523.30
Operculum, retina 361.32
  with detachment 361.01
Ophiasis 704.01
Ophthalmia — *see also* Conjunctivitis 372.30
  actinic rays 370.24
  allergic (acute) 372.05
    chronic 372.14
  blennorrhagic (neonatorum) 098.40
  catarrhal 372.03
  diphtheritic 032.81
  Egyptian 076.1
  electric, electrica 370.24
  gonococcal (neonatorum) 098.40
  metastatic 360.11
  migraine 346.8 ☑
  neonatorum, newborn 771.6
    gonococcal 098.40
  nodosa 360.14
  phlyctenular 370.31
    with ulcer (*see also* Ulcer, cornea) 370.00
  sympathetic 360.11
Ophthalmitis — *see* Ophthalmia
Ophthalmocele (congenital) 743.66
Ophthalmoneuromyelitis 341.0
Ophthalmopathy, infiltrative with thyrotoxicosis 242.0 ☑
Ophthalmoplegia — *see also* Strabismus 378.9
  anterior internuclear 378.86
  ataxia-areflexia syndrome 357.0
  bilateral 378.9
  diabetic 250.5 ☑ *[378.86]*
    due to secondary diabetes 249.5 ☑ *[378.86]*
  exophthalmic 242.0 ☑ *[376.22]*
  external 378.55
    progressive 378.72
    total 378.56
  internal (complete) (total) 367.52
  internuclear 378.86
  migraine 346.2 ☑
  painful 378.55
  Parinaud's 378.81
  progressive external 378.72
  supranuclear, progressive 333.0
  total (external) 378.56
    internal 367.52
  unilateral 378.9
Opisthognathism 524.00
Opisthorchiasis (felineus) (tenuicollis) (viverrini) 121.0
Opisthotonos, opisthotonus 781.0
Opitz's disease (congestive splenomegaly) 289.51
Opiumism — *see also* Dependence 304.0 ☑
Oppenheim's disease 358.8
Oppenheim-Urbach disease or syndrome (necrobiosis lipoidica diabeticorum) 250.8 ☑ *[709.3]*
  due to secondary diabetes 249.8 ☑ *[709.3]*
Opsoclonia 379.59
Optic nerve — *see* condition
Orbit — *see* condition
Orchioblastoma (M9071/3) 186.9
Orchitis (nonspecific) (septic) 604.90
  with abscess 604.0
  blennorrhagic (acute) 098.13
    chronic or duration of 2 months or over 098.33
  diphtheritic 032.89 *[604.91]*
  filarial 125.9 *[604.91]*
  gangrenous 604.99
  gonococcal (acute) 098.13
    chronic or duration of 2 months or over 098.33
  mumps 072.0
  parotidea 072.0
  suppurative 604.99
  syphilitic 095.8 *[604.91]*
  tuberculous (*see also* Tuberculosis) 016.5 ☑ *[608.81]*
Orf 051.2
Organic — *see also* condition
  heart — *see* Disease, heart

☑ **Additional Digit Required — Refer to the Tabular List for Digit Selection**   ▒ **Subterms under main terms may continue to next column or page**

2011 ICD-9-CM   ▶◀ Revised Text   ● New Line   ▲ Revised Code   October 2010 • Volume 2 — 217

☑ **Additional Digit Required** — Refer to the Tabular List for Digit Selection   ▽ **Subterms under main terms may continue to next column or page**

218 — Volume 2   ▶◀ Revised Text   ● New Line   ▲ Revised Code   2011 ICD-9-CM

Osteomyelitis (general) (infective) (localized) (neonatal) (purulent) (pyogenic) (septic) (staphylococcal) (streptococcal) (suppurative) (with periostitis) 730.2 ☑

Note — Use the following fifth-digit subclassification with category 730:

0	*site unspecified*
1	*shoulder region*
2	*upper arm*
3	*forearm*
4	*hand*
5	*pelvic region and thigh*
6	*lower leg*
7	*ankle and foot*
8	*other specified sites*
9	*multiple sites*

  acute or subacute 730.0 ☑
  chronic or old 730.1 ☑
  due to or associated with
    diabetes mellitus 250.8 ☑ [731.8]
      due to secondary diabetes 249.8 ☑ [731.8]
    tuberculosis (see also Tuberculosis, bone) 015.9 ☑ [730.8] ☑
      limb bones 015.5 ☑ [730.8] ☑
      specified bones NEC 015.7 ☑ [730.8] ☑
      spine 015.0 ☑ [730.8] ☑
    typhoid 002.0 [730.8] ☑
  Garré's 730.1 ☑
  jaw (acute) (chronic) (lower) (neonatal) (suppurative) (upper) 526.4
  nonsuppurating 730.1 ☑
  orbital 376.03
  petrous bone (see also Petrositis) 383.20
  Salmonella 003.24
  sclerosing, nonsuppurative 730.1 ☑
  sicca 730.1 ☑
  syphilitic 095.5
    congenital 090.0 [730.8] ☑
  tuberculous — see Tuberculosis, bone
  typhoid 002.0 [730.8] ☑
Osteomyelofibrosis 289.89
Osteomyelosclerosis 289.89
Osteonecrosis 733.40
  meaning osteomyelitis 730.1 ☑
Osteo-onycho-arthro dysplasia 756.89
Osteo-onychodysplasia, hereditary 756.89
Osteopathia
  condensans disseminata 756.53
  hyperostotica multiplex infantilis 756.59
  hypertrophica toxica 731.2
  striata 756.4
Osteopathy resulting from poliomyelitis — see also Poliomyelitis 045.9 ☑ [730.7] ☑
  familial dysplastic 731.2
Osteopecilia 756.53
Osteopenia 733.90
  borderline 733.90
Osteoperiostitis — see also Osteomyelitis 730.2 ☑
  ossificans toxica 731.2
  toxica ossificans 731.2
Osteopetrosis (familial) 756.52
Osteophyte — see Exostosis
Osteophytosis — see Exostosis
Osteopoikilosis 756.53
Osteoporosis (generalized) 733.00
  circumscripta 731.0
  disuse 733.03
  drug-induced 733.09
  idiopathic 733.02
  postmenopausal 733.01
  posttraumatic 733.7
  screening V82.81
  senile 733.01
  specified type NEC 733.09
Osteoporosis-osteomalacia syndrome 268.2
Osteopsathyrosis 756.51
Osteoradionecrosis, jaw 526.89

Osteosarcoma (M9180/3) — see also Neoplasm, bone, malignant
  chondroblastic (M9181/3) — see Neoplasm, bone, malignant
  fibroblastic (M9182/3) — see Neoplasm, bone, malignant
  in Paget's disease of bone (M9184/3) — see Neoplasm, bone, malignant
  juxtacortical (M9190/3) — see Neoplasm, bone, malignant
  parosteal (M9190/3) — see Neoplasm, bone, malignant
  telangiectatic (M9183/3) — see Neoplasm, bone, malignant
Osteosclerosis 756.52
  fragilis (generalisata) 756.52
Osteosclerotic anemia 289.89
Osteosis
  acromegaloid 757.39
  cutis 709.3
  parathyroid 252.01
  renal fibrocystic 588.0
Österreicher-Turner syndrome 756.89
Ostium
  atrioventriculare commune 745.69
  primum (arteriosum) (defect) (persistent) 745.61
  secundum (arteriosum) (defect) (patent) (persistent) 745.5
Ostrum-Furst syndrome 756.59
Os, uterus — see condition
Otalgia 388.70
  otogenic 388.71
  referred 388.72
Othematoma 380.31
Otitic hydrocephalus 348.2
Otitis 382.9
  with effusion 381.4
    purulent 382.4
    secretory 381.4
    serous 381.4
    suppurative 382.4
  acute 382.9
  adhesive (see also Adhesions, middle ear) 385.10
  chronic 382.9
    with effusion 381.3
    mucoid, mucous (simple) 381.20
    purulent 382.3
    secretory 381.3
    serous 381.10
    suppurative 382.3
  diffuse parasitic 136.8
  externa (acute) (diffuse) (hemorrhagica) 380.10
    actinic 380.22
    candidal 112.82
    chemical 380.22
    chronic 380.23
      mycotic — see Otitis, externa, mycotic
      specified type NEC 380.23
    circumscribed 380.10
    contact 380.22
    due to
      erysipelas 035 [380.13]
      impetigo 684 [380.13]
      seborrheic dermatitis 690.10 [380.13]
    eczematoid 380.22
    furuncular 680.0 [380.13]
    infective 380.10
      chronic 380.16
    malignant 380.14
    mycotic (chronic) 380.15
      due to
        aspergillosis 117.3 [380.15]
        moniliasis 112.82
        otomycosis 111.8 [380.15]
    reactive 380.22
    specified type NEC 380.22
    tropical 111.8 [380.15]
  insidiosa (see also Otosclerosis) 387.9
  interna (see also Labyrinthitis) 386.30
  media (hemorrhagic) (staphylococcal) (streptococcal) 382.9
    acute 382.9

Otitis — *continued*
  media — *continued*
    acute — *continued*
      with effusion 381.00
      allergic 381.04
        mucoid 381.05
        sanguinous 381.06
        serous 381.04
      catarrhal 381.00
      exudative 381.00
      mucoid 381.02
        allergic 381.05
      necrotizing 382.00
        with spontaneous rupture of ear drum 382.01
        in
          influenza ▶(see also Influenza)◀ 487.8 [382.02]
          measles 055.2
          scarlet fever 034.1 [382.02]
      nonsuppurative 381.00
      purulent 382.00
        with spontaneous rupture of ear drum 382.01
      sanguineous 381.03
        allergic 381.06
      secretory 381.01
      seromucinous 381.02
      serous 381.01
        allergic 381.04
      suppurative 382.00
        with spontaneous rupture of ear drum 382.01
        due to
          influenza ▶(see also Influenza)◀ 487.8 [382.02]
          scarlet fever 034.1 [382.02]
      transudative 381.00
    adhesive (see also Adhesions, middle ear) 385.10
    allergic 381.4
      acute 381.04
        mucoid 381.05
        sanguineous 381.06
        serous 381.04
      chronic 381.3
    catarrhal 381.4
      acute 381.00
      chronic (simple) 381.10
    chronic 382.9
      with effusion 381.3
      adhesive (see also Adhesions, middle ear) 385.10
      allergic 381.3
      atticoantral, suppurative (with posterior or superior marginal perforation of ear drum) 382.2
      benign suppurative (with anterior perforation of ear drum) 382.1
      catarrhal 381.10
      exudative 381.3
      mucinous 381.20
      mucoid, mucous (simple) 381.20
      mucosanguineous 381.29
      nonsuppurative 381.3
      purulent 382.3
      secretory 381.3
      seromucinous 381.3
      serosanguineous 381.19
      serous (simple) 381.10
      suppurative 382.3
        atticoantral (with posterior or superior marginal perforation of ear drum) 382.2
        benign (with anterior perforation of ear drum) 382.1
        tuberculous (see also Tuberculosis) 017.4 ☑
        tubotympanic 382.1
      transudative 381.3
    exudative 381.4
      acute 381.00
      chronic 381.3
    fibrotic (see also Adhesions, middle ear) 385.10
    mucoid, mucous 381.4

Otitis — *continued*
  media — *continued*
    mucoid, mucous — *continued*
      acute 381.02
      chronic (simple) 381.20
    mucosanguineous, chronic 381.29
    nonsuppurative 381.4
      acute 381.00
      chronic 381.3
    postmeasles 055.2
    purulent 382.4
      acute 382.00
        with spontaneous rupture of ear drum 382.01
      chronic 382.3
    sanguineous, acute 381.03
      allergic 381.06
    secretory 381.4
      acute or subacute 381.01
      chronic 381.3
    seromucinous 381.4
      acute or subacute 381.02
      chronic 381.3
    serosanguineous, chronic 381.19
    serous 381.4
      acute or subacute 381.01
      chronic (simple) 381.10
    subacute — see Otitis, media, acute
    suppurative 382.4
      acute 382.00
        with spontaneous rupture of ear drum 382.01
      chronic 382.3
        atticoantral 382.2
        benign 382.1
        tuberculous (see also Tuberculosis) 017.4 ☑
        tubotympanic 382.1
    transudative 381.4
      acute 381.00
      chronic 381.3
    tuberculous (see also Tuberculosis) 017.4 ☑
  postmeasles 055.2
Otoconia 386.8
Otolith syndrome 386.19
Otomycosis 111.8 [380.15]
  in
    aspergillosis 117.3 [380.15]
    moniliasis 112.82
Otopathy 388.9
Otoporosis — see also Otosclerosis 387.9
Otorrhagia 388.69
  traumatic — see nature of injury
Otorrhea 388.60
  blood 388.69
  cerebrospinal (fluid) 388.61
Otosclerosis (general) 387.9
  cochlear (endosteal) 387.2
  involving
    otic capsule 387.2
    oval window
      nonobliterative 387.0
      obliterative 387.1
    round window 387.2
  nonobliterative 387.0
  obliterative 387.1
  specified type NEC 387.8
Otospongiosis — see also Otosclerosis 387.9
Otto's disease or pelvis 715.35
Outburst, aggressive — see also Disturbance, conduct 312.0 ☑
  in children or adolescents 313.9
Outcome of delivery
  multiple birth NEC V27.9
    all liveborn V27.5
    all stillborn V27.7
    some liveborn V27.6
    unspecified V27.9
  single V27.9
    liveborn V27.0
    stillborn V27.1
  twins V27.9
    both liveborn V27.2
    both stillborn V27.4
    one liveborn, one stillborn V27.3

☑ Additional Digit Required — Refer to the Tabular List for Digit Selection

▽ Subterms under main terms may continue to next column or page

Outlet — see also condition
  syndrome (thoracic) 353.0
Outstanding ears (bilateral) 744.29
Ovalocytosis (congenital) (hereditary) — see
  also Elliptocytosis 282.1
Ovarian — see also condition
  pregnancy — see Pregnancy, ovarian
  remnant syndrome 620.8
  vein syndrome 593.4
Ovaritis (cystic) — see also Salpingo-oophoritis
  614.2
Ovary, ovarian — see condition
Overactive — see also Hyperfunction
  bladder 596.51
  eye muscle (see also Strabismus) 378.9
  hypothalamus 253.8
  thyroid (see also Thyrotoxicosis) 242.9 ☑
Overactivity, child 314.01
Overbite (deep) (excessive) (horizontal) (vertical) 524.29
Overbreathing — see also Hyperventilation
  786.01
Overconscientious personality 301.4
Overdevelopment — see also Hypertrophy
  breast (female) (male) 611.1
  nasal bones 738.0
  prostate, congenital 752.89
Overdistention — see Distention
Overdose overdosage (drug) 977.9
  specified drug or substance — see Table of
    Drugs and Chemicals
Overeating 783.6
  nonorganic origin 307.51
Overexertion (effects) (exhaustion) 994.5
Overexposure (effects) 994.9
  exhaustion 994.4
Overfeeding — see also Overeating 783.6
Overfill, endodontic 526.62
Overgrowth, bone NEC 733.99
Overhanging
  tooth restoration 525.62
  unrepairable, dental restorative materials
    525.62
Overheated (effects) (places) — see Heat
Overinhibited child 313.0
Overjet 524.29
  excessive horizontal 524.26
Overlaid, overlying (suffocation) 994.7
Overlap
  excessive horizontal 524.26
Overlapping toe (acquired) 735.8
  congenital (fifth toe) 755.66
Overload
  fluid 276.69 ▲
    due to transfusion (blood) (blood ●
      components) 276.61 ●
    iron, due to repeated red blood cell ●
      transfusions 275.02 ●
  potassium (K) 276.7
  sodium (Na) 276.0
  transfusion associated circulatory (TACO) ●
    276.61
Overnutrition — see also Hyperalimentation
  783.6
Overproduction — see also Hypersecretion
  ACTH 255.3
  cortisol 255.0
  growth hormone 253.0
  thyroid-stimulating hormone (TSH) 242.8 ☑
Overriding
  aorta 747.21
  finger (acquired) 736.29
    congenital 755.59
  toe (acquired) 735.8
    congenital 755.66
Oversize
  fetus (weight of 4500 grams or more) 766.0
    affecting management of pregnancy
      656.6 ☑
    causing disproportion 653.5 ☑
      with obstructed labor 660.1 ☑
        affecting fetus or newborn 763.1
Overstimulation, ovarian 256.1
Overstrained 780.79
  heart — see Hypertrophy, cardiac
Overweight — see also Obesity 278.02

Overwork 780.79
Oviduct — see condition
Ovotestis 752.7
Ovulation (cycle)
  failure or lack of 628.0
  pain 625.2
Ovum
  blighted 631
  donor V59.70
    over age 35 V59.73
      anonymous recipient V59.73
      designated recipient V59.74
    under age 35 V59.71
      anonymous recipient V59.71
      designated recipient V59.72
  dropsical 631
  pathologic 631
Owren's disease or syndrome (parahemophil-
  ia) — see also Defect, coagulation 286.3
Oxalosis 271.8
Oxaluria 271.8
Ox heart — see Hypertrophy, cardiac
OX syndrome 758.6
Oxycephaly, oxycephalic 756.0
  syphilitic, congenital 090.0
Oxyuriasis 127.4
Oxyuris vermicularis (infestation) 127.4
Ozena 472.0

P

Pacemaker syndrome 429.4
Pachyderma, pachydermia 701.8
  laryngis 478.5
  laryngitis 478.79
  larynx (verrucosa) 478.79
Pachydermatitis 701.8
Pachydermatocele (congenital) 757.39
  acquired 701.8
Pachydermatosis 701.8
Pachydermoperiostitis
  secondary 731.2
Pachydermoperiostosis
  primary idiopathic 757.39
  secondary 731.2
Pachymeningitis (adhesive) (basal) (brain)
  (cerebral) (cervical) (chronic) (circumscribed) (external) (fibrous) (hemorrhagic) (hypertrophic) (internal) (purulent)
  (spinal) (suppurative) — see also
  Meningitis 322.9
  gonococcal 098.82
Pachyonychia (congenital) 757.5
  acquired 703.8
Pachyperiosteodermia
  primary or idiopathic 757.39
  secondary 731.2
Pachyperiostosis
  primary or idiopathic 757.39
  secondary 731.2
Pacinian tumor (M9507/0) — see Neoplasm,
  skin, benign
Pads, knuckle or Garrod's 728.79
Paget's disease (osteitis deformans) 731.0
  with infiltrating duct carcinoma of the
    breast (M8541/3) — see Neoplasm,
    breast, malignant
  bone 731.0
    osteosarcoma in (M9184/3) — see Neo-
      plasm, bone, malignant
  breast (M8540/3) 174.0
  extramammary (M8542/3) (see also Neo-
    plasm, skin, malignant)
    anus 154.3
    skin 173.5
  malignant (M8540/3)
    breast 174.0
    specified site NEC (M8542/3) — see
      Neoplasm, skin, malignant
    unspecified site 174.0
  mammary (M8540/3) 174.0
  necrosis of bone 731.0
  nipple (M8540/3) 174.0
  osteitis deformans 731.0
Paget-Schroetter syndrome (intermittent
  venous claudication) 453.89
Pain(s) (see also Painful) 780.96

Pain(s) (see also Painful) — continued
  abdominal 789.0 ☑
  acute 338.19
    due to trauma 338.11
    postoperative 338.18
      post-thoracotomy 338.12
  adnexa (uteri) 625.9
  alimentary, due to vascular insufficiency
    557.9
  anginoid (see also Pain, precordial) 786.51
  anus 569.42
  arch 729.5
  arm 729.5
  axillary 729.5
  back (postural) 724.5
    low 724.2
      psychogenic 307.89
  bile duct 576.9
  bladder 788.99
  bone 733.90
  breast 611.71
    psychogenic 307.89
  broad ligament 625.9
  cancer associated 338.3
  cartilage NEC 733.90
  cecum 789.0 ☑
  cervicobrachial 723.3
  chest (central) 786.50
    atypical 786.59
    midsternal 786.51
    musculoskeletal 786.59
    noncardiac 786.59
    substernal 786.51
    wall (anterior) 786.52
  chronic 338.29
    associated with significant psychosocial
      dysfunction 338.4
    due to trauma 338.21
    postoperative 338.28
      post-thoracotomy 338.22
    syndrome 338.4
  coccyx 724.79
  colon 789.0 ☑
  common duct 576.9
  coronary — see Angina
  costochondral 786.52
  diaphragm 786.52
  due to (presence of) any device, implant, or
    graft classifiable to 996.0–996.5 —
    see Complications, due to (presence
    of) any device, implant, or graft clas-
    sified to 996.0–996.5 NEC
    malignancy (primary) (secondary) 338.3
  ear (see also Otalgia) 388.70
  epigastric, epigastrium 789.06
  extremity (lower) (upper) 729.5
  eye 379.91
  face, facial 784.0
    atypical 350.2
    nerve 351.8
  false (labor) 644.1 ☑
  female genital organ NEC 625.9
    psychogenic 307.89
  finger 729.5
  flank 789.0 ☑
  foot 729.5
  gallbladder 575.9
  gas (intestinal) 787.3
  gastric 536.8
  generalized 780.96
  genital organ
    female 625.9
    male 608.9
    psychogenic 307.89
  groin 789.0 ☑
  growing 781.99
  hand 729.5
  head (see also Headache) 784.0
  heart (see also Pain, precordial) 786.51
  infraorbital (see also Neuralgia, trigeminal)
    350.1
  intermenstrual 625.2
  jaw 784.92 ▲
  joint 719.40
    ankle 719.47
    elbow 719.42

Pain(s) (see also Painful) — continued
  joint — continued
    foot 719.47
    hand 719.44
    hip 719.45
    knee 719.46
    multiple sites 719.49
    pelvic region 719.45
    psychogenic 307.89
    shoulder (region) 719.41
    specified site NEC 719.48
    wrist 719.43
  kidney 788.0
  labor, false or spurious 644.1 ☑
  laryngeal 784.1
  leg 729.5
  limb 729.5
  low back 724.2
  lumbar region 724.2
  mandible, mandibular 784.92 ●
  mastoid (see also Otalgia) 388.70
  maxilla 784.92 ▲
  menstrual 625.3
  metacarpophalangeal (joint) 719.44
  metatarsophalangeal (joint) 719.47
  mouth 528.9
  muscle 729.1
    intercostal 786.59
  musculoskeletal (see also Pain, by site) 729.1
  nasal 478.19
  nasopharynx 478.29
  neck NEC 723.1
    psychogenic 307.89
  neoplasm related (acute) (chronic) 338.3
  nerve NEC 729.2
  neuromuscular 729.1
  nose 478.19
  ocular 379.91
  ophthalmic 379.91
  orbital region 379.91
  osteocopic 733.90
  ovary 625.9
    psychogenic 307.89
  over heart (see also Pain, precordial) 786.51
  ovulation 625.2
  pelvic (female) 625.9
    male NEC 789.0 ☑
      psychogenic 307.89
    psychogenic 307.89
  penis 607.9
    psychogenic 307.89
  pericardial (see also Pain, precordial) 786.51
  perineum
    female 625.9
    male 608.9
  pharynx 478.29
  pleura, pleural, pleuritic 786.52
  postoperative 338.18
    acute 338.18
    chronic 338.28
  post-thoracotomy 338.12
    acute 338.12
    chronic 338.22
  preauricular 388.70
  precordial (region) 786.51
    psychogenic 307.89
  premenstrual 625.4
  psychogenic 307.80
    cardiovascular system 307.89
    gastrointestinal system 307.89
    genitourinary system 307.89
    heart 307.89
    musculoskeletal system 307.89
    respiratory system 307.89
    skin 306.3
  radicular (spinal) (see also Radiculitis) 729.2
  rectum 569.42
  respiration 786.52
  retrosternal 786.51
  rheumatic NEC 729.0
    muscular 729.1
  rib 786.50
  root (spinal) (see also Radiculitis) 729.2
  round ligament (stretch) 625.9
  sacroiliac 724.6
  sciatic 724.3

☑ **Additional Digit Required** — Refer to the Tabular List for Digit Selection   ▽ **Subterms under main terms may continue to next column or page**

Pain(s) (*see also* Painful) — *continued*
scrotum 608.9
  psychogenic 307.89
seminal vesicle 608.9
sinus 478.19
skin 782.0
spermatic cord 608.9
spinal root (*see also* Radiculitis) 729.2
stomach 536.8
  psychogenic 307.89
substernal 786.51
temporomandibular (joint) 524.62
temporomaxillary joint 524.62
testis 608.9
  psychogenic 307.89
thoracic spine 724.1
  with radicular and visceral pain 724.4
throat 784.1
tibia 733.90
toe 729.5
tongue 529.6
tooth 525.9
total hip replacement 996.77
total knee replacement 996.77
trigeminal (*see also* Neuralgia, trigeminal) 350.1
tumor associated 338.3
umbilicus 789.05
ureter 788.0
urinary (organ) (system) 788.0
uterus 625.9
  psychogenic 307.89
vagina 625.9
vertebrogenic (syndrome) 724.5
vesical 788.99
vulva 625.9
xiphoid 733.90
Painful — *see also* Pain
arc syndrome 726.19
coitus
  female 625.0
  male 608.89
    psychogenic 302.76
ejaculation (semen) 608.89
  psychogenic 302.79
erection 607.3
feet syndrome 266.2
menstruation 625.3
  psychogenic 306.52
micturition 788.1
ophthalmoplegia 378.55
respiration 786.52
scar NEC 709.2
urination 788.1
wire sutures 998.89
Painters' colic 984.9
specified type of lead — *see* Table of Drugs and Chemicals
Palate — *see* condition
Palatoplegia 528.9
Palatoschisis — *see also* Cleft, palate 749.00
Palilalia 784.69
Palindromic arthritis — *see also* Rheumatism, palindromic 719.3 ☑
Palliative care V66.7
Pallor 782.61
temporal, optic disc 377.15
Palmar — *see also* condition
fascia — *see* condition
Palpable
cecum 569.89
kidney 593.89
liver 573.9
lymph nodes 785.6
ovary 620.8
prostate 602.9
spleen (*see also* Splenomegaly) 789.2
uterus 625.8
Palpitation (heart) 785.1
psychogenic 306.2
Palsy — *see also* Paralysis 344.9
atrophic diffuse 335.20
Bell's 351.0
  newborn 767.5
birth 767.7
brachial plexus 353.0

Palsy — *see also* Paralysis — *continued*
brachial plexus — *continued*
  fetus or newborn 767.6
brain (*see also* Palsy, cerebral)
  noncongenital or noninfantile 344.89
    late effect — *see* Late effect(s) (of) cerebrovascular disease
  syphilitic 094.89
    congenital 090.49
bulbar (chronic) (progressive) 335.22
  pseudo NEC 335.23
  supranuclear NEC 344.8 ☑
cerebral (congenital) (infantile) (spastic) 343.9
  athetoid 333.71
  diplegic 343.0
    late effect — *see* Late effect(s) (of) cerebrovascular disease
  hemiplegic 343.1
  monoplegic 343.3
  noncongenital or noninfantile 437.8
    late effect — *see* Late effect(s) (of) cerebrovascular disease
  paraplegic 343.0
  quadriplegic 343.2
  spastic, not congenital or infantile 344.89
  syphilitic 094.89
    congenital 090.49
  tetraplegic 343.2
cranial nerve (*see also* Disorder, nerve, cranial)
  multiple 352.6
creeping 335.21
divers' 993.3
Erb's (birth injury) 767.6
facial 351.0
  newborn 767.5
glossopharyngeal 352.2
Klumpke (-Déjérine) 767.6
lead 984.9
  specified type of lead — *see* Table of Drugs and Chemicals
median nerve (tardy) 354.0
peroneal nerve (acute) (tardy) 355.3
progressive supranuclear 333.0
pseudobulbar NEC 335.23
radial nerve (acute) 354.3
seventh nerve 351.0
  newborn 767.5
shaking (*see also* Parkinsonism) 332.0
spastic (cerebral) (spinal) 343.9
  hemiplegic 343.1
specified nerve NEC — *see* Disorder, nerve
supranuclear NEC 356.8
  progressive 333.0
ulnar nerve (tardy) 354.2
wasting 335.21
Paltauf-Sternberg disease 201.9 ☑
Paludism — *see* Malaria
Panama fever 084.0
Panaris (with lymphangitis) 681.9
finger 681.02
toe 681.11
Panaritium (with lymphangitis) 681.9
finger 681.02
toe 681.11
Panarteritis (nodosa) 446.0
brain or cerebral 437.4
Pancake heart 793.2
with cor pulmonale (chronic) 416.9
Pancarditis (acute) (chronic) 429.89
with
  rheumatic
    fever (active) (acute) (chronic) (subacute) 391.8
    inactive or quiescent 398.99
  rheumatic, acute 391.8
  chronic or inactive 398.99
Pancoast's syndrome or tumor (carcinoma, pulmonary apex) (M8010/3) 162.3
Pancoast-Tobias syndrome (M8010/3) (carcinoma, pulmonary apex) 162.3
Pancolitis 556.6
Pancreas, pancreatic — *see* condition
Pancreatitis 577.0

Pancreatitis — *continued*
acute (edematous) (hemorrhagic) (recurrent) 577.0
annular 577.0
apoplectic 577.0
calcerceous 577.0
chronic (infectious) 577.1
  recurrent 577.1
cystic 577.2
fibrous 577.8
gangrenous 577.0
hemorrhagic (acute) 577.0
interstitial (chronic) 577.1
  acute 577.0
malignant 577.0
mumps 072.3
painless 577.1
recurrent 577.1
relapsing 577.1
subacute 577.0
suppurative 577.0
syphilitic 095.8
Pancreatolithiasis 577.8
Pancytolysis 289.9
Pancytopenia (acquired) 284.1
with malformations 284.09
  congenital 284.09
Panencephalitis — *see also* Encephalitis
subacute, sclerosing 046.2
Panhematopenia 284.81
congenital 284.09
constitutional 284.09
splenic, primary 289.4
Panhemocytopenia 284.81
congenital 284.09
constitutional 284.09
Panhypogonadism 257.2
Panhypopituitarism 253.2
prepubertal 253.3
Panic (attack) (state) 300.01
reaction to exceptional stress (transient) 308.0
Panmyelopathy, familial constitutional 284.09
Panmyelophthisis 284.2
acquired (secondary) 284.81
congenital 284.2
idiopathic 284.9
Panmyelosis (acute) (M9951/1) 238.79
Panner's disease 732.3
capitellum humeri 732.3
head of humerus 732.3
tarsal navicular (bone) (osteochondrosis) 732.5
Panneuritis endemica 265.0 [357.4]
Panniculitis 729.30
back 724.8
knee 729.31
mesenteric 567.82
neck 723.6
nodular, nonsuppurative 729.30
sacral 724.8
specified site NEC 729.39
Panniculus adiposus (abdominal) 278.1
Pannus (corneal) 370.62
abdominal (symptomatic) 278.1
allergic eczematous 370.62
degenerativus 370.62
keratic 370.62
rheumatoid — *see* Arthritis, rheumatoid
trachomatosus, trachomatous (active) 076.1 [370.62]
  late effect 139.1
Panophthalmitis 360.02
Panotitis — *see* Otitis media
Pansinusitis (chronic) (hyperplastic) (nonpurulent) (purulent) 473.8
acute 461.8
due to fungus NEC 117.9
tuberculous (*see also* Tuberculosis) 012.8 ☑
Panuveitis 360.12
sympathetic 360.11
Panvalvular disease — *see* Endocarditis, mitral
Papageienkrankheit 073.9
Papanicolaou smear
anus 796.70

Papanicolaou smear — *continued*
anus — *continued*
  with
    atypical squamous cells
      cannot exclude high grade squamous intraepithelial lesion (ASC-H) 796.72
      of undetermined significance (ASC-US) 796.71
    cytologic evidence of malignancy 796.76
    high grade squamous intraepithelial lesion (HGSIL) 796.74
    low grade squamous intraepithelial lesion (LGSIL) 796.73
    glandular 796.70
    specified finding NEC 796.79
    unsatisfactory cytology 796.78
cervix (screening test) V76.2
  as part of gynecological examination V72.31
  for suspected malignant neoplasm V76.2
  no disease found V71.1
  inadequate cytology sample 795.08
  nonspecific abnormal finding 795.00
    with
      atypical squamous cells
        cannot exclude high grade squamous intraepithelial lesion (ASC-H) 795.02
        of undetermined significance (ASC-US) 795.01
      cytologic evidence of malignancy 795.06
      high grade squamous intraepithelial lesion (HGSIL) 795.04
      low grade squamous intraepithelial lesion (LGSIL) 795.03
    nonspecific finding NEC 795.09
  to confirm findings of recent normal smear following initial abnormal smear V72.32
  satisfactory smear but lacking transformation zone 795.07
  unsatisfactory cervical cytology 795.08
other specified site (*see also* Screening, malignant neoplasm)
  for suspected malignant neoplasm (*see also* Screening, malignant neoplasm)
  no disease found V71.1
  nonspecific abnormal finding 796.9
vagina V76.47
  with
    atypical squamous cells
      cannot exclude high grade squamous intraepithelial lesion (ASC-H) 795.12
      of undetermined significance (ASC-US) 795.11
    cytologic evidence of malignancy 795.16
    high grade squamous intraepithelial lesion (HGSIL) 795.14
    low grade squamous intraepithelial lesion (LGSIL) 795.13
    abnormal NEC 795.19
  following hysterectomy for malignant condition V67.01
  inadequate cytology sample 795.18
  unsatisfactory cytology 795.18
Papilledema 377.00
associated with
  decreased ocular pressure 377.02
  increased intracranial pressure 377.01
  retinal disorder 377.03
choked disc 377.00
infectional 377.00
Papillitis 377.31
anus 569.49
chronic lingual 529.4
necrotizing, kidney 584.7
optic 377.31
rectum 569.49
renal, necrotizing 584.7

☑ **Additional Digit Required** — Refer to the Tabular List for Digit Selection   ▽ **Subterms under main terms may continue to next column or page**

2011 ICD-9-CM   ▶◀ **Revised Text**   ● **New Line**   ▲ **Revised Code**   **Volume 2 — 221**

Pain(s) — Papillitis

Papillitis — continued
  tongue 529.0
Papilloma (M8050/0) — see also Neoplasm, by site, benign

> Note — Except where otherwise indicated, the morphological varieties of papilloma in the list below should be coded by site as for "Neoplasm, benign."

  acuminatum (female) (male) 078.11
  bladder (urinary) (transitional cell) (M8120/1) 236.7
    benign (M8120/0) 223.3
  choroid plexus (M9390/0) 225.0
    anaplastic type (M9390/3) 191.5
    malignant (M9390/3) 191.5
  ductal (M8503/0)
  dyskeratotic (M8052/0)
  epidermoid (M8052/0)
  hyperkeratotic (M8052/0)
  intracystic (M8504/0)
  intraductal (M8503/0)
  inverted (M8053/0)
  keratotic (M8052/0)
  parakeratotic (M8052/0)
  pinta (primary) 103.0
  renal pelvis (transitional cell) (M8120/1) 236.99
    benign (M8120/0) 223.1
  Schneiderian (M8121/0)
    specified site — see Neoplasm, by site, benign
    unspecified site 212.0
  serous surface (M8461/0)
    borderline malignancy (M8461/1)
      specified site — see Neoplasm, by site, uncertain behavior
      unspecified site 236.2
    specified site — see Neoplasm, by site, benign
    unspecified site 220
  squamous (cell) (M8052/0)
  transitional (cell) (M8120/0)
    bladder (urinary) (M8120/1) 236.7
    inverted type (M8121/1) — see Neoplasm, by site, uncertain behavior
    renal pelvis (M8120/1) 236.91
    ureter (M8120/1) 236.91
  ureter (transitional cell) (M8120/1) 236.91
    benign (M8120/0) 223.2
  urothelial (M8120/1) — see Neoplasm, by site, uncertain behavior
  verrucous (M8051/0)
  villous (M8261/1) — see Neoplasm, by site, uncertain behavior
  yaws, plantar or palmar 102.1
Papillomata, multiple, of yaws 102.1
Papillomatosis (M8060/0) — see also Neoplasm, by site, benign
  confluent and reticulate 701.8
  cutaneous 701.8
  ductal, breast 610.1
  Gougerot-Carteaud (confluent reticulate) 701.8
  intraductal (diffuse) (M8505/0) — see Neoplasm, by site, benign
  subareolar duct (M8506/0) 217
Papillon-Léage and Psaume syndrome (orodigitofacial dysostosis) 759.89
Papule 709.8
  carate (primary) 103.0
  fibrous, of nose (M8724/0) 216.3
  pinta (primary) 103.0
Papulosis
  lymphomatoid 709.8
  malignant 447.8
Papyraceous fetus 779.89
  complicating pregnancy 646.0 ☑
Paracephalus 759.7
Parachute mitral valve 746.5
Paracoccidioidomycosis 116.1
  mucocutaneous-lymphangitic 116.1
  pulmonary 116.1
  visceral 116.1
Paracoccidiomycosis — see Paracoccidioidomycosis
Paracusis 388.40

Paradentosis 523.5
Paradoxical facial movements 374.43
Paraffinoma 999.9
Paraganglioma (M8680/1)
  adrenal (M8700/0) 227.0
    malignant (M8700/3) 194.0
  aortic body (M8691/1) 237.3
    malignant (M8691/3) 194.6
  carotid body (M8692/1) 237.3
    malignant (M8692/3) 194.5
  chromaffin (M8700/0) (see also Neoplasm, by site, benign)
    malignant (M8700/3) — see Neoplasm, by site, malignant
  extra-adrenal (M8693/1)
    malignant (M8693/3)
      specified site — see Neoplasm, by site, malignant
      unspecified site 194.6
    specified site — see Neoplasm, by site, uncertain behavior
    unspecified site 237.3
  glomus jugulare (M8690/1) 237.3
    malignant (M8690/3) 194.6
  jugular (M8690/1) 237.3
    malignant (M8680/3)
      specified site — see Neoplasm, by site, malignant
      unspecified site 194.6
  nonchromaffin (M8693/1)
    malignant (M8693/3)
      specified site — see Neoplasm, by site, malignant
      unspecified site 194.6
    specified site — see Neoplasm, by site, uncertain behavior
    unspecified site 237.3
  parasympathetic (M8682/1)
    specified site — see Neoplasm, by site, uncertain behavior
    unspecified site 237.3
  specified site — see Neoplasm, by site, uncertain behavior
  sympathetic (M8681/1)
    specified site — see Neoplasm, by site, uncertain behavior
    unspecified site 237.3
  unspecified site 237.3
Parageusia 781.1
  psychogenic 306.7
Paragonimiasis 121.2
Paragranuloma, Hodgkin's (M9660/3) 201.0 ☑
Parahemophilia — see also Defect, coagulation 286.3
Parakeratosis 690.8
  psoriasiformis 696.2
  variegata 696.2
Paralysis, paralytic (complete) (incomplete) 344.9
  with
    broken
      back — see Fracture, vertebra, by site, with spinal cord injury
      neck — see Fracture, vertebra, cervical, with spinal cord injury
    fracture, vertebra — see Fracture, vertebra, by site, with spinal cord injury
    syphilis 094.89
  abdomen and back muscles 355.9
  abdominal muscles 355.9
  abducens (nerve) 378.54
  abductor 355.9
    lower extremity 355.8
    upper extremity 354.9
  accessory nerve 352.4
  accommodation 367.51
    hysterical 300.11
  acoustic nerve 388.5
  agitans 332.0
    arteriosclerotic 332.0
  alternating 344.89
    oculomotor 344.89
  amyotrophic 335.20
  ankle 355.8

Paralysis, paralytic — continued
  anterior serratus 355.9
  anus (sphincter) 569.49
  apoplectic (current episode) (see also Disease, cerebrovascular, acute) 436
    late effect — see Late effect(s) (of) cerebrovascular disease
  arm 344.40
    affecting
      dominant side 344.41
      nondominant side 344.42
    both 344.2
    hysterical 300.11
    late effect — see Late effect(s) (of) cerebrovascular disease
    psychogenic 306.0
    transient 781.4
    traumatic NEC (see also Injury, nerve, upper limb) 955.9
  arteriosclerotic (current episode) 437.0
    late effect — see Late effect(s) (of) cerebrovascular disease
  ascending (spinal), acute 357.0
  associated, nuclear 344.89
  asthenic bulbar 358.00
  ataxic NEC 334.9
    general 094.1
  athetoid 333.71
  atrophic 356.9
    infantile, acute (see also Poliomyelitis, with paralysis) 045.1 ☑
    muscle NEC 355.9
    progressive 335.21
    spinal (acute) (see also Poliomyelitis, with paralysis) 045.1 ☑
  attack (see also Disease, cerebrovascular, acute) 436
  axillary 353.0
  Babinski-Nageotte's 344.89
  Bell's 351.0
    newborn 767.5
  Benedikt's 344.89
  birth (injury) 767.7
    brain 767.0
    intracranial 767.0
    spinal cord 767.4
  bladder (sphincter) 596.53
    neurogenic 596.54
      with cauda equina syndrome 344.61
    puerperal, postpartum, childbirth 665.5 ☑
    sensory 596.54
      with cauda equina 344.61
    spastic 596.54
      with cauda equina 344.61
  bowel, colon, or intestine (see also Ileus) 560.1
  brachial plexus 353.0
    due to birth injury 767.6
    newborn 767.6
  brain
    congenital — see Palsy, cerebral
    current episode 437.8
    diplegia 344.2
    hemiplegia 342.9 ☑
      late effect — see Late effect(s) (of) cerebrovascular disease
    infantile — see Palsy, cerebral
    late effect — see Late effect(s) (of) cerebrovascular disease
    monoplegia (see also Monoplegia)
      late effect — see Late effect(s) (of) cerebrovascular disease
    paraplegia 344.1
    quadriplegia — see Quadriplegia
    syphilitic, congenital 090.49
    triplegia 344.89
  bronchi 519.19
  Brown-Séquard's 344.89
  bulbar (chronic) (progressive) 335.22
    infantile (see also Poliomyelitis, bulbar) 045.0 ☑
    poliomyelitic (see also Poliomyelitis, bulbar) 045.0 ☑
    pseudo 335.23
    supranuclear 344.89

Paralysis, paralytic — continued
  bulbospinal 358.00
  cardiac (see also Failure, heart) 428.9
  cerebral
    current episode 437.8
    spastic, infantile — see Palsy, cerebral
  cerebrocerebellar 437.8
    diplegic infantile 343.0
  cervical
    plexus 353.2
    sympathetic NEC 337.09
  Céstan-Chenais 344.89
  Charcôt-Marie-Tooth type 356.1
  childhood — see Palsy, cerebral
  Clark's 343.9
  colon (see also Ileus) 560.1
  compressed air 993.3
  compression
    arm NEC 354.9
    cerebral — see Paralysis, brain
    leg NEC 355.8
    lower extremity NEC 355.8
    upper extremity NEC 354.9
  congenital (cerebral) (spastic) (spinal) — see Palsy, cerebral
  conjugate movement (of eye) 378.81
    cortical (nuclear) (supranuclear) 378.81
  convergence 378.83
  cordis (see also Failure, heart) 428.9
  cortical (see also Paralysis, brain) 437.8
  cranial or cerebral nerve (see also Disorder, nerve, cranial) 352.9
  creeping 335.21
  crossed leg 344.89
  crutch 953.4
  deglutition 784.99
    hysterical 300.11
  dementia 094.1
  descending (spinal) NEC 335.9
  diaphragm (flaccid) 519.4
    due to accidental section of phrenic nerve during procedure 998.2
  digestive organs NEC 564.89
  diplegic — see Diplegia
  divergence (nuclear) 378.85
  divers' 993.3
  Duchenne's 335.22
  due to intracranial or spinal birth injury — see Palsy, cerebral
  embolic (current episode) (see also Embolism, brain) 434.1 ☑
    late effect — see Late effect(s) (of) cerebrovascular disease
  enteric (see also Ileus) 560.1
    with hernia — see Hernia, by site, with obstruction
  Erb (-Duchenne) (birth) (newborn) 767.6
  Erb's syphilitic spastic spinal 094.89
  esophagus 530.89
  essential, infancy (see also Poliomyelitis) 045.9 ☑
  extremity
    lower — see Paralysis, leg
    spastic (hereditary) 343.3
      noncongenital or noninfantile 344.1
    transient (cause unknown) 781.4
    upper — see Paralysis, arm
  eye muscle (extrinsic) 378.55
    intrinsic 367.51
  facial (nerve) 351.0
    birth injury 767.5
    congenital 767.5
    following operation NEC 998.2
    newborn 767.5
  familial 359.3
    periodic 359.3
    spastic 334.1
  fauces 478.29
  finger NEC 354.9
  foot NEC 355.8
  gait 781.2
  gastric nerve 352.3
  gaze 378.81
  general 094.1
    ataxic 094.1
    insane 094.1

☑ **Additional Digit Required** — Refer to the Tabular List for Digit Selection   ▽ **Subterms under main terms may continue to next column or page**

222 — Volume 2 · October 2010   ▶◀ Revised Text   ● New Line   ▲ Revised Code   **2011 ICD-9-CM**

Paralysis, paralytic — continued
general — continued
  juvenile 090.40
  progressive 094.1
  tabetic 094.1
glossopharyngeal (nerve) 352.2
glottis (see also Paralysis, vocal cord) 478.30
gluteal 353.4
Gubler (-Millard) 344.89
hand 354.9
  hysterical 300.11
  psychogenic 306.0
heart (see also Failure, heart) 428.9
hemifacial, progressive 349.89
hemiplegic — see Hemiplegia
hyperkalemic periodic (familial) 359.3
hypertensive (current episode) 437.8
hypoglossal (nerve) 352.5
hypokalemic periodic 359.3
Hyrtl's sphincter (rectum) 569.49
hysterical 300.11
ileus (see also Ileus) 560.1
infantile (see also Poliomyelitis) 045.9 ☑
  atrophic acute 045.1 ☑
  bulbar 045.0 ☑
  cerebral — see Palsy, cerebral
  paralytic 045.1 ☑
  progressive acute 045.9 ☑
  spastic — see Palsy, cerebral
  spinal 045.9 ☑
infective (see also Poliomyelitis) 045.9 ☑
inferior nuclear 344.9
insane, general or progressive 094.1
internuclear 378.86
interosseous 355.9
intestine (see also Ileus) 560.1
intracranial (current episode) (see also
  Paralysis, brain) 437.8
  due to birth injury 767.0
iris 379.49
  due to diphtheria (toxin) 032.81 [379.49]
ischemic, Volkmann's (complicating trauma)
  958.6
isolated sleep, recurrent
Jackson's 344.89
jake 357.7
Jamaica ginger (jake) 357.7
juvenile general 090.40
Klumpke (-Déjérine) (birth) (newborn) 767.6
labioglossal (laryngeal) (pharyngeal) 335.22
Landry's 357.0
laryngeal nerve (recurrent) (superior) (see
  also Paralysis, vocal cord) 478.30
larynx (see also Paralysis, vocal cord) 478.30
  due to diphtheria (toxin) 032.3
late effect
  due to
    birth injury, brain or spinal (cord) —
      see Palsy, cerebral
    edema, brain or cerebral — see
      Paralysis, brain
    lesion
      late effect — see Late effect(s) (of)
        cerebrovascular disease
      spinal (cord) — see Paralysis,
        spinal
lateral 335.24
lead 984.9
  specified type of lead — see Table of
    Drugs and Chemicals
left side — see Hemiplegia
leg 344.30
  affecting
    dominant side 344.31
    nondominant side 344.32
  both (see also Paraplegia) 344.1
  crossed 344.89
  hysterical 300.11
  psychogenic 306.0
  transient or transitory 781.4
    traumatic NEC (see also Injury, nerve,
      lower limb) 956.9
levator palpebrae superioris 374.31
limb NEC 344.5
  all four — see Quadriplegia
  quadriplegia — see Quadriplegia

Paralysis, paralytic — continued
lip 528.5
Lissauer's 094.1
local 355.9
lower limb (see also Paralysis, leg)
  both (see also Paraplegia) 344.1
lung 518.89
  newborn 770.89
median nerve 354.1
medullary (tegmental) 344.89
  tegmental 344.89
mesencephalic NEC 344.89
  tegmental 344.89
middle alternating 344.89
Millard-Gubler-Foville 344.89
monoplegic — see Monoplegia
motor NEC 344.9
  cerebral — see Paralysis, brain
  spinal — see Paralysis, spinal
multiple
  cerebral — see Paralysis, brain
  spinal — see Paralysis, spinal
muscle (flaccid) 359.9
  due to nerve lesion NEC 355.9
  eye (extrinsic) 378.55
    intrinsic 367.51
    oblique 378.51
  iris sphincter 364.89
  ischemic (complicating trauma) (Volk-
    mann's) 958.6
  pseudohypertrophic 359.1
muscular (atrophic) 359.9
  progressive 335.21
musculocutaneous nerve 354.9
musculospiral 354.9
nerve (see also Disorder, nerve)
  third or oculomotor (partial) 378.51
    total 378.52
  fourth or trochlear 378.53
  sixth or abducens 378.54
  seventh or facial 351.0
    birth injury 767.5
    due to
      injection NEC 999.9
      operation NEC 997.09
    newborn 767.5
  accessory 352.4
  auditory 388.5
  birth injury 767.7
  cranial or cerebral (see also Disorder,
    nerve, cranial) 352.9
  facial 351.0
    birth injury 767.5
    newborn 767.5
  laryngeal (see also Paralysis, vocal cord)
    478.30
  newborn 767.7
  phrenic 354.8
    newborn 767.7
  radial 354.3
    birth injury 767.6
    newborn 767.6
  syphilitic 094.89
  traumatic NEC (see also Injury, nerve, by
    site) 957.9
  trigeminal 350.9
  ulnar 354.2
newborn NEC 767.0
normokalemic periodic 359.3
obstetrical, newborn 767.7
ocular 378.9
oculofacial, congenital 352.6
oculomotor (nerve) (partial) 378.51
  alternating 344.89
  external bilateral 378.55
  total 378.52
olfactory nerve 352.0
palate 528.9
palatopharyngolaryngeal 352.6
paratrigeminal 350.9
periodic (familial) (hyperkalemic) (hypokalemic) (normokalemic) (potassium sensitive) (secondary) 359.3
peripheral
  autonomic nervous system — see Neu-
    ropathy, peripheral, autonomic
  nerve NEC 355.9

Paralysis, paralytic — continued
peroneal (nerve) 355.3
pharynx 478.29
phrenic nerve 354.8
plantar nerves 355.6
pneumogastric nerve 352.3
poliomyelitis (current) (see also Poliomyelitis, with paralysis) 045.1 ☑
  bulbar 045.0 ☑
popliteal nerve 355.3
pressure (see also Neuropathy, entrapment)
  355.9
progressive 335.21
  atrophic 335.21
  bulbar 335.22
  general 094.1
  hemifacial 349.89
  infantile, acute (see also Poliomyelitis)
    045.9 ☑
  multiple 335.20
pseudobulbar 335.23
pseudohypertrophic 359.1
  muscle 359.1
psychogenic 306.0
pupil, pupillary 379.49
quadriceps 355.8
quadriplegic (see also Quadriplegia)
  344.0 ☑
radial nerve 354.3
  birth injury 767.6
rectum (sphincter) 569.49
rectus muscle (eye) 378.55
recurrent
  isolated sleep 327.43
  laryngeal nerve (see also Paralysis, vocal
    cord) 478.30
respiratory (muscle) (system) (tract) 786.09
  center NEC 344.89
    fetus or newborn 770.87
  congenital 768.9
  newborn 768.9
right side — see Hemiplegia
Saturday night 354.3
saturnine 984.9
  specified type of lead — see Table of
    Drugs and Chemicals
sciatic nerve 355.0
secondary — see Paralysis, late effect
seizure (cerebral) (current episode) (see also
  Disease, cerebrovascular, acute) 436
  late effect — see Late effect(s) (of) cere-
    brovascular disease
senile NEC 344.9
serratus magnus 355.9
shaking (see also Parkinsonism) 332.0
shock (see also Disease, cerebrovascular,
  acute) 436
  late effect — see Late effect(s) (of) cere-
    brovascular disease
shoulder 354.9
soft palate 528.9
spasmodic — see Paralysis, spastic
spastic 344.9
  cerebral infantile — see Palsy, cerebral
  congenital (cerebral) — see Palsy, cere-
    bral
  familial 334.1
  hereditary 334.1
  infantile 343.9
  noncongenital or noninfantile, cerebral
    344.9
  syphilitic 094.0
    spinal 094.89
sphincter, bladder (see also Paralysis, bladder) 596.53
spinal (cord) NEC 344.1
  accessory nerve 352.4
  acute (see also Poliomyelitis) 045.9 ☑
  ascending acute 357.0
  atrophic (acute) (see also Poliomyelitis,
    with paralysis) 045.1 ☑
    spastic, syphilitic 094.89
  congenital NEC 343.9
  hemiplegic — see Hemiplegia
  hereditary 336.8
  infantile (see also Poliomyelitis) 045.9 ☑

Paralysis, paralytic — continued
spinal — continued
  late effect NEC 344.89
  monoplegic — see Monoplegia
  nerve 355.9
  progressive 335.10
  quadriplegic — see Quadriplegia
  spastic NEC 343.9
  traumatic — see Injury, spinal, by site
sternomastoid 352.4
stomach 536.3
  diabetic 250.6 ☑ [536.3]
    due to secondary diabetes
      249.6 ☑ [536.3]
  nerve (nondiabetic) 352.3
stroke (current episode) — see Infarct, brain
  late effect — see Late effect(s) (of) cere-
    brovascular disease
subscapularis 354.8
superior nuclear NEC 334.9
supranuclear 356.8
sympathetic
  cervical NEC 337.09
  nerve NEC (see also Neuropathy, periph-
    eral, autonomic) 337.9
  nervous system — see Neuropathy, pe-
    ripheral, autonomic
syndrome 344.9
  specified NEC 344.89
syphilitic spastic spinal (Erb's) 094.89
tabetic general 094.1
thigh 355.8
throat 478.29
  diphtheritic 032.0
  muscle 478.29
thrombotic (current episode) (see also
  Thrombosis, brain) 434.0 ☑
  late effect — see Late effect(s) (of) cere-
    brovascular disease
thumb NEC 354.9
tick (-bite) 989.5
Todd's (postepileptic transitory paralysis)
  344.89
toe 355.6
tongue 529.8
transient
  arm or leg NEC 781.4
  traumatic NEC (see also Injury, nerve, by
    site) 957.9
trapezius 352.4
traumatic, transient NEC (see also Injury,
  nerve, by site) 957.9
trembling (see also Parkinsonism) 332.0
triceps brachii 354.9
trigeminal nerve 350.9
trochlear nerve 378.53
ulnar nerve 354.2
upper limb (see also Paralysis, arm)
  both (see also Diplegia) 344.2
uremic — see Uremia
uveoparotitic 135
uvula 528.9
  hysterical 300.11
  postdiphtheritic 032.0
vagus nerve 352.3
vasomotor NEC 337.9
velum palati 528.9
vesical (see also Paralysis, bladder) 596.53
vestibular nerve 388.5
visual field, psychic 368.16
vocal cord 478.30
  bilateral (partial) 478.33
    complete 478.34
  complete (bilateral) 478.34
  unilateral (partial) 478.31
    complete 478.32
Volkmann's (complicating trauma) 958.6
wasting 335.21
Weber's 344.89
wrist NEC 354.9
Paramedial orifice, urethrovesical 753.8
Paramenia 626.9
Parametritis (chronic) — see also Disease,
  pelvis, inflammatory 614.4
acute 614.3
puerperal, postpartum, childbirth 670.8 ☑

☑ Additional Digit Required — Refer to the Tabular List for Digit Selection
▽ Subterms under main terms may continue to next column or page
2011 ICD-9-CM   ▶◀ Revised Text   ● New Line   ▲ Revised Code   Volume 2 — 223

Parametrium, parametric — see condition
Paramnesia — see also Amnesia 780.93
Paramolar 520.1
  causing crowding 524.31
Paramyloidosis 277.30
Paramyoclonus multiplex 333.2
Paramyotonia 359.29
  congenita (of von Eulenburg) 359.29
Paraneoplastic syndrome — see condition
Parangi — see also Yaws 102.9
Paranoia 297.1
  alcoholic 291.5
  querulans 297.8
  senile 290.20
Paranoid
  dementia (see also Schizophrenia) 295.3 ☑
    praecox (acute) 295.3 ☑
    senile 290.20
  personality 301.0
  psychosis 297.9
    alcoholic 291.5
    climacteric 297.2
    drug-induced 292.11
    involutional 297.2
    menopausal 297.2
    protracted reactive 298.4
    psychogenic 298.4
      acute 298.3
    senile 290.20
  reaction (chronic) 297.9
    acute 298.3
  schizophrenia (acute) (see also Schizophrenia) 295.3 ☑
  state 297.9
    alcohol-induced 291.5
    climacteric 297.2
    drug-induced 292.11
    due to or associated with
      arteriosclerosis (cerebrovascular) 290.42
      presenile brain disease 290.12
      senile brain disease 290.20
    involutional 297.2
    menopausal 297.2
    senile 290.20
    simple 297.0
    specified type NEC 297.8
  tendencies 301.0
  traits 301.0
  trends 301.0
  type, psychopathic personality 301.0
Paraparesis — see also Paraplegia 344.1
Paraphasia 784.3
Paraphilia — see also Deviation, sexual 302.9
Paraphimosis (congenital) 605
  chancroidal 099.0
Paraphrenia, paraphrenic (late) 297.2
  climacteric 297.2
  dementia (see also Schizophrenia) 295.3 ☑
  involutional 297.2
  menopausal 297.2
  schizophrenia (acute) (see also Schizophrenia) 295.3 ☑
Paraplegia 344.1
  with
    broken back — see Fracture, vertebra, by site, with spinal cord injury
    fracture, vertebra — see Fracture, vertebra, by site, with spinal cord injury
  ataxic — see Degeneration, combined, spinal cord
  brain (current episode) (see also Paralysis, brain) 437.8
  cerebral (current episode) (see also Paralysis, brain) 437.8
  congenital or infantile (cerebral) (spastic) (spinal) 343.0
  cortical — see Paralysis, brain
  familial spastic 334.1
  functional (hysterical) 300.11
  hysterical 300.11
  infantile 343.0
  late effect 344.1
  Pott's (see also Tuberculosis) 015.0 ☑ [730.88]

Paraplegia — continued
  psychogenic 306.0
  spastic
    Erb's spinal 094.89
    hereditary 334.1
    not infantile or congenital 344.1
  spinal (cord)
    traumatic NEC — see Injury, spinal, by site
  syphilitic (spastic) 094.89
  traumatic NEC — see Injury, spinal, by site
Paraproteinemia 273.2
  benign (familial) 273.1
  monoclonal 273.1
  secondary to malignant or inflammatory disease 273.1
Parapsoriasis 696.2
  en plaques 696.2
  guttata 696.2
  lichenoides chronica 696.2
  retiformis 696.2
  varioliformis (acuta) 696.2
Parascarlatina 057.8
Parasitic — see also condition
  disease NEC (see also Infestation, parasitic) 136.9
    contact V01.89
    exposure to V01.89
    intestinal NEC 129
    skin NEC 134.9
  stomatitis 112.0
  sycosis 110.0
    beard 110.0
    scalp 110.0
  twin 759.4
Parasitism NEC 136.9
  intestinal NEC 129
  skin NEC 134.9
  specified — see Infestation
Parasitophobia 300.29
Parasomnia 307.47
  alcohol induced 291.82
  drug induced 292.85
  nonorganic origin 307.47
  organic 327.40
    in conditions classified elsewhere 327.44
    other 327.49
Paraspadias 752.69
Paraspasm facialis 351.8
Parathyroid gland — see condition
Parathyroiditis (autoimmune) 252.1
Parathyroprival tetany 252.1
Paratrachoma 077.0
Paratyphilitis — see also Appendicitis 541
Paratyphoid (fever) — see Fever, paratyphoid
Paratyphus — see Fever, paratyphoid
Paraurethral duct 753.8
Para-urethritis 597.89
  gonococcal (acute) 098.0
    chronic or duration of 2 months or over 098.2
Paravaccinia NEC 051.9
  milkers' node 051.1
Paravaginitis — see also Vaginitis 616.10
Parencephalitis — see also Encephalitis 323.9
  late effect — see category 326
Parergasia 298.9
Paresis — see also Paralysis 344.9
  accommodation 367.51
  bladder (spastic) (sphincter) (see also Paralysis, bladder) 596.53
    tabetic 094.0
  bowel, colon, or intestine (see also Ileus) 560.1
  brain or cerebral — see Paralysis, brain
  extrinsic muscle, eye 378.55
  general 094.1
    arrested 094.1
    brain 094.1
    cerebral 094.1
    insane 094.1
    juvenile 090.40
      remission 090.49
    progressive 094.1
    remission (sustained) 094.1
    tabetic 094.1

Paresis — see also Paralysis — continued
  heart (see also Failure, heart) 428.9
  infantile (see also Poliomyelitis) 045.9 ☑
  insane 094.1
  juvenile 090.40
  late effect — see Paralysis, late effect
  luetic (general) 094.1
  peripheral progressive 356.9
  pseudohypertrophic 359.1
  senile NEC 344.9
  stomach 536.3
    diabetic 250.6 ☑ [536.3]
      due to secondary diabetes 249.6 ☑ [536.3]
  syphilitic (general) 094.1
    congenital 090.40
  transient, limb 781.4
  vesical (sphincter) NEC 596.53
Paresthesia — see also Disturbance, sensation 782.0
  Berger's (paresthesia of lower limb) 782.0
  Bernhardt 355.1
  Magnan's 782.0
Paretic — see condition
Parinaud's
  conjunctivitis 372.02
  oculoglandular syndrome 372.02
  ophthalmoplegia 378.81
  syndrome (paralysis of conjugate upward gaze) 378.81
Parkes Weber and Dimitri syndrome (encephalocutaneous angiomatosis) 759.6
Parkinson's disease, syndrome, or tremor — see Parkinsonism
Parkinsonism (arteriosclerotic) (idiopathic) (primary) 332.0
  associated with orthostatic hypotension (idiopathic) (symptomatic) 333.0
  due to drugs 332.1
  neuroleptic-induced 332.1
  secondary 332.1
  syphilitic 094.82
Parodontitis 523.40
Parodontosis 523.5
Paronychia (with lymphangitis) 681.9
  candidal (chronic) 112.3
  chronic 681.9
    candidal 112.3
    finger 681.02
    toe 681.11
  finger 681.02
  toe 681.11
  tuberculous (primary) (see also Tuberculosis) 017.0 ☑
Parorexia NEC 307.52
  hysterical 300.11
Parosmia 781.1
  psychogenic 306.7
Parotid gland — see condition
Parotiditis — see also Parotitis 527.2
  epidemic 072.9
  infectious 072.9
Parotitis 527.2
  allergic 527.2
  chronic 527.2
  epidemic (see also Mumps) 072.9
  infectious (see also Mumps) 072.9
  noninfectious 527.2
  nonspecific toxic 527.2
  not mumps 527.2
  postoperative 527.2
  purulent 527.2
  septic 527.2
  suppurative (acute) 527.2
  surgical 527.2
  toxic 527.2
Paroxysmal — see also condition
  dyspnea (nocturnal) 786.09
Parrot's disease (syphilitic osteochondritis) 090.0
Parrot fever 073.9
Parry's disease or syndrome (exophthalmic goiter) 242.0 ☑
Parry-Romberg syndrome 349.89
Parsonage-Aldren-Turner syndrome 353.5
Parsonage-Turner syndrome 353.5

Parson's disease (exophthalmic goiter) 242.0 ☑
Pars planitis 363.21
Particolored infant 757.39
Parturition — see Delivery
Parvovirus 079.83
  B19 079.83
  human 079.83
Passage
  false, urethra 599.4
  meconium noted during delivery 763.84
  of sounds or bougies (see also Attention to artificial opening) V55.9
Passive — see condition
Pasteurella septica 027.2
Pasteurellosis — see also Infection, Pasteurella 027.2
PAT (paroxysmal atrial tachycardia) 427.0
Patau's syndrome (trisomy D1) 758.1
Patch
  herald 696.3
Patches
  mucous (syphilitic) 091.3
    congenital 090.0
  smokers' (mouth) 528.6
Patellar — see condition
Patellofemoral syndrome 719.46
Patent — see also Imperfect closure
  atrioventricular ostium 745.69
  canal of Nuck 752.41
  cervix 622.5
    complicating pregnancy 654.5 ☑
      affecting fetus or newborn 761.0
  ductus arteriosus or Botalli 747.0
  Eustachian
    tube 381.7
    valve 746.89
  foramen
    Botalli 745.5
    ovale 745.5
  interauricular septum 745.5
  interventricular septum 745.4
  omphalomesenteric duct 751.0
  os (uteri) — see Patent, cervix
  ostium secundum 745.5
  urachus 753.7
  vitelline duct 751.0
Paternity testing V70.4
Paterson-Kelly syndrome or web (sideropenic dysphagia) 280.8
Paterson (-Brown) (-Kelly) syndrome (sideropenic dysphagia) 280.8
Paterson's syndrome (sideropenic dysphagia) 280.8
Pathologic, pathological — see also condition
  asphyxia 799.01
  drunkenness 291.4
  emotionality 301.3
  fracture — see Fracture, pathologic
  liar 301.7
  personality 301.9
  resorption, tooth 521.40
    external 521.42
    internal 521.41
    specified NEC 521.49
  sexuality (see also Deviation, sexual) 302.9
Pathology (of) — see also Disease
  periradicular, associated with previous endodontic treatment 526.69
Patterned motor discharge, idiopathic — see also Epilepsy 345.5 ☑
Patulous — see also Patent
  anus 569.49
  Eustachian tube 381.7
Pause, sinoatrial 427.81
Pavy's disease 593.6
Paxton's disease (white piedra) 111.2
Payr's disease or syndrome (splenic flexure syndrome) 569.89
PBA (pseudobulbar affect) 310.8
Pearls
  Elschnig 366.51
  enamel 520.2
Pearl-workers' disease (chronic osteomyelitis) — see also Osteomyelitis 730.1 ☑

☑ Additional Digit Required — Refer to the Tabular List for Digit Selection   ▽ Subterms under main terms may continue to next column or page

224 — Volume 2   ▶◀ Revised Text   ● New Line   ▲ Revised Code   2011 ICD-9-CM

Pectenitis 569.49
Pectenosis 569.49
Pectoral — *see* condition
Pectus
  carinatum (congenital) 754.82
    acquired 738.3
    rachitic (*see also* Rickets) 268.0
  excavatum (congenital) 754.81
    acquired 738.3
    rachitic (*see also* Rickets) 268.0
  recurvatum (congenital) 754.81
    acquired 738.3
Pedatrophia 261
Pederosis 302.2
Pediculosis (infestation) 132.9
  capitis (head louse) (any site) 132.0
  corporis (body louse) (any site) 132.1
  eyelid 132.0 *[373.6]*
  mixed (classifiable to more than one category in 132.0–132.2) 132.3
  pubis (pubic louse) (any site) 132.2
  vestimenti 132.1
  vulvae 132.2
Pediculus (infestation) — *see* Pediculosis
Pedophilia 302.2
Peg-shaped teeth 520.2
Pelade 704.01
Pel's crisis 094.0
Pel-Ebstein disease — *see* Disease, Hodgkin's
Pelger-Huët anomaly or syndrome (hereditary hyposegmentation) 288.2
Peliosis (rheumatica) 287.0
Pelizaeus-Merzbacher
  disease 330.0
  sclerosis, diffuse cerebral 330.0
Pellagra (alcoholic or with alcoholism) 265.2
  with polyneuropathy 265.2 *[357.4]*
Pellagra-cerebellar-ataxia-renal aminoaciduria syndrome 270.0
Pellegrini's disease (calcification, knee joint) 726.62
Pellegrini (-Stieda) disease or syndrome (calcification, knee joint) 726.62
Pellizzi's syndrome (pineal) 259.8
Pelvic — *see also* condition
  congestion-fibrosis syndrome 625.5
  kidney 753.3
Pelvioectasis 591
Pelviolithiasis 592.0
Pelviperitonitis
  female (*see also* Peritonitis, pelvic, female) 614.5
  male (*see also* Peritonitis) 567.21
Pelvis, pelvic — *see also* condition or type
  infantile 738.6
  Nägele's 738.6
  obliquity 738.6
  Robert's 755.69
Pemphigoid 694.5
  benign, mucous membrane 694.60
    with ocular involvement 694.61
  bullous 694.5
  cicatricial 694.60
    with ocular involvement 694.61
  juvenile 694.2
Pemphigus 694.4
  benign 694.5
    chronic familial 757.39
  Brazilian 694.4
  circinatus 694.0
  congenital, traumatic 757.39
  conjunctiva 694.61
  contagiosus 684
  erythematodes 694.4
  erythematosus 694.4
  foliaceus 694.4
  frambesiodes 694.4
  gangrenous (*see also* Gangrene) 785.4
  malignant 694.4
  neonatorum, newborn 684
  ocular 694.61
  papillaris 694.4
  seborrheic 694.4
  South American 694.4
  syphilitic (congenital) 090.0
  vegetans 694.4

Pemphigus — *continued*
  vulgaris 694.4
  wildfire 694.4
Pendred's syndrome (familial goiter with deaf-mutism) 243
Pendulous
  abdomen 701.9
    in pregnancy or childbirth 654.4 ☑
      affecting fetus or newborn 763.89
  breast 611.89
Penetrating wound — *see also* Wound, open, by site
  with internal injury — *see* Injury, internal, by site, with open wound
  eyeball 871.7
    with foreign body (nonmagnetic) 871.6
      magnetic 871.5
    ocular (*see also* Penetrating wound, eyeball) 871.7
    adnexa 870.3
      with foreign body 870.4
    orbit 870.3
      with foreign body 870.4
Penetration, pregnant uterus by instrument
  with
    abortion — *see* Abortion, by type, with damage to pelvic organs
    ectopic pregnancy (*see also* categories 633.0–633.9) 639.2
    molar pregnancy (*see also* categories 630–632) 639.2
  complication of delivery 665.1 ☑
    affecting fetus or newborn 763.89
  following
    abortion 639.2
    ectopic or molar pregnancy 639.2
Penfield's syndrome — *see also* Epilepsy 345.5 ☑
Penicilliosis of lung 117.3
Penis — *see* condition
Penitis 607.2
Pentalogy (of Fallot) 745.2
Penta X syndrome 758.81
Pentosuria (benign) (essential) 271.8
Peptic acid disease 536.8
Peregrinating patient V65.2
Perforated — *see* Perforation
Perforation, perforative (nontraumatic)
  antrum (*see also* Sinusitis, maxillary) 473.0
  appendix 540.0
    with peritoneal abscess 540.1
  atrial septum, multiple 745.5
  attic, ear 384.22
    healed 384.81
  bile duct, except cystic (*see also* Disease, biliary) 576.3
    cystic 575.4
  bladder (urinary) 596.6
    with
      abortion — *see* Abortion, by type, with damage to pelvic organs
      ectopic pregnancy (*see also* categories 633.0–633.9) 639.2
      molar pregnancy (*see also* categories 630–632) 639.2
    following
      abortion 639.2
      ectopic or molar pregnancy 639.2
    obstetrical trauma 665.5 ☑
  bowel 569.83
    with
      abortion — *see* Abortion, by type, with damage to pelvic organs
      ectopic pregnancy (*see also* categories 633.0–633.9) 639.2
      molar pregnancy (*see also* categories 630–632) 639.2
    fetus or newborn 777.6
    following
      abortion 639.2
      ectopic or molar pregnancy 639.2
    obstetrical trauma 665.5 ☑
  broad ligament
    with
      abortion — *see* Abortion, by type, with damage to pelvic organs

Perforation, perforative — *continued*
  broad ligament — *continued*
    with — *continued*
      ectopic pregnancy (*see also* categories 633.0–633.9) 639.2
      molar pregnancy (*see also* categories 630–632) 639.2
    following
      abortion 639.2
      ectopic or molar pregnancy 639.2
    obstetrical trauma 665.6 ☑
  by
    device, implant, or graft — *see* Complications, mechanical
    foreign body left accidentally in operation wound 998.4
    instrument (any) during a procedure, accidental 998.2
  cecum 540.0
    with peritoneal abscess 540.1
  cervix (uteri) (*see also* Injury, internal, cervix)
    with
      abortion — *see* Abortion, by type, with damage to pelvic organs
      ectopic pregnancy (*see also* categories 633.0–633.9) 639.2
      molar pregnancy (*see also* categories 630–632) 639.2
    following
      abortion 639.2
      ectopic or molar pregnancy 639.2
    obstetrical trauma 665.3 ☑
  colon 569.83
  common duct (bile) 576.3
  cornea (*see also* Ulcer, cornea) 370.00
    due to ulceration 370.06
  cystic duct 575.4
  diverticulum (*see also* Diverticula) 562.10
    small intestine 562.00
  duodenum, duodenal (ulcer) — *see* Ulcer, duodenum, with perforation
  ear drum — *see* Perforation, tympanum
  enteritis — *see* Enteritis
  esophagus 530.4
  ethmoidal sinus (*see also* Sinusitis, ethmoidal) 473.2
  foreign body (external site) (*see also* Wound, open, by site, complicated)
    internal site, by ingested object — *see* Foreign body
  frontal sinus (*see also* Sinusitis, frontal) 473.1
  gallbladder or duct (*see also* Disease, gallbladder) 575.4
  gastric (ulcer) — *see* Ulcer, stomach, with perforation
  heart valve — *see* Endocarditis
  ileum (*see also* Perforation, intestine) 569.83
  instrumental
    external — *see* Wound, open, by site
    pregnant uterus, complicating delivery 665.9 ☑
    surgical (accidental) (blood vessel) (nerve) (organ) 998.2
  intestine 569.83
    with
      abortion — *see* Abortion, by type, with damage to pelvic organs
      ectopic pregnancy (*see also* categories 633.0–633.9) 639.2
      molar pregnancy (*see also* categories 630–632) 639.2
    fetus or newborn 777.6
    obstetrical trauma 665.5 ☑
    ulcerative NEC 569.83
  jejunum, jejunal 569.83
    ulcer — *see* Ulcer, gastrojejunal, with perforation
  mastoid (antrum) (cell) 383.89
  maxillary sinus (*see also* Sinusitis, maxillary) 473.0
  membrana tympani — *see* Perforation, tympanum
  nasal
    septum 478.19
      congenital 748.1
      syphilitic 095.8

Perforation, perforative — *continued*
  nasal — *continued*
    sinus (*see also* Sinusitis) 473.9
      congenital 748.1
  palate (hard) 526.89
    soft 528.9
      syphilitic 095.8
    syphilitic 095.8
  palatine vault 526.89
    syphilitic 095.8
    congenital 090.5
  pelvic
    floor
      with
        abortion — *see* Abortion, by type, with damage to pelvic organs
        ectopic pregnancy (*see also* categories 633.0–633.9) 639.2
        molar pregnancy (*see also* categories 630–632) 639.2
      obstetrical trauma 664.1 ☑
    organ
      with
        abortion — *see* Abortion, by type, with damage to pelvic organs
        ectopic pregnancy (*see also* categories 633.0–633.9) 639.2
        molar pregnancy (*see also* categories 630–632) 639.2
      following
        abortion 639.2
        ectopic or molar pregnancy 639.2
      obstetrical trauma 665.5 ☑
  perineum — *see* Laceration, perineum
  periurethral tissue
    with
      abortion — *see* Abortion, by type, with damage to pelvic organs
      ectopic pregnancy (*see also* categories 630–632) 639.2
      molar pregnancy (*see also* categories 630–632) 639.2
  pharynx 478.29
  pylorus, pyloric (ulcer) — *see* Ulcer, stomach, with perforation
  rectum 569.49
  root canal space 526.61
  sigmoid 569.83
  sinus (accessory) (chronic) (nasal) (*see also* Sinusitis) 473.9
  sphenoidal sinus (*see also* Sinusitis, sphenoidal) 473.3
  stomach (due to ulcer) — *see* Ulcer, stomach, with perforation
  surgical (accidental) (by instrument) (blood vessel) (nerve) (organ) 998.2
  traumatic
    external — *see* Wound, open, by site
    eye (*see also* Penetrating wound, ocular) 871.7
    internal organ — *see* Injury, internal, by site
  tympanum (membrane) (persistent posttraumatic) (postinflammatory) 384.20
    with
      otitis media — *see* Otitis media
    attic 384.22
    central 384.21
    healed 384.81
    marginal NEC 384.23
    multiple 384.24
    pars flaccida 384.22
    total 384.25
    traumatic — *see* Wound, open, ear, drum
  typhoid, gastrointestinal 002.0
  ulcer — *see* Ulcer, by site, with perforation
  ureter 593.89
  urethra
    with
      abortion — *see* Abortion, by type, with damage to pelvic organs
      ectopic pregnancy (*see also* categories 633.0–633.9) 639.2

☑ Additional Digit Required — Refer to the Tabular List for Digit Selection   ▽ Subterms under main terms may continue to next column or page

2011 ICD-9-CM   ▶◀ Revised Text   ● New Line   ▲ Revised Code   Volume 2 — 225

☑ **Additional Digit Required** — Refer to the Tabular List for Digit Selection   ▽ **Subterms under main terms may continue to next column or page**

226 — Volume 2   ▶◀ Revised Text   ● New Line   ▲ Revised Code   2011 ICD-9-CM

Peritonitis — *continued*
  fibrinous 567.29
  fibrocaseous (*see also* Tuberculosis) 014.0 ☑
  fibropurulent 567.29
  general, generalized (acute) 567.21
  gonococcal 098.86
  in infective disease NEC 136.9 *[567.0]*
  meconium (newborn) 777.6
  pancreatic 577.8
  paroxysmal, benign 277.31
  pelvic
    female (acute) 614.5
      chronic NEC 614.7
        with adhesions 614.6
      puerperal, postpartum, childbirth 670.8 ☑
    male (acute) 567.21
  periodic (familial) 277.31
  phlegmonous 567.29
  pneumococcal 567.1
  postabortal 639.0
  proliferative, chronic 567.89
  puerperal, postpartum, childbirth 670.8 ☑
  purulent 567.29
  septic 567.29
  spontaneous bacterial 567.23
  staphylococcal 567.29
  streptococcal 567.29
  subdiaphragmatic 567.29
  subphrenic 567.29
  suppurative 567.29
  syphilitic 095.2
    congenital 090.0 *[567.0]*
  talc 998.7
  tuberculous (*see also* Tuberculosis) 014.0 ☑
  urine 567.89
Peritonsillar — *see* condition
Peritonsillitis 475
Perityphlitis — *see also* Appendicitis 541
Periureteritis 593.89
Periurethral — *see* condition
Periurethritis (gangrenous) 597.89
Periuterine — *see* condition
Perivaginitis — *see also* Vaginitis 616.10
Perivasculitis, retinal 362.18
Perivasitis (chronic) 608.4
Periventricular leukomalacia 779.7
Perivesiculitis (seminal) — *see also* Vesiculitis 608.0
Perlèche 686.8
  due to
    moniliasis 112.0
    riboflavin deficiency 266.0
Pernicious — *see* condition
Pernio, perniosis 991.5
Persecution
  delusion 297.9
  social V62.4
Perseveration (tonic) 784.69
Persistence, persistent (congenital) 759.89
  anal membrane 751.2
  arteria stapedia 744.04
  atrioventricular canal 745.69
  bloody ejaculate 792.2
  branchial cleft 744.41
  bulbus cordis in left ventricle 745.8
  canal of Cloquet 743.51
  capsule (opaque) 743.51
  cilioretinal artery or vein 743.51
  cloaca 751.5
  communication — *see* Fistula, congenital
  convolutions
    aortic arch 747.21
    fallopian tube 752.19
    oviduct 752.19
    uterine tube 752.19
  double aortic arch 747.21
  ductus
    arteriosus 747.0
    Botalli 747.0
  fetal
    circulation 747.83
    form of cervix (uteri) 752.49
    hemoglobin (hereditary) ("Swiss variety") 282.7
    pulmonary hypertension 747.83

Persistence, persistent — *continued*
  foramen
    Botalli 745.5
    ovale 745.5
  Gartner's duct 752.41
  hemoglobin, fetal (hereditary) (HPFH) 282.7
  hyaloid
    artery (generally incomplete) 743.51
    system 743.51
  hymen (tag)
    in pregnancy or childbirth 654.8 ☑
      causing obstructed labor 660.2 ☑
  lanugo 757.4
  left
    posterior cardinal vein 747.49
    root with right arch of aorta 747.21
    superior vena cava 747.49
  Meckel's diverticulum 751.0
  mesonephric duct 752.89
    fallopian tube 752.11
  mucosal disease (middle ear) (with posterior or superior marginal perforation of ear drum) 382.2
  nail(s), anomalous 757.5
  occiput, anterior or posterior 660.3 ☑
    fetus or newborn 763.1
  omphalomesenteric duct 751.0
  organ or site NEC — *see* Anomaly, specified type NEC
  ostium
    atrioventriculare commune 745.69
    primum 745.61
    secundum 745.5
  ovarian rests in fallopian tube 752.19
  pancreatic tissue in intestinal tract 751.5
  primary (deciduous)
    teeth 520.6
    vitreous hyperplasia 743.51
  pulmonary hypertension 747.83
  pupillary membrane 743.46
    iris 743.46
  Rhesus (Rh) titer ►◄(*see also* Complications, transfusion)◄ 999.70   ▲
  right aortic arch 747.21
  sinus
    urogenitalis 752.89
    venosus with imperfect incorporation in right auricle 747.49
  thymus (gland) 254.8
    hyperplasia 254.0
  thyroglossal duct 759.2
  thyrolingual duct 759.2
  truncus arteriosus or communis 745.0
  tunica vasculosa lentis 743.39
  umbilical sinus 753.7
  urachus 753.7
  vegetative state 780.03
  vitelline duct 751.0
  wolffian duct 752.89
Person (with)
  admitted for clinical research, as participant or control subject V70.7
  affected by
    family member
      currently on deployment (military) V61.01
      returned from deployment (military) (current or past conflict) V61.02
  awaiting admission to adequate facility elsewhere V63.2
  undergoing social agency investigation V63.8
  concern (normal) about sick person in family V61.49
  consulting on behalf of another V65.19
    pediatric
      pre-adoption visit for adoptive parents V65.11
      pre-birth visit for expectant parents V65.11
  currently deployed in theater or in support of military war, peacekeeping and humanitarian operations V62.21

Person — *continued*
  feared
    complaint in whom no diagnosis was made V65.5
    condition not demonstrated V65.5
  feigning illness V65.2
  healthy, accompanying sick person V65.0
  history of military war, peacekeeping and humanitarian deployment (current or past conflict) V62.22
  living (in)
    without
      adequate
        financial resources V60.2
        housing (heating) (space) V60.1
        housing (permanent) (temporary) V60.0
        material resources V60.2
        person able to render necessary care V60.4
        shelter V60.0
    alone V60.3
    boarding school V60.6
    residence remote from hospital or medical care facility V63.0
    residential institution V60.6
  medical services in home not available V63.1
  on waiting list V63.2
    undergoing social agency investigation V63.8
  sick or handicapped in family V61.49
  "worried well" V65.5
Personality
  affective 301.10
  aggressive 301.3
  amoral 301.7
  anancastic, anankastic 301.4
  antisocial 301.7
  asocial 301.7
  asthenic 301.6
  avoidant 301.82
  borderline 301.83
  change 310.1
  compulsive 301.4
  cycloid 301.13
  cyclothymic 301.13
  dependent 301.6
  depressive (chronic) 301.12
  disorder, disturbance NEC 301.9
    with
      antisocial disturbance 301.7
      pattern disturbance NEC 301.9
      sociopathic disturbance 301.7
      trait disturbance 301.9
  dual 300.14
  dyssocial 301.7
  eccentric 301.89
    "haltlose" type 301.89
  emotionally unstable 301.59
  epileptoid 301.3
  explosive 301.3
  fanatic 301.0
  histrionic 301.50
  hyperthymic 301.11
  hypomanic 301.11
  hypothymic 301.12
  hysterical 301.50
  immature 301.89
  inadequate 301.6
  labile 301.59
  masochistic 301.89
  morally defective 301.7
  multiple 300.14
  narcissistic 301.81
  obsessional 301.4
  obsessive-compulsive 301.4
  overconscientious 301.4
  paranoid 301.0
  passive (-dependent) 301.6
  passive-aggressive 301.84
  pathologic NEC 301.9
  pattern defect or disturbance 301.9
  pseudosocial 301.7
  psychoinfantile 301.59
  psychoneurotic NEC 301.89
  psychopathic 301.9

Personality — *continued*
  psychopathic — *continued*
    with
      amoral trend 301.7
      antisocial trend 301.7
      asocial trend 301.7
      pathologic sexuality (*see also* Deviation, sexual) 302.9
    mixed types 301.9
    schizoid 301.20
    type A 301.4
    unstable (emotional) 301.59
Perthes' disease (capital femoral osteochondrosis) 732.1
Pertussis — *see also* Whooping cough 033.9
  vaccination, prophylactic (against) V03.6
Peruvian wart 088.0
Perversion, perverted
  appetite 307.52
    hysterical 300.11
  function
    pineal gland 259.8
    pituitary gland 253.9
      anterior lobe
        deficient 253.2
        excessive 253.1
      posterior lobe 253.6
    placenta — *see* Placenta, abnormal
  sense of smell or taste 781.1
    psychogenic 306.7
  sexual (*see also* Deviation, sexual) 302.9
Pervious, congenital — *see also* Imperfect, closure
  ductus arteriosus 747.0
Pes (congenital) — *see also* Talipes 754.70
  abductus (congenital) 754.60
    acquired 736.79
  acquired NEC 736.79
    planus 734
  adductus (congenital) 754.79
    acquired 736.79
  cavus 754.71
    acquired 736.73
  planovalgus (congenital) 754.69
    acquired 736.79
  planus (acquired) (any degree) 734
    congenital 754.61
    rachitic 268.1
  valgus (congenital) 754.61
    acquired 736.79
  varus (congenital) 754.50
    acquired 736.79
Pest — *see also* Plague 020.9
Pestis — *see also* Plague 020.9
  bubonica 020.0
  fulminans 020.0
  minor 020.8
  pneumonica — *see* Plague, pneumonic
Petechial
  fever 036.0
  typhus 081.9
Petechia, petechiae 782.7
  fetus or newborn 772.6
Petges-Cléjat or Petges-Clégat syndrome (poikilodermatomyositis) 710.3
Petit's
  disease (*see also* Hernia, lumbar) 553.8
Petit mal (idiopathic) — *see also* Epilepsy 345.0 ☑
  status 345.2
Petrellidosis 117.6
Petrositis 383.20
  acute 383.21
  chronic 383.22
Peutz-Jeghers disease or syndrome 759.6
Peyronie's disease 607.85
Pfeiffer's disease 075
Phacentocele 379.32
  traumatic 921.3
Phacoanaphylaxis 360.19
Phacocele (old) 379.32
  traumatic 921.3
Phaehyphomycosis 117.8
Phagedena (dry) (moist) — *see also* Gangrene 785.4
  arteriosclerotic 440.24

☑ **Additional Digit Required** — Refer to the Tabular List for Digit Selection   ▽ **Subterms under main terms may continue to next column or page**

2011 ICD-9-CM   ►◄ Revised Text   ● New Line   ▲ Revised Code   October 2010 • Volume 2 — 227

Phagedena — *see also* Gangrene — *continued*
  geometric 686.09
  penis 607.89
  senile 440.2 ☑ *[785.4]*
  sloughing 785.4
  tropical (*see also* Ulcer, skin) 707.9
  vulva 616.50
Phagedenic — *see also* condition
  abscess (*see also* Abscess)
    chancroid 099.0
  bubo NEC 099.8
  chancre 099.0
  ulcer (tropical) (*see also* Ulcer, skin) 707.9
Phagomania 307.52
Phakoma 362.89
Phantom limb (syndrome) 353.6
Pharyngeal — *see also* condition
  arch remnant 744.41
  pouch syndrome 279.11
Pharyngitis (acute) (catarrhal) (gangrenous) (infective) (malignant) (membranous) (phlegmonous) (pneumococcal) (pseudomembranous) (simple) (staphylococcal) (subacute) (suppurative) (ulcerative) (viral) 462
  with influenza, flu, or grippe ▶(*see also* Influenza)◀ 487.1
  aphthous 074.0
  atrophic 472.1
  chlamydial 099.51
  chronic 472.1
  Coxsackie virus 074.0
  diphtheritic (membranous) 032.0
  follicular 472.1
  fusospirochetal 101
  gonococcal 098.6
  granular (chronic) 472.1
  herpetic 054.79
  hypertrophic 472.1
  infectional, chronic 472.1
  influenzal ▶(*see also* Influenza)◀ 487.1
  lymphonodular, acute 074.8
  septic 034.0
  streptococcal 034.0
  tuberculous (*see also* Tuberculosis) 012.8 ☑
  vesicular 074.0
Pharyngoconjunctival fever 077.2
Pharyngoconjunctivitis, viral 077.2
Pharyngolaryngitis (acute) 465.0
  chronic 478.9
  septic 034.0
Pharyngoplegia 478.29
Pharyngotonsillitis 465.8
  tuberculous 012.8 ☑
Pharyngotracheitis (acute) 465.8
  chronic 478.9
Pharynx, pharyngeal — *see* condition
Phase of life problem NEC V62.89
Phenomenon
  Arthus' 995.21
  flashback (drug) 292.89
  jaw-winking 742.8
  Jod-Basedow 242.8 ☑
  L. E. cell 710.0
  lupus erythematosus cell 710.0
  Pelger-Huët (hereditary hyposegmentation) 288.2
  Raynaud's (paroxysmal digital cyanosis) (secondary) 443.0
  Reilly's (*see also* Neuropathy, peripheral, autonomic) 337.9
  vasomotor 780.2
  vasospastic 443.9
  vasovagal 780.2
  Wenckebach's, heart block (second degree) 426.13
Phenylketonuria (PKU) 270.1
Phenylpyruvicaciduria 270.1
Pheochromoblastoma (M8700/3)
  specified site — *see* Neoplasm, by site, malignant
  unspecified site 194.0

Pheochromocytoma (M8700/0)
  malignant (M8700/3)
    specified site — *see* Neoplasm, by site, malignant
    unspecified site 194.0
  specified site — *see* Neoplasm, by site, benign
  unspecified site 227.0
Phimosis (congenital) 605
  chancroidal 099.0
  due to infection 605
Phlebectasia — *see also* Varicose, vein 454.9
  congenital NEC 747.60
  esophagus (*see also* Varix, esophagus) 456.1
    with hemorrhage (*see also* Varix, esophagus, bleeding) 456.0
Phlebitis (infective) (pyemic) (septic) (suppurative) 451.9
  antecubital vein 451.82
  arm NEC 451.84
    axillary vein 451.89
    basilic vein 451.82
    deep 451.83
    superficial 451.82
  axillary vein 451.89
  basilic vein 451.82
  blue 451.9
  brachial vein 451.83
  breast, superficial 451.89
  cavernous (venous) sinus — *see* Phlebitis, intracranial sinus
  cephalic vein 451.82
  cerebral (venous) sinus — *see* Phlebitis, intracranial sinus
  chest wall, superficial 451.89
  complicating pregnancy or puerperium 671.2 ☑
    affecting fetus or newborn 760.3
  cranial (venous) sinus — *see* Phlebitis, intracranial sinus
  deep (vessels) 451.19
    femoral vein 451.11
    specified vessel NEC 451.19
  due to implanted device — *see* Complications, due to (presence of) any device, implant, or graft classified to 996.0–996.5 NEC
  during or resulting from a procedure 997.2
  femoral vein (deep) (superficial) 451.11
  femoropopliteal 451.19
  following infusion, perfusion, or transfusion 999.2
  gouty 274.89 *[451.9]*
  hepatic veins 451.89
  iliac vein 451.81
  iliofemoral 451.11
  intracranial sinus (any) (venous) 325
    late effect — *see* category 326
    nonpyogenic 437.6
      in pregnancy or puerperium 671.5 ☑
  jugular vein 451.89
  lateral (venous) sinus — *see* Phlebitis, intracranial sinus
  leg 451.2
    deep (vessels) 451.19
      femoral vein 451.11
      specified vessel NEC 451.19
    superficial (vessels) 451.0
      femoral vein 451.11
  longitudinal sinus — *see* Phlebitis, intracranial sinus
  lower extremity 451.2
    deep (vessels) 451.19
      femoral vein 451.11
      specified vessel NEC 451.19
    migrans, migrating (superficial) 453.1
    superficial (vessels) 451.0
      femoral vein 451.11
  pelvic
    with
      abortion — *see* Abortion, by type, with sepsis
      ectopic pregnancy (*see also* categories 633.0–633.9) 639.0
      molar pregnancy (*see also* categories 630–632) 639.0

Phlebitis — *continued*
  pelvic — *continued*
    following
      abortion 639.0
      ectopic or molar pregnancy 639.0
    puerperal, postpartum 671.4 ☑
  popliteal vein 451.19
  portal (vein) 572.1
  postoperative 997.2
  pregnancy 671.2 ☑
    deep 671.3 ☑
    specified type NEC 671.5 ☑
    superficial 671.2 ☑
  puerperal, postpartum, childbirth 671.2 ☑
    deep 671.4 ☑
    lower extremities 671.2 ☑
    pelvis 671.4 ☑
    specified site NEC 671.5 ☑
    superficial 671.2 ☑
  radial vein 451.83
  retina 362.18
  saphenous (great) (long) 451.0
    accessory or small 451.0
  sinus (meninges) — *see* Phlebitis, intracranial sinus
  specified site NEC 451.89
  subclavian vein 451.89
  syphilitic 093.89
  tibial vein 451.19
  ulcer, ulcerative 451.9
    leg 451.2
      deep (vessels) 451.19
        femoral vein 451.11
        specified vessel NEC 451.19
      superficial (vessels) 451.0
        femoral vein 451.11
    lower extremity 451.2
      deep (vessels) 451.19
        femoral vein 451.11
        specified vessel NEC 451.19
      superficial (vessels) 451.0
  ulnar vein 451.83
  umbilicus 451.89
  upper extremity (*see also* Phlebitis, arm)
    deep (veins) 451.83
      brachial vein 451.83
      radial vein 451.83
      ulnar vein 451.83
    superficial (veins) 451.82
      antecubital vein 451.82
      basilica vein 451.82
      cephalic vein 451.82
  uterus (septic) (*see also* Endometritis) 615.9
  varicose (leg) (lower extremity) (*see also* Varicose, vein) 454.1
Phlebofibrosis 459.89
Phleboliths 459.89
Phlebosclerosis 459.89
Phlebothrombosis — *see* Thrombosis
Phlebotomus fever 066.0
Phlegmasia
  alba dolens (deep vessels) 451.19
    complicating pregnancy 671.3 ☑
    nonpuerperal 451.19
    puerperal, postpartum, childbirth 671.4 ☑
  cerulea dolens 451.19
Phlegm, choked on 933.1
Phlegmon — *see also* Abscess 682.9
  erysipelatous (*see also* Erysipelas) 035
  iliac 682.2
    fossa 540.1
  throat 478.29
Phlegmonous — *see* condition
Phlyctenulosis (allergic) (keratoconjunctivitis) (nontuberculous) 370.31
  cornea 370.31
    with ulcer (*see also* Ulcer, cornea) 370.00
  tuberculous (*see also* Tuberculosis) 017.3 ☑ *[370.31]*
Phobia, phobic (reaction) 300.20
  animal 300.29
  isolated NEC 300.29
  obsessional 300.3
  simple NEC 300.29
  social 300.23

Phobia, phobic — *continued*
  specified NEC 300.29
  state 300.20
Phocas' disease 610.1
Phocomelia 755.4
  lower limb 755.32
    complete 755.33
    distal 755.35
    proximal 755.34
  upper limb 755.22
    complete 755.23
    distal 755.25
    proximal 755.24
Phoria — *see also* Heterophoria 378.40
Phosphate-losing tubular disorder 588.0
Phosphatemia 275.3
Phosphaturia 275.3
Photoallergic response 692.72
Photocoproporphyria 277.1
Photodermatitis (sun) 692.72
  light other than sun 692.82
Photokeratitis 370.24
Photo-ophthalmia 370.24
Photophobia 368.13
Photopsia 368.15
Photoretinitis 363.31
Photoretinopathy 363.31
Photosensitiveness (sun) 692.72
  light other than sun 692.82
Photosensitization (skin) (sun) 692.72
  light other than sun 692.82
Phototoxic response 692.72
Phrenitis 323.9
Phrynoderma 264.8
Phthiriasis (pubis) (any site) 132.2
  with any infestation classifiable to 132.0, 132.1, 132.3
Phthirus infestation — *see* Phthiriasis
Phthisis — *see also* Tuberculosis 011.9 ☑
  bulbi (infectional) 360.41
  colliers' 011.4 ☑
  cornea 371.05
  eyeball (due to infection) 360.41
  millstone makers' 011.4 ☑
  miners' 011.4 ☑
  potters' 011.4 ☑
  sandblasters' 011.4 ☑
  stonemasons' 011.4 ☑
Phycomycosis 117.7
Physalopteriasis 127.7
Physical therapy NEC V57.1
  breathing exercises V57.0
Physiological cup, optic papilla
  borderline, glaucoma suspect 365.00
  enlarged 377.14
  glaucomatous 377.14
Phytobezoar 938
  intestine 936
  stomach 935.2
Pian — *see also* Yaws 102.9
Pianoma 102.1
Piarhemia, piarrhemia — *see also* Hyperlipemia 272.4
  bilharziasis 120.9
Pica 307.52
  hysterical 300.11
Pick's
  cerebral atrophy 331.11
    with dementia
      with behavioral disturbance 331.11 *[294.11]*
      without behavioral disturbance 331.11 *[294.10]*
  disease
    brain 331.11
      dementia in
        with behavioral disturbance 331.11 *[294.11]*
        without behavioral disturbance 331.11 *[294.10]*
    lipid histiocytosis 272.7
    liver (pericardial pseudocirrhosis of liver) 423.2
    pericardium (pericardial pseudocirrhosis of liver) 423.2

☑ **Additional Digit Required** — Refer to the Tabular List for Digit Selection   ▽ **Subterms under main terms may continue to next column or page**

Index   **Phagedena — Pick's**

228 — Volume 2 • October 2010   ▶◀ Revised Text   ● New Line   ▲ Revised Code   **2011 ICD-9-CM**

Pick's — *continued*
  polyserositis (pericardial pseudocirrhosis of liver) 423.2
  syndrome
    heart (pericardial pseudocirrhosis of liver) 423.2
    liver (pericardial pseudocirrhosis of liver) 423.2
  tubular adenoma (M8640/0)
    specified site — *see* Neoplasm, by site, benign
    unspecified site
      female 220
      male 222.0
Pick-Herxheimer syndrome (diffuse idiopathic cutaneous atrophy) 701.8
Pick-Niemann disease (lipid histiocytosis) 272.7
Pickwickian syndrome (cardiopulmonary obesity) 278.03 ▲
Piebaldism, classic 709.09
Piedra 111.2
  beard 111.2
    black 111.3
    white 111.2
  black 111.3
  scalp 111.3
    black 111.3
    white 111.2
  white 111.2
Pierre Marie-Bamberger syndrome (hypertrophic pulmonary osteoarthropathy) 731.2
Pierre Marie's syndrome (pulmonary hypertrophic osteoarthropathy) 731.2
Pierre Mauriac's syndrome (diabetes-dwarfism-obesity) 258.1
Pierre Robin deformity or syndrome (congenital) 756.0
Pierson's disease or osteochondrosis 732.1
Pigeon
  breast or chest (acquired) 738.3
    congenital 754.82
    rachitic (*see also* Rickets) 268.0
  breeders' disease or lung 495.2
  fanciers' disease or lung 495.2
  toe 735.8
Pigmentation (abnormal) 709.00
  anomaly 709.00
    congenital 757.33
    specified NEC 709.09
  conjunctiva 372.55
  cornea 371.10
    anterior 371.11
    posterior 371.13
    stromal 371.12
  lids (congenital) 757.33
    acquired 374.52
  limbus corneae 371.10
  metals 709.00
  optic papilla, congenital 743.57
  retina (congenital) (grouped) (nevoid) 743.53
    acquired 362.74
  scrotum, congenital 757.33
Piles — *see* Hemorrhoids
Pili
  annulati or torti (congenital) 757.4
  incarnati 704.8
Pill roller hand (intrinsic) 736.09
Pilomatrixoma (M8110/0) — *see* Neoplasm, skin, benign
Pilonidal — *see* condition
Pimple 709.8
PIN I (prostatic intraepithelial neoplasia I) 602.3
PIN II (prostatic intraepithelial neoplasia II) 602.3
PIN III (prostatic intraepithelial neoplasia III) 233.4
Pinched nerve — *see* Neuropathy, entrapment
Pineal body or gland — *see* condition
Pinealoblastoma (M9362/3) 194.4
Pinealoma (M9360/1) 237.1
  malignant (M9360/3) 194.4
Pineoblastoma (M9362/3) 194.4
Pineocytoma (M9361/1) 237.1

Pinguecula 372.51
Pingueculitis 372.34
Pinhole meatus — *see also* Stricture, urethra 598.9
Pink
  disease 985.0
  eye 372.03
  puffer 492.8
Pinkus' disease (lichen nitidus) 697.1
Pinpoint
  meatus (*see also* Stricture, urethra) 598.9
  os uteri (*see also* Stricture, cervix) 622.4
Pinselhaare (congenital) 757.4
Pinta 103.9
  cardiovascular lesions 103.2
  chancre (primary) 103.0
  erythematous plaques 103.1
  hyperchromic lesions 103.1
  hyperkeratosis 103.1
  lesions 103.9
    cardiovascular 103.2
    hyperchromic 103.1
    intermediate 103.1
    late 103.2
    mixed 103.3
    primary 103.0
    skin (achromic) (cicatricial) (dyschromic) 103.2
      hyperchromic 103.1
      mixed (achromic and hyperchromic) 103.3
  papule (primary) 103.0
  skin lesions (achromic) (cicatricial) (dyschromic) 103.2
    hyperchromic 103.1
    mixed (achromic and hyperchromic) 103.3
  vitiligo 103.2
Pintid 103.0
Pinworms (disease) (infection) (infestation) 127.4
Piry fever 066.8
Pistol wound — *see* Gunshot wound
Pitchers' elbow 718.82
Pithecoid pelvis 755.69
  with disproportion (fetopelvic) 653.2 ☑
    affecting fetus or newborn 763.1
    causing obstructed labor 660.1 ☑
Pithiatism 300.11
Pit, lip (mucus), **congenital** 750.25
Pitted — *see also* Pitting
  teeth 520.4
Pitting (edema) — *see also* Edema 782.3
  lip 782.3
  nail 703.8
    congenital 757.5
Pituitary gland — *see* condition
Pituitary snuff-takers' disease 495.8
Pityriasis 696.5
  alba 696.5
  capitis 690.11
  circinata (et maculata) 696.3
  Hebra's (exfoliative dermatitis) 695.89
  lichenoides et varioliformis 696.2
  maculata (et circinata) 696.3
  nigra 111.1
  pilaris 757.39
    acquired 701.1
    Hebra's 696.4
  rosea 696.3
  rotunda 696.3
  rubra (Hebra) 695.89
    pilaris 696.4
  sicca 690.18
  simplex 690.18
  specified type NEC 696.5
  streptogenes 696.5
  versicolor 111.0
    scrotal 111.0
Placenta, placental
  ablatio 641.2 ☑
    affecting fetus or newborn 762.1
  abnormal, abnormality 656.7 ☑
    with hemorrhage 641.8 ☑
      affecting fetus or newborn 762.1
    affecting fetus or newborn 762.2

Placenta, placental — *continued*
  abruptio 641.2 ☑
    affecting fetus or newborn 762.1
  accessory lobe — *see* Placenta, abnormal
  accreta (without hemorrhage) 667.0 ☑
    with hemorrhage 666.0 ☑
  adherent (without hemorrhage) 667.0 ☑
    with hemorrhage 666.0 ☑
  apoplexy — *see* Placenta, separation
  battledore — *see* Placenta, abnormal
  bilobate — *see* Placenta, abnormal
  bipartita — *see* Placenta, abnormal
  carneous mole 631
  centralis — *see* Placenta, previa
  circumvallata — *see* Placenta, abnormal
  cyst (amniotic) — *see* Placenta, abnormal
  deficiency — *see* Placenta, insufficiency
  degeneration — *see* Placenta, insufficiency
  detachment (partial) (premature) (with hemorrhage) 641.2 ☑
    affecting fetus or newborn 762.1
  dimidiata — *see* Placenta, abnormal
  disease 656.7 ☑
    affecting fetus or newborn 762.2
  duplex — *see* Placenta, abnormal
  dysfunction — *see* Placenta, insufficiency
  fenestrata — *see* Placenta, abnormal
  fibrosis — *see* Placenta, abnormal
  fleshy mole 631
  hematoma — *see* Placenta, abnormal
  hemorrhage NEC — *see* Placenta, separation
  hormone disturbance or malfunction — *see* Placenta, abnormal
  hyperplasia — *see* Placenta, abnormal
  increta (without hemorrhage) 667.0 ☑
    with hemorrhage 666.0 ☑
  infarction 656.7 ☑
    affecting fetus or newborn 762.2
  insertion, vicious — *see* Placenta, previa
  insufficiency
    affecting
      fetus or newborn 762.2
      management of pregnancy 656.5 ☑
  lateral — *see* Placenta, previa
  low implantation or insertion — *see* Placenta, previa
  low-lying — *see* Placenta, previa
  malformation — *see* Placenta, abnormal
  malposition — *see* Placenta, previa
  marginalis, marginata — *see* Placenta, previa
  marginal sinus (hemorrhage) (rupture) 641.2 ☑
    affecting fetus or newborn 762.1
  membranacea — *see* Placenta, abnormal
  multilobed — *see* Placenta, abnormal
  multipartita — *see* Placenta, abnormal
  necrosis — *see* Placenta, abnormal
  percreta (without hemorrhage) 667.0 ☑
    with hemorrhage 666.0 ☑
  polyp 674.4 ☑
  previa (central) (centralis) (complete) (lateral) (marginal) (marginalis) (partial) (partialis) (total) (with hemorrhage) 641.1 ☑
    without hemorrhage (before labor and delivery) (during pregnancy) 641.0 ☑
      affecting fetus or newborn 762.0
    noted
      before labor, without hemorrhage (with cesarean delivery) 641.0 ☑
      during pregnancy (without hemorrhage) 641.0 ☑
  retention (with hemorrhage) 666.0 ☑
    without hemorrhage 667.0 ☑
    fragments, complicating puerperium (delayed hemorrhage) 666.2 ☑
      without hemorrhage 667.1 ☑
    postpartum, puerperal 666.2 ☑
  separation (normally implanted) (partial) (premature) (with hemorrhage) 641.2 ☑
    affecting fetus or newborn 762.1

Placenta, placental — *continued*
  septuplex — *see* Placenta, abnormal
  small — *see* Placenta, insufficiency
  softening (premature) — *see* Placenta, abnormal
  spuria — *see* Placenta, abnormal
  succenturiata — *see* Placenta, abnormal
  syphilitic 095.8
  transfusion syndromes 762.3
  transmission of chemical substance — *see* Absorption, chemical, through placenta
  trapped (with hemorrhage) 666.0 ☑
    without hemorrhage 667.0 ☑
  trilobate — *see* Placenta, abnormal
  tripartita — *see* Placenta, abnormal
  triplex — *see* Placenta, abnormal
  varicose vessel — *see* Placenta, abnormal
  vicious insertion — *see* Placenta, previa
Placentitis
  affecting fetus or newborn 762.7
  complicating pregnancy 658.4 ☑
Plagiocephaly (skull) 754.0
Plague 020.9
  abortive 020.8
  ambulatory 020.8
  bubonic 020.0
  cellulocutaneous 020.1
  lymphatic gland 020.0
  pneumonic 020.5
    primary 020.3
    secondary 020.4
  pulmonary — *see* Plague, pneumonic
  pulmonic — *see* Plague, pneumonic
  septicemic 020.2
  tonsillar 020.9
    septicemic 020.2
  vaccination, prophylactic (against) V03.3
Planning, family V25.09
  contraception V25.9
  natural
    procreative V26.41
    to avoid pregnancy V25.04
  procreation V26.49
    natural V26.41
Plaque
  artery, arterial — *see* Arteriosclerosis
  calcareous — *see* Calcification
  Hollenhorst's (retinal) 362.33
  tongue 528.6
Plasma cell myeloma 203.0 ☑
Plasmacytoma, plasmocytoma (solitary) (M9731/1) 238.6
  benign (M9731/0) — *see* Neoplasm, by site, benign
  malignant (M9731/3) 203.8 ☑
Plasmacytopenia 288.59
Plasmacytosis 288.64
Plaster ulcer — *see also* Ulcer, pressure 707.00
Plateau iris syndrome 364.82
Platybasia 756.0
Platyonychia (congenital) 757.5
  acquired 703.8
Platypelloid pelvis 738.6
  with disproportion (fetopelvic) 653.2 ☑
    affecting fetus or newborn 763.1
    causing obstructed labor 660.1 ☑
      affecting fetus or newborn 763.1
  congenital 755.69
Platyspondylia 756.19
Plethora 782.62
  newborn 776.4
Pleuralgia 786.52
Pleura, pleural — *see* condition
Pleurisy (acute) (adhesive) (chronic) (costal) (diaphragmatic) (double) (dry) (fetid) (fibrinous) (fibrous) (interlobar) (latent) (lung) (old) (plastic) (primary) (residual) (sicca) (sterile) (subacute) (unresolved) (with adherent pleura) 511.0
  with
    effusion (without mention of cause) 511.9
      bacterial, nontuberculous 511.1
      nontuberculous NEC 511.9
        bacterial 511.1

☑ **Additional Digit Required** — Refer to the Tabular List for Digit Selection

▽ **Subterms under main terms may continue to next column or page**

Pleurisy — continued
- with — continued
  - effusion — continued
    - pneumococcal 511.1
    - specified type NEC 511.89
    - staphylococcal 511.1
    - streptococcal 511.1
    - tuberculous (see also Tuberculosis, pleura) 012.0 ☑
      - primary, progressive 010.1 ☑
    - influenza, flu, or grippe ▶(see also Influenza)◀ 487.1
    - tuberculosis — see Pleurisy, tuberculous
  - encysted 511.89
  - exudative (see also Pleurisy, with effusion) 511.9
    - bacterial, nontuberculous 511.1
  - fibrinopurulent 510.9
    - with fistula 510.0
  - fibropurulent 510.9
    - with fistula 510.0
  - hemorrhagic 511.89
  - influenzal ▶(see also Influenza)◀ 487.1
  - pneumococcal 511.0
    - with effusion 511.1
  - purulent 510.9
    - with fistula 510.0
  - septic 510.9
    - with fistula 510.0
  - serofibrinous (see also Pleurisy, with effusion) 511.9
    - bacterial, nontuberculous 511.1
  - seropurulent 510.9
    - with fistula 510.0
  - serous (see also Pleurisy, with effusion) 511.9
    - bacterial, nontuberculous 511.1
  - staphylococcal 511.0
    - with effusion 511.1
  - streptococcal 511.0
    - with effusion 511.1
  - suppurative 510.9
    - with fistula 510.0
  - traumatic (post) (current) 862.29
    - with open wound into cavity 862.39
  - tuberculous (with effusion) (see also Tuberculosis, pleura) 012.0 ☑
    - primary, progressive 010.1 ☑

Pleuritis sicca — see Pleurisy
Pleurobronchopneumonia — see also Pneumonia, broncho- 485
Pleurodynia 786.52
- epidemic 074.1
- viral 074.1
Pleurohepatitis 573.8
Pleuropericarditis — see also Pericarditis 423.9
- acute 420.90
Pleuropneumonia (acute) (bilateral) (double) (septic) — see Pneumonia 486
- chronic (see also Fibrosis, lung) 515
Pleurorrhea — see also Hydrothorax 511.89
Plexitis, brachial 353.0
Plica
- knee 727.83
- polonica 132.0
- syndrome 727.83
- tonsil 474.8
Plicae dysphonia ventricularis 784.49
Plicated tongue 529.5
- congenital 750.13
Plug
- bronchus NEC 519.19
- meconium (newborn) NEC 777.1
- mucus — see Mucus, plug
Plumbism 984.9
- specified type of lead — see Table of Drugs and Chemicals
Plummer's disease (toxic nodular goiter) 242.3 ☑
Plummer-Vinson syndrome (sideropenic dysphagia) 280.8
Pluricarential syndrome of infancy 260
Plurideficiency syndrome of infancy 260
Plus (and minus) hand (intrinsic) 736.09
PMDD (premenstrual dysphoric disorder) 625.4
PMS 625.4

Pneumathemia — see Air, embolism, by type
Pneumatic drill or hammer disease 994.9
Pneumatocele (lung) 518.89
- intracranial 348.89
- tension 492.0
Pneumatosis
- cystoides intestinalis 569.89
- peritonei 568.89
- pulmonum 492.8
Pneumaturia 599.84
Pneumoblastoma (M8981/3) — see Neoplasm, lung, malignant
Pneumocephalus 348.89
Pneumococcemia 038.2
Pneumococcus, pneumococcal — see condition
Pneumoconiosis (due to) (inhalation of) 505
- aluminum 503
- asbestos 501
- bagasse 495.1
- bauxite 503
- beryllium 503
- carbon electrode makers' 503
- coal
  - miners' (simple) 500
  - workers' (simple) 500
- cotton dust 504
- diatomite fibrosis 502
- dust NEC 504
  - inorganic 503
  - lime 502
  - marble 502
  - organic NEC 504
- fumes or vapors (from silo) 506.9
- graphite 503
- hard metal 503
- mica 502
- moldy hay 495.0
- rheumatoid 714.81
- silica NEC 502
  - and carbon 500
- silicate NEC 502
- talc 502
Pneumocystis carinii pneumonia 136.3
Pneumocystis jiroveci pneumonia 136.3
Pneumocystosis 136.3
- with pneumonia 136.3
Pneumoenteritis 025
Pneumohemopericardium — see also Pericarditis 423.9
Pneumohemothorax — see also Hemothorax 511.89
- traumatic 860.4
  - with open wound into thorax 860.5
Pneumohydropericardium — see also Pericarditis 423.9
Pneumohydrothorax — see also Hydrothorax 511.89
Pneumomediastinum 518.1
- congenital 770.2
- fetus or newborn 770.2
Pneumomycosis 117.9
Pneumonia (acute) (Alpenstich) (benign) (bilateral) (brain) (cerebral) (circumscribed) (congestive) (creeping) (delayed resolution) (double) (epidemic) (fever) (flash) (fulminant) (fungoid) (granulomatous) (hemorrhagic) (incipient) (infantile) (infectious) (infiltration) (insular) (intermittent) (latent) (lobe) (migratory) (newborn) (organized) (overwhelming) (primary) (progressive) (pseudolobar) (purulent) (resolved) (secondary) (senile) (septic) (suppurative) (terminal) (true) (unresolved) (vesicular) 486
- with influenza, flu, or grippe 487.0
  - due to   ●
    - identified (virus)   ●
      - avian 488.01   ●
      - novel H1N1 488.11   ●
- adenoviral 480.0
- adynamic 514
- alba 090.0
- allergic 518.3
- alveolar — see Pneumonia, lobar

Pneumonia — continued
- anaerobes 482.81
- anthrax 022.1 [484.5]
- apex, apical — see Pneumonia, lobar
- ascaris 127.0 [484.8]
- aspiration 507.0
  - due to
    - aspiration of microorganisms
      - bacterial 482.9
        - specified type NEC 482.89
      - specified organism NEC 483.8
        - bacterial NEC 482.89
      - viral 480.9
        - specified type NEC 480.8
    - food (regurgitated) 507.0
    - gastric secretions 507.0
    - milk 507.0
    - oils, essences 507.1
    - solids, liquids NEC 507.8
    - vomitus 507.0
  - fetal 770.18
    - due to
      - blood 770.16
      - clear amniotic fluid 770.14
      - meconium 770.12
      - postnatal stomach contents 770.86
  - newborn 770.18
    - due to
      - blood 770.16
      - clear amniotic fluid 770.14
      - meconium 770.12
      - postnatal stomach contents 770.86
- asthenic 514
- atypical (disseminated) (focal) (primary) 486
  - with influenza ▶(see also Influenza)◀ 487.0
- bacillus 482.9
  - specified type NEC 482.89
- bacterial 482.9
  - specified type NEC 482.89
- Bacteroides (fragilis) (oralis) (melaninogenicus) 482.81
- basal, basic, basilar — see Pneumonia, ▶by type◀
- bronchiolitis obliterans organized (BOOP) 516.8
- broncho-, bronchial (confluent) (croupous) (diffuse) (disseminated) (hemorrhagic) (involving lobes) (lobar) (terminal) 485
  - with influenza 487.0
    - due to   ●
      - identified (virus)   ●
        - avian 488.01   ●
        - novel H1N1 488.11   ●
  - allergic 518.3
  - aspiration (see also Pneumonia, aspiration) 507.0
  - bacterial 482.9
    - specified type NEC 482.89
  - capillary 466.19
    - with bronchospasm or obstruction 466.19
  - chronic (see also Fibrosis, lung) 515
  - congenital (infective) 770.0
  - diplococcal 481
  - Eaton's agent 483.0
  - Escherichia coli (E. coli) 482.82
  - Friedländer's bacillus 482.0
  - Hemophilus influenzae 482.2
  - hiberno-vernal 083.0 [484.8]
  - hypostatic 514
  - influenzal ▶(see also Influenza)◀ 487.0
  - inhalation (see also Pneumonia, aspiration) 507.0
    - due to fumes or vapors (chemical) 506.0
  - Klebsiella 482.0
  - lipid 507.1
    - endogenous 516.8
  - Mycoplasma (pneumoniae) 483.0
  - ornithosis 073.0
  - pleuropneumonia-like organisms (PPLO) 483.0

Pneumonia — continued
- broncho-, bronchial — continued
  - pneumococcal 481
  - Proteus 482.83
  - Pseudomonas 482.1
  - specified organism NEC 483.8
    - bacterial NEC 482.89
  - staphylococcal 482.40
    - aureus 482.41
    - methicillin
      - resistant (MRSA) 482.42
      - susceptible (MSSA) 482.41
    - specified type NEC 482.49
  - streptococcal — see Pneumonia, streptococcal
  - typhoid 002.0 [484.8]
  - viral, virus (see also Pneumonia, viral) 480.9
- Butyrivibrio (fibriosolvens) 482.81
- Candida 112.4
- capillary 466.19
  - with bronchospasm or obstruction 466.19
- caseous (see also Tuberculosis) 011.6 ☑
- catarrhal — see Pneumonia, broncho-
- central — see Pneumonia, lobar
- Chlamydia, chlamydial 483.1
  - pneumoniae 483.1
  - psittaci 073.0
  - specified type NEC 483.1
  - trachomatis 483.1
- cholesterol 516.8
- chronic (see also Fibrosis, lung) 515
- cirrhotic (chronic) (see also Fibrosis, lung) 515
- Clostridium (haemolyticum) (novyi) NEC 482.81
- confluent — see Pneumonia, broncho-
- congenital (infective) 770.0
  - aspiration 770.18
- croupous — see Pneumonia, lobar
- cryptogenic organizing 516.8   ●
- cytomegalic inclusion 078.5 [484.1]
- deglutition (see also Pneumonia, aspiration) 507.0
- desquamative interstitial 516.8
- diffuse — see Pneumonia, broncho-
- diplococcal, diplococcus (broncho-) (lobar) 481
- disseminated (focal) — see Pneumonia, broncho-
- due to
  - adenovirus 480.0
  - anaerobes 482.81
  - Bacterium anitratum 482.83
  - Chlamydia, chlamydial 483.1
    - pneumoniae 483.1
    - psittaci 073.0
    - specified type NEC 483.1
    - trachomatis 483.1
  - coccidioidomycosis 114.0
  - Diplococcus (pneumoniae) 481
  - Eaton's agent 483.0
  - Escherichia coli (E. coli) 482.82
  - Friedländer's bacillus 482.0
  - fumes or vapors (chemical) (inhalation) 506.0
  - fungus NEC 117.9 [484.7]
    - coccidioidomycosis 114.0
  - Hemophilus influenzae (H. influenzae) 482.2
  - Herellea 482.83
  - influenza ▶(see also Influenza)◀ 487.0
  - Klebsiella pneumoniae 482.0
  - Mycoplasma (pneumoniae) 483.0
  - parainfluenza virus 480.2
  - pleuropneumonia-like organism (PPLO) 483.0
  - Pneumococcus 481
  - Pneumocystis carinii 136.3
  - Pneumocystis jiroveci 136.3
  - Proteus 482.83
  - Pseudomonas 482.1
  - respiratory syncytial virus 480.1
  - rickettsia 083.9 [484.8]
  - SARS-associated coronavirus 480.3

☑ Additional Digit Required — Refer to the Tabular List for Digit Selection

▽ Subterms under main terms may continue to next column or page

▶◀ Revised Text   ● New Line   ▲ Revised Code

Pneumonia — *continued*
due to — *continued*
specified
bacteria NEC 482.89
organism NEC 483.8
virus NEC 480.8
Staphylococcus 482.40
aureus 482.41
methicillin
resistant (MRSA) 482.42
susceptible (MSSA) 482.41
specified type NEC 482.49
Streptococcus (*see also* Pneumonia, streptococcal)
pneumoniae 481
virus (*see also* Pneumonia, viral) 480.9
SARS-associated coronavirus 480.3
Eaton's agent 483.0
embolic, embolism — (*see* Embolism, pulmonary)
eosinophilic 518.3
Escherichia coli (E. coli) 482.82
Eubacterium 482.81
fibrinous — *see* Pneumonia, lobar
fibroid (chronic) (*see also* Fibrosis, lung) 515
fibrous (*see also* Fibrosis, lung) 515
Friedländer's bacillus 482.0
Fusobacterium (nucleatum) 482.81
gangrenous 513.0
giant cell (*see also* Pneumonia, viral) 480.9
gram-negative bacteria NEC 482.83
anaerobic 482.81
grippal ▶(*see also* Influenza)◀ 487.0
Hemophilus influenzae (bronchial) (lobar) 482.2
hypostatic (broncho-) (lobar) 514
in
actinomycosis 039.1
anthrax 022.1 [*484.5*]
aspergillosis 117.3 [*484.6*]
candidiasis 112.4
coccidioidomycosis 114.0
cytomegalic inclusion disease 078.5 [*484.1*]
histoplasmosis (*see also* Histoplasmosis) 115.95
infectious disease NEC 136.9 [*484.8*]
measles 055.1
mycosis, systemic NEC 117.9 [*484.7*]
nocardiasis, nocardiosis 039.1
ornithosis 073.0
pneumocystosis 136.3
psittacosis 073.0
Q fever 083.0 [*484.8*]
salmonellosis 003.22
toxoplasmosis 130.4
tularemia 021.2
typhoid (fever) 002.0 [*484.8*]
varicella 052.1
whooping cough (*see also* Whooping cough) 033.9 [*484.3*]
infective, acquired prenatally 770.0
influenzal (broncho) (lobar) (virus) ▶(*see also* Influenza)◀ 487.0
inhalation (*see also* Pneumonia, aspiration) 507.0
fumes or vapors (chemical) 506.0
interstitial 516.8
with influenzal ▶(*see also* Influenza)◀ 487.0
acute 136.3
chronic (*see also* Fibrosis, lung) 515
desquamative 516.8
hypostatic 514
lipoid 507.1
lymphoid 516.8
plasma cell 136.3
Pseudomonas 482.1
intrauterine (infective) 770.0
aspiration 770.18
blood 770.16
clear amniotic fluid 770.14
meconium 770.12
postnatal stomach contents 770.86
Klebsiella pneumoniae 482.0
Legionnaires' 482.84

Pneumonia — *continued*
lipid, lipoid (exogenous) (interstitial) 507.1
endogenous 516.8
lobar (diplococcal) (disseminated) (double) (interstitial) (pneumococcal, any type) 481
with influenza ▶(*see also* Influenza)◀ 487.0
bacterial 482.9
specified type NEC 482.89
chronic (*see also* Fibrosis, lung) 515
Escherichia coli (E. coli) 482.82
Friedländer's bacillus 482.0
Hemophilus influenzae (H. influenzae) 482.2
hypostatic 514
influenzal ▶(*see also* Influenza)◀ 487.0
Klebsiella 482.0
ornithosis 073.0
Proteus 482.83
Pseudomonas 482.1
psittacosis 073.0
specified organism NEC 483.8
bacterial NEC 482.89
staphylococcal 482.40
aureus 482.41
methicillin
resistant (MRSA) 482.42
susceptible (MSSA) 482.41
specified type NEC 482.49
streptococcal — *see* Pneumonia, streptococcal
viral, virus (*see also* Pneumonia, viral) 480.9
lobular (confluent) — *see* Pneumonia, broncho-
Löffler's 518.3
massive — *see* Pneumonia, lobar
meconium aspiration 770.12
metastatic NEC 038.8 [*484.8*]
methicillin resistant Staphylococcus aureus (MRSA) 482.42
methicillin susceptible Staphylococcus aureus (MSSA) 482.41
MRSA (methicillin resistant Staphylococcus aureus) 482.42
MSSA (methicillin susceptible Staphylococcus aureus) 482.41
multilobar — *see* Pneumonia, by type ●
Mycoplasma (pneumoniae) 483.0
necrotic 513.0
nitrogen dioxide 506.9
orthostatic 514
parainfluenza virus 480.2
parenchymatous (*see also* Fibrosis, lung) 515
passive 514
patchy — *see* Pneumonia, broncho-
Peptococcus 482.81
Peptostreptococcus 482.81
plasma cell 136.3
pleurolobar — *see* Pneumonia, lobar
pleuropneumonia-like organism (PPLO) 483.0
pneumococcal (broncho) (lobar) 481
Pneumocystis (carinii) (jiroveci) 136.3
postinfectional NEC 136.9 [*484.8*]
postmeasles 055.1
postoperative 997.39
primary atypical 486
Proprionibacterium 482.81
Proteus 482.83
Pseudomonas 482.1
psittacosis 073.0
radiation 508.0
respiratory syncytial virus 480.1
resulting from a procedure 997.39
rheumatic 390 [*517.1*]
Salmonella 003.22
SARS-associated coronavirus 480.3
segmented, segmental — *see* Pneumonia, broncho-
Serratia (marcescens) 482.83
specified
bacteria NEC 482.89
organism NEC 483.8
virus NEC 480.8

Pneumonia — *continued*
spirochetal 104.8 [*484.8*]
staphylococcal (broncho) (lobar) 482.40
aureus 482.41
methicillin
resistant 482.42
susceptible (MSSA) 482.41
specified type NEC 482.49
static, stasis 514
streptococcal (broncho) (lobar) NEC 482.30
Group
A 482.31
B 482.32
specified NEC 482.39
pneumoniae 481
specified type NEC 482.39
Streptococcus pneumoniae 481
traumatic (complication) (early) (secondary) 958.8
tuberculous (any) (*see also* Tuberculosis) 011.6 ☑
tularemic 021.2
TWAR agent 483.1
varicella 052.1
Veillonella 482.81
ventilator associated 997.31
viral, virus (broncho) (interstitial) (lobar) 480.9
with influenza, flu, or grippe ▶(*see also* Influenza)◀ 487.0
adenoviral 480.0
parainfluenza 480.2
respiratory syncytial 480.1
SARS-associated coronavirus 480.3
specified type NEC 480.8
white (congenital) 090.0
Pneumonic — *see* condition
Pneumonitis (acute) (primary) — *see also* Pneumonia 486
allergic 495.9
specified type NEC 495.8
aspiration 507.0
due to fumes or gases 506.0
fetal 770.18
due to
blood 770.16
clear amniotic fluid 770.14
meconium 770.12
postnatal stomach contents 770.86
newborn 770.18
due to
blood 770.16
clear amniotic fluid 770.14
meconium 770.12
postnatal stomach contents 770.86
obstetric 668.0 ☑
chemical 506.0
due to fumes or gases 506.0
cholesterol 516.8
chronic (*see also* Fibrosis, lung) 515
congenital rubella 771.0
crack 506.0
due to
crack (cocaine) 506.0
fumes or vapors 506.0
inhalation
food (regurgitated), milk, vomitus 507.0
oils, essences 507.1
saliva 507.0
solids, liquids NEC 507.8
toxoplasmosis (acquired) 130.4
congenital (active) 771.2 [*484.8*]
eosinophilic 518.3
fetal aspiration 770.18
due to
blood 770.16
clear amniotic fluid 770.14
meconium 770.12
postnatal stomach contents 770.86
hypersensitivity 495.9
interstitial (chronic) (*see also* Fibrosis, lung) 515
lymphoid 516.8

Pneumonitis — *see also* Pneumonia — *continued*
lymphoid, interstitial 516.8
meconium aspiration 770.12
postanesthetic
correct substance properly administered 507.0
obstetric 668.0 ☑
overdose or wrong substance given 968.4
specified anesthetic — *see* Table of Drugs and Chemicals
postoperative 997.3 ☑
obstetric 668.0 ☑
radiation 508.0
rubella, congenital 771.0
"ventilation" 495.7
ventilator associated 997.31
wood-dust 495.8
Pneumonoconiosis — *see* Pneumoconiosis
Pneumoparotid 527.8
Pneumopathy NEC 518.89
alveolar 516.9
specified NEC 516.8
due to dust NEC 504
parietoalveolar 516.9
specified condition NEC 516.8
Pneumopericarditis — *see also* Pericarditis 423.9
acute 420.90
Pneumopericardium — *see also* Pericarditis
congenital 770.2
fetus or newborn 770.2
traumatic (post) (*see also* Pneumothorax, traumatic) 860.0
with open wound into thorax 860.1
Pneumoperitoneum 568.89
fetus or newborn 770.2
Pneumophagia (psychogenic) 306.4
Pneumopleurisy, pneumopleuritis — *see also* Pneumonia 486
Pneumopyopericardium 420.99
Pneumopyothorax — *see also* Pyopneumothorax 510.9
with fistula 510.0
Pneumorrhagia 786.30   ▲
newborn 770.3
tuberculous (*see also* Tuberculosis, pulmonary) 011.9 ☑
Pneumosiderosis (occupational) 503
Pneumothorax (acute) (chronic) 512.8
congenital 770.2
due to operative injury of chest wall or lung 512.1
accidental puncture or laceration 512.1
fetus or newborn 770.2
iatrogenic 512.1
postoperative 512.1
spontaneous 512.8
fetus or newborn 770.2
tension 512.0
sucking 512.8
iatrogenic 512.1
postoperative 512.1
tense valvular, infectional 512.0
tension 512.0
iatrogenic 512.1
postoperative 512.1
spontaneous 512.0
traumatic 860.0
with
hemothorax 860.4
with open wound into thorax 860.5
open wound into thorax 860.1
tuberculous (*see also* Tuberculosis) 011.7 ☑
Pocket(s)
endocardial (*see also* Endocarditis) 424.90
periodontal 523.8
Podagra 274.01
Podencephalus 759.89
Poikilocytosis 790.09
Poikiloderma 709.09
Civatte's 709.09
congenital 757.33
vasculare atrophicans 696.2

☑ **Additional Digit Required** — Refer to the Tabular List for Digit Selection   ⓥᵉᵇˢ **Subterms under main terms may continue to next column or page**

2011 ICD-9-CM   ▶◀ **Revised Text**   ● **New Line**   ▲ **Revised Code**   October 2010 · Volume 2 — 231

Polyneuropathy — *continued*
in — *continued*
sarcoidosis 135 *[357.4]*
uremia 585.9 *[357.4]*
lead 357.7
nutritional 269.9 *[357.4]*
specified NEC 269.8 *[357.4]*
postherpetic 053.13
progressive 356.4
sensory (hereditary) 356.2
specified NEC 356.8
Polyonychia 757.5
Polyopia 368.2
refractive 368.15
Polyorchism, polyorchidism (three testes) 752.89
Polyorrhymenitis (peritoneal) — *see also* Polyserositis 568.82
pericardial 423.2
Polyostotic fibrous dysplasia 756.54
Polyotia 744.1
Polyphagia 783.6
Polypoid — *see* condition
Polyposis — *see also* Polyp
coli (adenomatous) (M8220/0) 211.3
adenocarcinoma in (M8220/3) 153.9
carcinoma in (M8220/3) 153.9
familial (M8220/0) 211.3
intestinal (adenomatous) (M8220/0) 211.3
multiple (M8221/0) — *see* Neoplasm, by site, benign
Polyp, polypus

Note — Polyps of organs or sites that do not appear in the list below should be coded to the residual category for diseases of the organ or site concerned.

accessory sinus 471.8
adenoid tissue 471.0
adenomatous (M8210/0) (*see also* Neoplasm, by site, benign)
adenocarcinoma in (M8210/3) — *see* Neoplasm, by site, malignant
carcinoma in (M8210/3) — *see* Neoplasm, by site, malignant
multiple (M8221/0) — *see* Neoplasm, by site, benign
antrum 471.8
anus, anal (canal) (nonadenomatous) 569.0
adenomatous 211.4
Bartholin's gland 624.6
bladder (M8120/1) 236.7
broad ligament 620.8
cervix (uteri) 622.7
adenomatous 219.0
in pregnancy or childbirth 654.6 ☑
affecting fetus or newborn 763.89
causing obstructed labor 660.2 ☑
mucous 622.7
nonneoplastic 622.7
choanal 471.0
cholesterol 575.6
clitoris 624.6
colon (M8210/0) (*see also* Polyp, adenomatous) 211.3
corpus uteri 621.0
dental 522.0
ear (middle) 385.30
endometrium 621.0
ethmoidal (sinus) 471.8
fallopian tube 620.8
female genital organs NEC 624.8
frontal (sinus) 471.8
gallbladder 575.6
gingiva 523.8
gum 523.8
labia 624.6
larynx (mucous) 478.4
malignant (M8000/3) — *see* Neoplasm, by site, malignant
maxillary (sinus) 471.8
middle ear 385.30
myometrium 621.0
nares
anterior 471.9
posterior 471.0
nasal (mucous) 471.9

Polyp, polypus — *continued*
nasal — *continued*
cavity 471.0
septum 471.9
nasopharyngeal 471.0
neoplastic (M8210/0) — *see* Neoplasm, by site, benign
nose (mucous) 471.9
oviduct 620.8
paratubal 620.8
pharynx 478.29
congenital 750.29
placenta, placental 674.4 ☑
prostate 600.20
with
other lower urinary tract symptoms (LUTS) 600.21
urinary
obstruction 600.21
retention 600.21
pudenda 624.6
pulp (dental) 522.0
rectosigmoid 211.4
rectum (nonadenomatous) 569.0
adenomatous 211.4
septum (nasal) 471.9
sinus (accessory) (ethmoidal) (frontal) (maxillary) (sphenoidal) 471.8
sphenoidal (sinus) 471.8
stomach (M8210/0) 211.1
tube, fallopian 620.8
turbinate, mucous membrane 471.8
ureter 593.89
urethra 599.3
uterine
ligament 620.8
tube 620.8
uterus (body) (corpus) (mucous) 621.0
in pregnancy or childbirth 654.1 ☑
affecting fetus or newborn 763.89
causing obstructed labor 660.2 ☑
vagina 623.7
vocal cord (mucous) 478.4
vulva 624.6
Polyradiculitis (acute) 357.0
Polyradiculoneuropathy (acute) (segmentally demyelinating) 357.0
Polysarcia 278.00
Polyserositis (peritoneal) 568.82
due to pericarditis 423.2
paroxysmal (familial) 277.31
pericardial 423.2
periodic (familial) 277.31
pleural — *see* Pleurisy
recurrent 277.31
tuberculous (*see also* Tuberculosis, polyserositis) 018.9 ☑
Polysialia 527.7
Polysplenia syndrome 759.0
Polythelia 757.6
Polytrichia — *see also* Hypertrichosis 704.1
Polyunguia (congenital) 757.5
acquired 703.8
Polyuria 788.42
Pompe's disease (glycogenosis II) 271.0
Pompholyx 705.81
Poncet's disease (tuberculous rheumatism) — *see also* Tuberculosis 015.9 ☑
Pond fracture — *see* Fracture, skull, vault
Ponos 085.0
Pons, pontine — *see* condition
Poor
aesthetics of existing restoration of tooth 525.67
contractions, labor 661.2 ☑
affecting fetus or newborn 763.7
fetal growth NEC 764.9 ☑
affecting management of pregnancy 656.5 ☑
incorporation
artificial skin graft 996.55
decellularized allodermis graft 996.55
obstetrical history V13.29
affecting management of current pregnancy V23.49
pre-term labor V23.41

Poor — *continued*
obstetrical history — *continued*
pre-term labor V13.21
sucking reflex (newborn) 796.1
vision NEC 369.9
Poradenitis, nostras 099.1
Porencephaly (congenital) (developmental) (true) 742.4
acquired 348.0
nondevelopmental 348.0
traumatic (post) 310.2
Porocephaliasis 134.1
Porokeratosis 757.39
disseminated superficial actinic (DSAP) 692.75
Poroma, eccrine (M8402/0) — *see* Neoplasm, skin, benign
Porphyria (acute) (congenital) (constitutional) (erythropoietic) (familial) (hepatica) (idiopathic) (idiosyncratic) (intermittent) (latent) (mixed hepatic) (photosensitive) (South African genetic) (Swedish) 277.1
acquired 277.1
cutaneatarda
hereditaria 277.1
symptomatica 277.1
due to drugs
correct substance properly administered 277.1
overdose or wrong substance given or taken 977.9
specified drug — *see* Table of Drugs and Chemicals
secondary 277.1
toxic NEC 277.1
variegata 277.1
Porphyrinuria (acquired) (congenital) (secondary) 277.1
Porphyruria (acquired) (congenital) 277.1
Portal — *see* condition
Port wine nevus or mark 757.32
Posadas-Wernicke disease 114.9
Position
fetus, abnormal (*see also* Presentation, fetal) 652.9 ☑
teeth, faulty (*see also* Anomaly, position tooth) 524.30
Positive
culture (nonspecific) 795.39
AIDS virus V08
blood 790.7
HIV V08
human immunodeficiency virus V08
nose 795.39
Staphylococcus — *see* Carrier (suspected) of, Staphylococcus
skin lesion NEC 795.39
spinal fluid 792.0
sputum 795.39
stool 792.1
throat 795.39
urine 791.9
wound 795.39
findings, anthrax 795.31
HIV V08
human immunodeficiency virus (HIV) V08
PPD 795.5
serology
AIDS virus V08
inconclusive 795.71
HIV V08
inconclusive 795.71
human immunodeficiency virus (HIV) V08
inconclusive 795.71
syphilis 097.1
with signs or symptoms — *see* Syphilis, by site and stage
false 795.6
skin test 795.7 ☑
tuberculin (without active tuberculosis) 795.5
VDRL 097.1
with signs or symptoms — *see* Syphilis, by site and stage
false 795.6

Positive — *continued*
Wassermann reaction 097.1
false 795.6
Postcardiotomy syndrome 429.4
Postcaval ureter 753.4
Postcholecystectomy syndrome 576.0
Postclimacteric bleeding 627.1
Postcommissurotomy syndrome 429.4
Postconcussional syndrome 310.2
Postcontusional syndrome 310.2
Postcricoid region — *see* condition
Post-dates (pregnancy) — *see* Pregnancy
Postencephalitic — *see also* condition
syndrome 310.8
Posterior — *see* condition
Posterolateral sclerosis (spinal cord) — *see* Degeneration, combined
Postexanthematous — *see* condition
Postfebrile — *see* condition
Postgastrectomy dumping syndrome 564.2
Posthemiplegic chorea 344.89
Posthemorrhagic anemia (chronic) 280.0
acute 285.1
newborn 776.5
Posthepatitis syndrome 780.79
Postherpetic neuralgia (intercostal) (syndrome) (zoster) 053.19
geniculate ganglion 053.11
ophthalmica 053.19
trigeminal 053.12
Posthitis 607.1
Postimmunization complication or reaction — *see* Complications, vaccination
Postinfectious — *see* condition
Postinfluenzal syndrome 780.79
Postlaminectomy syndrome 722.80
cervical, cervicothoracic 722.81
kyphosis 737.12
lumbar, lumbosacral 722.83
thoracic, thoracolumbar 722.82
Postleukotomy syndrome 310.0
Postlobectomy syndrome 310.0
Postmastectomy lymphedema (syndrome) 457.0
Postmaturity, postmature (fetus or newborn) (gestation period over 42 completed weeks) 766.22
affecting management of pregnancy
post-term pregnancy 645.1 ☑
prolonged pregnancy 645.2 ☑
syndrome 766.22
Postmeasles — *see also* condition
complication 055.8
specified NEC 055.79
Postmenopausal
endometrium (atrophic) 627.8
suppurative (see also Endometritis) 615.9
hormone replacement therapy V07.4
status (age related) (natural) V49.81
Postnasal drip 784.91
Postnatal — *see* condition
Postoperative — *see also* condition
confusion state 293.9
psychosis 293.9
status NEC (*see also* Status (post)) V45.89
Postpancreatectomy hyperglycemia 251.3
Postpartum — *see also* condition
anemia 648.2 ☑
cardiomyopathy 674.5 ☑
observation
immediately after delivery V24.0
routine follow-up V24.2
Postperfusion syndrome NEC 999.89
bone marrow 996.85
Postpoliomyelitic — *see* condition
Postsurgery status NEC — *see also* Status (post) V45.89
Post-term (pregnancy) 645.1 ☑
infant (gestation period over 40 completed weeks to 42 completed weeks) 766.21
Post-transplant lymphoproliferative disorder (PTLD) 238.77
Posttraumatic — *see* condition

⟱ Subterms under main terms may continue to next column or page

Polyneuropathy — Posttraumatic

Posttraumatic brain syndrome, nonpsychotic 310.2
Post-traumatic stress disorder (PTSD) 309.81
Post-typhoid abscess 002.0
Postures, hysterical 300.11
Postvaccinal reaction or complication — *see* Complications, vaccination
Postvagotomy syndrome 564.2
Postvalvulotomy syndrome 429.4
Postvasectomy sperm count V25.8
Potain's disease (pulmonary edema) 514
Potain's syndrome (gastrectasis with dyspepsia) 536.1
Pott's
  curvature (spinal) (*see also* Tuberculosis) 015.0 *[737.43]*
  disease or paraplegia (*see also* Tuberculosis) 015.0 *[730.88]*
  fracture (closed) 824.4
    open 824.5
  gangrene 440.24
  osteomyelitis (*see also* Tuberculosis) 015.0 *[730.88]*
  spinal curvature (*see also* Tuberculosis) 015.0 *[737.43]*
  tumor, puffy (*see also* Osteomyelitis) 730.2 ☑
Potter's
  asthma 502
  disease 753.0
  facies 754.0
  lung 502
  syndrome (with renal agenesis) 753.0
Pouch
  bronchus 748.3
  Douglas' — *see* condition
  esophagus, esophageal (congenital) 750.4
    acquired 530.6
  gastric 537.1
  Hartmann's (abnormal sacculation of gallbladder neck) 575.8
    of intestine V44.3
      attention to V55.3
  pharynx, pharyngeal (congenital) 750.27
Pouchitis 569.71
Poulet's disease 714.2
Poultrymen's itch 133.8
Poverty V60.2
PPE (palmar plantar erythrodysesthesia) 693.0
Prader-Labhart-Willi-Fanconi syndrome (hypogenital dystrophy with diabetic tendency) 759.81
Prader-Willi syndrome (hypogenital dystrophy with diabetic tendency) 759.81
Preachers' voice 784.49
Pre-AIDS — *see* Human immunodeficiency virus (disease) (illness) (infection)
Preauricular appendage 744.1
Prebetalipoproteinemia (acquired) (essential) (familial) (hereditary) (primary) (secondary) 272.1
  with chylomicronemia 272.3
Precipitate labor 661.3 ☑
  affecting fetus or newborn 763.6
Preclimacteric bleeding 627.0
  menorrhagia 627.0
Precocious
  adrenarche 259.1
  menarche 259.1
  menstruation 259.1 ▲
  pubarche 259.1
  puberty NEC 259.1
  sexual development NEC 259.1
  thelarche 259.1
Precocity, sexual (constitutional) (cryptogenic) (female) (idiopathic) (male) NEC 259.1
  with adrenal hyperplasia 255.2
Precordial pain 786.51
  psychogenic 307.89
Predeciduous teeth 520.2
Prediabetes, prediabetic 790.29
  complicating pregnancy, childbirth, or puerperium 648.8 ☑
    fetus or newborn 775.89
Predislocation status of hip, at birth — *see also* Subluxation, congenital, hip 754.32

Preeclampsia (mild) 642.4 ☑
  with pre-existing hypertension 642.7 ☑
  affecting fetus or newborn 760.0
  severe 642.5 ☑
  superimposed on pre-existing hypertensive disease 642.7 ☑
Preeruptive color change, teeth, tooth 520.8
Preexcitation 426.7
  atrioventricular conduction 426.7
  ventricular 426.7
Preglaucoma 365.00
Pregnancy (single) (uterine) (without sickness) V22.2

> Note — Use the following fifth-digit subclassification with categories 640–649, 651–679:
>
> 0   unspecified as to episode of care
>
> 1   delivered, with or without mention of antepartum condition
>
> 2   delivered, with mention of postpartum complication
>
> 3   antepartum condition or complication
>
> 4   postpartum condition or complication

  abdominal (ectopic) 633.00
    with intrauterine pregnancy 633.01
    affecting fetus or newborn 761.4
  abnormal NEC 646.9 ☑
  ampullar — *see* Pregnancy, tubal
  broad ligament — *see* Pregnancy, cornual
  cervical — *see* Pregnancy, cornual
  chemical 631
  combined (extrauterine and intrauterine) — *see* Pregnancy, cornual
  complicated (by)
    abnormal, abnormality NEC 646.9 ☑
      cervix 654.6 ☑
      cord (umbilical) 663.9 ☑
      glucose tolerance (conditions classifiable to 790.21–790.29) 648.8 ☑
      pelvic organs or tissues NEC 654.9 ☑
      pelvis (bony) 653.0 ☑
      perineum or vulva 654.8 ☑
      placenta, placental (vessel) 656.7 ☑
      position
        cervix 654.4 ☑
        placenta 641.1 ☑
          without hemorrhage 641.0 ☑
        uterus 654.4 ☑
      size, fetus 653.5 ☑
      uterus (congenital) 654.0 ☑
    abscess or cellulitis
      bladder 646.6 ☑
      genitourinary tract (conditions classifiable to 590, 595, 597, 599.0, 614.0–614.5, 614.7–614.9, 615) 646.6 ☑
      kidney 646.6 ☑
      urinary tract NEC 646.6 ☑
    adhesion, pelvic peritoneal 648.9 ☑
    air embolism 673.0 ☑
    albuminuria 646.2 ☑
      with hypertension — *see* Toxemia, of pregnancy
    amnionitis 658.4 ☑
    amniotic fluid embolism 673.1 ☑
    anemia (conditions classifiable to 280–285) 648.2 ☑
    appendicitis 648.9 ☑
    atrophy, yellow (acute) (liver) (subacute) 646.7 ☑
    bacilluria, asymptomatic 646.5 ☑
    bacteriuria, asymptomatic 646.5 ☑
    bariatric surgery status 649.2 ☑
    bicornis or bicornuate uterus 654.0 ☑
    biliary problems 646.8 ☑

Pregnancy — *continued*
  complicated — *continued*
    bone and joint disorders (conditions classifiable to 720–724 or conditions affecting lower limbs classifiable to 711–719, 725–738) 648.7 ☑
    breech presentation (buttocks) (complete) (frank) 652.2 ☑
      with successful version 652.1 ☑
    cardiovascular disease (conditions classifiable to 390–398, 410–429) 648.6 ☑
      congenital (conditions classifiable to 745–747) 648.5 ☑
    cerebrovascular disorders (conditions classifiable to 430–434, 436–437) 674.0 ☑
    cervicitis (conditions classifiable to 616.0) 646.6 ☑
    chloasma (gravidarum) 646.8 ☑
    cholelithiasis 646.8 ☑
    chorea (gravidarum) — *see* Eclampsia, pregnancy
    coagulation defect 649.3 ☑
    conjoined twins 678.1 ☑
    contraction, pelvis (general) 653.1 ☑
      inlet 653.2 ☑
      outlet 653.3 ☑
    convulsions (eclamptic) (uremic) 642.6 ☑
      with pre-existing hypertension 642.7 ☑
    current disease or condition (nonobstetric)
      abnormal glucose tolerance 648.8 ☑
      anemia 648.2 ☑
      bone and joint (lower limb) 648.7 ☑
      cardiovascular 648.6 ☑
        congenital 648.5 ☑
      cerebrovascular 674.0 ☑
      diabetes (conditions classifiable to 249 and 250) 648.0 ☑
      drug dependence 648.3 ☑
      female genital mutilation 648.9 ☑
      genital organ or tract 646.6 ☑
      gonorrheal 647.1 ☑
      hypertensive 642.2 ☑
        chronic kidney 642.2 ☑
        renal 642.1 ☑
      infectious 647.9 ☑
        specified type NEC 647.8 ☑
      liver 646.7 ☑
      malarial 647.4 ☑
      nutritional deficiency 648.9 ☑
      parasitic NEC 647.8 ☑
      periodontal disease 648.9 ☑
      renal 646.2 ☑
        hypertensive 642.1 ☑
      rubella 647.5 ☑
      specified condition NEC 648.9 ☑
      syphilitic 647.0 ☑
      thyroid 648.1 ☑
      tuberculous 647.3 ☑
      urinary 646.6 ☑
      venereal 647.2 ☑
      viral NEC 647.6 ☑
    cystitis 646.6 ☑
    cystocele 654.4 ☑
    death of fetus (near term) 656.4 ☑
      early pregnancy (before 22 completed weeks gestation) 632
    deciduitis 646.6 ☑
    decreased fetal movements 655.7 ☑
    diabetes (mellitus) (conditions classifiable to 249 and 250) 648.0 ☑
    disorders of liver 646.7 ☑
    displacement, uterus NEC 654.4 ☑
    disproportion — *see* Disproportion
    double uterus 654.0 ☑
    drug dependence (conditions classifiable to 304) 648.3 ☑
    dysplasia, cervix 654.6 ☑

Pregnancy — *continued*
  complicated — *continued*
    early onset of delivery (spontaneous) 644.2 ☑
    eclampsia, eclamptic (coma) (convulsions) (delirium) (nephritis) (uremia) 642.6 ☑
      with pre-existing hypertension 642.7 ☑
    edema 646.1 ☑
      with hypertension — *see* Toxemia, of pregnancy
    effusion, amniotic fluid 658.1 ☑
      delayed delivery following 658.2 ☑
    embolism
      air 673.0 ☑
      amniotic fluid 673.1 ☑
      blood-clot 673.2 ☑
      cerebral 674.0 ☑
      pulmonary NEC 673.2 ☑
      pyemic 673.3 ☑
      septic 673.3 ☑
    emesis (gravidarum) — *see* Pregnancy, complicated, vomiting
    endometritis (conditions classifiable to 615.0–615.9) 670.1 ☑
      decidual 646.6 ☑
    epilepsy 649.4 ☑
    excessive weight gain NEC 646.1 ☑
    face presentation 652.4 ☑
    failure, fetal head to enter pelvic brim 652.5 ☑
    false labor (pains) 644.1 ☑
    fatigue 646.8 ☑
    fatty metamorphosis of liver 646.7 ☑
    female genital mutilation 648.9 ☑
    fetal
      anemia 678.0 ☑
      complications from in utero procedure 679.1 ☑
      conjoined twins 678.1 ☑
      death (near term) 656.4 ☑
        early (before 22 completed weeks gestation) 632
      deformity 653.7 ☑
      distress 656.8 ☑
      hematologic conditions 678.0 ☑
      reduction of multiple fetuses reduced to single fetus 651.7 ☑
      thrombocytopenia 678.0 ☑
      twin to twin transfusion 678.0 ☑
    fibroid (tumor) (uterus) 654.1 ☑
    footling presentation 652.8 ☑
      with successful version 652.1 ☑
    gallbladder disease 646.8 ☑
    gastric banding status 649.2 ☑
    gastric bypass status for obesity
    genital herpes (asymptomatic) (history ● of) (inactive) 647.6 ☑ ●
    goiter 648.1 ☑
    gonococcal infection (conditions classifiable to 098) 647.1 ☑
    gonorrhea (conditions classifiable to 098) 647.1 ☑
    hemorrhage 641.9 ☑
      accidental 641.2 ☑
      before 22 completed weeks gestation NEC 640.9 ☑
      cerebrovascular 674.0 ☑
      due to
        afibrinogenemia or other coagulation defect (conditions classifiable to 286.0–286.9) 641.3 ☑
        leiomyoma, uterine 641.8 ☑
        marginal sinus (rupture) 641.2 ☑
        premature separation, placenta 641.2 ☑
        trauma 641.8 ☑
      early (before 22 completed weeks gestation) 640.9 ☑
      threatened abortion 640.0 ☑
      unavoidable 641.1 ☑

☑ **Additional Digit Required** — Refer to the Tabular List for Digit Selection   ▽ **Subterms under main terms may continue to next column or page**

234 — Volume 2 · October 2010   ►◄ **Revised Text**   ● **New Line**   ▲ **Revised Code**   **2011 ICD-9-CM**

Pregnancy — *continued*
  complicated — *continued*
    hepatitis (acute) (malignant) (subacute)
      646.7 ☑
      viral 647.6 ☑
    herniation of uterus 654.4 ☑
    high head at term 652.5 ☑
    hydatidiform mole (delivered) (undelivered) 630
    hydramnios 657.0 ☑
    hydrocephalic fetus 653.6 ☑
    hydrops amnii 657.0 ☑
    hydrorrhea 658.1 ☑
    hyperemesis (gravidarum) — *see* Hyperemesis, gravidarum
    hypertension — *see* Hypertension, complicating pregnancy
    hypertensive
      chronic kidney disease 642.2 ☑
      heart and chronic kidney disease 642.2 ☑
      heart and renal disease 642.2 ☑
      heart disease 642.2 ☑
      renal disease 642.2 ☑
    hypertensive heart and chronic kidney disease 642.2 ☑
    hyperthyroidism 648.1 ☑
    hypothyroidism 648.1 ☑
    hysteralgia 646.8 ☑
    icterus gravis 646.7 ☑
    incarceration, uterus 654.3 ☑
    incompetent cervix (os) 654.5 ☑
    infection 647.9 ☑
      amniotic fluid 658.4 ☑
      bladder 646.6 ☑
      genital organ (conditions classifiable to 614.0–614.5, 614.7–614.9, 615) 646.6 ☑
      kidney (conditions classifiable to 590.0–590.9) 646.6 ☑
      urinary (tract) 646.6 ☑
        asymptomatic 646.5 ☑
    infective and parasitic diseases NEC 647.8 ☑
    inflammation
      bladder 646.6 ☑
      genital organ (conditions classifiable to 614.0–614.5, 614.7–614.9, 615) 646.6 ☑
      urinary tract NEC 646.6 ☑
    insufficient weight gain 646.8 ☑
    intrauterine fetal death (near term) NEC 656.4 ☑
      early (before 22 completed weeks' gestation) 632
    malaria (conditions classifiable to 084) 647.4 ☑
    malformation, uterus (congenital) 654.0 ☑
    malnutrition (conditions classifiable to 260–269) 648.9 ☑
    malposition
      fetus — *see* Pregnancy, complicated, malpresentation
      uterus or cervix 654.4 ☑
    malpresentation 652.9 ☑
      with successful version 652.1 ☑
      in multiple gestation 652.6 ☑
      specified type NEC 652.8 ☑
    marginal sinus hemorrhage or rupture 641.2 ☑
    maternal complications from in utero procedure 679.0 ☑
    maternal drug abuse 648.4 ☑
    maternal obesity syndrome 646.1 ☑
    menstruation 640.8 ☑
    mental disorders (conditions classifiable to 290–303, 305.0, 305.2-305.9, 306–316, 317–319) 648.4 ☑
    mentum presentation 652.4 ☑
    missed
      abortion 632
      delivery (at or near term) 656.4 ☑
      labor (at or near term) 656.4 ☑

Pregnancy — *continued*
  complicated — *continued*
    necrosis
      genital organ or tract (conditions classifiable to 614.0–614.5, 614.7–614.9, 615) 646.6 ☑
      liver (conditions classifiable to 570) 646.7 ☑
      renal, cortical 646.2 ☑
    nephritis or nephrosis (conditions classifiable to 580–589) 646.2 ☑
      with hypertension 642.1 ☑
    nephropathy NEC 646.2 ☑
    neuritis (peripheral) 646.4 ☑
    nutritional deficiency (conditions classifiable to 260–269) 648.9 ☑
    obesity 649.1 ☑
      surgery status 649.2 ☑
    oblique lie or presentation 652.3 ☑
      with successful version 652.1 ☑
    obstetrical trauma NEC 665.9 ☑
    oligohydramnios NEC 658.0 ☑
    onset of contractions before 37 weeks 644.0 ☑
    oversize fetus 653.5 ☑
    papyraceous fetus 646.0 ☑
    patent cervix 654.5 ☑
    pelvic inflammatory disease (conditions classifiable to 614.0–614.5, 614.7–614.9, 615) 646.6 ☑
    pelvic peritoneal adhesion 648.9 ☑
    placenta, placental
      abnormality 656.7 ☑
      abruptio or ablatio 641.2 ☑
      detachment 641.2 ☑
      disease 656.7 ☑
      infarct 656.7 ☑
      low implantation 641.1 ☑
        without hemorrhage 641.0 ☑
      malformation 656.7 ☑
      malposition 641.1 ☑
        without hemorrhage 641.0 ☑
      marginal sinus hemorrhage 641.2 ☑
      previa 641.1 ☑
        without hemorrhage 641.0 ☑
      separation (premature) (undelivered) 641.2 ☑
    placentitis 658.4 ☑
    pneumonia 648.9 ☑   ●
    polyhydramnios 657.0 ☑
    postmaturity
      post-term 645.1 ☑
      prolonged 645.2 ☑
    prediabetes 648.8 ☑
    pre-eclampsia (mild) 642.4 ☑
      severe 642.5 ☑
      superimposed on pre-existing hypertensive disease 642.7 ☑
    premature rupture of membranes 658.1 ☑
      with delayed delivery 658.2 ☑
    previous
      infertility V23.0
      in utero procedure during previous pregnancy V23.86
      nonobstetric condition V23.89
      poor obstetrical history V23.49
      premature delivery V23.41
      trophoblastic disease (conditions classifiable to 630) V23.1
    prolapse, uterus 654.4 ☑
    proteinuria (gestational) 646.2 ☑
      with hypertension — *see* Toxemia, of pregnancy
    pruritus (neurogenic) 646.8 ☑
    psychosis or psychoneurosis 648.4 ☑
    ptyalism 646.8 ☑
    pyelitis (conditions classifiable to 590.0–590.9) 646.6 ☑
    renal disease or failure NEC 646.2 ☑
      with secondary hypertension 642.1 ☑
      hypertensive 642.2 ☑
    retention, retained dead ovum 631

Pregnancy — *continued*
  complicated — *continued*
    retroversion, uterus 654.3 ☑
    Rh immunization, incompatibility, or sensitization 656.1 ☑
    rubella (conditions classifiable to 056) 647.5 ☑
    rupture
      amnion (premature) 658.1 ☑
        with delayed delivery 658.2 ☑
      marginal sinus (hemorrhage) 641.2 ☑
      membranes (premature) 658.1 ☑
        with delayed delivery 658.2 ☑
      uterus (before onset of labor) 665.0 ☑
    salivation (excessive) 646.8 ☑
    salpingo–oophoritis (conditions classifiable to 614.0–614.2) 646.6 ☑
    septicemia (conditions classifiable to 038.0–038.9) 647.8 ☑
      postpartum 670.2 ☑
      puerperal 670.2 ☑
    smoking 649.0 ☑
    spasms, uterus (abnormal) 646.8 ☑
    specified condition NEC 646.8 ☑
    spotting 649.5 ☑
    spurious labor pains 644.1 ☑
    status post
      bariatric surgery 649.2 ☑
      gastric banding 649.2 ☑
      gastric bypass for obesity 649.2 ☑
      obesity surgery 649.2 ☑
    superfecundation 651.9 ☑
    superfetation 651.9 ☑
    syphilis (conditions classifiable to 090–097) 647.0 ☑
    threatened
      abortion 640.0 ☑
      premature delivery 644.2 ☑
      premature labor 644.0 ☑
    thrombophlebitis (superficial) 671.2 ☑
      deep 671.3 ☑
      septic 670.3 ☑
    thrombosis 671.2 ☑
      venous (superficial) 671.2 ☑
      deep 671.3 ☑
    thyroid dysfunction (conditions classifiable to 240–246) 648.1 ☑
    thyroiditis 648.1 ☑
    thyrotoxicosis 648.1 ☑
    tobacco use disorder 649.0 ☑
    torsion of uterus 654.4 ☑
    toxemia — *see* Toxemia, of pregnancy
    transverse lie or presentation 652.3 ☑
      with successful version 652.1 ☑
    trauma 648.9 ☑
      obstetrical 665.9 ☑
    tuberculosis (conditions classifiable to 010–018) 647.3 ☑
    tumor
      cervix 654.6 ☑
      ovary 654.4 ☑
      pelvic organs or tissue NEC 654.4 ☑
      uterus (body) 654.1 ☑
        cervix 654.6 ☑
      vagina 654.7 ☑
      vulva 654.8 ☑
    unstable lie 652.0 ☑
    uremia — *see* Pregnancy, complicated, renal disease
    urethritis 646.6 ☑
    vaginitis or vulvitis (conditions classifiable to 616.1) 646.6 ☑
    varicose
      placental vessels 656.7 ☑
      veins (legs) 671.0 ☑
        perineum 671.1 ☑
        vulva 671.1 ☑
    varicosity, labia or vulva 671.1 ☑
    venereal disease NEC (conditions classifiable to 099) 647.2 ☑
    venous complication 671.9 ☑

Pregnancy — *continued*
  complicated — *continued*
    viral disease NEC (conditions classifiable to 042, 050–055, 057–079, 795.05, 795.15, 796.75) 647.6 ☑
    vomiting (incoercible) (pernicious) (persistent) (uncontrollable) (vicious) 643.9 ☑
      due to organic disease or other cause 643.8 ☑
      early — *see* Hyperemesis, gravidarum
      late (after 22 completed weeks gestation) 643.2 ☑
    young maternal age 659.8 ☑
  complications NEC 646.9 ☑
  cornual 633.80
    with intrauterine pregnancy 633.81
    affecting fetus or newborn 761.4
  death, maternal NEC 646.9 ☑
  delivered — *see* Delivery
  ectopic (ruptured) NEC 633.90
    with intrauterine pregnancy 633.91
    abdominal — *see* Pregnancy, abdominal
    affecting fetus or newborn 761.4
    combined (extrauterine and intrauterine) — *see* Pregnancy, cornual
    ovarian — *see* Pregnancy, ovarian
    specified type NEC 633.80
      with intrauterine pregnancy 633.81
      affecting fetus or newborn 761.4
    tubal — *see* Pregnancy, tubal
  examination, pregnancy
    negative result V72.41
    not confirmed V72.40
    positive result V72.42
  extrauterine — *see* Pregnancy, ectopic
  fallopian — *see* Pregnancy, tubal
  false 300.11
    labor (pains) 644.1 ☑
  fatigue 646.8 ☑
  illegitimate V61.6
  incidental finding V22.2
  in double uterus 654.0 ☑
  interstitial — *see* Pregnancy, cornual
  intraligamentous — *see* Pregnancy, cornual
  intramural — *see* Pregnancy, cornual
  intraperitoneal — *see* Pregnancy, abdominal
  isthmian — *see* Pregnancy, tubal
  management affected by
    abnormal, abnormality
      fetus (suspected) 655.9 ☑
        specified NEC 655.8 ☑
      placenta 656.7 ☑
    advanced maternal age NEC 659.6 ☑
      multigravida 659.6 ☑
      primigravida 659.5 ☑
    antibodies (maternal)
      anti-c 656.1 ☑
      anti-d 656.1 ☑
      anti-e 656.1 ☑
      blood group (ABO) 656.2 ☑
        Rh(esus) 656.1 ☑
    appendicitis 648.9 ☑
    bariatric surgery status 649.2 ☑
    coagulation defect 649.3 ☑
    elderly multigravida 659.6 ☑
    elderly primigravida 659.5 ☑
    epilepsy 649.4 ☑
    fetal (suspected)
      abnormality 655.9 ☑
        abdominal 655.8 ☑
        acid-base balance 656.8 ☑
        cardiovascular 655.8 ☑
        facial 655.8 ☑
        gastrointestinal 655.8 ☑
        gentourinary 655.8 ☑
        heart rate or rhythm 659.7 ☑
        limb 655.8 ☑
        specified NEC 655.8 ☑
      acidemia 656.3 ☑
      anencephaly 655.0 ☑
      aneuploidy 655.1 ☑
      bradycardia 659.7 ☑

☑ Additional Digit Required — Refer to the Tabular List for Digit Selection   🔆 Subterms under main terms may continue to next column or page

2011 ICD-9-CM   ▶◀ Revised Text   ● New Line   ▲ Revised Code   October 2010 • Volume 2 — 235

Pregnancy — *continued*
  management affected by — *continued*
    fetal — *continued*
      central nervous system malformation 655.0 ☑
      chromosomal abnormalities (conditions classifiable to 758.0–758.9) 655.1 ☑
      damage from
        drugs 655.5 ☑
          obstetric, anesthetic, or sedative 655.5 ☑
        environmental toxins 655.8 ☑
        intrauterine contraceptive device 655.8 ☑
        maternal
          alcohol addiction 655.4 ☑
          disease NEC 655.4 ☑
          drug use 655.5 ☑
          listeriosis 655.4 ☑
          rubella 655.3 ☑
          toxoplasmosis 655.4 ☑
          viral infection 655.3 ☑
        radiation 655.6 ☑
      death (near term) 656.4 ☑
        early (before 22 completed weeks' gestation) 632
      distress 656.8 ☑
      excessive growth 656.6 ☑
      fetal-maternal hemorrhage 656.0 ☑
      growth retardation 656.5 ☑
      hereditary disease 655.2 ☑
      hereditary disease in family (possibly) affecting fetus 655.2 ☑
      hydrocephalus 655.0 ☑
      incompatibility, blood groups (ABO) 656.2 ☑
      intrauterine death 656.4 ☑
      poor growth 656.5 ☑
      Rh(esus) 656.1 ☑
      spina bifida (with myelomeningocele) 655.0 ☑
    gastric banding status 649.2 ☑
    gastric bypass status for obesity 649.2 ☑
    insufficient prenatal care V23.7
    intrauterine death 656.4 ☑
    isoimmunization (ABO) 656.2 ☑
      Rh(esus) 656.1 ☑
    large-for-dates fetus 656.6 ☑
    light-for-dates fetus 656.5 ☑
    meconium in liquor 656.8 ☑
    mental disorder (conditions classifiable to 290–303, 305.0, 305.2–305.9, 306–316, 317–319) 648.4 ☑
    multiparity (grand) 659.4 ☑
    obesity 649.1 ☑
      surgery status 649.2 ☑
    poor obstetric history V23.49
      pre-term labor V23.41
    postmaturity
      post-term 645.1 ☑
      prolonged 645.2 ☑
    post-term pregnancy 645.1 ☑
    previous
      abortion V23.2
        habitual 646.3 ☑
      cesarean delivery 654.2 ☑
      difficult delivery V23.49
      forceps delivery V23.49
      habitual abortions 646.3 ☑
      hemorrhage, antepartum or postpartum V23.49
      hydatidiform mole V23.1
      infertility V23.0
      in utero procedure during previous pregnancy V23.86
      malignancy NEC V23.89
      nonobstetrical conditions V23.8
      premature delivery V23.41
      recurrent pregnancy loss 646.3 ☑ ●
      trophoblastic disease (conditions in 630) V23.1
      vesicular mole V23.1
    prolonged pregnancy 645.2 ☑

Pregnancy — *continued*
  management affected by — *continued*
    recurrent pregnancy loss 646.3 ☑ ●
    small-for-dates fetus 656.5 ☑
    smoking 649.0 ☑
    spotting 649.5 ☑
    suspected conditions not found
      amniotic cavity and membrane problem V89.01
      cervical shortening V89.05
      fetal anomaly V89.03
      fetal growth problem V89.04
      oligohydramnios V89.01
      other specified problem NEC V89.09
      placental problem V89.02
      polyhydramnios V89.01
    tobacco use disorder 649.0 ☑
    venous complication 671.9 ☑
    young maternal age 659.8 ☑
  maternal death NEC 646.9 ☑
  mesometric (mural) — *see* Pregnancy, cornual
  molar 631
    hydatidiform (*see also* Hydatidiform mole) 630
    previous, affecting management of pregnancy V23.1
    previous, affecting management of pregnancy V23.49
  multiple NEC 651.9 ☑
    with fetal loss and retention of one or more fetus(es) 651.6 ☑
    affecting fetus or newborn 761.5
    following (elective) fetal reduction 651.7 ☑
    specified type NEC 651.8 ☑
      with fetal loss and retention of one or more fetus(es) 651.6 ☑
      following (elective) fetal reduction 651.7 ☑
  mural — *see* Pregnancy, cornual
  observation NEC V22.1
    first pregnancy V22.0
    high-risk V23.9
      specified problem NEC V23.89
  ovarian 633.20
    with intrauterine pregnancy 633.21
    affecting fetus or newborn 761.4
  possible, not (yet) confirmed V72.40
  postmature
    post-term 645.1 ☑
    prolonged 645.2 ☑
  post-term 645.1 ☑
  prenatal care only V22.1
    first pregnancy V22.0
    high-risk V23.9
      specified problem NEC V23.89
  prolonged 645.2 ☑
  quadruplet NEC 651.2 ☑
    with fetal loss and retention of one or more fetus(es) 651.5 ☑
    affecting fetus or newborn 761.5
    following (elective) fetal reduction 651.7 ☑
  quintuplet NEC 651.8 ☑
    with fetal loss and retention of one or more fetus(es) 651.6 ☑
    affecting fetus or newborn 761.5
    following (elective) fetal reduction 651.7 ☑
  resulting from
    assisted reproductive technology V23.85
    in vitro fertilization V23.85
  sextuplet NEC 651.8 ☑
    with fetal loss and retention of one or more fetus(es) 651.6 ☑
    affecting fetus or newborn 761.5
    following (elective) fetal reduction 651.7 ☑
  spurious 300.11
  superfecundation NEC 651.9 ☑
    with fetal loss and retention of one or more fetus(es) 651.6 ☑
    following (elective) fetal reduction 651.7 ☑

Pregnancy — *continued*
  superfetation NEC 651.9 ☑
    with fetal loss and retention of one or more fetus(es) 651.6 ☑
    following (elective) fetal reduction 651.7 ☑
  supervision (of) (for) (*see also* Pregnancy, management affected by)
    elderly
      multigravida V23.82
      primigravida V23.81
    high-risk V23.9
      insufficient prenatal care V23.7
      specified problem NEC V23.89
    multiparity V23.3
    normal NEC V22.1
      first V22.0
    poor
      obstetric history V23.49
        pre-term labor V23.41
      reproductive history V23.5
    previous
      abortion V23.2
      hydatidiform mole V23.1
      infertility V23.0
      neonatal death V23.5
      stillbirth V23.5
      trophoblastic disease V23.1
      vesicular mole V23.1
    specified problem NEC V23.89
    young
      multigravida V23.84
      primigravida V23.83
  triplet NEC 651.1 ☑
    with fetal loss and retention of one or more fetus(es) 651.4 ☑
    affecting fetus or newborn 761.5
    following (elective) fetal reduction 651.7 ☑
  tubal (with rupture) 633.10
    with intrauterine pregnancy 633.11
    affecting fetus or newborn 761.4
  twin NEC 651.0 ☑
    with fetal loss and retention of one fetus 651.3 ☑
    affecting fetus or newborn 761.5
    conjoined 678.1 ☑
    following (elective) fetal reduction 651.7 ☑
  unconfirmed V72.40
  undelivered (no other diagnosis) V22.2
    with false labor 644.1 ☑
    high-risk V23.9
      specified problem NEC V23.89
  unwanted NEC V61.7
Pregnant uterus — *see* condition
Preiser's disease (osteoporosis) 733.09
Prekwashiorkor 260
Preleukemia 238.75
Preluxation of hip, congenital — *see also* Subluxation, congenital, hip 754.32
Premature — *see also* condition
  beats (nodal) 427.60
    atrial 427.61
    auricular 427.61
    postoperative 997.1
    specified type NEC 427.69
    supraventricular 427.61
    ventricular 427.69
  birth NEC 765.1 ☑
  closure
    cranial suture 756.0
    fontanel 756.0
    foramen ovale 745.8
  contractions 427.60
    atrial 427.61
    auricular 427.61
    auriculoventricular 427.61
    heart (extrasystole) 427.60
    junctional 427.60
    nodal 427.60
    postoperative 997.1
    ventricular 427.69
  ejaculation 302.75
  infant NEC 765.1 ☑
    excessive 765.0 ☑

Premature — *see also* condition — *continued*
  infant — *continued*
    light-for-dates — *see* Light-for-dates
  labor 644.2 ☑
    threatened 644.0 ☑
  lungs 770.4
  menopause 256.31
  puberty 259.1
  rupture of membranes or amnion 658.1 ☑
    affecting fetus or newborn 761.1
    delayed delivery following 658.2 ☑
  senility (syndrome) 259.8
  separation, placenta (partial) — *see* Placenta, separation
  ventricular systole 427.69
Prematurity NEC 765.1 ☑
  extreme 765.0 ☑
Premenstrual syndrome 625.4
Premenstrual tension 625.4
Premolarization, cuspids 520.2
Premyeloma 273.1
Prenatal
  care, normal pregnancy V22.1
    first V22.0
  death, cause unknown — *see* Death, fetus
  screening — *see* Antenatal, screening
  teeth 520.6
Prepartum — *see* condition
Preponderance, left or right ventricular 429.3
Prepuce — *see* condition
PRES (posterior reversible encephalopathy syndrome) 348.39
Presbycardia 797
  hypertensive (*see also* Hypertension, heart) 402.90
Presbycusis 388.01
Presbyesophagus 530.89
Presbyophrenia 310.1
Presbyopia 367.4
Prescription of contraceptives NEC V25.02
  diaphragm V25.02
  oral (pill) V25.01
    emergency V25.03
    postcoital V25.03
    repeat V25.41
  repeat V25.40
    oral (pill) V25.41
Presenile — *see also* condition
  aging 259.8
  dementia (*see also* Dementia, presenile) 290.10
Presenility 259.8
Presentation, fetal
  abnormal 652.9 ☑
    with successful version 652.1 ☑
    before labor, affecting fetus or newborn 761.7
    causing obstructed labor 660.0 ☑
      affecting fetus or newborn, any, except breech 763.1
    in multiple gestation (one or more) 652.6 ☑
    specified NEC 652.8 ☑
  arm 652.7 ☑
    causing obstructed labor 660.0 ☑
  breech (buttocks) (complete) (frank) 652.2 ☑
    with successful version 652.1 ☑
      before labor, affecting fetus or newborn 761.7
    before labor, affecting fetus or newborn 761.7
  brow 652.4 ☑
    causing obstructed labor 660.0 ☑
  buttocks 652.2 ☑
  chin 652.4 ☑
  complete 652.2 ☑
  compound 652.8 ☑
  cord 663.0 ☑
  extended head 652.4 ☑
  face 652.4 ☑
    to pubes 652.8 ☑
  footling 652.8 ☑

☑ Additional Digit Required — Refer to the Tabular List for Digit Selection   ▽ Subterms under main terms may continue to next column or page

236 — Volume 2 · October 2010   ►◄ Revised Text   ● New Line   ▲ Revised Code   2011 ICD-9-CM

Index

Pregnancy — Presentation, fetal

Presentation, fetal — *continued*
  frank 652.2 ☑
  hand, leg, or foot NEC 652.8 ☑
  incomplete 652.8 ☑
  mentum 652.4 ☑
  multiple gestation (one fetus or more) 652.6 ☑
  oblique 652.3 ☑
    with successful version 652.1 ☑
  shoulder 652.8 ☑
    affecting fetus or newborn 763.1
  transverse 652.3 ☑
    with successful version 652.1 ☑
  umbilical cord 663.0 ☑
  unstable 652.0 ☑
Prespondylolisthesis (congenital) (lumbosacral) 756.11
Pressure
  area, skin ulcer (*see also* Ulcer, pressure) 707.00
  atrophy, spine 733.99
  birth, fetus or newborn NEC 767.9
  brachial plexus 353.0
  brain 348.4
    injury at birth 767.0
  cerebral — *see* Pressure, brain
  chest 786.59
  cone, tentorial 348.4
    injury at birth 767.0
  funis — *see* Compression, umbilical cord
  hyposystolic (*see also* Hypotension) 458.9
  increased
    intracranial 781.99
      due to
        benign intracranial hypertension 348.2
        hydrocephalus — *see* hydrocephalus
        injury at birth 767.8
    intraocular 365.00
  lumbosacral plexus 353.1
  mediastinum 519.3
  necrosis (chronic) (skin) (*see also* Decubitus) 707.00
  nerve — *see* Compression, nerve
  paralysis (*see also* Neuropathy, entrapment) 355.9
  pre-ulcer skin changes limited to persistent focal erythema (*see also* Ulcer, pressure) 707.21
  sore (chronic) (*see also* Ulcer, pressure) 707.00
  spinal cord 336.9
  ulcer (chronic) (*see also* Ulcer, pressure) 707.00
  umbilical cord — *see* Compression, umbilical cord
  venous, increased 459.89
Pre-syncope 780.2
Preterm infant NEC 765.1 ☑
  extreme 765.0 ☑
Priapism (penis) 607.3
Prickling sensation — *see also* Disturbance, sensation 782.0
Prickly heat 705.1
Primary — *see* condition
Primigravida, elderly
  affecting
    fetus or newborn 763.89
    management of pregnancy, labor, and delivery 659.5 ☑
Primipara, old
  affecting
    fetus or newborn 763.89
    management of pregnancy, labor, and delivery 659.5 ☑
Primula dermatitis 692.6
Primus varus (bilateral) (metatarsus) 754.52
PRIND (prolonged reversible ischemic neurologic deficit) 434.91
  history of (personal) V12.54
Pringle's disease (tuberous sclerosis) 759.5
Prinzmetal's angina 413.1
Prinzmetal-Massumi syndrome (anterior chest wall) 786.52
Prizefighter ear 738.7

Problem (with) V49.9
  academic V62.3
  acculturation V62.4
  adopted child V61.24
  aged
    in-law V61.3
    parent V61.3
    person NEC V61.8
  alcoholism in family V61.41
  anger reaction (*see also* Disturbance, conduct) 312.0 ☑
  behavioral V40.9
    specified NEC V40.3
  behavior, child 312.9
  betting V69.3
  biological child V61.23
  cardiorespiratory NEC V47.2
  career choice V62.29
  care of sick or handicapped person in family or household V61.49
  communication V40.1
  conscience regarding medical care V62.6
  delinquency (juvenile) 312.9
  diet, inappropriate V69.1
  digestive NEC V47.3
  ear NEC V41.3
  eating habits, inappropriate V69.1
  economic V60.2
    affecting care V60.9
      specified type NEC V60.89
  educational V62.3
  enuresis, child 307.6
  exercise, lack of V69.0
  eye NEC V41.1
  family V61.9
    specified circumstance NEC V61.8
  fear reaction, child 313.0
  feeding (elderly) (infant) 783.3
    newborn 779.31
    nonorganic 307.59
  fetal, affecting management of pregnancy 656.9 ☑
    specified type NEC 656.8 ☑
  financial V60.2
  foster child V61.25
  functional V41.9
    specified type NEC V41.8
  gambling V69.3
  genital NEC V47.5
  head V48.9
    deficiency V48.0
    disfigurement V48.6
    mechanical V48.2
    motor V48.2
    movement of V48.2
    sensory V48.4
    specified condition NEC V48.8
  hearing V41.2
  high-risk sexual behavior V69.2
  identity 313.82
  influencing health status NEC V49.89
  internal organ NEC V47.9
    deficiency V47.0
    mechanical or motor V47.1
  interpersonal NEC V62.81
  jealousy, child 313.3
  learning V40.0
  legal V62.5
  life circumstance NEC V62.89
  lifestyle V69.9
    specified NEC V69.8
  limb V49.9
    deficiency V49.0
    disfigurement V49.4
    mechanical V49.1
    motor V49.2
    movement, involving
      musculoskeletal system V49.1
      nervous system V49.2
    sensory V49.3
    specified condition NEC V49.5
  litigation V62.5
  living alone V60.3
  loneliness NEC V62.89
  marital V61.10

Problem — *continued*
  marital — *continued*
    involving
      divorce V61.03
      estrangement V61.09
      psychosexual disorder 302.9
      sexual function V41.7
    relationship V61.10
  mastication V41.6
  medical care, within family V61.49
  mental V40.9
    specified NEC V40.2
  mental hygiene, adult V40.9
  multiparity V61.5
  nail biting, child 307.9
  neck V48.9
    deficiency V48.1
    disfigurement V48.7
    mechanical V48.3
    motor V48.3
    movement V48.3
    sensory V48.5
    specified condition NEC V48.8
  neurological NEC 781.99
  none (feared complaint unfounded) V65.5
  occupational V62.29
  parent-child V61.20
    adopted child V61.24
    biological child V61.23
    foster child V61.25
    relationship V61.20
  partner V61.10
    relationship V61.10
  personal NEC V62.89
    interpersonal conflict NEC V62.81
  personality (*see also* Disorder, personality) 301.9
  phase of life V62.89
  placenta, affecting management of pregnancy 656.9 ☑
    specified type NEC 656.8 ☑
  poverty V60.2
  presence of sick or handicapped person in family or household V61.49
  psychiatric 300.9
  psychosocial V62.9
    specified type NEC V62.89
  relational NEC V62.81
  relationship, childhood 313.3
  religious or spiritual belief
    other than medical care V62.89
    regarding medical care V62.6
  self-damaging behavior V69.8
  sexual
    behavior, high-risk V69.2
    function NEC V41.7
  sibling
    relational V61.8
    relationship V61.8
  sight V41.0
  sleep disorder, child 307.40
  sleep, lack of V69.4
  smell V41.5
  speech V40.1
  spite reaction, child (*see also* Disturbance, conduct) 312.0 ☑
  spoiled child reaction (*see also* Disturbance, conduct) 312.1 ☑
  substance abuse in family V61.42
  swallowing V41.6
  tantrum, child (*see also* Disturbance, conduct) 312.1 ☑
  taste V41.5
  thumb sucking, child 307.9
  tic (child) 307.21
  trunk V48.9
    deficiency V48.1
    disfigurement V48.7
    mechanical V48.3
    motor V48.3
    movement V48.3
    sensory V48.5
    specified condition NEC V48.8
  unemployment V62.0
  urinary NEC V47.4
  voice production V41.4

Procedure (surgical) **not done** NEC V64.3
  because of
    contraindication V64.1
    patient's decision V64.2
      for reasons of conscience or religion V62.6
    specified reason NEC V64.3
Procidentia
  anus (sphincter) 569.1
  rectum (sphincter) 569.1
  stomach 537.89
  uteri 618.1
Proctalgia 569.42
  fugax 564.6
  spasmodic 564.6
    psychogenic 307.89
Proctitis 569.49
  amebic 006.8
  chlamydial 099.52
  gonococcal 098.7
  granulomatous 555.1
  idiopathic 556.2
    with ulcerative sigmoiditis 556.3
  tuberculous (*see also* Tuberculosis) 014.8 ☑
  ulcerative (chronic) (nonspecific) 556.2
    with ulcerative sigmoiditis 556.3
Proctocele
  female (without uterine prolapse) 618.04
    with uterine prolapse 618.4
      complete 618.3
      incomplete 618.2
  male 569.49
Proctocolitis, idiopathic 556.2
  with ulcerative sigmoiditis 556.3
Proctoptosis 569.1
Proctosigmoiditis 569.89
  ulcerative (chronic) 556.3
Proctospasm 564.6
  psychogenic 306.4
Prodromal-AIDS — *see* Human immunodeficiency virus (disease) (illness) (infection)
Profichet's disease or syndrome 729.90
Progeria (adultorum) (syndrome) 259.8
Prognathism (mandibular) (maxillary) 524.00
Progonoma (melanotic) (M9363/0) — *see* Neoplasm, by site, benign
Progressive — *see* condition
Prolapse, prolapsed
  anus, anal (canal) (sphincter) 569.1
  arm or hand, complicating delivery 652.7 ☑
    causing obstructed labor 660.0 ☑
      affecting fetus or newborn 763.1
    fetus or newborn 763.1
  bladder (acquired) (mucosa) (sphincter)
    congenital (female) (male) 756.71
    female (*see also* Cystocele, female) 618.01
    male 596.8
  breast implant (prosthetic) 996.54
  cecostomy 569.69
  cecum 569.89
  cervix, cervical (hypertrophied) 618.1
    anterior lip, obstructing labor 660.2 ☑
      affecting fetus or newborn 763.1
    congenital 752.49
    postpartal (old) 618.1
    stump 618.84
  ciliary body 871.1
  colon (pedunculated) 569.89
  colostomy 569.69
  conjunctiva 372.73
  cord — *see* Prolapse, umbilical cord
  disc (intervertebral) — *see* Displacement, intervertebral disc
  duodenum 537.89
  eye implant (orbital) 996.59
    lens (ocular) 996.53
  fallopian tube 620.4
  fetal extremity, complicating delivery 652.8 ☑
    causing obstructed labor 660.0 ☑
    fetus or newborn 763.1
  funis — *see* Prolapse, umbilical cord
  gastric (mucosa) 537.89
  genital, female 618.9
    specified NEC 618.89

☑ Additional Digit Required — Refer to the Tabular List for Digit Selection   ⟰ Subterms under main terms may continue to next column or page

2011 ICD-9-CM   ▶◀ Revised Text   ● New Line   ▲ Revised Code   Volume 2 — 237

Prolapse, prolapsed — continued
  globe 360.81
  ileostomy bud 569.69
  intervertebral disc — see Displacement, in-
     tervertebral disc
  intestine (small) 569.89
  iris 364.89
    traumatic 871.1
  kidney (see also Disease, renal) 593.0
    congenital 753.3
  laryngeal muscles or ventricle 478.79
  leg, complicating delivery 652.8 ☑
    causing obstructed labor 660.0 ☑
    fetus or newborn 763.1
  liver 573.8
  meatus urinarius 599.5
  mitral valve 424.0
  ocular lens implant 996.53
  organ or site, congenital NEC — see Malpo-
    sition, congenital
  ovary 620.4
  pelvic (floor), female 618.89
  perineum, female 618.89
  pregnant uterus 654.4 ☑
  rectum (mucosa) (sphincter) 569.1
    due to Trichuris trichiuria 127.3
  spleen 289.59
  stomach 537.89
  umbilical cord
    affecting fetus or newborn 762.4
    complicating delivery 663.0 ☑
  ureter 593.89
    with obstruction 593.4
  ureterovesical orifice 593.89
  urethra (acquired) (infected) (mucosa) 599.5
    congenital 753.8
  uterovaginal 618.4
    complete 618.3
    incomplete 618.2
    specified NEC 618.89
  uterus (first degree) (second degree) (third
    degree) (complete) (without vaginal
    wall prolapse) 618.1
    with mention of vaginal wall prolapse
     — see Prolapse, uterovaginal
    congenital 752.39   ▲
    in pregnancy or childbirth 654.4 ☑
     affecting fetus or newborn 763.1
     causing obstructed labor 660.2 ☑
      affecting fetus or newborn 763.1
    postpartal (old) 618.1
  uveal 871.1
  vagina (anterior) (posterior) (vault) (wall)
    (without uterine prolapse) 618.00
    with uterine prolapse 618.4
     complete 618.3
     incomplete 618.2
    paravaginal 618.02
    posthysterectomy 618.5
    specified NEC 618.09
  vitreous (humor) 379.26
    traumatic 871.1
  womb — see Prolapse, uterus
Prolapsus, female 618.9
Proliferative — see condition
Prolinemia 270.8
Prolinuria 270.8
Prolonged, prolongation
  bleeding time (see also Defect, coagulation)
    790.92
    "idiopathic" (in von Willebrand's disease)
     286.4
  coagulation time (see also Defect, coagula-
    tion) 790.92
  gestation syndrome 766.22
  labor 662.1 ☑
    affecting fetus or newborn 763.89
    first stage 662.0 ☑
    second stage 662.2 ☑
  pregnancy 645.2 ☑
  PR interval 426.11
  prothrombin time (see also Defect, coagula-
    tion) 790.92
  QT interval 794.31
    syndrome 426.82

Prolonged, prolongation — continued
  rupture of membranes (24 hours or more
    prior to onset of labor) 658.2 ☑
  uterine contractions in labor 661.4 ☑
    affecting fetus or newborn 763.7
Prominauris 744.29
Prominence
  auricle (ear) (congenital) 744.29
    acquired 380.32
  ischial spine or sacral promontory
    with disproportion (fetopelvic) 653.3 ☑
     affecting fetus or newborn 763.1
     causing obstructed labor 660.1 ☑
      affecting fetus or newborn 763.1
  nose (congenital) 748.1
    acquired 738.0
PROMM (proximal myotonic myotonia) 359.21
Pronation
  ankle 736.79
  foot 736.79
    congenital 755.67
Prophylactic
  administration of
    antibiotics, ▶long-term◀ V58.62
     short-term — omit code   ●
    antitoxin, any V07.2
    antivenin V07.2
    chemotherapeutic agent NEC V07.39
     fluoride V07.31
    diphtheria antitoxin V07.2
    drug V07.39
    exemestar (Aromasin) V07.52
    gamma globulin V07.2
    immune sera (gamma globulin) V07.2
    RhoGAM V07.2
    tetanus antitoxin V07.2
  chemotherapy NEC V07.39
    fluoride V07.31
  hormone replacement (postmenopausal)
    V07.4
  immunotherapy V07.2
  measure V07.9
    specified type NEC V07.8
  medication V07.39
  postmenopausal hormone replacement
    V07.4
  sterilization V25.2
Proptosis (ocular) — see also Exophthalmos
  376.30
  thyroid 242.0 ☑
Propulsion
  eyeball 360.81
Prosecution, anxiety concerning V62.5
Prosopagnosia 368.16
Prostate, prostatic — see condition
Prostatism 600.90
  with
    other lower urinary tract symptoms
     (LUTS) 600.91
    urinary
     obstruction 600.91
     retention 600.91
Prostatitis (congestive) (suppurative) 601.9
  acute 601.0
  cavitary 601.8
  chlamydial 099.54
  chronic 601.1
  diverticular 601.8
  due to Trichomonas (vaginalis) 131.03
  fibrous 600.90
    with
     other lower urinary tract symptoms
      (LUTS) 600.91
     urinary
      obstruction 600.91
      retention 600.91
  gonococcal (acute) 098.12
    chronic or duration of 2 months or over
     098.32
  granulomatous 601.8
  hypertrophic 600.00
    with
     other lower urinary tract symptoms
      (LUTS) 600.01
     urinary
      obstruction 600.01

Prostatitis — continued
  hypertrophic — continued
    with — continued
     urinary — continued
      retention 600.01
  specified type NEC 601.8
  subacute 601.1
  trichomonal 131.03
  tuberculous (see also Tuberculosis)
    016.5 ☑ [601.4]
Prostatocystitis 601.3
Prostatorrhea 602.8
Prostatoseminovesiculitis, trichomonal
  131.03
Prostration 780.79
  heat 992.5
    anhydrotic 992.3
    due to
     salt (and water) depletion 992.4
     water depletion 992.3
  nervous 300.5
  newborn 779.89
  senile 797
Protanomaly 368.51
Protanopia (anomalous trichromat) (complete)
  (incomplete) 368.51
Protection (against) (from) — see Prophylactic
Protein
  deficiency 260
  malnutrition 260
  sickness (prophylactic) (therapeutic) 999.5
Proteinemia 790.99
Proteinosis
  alveolar, lung or pulmonary 516.0
  lipid 272.8
  lipoid (of Urbach) 272.8
Proteinuria — see also Albuminuria 791.0
  Bence-Jones NEC 791.0
  gestational 646.2 ☑
    with hypertension — see Toxemia, of
     pregnancy
  orthostatic 593.6
  postural 593.6
Proteolysis, pathologic 286.6
Protocoproporphyria 277.1
Protoporphyria (erythrohepatic) (erythropoietic) 277.1
Protrusio acetabuli 718.65
Protrusion
  acetabulum (into pelvis) 718.65
  device, implant, or graft — see Complica-
    tions, mechanical
  ear, congenital 744.29
  intervertebral disc — see Displacement, in-
    tervertebral disc
  nucleus pulposus — see Displacement, in-
    tervertebral disc
Proud flesh 701.5
Prune belly (syndrome) 756.71
Prurigo (ferox) (gravis) (Hebra's) (hebrae) (mi-
  tis) (simplex) 698.2
  agria 698.3
  asthma syndrome 691.8
  Besnier's (atopic dermatitis) (infantile
    eczema) 691.8
  eczematodes allergicum 691.8
  estivalis (Hutchinson's) 692.72
  Hutchinson's 692.72
  nodularis 698.3
  psychogenic 306.3
Pruritus, pruritic 698.9
  ani 698.0
    psychogenic 306.3
  conditions NEC 698.9
    psychogenic 306.3
  due to Onchocerca volvulus 125.3
  ear 698.9
  essential 698.9
  genital organ(s) 698.1
    psychogenic 306.3
  gravidarum 646.8 ☑
  hiemalis 698.8
  neurogenic (any site) 306.3
  perianal 698.0
  psychogenic (any site) 306.3
  scrotum 698.1

Pruritus, pruritic — continued
  scrotum — continued
    psychogenic 306.3
  senile, senilis 698.8
  Trichomonas 131.9
  vulva, vulvae 698.1
    psychogenic 306.3
Psammocarcinoma (M8140/3) — see Neo-
  plasm, by site, malignant
Pseudarthrosis, pseudoarthrosis (bone)
  733.82
  joint following fusion V45.4
Pseudoacanthosis
  nigricans 701.8
Pseudoaneurysm — see Aneurysm
Pseudoangina (pectoris) — see Angina
Pseudoangioma 452
Pseudo-Argyll-Robertson pupil 379.45
Pseudoarteriosus 747.89
Pseudoarthrosis — see Pseudarthrosis
Pseudoataxia 799.89
Pseudobulbar affect (PBA) 310.8
Pseudobursa 727.89
Pseudocholera 025
Pseudochromidrosis 705.89
Pseudocirrhosis, liver, pericardial 423.2
Pseudocoarctation 747.21
Pseudocowpox 051.1
Pseudocoxalgia 732.1
Pseudocroup 478.75
Pseudocyesis 300.11
Pseudocyst
  lung 518.89
  pancreas 577.2
  retina 361.19
Pseudodementia 300.16
Pseudoelephantiasis neuroarthritica 757.0
Pseudoemphysema 518.89
Pseudoencephalitis
  superior (acute) hemorrhagic 265.1
Pseudoerosion cervix, congenital 752.49
Pseudoexfoliation, lens capsule 366.11
Pseudofracture (idiopathic) (multiple) (spon-
  taneous) (symmetrical) 268.2
Pseudoglanders 025
Pseudoglioma 360.44
Pseudogout — see Chondrocalcinosis
Pseudohallucination 780.1
Pseudohemianesthesia 782.0
Pseudohemophilia (Bernuth's) (hereditary)
  (typeB) 286.4
  type A 287.8
  vascular 287.8
Pseudohermaphroditism 752.7
  with chromosomal anomaly — see Anoma-
    ly, chromosomal
  adrenal 255.2
  female (without adrenocortical disorder)
    752.7
    with adrenocortical disorder 255.2
    adrenal 255.2
  male (without gonadal disorder) 752.7
    with
     adrenocortical disorder 255.2
     cleft scrotum 752.7
     feminizing testis 259.51
     gonadal disorder 257.9
    adrenal 255.2
Pseudohole, macula 362.54
Pseudo-Hurler's disease (mucolipidosis III)
  272.7
Pseudohydrocephalus 348.2
Pseudohypertrophic muscular dystrophy
  (Erb's) 359.1
Pseudohypertrophy, muscle 359.1
Pseudohypoparathyroidism 275.49
Pseudoinfluenza ▶— see also Influenza◀
  487.1
Pseudoinsomnia 307.49
Pseudoleukemia 288.8
  infantile 285.8
Pseudomembranous — see condition
Pseudomeningocele (cerebral) (infective)
  349.2
  postprocedural 997.01
  spinal 349.2

☑ Additional Digit Required — Refer to the Tabular List for Digit Selection   ☞ Subterms under main terms may continue to next column or page

Pseudomenstruation 626.8
Pseudomucinous
  cyst (ovary) (M8470/0) 220
  peritoneum 568.89
Pseudomyeloma 273.1
Pseudomyxoma peritonei (M8480/6) 197.6
Pseudoneuritis optic (nerve) 377.24
  papilla 377.24
    congenital 743.57
Pseudoneuroma — *see* Injury, nerve, by site
Pseudo-obstruction
  intestine (chronic) (idiopathic) (intermittent
    secondary) (primary) 564.89
    acute 560.89
Pseudopapilledema 377.24
Pseudoparalysis
  arm or leg 781.4
  atonic, congenital 358.8
Pseudopelade 704.09
Pseudophakia V43.1
Pseudopolycythemia 289.0
Pseudopolyposis, colon 556.4
Pseudoporencephaly 348.0
Pseudopseudohypoparathyroidism 275.49
Pseudopsychosis 300.16
Pseudopterygium 372.52
Pseudoptosis (eyelid) 374.34
Pseudorabies 078.89
Pseudoretinitis, pigmentosa 362.65
Pseudorickets 588.0
  senile (Pozzi's) 731.0
Pseudorubella 057.8
Pseudoscarlatina 057.8
Pseudosclerema 778.1
Pseudosclerosis (brain)
  Jakob's 046.19
  of Westphal (-Strümpell) (hepatolenticular
    degeneration) 275.1
  spastic 046.19
    with dementia
      with behavioral disturbance
        046.19 *[294.11]*
      without behavioral disturbance
        046.19 *[294.10]*
Pseudoseizure 780.39
  non-psychiatric 780.39
  psychiatric 300.11
Pseudotabes 799.89
  diabetic 250.6 ☑ *[337.1]*
    due to secondary diabetes
      249.6 ☑ *[337.1]*
Pseudotetanus — *see also* Convulsions 780.39
Pseudotetany 781.7
  hysterical 300.11
Pseudothalassemia 285.0
Pseudotrichinosis 710.3
Pseudotruncus arteriosus 747.29
Pseudotuberculosis, pasteurella (infection)
  027.2
Pseudotumor
  cerebri 348.2
  orbit (inflammatory) 376.11
Pseudo-Turner's syndrome 759.89
Pseudoxanthoma elasticum 757.39
Psilosis (sprue) (tropical) 579.1
  Monilia 112.89
  nontropical 579.0
  not sprue 704.00
Psittacosis 073.9
Psoitis 728.89
Psora NEC 696.1
Psoriasis 696.1
  any type, except arthropathic 696.1
  arthritic, arthropathic 696.0
  buccal 528.6
  flexural 696.1
  follicularis 696.1
  guttate 696.1
  inverse 696.1
  mouth 528.6
  nummularis 696.1
  psychogenic 316 *[696.1]*
  punctata 696.1
  pustular 696.1
  rupioides 696.1
  vulgaris 696.1

Psorospermiasis 136.4
Psorospermosis 136.4
  follicularis (vegetans) 757.39
Psychalgia 307.80
Psychasthenia 300.89
  compulsive 300.3
  mixed compulsive states 300.3
  obsession 300.3
Psychiatric disorder or problem NEC 300.9
Psychogenic — *see also* condition
  factors associated with physical conditions
    316
Psychoneurosis, psychoneurotic — *see also*
  Neurosis 300.9
  anxiety (state) 300.00
  climacteric 627.2
  compensation 300.16
  compulsion 300.3
  conversion hysteria 300.11
  depersonalization 300.6
  depressive type 300.4
  dissociative hysteria 300.15
  hypochondriacal 300.7
  hysteria 300.10
    conversion type 300.11
    dissociative type 300.15
  mixed NEC 300.89
  neurasthenic 300.5
  obsessional 300.3
  obsessive-compulsive 300.3
  occupational 300.89
  personality NEC 301.89
  phobia 300.20
  senile NEC 300.89
Psychopathic — *see also* condition
  constitution, posttraumatic 310.2
    with psychosis 293.9
  personality 301.9
    amoral trends 301.7
    antisocial trends 301.7
    asocial trends 301.7
    mixed types 301.7
  state 301.9
Psychopathy, sexual — *see also* Deviation,
  sexual 302.9
**Psychophysiologic, psychophysiological
  condition** — *see* Reaction, psychophysiologic
Psychose passionelle 297.8
Psychosexual identity disorder 302.6
  adult-life 302.85
  childhood 302.6
Psychosis 298.9
  acute hysterical 298.1
  affecting management of pregnancy,
    childbirth, or puerperium 648.4 ☑
  affective (*see also* Disorder, mood) 296.90

> *Note* — Use the following fifth-digit
> subclassification with categories
> 296.0–296.6:
>
> 0   unspecified
>
> 1   mild
>
> 2   moderate
>
> 3   severe, without mention of psy-
>   chotic behavior
>
> 4   severe, specified as with psychotic
>   behavior
>
> 5   in partial or unspecified remission
>
> 6   in full remission

    drug-induced 292.84
    due to or associated with physical condi-
      tion 293.83
    involutional 293.83
      recurrent episode 296.3 ☑
      single episode 296.2 ☑
    manic-depressive 296.80
      circular (alternating) 296.7
        currently depressed 296.5 ☑
        currently manic 296.4 ☑
      depressed type 296.2 ☑
        atypical 296.82
        recurrent episode 296.3 ☑

Psychosis — *continued*
  affective (*see also* Disorder, mood) — *contin-
    ued*
    manic-depressive — *continued*
      depressed type — *continued*
        single episode 296.2 ☑
      manic 296.0 ☑
        atypical 296.81
        recurrent episode 296.1 ☑
        single episode 296.0 ☑
      mixed type NEC 296.89
      specified type NEC 296.89
    senile 290.21
    specified type NEC 296.99
  alcoholic 291.9
    with
      anxiety 291.89
      delirium tremens 291.0
      delusions 291.5
      dementia 291.2
      hallucinosis 291.3
      jealousy 291.5
      mood disturbance 291.89
      paranoia 291.5
      persisting amnesia 291.1
      sexual dysfunction 291.89
      sleep disturbance 291.89
    amnestic confabulatory 291.1
    delirium tremens 291.0
    hallucinosis 291.3
    Korsakoff's, Korsakov's, Korsakow's 291.1
    paranoid type 291.5
    pathological intoxication 291.4
    polyneuritic 291.1
    specified type NEC 291.89
  alternating (*see also* Psychosis, manic-depres-
    sive, circular) 296.7
  anergastic (*see also* Psychosis, organic) 294.9
  arteriosclerotic 290.40
    with
      acute confusional state 290.41
      delirium 290.41
      delusions 290.42
      depressed mood 290.43
    depressed type 290.43
    paranoid type 290.42
    simple type 290.40
    uncomplicated 290.40
  atypical 298.9
    depressive 296.82
    manic 296.81
  borderline (schizophrenia) (*see also*
    Schizophrenia) 295.5
    of childhood (*see also* Psychosis, child-
      hood) 299.8 ☑
    prepubertal 299.8 ☑
  brief reactive 298.8
  childhood, with origin specific to 299.9 ☑

> *Note* — Use the following fifth-digit
> subclassification with category 299:
>
> 0   current or active state
>
> 1   residual state

    atypical 299.8 ☑
    specified type NEC 299.8 ☑
  circular (*see also* Psychosis, manic-depres-
    sive, circular) 296.7
  climacteric (*see also* Psychosis, involutional)
    298.8
  confusional 298.9
    acute 293.0
    reactive 298.2
    subacute 293.1
  depressive (*see also* Psychosis, affective)
    296.2 ☑
    atypical 296.82
    involutional 296.2 ☑
      with hypomania (bipolar II) 296.89
      recurrent episode 296.3 ☑
      single episode 296.2 ☑
    psychogenic 298.0
    reactive (emotional stress) (psychologi-
      cal trauma) 298.0
    recurrent episode 296.3 ☑
      with hypomania (bipolar II) 296.89

Psychosis — *continued*
  depressive (*see also* Psychosis, affective) —
    continued
    single episode 296.2 ☑
  disintegrative, childhood (*see also* Psychosis,
    childhood) 299.1 ☑
  drug 292.9
    with
      affective syndrome 292.84
      amnestic syndrome 292.83
      anxiety 292.89
      delirium 292.81
        withdrawal 292.0
      delusions 292.11
      dementia 292.82
      depressive state 292.84
      hallucinations 292.12
      hallucinosis 292.12
      mood disorder 292.84
      mood disturbance 292.84
      organic personality syndrome NEC
        292.89
      sexual dysfunction 292.89
      sleep disturbance 292.89
      withdrawal syndrome (and delirium)
        292.0
    affective syndrome 292.84
    delusions 292.11
    hallucinatory state 292.12
    hallucinosis 292.12
    paranoid state 292.11
    specified type NEC 292.89
    withdrawal syndrome (and delirium)
      292.0
  due to or associated with physical condition
    (*see also* Psychosis, organic) 293.9
  epileptic NEC 294.8
  excitation (psychogenic) (reactive) 298.1
  exhaustive (*see also* Reaction, stress, acute)
    308.9
  hypomanic (*see also* Psychosis, affective)
    296.0 ☑
    recurrent episode 296.1 ☑
    single episode 296.0 ☑
  hysterical 298.8
    acute 298.1
  in
    conditions classified elsewhere
      with
        delusions 293.81
        hallucinations 293.82
    pregnancy, childbirth, or puerperium
      648.4 ☑
  incipient 298.8
    schizophrenic (*see also* Schizophrenia)
      295.5 ☑
  induced 297.3
  infantile (*see also* Psychosis, childhood)
    299.0 ☑
  infective 293.9
    acute 293.0
    subacute 293.1
  interactional (childhood) (*see also* Psychosis,
    childhood) 299.1 ☑
  involutional 298.8
    depressive (*see also* Psychosis, affective)
      296.2 ☑
      recurrent episode 296.3 ☑
      single episode 296.2 ☑
    melancholic 296.2 ☑
      recurrent episode 296.3 ☑
      single episode 296.2 ☑
    paranoid state 297.2
    paraphrenia 297.2
  Korsakoff's, Korakov's, Korsakow's (nonalco-
    holic) 294.0
    alcoholic 291.1
  mania (phase) (*see also* Psychosis, affective)
    296.0 ☑
    recurrent episode 296.1 ☑
    single episode 296.0 ☑
  manic (*see also* Psychosis, affective) 296.0 ☑
    atypical 296.81
    recurrent episode 296.1 ☑
    single episode 296.0 ☑
  manic-depressive 296.80

☑ Additional Digit Required — Refer to the Tabular List for Digit Selection   �om Subterms under main terms may continue to next column or page

2011 ICD-9-CM   ▶◀ Revised Text   ● New Line   ▲ Revised Code   Volume 2 — 239

Psychosis — *continued*
  manic-depressive — *continued*
    circular 296.7
      currently
        depressed 296.5 ☑
        manic 296.4 ☑
      mixed 296.6 ☑
    depressive 296.2 ☑
      recurrent episode 296.3 ☑
        with hypomania (bipolar II)
          296.89
      single episode 296.2 ☑
    hypomanic 296.0 ☑
      recurrent episode 296.1 ☑
      single episode 296.0 ☑
    manic 296.0 ☑
      atypical 296.81
      recurrent episode 296.1 ☑
      single episode 296.0 ☑
    mixed NEC 296.89
    perplexed 296.89
    stuporous 296.89
  menopausal (*see also* Psychosis, involutional) 298.8
  mixed schizophrenic and affective (*see also* Schizophrenia) 295.7 ☑
  multi-infarct (cerebrovascular) (*see also* Psychosis, arteriosclerotic) 290.40
  organic NEC 294.9
    due to or associated with
      addiction
        alcohol (*see also* Psychosis, alcoholic) 291.9
        drug (*see also* Psychosis, drug) 292.9
      alcohol intoxication, acute (*see also* Psychosis, alcoholic) 291.9
      alcoholism (*see also* Psychosis, alcoholic) 291.9
      arteriosclerosis (cerebral) (*see also* Psychosis, arteriosclerotic) 290.40
      cerebrovascular disease
        acute (psychosis) 293.0
        arteriosclerotic (*see also* Psychosis, arteriosclerotic) 290.40
      childbirth — *see* Psychosis, puerperal
      dependence
        alcohol (*see also* Psychosis, alcoholic) 291.9
        drug 292.9
      disease
        alcoholic liver (*see also* Psychosis, alcoholic) 291.9
        brain
          arteriosclerotic (*see also* Psychosis, arteriosclerotic) 290.40
          cerebrovascular
            acute (psychosis) 293.0
            arteriosclerotic (*see also* Psychosis, arteriosclerotic) 290.40
          endocrine or metabolic 293.9
            acute (psychosis) 293.0
            subacute (psychosis) 293.1
          Jakob-Creutzfeldt 046.19
            with behavioral disturbance 046.19 [294.11]
            without behavioral disturbance 046.19 [294.10]
            familial 046.19
            iatrogenic 046.19
            specified NEC 046.19
            sporadic 046.19
            variant 046.11
              with dementia
                with behavioral disturbance 046.11 [294.11]
                without behavioral disturbance 046.11 [294.10]
        liver, alcoholic (*see also* Psychosis, alcoholic) 291.9

Psychosis — *continued*
  organic — *continued*
    due to or associated with — *continued*
      disorder
        cerebrovascular
          acute (psychosis) 293.0
        endocrine or metabolic 293.9
          acute (psychosis) 293.0
          subacute (psychosis) 293.1
      epilepsy
        with behavioral disturbance 345.9 ☑ [294.11]
        without behavioral disturbance 345.9 ☑ [294.10]
        transient (acute) 293.0
      Huntington's chorea
        with behavioral disturbance 333.4 [294.11]
        without behavioral disturbance 333.4 [294.10]
      infection
        brain 293.9
          acute (psychosis) 293.0
          chronic 294.8
          subacute (psychosis) 293.1
        intracranial NEC 293.9
          acute (psychosis) 293.0
          chronic 294.8
          subacute (psychosis) 293.1
      intoxication
        alcoholic (acute) (*see also* Psychosis, alcoholic) 291.9
        pathological 291.4
        drug (*see also* Psychosis, drug) 292.2
      ischemia
        cerebrovascular (generalized) (*see also* Psychosis, arteriosclerotic) 290.40
      Jakob-Creutzfeldt disease (syndrome) 046.19
        with behavioral disturbance 046.19 [294.11]
        without behavioral disturbance 046.19 [294.10]
        variant 046.11
          with dementia
            with behavioral disturbance 046.11 [294.11]
            without behavioral disturbance 046.11 [294.10]
      multiple sclerosis
        with behavioral disturbance 340 [294.11]
        without behavioral disturbance 340 [294.10]
      physical condition NEC 293.9
        with
          delusions 293.81
          hallucinations 293.82
      presenility 290.10
      puerperium — *see* Psychosis, puerperal
      sclerosis, multiple
        with behavioral disturbance 340 [294.11]
        without behavioral disturbance 340 [294.10]
      senility 290.20
      status epilepticus
        with behavioral disturbance 345.3 [294.11]
        without behavioral disturbance 345.3 [294.10]
      trauma
        brain (birth) (from electrical current) (surgical) 293.9
          acute (psychosis) 293.0
          chronic 294.8
          subacute (psychosis) 293.1
          unspecified physical condition 293.9

Psychosis — *continued*
  organic — *continued*
    due to or associated with — *continued*
      trauma — *continued*
        brain — *continued*
          unspecified physical condition — *continued*
            with
              delusion 293.81
              hallucinations 293.82
        infective 293.9
          acute (psychosis) 293.0
          subacute 293.1
        posttraumatic 293.9
          acute 293.0
          subacute 293.1
        specified type NEC 294.8
        transient 293.9
          with
            anxiety 293.84
            delusions 293.81
            depression 293.83
            hallucinations 293.82
          depressive type 293.83
          hallucinatory type 293.82
          paranoid type 293.81
          specified type NEC 293.89
  paranoic 297.1
  paranoid (chronic) 297.9
    alcoholic 291.5
    chronic 297.1
    climacteric 297.2
    involutional 297.2
    menopausal 297.2
    protracted reactive 298.4
    psychogenic 298.4
      acute 298.3
    schizophrenic (*see also* Schizophrenia) 295.3 ☑
    senile 290.20
  paroxysmal 298.9
    senile 290.20
  polyneuritic, alcoholic 291.1
  postoperative 293.9
  postpartum — *see* Psychosis, puerperal
  prepsychotic (*see also* Schizophrenia) 295.5 ☑
  presbyophrenic (type) 290.8
  presenile (*see also* Dementia, presenile) 290.10
  prison 300.16
  psychogenic 298.8
    depressive 298.0
    paranoid 298.4
      acute 298.3
  puerperal
    specified type — *see* categories 295-298 ☑
    unspecified type 293.89
      acute 293.0
      chronic 293.89
      subacute 293.1
  reactive (emotional stress) (psychological trauma) 298.8
    brief 298.8
    confusion 298.2
    depressive 298.0
    excitation 298.1
  schizo-affective (depressed) (excited) (*see also* Schizophrenia) 295.7 ☑
  schizophrenia, schizophrenic (*see also* Schizophrenia) 295.9 ☑
    borderline type 295.5 ☑
      of childhood (*see also* Psychosis, childhood) 299.8 ☑
    catatonic (excited) (withdrawn) 295.2 ☑
    childhood type (*see also* Psychosis, childhood) 299.9 ☑
    hebephrenic 295.1 ☑
    incipient 295.5 ☑
    latent 295.5 ☑
    paranoid 295.3 ☑
    prepsychotic 295.5 ☑
    prodromal 295.5 ☑
    pseudoneurotic 295.5 ☑

Psychosis — *continued*
  schizophrenia, schizophrenic (*see also* Schizophrenia) — *continued*
    pseudopsychopathic 295.5 ☑
    schizophreniform 295.4 ☑
    simple 295.0 ☑
    undifferentiated type 295.9 ☑
  schizophreniform 295.4 ☑
  senile NEC 290.20
    with
      delusional features 290.20
      depressive features 290.21
    depressed type 290.21
    paranoid type 290.20
    simple deterioration 290.20
    specified type — *see* categories 295-298 ☑
  shared 297.3
  situational (reactive) 298.8
  symbiotic (childhood) (*see also* Psychosis, childhood) 299.1 ☑
  toxic (acute) 293.9
Psychotic — *see also* condition 298.9
  episode 298.9
    due to or associated with physical conditions (*see also* Psychosis, organic) 293.9
Pterygium (eye) 372.40
  central 372.43
  colli 744.5
  double 372.44
  peripheral (stationary) 372.41
    progressive 372.42
  recurrent 372.45
Ptilosis 374.55
PTLD (post-transplant lymphoproliferative disorder) 238.77
Ptomaine (poisoning) — *see also* Poisoning, food 005.9
Ptosis (adiposa) 374.30
  breast 611.81
  cecum 569.89
  colon 569.89
  congenital (eyelid) 743.61
    specified site NEC — *see* Anomaly, specified type NEC
  epicanthus syndrome 270.2
  eyelid 374.30
    congenital 743.61
    mechanical 374.33
    myogenic 374.32
    paralytic 374.31
  gastric 537.5
  intestine 569.89
  kidney (*see also* Disease, renal) 593.0
    congenital 753.3
  liver 573.8
  renal (*see also* Disease, renal) 593.0
    congenital 753.3
  splanchnic 569.89
  spleen 289.59
  stomach 537.5
  viscera 569.89
PTP (posttransfusion purpura) 287.41 ●
PTSD (Post-traumatic stress disorder) 309.81
Ptyalism 527.7
  hysterical 300.11
  periodic 527.2
  pregnancy 646.8 ☑
  psychogenic 306.4
Ptyalolithiasis 527.5
Pubalgia 848.8
Pubarche, precocious 259.1
Pubertas praecox 259.1
Puberty V21.1
  abnormal 259.9
  bleeding 626.3
  delayed 259.0
  precocious (constitutional) (cryptogenic) (idiopathic) NEC 259.1
    due to
      adrenal
        cortical hyperfunction 255.2
        hyperplasia 255.2
      cortical hyperfunction 255.2
      ovarian hyperfunction 256.1

☑ Additional Digit Required — Refer to the Tabular List for Digit Selection   ▽ Subterms under main terms may continue to next column or page

240 — Volume 2 · October 2010   ▶◀ Revised Text   ● New Line   ▲ Revised Code   2011 ICD-9-CM

Puberty — continued
  precocious — continued
    due to — continued
      ovarian hyperfunction — continued
        estrogen 256.0
      pineal tumor 259.8
      testicular hyperfunction 257.0
    premature 259.1
    due to
      adrenal cortical hyperfunction 255.2
      pineal tumor 259.8
      pituitary (anterior) hyperfunction 253.1
Puckering, macula 362.56
Pudenda, pudendum — see condition
Puente's disease (simple glandular cheilitis) 528.5
Puerperal
  abscess
    areola 675.1 ☑
    Bartholin's gland 646.6 ☑
    breast 675.1 ☑
    cervix (uteri) 670.8 ☑
    fallopian tube 670.8 ☑
    genital organ 670.8 ☑
    kidney 646.6 ☑
    mammary 675.1 ☑
    mesosalpinx 670.8 ☑
    nabothian 646.6 ☑
    nipple 675.0 ☑
    ovary, ovarian 670.8 ☑
    oviduct 670.8 ☑
    parametric 670.8 ☑
    para-uterine 670.8 ☑
    pelvic 670.8 ☑
    perimetric 670.8 ☑
    periuterine 670.8 ☑
    retro-uterine 670.8 ☑
    subareolar 675.1 ☑
    suprapelvic 670.8 ☑
    tubal (ruptured) 670.8 ☑
    tubo-ovarian 670.8 ☑
    urinary tract NEC 646.6 ☑
    uterine, uterus 670.8 ☑
    vagina (wall) 646.6 ☑
    vaginorectal 646.6 ☑
    vulvovaginal gland 646.6 ☑
  accident 674.9 ☑
  adnexitis 670.8 ☑
  afibrinogenemia, or other coagulation defect 666.3 ☑
  albuminuria (acute) (subacute) 646.2 ☑
    pre-eclamptic 642.4 ☑
  anemia (conditions classifiable to 280–285) 648.2 ☑
  anuria 669.3 ☑
  apoplexy 674.0 ☑
  asymptomatic bacteriuria 646.5 ☑
  atrophy, breast 676.3 ☑
  blood dyscrasia 666.3 ☑
  caked breast 676.2 ☑
  cardiomyopathy 674.5 ☑
  cellulitis — see Puerperal, abscess
  cerebrovascular disorder (conditions classifiable to 430–434, 436–437) 674.0 ☑
  cervicitis (conditions classifiable to 616.0) 646.6 ☑
  coagulopathy (any) 666.3 ☑
  complications 674.9 ☑
    specified type NEC 674.8 ☑
  convulsions (eclamptic) (uremic) 642.6 ☑
    with pre-existing hypertension 642.7 ☑
  cracked nipple 676.1 ☑
  cystitis 646.6 ☑
  cystopyelitis 646.6 ☑
  deciduitis (acute) 670.8 ☑
  delirium NEC 293.9
  diabetes (mellitus) (conditions classifiable to 249 and 250) 648.0 ☑
  disease 674.9 ☑
    breast NEC 676.3 ☑
    cerebrovascular (acute) 674.0 ☑

Puerperal — continued
  disease — continued
    nonobstetric NEC (see also Pregnancy, complicated, current disease or condition) 648.9 ☑
    pelvis inflammatory 670.8 ☑
    renal NEC 646.2 ☑
    tubo-ovarian 670.8 ☑
    Valsuani's (progressive pernicious anemia) 648.2 ☑
  disorder
    lactation 676.9 ☑
      specified type NEC 676.8 ☑
    nonobstetric NEC (see also Pregnancy, complicated, current disease or condition) 648.9 ☑
  disruption
    cesarean wound 674.1 ☑
    episiotomy wound 674.2 ☑
    perineal laceration wound 674.2 ☑
  drug dependence (conditions classifiable to 304) 648.3 ☑
  eclampsia 642.6 ☑
    with pre-existing hypertension 642.7 ☑
  embolism (pulmonary) 673.2 ☑
    air 673.0 ☑
    amniotic fluid 673.1 ☑
    blood-clot 673.2 ☑
    brain or cerebral 674.0 ☑
    cardiac 674.8 ☑
    fat 673.8 ☑
    intracranial sinus (venous) 671.5 ☑
    pyemic 673.3 ☑
    septic 673.3 ☑
    spinal cord 671.5 ☑
  endometritis (conditions classifiable to 615.0–615.9) 670.1 ☑
  endophlebitis — see Puerperal, phlebitis
  endotrachelitis 646.6 ☑
  engorgement, breasts 676.2 ☑
  erysipelas 670.8 ☑
  failure
    lactation 676.4 ☑
    renal, acute 669.3 ☑
  fever 672 ▲
    meaning pyrexia (of unknown origin) 672.0 ☑
    meaning sepsis 670.2 ☑
  fissure, nipple 676.1 ☑
  fistula
    breast 675.1 ☑
    mammary gland 675.1 ☑
    nipple 675.0 ☑
  galactophoritis 675.2 ☑
  galactorrhea 676.6 ☑
  gangrene
    gas 670.8 ☑
      with sepsis 670.2 ☑
    uterus 670.8 ☑
  gonorrhea (conditions classifiable to 098) 647.1 ☑
  hematoma, subdural 674.0 ☑
  hematosalpinx, infectional 670.8 ☑
  hemiplegia, cerebral 674.0 ☑
  hemorrhage 666.1 ☑
    brain 674.0 ☑
    bulbar 674.0 ☑
    cerebellar 674.0 ☑
    cerebral 674.0 ☑
    cortical 674.0 ☑
    delayed (after 24 hours) (uterine) 666.2 ☑
    extradural 674.0 ☑
    internal capsule 674.0 ☑
    intracranial 674.0 ☑
    intrapontine 674.0 ☑
    meningeal 674.0 ☑
    pontine 674.0 ☑
    subarachnoid 674.0 ☑
    subcortical 674.0 ☑
    subdural 674.0 ☑
    uterine, delayed 666.2 ☑
    ventricular 674.0 ☑
  hemorrhoids 671.8 ☑

Puerperal — continued
  hepatorenal syndrome 674.8 ☑
  hypertrophy
    breast 676.3 ☑
    mammary gland 676.3 ☑
  induration breast (fibrous) 676.3 ☑
  infarction
    lung — see Puerperal, embolism
    pulmonary — see Puerperal, embolism
  infection
    Bartholin's gland 646.6 ☑
    breast 675.2 ☑
      with nipple 675.9 ☑
        specified type NEC 675.8 ☑
    cervix 646.6 ☑
    endocervix 646.6 ☑
    fallopian tube 670.8 ☑
    generalized 670.0 ☑
    genital tract (major) 670.0 ☑
      minor or localized 646.6 ☑
    kidney (bacillus coli) 646.6 ☑
    mammary gland 675.2 ☑
      with nipple 675.9 ☑
        specified type NEC 675.8 ☑
    nipple 675.0 ☑
      with breast 675.9 ☑
        specified type NEC 675.8 ☑
    ovary 670.8 ☑
    pelvic 670.8 ☑
    peritoneum 670.8 ☑
    renal 646.6 ☑
    tubo-ovarian 670.8 ☑
    urinary (tract) NEC 646.6 ☑
      asymptomatic 646.5 ☑
    uterus, uterine 670.8 ☑
    vagina 646.6 ☑
  inflammation (see also Puerperal, infection)
    areola 675.1 ☑
    Bartholin's gland 646.6 ☑
    breast 675.2 ☑
    broad ligament 670.8 ☑
    cervix (uteri) 646.6 ☑
    fallopian tube 670.8 ☑
    genital organs 670.8 ☑
      localized 646.6 ☑
    mammary gland 675.2 ☑
    nipple 675.0 ☑
    ovary 670.8 ☑
    oviduct 670.8 ☑
    pelvis 670.8 ☑
    periuterine 670.8 ☑
    tubal 670.8 ☑
    vagina 646.6 ☑
    vein — see Puerperal, phlebitis
  inversion, nipple 676.3 ☑
  ischemia, cerebral 674.0 ☑
  lymphangitis 670.8 ☑
    breast 675.2 ☑
  malaria (conditions classifiable to 084) 647.4 ☑
  malnutrition 648.9 ☑
  mammillitis 675.0 ☑
  mammitis 675.2 ☑
  mania 296.0 ☑
    recurrent episode 296.1 ☑
    single episode 296.0 ☑
  mastitis 675.2 ☑
    purulent 675.1 ☑
    retromammary 675.1 ☑
    submammary 675.1 ☑
  melancholia 296.2 ☑
    recurrent episode 296.3 ☑
    single episode 296.2 ☑
  mental disorder (conditions classifiable to 290–303, 305.0, 305.2–305.9, 306–316, 317–319) 648.4 ☑
  metritis (suppurative) 670.1 ☑
    septic 670.2 ☑
  metroperitonitis 670.8 ☑
  metrorrhagia 666.2 ☑
  metrosalpingitis 670.8 ☑
  metrovaginitis 670.8 ☑
  milk leg 671.4 ☑

Puerperal — continued
  monoplegia, cerebral 674.0 ☑
  necrosis
    kidney, tubular 669.3 ☑
    liver (acute) (subacute) (conditions classifiable to 570) 674.8 ☑
    ovary 670.8 ☑
    renal cortex 669.3 ☑
  nephritis or nephrosis (conditions classifiable to 580–589) 646.2 ☑
    with hypertension 642.1 ☑
  nutritional deficiency (conditions classifiable to 260–269) 648.9 ☑
  occlusion, precerebral artery 674.0 ☑
  oliguria 669.3 ☑
  oophoritis 670.8 ☑
  ovaritis 670.8 ☑
  paralysis
    bladder (sphincter) 665.5 ☑
    cerebral 674.0 ☑
  paralytic stroke 674.0 ☑
  parametritis 670.8 ☑
  paravaginitis 646.6 ☑
  pelviperitonitis 670.8 ☑
  perimetritis 670.8 ☑
  perimetrosalpingitis 670.8 ☑
  perinephritis 646.6 ☑
  perioophoritis 670.8 ☑
  periphlebitis — see Puerperal, phlebitis
  perisalpingitis 670.8 ☑
  peritoneal infection 670.8 ☑
  peritonitis (pelvic) 670.8 ☑
  perivaginitis 646.6 ☑
  phlebitis 671.2 ☑
    deep 671.4 ☑
    intracranial sinus (venous) 671.5 ☑
    pelvic 671.4 ☑
    specified site NEC 671.5 ☑
    superficial 671.2 ☑
  phlegmasia alba dolens 671.4 ☑
  placental polyp 674.4 ☑
  pneumonia, embolic — see Puerperal, embolism
  prediabetes 648.8 ☑
  pre-eclampsia (mild) 642.4 ☑
    with pre-existing hypertension 642.7 ☑
    severe 642.5 ☑
  psychosis, unspecified (see also Psychosis, puerperal) 293.89
  pyelitis 646.6 ☑
  pyelocystitis 646.6 ☑
  pyelohydronephrosis 646.6 ☑
  pyelonephritis 646.6 ☑
  pyelonephrosis 646.6 ☑
  pyemia 670.2 ☑
  pyocystitis 646.6 ☑
  pyohemia 670.2 ☑
  pyometra 670.8 ☑
  pyonephritis 646.6 ☑
  pyonephrosis 646.6 ☑
  pyo-oophoritis 670.8 ☑
  pyosalpingitis 670.8 ☑
  pyosalpinx 670.8 ☑
  pyrexia (of unknown origin) 672.0 ☑
  renal
    disease NEC 646.2 ☑
    failure, acute 669.3 ☑
  retention
    decidua (fragments) (with delayed hemorrhage) 666.2 ☑
      without hemorrhage 667.1 ☑
    placenta (fragments) (with delayed hemorrhage) 666.2 ☑
      without hemorrhage 667.1 ☑
    secundines (fragments) (with delayed hemorrhage) 666.2 ☑
      without hemorrhage 667.1 ☑
  retracted nipple 676.0 ☑
  rubella (conditions classifiable to 056) 647.5 ☑
  salpingitis 670.8 ☑
  salpingo-oophoritis 670.8 ☑
  salpingo-ovaritis 670.8 ☑
  salpingoperitonitis 670.8 ☑

☑ Additional Digit Required — Refer to the Tabular List for Digit Selection   ⬗ Subterms under main terms may continue to next column or page

2011 ICD-9-CM   ▶◀ Revised Text   ● New Line   ▲ Revised Code   October 2010 • Volume 2 — 241

Puberty — Puerperal

Puerperal — *continued*
  sapremia 670.2 ☑
  secondary perineal tear 674.2 ☑
  sepsis (pelvic) 670.2 ☑
  septicemia 670.2 ☑
  subinvolution (uterus) 674.8 ☑
  sudden death (cause unknown) 674.9 ☑
  suppuration — *see* Puerperal, abscess
  syphilis (conditions classifiable to 090–097)
      647.0 ☑
  tetanus 670.8 ☑
  thelitis 675.0 ☑
  thrombocytopenia 666.3 ☑
  thrombophlebitis (superficial) 671.2 ☑
      deep 671.4 ☑
      pelvic 671.4 ☑
      septic 670.3 ☑
      specified site NEC 671.5 ☑
  thrombosis (venous) — *see* Thrombosis,
      puerperal
  thyroid dysfunction (conditions classifiable
      to 240–246) 648.1 ☑
  toxemia (*see also* Toxemia, of pregnancy)
      642.4 ☑
      eclamptic 642.6 ☑
          with pre-existing hypertension
              642.7 ☑
      pre-eclamptic (mild) 642.4 ☑
          with
              convulsions 642.6 ☑
              pre-existing hypertension
                  642.7 ☑
          severe 642.5 ☑
  tuberculosis (conditions classifiable to
      010–018) 647.3 ☑
  uremia 669.3 ☑
  vaginitis (conditions classifiable to 616.1)
      646.6 ☑
  varicose veins (legs) 671.0 ☑
      vulva or perineum 671.1 ☑
  venous complication 671.9 ☑
  vulvitis (conditions classifiable to 616.1)
      646.6 ☑
  vulvovaginitis (conditions classifiable to
      616.1) 646.6 ☑
  white leg 671.4 ☑
Pulled muscle — *see* Sprain, by site
Pulmolithiasis 518.89
Pulmonary — *see* condition
Pulmonitis (unknown etiology) 486
Pulpitis (acute) (anachoretic) (chronic) (hyper-
      plastic) (putrescent) (suppurative) (ulcer-
      ative) 522.0
Pulpless tooth 522.9
Pulse
  alternating 427.89
      psychogenic 306.2
  bigeminal 427.89
  fast 785.0
  feeble, rapid, due to shock following injury
      958.4
  rapid 785.0
  slow 427.89
  strong 785.9
  trigeminal 427.89
  water-hammer (*see also* Insufficiency, aortic)
      424.1
  weak 785.9
Pulseless disease 446.7
Pulsus
  alternans or trigeminy 427.89
      psychogenic 306.2
Punch drunk 310.2
Puncta lacrimalia occlusion 375.52
Punctiform hymen 752.49
Puncture (traumatic) — *see also* Wound, open,
      by site
  accidental, complicating surgery 998.2
  bladder, nontraumatic 596.6
  by
      device, implant, or graft — *see* Compli-
          cations, mechanical
      foreign body
          internal organs (*see also* Injury, inter-
              nal, by site)

Puncture — *see also* Wound, open, by site —
      continued
  by — *continued*
      foreign body — *continued*
          internal organs (*see also* Injury, inter-
              nal, by site) — *continued*
              by ingested object — *see* Foreign
                  body
              left accidentally in operation wound
                  998.4
          instrument (any) during a procedure,
              accidental 998.2
      internal organs, abdomen, chest, or pelvis
          — *see* Injury, internal, by site
      kidney, nontraumatic 593.89
Pupil — *see* condition
Pupillary membrane 364.74
  persistent 743.46
Pupillotonia 379.46
  pseudotabetic 379.46
Purpura 287.2
  abdominal 287.0
  allergic 287.0
  anaphylactoid 287.0
  annularis telangiectodes 709.1
  arthritic 287.0
  autoerythrocyte sensitization 287.2
  autoimmune 287.0
  bacterial 287.0
  Bateman's (senile) 287.2
  capillary fragility (hereditary) (idiopathic)
      287.8
  cryoglobulinemic 273.2
  devil's pinches 287.2
  fibrinolytic (*see also* Fibrinolysis) 286.6
  fulminans, fulminous 286.6
  gangrenous 287.0
  hemorrhagic (*see also* Purpura, thrombocy-
      topenic) 287.39
      nodular 272.7
      nonthrombocytopenic 287.0
      thrombocytopenic 287.39
  Henoch's (purpura nervosa) 287.0
  Henoch-Schönlein (allergic) 287.0
  hypergammaglobulinemic (benign primary)
      (Waldenström's) 273.0
  idiopathic 287.31
      nonthrombocytopenic 287.0
      thrombocytopenic 287.31
  immune thrombocytopenic 287.31
  infectious 287.0
  malignant 287.0
  neonatorum 772.6
  nervosa 287.0
  newborn NEC 772.6
  nonthrombocytopenic 287.2
      hemorrhagic 287.0
      idiopathic 287.0
  nonthrombopenic 287.2
  peliosis rheumatica 287.0
  pigmentaria, progressiva 709.09
  posttransfusion ▶(PTP)◀ 287.41   ▲
      from whole blood (fresh) or blood   ●
          products 287.41   ●
  primary 287.0
  primitive 287.0
  red cell membrane sensitivity 287.2
  rheumatica 287.0
  Schönlein (-Henoch) (allergic) 287.0
  scorbutic 267
  senile 287.2
  simplex 287.2
  symptomatica 287.0
  telangiectasia annularis 709.1
  thrombocytopenic (*see also* Thrombocytope-
      nia) 287.30
      congenital 287.33
      essential 287.30
      hereditary 287.31
      idiopathic 287.31
      immune 287.31
      neonatal, transitory (*see also* Thrombo-
          cytopenia, neonatal transitory)
          776.1
      primary 287.30
      puerperal, postpartum 666.3 ☑

Purpura — *continued*
  thrombocytopenic (*see also* Thrombocytope-
      nia) — *continued*
      thrombotic 446.6
  thrombohemolytic (*see also* Fibrinolysis)
      286.6
  thrombopenic (*see also* Thrombocytopenia)
      287.30
      congenital 287.33
      essential 287.30
      thrombotic 446.6
          thrombocytic 446.6
          thrombocytopenic 446.6
  toxic 287.0
  variolosa 050.0
  vascular 287.0
  visceral symptoms 287.0
  Werlhof's (*see also* Purpura, thrombocy-
      topenic) 287.39
Purpuric spots 782.7
Purulent — *see* condition
Pus
  absorption, general — *see* Septicemia
  in
      stool 792.1
      urine 791.9
  tube (rupture) (*see also* Salpingo-oophoritis)
      614.2
Pustular rash 782.1
Pustule 686.9
  malignant 022.0
  nonmalignant 686.9
Putnam-Dana syndrome (subacute combined
      sclerosis with pernicious anemia)
      281.0 *[336.2]*
Putnam's disease (subacute combined sclero-
      sis with pernicious anemia) 281.0 *[336.2]*
Putrefaction, intestinal 569.89
Putrescent pulp (dental) 522.1
Pyarthritis — *see* Pyarthrosis
Pyarthrosis — *see also* Arthritis, pyogenic
      711.0 ☑
  tuberculous — *see* Tuberculosis, joint
Pycnoepilepsy, pycnolepsy (idiopathic) —
      see also Epilepsy 345.0 ☑
Pyelectasia 593.89
Pyelectasis 593.89
Pyelitis (congenital) (uremic) 590.80
  with
      abortion — *see* Abortion, by type, with
          specified complication NEC
      contracted kidney 590.00
      ectopic pregnancy (*see also* categories
          633.0–633.9) 639.8
      molar pregnancy (*see also* categories
          630–632) 639.8
  acute 590.10
      with renal medullary necrosis 590.11
  chronic 590.00
      with
          renal medullary necrosis 590.01
  complicating pregnancy, childbirth, or
      puerperium 646.6 ☑
      affecting fetus or newborn 760.1
  cystica 590.3
      following
          abortion 639.8
          ectopic or molar pregnancy 639.8
  gonococcal 098.19
      chronic or duration of 2 months or over
          098.39
  tuberculous (*see also* Tuberculosis)
      016.0 ☑ *[590.81]*
Pyelocaliectasia 593.89
Pyelocystitis — *see also* Pyelitis 590.80
Pyelohydronephrosis 591
Pyelonephritis — *see also* Pyelitis 590.80
  acute 590.10
      with renal medullary necrosis 590.11
  chronic 590.00
  syphilitic (late) 095.4
  tuberculous (*see also* Tuberculosis)
      016.0 ☑ *[590.81]*
Pyelonephrosis — *see also* Pyelitis 590.80
  chronic 590.00
Pyelophlebitis 451.89

Pyelo-ureteritis cystica 590.3
Pyemia, pyemic (purulent) — *see also* Sep-
      ticemia 038.9
  abscess — *see* Abscess
  arthritis (*see also* Arthritis, pyogenic)
      711.0 ☑
  Bacillus coli 038.42
  embolism (*see also* Septicemia) 415.12
  fever 038.9
  infection 038.9
  joint (*see also* Arthritis, pyogenic) 711.0 ☑
  liver 572.1
  meningococcal 036.2
  newborn 771.81
  phlebitis — *see* Phlebitis
  pneumococcal 038.2
  portal 572.1
  postvaccinal 999.39
  puerperal 670.2 ☑
  specified organism NEC 038.8
  staphylococcal 038.10
      aureus 038.11
          methicillin
              resistant 038.12
              susceptible 038.11
      specified organism NEC 038.19
  streptococcal 038.0
  tuberculous — *see* Tuberculosis, miliary
Pygopagus 759.4
Pykno-epilepsy, pyknolepsy (idiopathic) —
      see also Epilepsy 345.0 ☑
Pyle (-Cohn) disease (craniometaphyseal
      dysplasia) 756.89
Pylephlebitis (suppurative) 572.1
Pylethrombophlebitis 572.1
Pylethrombosis 572.1
Pyloritis — *see also* Gastritis 535.5 ☑
Pylorospasm (reflex) 537.81
  congenital or infantile 750.5
  neurotic 306.4
  newborn 750.5
  psychogenic 306.4
Pylorus, pyloric — *see* condition
Pyoarthrosis — *see* Pyarthrosis
Pyocele
  mastoid 383.00
  sinus (accessory) (nasal) (*see also* Sinusitis)
      473.9
  turbinate (bone) 473.9
  urethra (*see also* Urethritis) 597.0
Pyococcal dermatitis 686.00
Pyococcide, skin 686.00
Pyocolpos — *see also* Vaginitis 616.10
Pyocyaneus dermatitis 686.09
Pyocystitis — *see also* Cystitis 595.9
Pyoderma, pyodermia 686.00
  gangrenosum 686.01
  specified type NEC 686.09
  vegetans 686.8
Pyodermatitis 686.00
  vegetans 686.8
Pyogenic — *see* condition
Pyohemia — *see* Septicemia
Pyohydronephrosis — *see also* Pyelitis 590.80
Pyometra 615.9
Pyometritis — *see also* Endometritis 615.9
Pyometrium — *see also* Endometritis 615.9
Pyomyositis 728.0
  ossificans 728.19
  tropical (bungpagga) 040.81
Pyonephritis — *see also* Pyelitis 590.80
  chronic 590.00
Pyonephrosis (congenital) — *see also* Pyelitis
      590.80
  acute 590.10
Pyo-oophoritis — *see also* Salpingo-oophoritis
      614.2
Pyo-ovarium — *see also* Salpingo-oophoritis
      614.2
Pyopericarditis 420.99
Pyopericardium 420.99
Pyophlebitis — *see* Phlebitis
Pyopneumopericardium 420.99
Pyopneumothorax (infectional) 510.9
  with fistula 510.0

☑ **Additional Digit Required** — Refer to the Tabular List for Digit Selection   ⬇ **Subterms under main terms may continue to next column or page**

Pyopneumothorax — *continued*
  subdiaphragmatic (*see also* Peritonitis) 567.29
  subphrenic (*see also* Peritonitis) 567.29
  tuberculous (*see also* Tuberculosis, pleura) 012.0 ☑
Pyorrhea (alveolar) (alveolaris) 523.40
  degenerative 523.5
Pyosalpingitis — *see also* Salpingo-oophoritis 614.2
Pyosalpinx — *see also* Salpingo-oophoritis 614.2
Pyosepticemia — *see* Septicemia
Pyosis
  Corlett's (impetigo) 684
  Manson's (pemphigus contagiosus) 684
Pyothorax 510.9
  with fistula 510.0
  tuberculous (*see also* Tuberculosis, pleura) 012.0 ☑
Pyoureter 593.89
  tuberculous (*see also* Tuberculosis) 016.2 ☑
Pyramidopallidonigral syndrome 332.0
Pyrexia (of unknown origin) (P.U.O.) 780.60
  atmospheric 992.0
  during labor 659.2 ☑
  environmentally-induced newborn 778.4
  heat 992.0
  newborn, environmentally-induced 778.4
  puerperal 672.0 ☑
Pyroglobulinemia 273.8
Pyromania 312.33
Pyrosis 787.1
Pyrroloporphyria 277.1
Pyuria (bacterial) 791.9

Q

Q fever 083.0
  with pneumonia 083.0 *[484.8]*
Quadricuspid aortic valve 746.89
Quadrilateral fever 083.0
Quadriparesis — *see* Quadriplegia
  meaning muscle weakness 728.87
Quadriplegia 344.00
  with fracture, vertebra (process) — *see* Fracture, vertebra, cervical, with spinal cord injury
  brain (current episode) 437.8
  C1-C4
    complete 344.01
    incomplete 344.02
  C5-C7
    complete 344.03
    incomplete 344.04
  cerebral (current episode) 437.8
  congenital or infantile (cerebral) (spastic) (spinal) 343.2
  cortical 437.8
  embolic (current episode) (*see also* Embolism, brain) 434.1 ☑
  functional 780.72
  infantile (cerebral) (spastic) (spinal) 343.2
  newborn NEC 767.0
  specified NEC 344.09
  thrombotic (current episode) (*see also* Thrombosis, brain) 434.0 ☑
  traumatic — *see* Injury, spinal, cervical
Quadruplet
  affected by maternal complications of pregnancy 761.5
  healthy liveborn — *see* Newborn, multiple
  pregnancy (complicating delivery) NEC 651.8 ☑
    with fetal loss and retention of one or more fetus(es) 651.5 ☑
    following (elective) fetal reduction 651.7 ☑
Quarrelsomeness 301.3
Quartan
  fever 084.2
  malaria (fever) 084.2
Queensland fever 083.0
  coastal 083.0
  seven-day 100.89
Quervain's disease 727.04

Quervain's disease — *continued*
  thyroid (subacute granulomatous thyroiditis) 245.1
Queyrat's erythroplasia (M8080/2)
  specified site — *see* Neoplasm, skin, in situ
  unspecified site 233.5
Quincke's disease or edema — *see* Edema, angioneurotic
Quinquaud's disease (acne decalvans) 704.09
Quinsy (gangrenous) 475
Quintan fever 083.1
Quintuplet
  affected by maternal complications of pregnancy 761.5
  healthy liveborn — *see* Newborn, multiple
  pregnancy (complicating delivery) NEC 651.2 ☑
    with fetal loss and retention of one or more fetus(es) 651.6 ☑
    following (elective) fetal reduction 651.7 ☑
Quotidian
  fever 084.0
  malaria (fever) 084.0

R

Rabbia 071
Rabbit fever — *see also* Tularemia 021.9
Rabies 071
  contact V01.5
  exposure to V01.5
  inoculation V04.5
    reaction — *see* Complications, vaccination
  vaccination, prophylactic (against) V04.5
Rachischisis — *see also* Spina bifida 741.9 ☑
Rachitic — *see also* condition
  deformities of spine 268.1
  pelvis 268.1
    with disproportion (fetopelvic) 653.2 ☑
      affecting fetus or newborn 763.1
      causing obstructed labor 660.1 ☑
        affecting fetus or newborn 763.1
Rachitis, rachitism — *see also* Rickets
  acute 268.0
  fetalis 756.4
  renalis 588.0
  tarda 268.0
Racket nail 757.5
Radial nerve — *see* condition
Radiation effects or sickness — *see also* Effect, adverse, radiation
  cataract 366.46
  dermatitis 692.82
    sunburn (*see also* Sunburn) 692.71
Radiculitis (pressure) (vertebrogenic) 729.2
  accessory nerve 723.4
  anterior crural 724.4
  arm 723.4
  brachial 723.4
  cervical NEC 723.4
  due to displacement of intervertebral disc — *see* Neuritis, due to, displacement intervertebral disc
  leg 724.4
  lumbar NEC 724.4
  lumbosacral 724.4
  rheumatic 729.2
  syphilitic 094.89
  thoracic (with visceral pain) 724.4
Radiculomyelitis 357.0
  toxic, due to
    Clostridium tetani 037
    Corynebacterium diphtheriae 032.89
Radiculopathy — *see also* Radiculitis 729.2
Radioactive substances, adverse effect — *see* Effect, adverse, radioactive substance
Radiodermal burns (acute) (chronic) (occupational) — *see* Burn, by site
Radiodermatitis 692.82
Radionecrosis — *see* Effect, adverse, radiation
Radiotherapy session V58.0
Radium, adverse effect — *see* Effect, adverse, radioactive substance
Raeder-Harbitz syndrome (pulseless disease) 446.7

Rage — *see also* Disturbance, conduct 312.0 ☑
  meaning rabies 071
Rag sorters' disease 022.1
Raillietiniasis 123.8
Railroad neurosis 300.16
Railway spine 300.16
Raised — *see* Elevation
Raiva 071
Rake teeth, tooth 524.39
Rales 786.7
Ramifying renal pelvis 753.3
Ramsay Hunt syndrome (herpetic geniculate ganglionitis) 053.11
  meaning dyssynergia cerebellaris myoclonica 334.2
Ranke's primary infiltration — *see also* Tuberculosis 010.0 ☑
Ranula 527.6
  congenital 750.26
Rape
  adult 995.83
  alleged, observation or examination V71.5
  child 995.53
Rapid
  feeble pulse, due to shock, following injury 958.4
  heart (beat) 785.0
    psychogenic 306.2
  respiration 786.06
    psychogenic 306.1
  second stage (delivery) 661.3 ☑
    affecting fetus or newborn 763.6
  time-zone change syndrome 327.35
Rarefaction, bone 733.99
Rash 782.1
  canker 034.1
  diaper 691.0
  drug (internal use) 693.0
    contact 692.3
  ECHO 9 virus 078.89
  enema 692.89
  food (*see also* Allergy, food) 693.1
  heat 705.1
  napkin 691.0
  nettle 708.8
  pustular 782.1
  rose 782.1
    epidemic 056.9
    of infants 057.8
  scarlet 034.1
  serum (prophylactic) (therapeutic) 999.5
  toxic 782.1
  wandering tongue 529.1
Rasmussen's aneurysm — *see also* Tuberculosis 011.2 ☑
Rat-bite fever 026.9
  due to Streptobacillus moniliformis 026.1
  spirochetal (morsus muris) 026.0
Rathke's pouch tumor (M9350/1) 237.0
Raymond (-Céstan) syndrome 433.8 ☑
Raynaud's
  disease or syndrome (paroxysmal digital cyanosis) 443.0
  gangrene (symmetric) 443.0 *[785.4]*
  phenomenon (paroxysmal digital cyanosis) (secondary) 443.0
RDS 769
Reaction
  acute situational maladjustment (*see also* Reaction, adjustment) 309.9
  adaptation (*see also* Reaction, adjustment) 309.9
  adjustment 309.9
    with
      anxious mood 309.24
        with depressed mood 309.28
      conduct disturbance 309.3
        combined with disturbance of emotions 309.4
      depressed mood 309.0
        brief 309.0
          with anxious mood 309.28
        prolonged 309.1
      elective mutism 309.83
      mixed emotions and conduct 309.4
      mutism, elective 309.83

Reaction — *continued*
  adjustment — *continued*
    with — *continued*
      physical symptoms 309.82
      predominant disturbance (of)
        conduct 309.3
        emotions NEC 309.29
          mixed 309.28
        mixed, emotions and conduct 309.4
        specified type NEC 309.89
      specific academic or work inhibition 309.23
      withdrawal 309.83
    depressive 309.0
      with conduct disturbance 309.4
      brief 309.0
      prolonged 309.1
    specified type NEC 309.89
  adverse food NEC 995.7
  affective (*see also* Psychosis, affective) 296.90
    specified type NEC 296.99
  aggressive 301.3
    unsocialized (*see also* Disturbance, conduct) 312.0 ☑
  allergic (*see also* Allergy) 995.3
    drug, medicinal substance, and biological — *see* Allergy, drug
    due to correct medical substance ●
      properly administered 995.27 ●
    food — *see* Allergy, food
    serum 999.5
  anaphylactic — *see* Shock, anaphylactic
  anesthesia — *see* Anesthesia, complication
  anger 312.0 ☑
  antisocial 301.7
  antitoxin (prophylactic) (therapeutic) — *see* Complications, vaccination
  anxiety 300.00
  Arthus 995.21
  asthenic 300.5
  compulsive 300.3
  conversion (anesthetic) (autonomic) (hyperkinetic) (mixed paralytic) (paresthetic) 300.11
  deoxyribonuclease (DNA) (DNase) hypersensitivity NEC 287.2
  depressive 300.4
    acute 309.0
    affective (*see also* Psychosis, affective) 296.2 ☑
      recurrent episode 296.3 ☑
      single episode 296.2 ☑
    brief 309.0
    manic (*see also* Psychosis, affective) 296.80
    neurotic 300.4
    psychoneurotic 300.4
    psychotic 298.0
  dissociative 300.15
  drug NEC (*see also* Table of Drugs and Chemicals) 995.20
    allergic (*see also* Allergy, drug) 995.27
    correct substance properly administered 995.20
    obstetric anesthetic or analgesic NEC 668.9 ☑
      affecting fetus or newborn 763.5
      specified drug — *see* Table of Drugs and Chemicals
    overdose or poisoning 977.9
      specified drug — *see* Table of Drugs and Chemicals
    specific to newborn 779.4
    transmitted via placenta or breast milk — *see* Absorption, drug, through placenta
    withdrawal NEC 292.0
      infant of dependent mother 779.5
    wrong substance given or taken in error 977.9
      specified drug — *see* Table of Drugs and Chemicals
  dyssocial 301.7
  dystonic, acute, due to drugs 333.72

☑ **Additional Digit Required — Refer to the Tabular List for Digit Selection**   ⬙ **Subterms under main terms may continue to next column or page**

2011 ICD-9-CM   ▶◀ Revised Text   ● New Line   ▲ Revised Code   **October 2010 • Volume 2 — 243**

Reaction — *continued*
erysipeloid 027.1
fear 300.20
  child 313.0
fluid loss, cerebrospinal 349.0
food (*see also* Allergy, food)
  adverse NEC 995.7
  anaphylactic shock — *see* Anaphylactic shock, due to, food
foreign
  body NEC 728.82
    in operative wound (inadvertently left) 998.4
    due to surgical material intentionally left — *see* Complications, due to (presence of) any device, implant, or graft classified to 996.0–996.5 NEC
    substance accidentally left during a procedure (chemical) (powder) (talc) 998.7
    body or object (instrument) (sponge) (swab) 998.4
graft-versus-host (GVH) 279.50
grief (acute) (brief) 309.0
  prolonged 309.1
gross stress (*see also* Reaction, stress, acute) 308.9
group delinquent (*see also* Disturbance, conduct) 312.2 ☑
Herxheimer's 995.0
hyperkinetic (*see also* Hyperkinesia) 314.9
hypochondriacal 300.7
hypoglycemic, due to insulin 251.0
  therapeutic misadventure 962.3
hypomanic (*see also* Psychosis, affective) 296.0 ☑
  recurrent episode 296.1 ☑
  single episode 296.0 ☑
hysterical 300.10
  conversion type 300.11
  dissociative 300.15
id (bacterial cause) 692.89
immaturity NEC 301.89
  aggressive 301.3
  emotional instability 301.59
immunization — *see* Complications, vaccination
incompatibility
  blood group ▶(*see also* Complications, transfusion)◀ 999.80 ▲
    ABO ▶(due to transfusion of blood or blood products) (*see also* Complications, transfusion)◀ 999.60 ▲
    minor blood group 999.89
    non-ABO — *see also* Complications, transfusion 999.75 ●
    Rh ▶antigen (C) (c) (D) (E) (e)◀ (factor) (infusion) (transfusion) ▶(*see also* Complications, transfusion)◀ 999.70 ▲
inflammatory — *see* Infection
infusion — *see* Complications, infusion
inoculation (immune serum) — *see* Complications, vaccination
insulin 995.23
involutional
  paranoid 297.2
  psychotic (*see also* Psychosis, affective, depressive) 296.2 ☑
leukemoid (basophilic) (lymphocytic) (monocytic) (myelocytic) (neutrophilic) 288.62
LSD (*see also* Abuse, drugs, nondependent) 305.3 ☑
lumbar puncture 349.0
manic-depressive (*see also* Psychosis, affective) 296.80
  depressed 296.2 ☑
    recurrent episode 296.3 ☑
    single episode 296.2 ☑
  hypomanic 296.0 ☑
neurasthenic 300.5
neurogenic (*see also* Neurosis) 300.9

Reaction — *continued*
neurotic NEC 300.9
neurotic-depressive 300.4
nitritoid — *see* Crisis, nitritoid
obsessive compulsive 300.3
organic 293.9
  acute 293.0
  subacute 293.1
overanxious, child or adolescent 313.0
paranoid (chronic) 297.9
  acute 298.3
  climacteric 297.2
  involutional 297.2
  menopausal 297.2
  senile 290.20
  simple 297.0
passive
  aggressive 301.84
  dependency 301.6
personality (*see also* Disorder, personality) 301.9
phobic 300.20
postradiation — *see* Effect, adverse, radiation
psychogenic NEC 300.9
psychoneurotic (*see also* Neurosis) 300.9
  anxiety 300.00
  compulsive 300.3
  conversion 300.11
  depersonalization 300.6
  depressive 300.4
  dissociative 300.15
  hypochondriacal 300.7
  hysterical 300.10
    conversion type 300.11
    dissociative type 300.15
  neurasthenic 300.5
  obsessive 300.3
  obsessive-compulsive 300.3
  phobic 300.20
  tension state 300.9
psychophysiologic NEC (*see also* Disorder, psychosomatic) 306.9
  cardiovascular 306.2
  digestive 306.4
  endocrine 306.6
  gastrointestinal 306.4
  genitourinary 306.50
  heart 306.2
  hemic 306.8
  intestinal (large) (small) 306.4
  laryngeal 306.1
  lymphatic 306.8
  musculoskeletal 306.0
  pharyngeal 306.1
  respiratory 306.1
  skin 306.3
  special sense organs 306.7
psychosomatic (*see also* Disorder, psychosomatic) 306.9
psychotic (*see also* Psychosis) 298.9
  depressive 298.0
  due to or associated with physical condition (*see also* Psychosis, organic) 293.9
  involutional (*see also* Psychosis, affective) 296.2 ☑
    recurrent episode 296.3 ☑
    single episode 296.2 ☑
pupillary (myotonic) (tonic) 379.46
radiation — *see* Effect, adverse, radiation
runaway (*see also* Disturbance, conduct)
  socialized 312.2 ☑
  undersocialized, unsocialized 312.1 ☑
scarlet fever toxin — *see* Complications, vaccination
schizophrenic (*see also* Schizophrenia) 295.9 ☑
  latent 295.5 ☑
serological for syphilis — *see* Serology for syphilis
serum (prophylactic) (therapeutic) 999.5
  immediate 999.4
situational (*see also* Reaction, adjustment) 309.9
  acute, to stress 308.3

Reaction — *continued*
  situational (*see also* Reaction, adjustment) — *continued*
    adjustment (*see also* Reaction, adjustment) 309.9
  somatization (*see also* Disorder, psychosomatic) 306.9
  spinal puncture 349.0
  spite, child (*see also* Disturbance, conduct) 312.0 ☑
  stress, acute 308.9
    with predominant disturbance (of)
      consciousness 308.1
      emotions 308.0
      mixed 308.4
      psychomotor 308.2
      specified type NEC 308.3
    bone or cartilage — *see* Fracture, stress
  surgical procedure — *see* Complications, surgical procedure
  tetanus antitoxin — *see* Complications, vaccination
  toxin-antitoxin — *see* Complications, vaccination
  transfusion (blood) (bone marrow) (lymphocytes) (allergic) ▶(*see also* Complications, transfusion)◀ 999.80 ▲
  tuberculin skin test, nonspecific (without active tuberculosis) 795.5
    positive (without active tuberculosis) 795.5
  ultraviolet — *see* Effect, adverse, ultraviolet
  undersocialized, unsocialized (*see also* Disturbance, conduct)
    aggressive (type) 312.0 ☑
    unaggressive (type) 312.1 ☑
  vaccination (any) — *see* Complications, vaccination
  white graft (skin) 996.52
  withdrawing, child or adolescent 313.22
  x-ray — *see* Effect, adverse, x-rays
Reactive depression — *see also* Reaction, depressive 300.4
  neurotic 300.4
  psychoneurotic 300.4
  psychotic 298.0
Rebound tenderness 789.6 ☑
Recalcitrant patient V15.81
Recanalization, thrombus — *see* Thrombosis
Recession, receding
  chamber angle (eye) 364.77
  chin 524.06
  gingival (postinfective) (postoperative) 523.20
    generalized 523.25
    localized 523.24
    minimal 523.21
    moderate 523.22
    severe 523.23
Recklinghausen-Applebaum disease (hemochromatosis) 275.03 ▲
Recklinghausen's disease (M9540/1) 237.71
  bones (osteitis fibrosa cystica) 252.01
Reclus' disease (cystic) 610.1
Recrudescent typhus (fever) 081.1
Recruitment, auditory 388.44
Rectalgia 569.42
Rectitis 569.49
Rectocele
  female (without uterine prolapse) 618.04
    with uterine prolapse 618.4
      complete 618.3
      incomplete 618.2
  in pregnancy or childbirth 654.4 ☑
    causing obstructed labor 660.2 ☑
      affecting fetus or newborn 763.1
  male 569.49
  vagina, vaginal (outlet) 618.04
Rectosigmoiditis 569.89
  ulcerative (chronic) 556.3
Rectosigmoid junction — *see* condition
Rectourethral — *see* condition
Rectovaginal — *see* condition
Rectovesical — *see* condition
Rectum, rectal — *see* condition
Recurrent — *see* condition

Recurrent — *see* condition — *continued*
  pregnancy loss — *see* Pregnancy, management affected by, abortion, habitual ●
Red bugs 133.8
Red cedar asthma 495.8
Redness
  conjunctiva 379.93
  eye 379.93
  nose 478.19
Reduced ventilatory or vital capacity 794.2
Reduction
  function
    kidney (*see also* Disease, renal) 593.9
    liver 573.8
  ventilatory capacity 794.2
  vital capacity 794.2
Redundant, redundancy
  abdomen 701.9
  anus 751.5
  cardia 537.89
  clitoris 624.2
  colon (congenital) 751.5
  foreskin (congenital) 605
  intestine 751.5
  labia 624.3
  organ or site, congenital NEC — *see* Accessory
  panniculus (abdominal) 278.1
  prepuce (congenital) 605
  pylorus 537.89
  rectum 751.5
  scrotum 608.89
  sigmoid 751.5
  skin (of face) 701.9
    eyelids 374.30
  stomach 537.89
  uvula 528.9
  vagina 623.8
Reduplication — *see* Duplication
Referral
  adoption (agency) V68.89
  nursing care V63.8
  patient without examination or treatment V68.81
  social services V63.8
Reflex — *see also* condition
  blink, deficient 374.45
  hyperactive gag 478.29
  neurogenic bladder NEC 596.54
    atonic 596.54
      with cauda equina syndrome 344.61
  vasoconstriction 443.9
  vasovagal 780.2
Reflux 530.81
  acid 530.81
  esophageal 530.81
    with esophagitis 530.11
  esophagitis 530.11
  gastroesophageal 530.81
  mitral — *see* Insufficiency, mitral
  ureteral — *see* Reflux, vesicoureteral
  vesicoureteral 593.70
    with
      reflux nephropathy 593.73
        bilateral 593.72
        unilateral 593.71
Reformed gallbladder 576.0
Reforming, artificial openings — *see also* Attention to, artificial, opening V55.9
Refractive error — *see also* Error, refractive 367.9
Refsum's disease or syndrome (heredopathia atactica polyneuritiformis) 356.3
Refusal of
  food 307.59
    hysterical 300.11
  treatment because of, due to
    patient's decision NEC V64.2
    reason of conscience or religion V62.6
Regaud
  tumor (M8082/3) — *see* Neoplasm, nasopharynx, malignant
  type carcinoma (M8082/3) — *see* Neoplasm, nasopharynx, malignant
Regional — *see* condition

☑ **Additional Digit Required** — Refer to the Tabular List for Digit Selection

▽ **Subterms under main terms may continue to next column or page**

Regulation feeding (elderly) (infant) 783.3
   newborn 779.31
Regurgitated
   food, choked on 933.1
   stomach contents, choked on 933.1
Regurgitation 787.03
   aortic (valve) (see also Insufficiency, aortic)
      424.1
      congenital 746.4
      syphilitic 093.22
   food (see also Vomiting)
      with reswallowing — see Rumination
      newborn 779.33
   gastric contents — see Vomiting
   heart — see Endocarditis
   mitral (valve) (see also Insufficiency, mitral)
      congenital 746.6
   myocardial — see Endocarditis
   pulmonary (heart) (valve) (see also Endo-
      carditis, pulmonary) 424.3
   stomach — see Vomiting
   tricuspid — see Endocarditis, tricuspid
   valve, valvular — see Endocarditis
   vesicoureteral — see Reflux, vesicoureteral
Rehabilitation V57.9
   multiple types V57.89
   occupational V57.21
   specified type NEC V57.89
   speech (-language) V57.3
   vocational V57.22
Reichmann's disease or syndrome (gastrosuccorrhea) 536.8
Reifenstein's syndrome (hereditary familial
   hypogonadism, male) 259.52
Reilly's syndrome or phenomenon — see
   also Neuropathy, peripheral, autonomic
   337.9
Reimann's periodic disease 277.31
Reinsertion, contraceptive device V25.42 ●
   intrauterine V25.13 ●
Reiter's disease, syndrome, or urethritis
   099.3 [711.1] ☑
Rejection
   food, hysterical 300.11
   transplant 996.80
      bone marrow 996.85
      corneal 996.51
      organ (immune or nonimmune cause)
         996.80
         bone marrow 996.85
         heart 996.83
         intestines 996.87
         kidney 996.81
         liver 996.82
         lung 996.84
         pancreas 996.86
         specified NEC 996.89
      skin 996.52
         artificial 996.55
         decellularized allodermis 996.55
Relapsing fever 087.9
   Carter's (Asiatic) 087.0
   Dutton's (West African) 087.1
   Koch's 087.9
   louse-borne (epidemic) 087.0
   Novy's (American) 087.1
   Obermeyer's (European) 087.0
   Spirillum 087.9
   tick-borne (endemic) 087.1
Relaxation
   anus (sphincter) 569.49
      due to hysteria 300.11
   arch (foot) 734
      congenital 754.61
   back ligaments 728.4
   bladder (sphincter) 596.59
   cardio-esophageal 530.89
   cervix (see also Incompetency, cervix) 622.5
   diaphragm 519.4
   inguinal rings — see Hernia, inguinal
   joint (capsule) (ligament) (paralytic) (see also
      Derangement, joint) 718.90
      congenital 755.8
   lumbosacral joint 724.6
   pelvic floor 618.89
   pelvis 618.89

Relaxation — continued
   perineum 618.89
   posture 729.90
   rectum (sphincter) 569.49
   sacroiliac (joint) 724.6
   scrotum 608.89
   urethra (sphincter) 599.84
   uterus (outlet) 618.89
   vagina (outlet) 618.89
   vesical 596.59
Remains
   canal of Cloquet 743.51
   capsule (opaque) 743.51
Remittent fever (malarial) 084.6
Remnant
   canal of Cloquet 743.51
   capsule (opaque) 743.51
   cervix, cervical stump (acquired) (postoper-
      ative) 622.8
   cystic duct, postcholecystectomy 576.0
   fingernail 703.8
      congenital 757.5
   meniscus, knee 717.5
   thyroglossal duct 759.2
   tonsil 474.8
      infected 474.00
   urachus 753.7
Remote effect of cancer — see condition
Removal (of)
   catheter (urinary) (indwelling) V53.6
      from artificial opening — see Attention
         to, artificial, opening
      non-vascular V58.82
      vascular V58.81
   cerebral ventricle (communicating) shunt
      V53.01
   device (see also Fitting (of))
      contraceptive V25.12 ▲
         with reinsertion V25.13 ●
      fixation
         external V54.89
         internal V54.01
      traction V54.89
   drains V58.49
   dressing
      wound V58.30
         nonsurgical V58.30
         surgical V58.31
   ileostomy V55.2
   Kirschner wire V54.89
   nonvascular catheter V58.82
   pin V54.01
   plaster cast V54.89
   plate (fracture) V54.01
   rod V54.01
   screw V54.01
   splint, external V54.89
   staples V58.32
   subdermal implantable contraceptive
      V25.43
   sutures V58.32
   traction device, external V54.89
   vascular catheter V58.81
   wound packing V58.30
      nonsurgical V58.30
      surgical V58.31
Ren
   arcuatus 753.3
   mobile, mobilis (see also Disease, renal)
      593.0
      congenital 753.3
   unguliformis 753.3
Renal — see also condition
   glomerulohyalinosis-diabetic syndrome
      250.4 ☑ [581.81]
      due to secondary diabetes
         249.4 ☑ [581.81]
Rendu-Osler-Weber disease or syndrome
   (familial hemorrhagic telangiectasia)
   448.0
Reninoma (M8361/1) 236.91
Rénon-Delille syndrome 253.8
Repair
   pelvic floor, previous, in pregnancy or
      childbirth 654.4 ☑
      affecting fetus or newborn 763.89

Repair — continued
   scarred tissue V51.8
Replacement by artificial or mechanical de-
   vice or prosthesis of — see also Fitting
   (of)
   artificial skin V43.83
   bladder V43.5
   blood vessel V43.4
   breast V43.82
   eye globe V43.0
   heart
      with
         assist device V43.21
         fully implantable artificial heart
            V43.22
      valve V43.3
   intestine V43.89
   joint V43.60
      ankle V43.66
      elbow V43.62
      finger V43.69
      hip (partial) (total) V43.64
      knee V43.65
      shoulder V43.61
      specified NEC V43.69
      wrist V43.63
   kidney V43.89
   larynx V43.81
   lens V43.1
   limb(s) V43.7
   liver V43.89
   lung V43.89
   organ NEC V43.89
   pancreas V43.89
   skin (artificial) V43.83
   tissue NEC V43.89
Reprogramming
   cardiac pacemaker V53.31
Request for expert evidence V68.2
Reserve, decreased or low
   cardiac — see Disease, heart
   kidney (see also Disease, renal) 593.9
Residual — see also condition
   bladder 596.8
   foreign body — see Retention, foreign body
   state, schizophrenic (see also Schizophrenia)
      295.6 ☑
   urine 788.69
Resistance, resistant (to)
   activated protein C 289.81

> Note — use the following subclassifica-
> tion for categories V09.5, V09.7, V09.8,
> V09.9:
>
> 0   without mention of resistance to
>   multiple drugs
>
> 1   with resistance to multiple drugs
>
>   V09.5 quinolones and fluoro-
>   quinolones
>
>   V09.7 antimycobacterial agents
>
>   V09.8 specified drugs NEC
>
>   V09.9 unspecified drugs

   drugs by microorganisms V09.9 ☑
      Amikacin V09.4
      aminoglycosides V09.4
      Amodiaquine V09.5 ☑
      Amoxicillin V09.0
      Ampicillin V09.0
      antimycobacterial agents V09.7 ☑
      Azithromycin V09.2
      Azlocillin V09.0
      Aztreonam V09.1
      Bacampicillin V09.0
      Bacitracin V09.8 ☑
      Benznidazole V09.8 ☑
      B-lactam antibiotics V09.1
      Capreomycin V09.7 ☑
      Carbenicillin V09.0
      Cefaclor V09.1
      Cefadroxil V09.1
      Cefamandole V09.1
      Cefatetan V09.1
      Cefazolin V09.1

Resistance, resistant — continued
   drugs by microorganisms — continued
      Cefixime V09.1
      Cefonicid V09.1
      Cefoperazone V09.1
      Ceforanide V09.1
      Cefotaxime V09.1
      Cefoxitin V09.1
      Ceftazidime V09.1
      Ceftizoxime V09.1
      Ceftriaxone V09.1
      Cefuroxime V09.1
      Cephalexin V09.1
      Cephaloglycin V09.1
      Cephaloridine V09.1
      Cephalosporins V09.1
      Cephalothin V09.1
      Cephapirin V09.1
      Cephradine V09.1
      Chloramphenicol V09.8 ☑
      Chloroquine V09.5 ☑
      Chlorguanide V09.8 ☑
      Chlorproguanil V09.8 ☑
      Chlortetracycline V09.3
      Cinoxacin V09.5 ☑
      Ciprofloxacin V09.5 ☑
      Clarithromycin V09.2
      Clindamycin V09.8 ☑
      Clioquinol V09.5 ☑
      Clofazimine V09.7 ☑
      Cloxacillin V09.0
      Cyclacillin V09.0
      Cycloserine V09.7 ☑
      Dapsone [DZ] V09.7 ☑
      Demeclocycline V09.3
      Dicloxacillin V09.0
      Doxycycline V09.3
      Enoxacin V09.5 ☑
      Erythromycin V09.2
      Ethambutol [EMB] V09.7 ☑
      Ethionamide [ETA] V09.7 ☑
      fluoroquinolones V09.5 ☑
      Gentamicin V09.4
      Halofantrine V09.8 ☑
      Imipenem V09.1
      Iodoquinol V09.5 ☑
      Isoniazid [INH] V09.7 ☑
      Kanamycin V09.4
      macrolides V09.2
      Mafenide V09.6
      MDRO (multiple drug resistant organ-
         isms) NOS V09.91
      Mefloquine V09.8 ☑
      Melasoprol V09.8 ☑
      Methacycline V09.3
      Methenamine V09.8 ☑
      Methicillin — see Infection, Methicillin
         V09.0
      Metronidazole V09.8 ☑
      Mezlocillin V09.0
      Minocycline V09.3
      multiple drug resistant organisms NOS
         V09.91
      Nafcillin V09.0
      Nalidixic acid V09.5 ☑
      Natamycin V09.2
      Neomycin V09.4
      Netilmicin V09.4
      Nimorazole V09.8 ☑
      Nitrofurantoin V09.8 ☑
      Nitrofurtimox V09.8 ☑
      Norfloxacin V09.5 ☑
      Nystatin V09.2
      Ofloxacin V09.5 ☑
      Oleandomycin V09.2
      Oxacillin V09.0
      Oxytetracycline V09.3
      Para-amino salicylic acid [PAS] V09.7 ☑
      Paromomycin V09.4
      Penicillin (G) (V) (VK) V09.0
      penicillins V09.0
      Pentamidine V09.8 ☑
      Piperacillin V09.0
      Primaquine V09.5 ☑
      Proguanil V09.8 ☑

☑ Additional Digit Required — Refer to the Tabular List for Digit Selection   Ⓦ Subterms under main terms may continue to next column or page

2011 ICD-9-CM   ▶◀ Revised Text   ● New Line   ▲ Revised Code   October 2010 · Volume 2 — 245

Resistance, resistant — *continued*
  drugs by microorganisms — *continued*
    Pyrazinamide [PZA] V09.7 ☑
    Pyrimethamine/Sulfalene V09.8 ☑
    Pyrimethamine/Sulfadoxine V09.8 ☑
    Quinacrine V09.5 ☑
    Quinidine V09.8 ☑
    Quinine V09.8 ☑
    quinolones V09.5 ☑
    Rifabutin V09.7 ☑
    Rifampin [RIF] V09.7 ☑
    Rifamycin V09.7 ☑
    Rolitetracycline V09.3
    specified drugs NEC V09.8 ☑
    Spectinomycin V09.8 ☑
    Spiramycin V09.2
    Streptomycin [SM] V09.4
    Sulfacetamide V09.6
    Sulfacytine V09.6
    Sulfadiazine V09.6
    Sulfadoxine V09.6
    Sulfamethoxazole V09.6
    Sulfapyridine V09.6
    Sulfasalizine V09.6
    Sulfisoxazole V09.6
    sulfonamides V09.6
    Sulfoxone V09.7 ☑
    tetracycline V09.3
    tetracyclines V09.3
    Thiamphenicol V09.8 ☑
    Ticarcillin V09.0
    Tinidazole V09.8 ☑
    Tobramycin V09.4
    Triamphenicol V09.8 ☑
    Trimethoprim V09.8 ☑
    Vancomycin V09.8 ☑
  insulin 277.7
  thyroid hormone 246.8
Resorption
  biliary 576.8
    purulent or putrid (*see also* Cholecystitis)
      576.8
  dental (roots) 521.40
    alveoli 525.8
    pathological
      external 521.42
      internal 521.41
      specified NEC 521.49
  septic — *see* Septicemia
  teeth (roots) 521.40
    pathological
      external 521.42
      internal 521.41
      specified NEC 521.49
Respiration
  asymmetrical 786.09
  bronchial 786.09
  Cheyne-Stokes (periodic respiration) 786.04
  decreased, due to shock following injury
    958.4
  disorder of 786.00
    psychogenic 306.1
    specified NEC 786.09
  failure 518.81
    acute 518.81
    acute and chronic 518.84
    chronic 518.83
    newborn 770.84
  insufficiency 786.09
    acute 518.82
    newborn NEC 770.89
  Kussmaul (air hunger) 786.09
  painful 786.52
  periodic 786.09
    high altitude 327.22
  poor 786.09
    newborn NEC 770.89
  sighing 786.7
    psychogenic 306.1
  wheezing 786.07
Respiratory — *see also* condition
  distress 786.09
    acute 518.82
    fetus or newborn NEC 770.89
    syndrome (newborn) 769

Respiratory — *see also* condition —
    continued
  distress — *continued*
    syndrome — *continued*
      adult (following shock, surgery, or
        trauma) 518.5
      specified NEC 518.82
    failure 518.81
      acute 518.81
      acute and chronic 518.84
      chronic 518.83
Respiratory syncytial virus (RSV) 079.6
  bronchiolitis 466.11
  pneumonia 480.1
  vaccination, prophylactic (against) V04.82
Response
  photoallergic 692.72
  phototoxic 692.72
Restless legs syndrome (RLS) 333.94
Restlessness 799.29
**Restoration of organ continuity from previ-
  ous sterilization** (tuboplasty) (vasoplasty) V26.0
Rest, rests
  mesonephric duct 752.89
    fallopian tube 752.11
  ovarian, in fallopian tubes 752.19
  wolffian duct 752.89
Restriction of housing space V60.1
Restzustand, schizophrenic — *see also*
  Schizophrenia 295.6 ☑
Retained — *see* Retention
Retardation
  development, developmental, specific (*see
    also* Disorder, development, specific)
    315.9
  learning, specific 315.2
    arithmetical 315.1
    language (skills) 315.31
      expressive 315.31
      mixed receptive-expressive
        315.32
    mathematics 315.1
    reading 315.00
      phonological 315.39
      written expression 315.2
    motor 315.4
  endochondral bone growth 733.91
  growth (physical) in childhood 783.43
    due to malnutrition 263.2
  fetal (intrauterine) 764.9 ☑
    affecting management of pregnancy
      656.5 ☑
  intrauterine growth 764.9 ☑
    affecting management of pregnancy
      656.5 ☑
  mental 319
    borderline V62.89
    mild, IQ 50-70 317
    moderate, IQ 35-49 318.0
    profound, IQ under 20 318.2
    severe, IQ 20-34 318.1
  motor, specific 315.4
  physical 783.43
    child 783.43
    due to malnutrition 263.2
    fetus (intrauterine) 764.9 ☑
      affecting management of pregnancy
        656.5 ☑
  psychomotor NEC 307.9
  reading 315.00
Retching — *see* Vomiting
Retention, retained
  bladder (*see also* Retention, urine) 788.20
    psychogenic 306.53
  carbon dioxide 276.2
  cholelithiasis 997.4
  cyst — *see* Cyst
  dead
    fetus (after 22 completed weeks gesta-
      tion) 656.4 ☑
    early fetal death (before 22 complet-
      ed weeks gestation) 632
    ovum 631
  decidua (following delivery) (fragments)
    (with hemorrhage) 666.2 ☑

Retention, retained — *continued*
  decidua — *continued*
    without hemorrhage 667.1 ☑
  deciduous tooth 520.6
  dental root 525.3
  fecal (*see also* Constipation) 564.00
  fluid 276.69 ▲
  foreign body (*see also* Foreign body, re-
    tained)
    bone 733.99
    current trauma — *see* Foreign body, by
      site or type
    middle ear 385.83
    muscle 729.6
    soft tissue NEC 729.6
  gallstones 997.4
  gastric 536.8
  membranes (following delivery) (with
    hemorrhage) 666.2 ☑
    with abortion — *see* Abortion, by type
    without hemorrhage 667.1 ☑
  menses 626.8
  milk (puerperal) 676.2 ☑
  nitrogen, extrarenal 788.99
  placenta (total) (with hemorrhage) 666.0 ☑
    with abortion — *see* Abortion, by type
    without hemorrhage 667.0 ☑
    portions or fragments 666.2 ☑
      without hemorrhage 667.1 ☑
  products of conception
    early pregnancy (fetal death before 22
      completed weeks gestation) 632
    following
      abortion — *see* Abortion, by type
      delivery 666.2 ☑
        with hemorrhage 666.2 ☑
        without hemorrhage 667.1 ☑
  secundines (following delivery) (with hem-
    orrhage) 666.2 ☑
    with abortion — *see* Abortion, by type
    without hemorrhage 667.1 ☑
    complicating puerperium (delayed
      hemorrhage) 666.2 ☑
  smegma, clitoris 624.8
  urine NEC 788.20
    bladder, incomplete emptying 788.21
    due to
      benign prostatic hypertrophy
        (BPH) — *see* category 600
    due to
      benign prostatic hypertrophy (BPH)
        — *see* category 600
    psychogenic 306.53
    specified NEC 788.29
  water (in tissue) (*see also* Edema) 782.3
Reticulation, dust (occupational) 504
Reticulocytosis NEC 790.99
Reticuloendotheliosis
  acute infantile (M9722/3) 202.5 ☑
  leukemic (M9940/3) 202.4 ☑
  malignant (M9720/3) 202.3 ☑
  nonlipid (M9722/3) 202.5 ☑
Reticulohistiocytoma (giant cell) 277.89
Reticulohistiocytosis, multicentric 272.8
Reticulolymphosarcoma (diffuse) (M9613/3)
  200.8 ☑
  follicular (M9691/3) 202.0 ☑
  nodular (M9691/3) 202.0 ☑
Reticulosarcoma (M9640/3) 200.0 ☑
  nodular (M9642/3) 200.0 ☑
  pleomorphic cell type (M9641/3) 200.0 ☑
Reticulosis (skin)
  acute of infancy (M9722/3) 202.5 ☑
  familial hemophagocytic 288.4
  histiocytic medullary (M9721/3) 202.3 ☑
  lipomelanotic 695.89
  malignant (M9720/3) 202.3 ☑
  Sézary's (M9701/3) 202.2 ☑
Retina, retinal — *see* condition
Retinitis — *see also* Chorioretinitis 363.20
  albuminurica 585.9 [363.10]
  arteriosclerotic 440.8 [362.13]
  central angiospastic 362.41
  Coat's 362.12
  diabetic 250.5 ☑ [362.01]

Retinitis — *see also* Chorioretinitis —
    continued
  diabetic — *continued*
    due to secondary diabetes
      249.5 ☑ [362.01]
  disciformis 362.52
  disseminated 363.10
    metastatic 363.14
    neurosyphilitic 094.83
    pigment epitheliopathy 363.15
  exudative 362.12
  focal 363.00
    in histoplasmosis 115.92
      capsulatum 115.02
      duboisii 115.12
    juxtapapillary 363.05
    macular 363.06
    paramacular 363.06
    peripheral 363.08
    posterior pole NEC 363.07
  gravidarum 646.8 ☑
  hemorrhagica externa 362.12
  juxtapapillary (Jensen's) 363.05
  luetic — *see* Retinitis, syphilitic
  metastatic 363.14
  pigmentosa 362.74
  proliferans 362.29
  proliferating 362.29
  punctata albescens 362.76
  renal 585.9 [363.13]
  syphilitic (secondary) 091.51
    congenital 090.0 [363.13]
    early 091.51
    late 095.8 [363.13]
  syphilitica, central, recurrent 095.8 [363.13]
  tuberculous (*see also* Tuberculous)
    017.3 ☑ [363.13]
Retinoblastoma (M9510/3) 190.5
  differentiated type (M9511/3) 190.5
  undifferentiated type (M9512/3) 190.5
Retinochoroiditis — *see also* Chorioretinitis
  363.20
  central angiospastic 362.41
  disseminated 363.10
    metastatic 363.14
    neurosyphilitic 094.83
    pigment epitheliopathy 363.15
    syphilitic 094.83
  due to toxoplasmosis (acquired) (focal)
    130.2
  focal 363.00
    in histoplasmosis 115.92
      capsulatum 115.02
      duboisii 115.12
    juxtapapillary (Jensen's) 363.05
    macular 363.06
    paramacular 363.06
    peripheral 363.08
    posterior pole NEC 363.07
  juxtapapillaris 363.05
  syphilitic (disseminated) 094.83
Retinopathy (background) 362.10
  arteriosclerotic 440.8 [362.13]
  atherosclerotic 440.8 [362.13]
  central serous 362.41
  circinate 362.10
  Coat's 362.12
  diabetic 250.5 ☑ [362.01]
    due to secondary diabetes
      249.5 ☑ [362.01]
    nonproliferative 250.5 ☑ [362.03]
      due to secondary diabetes
        249.5 ☑ [362.03]
      mild 250.5 ☑ [362.04]
        due to secondary diabetes
          249.5 ☑ [362.04]
      moderate 250.5 ☑ [362.05]
        due to secondary diabetes
          249.5 ☑ [362.05]
      severe 250.5 ☑ [362.06]
        due to secondary diabetes
          249.5 ☑ [362.06]
    proliferative 250.5 ☑ [362.02]
      due to secondary diabetes
        249.5 ☑ [362.02]
  exudative 362.12

☑ **Additional Digit Required** — Refer to the Tabular List for Digit Selection   �ินᵛ **Subterms under main terms may continue to next column or page**

246 — Volume 2 · October 2010   ▶◀ **Revised Text**   ● **New Line**   ▲ **Revised Code**   **2011 ICD-9-CM**

Retinopathy — continued
  hypertensive 362.11
  nonproliferative
    diabetic 250.5 ☑ [362.03]
      due to secondary diabetes
        249.5 ☑ [362.03]
    mild 250.5 ☑ [362.04]
      due to secondary diabetes
        249.5 ☑ [362.04]
    moderate 250.5 ☑ [362.05]
      due to secondary diabetes
        249.5 ☑ [362.05]
    severe 250.5 ☑ [362.06]
      due to secondary diabetes
        249.5 ☑ [362.06]
  of prematurity 362.20
    cicatricial 362.21
    stage
      0 362.22
      1 362.23
      2 362.24
      3 362.25
      4 362.26
      5 362.27
  pigmentary, congenital 362.74
  proliferative 362.29
    diabetic 250.5 ☑ [362.02]
      due to secondary diabetes
        249.5 ☑ [362.02]
    sickle-cell 282.60 [362.29]
  solar 363.31
Retinoschisis 361.10
  bullous 361.12
  congenital 743.56
  flat 361.11
  juvenile 362.73
Retractile testis 752.52
Retraction
  cervix — see Retraction, uterus
  drum (membrane) 384.82
  eyelid 374.41
  finger 736.29
  head 781.0
  lid 374.41
  lung 518.89
  mediastinum 519.3
  nipple 611.79
    congenital 757.6
    puerperal, postpartum 676.0 ☑
  palmar fascia 728.6
  pleura (see also Pleurisy) 511.0
  ring, uterus (Bandl's) (pathological) 661.4 ☑
    affecting fetus or newborn 763.7
  sternum (congenital) 756.3
    acquired 738.3
    during respiration 786.9
  substernal 738.3
  supraclavicular 738.8
  syndrome (Duane's) 378.71
  uterus 621.6
  valve (heart) — see Endocarditis
Retrobulbar — see condition
Retrocaval ureter 753.4
Retrocecal — see also condition
  appendix (congenital) 751.5
Retrocession — see Retroversion
Retrodisplacement — see Retroversion
Retroflection, retroflexion — see Retroversion
Retrognathia, retrognathism (mandibular) (maxillary) 524.10
Retrograde
  ejaculation 608.87
  menstruation 626.8
Retroiliac ureter 753.4
Retroperineal — see condition
Retroperitoneal — see condition
Retroperitonitis 567.39
Retropharyngeal — see condition
Retroplacental — see condition
Retroposition — see Retroversion
Retroprosthetic membrane 996.51   ●
Retrosternal thyroid (congenital) 759.2
Retroversion, retroverted
  cervix — see Retroversion, uterus

Retroversion, retroverted — continued
  female NEC (see also Retroversion, uterus)
    621.6
  iris 364.70
  testis (congenital) 752.51
  uterus, uterine (acquired) (acute) (adherent)
    (any degree) (asymptomatic) (cervix)
    (postinfectional) (postpartal, old)
    621.6
    congenital 752.39   ▲
    in pregnancy or childbirth 654.3 ☑
      affecting fetus or newborn 763.89
      causing obstructed labor 660.2 ☑
        affecting fetus or newborn 763.1
Retrusion, premaxilla (developmental) 524.04
Rett's syndrome 330.8
Reverse, reversed
  peristalsis 787.4
Reye-Sheehan syndrome (postpartum pituitary necrosis) 253.2
Reye's syndrome 331.81
Rhabdomyolysis (idiopathic) 728.88
Rhabdomyoma (M8900/0) — see also Neoplasm, connective tissue, benign
  adult (M8904/0) — see Neoplasm, connective tissue, benign
  fetal (M8903/0) — see Neoplasm, connective tissue, benign
  glycogenic (M8904/0) — see Neoplasm, connective tissue, benign
Rhabdomyosarcoma (M8900/3) — see also Neoplasm, connective tissue, malignant
  alveolar (M8920/3) — see Neoplasm, connective tissue, malignant
  embryonal (M8910/3) — see Neoplasm, connective tissue, malignant
  mixed type (M8902/3) — see Neoplasm, connective tissue, malignant
  pleomorphic (M8901/3) — see Neoplasm, connective tissue, malignant
Rhabdosarcoma (M8900/3) — see Rhabdomyosarcoma
Rh ▶antigen (C) (c) (D) (E) (e)◀ (factor)
  hemolytic disease 773.0
  incompatibility, immunization, or sensitization
    affecting management of pregnancy
      656.1 ☑
    fetus or newborn 773.0
    transfusion reaction ▶(see also Complications, transfusion)◀
      999.70   ▲
  negative mother, affecting fetus or newborn
    773.0
  titer elevated ▶(see also Complications, transfusion)◀ 999.70   ▲
  transfusion reaction ▶(see also Complications, transfusion)◀ 999.70   ▲
Rhesus (factor) (Rh) incompatibility — see Rh, incompatibility
Rheumaticosis — see Rheumatism
Rheumatism, rheumatic (acute NEC) 729.0
  adherent pericardium 393
  arthritis
    acute or subacute — see Fever, rheumatic
    chronic 714.0
      spine 720.0
    articular (chronic) NEC (see also Arthritis)
      716.9 ☑
    acute or subacute — see Fever, rheumatic
  back 724.9
  blennorrhagic 098.59
  carditis — see Disease, heart, rheumatic
  cerebral — see Fever, rheumatic
  chorea (acute) — see Chorea, rheumatic
  chronic NEC 729.0
  coronary arteritis 391.9
    chronic 398.99
  degeneration, myocardium (see also Degeneration, myocardium, with rheumatic fever) 398.0
  desert 114.0
  febrile — see Fever, rheumatic
  fever — see Fever, rheumatic

Rheumatism, rheumatic — continued
  gonococcal 098.59
  gout 714.0   ▲
  heart
    disease (see also Disease, heart, rheumatic) 398.90
    failure (chronic) (congestive) (inactive) 398.91
  hemopericardium — see Rheumatic, pericarditis
  hydropericardium — see Rheumatic, pericarditis
  inflammatory (acute) (chronic) (subacute) — see Fever, rheumatic
  intercostal 729.0
    meaning Tietze's disease 733.6
  joint (chronic) NEC (see also Arthritis) 716.9 ☑
    acute — see Fever, rheumatic
  mediastinopericarditis — see Rheumatic, pericarditis
  muscular 729.0
  myocardial degeneration (see also Degeneration, myocardium, with rheumatic fever) 398.0
  myocarditis (chronic) (inactive) (with chorea) 398.0
    active or acute 391.2
      with chorea (acute) (rheumatic) (Sydenham's) 392.0
  myositis 729.1
  neck 724.9
  neuralgic 729.0
  neuritis (acute) (chronic) 729.2
  neuromuscular 729.0
  nodose — see Arthritis, nodosa
  nonarticular 729.0
  palindromic 719.30
    ankle 719.37
    elbow 719.32
    foot 719.37
    hand 719.34
    hip 719.35
    knee 719.36
    multiple sites 719.39
    pelvic region 719.35
    shoulder (region) 719.31
    specified site NEC 719.38
    wrist 719.33
  pancarditis, acute 391.8
    with chorea (acute) (rheumatic) (Sydenham's) 392.0
    chronic or inactive 398.99
  pericarditis (active) (acute) (with effusion) (with pneumonia) 391.0
    with chorea (acute) (rheumatic) (Sydenham's) 392.0
    chronic or inactive 393
  pericardium — see Rheumatic, pericarditis
  pleuropericarditis — see Rheumatic, pericarditis
  pneumonia 390 [517.1]
  pneumonitis 390 [517.1]
  pneumopericarditis — see Rheumatic, pericarditis
  polyarthritis
    acute or subacute — see Fever, rheumatic
    chronic 714.0
  polyarticular NEC (see also Arthritis) 716.9 ☑
  psychogenic 306.0
  radiculitis 729.2
  sciatic 724.3
  septic — see Fever, rheumatic
  spine 724.9
  subacute NEC 729.0
  torticollis 723.5
  tuberculous NEC (see also Tuberculosis) 015.9 ☑
  typhoid fever 002.0
Rheumatoid — see also condition
  lungs 714.81
Rhinitis (atrophic) (catarrhal) (chronic) (croupous) (fibrinous) (hyperplastic) (hypertrophic) (membranous) (purulent) (suppurative) (ulcerative) 472.0

Rhinitis — continued
  with
    hay fever (see also Fever, hay) 477.9
      with asthma (bronchial) 493.0 ☑
    sore throat — see Nasopharyngitis
  acute 460
  allergic (nonseasonal) (seasonal) (see also Fever, hay) 477.9
    with asthma (see also Asthma) 493.0 ☑
    due to food 477.1
  granulomatous 472.0
  infective 460
  obstructive 472.0
  pneumococcal 460
  syphilitic 095.8
    congenital 090.0
  tuberculous (see also Tuberculosis) 012.8 ☑
  vasomotor (see also Fever, hay) 477.9
Rhinoantritis (chronic) 473.0
  acute 461.0
Rhinodacryolith 375.57
Rhinolalia (aperta) (clausa) (open) 784.43
Rhinolith 478.19
  nasal sinus (see also Sinusitis) 473.9
Rhinomegaly 478.19
Rhinopharyngitis (acute) (subacute) — see also Nasopharyngitis 460
  chronic 472.2
  destructive ulcerating 102.5
  mutilans 102.5
Rhinophyma 695.3
Rhinorrhea 478.19
  cerebrospinal (fluid) 349.81
  paroxysmal (see also Fever, hay) 477.9
  spasmodic (see also Fever, hay) 477.9
Rhinosalpingitis 381.50
  acute 381.51
  chronic 381.52
Rhinoscleroma 040.1
Rhinosporidiosis 117.0
Rhinovirus infection 079.3
Rhizomelic chrondrodysplasia punctata 277.86
Rhizomelique, pseudopolyarthritic 446.5
Rhoads and Bomford anemia (refractory) 238.72
Rhus
  diversiloba dermatitis 692.6
  radicans dermatitis 692.6
  toxicodendron dermatitis 692.6
  venenata dermatitis 692.6
  verniciflua dermatitis 692.6
Rhythm
  atrioventricular nodal 427.89
  disorder 427.9
    coronary sinus 427.89
    ectopic 427.89
    nodal 427.89
  escape 427.89
  heart, abnormal 427.9
    fetus or newborn — see Abnormal, heart rate
  idioventricular 426.89
    accelerated 427.89
  nodal 427.89
  sleep, inversion 327.39
    nonorganic origin 307.45
Rhytidosis facialis 701.8
Rib — see also condition
  cervical 756.2
Riboflavin deficiency 266.0
Rice bodies — see also Loose, body, joint 718.1 ☑
  knee 717.6
Richter's hernia — see Hernia, Richter's
Ricinism 988.2
Rickets (active) (acute) (adolescent) (adult) (chest wall) (congenital) (current) (infantile) (intestinal) 268.0
  celiac 579.0
  fetal 756.4
  hemorrhagic 267
  hypophosphatemic with nephrotic-glycosuric dwarfism 270.0
  kidney 588.0
  late effect 268.1

☑ Additional Digit Required — Refer to the Tabular List for Digit Selection   ⓦ Subterms under main terms may continue to next column or page

2011 ICD-9-CM   ▶◀ Revised Text   ● New Line   ▲ Revised Code   October 2010 • Volume 2 — 247

Rickets — continued
  renal 588.0
  scurvy 267
  vitamin D-resistant 275.3
Rickettsial disease 083.9
  specified type NEC 083.8
Rickettsialpox 083.2
Rickettsiosis NEC 083.9
  specified type NEC 083.8
  tick-borne 082.9
    specified type NEC 082.8
  vesicular 083.2
Ricord's chancre 091.0
Riddoch's syndrome (visual disorientation) 368.16
Rider's
  bone 733.99
  chancre 091.0
Ridge, alveolus — see also condition
  edentulous
    atrophy 525.20
      mandible 525.20
        minimal 525.21
        moderate 525.22
        severe 525.23
      maxilla 525.20
        minimal 525.24
        moderate 525.25
        severe 525.26
    flabby 525.20
Ridged ear 744.29
Riedel's
  disease (ligneous thyroiditis) 245.3
  lobe, liver 751.69
  struma (ligneous thyroiditis) 245.3
  thyroiditis (ligneous) 245.3
Rieger's anomaly or syndrome (mesodermal dysgenesis, anterior ocular segment) 743.44
Riehl's melanosis 709.09
Rietti-Greppi-Micheli anemia or syndrome 282.49
Rieux's hernia — see Hernia, Rieux's
Rift Valley fever 066.3
Riga's disease (cachectic aphthae) 529.0
Riga-Fede disease (cachectic aphthae) 529.0
Riggs' disease (compound periodontitis) 523.40
Right middle lobe syndrome 518.0
Rigid, rigidity — see also condition
  abdominal 789.4 ☑
  articular, multiple congenital 754.89
  back 724.8
  cervix uteri
    in pregnancy or childbirth 654.6 ☑
      affecting fetus or newborn 763.89
      causing obstructed labor 660.2 ☑
        affecting fetus or newborn 763.1
  hymen (acquired) (congenital) 623.3
  nuchal 781.6
  pelvic floor
    in pregnancy or childbirth 654.4 ☑
      affecting fetus or newborn 763.89
      causing obstructed labor 660.2 ☑
        affecting fetus or newborn 763.1
  perineum or vulva
    in pregnancy or childbirth 654.8 ☑
      affecting fetus or newborn 763.89
      causing obstructed labor 660.2 ☑
        affecting fetus or newborn 763.1
  spine 724.8
  vagina
    in pregnancy or childbirth 654.7 ☑
      affecting fetus or newborn 763.89
      causing obstructed labor 660.2 ☑
        affecting fetus or newborn 763.1
Rigors 780.99
Riley-Day syndrome (familial dysautonomia) 742.8
RIND (reversible ischemic neurological deficit) 434.91
  history of (personal) V12.54
Ring(s)
  aorta 747.21
  Bandl's, complicating delivery 661.4 ☑
    affecting fetus or newborn 763.7

Ring(s) — continued
  contraction, complicating delivery 661.4 ☑
    affecting fetus or newborn 763.7
  esophageal (congenital) 750.3
  Fleischer (-Kayser) (cornea) 275.1 [371.14]
  hymenal, tight (acquired) (congenital) 623.3
  Kayser-Fleischer (cornea) 275.1 [371.14]
  retraction, uterus, pathological 661.4 ☑
    affecting fetus or newborn 763.7
  Schatzki's (esophagus) (congenital) (lower) 750.3
    acquired 530.3
  Soemmering's 366.51
  trachea, abnormal 748.3
  vascular (congenital) 747.21
  Vossius' 921.3
    late effect 366.21
Ringed hair (congenital) 757.4
Ringing in the ear — see also Tinnitus 388.30
Ringworm 110.9
  beard 110.0
  body 110.5
  Burmese 110.9
  corporeal 110.5
  foot 110.4
  groin 110.3
  hand 110.2
  honeycomb 110.0
  nails 110.1
  perianal (area) 110.3
  scalp 110.0
  specified site NEC 110.8
  Tokelau 110.5
Rise, venous pressure 459.89
Risk
  factor — see Problem
  falling
  suicidal 300.9
Ritter's disease (dermatitis exfoliativa neonatorum) 695.81
Rivalry, sibling 313.3
Rivalta's disease (cervicofacial actinomycosis) 039.3
River blindness 125.3 [360.13]
Robert's pelvis 755.69
  with disproportion (fetopelvic) 653.0 ☑
    affecting fetus or newborn 763.1
    causing obstructed labor 660.1 ☑
      affecting fetus or newborn 763.1
Robinson's (hidrotic) **ectodermal dysplasia** 757.31
Robin's syndrome 756.0
Robles' disease (onchocerciasis) 125.3 [360.13]
Rochalimea — see Rickettsial disease
Rocky Mountain fever (spotted) 082.0
Rodent ulcer (M8090/3) — see also Neoplasm, skin, malignant
  cornea 370.07
Roentgen ray, adverse effect — see Effect, adverse, x-ray
Roethel 056.9
Roger's disease (congenital interventricular septal defect) 745.4
Rokitansky's
  disease (see also Necrosis, liver) 570
  tumor 620.2
Rokitansky-Aschoff sinuses (mucosal outpouching of gallbladder) — see also Disease, gallbladder 575.8
Rokitansky-Kuster-Hauser syndrome (congenital absence vagina) 752.45 ▲
Rollet's chancre (syphilitic) 091.0
Rolling of head 781.0
Romano-Ward syndrome (prolonged QT interval syndrome) 426.82
Romanus lesion 720.1
Romberg's disease or syndrome 349.89
Roof, mouth — see condition
Rosacea 695.3
  acne 695.3
  keratitis 695.3 [370.49]
Rosary, rachitic 268.0
Rose
  cold 477.0
  fever 477.0
  rash 782.1

Rose — continued
  rash — continued
    epidemic 056.9
    of infants 057.8
Rosenbach's erysipelatoid or erysipeloid 027.1
Rosen-Castleman-Liebow syndrome (pulmonary proteinosis) 516.0
Rosenthal's disease (factor XI deficiency) 286.2
Roseola 057.8
  infantum, infantilis (see also Exanthem subitum) 058.10
Rossbach's disease (hyperchlorhydria) 536.8
  psychogenic 306.4
Rössle-Urbach-Wiethe lipoproteinosis 272.8
Ross river fever 066.3
Rostan's asthma (cardiac) — see also Failure, ventricular, left 428.1
Rot
  Barcoo (see also Ulcer, skin) 707.9
  knife-grinders' (see also Tuberculosis) 011.4 ☑
Rotation
  anomalous, incomplete or insufficient — see Malrotation
  cecum (congenital) 751.4
  colon (congenital) 751.4
  manual, affecting fetus or newborn 763.89
  spine, incomplete or insufficient 737.8
  tooth, teeth 524.35
  vertebra, incomplete or insufficient 737.8
Rot-Bernhardt disease 355.1
Röteln 056.9
Roth-Bernhardt disease or syndrome 355.1
Roth's disease or meralgia 355.1
Rothmund (-Thomson) syndrome 757.33
Rotor's disease or syndrome (idiopathic hyperbilirubinemia) 277.4
Rotundum ulcus — see Ulcer, stomach
Round
  back (with wedging of vertebrae) 737.10
    late effect of rickets 268.1
  hole, retina 361.31
    with detachment 361.01
  ulcer (stomach) — see Ulcer, stomach
  worms (infestation) (large) NEC 127.0
Roussy-Lévy syndrome 334.3
Routine postpartum follow-up V24.2
Roy (-Jutras) syndrome (acropachyderma) 757.39
Rubella (German measles) 056.9
  complicating pregnancy, childbirth, or puerperium 647.5 ☑
  complication 056.8
    neurological 056.00
      encephalomyelitis 056.01
      specified type NEC 056.09
    specified type NEC 056.79
  congenital 771.0
  contact V01.4
  exposure to V01.4
  maternal
    with suspected fetal damage affecting management of pregnancy 655.3 ☑
    affecting fetus or newborn 760.2
      manifest rubella in infant 771.0
  specified complications NEC 056.79
  vaccination, prophylactic (against) V04.3
Rubeola (measles) — see also Measles 055.9
  complicated 055.8
  meaning rubella (see also Rubella) 056.9
  scarlatinosis 057.8
Rubeosis iridis 364.42
  diabetica 250.5 ☑ [364.42]
    due to secondary diabetes 249.5 ☑ [364.42]
Rubinstein-Taybi's syndrome (brachydactylia, short stature and mental retardation) 759.89
Rudimentary (congenital) — see also Agenesis
  arm 755.22
  bone 756.9
  cervix uteri 752.43 ▲
  eye (see also Microphthalmos) 743.10
  fallopian tube 752.19

Rudimentary — see also Agenesis — continued
  leg 755.32
  lobule of ear 744.21
  patella 755.64
  respiratory organs in thoracopagus 759.4
  tracheal bronchus 748.3
  uterine horn 752.39   ▲
  uterus 752.39   ▲
    in male 752.7
    solid or with cavity 752.39   ▲
  vagina 752.45   ▲
Rud's syndrome (mental deficiency, epilepsy, and infantilism) 759.89
Ruiter-Pompen (-Wyers) syndrome (angiokeratoma corporis diffusum) 272.7
Ruled out condition — see also Observation, suspected V71.9
Rumination — see also Vomiting
  disorder 307.53
  neurotic 300.3
  obsessional 300.3
  psychogenic 307.53
Runaway reaction — see also Disturbance, conduct
  socialized 312.2 ☑
  undersocialized, unsocialized 312.1 ☑
Runeberg's disease (progressive pernicious anemia) 281.0
Runge's syndrome (postmaturity) 766.22
Runny nose 784.99
Rupia 091.3
  congenital 090.0
  tertiary 095.9
Rupture, ruptured 553.9
  abdominal viscera NEC 799.89
    obstetrical trauma 665.5 ☑
  abscess (spontaneous) — see Abscess, by site
  amnion — see Rupture, membranes
  aneurysm — see Aneurysm
  anus (sphincter) — see Laceration, anus
  aorta, aortic 441.5
    abdominal 441.3
    arch 441.1
    ascending 441.1
    descending 441.5
      abdominal 441.3
      thoracic 441.1
    syphilitic 093.0
    thoracoabdominal 441.6
    thorax, thoracic 441.1
    transverse 441.1
    traumatic (thoracic) 901.0
      abdominal 902.0
    valve or cusp (see also Endocarditis, aortic) 424.1
  appendix (with peritonitis) 540.0
    with peritoneal abscess 540.1
    traumatic — see Injury, internal, gastrointestinal tract
  arteriovenous fistula, brain (congenital) 430
  artery 447.2
    brain (see also Hemorrhage, brain) 431
    coronary (see also Infarct, myocardium) 410.9 ☑
    heart (see also Infarct, myocardium) 410.9 ☑
    pulmonary 417.8
    traumatic (complication) (see also Injury, blood vessel, by site) 904.9
  bile duct, except cystic (see also Disease, biliary) 576.3
    cystic 575.4
    traumatic — see Injury, internal, intraabdominal
  bladder (sphincter) 596.6
    with
      abortion — see Abortion, by type, with damage to pelvic organs
      ectopic pregnancy (see also categories 633.0–633.9) 639.2
      molar pregnancy (see also categories 630–632) 639.2
    following
      abortion 639.2

☑ **Additional Digit Required** — Refer to the Tabular List for Digit Selection   Subterms under main terms may continue to next column or page

248 — Volume 2 · October 2010   ▶◀ Revised Text   ● New Line   ▲ Revised Code   2011 ICD-9-CM

Rupture, ruptured — Rupture, ruptured

Rupture, ruptured — *continued*
  bladder — *continued*
    following — *continued*
      ectopic or molar pregnancy 639.2
    nontraumatic 596.6
    obstetrical trauma 665.5 ☑
    spontaneous 596.6
    traumatic — *see* Injury, internal, bladder
  blood vessel (*see also* Hemorrhage) 459.0
    brain (*see also* Hemorrhage, brain) 431
    heart (*see also* Infarct, myocardium) 410.9 ☑
    traumatic (complication) (*see also* Injury, blood vessel, by site) 904.9
  bone — *see* Fracture, by site
  bowel 569.89
    traumatic — *see* Injury, internal, intestine
  Bowman's membrane 371.31
  brain
    aneurysm (congenital) (*see also* Hemorrhage, subarachnoid) 430
      late effect — *see* Late effect(s) (of) cerebrovascular disease
      syphilitic 094.87
    hemorrhagic (*see also* Hemorrhage, brain) 431
    injury at birth 767.0
    syphilitic 094.89
  capillaries 448.9
  cardiac (*see also* Infarct, myocardium) 410.9 ☑
  cartilage (articular) (current) (*see also* Sprain, by site)
    knee — *see* Tear, meniscus
    semilunar — *see* Tear, meniscus
  cecum (with peritonitis) 540.0
    with peritoneal abscess 540.1
    traumatic 863.89
      with open wound into cavity 863.99
  cerebral aneurysm (congenital) (*see also* Hemorrhage, subarachnoid) 430
    late effect — *see* Late effect(s) (of) cerebrovascular disease
  cervix (uteri)
    with
      abortion — *see* Abortion, by type, with damage to pelvic organs
      ectopic pregnancy (*see also* categories 633.0–633.9) 639.2
      molar pregnancy (*see also* categories 630–632) 639.2
    following
      abortion 639.2
      ectopic or molar pregnancy 639.2
    obstetrical trauma 665.3 ☑
    traumatic — *see* Injury, internal, cervix
  chordae tendineae 429.5
  choroid (direct) (indirect) (traumatic) 363.63
  circle of Willis (*see also* Hemorrhage, subarachnoid) 430
    late effect — *see* Late effect(s) (of) cerebrovascular disease
  colon 569.89
    traumatic — *see* Injury, internal, colon
  cornea (traumatic) (*see also* Rupture, eye) due to ulcer 370.00
  coronary (artery) (thrombotic) (*see also* Infarct, myocardium) 410.9 ☑
  corpus luteum (infected) (ovary) 620.1
  cyst — *see* Cyst
  cystic duct (*see also* Disease, gallbladder) 575.4
  Descemet's membrane 371.33
    traumatic — *see* Rupture, eye
  diaphragm (*see also* Hernia, diaphragm)
    traumatic — *see* Injury, internal, diaphragm
  diverticulum
    bladder 596.3
    intestine (large) (*see also* Diverticula) 562.10
      small 562.00
  duodenal stump 537.89
  duodenum (ulcer) — *see* Ulcer, duodenum, with perforation

Rupture, ruptured — *continued*
  ear drum (*see also* Perforation, tympanum) 384.20
    with otitis media — *see* Otitis media
    traumatic — *see* Wound, open, ear
  esophagus 530.4
    traumatic 862.22
      with open wound into cavity 862.32
      cervical region — *see* Wound, open, esophagus
  eye (without prolapse of intraocular tissue) 871.0
    with
      exposure of intraocular tissue 871.1
      partial loss of intraocular tissue 871.2
      prolapse of intraocular tissue 871.1
    due to burn 940.5
  fallopian tube 620.8
    due to pregnancy — *see* Pregnancy, tubal
    traumatic — *see* Injury, internal, fallopian tube
  fontanel 767.3
  free wall (ventricle) (*see also* Infarct, myocardium) 410.9 ☑
  gallbladder or duct (*see also* Disease, gallbladder) 575.4
    traumatic — *see* Injury, internal, gallbladder
  gastric (*see also* Rupture, stomach) 537.89
    vessel 459.0
  globe (eye) (traumatic) — *see* Rupture, eye
  graafian follicle (hematoma) 620.0
  heart (auricle) (ventricle) (*see also* Infarct, myocardium) 410.9 ☑
    infectional 422.90
    traumatic — *see* Rupture, myocardium, traumatic
  hymen 623.8
  internal
    organ, traumatic (*see also* Injury, internal, by site)
      heart — *see* Rupture, myocardium, traumatic
      kidney — *see* Rupture, kidney
      liver — *see* Rupture, liver
      spleen — *see* Rupture, spleen, traumatic
    semilunar cartilage — *see* Tear, meniscus
  intervertebral disc — *see* Displacement, intervertebral disc
    traumatic (current) — *see* Dislocation, vertebra
  intestine 569.89
    traumatic — *see* Injury, internal, intestine
  intracranial, birth injury 767.0
  iris 364.76
    traumatic — *see* Rupture, eye
  joint capsule — *see* Sprain, by site
  kidney (traumatic) 866.03
    with open wound into cavity 866.13
    due to birth injury 767.8
    nontraumatic 593.89
  lacrimal apparatus (traumatic) 870.2
  lens (traumatic) 366.20
  ligament (*see also* Sprain, by site)
    with open wound — *see* Wound, open, by site
    old (*see also* Disorder, cartilage, articular) 718.0 ☑
  liver (traumatic) 864.04
    with open wound into cavity 864.14
    due to birth injury 767.8
    nontraumatic 573.8
  lymphatic (node) (vessel) 457.8
  marginal sinus (placental) (with hemorrhage) 641.2 ☑
    affecting fetus or newborn 762.1
  meaning hernia — *see* Hernia
  membrana tympani (*see also* Perforation, tympanum) 384.20
    with otitis media — *see* Otitis media
    traumatic — *see* Wound, open, ear

Rupture, ruptured — *continued*
  membranes (spontaneous)
    artificial
      delayed delivery following 658.3 ☑
        affecting fetus or newborn 761.1
        fetus or newborn 761.1
    delayed delivery following 658.2 ☑
      affecting fetus or newborn 761.1
    premature (less than 24 hours prior to onset of labor) 658.1 ☑
      affecting fetus or newborn 761.1
      delayed delivery following 658.2 ☑
        affecting fetus or newborn 761.1
  meningeal artery (*see also* Hemorrhage, subarachnoid) 430
    late effect — *see* Late effect(s) (of) cerebrovascular disease
  meniscus (knee) (*see also* Tear, meniscus)
    old (*see also* Derangement, meniscus) 717.5
      site other than knee — *see* Disorder, cartilage, articular
    site other than knee — *see* Sprain, by site
  mesentery 568.89
    traumatic — *see* Injury, internal, mesentery
  mitral — *see* Insufficiency, mitral
  muscle (traumatic) NEC (*see also* Sprain, by site)
    with open wound — *see* Wound, open, by site
    nontraumatic 728.83
  musculotendinous cuff (nontraumatic) (shoulder) 840.4
  mycotic aneurysm, causing cerebral hemorrhage (*see also* Hemorrhage, subarachnoid) 430
    late effect — *see* Late effect(s) (of) cerebrovascular disease
  myocardium, myocardial (*see also* Infarct, myocardium) 410.9 ☑
    traumatic 861.03
      with open wound into thorax 861.13
  nontraumatic (meaning hernia) (*see also* Hernia, by site) 553.9
  obstructed (*see also* Hernia, by site, with obstruction) 552.9
    gangrenous (*see also* Hernia, by site, with gangrene) 551.9
  operation wound (*see also* Dehiscence) 998.32
    internal 998.31
  ovary, ovarian 620.8
    corpus luteum 620.1
    follicle (graafian) 620.0
  oviduct 620.8
    due to pregnancy — *see* Pregnancy, tubal
  pancreas 577.8
    traumatic — *see* Injury, internal, pancreas
  papillary muscle (ventricular) 429.6
  pelvic
    floor, complicating delivery 664.1 ☑
    organ NEC — *see* Injury, pelvic, organs
  penis (traumatic) — *see* Wound, open, penis
  perineum 624.8
    during delivery (*see also* Laceration, perineum, complicating delivery) 664.4 ☑
  pharynx (nontraumatic) (spontaneous) 478.29
  pregnant uterus (before onset of labor) 665.0 ☑
  prostate (traumatic) — *see* Injury, internal, prostate
  pulmonary
    artery 417.8
    valve (heart) (*see also* Endocarditis, pulmonary) 424.3
    vein 417.8
    vessel 417.8
  pupil, sphincter 364.75
  pus tube (*see also* Salpingo-oophoritis) 614.2

Rupture, ruptured — *continued*
  pyosalpinx (*see also* Salpingo-oophoritis) 614.2
  rectum 569.49
    traumatic — *see* Injury, internal, rectum
  retina, retinal (traumatic) (without detachment) 361.30
    with detachment (*see also* Detachment, retina, with retinal defect) 361.00
  rotator cuff (capsule) (traumatic) 840.4
    nontraumatic, complete 727.61
  sclera 871.0
  semilunar cartilage, knee (*see also* Tear, meniscus) 836.2
    old (*see also* Derangement, meniscus) 717.5
  septum (cardiac) 410.8 ☑
  sigmoid 569.89
    traumatic — *see* Injury, internal, colon, sigmoid
  sinus of Valsalva 747.29
  spinal cord (*see also* Injury, spinal, by site)
    due to injury at birth 767.4
    fetus or newborn 767.4
    syphilitic 094.89
    traumatic (*see also* Injury, spinal, by site)
      with fracture — *see* Fracture, vertebra, by site, with spinal cord injury
  spleen 289.59
    congenital 767.8
    due to injury at birth 767.8
    malarial 084.9
    nontraumatic 289.59
    spontaneous 289.59
    traumatic 865.04
      with open wound into cavity 865.14
  splenic vein 459.0
  stomach 537.89
    due to injury at birth 767.8
    traumatic — *see* Injury, internal, stomach
    ulcer — *see* Ulcer, stomach, with perforation
  synovium 727.50
    specified site NEC 727.59
  tendon (traumatic) (*see also* Sprain, by site)
    with open wound — *see* Wound, open, by site
    Achilles 845.09
      nontraumatic 727.67
    ankle 845.09
      nontraumatic 727.68
    biceps (long head) 840.8
      nontraumatic 727.62
    foot 845.10
      interphalangeal (joint) 845.13
      metatarsophalangeal (joint) 845.12
      nontraumatic 727.68
      specified site NEC 845.19
      tarsometatarsal (joint) 845.11
    hand 842.10
      carpometacarpal (joint) 842.11
      interphalangeal (joint) 842.13
      metacarpophalangeal (joint) 842.12
      nontraumatic 727.63
        extensors 727.63
        flexors 727.64
      specified site NEC 842.19
    nontraumatic 727.60
      specified site NEC 727.69
    patellar 844.8
      nontraumatic 727.66
    quadriceps 844.8
      nontraumatic 727.65
    rotator cuff (capsule) 840.4
      nontraumatic, complete 727.61
    wrist 842.00
      carpal (joint) 842.01
      nontraumatic 727.63
        extensors 727.63
        flexors 727.64
      radiocarpal (joint) (ligament) 842.02
      radioulnar (joint), distal 842.09
      specified site NEC 842.09
  testis (traumatic) 878.2

☑ **Additional Digit Required** — Refer to the Tabular List for Digit Selection   ▽ **Subterms under main terms may continue to next column or page**

2011 ICD-9-CM   ▶◀ Revised Text   ● New Line   ▲ Revised Code   **Volume 2 — 249**

Rupture, ruptured — *continued*
  testis — *continued*
    complicated 878.3
    due to syphilis 095.8
  thoracic duct 457.8
  tonsil 474.8
  traumatic
    with open wound — *see* Wound, open,
        by site
    aorta — *see* Rupture, aorta, traumatic
    ear drum — *see* Wound, open, ear, drum
    external site — *see* Wound, open, by site
    eye 871.2
    globe (eye) — *see* Wound, open, eyeball
    internal organ (abdomen, chest, or
        pelvis) (*see also* Injury, internal,
        by site)
      heart — *see* Rupture, myocardium,
          traumatic
      kidney — *see* Rupture, kidney
      liver — *see* Rupture, liver
      spleen — *see* Rupture, spleen, trau-
          matic
    ligament, muscle, or tendon (*see also*
        Sprain, by site)
      with open wound — *see* Wound,
          open, by site

Rupture, ruptured — *continued*
  traumatic — *continued*
    meaning hernia — *see* Hernia
  tricuspid (heart) (valve) — *see* Endocarditis,
      tricuspid
  tube, tubal 620.8
    abscess (*see also* Salpingo-oophoritis)
        614.2
    due to pregnancy — *see* Pregnancy,
        tubal
  tympanum, tympanic (membrane) (*see also*
      Perforation, tympanum) 384.20
    with otitis media — *see* Otitis media
    traumatic — *see* Wound, open, ear,
        drum
  umbilical cord 663.8 ☑
    fetus or newborn 772.0
  ureter (traumatic) (*see also* Injury, internal,
      ureter) 867.2
    nontraumatic 593.89
  urethra 599.84
    with
      abortion — *see* Abortion, by type,
          with damage to pelvic organs
      ectopic pregnancy (*see also* cate-
          gories 633.0–633.9) 639.2

Rupture, ruptured — *continued*
  urethra — *continued*
    with — *continued*
      molar pregnancy (*see also* categories
          630–632) 639.2
    following
      abortion 639.2
      ectopic or molar pregnancy 639.2
    obstetrical trauma 665.5 ☑
    traumatic — *see* Injury, internal urethra
  uterosacral ligament 620.8
  uterus (traumatic) (*see also* Injury, internal,
      uterus)
    affecting fetus or newborn 763.89
    during labor 665.1 ☑
    nonpuerperal, nontraumatic 621.8
    nontraumatic 621.8
    pregnant (during labor) 665.1 ☑
      before labor 665.0 ☑
  vagina 878.6
    complicated 878.7
    complicating delivery — *see* Laceration,
        vagina, complicating delivery
  valve, valvular (heart) — *see* Endocarditis
  varicose vein — *see* Varicose, vein
  varix — *see* Varix
  vena cava 459.0

Rupture, ruptured — *continued*
  ventricle (free wall) (left) (*see also* Infarct,
      myocardium) 410.9 ☑
  vesical (urinary) 596.6
    traumatic — *see* Injury, internal, bladder
  vessel (blood) 459.0
    pulmonary 417.8
  viscus 799.89
  vulva 878.4
    complicated 878.5
    complicating delivery 664.0 ☑
Russell's dwarf (uterine dwarfism and cranio-
    facial dysostosis) 759.89
Russell's dysentery 004.8
Russell (-Silver) syndrome (congenital
    hemihypertrophy and short stature)
    759.89
Russian spring-summer type encephalitis
    063.0
Rust's disease (tuberculous spondylitis)
    015.0 ☑ *[720.81]*
Rustitskii's disease (multiple myeloma)
    (M9730/3) 203.0 ☑
Ruysch's disease (Hirschsprung's disease)
    751.3
Rytand-Lipsitch syndrome (complete atrioven-
    tricular block) 426.0

S

Saber
  shin 090.5
  tibia 090.5
Saccharomyces infection — *see also* Candidiasis 112.9
Saccharopinuria 270.7
Saccular — *see* condition
Sacculation
  aorta (nonsyphilitic) (*see also* Aneurysm, aorta) 441.9
    ruptured 441.5
    syphilitic 093.0
  bladder 596.3
  colon 569.89
  intralaryngeal (congenital) (ventricular) 748.3
  larynx (congenital) (ventricular) 748.3
  organ or site, congenital — *see* Distortion
  pregnant uterus, complicating delivery 654.4 ☑
    affecting fetus or newborn 763.1
      causing obstructed labor 660.2 ☑
        affecting fetus or newborn 763.1
  rectosigmoid 569.89
  sigmoid 569.89
  ureter 593.89
  urethra 599.2
  vesical 596.3
Sachs (-Tay) disease (amaurotic familial idiocy) 330.1
Sacks-Libman disease 710.0 *[424.91]*
Sac, lacrimal — *see* condition
Sacralgia 724.6
Sacralization
  fifth lumbar vertebra 756.15
  incomplete (vertebra) 756.15
Sacrodynia 724.6
Sacroiliac joint — *see* condition
Sacroiliitis NEC 720.2
Sacrum — *see* condition
Saddle
  back 737.8
  embolus, aorta 444.0
  nose 738.0
    congenital 754.0
    due to syphilis 090.5
Sadism (sexual) 302.84
Saemisch's ulcer 370.04
Saenger's syndrome 379.46
Sago spleen 277.39
Sailors' skin 692.74
Saint
  Anthony's fire (*see also* Erysipelas) 035
  Guy's dance — *see* Chorea
  Louis-type encephalitis 062.3
  triad (*see also* Hernia, diaphragm) 553.3
  Vitus' dance — *see* Chorea
Salicylism
  correct substance properly administered 535.4 ☑
  overdose or wrong substance given or taken 965.1
Salivary duct or gland — *see also* condition
  virus disease 078.5
Salivation (excessive) — *see also* Ptyalism 527.7
Salmonella (aertrycke) (choleraesuis) (enteritidis) (gallinarum) (suipestifer) (typhimurium) — *see also* Infection, Salmonella 003.9
  arthritis 003.23
  carrier (suspected) of V02.3
  meningitis 003.21
  osteomyelitis 003.24
  pneumonia 003.22
  septicemia 003.1
  typhosa 002.0
    carrier (suspected) of V02.1
Salmonellosis 003.0
  with pneumonia 003.22
Salpingitis (catarrhal) (fallopian tube) (nodular) (pseudofollicular) (purulent) (septic) — *see also* Salpingo-oophoritis 614.2
  ear 381.50

Salpingitis — *see also* Salpingo-oophoritis — *continued*
  ear — *continued*
    acute 381.51
    chronic 381.52
    Eustachian (tube) 381.50
      acute 381.51
      chronic 381.52
  follicularis 614.1
  gonococcal (chronic) 098.37
    acute 098.17
  interstitial, chronic 614.1
  isthmica nodosa 614.1
  old — *see* Salpingo-oophoritis, chronic
  puerperal, postpartum, childbirth 670.8 ☑
  specific (chronic) 098.37
    acute 098.17
  tuberculous (acute) (chronic) (*see also* Tuberculosis) 016.6 ☑
  venereal (chronic) 098.37
    acute 098.17
Salpingocele 620.4
Salpingo-oophoritis (catarrhal) (purulent) (ruptured) (septic) (suppurative) 614.2
  acute 614.0
    with
      abortion — *see* Abortion, by type, with sepsis
      ectopic pregnancy (*see also* categories 633.0–633.9) 639.0
      molar pregnancy (*see also* categories 630–632) 639.0
    following
      abortion 639.0
      ectopic or molar pregnancy 639.0
    gonococcal 098.17
    puerperal, postpartum, childbirth 670.8 ☑
    tuberculous (*see also* Tuberculosis) 016.6 ☑
  chronic 614.1
    gonococcal 098.37
    tuberculous (see also Tuberculosis) 016.6 ☑
  complicating pregnancy 646.6 ☑
    affecting fetus or newborn 760.8
  gonococcal (chronic) 098.37
    acute 098.17
  old — *see* Salpingo-oophoritis, chronic
  puerperal 670.8 ☑
  specific — *see* Salpingo-oophoritis, gonococcal
  subacute (*see also* Salpingo-oophoritis, acute) 614.0
  tuberculous (acute) (chronic) (*see also* Tuberculosis) 016.6 ☑
  venereal — *see* Salpingo-oophoritis, gonococcal
Salpingo-ovaritis — *see also* Salpingo-oophoritis 614.2
Salpingoperitonitis — *see also* Salpingo-oophoritis 614.2
Salt-losing
  nephritis (*see also* Disease, renal) 593.9
  syndrome (*see also* Disease, renal) 593.9
Salt-rheum — *see also* Eczema 692.9
Salzmann's nodular dystrophy 371.46
Sampling
  chorionic villus V28.89
Sampson's cyst or tumor 617.1
Sandblasters'
  asthma 502
  lung 502
Sander's disease (paranoia) 297.1
Sandfly fever 066.0
Sandhoff's disease 330.1
Sanfilippo's syndrome (mucopolysaccharidosis III) 277.5
Sanger-Brown's ataxia 334.2
San Joaquin Valley fever 114.0
Sao Paulo fever or typhus 082.0
Saponification, mesenteric 567.89
Sapremia — *see* Septicemia
Sarcocele (benign)
  syphilitic 095.8
    congenital 090.5

Sarcoepiplocele — *see also* Hernia 553.9
Sarcoepiplomphalocele — *see also* Hernia, umbilicus 553.1
Sarcoid (any site) 135
  with lung involvement 135 *[517.8]*
  Boeck's 135
  Darier-Roussy 135
  Spiegler-Fendt 686.8
Sarcoidosis 135
  cardiac 135 *[425.8]*
  lung 135 *[517.8]*
Sarcoma (M8800/3) — *see also* Neoplasm, connective tissue, malignant
  alveolar soft part (M9581/3) — *see* Neoplasm, connective tissue, malignant
  ameloblastic (M9330/3) 170.1
    upper jaw (bone) 170.0
  botryoid (M8910/3) — *see* Neoplasm, connective tissue, malignant
  botryoides (M8910/3) — *see* Neoplasm, connective tissue, malignant
  cerebellar (M9480/3) 191.6
    circumscribed (arachnoidal) (M9471/3) 191.6
  circumscribed (arachnoidal) cerebellar (M9471/3) 191.6
  clear cell, of tendons and aponeuroses (M9044/3) — *see* Neoplasm, connective tissue, malignant
  embryonal (M8991/3) — *see* Neoplasm, connective tissue, malignant
  endometrial (stromal) (M8930/3) 182.0
    isthmus 182.1
  endothelial (M9130/3) (*see also* Neoplasm, connective tissue, malignant)
    bone (M9260/3) — *see* Neoplasm, bone, malignant
  epithelioid cell (M8804/3) — *see* Neoplasm, connective tissue, malignant
  Ewing's (M9260/3) — *see* Neoplasm, bone, malignant
  follicular dendritic cell 202.9 ☑
  germinoblastic (diffuse) (M9632/3) 202.8 ☑
    follicular (M9697/3) 202.0 ☑
  giant cell (M8802/3) (*see also* Neoplasm, connective tissue, malignant)
    bone (M9250/3) — *see* Neoplasm, bone, malignant
  glomoid (M8710/3) — *see* Neoplasm, connective tissue, malignant
  granulocytic (M9930/3) 205.3 ☑
  hemangioendothelial (M9130/3) — *see* Neoplasm, connective tissue, malignant
  hemorrhagic, multiple (M9140/3) — *see* Kaposi's, sarcoma
  Hodgkin's (M9662/3) 201.2 ☑
  immunoblastic (M9612/3) 200.8 ☑
  interdigitating dendritic cell 202.9 ☑
  Kaposi's (M9140/3) — *see* Kaposi's, sarcoma
  Kupffer cell (M9124/3) 155.0
  Langerhans cell 202.9 ☑
  leptomeningeal (M9530/3) — *see* Neoplasm, meninges, malignant
  lymphangioendothelial (M9170/3) — *see* Neoplasm, connective tissue, malignant
  lymphoblastic (M9630/3) 200.1 ☑
  lymphocytic (M9620/3) 200.1 ☑
  mast cell (M9740/3) 202.6 ☑
  melanotic (M8720/3) — *see* Melanoma
  meningeal (M9530/3) — *see* Neoplasm, meninges, malignant
  meningothelial (M9530/3) — *see* Neoplasm, meninges, malignant
  mesenchymal (M8800/3) (*see also* Neoplasm, connective tissue, malignant)
    mixed (M8990/3) — *see* Neoplasm, connective tissue, malignant
  mesothelial (M9050/3) — *see* Neoplasm, by site, malignant
  monstrocellular (M9481/3)
    specified site — *see* Neoplasm, by site, malignant
    unspecified site 191.9
  myeloid (M9930/3) 205.3 ☑

Sarcoma — *see also* Neoplasm, connective tissue, malignant — *continued*
  neurogenic (M9540/3) — *see* Neoplasm, connective tissue, malignant
  odontogenic (M9270/3) 170.1
    upper jaw (bone) 170.0
  osteoblastic (M9180/3) — *see* Neoplasm, bone, malignant
  osteogenic (M9180/3) (*see also* Neoplasm, bone, malignant)
    juxtacortical (M9190/3) — *see* Neoplasm, bone, malignant
    periosteal (M9190/3) — *see* Neoplasm, bone, malignant
  periosteal (M8812/3) (*see also* Neoplasm, bone, malignant)
    osteogenic (M9190/3) — *see* Neoplasm, bone, malignant
  plasma cell (M9731/3) 203.8 ☑
  pleomorphic cell (M8802/3) — *see* Neoplasm, connective tissue, malignant
  reticuloendothelial (M9720/3) 202.3 ☑
  reticulum cell (M9640/3) 200.0 ☑
    nodular (M9642/3) 200.0 ☑
    pleomorphic cell type (M9641/3) 200.0 ☑
  round cell (M8803/3) — *see* Neoplasm, connective tissue, malignant
  small cell (M8803/3) — *see* Neoplasm, connective tissue, malignant
  spindle cell (M8801/3) — *see* Neoplasm, connective tissue, malignant
  stromal (endometrial) (M8930/3) 182.0
    isthmus 182.1
  synovial (M9040/3) (*see also* Neoplasm, connective tissue, malignant)
    biphasic type (M9043/3) — *see* Neoplasm, connective tissue, malignant
    epithelioid cell type (M9042/3) — *see* Neoplasm, connective tissue, malignant
    spindle cell type (M9041/3) — *see* Neoplasm, connective tissue, malignant
Sarcomatosis
  meningeal (M9539/3) — *see* Neoplasm, meninges, malignant
  specified site NEC (M8800/3) — *see* Neoplasm, connective tissue, malignant
  unspecified site (M8800/6) 171.9
Sarcosinemia 270.8
Sarcosporidiosis 136.5
Satiety, early 780.94
Satisfactory smear but lacking transformation zone
  anal 796.77
  cervical 795.07
Saturnine — *see* condition
Saturnism 984.9
  specified type of lead — *see* Table of Drugs and Chemicals
Satyriasis 302.89
Sauriasis — *see* Ichthyosis
Sauriderma 757.39
Sauriosis — *see* Ichthyosis
Savill's disease (epidemic exfoliative dermatitis) 695.89
SBE (subacute bacterial endocarditis) 421.0
Scabies (any site) 133.0
Scabs 782.8
Scaglietti-Dagnini syndrome (acromegalic macrospondylitis) 253.0
Scald, scalded — *see also* Burn, by site
  skin syndrome 695.81
Scalenus anticus (anterior) syndrome 353.0
Scales 782.8
Scalp — *see* condition
Scaphocephaly 756.0
Scaphoiditis, tarsal 732.5
Scapulalgia 733.90
Scapulohumeral myopathy 359.1
Scarabiasis 134.1
Scarlatina 034.1
  anginosa 034.1
  maligna 034.1

☑ Additional Digit Required — Refer to the Tabular List for Digit Selection   ⩗ Subterms under main terms may continue to next column or page

2011 ICD-9-CM   ▶◀ Revised Text   ● New Line   ▲ Revised Code   Volume 2 — 251

Scarlatina — continued
  myocarditis, acute 034.1 *[422.0]*
    old (see also Myocarditis) 429.0
  otitis media 034.1 *[382.02]*
  ulcerosa 034.1
Scarlatinella 057.8
Scarlet fever (albuminuria) (angina) (convulsions) (lesions of lid) (rash) 034.1
Scar, scarring — see also Cicatrix 709.2
  adherent 709.2
  atrophic 709.2
  cervix
    in pregnancy or childbirth 654.6 ☑
      affecting fetus or newborn 763.89
      causing obstructed labor 660.2 ☑
        affecting fetus or newborn 763.1
  cheloid 701.4
  chorioretinal 363.30
    disseminated 363.35
    macular 363.32
    peripheral 363.34
    posterior pole NEC 363.33
  choroid (see also Scar, chorioretinal) 363.30
  compression, pericardial 423.9
  congenital 757.39
  conjunctiva 372.64
  cornea 371.00
    xerophthalmic 264.6
  due to previous cesarean delivery, complicating pregnancy or childbirth 654.2 ☑
    affecting fetus or newborn 763.89
  duodenal (bulb) (cap) 537.3
  hypertrophic 701.4
  keloid 701.4
  labia 624.4
  lung (base) 518.89
  macula 363.32
    disseminated 363.35
    peripheral 363.34
  muscle 728.89
  myocardium, myocardial 412
  painful 709.2
  papillary muscle 429.81
  posterior pole NEC 363.33
    macular — see Scar, macula
  postnecrotic (hepatic) (liver) 571.9
  psychic V15.49
  retina (see also Scar, chorioretinal) 363.30
  trachea 478.9
  uterus 621.8
    in pregnancy or childbirth NEC 654.9 ☑
      affecting fetus or newborn 763.89
      due to previous cesarean delivery 654.2 ☑
  vulva 624.4
Schamberg's disease, dermatitis, or dermatosis (progressive pigmentary dermatosis) 709.09
Schatzki's ring (esophagus) (lower) (congenital) 750.3
  acquired 530.3
Schaufenster krankheit 413.9
Schaumann's
  benign lymphogranulomatosis 135
  disease (sarcoidosis) 135
  syndrome (sarcoidosis) 135
Scheie's syndrome (mucopolysaccharidosis IS) 277.5
Schenck's disease (sporotrichosis) 117.1
Scheuermann's disease or osteochondrosis 732.0
Scheuthauer-Marie-Sainton syndrome (cleidocranialis dysostosis) 755.59
Schilder (-Flatau) disease 341.1
Schilling-type monocytic leukemia (M9890/3) 206.9 ☑
Schimmelbusch's disease, cystic mastitis, or hyperplasia 610.1
Schirmer's syndrome (encephalocutaneous angiomatosis) 759.6
Schistocelia 756.79
Schistoglossia 750.13
Schistosoma infestation — see Infestation, Schistosoma
Schistosomiasis 120.9

Schistosomiasis — continued
  Asiatic 120.2
  bladder 120.0
  chestermani 120.8
  colon 120.1
  cutaneous 120.3
  due to
    S. hematobium 120.0
    S. japonicum 120.2
    S. mansoni 120.1
    S. mattheii 120.8
  eastern 120.2
  genitourinary tract 120.0
  intestinal 120.1
  lung 120.2
  Manson's (intestinal) 120.1
  Oriental 120.2
  pulmonary 120.2
  specified type NEC 120.8
  vesical 120.0
Schizencephaly 742.4
Schizo-affective psychosis — see also Schizophrenia 295.7 ☑
Schizodontia 520.2
Schizoid personality 301.20
  introverted 301.21
  schizotypal 301.22
Schizophrenia, schizophrenic (reaction) 295.9 ☑

> Note — Use the following fifth-digit subclassification with category 295:
>
> 0   unspecified
> 1   subchronic
> 2   chronic
> 3   subchronic with acute exacerbation
> 4   chronic with acute exacerbation
> 5   in remission

  acute (attack) NEC 295.8 ☑
    episode 295.4 ☑
  atypical form 295.8 ☑
  borderline 295.5 ☑
  catalepsy 295.2 ☑
  catatonic (type) (acute) (excited) (withdrawn) 295.2 ☑
  childhood (type) (see also Psychosis, childhood) 299.9 ☑
  chronic NEC 295.6 ☑
  coenesthesiopathic 295.8 ☑
  cyclic (type) 295.7 ☑
  disorganized (type) 295.1 ☑
  flexibilitas cerea 295.2 ☑
  hebephrenic (type) (acute) 295.1 ☑
  incipient 295.5 ☑
  latent 295.5 ☑
  paranoid (type) (acute) 295.3 ☑
  paraphrenic (acute) 295.3 ☑
  prepsychotic 295.5 ☑
  primary (acute) 295.0 ☑
  prodromal 295.5 ☑
  pseudoneurotic 295.5 ☑
  pseudopsychopathic 295.5 ☑
  reaction 295.9 ☑
  residual type (state) 295.6 ☑
  restzustand 295.6 ☑
  schizo-affective (type) (depressed) (excited) 295.7 ☑
  schizophreniform type 295.4 ☑
  simple (type) (acute) 295.0 ☑
  simplex (acute) 295.0 ☑
  specified type NEC 295.8 ☑
  syndrome of childhood NEC (see also Psychosis, childhood) 299.9 ☑
  undifferentiated type 295.9 ☑
    acute 295.8 ☑
    chronic 295.6 ☑
Schizothymia 301.20
  introverted 301.21
  schizotypal 301.22
Schlafkrankheit 086.5

Schlatter-Osgood disease (osteochondrosis, tibial tubercle) 732.4
Schlatter's tibia (osteochondrosis) 732.4
Schloffer's tumor — see also Peritonitis 567.29
Schmidt's syndrome
  sphallo-pharyngo-laryngeal hemiplegia 352.6
  thyroid-adrenocortical insufficiency 258.1
  vagoaccessory 352.6
Schmincke
  carcinoma (M8082/3) — see Neoplasm, nasopharynx, malignant
  tumor (M8082/3) — see Neoplasm, nasopharynx, malignant
Schmitz (-Stutzer) dysentery 004.0
Schmorl's disease or nodes 722.30
  lumbar, lumbosacral 722.32
  specified region NEC 722.39
  thoracic, thoracolumbar 722.31
Schneiderian
  carcinoma (M8121/3)
    specified site — see Neoplasm, by site, malignant
    unspecified site 160.0
  papilloma (M8121/0)
    specified site — see Neoplasm, by site, benign
    unspecified site 212.0
Schneider's syndrome 047.9
Schnitzler syndrome 273.1
Schoffer's tumor — see also Peritonitis 567.29
Scholte's syndrome (malignant carcinoid) 259.2
Scholz's disease 330.0
Scholz (-Bielschowsky-Henneberg) syndrome 330.0
Schönlein (-Henoch) disease (primary) (purpura) (rheumatic) 287.0
School examination V70.3
  following surgery V67.09
Schottmüller's disease — see also Fever, paratyphoid 002.9
Schroeder's syndrome (endocrine-hypertensive) 255.3
Schüller-Christian disease or syndrome (chronic histiocytosis X) 277.89
Schultz's disease or syndrome (agranulocytosis) 288.09
Schultze's acroparesthesia, simple 443.89
Schwalbe-Ziehen-Oppenheimer disease 333.6
Schwannoma (M9560/0) — see also Neoplasm, connective tissue, benign
  malignant (M9560/3) — see Neoplasm, connective tissue, malignant
Schwannomatosis 237.73 ●
Schwartz-Bartter syndrome (inappropriate secretion of antidiuretic hormone) 253.6
Schwartz (-Jampel) syndrome 359.23
Schweninger-Buzzi disease (macular atrophy) 701.3
Sciatic — see condition
Sciatica (infectional) 724.3
  due to
    displacement of intervertebral disc 722.10
    herniation, nucleus pulposus 722.10
  wallet 724.3
Scimitar syndrome (anomalous venous drainage, right lung to inferior vena cava) 747.49
Sclera — see condition
Sclerectasia 379.11
Scleredema
  adultorum 710.1
  Buschke's 710.1
  newborn 778.1
Sclerema
  adiposum (newborn) 778.1
  adultorum 710.1
  edematosum (newborn) 778.1
  neonatorum 778.1
  newborn 778.1
Scleriasis — see Scleroderma
Scleritis 379.00
  with corneal involvement 379.05

Scleritis — continued
  anterior (annular) (localized) 379.03
  brawny 379.06
  granulomatous 379.09
  posterior 379.07
  specified NEC 379.09
  suppurative 379.09
  syphilitic 095.0
  tuberculous (nodular) (see also Tuberculosis) 017.3 ☑ *[379.09]*
Sclerochoroiditis — see also Scleritis 379.00
Scleroconjunctivitis — see also Scleritis 379.00
Sclerocystic ovary (syndrome) 256.4
Sclerodactylia 701.0
Scleroderma, sclerodermia (acrosclerotic) (diffuse) (generalized) (progressive) (pulmonary) 710.1
  circumscribed 701.0
  linear 701.0
  localized (linear) 701.0
  newborn 778.1
Sclerokeratitis 379.05
  meaning sclerosing keratitis 370.54
  tuberculous (see also Tuberculosis) 017.3 ☑ *[379.09]*
Scleromalacia
  multiple 731.0
  perforans 379.04
Scleroma, trachea 040.1
Scleromyxedema 701.8
Scleroperikeratitis 379.05
Sclerose en plaques 340
Sclerosis, sclerotic
  adrenal (gland) 255.8
  Alzheimer's 331.0
    with dementia — see Alzheimer's, dementia
  amyotrophic (lateral) 335.20
  annularis fibrosi
    aortic 424.1
    mitral 424.0
  aorta, aortic 440.0
    valve (see also Endocarditis, aortic) 424.1
  artery, arterial, arteriolar, arteriovascular — see Arteriosclerosis
  ascending multiple 340
  Baló's (concentric) 341.1
  basilar — see Sclerosis, brain
  bone (localized) NEC 733.99
  brain (general) (lobular) 348.89
    Alzheimer's — see Alzheimer's, dementia
    artery, arterial 437.0
    atrophic lobar 331.0
      with dementia
        with behavioral disturbance 331.0 *[294.11]*
        without behavioral disturbance 331.0 *[294.10]*
    diffuse 341.1
      familial (chronic) (infantile) 330.0
      infantile (chronic) (familial) 330.0
      Pelizaeus-Merzbacher type 330.0
    disseminated 340
    hereditary 334.2
    hippocampal 348.81
    infantile (degenerative) (diffuse) 330.0
    insular 340
    Krabbe's 330.0
    mesial temporal 348.81
    miliary 340
    multiple 340
    Pelizaeus-Merzbacher 330.0
    progressive familial 330.0
    senile 437.0
    temporal 348.81
      mesial 348.81
    tuberous 759.5
  bulbar, progressive 340
  bundle of His 426.50
    left 426.3
    right 426.4
  cardiac — see Arteriosclerosis, coronary
  cardiorenal (see also Hypertension, cardiorenal) 404.90

☑ Additional Digit Required — Refer to the Tabular List for Digit Selection   ▽ Subterms under main terms may continue to next column or page

252 — Volume 2 • October 2010   ▶◀ Revised Text   ● New Line   ▲ Revised Code   2011 ICD-9-CM

Sclerosis, sclerotic — *continued*
  cardiovascular (*see also* Disease, cardiovascular) 429.2
    renal (*see also* Hypertension, cardiorenal) 404.90
  centrolobar, familial 330.0
  cerebellar — *see* Sclerosis, brain
  cerebral — *see* Sclerosis, brain
  cerebrospinal 340
    disseminated 340
    multiple 340
  cerebrovascular 437.0
  choroid 363.40
    diffuse 363.56
  combined (spinal cord) (*see also* Degeneration, combined)
    multiple 340
  concentric, Baló's 341.1
  cornea 370.54
  coronary (artery) — *see* Arteriosclerosis, coronary
  corpus cavernosum
    female 624.8
    male 607.89
  Dewitzky's
    aortic 424.1
    mitral 424.0
  diffuse NEC 341.1
  disease, heart — *see* Arteriosclerosis, coronary
  disseminated 340
  dorsal 340
  dorsolateral (spinal cord) — *see* Degeneration, combined
  endometrium 621.8
  extrapyramidal 333.90
  eye, nuclear (senile) 366.16
  Friedreich's (spinal cord) 334.0
  funicular (spermatic cord) 608.89
  gastritis 535.4 ☑
  general (vascular) — *see* Arteriosclerosis
  gland (lymphatic) 457.8
  hepatic 571.9
  hereditary
    cerebellar 334.2
    spinal 334.0
  hippocampal 348.81
  idiopathic cortical (Garré's) (*see also* Osteomyelitis) 730.1 ☑
  ilium, piriform 733.5
  insular 340
    pancreas 251.8
  Islands of Langerhans 251.8
  kidney — *see* Sclerosis, renal
  larynx 478.79
  lateral 335.24
    amyotrophic 335.20
    descending 335.24
    primary 335.24
    spinal 335.24
  liver 571.9
  lobar, atrophic (of brain) 331.0
    with dementia
      with behavioral disturbance 331.0 *[294.11]*
      without behavioral disturbance 331.0 *[294.10]*
  lung (*see also* Fibrosis, lung) 515
  mastoid 383.1
  mesial temporal 348.81
  mitral — *see* Endocarditis, mitral
  Mönckeberg's (medial) (*see also* Arteriosclerosis, extremities) 440.20
  multiple (brain stem) (cerebral) (generalized) (spinal cord) 340
  myocardium, myocardial — *see* Arteriosclerosis, coronary
  nuclear (senile), eye 366.16
  ovary 620.8
  pancreas 577.8
  penis 607.89
  peripheral arteries (*see also* Arteriosclerosis, extremities) 440.20
  plaques 340
  pluriglandular 258.8
  polyglandular 258.8

Sclerosis, sclerotic — *continued*
  posterior (spinal cord) (syphilitic) 094.0
  posterolateral (spinal cord) — *see* Degeneration, combined
  prepuce 607.89
  primary lateral 335.24
  progressive systemic 710.1
  pulmonary (*see also* Fibrosis, lung) 515
    artery 416.0
    valve (heart) (*see also* Endocarditis, pulmonary) 424.3
  renal 587
    with
      cystine storage disease 270.0
      hypertension (*see also* Hypertension, kidney) 403.90
      hypertensive heart disease (conditions classifiable to 402) (*see also* Hypertension, cardiorenal) 404.90
      arteriolar (hyaline) (*see also* Hypertension, kidney) 403.90
      hyperplastic (*see also* Hypertension, kidney) 403.90
  retina (senile) (vascular) 362.17
  rheumatic
    aortic valve 395.9
    mitral valve 394.9
  Schilder's 341.1
  senile — *see* Arteriosclerosis
  spinal (cord) (general) (progressive) (transverse) 336.8
    ascending 357.0
    combined (*see also* Degeneration, combined)
      multiple 340
      syphilitic 094.89
    disseminated 340
    dorsolateral — *see* Degeneration, combined
    hereditary (Friedreich's) (mixed form) 334.0
    lateral (amyotrophic) 335.24
    multiple 340
    posterior (syphilitic) 094.0
  stomach 537.89
  subendocardial, congenital 425.3
  systemic (progressive) 710.1
    with lung involvement 710.1 *[517.2]*
  temporal 348.81
    mesial 348.81
  tricuspid (heart) (valve) — *see* Endocarditis, tricuspid
  tuberous (brain) 759.5
  tympanic membrane (*see also* Tympanosclerosis) 385.00
  valve, valvular (heart) — *see* Endocarditis
  vascular — *see* Arteriosclerosis
  vein 459.89
Sclerotenonitis 379.07
Sclerotitis — *see also* Scleritis 379.00
  syphilitic 095.0
  tuberculous (*see also* Tuberculosis) 017.3 ☑ *[379.09]*
Scoliosis (acquired) (postural) 737.30
  congenital 754.2
  due to or associated with
    Charcôt-Marie-Tooth disease 356.1 *[737.43]*
    mucopolysaccharidosis 277.5 *[737.43]*
    neurofibromatosis 237.71 *[737.43]*
    osteitis
      deformans 731.0 *[737.43]*
      fibrosa cystica 252.01 *[737.43]*
    osteoporosis (*see also* Osteoporosis) 733.00 *[737.43]*
    poliomyelitis 138 *[737.43]*
    radiation 737.33
    tuberculosis (*see also* Tuberculosis) 015.0 ☑ *[737.43]*
  idiopathic 737.30
    infantile
      progressive 737.32
      resolving 737.31
  paralytic 737.39
  rachitic 268.1

Scoliosis — *continued*
  sciatic 724.3
  specified NEC 737.39
  thoracogenic 737.34
  tuberculous (*see also* Tuberculosis) 015.0 ☑ *[737.43]*
Scoliotic pelvis 738.6
  with disproportion (fetopelvic) 653.0 ☑
    affecting fetus or newborn 763.1
    causing obstructed labor 660.1 ☑
      affecting fetus or newborn 763.1
Scorbutus, scorbutic 267
  anemia 281.8
Scotoma (ring) 368.44
  arcuate 368.43
  Bjerrum 368.43
  blind spot area 368.42
  central 368.41
  centrocecal 368.41
  paracecal 368.42
  paracentral 368.41
  scintillating 368.12
  Seidel 368.43
Scratch — *see* Injury, superficial, by site
Scratchy throat 784.99
Screening (for) V82.9
  alcoholism V79.1
  anemia, deficiency NEC V78.1
    iron V78.0
  anomaly, congenital V82.89
  antenatal, of mother V28.9
    alphafetoprotein levels, raised V28.1
    based on amniocentesis V28.2
      chromosomal anomalies V28.0
      raised alphafetoprotein levels V28.1
    fetal growth retardation using ultrasonics V28.4
      ultrasonics V28.4
    genomic V28.89
    isoimmunization V28.5
    malformations using ultrasonics V28.3
    proteomic V28.89
    raised alphafetoprotein levels V28.1
    risk
      pre-term labor V28.82
    specified condition NEC V28.89
    Streptococcus B V28.6
  arterial hypertension V81.1
  arthropod-borne viral disease NEC V73.5
  asymptomatic bacteriuria V81.5
  bacterial
    and spirochetal sexually transmitted diseases V74.5
    conjunctivitis V74.4
    disease V74.9
      sexually transmitted V74.5
      specified condition NEC V74.8
  bacteriuria, asymptomatic V81.5
  blood disorder NEC V78.9
    specified type NEC V78.8
  bronchitis, chronic V81.3
  brucellosis V74.8
  cancer — *see* Screening, malignant neoplasm
  cardiovascular disease NEC V81.2
  cataract V80.2
  Chagas' disease V75.3
  chemical poisoning V82.5
  cholera V74.0
  cholesterol level V77.91
  chromosomal
    anomalies
      by amniocentesis, antenatal V28.0
      maternal postnatal V82.4
    athletes V70.3
  colonoscopy V76.51   ●
  condition
    cardiovascular NEC V81.2
    eye NEC V80.2
    genitourinary NEC V81.6
    neurological NEC V80.09
    respiratory NEC V81.4
    skin V82.0
    specified NEC V82.89
  congenital
    anomaly V82.89

Screening — *continued*
  congenital — *continued*
    anomaly — *continued*
      eye V80.2
    dislocation of hip V82.3
    eye condition or disease V80.2
  conjunctivitis, bacterial V74.4
  contamination NEC (*see also* Poisoning) V82.5
  coronary artery disease V81.0
  cystic fibrosis V77.6
  deficiency anemia NEC V78.1
    iron V78.0
  dengue fever V73.5
  depression V79.0
  developmental handicap V79.9
    in early childhood V79.3
    specified type NEC V79.8
  diabetes mellitus V77.1
  diphtheria V74.3
  disease or disorder V82.9
    bacterial V74.9
      specified NEC V74.8
    blood V78.9
      specified type NEC V78.8
    blood-forming organ V78.9
      specified type NEC V78.8
    cardiovascular NEC V81.2
      hypertensive V81.1
      ischemic V81.0
    Chagas' V75.3
    chlamydial V73.98
      specified NEC V73.88
    ear NEC V80.3
    endocrine NEC V77.99
    eye NEC V80.2
    genitourinary NEC V81.6
    heart NEC V81.2
      hypertensive V81.1
      ischemic V81.0
    HPV (human papillomavirus) V73.81
    human papillomavirus V73.81
    immunity NEC V77.99
    infectious NEC V75.9
    lipoid NEC V77.91
    mental V79.9
      specified type NEC V79.8
    metabolic NEC V77.99
      inborn NEC V77.7
    neurological NEC V80.09
    nutritional NEC V77.99
    rheumatic NEC V82.2
    rickettsial V75.0
    sexually transmitted V74.5
      bacterial V74.5
      spirochetal V74.5
    sickle-cell V78.2
      trait V78.2
    specified type NEC V82.89
    thyroid V77.0
    vascular NEC V81.2
      ischemic V81.0
    venereal V74.5
    viral V73.99
      arthropod-borne NEC V73.5
      specified type NEC V73.89
  dislocation of hip, congenital V82.3
  drugs in athletes V70.3
  elevated titer V82.9
  emphysema (chronic) V81.3
  encephalitis, viral (mosquito or tick borne) V73.5
  endocrine disorder NEC V77.99
  eye disorder NEC V80.2
    congenital V80.2
  fever
    dengue V73.5
    hemorrhagic V73.5
    yellow V73.4
  filariasis V75.6
  galactosemia V77.4
  genetic V82.79
    disease carrier status V82.71
  genitourinary condition NEC V81.6
  glaucoma V80.1
  gonorrhea V74.5

☑ **Additional Digit Required** — Refer to the Tabular List for Digit Selection   ▽ **Subterms under main terms may continue to next column or page**

2011 ICD-9-CM   ▶◀ **Revised Text**   ● **New Line**   ▲ **Revised Code**   October 2010 · Volume 2 — 253

☑ **Additional Digit Required — Refer to the Tabular List for Digit Selection**   ▽ **Subterms under main terms may continue to next column or page**

254 — Volume 2 • October 2010   ▶◀ **Revised Text**   ● **New Line**   ▲ **Revised Code**   2011 ICD-9-CM

Separation — *continued*
  apophysis, traumatic — *see* Fracture, by site
  choroid 363.70
    hemorrhagic 363.72
    serous 363.71
  costochondral (simple) (traumatic) — *see* Dislocation, costochondral
  delayed
    umbilical cord 779.83
  epiphysis, epiphyseal
    nontraumatic 732.9
      upper femoral 732.2
    traumatic — *see* Fracture, by site
  fracture — *see* Fracture, by site
  infundibulum cardiac from right ventricle by a partition 746.83
  joint (current) (traumatic) — *see* Dislocation, by site
  placenta (normally implanted) — *see* Placenta, separation
  pubic bone, obstetrical trauma 665.6 ☑
  retina, retinal (*see also* Detachment, retina) 361.9
    layers 362.40
      sensory (*see also* Retinoschisis) 361.10
    pigment epithelium (exudative) 362.42
      hemorrhagic 362.43
  sternoclavicular (traumatic) — *see* Dislocation, sternoclavicular
  symphysis pubis, obstetrical trauma 665.6 ☑
  tracheal ring, incomplete (congenital) 748.3
Sepsis (generalized) 995.91
  with
    abortion — *see* Abortion, by type, with sepsis
    acute organ dysfunction 995.92
    ectopic pregnancy (*see also* categories 633.0–633.9) 639.0
    molar pregnancy (*see also* categories 630–632) 639.0
    multiple organ dysfunction (MOD) 995.92
  buccal 528.3
  complicating labor 659.3 ☑
  dental (pulpal origin) 522.4
  female genital organ NEC 614.9
  fetus (intrauterine) 771.81
  following
    abortion 639.0
    ectopic or molar pregnancy 639.0
    infusion, perfusion, or transfusion 999.39
  Friedländer's 038.49
  intraocular 360.00
  localized
    in operation wound 998.59
    skin (*see also* Abscess) 682.9
  malleus 024
  nadir 038.9
  newborn (organism unspecified) NEC 771.81
  oral 528.3
  puerperal, postpartum, childbirth (pelvic) 670.2 ☑
  resulting from infusion, injection, transfusion, or vaccination 999.39
  severe 995.92
  skin, localized (*see also* Abscess) 682.9
  umbilical (newborn) (organism unspecified) 771.89
    tetanus 771.3
  urinary 599.0
    meaning sepsis 995.91
    meaning urinary tract infection 599.0
Septate — *see also* Septum
Septic — *see also* condition
  adenoids 474.01
    and tonsils 474.02
  arm (with lymphangitis) 682.3
  embolus — *see* Embolism
  finger (with lymphangitis) 681.00
  foot (with lymphangitis) 682.7
  gallbladder (*see also* Cholecystitis) 575.8
  hand (with lymphangitis) 682.4
  joint (*see also* Arthritis, septic) 711.0 ☑
  kidney (*see also* Infection, kidney) 590.9

Septic — *see also* condition — *continued*
  leg (with lymphangitis) 682.6
  mouth 528.3
  nail 681.9
    finger 681.02
    toe 681.11
  shock (endotoxic) 785.52
  sore (*see also* Abscess) 682.9
    throat 034.0
      milk-borne 034.0
      streptococcal 034.0
  spleen (acute) 289.59
  teeth (pulpal origin) 522.4
  throat 034.0
  thrombus — *see* Thrombosis
  toe (with lymphangitis) 681.10
  tonsils 474.00
    and adenoids 474.02
  umbilical cord (newborn) (organism unspecified) 771.89
  uterus (*see also* Endometritis) 615.9
Septicemia, septicemic (generalized) (suppurative) 038.9
  with
    abortion — *see* Abortion, by type, with sepsis
    ectopic pregnancy (*see also* categories 633.0–633.9) 639.0
    molar pregnancy (*see also* categories 630–632) 639.0
  Aerobacter aerogenes 038.49
  anaerobic 038.3
  anthrax 022.3
  Bacillus coli 038.42
  Bacteroides 038.3
  Clostridium 038.3
  complicating labor 659.3 ☑
  cryptogenic 038.9
  enteric gram-negative bacilli 038.40
  Enterobacter aerogenes 038.49
  Erysipelothrix (insidiosa) (rhusiopathiae) 027.1
  Escherichia coli 038.42
  following
    abortion 639.0
    ectopic or molar pregnancy 639.0
    infusion, injection, transfusion, or vaccination 999.39
  Friedländer's (bacillus) 038.49
  gangrenous 038.9
  gonococcal 098.89
  gram-negative (organism) 038.40
    anaerobic 038.3
  Hemophilus influenzae 038.41
  herpes (simplex) 054.5
  herpetic 054.5
  Listeria monocytogenes 027.0
  meningeal — *see* Meningitis
  meningococcal (chronic) (fulminating) 036.2
  methicillin
    resistant Staphylococcus aureus (MRSA) 038.12
    susceptible Staphylococcus aureus (MSSA) 038.11
  MRSA (methicillin resistant Staphylococcus aureus) 038.12
  MSSA (methicillin susceptible Staphylococcus aureus) 038.11
  navel, newborn (organism unspecified) 771.89
  newborn (organism unspecified) 771.81
  plague 020.2
  pneumococcal 038.2
  postabortal 639.0
  postoperative 998.59
  Proteus vulgaris 038.49
  Pseudomonas (aeruginosa) 038.43
  puerperal, postpartum 670.2 ☑
  Salmonella (aertrycke) (callinarum) (choleraesuis) (enteritidis) (suipestifer) 003.1
  Serratia 038.44
  Shigella (*see also* Dysentery, bacillary) 004.9
  specified organism NEC 038.8
  staphylococcal 038.10
    aureus 038.11

Septicemia, septicemic — *continued*
  staphylococcal — *continued*
    aureus — *continued*
      methicillin
        resistant (MRSA) 038.12
        susceptible (MSSA) 038.11
      specified organism NEC 038.19
  streptococcal (anaerobic) 038.0
  Streptococcus pneumoniae 038.2
  suipestifer 003.1
  umbilicus, newborn (organism unspecified) 771.89
  viral 079.99
  Yersinia enterocolitica 038.49
Septum, septate (congenital) — *see also* Anomaly, specified type NEC
  anal 751.2
  aqueduct of Sylvius 742.3
    with spina bifida (*see also* Spina bifida) 741.0 ☑
  hymen 752.49
  uterus (*see also* Double, uterus) ▶(complete) (partial)◀ 752.35 ▲
  vagina
    in pregnancy or childbirth 654.7 ☑
      affecting fetus or newborn 763.89
      causing obstructed labor 660.2 ☑
        affecting fetus or newborn 763.1
    longitudinal (with or without obstruc-● tion) 752.47 ●
    transverse 752.46 ●
Sequestration
  lung (congenital) (extralobar) (intralobar) 748.5
  orbit 376.10
  pulmonary artery (congenital) 747.3
  splenic 289.52
Sequestrum
  bone (*see also* Osteomyelitis) 730.1 ☑
    jaw 526.4
  dental 525.8
  jaw bone 526.4
  sinus (accessory) (nasal) (*see also* Sinusitis) 473.9
    maxillary 473.0
Sequoiosis asthma 495.8
Serology for syphilis
  doubtful
    with signs or symptoms — *see* Syphilis, by site and stage
    follow-up of latent syphilis — *see* Syphilis, latent
  false positive 795.6
  negative, with signs or symptoms — *see* Syphilis, by site and stage
  positive 097.1
    with signs or symptoms — *see* Syphilis, by site and stage
    false 795.6
    follow-up of latent syphilis — *see* Syphilis, latent
    only finding — *see* Syphilis, latent
  reactivated 097.1
Seroma (postoperative) (non-infected) 998.13
  infected 998.51
  post-traumatic 729.91
Seropurulent — *see* condition
Serositis, multiple 569.89
  pericardial 423.2
  peritoneal 568.82
  pleural — *see* Pleurisy
Serotonin syndrome 333.99
Serous — *see* condition
Sertoli cell
  adenoma (M8640/0)
    specified site — *see* Neoplasm, by site, benign
    unspecified site
      female 220
      male 222.0
  carcinoma (M8640/3)
    specified site — *see* Neoplasm, by site, malignant
    unspecified site 186.9
  syndrome (germinal aplasia) 606.0

Sertoli cell — *continued*
  tumor (M8640/0)
    with lipid storage (M8641/0)
      specified site — *see* Neoplasm, by site, benign
      unspecified site
        female 220
        male 222.0
    specified site — *see* Neoplasm, by site, benign
    unspecified site
      female 220
      male 222.0
Sertoli-Leydig cell tumor (M8631/0)
  specified site — *see* Neoplasm, by site, benign
  unspecified site
    female 220
    male 222.0
Serum
  allergy, allergic reaction 999.5
    shock 999.4
  arthritis 999.5 [713.6]
  complication or reaction NEC 999.5
  disease NEC 999.5
  hepatitis 070.3 ☑
  intoxication 999.5
  jaundice (homologous) — *see* Hepatitis, viral, type B
  neuritis 999.5
  poisoning NEC 999.5
  rash NEC 999.5
  reaction NEC 999.5
  sickness NEC 999.5
Sesamoiditis 733.99
Seven-day fever 061
  of
    Japan 100.89
    Queensland 100.89
Sever's disease or osteochondrosis (calcaneum) 732.5
Sex chromosome mosaics 758.81
Sex reassignment surgery status (*see also* Trans-sexualism) 302.50
Sextuplet
  affected by maternal complications of pregnancy 761.5
  healthy liveborn — *see* Newborn, multiple
  pregnancy (complicating delivery) NEC 651.8 ☑
    with fetal loss and retention of one or more fetus(es) 651.6 ☑
    following (elective) fetal reduction 651.7 ☑
Sexual
  anesthesia 302.72
  deviation (*see also* Deviation, sexual) 302.9
  disorder (*see also* Deviation, sexual) 302.9
  frigidity (female) 302.72
  function, disorder of (psychogenic) 302.70
    specified type NEC 302.79
  immaturity (female) (male) 259.0
  impotence 607.84
    organic origin NEC 607.84
    psychogenic 302.72
  precocity (constitutional) (cryptogenic) (female) (idiopathic) (male) NEC 259.1
    with adrenal hyperplasia 255.2
  sadism 302.84
Sexuality, pathological — *see also* Deviation, sexual 302.9
Sézary's disease, reticulosis, or syndrome (M9701/3) 202.2 ☑
Shadow, lung 793.1
Shaken infant syndrome 995.55
Shaking
  head (tremor) 781.0
  palsy or paralysis (*see also* Parkinsonism) 332.0
Shallowness, acetabulum 736.39
Shaver's disease or syndrome (bauxite pneumoconiosis) 503
Shearing
  artificial skin graft 996.55
  decellularized allodermis graft 996.55
Sheath (tendon) — *see* condition

☑ **Additional Digit Required** — Refer to the Tabular List for Digit Selection

▽ **Subterms under main terms may continue to next column or page**

Shedding
nail 703.8
teeth, premature, primary (deciduous) 520.6
Sheehan's disease or syndrome (postpartum pituitary necrosis) 253.2
Shelf, rectal 569.49
Shell
shock (current) (*see also* Reaction, stress, acute) 308.9
lasting state 300.16
teeth 520.5
Shield kidney 753.3
Shifting
pacemaker 427.89
sleep-work schedule (affecting sleep) 327.36
Shift, mediastinal 793.2
Shiga's
bacillus 004.0
dysentery 004.0
Shigella (dysentery) — *see also* Dysentery, bacillary 004.9
carrier (suspected) of V02.3
Shigellosis — *see also* Dysentery, bacillary 004.9
Shingles — *see also* Herpes, zoster 053.9
eye NEC 053.29
Shin splints 844.9
Shipyard eye or disease 077.1
Shirodkar suture, in pregnancy 654.5 ☑
Shock 785.50
with
abortion — *see* Abortion, by type, with shock
ectopic pregnancy (*see also* categories 633.0–633.9) 639.5
molar pregnancy (*see also* categories 630–632) 639.5
allergic — *see* Shock, anaphylactic
anaclitic 309.21
anaphylactic 995.0
chemical — *see* Table of Drugs and Chemicals
correct medicinal substance properly administered 995.0
drug or medicinal substance
correct substance properly administered 995.0
overdose or wrong substance given or taken 977.9
specified drug — *see* Table of Drugs and Chemicals
following sting(s) 989.5
food — *see* Anaphylactic shock, due to, food
immunization 999.4
serum 999.4
anaphylactoid — *see* Shock, anaphylactic
anesthetic
correct substance properly administered 995.4
overdose or wrong substance given 968.4
specified anesthetic — *see* Table of Drugs and Chemicals
birth, fetus or newborn NEC 779.89
cardiogenic 785.51
chemical substance — *see* Table of Drugs and Chemicals
circulatory 785.59
complicating
abortion — *see* Abortion, by type, with shock
ectopic pregnancy (*see also* categories 633.0–633.9) 639.5
labor and delivery 669.1 ☑
molar pregnancy (*see also* categories 630–632) 639.5
culture 309.29
due to
drug 995.0
correct substance properly administered 995.0
overdose or wrong substance given or taken 977.9
specified drug — *see* Table of Drugs and Chemicals

Shock — *continued*
due to — *continued*
food — *see* Anaphylactic shock, due to, food
during labor and delivery 669.1 ☑
electric 994.8
from electroshock gun (taser) 994.8
endotoxic 785.52
due to surgical procedure 998.0
following
abortion 639.5
ectopic or molar pregnancy 639.5
injury (immediate) (delayed) 958.4
labor and delivery 669.1 ☑
gram-negative 785.52
hematogenic 785.59
hemorrhagic
due to
disease 785.59
surgery (intraoperative) (postoperative) 998.0
trauma 958.4
hypovolemic NEC 785.59
surgical 998.0
traumatic 958.4
insulin 251.0
therapeutic misadventure 962.3
kidney 584.5
traumatic (following crushing) 958.5
lightning 994.0
lung 518.5
nervous (*see also* Reaction, stress, acute) 308.9
obstetric 669.1 ☑
with
abortion — *see* Abortion, by type, with shock
ectopic pregnancy (*see also* categories 633.0–633.9) 639.5
molar pregnancy (*see also* categories 630–632) 639.5
following
abortion 639.5
ectopic or molar pregnancy 639.5
paralysis, paralytic (*see also* Disease, cerebrovascular, acute) 436
late effect — *see* Late effect(s) (of) cerebrovascular disease
pleural (surgical) 998.0
due to trauma 958.4
postoperative 998.0
with
abortion — *see* Abortion, by type, with shock
ectopic pregnancy (*see also* categories 633.0–633.9) 639.5
molar pregnancy (*see also* categories 630–632) 639.5
following
abortion 639.5
ectopic or molar pregnancy 639.5
psychic (*see also* Reaction, stress, acute) 308.9
past history (of) V15.49
psychogenic (*see also* Reaction, stress, acute) 308.9
septic 785.52
with
abortion — *see* Abortion, by type, with shock
ectopic pregnancy (*see also* categories 633.0–633.9) 639.5
molar pregnancy (*see also* categories 630–632) 639.5
due to
surgical procedure 998.0
transfusion NEC 999.89
bone marrow 996.85
following
abortion 639.5
ectopic or molar pregnancy 639.5
surgical procedure 998.0
transfusion NEC 999.89
bone marrow 996.85
spinal (*see also* Injury, spinal, by site)

Shock — *continued*
spinal (*see also* Injury, spinal, by site) — *continued*
with spinal bone injury — *see* Fracture, vertebra, by site, with spinal cord injury
surgical 998.0
therapeutic misadventure NEC (*see also* Complications) 998.89
thyroxin 962.7
toxic 040.82
transfusion — *see* Complications, transfusion
traumatic (immediate) (delayed) 958.4
Shoemakers' chest 738.3
Short, shortening, shortness
Achilles tendon (acquired) 727.81
arm 736.89
congenital 755.20
back 737.9
bowel syndrome 579.3
breath 786.05
cervical, cervix 649.7 ☑
gravid uterus 649.7 ☑
non-gravid uterus 622.5
acquired 622.5
congenital 752.49
chain acyl CoA dehydrogenase deficiency (SCAD) 277.85
common bile duct, congenital 751.69
cord (umbilical) 663.4 ☑
affecting fetus or newborn 762.6
cystic duct, congenital 751.69
esophagus (congenital) 750.4
femur (acquired) 736.81
congenital 755.34
frenulum linguae 750.0
frenum, lingual 750.0
hamstrings 727.81
hip (acquired) 736.39
congenital 755.63
leg (acquired) 736.81
congenital 755.30
metatarsus (congenital) 754.79
acquired 736.79
organ or site, congenital NEC — *see* Distortion
palate (congenital) 750.26
P-R interval syndrome 426.81
radius (acquired) 736.09
congenital 755.26
round ligament 629.89
sleeper 307.49
stature, constitutional (hereditary) (idiopathic) 783.43
tendon 727.81
Achilles (acquired) 727.81
congenital 754.79
congenital 756.89
thigh (acquired) 736.81
congenital 755.34
tibialis anticus 727.81
umbilical cord 663.4 ☑
affecting fetus or newborn 762.6
urethra 599.84
uvula (congenital) 750.26
vagina 623.8
Shortsightedness 367.1
Shoshin (acute fulminating beriberi) 265.0
Shoulder — *see* condition
Shovel-shaped incisors 520.2
Shower, thromboembolic — *see* Embolism
Shunt (status)
aortocoronary bypass V45.81
arterial-venous (dialysis) V45.11
arteriovenous, pulmonary (acquired) 417.0
congenital 747.3
traumatic (complication) 901.40
cerebral ventricle (communicating) in situ V45.2
coronary artery bypass V45.81
surgical, prosthetic, with complications — *see* Complications, shunt
vascular NEC V45.89
Shutdown
renal 586

Shutdown — *continued*
renal — *continued*
with
abortion — *see* Abortion, by type, with renal failure
ectopic pregnancy (*see also* categories 633.0–633.9) 639.3
molar pregnancy (*see also* categories 630–632) 639.3
complicating
abortion 639.3
ectopic or molar pregnancy 639.3
following labor and delivery 669.3 ☑
Shwachman's syndrome 288.02
Shy-Drager syndrome (orthostatic hypotension with multisystem degeneration) 333.0
Sialadenitis (any gland) (chronic) (suppurative) 527.2
epidemic — *see* Mumps
Sialadenosis, periodic 527.2
Sialaporia 527.7
Sialectasia 527.8
Sialitis 527.2
Sialoadenitis — *see also* Sialadenitis 527.2
Sialoangitis 527.2
Sialodochitis (fibrinosa) 527.2
Sialodocholithiasis 527.5
Sialolithiasis 527.5
Sialorrhea — *see also* Ptyalism 527.7
periodic 527.2
Sialosis 527.8
rheumatic 710.2
Siamese twin 759.4
complicating pregnancy 678.1 ☑
Sicard's syndrome 352.6
Sicca syndrome (keratoconjunctivitis) 710.2
Sick 799.9
cilia syndrome 759.89
or handicapped person in family V61.49
Sickle-cell
anemia (see also Disease, sickle-cell) 282.60
disease (see also Disease, sickle-cell) 282.60
hemoglobin
C disease (without crisis) 282.63
with
crisis 282.64
vaso-occlusive pain 282.64
D disease (without crisis) 282.68
with crisis 282.69
E disease (without crisis) 282.68
with crisis 282.69
thalassemia (without crisis) 282.41
with
crisis 282.42
vaso-occlusive pain 282.42
trait 282.5
Sicklemia — *see also* Disease, sickle-cell 282.60
trait 282.5
Sickness
air (travel) 994.6
airplane 994.6
alpine 993.2
altitude 993.2
Andes 993.2
aviators' 993.2
balloon 993.2
car 994.6
compressed air 993.3
decompression 993.3
green 280.9
harvest 100.89
milk 988.8
morning 643.0 ☑
motion 994.6
mountain 993.2
acute 289.0
protein (*see also* Complications, vaccination) 999.5
radiation NEC 990
roundabout (motion) 994.6
sea 994.6
serum NEC 999.5
sleeping (African) 086.5
by Trypanosoma 086.5
gambiense 086.3

☑ **Additional Digit Required — Refer to the Tabular List for Digit Selection**   ▼ **Subterms under main terms may continue to next column or page**

256 — Volume 2   ▶◀ **Revised Text**   ● **New Line**   ▲ **Revised Code**   **2011 ICD-9-CM**

Sickness — *continued*
  sleeping — *continued*
    by Trypanosoma — *continued*
      rhodesiense 086.4
      Gambian 086.3
      late effect 139.8
      Rhodesian 086.4
  sweating 078.2
  swing (motion) 994.6
  train (railway) (travel) 994.6
  travel (any vehicle) 994.6
Sick sinus syndrome 427.81
Sideropenia — *see also* Anemia, iron deficiency 280.9
Siderosis (lung) (occupational) 503
  cornea 371.15
  eye (bulbi) (vitreous) 360.23
  lens 360.23
Siegal-Cattan-Mamou disease (periodic) 277.31
Siemens' syndrome
  ectodermal dysplasia 757.31
  keratosis follicularis spinulosa (decalvans) 757.39
Sighing respiration 786.7
Sigmoid
  flexure — *see* condition
  kidney 753.3
Sigmoiditis — *see* Enteritis
Silfverskiöld's syndrome 756.50
Silicosis, silicotic (complicated) (occupational) (simple) 502
  fibrosis, lung (confluent) (massive) (occupational) 502
  non-nodular 503
  pulmonum 502
Silicotuberculosis — *see also* Tuberculosis 011.4 ☑
Silo fillers' disease 506.9
Silver's syndrome (congenital hemihypertrophy and short stature) 759.89
Silver wire arteries, retina 362.13
Silvestroni-Bianco syndrome (thalassemia minima) 282.49
Simian crease 757.2
Simmonds' cachexia or disease (pituitary cachexia) 253.2
Simons' disease or syndrome (progressive lipodystrophy) 272.6
Simple, simplex — *see* condition
Sinding-Larsen disease (juvenile osteopathia patellae) 732.4
Singapore hemorrhagic fever 065.4
Singers' node or nodule 478.5
Single
  atrium 745.69
  coronary artery 746.85
  umbilical artery 747.5
  ventricle 745.3
Singultus 786.8
  epidemicus 078.89
Sinus — *see also* Fistula
  abdominal 569.81
  arrest 426.6
  arrhythmia 427.89
  bradycardia 427.89
    chronic 427.81
  branchial cleft (external) (internal) 744.41
  coccygeal (infected) 685.1
    with abscess 685.0
  dental 522.7
  dermal (congenital) 685.1
    with abscess 685.0
  draining — *see* Fistula
  infected, skin NEC 686.9
  marginal, ruptured or bleeding 641.2 ☑
    affecting fetus or newborn 762.1
  pause 426.6
  pericranii 742.0
  pilonidal (infected) (rectum) 685.1
    with abscess 685.0
  preauricular 744.46
  rectovaginal 619.1
  sacrococcygeal (dermoid) (infected) 685.1
    with abscess 685.0

Sinus — *see also* Fistula — *continued*
  skin
    infected NEC 686.9
    noninfected — *see* Ulcer, skin
  tachycardia 427.89
  tarsi syndrome 726.79
  testis 608.89
  tract (postinfectional) — *see* Fistula
  urachus 753.7
Sinuses, Rokitansky-Aschoff — *see also* Disease, gallbladder 575.8
Sinusitis (accessory) (nasal) (hyperplastic) (nonpurulent) (purulent) (chronic) 473.9
  with influenza, flu, or grippe ▶(*see also* Influenza)◀ 487.1
  acute 461.9
    ethmoidal 461.2
    frontal 461.1
    maxillary 461.0
    specified type NEC 461.8
    sphenoidal 461.3
  allergic (*see also* Fever, hay) 477.9
  antrum — *see* Sinusitis, maxillary
  due to
    fungus, any sinus 117.9
    high altitude 993.1
  ethmoidal 473.2
    acute 461.2
  frontal 473.1
    acute 461.1
  influenzal ▶(*see also* Influenza)◀ 487.1
  maxillary 473.0
    acute 461.0
  specified site NEC 473.8
  sphenoidal 473.3
    acute 461.3
  syphilitic, any sinus 095.8
  tuberculous, any sinus (*see also* Tuberculosis) 012.8 ☑
Sinusitis-bronchiectasis-situs inversus (syndrome) (triad) 759.3
Sioloangitis 527.2
Sipple's syndrome (medullary thyroid carcinoma-pheochromocytoma) 258.02
Sirenomelia 759.89
Siriasis 992.0
Sirkari's disease 085.0
SIRS (systemic inflammatory response syndrome) 995.90
  due to
    infectious process 995.91
      with acute organ dysfunction 995.92
    non-infectious process 995.93
      with acute organ dysfunction 995.94
Siti 104.0
Sitophobia 300.29
Situational
  disturbance (transient) (*see also* Reaction, adjustment) 309.9
    acute 308.3
  maladjustment, acute (*see also* Reaction, adjustment) 309.9
  reaction (*see also* Reaction, adjustment) 309.9
    acute 308.3
Situation, psychiatric 300.9
Situs inversus or transversus 759.3
  abdominalis 759.3
  thoracis 759.3
Sixth disease
  due to
    human herpesvirus 6 058.11
    human herpesvirus 7 058.12
Sjögren-Larsson syndrome (ichthyosis congenita) 757.1
Sjögren (-Gougerot) syndrome or disease (keratoconjunctivitis sicca) 710.2
  with lung involvement 710.2 [517.8]
SJS-TEN (Stevens-Johnson syndrome - toxic epidermal necrolysis overlap syndrome) 695.14
Skeletal — *see* condition
Skene's gland — *see* condition
Skenitis — *see also* Urethritis 597.89
  gonorrheal (acute) 098.0

Skenitis — *see also* Urethritis — *continued*
  gonorrheal — *continued*
    chronic or duration of 2 months or over 098.2
Skerljevo 104.0
Skevas-Zerfus disease 989.5
Skin — *see also* condition
  donor V59.1
  hidebound 710.9
SLAP lesion (superior glenoid labrum) 840.7
Slate-dressers' lung 502
Slate-miners' lung 502
Sleep
  deprivation V69.4
  disorder 780.50
    with apnea — *see* Apnea, sleep
    child 307.40
    movement, unspecified 780.58
    nonorganic origin 307.40
      specified type NEC 307.49
  disturbance 780.50
    with apnea — *see* Apnea, sleep
    nonorganic origin 307.40
      specified type NEC 307.49
  drunkenness 307.47
  movement disorder, unspecified 780.58
  paroxysmal (*see also* Narcolepsy) 347.00
  related movement disorder, unspecified 780.58
  rhythm inversion 327.39
    nonorganic origin 307.45
  walking 307.46
    hysterical 300.13
Sleeping sickness 086.5
  late effect 139.8
Sleeplessness — *see also* Insomnia 780.52
  menopausal 627.2
  nonorganic origin 307.41
Slipped, slipping
  epiphysis (postinfectional) 732.9
    traumatic (old) 732.9
      current — *see* Fracture, by site
      upper femoral (nontraumatic) 732.2
  intervertebral disc — *see* Displacement, intervertebral disc
  ligature, umbilical 772.3
  patella 717.89
  rib 733.99
  sacroiliac joint 724.6
  tendon 727.9
  ulnar nerve, nontraumatic 354.2
  vertebra NEC (*see also* Spondylolisthesis) 756.12
Slocumb's syndrome 255.3
Sloughing (multiple) (skin) 686.9
  abscess — *see* Abscess, by site
  appendix 543.9
  bladder 596.8
  fascia 728.9
  graft — *see* Complications, graft
  phagedena (*see also* Gangrene) 785.4
  reattached extremity (*see also* Complications, reattached extremity) 996.90
  rectum 569.49
  scrotum 608.89
  tendon 727.9
  transplanted organ (*see also* Rejection, transplant, organ, by site) 996.80
  ulcer (*see also* Ulcer, skin) 707.9
Slow
  feeding newborn 779.31
  fetal, growth NEC 764.9 ☑
    affecting management of pregnancy 656.5 ☑
Slowing
  heart 427.89
  urinary stream 788.62
Sluder's neuralgia or syndrome 337.09
Slurred, slurring, speech 784.59
Small-for-dates — *see also* Light-for-dates 764.0 ☑
  affecting management of pregnancy 656.5 ☑
Smallpox 050.9
  contact V01.3
  exposure to V01.3

Smallpox — *continued*
  hemorrhagic (pustular) 050.0
  malignant 050.0
  modified 050.2
  vaccination
    complications — *see* Complications, vaccination
    prophylactic (against) V04.1
Small, smallness
  cardiac reserve — *see* Disease, heart
  for dates
    fetus or newborn 764.0 ☑
      with malnutrition 764.1 ☑
      affecting management of pregnancy 656.5 ☑
    infant, term 764.0 ☑
      with malnutrition 764.1 ☑
      affecting management of pregnancy 656.5 ☑
  introitus, vagina 623.3
  kidney, unknown cause 589.9
    bilateral 589.1
    unilateral 589.0
  ovary 620.8
  pelvis
    with disproportion (fetopelvic) 653.1 ☑
      affecting fetus or newborn 763.1
    causing obstructed labor 660.1 ☑
      affecting fetus or newborn 763.1
  placenta — *see* Placenta, insufficiency
  uterus 621.8
  white kidney 582.9
Smearing, fecal 787.62   ●
Smith's fracture (separation) (closed) 813.41
  open 813.51
Smith-Lemli Opitz syndrome (cerebrohepatorenal syndrome) 759.89
Smith-Magenis syndrome 758.33
Smith-Strang disease (oasthouse urine) 270.2
Smokers'
  bronchitis 491.0
  cough 491.0
  syndrome (*see also* Abuse, drugs, nondependent) 305.1
  throat 472.1
  tongue 528.6
Smoking complicating pregnancy, childbirth, or the puerperium 649.0 ☑
Smothering spells 786.09
Snaggle teeth, tooth 524.39
Snapping
  finger 727.05
  hip 719.65
  jaw 524.69
    temporomandibular joint sounds on opening or closing 524.64
  knee 717.9
  thumb 727.05
Sneddon-Wilkinson disease or syndrome (subcorneal pustular dermatosis) 694.1
Sneezing 784.99
  intractable 478.19
Sniffing
  cocaine (*see also* Dependence) 304.2 ☑
  ether (*see also* Dependence) 304.6 ☑
  glue (airplane) (*see also* Dependence) 304.6 ☑
Snoring 786.09
Snow blindness 370.24
Snuffles (nonsyphilitic) 460
  syphilitic (infant) 090.0
Social migrant V60.0
Sodoku 026.0
Soemmering's ring 366.51
Soft — *see also* condition
  enlarged prostate 600.00
    with
      other lower urinary tract symptoms (LUTS) 600.01
      urinary
        obstruction 600.01
        retention 600.01
  nails 703.8
Softening
  bone 268.2
  brain (necrotic) (progressive) 348.89   ▲

☑ **Additional Digit Required** — Refer to the Tabular List for Digit Selection   ▽ **Subterms under main terms may continue to next column or page**

2011 ICD-9-CM   ▶◀ **Revised Text**   ● **New Line**   ▲ **Revised Code**   **October 2010 · Volume 2 — 257**

Softening — *continued*
- brain — *continued*
  - arteriosclerotic 437.0
  - congenital 742.4
  - due to cerebrovascular accident 438.89●
  - embolic (*see also* Embolism, brain)
    - 434.1 ☑
  - hemorrhagic (*see also* Hemorrhage, brain) 431
  - occlusive 434.9 ☑
  - thrombotic (*see also* Thrombosis, brain) 434.0 ☑
- cartilage 733.92
- cerebellar — *see* Softening, brain
- cerebral — *see* Softening, brain
- cerebrospinal — *see* Softening, brain
- myocardial, heart (*see also* Degeneration, myocardial) 429.1
- nails 703.8
- spinal cord 336.8
- stomach 537.89

Soiling, fecal 787.62   ●

Solar fever 061

Soldier's
- heart 306.2
- patches 423.1

Solitary
- cyst
  - bone 733.21
  - kidney 593.2
- kidney (congenital) 753.0
- tubercle, brain (*see also* Tuberculosis, brain) 013.2 ☑
- ulcer, bladder 596.8

Somatization reaction, somatic reaction — *see also* Disorder, psychosomatic 306.9
- disorder 300.81

Somatoform disorder 300.82
- atypical 300.82
- severe 300.81
- undifferentiated 300.82

Somnambulism 307.46
- hysterical 300.13

Somnolence 780.09
- nonorganic origin 307.43
- periodic 349.89

Sonne dysentery 004.3

Soor 112.0

Sore
- Delhi 085.1
- desert (*see also* Ulcer, skin) 707.9
- eye 379.99
- Lahore 085.1
- mouth 528.9
  - canker 528.2
  - due to dentures 528.9
- muscle 729.1
- Naga (*see also* Ulcer, skin) 707.9
- oriental 085.1
- pressure (*see also* Ulcer, pressure) 707.00
  - with gangrene (*see also* Ulcer, pressure) 707.00 [785.4]
- skin NEC 709.9
- soft 099.0
- throat 462
  - with influenza, flu, or grippe ▶(*see also* Influenza)◀ 487.1
  - acute 462
  - chronic 472.1
  - clergyman's 784.49
  - coxsackie (virus) 074.0
  - diphtheritic 032.0
  - epidemic 034.0
  - gangrenous 462
  - herpetic 054.79
  - influenzal ▶(*see also* Influenza)◀ 487.1
  - malignant 462
  - purulent 462
  - putrid 462
  - septic 034.0
  - streptococcal (ulcerative) 034.0
  - ulcerated 462
  - viral NEC 462
    - Coxsackie 074.0
- tropical (*see also* Ulcer, skin) 707.9
- veldt (*see also* Ulcer, skin) 707.9

Sotos' syndrome (cerebral gigantism) 253.0

Sounds
- friction, pleural 786.7
- succussion, chest 786.7
- temporomandibular joint
  - on opening or closing 524.64

South African cardiomyopathy syndrome 425.2

South American
- blastomycosis 116.1
- trypanosomiasis — *see* Trypanosomiasis

Southeast Asian hemorrhagic fever 065.4

Spacing, teeth, abnormal 524.30
- excessive 524.32

Spade-like hand (congenital) 754.89

Spading nail 703.8
- congenital 757.5

Spanemia 285.9

Spanish collar 605

Sparganosis 123.5

Spasmodic — *see* condition

Spasmophilia — *see also* Tetany 781.7

Spasm, spastic, spasticity — *see* condition 781.0
- accommodation 367.53
- ampulla of Vater (*see also* Disease, gallbladder) 576.8
- anus, ani (sphincter) (reflex) 564.6
  - psychogenic 306.4
- artery NEC 443.9
  - basilar 435.0
  - carotid 435.8
  - cerebral 435.9
    - specified artery NEC 435.8
  - retinal (*see also* Occlusion, retinal, artery) 362.30
  - vertebral 435.1
  - vertebrobasilar 435.3
- Bell's 351.0
- bladder (sphincter, external or internal) 596.8
- bowel 564.9
  - psychogenic 306.4
- bronchus, bronchiole 519.11
- cardia 530.0
- cardiac — *see* Angina
- carpopedal (*see also* Tetany) 781.7
- cecum 564.9
  - psychogenic 306.4
- cerebral (arteries) (vascular) 435.9
  - specified artery NEC 435.8
- cerebrovascular 435.9
- cervix, complicating delivery 661.4 ☑
  - affecting fetus or newborn 763.7
- ciliary body (of accommodation) 367.53
- colon 564.1
  - psychogenic 306.4
- common duct (*see also* Disease, biliary) 576.8
- compulsive 307.22
- conjugate 378.82
- convergence 378.84
- coronary (artery) — *see* Angina
- diaphragm (reflex) 786.8
  - psychogenic 306.1
- duodenum, duodenal (bulb) 564.89
- esophagus (diffuse) 530.5
  - psychogenic 306.4
- facial 351.8
- fallopian tube 620.8
- gait 781.2
- gastrointestinal (tract) 536.8
  - psychogenic 306.4
- glottis 478.75
  - hysterical 300.11
  - psychogenic 306.1
    - specified as conversion reaction 300.11
  - reflex through recurrent laryngeal nerve 478.75
- habit 307.20
  - chronic 307.22
  - transient (of childhood) 307.21
- heart — *see* Angina
- hourglass — *see* Contraction, hourglass
- hysterical 300.11

Spasm, spastic, spasticity — *see also* condition — *continued*
- infantile (*see also* Epilepsy) 345.6 ☑
- internal oblique, eye 378.51
- intestinal 564.9
  - psychogenic 306.4
- larynx, laryngeal 478.75
  - hysterical 300.11
  - psychogenic 306.1
    - specified as conversion reaction 300.11
- levator palpebrae superioris 333.81
- lightning (*see also* Epilepsy) 345.6 ☑
- mobile 781.0
- muscle 728.85
  - back 724.8
  - psychogenic 306.0
- nerve, trigeminal 350.1
- nervous 306.0
- nodding 307.3
  - infantile (*see also* Epilepsy) 345.6 ☑
- occupational 300.89
- oculogyric 378.87
- ophthalmic artery 362.30
- orbicularis 781.0
- perineal 625.8
- peroneo-extensor (*see also* Flat, foot) 734
- pharynx (reflex) 478.29
  - hysterical 300.11
  - psychogenic 306.1
    - specified as conversion reaction 300.11
- pregnant uterus, complicating delivery 661.4 ☑
- psychogenic 306.0
- pylorus 537.81
  - adult hypertrophic 537.0
  - congenital or infantile 750.5
  - psychogenic 306.4
- rectum (sphincter) 564.6
  - psychogenic 306.4
- retinal artery NEC (*see also* Occlusion, retina, artery) 362.30
- sacroiliac 724.6
- salaam (infantile) (*see also* Epilepsy) 345.6 ☑
- saltatory 781.0
- sigmoid 564.9
  - psychogenic 306.4
- sphincter of Oddi (*see also* Disease, gallbladder) 576.5
- stomach 536.8
  - neurotic 306.4
- throat 478.29
  - hysterical 300.11
  - psychogenic 306.1
    - specified as conversion reaction 300.11
- tic 307.20
  - chronic 307.22
  - transient (of childhood) 307.21
- tongue 529.8
- torsion 333.6
- trigeminal nerve 350.1
  - postherpetic 053.12
- ureter 593.89
- urethra (sphincter) 599.84
- uterus 625.8
  - complicating labor 661.4 ☑
  - affecting fetus or newborn 763.7
- vagina 625.1
  - psychogenic 306.51
- vascular NEC 443.9
- vasomotor NEC 443.9
- vein NEC 459.89
- vesical (sphincter, external or internal) 596.8
- viscera 789.0 ☑

Spasmus nutans 307.3

Spastic — *see also* Spasm
- child 343.9

Spasticity — *see also* Spasm
- cerebral, child 343.9

Speakers' throat 784.49

Specific, specified — *see* condition

Speech
- defect, disorder, disturbance, impediment NEC 784.59
  - psychogenic 307.9
- (language) therapy V57.3

Spells 780.39
- breath-holding 786.9

Spencer's disease (epidemic vomiting) 078.82

Spens' syndrome (syncope with heart block) 426.9

Spermatic cord — *see* condition

Spermatocele 608.1
- congenital 752.89

Spermatocystitis 608.4

Spermatocytoma (M9063/3)
- specified site — *see* Neoplasm, by site, malignant
- unspecified site 186.9

Spermatorrhea 608.89

Sperm counts
- fertility testing V26.21
- following sterilization reversal V26.22
- postvasectomy V25.8

Sphacelus — *see also* Gangrene 785.4

Sphenoidal — *see* condition

Sphenoiditis (chronic) — *see also* Sinusitis, sphenoidal 473.3

Sphenopalatine ganglion neuralgia 337.09

Sphericity, increased, lens 743.36

Spherocytosis (congenital) (familial) (hereditary) 282.0
- hemoglobin disease 282.7
- sickle-cell (disease) 282.60

Spherophakia 743.36

Sphincter — *see* condition

Sphincteritis, sphincter of Oddi — *see also* Cholecystitis 576.8

Sphingolipidosis 272.7

Sphingolipodystrophy 272.7

Sphingomyelinosis 272.7

Spicule tooth 520.2

Spider
- finger 755.59
- nevus 448.1
- vascular 448.1

Spiegler-Fendt sarcoid 686.8

Spielmeyer-Stock disease 330.1

Spielmeyer-Vogt disease 330.1

Spina bifida (aperta) 741.9 ☑

Note — Use the following fifth-digit subclassification with category 741:
0   unspecified region
1   cervical region
2   dorsal [thoracic} region
3   lumbar region

- with hydrocephalus 741.0 ☑
  - fetal (suspected), affecting management of pregnancy 655.0 ☑
- occulta 756.17

Spindle, Krukenberg's 371.13

Spine, spinal — *see* condition

Spiradenoma (eccrine) (M8403/0) — *see* Neoplasm, skin, benign

Spirillosis NEC — *see also* Fever, relapsing 087.9

Spirillum minus 026.0

Spirillum obermeieri infection 087.0

Spirochetal — *see* condition

Spirochetosis 104.9
- arthritic, arthritica 104.9 [711.8] ☑
- bronchopulmonary 104.8
- icterohemorrhagica 100.0
- lung 104.8

Spitting blood — *see also* Hemoptysis 786.30   ▲

Splanchnomegaly 569.89

Splanchnoptosis 569.89

Spleen, splenic — *see also* condition
- agenesis 759.0
- flexure syndrome 569.89
- neutropenia syndrome 289.53
- sequestration syndrome 289.52

Splenectasis — *see also* Splenomegaly 789.2

☑ **Additional Digit Required** — Refer to the Tabular List for Digit Selection   ▽ **Subterms under main terms may continue to next column or page**

258 — Volume 2 · October 2010   ▶◀ **Revised Text**   ● **New Line**   ▲ **Revised Code**   2011 ICD-9-CM

Splenitis (interstitial) (malignant) (nonspecific) 289.59
  malarial (*see also* Malaria) 084.6
  tuberculous (*see also* Tuberculosis) 017.7 ☑
Splenocele 289.59
Splenomegalia — *see* Splenomegaly
Splenomegalic — *see* condition
Splenomegaly 789.2
  Bengal 789.2
  cirrhotic 289.51
  congenital 759.0
  congestive, chronic 289.51
  cryptogenic 789.2
  Egyptian 120.1
  Gaucher's (cerebroside lipidosis) 272.7
  idiopathic 789.2
  malarial (*see also* Malaria) 084.6
  neutropenic 289.53
  Niemann-Pick (lipid histiocytosis) 272.7
  siderotic 289.51
  syphilitic 095.8
    congenital 090.0
  tropical (Bengal) (idiopathic) 789.2
Splenopathy 289.50
Splenopneumonia — *see* Pneumonia
Splenoptosis 289.59
Splinter — *see* Injury, superficial, by site
Split, splitting
  heart sounds 427.89
  lip, congenital (*see also* Cleft, lip) 749.10
  nails 703.8
  urinary stream 788.61
Spoiled child reaction — *see also* Disturbance, conduct 312.1 ☑
Spondylarthritis — *see also* Spondylosis 721.90
Spondylarthrosis — *see also* Spondylosis 721.90
Spondylitis 720.9
  ankylopoietica 720.0
  ankylosing (chronic) 720.0
  atrophic 720.9
    ligamentous 720.9
  chronic (traumatic) (*see also* Spondylosis) 721.90
  deformans (chronic) (*see also* Spondylosis) 721.90
  gonococcal 098.53
  gouty 274.00
  hypertrophic (*see also* Spondylosis) 721.90
  infectious NEC 720.9
  juvenile (adolescent) 720.0
  Kümmell's 721.7
  Marie-Strümpell (ankylosing) 720.0
  muscularis 720.9
  ossificans ligamentosa 721.6
  osteoarthritica (*see also* Spondylosis) 721.90
  posttraumatic 721.7
  proliferative 720.0
  rheumatoid 720.0
  rhizomelica 720.0
  sacroiliac NEC 720.2
  senescent (*see also* Spondylosis) 721.90
  senile (*see also* Spondylosis) 721.90
  static (*see also* Spondylosis) 721.90
  traumatic (chronic) (*see also* Spondylosis) 721.90
  tuberculous (*see also* Tuberculosis) 015.0 ☑ *[720.81]*
  typhosa 002.0 *[720.81]*
Spondyloarthrosis — *see also* Spondylosis 721.90
Spondylolisthesis (congenital) (lumbosacral) 756.12
  with disproportion (fetopelvic) 653.3 ☑
    affecting fetus or newborn 763.1
    causing obstructed labor 660.1 ☑
      affecting fetus or newborn 763.1
  acquired 738.4
  degenerative 738.4
  traumatic 738.4
    acute (lumbar) — *see* Fracture, vertebra, lumbar
      site other than lumbosacral — *see* Fracture, vertebra, by site
Spondylolysis (congenital) 756.11

Spondylolysis — *continued*
  acquired 738.4
  cervical 756.19
  lumbosacral region 756.11
    with disproportion (fetopelvic) 653.3 ☑
      affecting fetus or newborn 763.1
      causing obstructed labor 660.1 ☑
        affecting fetus or newborn 763.1
Spondylopathy
  inflammatory 720.9
    specified type NEC 720.89
  traumatic 721.7
Spondylose rhizomelique 720.0
Spondylosis 721.90
  with
    disproportion 653.3 ☑
      affecting fetus or newborn 763.1
      causing obstructed labor 660.1 ☑
        affecting fetus or newborn 763.1
    myelopathy NEC 721.91
  cervical, cervicodorsal 721.0
    with myelopathy 721.1
  inflammatory 720.9
  lumbar, lumbosacral 721.3
    with myelopathy 721.42
  sacral 721.3
    with myelopathy 721.42
  thoracic 721.2
    with myelopathy 721.41
  traumatic 721.7
Sponge
  divers' disease 989.5
  inadvertently left in operation wound 998.4
  kidney (medullary) 753.17
Spongioblastoma (M9422/3)
  multiforme (M9440/3)
    specified site — *see* Neoplasm, by site, malignant
    unspecified site 191.9
  polare (M9423/3)
    specified site — *see* Neoplasm, by site, malignant
    unspecified site 191.9
  primitive polar (M9443/3)
    specified site — *see* Neoplasm, by site, malignant
    unspecified site 191.9
  specified site — *see* Neoplasm, by site, malignant
  unspecified site 191.9
Spongiocytoma (M9400/3)
  specified site — *see* Neoplasm, by site, malignant
  unspecified site 191.9
Spongioneuroblastoma (M9504/3) — *see* Neoplasm, by site, malignant
Spontaneous — *see also* condition
  fracture — *see* Fracture, pathologic
Spoon nail 703.8
  congenital 757.5
Sporadic — *see* condition
Sporotrichosis (bones) (cutaneous) (disseminated) (epidermal) (lymphatic) (lymphocutaneous) (mucous membranes) (pulmonary) (skeletal) (visceral) 117.1
Sporotrichum schenckii infection 117.1
Spots, spotting
  atrophic (skin) 701.3
  Bitôt's (in the young child) 264.1
  café au lait 709.09
  cayenne pepper 448.1
  complicating pregnancy 649.5 ☑
  cotton wool (retina) 362.83
  de Morgan's (senile angiomas) 448.1
  Fúchs' black (myopic) 360.21
  intermenstrual
    irregular 626.6
    regular 626.5
  interpalpebral 372.53
  Koplik's 055.9
  liver 709.09
  Mongolian (pigmented) 757.33
  of pregnancy 649.5 ☑
  purpuric 782.7
  ruby 448.1
Spotted fever — *see* Fever, spotted

Sprain, strain (joint) (ligament) (muscle) (tendon) 848.9
  abdominal wall (muscle) 848.8
  Achilles tendon 845.09
  acromioclavicular 840.0
  ankle 845.00
    and foot 845.00
  anterior longitudinal, cervical 847.0
  arm 840.9
    upper 840.9
      and shoulder 840.9
  astragalus 845.00
  atlanto-axial 847.0
  atlanto-occipital 847.0
  atlas 847.0
  axis 847.0
  back (*see also* Sprain, spine) 847.9
  breast bone 848.40
  broad ligament — *see* Injury, internal, broad ligament
  calcaneofibular 845.02
  carpal 842.01
  carpometacarpal 842.11
  cartilage
    costal, without mention of injury to sternum 848.3
      involving sternum 848.42
    ear 848.8
    knee 844.9
      with current tear (*see also* Tear, meniscus) 836.2
    semilunar (knee) 844.8
      with current tear (*see also* Tear, meniscus) 836.2
    septal, nose 848.0
    thyroid region 848.2
    xiphoid 848.49
  cervical, cervicodorsal, cervicothoracic 847.0
  chondrocostal, without mention of injury to sternum 848.3
    involving sternum 848.42
  chondrosternal 848.42
  chronic (joint) — *see* Derangement, joint
  clavicle 840.9
  coccyx 847.4
  collar bone 840.9
  collateral, knee (medial) (tibial) 844.1
    lateral (fibular) 844.0
    recurrent or old 717.89
      lateral 717.81
      medial 717.82
  coracoacromial 840.8
  coracoclavicular 840.1
  coracohumeral 840.2
  coracoid (process) 840.9
  coronary, knee 844.8
  costal cartilage, without mention of injury to sternum 848.3
    involving sternum 848.42
  cricoarytenoid articulation 848.2
  cricothyroid articulation 848.2
  cruciate
    knee 844.2
    old 717.89
      anterior 717.83
      posterior 717.84
  deltoid
    ankle 845.01
    shoulder 840.8
  dorsal (spine) 847.1
  ear cartilage 848.8
  elbow 841.9
    and forearm 841.9
    specified site NEC 841.8
  femur (proximal end) 843.9
    distal end 844.9
  fibula (proximal end) 844.9
    distal end 845.00
  fibulocalcaneal 845.02
  finger(s) 842.10
  foot 845.10
    and ankle 845.00
  forearm 841.9
    and elbow 841.9
    specified site NEC 841.8

Sprain, strain — *continued*
  glenoid (shoulder) (*see also* SLAP lesion) 840.8
  hand 842.10
  hip 843.9
    and thigh 843.9
  humerus (proximal end) 840.9
    distal end 841.9
  iliofemoral 843.0
  infraspinatus 840.3
  innominate
    acetabulum 843.9
    pubic junction 848.5
    sacral junction 846.1
  internal
    collateral, ankle 845.01
    semilunar cartilage 844.8
      with current tear (*see also* Tear, meniscus) 836.2
      old 717.5
  interphalangeal
    finger 842.13
    toe 845.13
  ischiocapsular 843.1
  jaw (cartilage) (meniscus) 848.1
    old 524.69
  knee 844.9
    and leg 844.9
    old 717.5
      collateral
        lateral 717.81
        medial 717.82
      cruciate
        anterior 717.83
        posterior 717.84
  late effect — *see* Late, effects (of), sprain
  lateral collateral, knee 844.0
    old 717.81
  leg 844.9
    and knee 844.9
  ligamentum teres femoris 843.8
  low back 846.9
  lumbar (spine) 847.2
  lumbosacral 846.0
    chronic or old 724.6
  mandible 848.1
    old 524.69
  maxilla 848.1
  medial collateral, knee 844.1
    old 717.82
  meniscus
    jaw 848.1
      old 524.69
    knee 844.8
      with current tear (*see also* Tear, meniscus) 836.2
      old 717.5
    mandible 848.1
      old 524.69
    specified site NEC 848.8
  metacarpal 842.10
    distal 842.12
    proximal 842.11
  metacarpophalangeal 842.12
  metatarsal 845.10
  metatarsophalangeal 845.12
  midcarpal 842.19
  midtarsal 845.19
  multiple sites, except fingers alone or toes alone 848.8
  neck 847.0
  nose (septal cartilage) 848.0
  occiput from atlas 847.0
  old — *see* Derangement, joint
  orbicular, hip 843.8
  patella(r) 844.8
    old 717.89
  pelvis 848.5
  phalanx
    finger 842.10
    toe 845.10
  radiocarpal 842.02
  radiohumeral 841.2
  radioulnar 841.9
    distal 842.09
  radius, radial (proximal end) 841.9

☑ Additional Digit Required — Refer to the Tabular List for Digit Selection   ᴺᴱᵂ Subterms under main terms may continue to next column or page

2011 ICD-9-CM   ▶◀ Revised Text   ● New Line   ▲ Revised Code   Volume 2 — 259

Sprain, strain — continued
  radius, radial — continued
    and ulna 841.9
      distal 842.09
      collateral 841.0
      distal end 842.00
    recurrent — see Sprain, by site
    rib (cage), without mention of injury to
        sternum 848.3
      involving sternum 848.42
    rotator cuff (capsule) 840.4
    round ligament (see also Injury, internal,
        round ligament)
      femur 843.8
    sacral (spine) 847.3
    sacrococcygeal 847.3
    sacroiliac (region) 846.9
      chronic or old 724.6
      ligament 846.1
      specified site NEC 846.8
    sacrospinatus 846.2
    sacrospinous 846.2
    sacrotuberous 846.3
    scaphoid bone, ankle 845.00
    scapula(r) 840.9
    semilunar cartilage (knee) 844.8
      with current tear (see also Tear, menis-
          cus) 836.2
      old 717.5
    septal cartilage (nose) 848.0
    shoulder 840.9
      and arm, upper 840.9
      blade 840.9
    specified site NEC 848.8
    spine 847.9
      cervical 847.0
      coccyx 847.4
      dorsal 847.1
      lumbar 847.2
      lumbosacral 846.0
        chronic or old 724.6
      sacral 847.3
      sacroiliac (see also Sprain, sacroiliac)
          846.9
        chronic or old 724.6
      thoracic 847.1
    sternoclavicular 848.41
    sternum 848.40
    subglenoid (see also SLAP lesion) 840.8
    subscapularis 840.5
    supraspinatus 840.6
    symphysis
      jaw 848.1
        old 524.69
      mandibular 848.1
        old 524.69
      pubis 848.5
    talofibular 845.09
    tarsal 845.10
    tarsometatarsal 845.11
    temporomandibular 848.1
      old 524.69
    teres
      ligamentum femoris 843.8
      major or minor 840.8
    thigh (proximal end) 843.9
      and hip 843.9
      distal end 844.9
    thoracic (spine) 847.1
    thorax 848.8
    thumb 842.10
    thyroid cartilage or region 848.2
    tibia (proximal end) 844.9
      distal end 845.00
    tibiofibular
      distal 845.03
      superior 844.3
    toe(s) 845.10
    trachea 848.8
    trapezoid 840.8
    ulna, ulnar (proximal end) 841.9
      collateral 841.1
      distal end 842.00
    ulnohumeral 841.3
    vertebrae (see also Sprain, spine) 847.9

Sprain, strain — continued
  vertebrae (see also Sprain, spine) — contin-
      ued
    cervical, cervicodorsal, cervicothoracic
        847.0
    wrist (cuneiform) (scaphoid) (semilunar)
        842.00
    xiphoid cartilage 848.49
Sprengel's deformity (congenital) 755.52
Spring fever 309.23
Sprue 579.1
  celiac 579.0
  idiopathic 579.0
  meaning thrush 112.0
  nontropical 579.0
  tropical 579.1
Spur — see also Exostosis
  bone 726.91
    calcaneal 726.73
  calcaneal 726.73
  iliac crest 726.5
  nose (septum) 478.19
    bone 726.91
  septal 478.19
Spuria placenta — see Placenta, abnormal
Spurway's syndrome (brittle bones and blue
    sclera) 756.51
Sputum, abnormal (amount) (color) (exces-
    sive) (odor) (purulent) 786.4
  bloody 786.30   ▲
Squamous — see also condition
  cell metaplasia
    bladder 596.8
    cervix — see condition
  epithelium in
    cervical canal (congenital) 752.49
    uterine mucosa (congenital)
        752.39   ▲
  metaplasia
    bladder 596.8
    cervix — see condition
Squashed nose 738.0
  congenital 754.0
Squeeze, divers' 993.3
Squint — see also Strabismus 378.9
  accommodative (see also Esotropia) 378.00
  concomitant (see also Heterotropia) 378.30
Stab — see also Wound, open, by site
  internal organs — see Injury, internal, by
      site, with open wound
Staggering gait 781.2
  hysterical 300.11
Staghorn calculus 592.0
Stain, staining
  meconium 779.84
  port wine 757.32
  tooth, teeth (hard tissues) 521.7
    due to
      accretions 523.6
      deposits (betel) (black) (green) (ma-
          teria alba) (orange) (tobacco)
          523.6
      metals (copper) (silver) 521.7
      nicotine 523.6
      pulpal bleeding 521.7
      tobacco 523.6
Stälh's
  ear 744.29
  pigment line (cornea) 371.11
Stälhi's pigment lines (cornea) 371.11
Stammering ►— see also Disorder, fluency◄
    315.35   ▲
Standstill
  atrial 426.6
  auricular 426.6
  cardiac (see also Arrest, cardiac) 427.5
  sinoatrial 426.6
  sinus 426.6
  ventricular (see also Arrest, cardiac) 427.5
Stannosis 503
Stanton's disease (melioidosis) 025
Staphylitis (acute) (catarrhal) (chronic) (gan-
    grenous) (membranous) (suppurative)
    (ulcerative) 528.3
Staphylococcemia 038.10
  aureus 038.11

Staphylococcemia — continued
  specified organism NEC 038.19
Staphylococcus, staphylococcal — see condi-
    tion
Staphyloderma (skin) 686.00
Staphyloma 379.11
  anterior, localized 379.14
  ciliary 379.11
  cornea 371.73
  equatorial 379.13
  posterior 379.12
  posticum 379.12
  ring 379.15
  sclera NEC 379.11
Starch eating 307.52
Stargardt's disease 362.75
Starvation (inanition) (due to lack of food)
    994.2
  edema 262
  voluntary NEC 307.1
Stasis
  bile (duct) (see also Disease, biliary) 576.8
  bronchus (see also Bronchitis) 490
  cardiac (see also Failure, heart) 428.0
  cecum 564.89
  colon 564.89
  dermatitis (see also Varix, with stasis dermati-
      tis) 454.1
  duodenal 536.8
  eczema (see also Varix, with stasis dermati-
      tis) 454.1
  edema (see also Hypertension, venous)
      459.30
  foot 991.4
  gastric 536.3
  ileocecal coil 564.89
  ileum 564.89
  intestinal 564.89
  jejunum 564.89
  kidney 586
  liver 571.9
    cirrhotic — see Cirrhosis, liver
  lymphatic 457.8
  pneumonia 514
  portal 571.9
  pulmonary 514
  rectal 564.89
  renal 586
    tubular 584.5
  stomach 536.3
  ulcer
    with varicose veins 454.0
    without varicose veins 459.81
  urine NEC (see also Retention, urine) 788.20
  venous 459.81
State
  affective and paranoid, mixed, organic psy-
      chotic 294.8
  agitated 307.9
    acute reaction to stress 308.2
  anxiety (neurotic) (see also Anxiety) 300.00
    specified type NEC 300.09
  apprehension (see also Anxiety) 300.00
    specified type NEC 300.09
  climacteric, female 627.2
    following induced menopause 627.4
  clouded
    epileptic (see also Epilepsy) 345.9 ☑
    paroxysmal (idiopathic) (see also Epilep-
        sy) 345.9 ☑
  compulsive (mixed) (with obsession) 300.3
  confusional 298.9
    acute 293.0
      with
        arteriosclerotic dementia 290.41
        presenile brain disease 290.11
        senility 290.3
      alcoholic 291.0
      drug-induced 292.81
    epileptic 293.0
    postoperative 293.9
    reactive (emotional stress) (psychologi-
        cal trauma) 298.2
    subacute 293.1
  constitutional psychopathic 301.9
  convulsive (see also Convulsions) 780.39

State — continued
  depressive NEC 311
    induced by drug 292.84
    neurotic 300.4
  dissociative 300.15
  hallucinatory 780.1
    induced by drug 292.12
  hypercoagulable (primary) 289.81
    secondary 289.82
  hyperdynamic beta-adrenergic circulatory
      429.82
  locked-in 344.81
  menopausal 627.2
    artificial 627.4
    following induced menopause 627.4
  neurotic NEC 300.9
    with depersonalization episode 300.6
  obsessional 300.3
  oneiroid (see also Schizophrenia) 295.4 ☑
  panic 300.01
  paranoid 297.9
    alcohol-induced 291.5
    arteriosclerotic 290.42
    climacteric 297.2
    drug-induced 292.11
    in
      presenile brain disease 290.12
      senile brain disease 290.20
    involutional 297.2
    menopausal 297.2
    senile 290.20
    simple 297.0
  postleukotomy 310.0
  pregnant (see also Pregnancy) V22.2
  psychogenic, twilight 298.2
  psychotic, organic (see also Psychosis, organ-
      ic) 294.9
    mixed paranoid and affective 294.8
    senile or presenile NEC 290.9
    transient NEC 293.9
      with
        anxiety 293.84
        delusions 293.81
        depression 293.83
        hallucinations 293.82
  residual schizophrenic (see also
      Schizophrenia) 295.6 ☑
  tension (see also Anxiety) 300.9
  transient organic psychotic 293.9
    anxiety type 293.84
    depressive type 293.83
    hallucinatory type 293.83
    paranoid type 293.81
    specified type NEC 293.89
  twilight
    epileptic 293.0
    psychogenic 298.2
  vegetative (persistent) 780.03
Status (post)
  absence
    epileptic (see also Epilepsy) 345.2
    of organ, acquired (postsurgical) — see
        Absence, by site, acquired
  administration of tPA(rtPA) in a different
      institution within the last 24 hours
      prior to admission to facility V45.88
  anastomosis of intestine (for bypass) V45.3
  anginosus 413.9
  angioplasty, percutaneous transluminal
      coronary V45.82
  ankle prosthesis V43.66
  aortocoronary bypass or shunt V45.81
  arthrodesis V45.4
  artificially induced condition NEC V45.89
  artificial opening (of) V44.9
    gastrointestinal tract NEC V44.4
    specified site NEC V44.8
    urinary tract NEC V44.6
    vagina V44.7
  aspirator V46.0
  asthmaticus (see also Asthma) 493.9 ☑
  awaiting organ transplant V49.83
  bariatric surgery V45.86
    complicating pregnancy, childbirth, or
        the puerperium 649.2 ☑
  bed confinement V49.84

☑ **Additional Digit Required** — Refer to the Tabular List for Digit Selection   ▽ **Subterms under main terms may continue to next column or page**

Status — *continued*
breast
  correction V43.82
  implant removal V45.83
  reconstruction V43.82
cardiac
  device (in situ) V45.00
    carotid sinus V45.09
      fitting or adjustment V53.39
    defibrillator, automatic implantable
      ▶(with synchronous cardiac
      pacemaker)◀ V45.02
    pacemaker V45.01
      fitting or adjustment V53.31
carotid sinus stimulator V45.09
cataract extraction V45.61
chemotherapy V66.2
  current V58.69
circumcision, female 629.20
clitorectomy (female genital mutilation type I) 629.21
  with excision of labia minora (female genital mutilation type II) 629.22
colonization — *see* Carrier (suspected) of
colostomy V44.3
contraceptive device V45.59
  intrauterine V45.51
  subdermal V45.52
convulsivus idiopathicus (*see also* Epilepsy) 345.3
coronary artery bypass or shunt V45.81
cutting
  female genital 629.20
    specified NEC 629.29
    type I 629.21
    type II 629.22
    type III 629.23
    type IV 629.29
cystostomy V44.50
  appendico-vesicostomy V44.52
  cutaneous-vesicostomy V44.51
  specified type NEC V44.59
defibrillator, automatic implantable cardiac
  ▶(with synchronous cardiac pacemaker)◀ V45.02
delinquent immunization V15.83
dental crowns V45.84
dental fillings V45.84
dental restoration V45.84
dental sealant V49.82
dialysis (hemo) (peritoneal) V45.11
donor V59.9
do not resuscitate V49.86 ●
drug therapy or regimen V67.59
  high-risk medication NEC V67.51
elbow prosthesis V43.62
embedded ●
  fragment — *see* Foreign body, retained ●
  splinter — *see* Foreign body, retained ●
enterostomy V44.4
epileptic, epilepticus (absence) (grand mal) (*see also* Epilepsy) 345.3
  focal motor 345.7 ☑
  partial 345.7 ☑
  petit mal 345.2
  psychomotor 345.7 ☑
  temporal lobe 345.7 ☑
estrogen receptor
  negative [ER-] V86.1
  positive [ER+] V86.0
eye (adnexa) surgery V45.69
female genital
  cutting 629.20
    specified NEC 629.29
    type I 629.21
    type II 629.22
    type III 629.23
    type IV 629.29
  mutilation 629.20
    type I 629.21
    type II 629.22
    type III 629.23
    type IV 629.29
filtering bleb (eye) (postglaucoma) V45.69
  with rupture or complication 997.99

Status — *continued*
filtering bleb — *continued*
  postcataract extraction (complication) 997.99
finger joint prosthesis V43.69
foster care V60.81
gastric
  banding V45.86
    complicating pregnancy, childbirth, or the puerperium 649.2 ☑
  bypass for obesity V45.86
    complicating pregnancy, childbirth, or the puerperium 649.2 ☑
gastrostomy V44.1
grand mal 345.3
heart valve prosthesis V43.3
hemodialysis V45.11
hip prosthesis (joint) (partial) (total) V43.64
hysterectomy V88.01
  partial with remaining cervical stump V88.02
  total V88.01
ileostomy V44.2
infibulation (female genital mutilation type III) 629.23
insulin pump V45.85
intestinal bypass V45.3
intrauterine contraceptive device V45.51
jejunostomy V44.4
knee joint prosthesis V43.65
lacunaris 437.8
lacunosis 437.8
lapsed immunization schedule V15.83
low birth weight V21.30
  less than 500 grams V21.31
  1000–1499 grams V21.33
  1500–1999 grams V21.34
  2000–2500 grams V21.35
  500–999 grams V21.32
lymphaticus 254.8
malignant neoplasm, ablated or excised — *see* History, malignant neoplasm
marmoratus 333.79
military deployment V62.22
mutilation, female 629.20
  type I 629.21
  type II 629.22
  type III 629.23
  type IV 629.29
nephrostomy V44.6
neuropacemaker NEC V45.89
  brain V45.89
  carotid sinus V45.09
  neurologic NEC V45.89
obesity surgery V45.86
  complicating pregnancy, childbirth, or the puerperium 649.2 ☑
organ replacement
  by artificial or mechanical device or prosthesis of
    artery V43.4
    artificial skin V43.83
    bladder V43.5
    blood vessel V43.4
    breast V43.82
    eye globe V43.0
    heart
      assist device V43.21
      fully implantable artificial heart V43.22
      valve V43.3
    intestine V43.89
    joint V43.60
      ankle V43.66
      elbow V43.62
      finger V43.69
      hip (partial) (total) V43.64
      knee V43.65
      shoulder V43.61
      specified NEC V43.69
      wrist V43.63
    kidney V43.89
    larynx V43.81
    lens V43.1
    limb(s) V43.7
    liver V43.89

Status — *continued*
organ replacement — *continued*
  by artificial or mechanical device or prosthesis of — *continued*
    lung V43.89
    organ NEC V43.89
    pancreas V43.89
    skin (artificial) V43.83
    tissue NEC V43.89
    vein V43.4
  by organ transplant (heterologous) (homologous) — *see* Status, transplant
pacemaker
  brain V45.89
  cardiac V45.01
  carotid sinus V45.09
  neurologic NEC V45.89
  specified site NEC V45.89
percutaneous transluminal coronary angioplasty V45.82
peritoneal dialysis V45.11
petit mal 345.2
physical restraints V49.87 ●
postcommotio cerebri 310.2
postmenopausal (age related) (natural) V49.81
postoperative NEC V45.89
postpartum NEC V24.2
  care immediately following delivery V24.0
  routine follow-up V24.2
postsurgical NEC V45.89
renal dialysis V45.11
  noncompliance V45.12
respirator [ventilator] V46.11
  encounter
    during
      mechanical failure V46.14
      power failure V46.12
    for weaning V46.13
retained foreign body — *see* Foreign ●
  body, retained ●
reversed jejunal transposition (for bypass) V45.3
sex reassignment surgery (*see also* Transsexualism) 302.50
shoulder prosthesis V43.61
shunt
  aortocoronary bypass V45.81
  arteriovenous (for dialysis) V45.11
  cerebrospinal fluid V45.2
  vascular NEC V45.89
    aortocoronary (bypass) V45.81
  ventricular (communicating) (for drainage) V45.2
sterilization
  tubal ligation V26.51
  vasectomy V26.52
subdermal contraceptive device V45.52
thymicolymphaticus 254.8
thymicus 254.8
thymolymphaticus 254.8
tooth extraction 525.10
tracheostomy V44.0
transplant
  blood vessel V42.89
  bone V42.4
    marrow V42.81
  cornea V42.5
  heart V42.1
    valve V42.2
  intestine V42.84
  kidney V42.0
  liver V42.7
  lung V42.6
  organ V42.9
    removal (due to complication, failure, rejection or infection) V45.87
    specified site NEC V42.89
  pancreas V42.83
  peripheral stem cells V42.82
  skin V42.3
  stem cells, peripheral V42.82
  tissue V42.9
    specified type NEC V42.89

Status — *continued*
transplant — *continued*
  vessel, blood V42.89
tubal ligation V26.51
underimmunization V15.83
ureterostomy V44.6
urethrostomy V44.6
vagina, artificial V44.7
vascular shunt NEC V45.89
  aortocoronary (bypass) V45.81
vasectomy V26.52
ventilator [respirator] V46.11
  encounter
    during
      mechanical failure V46.14
      power failure V46.12
    for weaning V46.13
wheelchair confinement V46.3
wrist prosthesis V43.63
Stave fracture — *see* Fracture, metacarpus, metacarpal bone(s)
Steal
subclavian artery 435.2
vertebral artery 435.1
Stealing, solitary, child problem — *see also* Disturbance, conduct 312.1 ☑
Steam burn — *see* Burn, by site
Steatocystoma multiplex 706.2
Steatoma (infected) 706.2
eyelid (cystic) 374.84
  infected 373.13
Steatorrhea (chronic) 579.8
with lacteal obstruction 579.2
idiopathic 579.0
  adult 579.0
  infantile 579.0
pancreatic 579.4
primary 579.0
secondary 579.8
specified cause NEC 579.8
tropical 579.1
Steatosis 272.8
heart (*see also* Degeneration, myocardial) 429.1
kidney 593.89
liver 571.8
Steele-Richardson (-Olszewski) Syndrome 333.0
Steinbrocker's syndrome — *see also* Neuropathy, peripheral, autonomic 337.9
Steinert's disease 359.21
Stein-Leventhal syndrome (polycystic ovary) 256.4
Stein's syndrome (polycystic ovary) 256.4
STEMI (ST elevation myocardial infarction — *see also* — Infarct, myocardium, ST elevation 410.9 ☑
Stenocardia — *see also* Angina 413.9
Stenocephaly 756.0
Stenosis (cicatricial) — *see also* Stricture
ampulla of Vater 576.2
  with calculus, cholelithiasis, or stones — *see* Choledocholithiasis
anus, anal (canal) (sphincter) 569.2
  congenital 751.2
aorta (ascending) 747.22
  arch 747.10
  arteriosclerotic 440.0
  calcified 440.0
aortic (valve) 424.1
  with
    mitral (valve)
      insufficiency or incompetence 396.2
      stenosis or obstruction 396.0
  atypical 396.0
  congenital 746.3
  rheumatic 395.0
    with
      insufficiency, incompetency or regurgitation 395.2
      with mitral (valve) disease 396.8
    mitral (valve)
      disease (stenosis) 396.0

Stenosis — *see also* Stricture — *continued*
aortic — *continued*
  rheumatic — *continued*
    with — *continued*
      mitral — *continued*
        insufficiency or incompetence 396.2
        stenosis or obstruction 396.0
  specified cause, except rheumatic 424.1
  syphilitic 093.22
aqueduct of Sylvius (congenital) 742.3
  with spina bifida (*see also* Spina bifida) 741.0 ☑
  acquired 331.4
artery NEC (*see also* Arteriosclerosis) 447.1
  basilar — *see* Narrowing, artery, basilar
  carotid (common) (internal) — *see* Narrowing, artery, carotid
  celiac 447.4
  cerebral 437.0
    due to
      embolism (*see also* Embolism, brain) 434.1 ☑
      thrombus (*see also* Thrombosis, brain) 434.0 ☑
  extremities 440.20
  precerebral — *see* Narrowing, artery, precerebral
  pulmonary (congenital) 747.3
    acquired 417.8
  renal 440.1
  vertebral — *see* Narrowing, artery, vertebral
bile duct or biliary passage (*see also* Obstruction, biliary) 576.2
  congenital 751.61
bladder neck (acquired) 596.0
  congenital 753.6
brain 348.89
bronchus 519.19
  syphilitic 095.8
cardia (stomach) 537.89
  congenital 750.7
cardiovascular (*see also* Disease, cardiovascular) 429.2
carotid artery — *see* Narrowing, artery, carotid
cervix, cervical (canal) 622.4
  congenital 752.49
  in pregnancy or childbirth 654.6 ☑
    affecting fetus or newborn 763.89
    causing obstructed labor 660.2 ☑
      affecting fetus or newborn 763.1
colon (*see also* Obstruction, intestine) 560.9
  congenital 751.2
colostomy 569.62
common bile duct (*see also* Obstruction, biliary) 576.2
  congenital 751.61
coronary (artery) — *see* Arteriosclerosis, coronary
cystic duct (*see also* Obstruction, gallbladder) 575.2
  congenital 751.61
due to (presence of) any device, implant, or graft classifiable to 996.0–996.5 — *see* Complications, due to (presence of) any device, implant, or graft classified to 996.0–996.5 NEC
duodenum 537.3
  congenital 751.1
ejaculatory duct NEC 608.89
endocervical os — *see* Stenosis, cervix
enterostomy 569.62
esophagostomy 530.87
esophagus 530.3
  congenital 750.3
  syphilitic 095.8
    congenital 090.5
external ear canal 380.50
  secondary to
    inflammation 380.53
    surgery 380.52
    trauma 380.51
gallbladder (*see also* Obstruction, gallbladder) 575.2

Stenosis — *see also* Stricture — *continued*
glottis 478.74
heart valve (acquired) (*see also* Endocarditis)
  congenital NEC 746.89
    aortic 746.3
    mitral 746.5
    pulmonary 746.02
    tricuspid 746.1
hepatic duct (*see also* Obstruction, biliary) 576.2
hymen 623.3
hypertrophic subaortic (idiopathic) 425.1
infundibulum cardiac 746.83
intestine (*see also* Obstruction, intestine) 560.9
  congenital (small) 751.1
    large 751.2
lacrimal
  canaliculi 375.53
  duct 375.56
    congenital 743.65
  punctum 375.52
    congenital 743.65
  sac 375.54
    congenital 743.65
lacrimonasal duct 375.56
  congenital 743.65
  neonatal 375.55
larynx 478.74
  congenital 748.3
  syphilitic 095.8
    congenital 090.5
mitral (valve) (chronic) (inactive) 394.0
  with
    aortic (valve)
      disease (insufficiency) 396.1
      insufficiency or incompetence 396.1
      stenosis or obstruction 396.0
    incompetency, insufficiency or regurgitation 394.2
    with aortic valve disease 396.8
  active or acute 391.1
    with chorea (acute) (rheumatic) (Sydenham's) 392.0
  congenital 746.5
  specified cause, except rheumatic 424.0
  syphilitic 093.21
myocardium, myocardial (*see also* Degeneration, myocardial) 429.1
  hypertrophic subaortic (idiopathic) 425.1
nares (anterior) (posterior) 478.19
  congenital 748.0
nasal duct 375.56
  congenital 743.65
nasolacrimal duct 375.56
  congenital 743.65
  neonatal 375.55
organ or site, congenital NEC — *see* Atresia
papilla of Vater 576.2
  with calculus, cholelithiasis, or stones — *see* Choledocholithiasis
pulmonary (artery) (congenital) 747.3
  with ventricular septal defect, dextraposition of aorta and hypertrophy of right ventricle 745.2
  acquired 417.8
  infundibular 746.83
  in tetralogy of Fallot 745.2
  subvalvular 746.83
  valve (*see also* Endocarditis, pulmonary) 424.3
    congenital 746.02
  vein 747.49
    acquired 417.8
  vessel NEC 417.8
pulmonic (congenital) 746.02
  infundibular 746.83
  subvalvular 746.83
pylorus (hypertrophic) 537.0
  adult 537.0
  congenital 750.5
  infantile 750.5
rectum (sphincter) (*see also* Stricture, rectum) 569.2
renal artery 440.1

Stenosis — *see also* Stricture — *continued*
salivary duct (any) 527.8
sphincter of Oddi (*see also* Obstruction, biliary) 576.2
spinal 724.00
  cervical 723.0
  lumbar, lumbosacral ►(without neurogenic claudication)◄ 724.02
    with neurogenic claudication 724.03 ●
  nerve (root) NEC 724.9
  specified region NEC 724.09
  thoracic, thoracolumbar 724.01
stomach, hourglass 537.6
subaortic 746.81
  hypertrophic (idiopathic) 425.1
supra (valvular)-aortic 747.22
trachea 519.19
  congenital 748.3
  syphilitic 095.8
  tuberculous (*see also* Tuberculosis) 012.8 ☑
tracheostomy 519.02
tricuspid (valve) (*see also* Endocarditis, tricuspid) 397.0
  congenital 746.1
  nonrheumatic 424.2
tubal 628.2
ureter (*see also* Stricture, ureter) 593.3
  congenital 753.29
urethra (*see also* Stricture, urethra) 598.9
vagina 623.2
  congenital 752.49
  in pregnancy or childbirth 654.7 ☑
    affecting fetus or newborn 763.89
    causing obstructed labor 660.2 ☑
      affecting fetus or newborn 763.1
valve (cardiac) (heart) (*see also* Endocarditis) 424.90
  congenital NEC 746.89
    aortic 746.3
    mitral 746.5
    pulmonary 746.02
    tricuspid 746.1
    urethra 753.6
valvular (*see also* Endocarditis) 424.90
  congenital NEC 746.89
    urethra 753.6
vascular graft or shunt 996.1
  atherosclerosis — *see* Arteriosclerosis, extremities
  embolism 996.74
  occlusion NEC 996.74
  thrombus 996.74
vena cava (inferior) (superior) 459.2
  congenital 747.49
ventricular shunt 996.2
vulva 624.8

Stercolith — *see also* Fecalith 560.32 ▲
  appendix 543.9
Stercoraceous, stercoral ulcer 569.82
anus or rectum 569.41
Stereopsis, defective
with fusion 368.33
without fusion 368.32
Stereotypes NEC 307.3
Sterility
female — *see* Infertility, female
male (*see also* Infertility, male) 606.9
Sterilization, admission for V25.2
status
  tubal ligation V26.51
  vasectomy V26.52
Sternalgia — *see also* Angina 413.9
Sternopagus 759.4
Sternum bifidum 756.3
Sternutation 784.99
Steroid
effects (adverse) (iatrogenic)
  cushingoid
    correct substance properly administered 255.0
    overdose or wrong substance given or taken 962.0
  diabetes — *see* Diabetes, secondary

Steroid — *continued*
effects — *continued*
  diabetes — *see* Diabetes, secondary — *continued*
    correct substance properly administered 251.8
    overdose or wrong substance given or taken 962.0
  due to
    correct substance properly administered 255.8
    overdose or wrong substance given or taken 962.0
  fever
    correct substance properly administered 780.60
    overdose or wrong substance given or taken 962.0
  withdrawal
    correct substance properly administered 255.41
    overdose or wrong substance given or taken 962.0
responder 365.03
Stevens-Johnson disease or syndrome (erythema multiforme exudativum) 695.13
toxic epidermal necrolysis overlap (SJS-TEN overlap syndrome) 695.14
Stewart-Morel syndrome (hyperostosis frontalis interna) 733.3
Sticker's disease (erythema infectiosum) 057.0
Stickler syndrome 759.89
Sticky eye 372.03
Stieda's disease (calcification, knee joint) 726.62
Stiff
back 724.8
neck (*see also* Torticollis) 723.5
Stiff-baby 759.89
Stiff-man syndrome 333.91
Stiffness, joint NEC 719.50
ankle 719.57
back 724.8
elbow 719.52
finger 719.54
hip 719.55
knee 719.56
multiple sites 719.59
sacroiliac 724.6
shoulder 719.51
specified site NEC 719.58
spine 724.9
surgical fusion V45.4
wrist 719.53
Stigmata, congenital syphilis 090.5
Stillbirth, stillborn NEC 779.9
Still's disease or syndrome 714.30
adult onset 714.2
Stiller's disease (asthenia) 780.79
Still-Felty syndrome (rheumatoid arthritis with splenomegaly and leukopenia) 714.1
Stilling-Türk-Duane syndrome (ocular retraction syndrome) 378.71
Stimulation, ovary 256.1
Sting (animal) (bee) (fish) (insect) (jellyfish) (Portuguese man-o-war) (wasp) (venomous) 989.5
anaphylactic shock or reaction 989.5
plant 692.6
Stippled epiphyses 756.59
Stitch
abscess 998.59
burst (in external operation wound) (*see also* Dehiscence) 998.32
  internal 998.31
in back 724.5
Stojano's (subcostal) **syndrome** 098.86
Stokes-Adams syndrome (syncope with heart block) 426.9
Stokes' disease (exophthalmic goiter) 242.0 ☑
Stokvis' (-Talma) disease (enterogenous cyanosis) 289.7
Stomach — *see* condition
Stoma malfunction
colostomy 569.62

☑ **Additional Digit Required** — Refer to the Tabular List for Digit Selection   ▽ **Subterms under main terms may continue to next column or page**

262 — Volume 2 · October 2010   ►◄ Revised Text   ● New Line   ▲ Revised Code   2011 ICD-9-CM

Stoma malfunction — *continued*
  cystostomy 997.5
  enterostomy 569.62
  esophagostomy 530.87
  gastrostomy 536.42
  ileostomy 569.62
  nephrostomy 997.5
  tracheostomy 519.02
  ureterostomy 997.5
Stomatitis 528.00
  angular 528.5
    due to dietary or vitamin deficiency
      266.0
  aphthous 528.2
  bovine 059.11
  candidal 112.0
  catarrhal 528.00
  denture 528.9
  diphtheritic (membranous) 032.0
  due to
    dietary deficiency 266.0
    thrush 112.0
    vitamin deficiency 266.0
  epidemic 078.4
  epizootic 078.4
  follicular 528.00
  gangrenous 528.1
  herpetic 054.2
  herpetiformis 528.2
  malignant 528.00
  membranous acute 528.00
  monilial 112.0
  mycotic 112.0
  necrotic 528.1
    ulcerative 101
  necrotizing ulcerative 101
  parasitic 112.0
  septic 528.00
  specified NEC 528.09
  spirochetal 101
  suppurative (acute) 528.00
  ulcerative 528.00
    necrotizing 101
  ulceromembranous 101
  vesicular 528.00
    with exanthem 074.3
  Vincent's 101
Stomatocytosis 282.8
Stomatomycosis 112.0
Stomatorrhagia 528.9
Stone(s) — *see also* Calculus
  bladder 594.1
    diverticulum 594.0
  cystine 270.0
  heart syndrome (*see also* Failure, ventricular,
    left) 428.1
  kidney 592.0
  prostate 602.0
  pulp (dental) 522.2
  renal 592.0
  salivary duct or gland (any) 527.5
  ureter 592.1
  urethra (impacted) 594.2
  urinary (duct) (impacted) (passage) 592.9
    bladder 594.1
      diverticulum 594.0
    lower tract NEC 594.9
    specified site 594.8
  xanthine 277.2
Stonecutters' lung 502
  tuberculous (*see also* Tuberculosis) 011.4 ☑
Stonemasons'
  asthma, disease, or lung 502
    tuberculous (*see also* Tuberculosis)
      011.4 ☑
  phthisis (*see also* Tuberculosis) 011.4 ☑
Stoppage
  bowel (*see also* Obstruction, intestine) 560.9
  heart (*see also* Arrest, cardiac) 427.5
  intestine (*see also* Obstruction, intestine)
    560.9
  urine NEC (*see also* Retention, urine) 788.20
Storm, thyroid (apathetic) — *see also* Thyrotoxicosis 242.9 ☑
Strabismus (alternating) (congenital) (nonparalytic) 378.9

Strabismus — *continued*
  concomitant (*see also* Heterotropia) 378.30
    convergent (*see also* Esotropia) 378.00
    divergent (*see also* Exotropia) 378.10
  convergent (*see also* Esotropia) 378.00
  divergent (*see also* Exotropia) 378.10
  due to adhesions, scars — *see* Strabismus,
    mechanical
  in neuromuscular disorder NEC 378.73
    intermittent 378.20
      vertical 378.31
  latent 378.40
    convergent (esophoria) 378.41
    divergent (exophoria) 378.42
    vertical 378.43
  mechanical 378.60
    due to
      Brown's tendon sheath syndrome
        378.61
      specified musculofascial disorder
        NEC 378.62
  paralytic 378.50
    third or oculomotor nerve (partial)
      378.51
      total 378.52
    fourth or trochlear nerve 378.53
    sixth or abducens nerve 378.54
  specified type NEC 378.73
  vertical (hypertropia) 378.31
Strain — *see also* Sprain, by site
  eye NEC 368.13
  heart — *see* Disease, heart
  meaning gonorrhea — *see* Gonorrhea
  on urination 788.65
  physical NEC V62.89
  postural 729.90
  psychological NEC V62.89
Strands
  conjunctiva 372.62
  vitreous humor 379.25
Strangulation, strangulated 994.7
  appendix 543.9
  asphyxiation or suffocation by 994.7
  bladder neck 596.0
  bowel — *see* Strangulation, intestine
  colon — *see* Strangulation, intestine
  cord (umbilical) — *see* Compression, umbil-
    ical cord
  due to birth injury 767.8
  food or foreign body (*see also* Asphyxia,
    food) 933.1
  hemorrhoids 455.8
    external 455.5
    internal 455.2
  hernia (*see also* Hernia, by site, with obstruc-
    tion)
    gangrenous — *see* Hernia, by site, with
      gangrene
  intestine (large) (small) 560.2
    with hernia (*see also* Hernia, by site, with
      obstruction)
      gangrenous — *see* Hernia, by site,
        with gangrene
    congenital (small) 751.1
    large 751.2
  mesentery 560.2
  mucus (*see also* Asphyxia, mucus) 933.1
    newborn 770.18
  omentum 560.2
  organ or site, congenital NEC — *see* Atresia
  ovary 620.8
    due to hernia 620.4
  penis 607.89
    foreign body 939.3
  rupture (*see also* Hernia, by site, with obstruc-
    tion) 552.9
    gangrenous (*see also* Hernia, by site, with
      gangrene) 551.9
  stomach, due to hernia (*see also* Hernia, by
    site, with obstruction) 552.9
    with gangrene (*see also* Hernia, by site,
      with gangrene) 551.9
  umbilical cord — *see* Compression, umbili-
    cal cord
  vesicourethral orifice 596.0
Strangury 788.1

Strawberry
  gallbladder (*see also* Disease, gallbladder)
    575.6
  mark 757.32
  tongue (red) (white) 529.3
Straw itch 133.8
Streak, ovarian 752.0
Strephosymbolia 315.01
  secondary to organic lesion 784.69
Streptobacillary fever 026.1
Streptobacillus moniliformis 026.1
Streptococcemia 038.0
Streptococcicosis — *see* Infection, streptococ-
  cal
Streptococcus, streptococcal — *see* condition
Streptoderma 686.00
Streptomycosis — *see* Actinomycosis
Streptothricosis — *see* Actinomycosis
Streptothrix — *see* Actinomycosis
Streptotrichosis — *see* Actinomycosis
Stress 308.9
  fracture — *see* Fracture, stress
  polycythemia 289.0
  reaction (gross) (*see also* Reaction, stress,
    acute) 308.9
Stretching, nerve — *see* Injury, nerve, by site
Striae (albicantes) (atrophicae) (cutis distensae)
  (distensae) 701.3
Striations of nails 703.8
Stricture — *see also* Stenosis 799.89
  ampulla of Vater 576.2
    with calculus, cholelithiasis, or stones —
      see Choledocholithiasis
  anus (sphincter) 569.2
    congenital 751.2
    infantile 751.2
  aorta (ascending) 747.22
    arch 747.10
    arteriosclerotic 440.0
    calcified 440.0
  aortic (valve) (*see also* Stenosis, aortic) 424.1
    congenital 746.3
  aqueduct of Sylvius (congenital) 742.3
    with spina bifida (*see also* Spina bifida)
      741.0 ☑
    acquired 331.4
  artery 447.1
    basilar — *see* Narrowing, artery, basilar
    carotid (common) (internal) — *see* Nar-
      rowing, artery, carotid
    celiac 447.4
    cerebral 437.0
      congenital 747.81
      due to
        embolism (*see also* Embolism,
          brain) 434.1 ☑
        thrombus (*see also* Thrombosis,
          brain) 434.0 ☑
    congenital (peripheral) 747.60
      cerebral 747.81
      coronary 746.85
      gastrointestinal 747.61
      lower limb 747.64
      renal 747.62
      retinal 743.58
      specified NEC 747.69
      spinal 747.82
      umbilical 747.5
      upper limb 747.63
    coronary — *see* Arteriosclerosis, coro-
      nary
      congenital 746.85
    precerebral — *see* Narrowing, artery,
      precerebral NEC
    pulmonary (congenital) 747.3
      acquired 417.8
      renal 440.1
    vertebral — *see* Narrowing, artery, verte-
      bral
  auditory canal (congenital) (external) 744.02
    acquired (*see also* Stricture, ear canal,
      acquired) 380.50
  bile duct or passage (any) (postoperative)
    (*see also* Obstruction, biliary) 576.2
    congenital 751.61
  bladder 596.8

Stricture — *see also* Stenosis — *continued*
  bladder — *continued*
    congenital 753.6
    neck 596.0
      congenital 753.6
  bowel (*see also* Obstruction, intestine) 560.9
  brain 348.89
  bronchus 519.19
    syphilitic 095.8
  cardia (stomach) 537.89
    congenital 750.7
  cardiac (*see also* Disease, heart)
    orifice (stomach) 537.89
  cardiovascular (*see also* Disease, cardiovas-
    cular) 429.2
  carotid artery — *see* Narrowing, artery,
    carotid
  cecum (*see also* Obstruction, intestine) 560.9
  cervix, cervical (canal) 622.4
    congenital 752.49
    in pregnancy or childbirth 654.6 ☑
      affecting fetus or newborn 763.89
      causing obstructed labor 660.2 ☑
        affecting fetus or newborn 763.1
  colon (*see also* Obstruction, intestine) 560.9
    congenital 751.2
  colostomy 569.62
  common bile duct (*see also* Obstruction,
    biliary) 576.2
    congenital 751.61
  coronary (artery) — *see* Arteriosclerosis,
    coronary
    congenital 746.85
  cystic duct (*see also* Obstruction, gallblad-
    der) 575.2
    congenital 751.61
  cystostomy 997.5
  digestive organs NEC, congenital 751.8
  duodenum 537.3
    congenital 751.1
  ear canal (external) (congenital) 744.02
    acquired 380.50
      secondary to
        inflammation 380.53
        surgery 380.52
        trauma 380.51
  ejaculatory duct 608.85
  enterostomy 569.62
  esophagostomy 530.87
  esophagus (corrosive) (peptic) 530.3
    congenital 750.3
    syphilitic 095.8
      congenital 090.5
  eustachian tube (*see also* Obstruction, Eu-
    stachian tube) 381.60
    congenital 744.24
  fallopian tube 628.2
    gonococcal (chronic) 098.37
      acute 098.17
    tuberculous (*see also* Tuberculosis)
      016.6 ☑
  gallbladder (*see also* Obstruction, gallblad-
    der) 575.2
    congenital 751.69
  glottis 478.74
  heart (*see also* Disease, heart)
    congenital NEC 746.89
    valve (*see also* Endocarditis)
      congenital NEC 746.89
        aortic 746.3
        mitral 746.5
        pulmonary 746.02
        tricuspid 746.1
  hepatic duct (*see also* Obstruction, biliary)
    576.2
  hourglass, of stomach 537.6
  hymen 623.3
  hypopharynx 478.29
  intestine (*see also* Obstruction, intestine)
    560.9
    congenital (small) 751.1
      large 751.2
    ischemic 557.1
  lacrimal
    canaliculi 375.53
      congenital 743.65

Index

Stricture — Subnormal, subnormality

Stricture — see also Stenosis — continued
- lacrimal — continued
  - punctum 375.52
    - congenital 743.65
  - sac 375.54
    - congenital 743.65
- lacrimonasal duct 375.56
  - congenital 743.65
  - neonatal 375.55
- larynx 478.79
  - congenital 748.3
  - syphilitic 095.8
    - congenital 090.5
- lung 518.89
- meatus
  - ear (congenital) 744.02
    - acquired (see also Stricture, ear canal, acquired) 380.50
  - osseous (congenital) (ear) 744.03
    - acquired (see also Stricture, ear canal, acquired) 380.50
  - urinarius (see also Stricture, urethra) 598.9
    - congenital 753.6
- mitral (valve) (see also Stenosis, mitral) 394.0
  - congenital 746.5
  - specified cause, except rheumatic 424.0
- myocardium, myocardial (see also Degeneration, myocardial) 429.1
  - hypertrophic subaortic (idiopathic) 425.1
- nares (anterior) (posterior) 478.19
  - congenital 748.0
- nasal duct 375.56
  - congenital 743.65
  - neonatal 375.55
- nasolacrimal duct 375.56
  - congenital 743.65
  - neonatal 375.55
- nasopharynx 478.29
  - syphilitic 095.8
- nephrostomy 997.5
- nose 478.19
  - congenital 748.0
- nostril (anterior) (posterior) 478.19
  - congenital 748.0
- organ or site, congenital NEC — see Atresia
- osseous meatus (congenital) (ear) 744.03
  - acquired (see also Stricture, ear canal, acquired) 380.50
- os uteri (see also Stricture, cervix) 622.4
- oviduct — see Stricture, fallopian tube
- pelviureteric junction 593.3
- pharynx (dilation) 478.29
- prostate 602.8
- pulmonary, pulmonic
  - artery (congenital) 747.3
    - acquired 417.8
    - noncongenital 417.8
  - infundibulum (congenital) 746.83
  - valve (see also Endocarditis, pulmonary) 424.3
    - congenital 746.02
  - vein (congenital) 747.49
    - acquired 417.8
  - vessel NEC 417.8
- punctum lacrimale 375.52
  - congenital 743.65
- pylorus (hypertrophic) 537.0
  - adult 537.0
  - congenital 750.5
  - infantile 750.5
- rectosigmoid 569.89
- rectum (sphincter) 569.2
  - congenital 751.2
  - due to
    - chemical burn 947.3
    - irradiation 569.2
    - lymphogranuloma venereum 099.1
  - gonococcal 098.7
  - inflammatory 099.1
  - syphilitic 095.8
  - tuberculous (see also Tuberculosis) 014.8 ☑
- renal artery 440.1
- salivary duct or gland (any) 527.8

Stricture — see also Stenosis — continued
- sigmoid (flexure) (see also Obstruction, intestine) 560.9
- spermatic cord 608.85
- stoma (following) (of)
  - colostomy 569.62
  - cystostomy 997.5
  - enterostomy 569.62
  - esophagostomy 530.87
  - gastrostomy 536.42
  - ileostomy 569.62
  - nephrostomy 997.5
  - tracheostomy 519.02
  - ureterostomy 997.5
- stomach 537.89
  - congenital 750.7
  - hourglass 537.6
- subaortic 746.81
  - hypertrophic (acquired) (idiopathic) 425.1
- subglottic 478.74
- syphilitic NEC 095.8
- tendon (sheath) 727.81
- trachea 519.19
  - congenital 748.3
  - syphilitic 095.8
  - tuberculous (see also Tuberculosis) 012.8 ☑
- tracheostomy 519.02
- tricuspid (valve) (see also Endocarditis, tricuspid) 397.0
  - congenital 746.1
  - nonrheumatic 424.2
- tunica vaginalis 608.85
- ureter (postoperative) 593.3
  - congenital 753.29
  - tuberculous (see also Tuberculosis) 016.2 ☑
- ureteropelvic junction 593.3
  - congenital 753.21
- ureterovesical orifice 593.3
  - congenital 753.22
- urethra (anterior) (meatal) (organic) (posterior) (spasmodic) 598.9
  - associated with schistosomiasis (see also Schistosomiasis) 120.9 [598.01]
  - congenital (valvular) 753.6
  - due to
    - infection 598.00
      - syphilis 095.8 [598.01]
    - trauma 598.1
  - gonococcal 098.2 [598.01]
  - gonorrheal 098.2 [598.01]
  - infective 598.00
  - late effect of injury 598.1
  - postcatheterization 598.2
  - postobstetric 598.1
  - postoperative 598.2
  - specified cause NEC 598.8
  - syphilitic 095.8 [598.01]
  - traumatic 598.1
  - valvular, congenital 753.6
- urinary meatus (see also Stricture, urethra) 598.9
  - congenital 753.6
- uterus, uterine 621.5
  - os (external) (internal) — see Stricture, cervix
- vagina (outlet) 623.2
  - congenital 752.49
- valve (cardiac) (heart) (see also Endocarditis) 424.90
  - congenital (cardiac) (heart) NEC 746.89
    - aortic 746.3
    - mitral 746.5
    - pulmonary 746.02
    - tricuspid 746.1
    - urethra 753.6
- valvular (see also Endocarditis) 424.90
- vascular graft or shunt 996.1
  - atherosclerosis — see Arteriosclerosis, extremities
  - embolism 996.74
  - occlusion NEC 996.74
  - thrombus 996.74
- vas deferens 608.85

Stricture — see also Stenosis — continued
- vas deferens — continued
  - congenital 752.89
  - vein 459.2
  - vena cava (inferior) (superior) NEC 459.2
    - congenital 747.49
  - ventricular shunt 996.2
  - vesicourethral orifice 596.0
    - congenital 753.6
  - vulva (acquired) 624.8
- **Stridor** 786.1
  - congenital (larynx) 748.3
- **Stridulous** — see condition
- **Strippling of nails** 703.8
- **Stroke** 434.91
  - apoplectic (see also Disease, cerebrovascular, acute) 436
  - brain — see Infarct, brain
  - embolic 434.11
  - epileptic — see Epilepsy
  - healed or old V12.54
  - heart — see Disease, heart
  - heat 992.0
  - hemorrhagic — see Hemorrhage, brain
  - iatrogenic 997.02
  - in evolution 434.91
  - ischemic 434.91
  - late effect — see Late effect(s) (of) cerebrovascular disease
  - lightning 994.0
  - paralytic — see Infarct, brain
  - postoperative 997.02
  - progressive 435.9
  - thrombotic 434.01
- **Stromatosis, endometrial** (M8931/1) 236.0
- **Strong pulse** 785.9
- **Strongyloides stercoralis infestation** 127.2
- **Strongyloidiasis** 127.2
- **Strongyloidosis** 127.2
- **Strongylus** (gibsoni) infestation 127.7
- **Strophulus** (newborn) 779.89
  - pruriginosus 698.2
- **Struck by lightning** 994.0
- **Struma** — see also Goiter 240.9
  - fibrosa 245.3
  - Hashimoto (struma lymphomatosa) 245.2
  - lymphomatosa 245.2
  - nodosa (simplex) 241.9
    - endemic 241.9
    - multinodular 241.1
    - sporadic 241.9
    - toxic or with hyperthyroidism 242.3 ☑
      - multinodular 242.2 ☑
      - uninodular 242.1 ☑
    - toxicosa 242.3 ☑
      - multinodular 242.2 ☑
      - uninodular 242.1 ☑
    - uninodular 241.0
  - ovarii (M9090/0) 220
    - and carcinoid (M9091/1) 236.2
    - malignant (M9090/3) 183.0
  - Riedel's (ligneous thyroiditis) 245.3
  - scrofulous (see also Tuberculosis) 017.2 ☑
  - tuberculous (see also Tuberculosis) 017.2 ☑
    - abscess 017.2 ☑
    - adenitis 017.2 ☑
    - lymphangitis 017.2 ☑
    - ulcer 017.2 ☑
- **Strumipriva cachexia** — see also Hypothyroidism 244.9
- **Strümpell-Marie disease or spine** (ankylosing spondylitis) 720.0
- **Strümpell-Westphal pseudosclerosis** (hepatolenticular degeneration) 275.1
- **Stuart's disease** (congenital factor X deficiency) — see also Defect, coagulation 286.3
- **Stuart-Prower factor deficiency** (congenital factor X deficiency) — see also Defect, coagulation 286.3
- **Students' elbow** 727.2
- **Stuffy nose** 478.19
- **Stump** — see also Amputation
  - cervix, cervical (healed) 622.8
- **Stupor** 780.09
  - catatonic (see also Schizophrenia) 295.2 ☑

Stupor — continued
- circular (see also Psychosis, manic-depressive, circular) 296.7
  - manic 296.89
  - manic-depressive (see also Psychosis, affective) 296.89
  - mental (anergic) (delusional) 298.9
  - psychogenic 298.8
  - reaction to exceptional stress (transient) 308.2
  - traumatic NEC (see also Injury, intracranial)
    - with spinal (cord)
      - lesion — see Injury, spinal, by site
      - shock — see Injury, spinal, by site
- **Sturge (-Weber) (-Dimitri) disease or syndrome** (encephalocutaneous angiomatosis) 759.6
- **Sturge-Kalischer-Weber syndrome** (encephalocutaneous angiomatosis) 759.6
- **Stuttering** 315.35   ▲
  - adult onset 307.0   ●
  - childhood onset 315.35   ●
  - due to late effect of cerebrovascular disease (see also Late effect(s) (of) cerebrovascular disease) 438.14
  - in conditions classified elsewhere 784.52 ●
- **Sty, stye** 373.11
  - external 373.11
  - internal 373.12
  - meibomian 373.12
- **Subacidity, gastric** 536.8
  - psychogenic 306.4
- **Subacute** — see condition
- **Subarachnoid** — see condition
- **Subclavian steal syndrome** 435.2
- **Subcortical** — see condition
- **Subcostal syndrome** 098.86
  - nerve compression 354.8
- **Subcutaneous, subcuticular** — see condition
- **Subdelirium** 293.1
- **Subdural** — see condition
- **Subendocardium** — see condition
- **Subependymoma** (M9383/1) 237.5
- **Suberosis** 495.3
- **Subglossitis** — see Glossitis
- **Subhemophilia** 286.0
- **Subinvolution** (uterus) 621.1
  - breast (postlactational) (postpartum) 611.89
  - chronic 621.1
  - puerperal, postpartum 674.8 ☑
- **Sublingual** — see condition
- **Sublinguitis** 527.2
- **Subluxation** — see also Dislocation, by site
  - congenital NEC (see also Malposition, congenital)
    - hip (unilateral) 754.32
      - with dislocation of other hip 754.35
      - bilateral 754.33
    - joint
      - lower limb 755.69
      - shoulder 755.59
      - upper limb 755.59
    - lower limb (joint) 755.69
    - shoulder (joint) 755.59
    - upper limb (joint) 755.59
  - lens 379.32
    - anterior 379.33
    - posterior 379.34
  - radial head 832.2
  - rotary, cervical region of spine — see Fracture, vertebra, cervical
- **Submaxillary** — see condition
- **Submersion** (fatal) (nonfatal) 994.1
- **Submissiveness** (undue), in child 313.0
- **Submucous** — see condition
- **Subnormal, subnormality**
  - accommodation (see also Disorder, accommodation) 367.9
  - mental (see also Retardation, mental) 319
    - mild 317
    - moderate 318.0
    - profound 318.2
    - severe 318.1
  - temperature (accidental) 991.6
    - not associated with low environmental temperature 780.99

Subphrenic — *see* condition

Subscapular nerve — *see* condition

Subseptus uterus 752.35 ▲

Subsiding appendicitis 542

Substance abuse in family V61.42

Substernal thyroid — *see also* Goiter 240.9
  congenital 759.2

Substitution disorder 300.11

Subtentorial — *see* condition

Subtertian
  fever 084.0
  malaria (fever) 084.0

Subthyroidism (acquired) — *see also* Hypothyroidism 244.9
  congenital 243

Succenturiata placenta — *see* Placenta, abnormal

Succussion sounds, chest 786.7

Sucking thumb, child 307.9

Sudamen 705.1

Sudamina 705.1

Sudanese kala-azar 085.0

Sudden
  death, cause unknown (less than 24 hours) 798.1
    cardiac (SCD)
      family history of V17.41
      personal history of, successfully resuscitated V12.53
    during childbirth 669.9 ☑
    infant 798.0
    puerperal, postpartum 674.9 ☑
  hearing loss NEC 388.2
  heart failure (*see also* Failure, heart) 428.9
  infant death syndrome 798.0

Sudeck's atrophy, disease, or syndrome 733.7

SUDS (sudden unexplained death) 798.2

Suffocation — *see also* Asphyxia 799.01
  by
    bed clothes 994.7
    bunny bag 994.7
    cave-in 994.7
    constriction 994.7
    drowning 994.1
    inhalation
      food or foreign body (*see also* Asphyxia, food or foreign body) 933.1
      oil or gasoline (*see also* Asphyxia, food or foreign body) 933.1
    overlying 994.7
    plastic bag 994.7
    pressure 994.7
    strangulation 994.7
  during birth 768.1
  mechanical 994.7

Sugar
  blood
    high 790.29
    low 251.2
  in urine 791.5

Suicide, suicidal (attempted)
  by poisoning — *see* Table of Drugs and Chemicals
  ideation V62.84
  risk 300.9
  tendencies 300.9
  trauma NEC (*see also* nature and site of injury) 959.9

Suipestifer infection — *see also* Infection, Salmonella 003.9

Sulfatidosis 330.0

Sulfhemoglobinemia, sulphemoglobinemia (acquired) (congenital) 289.7

Sumatran mite fever 081.2

Summer — *see* condition

Sunburn 692.71
  first degree 692.71
  second degree 692.76
  third degree 692.77
  dermatitis 692.71
  due to
    other ultraviolet radiation 692.82
    tanning bed 692.82

SUNCT (short lasting unilateral neuralgiform headache with conjunctival injection and tearing) 339.05

Sunken
  acetabulum 718.85
  fontanels 756.0

Sunstroke 992.0

Superfecundation 651.9 ☑
  with fetal loss and retention of one or more fetus(es) 651.6 ☑
  following (elective) fetal reduction 651.7 ☑

Superfetation 651.9 ☑
  with fetal loss and retention of one or more fetus(es) 651.6 ☑
  following (elective) fetal reduction 651.7 ☑

Superinvolution uterus 621.8

Supernumerary (congenital)
  aortic cusps 746.89
  auditory ossicles 744.04
  bone 756.9
  breast 757.6
  carpal bones 755.56
  cusps, heart valve NEC 746.89
    mitral 746.5
    pulmonary 746.09
  digit(s) 755.00
    finger 755.01
    toe 755.02
  ear (lobule) 744.1
  fallopian tube 752.19
  finger 755.01
  hymen 752.49
  kidney 753.3
  lacrimal glands 743.64
  lacrimonasal duct 743.65
  lobule (ear) 744.1
  mitral cusps 746.5
  muscle 756.82
  nipples 757.6
  organ or site NEC — *see* Accessory
  ossicles, auditory 744.04
  ovary 752.0
  oviduct 752.19
  pulmonic cusps 746.09
  rib 756.3
    cervical or first 756.2
      syndrome 756.2
  roots (of teeth) 520.2
  spinal vertebra 756.19
  spleen 759.0
  tarsal bones 755.67
  teeth 520.1
    causing crowding 524.31
  testis 752.89
  thumb 755.01
  toe 755.02
  uterus 752.2
  vagina 752.49
  vertebra 756.19

Supervision (of)
  contraceptive method previously prescribed V25.40
    intrauterine device V25.42
    oral contraceptive (pill) V25.41
    specified type NEC V25.49
    subdermal implantable contraceptive V25.43
  dietary (for) V65.3
    allergy (food) V65.3
    colitis V65.3
    diabetes mellitus V65.3
    food allergy intolerance V65.3
    gastritis V65.3
    hypercholesterolemia V65.3
    hypoglycemia V65.3
    intolerance (food) V65.3
    obesity V65.3
    specified NEC V65.3
  lactation V24.1
  newborn health
    8 to 28 days old V20.32
    under 8 days old V20.31
  pregnancy — *see* Pregnancy, supervision of

Supplemental teeth 520.1
  causing crowding 524.31

Suppression
  binocular vision 368.31
  lactation 676.5 ☑
  menstruation 626.8
  ovarian secretion 256.39
  renal 586
  urinary secretion 788.5
  urine 788.5

Suppuration, suppurative — *see also* condition
  accessory sinus (chronic) (*see also* Sinusitis) 473.9
  adrenal gland 255.8
  antrum (chronic) (*see also* Sinusitis, maxillary) 473.0
  bladder (*see also* Cystitis) 595.89
  bowel 569.89
  brain 324.0
    late effect 326
  breast 611.0
    puerperal, postpartum 675.1 ☑
  dental periosteum 526.5
  diffuse (skin) 686.00
  ear (middle) (*see also* Otitis media) 382.4
    external (*see also* Otitis, externa) 380.10
    Internal 386.33
  ethmoidal (sinus) (chronic) (*see also* Sinusitis, ethmoidal) 473.2
  fallopian tube (*see also* Salpingo-oophoritis) 614.2
  frontal (sinus) (chronic) (*see also* Sinusitis, frontal) 473.1
  gallbladder (*see also* Cholecystitis, acute) 575.0
  gum 523.30
  hernial sac — *see* Hernia, by site
  intestine 569.89
  joint (*see also* Arthritis, suppurative) 711.0 ☑
  labyrinthine 386.33
  lung 513.0
  mammary gland 611.0
    puerperal, postpartum 675.1 ☑
  maxilla, maxillary 526.4
    sinus (chronic) (*see also* Sinusitis, maxillary) 473.0
  muscle 728.0
  nasal sinus (chronic) (*see also* Sinusitis) 473.9
  pancreas 577.0
  parotid gland 527.2
  pelvis, pelvic
    female (*see also* Disease, pelvis, inflammatory) 614.4
      acute 614.3
    male (*see also* Peritonitis) 567.21
  pericranial (*see also* Osteomyelitis) 730.2 ☑
  salivary duct or gland (any) 527.2
  sinus (nasal) (*see also* Sinusitis) 473.9
  sphenoidal (sinus) (chronic) (*see also* Sinusitis, sphenoidal) 473.3
  thymus (gland) 254.1
  thyroid (gland) 245.0
  tonsil 474.8
  uterus (*see also* Endometritis) 615.9
  vagina 616.10
  wound (*see also* Wound, open, by site, complicated)
    dislocation — *see* Dislocation, by site, compound
    fracture — *see* Fracture, by site, open
    scratch or other superficial injury — *see* Injury, superficial, by site

Supraeruption, teeth 524.34

Supraglottitis 464.50
  with obstruction 464.51

Suprapubic drainage 596.8

Suprarenal (gland) — *see* condition

Suprascapular nerve — *see* condition

Suprasellar — *see* condition

Supraspinatus syndrome 726.10

Surfer knots 919.8
  infected 919.9

Surgery
  cosmetic NEC V50.1
    breast reconstruction following mastectomy V51.0

Surgery — *continued*
  cosmetic — *continued*
    following healed injury or operation V51.8
    hair transplant V50.0
    elective V50.9
      breast
        augmentation or reduction V50.1
        reconstruction following mastectomy V51.0
      circumcision, ritual or routine (in absence of medical indication) V50.2
      cosmetic NEC V50.1
      ear piercing V50.3
      face-lift V50.1
      following healed injury or operation V51.8
      hair transplant V50.0
    not done because of
      contraindication V64.1
      patient's decision V64.2
      specified reason NEC V64.3
    plastic
      breast
        augmentation or reduction V50.1
        reconstruction following mastectomy V51.0
        cosmetic V50.1
      face-lift V50.1
      following healed injury or operation V51.8
      repair of scarred tissue (following healed injury or operation) V51.8
      specified type NEC V50.8
    previous, in pregnancy and childbirth
      cervix 654.6 ☑
        affecting fetus or newborn (*see also* Newborn, affected by) 760.63
        causing obstructed labor 660.2 ☑
          affecting fetus or newborn 763.1
      pelvic soft tissues NEC 654.9 ☑
        affecting fetus or newborn (*see also* Newborn, affected by) 760.63
        causing obstructed labor 660.2 ☑
          affecting fetus or newborn 763.1
      perineum or vulva 654.8 ☑
      uterus NEC 654.9 ☑
        affecting fetus or newborn (*see also* Newborn, affected by) 760.63
        causing obstructed labor 660.2 ☑
          affecting fetus or newborn 763.1
        due to previous cesarean delivery 654.2 ☑
      vagina 654.7 ☑

Surgical
  abortion — *see* Abortion, legal
  emphysema 998.81
  kidney (*see also* Pyelitis) 590.80
  operation NEC 799.9
  procedures, complication or misadventure — *see* Complications, surgical procedure
  shock 998.0

Survey
  fetal anatomic V28.81

Susceptibility
  genetic
    to
      MEN (multiple endocrine neoplasia) V84.81
      neoplasia
        multiple endocrine (MEN) V84.81
      neoplasm
        malignant, of
          breast V84.01
          endometrium V84.04
          other V84.09
          ovary V84.02
          prostate V84.03
        specified disease V84.89

Suspected condition, ruled out — *see also* Observation, suspected V71.9
  specified condition NEC V71.89

Suspended uterus, in pregnancy or childbirth 654.4 ☑

☑ **Additional Digit Required** — Refer to the Tabular List for Digit Selection   ⌖ **Subterms under main terms may continue to next column or page**

2011 ICD-9-CM   ▶◀ Revised Text   ● New Line   ▲ Revised Code   **October 2010 · Volume 2 — 265**

Suspended uterus, in pregnancy or childbirth — *continued*
- affecting fetus or newborn 763.89
- causing obstructed labor 660.2 ☑
  - affecting fetus or newborn 763.1

Sutton and Gull's disease (arteriolar nephrosclerosis) — *see also* Hypertension, kidney 403.90

Sutton's disease 709.09

Suture
- burst (in external operation wound) (*see also* Dehiscence) 998.32
  - internal 998.31
- inadvertently left in operation wound 998.4
- removal V58.32
- Shirodkar, in pregnancy (with or without cervical incompetence) 654.5 ☑

Swab inadvertently left in operation wound 998.4

Swallowed, swallowing
- difficulty (*see also* Dysphagia) 787.20
- foreign body NEC (*see also* Foreign body) 938

Swamp fever 100.89

Swan neck hand (intrinsic) 736.09

Sweat(s), sweating
- disease or sickness 078.2
- excessive (*see also* Hyperhidrosis) 780.8
- fetid 705.89
- fever 078.2
- gland disease 705.9
  - specified type NEC 705.89
- miliary 078.2
- night 780.8

Sweeley-Klionsky disease (angiokeratoma corporis diffusum) 272.7

Sweet's syndrome (acute febrile neutrophilic dermatosis) 695.89

Swelling 782.3
- abdominal (not referable to specific organ) 789.3 ☑
- adrenal gland, cloudy 255.8
- ankle 719.07
- anus 787.99
- arm 729.81
- breast 611.72
- Calabar 125.2
- cervical gland 785.6
- cheek 784.2
- chest 786.6
- ear 388.8
- epigastric 789.3 ☑
- extremity (lower) (upper) 729.81
- eye 379.92
- female genital organ 625.8
- finger 729.81
- foot 729.81
- glands 785.6
- gum 784.2
- hand 729.81
- head 784.2
- inflammatory — *see* Inflammation
- joint (*see also* Effusion, joint) 719.0 ☑
  - tuberculous — *see* Tuberculosis, joint
- kidney, cloudy 593.89
- leg 729.81
- limb 729.81
- liver 573.8
- lung 786.6
- lymph nodes 785.6
- mediastinal 786.6
- mouth 784.2
- muscle (limb) 729.81
- neck 784.2
- nose or sinus 784.2
- palate 784.2
- pelvis 789.3 ☑
- penis 607.83
- perineum 625.8
- rectum 787.99
- scrotum 608.86
- skin 782.2
- splenic (*see also* Splenomegaly) 789.2
- substernal 786.6
- superficial, localized (skin) 782.2
- testicle 608.86

Swelling — *continued*
- throat 784.2
- toe 729.81
- tongue 784.2
- tubular (*see also* Disease, renal) 593.9
- umbilicus 789.3 ☑
- uterus 625.8
- vagina 625.8
- vulva 625.8
- wandering, due to Gnathostoma (spinigerum) 128.1
- white — *see* Tuberculosis, arthritis

Swift's disease 985.0

Swimmers'
- ear (acute) 380.12
- itch 120.3

Swimming in the head 780.4

Swollen — *see also* Swelling
- glands 785.6

Swyer-James syndrome (unilateral hyperlucent lung) 492.8

Swyer's syndrome (XY pure gonadal dysgenesis) 752.7

Sycosis 704.8
- barbae (not parasitic) 704.8
- contagiosa 110.0
- lupoid 704.8
- mycotic 110.0
- parasitic 110.0
- vulgaris 704.8

Sydenham's chorea — *see* Chorea, Sydenham's

Sylvatic yellow fever 060.0

Sylvest's disease (epidemic pleurodynia) 074.1

Symblepharon 372.63
- congenital 743.62

Symonds' syndrome 348.2

Sympathetic — *see* condition

Sympatheticotonia — *see also* Neuropathy, peripheral, autonomic 337.9

Sympathicoblastoma (M9500/3)
- specified site — *see* Neoplasm, by site, malignant
- unspecified site 194.0

Sympathicogonioma (M9500/3) — *see* Sympathicoblastoma

Sympathoblastoma (M9500/3) — *see* Sympathicoblastoma

Sympathogonioma (M9500/3) — *see* Sympathicoblastoma

Symphalangy — *see also* Syndactylism 755.10

Symptoms, specified (general) NEC 780.99
- abdomen NEC 789.9
- bone NEC 733.90
- breast NEC 611.79
- cardiac NEC 785.9
- cardiovascular NEC 785.9
- chest NEC 786.9
- cognition 799.59 ●
- development NEC 783.9
- digestive system NEC 787.99
- emotional state NEC 799.29
- eye NEC 379.99
- gastrointestinal tract NEC 787.99
- genital organs NEC
  - female 625.9
  - male 608.9
- head and neck NEC 784.99
- heart NEC 785.9
- jaw 784.92 ●
- joint NEC 719.60
  - ankle 719.67
  - elbow 719.62
  - foot 719.67
  - hand 719.64
  - hip 719.65
  - knee 719.66
  - multiple sites 719.69
  - pelvic region 719.65
  - shoulder (region) 719.61
  - specified site NEC 719.68
  - temporomandibular 524.69 ●
  - wrist 719.63
- larynx NEC 784.99
- limbs NEC 729.89
- lymphatic system NEC 785.9

Symptoms, specified — *continued*
- maxilla 784.92 ●
- menopausal 627.2
- metabolism NEC 783.9
- mouth NEC 528.9
- muscle NEC 728.9
- musculoskeletal NEC 781.99
  - limbs NEC 729.89
- nervous system NEC 781.99
- neurotic NEC 300.9
- nutrition, metabolism, and development NEC 783.9
- pelvis NEC 789.9
  - female 625.9
- peritoneum NEC 789.9
- respiratory system NEC 786.9
- skin and integument NEC 782.9
- subcutaneous tissue NEC 782.9
- throat NEC 784.9
- tonsil NEC 784.99
- urinary system NEC 788.99
- vascular NEC 785.9

Sympus 759.89

Synarthrosis 719.80
- ankle 719.87
- elbow 719.82
- foot 719.87
- hand 719.84
- hip 719.85
- knee 719.86
- multiple sites 719.89
- pelvic region 719.85
- shoulder (region) 719.81
- specified site NEC 719.88
- wrist 719.83

Syncephalus 759.4

Synchondrosis 756.9
- abnormal (congenital) 756.9
- ischiopubic (van Neck's) 732.1

Synchysis (senile) (vitreous humor) 379.21
- scintillans 379.22

Syncope (near) (pre-) 780.2
- anginosa 413.9
- bradycardia 427.89
- cardiac 780.2
- carotid sinus 337.01
- complicating delivery 669.2 ☑
- due to lumbar puncture 349.0
- fatal 798.1
- heart 780.2
- heat 992.1
- laryngeal 786.2
- tussive 786.2
- vasoconstriction 780.2
- vasodepressor 780.2
- vasomotor 780.2
- vasovagal 780.2

Syncytial infarct — *see* Placenta, abnormal

Syndactylism, syndactyly (multiple sites) 755.10
- fingers (without fusion of bone) 755.11
  - with fusion of bone 755.12
- toes (without fusion of bone) 755.13
  - with fusion of bone 755.14

Syndrome — *see also* Disease
- with 5q deletion 238.74
- 5q minus 238.74
- abdominal
  - acute 789.0 ☑
  - migraine 346.2 ☑
  - muscle deficiency 756.79
- Abercrombie's (amyloid degeneration) 277.39
- abnormal innervation 374.43
- abstinence
  - alcohol 291.81
  - drug 292.0
  - neonatal 779.5
- Abt-Letterer-Siwe (acute histiocytosis X) (M9722/3) 202.5 ☑
- Achard-Thiers (adrenogenital) 255.2
- acid pulmonary aspiration 997.39
  - obstetric (Mendelson's) 668.0 ☑
- acquired immune deficiency 042
- acquired immunodeficiency 042
- acrocephalosyndactylism 755.55

Syndrome — *see also* Disease — *continued*
- acute abdominal 789.0 ☑
- acute chest 517.3
- acute coronary 411.1
- Adair-Dighton (brittle bones and blue sclera, deafness) 756.51
- Adams-Stokes (-Morgagni) (syncope with heart block) 426.9
- Addisonian 255.41
- Adie (-Holmes) (pupil) 379.46
- adiposogenital 253.8
- adrenal
  - hemorrhage 036.3
  - meningococcic 036.3
- adrenocortical 255.3
- adrenogenital (acquired) (congenital) 255.2
  - feminizing 255.2
  - iatrogenic 760.79
  - virilism (acquired) (congenital) 255.2
- affective organic NEC 293.89
  - drug-induced 292.84
- afferent loop NEC 537.89
- African macroglobulinemia 273.3
- Ahumada-Del Castillo (nonpuerperal galactorrhea and amenorrhea) 253.1
- air blast concussion — *see* Injury, internal, by site
- Alagille 759.89
- Albright (-Martin) (pseudohypoparathyroidism) 275.49
- Albright-McCune-Sternberg (osteitis fibrosa disseminata) 756.59
- alcohol withdrawal 291.81
- Alder's (leukocyte granulation anomaly) 288.2
- Aldrich (-Wiskott) (eczema-thrombocytopenia) 279.12
- Alibert-Bazin (mycosis fungoides) (M9700/3) 202.1 ☑
- Alice in Wonderland 293.89
- alien hand 781.8
- Allen-Masters 620.6
- Alligator baby (ichthyosis congenita) 757.1
- Alport's (hereditary hematuria-nephropathy-deafness) 759.89
- Alvarez (transient cerebral ischemia) 435.9
- alveolar capillary block 516.3
- Alzheimer's 331.0
  - with dementia — *see* Alzheimer's, dementia
- amnestic (confabulatory) 294.0
  - alcohol-induced persisting 291.1
  - drug-induced 292.83
  - posttraumatic 294.0
- amotivational 292.89
- amyostatic 275.1
- amyotrophic lateral sclerosis 335.20
- androgen insensitivity 259.51
  - partial 259.52
- Angelman 759.89
- angina (*see also* Angina) 413.9
- ankyloglossia superior 750.0
- anterior
  - chest wall 786.52
  - compartment (tibial) 958.8
  - spinal artery 433.8 ☑
    - compression 721.1
  - tibial (compartment) 958.8
- antibody deficiency 279.00
  - agammaglobulinemic 279.00
  - congenital 279.04
  - hypogammaglobulinemic 279.00
- anticardiolipin antibody 289.81
- antimongolism 758.39
- antiphospholipid antibody 289.81
- Anton (-Babinski) (hemiasomatognosia) 307.9
- anxiety (*see also* Anxiety) 300.00
  - organic 293.84
- aortic
  - arch 446.7
  - bifurcation (occlusion) 444.0
  - ring 747.21
- Apert's (acrocephalosyndactyly) 755.55
- Apert-Gallais (adrenogenital) 255.2
- aphasia-apraxia-alexia 784.69

Syndrome — Syndrome

Syndrome — *see also* Disease — *continued*
apical ballooning 429.83
"approximate answers" 300.16
arcuate ligament (-celiac axis) 447.4
arcus aortae 446.7
arc welders' 370.24
argentaffin, argintaffinoma 259.2
Argonz-Del Castillo (nonpuerperal galactor-
    rhea and amenorrhea) 253.1
Argyll Robertson's (syphilitic) 094.89
    nonsyphilitic 379.45
Armenian 277.31
arm-shoulder (*see also* Neuropathy, periph-
    eral, autonomic) 337.9
Arnold-Chiari (*see also* Spina bifida) 741.0 ☑
    type I 348.4
    type II 741.0 ☑
    type III 742.0
    type IV 742.2
Arrillaga-Ayerza (pulmonary artery sclerosis
    with pulmonary hypertension) 416.0
arteriomesenteric duodenum occlusion
    537.89
arteriovenous steal 996.73
arteritis, young female (obliterative brachio-
    cephalic) 446.7
aseptic meningitis — *see* Meningitis, aseptic
Asherman's 621.5
Asperger's 299.8 ☑
asphyctic (*see also* Anxiety) 300.00
aspiration, of newborn (massive) 770.18
    meconium 770.12
ataxia-telangiectasia 334.8
Audry's (acropachyderma) 757.39
auriculotemporal 350.8
autoimmune lymphoproliferative (ALPS)
    279.41
autosomal (*see also* Abnormal, autosomes
    NEC)
    deletion 758.39
        5p 758.31
        22q11.2 758.32
Avellis' 344.89
Axenfeld's 743.44
Ayerza (-Arrillaga) (pulmonary artery sclero-
    sis with pulmonary hypertension)
    416.0
Baader's (erythema multiforme exudativum)
    695.19
Baastrup's 721.5
Babinski (-Vaquez) (cardiovascular syphilis)
    093.89
Babinski-Fröhlich (adiposogenital dystro-
    phy) 253.8
Babinski-Nageotte 344.89
Bagratuni's (temporal arteritis) 446.5
Bakwin-Krida (craniometaphyseal dysplasia)
    756.89
Balint's (psychic paralysis of visual disorien-
    tation) 368.16
Ballantyne (-Runge) (postmaturity) 766.22
ballooning posterior leaflet 424.0
Banti's — *see* Cirrhosis, liver
Bardet-Biedl (obesity, polydactyly, and
    mental retardation) 759.89
Bard-Pic's (carcinoma, head of pancreas)
    157.0
Barlow (-Möller) (infantile scurvy) 267
Barlow's (mitral valve prolapse) 424.0
Baron Munchausen's 301.51
Barré-Guillain 357.0
Barré-Liéou (posterior cervical sympathetic)
    723.2
Barrett's (chronic peptic ulcer of esophagus)
    530.85
Bársony-Polgár (corkscrew esophagus)
    530.5
Bársony-Teschendorf (corkscrew esophagus)
    530.5
Barth 759.89
Bartter's (secondary hyperaldosteronism
    with juxtaglomerular hyperplasia)
    255.13
basal cell nevus 759.89
Basedow's (exophthalmic goiter) 242.0 ☑
basilar artery 435.0

Syndrome — *see also* Disease — *continued*
basofrontal 377.04
Bassen-Kornzweig (abetalipoproteinemia)
    272.5
Batten-Steinert 359.21
battered
    adult 995.81
    baby or child 995.54
    spouse 995.81
Baumgarten-Cruveilhier (cirrhosis of liver)
    571.5
Beals 759.82
Bearn-Kunkel (-Slater) (lupoid hepatitis)
    571.49
Beau's (*see also* Degeneration, myocardial)
    429.1
Bechterew-Strümpell-Marie (ankylosing
    spondylitis) 720.0
Beck's (anterior spinal artery occlusion)
    433.8 ☑
Beckwith (-Wiedemann) 759.89
Behçet's 136.1
Bekhterev-Strümpell-Marie (ankylosing
    spondylitis) 720.0
Benedikt's 344.89
Béquez César (-Steinbrinck-Chédiak-Higashi)
    (congenital gigantism of peroxidase
    granules) 288.2
Bernard-Horner (*see also* Neuropathy, periph-
    eral, autonomic) 337.9
Bernard-Sergent (acute adrenocortical insuf-
    ficiency) 255.41
Bernhardt-Roth 355.1
Bernheim's (*see also* Failure, heart) 428.0
Bertolotti's (sacralization of fifth lumbar
    vertebra) 756.15
Besnier-Boeck-Schaumann (sarcoidosis) 135
Bianchi's (aphasia-apraxia-alexia syndrome)
    784.69
Biedl-Bardet (obesity, polydactyly, and
    mental retardation) 759.89
Biemond's (obesity, polydactyly, and mental
    retardation) 759.89
big spleen 289.4
bilateral polycystic ovarian 256.4
Bing-Horton's 339.00
Biörck (-Thorson) (malignant carcinoid)
    259.2
Birt-Hogg-Dube 759.89
Blackfan-Diamond (congenital hypoplastic
    anemia) 284.01
black lung 500
black widow spider bite 989.5
bladder neck (*see also* Incontinence, urine)
    788.30
blast (concussion) — *see* Blast, injury
blind loop (postoperative) 579.2
Bloch-Siemens (incontinentia pigmenti)
    757.33
Bloch-Sulzberger (incontinentia pigmenti)
    757.33
Bloom (-Machacek) (-Torre) 757.39
Blount-Barber (tibia vara) 732.4
blue
    bloater 491.20
        with
            acute bronchitis 491.22
            exacerbation (acute) 491.21
    diaper 270.0
    drum 381.02
    sclera 756.51
    toe 445.02
Boder-Sedgwick (ataxia-telangiectasia)
    334.8
Boerhaave's (spontaneous esophageal rup-
    ture) 530.4
Bonnevie-Ullrich 758.6
Bonnier's 386.19
Borjeson-Forssman-Lehmann 759.89
Bouillaud's (rheumatic heart disease) 391.9
Bourneville (-Pringle) (tuberous sclerosis)
    759.5
Bouveret (-Hoffmann) (paroxysmal tachycar-
    dia) 427.2
brachial plexus 353.0

Syndrome — *see also* Disease — *continued*
Brachman-de Lange (Amsterdam dwarf,
    mental retardation, and brachy-
    cephaly) 759.89
bradycardia-tachycardia 427.81
Brailsford-Morquio (dystrophy) (mu-
    copolysaccharidosis IV) 277.5
brain (acute) (chronic) (nonpsychotic) (or-
    ganic) (with behavioral reaction)
    (with neurotic reaction) 310.9
    with
        presenile brain disease (*see also* De-
            mentia, presenile) 290.10
        psychosis, psychotic reaction (*see al-
            so* Psychosis, organic) 294.9
    chronic alcoholic 291.2
    congenital (*see also* Retardation, mental)
        319
    postcontusional 310.2
    posttraumatic
        nonpsychotic 310.2
        psychotic 293.9
            acute 293.0
            chronic (*see also* Psychosis, organ-
                ic) 294.8
            subacute 293.1
    psycho-organic (*see also* Syndrome,
        psycho-organic) 310.9
    psychotic (*see also* Psychosis, organic)
        294.9
    senile (*see also* Dementia, senile) 290.0
branchial arch 744.41
Brandt's (acrodermatitis enteropathica)
    686.8
Brennemann's 289.2
Briquet's 300.81
Brissaud-Meige (infantile myxedema) 244.9
broad ligament laceration 620.6
Brock's (atelectasis due to enlarged lymph
    nodes) 518.0
broken heart 429.83
Brown-Séquard 344.89
brown spot 756.59
Brown's tendon sheath 378.61
Brugada 746.89
Brugsch's (acropachyderma) 757.39
bubbly lung 770.7
Budd-Chiari (hepatic vein thrombosis) 453.0
Büdinger-Ludloff-Läwen 717.89
bulbar 335.22
    lateral (*see also* Disease, cerebrovascular,
        acute) 436
Bullis fever 082.8
bundle of Kent (anomalous atrioventricular
    excitation) 426.7
Bürger-Grütz (essential familial hyper-
    lipemia) 272.3
Burke's (pancreatic insufficiency and
    chronic neutropenia) 577.8
Burnett's (milk-alkali) 275.42
Burnier's (hypophyseal dwarfism) 253.3
burning feet 266.2
Bywaters' 958.5
Caffey's (infantile cortical hyperostosis)
    756.59
Calvé-Legg-Perthes (osteochondrosis,
    femoral capital) 732.1
Caplan (-Colinet) syndrome 714.81
capsular thrombosis (*see also* Thrombosis,
    brain) 434.0 ☑
carbohydrate-deficient glycoprotein (CDGS)
    271.8
carcinogenic thrombophlebitis 453.1
carcinoid 259.2
cardiac asthma (*see also* Failure, ventricular,
    left) 428.1
cardiacos negros 416.0
cardiofaciocutaneous 759.89
cardiopulmonary obesity 278.03 ▲
cardiorenal (*see also* Hypertension, cardiore-
    nal) 404.90
cardiorespiratory distress (idiopathic),
    newborn 769
cardiovascular renal (*see also* Hypertension,
    cardiorenal) 404.90

Syndrome — *see also* Disease — *continued*
cardiovasorenal 272.7
Carini's (ichthyosis congenita) 757.1
carotid
    artery (internal) 435.8
    body or sinus 337.01
carpal tunnel 354.0
Carpenter's 759.89
Cassidy (-Scholte) (malignant carcinoid)
    259.2
cat-cry 758.31
cauda equina 344.60
causalgia 355.9
    lower limb 355.71
    upper limb 354.4
cavernous sinus 437.6
celiac 579.0
    artery compression 447.4
    axis 447.4
central pain 338.0
cerebellomedullary malformation (*see also*
    Spina bifida) 741.0 ☑
cerebral gigantism 253.0
cerebrohepatorenal 759.89
cervical (root) (spine) NEC 723.8
    disc 722.71
    posterior, sympathetic 723.2
    rib 353.0
    sympathetic paralysis 337.09
    traumatic (acute) NEC 847.0
cervicobrachial (diffuse) 723.3
cervicocranial 723.2
cervicodorsal outlet 353.2
Céstan (-Raymond) 433.8 ☑
Céstan's 344.89
Céstan-Chenais 344.89
chancriform 114.1
Charcôt's (intermittent claudication) 443.9
    angina cruris 443.9
    due to atherosclerosis 440.21
Charcôt-Marie-Tooth 356.1
Charcôt-Weiss-Baker 337.01
CHARGE association 759.89
Cheadle (-Möller) (-Barlow) (infantile scurvy)
    267
Chédiak-Higashi (-Steinbrinck) (congenital
    gigantism of peroxidase granules)
    288.2
chest wall 786.52
Chiari's (hepatic vein thrombosis) 453.0
Chiari-Frommel 676.6 ☑
chiasmatic 368.41
Chilaiditi's (subphrenic displacement, colon)
    751.4
chondroectodermal dysplasia 756.55
chorea-athetosis-agitans 275.1
Christian's (chronic histiocytosis X) 277.89
chromosome 4 short arm deletion 758.39
chronic pain 338.4
Churg-Strauss 446.4
Clarke-Hadfield (pancreatic infantilism)
    577.8
Claude's 352.6
Claude Bernard-Horner (*see also* Neuropa-
    thy, peripheral, autonomic) 337.9
Clérambault's
    automatism 348.89
    erotomania 297.8
Clifford's (postmaturity) 766.22
climacteric 627.2
Clouston's (hidrotic ectodermal dysplasia)
    757.31
clumsiness 315.4
Cockayne's (microencephaly and dwarfism)
    759.89
Cockayne-Weber (epidermolysis bullosa)
    757.39
Coffin-Lowry 759.89
Cogan's (nonsyphilitic interstitial keratitis)
    370.52
cold injury (newborn) 778.2
Collet (-Sicard) 352.6
combined immunity deficiency 279.2
compartment(al) (anterior) (deep) (posteri-
    or) 958.8

☑ **Additional Digit Required** — Refer to the Tabular List for Digit Selection   ▽ **Subterms under main terms may continue to next column or page**

2011 ICD-9-CM   ►◄ Revised Text   ● New Line   ▲ Revised Code   October 2010 · Volume 2 — 267

Syndrome — *see also* Disease — *continued*

compartment — *continued*
  nontraumatic
    abdomen 729.73
    arm 729.71
    buttock 729.72
    fingers 729.71
    foot 729.72
    forearm 729.71
    hand 729.71
    hip 729.72
    leg 729.72
    lower extremity 729.72
    shoulder 729.71
    specified site NEC 729.79
    thigh 729.72
    toes 729.72
    upper extremity 729.71
    wrist 729.71
  post-surgical (*see also* Syndrome, compartment, non-traumatic) 998.89
  traumatic 958.90
    adomen 958.93
    arm 958.91
    buttock 958.92
    fingers 958.91
    foot 958.92
    forearm 958.91
    hand 958.91
    hip 958.92
    leg 958.92
    lower extremity 958.92
    shoulder 958.91
    specified site NEC 958.99
    thigh 958.92
    tibial 958.92
    toes 958.92
    upper extremity 958.91
    wrist 958.91
complex regional pain — *see also* Dystrophy, sympathetic
  type I — *see* Dystrophy, sympathetic (posttraumatic) (reflex)
  type II — *see* Causalgia
compression 958.5
  cauda equina 344.60
    with neurogenic bladder 344.61
concussion 310.2
congenital
  affecting more than one system 759.7
    specified type NEC 759.89
  congenital central alveolar hypoventilation 327.25
  facial diplegia 352.6
  muscular hypertrophy-cerebral 759.89
congestion-fibrosis (pelvic) 625.5
conjunctivourethrosynovial 099.3
Conn (-Louis) (primary aldosteronism) 255.12
Conradi (-Hünermann) (chondrodysplasia calcificans congenita) 756.59
conus medullaris 336.8
Cooke-Apert-Gallais (adrenogenital) 255.2
Cornelia de Lange's (Amsterdam dwarf, mental retardation, and brachycephaly) 759.8 ☑
coronary insufficiency or intermediate 411.1
cor pulmonale 416.9
corticosexual 255.2
Costen's (complex) 524.60
costochondral junction 733.6
costoclavicular 353.0
costovertebral 253.0
Cotard's (paranoia) 297.1
Cowden 759.6
craniovertebral 723.2
Creutzfeldt-Jakob 046.19
  with dementia
    with behavioral disturbance 046.19 [294.11]
    without behavioral disturbance 046.19 [294.10]
  variant 046.11
    with dementia
      with behavioral disturbance 046.11 [294.11]

Syndrome — *see also* Disease — *continued*

Creutzfeldt-Jakob — *continued*
  variant — *continued*
    with dementia — *continued*
      without behavioral disturbance 046.11 [294.10]
crib death 798.0
cricopharyngeal 787.20
cri-du-chat 758.31
Crigler-Najjar (congenital hyperbilirubinemia) 277.4
crocodile tears 351.8
Cronkhite-Canada 211.3
croup 464.4
CRST (cutaneous systemic sclerosis) 710.1
crush 958.5
crushed lung (*see also* Injury, internal, lung) 861.20
Cruveilhier-Baumgarten (cirrhosis of liver) 571.5
cubital tunnel 354.2
Cuiffini-Pancoast (M8010/3) (carcinoma, pulmonary apex) 162.3
Curschmann (-Batten) (-Steinert) 359.21
Cushing's (iatrogenic) (idiopathic) (pituitary basophilism) (pituitary-dependent) 255.0
  overdose or wrong substance given or taken 962.0
Cyriax's (slipping rib) 733.99
cystic duct stump 576.0
Da Costa's (neurocirculatory asthenia) 306.2
Dameshek's (erythroblastic anemia) 282.49
Dana-Putnam (subacute combined sclerosis with pernicious anemia) 281.0 [336.2]
Danbolt (-Closs) (acrodermatitis enteropathica) 686.8
Dandy-Walker (atresia, foramen of Magendie) 742.3
  with spina bifida (*see also* Spina bifida) 741.0 ☑
Danlos' 756.83
Davies-Colley (slipping rib) 733.99
dead fetus 641.3 ☑
defeminization 255.2
defibrination (*see also* Fibrinolysis) 286.6
Degos' 447.8
Deiters' nucleus 386.19
Déjérine-Roussy 338.0
Déjérine-Thomas 333.0
de Lange's (Amsterdam dwarf, mental retardation, and brachycephaly) (Cornelia) 759.89
Del Castillo's (germinal aplasia) 606.0
deletion chromosomes 758.39
delusional
  induced by drug 292.11
dementia-aphonia, of childhood (*see also* Psychosis, childhood) 299.1 ☑
demyelinating NEC 341.9
denial visual hallucination 307.9
depersonalization 300.6
de Quervain's 259.51
Dercum's (adiposis dolorosa) 272.8
de Toni-Fanconi (-Debré) (cystinosis) 270.0
diabetes-dwarfism-obesity (juvenile) 258.1
diabetes mellitus-hypertension-nephrosis 250.4 [581.81]
  due to secondary diabetes 249.4 [581.81]
diabetes mellitus in newborn infant 775.1
diabetes-nephrosis 250.4 ☑ [581.81]
  due to secondary diabetes 249.4 [581.81]
diabetic amyotrophy 250.6 ☑ [353.5]
  due to secondary diabetes 249.6 ☑ [353.5]
Diamond-Blackfan (congenital hypoplastic anemia) 284.01
Diamond-Gardener (autoerythrocyte sensitization) 287.2
DIC (diffuse or disseminated intravascular coagulopathy) (*see also* Fibrinolysis) 286.6
diencephalohypophyseal NEC 253.8
diffuse cervicobrachial 723.3

Syndrome — *see also* Disease — *continued*

diffuse obstructive pulmonary 496
DiGeorge's (thymic hypoplasia) 279.11
Dighton's 756.51
Di Guglielmo's (erythremic myelosis) (M9841/3) 207.0 ☑
disequilibrium 276.9
disseminated platelet thrombosis 446.6
Ditthomska 307.81
Doan-Wiseman (primary splenic neutropenia) 289.53
Döhle body-panmyelopathic 288.2
Donohue's (leprechaunism) 259.8
dorsolateral medullary (*see also* Disease, cerebrovascular, acute) 436
double athetosis 333.71
double whammy 360.81
Down's (mongolism) 758.0
Dresbach's (elliptocytosis) 282.1
Dressler's (postmyocardial infarction) 411.0
  hemoglobinuria 283.2
  postcardiotomy 429.4
drug withdrawal, infant, of dependent mother 779.5
dry skin 701.1
  eye 375.15
DSAP (disseminated superficial actinic porokeratosis) 692.75
Duane's (retraction) 378.71
Duane-Stilling-Türk (ocular retraction syndrome) 378.71
Dubin-Johnson (constitutional hyperbilirubinemia) 277.4
Dubin-Sprinz (constitutional hyperbilirubinemia) 277.4
Duchenne's 335.22
due to abnormality
  autosomal NEC (*see also* Abnormal, autosomes NEC) 758.5
    13 758.1
    18 758.2
    21 or 22 758.0
    D1 758.1
    E3 758.2
    G 758.0
  chromosomal 758.89
    sex 758.81
dumping 564.2
  nonsurgical 536.8
Duplay's 726.2
Dupré's (meningism) 781.6
Dyke-Young (acquired macrocytic hemolytic anemia) 283.9
dyspraxia 315.4
dystocia, dystrophia 654.9 ☑
Eagle-Barret 756.71
Eales' 362.18
Eaton-Lambert (*see also* Neoplasm, by site, malignant) 199.1 [358.1]
Ebstein's (downward displacement, tricuspid valve into right ventricle) 746.2
ectopic ACTH secretion 255.0
eczema-thrombocytopenia 279.12
Eddowes' (brittle bones and blue sclera) 756.51
Edwards' 758.2
efferent loop 537.89
effort (aviators') (psychogenic) 306.2
Ehlers-Danlos 756.83
Eisenmenger's (ventricular septal defect) 745.4
Ekbom's (restless legs) 333.94
Ekman's (brittle bones and blue sclera) 756.51
electric feet 266.2
Elephant man 237.71
Ellison-Zollinger (gastric hypersecretion with pancreatic islet cell tumor) 251.5
Ellis-van Creveld (chondroectodermal dysplasia) 756.55
embryonic fixation 270.2
empty sella (turcica) 253.8
endocrine-hypertensive 255.3
Engel-von Recklinghausen (osteitis fibrosa cystica) 252.01
enteroarticular 099.3

Syndrome — *see also* Disease — *continued*

entrapment — *see* Neuropathy, entrapment
eosinophilia myalgia 710.5
epidemic vomiting 078.82
Epstein's — *see* Nephrosis
Erb (-Oppenheim)-Goldflam 358.00
Erdheim's (acromegalic macrospondylitis) 253.0
Erdheim-Chester 277.89
Erlacher-Blount (tibia vara) 732.4
erythrocyte fragmentation 283.19
euthyroid sick 790.94
Evans' (thrombocytopenic purpura) 287.32
excess cortisol, iatrogenic 255.0
exhaustion 300.5
extrapyramidal 333.90
eyelid-malar-mandible 756.0
eye retraction 378.71
Faber's (achlorhydric anemia) 280.9
Fabry (-Anderson) (angiokeratoma corporis diffusum) 272.7
facet 724.8
Fallot's 745.2
falx (*see also* Hemorrhage, brain) 431
familial eczema-thrombocytopenia 279.12
Fanconi (-de Toni) (-Debré) (cystinosis) 270.0
Fanconi's (anemia) (congenital pancytopenia) 284.09
Farber (-Uzman) (disseminated lipogranulomatosis) 272.8
fatigue NEC 300.5
  chronic 780.71
faulty bowel habit (idiopathic megacolon) 564.7
FDH (focal dermal hypoplasia) 757.39
fecal reservoir 560.39
Feil-Klippel (brevicollis) 756.16
Felty's (rheumatoid arthritis with splenomegaly and leukopenia) 714.1
fertile eunuch 257.2
fetal alcohol 760.71
  late effect 760.71
fibrillation-flutter 427.32
fibrositis (periarticular) 729.0
Fiedler's (acute isolated myocarditis) 422.91
Fiessinger-Leroy (-Reiter) 099.3
Fiessinger-Rendu (erythema multiforme exudativum) 695.19
first arch 756.0
Fisher's 357.0
fish odor 270.8
Fitz's (acute hemorrhagic pancreatitis) 577.0
Fitz-Hugh and Curtis 098.86
  due to
    Chlamydia trachomatis 099.56
    Neisseria gonorrhoeae (gonococcal peritonitis) 098.86
Flajani (-Basedow) (exophthalmic goiter) 242.0 ☑
flat back
  acquired 737.29
  postprocedural 738.5
floppy
  infant 781.99
  iris 364.81
  valve (mitral) 424.0
flush 259.2
Foix-Alajouanine 336.1
Fong's (hereditary osteo-onychodysplasia) 756.89
foramen magnum 348.4
Forbes-Albright (nonpuerperal amenorrhea and lactation associated with pituitary tumor) 253.1
Foster-Kennedy 377.04
Foville's (peduncular) 344.89
fragile X 759.83
Franceschetti's (mandibulofacial dysostosis) 756.0
Fraser's 759.89
Freeman-Sheldon 759.89
Frey's (auriculotemporal) 705.22
Friderichsen-Waterhouse 036.3
Friedrich-Erb-Arnold (acropachyderma) 757.39
Fröhlich's (adiposogenital dystrophy) 253.8

☑ **Additional Digit Required** — Refer to the Tabular List for Digit Selection   ▽ **Subterms under main terms may continue to next column or page**

268 — Volume 2   ▶◀ Revised Text   ● New Line   ▲ Revised Code   2011 ICD-9-CM

Syndrome — *see also* Disease — *continued*
Froin's 336.8
Frommel-Chiari 676.6 ☑
frontal lobe 310.0
Fukuhara 277.87
Fuller Albright's (osteitis fibrosa dissemina-
    ta) 756.59
functional
    bowel 564.9
    prepubertal castrate 752.89
Gaisböck's (polycythemia hypertonica)
    289.0
ganglion (basal, brain) 333.90
    geniculi 351.1
Ganser's, hysterical 300.16
Gardner-Diamond (autoerythrocyte sensiti-
    zation) 287.2
gastroesophageal junction 530.0
gastroesophageal laceration-hemorrhage
    530.7
gastrojejunal loop obstruction 537.89
Gayet-Wernicke's (superior hemorrhagic
    polioencephalitis) 265.1
Gee-Herter-Heubner (nontropical sprue)
    579.0
Gélineau's (*see also* Narcolepsy) 347.00
genito-anorectal 099.1
Gerhardt's (vocal cord paralysis) 478.30
Gerstmann's (finger agnosia) 784.69
Gerstmann-Sträussler-Scheinker (GSS)
    046.71
Gianotti Crosti 057.8
    due to known virus — *see* Infection,
        virus
    due to unknown virus 057.8
Gilbert's 277.4
Gilford (-Hutchinson) (progeria) 259.8
Gilles de la Tourette's 307.23
Gillespie's (dysplasia oculodentodigitalis)
    759.89
Glénard's (enteroptosis) 569.89
Glinski-Simmonds (pituitary cachexia) 253.2
glucuronyl transferase 277.4
glue ear 381.20
Goldberg (-Maxwell) (-Morris) (testicular
    feminization) 259.51
Goldenhar's (oculoauriculovertebral dyspla-
    sia) 756.0
Goldflam-Erb 358.00
Goltz-Gorlin (dermal hypoplasia) 757.39
Good's 279.06
Goodpasture's (pneumorenal) 446.21
Gopalan's (burning feet) 266.2
Gorlin's 759.89
Gorlin-Chaudhry-Moss 759.89
Gougerot-Blum (pigmented purpuric
    lichenoid dermatitis) 709.1
Gougerot-Carteaud (confluent reticulate
    papillomatosis) 701.8
Gougerot (-Houwer)-Sjögren (keratoconjunc-
    tivitis sicca) 710.2
Gouley's (constrictive pericarditis) 423.2
Gowers' (vasovagal attack) 780.2
Gowers-Paton-Kennedy 377.04
Gradenigo's 383.02
gray or grey (chloramphenicol) (newborn)
    779.4
Greig's (hypertelorism) 756.0
GSS (Gerstmann-Sträussler-Scheinker)
    046.71
Gubler-Millard 344.89
Guérin-Stern (arthrogryposis multiplex
    congenita) 754.89
Guillain-Barré (-Strohl) 357.0
Gunn's (jaw-winking syndrome) 742.8
Günther's (congenital erythropoietic por-
    phyria) 277.1
gustatory sweating 350.8
H₃O 759.81
Hadfield-Clarke (pancreatic infantilism)
    577.8
Haglund-Läwen-Fründ 717.89
hairless women 257.8
hair tourniquet (*see also* Injury, superficial,
    by site)
    finger 915.8

Syndrome — *see also* Disease — *continued*
hair tourniquet (*see also* Injury, superficial,
    by site) — *continued*
    finger — *continued*
        infected 915.9
        penis 911.8
            infected 911.9
        toe 917.8
            infected 917.9
Hallermann-Streiff 756.0
Hallervorden-Spatz 333.0
Hamman's (spontaneous mediastinal em-
    physema) 518.1
Hamman-Rich (diffuse interstitial pulmonary
    fibrosis) 516.3
hand-foot 693.0
Hand-Schüller-Christian (chronic histiocyto-
    sis X) 277.89
Hanot-Chauffard (-Troisier) (bronze dia-
    betes) 275.01   ▲
Harada's 363.22
Hare's (M8010/3) (carcinoma, pulmonary
    apex) 162.3
Harkavy's 446.0
harlequin color change 779.89
Harris' (organic hyperinsulinism) 251.1
Hart's (pellagra-cerebellar ataxia-renal
    aminoaciduria) 270.0
Hayem-Faber (achlorhydric anemia) 280.9
Hayem-Widal (acquired hemolytic jaundice)
    283.9
headache — *see* Headache, syndrome
Heberden's (angina pectoris) 413.9
Hedinger's (malignant carcinoid) 259.2
Hegglin's 288.2
Heller's (infantile psychosis) (*see also* Psy-
    chosis, childhood) 299.1 ☑
H.E.L.L.P 642.5 ☑
hemolytic-uremic (adult) (child) 283.11
hemophagocytic 288.4
    infection-associated 288.4
Hench-Rosenberg (palindromic arthritis)
    (*see also* Rheumatism, palindromic)
    719.3 ☑
Henoch-Schönlein (allergic purpura) 287.0
hepatic flexure 569.89
hepatorenal 572.4
    due to a procedure 997.4
    following delivery 674.8 ☑
hepatourologic 572.4
Herrick's (hemoglobin S disease) 282.61
Herter (-Gee) (nontropical sprue) 579.0
Heubner-Herter (nontropical sprue) 579.0
Heyd's (hepatorenal) 572.4
HHHO 759.81
high grade myelodysplastic 238.73
    with 5q deletion 238.73
Hilger's 337.09
histiocytic 288.4
Hoffa (-Kastert) (liposynovitis prepatellaris)
    272.8
Hoffmann's 244.9 [359.5]
Hoffmann-Bouveret (paroxysmal tachycar-
    dia) 427.2
Hoffmann-Werdnig 335.0
Holländer-Simons (progressive lipodystro-
    phy) 272.6
Holmes' (visual disorientation) 368.16
Holmes-Adie 379.46
Hoppe-Goldflam 358.00
Horner's (*see also* Neuropathy, peripheral,
    autonomic) 337.9
    traumatic — *see* Injury, nerve, cervical
        sympathetic
hospital addiction 301.51
hungry bone 275.5
Hunt's (herpetic geniculate ganglionitis)
    053.11
    dyssynergia cerebellaris myoclonica
        334.2
Hunter (-Hurler) (mucopolysaccharidosis II)
    277.5
hunterian glossitis 529.4
Hurler (-Hunter) (mucopolysaccharidosis II)
    277.5
Hutchinson-Boeck (sarcoidosis) 135

Syndrome — *see also* Disease — *continued*
Hutchinson-Gilford (progeria) 259.8
Hutchinson's incisors or teeth 090.5
hydralazine
    correct substance properly administered
        695.4
    overdose or wrong substance given or
        taken 972.6
hydraulic concussion (abdomen) (*see also*
    Injury, internal, abdomen) 868.00
hyperabduction 447.8
hyperactive bowel 564.9
hyperaldosteronism with hypokalemic alka-
    losis (Bartter's) 255.13
hypercalcemic 275.42
hypercoagulation NEC 289.89
hypereosinophilic (idiopathic) 288.3
hyperkalemic 276.7
hyperkinetic (*see also* Hyperkinesia)
    heart 429.82
hyperlipemia-hemolytic anemia-icterus
    571.1
hypermobility 728.5
hypernatremia 276.0
hyperosmolarity 276.0
hyperperfusion 997.01
hypersomnia-bulimia 349.89
hypersplenic 289.4
hypersympathetic (*see also* Neuropathy,
    peripheral, autonomic) 337.9
hypertransfusion, newborn 776.4
hyperventilation, psychogenic 306.1
hyperviscosity (of serum) NEC 273.3
    polycythemic 289.0
    sclerothymic 282.8
hypoglycemic (familial) (neonatal) 251.2
    functional 251.1
hypokalemic 276.8
hypophyseal 253.8
hypophyseothalamic 253.8
hypopituitarism 253.2
hypoplastic left heart 746.7
hypopotassemia 276.8
hyposmolality 276.1
hypotension, maternal 669.2 ☑
hypothenar hammer 443.89
hypotonia-hypomentia-hypogonadism-
    obesity 759.81
ICF (intravascular coagulation-fibrinolysis)
    (*see also* Fibrinolysis) 286.6
idiopathic cardiorespiratory distress, new-
    born 769
idiopathic nephrotic (infantile) 581.9
iliotibial band 728.89
Imerslund (-Gräsbeck) (anemia due to famil-
    ial selective vitamin B₁₂ malabsorp-
    tion) 281.1
immobility (paraplegic) 728.3
immunity deficiency, combined 279.2
impending coronary 411.1
impingement
    shoulder 726.2
    vertebral bodies 724.4
inappropriate secretion of antidiuretic hor-
    mone (ADH) 253.6
incomplete
    mandibulofacial 756.0
infant
    death, sudden (SIDS) 798.0
    Hercules 255.2
    of diabetic mother 775.0
    shaken 995.55
infantilism 253.3
inferior vena cava 459.2
influenza-like ►(*see also* Influenza)◄ 487.1
inspissated bile, newborn 774.4
insufficient sleep 307.44
intermediate coronary (artery) 411.1
internal carotid artery (*see also* Occlusion,
    artery, carotid) 433.1 ☑
interspinous ligament 724.8
intestinal
    carcinoid 259.2
    gas 787.3
    knot 560.2
intraoperative floppy iris (IFIS) 364.81

Syndrome — *see also* Disease — *continued*
intravascular
    coagulation-fibrinolysis (ICF) (*see also*
        Fibrinolysis) 286.6
    coagulopathy (*see also* Fibrinolysis) 286.6
inverted Marfan's 759.89
IRDS (idiopathic respiratory distress, new-
    born) 769
irritable
    bowel 564.1
    heart 306.2
    weakness 300.5
ischemic bowel (transient) 557.9
    chronic 557.1
    due to mesenteric artery insufficiency
        557.1
Itsenko-Cushing (pituitary basophilism)
    255.0
IVC (intravascular coagulopathy) (*see also*
    Fibrinolysis) 286.6
Ivemark's (asplenia with congenital heart
    disease) 759.0
Jaccoud's 714.4
Jackson's 344.89
Jadassohn-Lewandowski (pachyonchia
    congenita) 757.5
Jaffe-Lichtenstein (-Uehlinger) 252.01
Jahnke's (encephalocutaneous angiomato-
    sis) 759.6
Jakob-Creutzfeldt 046.19
    with dementia
        with behavioral disturbance
            046.19 [294.11]
        without behavioral disturbance
            046.19 [294.10]
    variant 046.11
        with dementia
            with behavioral disturbance
                046.11 [294.11]
            without behavioral disturbance
                046.11 [294.10]
Jaksch's (pseudoleukemia infantum) 285.8
Jaksch-Hayem (-Luzet) (pseudoleukemia
    infantum) 285.8
jaw-winking 742.8
jejunal 564.2
Jervell-Lange-Nielsen 426.82
jet lag 327.35
Jeune's (asphyxiating thoracic dystrophy of
    newborn) 756.4
Job's (chronic granulomatous disease) 288.1
Jordan's 288.2
Joseph-Diamond-Blackfan (congenital hy-
    poplastic anemia) 284.01
Joubert 759.89
jugular foramen 352.6
Kabuki 759.89
Kahler's (multiple myeloma) (M9730/3)
    203.0 ☑
Kalischer's (encephalocutaneous angiomato-
    sis) 759.6
Kallmann's (hypogonadotropic hypogo-
    nadism with anosmia) 253.4
Kanner's (autism) (*see also* Psychosis, child-
    hood) 299.0 ☑
Kartagener's (sinusitis, bronchiectasis, situs
    inversus) 759.3
Kasabach-Merritt (capillary hemangioma
    associated with thrombocytopenic
    purpura) 287.39
Kast's (dyschondroplasia with heman-
    giomas) 756.4
Kaznelson's (congenital hypoplastic anemia)
    284.01
Kearns-Sayre 277.87
Kelly's (sideropenic dysphagia) 280.8
Kimmelstiel-Wilson (intercapillary
    glomerulosclerosis) 250.4 ☑ [581.81]
    due to secondary diabetes
        249.4 ☑ [581.81]
Klauder's (erythema multiforme exuda-
    tivum) 695.19
Kleine-Levin 327.13
Klein-Waardenburg (ptosis-epicanthus)
    270.2
Klinefelter's 758.7

☑ Additional Digit Required — Refer to the Tabular List for Digit Selection   ▽ Subterms under main terms may continue to next column or page

2011 ICD-9-CM   ►◄ Revised Text   ● New Line   ▲ Revised Code   October 2010 • Volume 2 — 269

☑ **Additional Digit Required** — **Refer to the Tabular List for Digit Selection**   ▽ **Subterms under main terms may continue to next column or page**

Syndrome — see also Disease — continued
Oppenheim-Urbach — continued
due to secondary diabetes
249.8 ☑ [709.3]
oral-facial-digital 759.89
organic
affective NEC 293.83
drug-induced 292.84
anxiety 293.84
delusional 293.81
alcohol-induced 291.5
drug-induced 292.11
due to or associated with
arteriosclerosis 290.42
presenile brain disease 290.12
senility 290.20
depressive 293.83
drug-induced 292.84
due to or associated with
arteriosclerosis 290.43
presenile brain disease 290.13
senile brain disease 290.21
hallucinosis 293.82
drug-induced 292.84
organic affective 293.83
induced by drug 292.84
organic personality 310.1
induced by drug 292.89
Ormond's 593.4
orodigitofacial 759.89
orthostatic hypotensive-dysautonomic
dyskinetic 333.0
Osler-Weber-Rendu (familial hemorrhagic
telangiectasia) 448.0
osteodermopathic hyperostosis 757.39
osteoporosis-osteomalacia 268.2
Österreicher-Turner (hereditary osteo-onychodysplasia) 756.89
os trigonum 755.69
Ostrum-Furst 756.59
otolith 386.19
otopalatodigital 759.89
outlet (thoracic) 353.0
ovarian remnant 620.8
Owren's (see also Defect, coagulation) 286.3
OX 758.6
pacemaker 429.4
Paget-Schroetter (intermittent venous
claudication) 453.89
pain (see also Pain)
central 338.0
chronic 338.4
complex regional 355.9
type I 337.20
lower limb 337.22
specified site NEC 337.29
upper limb 337.21
type II
lower limb 355.71
upper limb 354.4
myelopathic 338.0
thalamic (hyperesthetic) 338.0
painful
apicocostal vertebral (M8010/3) 162.3
arc 726.19
bruising 287.2
feet 266.2
Pancoast's (carcinoma, pulmonary apex)
(M8010/3) 162.3
panhypopituitary (postpartum) 253.2
papillary muscle 429.81
with myocardial infarction 410.8 ☑
Papillon-Léage and Psaume (orodigitofacial
dysostosis) 759.89
parabiotic (transfusion)
donor (twin) 772.0
recipient (twin) 776.4
paralysis agitans 332.0
paralytic 344.9
specified type NEC 344.89
paraneoplastic — see condition
Parinaud's (paralysis of conjugate upward
gaze) 378.81
oculoglandular 372.02
Parkes Weber and Dimitri (encephalocutaneous angiomatosis) 759.6

Syndrome — see also Disease — continued
Parkinson's (see also Parkinsonism) 332.0
parkinsonian (see also Parkinsonism) 332.0
Parry's (exophthalmic goiter) 242.0 ☑
Parry-Romberg 349.89
Parsonage-Aldren-Turner 353.5
Parsonage-Turner 353.5
Patau's (trisomy D1) 758.1
patella clunk 719.66
patellofemoral 719.46
Paterson (-Brown) (-Kelly) (sideropenic dysphagia) 280.8
Payr's (splenic flexure syndrome) 569.89
pectoral girdle 447.8
pectoralis minor 447.8
Pelger-Huët (hereditary hyposegmentation)
288.2
pellagra-cerebellar ataxia-renal
aminoaciduria 270.0
pellagroid 265.2
Pellegrini-Stieda 726.62
Pellizzi's (pineal) 259.8
Pendred's (familial goiter with deaf-mutism)
243
Penfield's (see also Epilepsy) 345.5 ☑
Penta X 758.81
peptic ulcer — see Ulcer, peptic 533.9 ☑
perabduction 447.8
periodic 277.31
periurethral fibrosis 593.4
persistent fetal circulation 747.83
Petges-Cléjat (poikilodermatomyositis)
710.3
Peutz-Jeghers 759.6
Pfeiffer (acrocephalosyndactyly) 755.55
phantom limb 353.6
pharyngeal pouch 279.11
Pick's (pericardial pseudocirrhosis of liver)
423.2
heart 423.2
liver 423.2
Pick-Herxheimer (diffuse idiopathic cutaneous atrophy) 701.8
Pickwickian (cardiopulmonary obesity)
278.03 ▲
PIE (pulmonary infiltration with eosinophilia) 518.3
Pierre Marie-Bamberger (hypertrophic pulmonary osteoarthropathy) 731.2
Pierre Mauriac's (diabetes-dwarfism-obesity)
258.1
Pierre Robin 756.0
pigment dispersion, iris 364.53
pineal 259.8
pink puffer 492.8
pituitary 253.0
placental
dysfunction 762.2
insufficiency 762.2
transfusion 762.3
plantar fascia 728.71
plateau iris 364.82
plica knee 727.83
Plummer-Vinson (sideropenic dysphagia)
280.8
pluricarential of infancy 260
plurideficiency of infancy 260
pluriglandular (compensatory) 258.8
Poland 756.81 ●
polycarential of infancy 260
polyglandular 258.8
polysplenia 759.0
pontine 433.8 ☑
popliteal
artery entrapment 447.8
web 756.89
postartificial menopause 627.4
postcardiac injury
postcardiotomy 429.4
postmyocardial infarction 411.0
postcardiotomy 429.4
postcholecystectomy 576.0
postcommissurotomy 429.4
postconcussional 310.2
postcontusional 310.2

Syndrome — see also Disease — continued
postencephalitic 310.8
posterior
cervical sympathetic 723.2
fossa compression 348.4
inferior cerebellar artery (see also Disease, cerebrovascular, acute) 436
reversible encephalopathy (PRES) 348.39
postgastrectomy (dumping) 564.2
post-gastric surgery 564.2
posthepatitis 780.79
postherpetic (neuralgia) (zoster) 053.19
geniculate ganglion 053.11
ophthalmica 053.19
postimmunization — see Complications,
vaccination
postinfarction 411.0
postinfluenza (asthenia) 780.79
postirradiation 990
postlaminectomy 722.80
cervical, cervicothoracic 722.81
lumbar, lumbosacral 722.83
thoracic, thoracolumbar 722.82
postleukotomy 310.0
postlobotomy 310.0
postmastectomy lymphedema 457.0
postmature (of newborn) 766.22
postmyocardial infarction 411.0
postoperative NEC 998.9
blind loop 579.2
postpartum panhypopituitary 253.2
postperfusion NEC 999.89
bone marrow 996.85
postpericardiotomy 429.4
postphlebitic (asymptomatic) 459.10
with
complications NEC 459.19
inflammation 459.12
and ulcer 459.13
stasis dermatitis 459.12
with ulcer 459.13
ulcer 459.11
with inflammation 459.13
postpolio (myelitis) 138
postvagotomy 564.2
postvalvulotomy 429.4
postviral (asthenia) NEC 780.79
Potain's (gastrectasis with dyspepsia) 536.1
potassium intoxication 276.7
Potter's 753.0
Prader (-Labhart) -Willi (-Fanconi) 759.81
preinfarction 411.1
preleukemic 238.75
premature senility 259.8
premenstrual 625.4
premenstrual tension 625.4
pre ulcer 536.9
Prinzmetal-Massumi (anterior chest wall
syndrome) 786.52
Profichet's 729.90
progeria 259.8
progressive pallidal degeneration 333.0
prolonged gestation 766.22
Proteus (dermal hypoplasia) 757.39
prune belly 756.71
prurigo-asthma 691.8
pseudocarpal tunnel (sublimis) 354.0
pseudohermaphroditism-virilism-hirsutism
255.2
pseudoparalytica 358.00
pseudo-Turner's 759.89
psycho-organic 293.9
acute 293.0
anxiety type 293.84
depressive type 293.83
hallucinatory type 293.82
nonpsychotic severity 310.1
specified focal (partial) NEC 310.8
paranoid type 293.81
specified type NEC 293.89
subacute 293.1
pterygolymphangiectasia 758.6
ptosis-epicanthus 270.2
pulmonary
arteriosclerosis 416.0
hypoperfusion (idiopathic) 769

Syndrome — see also Disease — continued
pulmonary — continued
renal (hemorrhagic) 446.21
pulseless 446.7
Putnam-Dana (subacute combined sclerosis
with pernicious anemia) 281.0 [336.2]
pyloroduodenal 537.89
pyramidopallidonigral 332.0
pyriformis 355.0
QT interval prolongation 426.82
radicular NEC 729.2
lower limbs 724.4
upper limbs 723.4
newborn 767.4
Raeder-Harbitz (pulseless disease) 446.7
Ramsay Hunt's
dyssynergia cerebellaris myoclonica
334.2
herpetic geniculate ganglionitis 053.11
rapid time-zone change 327.35
Raymond (-Céstan) 433.8 ☑
Raynaud's (paroxysmal digital cyanosis)
443.0
RDS (respiratory distress syndrome, newborn) 769
Refsum's (heredopathia atactica polyneuritiformis) 356.3
Reichmann's (gastrosuccorrhea) 536.8
Reifenstein's (hereditary familial hypogonadism, male) 259.52
Reilly's (see also Neuropathy, peripheral,
autonomic) 337.9
Reiter's 099.3
renal glomerulohyalinosis-diabetic
250.4 ☑ [581.81]
due to secondary diabetes
249.4 ☑ [581.81]
Rendu-Osler-Weber (familial hemorrhagic
telangiectasia) 448.0
renofacial (congenital biliary fibroan-
giomatosis) 753.0
Rénon-Delille 253.8
respiratory distress (idiopathic) (newborn)
769
adult (following shock, surgery, or trauma) 518.5
specified NEC 518.82
type II 770.6
restless legs (RLS) 333.94
retinoblastoma (familial) 190.5
retraction (Duane's) 378.71
retroperitoneal fibrosis 593.4
retroviral seroconversion (acute) V08
Rett's 330.8
Reye's 331.81
Reye-Sheehan (postpartum pituitary
necrosis) 253.2
Riddoch's (visual disorientation) 368.16
Ridley's (see also Failure, ventricular, left)
428.1
Rieger's (mesodermal dysgenesis, anterior
ocular segment) 743.44
Rietti-Greppi-Micheli (thalassemia minor)
282.49
right ventricular obstruction — see Failure,
heart
Riley Day (familial dysautonomia) 742.8
Robin's 756.0
Rokitansky-Kuster-Hauser (congenital ab-
sence, vagina) 752.45 ▲
Romano-Ward (prolonged QT interval syn-
drome) 426.82
Romberg's 349.89
Rosen-Castleman-Liebow (pulmonary pro-
teinosis) 516.0
rotator cuff, shoulder 726.10
Roth's 355.1
Rothmund's (congenital poikiloderma)
757.33
Rotor's (idiopathic hyperbilirubinemia)
277.4
Roussy-Lévy 334.3
Roy (-Jutras) (acropachyderma) 757.39
rubella (congenital) 771.0

☑ Additional Digit Required — Refer to the Tabular List for Digit Selection ▽ Subterms under main terms may continue to next column or page

2011 ICD-9-CM ▶◀ Revised Text ● New Line ▲ Revised Code October 2010 • Volume 2 — 271

☑ **Additional Digit Required** — Refer to the Tabular List for Digit Selection   ▽ **Subterms under main terms may continue to next column or page**

272 — Volume 2 · October 2010   ▶◀ Revised Text   ● New Line   ▲ Revised Code   **2011 ICD-9-CM**

☑ **Additional Digit Required** — Refer to the Tabular List for Digit Selection   🔲 **Subterms under main terms may continue to next column or page**

2011 ICD-9-CM   ▶◀ **Revised Text**   ● **New Line**   ▲ **Revised Code**   October 2010 · Volume 2 — 273

Index

Syphilis, syphilitic — Syphilis, syphilitic

Syphilis, syphilitic — *continued*
coronary — *continued*
   sclerosis 093.89
coryza 095.8
  congenital 090.0
cranial nerve 094.89
cutaneous — *see* Syphilis, skin
dacryocystitis 095.8
degeneration, spinal cord 094.89
d'emblée 095.8
dementia 094.1
  paralytica 094.1
    juvenilis 090.40
destruction of bone 095.5
dilatation, aorta 093.0
due to blood transfusion 097.9
dura mater 094.89
ear 095.8
  inner 095.8
    nerve (eighth) 094.86
    neurorecurrence 094.86
early NEC 091.0
  cardiovascular 093.9
  central nervous system 094.9
    paresis 094.1
    tabes 094.0
  latent (without manifestations) (less
    than 2 years after infection) 092.9
    negative spinal fluid test 092.9
    serological relapse following treat-
      ment 092.0
    serology positive 092.9
  paresis 094.1
  relapse (treated, untreated) 091.7
  skin 091.3
  symptomatic NEC 091.89
    extragenital chancre 091.2
    primary, except extragenital chancre
      091.0
    secondary (*see also* Syphilis, sec-
      ondary) 091.3
      relapse (treated, untreated) 091.7
  tabes 094.0
  ulcer 091.3
eighth nerve 094.86
endemic, nonvenereal 104.0
endocarditis 093.20
  aortic 093.22
  mitral 093.21
  pulmonary 093.24
  tricuspid 093.23
epididymis (late) 095.8
epiglottis 095.8
epiphysitis (congenital) 090.0
esophagus 095.8
Eustachian tube 095.8
exposure to V01.6
eye 095.8 *[363.13]*
  neuromuscular mechanism 094.85
eyelid 095.8 *[373.5]*
  with gumma 095.8 *[373.5]*
  ptosis 094.89
fallopian tube 095.8
fracture 095.5
gallbladder (late) 095.8
gastric 095.8
  crisis 094.0
  polyposis 095.8
general 097.9
  paralysis 094.1
    juvenile 090.40
genital (primary) 091.0
glaucoma 095.8
gumma (late) NEC 095.9
  cardiovascular system 093.9
  central nervous system 094.9
  congenital 090.5
  heart or artery 093.89
heart 093.89
  block 093.89
  decompensation 093.89
  disease 093.89
  failure 093.89
  valve (*see also* Syphilis, endocarditis)
    093.20
hemianesthesia 094.89

Syphilis, syphilitic — *continued*
hemianopsia 095.8
hemiparesis 094.89
hemiplegia 094.89
hepatic artery 093.89
hepatitis 095.3
hepatomegaly 095.3
  congenital 090.0
hereditaria tarda (*see also* Syphilis, congenital, late) 090.7
hereditary (*see also* Syphilis, congenital)
  090.9
  interstitial keratitis 090.3
  Hutchinson's teeth 090.5
hyalitis 095.8
inactive — *see* Syphilis, latent
infantum NEC (*see also* Syphilis, congenital)
  090.9
inherited — *see* Syphilis, congenital
internal ear 095.8
intestine (late) 095.8
iris, iritis (secondary) 091.52
  late 095.8 *[364.11]*
joint (late) 095.8
keratitis (congenital) (early) (interstitial)
  (late) (parenchymatous) (punctata
  profunda) 090.3
kidney 095.4
lacrimal apparatus 095.8
laryngeal paralysis 095.8
larynx 095.8
late 097.0
  cardiovascular 093.9
  central nervous system 094.9
  latent or 2 years or more after infection
    (without manifestations) 096
    negative spinal fluid test 096
    serology positive 096
  paresis 094.1
  specified site NEC 095.8
  symptomatic or with symptoms 095.9
  tabes 094.0
latent 097.1
  central nervous system 094.9
  date of infection unspecified 097.1
  early or less than 2 years after infection
    092.9
  late or 2 years or more after infection 096
  serology
    doubtful
      follow-up of latent syphilis 097.1
        central nervous system 094.9
        date of infection unspecified
          097.1
        early or less than 2 years after
          infection 092.9
        late or 2 years or more after
          infection 096
    positive, only finding 097.1
      date of infection unspecified
        097.1
      early or less than 2 years after in-
        fection 097.1
      late or 2 years or more after infec-
        tion 097.1
lens 095.8
leukoderma 091.3
  late 095.8
lienis 095.8
lip 091.3
  chancre 091.2
  late 095.8
  primary 091.2
Lissauer's paralysis 094.1
liver 095.3
  secondary 091.62
locomotor ataxia 094.0
lung 095.1
lymphadenitis (secondary) 091.4
lymph gland (early) (secondary) 091.4
  late 095.8
macular atrophy of skin 091.3
  striated 095.8
maternal, affecting fetus or newborn 760.2
  manifest syphilis in newborn — *see*
    Syphilis, congenital

Syphilis, syphilitic — *continued*
mediastinum (late) 095.8
meninges (adhesive) (basilar) (brain) (spinal
  cord) 094.2
meningitis 094.2
  acute 091.81
  congenital 090.42
meningoencephalitis 094.2
meningovascular 094.2
  congenital 090.49
mesarteritis 093.89
  brain 094.89
  spine 094.89
middle ear 095.8
mitral stenosis 093.21
monoplegia 094.89
mouth (secondary) 091.3
  late 095.8
mucocutaneous 091.3
  late 095.8
mucous
  membrane 091.3
    late 095.8
  patches 091.3
    congenital 090.0
mulberry molars 090.5
muscle 095.6
myocardium 093.82
myositis 095.6
nasal sinus 095.8
neonatorum NEC (*see also* Syphilis, congenital) 090.9
nerve palsy (any cranial nerve) 094.89
nervous system, central 094.9
neuritis 095.8
  acoustic nerve 094.86
neurorecidive of retina 094.83
neuroretinitis 094.85
newborn (*see also* Syphilis, congenital) 090.9
nodular superficial 095.8
nonvenereal, endemic 104.0
nose 095.8
  saddle back deformity 090.5
  septum 095.8
    perforated 095.8
occlusive arterial disease 093.89
ophthalmic 095.8 *[363.13]*
ophthalmoplegia 094.89
optic nerve (atrophy) (neuritis) (papilla)
  094.84
orbit (late) 095.8
orchitis 095.8
organic 097.9
osseous (late) 095.5
osteochondritis (congenital) 090.0
osteoporosis 095.5
ovary 095.8
oviduct 095.8
palate 095.8
  gumma 095.8
  perforated 090.5
pancreas (late) 095.8
pancreatitis 095.8
paralysis 094.89
  general 094.1
  juvenile 090.40
paraplegia 094.89
paresis (general) 094.1
  juvenile 090.40
paresthesia 094.89
Parkinson's disease or syndrome 094.82
paroxysmal tachycardia 093.89
pemphigus (congenital) 090.0
penis 091.0
  chancre 091.0
  late 095.8
pericardium 093.81
perichondritis, larynx 095.8
periosteum 095.5
  congenital 090.0
  early 091.61
  secondary 091.61
peripheral nerve 095.8
petrous bone (late) 095.5
pharynx 095.8
  secondary 091.3

Syphilis, syphilitic — *continued*
pituitary (gland) 095.8
placenta 095.8
pleura (late) 095.8
pneumonia, white 090.0
pontine (lesion) 094.89
portal vein 093.89
primary NEC 091.2
  anal 091.1
  and secondary (*see also* Syphilis, sec-
    ondary) 091.9
  cardiovascular 093.9
  central nervous system 094.9
  extragenital chancre NEC 091.2
  fingers 091.2
  genital 091.0
  lip 091.2
  specified site NEC 091.2
  tonsils 091.2
prostate 095.8
psychosis (intracranial gumma) 094.89
ptosis (eyelid) 094.89
pulmonary (late) 095.1
  artery 093.89
pulmonum 095.1
pyelonephritis 095.4
recently acquired, symptomatic NEC 091.89
rectum 095.8
respiratory tract 095.8
retina
  late 094.83
  neurorecidive 094.83
retrobulbar neuritis 094.85
salpingitis 095.8
sclera (late) 095.0
sclerosis
  cerebral 094.89
  coronary 093.89
  multiple 094.89
  subacute 094.89
scotoma (central) 095.8
scrotum 095.8
secondary (and primary) 091.9
  adenopathy 091.4
  anus 091.3
  bone 091.61
  cardiovascular 093.9
  central nervous system 094.9
  chorioretinitis, choroiditis 091.51
  hepatitis 091.62
  liver 091.62
  lymphadenitis 091.4
  meningitis, acute 091.81
  mouth 091.3
  mucous membranes 091.3
  periosteum 091.61
  periostitis 091.61
  pharynx 091.3
  relapse (treated) (untreated) 091.7
  skin 091.3
  specified form NEC 091.89
  tonsil 091.3
  ulcer 091.3
  viscera 091.69
  vulva 091.3
seminal vesicle (late) 095.8
seronegative
  with signs or symptoms — *see* Syphilis,
    by site or stage
seropositive
  with signs or symptoms — *see* Syphilis,
    by site and stage
  follow-up of latent syphilis — *see*
    Syphilis, latent
  only finding — *see* Syphilis, latent
seventh nerve (paralysis) 094.89
sinus 095.8
sinusitis 095.8
skeletal system 095.5
skin (early) (secondary) (with ulceration)
  091.3
  late or tertiary 095.8
small intestine 095.8
spastic spinal paralysis 094.0
spermatic cord (late) 095.8
spinal (cord) 094.89

☑ **Additional Digit Required** — Refer to the Tabular List for Digit Selection   ▽ **Subterms under main terms may continue to next column or page**

274 — Volume 2   ▶◀ Revised Text   ● New Line   ▲ Revised Code   **2011 ICD-9-CM**

Syphilis, syphilitic — *continued*
  spinal — *continued*
    with
      paresis 094.1
      tabes 094.0
  spleen 095.8
  splenomegaly 095.8
  spondylitis 095.5
  staphyloma 095.8
  stigmata (congenital) 090.5
  stomach 095.8
  synovium (late) 095.7
  tabes dorsalis (early) (late) 094.0
    juvenile 090.40
  tabetic type 094.0
    juvenile 090.40
  taboparesis 094.1
    juvenile 090.40
  tachycardia 093.89
  tendon (late) 095.7
  tertiary 097.0
    with symptoms 095.8
    cardiovascular 093.9
    central nervous system 094.9
    multiple NEC 095.8
    specified site NEC 095.8
  testis 095.8
  thorax 095.8
  throat 095.8
  thymus (gland) 095.8
  thyroid (late) 095.8
  tongue 095.8
  tonsil (lingual) 095.8
    primary 091.2
    secondary 091.3
  trachea 095.8
  tricuspid valve 093.23
  tumor, brain 094.89
  tunica vaginalis (late) 095.8
  ulcer (any site) (early) (secondary) 091.3
    late 095.9
      perforating 095.9
        foot 094.0
  urethra (stricture) 095.8
  urogenital 095.8
  uterus 095.8
  uveal tract (secondary) 091.50
    late 095.8 [363.13]
  uveitis (secondary) 091.50
    late 095.8 [363.13]
  uvula (late) 095.8
    perforated 095.8
  vagina 091.0
    late 095.8
  valvulitis NEC 093.20
  vascular 093.89
    brain or cerebral 094.89
  vein 093.89
    cerebral 094.89
  ventriculi 095.8
  vesicae urinariae 095.8
  viscera (abdominal) 095.2
    secondary 091.69
  vitreous (hemorrhage) (opacities) 095.8
  vulva 091.0
    late 095.8
    secondary 091.3
Syphiloma 095.9
  cardiovascular system 093.9
  central nervous system 094.9
  circulatory system 093.9
  congenital 090.5
Syphilophobia 300.29
Syringadenoma (M8400/0) — *see also* Neoplasm, skin, benign
  papillary (M8406/0) — *see* Neoplasm, skin, benign
Syringobulbia 336.0
Syringocarcinoma (M8400/3) — *see* Neoplasm, skin, malignant
Syringocystadenoma (M8400/0) — *see also* Neoplasm, skin, benign
  papillary (M8406/0) — *see* Neoplasm, skin, benign
Syringocystoma (M8407/0) — *see* Neoplasm, skin, benign

Syringoma (M8407/0) — *see also* Neoplasm, skin, benign
  chondroid (M8940/0) — *see* Neoplasm, by site, benign
Syringomyelia 336.0
Syringomyelitis 323.9
  late effect — *see* category 326
Syringomyelocele — *see also* Spina bifida 741.9 ☑
Syringopontia 336.0
  disease, combined — *see* Degeneration, combined
  fibrosclerosing syndrome 710.8
  inflammatory response syndrome (SIRS) 995.90
    due to
      infectious process 995.91
        with organ dysfunction 995.92
      non-infectious process 995.93
        with organ dysfunction 995.94
  lupus erythematosus 710.0
    inhibitor 286.5
System, systemic — *see also* condition
  disease, combined — *see* Degeneration, combined
  fibrosclerosing syndrome 710.8
  inflammatory response syndrome (SIRS) 995.90
    due to
      infectious process 995.91
        with acute organ dysfunction 995.92
      non-infectious process 995.93
        with acute organ dysfunction 995.94
  lupus erythematosus 710.0
    inhibitor 286.5

T

Tab — *see* Tag
Tabacism 989.84
Tabacosis 989.84
Tabardillo 080
  flea-borne 081.0
  louse-borne 080
Tabes, tabetic
  with
    central nervous system syphilis 094.0
    Charcôt's joint 094.0 [713.5]
    cord bladder 094.0
    crisis, viscera (any) 094.0
    paralysis, general 094.1
    paresis (general) 094.1
    perforating ulcer 094.0
  arthropathy 094.0 [713.5]
  bladder 094.0
  bone 094.0
  cerebrospinal 094.0
  congenital 090.40
  conjugal 094.0
  dorsalis 094.0
    neurosyphilis 094.0
  early 094.0
  juvenile 090.40
  latent 094.0
  mesenterica (*see also* Tuberculosis) 014.8 ☑
  paralysis insane, general 094.1
  peripheral (nonsyphilitic) 799.89
  spasmodic 094.0
    not dorsal or dorsalis 343.9
  syphilis (cerebrospinal) 094.0
Taboparalysis 094.1
Taboparesis (remission) 094.1
  with
    Charcôt's joint 094.1 [713.5]
    cord bladder 094.1
    perforating ulcer 094.1
  juvenile 090.40
Tache noir 923.20
Tachyalimentation 579.3
Tachyarrhythmia, tachyrhythmia — *see also* Tachycardia
  paroxysmal with sinus bradycardia 427.81
Tachycardia 785.0
  atrial 427.89
  auricular 427.89

Tachycardia — *continued*
  AV nodal re-entry (re-entrant) 427.89
  junctional ectopic 427.0
  newborn 779.82
  nodal 427.89
    nonparoxysmal atrioventricular 426.89
    nonparoxysmal atrioventricular (nodal) 426.89
  nonsustained 427.2
  paroxysmal 427.2
    with sinus bradycardia 427.81
    atrial (PAT) 427.0
      psychogenic 316 [427.0]
    atrioventricular (AV) 427.0
      psychogenic 316 [427.0]
    essential 427.2
    junctional 427.0
    nodal 427.0
    psychogenic 316 [427.2]
      atrial 316 [427.0]
      supraventricular 316 [427.0]
      ventricular 316 [427.1]
    supraventricular 427.0
      psychogenic 316 [427.0]
    ventricular 427.1
      psychogenic 316 [427.1]
  postoperative 997.1
  psychogenic 306.2
  sick sinus 427.81
  sinoauricular 427.89
  sinus 427.89
  supraventricular 427.89
  sustained 427.2
    supraventricular 427.0
    ventricular 427.1
  ventricular (paroxysmal) 427.1
    psychogenic 316 [427.1]
Tachygastria 536.8
Tachypnea 786.06
  hysterical 300.11
  newborn (idiopathic) (transitory) 770.6
  psychogenic 306.1
  transitory, of newborn 770.6
TACO (transfusion associated circulatory ● overload) 276.61 ●
Taenia (infection) (infestation) — *see also* Infestation, taenia 123.3
  diminuta 123.6
  echinococcal infestation (*see also* Echinococcus) 122.9
  nana 123.6
  saginata infestation 123.2
  solium (intestinal form) 123.0
    larval form 123.1
Taeniasis (intestine) — *see also* Infestation, taenia 123.3
  saginata 123.2
  solium 123.0
Taenzer's disease 757.4
Tag (hypertrophied skin) (infected) 701.9
  adenoid 474.8
  anus 455.9
  endocardial (*see also* Endocarditis) 424.90
  hemorrhoidal 455.9
  hymen 623.8
  perineal 624.8
  preauricular 744.1
  rectum 455.9
  sentinel 455.9
  skin 701.9
    accessory 757.39
    anus 455.9
    congenital 757.39
    preauricular 744.1
    rectum 455.9
  tonsil 474.8
  urethra, urethral 599.84
  vulva 624.8
Tahyna fever 062.5
Takayasu (-Onishi) disease or syndrome (pulseless disease) 446.7
Takotsubo syndrome 429.83
Talc granuloma 728.82
  in operation wound 998.7
Talcosis 502
Talipes (congenital) 754.70

Talipes — *continued*
  acquired NEC 736.79
    planus 734
  asymmetric 754.79
    acquired 736.79
  calcaneovalgus 754.62
    acquired 736.76
  calcaneovarus 754.59
    acquired 736.76
  calcaneus 754.79
    acquired 736.76
  cavovarus 754.59
    acquired 736.75
  cavus 754.71
    acquired 736.73
  equinovalgus 754.69
    acquired 736.72
  equinovarus 754.51
    acquired 736.71
  equinus 754.79
    acquired, NEC 736.72
  percavus 754.71
    acquired 736.73
  planovalgus 754.69
    acquired 736.79
  planus (acquired) (any degree) 734
    congenital 754.61
    due to rickets 268.1
  valgus 754.60
    acquired 736.79
  varus 754.50
    acquired 736.79
Talma's disease 728.85
Talon noir 924.20
  hand 923.20
  heel 924.20
  toe 924.3
Tamponade heart (Rose's) — *see also* Pericarditis 423.3
Tanapox 059.21
Tangier disease (familial high-density lipoprotein deficiency) 272.5
Tank ear 380.12
Tantrum (childhood) — *see also* Disturbance, conduct 312.1 ☑
Tapeworm (infection) (infestation) — *see also* Infestation, tapeworm 123.9
Tapia's syndrome 352.6
Tarantism 297.8
Target-oval cell anemia 282.49
Tarlov's cyst 355.9
Tarral-Besnier disease (pityriasis rubra pilaris) 696.4
Tarsalgia 729.2
Tarsal tunnel syndrome 355.5
Tarsitis (eyelid) 373.00
  syphilitic 095.8 [373.00]
  tuberculous (*see also* Tuberculosis) 017.0 ☑ [373.4]
Tartar (teeth) 523.6
Tattoo (mark) 709.09
Taurodontism 520.2
Taussig-Bing defect, heart, or syndrome (transposition, aorta and overriding pulmonary artery) 745.11
Taybi's syndrome (otopalatodigital) 759.89
Tay's choroiditis 363.41
Taylor's
  disease (diffuse idiopathic cutaneous atrophy) 701.8
  syndrome 625.5
Tay-Sachs
  amaurotic familial idiocy 330.1
  disease 330.1
TBI (traumatic brain injury) — *see also* Injury, intracranial 854.0 ☑
  with skull fracture — *see* Fracture, skull, by site
Tear stone 375.57
Tear, torn (traumatic) — *see also* Wound, open, by site
  anus, anal (sphincter) 863.89
    with open wound in cavity 863.99
    complicating delivery (healed) (old) 654.8 ☑
      with mucosa 664.3 ☑

☑ **Additional Digit Required** — Refer to the Tabular List for Digit Selection   ▽ **Subterms under main terms may continue to next column or page**

2011 ICD-9-CM   ▶◀ Revised Text   ● New Line   ▲ Revised Code   October 2010 · Volume 2 — 275

Tear, torn — *see also* Wound, open, by site — *continued*

anus, anal — *continued*

complicating delivery — *continued*

not associated with third-degree perineal laceration 664.6 ☑

nontraumatic, nonpuerperal (healed) (old) 569.43

articular cartilage, old (*see also* Disorder, cartilage, articular) 718.0 ☑

bladder

with

abortion — *see* Abortion, by type, with damage to pelvic organs

ectopic pregnancy (*see also* categories 633.0–633.9) 639.2

molar pregnancy (*see also* categories 630–632) 639.2

following

abortion 639.2

ectopic or molar pregnancy 639.2

obstetrical trauma 665.5 ☑

bowel

with

abortion — *see* Abortion, by type, with damage to pelvic organs

ectopic pregnancy (*see also* categories 633.0–633.9) 639.2

molar pregnancy (*see also* categories 630–632) 639.2

following

abortion 639.2

ectopic or molar pregnancy 639.2

obstetrical trauma 665.5 ☑

broad ligament

with

abortion — *see* Abortion, by type, with damage to pelvic organs

ectopic pregnancy (*see also* categories 633.0–633.9) 639.2

molar pregnancy (*see also* categories 630–632) 639.2

following

abortion 639.2

ectopic or molar pregnancy 639.2

obstetrical trauma 665.6 ☑

bucket handle (knee) (meniscus) — *see* Tear, meniscus

capsule

joint — *see* Sprain, by site

spleen — *see* Laceration, spleen, capsule

cartilage (*see also* Sprain, by site)

articular, old (*see also* Disorder, cartilage, articular) 718.0 ☑

knee — *see* Tear, meniscus

semilunar (knee) (current injury) — *see* Tear, meniscus

cervix

with

abortion — *see* Abortion, by type, with damage to pelvic organs

ectopic pregnancy (*see also* categories 633.0–633.9) 639.2

molar pregnancy (*see also* categories 630–632) 639.2

following

abortion 639.2

ectopic or molar pregnancy 639.2

obstetrical trauma (current) 665.3 ☑

old 622.3

dural 349.31

accidental puncture or laceration during a procedure 349.31

incidental (inadvertent) 349.31

nontraumatic NEC 349.39

internal organ (abdomen, chest, or pelvis) — *see* Injury, internal, by site

ligament (*see also* Sprain, by site)

with open wound — *see* Wound, open by site

meniscus (knee) (current injury) 836.2

bucket handle 836.0

old 717.0

lateral 836.1

anterior horn 836.1

old 717.42

Tear, torn — *see also* Wound, open, by site — *continued*

meniscus — *continued*

lateral — *continued*

bucket handle 836.1

old 717.41

old 717.40

posterior horn 836.1

old 717.43

specified site NEC 836.1

old 717.49

medial 836.0

anterior horn 836.0

old 717.1

bucket handle 836.0

old 717.0

old 717.3

posterior horn 836.0

old 717.2

old NEC 717.5

site other than knee — *see* Sprain, by site

muscle (*see also* Sprain, by site)

with open wound — *see* Wound, open by site

pelvic

floor, complicating delivery 664.1 ☑

organ NEC

with

abortion — *see* Abortion, by type, with damage to pelvic organs

ectopic pregnancy (*see also* categories 633.0–633.9) 639.2

molar pregnancy (*see also* categories 630–632) 639.2

following

abortion 639.2

ectopic or molar pregnancy 639.2

obstetrical trauma 665.5 ☑

perineum (*see also* Laceration, perineum)

obstetrical trauma 665.5 ☑

periurethral tissue

with

abortion — *see* Abortion, by type, with damage to pelvic organs

ectopic pregnancy (*see also* categories 633.0–633.9) 639.2

molar pregnancy (*see also* categories 630–632) 639.2

following

abortion 639.2

ectopic or molar pregnancy 639.2

obstetrical trauma 664.8 ☑   ▲

rectovaginal septum — *see* Laceration, rectovaginal septum

retina, retinal (recent) (with detachment) 361.00

without detachment 361.30

dialysis (juvenile) (with detachment) 361.04

giant (with detachment) 361.03

horseshoe (without detachment) 361.32

multiple (with detachment) 361.02

without detachment 361.33

old

delimited (partial) 361.06

partial 361.06

total or subtotal 361.07

partial (without detachment)

giant 361.03

multiple defects 361.02

old (delimited) 361.06

single defect 361.01

round hole (without detachment) 361.31

single defect (with detachment) 361.01

total or subtotal (recent) 361.05

old 361.07

rotator cuff (traumatic) 840.4

current injury 840.4

degenerative 726.10

nontraumatic 727.61

semilunar cartilage, knee (*see also* Tear, meniscus) 836.2

old 717.5

tendon (*see also* Sprain, by site)

Tear, torn — *see also* Wound, open, by site — *continued*

tendon (*see also* Sprain, by site) — *continued*

with open wound — *see* Wound, open by site

tentorial, at birth 767.0

umbilical cord

affecting fetus or newborn 772.0

complicating delivery 663.8 ☑

urethra

with

abortion — *see* Abortion, by type, with damage to pelvic organs

ectopic pregnancy (*see also* categories 633.0–633.9) 639.2

molar pregnancy (*see also* categories 630–632) 639.2

following

abortion 639.2

ectopic or molar pregnancy 639.2

obstetrical trauma 665.5 ☑

uterus — *see* Injury, internal, uterus

vagina — *see* Laceration, vagina

vessel, from catheter 998.2

vulva, complicating delivery 664.0 ☑

Teething 520.7

syndrome 520.7

Teeth, tooth — *see also* condition

grinding 306.8

prenatal 520.6

Tegmental syndrome 344.89

Telangiectasia, telangiectasis (verrucous) 448.9

ataxic (cerebellar) 334.8

familial 448.0

hemorrhagic, hereditary (congenital) (senile) 448.0

hereditary hemorrhagic 448.0

retina 362.15

spider 448.1

Telecanthus (congenital) 743.63

Telescoped bowel or intestine — *see also* Intussusception 560.0

Teletherapy, adverse effect NEC 990

Telogen effluvium 704.02

Temperature

body, high (of unknown origin) (*see also* Pyrexia) 780.60

cold, trauma from 991.9

newborn 778.2

specified effect NEC 991.8

high

body (of unknown origin) (*see also* Pyrexia) 780.60

trauma from — *see* Heat

Temper tantrum (childhood) — *see also* Disturbance, conduct 312.1 ☑

Temple — *see* condition

Temporal — *see also* condition

lobe syndrome 310.0

Temporomandibular joint-pain-dysfunction syndrome 524.60

Temporosphenoidal — *see* condition

Tendency

bleeding (*see also* Defect, coagulation) 286.9

homosexual, ego-dystonic 302.0

paranoid 301.0

suicide 300.9

Tenderness

abdominal (generalized) (localized) 789.6 ☑

rebound 789.6 ☑

skin 782.0

Tendinitis, tendonitis — *see also* Tenosynovitis 726.90

Achilles 726.71

adhesive 726.90

shoulder 726.0

calcific 727.82

shoulder 726.11

gluteal 726.5

patellar 726.64

peroneal 726.79

pes anserinus 726.61

psoas 726.5

tibialis (anterior) (posterior) 726.72

Tendinitis, tendonitis — *see also* Tenosynovitis — *continued*

trochanteric 726.5

Tendon — *see* condition

Tendosynovitis — *see* Tenosynovitis

Tendovaginitis — *see* Tenosynovitis

Tenesmus 787.99

rectal 787.99

vesical 788.99

Tenia — *see* Taenia

Teniasis — *see* Taeniasis

Tennis elbow 726.32

Tenonitis — *see also* Tenosynovitis

eye (capsule) 376.04

Tenontosynovitis — *see* Tenosynovitis

Tenontothecitis — *see* Tenosynovitis

Tenophyte 727.9

Tenosynovitis (*see also* Synovitis) 727.00

adhesive 726.90

shoulder 726.0

ankle 727.06

bicipital (calcifying) 726.12

buttock 727.09

due to crystals — *see* Arthritis, due to crystals

elbow 727.09

finger 727.05

foot 727.06

gonococcal 098.51

hand 727.05

hip 727.09

knee 727.09

radial styloid 727.04

shoulder 726.10

adhesive 726.0

specified NEC 727.09

spine 720.1

supraspinatus 726.10

toe 727.06

tuberculous — *see* Tuberculosis, tenosynovitis

wrist 727.05

Tenovaginitis — *see* Tenosynovitis

Tension

arterial, high (*see also* Hypertension) 401.9

without diagnosis of hypertension 796.2

headache 307.81

intraocular (elevated) 365.00

nervous 799.21

ocular (elevated) 365.00

pneumothorax 512.0

iatrogenic 512.1

postoperative 512.1

spontaneous 512.0

premenstrual 625.4

state 300.9

Tentorium — *see* condition

Teratencephalus 759.89

Teratism 759.7

Teratoblastoma (malignant) (M9080/3) — *see* Neoplasm, by site, malignant

Teratocarcinoma (M9081/3) — *see also* Neoplasm, by site, malignant

liver 155.0

Teratoma (solid) (M9080/1) — *see also* Neoplasm, by site, uncertain behavior

adult (cystic) (M9080/0) — *see* Neoplasm, by site, benign

and embryonal carcinoma, mixed (M9081/3) — *see* Neoplasm, by site, malignant

benign (M9080/0) — *see* Neoplasm, by site, benign

combined with choriocarcinoma (M9101/3) — *see* Neoplasm, by site, malignant

cystic (adult) (M9080/0) — *see* Neoplasm, by site, benign

differentiated type (M9080/0) — *see* Neoplasm, by site, benign

embryonal (M9080/3) (*see also* Neoplasm, by site, malignant)

liver 155.0

fetal

sacral, causing fetopelvic disproportion 653.7 ☑

immature (M9080/3) — *see* Neoplasm, by site, malignant

☑ **Additional Digit Required** — Refer to the Tabular List for Digit Selection   ▽ **Subterms under main terms may continue to next column or page**

276 — Volume 2 • October 2010   ▶◀ **Revised Text**   ● **New Line**   ▲ **Revised Code**   2011 ICD-9-CM

Tear, torn — Teratoma

Teratoma — *see also* Neoplasm, by site, uncertain behavior — *continued*
  liver (M9080/3) 155.0
    adult, benign, cystic, differentiated type or mature (M9080/0) 211.5
  malignant (M9080/3) (*see also* Neoplasm, by site, malignant)
    anaplastic type (M9082/3) — *see* Neoplasm, by site, malignant
    intermediate type (M9083/3) — *see* Neoplasm, by site, malignant
    liver (M9080/3) 155.0
    trophoblastic (M9102/3)
      specified site — *see* Neoplasm, by site, malignant
      unspecified site 186.9
    undifferentiated type (M9082/3) — *see* Neoplasm, by site, malignant
  mature (M9080/0) — *see* Neoplasm, by site, benign
    malignant (M9080/3) — *see* Neoplasm, by site, malignant
  ovary (M9080/0) 220
    embryonal, immature, or malignant (M9080/3) 183.0
  suprasellar (M9080/3) — *see* Neoplasm, by site, malignant
  testis (M9080/3) 186.9
    adult, benign, cystic, differentiated type or mature (M9080/0) 222.0
    undescended 186.0
Terminal care V66.7
Termination
  anomalous (*see also* Malposition, congenital)
    portal vein 747.49
    right pulmonary vein 747.42
  pregnancy (legal) (therapeutic) — *see* Abortion, legal 635.9 ☑
    fetus NEC 779.6
    illegal (*see also* Abortion, illegal) 636.9 ☑
Ternidens diminutus infestation 127.7
Terrors, night (child) 307.46
Terry's syndrome (*see also* Retinopathy of prematurity) 362.21
Tertiary — *see* condition
Tessellated fundus, retina (tigroid) 362.89
Test(s)
  adequacy
    hemodialysis V56.31
    peritoneal dialysis V56.32
  AIDS virus V72.69
  allergen V72.7
  bacterial disease NEC (*see also* Screening, by name of disease) V74.9
  basal metabolic rate V72.69
  blood
    alcohol V70.4
    drug V70.4
      for therapeutic drug monitoring V58.83
      for routine general physical examination V72.62
      prior to treatment or procedure V72.63
    typing V72.86
      Rh typing V72.86
  developmental, infant or child V20.2
  Dick V74.8
  fertility V26.21
  genetic
    female V26.32
    for genetic disease carrier status
      female V26.31
      male V26.34
    male V26.39
  hearing V72.19
    following failed hearing screening V72.11
    routine, for infant and child V20.2
  HIV V72.69
  human immunodeficiency virus V72.69
  immunity status V72.61
  Kveim V82.89
  laboratory V72.60
    for medicolegal reason V70.4

Test(s) — *continued*
  laboratory — *continued*
    ordered as part of a routine general medical examination V72.62
    pre-operative V72.63
    pre-procedural V72.63
    specified NEC V72.69
  male partner of ▶female with recurrent pregnancy loss◀ V26.35
  Mantoux (for tuberculosis) V74.1
  mycotic organism V75.4
  nuchal translucency V28.89
  parasitic agent NEC V75.8
  paternity V70.4
  peritoneal equilibration V56.32
  pregnancy
    negative result V72.41
    positive result V72.42
      first pregnancy V72.42
    unconfirmed V72.40
  preoperative V72.84
    cardiovascular V72.81
    respiratory V72.82
    specified NEC V72.83
  procreative management NEC V26.29
    genetic disease carrier status
      female V26.31
      male V26.34
  Rh typing V72.86
  sarcoidosis V82.89
  Schick V74.3
  Schultz-Charlton V74.8
  skin, diagnostic
    allergy V72.7
    bacterial agent NEC (*see also* Screening, by name of disease) V74.9
    Dick V74.8
    hypersensitivity V72.7
    Kveim V82.89
    Mantoux V74.1
    mycotic organism V75.4
    parasitic agent NEC V75.8
    sarcoidosis V82.89
    Schick V74.3
    Schultz-Charlton V74.8
    tuberculin V74.1
  specified type NEC V72.85
  tuberculin V74.1
  vision V72.0
    routine, for infant and child V20.2
  Wassermann
    positive (*see also* Serology for syphilis, positive) 097.1
    false 795.6
Testicle, testicular, testis — *see also* condition
  feminization (syndrome) 259.51
Tetanus, tetanic (cephalic) (convulsions) 037
  with
    abortion — *see* Abortion, by type, with sepsis
    ectopic pregnancy (*see also* categories 633.0–633.9) 639.0
    molar pregnancy — *see* categories 630–632 639.0
  following
    abortion 639.0
    ectopic or molar pregnancy 639.0
  inoculation V03.7
    reaction (due to serum) — *see* Complications, vaccination
  neonatorum 771.3
  puerperal, postpartum, childbirth 670.8 ☑
Tetany, tetanic 781.7
  alkalosis 276.3
  associated with rickets 268.0
  convulsions 781.7
    hysterical 300.11
  functional (hysterical) 300.11
  hyperkinetic 781.7
    hysterical 300.11
  hyperpnea 786.01
    hysterical 300.11
    psychogenic 306.1
  hyperventilation 786.01
    hysterical 300.11
    psychogenic 306.1

Tetany, tetanic — *continued*
  hypocalcemic, neonatal 775.4
  hysterical 300.11
  neonatal 775.4
  parathyroid (gland) 252.1
  parathyroprival 252.1
  postoperative 252.1
  postthyroidectomy 252.1
  pseudotetany 781.7
    hysterical 300.11
  psychogenic 306.1
    specified as conversion reaction 300.11
Tetralogy of Fallot 745.2
Tetraplegia — *see* Quadriplegia
Thailand hemorrhagic fever 065.4
Thalassanemia 282.49
Thalassemia (alpha) (beta) (disease) (Hb-C) (Hb-D) (Hb-E) (Hb-H) (Hb-I) (high fetal gene) (high fetal hemoglobin) (intermedia) (major) (minima) (minor) (mixed) (trait) (with other hemoglobinopathy) 282.49
  Hb-S (without crisis) 282.41
    with
      crisis 282.42
      vaso-occlusive pain 282.42
  sickle-cell (without crisis) 282.41
    with
      crisis 282.42
      vaso-occlusive pain 282.42
Thalassemic variants 282.49
Thaysen-Gee disease (nontropical sprue) 579.0
Thecoma (M8600/0) 220
  malignant (M8600/3) 183.0
Thelarche, precocious 259.1
Thelitis 611.0
  puerperal, postpartum 675.0 ☑
Therapeutic — *see* condition
Therapy V57.9
  blood transfusion, without reported diagnosis V58.2
  breathing V57.0
  chemotherapy, antineoplastic V58.11
    fluoride V07.31
    prophylactic NEC V07.39
  dialysis (intermittent) (treatment)
    extracorporeal V56.0
    peritoneal V56.8
    renal V56.0
    specified type NEC V56.8
  exercise NEC V57.1
    breathing V57.0
  extracorporeal dialysis (renal) V56.0
  fluoride prophylaxis V07.31
  hemodialysis V56.0
  hormone replacement (postmenopausal) V07.4
  immunotherapy antineoplastic V58.12
  long term oxygen therapy V46.2
  occupational V57.21
  orthoptic V57.4
  orthotic V57.81
  peritoneal dialysis V56.8
  physical NEC V57.1
  postmenopausal hormone replacement V07.4
  radiation V58.0
  speech (-language) V57.3
  vocational V57.22
Thermalgesia 782.0
Thermalgia 782.0
Thermanalgesia 782.0
Thermanesthesia 782.0
Thermic — *see* condition
Thermography (abnormal) 793.99
  breast 793.89
Thermoplegia 992.0
Thesaurismosis
  amyloid 277.39
  bilirubin 277.4
  calcium 275.40
  cystine 270.0
  glycogen (*see also* Disease, glycogen storage) 271.0
  kerasin 272.7

Thesaurismosis — *continued*
  lipoid 272.7
  melanin 255.41
  phosphatide 272.7
  urate 274.9
Thiaminic deficiency 265.1
  with beriberi 265.0
Thibierge-Weissenbach syndrome (cutaneous systemic sclerosis) 710.1
Thickened endometrium 793.5
Thickening
  bone 733.99
    extremity 733.99
  breast 611.79
  hymen 623.3
  larynx 478.79
  nail 703.8
    congenital 757.5
  periosteal 733.99
  pleura (*see also* Pleurisy) 511.0
  skin 782.8
  subepiglottic 478.79
  tongue 529.8
  valve, heart — *see* Endocarditis
Thiele syndrome 724.6
Thigh — *see* condition
Thinning vertebra — *see also* Osteoporosis 733.00
Thirst, excessive 783.5
  due to deprivation of water 994.3
Thomsen's disease 359.22
Thomson's disease (congenital poikiloderma) 757.33
Thoracic — *see also* condition
  kidney 753.3
  outlet syndrome 353.0
  stomach — *see* Hernia, diaphragm
Thoracogastroschisis (congenital) 759.89
Thoracopagus 759.4
Thoracoschisis 756.3
Thoracoscopic surgical procedure converted to open procedure V64.42
Thorax — *see* condition
Thorn's syndrome — *see also* Disease, renal 593.9
Thornwaldt's, Tornwaldt's
  bursitis (pharyngeal) 478.29
  cyst 478.26
  disease (pharyngeal bursitis) 478.29
Thorson-Biörck syndrome (malignant carcinoid) 259.2
Threadworm (infection) (infestation) 127.4
Threatened
  abortion or miscarriage 640.0 ☑
    with subsequent abortion (*see also* Abortion, spontaneous) 634.9 ☑
    affecting fetus 762.1
  labor 644.1 ☑
    affecting fetus or newborn 761.8
    premature 644.0 ☑
  miscarriage 640.0 ☑
    affecting fetus 762.1
  premature
    delivery 644.2 ☑
      affecting fetus or newborn 761.8
    labor 644.0 ☑
      before 22 completed weeks gestation 640.0 ☑
Three-day fever 066.0
Threshers' lung 495.0
Thrix annulata (congenital) 757.4
Throat — *see* condition
Thrombasthenia (Glanzmann's) (hemorrhagic) (hereditary) 287.1
Thromboangiitis 443.1
  obliterans (general) 443.1
    cerebral 437.1
    vessels
      brain 437.1
      spinal cord 437.1
Thromboarteritis — *see* Arteritis
Thromboasthenia (Glanzmann's) (hemorrhagic) (hereditary) 287.1
Thrombocytasthenia (Glanzmann's) 287.1
Thrombocythemia (primary) (M9962/1) 238.71
  essential 238.71

☑ **Additional Digit Required** — Refer to the Tabular List for Digit Selection

▿ **Subterms under main terms may continue to next column or page**

Thrombocythemia — *continued*
  hemorrhagic 238.71
  idiopathic (hemorrhagic) (M9962/1) 238.71
Thrombocytopathy (dystrophic) (granu-
    lopenic) 287.1
Thrombocytopenia, thrombocytopenic 287.5
  with
      absent radii (TAR) syndrome
      giant hemangioma
  amegakaryocytic, congenital 287.33
  congenital 287.33
  cyclic 287.39
  dilutional 287.49   ▲
  due to
      drugs 287.49   ▲
      extracorporeal circulation of blood
          287.49   ▲
      massive blood transfusion 287.49   ▲
      platelet alloimmunization 287.49   ▲
  essential 287.30
  fetal 678.0 ☑
  heparin-induced (HIT) 289.84
  hereditary 287.33
  Kasabach-Merritt 287.39
  neonatal, transitory 776.1
      due to
          exchange transfusion 776.1
          idiopathic maternal thrombocytope-
              nia 776.1
          isoimmunization 776.1
  primary 287.30
  puerperal, postpartum 666.3 ☑
  purpura (*see also* Purpura, thrombocy-
      topenic) 287.30
      thrombotic 446.6
  secondary ▶NEC◀ 287.49   ▲
  sex-linked 287.39
Thrombocytosis 238.71
  essential 238.71
  primary 238.71
Thromboembolism — *see* Embolism
Thrombopathy (Bernard-Soulier) 287.1
  constitutional 286.4
  Willebrand-Jürgens (angiohemophilia) 286.4
Thrombopenia — *see also* Thrombocytopenia
    287.5
Thrombophlebitis 451.9
  antecubital vein 451.82
  antepartum (superficial) 671.2 ☑
      affecting fetus or newborn 760.3
      deep 671.3 ☑
  arm 451.89
      deep 451.83
      superficial 451.82
  breast, superficial 451.89
  cavernous (venous) sinus — *see* Throm-
      bophlebitis, intracranial venous sinus
  cephalic vein 451.82
  cerebral (sinus) (vein) 325
      late effect — *see* category 326
      nonpyogenic 437.6
          in pregnancy or puerperium 671.5 ☑
          late effect — *see* Late effect(s) (of)
              cerebrovascular disease
  due to implanted device — *see* Complica-
      tions, due to (presence of) any de-
      vice, implant or graft classified to
      996.0–996.5 NEC
  during or resulting from a procedure NEC
      997.2
  femoral 451.11
  femoropopliteal 451.19
  following infusion, perfusion, or transfusion
      999.2
  hepatic (vein) 451.89
  idiopathic, recurrent 453.1
  iliac vein 451.81
  iliofemoral 451.11
  intracranial venous sinus (any) 325
      late effect — *see* category 326
      nonpyogenic 437.6
          in pregnancy or puerperium 671.5 ☑
          late effect — *see* Late effect(s) (of)
              cerebrovascular disease
  jugular vein 451.89

Thrombophlebitis — *continued*
  lateral (venous) sinus — *see* Throm-
      bophlebitis, intracranial venous sinus
  leg 451.2
      deep (vessels) 451.19
          femoral 451.11
          specified vessel NEC 451.19
      superficial (vessels) 451.0
          femoral vein 451.11
  longitudinal (venous) sinus — *see* Throm-
      bophlebitis, intracranial venous sinus
  lower extremity 451.2
      deep (vessels) 451.19
          femoral 451.11
          specified vessel NEC 451.19
      superficial (vessels) 451.0
  migrans, migrating 453.1
  pelvic
      with
          abortion — *see* Abortion, by type,
              with sepsis
          ectopic pregnancy (*see also* cate-
              gories 633.0–633.9) 639.0
          molar pregnancy (*see also* categories
              630–632) 639.0
      following
          abortion 639.0
          ectopic or molar pregnancy 639.0
      puerperal 671.4 ☑
  popliteal vein 451.19
  portal (vein) 572.1
  postoperative 997.2
  pregnancy (superficial) 671.2 ☑
      affecting fetus or newborn 760.3
      deep 671.3 ☑
  puerperal, postpartum, childbirth (extremi-
      ties) (superficial) 671.2 ☑
      deep 671.4 ☑
      pelvic 671.4 ☑
      septic 670.3 ☑
      specified site NEC 671.5 ☑
  radial vein 451.83
  saphenous (greater) (lesser) 451.0
  sinus (intracranial) — *see* Thrombophlebitis,
      intracranial venous sinus
  specified site NEC 451.89
  tibial vein 451.19

Thrombosis, thrombotic (maranic) (multiple)
    (progressive) (vein) (vessel) 453.9
  with childbirth or during the puerperium
      — *see* Thrombosis, puerperal, post-
      partum
  antepartum — *see* Thrombosis, pregnancy
  aorta, aortic 444.1
      abdominal 444.0
      bifurcation 444.0
      saddle 444.0
      terminal 444.0
      thoracic 444.1
      valve — *see* Endocarditis, aortic
  apoplexy (*see also* Thrombosis, brain)
      434.0 ☑
      late effect — *see* Late effect(s) (of) cere-
          brovascular disease
  appendix, septic — *see* Appendicitis, acute
  arteriolar-capillary platelet, disseminated
      446.6
  artery, arteries (postinfectional) 444.9
      auditory, internal 433.8 ☑
      basilar (*see also* Occlusion, artery, basilar)
          433.0 ☑
      carotid (common) (internal) (*see also*
          Occlusion, artery, carotid)
          433.1 ☑
          with other precerebral artery
              433.3 ☑
      cerebellar (anterior inferior) (posterior
          inferior) (superior) 433.8 ☑
      cerebral (*see also* Thrombosis, brain)
          434.0 ☑
      choroidal (anterior) 433.8 ☑
      communicating posterior 433.8 ☑
      coronary (*see also* Infarct, myocardium)
          410.9 ☑
          without myocardial infarction 411.81
          due to syphilis 093.89

Thrombosis, thrombotic — *continued*
  artery, arteries — *continued*
      coronary (*see also* Infarct, myocardium)
          — *continued*
          healed or specified as old 412
      extremities 444.22
          lower 444.22
          upper 444.21
      femoral 444.22
      hepatic 444.89
      hypophyseal 433.8 ☑
      meningeal, anterior or posterior
          433.8 ☑
      mesenteric (with gangrene) 557.0
      ophthalmic (*see also* Occlusion, retina)
          362.30
      pontine 433.8 ☑
      popliteal 444.22
      precerebral — *see* Occlusion, artery,
          precerebral NEC
      pulmonary 415.19
          iatrogenic 415.11
          personal history of V12.51
          postoperative 415.11
          septic 415.12
      renal 593.81
      retinal (*see also* Occlusion, retina) 362.30
      specified site NEC 444.89
      spinal, anterior or posterior 433.8 ☑
      traumatic (complication) (early) (*see also*
          Injury, blood vessel, by site) 904.9
      vertebral (*see also* Occlusion, artery, ver-
          tebral) 433.2 ☑
          with other precerebral artery
              433.3 ☑
  atrial (endocardial) 424.90
      without endocarditis 429.89
      due to syphilis 093.89
  auricular (*see also* Infarct, myocardium)
      410.9 ☑
  axillary (acute) (vein) 453.84
      chronic 453.74
      personal history of V12.51
  basilar (artery) (*see also* Occlusion, artery,
      basilar) 433.0 ☑
  bland NEC 453.9
  brain (artery) (stem) 434.0 ☑
      due to syphilis 094.89
      iatrogenic 997.02
      late effect — *see* Late effect(s) (of) cere-
          brovascular disease
      postoperative 997.02
      puerperal, postpartum, childbirth
          674.0 ☑
      sinus (*see also* Thrombosis, intracranial
          venous sinus) 325
  capillary 448.9
      arteriolar, generalized 446.6
  cardiac (*see also* Infarct, myocardium)
      410.9 ☑
      due to syphilis 093.89
      healed or specified as old 412
      valve — *see* Endocarditis
  carotid (artery) (common) (internal) (*see also*
      Occlusion, artery, carotid) 433.1 ☑
      with other precerebral artery 433.3 ☑
  cavernous sinus (venous) — *see* Thrombosis,
      intracranial venous sinus
  cerebellar artery (anterior inferior) (posterior
      inferior) (superior) 433.8 ☑
      late effect — *see* Late effect(s) (of) cere-
          brovascular disease
  cerebral (arteries) (*see also* Thrombosis,
      brain) 434.0 ☑
      late effect — *see* Late effect(s) (of) cere-
          brovascular disese
  coronary (artery) (*see also* Infarct, myocardi-
      um) 410.9 ☑
      without myocardial infarction 411.81
      due to syphilis 093.89
      healed or specified as old 412
  corpus cavernosum 607.82
  cortical (*see also* Thrombosis, brain) 434.0 ☑

Thrombosis, thrombotic — *continued*
  due to (presence of) any device, implant, or
      graft classifiable to 996.0–996.5 —
      see Complications, due to (presence
      of) any device, implant, or graft clas-
      sified to 996.0–996.5 NEC
  effort 453.89
  endocardial — *see* Infarct, myocardium
  eye (*see also* Occlusion, retina) 362.30
  femoral (vein) 453.6
      with inflammation or phlebitis 451.11
      artery 444.22
      deep 453.41
      personal history of V12.51
  genital organ, male 608.83
  heart (chamber) (*see also* Infarct, myocardi-
      um) 410.9 ☑
  hepatic (vein) 453.0
      artery 444.89
      infectional or septic 572.1
  iliac ▶(acute)◀ (vein) 453.89
      with inflammation or phlebitis 451.81
      artery (common) (external) (internal)
          444.81
      chronic 453.79   ●
      personal history of V12.51
  inflammation, vein — *see* Thrombophlebitis
  internal carotid artery (*see also* Occlusion,
      artery, carotid) 433.1 ☑
      with other precerebral artery 433.3 ☑
  intestine (with gangrene) 557.0
  intracranial (*see also* Thrombosis, brain)
      434.0 ☑
      venous sinus (any) 325
          nonpyogenic origin 437.6
              in pregnancy or puerperium
                  671.5 ☑
  intramural (*see also* Infarct, myocardium)
      410.9 ☑
      without
          cardiac condition 429.89
          coronary artery disease 429.89
          myocardial infarction 429.89
      healed or specified as old 412
  jugular (bulb)
      external ▶(acute)◀ 453.89   ▲
          chronic 453.79
      internal ▶(acute)◀ 453.86   ▲
          chronic 453.76
  kidney 593.81
      artery 593.81
  lateral sinus (venous) — *see* Thrombosis,
      intracranial venous sinus
  leg (*see also* Thrombosis, lower extremity)
      453.6
      with inflammation or phlebitis — *see*
          Thrombophlebitis
      deep (vessels) 453.40
          acute 453.40
              lower distal 453.42
              upper (proximal) 453.41
          chronic 453.50
              lower (distal) 453.52
              upper (proximal) 453.51
          lower (distal) 453.42
          upper (proximal) 453.41
      personal history of V12.51
      superficial (vessels) 453.6
  liver (venous) 453.0
      artery 444.89
      infectional or septic 572.1
      portal vein 452
  longitudinal sinus (venous) — *see* Thrombo-
      sis, intracranial venous sinus
  lower extremity (superficial) 453.6
      deep vessels 453.40
          acute 453.40
              calf 453.42
              distal (lower leg) 453.42
              femoral 453.41
              iliac 453.41
              lower leg 453.42
              peroneal 453.42
              popliteal 453.41
              proximal (upper leg) 453.41
              thigh 453.41

Thrombosis, thrombotic — *continued*
  lower extremity — *continued*
    deep vessels — *continued*
      acute — *continued*
        tibial 453.42
        chronic 453.50
          calf 453.52
          distal (lower leg) 453.52
          femoral 453.51
          iliac 453.51
          lower leg 453.52
          peroneal 453.52
          popliteal 453.51
          proximal (upper leg) 453.51
          thigh 453.51
          tibial 453.52
      personal history of V12.51
      saphenous (greater) (lesser) 453.6
      superficial 453.6
  lung 415.19
    iatrogenic 415.11
    personal history of V12.51
    postoperative 415.11
    septic 415.12
  marantic, dural sinus 437.6
  meninges (brain) (*see also* Thrombosis, brain) 434.0 ☑
  mesenteric (artery) (with gangrene) 557.0
    vein (inferior) (superior) 557.0
  mitral — *see* Insufficiency, mitral
  mural (heart chamber) (*see also* Infarct, myocardium) 410.9 ☑
    without
      cardiac condition 429.89
      coronary artery disease 429.89
      myocardial infarction 429.89
    due to syphilis 093.89
    following myocardial infarction 429.79
    healed or specified as old 412
  omentum (with gangrene) 557.0
  ophthalmic (artery) (*see also* Occlusion, retina) 362.30
  pampiniform plexus (male) 608.83
    female 620.8
  parietal (*see also* Infarct, myocardium) 410.9 ☑
  penis, penile 607.82
  peripheral arteries 444.22
    lower 444.22
    upper 444.21
  platelet 446.6
  portal 452
    due to syphilis 093.89
    infectional or septic 572.1
  precerebral artery (*see also* Occlusion, artery, precerebral NEC)
  pregnancy 671.2 ☑
    deep (vein) 671.3 ☑
    superficial (vein) 671.2 ☑
  puerperal, postpartum, childbirth 671.2 ☑
    brain (artery) 674.0 ☑
      venous 671.5 ☑
    cardiac 674.8 ☑
    cerebral (artery) 674.0 ☑
      venous 671.5 ☑
    deep (vein) 671.4 ☑
    intracranial sinus (nonpyogenic) (venous) 671.5 ☑
    pelvic 671.4 ☑
    pulmonary (artery) 673.2 ☑
    specified site NEC 671.5 ☑
    superficial 671.2 ☑
  pulmonary (artery) (vein) 415.19
    iatrogenic 415.11
    personal history of V12.51
    postoperative 415.11
    septic 415.12
  renal (artery) 593.81
    vein 453.3
  resulting from presence of shunt or other internal prosthetic device — *see* Complications, due to (presence of) any device, implant, or graft classified to 996.0–996.5 NEC
  retina, retinal (artery) 362.30
    arterial branch 362.32

Thrombosis, thrombotic — *continued*
  retina, retinal — *continued*
    central 362.31
    partial 362.33
    vein
      central 362.35
      tributary (branch) 362.36
  saphenous vein (greater) (lesser) 453.6
  scrotum 608.83
  seminal vesicle 608.83
  sigmoid (venous) sinus — *see* Thrombosis, intracranial venous sinus 325
  silent NEC 453.9
  sinus, intracranial (venous) (any) (*see also* Thrombosis, intracranial venous sinus) 325
  softening, brain (*see also* Thrombosis, brain) 434.0 ☑
  specified site NEC (acute) 453.89
    chronic 453.79
  spermatic cord 608.83
  spinal cord 336.1
    due to syphilis 094.89
    in pregnancy or puerperium 671.5 ☑
    pyogenic origin 324.1
      late effect — *see* category 326
  spleen, splenic 289.59
    artery 444.89
  testis 608.83
  traumatic (complication) (early) (*see also* Injury, blood vessel, by site) 904.9
  tricuspid — *see* Endocarditis, tricuspid
  tumor — *see* Neoplasm, by site
  tunica vaginalis 608.83
  umbilical cord (vessels) 663.6 ☑
    affecting fetus or newborn 762.6
  upper extremity 453.83
    acute 453.83
      deep 453.82
      superficial 453.81
    chronic 453.73
      deep 453.72
      superficial 453.71
  vas deferens 608.83
  vein
    antecubital ►◄ (acute)◄ 453.81   ▲
      chronic 453.71
    axillary ►◄ (acute)◄ 453.84   ▲
      chronic 453.74
    basilic ►◄ (acute)◄ 453.81   ▲
      chronic 453.71
    brachial ►◄ (acute)◄ 453.82   ▲
      chronic 453.72
    brachiocephalic (innominate) ►◄ (acute)◄ 453.87   ▲
      chronic 453.77
    cephalic ►◄ (acute)◄ 453.81   ▲
      chronic 453.71
    deep 453.40
      personal history of V12.51
    internal jugular ►◄ (acute)◄ 453.86   ▲
      chronic 453.76
    lower extremity — *see* Thrombosis, lower extremity
    personal history of V12.51
    radial ►◄ (acute)◄ 453.82   ▲
      chronic 453.72
    saphenous (greater) (lesser) 453.6
    specified site NEC ►◄ (acute)◄ 453.89   ▲
      chronic 453.79
    subclavian ►◄ (acute)◄ 453.85   ▲
      chronic 453.75
    superior vena cava ►◄ (acute)◄ 453.87   ▲
      chronic 453.77
    thoracic ►◄ (acute)◄ 453.87   ▲
      chronic 453.77
    ulnar ►◄ (acute)◄ 453.82   ▲
      chronic 453.72
    upper extremity — *see* Thrombosis, upper extremity
  vena cava
    inferior 453.2
    personal history of V12.51
    superior ►◄ (acute)◄ 453.87   ▲

Thrombosis, thrombotic — *continued*
  vena cava — *continued*
    superior — *continued*
      chronic 453.77
Thrombus — *see* Thrombosis
Thrush 112.0
  newborn 771.7
Thumb — *see also* condition
  gamekeeper's 842.12
  sucking (child problem) 307.9
Thygeson's superficial punctate keratitis 370.21
Thymergasia — *see also* Psychosis, affective 296.80
Thymitis 254.8
Thymoma (benign) (M8580/0) 212.6
  malignant (M8580/3) 164.0
Thymus, thymic (gland) — *see* condition
Thyrocele — *see also* Goiter 240.9
Thyroglossal — *see also* condition
  cyst 759.2
  duct, persistent 759.2
Thyroid (body) (gland) — *see also* condition
  hormone resistance 246.8
  lingual 759.2
Thyroiditis 245.9
  acute (pyogenic) (suppurative) 245.0
    nonsuppurative 245.0
  autoimmune 245.2
  chronic (nonspecific) (sclerosing) 245.8
    fibrous 245.3
    lymphadenoid 245.2
    lymphocytic 245.2
    lymphoid 245.2
  complicating pregnancy, childbirth, or puerperium 648.1 ☑
  de Quervain's (subacute granulomatous) 245.1
  fibrous (chronic) 245.3
  giant (cell) (follicular) 245.1
  granulomatous (de Quervain's) (subacute) 245.1
  Hashimoto's (struma lymphomatosa) 245.2
  iatrogenic 245.4
  invasive (fibrous) 245.3
  ligneous 245.3
  lymphocytic (chronic) 245.2
  lymphoid 245.2
  lymphomatous 245.2
  pseudotuberculous 245.1
  pyogenic 245.0
  radiation 245.4
  Riedel's (ligneous) 245.3
  subacute 245.1
  suppurative 245.0
  tuberculous (*see also* Tuberculosis) 017.5 ☑
  viral 245.1
  woody 245.3
Thyrolingual duct, persistent 759.2
Thyromegaly 240.9
Thyrotoxic
  crisis or storm (*see also* Thyrotoxicosis) 242.9 ☑
  heart failure (*see also* Thyrotoxicosis) 242.9 ☑ *[425.7]*
Thyrotoxicosis 242.9 ☑   ▲

Note — *Use the following fifth-digit subclassification with category 242:*

0 *without mention of thyrotoxic crisis or storm*

1 *with mention of thyrotoxic crisis or storm*

  with
    goiter (diffuse) 242.0 ☑
      adenomatous 242.3 ☑
        multinodular 242.2 ☑
        uninodular 242.1 ☑
      nodular 242.3 ☑
        multinodular 242.2 ☑
        uninodular 242.1 ☑
    infiltrative
      dermopathy 242.0 ☑
      ophthalmopathy 242.0 ☑
    thyroid acropachy 242.0 ☑

Thyrotoxicosis — *continued*
  complicating pregnancy, childbirth, or puerperium 648.1 ☑
  due to
    ectopic thyroid nodule 242.4 ☑
    ingestion of (excessive) thyroid material 242.8 ☑
    specified cause NEC 242.8 ☑
  factitia 242.8 ☑
  heart 242.9 ☑ *[425.7]*
  neonatal (transient) 775.3
TIA (transient ischemic attack) 435.9
  with transient neurologic deficit 435.9
  late effect — *see* Late effect(s) (of) cerebrovascular disease
Tibia vara 732.4
Tic 307.20
  breathing 307.20
  child problem 307.21
  compulsive 307.22
  convulsive 307.20
  degenerative (generalized) (localized) 333.3
    facial 351.8
  douloureux (*see also* Neuralgia, trigeminal) 350.1
    atypical 350.2
  habit 307.20
    chronic (motor or vocal) 307.22
    transient (of childhood) 307.21
  lid 307.20
    transient (of childhood) 307.21
  motor-verbal 307.23
  occupational 300.89
  orbicularis 307.20
    transient (of childhood) 307.21
  organic origin 333.3
  postchoreic — *see* Chorea
  psychogenic 307.20
    compulsive 307.22
  salaam 781.0
  spasm 307.20
    chronic (motor or vocal) 307.22
    transient (of childhood) 307.21
Tick-bite fever NEC 066.1
  African 087.1
  Colorado (virus) 066.1
  Rocky Mountain 082.0
Tick (-borne) fever NEC 066.1
  American mountain 066.1
  Colorado 066.1
  hemorrhagic NEC 065.3
    Crimean 065.0
    Kyasanur Forest 065.2
    Omsk 065.1
  mountain 066.1
  nonexanthematous 066.1
Tick paralysis 989.5
Tics and spasms, compulsive 307.22
Tietze's disease or syndrome 733.6
Tight, tightness
  anus 564.89
  chest 786.59
  fascia (lata) 728.9
  foreskin (congenital) 605
  hymen 623.3
  introitus (acquired) (congenital) 623.3
  rectal sphincter 564.89
  tendon 727.81
    Achilles (heel) 727.81
  urethral sphincter 598.9
Tilting vertebra 737.9
Timidity, child 313.21
Tinea (intersecta) (tarsi) 110.9
  amiantacea 110.0
  asbestina 110.0
  barbae 110.0
  beard 110.0
  black dot 110.0
  blanca 111.2
  capitis 110.0
  corporis 110.5
  cruris 110.3
  decalvans 704.09
  flava 111.0
  foot 110.4
  furfuracea 111.0

☑ **Additional Digit Required — Refer to the Tabular List for Digit Selection**   ▽ **Subterms under main terms may continue to next column or page**

2011 ICD-9-CM   ►◄ **Revised Text**   ● **New Line**   ▲ **Revised Code**   **October 2010 • Volume 2 — 279**

Tinea — continued
  imbricata (Tokelau) 110.5
  lepothrix 039.0
  manuum 110.2
  microsporic (see also Dermatophytosis)
      110.9
  nigra 111.1
  nodosa 111.2
  pedis 110.4
  scalp 110.0
  specified site NEC 110.8
  sycosis 110.0
  tonsurans 110.0
  trichophytic (see also Dermatophytosis)
      110.9
  unguium 110.1
  versicolor 111.0
Tingling sensation — see also Disturbance,
    sensation 782.0
Tin-miners' lung 503
Tinnitus (aurium) 388.30
  audible 388.32
  objective 388.32
  subjective 388.31
Tipped, teeth 524.33
Tipping
  pelvis 738.6
    with disproportion (fetopelvic) 653.0 ☑
      affecting fetus or newborn 763.1
      causing obstructed labor 660.1 ☑
        affecting fetus or newborn 763.1
  teeth 524.33
Tiredness 780.79
Tissue — see condition
Tobacco
  abuse (affecting health) NEC (see also Abuse,
      drugs, nondependent) 305.1
  heart 989.84
  use disorder complicating pregnancy,
      childbirth, or the puerperium
      649.0 ☑
Tobias' syndrome (carcinoma, pulmonary
    apex) (M8010/3) 162.3
Tocopherol deficiency 269.1
Todd's
  cirrhosis — see Cirrhosis, biliary
  paralysis (postepileptic transitory paralysis)
      344.89
Toe — see condition
Toilet, artificial opening — see also Attention
    to, artificial, opening V55.9
Tokelau ringworm 110.5
Tollwut 071
Tolosa-Hunt syndrome 378.55
Tommaselli's disease
  correct substance properly administered
      599.70
  overdose or wrong substance given or taken
      961.4
Tongue — see also condition
  worms 134.1
Tongue tie 750.0
Tonic pupil 379.46
Tonsil — see condition
Tonsillitis (acute) (catarrhal) (croupous) (follic-
    ular) (gangrenous) (infective) (lacunar)
    (lingual) (malignant) (membranous)
    (phlegmonous) (pneumococcal) (pseu-
    domembranous) (purulent) (septic)
    (staphylococcal) (subacute) (suppura-
    tive) (toxic) (ulcerative) (vesicular) (viral)
    463
  with influenza, flu, or grippe ▶(see also In-
      fluenza)◀ 487.1
  chronic 474.00
  diphtheritic (membranous) 032.0
  hypertrophic 474.00
  influenzal ▶(see also Influenza)◀ 487.1
  parenchymatous 475
  streptococcal 034.0
  tuberculous (see also Tuberculosis) 012.8 ☑
  Vincent's 101
Tonsillopharyngitis 465.8
Toothache 525.9
Tooth, teeth — see condition

Topagnosis 782.0
Tophi (gouty) 274.03
  ear 274.81
  heart 274.82
  specified site NEC 274.82
TORCH infection — see also Infection, congen-
    ital 760.2
Torn — see Tear, torn
Tornwaldt's bursitis (disease) (pharyngeal
    bursitis) 478.29
  cyst 478.26
Torpid liver 573.9
Torsion
  accessory tube 620.5
  adnexa (female) 620.5
  aorta (congenital) 747.29
    acquired 447.1
  appendix
    epididymis 608.24
    testis 608.23
  bile duct 576.8
    with calculus, choledocholithiasis or
        stones — see Choledocholithiasis
    congenital 751.69
  bowel, colon, or intestine 560.2
  cervix — see Malposition, uterus
  duodenum 537.3
  dystonia — see Dystonia, torsion
  epididymis 608.24
    appendix 608.24
  fallopian tube 620.5
  gallbladder (see also Disease, gallbladder)
      575.8
    congenital 751.69
  gastric 537.89
  hydatid of Morgagni (female) 620.5
  kidney (pedicle) 593.89
  Meckel's diverticulum (congenital) 751.0
  mesentery 560.2
  omentum 560.2
  organ or site, congenital NEC — see
      Anomaly, specified type NEC
  ovary (pedicle) 620.5
    congenital 752.0
  oviduct 620.5
  penis 607.89
    congenital 752.69
  renal 593.89
  spasm — see Dystonia, torsion
  spermatic cord 608.22
    extravaginal 608.21
    intravaginal 608.22
  spleen 289.59
  testicle, testis 608.20
    appendix 608.23
  tibia 736.89
  umbilical cord — see Compression, umbili-
      cal cord
  uterus (see also Malposition, uterus) 621.6
Torticollis (intermittent) (spastic) 723.5
  congenital 754.1
    sternomastoid 754.1
  due to birth injury 767.8
  hysterical 300.11
  ocular 781.93
  psychogenic 306.0
    specified as conversion reaction 300.11
  rheumatic 723.5
  rheumatoid 714.0
  spasmodic 333.83
  traumatic, current NEC 847.0
Tortuous
  artery 447.1
  fallopian tube 752.19
  organ or site, congenital NEC — see Distor-
      tion
  renal vessel (congenital) 747.62
  retina vessel (congenital) 743.58
    acquired 362.17
  ureter 593.4
  urethra 599.84
  vein — see Varicose, vein
Torula, torular (infection) 117.5
  histolytica 117.5
  lung 117.5
Torulosis 117.5

Torus
  fracture
    fibula 823.41
      with tibia 823.42
    humerus 812.49
    radius (alone) 813.45
      with ulna 813.47
    tibia 823.40
      with fibula 823.42
    ulna (alone) 813.46
      with radius 813.47
  mandibularis 526.81
  palatinus 526.81
Touch, vitreous 997.99
Touraine-Solente-Golé syndrome
    (acropachyderma) 757.39
Touraine's syndrome (hereditary osteo-ony-
    chodysplasia) 756.89
Tourette's disease (motor-verbal tic) 307.23
Tower skull 756.0
  with exophthalmos 756.0
Toxemia 799.89
  with
    abortion — see Abortion, by type, with
        toxemia
  bacterial — see Septicemia
  biliary (see also Disease, biliary) 576.8
  burn — see Burn, by site
  congenital NEC 779.89
  eclamptic 642.6 ☑
    with pre-existing hypertension 642.7 ☑
  erysipelatous (see also Erysipelas) 035
  fatigue 799.89
  fetus or newborn NEC 779.89
  food (see also Poisoning, food) 005.9
  gastric 537.89
  gastrointestinal 558.2
  intestinal 558.2
  kidney (see also Disease, renal) 593.9
  lung 518.89
  malarial NEC (see also Malaria) 084.6
  maternal (of pregnancy), affecting fetus or
      newborn 760.0
  myocardial — see Myocarditis, toxic
  of pregnancy (mild) (pre-eclamptic)
      642.4 ☑
    with
      convulsions 642.6 ☑
      pre-existing hypertension 642.7 ☑
    affecting fetus or newborn 760.0
    severe 642.5 ☑
  pre-eclamptic — see Toxemia, of pregnancy
  puerperal, postpartum — see Toxemia, of
      pregnancy
  pulmonary 518.89
  renal (see also Disease, renal) 593.9
  septic (see also Septicemia) 038.9
  small intestine 558.2
  staphylococcal 038.10
    aureus 038.11
    due to food 005.0
    specified organism NEC 038.19
  stasis 799.89
  stomach 537.89
  uremic (see also Uremia) 586
  urinary 586
Toxemica cerebropathia psychica (nonalco-
    holic) 294.0
  alcoholic 291.1
Toxic (poisoning) — see also condition
  from drug or poison — see Table of Drugs
      and Chemicals
  oil syndrome 710.5
  shock syndrome 040.82
  thyroid (gland) (see also Thyrotoxicosis)
      242.9 ☑
Toxicemia — see Toxemia
Toxicity
  dilantin
    asymptomatic 796.0
    symptomatic — see Table of Drugs and
        Chemicals
  drug
    asymptomatic 796.0
    symptomatic — see Table of Drugs and
        Chemicals

Toxicity — continued
  fava bean 282.2
  from drug or poison
    asymptomatic 796.0
    symptomatic — see Table of Drugs and
        Chemicals
Toxicosis — see also Toxemia 799.89
  capillary, hemorrhagic 287.0
Toxinfection 799.89
  gastrointestinal 558.2
Toxocariasis 128.0
Toxoplasma infection, generalized 130.9
Toxoplasmosis (acquired) 130.9
  with pneumonia 130.4
  congenital, active 771.2
  disseminated (multisystemic) 130.8
  maternal
    with suspected damage to fetus affect-
        ing management of pregnancy
        655.4 ☑
    affecting fetus or newborn 760.2
      manifest toxoplasmosis in fetus or
          newborn 771.2
  multiple sites 130.8
  multisystemic disseminated 130.8
  specified site NEC 130.7
Trabeculation, bladder 596.8
Trachea — see condition
Tracheitis (acute) (catarrhal) (infantile) (mem-
    branous) (plastic) (pneumococcal) (sep-
    tic) (suppurative) (viral) 464.10
  with
    bronchitis 490
      acute or subacute 466.0
      chronic 491.8
      tuberculosis — see Tuberculosis,
          pulmonary
    laryngitis (acute) 464.20
      with obstruction 464.21
      chronic 476.1
      tuberculous (see also Tuberculosis,
          larynx) 012.3 ☑
    obstruction 464.11
  chronic 491.8
    with
      bronchitis (chronic) 491.8
      laryngitis (chronic) 476.1
    due to external agent — see Condition,
        respiratory, chronic, due to
  diphtheritic (membranous) 032.3
    due to external agent — see Inflamma-
        tion, respiratory, upper, due to
  edematous 464.11
  influenzal ▶(see also Influenza)◀ 487.1
  streptococcal 034.0
  syphilitic 095.8
  tuberculous (see also Tuberculosis) 012.8 ☑
Trachelitis (nonvenereal) — see also Cervicitis
    616.0
  trichomonal 131.09
Tracheobronchial — see condition
Tracheobronchitis — see also Bronchitis 490
  acute or subacute 466.0
    with bronchospasm or obstruction 466.0
  chronic 491.8
  influenzal ▶(see also Influenza)◀ 487.1
  senile 491.8
Tracheobronchomegaly (congenital) 748.3
  with bronchiectasis 494.0
    with (acute) exacerbation 494.1
  acquired 519.19
    with bronchiectasis 494.0
      with (acute) exacerbation 494.1
Tracheobronchopneumonitis — see Pneumo-
    nia, broncho
Tracheocele (external) (internal) 519.19
  congenital 748.3
Tracheomalacia 519.19
  congenital 748.3
Tracheopharyngitis (acute) 465.8
  chronic 478.9
    due to external agent — see Condition,
        respiratory, chronic, due to
    due to external agent — see Inflammation,
        respiratory, upper, due to
Tracheostenosis 519.19

☑ **Additional Digit Required** — Refer to the Tabular List for Digit Selection   🕮 **Subterms under main terms may continue to next column or page**

280 — Volume 2 · October 2010   ▶◀ **Revised Text**   ● **New Line**   ▲ **Revised Code**   **2011 ICD-9-CM**

Tracheostenosis — *continued*
congenital 748.3
Tracheostomy
attention to V55.0
complication 519.00
granuloma 519.09
hemorrhage 519.09
infection 519.01
malfunctioning 519.02
obstruction 519.09
sepsis 519.01
status V44.0
stenosis 519.02
Trachoma, trachomatous 076.9
active (stage) 076.1
contraction of conjunctiva 076.1
dubium 076.0
healed or late effect 139.1
initial (stage) 076.0
Türck's (chronic catarrhal laryngitis) 476.0
Trachyphonia 784.49
Training
insulin pump V65.46
orthoptic V57.4
orthotic V57.81
Train sickness 994.6
Trait
hemoglobin
abnormal NEC 282.7
with thalassemia 282.49
C (*see also* Disease, hemoglobin, C) 282.7
with elliptocytosis 282.7
S (Hb-S) 282.5
Lepore 282.49
with other abnormal hemoglobin NEC 282.49
paranoid 301.0
sickle-cell 282.5
with
elliptocytosis 282.5
spherocytosis 282.5
Traits, paranoid 301.0
Tramp V60.0
Trance 780.09
hysterical 300.13
Transaminasemia 790.4
Transfusion, blood
without reported diagnosis V58.2
donor V59.01
stem cells V59.02
fetal twin to twin 678.0 ☑
incompatible ▶(*see also* Complications, transfusion)◀ 999.80 ▲
ABO ▶(*see also* Complications, transfusion)◀ 999.60 ▲
minor blood group 999.89
non-ABO (*see also* Complications, transfusion) 999.75 ●
Rh (antigen) (C) (c) (D) (E) (e) (*see also* ●
Complications, transfusion) ●
999.70 ●
reaction or complication — *see* Complications, transfusion
related acute lung injury (TRALI) 518.7
syndrome
fetomaternal 772.0
twin-to-twin
blood loss (donor twin) 772.0
recipient twin 776.4
twin to twin fetal 678.0 ☑
Transient — *see also* condition
alteration of awareness 780.02
blindness 368.12
deafness (ischemic) 388.02
global amnesia 437.7
hyperglycemia (post-procedural) 790.29
hypoglycemia (post-procedural) 251.2
person (homeless) NEC V60.0
Transitional, lumbosacral joint of vertebra 756.19
Translocation
autosomes NEC 758.5
13-15 758.1
16-18 758.2
21 or 22 758.0
balanced in normal individual 758.4

Translocation — *continued*
autosomes — *continued*
D₁ 758.1 → D_1 758.1
E₃ 758.2 → E_3 758.2
G 758.0
balanced autosomal in normal individual 758.4
chromosomes NEC 758.89
Down's syndrome 758.0
Translucency, iris 364.53
Transmission of chemical substances through the placenta (affecting fetus or newborn) 760.70
alcohol 760.71
anticonvulsants 760.77
antifungals 760.74
anti-infective agents 760.74
antimetabolics 760.78
cocaine 760.75
"crack" 760.75
diethylstilbestrol [DES] 760.76
hallucinogenic agents 760.73
medicinal agents NEC 760.79
narcotics 760.72
obstetric anesthetic or analgesic drug 763.5
specified agent NEC 760.79
suspected, affecting management of pregnancy 655.5 ☑
Transplant(ed)
bone V42.4
marrow V42.81
complication (*see also* Complications, due to (presence of) any device, implant, or graft classified to 996.0–996.5 NEC)
bone marrow 996.85
corneal graft NEC 996.79
infection or inflammation 996.69
reaction 996.51
rejection 996.51
organ (failure) (immune or nonimmune cause) (infection) (rejection) 996.80
bone marrow 996.85
heart 996.83
intestines 996.87
kidney 996.81
liver 996.82
lung 996.84
pancreas 996.86
specified NEC 996.89
previously removed due to complication, failure, rejection or infection V45.87
removal status V45.87
skin NEC 996.79
infection or inflammation 996.69
rejection 996.52
artificial 996.55
decellularized allodermis 996.55
cornea V42.5
hair V50.0
heart V42.1
valve V42.2
intestine V42.84
kidney V42.0
liver V42.7
lung V42.6
organ V42.9
specified NEC V42.89
pancreas V42.83
peripheral stem cells V42.82
skin V42.3
stem cells, peripheral V42.82
tissue V42.9
specified NEC V42.89
Transplants, ovarian, endometrial 617.1
Transposed — *see* Transposition
Transposition (congenital) — *see also* Malposition, congenital
abdominal viscera 759.3
aorta (dextra) 745.11
appendix 751.5
arterial trunk 745.10
colon 751.5
great vessels (complete) 745.10

Transposition — *see also* Malposition, congenital — *continued*
great vessels — *continued*
both originating from right ventricle 745.11
corrected 745.12
double outlet right ventricle 745.11
incomplete 745.11
partial 745.11
specified type NEC 745.19
heart 746.87
with complete transposition of viscera 759.3
intestine (large) (small) 751.5
pulmonary veins 747.49
reversed jejunal (for bypass) (status) V45.3
scrotal 752.81
stomach 750.7
with general transposition of viscera 759.3
teeth, tooth 524.30
vessels (complete) 745.10
partial 745.11
viscera (abdominal) (thoracic) 759.3
Trans-sexualism 302.50
with
asexual history 302.51
heterosexual history 302.53
homosexual history 302.52
Transverse — *see also* condition
arrest (deep), in labor 660.3 ☑
affecting fetus or newborn 763.1
lie 652.3 ☑
before labor, affecting fetus or newborn 761.7
causing obstructed labor 660.0 ☑
affecting fetus or newborn 763.1
during labor, affecting fetus or newborn 763.1
Transvestism, transvestitism (transvestic fetishism) 302.3
Trapped placenta (with hemorrhage) 666.0 ☑
without hemorrhage 667.0 ☑
Traumatic — *see also* condition
brain injury (TBI) (*see also* Injury, intracranial) 854.0 ☑
with skull fracture — *see* Fracture, skull, by site
Trauma, traumatism — *see also* Injury, by site 959.9
birth — *see* Birth, injury NEC
causing hemorrhage of pregnancy or delivery 641.8 ☑
complicating
abortion — *see* Abortion, by type, with damage to pelvic organs
ectopic pregnancy (*see also* categories 633.0–633.9) 639.2
molar pregnancy (*see also* categories 630–632) 639.2
during delivery NEC 665.9 ☑
following
abortion 639.2
ectopic or molar pregnancy 639.2
maternal, during pregnancy, affecting fetus or newborn 760.5
neuroma — *see* Injury, nerve, by site
previous major, affecting management of pregnancy, childbirth, or puerperium V23.89
psychic (current) (*see also* Reaction, adjustment)
previous (history) V15.49
psychologic, previous (affecting health) V15.49
transient paralysis — *see* Injury, nerve, by site
Treacher Collins' syndrome (incomplete facial dysostosis) 756.0
Treitz's hernia — *see* Hernia, Treitz's
Trematode infestation NEC 121.9
Trematodiasis NEC 121.9
Trembles 988.8
Trembling paralysis — *see also* Parkinsonism 332.0
Tremor 781.0

Tremor — *continued*
essential (benign) 333.1
familial 333.1
flapping (liver) 572.8
hereditary 333.1
hysterical 300.11
intention 333.1
medication-induced postural 333.1
mercurial 985.0
muscle 728.85
Parkinson's (*see also* Parkinsonism) 332.0
psychogenic 306.0
specified as conversion reaction 300.11
senilis 797
specified type NEC 333.1
Trench
fever 083.1
foot 991.4
mouth 101
nephritis — *see* Nephritis, acute
Treponema pallidum infection — *see also* Syphilis 097.9
Treponematosis 102.9
due to
T. pallidum — *see* Syphilis
T. pertenue (yaws) (*see also* Yaws) 102.9
Triad
Kartagener's 759.3
Reiter's (complete) (incomplete) 099.3
Saint's (*see also* Hernia, diaphragm) 553.3
Trichiasis 704.2
cicatricial 704.2
eyelid 374.05
with entropion (*see also* Entropion) 374.00
Trichinella spiralis (infection) (infestation) 124
Trichinelliasis 124
Trichinellosis 124
Trichiniasis 124
Trichinosis 124
Trichobezoar 938
intestine 936
stomach 935.2
Trichocephaliasis 127.3
Trichocephalosis 127.3
Trichocephalus infestation 127.3
Trichoclasis 704.2
Trichoepithelioma (M8100/0) — *see also* Neoplasm, skin, benign
breast 217
genital organ NEC — *see* Neoplasm, by site, benign
malignant (M8100/3) — *see* Neoplasm, skin, malignant
Trichofolliculoma (M8101/0) — *see* Neoplasm, skin, benign
Tricholemmoma (M8102/0) — *see* Neoplasm, skin, benign
Trichomatosis 704.2
Trichomoniasis 131.9
bladder 131.09
cervix 131.09
intestinal 007.3
prostate 131.03
seminal vesicle 131.09
specified site NEC 131.8
urethra 131.02
urogenitalis 131.00
vagina 131.01
vulva 131.01
vulvovaginal 131.01
Trichomycosis 039.0
axillaris 039.0
nodosa 111.2
nodularis 111.2
rubra 039.0
Trichonocardiosis (axillaris) (palmellina) 039.0
Trichonodosis 704.2
Trichophytide — *see* Dermatophytosis
Trichophytid, trichophyton infection — *see also* Dermatophytosis 110.9
Trichophytobezoar 938
intestine 936
stomach 935.2
Trichophytosis — *see* Dermatophytosis
Trichoptilosis 704.2

☑ **Additional Digit Required** — Refer to the Tabular List for Digit Selection   ▽ **Subterms under main terms may continue to next column or page**

2011 ICD-9-CM   ▶◀ Revised Text   ● New Line   ▲ Revised Code   October 2010 • Volume 2 — 281

Trichorrhexis (nodosa) 704.2
Trichosporosis nodosa 111.2
Trichstasis spinulosa (congenital) 757.4
Trichostrongyliasis (small intestine) 127.6
Trichostrongylosis 127.6
Trichostrongylus (instabilis) infection 127.6
Trichotillomania 312.39
Trichromat, anomalous (congenital) 368.59
Trichromatopsia, anomalous (congenital) 368.59
Trichuriasis 127.3
Trichuris trichiuria (any site) (infection) (infestation) 127.3
Tricuspid (valve) — see condition
Trifid — see also Accessory
  kidney (pelvis) 753.3
  tongue 750.13
Trigeminal neuralgia — see also Neuralgia, trigeminal 350.1
Trigeminoencephaloangiomatosis 759.6
Trigeminy 427.89
  postoperative 997.1
Trigger finger (acquired) 727.03
  congenital 756.89
Trigonitis (bladder) (chronic) (pseudomembranous) 595.3
  tuberculous (see also Tuberculosis) 016.1 ☑
Trigonocephaly 756.0
Trihexosidosis 272.7
Trilobate placenta — see Placenta, abnormal
Trilocular heart 745.8
Trimethylaminuria 270.8
Tripartita placenta — see Placenta, abnormal
Triple — see also Accessory
  kidneys 753.3
  uteri 752.2
  X female 758.81
Triplegia 344.89
  congenital or infantile 343.8
Triplet
  affected by maternal complications of pregnancy 761.5
  healthy liveborn — see Newborn, multiple
  pregnancy (complicating delivery) NEC 651.1 ☑
    with fetal loss and retention of one or more fetus(es) 651.4 ☑
    following (elective) fetal reduction 651.7 ☑
Triplex placenta — see Placenta, abnormal
Triplication — see Accessory
Trismus 781.0
  neonatorum 771.3
  newborn 771.3
Trisomy (syndrome) NEC 758.5
  13 (partial) 758.1
  16-18 758.2
  18 (partial) 758.2
  21 (partial) 758.0
  22 758.0
  autosomes NEC 758.5
  D$_1$ 758.1
  E$_3$ 758.2
  G (group) 758.0
  group D$_1$ 758.1
  group E 758.2
  group G 758.0
Tritanomaly 368.53
Tritanopia 368.53
Troisier-Hanot-Chauffard syndrome (bronze diabetes) 275.01 ▲
Trombidiosis 133.8
Trophedema (hereditary) 757.0
  congenital 757.0
Trophoblastic disease — see also Hydatidiform mole 630
  previous, affecting management of pregnancy V23.1
Tropholymphedema 757.0
Trophoneurosis NEC 356.9
  arm NEC 354.9
  disseminated 710.1
  facial 349.89
  leg NEC 355.8
  lower extremity NEC 355.8
  upper extremity NEC 354.9

Tropical — see also condition
  maceration feet (syndrome) 991.4
  wet foot (syndrome) 991.4
Trouble — see also Disease
  bowel 569.9
  heart — see Disease, heart
  intestine 569.9
  kidney (see also Disease, renal) 593.9
  nervous 799.21
  sinus (see also Sinusitis) 473.9
Trousseau's syndrome (thrombophlebitis migrans) 453.1
Truancy, childhood — see also Disturbance, conduct
  socialized 312.2 ☑
  undersocialized, unsocialized 312.1 ☑
Truncus
  arteriosus (persistent) 745.0
  common 745.0
  communis 745.0
Trunk — see condition
Trychophytide — see Dermatophytosis
Trypanosoma infestation — see Trypanosomiasis
Trypanosomiasis 086.9
  with meningoencephalitis 086.9 [323.2]
  African 086.5
    due to Trypanosoma 086.5
      gambiense 086.3
      rhodesiense 086.4
  American 086.2
    with
      heart involvement 086.0
      other organ involvement 086.1
    without mention of organ involvement 086.2
  Brazilian — see Trypanosomiasis, American
  Chagas' — see Trypanosomiasis, American
  due to Trypanosoma
    cruzi — see Trypanosomiasis, American
    gambiense 086.3
    rhodesiense 086.4
  gambiensis, Gambian 086.3
  North American — see Trypanosomiasis, American
  rhodesiensis, Rhodesian 086.4
  South American — see Trypanosomiasis, American
T-shaped incisors 520.2
Tsutsugamushi fever 081.2
Tubercle — see also Tuberculosis
  brain, solitary 013.2 ☑
  Darwin's 744.29
  epithelioid noncaseating 135
  Ghon, primary infection 010.0 ☑
Tuberculid, tuberculide (indurating) (lichenoid) (miliary) (papulonecrotic) (primary) (skin) (subcutaneous) — see also Tuberculosis 017.0 ☑
Tuberculoma — see also Tuberculosis
  brain (any part) 013.2 ☑
  meninges (cerebral) (spinal) 013.1 ☑
  spinal cord 013.4 ☑

Tuberculosis, tubercular, tuberculous (calcification) (calcified) (caseous) (chromogenic acid-fast bacilli) (congenital) (degeneration) (disease) (fibrocaseous) (fistula) (gangrene) (interstitial) (isolated circumscribed lesions) (necrosis) (parenchymatous) (ulcerative) 011.9 ☑

> Note — Use the following fifth-digit subclassification with categories 010–018:
>
> 0   unspecified
>
> 1   bacteriological or histological examination not done
>
> 2   bacteriological or histological examination unknown (at present)
>
> 3   tubercle bacilli found (in sputum) by microscopy
>
> 4   tubercle bacilli not found (in sputum) by microscopy, but found by bacterial culture
>
> 5   tubercle bacilli not found by bacteriological examination, but tuberculosis confirmed histologically
>
> 6   tubercle bacilli not found by bacteriological or histological examination, but tuberculosis confirmed by other methods [inoculation of animals]
>
> For tuberculous conditions specified as late effects or sequelae, see category 137.

  abdomen 014.8 ☑
    lymph gland 014.8 ☑
  abscess 011.9 ☑
    arm 017.9 ☑
    bone (see also Osteomyelitis, due to, tuberculosis) 015.9 ☑ [730.8]
      hip 015.1 ☑ [730.85]
      knee 015.2 ☑ [730.86]
      sacrum 015.0 ☑ [730.88]
      specified site NEC 015.7 ☑ [730.88]
      spinal 015.0 ☑ [730.88]
      vertebra 015.0 ☑ [730.88]
    brain 013.3 ☑
    breast 017.9 ☑
    Cowper's gland 016.5 ☑
    dura (mater) 013.8 ☑
      brain 013.3 ☑
      spinal cord 013.5 ☑
    epidural 013.8 ☑
      brain 013.3 ☑
      spinal cord 013.5 ☑
    frontal sinus — see Tuberculosis, sinus
    genital organs NEC 016.9 ☑
      female 016.7 ☑
      male 016.5 ☑
    genitourinary NEC 016.9 ☑
    gland (lymphatic) — see Tuberculosis, lymph gland
    hip 015.1 ☑
    iliopsoas 015.0 ☑ [730.88]
    intestine 014.8 ☑
    ischiorectal 014.8 ☑
    joint 015.9 ☑
      hip 015.1 ☑
      knee 015.2 ☑
      specified joint NEC 015.8 ☑
      vertebral 015.0 ☑ [730.88]
    kidney 016.0 ☑ [590.81]
    knee 015.2 ☑
    lumbar 015.0 ☑ [730.88]
    lung 011.2 ☑
      primary, progressive 010.8 ☑
    meninges (cerebral) (spinal) 013.0 ☑
    pelvic 016.9 ☑
      female 016.7 ☑
      male 016.5 ☑
    perianal 014.8 ☑
      fistula 014.8 ☑
    perinephritic 016.0 ☑ [590.81]

Tuberculosis, tubercular, tuberculous — continued
  abscess — continued
    perineum 017.9 ☑
    perirectal 014.8 ☑
    psoas 015.0 ☑ [730.88]
    rectum 014.8 ☑
    retropharyngeal 012.8 ☑
    sacrum 015.0 ☑ [730.88]
    scrofulous 017.2 ☑
    scrotum 016.5 ☑
    skin 017.0 ☑
      primary 017.0 ☑
    spinal cord 013.5 ☑
    spine or vertebra (column) 015.0 ☑ [730.88]
    strumous 017.2 ☑
    subdiaphragmatic 014.8 ☑
    testis 016.5 ☑
    thigh 017.9 ☑
    urinary 016.3 ☑
      kidney 016.0 ☑ [590.81]
    uterus 016.7 ☑
  accessory sinus — see Tuberculosis, sinus
  Addison's disease 017.6 ☑
  adenitis (see also Tuberculosis, lymph gland) 017.2 ☑
  adenoids 012.8 ☑
  adenopathy (see also Tuberculosis, lymph gland) 017.2 ☑
    tracheobronchial 012.1 ☑
      primary progressive 010.8 ☑
  adherent pericardium 017.9 ☑ [420.0]
  adnexa (uteri) 016.7 ☑
  adrenal (capsule) (gland) 017.6 ☑
  air passage NEC 012.8 ☑
  alimentary canal 014.8 ☑
  anemia 017.9 ☑
  ankle (joint) 015.8 ☑
    bone 015.5 ☑ [730.87]
  anus 014.8 ☑
  apex (see also Tuberculosis, pulmonary) 011.9 ☑
  apical (see also Tuberculosis, pulmonary) 011.9 ☑
  appendicitis 014.8 ☑
  appendix 014.8 ☑
  arachnoid 013.0 ☑
  artery 017.9 ☑
  arthritis (chronic) (synovial) 015.9 ☑ [711.40]
    ankle 015.8 ☑ [730.87]
    hip 015.1 ☑ [711.45]
    knee 015.2 ☑ [711.46]
    specified site NEC 015.8 ☑ [711.48]
    spine or vertebra (column) 015.0 ☑ [720.81]
    wrist 015.8 ☑ [730.83]
  articular — see Tuberculosis, joint
  ascites 014.0 ☑
  asthma (see also Tuberculosis, pulmonary) 011.9 ☑
  axilla, axillary 017.2 ☑
    gland 017.2 ☑
  bilateral (see also Tuberculosis, pulmonary) 011.9 ☑
  bladder 016.1 ☑
  bone (see also Osteomyelitis, due to, tuberculosis) 015.9 ☑ [730.8]
    hip 015.1 ☑ [730.85]
    knee 015.2 ☑ [730.86]
    limb NEC 015.5 ☑ [730.88]
    sacrum 015.0 ☑ [730.88]
    specified site NEC 015.7 ☑ [730.88]
    spinal or vertebral column 015.0 ☑ [730.88]
  bowel 014.8 ☑
    miliary 018.9 ☑
  brain 013.2 ☑
  breast 017.9 ☑
  broad ligament 016.7 ☑
  bronchi, bronchial, bronchus 011.3 ☑
    ectasia, ectasis 011.5 ☑
    fistula 011.3 ☑

Tuberculosis, tubercular, tuberculous — *continued*
  bronchi, bronchial, bronchus — *continued*
    fistula — *continued*
      primary, progressive 010.8 ☑
    gland 012.1 ☑
      primary, progressive 010.8 ☑
      isolated 012.2 ☑
    lymph gland or node 012.1 ☑
      primary, progressive 010.8 ☑
  bronchiectasis 011.5 ☑
  bronchitis 011.3 ☑
  bronchopleural 012.0 ☑
  bronchopneumonia, bronchopneumonic 011.6 ☑
  bronchorrhagia 011.3 ☑
  bronchotracheal 011.3 ☑
    isolated 012.2 ☑
  bronchus — *see* Tuberculosis, bronchi
  bronze disease (Addison's) 017.6 ☑
  buccal cavity 017.9 ☑
  bulbourethral gland 016.5 ☑
  bursa (*see also* Tuberculosis, joint) 015.9 ☑
  cachexia NEC (*see also* Tuberculosis, pulmonary) 011.9 ☑
  cardiomyopathy 017.9 ☑ *[425.8]*
  caries (*see also* Tuberculosis, bone) 015.9 ☑ *[730.8]*
  cartilage (*see also* Tuberculosis, bone) 015.9 ☑ *[730.8]*
    intervertebral 015.0 ☑ *[730.88]*
  catarrhal (*see also* Tuberculosis, pulmonary) 011.9 ☑
  cecum 014.8 ☑
  cellular tissue (primary) 017.0 ☑
  cellulitis (primary) 017.0 ☑
  central nervous system 013.9 ☑
    specified site NEC 013.8 ☑
  cerebellum (current) 013.2 ☑
  cerebral (current) 013.2 ☑
    meninges 013.0 ☑
  cerebrospinal 013.6 ☑
    meninges 013.0 ☑
  cerebrum (current) 013.2 ☑
  cervical 017.2 ☑
    gland 017.2 ☑
    lymph nodes 017.2 ☑
  cervicitis (uteri) 016.7 ☑
  cervix 016.7 ☑
  chest (*see also* Tuberculosis, pulmonary) 011.9 ☑
  childhood type or first infection 010.0 ☑
  choroid 017.3 ☑ *[363.13]*
  choroiditis 017.3 ☑ *[363.13]*
  ciliary body 017.3 ☑ *[364.11]*
  colitis 014.8 ☑
  colliers' 011.4 ☑
  colliquativa (primary) 017.0 ☑
  colon 014.8 ☑
    ulceration 014.8 ☑
  complex, primary 010.0 ☑
  complicating pregnancy, childbirth, or puerperium 647.3 ☑
    affecting fetus or newborn 760.2
  congenital 771.2
  conjunctiva 017.3 ☑ *[370.31]*
  connective tissue 017.9 ☑
    bone — *see* Tuberculosis, bone
  contact V01.1
  converter (tuberculin skin test) (without disease) 795.5
  cornea (ulcer) 017.3 ☑ *[370.31]*
  Cowper's gland 016.5 ☑
  coxae 015.1 ☑ *[730.85]*
  coxalgia 015.1 ☑ *[730.85]*
  cul-de-sac of Douglas 014.8 ☑
  curvature, spine 015.0 ☑ *[737.40]*
  cutis (colliquativa) (primary) 017.0 ☑
  cystitis 016.1 ☑
  cyst, ovary 016.6 ☑
  dacryocystitis 017.3 ☑ *[375.32]*
  dactylitis 015.5 ☑
  diarrhea 014.8 ☑

Tuberculosis, tubercular, tuberculous — *continued*
  diffuse (*see also* Tuberculosis, miliary) 018.9 ☑
    lung — *see* Tuberculosis, pulmonary
    meninges 013.0 ☑
  digestive tract 014.8 ☑
  disseminated (*see also* Tuberculosis, miliary) 018.9 ☑
    meninges 013.0 ☑
  duodenum 014.8 ☑
  dura (mater) 013.9 ☑
    abscess 013.8 ☑
      cerebral 013.3 ☑
      spinal 013.5 ☑
  dysentery 014.8 ☑
  ear (inner) (middle) 017.4 ☑
    bone 015.6 ☑
    external (primary) 017.0 ☑
    skin (primary) 017.0 ☑
  elbow 015.9 ☑
  emphysema — *see* Tuberculosis, pulmonary
  empyema 012.0 ☑
  encephalitis 013.6 ☑
  endarteritis 017.9 ☑
  endocarditis (any valve) 017.9 ☑ *[424.91]*
  endocardium (any valve) 017.9 ☑ *[424.91]*
  endocrine glands NEC 017.9 ☑
  endometrium 016.7 ☑
  enteric, enterica 014.8 ☑
  enteritis 014.8 ☑
  enterocolitis 014.8 ☑
  epididymis 016.4 ☑
  epididymitis 016.4 ☑
  epidural abscess 013.8 ☑
    brain 013.3 ☑
    spinal cord 013.5 ☑
  epiglottis 012.3 ☑
  episcleritis 017.3 ☑ *[379.00]*
  erythema (induratum) (nodosum) (primary) 017.1 ☑
  esophagus 017.8 ☑
  Eustachian tube 017.4 ☑
  exposure to V01.1
  exudative 012.0 ☑
    primary, progressive 010.1 ☑
  eye 017.3 ☑
  eyelid (primary) 017.0 ☑
    lupus 017.0 ☑ *[373.4]*
  fallopian tube 016.6 ☑
  fascia 017.9 ☑
  fauces 012.8 ☑
  finger 017.9 ☑
  first infection 010.0 ☑
  fistula, perirectal 014.8 ☑
  Florida 011.6 ☑
  foot 017.9 ☑
  funnel pelvis 137.3
  gallbladder 017.9 ☑
  galloping (*see also* Tuberculosis, pulmonary) 011.9 ☑
  ganglionic 015.9 ☑
  gastritis 017.9 ☑
  gastrocolic fistula 014.8 ☑
  gastroenteritis 014.8 ☑
  gastrointestinal tract 014.8 ☑
  general, generalized 018.9 ☑
    acute 018.0 ☑
    chronic 018.8 ☑
  genital organs NEC 016.9 ☑
    female 016.7 ☑
    male 016.5 ☑
  genitourinary NEC 016.9 ☑
  genu 015.2 ☑
  glandulae suprarenalis 017.6 ☑
  glandular, general 017.2 ☑
  glottis 012.3 ☑
  grinders' 011.4 ☑
  groin 017.2 ☑
  gum 017.9 ☑
  hand 017.9 ☑
  heart 017.9 ☑ *[425.8]*
  hematogenous — *see* Tuberculosis, miliary

Tuberculosis, tubercular, tuberculous — *continued*
  hemoptysis (*see also* Tuberculosis, pulmonary) 011.9 ☑
  hemorrhage NEC (*see also* Tuberculosis, pulmonary) 011.9 ☑
  hemothorax 012.0 ☑
  hepatitis 017.9 ☑
  hilar lymph nodes 012.1 ☑
    primary, progressive 010.8 ☑
  hip (disease) (joint) 015.1 ☑
    bone 015.1 ☑ *[730.85]*
  hydrocephalus 013.8 ☑
  hydropneumothorax 012.0 ☑
  hydrothorax 012.0 ☑
  hypoadrenalism 017.6 ☑
  hypopharynx 012.8 ☑
  ileocecal (hyperplastic) 014.8 ☑
  ileocolitis 014.8 ☑
  ileum 014.8 ☑
  iliac spine (superior) 015.0 ☑ *[730.88]*
  incipient NEC (*see also* Tuberculosis, pulmonary) 011.9 ☑
  indurativa (primary) 017.1 ☑
  infantile 010.0 ☑
  infection NEC 011.9 ☑
    without clinical manifestation 010.0 ☑
  infraclavicular gland 017.2 ☑
  inguinal gland 017.2 ☑
  inguinalis 017.2 ☑
  intestine (any part) 014.8 ☑
  iris 017.3 ☑ *[364.11]*
  iritis 017.3 ☑ *[364.11]*
  ischiorectal 014.8 ☑
  jaw 015.7 ☑ *[730.88]*
  jejunum 014.8 ☑
  joint 015.9 ☑
    hip 015.1 ☑
    knee 015.2 ☑
    specified site NEC 015.8 ☑
    vertebral 015.0 ☑ *[730.88]*
  keratitis 017.3 ☑ *[370.31]*
    interstitial 017.3 ☑ *[370.59]*
  keratoconjunctivitis 017.3 ☑ *[370.31]*
  kidney 016.0 ☑
  knee (joint) 015.2 ☑
  kyphoscoliosis 015.0 ☑ *[737.43]*
  kyphosis 015.0 ☑ *[737.41]*
  lacrimal apparatus, gland 017.3 ☑
  laryngitis 012.3 ☑
  larynx 012.3 ☑
  leptomeninges, leptomeningitis (cerebral) (spinal) 013.0 ☑
  lichenoides (primary) 017.0 ☑
  linguae 017.9 ☑
  lip 017.9 ☑
  liver 017.9 ☑
  lordosis 015.0 ☑ *[737.42]*
  lung — *see* Tuberculosis, pulmonary
  luposa 017.0 ☑
    eyelid 017.0 ☑ *[373.4]*
  lymphadenitis — *see* Tuberculosis, lymph gland
  lymphangitis — *see* Tuberculosis, lymph gland
  lymphatic (gland) (vessel) — *see* Tuberculosis, lymph gland
  lymph gland or node (peripheral) 017.2 ☑
    abdomen 014.8 ☑
    bronchial 012.1 ☑
      primary, progressive 010.8 ☑
    cervical 017.2 ☑
    hilar 012.1 ☑
      primary, progressive 010.8 ☑
    intrathoracic 012.1 ☑
      primary, progressive 010.8 ☑
    mediastinal 012.1 ☑
      primary, progressive 010.8 ☑
    mesenteric 014.8 ☑
    peripheral 017.2 ☑
    retroperitoneal 014.8 ☑
    tracheobronchial 012.1 ☑
      primary, progressive 010.8 ☑

Tuberculosis, tubercular, tuberculous — *continued*
  malignant NEC (*see also* Tuberculosis, pulmonary) 011.9 ☑
  mammary gland 017.9 ☑
  marasmus NEC (*see also* Tuberculosis, pulmonary) 011.9 ☑
  mastoiditis 015.6 ☑
  maternal, affecting fetus or newborn 760.2
  mediastinal (lymph) gland or node 012.1 ☑
    primary, progressive 010.8 ☑
  mediastinitis 012.8 ☑
    primary, progressive 010.8 ☑
  mediastinopericarditis 017.9 ☑ *[420.0]*
  mediastinum 012.8 ☑
    primary, progressive 010.8 ☑
  medulla 013.9 ☑
    brain 013.2 ☑
    spinal cord 013.4 ☑
  melanosis, Addisonian 017.6 ☑
  membrane, brain 013.0 ☑
  meninges (cerebral) (spinal) 013.0 ☑
  meningitis (basilar) (brain) (cerebral) (cerebrospinal) (spinal) 013.0 ☑
  meningoencephalitis 013.0 ☑
  mesentery, mesenteric 014.8 ☑
    lymph gland or node 014.8 ☑
  miliary (any site) 018.9 ☑
    acute 018.0 ☑
    chronic 018.8 ☑
    specified type NEC 018.8 ☑
  millstone makers' 011.4 ☑
  miners' 011.4 ☑
  moulders' 011.4 ☑
  mouth 017.9 ☑
  multiple 018.9 ☑
    acute 018.0 ☑
    chronic 018.8 ☑
  muscle 017.9 ☑
  myelitis 013.6 ☑
  myocarditis 017.9 ☑ *[422.0]*
  myocardium 017.9 ☑ *[422.0]*
  nasal (passage) (sinus) 012.8 ☑
  nasopharynx 012.8 ☑
  neck gland 017.2 ☑
  nephritis 016.0 ☑ *[583.81]*
  nerve 017.9 ☑
  nose (septum) 012.8 ☑
  ocular 017.3 ☑
  old NEC 137.0
    without residuals V12.01
  omentum 014.8 ☑
  oophoritis (acute) (chronic) 016.6 ☑
  optic 017.3 ☑ *[377.39]*
    nerve trunk 017.3 ☑ *[377.39]*
    papilla, papillae 017.3 ☑ *[377.39]*
  orbit 017.3 ☑
  orchitis 016.5 ☑ *[608.81]*
  organ, specified NEC 017.9 ☑
  orificialis (primary) 017.0 ☑
  osseous (*see also* Tuberculosis, bone) 015.9 ☑ *[730.8]*
  osteitis (*see also* Tuberculosis, bone) 015.9 ☑ *[730.8]*
  osteomyelitis (*see also* Tuberculosis, bone) 015.9 ☑ *[730.8]*
  otitis (media) 017.4 ☑
  ovaritis (acute) (chronic) 016.6 ☑
  ovary (acute) (chronic) 016.6 ☑
  oviducts (acute) (chronic) 016.6 ☑
  pachymeningitis 013.0 ☑
  palate (soft) 017.9 ☑
  pancreas 017.9 ☑
  papulonecrotic (primary) 017.0 ☑
  parathyroid glands 017.9 ☑
  paronychia (primary) 017.0 ☑
  parotid gland or region 017.9 ☑
  pelvic organ NEC 016.9 ☑
    female 016.7 ☑
    male 016.5 ☑
  pelvis (bony) 015.7 ☑ *[730.85]*
  penis 016.5 ☑
  peribronchitis 011.3 ☑

☑ **Additional Digit Required — Refer to the Tabular List for Digit Selection**   ▼ Subterms under main terms may continue to next column or page

Index · Tuberculosis, tubercular, tuberculous — Tumor

Tuberculosis, tubercular, tuberculous — *continued*
- pericarditis 017.9 ✓ [420.0]
- pericardium 017.9 ✓ [420.0]
- perichondritis, larynx 012.3 ✓
- perineum 017.9 ✓
- periostitis (*see also* Tuberculosis, bone) 015.9 ✓ [730.8]
- periphlebitis 017.9 ✓
  - eye vessel 017.3 ✓ [362.18]
  - retina 017.3 ✓ [362.18]
- perirectal fistula 014.8 ✓
- peritoneal gland 014.8 ✓
- peritoneum 014.0 ✓
- peritonitis 014.0 ✓
- pernicious NEC (*see also* Tuberculosis, pulmonary) 011.9 ✓
- pharyngitis 012.8 ✓
- pharynx 012.8 ✓
- phlyctenulosis (conjunctiva) 017.3 ✓ [370.31]
- phthisis NEC (*see also* Tuberculosis, pulmonary) 011.9 ✓
- pituitary gland 017.9 ✓
- placenta 016.7 ✓
- pleura, pleural, pleurisy, pleuritis (fibrinous) (obliterative) (purulent) (simple plastic) (with effusion) 012.0 ✓
  - primary, progressive 010.1 ✓
- pneumonia, pneumonic 011.6 ✓
- pneumothorax 011.7 ✓
- polyserositis 018.9 ✓
  - acute 018.0 ✓
  - chronic 018.8 ✓
- potters' 011.4 ✓
- prepuce 016.5 ✓
- primary 010.9 ✓
  - complex 010.0 ✓
  - complicated 010.8 ✓
    - with pleurisy or effusion 010.1 ✓
  - progressive 010.8 ✓
    - with pleurisy or effusion 010.1 ✓
  - skin 017.0 ✓
- proctitis 014.8 ✓
- prostate 016.5 ✓ [601.4]
- prostatitis 016.5 ✓ [601.4]
- pulmonaris (*see also* Tuberculosis, pulmonary) 011.9 ✓
- pulmonary (artery) (incipient) (malignant) (multiple round foci) (pernicious) (reinfection stage) 011.9 ✓
  - cavitated or with cavitation 011.2 ✓
    - primary, progressive 010.8 ✓
  - childhood type or first infection 010.0 ✓
  - chromogenic acid-fast bacilli 795.39
  - fibrosis or fibrotic 011.4 ✓
  - infiltrative 011.0 ✓
    - primary, progressive 010.9 ✓
  - nodular 011.1 ✓
  - specified NEC 011.8 ✓
  - sputum positive only 795.39
  - status following surgical collapse of lung NEC 011.9 ✓
- pyelitis 016.0 ✓ [590.81]
- pyelonephritis 016.0 ✓ [590.81]
- pyemia — *see* Tuberculosis, miliary
- pyonephrosis 016.0 ✓
- pyopneumothorax 012.0 ✓
- pyothorax 012.0 ✓
- rectum (with abscess) 014.8 ✓
  - fistula 014.8 ✓
- reinfection stage (*see also* Tuberculosis, pulmonary) 011.9 ✓
- renal 016.0 ✓
- renis 016.0 ✓
- reproductive organ 016.7 ✓
- respiratory NEC (*see also* Tuberculosis, pulmonary) 011.9 ✓
  - specified site NEC 012.8 ✓
- retina 017.3 ✓ [363.13]
- retroperitoneal (lymph gland or node) 014.8 ✓
  - gland 014.8 ✓
- retropharyngeal abscess 012.8 ✓

Tuberculosis, tubercular, tuberculous — *continued*
- rheumatism 015.9 ✓
- rhinitis 012.8 ✓
- sacroiliac (joint) 015.8 ✓
- sacrum 015.0 ✓ [730.88]
- salivary gland 017.9 ✓
- salpingitis (acute) (chronic) 016.6 ✓
- sandblasters' 011.4 ✓
- sclera 017.3 ✓ [379.09]
- scoliosis 015.0 ✓ [737.43]
- scrofulous 017.2 ✓
- scrotum 016.5 ✓
- seminal tract or vesicle 016.5 ✓ [608.81]
- senile NEC (*see also* Tuberculosis, pulmonary) 011.9 ✓
- septic NEC (*see also* Tuberculosis, miliary) 018.9 ✓
- shoulder 015.8 ✓
  - blade 015.7 ✓ [730.8]
- sigmoid 014.8 ✓
- sinus (accessory) (nasal) 012.8 ✓
  - bone 015.7 ✓ [730.88]
  - epididymis 016.4 ✓
- skeletal NEC (*see also* Osteomyelitis, due to tuberculosis) 015.9 ✓ [730.8]
- skin (any site) (primary) 017.0 ✓
- small intestine 014.8 ✓
- soft palate 017.9 ✓
- spermatic cord 016.5 ✓
- spinal
  - column 015.0 ✓ [730.88]
  - cord 013.4 ✓
  - disease 015.0 ✓ [730.88]
  - medulla 013.4 ✓
  - membrane 013.0 ✓
  - meninges 013.0 ✓
- spine 015.0 ✓ [730.88]
- spleen 017.7 ✓
- splenitis 017.7 ✓
- spondylitis 015.0 ✓ [720.81]
- spontaneous pneumothorax — *see* Tuberculosis, pulmonary
- sternoclavicular joint 015.8 ✓
- stomach 017.9 ✓
- stonemasons' 011.4 ✓
- struma 017.2 ✓
- subcutaneous tissue (cellular) (primary) 017.0 ✓
- subcutis (primary) 017.0 ✓
- subdeltoid bursa 017.9 ✓
- submaxillary 017.9 ✓
  - region 017.9 ✓
- supraclavicular gland 017.2 ✓
- suprarenal (capsule) (gland) 017.6 ✓
- swelling, joint (*see also* Tuberculosis, joint) 015.9 ✓
- symphysis pubis 015.7 ✓ [730.88]
- synovitis 015.9 ✓ [727.01]
  - hip 015.1 ✓ [727.01]
  - knee 015.2 ✓ [727.01]
  - specified site NEC 015.8 ✓ [727.01]
  - spine or vertebra 015.0 ✓ [727.01]
- systemic — *see* Tuberculosis, miliary
- tarsitis (eyelid) 017.0 ✓ [373.4]
  - ankle (bone) 015.5 ✓ [730.87]
- tendon (sheath) — *see* Tuberculosis, tenosynovitis
- tenosynovitis 015.9 ✓ [727.01]
  - hip 015.1 ✓ [727.01]
  - knee 015.2 ✓ [727.01]
  - specified site NEC 015.8 ✓ [727.01]
  - spine or vertebra 015.0 ✓ [727.01]
- testis 016.5 ✓ [608.81]
- throat 012.8 ✓
- thymus gland 017.9 ✓
- thyroid gland 017.5 ✓
- toe 017.9 ✓
- tongue 017.9 ✓
- tonsil (lingual) 012.8 ✓
- tonsillitis 012.8 ✓
- trachea, tracheal 012.8 ✓
  - gland 012.1 ✓

Tuberculosis, tubercular, tuberculous — *continued*
- trachea, tracheal — *continued*
  - gland — *continued*
    - primary, progressive 010.8 ✓
    - isolated 012.2 ✓
  - tracheobronchial 011.3 ✓
    - glandular 012.1 ✓
      - primary, progressive 010.8 ✓
      - isolated 012.2 ✓
    - lymph gland or node 012.1 ✓
      - primary, progressive 010.8 ✓
- tubal 016.6 ✓
- tunica vaginalis 016.5 ✓
- typhlitis 014.8 ✓
- ulcer (primary) (skin) 017.0 ✓
  - bowel or intestine 014.8 ✓
  - specified site NEC — *see* Tuberculosis, by site
  - unspecified site — *see* Tuberculosis, pulmonary
- ureter 016.2 ✓
- urethra, urethral 016.3 ✓
- urinary organ or tract 016.3 ✓
  - kidney 016.0 ✓
- uterus 016.7 ✓
- uveal tract 017.3 ✓ [363.13]
- uvula 017.9 ✓
- vaccination, prophylactic (against) V03.2
- vagina 016.7 ✓
- vas deferens 016.5 ✓
- vein 017.9 ✓
- verruca (primary) 017.0 ✓
- verrucosa (cutis) (primary) 017.0 ✓
- vertebra (column) 015.0 ✓ [730.88]
- vesiculitis 016.5 ✓ [608.81]
- viscera NEC 014.8 ✓
- vulva 016.7 ✓ [616.51]
- wrist (joint) 015.8 ✓
  - bone 015.5 ✓ [730.83]

Tuberculum
- auriculae 744.29
- occlusal 520.2
- paramolare 520.2

Tuberosity
- jaw, excessive 524.07
- maxillary, entire 524.07

Tuberous sclerosis (brain) 759.5

Tube, tubal, tubular — *see also* condition
- ligation, admission for V25.2

Tubo-ovarian — *see* condition

Tuboplasty, after previous sterilization V26.0

Tubotympanitis 381.10

Tularemia 021.9
- with
  - conjunctivitis 021.3
  - pneumonia 021.2
- bronchopneumonic 021.2
- conjunctivitis 021.3
- cryptogenic 021.1
- disseminated 021.8
- enteric 021.1
- generalized 021.8
- glandular 021.8
- intestinal 021.1
- oculoglandular 021.3
- ophthalmic 021.3
- pneumonia 021.2
- pulmonary 021.2
- specified NEC 021.8
- typhoidal 021.1
- ulceroglandular 021.0
- vaccination, prophylactic (against) V03.4

Tularensis conjunctivitis 021.3

Tumefaction — *see also* Swelling
- liver (*see also* Hypertrophy, liver) 789.1

Tumor (M8000/1) — *see also* Neoplasm, by site, unspecified nature
- Abrikossov's (M9580/0) (*see also* Neoplasm, connective tissue, benign)
  - malignant (M9580/3) — *see* Neoplasm, connective tissue, malignant
- acinar cell (M8550/1) — *see* Neoplasm, by site, uncertain behavior

Tumor — *see also* Neoplasm, by site, unspecified nature — *continued*
- acinic cell (M8550/1) — *see* Neoplasm, by site, uncertain behavior
- adenomatoid (M9054/0) (*see also* Neoplasm, by site, benign)
  - odontogenic (M9300/0) 213.1
    - upper jaw (bone) 213.0
- adnexal (skin) (M8390/0) — *see* Neoplasm, skin, benign
- adrenal
  - cortical (benign) (M8370/0) 227.0
    - malignant (M8370/3) 194.0
  - rest (M8671/0) — *see* Neoplasm, by site, benign
- alpha cell (M8152/0)
  - malignant (M8152/3)
    - pancreas 157.4
    - specified site NEC — *see* Neoplasm, by site, malignant
    - unspecified site 157.4
  - pancreas 211.7
  - specified site NEC — *see* Neoplasm, by site, benign
  - unspecified site 211.7
- aneurysmal (*see also* Aneurysm) 442.9
- aortic body (M8691/1) 237.3
  - malignant (M8691/3) 194.6
- argentaffin (M8241/1) — *see* Neoplasm, by site, uncertain behavior
- basal cell (M8090/1) (*see also* Neoplasm, skin, uncertain behavior)
- benign (M8000/0) — *see* Neoplasm, by site, benign
- beta cell (M8151/0)
  - malignant (M8151/3)
    - pancreas 157.4
    - specified site — *see* Neoplasm, by site, malignant
    - unspecified site 157.4
  - pancreas 211.7
  - specified site NEC — *see* Neoplasm, by site, benign
  - unspecified site 211.7
- blood — *see* Hematoma
- Brenner (M9000/0) 220
  - borderline malignancy (M9000/1) 236.2
  - malignant (M9000/3) 183.0
  - proliferating (M9000/1) 236.2
- Brooke's (M8100/0) — *see* Neoplasm, skin, benign
- brown fat (M8880/0) — *see* Lipoma, by site
- Burkitt's (M9750/3) 200.2 ✓
- calcifying epithelial odontogenic (M9340/0) 213.1
  - upper jaw (bone) 213.0
- carcinoid (M8240/1) 209.60
  - benign 209.60
    - appendix 209.51
    - ascending colon 209.53
    - bronchus 209.61
    - cecum 209.52
    - colon 209.50
    - descending colon 209.55
    - duodenum 209.41
    - foregut 209.65
    - hindgut 209.67
    - ileum 209.43
    - jejunum 209.42
    - kidney 209.64
    - large intestine 209.50
    - lung 209.61
    - midgut 209.66
    - rectum 209.57
    - sigmoid colon 209.56
    - small intestine 209.40
    - specified NEC 209.69
    - stomach 209.63
    - thymus 209.62
    - transverse colon 209.54
  - malignant (of) 209.20
    - appendix 209.11
    - ascending colon 209.13
    - bronchus 209.21
    - cecum 209.12
    - colon 209.10

Tumor — see also Neoplasm, by site, unspecified nature — continued
  carcinoid — continued
    malignant — continued
      descending colon 209.15
      duodenum 209.01
      foregut 209.25
      hindgut 209.27
      ileum 209.03
      jejunum 209.02
      kidney 209.24
      large intestine 209.10
      lung 209.21
      midgut 209.26
      rectum 209.17
      sigmoid colon 209.16
      small intestine 209.00
      specified NEC 209.29
      stomach 209.23
      thymus 209.22
      transverse colon 209.14
    secondary — see Tumor, neuroendocrine, secondary
  carotid body (M8692/1) 237.3
    malignant (M8692/3) 194.5
  Castleman's (mediastinal lymph node hyperplasia) 785.6
  cells (M8001/1) (see also Neoplasm, by site, unspecified nature)
    benign (M8001/0) — see Neoplasm, by site, benign
    malignant (M8001/3) — see Neoplasm, by site, malignant
    uncertain whether benign or malignant (M8001/1) — see Neoplasm, by site, uncertain nature
  cervix
    in pregnancy or childbirth 654.6 ☑
      affecting fetus or newborn 763.89
      causing obstructed labor 660.2 ☑
        affecting fetus or newborn 763.1
  chondromatous giant cell (M9230/0) — see Neoplasm, bone, benign
  chromaffin (M8700/0) (see also Neoplasm, by site, benign)
    malignant (M8700/3) — see Neoplasm, by site, malignant
  Cock's peculiar 706.2
  Codman's (benign chondroblastoma) (M9230/0) — see Neoplasm, bone, benign
  dentigerous, mixed (M9282/0) 213.1
    upper jaw (bone) 213.0
  dermoid (M9084/0) — see Neoplasm, by site, benign
    with malignant transformation (M9084/3) 183.0
  desmoid (extra-abdominal) (M8821/1) (see also Neoplasm, connective tissue, uncertain behavior)
    abdominal (M8822/1) — see Neoplasm, connective tissue, uncertain behavior
  embryonal (mixed) (M9080/1) (see also Neoplasm, by site, uncertain behavior)
    liver (M9080/3) 155.0
  endodermal sinus (M9071/3)
    specified site — see Neoplasm, by site, malignant
    unspecified site
      female 183.0
      male 186.9
  epithelial
    benign (M8010/0) — see Neoplasm, by site, benign
    malignant (M8010/3) — see Neoplasm, by site, malignant
  Ewing's (M9260/3) — see Neoplasm, bone, malignant
  fatty — see Lipoma
  fetal, causing disproportion 653.7 ☑
    causing obstructed labor 660.1 ☑
  fibroid (M8890/0) — see Leiomyoma

Tumor — see also Neoplasm, by site, unspecified nature — continued
  G cell (M8153/1)
    malignant (M8153/3)
      pancreas 157.4
      specified site NEC — see Neoplasm, by site, malignant
      unspecified site 157.4
    specified site — see Neoplasm, by site, uncertain behavior
    unspecified site 235.5
  giant cell (type) (M8003/1) (see also Neoplasm, by site, unspecified nature)
    bone (M9250/1) 238.0
      malignant (M9250/3) — see Neoplasm, bone, malignant
    chondromatous (M9230/0) — see Neoplasm, bone, benign
    malignant (M8003/3) — see Neoplasm, by site, malignant
    peripheral (gingiva) 523.8
    soft parts (M9251/1) (see also Neoplasm, connective tissue, uncertain behavior)
      malignant (M9251/3) — see Neoplasm, connective tissue, malignant
    tendon sheath 727.02
  glomus (M8711/0) (see also Hemangioma, by site)
    jugulare (M8690/1) 237.3
      malignant (M8690/3) 194.6
  gonadal stromal (M8590/1) — see Neoplasm, by site, uncertain behavior
  granular cell (M9580/0) (see also Neoplasm, connective tissue, benign)
    malignant (M9580/3) — see Neoplasm, connective tissue, malignant
  granulosa cell (M8620/1) 236.2
    malignant (M8620/3) 183.0
  granulosa cell-theca cell (M8621/1) 236.2
    malignant (M8621/3) 183.0
  Grawitz's (hypernephroma) (M8312/3) 189.0
  hazard-crile (M8350/3) 193
  hemorrhoidal — see Hemorrhoids
  hilar cell (M8660/0) 220
  Hürthle cell (benign) (M8290/0) 226
    malignant (M8290/3) 193
  hydatid (see also Echinococcus) 122.9
  hypernephroid (M8311/1) (see also Neoplasm, by site, uncertain behavior)
  interstitial cell (M8650/1) (see also Neoplasm, by site, uncertain behavior)
    benign (M8650/0) — see Neoplasm, by site, benign
    malignant (M8650/3) — see Neoplasm, by site, malignant
  islet cell (M8150/0)
    malignant (M8150/3)
      pancreas 157.4
      specified site — see Neoplasm, by site, malignant
      unspecified site 157.4
    pancreas 211.7
    specified site NEC — see Neoplasm, by site, benign
    unspecified site 211.7
  juxtaglomerular (M8361/1) 236.91
  Krukenberg's (M8490/6) 198.6
  Leydig cell (M8650/1)
    benign (M8650/0)
      specified site — see Neoplasm, by site, benign
      unspecified site
        female 220
        male 222.0
    malignant (M8650/3)
      specified site — see Neoplasm, by site, malignant
      unspecified site
        female 183.0
        male 186.9
    specified site — see Neoplasm, by site, uncertain behavior
    unspecified site
      female 236.2

Tumor — see also Neoplasm, by site, unspecified nature — continued
  Leydig cell — continued
    unspecified site — continued
      male 236.4
  lipid cell, ovary (M8670/0) 220
  lipoid cell, ovary (M8670/0) 220
  lymphomatous, benign (M9590/0) (see also Neoplasm, by site, benign)
  lysis syndrome (following antineoplastic drug therapy) (spontaneous) 277.88
  Malherbe's (M8110/0) — see Neoplasm, skin, benign
  malignant (M8000/3) (see also Neoplasm, by site, malignant)
    fusiform cell (type) (M8004/3) — see Neoplasm, by site, malignant
    giant cell (type) (M8003/3) — see Neoplasm, by site, malignant
    mixed NEC (M8940/3) — see Neoplasm, by site, malignant
    small cell (type) (M8002/3) — see Neoplasm, by site, malignant
    spindle cell (type) (M8004/3) — see Neoplasm, by site, malignant
  mast cell (M9740/1) 238.5
    malignant (M9740/3) 202.6 ☑
  melanotic, neuroectodermal (M9363/0) — see Neoplasm, by site, benign
  Merkel cell — see Carcinoma, Merkel cell
  mesenchymal
    malignant (M8800/3) — see Neoplasm, connective tissue, malignant
    mixed (M8990/1) — see Neoplasm, connective tissue, uncertain behavior
  mesodermal, mixed (M8951/3) (see also Neoplasm, by site, malignant)
    liver 155.0
  mesonephric (M9110/1) (see also Neoplasm, by site, uncertain behavior)
    malignant (M9110/3) — see Neoplasm, by site, malignant
  metastatic
    from specified site (M8000/3) — see Neoplasm, by site, malignant
    to specified site (M8000/6) — see Neoplasm, by site, malignant, secondary
  mixed NEC (M8940/0) (see also Neoplasm, by site, benign)
    malignant (M8940/3) — see Neoplasm, by site, malignant
  mucocarcinoid, malignant (M8243/3) — see Neoplasm, by site, malignant
  mucoepidermoid (M8430/1) — see Neoplasm, by site, uncertain behavior
  Müllerian, mixed (M8950/3) — see Neoplasm, by site, malignant
  myoepithelial (M8982/0) — see Neoplasm, by site, benign
  neuroendocrine 209.60
    malignant poorly differentiated 209.30
    secondary 209.70
      bone 209.73
      distant lymph nodes 209.71
      liver 209.72
      peritoneum 209.74
      site specified NEC 209.79
  neurogenic olfactory (M9520/3) 160.0
  nonencapsulated sclerosing (M8350/3) 193
  odontogenic (M9270/1) 238.0
    adenomatoid (M9300/0) 213.1
      upper jaw (bone) 213.0
    benign (M9270/0) 213.1
      upper jaw (bone) 213.0
    calcifying epithelial (M9340/0) 213.1
      upper jaw (bone) 213.0
    malignant (M9270/3) 170.1
      upper jaw (bone) 170.0
    squamous (M9312/0) 213.1
      upper jaw (bone) 213.0
  ovarian stromal (M8590/1) 236.2
  ovary
    in pregnancy or childbirth 654.4 ☑
      affecting fetus or newborn 763.89

Tumor — see also Neoplasm, by site, unspecified nature — continued
  ovary — continued
    in pregnancy or childbirth — continued
      causing obstructed labor 660.2 ☑
        affecting fetus or newborn 763.1
  pacinian (M9507/0) — see Neoplasm, skin, benign
  Pancoast's (M8010/3) 162.3
  papillary — see Papilloma
  pelvic, in pregnancy or childbirth 654.9 ☑
    affecting fetus or newborn 763.89
    causing obstructed labor 660.2 ☑
      affecting fetus or newborn 763.1
  phantom 300.11
  plasma cell (M9731/1) 238.6
    benign (M9731/0) — see Neoplasm, by site, benign
    malignant (M9731/3) 203.8 ☑
  polyvesicular vitelline (M9071/3)
    specified site — see Neoplasm, by site, malignant
    unspecified site
      female 183.0
      male 186.9
  Pott's puffy (see also Osteomyelitis) 730.2 ☑
  Rathke's pouch (M9350/1) 237.0
  regaud's (M8082/3) — see Neoplasm, nasopharynx, malignant
  rete cell (M8140/0) 222.0
  retinal anlage (M9363/0) — see Neoplasm, by site, benign
  Rokitansky's 620.2
  salivary gland type, mixed (M8940/0) (see also Neoplasm, by site, benign)
    malignant (M8940/3) — see Neoplasm, by site, malignant
  Sampson's 617.1
  Schloffer's (see also Peritonitis) 567.29
  Schmincke (M8082/3) — see Neoplasm, nasopharynx, malignant
  sebaceous (see also Cyst, sebaceous) 706.2
  secondary (M8000/6) — see Neoplasm, by site, secondary
    carcinoid — see Tumor, neuroendocrine, secondary
    neuroendocrine — see Tumor, neuroendocrine, secondary
  Sertoli cell (M8640/0)
    with lipid storage (M8641/0)
      specified site — see Neoplasm, by site, benign
      unspecified site
        female 220
        male 222.0
    specified site — see Neoplasm, by site, benign
    unspecified site
      female 220
      male 222.0
  Sertoli-Leydig cell (M8631/0)
    specified site, — see Neoplasm, by site, benign
    unspecified site
      female 220
      male 222.0
  sex cord (-stromal) (M8590/1) — see Neoplasm, by site, uncertain behavior
  skin appendage (M8390/0) — see Neoplasm, skin, benign
  soft tissue
    benign (M8800/0) — see Neoplasm, connective tissue, benign
    malignant (M8800/3) — see Neoplasm, connective tissue, malignant
  sternomastoid 754.1
  stromal
    abdomen
      benign 215.5
      malignant NEC 171.5
      uncertain behavior 238.1
    digestive system 238.1
      benign 215.5
      malignant NEC 171.5
      uncertain behavior 238.1

☑ Additional Digit Required — Refer to the Tabular List for Digit Selection   ▽ Subterms under main terms may continue to next column or page

2011 ICD-9-CM   ▶◀ Revised Text   ● New Line   ▲ Revised Code   Volume 2 — 285

Index

Tumor — Ulcer, ulcerated, ulcerating

Tumor — *see also* Neoplasm, by site, unspecified nature — *continued*
stromal — *continued*
endometrium (endometrial) 236.0 ●
gastric 238.1
benign 215.5
malignant 151.9
uncertain behavior 238.1
gastrointestinal 238.1
benign 215.5
malignant NEC 171.5
uncertain behavior 238.1
intestine (small) 238.1
benign 215.5
malignant 152.9
uncertain behavior 238.1
stomach 238.1
benign 215.5
malignant 151.9
uncertain behavior 238.1
superior sulcus (lung) (pulmonary) (syndrome) (M8010/3) 162.3
suprasulcus (M8010/3) 162.3
sweat gland (M8400/1) (*see also* Neoplasm, skin, uncertain behavior)
benign (M8400/0) — *see* Neoplasm, skin, benign
malignant (M8400/3) — *see* Neoplasm, skin, malignant
syphilitic brain 094.89
congenital 090.49
testicular stromal (M8590/1) 236.4
theca cell (M8600/0) 220
theca cell-granulosa cell (M8621/1) 236.2
theca-lutein (M8610/0) 220
turban (M8200/0) 216.4
uterus
in pregnancy or childbirth 654.1 ☑
affecting fetus or newborn 763.89
causing obstructed labor 660.2 ☑
affecting fetus or newborn 763.1
vagina
in pregnancy or childbirth 654.7 ☑
affecting fetus or newborn 763.89
causing obstructed labor 660.2 ☑
affecting fetus or newborn 763.1
varicose (*see also* Varicose, vein) 454.9
von Recklinghausen's (M9540/1) 237.71
vulva
in pregnancy or childbirth 654.8 ☑
affecting fetus or newborn 763.89
causing obstructed labor 660.2 ☑
affecting fetus or newborn 763.1
Warthin's (salivary gland) (M8561/0) 210.2
white (*see also* Tuberculosis, arthritis)
White-Darier 757.39
Wilms' (nephroblastoma) (M8960/3) 189.0
yolk sac (M9071/3)
specified site — *see* Neoplasm, by site, malignant
unspecified site
female 183.0
male 186.9
Tumorlet (M8040/1) — *see* Neoplasm, by site, uncertain behavior
Tungiasis 134.1
Tunica vasculosa lentis 743.39
Tunnel vision 368.45
Turban tumor (M8200/0) 216.4
Türck's trachoma (chronic catarrhal laryngitis) 476.0
Türk's syndrome (ocular retraction syndrome) 378.71
Turner's
hypoplasia (tooth) 520.4
syndrome 758.6
tooth 520.4
Turner-Kieser syndrome (hereditary osteo-onychodysplasia) 756.89
Turner-Varny syndrome 758.6
Turricephaly 756.0
Tussis convulsiva — *see also* Whooping cough 033.9
Twiddler's syndrome (due to)
automatic implantable defibrillator 996.04
pacemaker 996.01

Twin
affected by maternal complications of pregnancy 761.5
conjoined 759.4
fetal 678.1 ☑
healthy liveborn — *see* Newborn, twin
pregnancy (complicating delivery) NEC 651.0 ☑
with fetal loss and retention of one fetus 651.3 ☑
conjoined 678.1 ☑
following (elective) fetal reduction
Twinning, teeth 520.2
Twist, twisted
bowel, colon, or intestine 560.2
hair (congenital) 757.4
mesentery 560.2
omentum 560.2
organ or site, congenital NEC — *see* Anomaly, specified type NEC
ovarian pedicle 620.5
congenital 752.0
umbilical cord — *see* Compression, umbilical cord
Twitch 781.0
Tylosis 700
buccalis 528.6
gingiva 523.8
linguae 528.6
palmaris et plantaris 757.39
Tympanism 787.3
Tympanites (abdominal) (intestine) 787.3
Tympanitis — *see* Myringitis
Tympanosclerosis 385.00
involving
combined sites NEC 385.09
with tympanic membrane 385.03
tympanic membrane 385.01
with ossicles 385.02
and middle ear 385.03
Tympanum — *see* condition
Tympany
abdomen 787.3
chest 786.7
Typhlitis — *see also* Appendicitis 541
Typhoenteritis 002.0
Typhogastric fever 002.0
Typhoid (abortive) (ambulant) (any site) (fever) (hemorrhagic) (infection) (intermittent) (malignant) (rheumatic) 002.0
with pneumonia 002.0 [484.8]
abdominal 002.0
carrier (suspected) of V02.1
cholecystitis (current) 002.0
clinical (Widal and blood test negative) 002.0
endocarditis 002.0 [421.1]
inoculation reaction — *see* Complications, vaccination
meningitis 002.0 [320.7]
mesenteric lymph nodes 002.0
myocarditis 002.0 [422.0]
osteomyelitis (*see also* Osteomyelitis, due to, typhoid) 002.0 [730.8] ☑
perichondritis, larynx 002.0 [478.71]
pneumonia 002.0 [484.8]
spine 002.0 [720.81]
ulcer (perforating) 002.0
vaccination, prophylactic (against) V03.1
Widal negative 002.0
Typhomalaria (fever) — *see also* Malaria 084.6
Typhomania 002.0
Typhoperitonitis 002.0
Typhus (fever) 081.9
abdominal, abdominalis 002.0
African tick 082.1
amarillic (*see also* Fever, Yellow) 060.9
brain 081.9
cerebral 081.9
classical 080
endemic (flea-borne) 081.0
epidemic (louse-borne) 080
exanthematic NEC 080
exanthematicus SAI 080
brillii SAI 081.1
Mexicanus SAI 081.0

Typhus — *continued*
exanthematicus SAI — *continued*
pediculo vestimenti causa 080
typhus murinus 081.0
flea-borne 081.0
Indian tick 082.1
Kenya tick 082.1
louse-borne 080
Mexican 081.0
flea-borne 081.0
louse-borne 080
tabardillo 080
mite-borne 081.2
murine 081.0
North Asian tick-borne 082.2
petechial 081.9
Queensland tick 082.3
rat 081.0
recrudescent 081.1
recurrent (*see also* Fever, relapsing) 087.9
São Paulo 082.0
scrub (China) (India) (Malaya) (New Guinea) 081.2
shop (of Malaya) 081.0
Siberian tick 082.2
tick-borne NEC 082.9
tropical 081.2
vaccination, prophylactic (against) V05.8
Tyrosinemia 270.2
neonatal 775.89
Tyrosinosis (Medes) (Sakai) 270.2
Tyrosinuria 270.2
Tyrosyluria 270.2

U

Uehlinger's syndrome (acropachyderma) 757.39
Uhl's anomaly or disease (hypoplasia of myocardium, right ventricle) 746.84
Ulcerosa scarlatina 034.1
Ulcer, ulcerated, ulcerating, ulceration, ulcerative 707.9
with gangrene 707.9 [785.4]
abdomen (wall) (*see also* Ulcer, skin) 707.8
ala, nose 478.19
alveolar process 526.5
amebic (intestine) 006.9
skin 006.6
anastomotic — *see* Ulcer, gastrojejunal
anorectal 569.41
antral — *see* Ulcer, stomach
anus (sphincter) (solitary) 569.41
varicose — *see* Varicose, ulcer, anus
aorta — *see* Aneuysm
aphthous (oral) (recurrent) 528.2
genital organ(s)
female 616.50
male 608.89
mouth 528.2
arm (*see also* Ulcer, skin) 707.8
arteriosclerotic plaque — *see* Arteriosclerosis, by site
artery NEC 447.2
without rupture 447.8
atrophic NEC — *see* Ulcer, skin
Barrett's (chronic peptic ulcer of esophagus) 530.85
bile duct 576.8
bladder (solitary) (sphincter) 596.8
bilharzial (*see also* Schistosomiasis) 120.9 [595.4]
submucosal (*see also* Cystitis) 595.1
tuberculous (*see also* Tuberculosis) 016.1 ☑
bleeding NEC — *see* Ulcer, peptic, with hemorrhage
bone 730.9 ☑
bowel (*see also* Ulcer, intestine) 569.82
breast 611.0
bronchitis 491.8
bronchus 519.19
buccal (cavity) (traumatic) 528.9
burn (acute) — *see* Ulcer, duodenum
Buruli 031.1
buttock (*see also* Ulcer, skin) 707.8

Ulcer, ulcerated, ulcerating, ulceration, ulcerative — *continued*
buttock (*see also* Ulcer, skin) — *continued*
decubitus (*see also* Ulcer, pressure) 707.00
cancerous (M8000/3) — *see* Neoplasm, by site, malignant
cardia — *see* Ulcer, stomach
cardio-esophageal (peptic) 530.20
with bleeding 530.21
cecum (*see also* Ulcer, intestine) 569.82
cervix (uteri) (trophic) 622.0
with mention of cervicitis 616.0
chancroidal 099.0
chest (wall) (*see also* Ulcer, skin) 707.8
Chiclero 085.4
chin (pyogenic) (*see also* Ulcer, skin) 707.8
chronic (cause unknown) (*see also* Ulcer, skin)
penis 607.89
Cochin-China 085.1
colitis — *see* Colitis, ulcerative
colon (*see also* Ulcer, intestine) 569.82
conjunctiva (acute) (postinfectional) 372.00
cornea (infectional) 370.00
with perforation 370.06
annular 370.02
catarrhal 370.01
central 370.03
dendritic 054.42
marginal 370.01
mycotic 370.05
phlyctenular, tuberculous (*see also* Tuberculosis) 017.3 ☑ [370.31]
ring 370.02
rodent 370.07
serpent, serpiginous 370.04
superficial marginal 370.01
tuberculous (*see also* Tuberculosis) 017.3 ☑ [370.31]
corpus cavernosum (chronic) 607.89
crural — *see* Ulcer, lower extremity
Curling's — *see* Ulcer, duodenum
Cushing's — *see* Ulcer, peptic
cystitis (interstitial) 595.1
decubitus (unspecified site) (*see also* Ulcer, pressure) 707.00
with gangrene 707.00 [785.4]
ankle 707.06
back
lower 707.03
upper 707.02
buttock 707.05
coccyx 707.03
elbow 707.01
head 707.09
heel 707.07
hip 707.04
other site 707.09
sacrum 707.03
shoulder blades 707.02
dendritic 054.42
diabetes, diabetic (mellitus) 250.8 ☑ [707.9]
due to secondary diabetes 249.8 ☑ [707.9]
lower limb 250.8 ☑ [707.10]
ankle 250.8 ☑ [707.13]
due to secondary diabetes 249.8 ☑ [707.13]
calf 250.8 ☑ [707.12]
due to secondary diabetes 249.8 ☑ [707.12]
due to secondary diabetes 249.8 ☑ [707.10]
foot 250.8 ☑ [707.15]
due to secondary diabetes 249.8 ☑ [707.15]
heel 250.8 ☑ [707.14]
due to secondary diabetes 249.8 ☑ [707.14]
knee 250.8 ☑ [707.19]
due to secondary diabetes 249.8 ☑ [707.19]
specified site NEC 250.8 ☑ [707.19]

☑ **Additional Digit Required** — Refer to the Tabular List for Digit Selection ▽ **Subterms under main terms may continue to next column or page**

286 — Volume 2 · October 2010 ▶◀ **Revised Text** ● **New Line** ▲ **Revised Code** 2011 ICD-9-CM

Ulcer, ulcerated, ulcerating, ulceration, ulcerative — *continued*
diabetes, diabetic — *continued*
  lower limb — *continued*
    specified site — *continued*
      due to secondary diabetes
        249.8 ☑ *[707.19]*
    thigh 250.8 ☑ *[707.11]*
      due to secondary diabetes
        249.8 ☑ *[707.11]*
    toes 250.8 ☑ *[707.15]*
      due to secondary diabetes
        249.8 ☑ *[707.15]*
    specified site NEC 250.8 ☑ *[707.8]*
      due to secondary diabetes
        249.8 ☑ *[707.8]*
Dieulafoy — *see* Lesion, Dieulafoy
due to
  infection NEC — *see* Ulcer, skin
  radiation, radium — *see* Ulcer, by site
  trophic disturbance (any region) — *see*
    Ulcer, skin
  x-ray — *see* Ulcer, by site
duodenum, duodenal (eroded) (peptic)
  532.9 ☑

> Note — Use the following fifth-digit
> subclassification with categories
> 531–534:
>
> 0   *without mention of obstruction*
>
> 1   *with obstruction*

  with
    hemorrhage (chronic) 532.4 ☑
      and perforation 532.6 ☑
    perforation (chronic) 532.5 ☑
      and hemorrhage 532.6 ☑
  acute 532.3 ☑
    with
      hemorrhage 532.0 ☑
        and perforation 532.2 ☑
      perforation 532.1 ☑
        and hemorrhage 532.2 ☑
  bleeding (recurrent) — *see* Ulcer, duode-
    num, with hemorrhage
  chronic 532.7 ☑
    with
      hemorrhage 532.4 ☑
        and perforation 532.6 ☑
      perforation 532.5 ☑
        and hemorrhage 532.6 ☑
  penetrating — *see* Ulcer, duodenum,
    with perforation
  perforating — *see* Ulcer, duodenum,
    with perforation
dysenteric NEC 009.0
elusive 595.1
endocarditis (any valve) (acute) (chronic)
  (subacute) 421.0
enteritis — *see* Colitis, ulcerative
enterocolitis 556.0
epiglottis 478.79
esophagus (peptic) 530.20
  with bleeding 530.21
  due to ingestion
    aspirin 530.20
    chemicals 530.20
    medicinal agents 530.20
  fungal 530.20
  infectional 530.20
  varicose (*see also* Varix, esophagus) 456.1
    bleeding (*see also* Varix, esophagus,
      bleeding) 456.0
eye NEC 360.00
  dendritic 054.42
eyelid (region) 373.01
face (*see also* Ulcer, skin) 707.8
fauces 478.29
Fenwick (-Hunner) (solitary) (*see also* Cystitis) 595.1
fistulous NEC — *see* Ulcer, skin
foot (indolent) (*see also* Ulcer, lower extremity) 707.15
  perforating 707.15
    leprous 030.1
    syphilitic 094.0

Ulcer, ulcerated, ulcerating, ulceration, ulcerative — *continued*
foot (*see also* Ulcer, lower extremity) —
  continued
  trophic 707.15
  varicose 454.0
    inflamed or infected 454.2
frambesial, initial or primary 102.0
gallbladder or duct 575.8
gall duct 576.8
gangrenous (*see also* Gangrene) 785.4
gastric — *see* Ulcer, stomach
gastrocolic — *see* Ulcer, gastrojejunal
gastroduodenal — *see* Ulcer, peptic
gastroesophageal — *see* Ulcer, stomach
gastrohepatic — *see* Ulcer, stomach
gastrointestinal — *see* Ulcer, gastrojejunal
gastrojejunal (eroded) (peptic) 534.9 ☑

> Note — Use the following fifth-digit
> subclassification with categories
> 531–534:
>
> 0   *without mention of obstruction*
>
> 1   *with obstruction*

  with
    hemorrhage (chronic) 534.4 ☑
      and perforation 534.6 ☑
    perforation 534.5 ☑
      and hemorrhage 534.6 ☑
  acute 534.3 ☑
    with
      hemorrhage 534.0 ☑
        and perforation 534.2 ☑
      perforation 534.1 ☑
        and hemorrhage 534.2 ☑
  bleeding (recurrent) — *see* Ulcer, gastro-
    jejunal, with hemorrhage
  chronic 534.7 ☑
    with
      hemorrhage 534.4 ☑
        and perforation 534.6 ☑
      perforation 534.5 ☑
        and hemorrhage 534.6 ☑
  penetrating — *see* Ulcer, gastrojejunal,
    with perforation
  perforating — *see* Ulcer, gastrojejunal,
    with perforation
gastrojejunocolic — *see* Ulcer, gastrojejunal
genital organ
  female 629.89
  male 608.89
gingiva 523.8
gingivitis 523.10
glottis 478.79
granuloma of pudenda 099.2
groin (*see also* Ulcer, skin) 707.8
gum 523.8
gumma, due to yaws 102.4
hand (*see also* Ulcer, skin) 707.8
hard palate 528.9
heel (*see also* Ulcer, lower extremity) 707.14
  decubitus (*see also* Ulcer, pressure)
    707.07
hemorrhoids 455.8
  external 455.5
  internal 455.2
hip (*see also* Ulcer, skin) 707.8
  decubitus (*see also* Ulcer, pressure)
    707.04
Hunner's 595.1
hypopharynx 478.29
hypopyon (chronic) (subacute) 370.04
hypostaticum — *see* Ulcer, varicose
ileocolitis 556.1
ileum (*see also* Ulcer, intestine) 569.82
intestine, intestinal 569.82
  with perforation 569.83
  amebic 006.9
  duodenal — *see* Ulcer, duodenum
  granulocytopenic (with hemorrhage)
    288.09
  marginal 569.82
  perforating 569.83
  small, primary 569.82
  stercoraceous 569.82

Ulcer, ulcerated, ulcerating, ulceration, ulcerative — *continued*
intestine, intestinal — *continued*
  stercoral 569.82
  tuberculous (*see also* Tuberculosis)
    014.8 ☑
  typhoid (fever) 002.0
  varicose 456.8
ischemic 707.9
  lower extremity (*see also* Ulcer, lower
    extremity) 707.10
    ankle 707.13
    calf 707.12
    foot 707.15
    heel 707.14
    knee 707.19
    specified site NEC 707.19
    thigh 707.11
    toes 707.15
jejunum, jejunal — *see* Ulcer, gastrojejunal
keratitis (*see also* Ulcer, cornea) 370.00
knee — *see* Ulcer, lower extremity
labium (majus) (minus) 616.50
laryngitis (*see also* Laryngitis) 464.00
  with obstruction 464.01
larynx (aphthous) (contact) 478.79
  diphtheritic 032.3
leg — *see* Ulcer, lower extremity
lip 528.5
Lipschütz's 616.50
lower extremity (atrophic) (chronic) (neurogenic) (perforating) (pyogenic)
  (trophic) (tropical) 707.10
  with gangrene (*see also* Ulcer, lower ex-
    tremity) 707.10 *[785.4]*
    arteriosclerotic 440.24
  ankle 707.13
    arteriosclerotic 440.23
      with gangrene 440.24
  calf 707.12
  decubitus (*see also* Ulcer, pressure)
    707.00
    with gangrene 707.00 *[785.4]*
    ankle 707.06
    buttock 707.05
    heel 707.07
    hip 707.04
  foot 707.15
  heel 707.14
  knee 707.19
  specified site NEC 707.19
  thigh 707.11
  toes 707.15
  varicose 454.0
    inflamed or infected 454.2
luetic — *see* Ulcer, syphilitic
lung 518.89
  tuberculous (*see also* Tuberculosis)
    011.2 ☑
malignant (M8000/3) — *see* Neoplasm, by
  site, malignant
marginal NEC — *see* Ulcer, gastrojejunal
meatus (urinarius) 597.89
Meckel's diverticulum 751.0
Meleney's (chronic undermining) 686.09
Mooren's (cornea) 370.07
mouth (traumatic) 528.9
mycobacterial (skin) 031.1
nasopharynx 478.29
navel cord (newborn) 771.4
neck (*see also* Ulcer, skin) 707.8
  uterus 622.0
neurogenic NEC — *see* Ulcer, skin
nose, nasal (infectional) (passage) 478.19
  septum 478.19
    varicose 456.8
  skin — *see* Ulcer, skin
  spirochetal NEC 104.8
oral mucosa (traumatic) 528.9
palate (soft) 528.9
penetrating NEC — *see* Ulcer, peptic, with
  perforation
penis (chronic) 607.89

Ulcer, ulcerated, ulcerating, ulceration, ulcerative — *continued*
peptic (site unspecified) 533.9 ☑

> Note — Use the following fifth-digit
> subclassification with categories
> 531–534:
>
> 0   *without mention of obstruction*
>
> 1   *with obstruction*

  with
    hemorrhage 533.4 ☑
      and perforation 533.6 ☑
    perforation (chronic) 533.5 ☑
      and hemorrhage 533.6 ☑
  acute 533.3 ☑
    with
      hemorrhage 533.0 ☑
        and perforation 533.2 ☑
      perforation 533.1 ☑
        and hemorrhage 533.2 ☑
  bleeding (recurrent) — *see* Ulcer, peptic,
    with hemorrhage
  chronic 533.7 ☑
    with
      hemorrhage 533.4 ☑
        and perforation 533.6 ☑
      perforation 533.5 ☑
        and hemorrhage 533.6 ☑
  penetrating — *see* Ulcer, peptic, with
    perforation
  perforating NEC (*see also* Ulcer, peptic, with
    perforation) 533.5 ☑
  skin 707.9
perineum (*see also* Ulcer, skin) 707.8
peritonsillar 474.8
phagedenic (tropical) NEC — *see* Ulcer, skin
pharynx 478.29
phlebitis — *see* Phlebitis
plaster (*see also* Ulcer, pressure) 707.00
popliteal space — *see* Ulcer, lower extremity
postpyloric — *see* Ulcer, duodenum
prepuce 607.89
prepyloric — *see* Ulcer, stomach
pressure 707.00
  with
    abrasion, blister, partial thickness
      skin loss involving epidermis
      and/or dermis 707.22
    full thickness skin loss involving
      damage or necrosis of subcu-
      taneous tissue 707.23
    gangrene 707.00 *[785.4]*
    necrosis of soft tissue through to un-
      derlying muscle, tendon, or
      bone 707.24
  ankle 707.06
  back
    lower 707.03
    upper 707.02
  buttock 707.05
  coccyx 707.03
  elbow 707.01
  head 707.09
  healed — omit code
  healing — code to Ulcer, pressure, by
    stage
  heel 707.07
  hip 707.04
  other site 707.09
  sacrum 707.03
  shoulder blades 707.02
  stage
    I (healing) 707.21
    II (healing) 707.22
    III (healing) 707.23
    IV (healing) 707.24
    unspecified (healing) 707.20
  unstageable 707.25
primary of intestine 569.82
  with perforation 569.83
proctitis 556.2
  with ulcerative sigmoiditis 556.3
prostate 601.8
pseudopeptic — *see* Ulcer, peptic
pyloric — *see* Ulcer, stomach

☑ **Additional Digit Required — Refer to the Tabular List for Digit Selection**   **Subterms under main terms may continue to next column or page**

2011 ICD-9-CM   ▶◀ **Revised Text**   ● **New Line**   ▲ **Revised Code**   **Volume 2 — 287**

Ulcer, ulcerated, ulcerating, ulceration, ulcerative — *continued*
rectosigmoid 569.82
  with perforation 569.83
rectum (sphincter) (solitary) 569.41
  stercoraceous, stercoral 569.41
  varicose — *see* Varicose, ulcer, anus
retina (*see also* Chorioretinitis) 363.20
rodent (M8090/3) (*see also* Neoplasm, skin, malignant)
  cornea 370.07
round — *see* Ulcer, stomach
sacrum (region) (*see also* Ulcer, skin) 707.8
Saemisch's 370.04
scalp (*see also* Ulcer, skin) 707.8
sclera 379.09
scrofulous (*see also* Tuberculosis) 017.2 ☑
scrotum 608.89
  tuberculous (*see also* Tuberculosis) 016.5 ☑
  varicose 456.4
seminal vesicle 608.89
sigmoid 569.82
  with perforation 569.83
skin (atrophic) (chronic) (neurogenic) (non-healing) (perforating) (pyogenic) (trophic) 707.9
  with gangrene 707.9 [785.4]
  amebic 006.6
  decubitus (*see also* Ulcer, pressure) 707.00
    with gangrene 707.00 [785.4]
  in granulocytopenia 288.09
  lower extremity (*see also* Ulcer, lower extremity) 707.10
    with gangrene 707.10 [785.4]
    arteriosclerotic 440.24
    ankle 707.13
    arteriosclerotic 440.23
      with gangrene 440.24
    calf 707.12
    foot 707.15
    heel 707.14
    knee 707.19
    specified site NEC 707.19
    thigh 707.11
    toes 707.15
  mycobacterial 031.1
  syphilitic (early) (secondary) 091.3
  tuberculous (primary) (*see also* Tuberculosis) 017.0 ☑
  varicose — *see* Ulcer, varicose
sloughing NEC — *see* Ulcer, skin
soft palate 528.9
solitary, anus or rectum (sphincter) 569.41
sore throat 462
  streptococcal 034.0
spermatic cord 608.89
spine (tuberculous) 015.0 ☑ [730.88]
stasis (leg) (venous) 454.0
  with varicose veins 454.0
  without varicose veins 459.81
  inflamed or infected 454.2
stercoral, stercoraceous 569.82
  with perforation 569.83
  anus or rectum 569.41
stomach (eroded) (peptic) (round) 531.9 ☑

> Note — Use the following fifth-digit subclassification with categories 531–534:
>
> 0   without mention of obstruction
> 1   with obstruction

  with
    hemorrhage 531.4 ☑
      and perforation 531.6 ☑
    perforation (chronic) 531.5 ☑
      and hemorrhage 531.6 ☑
  acute 531.3 ☑
    with
      hemorrhage 531.0 ☑
        and perforation 531.2 ☑
      perforation 531.1 ☑
        and hemorrhage 531.2 ☑

Ulcer, ulcerated, ulcerating, ulceration, ulcerative — *continued*
stomach — *continued*
  bleeding (recurrent) — *see* Ulcer, stomach, with hemorrhage
  chronic 531.7 ☑
    with
      hemorrhage 531.4 ☑
        and perforation 531.6 ☑
      perforation 531.5 ☑
        and hemorrhage 531.6 ☑
    penetrating — *see* Ulcer, stomach, with perforation
    perforating — *see* Ulcer, stomach, with perforation
stoma, stomal — *see* Ulcer, gastrojejunal
stomatitis 528.00
stress — *see* Ulcer, peptic
strumous (tuberculous) (*see also* Tuberculosis) 017.2 ☑
submental (*see also* Ulcer, skin) 707.8
submucosal, bladder 595.1
syphilitic (any site) (early) (secondary) 091.3
  late 095.9
  perforating 095.9
    foot 094.0
testis 608.89
thigh — *see* Ulcer, lower extremity
throat 478.29
  diphtheritic 032.0
toe — *see* Ulcer, lower extremity
tongue (traumatic) 529.0
tonsil 474.8
  diphtheritic 032.0
trachea 519.19
trophic — *see* Ulcer, skin
tropical NEC (*see also* Ulcer, skin) 707.9
tuberculous — *see* Tuberculosis, ulcer
tunica vaginalis 608.89
turbinate 730.9 ☑
typhoid (fever) 002.0
  perforating 002.0
umbilicus (newborn) 771.4
unspecified site NEC — *see* Ulcer, skin
urethra (meatus) (*see also* Urethritis) 597.89
uterus 621.8
  cervix 622.0
    with mention of cervicitis 616.0
  neck 622.0
    with mention of cervicitis 616.0
vagina 616.89
valve, heart 421.0
varicose (lower extremity, any part) 454.0
  anus — *see* Varicose, ulcer, anus
  broad ligament 456.5
  esophagus (*see also* Varix, esophagus) 456.1
    bleeding (*see also* Varix, esophagus, bleeding) 456.0
  inflamed or infected 454.2
  nasal septum 456.8
  perineum 456.6
  rectum — *see* Varicose, ulcer, anus
  scrotum 456.4
  specified site NEC 456.8
  sublingual 456.3
  vulva 456.6
vas deferens 608.89
vesical (*see also* Ulcer, bladder) 596.8
vulva (acute) (infectional) 616.50
  Behçet's syndrome 136.1 [616.51]
  herpetic 054.12
  tuberculous 016.7 ☑ [616.51]
vulvobuccal, recurring 616.50
x-ray — *see* Ulcer, by site
yaws 102.4
Ulcus — *see also* Ulcer
cutis tuberculosum (*see also* Tuberculosis) 017.0 ☑
duodeni — *see* Ulcer, duodenum
durum 091.0
  extragenital 091.2
gastrojejunale — *see* Ulcer, gastrojejunal
hypostaticum — *see* Ulcer, varicose
molle (cutis) (skin) 099.0
serpens corneae (pneumococcal) 370.04

Ulcus — *see also* Ulcer — *continued*
ventriculi — *see* Ulcer, stomach
Ulegyria 742.4
Ulerythema
  acneiforma 701.8
  centrifugum 695.4
  ophryogenes 757.4
Ullrich-Feichtiger syndrome 759.89
Ullrich (-Bonnevie) (-Turner) syndrome 758.6
Ulnar — *see* condition
Ulorrhagia 523.8
Ulorrhea 523.8
Umbilicus, umbilical — *see also* condition
  cord necrosis, affecting fetus or newborn 762.6
Unacceptable
  existing dental restoration
    contours 525.65
    morphology 525.65
Unavailability of medical facilities (at) V63.9
  due to
    investigation by social service agency V63.8
    lack of services at home V63.1
    remoteness from facility V63.0
    waiting list V63.2
    home V63.1
  outpatient clinic V63.0
  specified reason NEC V63.8
Uncinaria americana infestation 126.1
Uncinariasis (*see also* Ancylostomiasis) 126.9
Unconscious, unconsciousness 780.09
Underdevelopment — *see also* Undeveloped
  sexual 259.0
Underfill, endodontic 526.63
Undernourishment 269.9
Undernutrition 269.9
Under observation — *see* Observation
Underweight 783.22
  for gestational age — *see* Light-for-dates
Underwood's disease (sclerema neonatorum) 778.1
Undescended — *see also* Malposition, congenital
  cecum 751.4
  colon 751.4
  testis 752.51
Undetermined diagnosis or cause 799.9
Undeveloped, undevelopment — *see also* Hypoplasia
  brain (congenital) 742.1
  cerebral (congenital) 742.1
  fetus or newborn 764.9 ☑
  heart 746.89
  lung 748.5
  testis 257.2
  uterus 259.0
Undiagnosed (disease) 799.9
Undulant fever — *see also* Brucellosis 023.9
Unemployment, anxiety concerning V62.0
Unequal leg (acquired) (length) 736.81
  congenital 755.30
Unerupted teeth, tooth 520.6
Unextracted dental root 525.3
Unguis incarnatus 703.0
Unicornis uterus 752.33 ▲
Unicornuate uterus (with or without a separate uterine horn) 752.33 ●
Unicorporeus uterus 752.39 ▲
Uniformis uterus 752.39 ▲
Unilateral — *see also* condition
  development, breast 611.89
  organ or site, congenital NEC — *see* Agenesis
  vagina 752.49
Unilateralis uterus 752.39 ▲
Unilocular heart 745.8
Uninhibited bladder 596.54
  with cauda equina syndrome 344.61
  neurogenic — *see also* Neurogenic, bladder 596.54
Union, abnormal — *see also* Fusion
  divided tendon 727.89
  larynx and trachea 748.3
Universal
  joint, cervix 620.6

Universal — *continued*
  mesentery 751.4
Unknown
  cause of death 799.9
  diagnosis 799.9
Unna's disease (seborrheic dermatitis) 690.10
Unresponsiveness, adrenocorticotropin (ACTH) 255.41
Unsatisfactory
  cytology smear
    anal 796.78
    cervical 795.08
    vaginal 795.18
  restoration, tooth (existing) 525.60
    specified NEC 525.69
Unsoundness of mind — *see also* Psychosis 298.9
Unspecified cause of death 799.9
Unstable
  back NEC 724.9
  colon 569.89
  joint — *see* Instability, joint
  lie 652.0 ☑
    affecting fetus or newborn (before labor) 761.7
    causing obstructed labor 660.0 ☑
      affecting fetus or newborn 763.1
  lumbosacral joint (congenital) 756.19
    acquired 724.6
  sacroiliac 724.6
  spine NEC 724.9
Untruthfulness, child problem — *see also* Disturbance, conduct 312.0 ☑
Unverricht (-Lundborg) disease, syndrome, or epilepsy 345.1 ☑
Unverricht-Wagner syndrome (dermatomyositis) 710.3
Upper respiratory — *see* condition
Upset
  gastric 536.8
    psychogenic 306.4
  gastrointestinal 536.8
    psychogenic 306.4
    virus (*see also* Enteritis, viral) 008.8
  intestinal (large) (small) 564.9
    psychogenic 306.4
  menstruation 626.9
  mental 300.9
  stomach 536.8
    psychogenic 306.4
Urachus — *see also* condition
  patent 753.7
  persistent 753.7
Uratic arthritis 274.00
Urbach's lipoid proteinosis 272.8
Urbach-Oppenheim disease or syndrome (necrobiosis lipoidica diabeticorum) 250.8 ☑ [709.3]
  due to secondary diabetes 249.8 ☑ [709.3]
Urbach-Wiethe disease or syndrome (lipoid proteinosis) 272.8
Urban yellow fever 060.1
Urea, blood, high — *see* Uremia
Uremia, uremic (absorption) (amaurosis) (amblyopia) (aphasia) (apoplexy) (coma) (delirium) (dementia) (dropsy) (dyspnea) (fever) (intoxication) (mania) (paralysis) (poisoning) (toxemia) (vomiting) 586
  with
    abortion — *see* Abortion, by type, with renal failure
    ectopic pregnancy (*see also* categories 633.0–633.9) 639.3
    hypertension (*see also* Hypertension, kidney) 403.91
    molar pregnancy (*see also* categories 630–632) 639.3
  chronic 585.9
  complicating
    abortion 639.3
    ectopic or molar pregnancy 639.3
    hypertension (*see also* Hypertension, kidney) 403.91
    labor and delivery 669.3 ☑
  congenital 779.89
  extrarenal 788.99

☑ **Additional Digit Required** — **Refer to the Tabular List for Digit Selection**

▽ **Subterms under main terms may continue to next column or page**

Uremia, uremic — *continued*
  hypertensive (chronic) (*see also* Hypertension, kidney) 403.91
  maternal NEC, affecting fetus or newborn 760.1
  neuropathy 585.9 *[357.4]*
  pericarditis 585.9 *[420.0]*
  prerenal 788.99
  pyelitic (*see also* Pyelitis) 590.80
Ureteralgia 788.0
Ureterectasis 593.89
Ureteritis 593.89
  cystica 590.3
  due to calculus 592.1
  gonococcal (acute) 098.19
    chronic or duration of 2 months or over 098.39
  nonspecific 593.89
Ureterocele (acquired) 593.89
  congenital 753.23
Ureterolith 592.1
Ureterolithiasis 592.1
Ureterostomy status V44.6
  with complication 997.5
Ureter, ureteral — *see* condition
Urethralgia 788.99
Urethra, urethral — *see* condition
Urethritis (abacterial) (acute) (allergic) (anterior) (chronic) (nonvenereal) (posterior) (recurrent) (simple) (subacute) (ulcerative) (undifferentiated) 597.80
  diplococcal (acute) 098.0
    chronic or duration of 2 months or over 098.2
  due to Trichomonas (vaginalis) 131.02
  gonococcal (acute) 098.0
    chronic or duration of 2 months or over 098.2
  nongonococcal (sexually transmitted) 099.40
    Chlamydia trachomatis 099.41
    Reiter's 099.3
    specified organism NEC 099.49
  nonspecific (sexually transmitted) (*see also* Urethritis, nongonococcal) 099.40
  not sexually transmitted 597.80
  Reiter's 099.3
  trichomonal or due to Trichomonas (vaginalis) 131.02
  tuberculous (*see also* Tuberculosis) 016.3 ☑
  venereal NEC (*see also* Urethritis, nongonococcal) 099.40
Urethrocele
  female 618.03
    with uterine prolapse 618.4
      complete 618.3
      incomplete 618.2
  male 599.5
Urethrolithiasis 594.2
Urethro-oculoarticular syndrome 099.3
Urethro-oculosynovial syndrome 099.3
Urethrorectal — *see* condition
Urethrorrhagia 599.84
Urethrorrhea 788.7

Urethrostomy status V44.6
  with complication 997.5
Urethrotrigonitis 595.3
Urethrovaginal — *see* condition
Urgency
  fecal 787.63
  hypertensive — *see* Hypertension
Urhidrosis, uridrosis 705.89
Uric acid
  diathesis 274.9
  in blood 790.6
Uricacidemia 790.6
Uricemia 790.6
Uricosuria 791.9
Urination
  frequent 788.41
  painful 788.1
  urgency 788.63
Urinemia — *see* Uremia
Urine, urinary — *see also* condition
  abnormality NEC 788.69
  blood in (*see also* Hematuria) 599.70
  discharge, excessive 788.42
  enuresis 788.30
    nonorganic origin 307.6
  extravasation 788.8
  frequency 788.41
  hesitancy 788.64
  incontinence 788.30
    active 788.30
    female 788.30
      stress 625.6
        and urge 788.33
    male 788.30
      stress 788.32
        and urge 788.33
    mixed (stress and urge) 788.33
    neurogenic 788.39
    nonorganic origin 307.6
    overflow 788.38
    stress (female) 625.6
      male NEC 788.32
  intermittent stream 788.61
  pus in 791.9
  retention or stasis NEC 788.20
    bladder, incomplete emptying 788.21
    psychogenic 306.53
    specified NEC 788.29
  secretion
    deficient 788.5
    excessive 788.42
    frequency 788.41
  strain 788.65
  stream
    intermittent 788.61
    slowing 788.62
    splitting 788.61
    weak 788.62
  urgency 788.63
Urinoma NEC 599.9
  bladder 596.8
  kidney 593.89
  renal 593.89
  ureter 593.89

Urinoma — *continued*
  urethra 599.84
Uroarthritis, infectious 099.3
Urodialysis 788.5
● **Urolithiasis** 592.9
● **Uronephrosis** 593.89
● **Uropathy** 599.9
  obstructive 599.60
Urosepsis 599.0
  meaning sepsis 995.91
  meaning urinary tract infection 599.0
Urticaria 708.9
  with angioneurotic edema 995.1
    hereditary 277.6
  allergic 708.0
  cholinergic 708.5
  chronic 708.8
  cold, familial 708.2
  dermatographic 708.3
  due to
    cold or heat 708.2
    drugs 708.0
    food 708.0
    inhalants 708.0
    plants 708.8
    serum 999.5
  factitial 708.3
  giant 995.1
    hereditary 277.6
  gigantea 995.1
    hereditary 277.6
  idiopathic 708.1
  larynx 995.1
    hereditary 277.6
  neonatorum 778.8
  nonallergic 708.1
  papulosa (Hebra) 698.2
  perstans hemorrhagica 757.39
  pigmentosa 757.33
  recurrent periodic 708.8
  serum 999.5
  solare 692.72
  specified type NEC 708.8
  thermal (cold) (heat) 708.2
  vibratory 708.4
Urticarioides acarodermatitis 133.9
Use of
  agents affecting estrogen receptors and estrogen levels NEC V07.59 ●
  anastrozole (Arimidex) V07.52 ●
  aromatase inhibitors V07.52 ●
  estrogen receptor downregulators V07.59 ●
  exemestane (Aromasin) V07.52 ●
  fulvestrant (Faslodex) V07.59 ●
  gonadotropin-releasing hormone (GnRH) agonist V07.59 ●
  goserelin acetate (Zoladex) V07.59 ●
  letrozole (Femara) V07.52 ●
  leuprolide acetate (leuprorelin) (Lupron) V07.59 ●
  megestrol acetate (Megace) V07.59 ●
  methadone 304.00
  nonprescribed drugs (*see also* Abuse, drugs, nondependent) 305.9 ☑

Use of — *continued*
  patent medicines (*see also* Abuse, drugs, nondependent) 305.9 ☑
  raloxifene (Evista) V07.51 ●
  selective estrogen receptor modulators (SERMs) V07.51 ●
  tamoxifen (Nolvadex) V07.51 ●
  toremifene (Fareston) V07.51 ●
Usher-Senear disease (pemphigus erythematosus) 694.4
Uta 085.5
Uterine size-date discrepancy 649.6 ☑
Uteromegaly 621.2
Uterovaginal — *see* condition
Uterovesical — *see* condition
Uterus — ►*see also*◄ condition
  with only one functioning horn 752.33 ●
Utriculitis (utriculus prostaticus) 597.89
Uveal — *see* condition
Uveitis (anterior) — *see also* Iridocyclitis 364.3
  acute or subacute 364.00
    due to or associated with
      gonococcal infection 098.41
      herpes (simplex) 054.44
        zoster 053.22
    primary 364.01
    recurrent 364.02
    secondary (noninfectious) 364.04
      infectious 364.03
  allergic 360.11
  chronic 364.10
    due to or associated with
      sarcoidosis 135 *[364.11]*
      tuberculosis (*see also* Tuberculosis) 017.3 ☑ *[364.11]*
  due to
    operation 360.11
    toxoplasmosis (acquired) 130.2
      congenital (active) 771.2
  granulomatous 364.10
  heterochromic 364.21
  lens-induced 364.23
  nongranulomatous 364.00
  posterior 363.20
    disseminated — *see* Chorioretinitis, disseminated
    focal — *see* Chorioretinitis, focal
  recurrent 364.02
  sympathetic 360.11
  syphilitic (secondary) 091.50
    congenital 090.0 *[363.13]*
    late 095.8 *[363.13]*
  tuberculous (*see also* Tuberculosis) 017.3 ☑ *[364.11]*
Uveoencephalitis 363.22
Uveokeratitis — *see also* Iridocyclitis 364.3
Uveoparotid fever 135
Uveoparotitis 135
Uvula — *see* condition
Uvulitis (acute) (catarrhal) (chronic) (gangrenous) (membranous) (suppurative) (ulcerative) 528.3

☑ Additional Digit Required — Refer to the Tabular List for Digit Selection   ⩗ Subterms under main terms may continue to next column or page

2011 ICD-9-CM   ►◄ Revised Text   ● New Line   ▲ Revised Code   October 2010 • Volume 2 — **289**

V

Vaccination
complication or reaction — see Complications, vaccination
delayed V64.00
not carried out V64.00
  because of
    acute illness V64.01
    allergy to vaccine or component V64.04
    caregiver refusal V64.05
    chronic illness V64.02
    guardian refusal V64.05
    immune compromised state V64.03
    parent refusal V64.05
    patient had disease being vaccinated against V64.08
    patient refusal V64.06
    reason NEC V64.09
    religious reasons V64.07
prophylactic (against) V05.9
  arthropod-borne viral
    disease NEC V05.1
    encephalitis V05.0
  chickenpox V05.4
  cholera (alone) V03.0
    with typhoid-paratyphoid (cholera + TAB) V06.0
  common cold V04.7
  diphtheria (alone) V03.5
    with
      poliomyelitis (DTP+ polio) V06.3
      tetanus V06.5
        pertussis combined (DTP) (DTaP) V06.1
        typhoid-paratyphoid (DTP + TAB) V06.2
  disease (single) NEC V05.9
    bacterial NEC V03.9
      specified type NEC V03.89
    combination NEC V06.9
      specified type NEC V06.8
    specified type NEC V05.8
  encephalitis, viral, arthropod-borne V05.0
  Hemophilus influenzae, type B [Hib] V03.81
  hepatitis, viral V05.3
  influenza V04.81
    with
      Streptococcus pneumoniae [pneumococcus] V06.6
  leishmaniasis V05.2
  measles (alone) V04.2
    with mumps-rubella (MMR) V06.4
  mumps (alone) V04.6
    with measles and rubella (MMR) V06.4
  pertussis alone V03.6
  plague V03.3
  poliomyelitis V04.0
    with diphtheria-tetanus-pertussis (DTP + polio) V06.3
  rabies V04.5
  respiratory syncytial virus (RSV) V04.82
  rubella (alone) V04.3
    with measles and mumps (MMR) V06.4
  smallpox V04.1
  Streptococcus pneumoniae [pneumococcus] V03.82
    with
      influenza V06.6
  tetanus toxoid (alone) V03.7
    with diphtheria [Td] [DT] V06.5
      with
        pertussis (DTP) (DTaP) V06.1
          with poliomyelitis (DTP+polio) V06.3
  tuberculosis (BCG) V03.2
  tularemia V03.4
  typhoid-paratyphoid (TAB) (alone) V03.1
    with diphtheria-tetanus-pertussis (TAB + DTP) V06.2
  varicella V05.4

Vaccination — continued
prophylactic — continued
  viral
    disease NEC V04.89
    encephalitis, arthropod-borne V05.0
    hepatitis V05.3
    yellow fever V04.4
Vaccinia (generalized) 999.0
without vaccination 051.02
congenital 771.2
conjunctiva 999.39
eyelids 999.0 *[373.5]*
localized 999.39
nose 999.39
not from vaccination 051.02
  eyelid 051.02 *[373.5]*
sine vaccinatione 051.02
Vacuum
extraction of fetus or newborn 763.3
in sinus (accessory) (nasal) (see also Sinusitis) 473.9
Vagabond V60.0
Vagabondage V60.0
Vagabonds' disease 132.1
Vaginalitis (tunica) 608.4
Vagina, vaginal — see also condition
high risk human papillomavirus (HPV) DNA test positive 795.15
low risk human papillomavirus (HPV) DNA test positive 795.19
Vaginismus (reflex) 625.1
functional 306.51
hysterical 300.11
psychogenic 306.51
Vaginitis (acute) (chronic) (circumscribed) (diffuse) (emphysematous) (Hemophilus vaginalis) (nonspecific) (nonvenereal) (ulcerative) 616.10
with
  abortion — see Abortion, by type, with sepsis
  ectopic pregnancy (see also categories 633–633.9) 639.0
  molar pregnancy (see also categories 630–632) 639.0
adhesive, congenital 752.49
atrophic, postmenopausal 627.3
bacterial 616.10
blennorrhagic (acute) 098.0
  chronic or duration of 2 months or over 098.2
candidal 112.1
chlamydial 099.53
complicating pregnancy or puerperium 646.6 ☑
  affecting fetus or newborn 760.8
congenital (adhesive) 752.49
due to
  C. albicans 112.1
  Trichomonas (vaginalis) 131.01
following
  abortion 639.0
  ectopic or molar pregnancy 639.0
gonococcal (acute) 098.0
  chronic or duration of 2 months or over 098.2
granuloma 099.2
Monilia 112.1
mycotic 112.1
pinworm 127.4 *[616.11]*
postirradiation 616.10
postmenopausal atrophic 627.3
senile (atrophic) 627.3
syphilitic (early) 091.0
  late 095.8
trichomonal 131.01
tuberculous (see also Tuberculosis) 016.7 ☑
venereal NEC 099.8
Vaginosis — see Vaginitis
Vagotonia 352.3
Vagrancy V60.0
VAIN I (vaginal intraepithelial neoplasia I) 623.0
VAIN II (vaginal intraepithelial neoplasia II) 623.0
VAIN III (vaginal intraepithelial neoplasia III) 233.31

Vallecula — see condition
Valley fever 114.0
Valsuani's disease (progressive pernicious anemia, puerperal) 648.2 ☑
Valve, valvular (formation) — see also condition
cerebral ventricle (communicating) in situ V45.2
cervix, internal os 752.49
colon 751.5
congenital NEC — see Atresia
formation, congenital NEC — see Atresia
heart defect — see Anomaly, heart, valve
ureter 753.29
  pelvic junction 753.21
  vesical orifice 753.22
urethra 753.6
Valvulitis (chronic) — see also Endocarditis 424.90
rheumatic (chronic) (inactive) (with chorea) 397.9
  active or acute (aortic) (mitral) (pulmonary) (tricuspid) 391.1
syphilitic NEC 093.20
  aortic 093.22
  mitral 093.21
  pulmonary 093.24
  tricuspid 093.23
Valvulopathy — see Endocarditis
van Bogaert-Nijssen (-Peiffer) disease 330.0
van Bogaert's leukoencephalitis (sclerosing) (subacute) 046.2
van Buchem's syndrome (hyperostosis corticalis) 733.3
Vancomycin (glycopeptide)
intermediate staphylococcus aureus (VISA/GISA) V09.8 ☑
resistant
  enterococcus (VRE) V09.8 ☑
  staphylococcus aureus (VRSA/GRSA) V09.8 ☑
van Creveld-von Gierke disease (glycogenosis I) 271.0
van den Bergh's disease (enterogenous cyanosis) 289.7
van der Hoeve-Halbertsma-Waardenburg syndrome (ptosis-epicanthus) 270.2
van der Hoeve-Waardenburg-Gualdi syndrome (ptosis epicanthus) 270.2
van der Hoeve's syndrome (brittle bones and blue sclera, deafness) 756.51
Vanillism 692.89
Vanishing lung 492.0
Vanishing twin 651.33
van Neck (-Odelberg) disease or syndrome (juvenile osteochondrosis) 732.1
Vapor asphyxia or suffocation NEC 987.9
specified agent — see Table of Drugs and Chemicals
Vaquez's disease (M9950/1) 238.4
Vaquez-Osler disease (polycythemia vera) (M9950/1) 238.4
Variance, lethal ball, prosthetic heart valve 996.02
Variants, thalassemic 282.49
Variations in hair color 704.3
Varicella 052.9
with
  complication 052.8
    specified NEC 052.7
  pneumonia 052.1
  vaccination and inoculation (prophylactic) V05.4
exposure to V01.71
vaccination and inoculation (against) (prophylactic) V05.4
Varices — see Varix
Varicocele (scrotum) (thrombosed) 456.4
ovary 456.5
perineum 456.6
spermatic cord (ulcerated) 456.4
Varicose
aneurysm (ruptured) (see also Aneurysm) 442.9
dermatitis (lower extremity) — see Varicose, vein, inflamed or infected

Varicose — continued
eczema — see Varicose, vein
phlebitis — see Varicose, vein, inflamed or infected
placental vessel — see Placenta, abnormal
tumor — see Varicose, vein
ulcer (lower extremity, any part) 454.0
  anus 455.8
    external 455.5
    internal 455.2
  esophagus (see also Varix, esophagus) 456.1
    bleeding (see also Varix, esophagus, bleeding) 456.0
  inflamed or infected 454.2
  nasal septum 456.8
  perineum 456.6
  rectum — see Varicose, ulcer, anus
  scrotum 456.4
  specified site NEC 456.8
vein (lower extremity) (ruptured) (see also Varix) 454.9
  with
    complications NEC 454.8
    edema 454.8
    inflammation or infection 454.1
      ulcerated 454.2
    pain 454.8
    stasis dermatitis 454.1
      with ulcer 454.2
    swelling 454.8
    ulcer 454.0
      inflamed or infected 454.2
  anus — see Hemorrhoids
  broad ligament 456.5
  congenital (peripheral) 747.60
    gastrointestinal 747.61
    lower limb 747.64
    renal 747.62
    specified NEC 747.69
    upper limb 747.63
  esophagus (ulcerated) (see also Varix, esophagus) 456.1
    bleeding (see also Varix, esophagus, bleeding) 456.0
  inflamed or infected 454.1
    with ulcer 454.2
  in pregnancy or puerperium 671.0 ☑
    vulva or perineum 671.1 ☑
  nasal septum (with ulcer) 456.8
  pelvis 456.5
  perineum 456.6
    in pregnancy, childbirth, or puerperium 671.1 ☑
  rectum — see Hemorrhoids
  scrotum (ulcerated) 456.4
  specified site NEC 456.8
  sublingual 456.3
  ulcerated 454.0
    inflamed or infected 454.2
  umbilical cord, affecting fetus or newborn 762.6
  urethra 456.8
  vulva 456.6
    in pregnancy, childbirth, or puerperium 671.1 ☑
vessel (see also Varix)
  placenta — see Placenta, abnormal
Varicosis, varicosities, varicosity — see also Varix 454.9
Variola 050.9
hemorrhagic (pustular) 050.0
major 050.0
minor 050.1
modified 050.2
Varioloid 050.2
Variolosa, purpura 050.0
Varix (lower extremity) (ruptured) 454.9
with
  complications NEC 454.8
  edema 454.8
  inflammation or infection 454.1
    with ulcer 454.2
  pain 454.8
  stasis dermatitis 454.1
    with ulcer 454.2

☑ Additional Digit Required — Refer to the Tabular List for Digit Selection   Subterms under main terms may continue to next column or page

Varix — *continued*
  with — *continued*
    swelling 454.8
    ulcer 454.0
      with inflammation or infection 454.2
  aneurysmal (*see also* Aneurysm) 442.9
  anus — *see* Hemorrhoids
  arteriovenous (congenital) (peripheral) NEC
      747.60
    gastrointestinal 747.61
    lower limb 747.64
    renal 747.62
    specified NEC 747.69
    spinal 747.82
    upper limb 747.63
  bladder 456.5
  broad ligament 456.5
  congenital (peripheral) 747.60
  esophagus (ulcerated) 456.1
    bleeding 456.0
      in
        cirrhosis of liver 571.5 *[456.20]*
        portal hypertension
            572.3 *[456.20]*
    congenital 747.69
      in
        cirrhosis of liver 571.5 *[456.21]*
          with bleeding 571.5 *[456.20]*
        portal hypertension
            572.3 *[456.21]*
          with bleeding 572.3 *[456.20]*
  gastric 456.8
  inflamed or infected 454.1
    ulcerated 454.2
  in pregnancy or puerperium 671.0 ☑
    perineum 671.1 ☑
    vulva 671.1 ☑
  labia (majora) 456.6
  orbit 456.8
    congenital 747.69
  ovary 456.5
  papillary 448.1
  pelvis 456.5
  perineum 456.6
    in pregnancy or puerperium 671.1 ☑
  pharynx 456.8
  placenta — *see* Placenta, abnormal
  prostate 456.8
  rectum — *see* Hemorrhoids
  renal papilla 456.8
  retina 362.17
  scrotum (ulcerated) 456.4
  sigmoid colon 456.8
  specified site NEC 456.8
  spinal (cord) (vessels) 456.8
  spleen, splenic (vein) (with phlebolith) 456.8
  sublingual 456.3
  ulcerated 454.0
    inflamed or infected 454.2
  umbilical cord, affecting fetus or newborn
      762.6
  uterine ligament 456.5
  vocal cord 456.8
  vulva 456.6
    in pregnancy, childbirth, or puerperium
        671.1 ☑
Vasa previa 663.5 ☑
  affecting fetus or newborn 762.6
  hemorrhage from, affecting fetus or new-
      born 772.0
Vascular — *see also* condition
  loop on papilla (optic) 743.57
  sheathing, retina 362.13
  spasm 443.9
  spider 448.1
Vascularity, pulmonary, congenital 747.3
Vascularization
  choroid 362.16
  cornea 370.60
    deep 370.63
    localized 370.61
  retina 362.16
  subretinal 362.16
Vasculitis 447.6
  allergic 287.0
  cryoglobulinemic 273.2

Vasculitis — *continued*
  disseminated 447.6
  kidney 447.8
  leukocytoclastic 446.29
  nodular 695.2
  retinal 362.18
  rheumatic — *see* Fever, rheumatic
Vasculopathy
  cardiac allograft 996.83
Vas deferens — *see* condition
Vas deferentitis 608.4
Vasectomy, admission for V25.2
Vasitis 608.4
  nodosa 608.4
  scrotum 608.4
  spermatic cord 608.4
  testis 608.4
  tuberculous (*see also* Tuberculosis) 016.5 ☑
  tunica vaginalis 608.4
  vas deferens 608.4
Vasodilation 443.9
Vasomotor — *see* condition
Vasoplasty, after previous sterilization V26.0
Vasoplegia, splanchnic — *see also* Neuropa-
      thy, peripheral, autonomic 337.9
Vasospasm 443.9
  cerebral (artery) 435.9
    with transient neurologic deficit 435.9
  coronary 413.1
  nerve
    arm NEC 354.9
    autonomic 337.9
    brachial plexus 353.0
    cervical plexus 353.2
    leg NEC 355.8
    lower extremity NEC 355.8
    peripheral NEC 355.9
    spinal NEC 355.9
    sympathetic 337.9
    upper extremity NEC 354.9
  peripheral NEC 443.9
  retina (artery) (*see also* Occlusion, retinal,
      artery) 362.30
Vasospastic — *see* condition
Vasovagal attack (paroxysmal) 780.2
  psychogenic 306.2
Vater's ampulla — *see* condition
VATER syndrome 759.89
vCJD (variant Creutzfeldt-Jakob disease) 046.11
Vegetation, vegetative
  adenoid (nasal fossa) 474.2
  consciousness (persistent) 780.03
  endocarditis (acute) (any valve) (chronic)
      (subacute) 421.0
  heart (mycotic) (valve) 421.0
  state (persistent) 780.03
Veil
  Jackson's 751.4
  over face (causing asphyxia) 768.9
Vein, venous — *see* condition
Veldt sore — *see also* Ulcer, skin 707.9
Velo-cardio-facial syndrome 758.32
Velpeau's hernia — *see* Hernia, femoral
Venereal
  balanitis NEC 099.8
  bubo 099.1
  disease 099.9
    specified nature or type NEC 099.8
  granuloma inguinale 099.2
  lymphogranuloma (Durand-Nicolas-Favre),
      any site 099.1
  salpingitis 098.37
  urethritis (*see also* Urethritis, nongonococ-
      cal) 099.40
  vaginitis NEC 099.8
  warts 078.11
Vengefulness, in child — *see also* Disturbance,
      conduct 312.0 ☑
Venofibrosis 459.89
Venom, venomous
  bite or sting (animal or insect) 989.5
  poisoning 989.5
Venous — *see* condition
Ventouse delivery NEC 669.5 ☑
  affecting fetus or newborn 763.3
Ventral — *see* condition

Ventricle, ventricular — *see also* condition
  escape 427.69
  standstill (*see also* Arrest, cardiac) 427.5
Ventriculitis, cerebral — *see also* Meningitis
      322.9
Ventriculostomy status V45.2
Verbiest's syndrome (claudicatio intermittens
      spinalis) 435.1
Vernet's syndrome 352.6
Verneuil's disease (syphilitic bursitis) 095.7
Verruca (filiformis) 078.10
  acuminata (any site) 078.11
  necrogenica (primary) (*see also* Tuberculosis)
      017.0 ☑
  peruana 088.0
  peruviana 088.0
  plana (juvenilis) 078.19
  plantaris 078.12
  seborrheica 702.19
    inflamed 702.11
  senilis 702.0
  tuberculosa (primary) (*see also* Tuberculosis)
      017.0 ☑
  venereal 078.11
  viral 078.10
    specified NEC 078.19
  vulgaris 078.10
Verrucosities — *see also* Verruca 078.10
Verrucous endocarditis (acute) (any valve)
      (chronic) (subacute) 710.0 *[424.91]*
  nonbacterial 710.0 *[424.91]*
Verruga
  peruana 088.0
  peruviana 088.0
Verse's disease (calcinosis intervertebralis)
      275.49 *[722.90]*
Version
  before labor, affecting fetus or newborn
      761.7
  cephalic (correcting previous malposition)
      652.1 ☑
    affecting fetus or newborn 763.1
  cervix — *see* Version, uterus
  uterus (postinfectional) (postpartal, old) (*see*
      also Malposition, uterus) 621.6
    forward — *see* Anteversion, uterus
    lateral — *see* Lateroversion, uterus
Vertebra, vertebral — *see* condition
Vertigo 780.4
  auditory 386.19
  aural 386.19
  benign paroxysmal positional 386.11
  central origin 386.2
  cerebral 386.2
  Dix and Hallpike (epidemic) 386.12
  endemic paralytic 078.81
  epidemic 078.81
    Dix and Hallpike 386.12
    Gerlier's 078.81
    Pedersen's 386.12
    vestibular neuronitis 386.12
  epileptic — *see* Epilepsy
  Gerlier's (epidemic) 078.81
  hysterical 300.11
  labyrinthine 386.10
  laryngeal 786.2
  malignant positional 386.2
  Ménière's (*see also* Disease, Ménière's)
      386.00
  menopausal 627.2
  otogenic 386.19
  paralytic 078.81
  paroxysmal positional, benign 386.11
  Pedersen's (epidemic) 386.12
  peripheral 386.10
    specified type NEC 386.19
  positional
    benign paroxysmal 386.11
    malignant 386.2
Verumontanitis (chronic) — *see also* Urethritis
      597.89
Vesania — *see also* Psychosis 298.9
Vesical — *see* condition
Vesicle
  cutaneous 709.8
  seminal — *see* condition

Vesicle — *continued*
  skin 709.8
Vesicocolic — *see* condition
Vesicoperineal — *see* condition
Vesicorectal — *see* condition
Vesicourethrorectal — *see* condition
Vesicovaginal — *see* condition
Vesicular — *see* condition
Vesiculitis (seminal) 608.0
  amebic 006.8
  gonorrheal (acute) 098.14
    chronic or duration of 2 months or over
        098.34
  trichomonal 131.09
  tuberculous (*see also* Tuberculosis)
      016.5 ☑ *[608.81]*
Vestibulitis (ear) — *see also* Labyrinthitis
      386.30
  nose (external) 478.19
  vulvar 625.71
Vestibulopathy, acute peripheral (recurrent)
      386.12
Vestige, vestigial — *see also* Persistence
  branchial 744.41
  structures in vitreous 743.51
Vibriosis NEC 027.9
Vidal's disease (lichen simplex chronicus)
      698.3
Video display tube syndrome 723.8
Vienna-type encephalitis 049.8
Villaret's syndrome 352.6
Villous — *see* condition
VIN I (vulvar intraepithelial neoplasia I) 624.01
VIN II (vulvar intraepithelial neoplasia II) 624.02
VIN III (vulvar intraepithelial neoplasia III)
      233.32
Vincent's
  angina 101
  bronchitis 101
  disease 101
  gingivitis 101
  infection (any site) 101
  laryngitis 101
  stomatitis 101
  tonsillitis 101
Vinson-Plummer syndrome (sideropenic
      dysphagia) 280.8
Viosterol deficiency — *see also* Deficiency,
      calciferol 268.9
Virchow's disease 733.99
Viremia 790.8
Virilism (adrenal) (female) NEC 255.2
  with
    3-beta-hydroxysteroid dehydrogenase
        defect 255.2
    11-hydroxylase defect 255.2
    21-hydroxylase defect 255.2
    adrenal
      hyperplasia 255.2
      insufficiency (congenital) 255.2
    cortical hyperfunction 255.2
Virilization (female) (suprarenal) — *see also*
      Virilism 255.2
  isosexual 256.4
Virulent bubo 099.0
Virus, viral — *see also* condition
  infection NEC (*see also* Infection, viral)
      079.99
  septicemia 079.99
  yaba monkey tumor 059.22
VISA (vancomycin intermediate staphylococcus
      aureus) V09.8 ☑
Viscera, visceral — *see* condition
Visceroptosis 569.89
Visible peristalsis 787.4
Vision, visual
  binocular, suppression 368.31
  blurred, blurring 368.8
    hysterical 300.11
  defect, defective (*see also* Impaired, vision)
      369.9
  disorientation (syndrome) 368.16
  disturbance NEC (*see also* Disturbance, vi-
      sion) 368.9
    hysterical 300.11
  examination V72.0

☑ **Additional Digit Required** — **Refer to the Tabular List for Digit Selection**   ▽ **Subterms under main terms may continue to next column or page**

Vision, visual — *continued*
field, limitation 368.40
fusion, with defective steropsis 368.33
hallucinations 368.16
halos 368.16
loss 369.9
both eyes (*see also* Blindness, both eyes) 369.3
complete (*see also* Blindness, both eyes) 369.00
one eye 369.8
sudden 368.16
low (both eyes) 369.20
one eye (other eye normal) (*see also* Impaired, vision) 369.70
blindness, other eye 369.10
perception, simultaneous without fusion 368.32
tunnel 368.45
Vitality, lack or want of 780.79
newborn 779.89
Vitamin deficiency NEC — *see also* Deficiency, vitamin 269.2
Vitelline duct, persistent 751.0
Vitiligo 709.01
due to pinta (carate) 103.2
eyelid 374.53
vulva 624.8
Vitium cordis — *see* Disease, heart
Vitreous — *see also* condition
touch syndrome 997.99
VLCAD (long chain/very long chain acyl CoA dehydrogenase deficiency, LCAD) 277.85
Vocal cord — *see* condition
Vocational rehabilitation V57.22
Vogt's (Cecile) disease or syndrome 333.7 ☑
Vogt-Koyanagi syndrome 364.24
Vogt-Spielmeyer disease (amaurotic familial idiocy) 330.1
Voice
change (*see also* Dysphonia) 784.49
loss (*see also* Aphonia) 784.41
Volhard-Fahr disease (malignant nephrosclerosis) 403.00
Volhynian fever 083.1
Volkmann's ischemic contracture or paralysis (complicating trauma) 958.6
Voluntary starvation 307.1
Volvulus (bowel) (colon) (intestine) 560.2
with
hernia (*see also* Hernia, by site, with obstruction)
gangrenous — *see* Hernia, by site, with gangrene
perforation 560.2
congenital 751.5
duodenum 537.3
fallopian tube 620.5
oviduct 620.5
stomach (due to absence of gastrocolic ligament) 537.89
Vomiting 787.03
with nausea 787.01
allergic 535.4 ☑
asphyxia 933.1
bilious (cause unknown) 787.04
following gastrointestinal surgery 564.3
newborn 779.32
blood (*see also* Hematemesis) 578.0
causing asphyxia, choking, or suffocation (*see also* Asphyxia, food) 933.1
cyclical 536.2
associated with migraine 346.2 ☑
psychogenic 306.4
epidemic 078.82
fecal matter 569.87
following gastrointestinal surgery 564.3
functional 536.8
psychogenic 306.4
habit 536.2
hysterical 300.11
nervous 306.4
neurotic 306.4
newborn 779.33
bilious 779.32
of or complicating pregnancy 643.9 ☑

Vomiting — *continued*
of or complicating pregnancy — *continued*
due to
organic disease 643.8 ☑
specific cause NEC 643.8 ☑
early — *see* Hyperemesis, gravidarum
late (after 22 completed weeks of gestation) 643.2 ☑
pernicious or persistent 536.2
complicating pregnancy — *see* Hyperemesis, gravidarum
psychogenic 306.4
physiological 787.03
bilious 787.04
psychic 306.4
psychogenic 307.54
stercoral 569.89
uncontrollable 536.2
psychogenic 306.4
uremic — *see* Uremia
winter 078.82
von Bechterew (-Strumpell) disease or syndrome (ankylosing spondylitis) 720.0
von Bezold's abscess 383.01
von Economo's disease (encephalitis lethargica) 049.8
von Eulenburg's disease (congenital paramyotonia) 359.29
von Gierke's disease (glycogenosis I) 271.0
von Gies' joint 095.8
von Graefe's disease or syndrome 378.72
von Hippel (-Lindau) disease or syndrome (retinocerebral angiomatosis) 759.6
von Jaksch's anemia or disease (pseudoleukemia infantum) 285.8
von Recklinghausen-Applebaum disease (hemochromatosis) ►— *see also* Hemochromatosis◄ 275.03 ▲
von Recklinghausen's
disease or syndrome (nerves) (skin) (M9540/1) 237.71
bones (osteitis fibrosa cystica) 252.01
tumor (M9540/1) 237.71
von Schroetter's syndrome (intermittent venous claudication) 453.89
von Willebrand (-Jürgens) (-Minot) disease or syndrome (angiohemophilia) 286.4
von Zambusch's disease (lichen sclerosus et atrophicus) 701.0
Voorhoeve's disease or dyschondroplasia 756.4
Vossius' ring 921.3
late effect 366.21
Voyeurism 302.82
VRE (vancomycin resistant enterococcus) V09.8 ☑
Vrolik's disease (osteogenesis imperfecta) 756.51
VRSA (vancomycin resistant staphylococcus aureus) V09.8 ☑
Vulva — *see* condition
Vulvismus 625.1
Vulvitis (acute) (allergic) (chronic) (gangrenous) (hypertrophic) (intertriginous) 616.10
with
abortion — *see* Abortion, by type, with sepsis
ectopic pregnancy (*see also* categories 633.0–633.9) 639.0
molar pregnancy (*see also* categories 630–632) 639.0
adhesive, congenital 752.49
blennorrhagic (acute) 098.0
chronic or duration of 2 months or over 098.2
chlamydial 099.53
complicating pregnancy or puerperium 646.6 ☑
due to Ducrey's bacillus 099.0
following
abortion 639.0
ectopic or molar pregnancy 639.0
gonococcal (acute) 098.0

Vulvitis — *continued*
gonococcal — *continued*
chronic or duration of 2 months or over 098.2
herpetic 054.11
leukoplakic 624.09
monilial 112.1
puerperal, postpartum, childbirth 646.6 ☑
syphilitic (early) 091.0
late 095.8
trichomonal 131.01
Vulvodynia 625.70
specified NEC 625.79
Vulvorectal — *see* condition
Vulvovaginitis — *see also* Vulvitis 616.10
amebic 006.8
chlamydial 099.53
gonococcal (acute) 098.0
chronic or duration of 2 months or over 098.2
herpetic 054.11
monilial 112.1
trichomonal (Trichomonas vaginalis) 131.01

W

Waardenburg-Klein syndrome (ptosis-epicanthus) 270.2
Waardenburg's syndrome 756.89
meaning ptosis-epicanthus 270.2
Wagner's disease (colloid milium) 709.3
Wagner (-Unverricht) syndrome (dermatomyositis) 710.3
Waiting list, person on V63.2
undergoing social agency investigation V63.8
Wakefulness disorder — *see also* Hypersomnia 780.54
nonorganic origin 307.43
Waldenström's
disease (osteochondrosis, capital femoral) 732.1
hepatitis (lupoid hepatitis) 571.49
hypergammaglobulinemia 273.0
macroglobulinemia 273.3
purpura, hypergammaglobulinemic 273.0
syndrome (macroglobulinemia) 273.3
Waldenström-Kjellberg syndrome (sideropenic dysphagia) 280.8
Walking
difficulty 719.7
psychogenic 307.9
sleep 307.46
hysterical 300.13
Wall, abdominal — *see* condition
Wallenberg's syndrome (posterior inferior cerebellar artery) — *see also* Disease, cerebrovascular, acute 436
Wallgren's
disease (obstruction of splenic vein with collateral circulation) 459.89
meningitis (*see also* Meningitis, aseptic) 047.9
Wandering
acetabulum 736.39
gallbladder 751.69
kidney, congenital 753.3
organ or site, congenital NEC — *see* Malposition, congenital
pacemaker (atrial) (heart) 427.89
spleen 289.59
Wardrop's disease (with lymphangitis) 681.9
finger 681.02
toe 681.11
War neurosis 300.16
Wart (digitate) (filiform) (infectious) (viral) 078.10
common 078.19
external genital organs (venereal) 078.11
fig 078.19
flat 078.19
genital 078.11
Hassall-Henle's (of cornea) 371.41
Henle's (of cornea) 371.41
juvenile 078.19
moist 078.10
Peruvian 088.0

Wart — *continued*
plantar 078.12
prosector (*see also* Tuberculosis) 017.0 ☑
seborrheic 702.19
inflamed 702.11
senile 702.0
specified NEC 078.19
syphilitic 091.3
tuberculous (*see also* Tuberculosis) 017.0 ☑
venereal (female) (male) 078.11
Warthin's tumor (salivary gland) (M8561/0) 210.2
Washerwoman's itch 692.4
Wassilieff's disease (leptospiral jaundice) 100.0
Wasting
disease 799.4
due to malnutrition 261
extreme (due to malnutrition) 261
muscular NEC 728.2
palsy, paralysis 335.21
pelvic muscle 618.83
Water
clefts 366.12
deprivation of 994.3
in joint (*see also* Effusion, joint) 719.0 ☑
intoxication 276.69 ▲
itch 120.3
lack of 994.3
loading 276.69 ▲
on
brain — *see* Hydrocephalus
chest 511.89
poisoning 276.69 ▲
Waterbrash 787.1
Water-hammer pulse — *see also* Insufficiency, aortic 424.1
Waterhouse (-Friderichsen) disease or syndrome 036.3
Water-losing nephritis 588.89
Watermelon stomach 537.82
with hemorrhage 537.83
without hemorrhage 537.82
Wax in ear 380.4
Waxy
degeneration, any site 277.39
disease 277.39
kidney 277.39 [583.81]
liver (large) 277.39
spleen 277.39
Weak, weakness (generalized) 780.79
arches (acquired) 734
congenital 754.61
bladder sphincter 596.59
congenital 779.89
eye muscle — *see* Strabismus
facial 781.94
foot (double) — *see* Weak, arches
heart, cardiac (*see also* Failure, heart) 428.9
congenital 746.9
mind 317
muscle (generalized) 728.87
myocardium (*see also* Failure, heart) 428.9
newborn 779.89
pelvic fundus
pubocervical tissue 618.81
rectovaginal tissue 618.82
pulse 785.9
senile 797
urinary stream 788.62
valvular — *see* Endocarditis
Wear, worn, tooth, teeth (approximal) (hard tissues) (interproximal) (occlusal) — *see also* Attrition, teeth 521.10
Weather, weathered
effects of
cold NEC 991.9
specified effect NEC 991.8
hot (*see also* Heat) 992.9
skin 692.74
Weber-Christian disease or syndrome (nodular nonsuppurative panniculitis) 729.30
Weber-Cockayne syndrome (epidermolysis bullosa) 757.39
Weber-Dimitri syndrome 759.6

Note — For fracture with open wound, see Fracture.

For laceration, traumatic rupture, tear or penetrating wound of internal organs, such as heart, lung, liver, kidney, pelvic organs, etc., whether or not accompanied by open wound or fracture in the same region, see Injury, internal.

For contused wound, see Contusion. For crush injury, see Crush. For abrasion, insect bite (nonvenomous), blister, or scratch, see Injury, superficial.

Complicated includes wounds with:

  delayed healing

  delayed treatment

  foreign body

  primary infection

For late effect of open wound, see Late, effect, wound, open, by site.

☑ **Additional Digit Required** — Refer to the Tabular List for Digit Selection
▽ **Subterms under main terms may continue to next column or page**

294 — Volume 2 • October 2010   ►◄ Revised Text   ● New Line   ▲ Revised Code   2011 ICD-9-CM

Wound, open — *continued*
  costal region — *continued*
    complicated 875.1
  Descemet's membrane (*see also* Wound, open, intraocular) 871.9
  digit(s)
    foot 893.0
      with tendon involvement 893.2
      complicated 893.1
    hand 883.0
      with tendon involvement 883.2
      complicated 883.1
  drumhead, ear 872.61
    complicated 872.71
  ear 872.8
    canal 872.02
      complicated 872.12
    complicated 872.9
    drum 872.61
      complicated 872.71
    external 872.00
      complicated 872.10
    multiple sites 872.69
      complicated 872.79
    ossicles (incus) (malleus) (stapes) 872.62
      complicated 872.72
    specified part NEC 872.69
      complicated 872.79
  elbow 881.01
    with tendon involvement 881.21
    complicated 881.11
  epididymis 878.2
    complicated 878.3
  epigastric region 879.2
    complicated 879.3
  epiglottis 874.01
    complicated 874.11
  esophagus (cervical) 874.4
    complicated 874.5
    thoracic — *see* Injury, internal, esophagus
  Eustachian tube 872.63
    complicated 872.73
  extremity
    lower (multiple) NEC 894.0
      with tendon involvement 894.2
      complicated 894.1
    upper (multiple) NEC 884.0
      with tendon involvement 884.2
      complicated 884.1
  eye(s) (globe) — *see* Wound, open, intraocular
  eyeball NEC 871.9
    laceration (*see also* Laceration, eyeball) 871.4
    penetrating (*see also* Penetrating wound, eyeball) 871.7
  eyebrow 873.42
    complicated 873.52
  eyelid NEC 870.8
    laceration — *see* Laceration, eyelid
  face 873.40
    complicated 873.50
    multiple sites 873.49
      complicated 873.59
    specified part NEC 873.49
      complicated 873.59
  fallopian tube — *see* Injury, internal, fallopian tube
  finger(s) (nail) (subungual) 883.0
    with tendon involvement 883.2
    complicated 883.1
  flank 879.4
    complicated 879.5
  foot (any part except toe(s) alone) 892.0
    with tendon involvement 892.2
    complicated 892.1
  forearm 881.00
    with tendon involvement 881.20
    complicated 881.10
  forehead 873.42
    complicated 873.52
  genital organs (external) NEC 878.8
    complicated 878.9
    internal — *see* Injury, internal, by site

Wound, open — *continued*
  globe (eye) (*see also* Wound, open, eyeball) 871.9
  groin 879.4
    complicated 879.5
  gum(s) 873.62
    complicated 873.72
  hand (except finger(s) alone) 882.0
    with tendon involvement 882.2
    complicated 882.1
  head NEC 873.8
    with intracranial injury — *see* Injury, intracranial
      due to or associated with skull fracture — *see* Fracture, skull
    complicated 873.9
    scalp — *see* Wound, open, scalp
  heel 892.0
    with tendon involvement 892.2
    complicated 892.1
  high-velocity (grease gun) — *see* Wound, open, complicated, by site
  hip 890.0
    with tendon involvement 890.2
    complicated 890.1
  hymen 878.6
    complicated 878.7
  hypochondrium 879.4
    complicated 879.5
  hypogastric region 879.2
    complicated 879.3
  iliac (region) 879.4
    complicated 879.5
  incidental to
    dislocation — *see* Dislocation, open, by site
    fracture — *see* Fracture, open, by site
    intracranial injury — *see* Injury, intracranial, with open intracranial wound
    nerve injury — *see* Injury, nerve, by site
  inguinal region 879.4
    complicated 879.5
  instep 892.0
    with tendon involvement 892.2
    complicated 892.1
  interscapular region 876.0
    complicated 876.1
  intracranial — *see* Injury, intracranial, with open intracranial wound
  intraocular 871.9
    with
      partial loss (of intraocular tissue) 871.2
      prolapse or exposure (of intraocular tissue) 871.1
      without prolapse (of intraocular tissue) 871.0
    laceration (*see also* Laceration, eyeball) 871.4
    penetrating 871.7
      with foreign body (nonmagnetic) 871.6
        magnetic 871.5
  iris (*see also* Wound, open, eyeball) 871.9
  jaw (fracture not involved) 873.44
    with fracture — *see* Fracture, jaw
    complicated 873.54
  knee 891.0
    with tendon involvement 891.2
    complicated 891.1
  labium (majus) (minus) 878.4
    complicated 878.5
  lacrimal apparatus, gland, or sac 870.8
    with laceration of eyelid 870.2
  larynx 874.01
    with trachea 874.00
      complicated 874.10
    complicated 874.11
  leg (multiple) 891.0
    with tendon involvement 891.2
    complicated 891.1
    lower 891.0
      with tendon involvement 891.2
      complicated 891.1
    thigh 890.0

Wound, open — *continued*
  leg — *continued*
    thigh — *continued*
      with tendon involvement 890.2
      complicated 890.1
    upper 890.0
      with tendon involvement 890.2
      complicated 890.1
  lens (eye) (alone) (*see also* Cataract, traumatic) 366.20
    with involvement of other eye structures — *see* Wound, open, eyeball
  limb
    lower (multiple) NEC 894.0
      with tendon involvement 894.2
      complicated 894.1
    upper (multiple) NEC 884.0
      with tendon involvement 884.2
      complicated 884.1
  lip 873.43
    complicated 873.53
  loin 876.0
    complicated 876.1
  lumbar region 876.0
    complicated 876.1
  malar region 873.41
    complicated 873.51
  mastoid region 873.49
    complicated 873.59
  mediastinum — *see* Injury, internal, mediastinum
  midthoracic region 875.0
    complicated 875.1
  mouth 873.60
    complicated 873.70
    floor 873.64
      complicated 873.74
    multiple sites 873.69
      complicated 873.79
    specified site NEC 873.69
      complicated 873.79
  multiple, unspecified site(s) 879.8

> *Note* — *Multiple open wounds of sites classifiable to the same four-digit category should be classified to that category unless they are in different limbs.*
>
> *Multiple open wounds of sites classifiable to different four-digit categories, or to different limbs, should be coded separately.*

    complicated 879.9
    lower limb(s) (one or both) (sites classifiable to more than one three-digit category in 890 to 893) 894.0
      with tendon involvement 894.2
      complicated 894.1
    upper limb(s) (one or both) (sites classifiable to more than one three-digit category in 880 to 883) 884.0
      with tendon involvement 884.2
      complicated 884.1
  muscle — *see* Sprain, by site
  nail
    finger(s) 883.0
      complicated 883.1
    thumb 883.0
      complicated 883.1
    toe(s) 893.0
      complicated 893.1
  nape (neck) 874.8
    complicated 874.9
    specified part NEC 874.8
      complicated 874.9
  nasal (*see also* Wound, open, nose)
    cavity 873.22
      complicated 873.32
    septum 873.21
      complicated 873.31
    sinuses 873.23
      complicated 873.33
  nasopharynx 873.22
    complicated 873.32
  neck 874.8
    complicated 874.9

Wound, open — *continued*
  neck — *continued*
    nape 874.8
      complicated 874.9
    specified part NEC 874.8
      complicated 874.9
  nerve — *see* Injury, nerve, by site
  non-healing surgical 998.83
  nose 873.20
    complicated 873.30
    multiple sites 873.29
      complicated 873.39
    septum 873.21
      complicated 873.31
    sinuses 873.23
      complicated 873.33
  occipital region — *see* Wound, open, scalp
  ocular NEC 871.9
    adnexa 870.9
      specified region NEC 870.8
    laceration (*see also* Laceration, ocular) 871.4
    muscle (extraocular) 870.3
      with foreign body 870.4
      eyelid 870.1
      intraocular — *see* Wound, open, eyeball
    penetrating (*see also* Penetrating wound, ocular) 871.7
  orbit 870.8
    penetrating 870.3
      with foreign body 870.4
  orbital region 870.9
  ovary — *see* Injury, internal, pelvic organs
  palate 873.65
    complicated 873.75
  palm 882.0
    with tendon involvement 882.2
    complicated 882.1
  parathyroid (gland) 874.2
    complicated 874.3
  parietal region — *see* Wound, open, scalp
  pelvic floor or region 879.6
    complicated 879.7
  penis 878.0
    complicated 878.1
  perineum 879.6
    complicated 879.7
  periocular area 870.8
    laceration of skin 870.0
  pharynx 874.4
    complicated 874.5
  pinna 872.01
    complicated 872.11
  popliteal space 891.0
    with tendon involvement 891.2
    complicated 891.1
  prepuce 878.0
    complicated 878.1
  pubic region 879.2
    complicated 879.3
  pudenda 878.8
    complicated 878.9
  rectovaginal septum 878.8
    complicated 878.9
  sacral region 877.0
    complicated 877.1
  sacroiliac region 877.0
    complicated 877.1
  salivary (ducts) (glands) 873.69
    complicated 873.79
  scalp 873.0
    complicated 873.1
  scalpel, fetus or newborn 767.8
  scapular region 880.01
    with tendon involvement 880.21
    complicated 880.11
    involving other sites of upper arm 880.09
      with tendon involvement 880.29
      complicated 880.19
  sclera (*see also* Wound, open, intraocular) 871.9
  scrotum 878.2
    complicated 878.3
  seminal vesicle — *see* Injury, internal, pelvic organs

☑ Additional Digit Required — Refer to the Tabular List for Digit Selection   ⚐ Subterms under main terms may continue to next column or page

2011 ICD-9-CM   ▶◀ Revised Text   ● New Line   ▲ Revised Code   Volume 2 — 295

Wound, open — *continued*
shin 891.0
　with tendon involvement 891.2
　complicated 891.1
shoulder 880.00
　with tendon involvement 880.20
　complicated 880.10
　involving other sites of upper arm 880.09
　　with tendon involvement 880.29
　　complicated 880.19
skin NEC 879.8
　complicated 879.9
skull (*see also* Injury, intracranial, with open intracranial wound)
　with skull fracture — *see* Fracture, skull
spermatic cord (scrotal) 878.2
　complicated 878.3
　pelvic region — *see* Injury, internal, spermatic cord
spinal cord — *see* Injury, spinal
sternal region 875.0
　complicated 875.1
subconjunctival — *see* Wound, open, intraocular
subcutaneous NEC 879.8
　complicated 879.9
submaxillary region 873.44
　complicated 873.54
submental region 873.44
　complicated 873.54
subungual
　finger(s) (thumb) — *see* Wound, open, finger
　toe(s) — *see* Wound, open, toe
supraclavicular region 874.8
　complicated 874.9
supraorbital 873.42
　complicated 873.52
surgical, non-healing 998.83
temple 873.49
　complicated 873.59
temporal region 873.49
　complicated 873.59
testis 878.2
　complicated 878.3
thigh 890.0
　with tendon involvement 890.2
　complicated 890.1
thorax, thoracic (external) 875.0
　complicated 875.1
throat 874.8
　complicated 874.9
thumb (nail) (subungual) 883.0
　with tendon involvement 883.2
　complicated 883.1
thyroid (gland) 874.2
　complicated 874.3
toe(s) (nail) (subungual) 893.0
　with tendon involvement 893.2
　complicated 893.1
tongue 873.64
　complicated 873.74
tonsil — *see* Wound, open, neck
trachea (cervical region) 874.02
　with larynx 874.00
　　complicated 874.10
　complicated 874.12
　intrathoracic — *see* Injury, internal, trachea
trunk (multiple) NEC 879.6
　complicated 879.7
　specified site NEC 879.6

Wound, open — *continued*
trunk — *continued*
　specified site — *continued*
　　complicated 879.7
　tunica vaginalis 878.2
　　complicated 878.3
　tympanic membrane 872.61
　　complicated 872.71
　tympanum 872.61
　　complicated 872.71
　umbilical region 879.2
　　complicated 879.3
　ureter — *see* Injury, internal, ureter
　urethra — *see* Injury, internal, urethra
　uterus — *see* Injury, internal, uterus
　uvula 873.69
　　complicated 873.79
　vagina 878.6
　　complicated 878.7
　vas deferens — *see* Injury, internal, vas deferens
　vitreous (humor) 871.2
　vulva 878.4
　　complicated 878.5
　wrist 881.02
　　with tendon involvement 881.22
　　complicated 881.12
Wright's syndrome (hyperabduction) 447.8
　pneumonia 390 *[517.1]*
Wringer injury — *see* Crush injury, by site
Wrinkling of skin 701.8
Wrist — *see also* condition
　drop (acquired) 736.05
Wrong drug (given in error) NEC 977.9
　specified drug or substance — *see* Table of Drugs and Chemicals
Wry neck — *see also* Torticollis
　congenital 754.1
Wuchereria infestation 125.0
　bancrofti 125.0
　Brugia malayi 125.1
　malayi 125.1
Wuchereriasis 125.0
Wuchereriosis 125.0
Wuchernde struma langhans (M8332/3) 193

X

Xanthelasma 272.2
　eyelid 272.2 *[374.51]*
　palpebrarum 272.2 *[374.51]*
Xanthelasmatosis (essential) 272.2
Xanthelasmoidea 757.33
Xanthine stones 277.2
Xanthinuria 277.2
Xanthofibroma (M8831/0) — *see* Neoplasm, connective tissue, benign
Xanthoma(s), xanthomatosis 272.2
　with
　　hyperlipoproteinemia
　　　type I 272.3
　　　type III 272.2
　　　type IV 272.1
　　　type V 272.3
　bone 272.7
　craniohypophyseal 277.89
　cutaneotendinous 272.7
　diabeticorum 250.8 ☑ *[272.2]*
　　due to secondary diabetes 249.8 ☑ *[272.2]*
　disseminatum 272.7
　eruptive 272.2

Xanthoma(s), xanthomatosis — *continued*
　eyelid 272.2 *[374.51]*
　familial 272.7
　hereditary 272.7
　hypercholesterinemic 272.0
　hypercholesterolemic 272.0
　hyperlipemic 272.4
　hyperlipidemic 272.4
　infantile 272.7
　joint 272.7
　juvenile 272.7
　multiple 272.7
　multiplex 272.7
　primary familial 272.7
　tendon (sheath) 272.7
　tuberosum 272.2
　tuberous 272.2
　tubo-eruptive 272.2
Xanthosis 709.09
　surgical 998.81
Xenophobia 300.29
Xeroderma (congenital) 757.39
　acquired 701.1
　　eyelid 373.33
　eyelid 373.33
　pigmentosum 757.33
　vitamin A deficiency 264.8
Xerophthalmia 372.53
　vitamin A deficiency 264.7
Xerosis
　conjunctiva 372.53
　　with Bitôt's spot 372.53
　　　vitamin A deficiency 264.1
　　vitamin A deficiency 264.0
　cornea 371.40
　　with corneal ulceration 370.00
　　　vitamin A deficiency 264.3
　　vitamin A deficiency 264.2
　cutis 706.8
　skin 706.8
Xerostomia 527.7
Xiphodynia 733.90
Xiphoidalgia 733.90
Xiphoiditis 733.99
Xiphopagus 759.4
XO syndrome 758.6
X-ray
　effects, adverse, NEC 990
　of chest
　　for suspected tuberculosis V71.2
　　routine V72.5
XXX syndrome 758.81
XXXXY syndrome 758.81
XXY syndrome 758.7
Xyloketosuria 271.8
Xylosuria 271.8
Xylulosuria 271.8
XYY syndrome 758.81

Y

Yaba monkey tumor virus 059.22
Yawning 786.09
　psychogenic 306.1
Yaws 102.9
　bone or joint lesions 102.6
　butter 102.1
　chancre 102.0
　cutaneous, less than five years after infection 102.2

Yaws — *continued*
　early (cutaneous) (macular) (maculopapular) (micropapular) (papular) 102.2
　　frambeside 102.2
　　skin lesions NEC 102.2
　eyelid 102.9 *[373.4]*
　ganglion 102.6
　gangosis, gangosa 102.5
　gumma, gummata 102.4
　　bone 102.6
　gummatous
　　frambeside 102.4
　　osteitis 102.6
　　periostitis 102.6
　hydrarthrosis 102.6
　hyperkeratosis (early) (late) (palmar) (plantar) 102.3
　initial lesions 102.0
　joint lesions 102.6
　juxta-articular nodules 102.7
　late nodular (ulcerated) 102.4
　latent (without clinical manifestations) (with positive serology) 102.8
　mother 102.0
　mucosal 102.7
　multiple papillomata 102.1
　nodular, late (ulcerated) 102.4
　osteitis 102.6
　papilloma, papillomata (palmar) (plantar) 102.1
　periostitis (hypertrophic) 102.6
　ulcers 102.4
　wet crab 102.1
Yeast infection — *see also* Candidiasis 112.9
Yellow
　atrophy (liver) 570
　　chronic 571.8
　　resulting from administration of blood, plasma, serum, or other biological substance (within 8 months of administration) — *see* Hepatitis, viral
　fever — *see* Fever, yellow
　jack (*see also* Fever, yellow) 060.9
　jaundice (*see also* Jaundice) 782.4
　vernix syndrome 762.2
Yersinia septica 027.8

Z

Zagari's disease (xerostomia) 527.7
Zahorsky's disease (exanthema subitum) (*see also* Exanthem subitum) 058.10
　syndrome (herpangina) 074.0
Zellweger syndrome 277.86
Zenker's diverticulum (esophagus) 530.6
Ziehen-Oppenheim disease 333.6
Zieve's syndrome (jaundice, hyperlipemia, and hemolytic anemia) 571.1
Zika fever 066.3
Zollinger-Ellison syndrome (gastric hypersecretion with pancreatic islet cell tumor) 251.5
Zona — *see also* Herpes, zoster 053.9
Zoophilia (erotica) 302.1
Zoophobia 300.29
Zoster (herpes) — *see also* Herpes, zoster 053.9
Zuelzer (-Ogden) anemia or syndrome (nutritional megaloblastic anemia) 281.2
Zygodactyly — *see also* Syndactylism 755.10
Zygomycosis 117.7
Zymotic — *see* condition

☑ Additional Digit Required — Refer to the Tabular List for Digit Selection　　　　　　　⍦ Subterms under main terms may continue to next column or page

SECTION 2

Alphabetic Index to Poisoning and External Causes of Adverse Effects of Drugs and Other Chemical Substances

TABLE OF DRUGS AND CHEMICALS

This table contains a classification of drugs and other chemical substances to identify poisoning states and external causes of adverse effects.

Each of the listed substances in the table is assigned a code according to the poisoning classification (960-989). These codes are used when there is a statement of poisoning, overdose, wrong substance given or taken, or intoxication.

The table also contains a listing of external causes of adverse effects. An adverse effect is a pathologic manifestation due to ingestion or exposure to drugs or other chemical substances (e.g., dermatitis, hypersensitivity reaction, aspirin gastritis). The adverse effect is to be identified by the appropriate code found in Section 1, Index to Diseases and Injuries. An external cause code can then be used to identify the circumstances involved. The table headings pertaining to external causes are defined below:

Accidental poisoning (E850-E869) — accidental overdose of drug, wrong substance given or taken, drug taken inadvertently, accidents in the usage of drugs and biologicals in medical and surgical procedures, and to show external causes of poisonings classifiable to 980-989.

Therapeutic use (E930-E949) — a correct substance properly administered in therapeutic or prophylactic dosage as the external cause of adverse effects.

Suicide attempt (E950-E952) — instances in which self-inflicted injuries or poisonings are involved.

Assault (E961-E962) — injury or poisoning inflicted by another person with the intent to injure or kill.

Undetermined (E980-E982) — to be used when the intent of the poisoning or injury cannot be determined whether it was intentional or accidental.

The American Hospital Formulary Service list numbers are included in the table to help classify new drugs not identified in the table by name. The AHFS list numbers are keyed to the continually revised American Hospital Formulary Service (AHFS).* These listings are found in the table under the main term **Drug**.

Excluded from the table are radium and other radioactive substances. The classification of adverse effects and complications pertaining to these substances will be found in Section 1, Index to Diseases and Injuries, and Section 3, Index to External Causes of Injuries.

Although certain substances are indexed with one or more subentries, the majority are listed according to one use or state. It is recognized that many substances may be used in various ways, in medicine and in industry, and may cause adverse effects whatever the state of the agent (solid, liquid, or fumes arising from a liquid). In cases in which the reported data indicates a use or state not in the table, or which is clearly different from the one listed, an attempt should be made to classify the substance in the form which most nearly expresses the reported facts.

*American Hospital Formulary Service, 2 vol. (Washington, D.C.: American Society of Hospital Pharmacists, 1959-)

☑ Additional Digit Required — Refer to the Tabular List for Digit Selection ⬇ Subterms under main terms may continue to next column or page

2011 ICD-9-CM ▶◀ Revised Text ● New Line ▲ Revised Code Volume 2 — 297

Index
1-propanol — Aliphatic thiocyanates

	Poisoning	Accident	Therapeutic Use	Suicide Attempt	Assault	Undetermined
1-propanol	980.3	E860.4	—	E950.9	E962.1	E980.9
2-propanol	980.2	E860.3	—	E950.9	E962.1	E980.9
2,4-D (dichlorophenoxyacetic acid)	989.4	E863.5	—	E950.6	E962.1	E980.7
2,4-toluene diiso-cyanate	983.0	E864.0	—	E950.7	E962.1	E980.6
2,4,5-T (trichlorophenoxy-acetic acid)	989.2	E863.5	—	E950.6	E962.1	E980.7
14-hydroxydihydromorphi-none	965.09	E850.2	E935.2	E950.0	E962.0	E980.0
ABOB	961.7	E857	E931.7	E950.4	E962.0	E980.4
Abrus (seed)	988.2	E865.3	—	E950.9	E962.1	E980.9
Absinthe	980.0	E860.1	—	E950.9	E962.1	E980.9
beverage	980.0	E860.0	—	E950.9	E962.1	E980.9
Acenocoumarin, aceno-coumarol	964.2	E858.2	E934.2	E950.4	E962.0	E980.4
Acepromazine	969.1	E853.0	E939.1	E950.3	E962.0	E980.3
Acetal	982.8	E862.4	—	E950.9	E962.1	E980.9
Acetaldehyde (vapor)	987.8	E869.8	—	E952.8	E962.2	E982.8
liquid	989.89	E866.8	—	E950.9	E962.1	E980.9
Acetaminophen	965.4	E850.4	E935.4	E950.0	E962.0	E980.0
Acetaminosalol	965.1	E850.3	E935.3	E950.0	E962.0	E980.0
Acetanilid(e)	965.4	E850.4	E935.4	E950.0	E962.0	E980.0
Acetarsol, acetarsone	961.1	E857	E931.1	E950.4	E962.0	E980.4
Acetazolamide	974.2	E858.5	E944.2	E950.4	E962.0	E980.4
Acetic						
acid	983.1	E864.1	—	E950.7	E962.1	E980.6
with sodium acetate (ointment)	976.3	E858.7	E946.3	E950.4	E962.0	E980.4
irrigating solution	974.5	E858.5	E944.5	E950.4	E962.0	E980.4
lotion	976.2	E858.7	E946.2	E950.4	E962.0	E980.4
anhydride	983.1	E864.1	—	E950.7	E962.1	E980.6
ether	982.8	E862.4	—	E950.9	E962.1	E980.9
Acetohexamide	962.3	E858.0	E932.3	E950.4	E962.0	E980.4
Acetomenaphthone	964.3	E858.2	E934.3	E950.4	E962.0	E980.4
Acetomorphine	965.01	E850.0	E935.0	E950.0	E962.0	E980.0
Acetone (oils) (vapor)	982.8	E862.4	—	E950.9	E962.1	E980.9
Acetophenazine (maleate)	969.1	E853.0	E939.1	E950.3	E962.0	E980.3
Acetophenetidin	965.4	E850.4	E935.4	E950.0	E962.0	E980.0
Acetophenone	982.0	E862.4	—	E950.9	E962.1	E980.9
Acetorphine	965.09	E850.2	E935.2	E950.0	E962.0	E980.0
Acetosulfone (sodium)	961.8	E857	E931.8	E950.4	E962.0	E980.4
Acetrizoate (sodium)	977.8	E858.8	E947.8	E950.4	E962.0	E980.4
Acetylcarbromal	967.3	E852.2	E937.3	E950.2	E962.0	E980.2
Acetylcholine (chloride)	971.0	E855.3	E941.0	E950.4	E962.0	E980.4
Acetylcysteine	975.5	E858.6	E945.5	E950.4	E962.0	E980.4
Acetyldigitoxin	972.1	E858.3	E942.1	E950.4	E962.0	E980.4
Acetyldihydrocodeine	965.09	E850.2	E935.2	E950.0	E962.0	E980.0
Acetyldihydrocodeinone	965.09	E850.2	E935.2	E950.0	E962.0	E980.0
Acetylene (gas) (industrial)	987.1	E868.1	—	E951.8	E962.2	E981.8
incomplete combustion of — see Carbon monoxide, fuel, utility						
tetrachloride (vapor)	982.3	E862.4	—	E950.9	E962.1	E980.9
Acetyliodosalicylic acid	965.1	E850.3	E935.3	E950.0	E962.0	E980.0
Acetylphenylhydrazine	965.8	E850.8	E935.8	E950.0	E962.0	E980.0
Acetylsalicylic acid	965.1	E850.3	E935.3	E950.0	E962.0	E980.0
Achromycin	960.4	E856	E930.4	E950.4	E962.0	E980.4
ophthalmic preparation	976.5	E858.7	E946.5	E950.4	E962.0	E980.4
topical NEC	976.0	E858.7	E946.0	E950.4	E962.0	E980.4
Acidifying agents	963.2	E858.1	E933.2	E950.4	E962.0	E980.4
Acids (corrosive) NEC	983.1	E864.1	—	E950.7	E962.1	E980.6
Aconite (wild)	988.2	E865.4	—	E950.9	E962.1	E980.9
Aconitine (liniment)	976.8	E858.7	E946.8	E950.4	E962.0	E980.4
Aconitum ferox	988.2	E865.4	—	E950.9	E962.1	E980.9
Acridine	983.0	E864.0	—	E950.7	E962.1	E980.6
vapor	987.8	E869.8	—	E952.8	E962.2	E982.8
Acriflavine	961.9	E857	E931.9	E950.4	E962.0	E980.4
Acrisorcin	976.0	E858.7	E946.0	E950.4	E962.0	E980.4
Acrolein (gas)	987.8	E869.8	—	E952.8	E962.2	E982.8
liquid	989.89	E866.8	—	E950.9	E962.1	E980.9
Actaea spicata	988.2	E865.4	—	E950.9	E962.1	E980.9
Acterol	961.5	E857	E931.5	E950.4	E962.0	E980.4
ACTH	962.4	E858.0	E932.4	E950.4	E962.0	E980.4
Acthar	962.4	E858.0	E932.4	E950.4	E962.0	E980.4
Actinomycin (C) (D)	960.7	E856	E930.7	E950.4	E962.0	E980.4
Adalin (acetyl)	967.3	E852.2	E937.3	E950.2	E962.0	E980.2
Adenosine (phosphate)	977.8	E858.8	E947.8	E950.4	E962.0	E980.4
ADH	962.5	E858.0	E932.5	E950.4	E962.0	E980.4
Adhesives	989.89	E866.6	—	E950.9	E962.1	E980.9
Adicillin	960.0	E856	E930.0	E950.4	E962.0	E980.4
Adiphenine	975.1	E855.6	E945.1	E950.4	E962.0	E980.4
Adjunct, pharmaceutical	977.4	E858.8	E947.4	E950.4	E962.0	E980.4
Adrenal (extract, cortex or medulla) (glucocorticoids) (hormones) (mineralocorti-coids)	962.0	E858.0	E932.0	E950.4	E962.0	E980.4
ENT agent	976.6	E858.7	E946.6	E950.4	E962.0	E980.4
ophthalmic preparation	976.5	E858.7	E946.5	E950.4	E962.0	E980.4
topical NEC	976.0	E858.7	E946.0	E950.4	E962.0	E980.4
Adrenalin	971.2	E855.5	E941.2	E950.4	E962.0	E980.4
Adrenergic blocking agents	971.3	E855.6	E941.3	E950.4	E962.0	E980.4
Adrenergics	971.2	E855.5	E941.2	E950.4	E962.0	E980.4
Adrenochrome (derivatives)	972.8	E858.3	E942.8	E950.4	E962.0	E980.4
Adrenocorticotropic hormone	962.4	E858.0	E932.4	E950.4	E962.0	E980.4
Adrenocorticotropin	962.4	E858.0	E932.4	E950.4	E962.0	E980.4
Adriamycin	960.7	E856	E930.7	E950.4	E962.0	E980.4
Aerosol spray — see Sprays						
Aerosporin	960.8	E856	E930.8	E950.4	E962.0	E980.4
ENT agent	976.6	E858.7	E946.6	E950.4	E962.0	E980.4
ophthalmic preparation	976.5	E858.7	E946.5	E950.4	E962.0	E980.4
topical NEC	976.0	E858.7	E946.0	E950.4	E962.0	E980.4
Aethusa cynapium	988.2	E865.4	—	E950.9	E962.1	E980.9
Afghanistan black	969.6	E854.1	E939.6	E950.3	E962.0	E980.3
Aflatoxin	989.7	E865.9	—	E950.9	E962.1	E980.9
African boxwood	988.2	E865.4	—	E950.9	E962.1	E980.9
Agar (-agar)	973.3	E858.4	E943.3	E950.4	E962.0	E980.4
Agricultural agent NEC	989.89	E863.9	—	E950.6	E962.1	E980.7
Agrypnal	967.0	E851	E937.0	E950.1	E962.0	E980.1
Air contaminant(s), source or type not specified	987.9	E869.9	—	E952.9	E962.2	E982.9
specified type — see specific substance						
Akee	988.2	E865.4	—	E950.9	E962.1	E980.9
Akrinol	976.0	E858.7	E946.0	E950.4	E962.0	E980.4
Alantolactone	961.6	E857	E931.6	E950.4	E962.0	E980.4
Albamycin	960.8	E856	E930.8	E950.4	E962.0	E980.4
Albumin (normal human serum)	964.7	E858.2	E934.7	E950.4	E962.0	E980.4
Albuterol	975.7	E858.6	E945.7	E950.4	E962.0	E980.4
Alcohol	980.9	E860.9	—	E950.9	E962.1	E980.9
absolute	980.0	E860.1	—	E950.9	E962.1	E980.9
beverage	980.0	E860.0	E947.8	E950.9	E962.1	E980.9
amyl	980.3	E860.4	—	E950.9	E962.1	E980.9
antifreeze	980.1	E860.2	—	E950.9	E962.1	E980.9
butyl	980.3	E860.4	—	E950.9	E962.1	E980.9
dehydrated	980.0	E860.1	—	E950.9	E962.1	E980.9
beverage	980.0	E860.0	E947.8	E950.9	E962.1	E980.9
denatured	980.0	E860.1	—	E950.9	E962.1	E980.9
deterrents	977.3	E858.8	E947.3	E950.4	E962.0	E980.4
diagnostic (gastric function)	977.8	E858.8	E947.8	E950.4	E962.0	E980.4
ethyl	980.0	E860.1	—	E950.9	E962.1	E980.9
beverage	980.0	E860.0	E947.8	E950.9	E962.1	E980.9
grain	980.0	E860.1	—	E950.9	E962.1	E980.9
beverage	980.0	E860.0	E947.8	E950.9	E962.1	E980.9
industrial	980.9	E860.9	—	E950.9	E962.1	E980.9
isopropyl	980.2	E860.3	—	E950.9	E962.1	E980.9
methyl	980.1	E860.2	—	E950.9	E962.1	E980.9
preparation for consumption	980.0	E860.0	E947.8	E950.9	E962.1	E980.9
propyl	980.3	E860.4	—	E950.9	E962.1	E980.9
secondary	980.2	E860.3	—	E950.9	E962.1	E980.9
radiator	980.1	E860.2	—	E950.9	E962.1	E980.9
rubbing	980.2	E860.3	—	E950.9	E962.1	E980.9
specified type NEC	980.8	E860.8	—	E950.9	E962.1	E980.9
surgical	980.9	E860.9	—	E950.9	E962.1	E980.9
vapor (from any type of alcohol)	987.8	E869.8	—	E952.8	E962.2	E982.8
wood	980.1	E860.2	—	E950.9	E962.1	E980.9
Alcuronium chloride	975.2	E858.6	E945.2	E950.4	E962.0	E980.4
Aldactone	974.4	E858.5	E944.4	E950.4	E962.0	E980.4
Aldicarb	989.3	E863.2	—	E950.6	E962.1	E980.7
Aldomet	972.6	E858.3	E942.6	E950.4	E962.0	E980.4
Aldosterone	962.0	E858.0	E932.0	E950.4	E962.0	E980.4
Aldrin (dust)	989.2	E863.0	—	E950.6	E962.1	E980.7
Algeldrate	973.0	E858.4	E943.0	E950.4	E962.0	E980.4
Alidase	963.4	E858.1	E933.4	E950.4	E962.0	E980.4
Aliphatic thiocyanates	989.0	E866.8	—	E950.9	E962.1	E980.9

Nontherapeutic use substance

Subterms under main terms may continue to next column or page

		External Cause (E-Code)			
	Poisoning	Accident	Therapeutic Use	Suicide Attempt	Assault	Undetermined
Alkaline antiseptic solution (aromatic)	976.6	E858.7	E946.6	E950.4	E962.0	E980.4
Alkalinizing agents (medicinal)	963.3	E858.1	E933.3	E950.4	E962.0	E980.4
Alkalis, caustic	983.2	E864.2	—	E950.7	E962.1	E980.6
Alkalizing agents (medicinal)	963.3	E858.1	E933.3	E950.4	E962.0	E980.4
Alka-seltzer	965.1	E850.3	E935.3	E950.0	E962.0	E980.0
Alkavervir	972.6	E858.3	E942.6	E950.4	E962.0	E980.4
Allegron	969.05	E854.0	E939.0	E950.3	E962.0	E980.3
Alleve — Naproxen						
Allobarbital, allobarbitone	967.0	E851	E937.0	E950.1	E962.0	E980.1
Allopurinol	974.7	E858.5	E944.7	E950.4	E962.0	E980.4
Allylestrenol	962.2	E858.0	E932.2	E950.4	E962.0	E980.4
Allylisopropylacetylurea	967.8	E852.8	E937.8	E950.2	E962.0	E980.2
Allylisopropylmalonylurea	967.0	E851	E937.0	E950.1	E962.0	E980.1
Allyltribromide	967.3	E852.2	E937.3	E950.2	E962.0	E980.2
Aloe, aloes, aloin	973.1	E858.4	E943.1	E950.4	E962.0	E980.4
Alosetron	973.8	E858.4	E943.8	E950.4	E962.0	E980.4
Aloxidone	966.0	E855.0	E936.0	E950.4	E962.0	E980.4
Aloxiprin	965.1	E850.3	E935.3	E950.0	E962.0	E980.0
Alpha-1 blockers	971.3	E855.6	E941.3	E950.4	E962.0	E980.4
Alpha amylase	963.4	E858.1	E933.4	E950.4	E962.0	E980.4
Alphaprodine (hydrochloride)	965.09	E850.2	E935.2	E950.0	E962.0	E980.0
Alpha tocopherol	963.5	E858.1	E933.5	E950.4	E962.0	E980.4
Alseroxylon	972.6	E858.3	E942.6	E950.4	E962.0	E980.4
Alum (ammonium) (potassium)	983.2	E864.2	—	E950.7	E962.1	E980.6
medicinal (astringent) NEC	976.2	E858.7	E946.2	E950.4	E962.0	E980.4
Aluminium, aluminum (gel) (hydroxide)	973.0	E858.4	E943.0	E950.4	E962.0	E980.4
acetate solution	976.2	E858.7	E946.2	E950.4	E962.0	E980.4
aspirin	965.1	E850.3	E935.3	E950.0	E962.0	E980.0
carbonate	973.0	E858.4	E943.0	E950.4	E962.0	E980.4
glycinate	973.0	E858.4	E943.0	E950.4	E962.0	E980.4
nicotinate	972.2	E858.3	E942.2	E950.4	E962.0	E980.4
ointment (surgical) (topical)	976.3	E858.7	E946.3	E950.4	E962.0	E980.4
phosphate	973.0	E858.4	E943.0	E950.4	E962.0	E980.4
subacetate	976.2	E858.7	E946.2	E950.4	E962.0	E980.4
topical NEC	976.3	E858.7	E946.3	E950.4	E962.0	E980.4
Alurate	967.0	E851	E937.0	E950.1	E962.0	E980.1
Alverine (citrate)	975.1	E858.6	E945.1	E950.4	E962.0	E980.4
Alvodine	965.09	E850.2	E935.2	E950.0	E962.0	E980.0
Amanita phalloides	988.1	E865.5	—	E950.9	E962.1	E980.9
Amantadine (hydrochloride)	966.4	E855.0	E936.4	E950.4	E962.0	E980.4
Ambazone	961.9	E857	E931.9	E950.4	E962.0	E980.4
Ambenonium	971.0	E855.3	E941.0	E950.4	E962.0	E980.4
Ambutonium bromide	971.1	E855.4	E941.1	E950.4	E962.0	E980.4
Ametazole	977.8	E858.8	E947.8	E950.4	E962.0	E980.4
Amethocaine (infiltration) (topical)	968.5	E855.2	E938.5	E950.4	E962.0	E980.4
nerve block (peripheral) (plexus)	968.6	E855.2	E938.6	E950.4	E962.0	E980.4
spinal	968.7	E855.2	E938.7	E950.4	E962.0	E980.4
Amethopterin	963.1	E858.1	E933.1	E950.4	E962.0	E980.4
Amfepramone	977.0	E858.8	E947.0	E950.4	E962.0	E980.4
Amidon	965.02	E850.1	E935.1	E950.0	E962.0	E980.0
Amidopyrine	965.5	E850.5	E935.5	E950.0	E962.0	E980.0
Aminacrine	976.0	E858.7	E946.0	E950.4	E962.0	E980.4
Aminitrozole	961.5	E857	E931.5	E950.4	E962.0	E980.4
Aminoacetic acid	974.5	E858.5	E944.5	E950.4	E962.0	E980.4
Amino acids	974.5	E858.5	E944.5	E950.4	E962.0	E980.4
Aminocaproic acid	964.4	E858.2	E934.4	E950.4	E962.0	E980.4
Aminoethylisothiourium	963.8	E858.1	E933.8	E950.4	E962.0	E980.4
Aminoglutethimide	966.3	E855.0	E936.3	E950.4	E962.0	E980.4
Aminometradine	974.3	E858.5	E944.3	E950.4	E962.0	E980.4
Aminopentamide	971.1	E855.4	E941.1	E950.4	E962.0	E980.4
Aminophenazone	965.5	E850.5	E935.5	E950.0	E962.0	E980.0
Aminophenol	983.0	E864.0	—	E950.7	E962.1	E980.6
Aminophenylpyridone	969.5	E853.8	E939.5	E950.3	E962.0	E980.3
Aminophyllin	975.7	E858.6	E945.7	E950.4	E962.0	E980.4
Aminopterin	963.1	E858.1	E933.1	E950.4	E962.0	E980.4
Aminopyrine	965.5	E850.5	E935.5	E950.0	E962.0	E980.0
Aminosalicylic acid	961.8	E857	E931.8	E950.4	E962.0	E980.4
Amiphenazole	970.1	E854.3	E940.1	E950.4	E962.0	E980.4
Amiquinsin	972.6	E858.3	E942.6	E950.4	E962.0	E980.4

		External Cause (E-Code)			
	Poisoning	Accident	Therapeutic Use	Suicide Attempt	Assault	Undetermined
Amisometradine	974.3	E858.5	E944.3	E950.4	E962.0	E980.4
Amitriptyline	969.05	E854.0	E939.0	E950.3	E962.0	E980.3
Ammonia (fumes) (gas) (vapor)	987.8	E869.8	—	E952.8	E962.2	E982.8
liquid (household) NEC	983.2	E861.4	—	E950.7	E962.1	E980.6
spirit, aromatic	970.89 ▲	E854.3	E940.8	E950.4	E962.0	E980.4
Ammoniated mercury	976.0	E858.7	E946.0	E950.4	E962.0	E980.4
Ammonium						
carbonate	983.2	E864.2	—	E950.7	E962.1	E980.6
chloride (acidifying agent)	963.2	E858.1	E933.2	E950.4	E962.0	E980.4
expectorant	975.5	E858.6	E945.5	E950.4	E962.0	E980.4
compounds (household) NEC	983.2	E861.4	—	E950.7	E962.1	E980.6
fumes (any usage)	987.8	E869.8	—	E952.8	E962.2	E982.8
industrial	983.2	E864.2	—	E950.7	E962.1	E980.6
ichthyosulfonate	976.4	E858.7	E946.4	E950.4	E962.0	E980.4
mandelate	961.9	E857	E931.9	E950.4	E962.0	E980.4
Amobarbital	967.0	E851	E937.0	E950.1	E962.0	E980.1
Amodiaquin(e)	961.4	E857	E931.4	E950.4	E962.0	E980.4
Amopyroquin(e)	961.4	E857	E931.4	E950.4	E962.0	E980.4
Amphenidone	969.5	E853.8	E939.5	E950.3	E962.0	E980.3
Amphetamine	969.72	E854.2	E939.7	E950.3	E962.0	E980.3
Amphomycin	960.8	E856	E930.8	E950.4	E962.0	E980.4
Amphotericin B	960.1	E856	E930.1	E950.4	E962.0	E980.4
topical	976.0	E858.7	E946.0	E950.4	E962.0	E980.4
Ampicillin	960.0	E856	E930.0	E950.4	E962.0	E980.4
Amprotropine	971.1	E855.4	E941.1	E950.4	E962.0	E980.4
Amygdalin	977.8	E858.8	E947.8	E950.4	E962.0	E980.4
Amyl						
acetate (vapor)	982.8	E862.4	—	E950.9	E962.1	E980.9
alcohol	980.3	E860.4	—	E950.9	E962.1	E980.9
nitrite (medicinal)	972.4	E858.3	E942.4	E950.4	E962.0	E980.4
Amylase (alpha)	963.4	E858.1	E933.4	E950.4	E962.0	E980.4
Amylene hydrate	980.8	E860.8	—	E950.9	E962.1	E980.9
Amylobarbitone	967.0	E851	E937.0	E950.1	E962.0	E980.1
Amylocaine	968.9	E855.2	E938.9	E950.4	E962.0	E980.4
infiltration (subcutaneous)	968.5	E855.2	E938.5	E950.4	E962.0	E980.4
nerve block (peripheral) (plexus)	968.6	E855.2	E938.6	E950.4	E962.0	E980.4
spinal	968.7	E855.2	E938.7	E950.4	E962.0	E980.4
topical (surface)	968.5	E855.2	E938.5	E950.4	E962.0	E980.4
Amytal (sodium)	967.0	E851	E937.0	E950.1	E962.0	E980.1
Analeptics	970.0	E854.3	E940.0	E950.4	E962.0	E980.4
Analgesics	965.9	E850.9	E935.9	E950.0	E962.0	E980.0
aromatic NEC	965.4	E850.4	E935.4	E950.0	E962.0	E980.0
non-narcotic NEC	965.7	E850.7	E935.7	E950.0	E962.0	E980.0
specified NEC	965.8	E850.8	E935.8	E950.0	E962.0	E980.0
Anamirta cocculus	988.2	E865.3	—	E950.9	E962.1	E980.9
Ancillin	960.0	E856	E930.0	E950.4	E962.0	E980.4
Androgens (anabolic congeners)	962.1	E858.0	E932.1	E950.4	E962.0	E980.4
Androstalone	962.1	E858.0	E932.1	E950.4	E962.0	E980.4
Androsterone	962.1	E858.0	E932.1	E950.4	E962.0	E980.4
Anemone pulsatilla	988.2	E865.4	—	E950.9	E962.1	E980.9
Anesthesia, anesthetic (general) NEC	968.4	E855.1	E938.4	E950.4	E962.0	E980.4
block (nerve) (plexus)	968.6	E855.2	E938.6	E950.4	E962.0	E980.4
gaseous NEC	968.2	E855.1	E938.2	E950.4	E962.0	E980.4
halogenated hydrocarbon derivatives NEC	968.2	E855.1	E938.2	E950.4	E962.0	E980.4
infiltration (intradermal) (subcutaneous) (submucosal)	968.5	E855.2	E938.5	E950.4	E962.0	E980.4
intravenous	968.3	E855.1	E938.3	E950.4	E962.0	E980.4
local NEC	968.9	E855.2	E938.9	E950.4	E962.0	E980.4
nerve blocking (peripheral) (plexus)	968.6	E855.2	E938.6	E950.4	E962.0	E980.4
rectal NEC	968.3	E855.1	E938.3	E950.4	E962.0	E980.4
spinal	968.7	E855.2	E938.7	E950.4	E962.0	E980.4
surface	968.5	E855.2	E938.5	E950.4	E962.0	E980.4
topical	968.5	E855.2	E938.5	E950.4	E962.0	E980.4
Aneurine	963.5	E858.1	E933.5	E950.4	E962.0	E980.4
Anginine — see Glyceryl trinitrate						
Angio-Conray	977.8	E858.8	E947.8	E950.4	E962.0	E980.4
Angiotensin	971.2	E855.5	E941.2	E950.4	E962.0	E980.4
Anhydrohydroxyprogesterone	962.2	E858.0	E932.2	E950.4	E962.0	E980.4
Anhydron	974.3	E858.5	E944.3	E950.4	E962.0	E980.4
Anileridine	965.09	E850.2	E935.2	E950.0	E962.0	E980.0

Nontherapeutic use substance

Subterms under main terms may continue to next column or page

Index — Aniline — Aristocort

	Poisoning	External Cause (E-Code) Accident	Therapeutic Use	Suicide Attempt	Assault	Undetermined
Aniline (dye) (liquid)	983.0	E864.0	—	E950.7	E962.1	E980.6
analgesic	965.4	E850.4	E935.4	E950.0	E962.0	E980.0
derivatives, therapeutic NEC	965.4	E850.4	E935.4	E950.0	E962.0	E980.0
vapor	987.8	E869.8	—	E952.8	E962.2	E982.8
Aniscoropine	971.1	E855.4	E941.1	E950.4	E962.0	E980.4
Anisindione	964.2	E858.2	E934.2	E950.4	E962.0	E980.4
Anorexic agents	977.0	E858.8	E947.0	E950.4	E962.0	E980.4
Ant (bite) (sting)	—	E905.5	—	E950.9	E962.1	E980.9
Antabuse	977.3	E858.8	E947.3	E950.4	E962.0	E980.4
Antacids	973.0	E858.4	E943.0	E950.4	E962.0	E980.4
Antazoline	963.0	E858.1	E933.0	E950.4	E962.0	E980.4
Anthralin	976.4	E858.7	E946.4	E950.4	E962.0	E980.4
Anthramycin	960.7	E856	E930.7	E950.4	E962.0	E980.4
Antiadrenergics	971.3	E855.6	E941.3	E950.4	E962.0	E980.4
Antiallergic agents	963.0	E858.1	E933.0	E950.4	E962.0	E980.4
Antianemic agents NEC	964.1	E858.2	E934.1	E950.4	E962.0	E980.4
Antiaris toxicaria	988.2	E865.4	—	E950.9	E962.1	E980.9
Antiarteriosclerotic agents	972.2	E858.3	E942.2	E950.4	E962.0	E980.4
Antiasthmatics	975.7	E858.6	E945.7	E950.4	E962.0	E980.4
Antibiotics	960.9	E856	E930.9	E950.4	E962.0	E980.4
antifungal	960.1	E856	E930.1	E950.4	E962.0	E980.4
antimycobacterial	960.6	E856	E930.6	E950.4	E962.0	E980.4
antineoplastic	960.7	E856	E930.7	E950.4	E962.0	E980.4
cephalosporin (group)	960.5	E856	E930.5	E950.4	E962.0	E980.4
chloramphenicol (group)	960.2	E856	E930.2	E950.4	E962.0	E980.4
macrolides	960.3	E856	E930.3	E950.4	E962.0	E980.4
specified NEC	960.8	E856	E930.8	E950.4	E962.0	E980.4
tetracycline (group)	960.4	E856	E930.4	E950.4	E962.0	E980.4
Anticancer agents NEC	963.1	E858.1	E933.1	E950.4	E962.0	E980.4
antibiotics	960.7	E856	E930.7	E950.4	E962.0	E980.4
Anticholinergics	971.1	E855.4	E941.1	E950.4	E962.0	E980.4
Anticholinesterase (organophosphorus) (reversible)	971.0	E855.3	E941.0	E950.4	E962.0	E980.4
Anticoagulants	964.2	E858.2	E934.2	E950.4	E962.0	E980.4
antagonists	964.5	E858.2	E934.5	E950.4	E962.0	E980.4
Anti-common cold agents NEC	975.6	E858.6	E945.6	E950.4	E962.0	E980.4
Anticonvulsants NEC	966.3	E855.0	E936.3	E950.4	E962.0	E980.4
Antidepressants	969.00	E854.0	E939.0	E950.3	E962.0	E980.3
monoamine oxidase inhibitors (MAOI)	969.01	E854.0	E939.0	E950.3	E962.0	E980.3
specified type NEC	969.09	E854.0	E939.0	E950.3	E962.0	E980.3
SSNRI (selective serotonin and norepinephrine reuptake inhibitors)	969.02	E854.0	E939.0	E950.3	E962.0	E980.3
SSRI (selective serotonin reuptake inhibitors)	969.03	E854.0	E939.0	E950.3	E962.0	E980.3
tetracyclic	969.04	E854.0	E939.0	E950.3	E962.0	E980.3
tricyclic	969.05	E854.0	E939.0	E950.3	E962.0	E980.3
Antidiabetic agents	962.3	E858.0	E932.3	E950.4	E962.0	E980.4
Antidiarrheal agents	973.5	E858.4	E943.5	E950.4	E962.0	E980.4
Antidiuretic hormone	962.5	E858.0	E932.5	E950.4	E962.0	E980.4
Antidotes NEC	977.2	E858.8	E947.2	E950.4	E962.0	E980.4
Antiemetic agents	963.0	E858.1	E933.0	E950.4	E962.0	E980.4
Antiepilepsy agent NEC	966.3	E855.0	E936.3	E950.4	E962.0	E980.4
Antifertility pills	962.2	E858.0	E932.2	E950.4	E962.0	E980.4
Antiflatulents	973.8	E858.4	E943.8	E950.4	E962.0	E980.4
Antifreeze	989.89	E866.8	—	E950.9	E962.1	E980.9
alcohol	980.1	E860.2	—	E950.9	E962.1	E980.9
ethylene glycol	982.8	E862.4	—	E950.9	E962.1	E980.9
Antifungals (nonmedicinal) (sprays)	989.4	E863.6	—	E950.6	E962.1	E980.7
medicinal NEC	961.9	E857	E931.9	E950.4	E962.0	E980.4
antibiotic	960.1	E856	E930.1	E950.4	E962.0	E980.4
topical	976.0	E858.7	E946.0	E950.4	E962.0	E980.4
Antigastric secretion agents	973.0	E858.4	E943.0	E950.4	E962.0	E980.4
Antihelmintics	961.6	E857	E931.6	E950.4	E962.0	E980.4
Antihemophilic factor (human)	964.7	E858.2	E934.7	E950.4	E962.0	E980.4
Antihistamine	963.0	E858.1	E933.0	E950.4	E962.0	E980.4
Antihypertensive agents NEC	972.6	E858.3	E942.6	E950.4	E962.0	E980.4
Anti-infectives NEC	961.9	E857	E931.9	E950.4	E962.0	E980.4
antibiotics	960.9	E856	E930.9	E950.4	E962.0	E980.4
specified NEC	960.8	E856	E930.8	E950.4	E962.0	E980.4
antihelmintic	961.6	E857	E931.6	E950.4	E962.0	E980.4
antimalarial	961.4	E857	E931.4	E950.4	E962.0	E980.4
antimycobacterial NEC	961.8	E857	E931.8	E950.4	E962.0	E980.4
Anti-infectives — continued						
antimycobacterial — continued						
antibiotics	960.6	E856	E930.6	E950.4	E962.0	E980.4
antiprotozoal NEC	961.5	E857	E931.5	E950.4	E962.0	E980.4
blood	961.4	E857	E931.4	E950.4	E962.0	E980.4
antiviral	961.7	E857	E931.7	E950.4	E962.0	E980.4
arsenical	961.1	E857	E931.1	E950.4	E962.0	E980.4
ENT agents	976.6	E858.7	E946.6	E950.4	E962.0	E980.4
heavy metals NEC	961.2	E857	E931.2	E950.4	E962.0	E980.4
local	976.0	E858.7	E946.0	E950.4	E962.0	E980.4
ophthalmic preparation	976.5	E858.7	E946.5	E950.4	E962.0	E980.4
topical NEC	976.0	E858.7	E946.0	E950.4	E962.0	E980.4
Anti-inflammatory agents (topical)	976.0	E858.7	E946.0	E950.4	E962.0	E980.4
Antiknock (tetraethyl lead)	984.1	E862.1	—	E950.9	E962.1	E980.9
Antilipemics	972.2	E858.3	E942.2	E950.4	E962.0	E980.4
Antimalarials	961.4	E857	E931.4	E950.4	E962.0	E980.4
Antimony (compounds) (vapor) NEC	985.4	E866.2	—	E950.9	E962.1	E980.9
anti-infectives	961.2	E857	E931.2	E950.4	E962.0	E980.4
pesticides (vapor)	985.4	E863.4	—	E950.6	E962.2	E980.7
potassium tartrate	961.2	E857	E931.2	E950.4	E962.0	E980.4
tartrated	961.2	E857	E931.2	E950.4	E962.0	E980.4
Antimuscarinic agents	971.1	E855.4	E941.1	E950.4	E962.0	E980.4
Antimycobacterials NEC	961.8	E857	E931.8	E950.4	E962.0	E980.4
antibiotics	960.6	E856	E930.6	E950.4	E962.0	E980.4
Antineoplastic agents	963.1	E858.1	E933.1	E950.4	E962.0	E980.4
antibiotics	960.7	E856	E930.7	E950.4	E962.0	E980.4
Anti-Parkinsonism agents	966.4	E855.0	E936.4	E950.4	E962.0	E980.4
Antiphlogistics	965.69	E850.6	E935.6	E950.0	E962.0	E980.0
Antiprotozoals NEC	961.5	E857	E931.5	E950.4	E962.0	E980.4
blood	961.4	E857	E931.4	E950.4	E962.0	E980.4
Antipruritics (local)	976.1	E858.7	E946.1	E950.4	E962.0	E980.4
Antipsychotic agents NEC	969.3	E853.8	E939.3	E950.3	E962.0	E980.3
Antipyretics	965.9	E850.9	E935.9	E950.0	E962.0	E980.0
specified NEC	965.8	E850.8	E935.8	E950.0	E962.0	E980.0
Antipyrine	965.5	E850.5	E935.5	E950.0	E962.0	E980.0
Antirabies serum (equine)	979.9	E858.8	E949.9	E950.4	E962.0	E980.4
Antirheumatics	965.69	E850.6	E935.6	E950.0	E962.0	E980.0
Antiseborrheics	976.4	E858.7	E946.4	E950.4	E962.0	E980.4
Antiseptics (external) (medicinal)	976.0	E858.7	E946.0	E950.4	E962.0	E980.4
Antistine	963.0	E858.1	E933.0	E950.4	E962.0	E980.4
Antithyroid agents	962.8	E858.0	E932.8	E950.4	E962.0	E980.4
Antitoxin, any	979.9	E858.8	E949.9	E950.4	E962.0	E980.4
Antituberculars	961.8	E857	E931.8	E950.4	E962.0	E980.4
antibiotics	960.6	E856	E930.6	E950.4	E962.0	E980.4
Antitussives	975.4	E858.6	E945.4	E950.4	E962.0	E980.4
Antivaricose agents (sclerosing)	972.7	E858.3	E942.7	E950.4	E962.0	E980.4
Antivenin (crotaline) (spiderbite)	979.9	E858.8	E949.9	E950.4	E962.0	E980.4
Antivert	963.0	E858.1	E933.0	E950.4	E962.0	E980.4
Antivirals NEC	961.7	E857	E931.7	E950.4	E962.0	E980.4
Ant poisons — see Pesticides						
Antrol	989.4	E863.4	—	E950.6	E962.1	E980.7
fungicide	989.4	E863.6	—	E950.6	E962.1	E980.7
Apomorphine hydrochloride (emetic)	973.6	E858.4	E943.6	E950.4	E962.0	E980.4
Appetite depressants, central	977.0	E858.8	E947.0	E950.4	E962.0	E980.4
Apresoline	972.6	E858.3	E942.6	E950.4	E962.0	E980.4
Aprobarbital, aprobarbitone	967.0	E851	E937.0	E950.1	E962.0	E980.1
Apronalide	967.8	E852.8	E937.8	E950.2	E962.0	E980.2
Aqua fortis	983.1	E864.1	—	E950.7	E962.1	E980.6
Arachis oil (topical)	976.3	E858.7	E946.3	E950.4	E962.0	E980.4
cathartic	973.2	E858.4	E943.2	E950.4	E962.0	E980.4
Aralen	961.4	E857	E931.4	E950.4	E962.0	E980.4
Arginine salts	974.5	E858.5	E944.5	E950.4	E962.0	E980.4
Argyrol	976.0	E858.7	E946.0	E950.4	E962.0	E980.4
ENT agent	976.6	E858.7	E946.6	E950.4	E962.0	E980.4
ophthalmic preparation	976.5	E858.7	E946.5	E950.4	E962.0	E980.4
Aristocort	962.0	E858.0	E932.0	E950.4	E962.0	E980.4
ENT agent	976.6	E858.7	E946.6	E950.4	E962.0	E980.4
ophthalmic preparation	976.5	E858.7	E946.5	E950.4	E962.0	E980.4
topical NEC	976.0	E858.7	E946.0	E950.4	E962.0	E980.4

Nontherapeutic use substance

▼ Subterms under main terms may continue to next column or page

	Poisoning	Accident	Therapeutic Use	Suicide Attempt	Assault	Undetermined
Aromatics, corrosive	983.0	E864.0	—	E950.7	E962.1	E980.6
disinfectants	983.0	E861.4	—	E950.7	E962.1	E980.6
Arsenate of lead (insecticide)	985.1	E863.4	—	E950.8	E962.1	E980.8
herbicide	985.1	E863.5	—	E950.8	E962.1	E980.8
Arsenic, arsenicals (compounds) (dust) (fumes) (vapor) NEC	985.1	E866.3	—	E950.8	E962.1	E980.8
anti-infectives	961.1	E857	E931.1	E950.4	E962.0	E980.4
pesticide (dust) (fumes)	985.1	E863.4	—	E950.8	E962.1	E980.8
Arsine (gas)	985.1	E866.3	—	E950.8	E962.1	E980.8
Arsphenamine (silver)	961.1	E857	E931.1	E950.4	E962.0	E980.4
Arsthinol	961.1	E857	E931.1	E950.4	E962.0	E980.4
Artane	971.1	E855.4	E941.1	E950.4	E962.0	E980.4
Arthropod (venomous) NEC	989.5	E905.5		E950.9	E962.1	E980.9
Asbestos	989.81	E866.8	—	E950.9	E962.1	E980.9
Ascaridole	961.6	E857	E931.6	E950.4	E962.0	E980.4
Ascorbic acid	963.5	E858.1	E933.5	E950.4	E962.0	E980.4
Asiaticoside	976.0	E858.7	E946.0	E950.4	E962.0	E980.4
Aspldlum (oleoresin)	961.6	E857	E931.6	E950.4	E962.0	E980.4
Aspirin	965.1	E850.3	E935.3	E950.0	E962.0	E980.0
Astringents (local)	976.2	E858.7	E946.2	E950.4	E962.0	E980.4
Atabrine	961.3	E857	E931.3	E950.4	E962.0	E980.4
Ataractics	969.5	E853.8	E939.5	E950.3	E962.0	E980.3
Atonia drug, intestinal	973.3	E858.4	E943.3	E950.4	E962.0	E980.4
Atophan	974.7	E858.5	E944.7	E950.4	E962.0	E980.4
Atropine	971.1	E855.4	E941.1	E950.4	E962.0	E980.4
Attapulgite	973.5	E858.4	E943.5	E950.4	E962.0	E980.4
Attenuvax	979.4	E858.8	E949.4	E950.4	E962.0	E980.4
Aureomycin	960.4	E856	E930.4	E950.4	E962.0	E980.4
ophthalmic preparation	976.5	E858.7	E946.5	E950.4	E962.0	E980.4
topical NEC	976.0	E858.7	E946.0	E950.4	E962.0	E980.4
Aurothioglucose	965.69	E850.6	E935.6	E950.0	E962.0	E980.0
Aurothioglycanide	965.69	E850.6	E935.6	E950.0	E962.0	E980.0
Aurothiomalate	965.69	E850.6	E935.6	E950.0	E962.0	E980.0
Automobile fuel	981	E862.1	—	E950.9	E962.1	E980.9
Autonomic nervous system agents NEC	971.9	E855.9	E941.9	E950.4	E962.0	E980.4
Avlosulfon	961.8	E857	E931.8	E950.4	E962.0	E980.4
Avomine	967.8	E852.8	E937.8	E950.2	E962.0	E980.2
Azacyclonol	969.5	E853.8	E939.5	E950.3	E962.0	E980.3
Azapetine	971.3	E855.6	E941.3	E950.4	E962.0	E980.4
Azaribine	963.1	E858.1	E933.1	E950.4	E962.0	E980.4
Azaserine	960.7	E856	E930.7	E950.4	E962.0	E980.4
Azathioprine	963.1	E858.1	E933.1	E950.4	E962.0	E980.4
Azosulfamide	961.0	E857	E931.0	E950.4	E962.0	E980.4
Azulfidine	961.0	E857	E931.0	E950.4	E962.0	E980.4
Azuresin	977.8	E858.8	E947.8	E950.4	E962.0	E980.4
Bacimycin	976.0	E858.7	E946.0	E950.4	E962.0	E980.4
ophthalmic preparation	976.5	E858.7	E946.5	E950.4	E962.0	E980.4
Bacitracin	960.8	E856	E930.8	E950.4	E962.0	E980.4
ENT agent	976.6	E858.7	E946.6	E950.4	E962.0	E980.4
ophthalmic preparation	976.5	E858.7	E946.5	E950.4	E962.0	E980.4
topical NEC	976.0	E858.7	E946.0	E950.4	E962.0	E980.4
Baking soda	963.3	E858.1	E933.3	E950.4	E962.0	E980.4
BAL	963.8	E858.1	E933.8	E950.4	E962.0	E980.4
Bamethan (sulfate)	972.5	E858.3	E942.5	E950.4	E962.0	E980.4
Bamipine	963.0	E858.1	E933.0	E950.4	E962.0	E980.4
Baneberry	988.2	E865.4	—	E950.9	E962.1	E980.9
Banewort	988.2	E865.4	—	E950.9	E962.1	E980.9
Barbenyl	967.0	E851	E937.0	E950.1	E962.0	E980.1
Barbital, barbitone	967.0	E851	E937.0	E950.1	E962.0	E980.1
Barbiturates, barbituric acid	967.0	E851	E937.0	E950.1	E962.0	E980.1
anesthetic (intravenous)	968.3	E855.1	E938.3	E950.4	E962.0	E980.4
Barium (carbonate) (chloride) (sulfate)	985.8	E866.4	—	E950.9	E962.1	E980.9
diagnostic agent	977.8	E858.8	E947.8	E950.4	E962.0	E980.4
pesticide	985.8	E863.4	—	E950.6	E962.1	E980.7
rodenticide	985.8	E863.7	—	E950.6	E962.1	E980.7
Barrier cream	976.3	E858.7	E946.3	E950.4	E962.0	E980.4
Battery acid or fluid	983.1	E864.1	—	E950.7	E962.1	E980.6
Bay rum	980.8	E860.8	—	E950.9	E962.1	E980.9
BCG vaccine	978.0	E858.8	E948.0	E950.4	E962.0	E980.4
Bearsfoot	988.2	E865.4	—	E950.9	E962.1	E980.9
Beclamide	966.3	E855.0	E936.3	E950.4	E962.0	E980.4
Bee (sting) (venom)	989.5	E905.3	—	E950.9	E962.1	E980.9
Belladonna (alkaloids)	971.1	E855.4	E941.1	E950.4	E962.0	E980.4
Bemegride	970.0	E854.3	E940.0	E950.4	E962.0	E980.4
Benactyzine	969.8	E855.8	E939.8	E950.3	E962.0	E980.3
Benadryl	963.0	E858.1	E933.0	E950.4	E962.0	E980.4
Bendrofluazide	974.3	E858.5	E944.3	E950.4	E962.0	E980.4
Bendroflumethiazide	974.3	E858.5	E944.3	E950.4	E962.0	E980.4
Benemid	974.7	E858.5	E944.7	E950.4	E962.0	E980.4
Benethamine penicillin G	960.0	E856	E930.0	E950.4	E962.0	E980.4
Benisone	976.0	E858.7	E946.0	E950.4	E962.0	E980.4
Benoquin	976.8	E858.7	E946.8	E950.4	E962.0	E980.4
Benoxinate	968.5	E855.2	E938.5	E950.4	E962.0	E980.4
Bentonite	976.3	E858.7	E946.3	E950.4	E962.0	E980.4
Benzalkonium (chloride)	976.0	E858.7	E946.0	E950.4	E962.0	E980.4
ophthalmic preparation	976.5	E858.7	E946.5	E950.4	E962.0	E980.4
Benzamidosalicylate (calcium)	961.8	E857	E931.8	E950.4	E962.0	E980.4
Benzathine penicillin	960.0	E856	E930.0	E950.4	E962.0	E980.4
Benzcarbimine	963.1	E858.1	E933.1	E950.4	E962.0	E980.4
Benzedrex	971.2	E855.5	E941.2	E950.4	E962.0	E980.4
Benzedrine (amphetamine)	969.72	E854.2	E939.7	E950.3	E962.0	E980.3
Benzene (acetyl) (dimethyl) (methyl) (solvent) (vapor)	982.0	E862.4	—	E950.9	E962.1	E980.9
hexachloride (gamma) (insecticide) (vapor)	989.2	E863.0	—	E950.6	E962.1	E980.7
Benzethonium	976.0	E858.7	E946.0	E950.4	E962.0	E980.4
Benzhexol (chloride)	966.4	E855.0	E936.4	E950.4	E962.0	E980.4
Benzilonium	971.1	E855.4	E941.1	E950.4	E962.0	E980.4
Benzin(e) — see Ligroin						
Benziodarone	972.4	E858.3	E942.4	E950.4	E962.0	E980.4
Benzocaine	968.5	E855.2	E938.5	E950.4	E962.0	E980.4
Benzodiapin	969.4	E853.2	E939.4	E950.3	E962.0	E980.3
Benzodiazepines (tranquilizers) NEC	969.4	E853.2	E939.4	E950.3	E962.0	E980.3
Benzoic acid (with salicylic acid) (anti-infective)	976.0	E858.7	E946.0	E950.4	E962.0	E980.4
Benzoin	976.3	E858.7	E946.3	E950.4	E962.0	E980.4
Benzol (vapor)	982.0	E862.4	—	E950.9	E962.1	E980.9
Benzomorphan	965.09	E850.2	E935.2	E950.0	E962.0	E980.0
Benzonatate	975.4	E858.6	E945.4	E950.4	E962.0	E980.4
Benzothiadiazides	974.3	E858.5	E944.3	E950.4	E962.0	E980.4
Benzoylpas	961.8	E857	E931.8	E950.4	E962.0	E980.4
Benzperidol	969.5	E853.8	E939.5	E950.3	E962.0	E980.3
Benzphetamine	977.0	E858.8	E947.0	E950.4	E962.0	E980.4
Benzpyrinium	971.0	E855.3	E941.0	E950.4	E962.0	E980.4
Benzquinamide	963.0	E858.1	E933.0	E950.4	E962.0	E980.4
Benzthiazide	974.3	E858.5	E944.3	E950.4	E962.0	E980.4
Benztropine	971.1	E855.4	E941.1	E950.4	E962.0	E980.4
Benzyl						
acetate	982.8	E862.4	—	E950.9	E962.1	E980.9
benzoate (anti-infective)	976.0	E858.7	E946.0	E950.4	E962.0	E980.4
morphine	965.09	E850.2	E935.2	E950.0	E962.0	E980.0
penicillin	960.0	E856	E930.0	E950.4	E962.0	E980.4
Bephenium hydroxynapthoate	961.6	E857	E931.6	E950.4	E962.0	E980.4
Bergamot oil	989.89	E866.8	—	E950.9	E962.1	E980.9
Berries, poisonous	988.2	E865.3	—	E950.9	E962.1	E980.9
Beryllium (compounds) (fumes)	985.3	E866.4	—	E950.9	E962.1	E980.9
Beta-carotene	976.3	E858.7	E946.3	E950.4	E962.0	E980.4
Beta-Chlor	967.1	E852.0	E937.1	E950.2	E962.0	E980.2
Betamethasone	962.0	E858.0	E932.0	E950.4	E962.0	E980.4
topical	976.0	E858.7	E946.0	E950.4	E962.0	E980.4
Betazole	977.8	E858.8	F947.8	E950.4	E962.0	E980.4
Bethanechol	971.0	E855.3	E941.0	E950.4	E962.0	E980.4
Bethanidine	972.6	E858.3	E942.6	E950.4	E962.0	E980.4
Betula oil	976.3	E858.7	E946.3	E950.4	E962.0	E980.4
Bhang	969.6	E854.1	E939.6	E950.3	E962.0	E980.3
Bialamicol	961.5	E857	E931.5	E950.4	E962.0	E980.4
Bichloride of mercury — see Mercury, chloride						
Bichromates (calcium) (crystals) (potassium) (sodium)	983.9	E864.3	—	E950.7	E962.1	E980.6
fumes	987.8	E869.8	—	E952.8	E962.2	E982.8
Biguanide derivatives, oral	962.3	E858.0	E932.3	E950.4	E962.0	E980.4
Biligrafin	977.8	E858.8	E947.8	E950.4	E962.0	E980.4
Bilopaque	977.8	E858.8	E947.8	E950.4	E962.0	E980.4
Bioflavonoids	972.8	E858.3	E942.8	E950.4	E962.0	E980.4
Biological substance NEC	979.9	E858.8	E949.9	E950.4	E962.0	E980.4
Biperiden	966.4	E855.0	E936.4	E950.4	E962.0	E980.4
Bisacodyl	973.1	E858.4	E943.1	E950.4	E962.0	E980.4
Bishydroxycoumarin	964.2	E858.2	E934.2	E950.4	E962.0	E980.4

Nontherapeutic use substance

▽ Subterms under main terms may continue to next column or page

Bismarsen

Table of Drugs and Chemicals

Index

Bismarsen — Camphor

302 — Volume 2

2011 ICD-9-CM

	Poisoning	Accident	Therapeutic Use	Suicide Attempt	Assault	Undetermined
Bismarsen	961.1	E857	E931.1	E950.4	E962.0	E980.4
Bismuth (compounds)						
NEC	985.8	E866.4	—	E950.9	E962.1	E980.9
anti-infectives	961.2	E857	E931.2	E950.4	E962.0	E980.4
subcarbonate	973.5	E858.4	E943.5	E950.4	E962.0	E980.4
sulfarsphenamine	961.1	E857	E931.1	E950.4	E962.0	E980.4
Bisphosphonates						
intravenous	963.1	E858.1	E933.7	E950.4	E962.0	E980.4
oral	963.1	E858.1	E933.6	E950.4	E962.0	E980.4
Bithionol	961.6	E857	E931.6	E950.4	E962.0	E980.4
Bitter almond oil	989.0	E866.8	—	E950.9	E962.1	E980.9
Bittersweet	988.2	E865.4	—	E950.9	E962.1	E930.9
Black						
flag	989.4	E863.4	—	E950.6	E962.1	E980.7
henbane	988.2	E865.4	—	E950.9	E962.1	E980.9
leaf (40)	989.4	E863.4	—	E950.6	E962.1	E980.7
widow spider (bite)	989.5	E905.1	—	E950.9	E962.1	E980.9
antivenin	979.9	E858.8	E949.9	E950.4	E962.0	E980.4
Blast furnace gas (carbon monoxide from)	986	E868.8	—	E952.1	E962.2	E982.1
Bleach NEC	983.9	E864.3	—	E950.7	E962.1	E980.6
Bleaching solutions	983.9	E864.3	—	E950.7	E962.1	E980.6
Bleomycin (sulfate)	960.7	E856	E930.7	E950.4	E962.0	E980.4
Blockain	968.9	E855.2	E938.9	E950.4	E962.0	E980.4
infiltration (subcutaneous)	968.5	E855.2	E938.5	E950.4	E962.0	E980.4
nerve block (peripheral) (plexus)	968.6	E855.2	E938.6	E950.4	E962.0	E980.4
topical (surface)	968.5	E855.2	E938.5	E950.4	E962.0	E980.4
Blood (derivatives) (natural) (plasma) (whole)	964.7	E858.2	E934.7	E950.4	E962.0	E980.4
affecting agent	964.9	E858.2	E934.9	E950.4	E962.0	E980.4
specified NEC	964.8	E858.2	E934.8	E950.4	E962.0	E980.4
substitute (macromolecular)	964.8	E858.2	E934.8	E950.4	E962.0	E980.4
Blue velvet	965.09	E850.2	E935.2	E950.0	E962.0	E980.0
Bone meal	989.89	E866.5	—	E950.9	E962.1	E980.9
Bonine	963.0	E858.1	E933.0	E950.4	E962.0	E980.4
Boracic acid	976.0	E858.7	E946.0	E950.4	E962.0	E980.4
ENT agent	976.6	E858.7	E946.6	E950.4	E962.0	E980.4
ophthalmic preparation	976.5	E858.7	E946.5	E950.4	E962.0	E980.4
Borate (cleanser) (sodium)	989.6	E861.3	—	E950.9	E962.1	E980.9
Borax (cleanser)	989.6	E861.3	—	E950.9	E962.1	E980.9
Boric acid	976.0	E858.7	E946.0	E950.4	E962.0	E980.4
ENT agent	976.6	E858.7	E946.6	E950.4	E962.0	E980.4
ophthalmic preparation	976.5	E858.7	E946.5	E950.4	E962.0	E980.4
Boron hydride NEC	989.89	E866.8	—	E950.9	E962.1	E980.9
fumes or gas	987.8	E869.8	—	E952.8	E962.2	E982.8
Botox	975.3	E858.6	E945.3	E950.4	E962.0	E980.4
Brake fluid vapor	987.8	E869.8	—	E952.8	E962.2	E982.8
Brass (compounds) (fumes)	985.8	E866.4	—	E950.9	E962.1	E980.9
Brasso	981	E861.3	—	E950.9	E962.1	E980.9
Bretylium (tosylate)	972.6	E858.3	E942.6	E950.4	E962.0	E980.4
Brevital (sodium)	968.3	E855.1	E938.3	E950.4	E962.0	E980.4
British antilewisite	963.8	E858.1	E933.8	E950.4	E962.0	E980.4
Bromal (hydrate)	967.3	E852.2	E937.3	E950.2	E962.0	E980.2
Bromelains	963.4	E858.1	E933.4	E950.4	E962.0	E980.4
Bromides NEC	967.3	E852.2	E937.3	E950.2	E962.0	E980.2
Bromine (vapor)	987.8	E869.8	—	E952.8	E962.2	E982.8
compounds (medicinal)	967.3	E852.2	E937.3	E950.2	E962.0	E980.2
Bromisovalum	967.3	E852.2	E937.3	E950.2	E962.0	E980.2
Bromobenzyl cyanide	987.5	E869.3	—	E952.8	E962.2	E982.8
Bromodiphenhydramine	963.0	E858.1	E933.0	E950.4	E962.0	E980.4
Bromoform	967.3	E852.2	E937.3	E950.2	E962.0	E980.2
Bromophenol blue reagent	977.8	E858.8	E947.8		E962.0	E980.4
Bromosalicylhydroxamic acid	961.8	E857	E931.8	E950.4	E962.0	E980.4
Bromo-seltzer	965.4	E850.4	E935.4	E950.0	E962.0	E980.0
Brompheniramine	963.0	E858.1	E933.0	E950.4	E962.0	E980.4
Bromural	967.3	E852.2	E937.3	E950.2	E962.0	E980.2
Brown spider (bite) (venom)	989.5	E905.1	—	E950.9	E962.1	E980.9
Brucia	988.2	E865.3	—	E950.9	E962.1	E980.9
Brucine	989.1	E863.7	—	E950.6	E962.1	E980.7
Brunswick green — *see* Copper						
Bruten — *see* Ibuprofen						
Bryonia (alba) (dioica)	988.2	E865.4	—	E950.9	E962.1	E980.9
Buclizine	969.5	E853.8	E939.5	E950.3	E962.0	E980.3

	Poisoning	Accident	Therapeutic Use	Suicide Attempt	Assault	Undetermined
Bufferin	965.1	E850.3	E935.3	E950.0	E962.0	E980.0
Bufotenine	969.6	E854.1	E939.6	E950.3	E962.0	E980.3
Buphenine	971.2	E855.5	E941.2	E950.4	E962.0	E980.4
Bupivacaine	968.9	E855.2	E938.9	E950.4	E962.0	E980.4
infiltration (subcutaneous)	968.5	E855.2	E938.5	E950.4	E962.0	E980.4
nerve block (peripheral) (plexus)	968.6	E855.2	E938.6	E950.4	E962.0	E980.4
Busulfan	963.1	E858.1	E933.1	E950.4	E962.0	E980.4
Butabarbital (sodium)	967.0	E851	E937.0	E950.1	E962.0	E980.1
Butabarbitone	967.0	E851	E937.0	E950.1	E962.0	E980.1
Butabarpal	967.0	E851	E937.0	E950.1	E962.0	E980.1
Butacaine	968.5	E855.2	E938.5	E950.4	E962.0	E980.4
Butallylonal	967.0	E851	E937.0	E950.1	E962.0	E980.1
Butane (distributed in mobile container)	987.0	E868.0	—	E951.1	E962.2	E981.1
distributed through pipes	987.0	E867	—	E951.0	E962.2	E981.0
incomplete combustion of — see Carbon monoxide, butane						
Butanol	980.3	E860.4	—	E950.9	E962.1	E980.9
Butanone	982.8	E862.4	—	E950.9	E962.1	E980.9
Butaperazine	969.1	E853.0	E939.1	E950.3	E962.0	E980.3
Butazolidin	965.5	E850.5	E935.5	E950.0	E962.0	E980.0
Butethal	967.0	E851	E937.0	E950.1	E962.0	E980.1
Butethamate	971.1	E855.4	E941.1	E950.4	E962.0	E980.4
Buthalitone (sodium)	968.3	E855.1	E938.3	E950.4	E962.0	E980.4
Butisol (sodium)	967.0	E851	E937.0	E950.1	E962.0	E980.1
Butobarbital, butobarbitone	967.0	E851	E937.0	E950.1	E962.0	E980.1
Butriptyline	969.05	E854.0	E939.0	E950.3	E962.0	E980.3
Buttercups	988.2	E865.4	—	E950.9	E962.1	E980.9
Butter of antimony — *see* Antimony						
Butyl						
acetate (secondary)	982.8	E862.4	—	E950.9	E962.1	E980.9
alcohol	980.3	E860.4	—	E950.9	E962.1	E980.9
carbinol	980.8	E860.8	—	E950.9	E962.1	E980.9
carbitol	982.8	E862.4	—	E950.9	E962.1	E980.9
cellosolve	982.8	E862.4	—	E950.9	E962.1	E980.9
chloral (hydrate)	967.1	E852.0	E937.1	E950.2	E962.0	E980.2
formate	982.8	E862.4	—	E950.9	E962.1	E980.9
scopolammonium bromide	971.1	E855.4	E941.1	E950.4	E962.0	E980.4
Butyn	968.5	E855.2	E938.5	E950.4	E962.0	E980.4
Butyrophenone (-based tranquilizers)	969.2	E853.1	E939.2	E950.3	E962.0	E980.3
Cacodyl, cacodylic acid — *see* Arsenic						
Cactinomycin	960.7	E856	E930.7	E950.4	E962.0	E980.4
Cade oil	976.4	E858.7	E946.4	E950.4	E962.0	E980.4
Cadmium (chloride) (compounds) (dust) (fumes) (oxide)	985.5	E866.4	—	E950.9	E962.1	E980.9
sulfide (medicinal) NEC	976.4	E858.7	E946.4	E950.4	E962.0	E980.4
Caffeine	969.71	E854.2	E939.7	E950.3	E962.0	E980.3
Calabar bean	988.2	E865.4	—	E950.9	E962.1	E980.9
Caladium seguinium	988.2	E865.4	—	E950.9	E962.1	E980.9
Calamine (liniment) (lotion)	976.3	E858.7	E946.3	E950.4	E962.0	E980.4
Calciferol	963.5	E858.1	E933.5	E950.4	E962.0	E980.4
Calcium (salts) NEC	974.5	E858.5	E944.5	E950.4	E962.0	E980.4
acetylsalicylate	965.1	E850.3	E935.3	E950.0	E962.0	E980.0
benzamidosalicylate	961.8	E857	E931.8	E950.4	E962.0	E980.4
carbaspirin	965.1	E850.3	E935.3	E950.0	E962.0	E980.0
carbimide (citrated)	977.3	E858.8	E947.3	E950.4	E962.0	E980.4
carbonate (antacid)	973.0	E858.4	E943.0	E950.4	E962.0	E980.4
cyanide (citrated)	977.3	E858.8	E947.3	E950.4	E962.0	E980.4
dioctyl sulfosuccinate	973.2	E858.4	E943.2	E950.4	E962.0	E980.4
disodium edathamil	963.8	E858.1	E933.8	E950.4	E962.0	E980.4
disodium edetate	963.8	E858.1	E933.8	E950.4	E962.0	E980.4
EDTA	963.8	E858.1	E933.8	E950.4	E962.0	E980.4
hydrate, hydroxide	983.2	E864.2	—	E950.7	E962.1	E980.6
mandelate	961.9	E857	E931.9	E950.4	E962.0	E980.4
oxide	983.2	E864.2	—	E950.7	E962.1	E980.6
Calomel — *see* Mercury, chloride						
Caloric agents NEC	974.5	E858.5	E944.5	E950.4	E962.0	E980.4
Calusterone	963.1	E858.1	E933.1	E950.4	E962.0	E980.4
Camoquin	961.4	E857	E931.4	E950.4	E962.0	E980.4
Camphor (oil)	976.1	E858.7	E946.1	E950.4	E962.0	E980.4

Nontherapeutic use substance

Subterms under main terms may continue to next column or page

▶◀ Revised Text   ● New Line   ▲ Revised Code

	Poisoning	Accident	Therapeutic Use	Suicide Attempt	Assault	Undetermined
Candeptin	976.0	E858.7	E946.0	E950.4	E962.0	E980.4
Candicidin	976.0	E858.7	E946.0	E950.4	E962.0	E980.4
Cannabinols	969.6	E854.1	E939.6	E950.3	E962.0	E980.3
Cannabis (derivatives) (indica) (sativa)	969.6	E854.1	E939.6	E950.3	E962.0	E980.3
Canned heat	980.1	E860.2	—	E950.9	E962.1	E980.9
Cantharides, cantharidin, cantharis	976.8	E858.7	E946.8	E950.4	E962.0	E980.4
Capillary agents	972.8	E858.3	E942.8	E950.4	E962.0	E980.4
Capreomycin	960.6	E856	E930.6	E950.4	E962.0	E980.4
Captodiame, captodiamine	969.5	E853.8	E939.5	E950.3	E962.0	E980.3
Caramiphen (hydrochloride)	971.1	E855.4	E941.1	E950.4	E962.0	E980.4
Carbachol	971.0	E855.3	E941.0	E950.4	E962.0	E980.4
Carbacrylamine resins	974.5	E858.5	E944.5	E950.4	E962.0	E980.4
Carbamate (sedative)	967.8	E852.8	E937.8	E950.2	E962.0	E980.2
herbicide	989.3	E863.5	—	E950.6	E962.1	E980.7
insecticide	989.3	E863.2	—	E950.6	E962.1	E980.7
Carbamazepine	966.3	E855.0	E936.3	E950.4	E962.0	E980.4
Carbamic esters	967.8	E852.8	E937.8	E950.2	E962.0	E980.2
Carbamide	974.4	E858.5	E944.4	E950.4	E962.0	E980.4
topical	976.8	E858.7	E946.8	E950.4	E962.0	E980.4
Carbamylcholine chloride	971.0	E855.3	E941.0	E950.4	E962.0	E980.4
Carbarsone	961.1	E857	E931.1	E950.4	E962.0	E980.4
Carbaryl	989.3	E863.2	—	E950.6	E962.1	E980.7
Carbaspirin	965.1	E850.3	E935.3	E950.0	E962.0	E980.0
Carbazochrome	972.8	E858.3	E942.8	E950.4	E962.0	E980.4
Carbenicillin	960.0	E856	E930.0	E950.4	E962.0	E980.4
Carbenoxolone	973.8	E858.4	E943.8	E950.4	E962.0	E980.4
Carbetapentane	975.4	E858.6	E945.4	E950.4	E962.0	E980.4
Carbimazole	962.8	E858.0	E932.8	E950.4	E962.0	E980.4
Carbinol	980.1	E860.2	—	E950.9	E962.1	E980.9
Carbinoxamine	963.0	E858.1	E933.0	E950.4	E962.0	E980.4
Carbitol	982.8	E862.4	—	E950.9	E962.1	E980.9
Carbocaine	968.9	E855.2	E938.9	E950.4	E962.0	E980.4
infiltration (subcutaneous)	968.5	E855.2	E938.5	E950.4	E962.0	E980.4
nerve block (peripheral) (plexus)	968.6	E855.2	E938.6	E950.4	E962.0	E980.4
topical (surface)	968.5	E855.2	E938.5	E950.4	E962.0	E980.4
Carbol-fuchsin solution	976.0	E858.7	E946.0	E950.4	E962.0	E980.4
Carbolic acid — see also Phenol)	983.0	E864.0	—	E950.7	E962.1	E980.6
Carbomycin	960.8	E856	E930.8	E950.4	E962.0	E980.4
Carbon						
bisulfide (liquid) (vapor)	982.2	E862.4	—	E950.9	E962.1	E980.9
dioxide (gas)	987.8	E869.8	—	E952.8	E962.2	E982.8
disulfide (liquid) (vapor)	982.2	E862.4	—	E950.9	E962.1	E980.9
monoxide (from incomplete combustion of) (in)						
NEC	986	E868.9	—	E952.1	E962.2	E982.1
blast furnace gas	986	E868.8	—	E952.1	E962.2	E982.1
butane (distributed in mobile container)	986	E868.0	—	E951.1	E962.2	E981.1
distributed through pipes	986	E867	—	E951.0	E962.2	E981.0
charcoal fumes	986	E868.3	—	E952.1	E962.2	E982.1
coal						
gas (piped)	986	E867	—	E951.0	E962.2	E981.0
solid (in domestic stoves, fireplaces)	986	E868.3	—	E952.1	E962.2	E982.1
coke (in domestic stoves, fireplaces)	986	E868.3	—	E952.1	E962.2	E982.1
exhaust gas (motor) not in transit	986	E868.2	—	E952.0	E962.2	E982.0
combustion engine, any not in watercraft	986	E868.2	—	E952.0	E962.2	E982.0
farm tractor, not in transit	986	E868.2	—	E952.0	E962.2	E982.0
gas engine	986	E868.2	—	E952.0	E962.2	E982.0
motor pump	986	E868.2	—	E952.0	E962.2	E982.0
motor vehicle, not in transit	986	E868.2	—	E952.0	E962.2	E982.0
fuel (in domestic use)	986	E868.3	—	E952.1	E962.2	E982.1
gas (piped)	986	E867	—	E951.0	E962.2	E981.0
in mobile container	986	E868.0	—	E951.1	E962.2	E981.1
utility	986	E868.1	—	E951.8	E962.2	E981.1
in mobile container	986	E868.0	—	E951.1	E962.2	E981.1
piped (natural)	986	E867	—	E951.0	E962.2	E981.0
illuminating gas	986	E868.1	—	E951.8	E962.2	E981.8

	Poisoning	Accident	Therapeutic Use	Suicide Attempt	Assault	Undetermined
Carbon — continued						
monoxide — continued						
industrial fuels or gases, any	986	E868.8	—	E952.1	E962.2	E982.1
kerosene (in domestic stoves, fireplaces)	986	E868.3	—	E952.1	E962.2	E982.1
kiln gas or vapor	986	E868.8	—	E952.1	E962.2	E982.1
motor exhaust gas, not in transit	986	E868.2	—	E952.0	E962.2	E982.0
piped gas (manufactured) (natural)	986	E867	—	E951.0	E962.2	E981.0
producer gas	986	E868.8	—	E952.1	E962.2	E982.1
propane (distributed in mobile container)	986	E868.0	—	E951.1	E962.2	E981.1
distributed through pipes	986	E867	—	E951.0	E962.2	E981.0
specified source NEC	986	E868.8	—	E952.1	E962.2	E982.1
stove gas	986	E868.1	—	E951.8	E962.2	E981.8
piped	986	E867	—	E951.0	E962.2	E981.0
utility gas	986	E868.1	—	E951.8	E962.2	E981.8
piped	986	E867	—	E951.0	E962.2	E981.0
water gas	986	E868.1	—	E951.8	E962.2	E981.8
wood (in domestic stoves, fireplaces)	986	E868.3	—	E952.1	E962.2	E982.1
tetrachloride (vapor) NEC	987.8	E869.8	—	E952.8	E962.2	E982.8
liquid (cleansing agent)						
NEC	982.1	E861.3	—	E950.9	E962.1	E980.9
solvent	982.1	E862.4	—	E950.9	E962.1	E980.9
Carbonic acid (gas)	987.8	E869.8	—	E952.8	E962.2	E982.8
anhydrase inhibitors	974.2	E858.5	E944.2	E950.4	E962.0	E980.4
Carbowax	976.3	E858.7	E946.3	E950.4	E962.0	E980.4
Carbrital	967.0	E851	E937.0	E950.1	E962.0	E980.1
Carbromal (derivatives)	967.3	E852.2	E937.3	E950.2	E962.0	E980.2
Cardiac						
depressants	972.0	E858.3	E942.0	E950.4	E962.0	E980.4
rhythm regulators	972.0	E858.3	E942.0	E950.4	E962.0	E980.4
Cardiografin	977.8	E858.8	E947.8	E950.4	E962.0	E980.4
Cardio-green	977.8	E858.8	E947.8	E950.4	E962.0	E980.4
Cardiotonic glycosides	972.1	E858.3	E942.1	E950.4	E962.0	E980.4
Cardiovascular agents						
NEC	972.9	E858.3	E942.9	E950.4	E962.0	E980.4
Cardrase	974.2	E858.5	E944.2	E950.4	E962.0	E980.4
Carfusin	976.0	E858.7	E946.0	E950.4	E962.0	E980.4
Carisoprodol	968.0	E855.1	E938.0	E950.4	E962.0	E980.4
Carmustine	963.1	E858.1	E933.1	E950.4	E962.0	E980.4
Carotene	963.5	E858.1	E933.5	E950.4	E962.0	E980.4
Carphenazine (maleate)	969.1	E853.0	E939.1	E950.3	E962.0	E980.3
Carter's Little Pills	973.1	E858.4	E943.1	E950.4	E962.0	E980.4
Cascara (sagrada)	973.1	E858.4	E943.1	E950.4	E962.0	E980.4
Cassava	988.2	E865.4	—	E950.9	E962.1	E980.9
Castellani's paint	976.0	E858.7	E946.0	E950.4	E962.0	E980.4
Castor						
bean	988.2	E865.3	—	E950.9	E962.1	E980.9
oil	973.1	E858.4	E943.1	E950.4	E962.0	E980.4
Caterpillar (sting)	989.5	E905.5	—	E950.9	E962.1	E980.9
Catha (edulis)	970.89 ▲	E854.3	E940.8	E950.4	E962.0	E980.4
Cathartics NEC	973.3	E858.4	E943.3	E950.4	E962.0	E980.4
contact	973.1	E858.4	E943.1	E950.4	E962.0	E980.4
emollient	973.2	E858.4	E943.2	E950.4	E962.0	E980.4
intestinal irritants	973.1	E858.4	E943.1	E950.4	E962.0	E980.4
saline	973.3	E858.4	E943.3	E950.4	E962.0	E980.4
Cathomycin	960.8	E856	E930.8	E950.4	E962.0	E980.4
Caustic(s)	983.9	E864.4	—	E950.7	E962.1	E980.6
alkali	983.2	E864.2	—	E950.7	E962.1	E980.6
hydroxide	983.2	E864.2	—	E950.7	E962.1	E980.6
potash	983.2	E864.2	—	E950.7	E962.1	E980.6
soda	983.2	E864.2	—	E950.7	E962.1	E980.6
specified NEC	983.9	E864.3	—	E950.7	E962.1	E980.6
Ceepryn	976.0	E858.7	E946.0	E950.4	E962.0	E980.4
ENT agent	976.6	E858.7	E946.6	E950.4	E962.0	E980.4
lozenges	976.6	E858.7	E946.6	E950.4	E962.0	E980.4
Celestone	962.0	E858.0	E932.0	E950.4	E962.0	E980.4
topical	976.0	E858.7	E946.0	E950.4	E962.0	E980.4
Cellosolve	982.8	E862.4	—	E950.9	E962.1	E980.9
Cell stimulants and proliferants	976.8	E858.7	E946.8	E950.4	E962.0	E980.4
Cellulose derivatives, cathartic	973.3	E858.4	E943.3	E950.4	E962.0	E980.4
nitrates (topical)	976.3	E858.7	E946.3	E950.4	E962.0	E980.4
Centipede (bite)	989.5	E905.4	—	E950.9	E962.1	E980.9
Central nervous system						
depressants	968.4	E855.1	E938.4	E950.4	E962.0	E980.4

Central nervous system — continued	Poisoning	Accident	Therapeutic Use	Suicide Attempt	Assault	Undetermined
depressants — continued						
anesthetic (general)						
NEC	968.4	E855.1	E938.4	E950.4	E962.0	E980.4
gases NEC	968.2	E855.1	E938.2	E950.4	E962.0	E980.4
intravenous	968.3	E855.1	E938.3	E950.4	E962.0	E980.4
barbiturates	967.0	E851	E937.0	E950.1	E962.0	E980.1
bromides	967.3	E852.2	E937.3	E950.2	E962.0	E980.2
cannabis sativa	969.6	E854.1	E939.6	E950.3	E962.0	E980.3
chloral hydrate	967.1	E852.0	E937.1	E950.2	E962.0	E980.2
hallucinogenics	969.6	E854.1	E939.6	E950.3	E962.0	E980.3
hypnotics	967.9	E852.9	E937.9	E950.2	E962.0	E980.2
specified NEC	967.8	E852.8	E937.8	E950.2	E962.0	E980.2
muscle relaxants	968.0	E855.1	E938.0	E950.4	E962.0	E980.4
paraldehyde	967.2	E852.1	E937.2	E950.2	E962.0	E980.2
sedatives	967.9	E852.9	E937.9	E950.2	E962.0	E980.2
mixed NEC	967.6	E852.5	E937.6	E950.2	E962.0	E980.2
specified NEC	967.8	E852.8	E937.8	E950.2	E962.0	E980.2
muscle-tone depressants	—	—	—	—	—	E980.4
stimulants	970.9	E854.3	E940.9	E950.4	E962.0	E980.4
amphetamines	969.72	E854.2	E939.7	E950.3	E962.0	E980.3
analeptics	970.0	E854.3	E940.0	E950.4	E962.0	E980.4
antidepressants	969.00	E854.0	E939.0	E950.3	E962.0	E980.3
opiate antagonists	970.1	E854.3	E940.1	E950.4	E962.0	E980.4
specified NEC	970.89▲	E854.3	E940.8	E950.4	E962.0	E980.4
Cephalexin	960.5	E856	E930.5	E950.4	E962.0	E980.4
Cephaloglycin	960.5	E856	E930.5	E950.4	E962.0	E980.4
Cephaloridine	960.5	E856	E930.5	E950.4	E962.0	E980.4
Cephalosporins NEC	960.5	E856	E930.5	E950.4	E962.0	E980.4
N (adicillin)	960.0	E856	E930.0	E950.4	E962.0	E980.4
Cephalothin (sodium)	960.5	E856	E930.5	E950.4	E962.0	E980.4
Cerbera (odallam)	988.2	E865.4	—	E950.9	E962.1	E980.9
Cerberin	972.1	E858.3	E942.1	E950.4	E962.0	E980.4
Cerebral stimulants	970.9	E854.3	E940.9	E950.4	E962.0	E980.4
psychotherapeutic	969.79	E854.2	E939.7	E950.3	E962.0	E980.3
specified NEC	970.89▲	E854.3	E940.8	E950.4	E962.0	E980.4
Cetalkonium (chloride)	976.0	E858.7	E946.0	E950.4	E962.0	E980.4
Cetoxime	963.0	E858.1	E933.0	E950.4	E962.0	E980.4
Cetrimide	976.2	E858.7	E946.2	E950.4	E962.0	E980.4
Cetylpyridinium	976.0	E858.7	E946.0	E950.4	E962.0	E980.4
ENT agent	976.6	E858.7	E946.6	E950.4	E962.0	E980.4
lozenges	976.6	E858.7	E946.6	E950.4	E962.0	E980.4
Cevadilla — see Sabadilla						
Cevitamic acid	963.5	E858.1	E933.5	E950.4	E962.0	E980.4
Chalk, precipitated	973.0	E858.4	E943.0	E950.4	E962.0	E980.4
Charcoal						
fumes (carbon monoxide)	986	E868.3	—	E952.1	E962.2	E982.1
industrial	986	E868.8	—	E952.1	E962.2	E982.1
medicinal (activated)	973.0	E858.4	E943.0	E950.4	E962.0	E980.4
Chelating agents NEC	977.2	E858.8	E947.2	E950.4	E962.0	E980.4
Chelidonium majus	988.2	E865.4	—	E950.9	E962.1	E980.9
Chemical substance	989.9	E866.9	—	E950.9	E962.1	E980.9
specified NEC	989.89	E866.8	—	E950.9	E962.1	E980.9
Chemotherapy, antineoplastic	963.1	E858.1	E933.1	E950.4	E962.0	E980.4
Chenopodium (oil)	961.6	E857	E931.6	E950.4	E962.0	E980.4
Cherry laurel	988.2	E865.4	—	E950.9	E962.1	E980.9
Chiniofon	961.3	E857	E931.3	E950.4	E962.0	E980.4
Chlophedianol	975.4	E858.6	E945.4	E950.4	E962.0	E980.4
Chloral (betaine) (formamide) (hydrate)	967.1	E852.0	E937.1	E950.2	E962.0	E980.2
Chloralamide	967.1	E852.0	E937.1	E950.2	E962.0	E980.2
Chlorambucil	963.1	E858.1	E933.1	E950.4	E962.0	E980.4
Chloramphenicol	960.2	E856	E930.2	E950.4	E962.0	E980.4
ENT agent	976.6	E858.7	E946.6	E950.4	E962.0	E980.4
ophthalmic preparation	976.5	E858.7	E946.5	E950.4	E962.0	E980.4
topical NEC	976.0	E858.7	E946.0	E950.4	E962.0	E980.4
Chlorate(s) (potassium) (sodium) NEC	983.9	E864.3	—	E950.7	E962.1	E980.6
herbicides	989.4	E863.5	—	E950.6	E962.1	E980.7
Chlorcyclizine	963.0	E858.1	E933.0	E950.4	E962.0	E980.4
Chlordan(e) (dust)	989.2	E863.0	—	E950.6	E962.1	E980.7
Chlordantoin	976.0	E858.7	E946.0	E950.4	E962.0	E980.4
Chlordiazepoxide	969.4	E853.2	E939.4	E950.3	E962.0	E980.3
Chloresium	976.8	E858.7	E946.8	E950.4	E962.0	E980.4
Chlorethiazol	967.1	E852.0	E937.1	E950.2	E962.0	E980.2
Chlorethyl — see Ethyl, chloride						
Chloretone	967.1	E852.0	E937.1	E950.2	E962.0	E980.2
Chlorex	982.3	E862.4	—	E950.9	E962.1	E980.9

	Poisoning	Accident	Therapeutic Use	Suicide Attempt	Assault	Undetermined
Chlorhexadol	967.1	E852.0	E937.1	E950.2	E962.0	E980.2
Chlorhexidine (hydrochloride)	976.0	E858.7	E946.0	E950.4	E962.0	E980.4
Chlorhydroxyquinolin	976.0	E858.7	E946.0	E950.4	E962.0	E980.4
Chloride of lime (bleach)	983.9	E864.3	—	E950.7	E962.1	E980.6
Chlorinated						
camphene	989.2	E863.0	—	E950.6	E962.1	E980.7
diphenyl	989.89	E866.8	—	E950.9	E962.1	E980.9
hydrocarbons NEC	989.2	E863.0	—	E950.6	E962.1	E980.7
solvent	982.3	E862.4	—	E950.9	E962.1	E980.9
lime (bleach)	983.9	E864.3	—	E950.7	E962.1	E980.6
naphthalene — see Naphthalene						
pesticides NEC	989.2	E863.0	—	E950.6	E962.1	E980.7
soda — see Sodium, hypochlorite						
Chlorine (fumes) (gas)	987.6	E869.8	—	E952.8	E962.2	E982.8
bleach	983.9	E864.3	—	E950.7	E962.1	E980.6
compounds NEC	983.9	E864.3	—	E950.7	E962.1	E980.6
disinfectant	983.9	E861.4	—	E950.7	E962.1	E980.6
releasing agents NEC	983.9	E864.3	—	E950.7	E962.1	E980.6
Chlorisondamine	972.3	E858.3	E942.3	E950.4	E962.0	E980.4
Chlormadinone	962.2	E858.0	E932.2	E950.4	E962.0	E980.4
Chlormerodrin	974.0	E858.5	E944.0	E950.4	E962.0	E980.4
Chlormethiazole	967.1	E852.0	E937.1	E950.2	E962.0	E980.2
Chlormethylenecycline	960.4	E856	E930.4	E950.4	E962.0	E980.4
Chlormezanone	969.5	E853.8	E939.5	E950.3	E962.0	E980.3
Chloroacetophenone	987.5	E869.3	—	E952.8	E962.2	E982.8
Chloroaniline	983.0	E864.0	—	E950.7	E962.1	E980.6
Chlorobenzene, chlorobenzol	982.0	E862.4	—	E950.9	E962.1	E980.9
Chlorobutanol	967.1	E852.0	E937.1	E950.2	E962.0	E980.2
Chlorodinitrobenzene	983.0	E864.0	—	E950.7	E962.1	E980.6
dust or vapor	987.8	E869.8	—	E952.8	E962.2	E982.8
Chloroethane — see Ethyl, chloride						
Chloroform (fumes) (vapor)	987.8	E869.8	—	E952.8	E962.2	E982.8
anesthetic (gas)	968.2	E855.1	E938.2	E950.4	E962.0	E980.4
liquid NEC	968.4	E855.1	E938.4	E950.4	E962.0	E980.4
solvent	982.3	E862.4	—	E950.9	E962.1	E980.9
Chloroguanide	961.4	E857	E931.4	E950.4	E962.0	E980.4
Chloromycetin	960.2	E856	E930.2	E950.4	E962.0	E980.4
ENT agent	976.6	E858.7	E946.6	E950.4	E962.0	E980.4
ophthalmic preparation	976.5	E858.7	E946.5	E950.4	E962.0	E980.4
otic solution	976.6	E858.7	E946.6	E950.4	E962.0	E980.4
topical NEC	976.0	E858.7	E946.0	E950.4	E962.0	E980.4
Chloronitrobenzene	983.0	E864.0	—	E950.7	E962.1	E980.6
dust or vapor	987.8	E869.8	—	E952.8	E962.2	E982.8
Chlorophenol	983.0	E864.0	—	E950.7	E962.1	E980.6
Chlorophenothane	989.2	E863.0	—	E950.6	E962.1	E980.7
Chlorophyll (derivatives)	976.8	E858.7	E946.8	E950.4	E962.0	E980.4
Chloropicrin (fumes)	987.8	E869.8	—	E952.8	E962.2	E982.8
fumigant	989.4	E863.8	—	E950.6	E962.1	E980.7
fungicide	989.4	E863.6	—	E950.6	E962.1	E980.7
pesticide (fumes)	989.4	E863.4	—	E950.6	E962.1	E980.7
Chloroprocaine	968.9	E855.2	E938.9	E950.4	E962.0	E980.4
infiltration (subcutaneous)	968.5	E855.2	E938.5	E950.4	E962.0	E980.4
nerve block (peripheral) (plexus)	968.6	E855.2	E938.6	E950.4	E962.0	E980.4
Chloroptic	976.5	E858.7	E946.5	E950.4	E962.0	E980.4
Chloropurine	963.1	E858.1	E933.1	E950.4	E962.0	E980.4
Chloroquine (hydrochloride) (phosphate)	961.4	E857	E931.4	E950.4	E962.0	E980.4
Chlorothen	963.0	E858.1	E933.0	E950.4	E962.0	E980.4
Chlorothiazide	974.3	E858.5	E944.3	E950.4	E962.0	E980.4
Chlorotrianisene	962.2	E858.0	E932.2	E950.4	E962.0	E980.4
Chlorovinyldichloroarsine	985.1	E866.3	—	E950.8	E962.1	E980.8
Chloroxylenol	976.0	E858.7	E946.0	E950.4	E962.0	E980.4
Chlorphenesin (carbamate)	968.0	E855.1	E938.0	E950.4	E962.0	E980.4
topical (antifungal)	976.0	E858.7	E946.0	E950.4	E962.0	E980.4
Chlorpheniramine	963.0	E858.1	E933.0	E950.4	E962.0	E980.4
Chlorphenoxamine	966.4	E855.0	E936.4	E950.4	E962.0	E980.4
Chlorphentermine	977.0	E858.8	E947.0	E950.4	E962.0	E980.4
Chlorproguanil	961.4	E857	E931.4	E950.4	E962.0	E980.4
Chlorpromazine	969.1	E853.0	E939.1	E950.3	E962.0	E980.3
Chlorpropamide	962.3	E858.0	E932.3	E950.4	E962.0	E980.4
Chlorprothixene	969.3	E853.8	E939.3	E950.3	E962.0	E980.3
Chlorquinaldol	976.0	E858.7	E946.0	E950.4	E962.0	E980.4

Nontherapeutic use substance

⬇ Subterms under main terms may continue to next column or page

	Poisoning	Accident	Therapeutic Use	Suicide Attempt	Assault	Undetermined
External Cause (E-Code)						
Chlortetracycline	960.4	E856	E930.4	E950.4	E962.0	E980.4
Chlorthalidone	974.4	E858.5	E944.4	E950.4	E962.0	E980.4
Chlortrianisene	962.2	E858.0	E932.2	E950.4	E962.0	E980.4
Chlor-Trimeton	963.0	E858.1	E933.0	E950.4	E962.0	E980.4
Chlorzoxazone	968.0	E855.1	E938.0	E950.4	E962.0	E980.4
Choke damp	987.8	E869.8	—	E952.8	E962.2	E982.8
Cholebrine	977.8	E858.8	E947.8	E950.4	E962.0	E980.4
Cholera vaccine	978.2	E858.8	E948.2	E950.4	E962.0	E980.4
Cholesterol-lowering agents	972.2	E858.3	E942.2	E950.4	E962.0	E980.4
Cholestyramine (resin)	972.2	E858.3	E942.2	E950.4	E962.0	E980.4
Cholic acid	973.4	E858.4	E943.4	E950.4	E962.0	E980.4
Choline						
dihydrogen citrate	977.1	E858.8	E947.1	E950.4	E962.0	E980.4
salicylate	965.1	E850.3	E935.3	E950.0	E962.0	E980.0
theophyllinate	974.1	E858.5	E944.1	E950.4	E962.0	E980.4
Cholinergics	971.0	E855.3	E941.0	E950.4	E962.0	E980.4
Cholografin	977.8	E858.8	E947.8	E950.4	E962.0	E980.4
Chorionic gonadotropin	962.4	E858.0	E932.4	E950.4	E962.0	E980.4
Chromates	983.9	E864.3	—	E950.7	E962.1	E980.6
dust or mist	987.8	E869.8	—	E952.8	E962.2	E982.8
lead	984.0	E866.0	—	E950.9	E962.1	E980.9
paint	984.0	E861.5	—	E950.9	E962.1	E980.9
Chromic acid	983.9	E864.3	—	E950.7	E962.1	E980.6
dust or mist	987.8	E869.8	—	E952.8	E962.2	E982.8
Chromium	985.6	E866.4	—	E950.9	E962.1	E980.9
compounds — see Chromates						
Chromonar	972.4	E858.3	E942.4	E950.4	E962.0	E980.4
Chromyl chloride	983.9	E864.3	—	E950.7	E962.1	E980.6
Chrysarobin (ointment)	976.4	E858.7	E946.4	E950.4	E962.0	E980.4
Chrysazin	973.1	E858.4	E943.1	E950.4	E962.0	E980.4
Chymar	963.4	E858.1	E933.4	E950.4	E962.0	E980.4
ophthalmic preparation	976.5	E858.7	E946.5	E950.4	E962.0	E980.4
Chymotrypsin	963.4	E858.1	E933.4	E950.4	E962.0	E980.4
ophthalmic preparation	976.5	E858.7	E946.5	E950.4	E962.0	E980.4
Cicuta maculata or virosa	988.2	E865.4	—	E950.9	E962.1	E980.9
Cigarette lighter fluid	981	E862.1	—	E950.9	E962.1	E980.9
Cinchocaine (spinal)	968.7	E855.2	E938.7	E950.4	E962.0	E980.4
topical (surface)	968.5	E855.2	E938.5	E950.4	E962.0	E980.4
Cinchona	961.4	E857	E931.4	E950.4	E962.0	E980.4
Cinchonine alkaloids	961.4	E857	E931.4	E950.4	E962.0	E980.4
Cinchophen	974.7	E858.5	E944.7	E950.4	E962.0	E980.4
Cinnarizine	963.0	E858.1	E933.0	E950.4	E962.0	E980.4
Citanest	968.9	E855.2	E938.9	E950.4	E962.0	E980.4
infiltration (subcutaneous)	968.5	E855.2	E938.5	E950.4	E962.0	E980.4
nerve block (peripheral) (plexus)	968.6	E855.2	E938.6	E950.4	E962.0	E980.4
Citric acid	989.89	E866.8	—	E950.9	E962.1	E980.9
Citrovorum factor	964.1	E858.2	E934.1	E950.4	E962.0	E980.4
Claviceps purpurea	988.2	E865.4	—	E950.9	E962.1	E980.9
Cleaner, cleansing agent NEC	989.89	E861.3	—	E950.9	E962.1	E980.9
of paint or varnish	982.8	E862.9	—	E950.9	E962.1	E980.9
Clematis vitalba	988.2	E865.4	—	E950.9	E962.1	E980.9
Clemizole	963.0	E858.1	E933.0	E950.4	E962.0	E980.4
penicillin	960.0	E856	E930.0	E950.4	E962.0	E980.4
Clidinium	971.1	E855.4	E941.1	E950.4	E962.0	E980.4
Clindamycin	960.8	E856	E930.8	E950.4	E962.0	E980.4
Cliradon	965.09	E850.2	E935.2	E950.0	E962.0	E980.0
Clocortolone	962.0	E858.0	E932.0	E950.4	E962.0	E980.4
Clofedanol	975.4	E858.6	E945.4	E950.4	E962.0	E980.4
Clofibrate	972.2	E858.3	E942.2	E950.4	E962.0	E980.4
Clomethiazole	967.1	E852.0	E937.1	E950.2	E962.0	E980.2
Clomiphene	977.8	E858.8	E947.8	E950.4	E962.0	E980.4
Clonazepam	969.4	E853.2	E939.4	E950.3	E962.0	E980.3
Clonidine	972.6	E858.3	E942.6	E950.4	E962.0	E980.4
Clopamide	974.3	E858.5	E944.3	E950.4	E962.0	E980.4
Clorazepate	969.4	E853.2	E939.4	E950.3	E962.0	E980.3
Clorexolone	974.4	E858.5	E944.4	E950.4	E962.0	E980.4
Clorox (bleach)	983.9	E864.3	—	E950.7	E962.1	E980.6
Clortermine	977.0	E858.8	E947.0	E950.4	E962.0	E980.4
Clotrimazole	976.0	E858.7	E946.0	E950.4	E962.0	E980.4
Cloxacillin	960.0	E856	E930.0	E950.4	E962.0	E980.4
Coagulants NEC	964.5	E858.2	E934.5	E950.4	E962.0	E980.4
Coal (carbon monoxide from) — see also Carbon, monoxide, coal						
oil — see Kerosene						
tar NEC	983.0	E864.0	—	E950.7	E962.1	E980.6

	Poisoning	Accident	Therapeutic Use	Suicide Attempt	Assault	Undetermined
External Cause (E-Code)						
Coal — see also Carbon, monoxide, coal — continued						
tar — continued						
fumes	987.8	E869.8	—	E952.8	E962.2	E982.8
medicinal (ointment)	976.4	E858.7	E946.4	E950.4	E962.0	E980.4
analgesics NEC	965.5	E850.5	E935.5	E950.0	E962.0	E980.0
naphtha (solvent)	981	E862.0	—	E950.9	E962.1	E980.9
Cobalt (fumes) (industrial)	985.8	E866.4	—	E950.9	E962.1	E980.9
Cobra (venom)	989.5	E905.0	—	E950.9	E962.1	E980.9
Coca (leaf)	970.81 ▲	E854.3	E940.8	E950.4	E962.0	E980.4
Cocaine (hydrochloride) (salt)	970.81 ▲	E854.3	E940.8	E950.4	E962.0	E980.4
topical anesthetic	968.5	E855.2	E938.5	E950.4	E962.0	E980.4
Coccidioidin	977.8	E858.8	E947.8	E950.4	E962.0	E980.4
Cocculus indicus	988.2	E865.3	—	E950.9	E962.1	E980.9
Cochineal	989.89	E866.8	—	E950.9	E962.1	E980.9
medicinal products	977.4	E858.8	E947.4	E950.4	E962.0	E980.4
Codeine	965.09	E850.2	E935.2	E950.0	E962.0	E980.0
Coffee	989.89	E866.8	—	E950.9	E962.1	E980.9
Cogentin	971.1	E855.4	E941.1	E950.4	E962.0	E980.4
Coke fumes or gas (carbon monoxide)	986	E868.3	—	E952.1	E962.2	E982.1
industrial use	986	E868.8	—	E952.1	E962.2	E982.1
Colace	973.2	E858.4	E943.2	E950.4	E962.0	E980.4
Colchicine	974.7	E858.5	E944.7	E950.4	E962.0	E980.4
Colchicum	988.2	E865.3	—	E950.9	E962.1	E980.9
Cold cream	976.3	E858.7	E946.3	E950.4	E962.0	E980.4
Colestipol	972.2	E858.3	E942.2	E950.4	E962.0	E980.4
Colistimethate	960.8	E856	E930.8	E950.4	E962.0	E980.4
Colistin	960.8	E856	E930.8	E950.4	E962.0	E980.4
Collagen	977.8	E866.8	E947.8	E950.9	E962.1	E980.9
Collagenase	976.8	E858.7	E946.8	E950.4	E962.0	E980.4
Collodion (flexible)	976.3	E858.7	E946.3	E950.4	E962.0	E980.4
Colocynth	973.1	E858.4	E943.1	E950.4	E962.0	E980.4
Coloring matter — see Dye(s)						
Combustion gas — see Carbon, monoxide						
Compazine	969.1	E853.0	E939.1	E950.3	E962.0	E980.3
Compound						
42 (warfarin)	989.4	E863.7	—	E950.6	E962.1	E980.7
269 (endrin)	989.2	E863.0	—	E950.6	E962.1	E980.7
497 (dieldrin)	989.2	E863.0	—	E950.6	E962.1	E980.7
1080 (sodium fluoroacetate)	989.4	E863.7	—	E950.6	E962.1	E980.7
3422 (parathion)	989.3	E863.1	—	E950.6	E962.1	E980.7
3911 (phorate)	989.3	E863.1	—	E950.6	E962.1	E980.7
3956 (toxaphene)	989.2	E863.0	—	E950.6	E962.1	E980.7
4049 (malathion)	989.3	E863.1	—	E950.6	E962.1	E980.7
4124 (dicapthon)	989.4	E863.4	—	E950.6	E962.1	E980.7
E (cortisone)	962.0	E858.0	E932.0	E950.4	E962.0	E980.4
F (hydrocortisone)	962.0	E858.0	E932.0	E950.4	E962.0	E980.4
Congo red	977.8	E858.8	E947.8	E950.4	E962.0	E980.4
Coniine, conine	965.7	E850.7	E935.7	E950.0	E962.0	E980.0
Conium (maculatum)	988.2	E865.4	—	E950.9	E962.1	E980.9
Conjugated estrogens (equine)	962.2	E858.0	E932.2	E950.4	E962.0	E980.4
Contac	975.6	E858.6	E945.6	E950.4	E962.0	E980.4
Contact lens solution	976.5	E858.7	E946.5	E950.4	E962.0	E980.4
Contraceptives (oral)	962.2	E858.0	E932.2	E950.4	E962.0	E980.4
vaginal	976.8	E858.7	E946.8	E950.4	E962.0	E980.4
Contrast media (roentgenographic)	977.8	E858.8	E947.8	E950.4	E962.0	E980.4
Convallaria majalis	988.2	E865.4	—	E950.9	E962.1	E980.9
Copper (dust) (fumes) (salts) NEC	985.8	E866.4	—	E950.9	E962.1	E980.9
arsenate, arsenite	985.1	E866.3	—	E950.8	E962.1	E980.8
insecticide	985.1	E863.4	—	E950.6	E962.1	E980.7
emetic	973.6	E858.4	E943.6	E950.4	E962.0	E980.4
fungicide	985.8	E863.6	—	E950.6	E962.1	E980.7
insecticide	985.8	E863.4	—	E950.6	E962.1	E980.7
oleate	976.0	E858.7	E946.0	E950.4	E962.0	E980.4
sulfate	983.9	E864.3	—	E950.7	E962.1	E980.6
cupric	973.6	E858.4	E943.6	E950.4	E962.0	E980.4
cuprous	983.9	E864.3	—	E950.7	E962.1	E980.6
fungicide	983.9	E863.6	—	E950.7	E962.1	E980.6
Copperhead snake (bite) (venom)	989.5	E905.0	—	E950.9	E962.1	E980.9
Coral (sting)	989.5	E905.6	—	E950.9	E962.1	E980.9
snake (bite) (venom)	989.5	E905.0	—	E950.9	E962.1	E980.9
Cordran	976.0	E858.7	E946.0	E950.4	E962.0	E980.4
Corn cures	976.4	E858.7	E946.4	E950.4	E962.0	E980.4
Cornhusker's lotion	976.3	E858.7	E946.3	E950.4	E962.0	E980.4

Nontherapeutic use substance

▽ Subterms under main terms may continue to next column or page

	Poisoning	Accident	Therapeutic Use	Suicide Attempt	Assault	Undetermined
External Cause (E-Code)						
Corn starch	976.3	E858.7	E946.3	E950.4	E962.0	E980.4
Corrosive	983.9	E864.4	—	E950.7	E962.1	E980.6
acids NEC	983.1	E864.1	—	E950.7	E962.1	E980.6
aromatics	983.0	E864.0	—	E950.7	E962.1	E980.6
disinfectant	983.0	E861.4	—	E950.7	E962.1	E980.6
fumes NEC	987.9	E869.9	—	E952.9	E962.2	E982.9
specified NEC	983.9	E864.3	—	E950.7	E962.1	E980.6
sublimate — see Mercury, chloride						
Cortate	962.0	E858.0	E932.0	E950.4	E962.0	E980.4
Cort-Dome	962.0	E858.0	E932.0	E950.4	E962.0	E980.4
ENT agent	976.6	E858.7	E946.6	E950.4	E962.0	E980.4
ophthalmic preparation	976.5	E858.7	E946.5	E950.4	E962.0	E980.4
topical NEC	976.0	E858.7	E946.0	E950.4	E962.0	E980.4
Cortef	962.0	E858.0	E932.0	E950.4	E962.0	E980.4
ENT agent	976.6	E858.7	E946.6	E950.4	E962.0	E980.4
ophthalmic preparation	976.5	E858.7	E946.5	E950.4	E962.0	E980.4
topical NEC	976.0	E858.7	E946.0	E950.4	E962.0	E980.4
Corticosteroids (fluorinated)	962.0	E858.0	E932.0	E950.4	E962.0	E980.4
ENT agent	976.6	E858.7	E946.6	E950.4	E962.0	E980.4
ophthalmic preparation	976.5	E858.7	E946.5	E950.4	E962.0	E980.4
topical NEC	976.0	E858.7	E946.0	E950.4	E962.0	E980.4
Corticotropin	962.4	E858.0	E932.4	E950.4	E962.0	E980.4
Cortisol	962.0	E858.0	E932.0	E950.4	E962.0	E980.4
ENT agent	976.6	E858.7	E946.6	E950.4	E962.0	E980.4
ophthalmic preparation	976.5	E858.7	E946.5	E950.4	E962.0	E980.4
topical NEC	976.0	E858.7	E946.0	E950.4	E962.0	E980.4
Cortisone derivatives (acetate)	962.0	E858.0	E932.0	E950.4	E962.0	E980.4
ENT agent	976.6	E858.7	E946.6	E950.4	E962.0	E980.4
ophthalmic preparation	976.5	E858.7	E946.5	E950.4	E962.0	E980.4
topical NEC	976.0	E858.7	E946.0	E950.4	E962.0	E980.4
Cortogen	962.0	E858.0	E932.0	E950.4	E962.0	E980.4
ENT agent	976.6	E858.7	E946.6	E950.4	E962.0	E980.4
ophthalmic preparation	976.5	E858.7	E946.5	E950.4	E962.0	E980.4
Cortone	962.0	E858.0	E932.0	E950.4	E962.0	E980.4
ENT agent	976.6	E858.7	E946.6	E950.4	E962.0	E980.4
ophthalmic preparation	976.5	E858.7	E946.5	E950.4	E962.0	E980.4
Cortril	962.0	E858.0	E932.0	E950.4	E962.0	E980.4
ENT agent	976.6	E858.7	E946.6	E950.4	E962.0	E980.4
ophthalmic preparation	976.5	E858.7	E946.5	E950.4	E962.0	E980.4
topical NEC	976.0	E858.7	E946.0	E950.4	E962.0	E980.4
Cosmetics	989.89	E866.7	—	E950.9	E962.1	E980.9
Cosyntropin	977.8	E858.8	E947.8	E950.4	E962.0	E980.4
Cotarnine	964.5	E858.2	E934.5	E950.4	E962.0	E980.4
Cottonseed oil	976.3	E858.7	E946.3	E950.4	E962.0	E980.4
Cough mixtures (antitussives)	975.4	E858.6	E945.4	E950.4	E962.0	E980.4
containing opiates	965.09	E850.2	E935.2	E950.0	E962.0	E980.0
expectorant	975.5	E858.6	E945.5	E950.4	E962.0	E980.4
Coumadin	964.2	E858.2	E934.2	E950.4	E962.0	E980.4
rodenticide	989.4	E863.7	—	E950.6	E962.1	E980.7
Coumarin	964.2	E858.2	E934.2	E950.4	E962.0	E980.4
Coumetarol	964.2	E858.2	E934.2	E950.4	E962.0	E980.4
Cowbane	988.2	E865.4	—	E950.9	E962.1	E980.9
Cozyme	963.5	E858.1	E933.5	E950.4	E962.0	E980.4
Crack	970.81 ▲	E854.3	E940.8	E950.4	E962.0	E980.4
Creolin	983.0	E864.0	—	E950.7	E962.1	E980.6
disinfectant	983.0	E861.4	—	E950.7	E962.1	E980.6
Creosol (compound)	983.0	E864.0	—	E950.7	E962.1	E980.6
Creosote (beechwood) (coal tar)	983.0	E864.0	—	E950.7	E962.1	E980.6
medicinal (expectorant)	975.5	E858.6	E945.5	E950.4	E962.0	E980.4
syrup	975.5	E858.6	E945.5	E950.4	E962.0	E980.4
Cresol	983.0	E864.0	—	E950.7	E962.1	E980.6
disinfectant	983.0	E861.4	—	E950.7	E962.1	E980.6
Cresylic acid	983.0	E864.0	—	E950.7	E962.1	E980.6
Cropropamide	965.7	E850.7	E935.7	E950.0	E962.0	E980.0
with crotethamide	970.0	E854.3	E940.0	E950.4	E962.0	E980.4
Crotamiton	976.0	E858.7	E946.0	E950.4	E962.0	E980.4
Crotethamide	965.7	E850.7	E935.7	E950.0	E962.0	E980.0
with cropropamide	970.0	E854.3	E940.0	E950.4	E962.0	E980.4
Croton (oil)	973.1	E858.4	E943.1	E950.4	E962.0	E980.4
chloral	967.1	E852.0	E937.1	E950.2	E962.0	E980.2
Crude oil	981	E862.1	—	E950.9	E962.1	E980.9
Cryogenine	965.8	E850.8	E935.8	E950.0	E962.0	E980.0
Cryolite (pesticide)	989.4	E863.4	—	E950.6	E962.1	E980.7
Cryptenamine	972.6	E858.3	E942.6	E950.4	E962.0	E980.4
Crystal violet	976.0	E858.7	E946.0	E950.4	E962.0	E980.4
Cuckoopint	988.2	E865.4	—	E950.9	E962.1	E980.9
Cumetharol	964.2	E858.2	E934.2	E950.4	E962.0	E980.4

	Poisoning	Accident	Therapeutic Use	Suicide Attempt	Assault	Undetermined
External Cause (E-Code)						
Cupric sulfate	973.6	E858.4	E943.6	E950.4	E962.0	E980.4
Cuprous sulfate	983.9	E864.3	—	E950.7	E962.1	E980.6
Curare, curarine	975.2	E858.6	E945.2	E950.4	E962.0	E980.4
Cyanic acid — see Cyanide(s)						
Cyanide(s) (compounds) (hydrogen) (potassium) (sodium) NEC	989.0	E866.8	—	E950.9	E962.1	E980.9
dust or gas (inhalation) NEC	987.7	E869.8	—	E952.8	E962.2	E982.8
fumigant	989.0	E863.8	—	E950.6	E962.1	E980.7
mercuric — see Mercury						
pesticide (dust) (fumes)	989.0	E863.4	—	E950.6	E962.1	E980.7
Cyanocobalamin	964.1	E858.2	E934.1	E950.4	E962.0	E980.4
Cyanogen (chloride) (gas) NEC	987.8	E869.8	—	E952.8	E962.2	E982.8
Cyclaine	968.5	E855.2	E938.5	E950.4	E962.0	E980.4
Cyclamen europaeum	988.2	E865.4	—	E950.9	E962.1	E980.9
Cyclandelate	972.5	E858.3	E942.5	E950.4	E962.0	E980.4
Cyclazocine	965.09	E850.2	E935.2	E950.0	E962.0	E980.0
Cyclizine	963.0	E858.1	E933.0	E950.4	E962.0	E980.4
Cyclobarbital, cyclobarbitone	967.0	E851	E937.0	E950.1	E962.0	E980.1
Cycloguanil	961.4	E857	E931.4	E950.4	E962.0	E980.4
Cyclohexane	982.0	E862.4	—	E950.9	E962.1	E980.9
Cyclohexanol	980.8	E860.8	—	E950.9	E962.1	E980.9
Cyclohexanone	982.8	E862.4	—	E950.9	E962.1	E980.9
Cyclomethycaine	968.5	E855.2	E938.5	E950.4	E962.0	E980.4
Cyclopentamine	971.2	E855.5	E941.2	E950.4	E962.0	E980.4
Cyclopenthiazide	974.3	E858.5	E944.3	E950.4	E962.0	E980.4
Cyclopentolate	971.1	E855.4	E941.1	E950.4	E962.0	E980.4
Cyclophosphamide	963.1	E858.1	E933.1	E950.4	E962.0	E980.4
Cyclopropane	968.2	E855.1	E938.2	E950.4	E962.0	E980.4
Cycloserine	960.6	E856	E930.6	E950.4	E962.0	E980.4
Cyclothiazide	974.3	E858.5	E944.3	E950.4	E962.0	E980.4
Cycrimine	966.4	E855.0	E936.4	E950.4	E962.0	E980.4
Cymarin	972.1	E858.3	E942.1	E950.4	E962.0	E980.4
Cyproheptadine	963.0	E858.1	E933.0	E950.4	E962.0	E980.4
Cyprolidol	969.09	E854.0	E939.0	E950.3	E962.0	E980.3
Cytarabine	963.1	E858.1	E933.1	E950.4	E962.0	E980.4
Cytisus						
laburnum	988.2	E865.4	—	E950.9	E962.1	E980.9
scoparius	988.2	E865.4	—	E950.9	E962.1	E980.9
Cytomel	962.7	E858.0	E932.7	E950.4	E962.0	E980.4
Cytosine (antineoplastic)	963.1	E858.1	E933.1	E950.4	E962.0	E980.4
Cytoxan	963.1	E858.1	E933.1	E950.4	E962.0	E980.4
Dacarbazine	963.1	E858.1	E933.1	E950.4	E962.0	E980.4
Dactinomycin	960.7	E856	E930.7	E950.4	E962.0	E980.4
DADPS	961.8	E857	E931.8	E950.4	E962.0	E980.4
Dakin's solution (external)	976.0	E858.7	E946.0	E950.4	E962.0	E980.4
Dalmane	969.4	E853.2	E939.4	E950.3	E962.0	E980.3
DAM	977.2	E858.8	E947.2	E950.4	E962.0	E980.4
Danilone	964.2	E858.2	E934.2	E950.4	E962.0	E980.4
Danthron	973.1	E858.4	E943.1	E950.4	E962.0	E980.4
Dantrolene	975.2	E858.6	E945.2	E950.4	E962.0	E980.4
Daphne (gnidium) (mezereum)	988.2	E865.4	—	E950.9	E962.1	E980.9
berry	988.2	E865.3	—	E950.9	E962.1	E980.9
Dapsone	961.8	E857	E931.8	E950.4	E962.0	E980.4
Daraprim	961.4	E857	E931.4	E950.4	E962.0	E980.4
Darnel	988.2	E865.3	—	E950.9	E962.1	E980.9
Darvon	965.8	E850.8	E935.8	E950.0	E962.0	E980.0
Daunorubicin	960.7	E856	E930.7	E950.4	E962.0	E980.4
DBI	962.3	E858.0	E932.3	E950.4	E962.0	E980.4
D-Con (rodenticide)	989.4	E863.7	—	E950.6	E962.1	E980.7
DDS	961.8	E857	E931.8	E950.4	E962.0	E980.4
DDT	989.2	E863.0	—	E950.6	E962.1	E980.7
Deadly nightshade	988.2	E865.4	—	E950.9	E962.1	E980.9
berry	988.2	E865.3	—	E950.9	E962.1	E980.9
Deanol	969.79	E854.2	E939.7	E950.3	E962.0	E980.3
Debrisoquine	972.6	E858.3	E942.6	E950.4	E962.0	E980.4
Decaborane	989.89	E866.8	—	E950.9	E962.1	E980.9
fumes	987.8	E869.8	—	E952.8	E962.2	E982.8
Decadron	962.0	E858.0	E932.0	E950.4	E962.0	E980.4
ENT agent	976.6	E858.7	E946.6	E950.4	E962.0	E980.4
ophthalmic preparation	976.5	E858.7	E946.5	E950.4	E962.0	E980.4
topical NEC	976.0	E858.7	E946.0	E950.4	E962.0	E980.4
Decahydronaphthalene	982.0	E862.4	—	E950.9	E962.1	E980.9
Decalin	982.0	E862.4	—	E950.9	E962.1	E980.9
Decamethonium	975.2	E858.6	E945.2	E950.4	E962.0	E980.4
Decholin	973.4	E858.4	E943.4	E950.4	E962.0	E980.4
sodium (diagnostic)	977.8	E858.8	E947.8	E950.4	E962.0	E980.4

▼ Subterms under main terms may continue to next column or page

►◄ Revised Text　　●　New Line　　▲　Revised Code

		External Cause (E-Code)			
Poisoning	Accident	Therapeutic Use	Suicide Attempt	Assault	Undetermined

Substance	Poisoning	Accident	Therapeutic Use	Suicide Attempt	Assault	Undetermined
Declomycin	960.4	E856	E930.4	E950.4	E962.0	E980.4
Deferoxamine	963.8	E858.1	E933.8	E950.4	E962.0	E980.4
Dehydrocholic acid	973.4	E858.4	E943.4	E950.4	E962.0	E980.4
Dekalin	982.0	E862.4	—	E950.9	E962.1	E980.9
Delalutin	962.2	E858.0	E932.2	E950.4	E962.0	E980.4
Delphinium	988.2	E865.3	—	E950.9	E962.1	E980.9
Deltasone	962.0	E858.0	E932.0	E950.4	E962.0	E980.4
Deltra	962.0	E858.0	E932.0	E950.4	E962.0	E980.4
Delvinal	967.0	E851	E937.0	E950.1	E962.0	E980.1
Demecarium (bromide)	971.0	E855.3	E941.0	E950.4	E962.0	E980.4
Demeclocycline	960.4	E856	E930.4	E950.4	E962.0	E980.4
Demecolcine	963.1	E858.1	E933.1	E950.4	E962.0	E980.4
Demelanizing agents	976.8	E858.7	E946.8	E950.4	E962.0	E980.4
Demerol	965.09	E850.2	E935.2	E950.0	E962.0	E980.0
Demethylchlortetracy- cline	960.4	E856	E930.4	E950.4	E962.0	E980.4
Demethyltetracycline	960.4	E856	E930.4	E950.4	E962.0	E980.4
Demeton	989.3	E863.1	—	E950.6	E962.1	E980.7
Demulcents	976.3	E858.7	E946.3	E950.4	E962.0	E980.4
Demulen	962.2	E858.0	E932.2	E950.4	E962.0	E980.4
Denatured alcohol	980.0	E860.1	—	E950.9	E962.1	E980.9
Dendrid	976.5	E858.7	E946.5	E950.4	E962.0	E980.4
Dental agents, topical	976.7	E858.7	E946.7	E950.4	E962.0	E980.4
Deodorant spray (feminine hygiene)	976.8	E858.7	E946.8	E950.4	E962.0	E980.4
Deoxyribonuclease	963.4	E858.1	E933.4	E950.4	E962.0	E980.4
Depressants						
appetite, central	977.0	E858.8	E947.0	E950.4	E962.0	E980.4
cardiac	972.0	E858.3	E942.0	E950.4	E962.0	E980.4
central nervous system (anes- thetic)	968.4	E855.1	E938.4	E950.4	E962.0	E980.4
psychotherapeutic	969.5	E853.9	E939.5	E950.3	E962.0	E980.3
Dequalinium	976.0	E858.7	E946.0	E950.4	E962.0	E980.4
Dermolate	976.2	E858.7	E946.2	E950.4	E962.0	E980.4
DES	962.2	E858.0	E932.2	E950.4	E962.0	E980.4
Desenex	976.0	E858.7	E946.0	E950.4	E962.0	E980.4
Deserpidine	972.6	E858.3	E942.6	E950.4	E962.0	E980.4
Desipramine	969.05	E854.0	E939.0	E950.3	E962.0	E980.3
Deslanoside	972.1	E858.3	E942.1	E950.4	E962.0	E980.4
Desocodeine	965.09	E850.2	E935.2	E950.0	E962.0	E980.0
Desomorphine	965.09	E850.2	E935.2	E950.0	E962.0	E980.0
Desonide	976.0	E858.7	E946.0	E950.4	E962.0	E980.4
Desoxycorticosterone derivatives	962.0	E858.0	E932.0	E950.4	E962.0	E980.4
Desoxyephedrine	969.72	E854.2	E939.7	E950.3	E962.0	E980.3
DET	969.6	E854.1	E939.6	E950.3	E962.0	E980.3
Detergents (ingested) (synthet- ic)	989.6	E861.0	—	E950.9	E962.1	E980.9
ENT agent	976.6	E858.7	E946.6	E950.4	E962.0	E980.4
external medication	976.2	E858.7	E946.2	E950.4	E962.0	E980.4
ophthalmic preparation	976.5	E858.7	E946.5	E950.4	E962.0	E980.4
topical NEC	976.0	E858.7	E946.0	E950.4	E962.0	E980.4
Deterrent, alcohol	977.3	E858.8	E947.3	E950.4	E962.0	E980.4
Detrothyronine	962.7	E858.0	E932.7	E950.4	E962.0	E980.4
Dettol (external medica- tion)	976.0	E858.7	E946.0	E950.4	E962.0	E980.4
Dexamethasone	962.0	E858.0	E932.0	E950.4	E962.0	E980.4
Dexamphetamine	969.72	E854.2	E939.7	E950.3	E962.0	E980.3
Dexedrine	969.72	E854.2	E939.7	E950.3	E962.0	E980.3
Dexpanthenol	963.5	E858.1	E933.5	E950.4	E962.0	E980.4
Dextran	964.8	E858.2	E934.8	E950.4	E962.0	E980.4
Dextriferron	964.0	E858.2	E934.0	E950.4	E962.0	E980.4
Dextroamphetamine	969.72	E854.2	E939.7	E950.3	E962.0	E980.3
Dextro calcium pantothen- ate	963.5	E858.1	E933.5	E950.4	E962.0	E980.4
Dextromethorphan	975.4	E858.6	E945.4	E950.4	E962.0	E980.4
Dextromoramide	965.09	E850.2	E935.2	E950.0	E962.0	E980.0
Dextro pantothenyl alco- hol	963.5	E858.1	E933.5	E950.4	E962.0	E980.4
topical	976.8	E858.7	E946.8	E950.4	E962.0	E980.4
Dextropropoxyphene (hy- drochloride)	965.8	E850.8	E935.8	E950.0	E962.0	E980.0
Dextrorphan	965.09	E850.2	E935.2	E950.0	E962.0	E980.0
Dextrose NEC	974.5	E858.5	E944.5	E950.4	E962.0	E980.4
Dextrothyroxin	962.7	E858.0	E932.7	E950.4	E962.0	E980.4
DFP	971.0	E855.3	E941.0	E950.4	E962.0	E980.4
DHE-45	972.9	E858.3	E942.9	E950.4	E962.0	E980.4
Diabinese	962.3	E858.0	E932.3	E950.4	E962.0	E980.4
Diacetyl monoxime	977.2	E858.8	E947.2	E950.4	E962.0	E980.4
Diacetylmorphine	965.01	E850.0	E935.0	E950.0	E962.0	E980.0
Diagnostic agents	977.8	E858.8	E947.8	E950.4	E962.0	E980.4
Dial (soap)	976.2	E858.7	E946.2	E950.4	E962.0	E980.4
Dial — continued						
sedative	967.0	E851	E937.0	E950.1	E962.0	E980.1
Diallylbarbituric acid	967.0	E851	E937.0	E950.1	E962.0	E980.1
Diaminodiphenylsulfone	961.8	E857	E931.8	E950.4	E962.0	E980.4
Diamorphine	965.01	E850.0	E935.0	E950.0	E962.0	E980.0
Diamox	974.2	E858.5	E944.2	E950.4	E962.0	E980.4
Diamthazole	976.0	E858.7	E946.0	E950.4	E962.0	E980.4
Diaphenylsulfone	961.8	E857	E931.8	E950.4	E962.0	E980.4
Diasone (sodium)	961.8	E857	E931.8	E950.4	E962.0	E980.4
Diazepam	969.4	E853.2	E939.4	E950.3	E962.0	E980.3
Diazinon	989.3	E863.1	—	E950.6	E962.1	E980.7
Diazomethane (gas)	987.8	E869.8	—	E952.8	E962.2	E982.8
Diazoxide	972.5	E858.3	E942.5	E950.4	E962.0	E980.4
Dibenamine	971.3	E855.6	E941.3	E950.4	E962.0	E980.4
Dibenzheptropine	963.0	E858.1	E933.0	E950.4	E962.0	E980.4
Dibenzyline	971.3	E855.6	E941.3	E950.4	E962.0	E980.4
Diborane (gas)	987.8	E869.8	—	E952.8	E962.2	E982.8
Dibromomannitol	963.1	E858.1	E933.1	E950.4	E962.0	E980.4
Dibucaine (spinal)	968.7	E855.2	E938.7	E950.4	E962.0	E980.4
topical (surface)	968.5	E855.2	E938.5	E950.4	E962.0	E980.4
Dibunate sodium	975.4	E858.6	E945.4	E950.4	E962.0	E980.4
Dibutoline	971.1	E855.4	E941.1	E950.4	E962.0	E980.4
Dicapthon	989.4	E863.4	—	E950.6	E962.1	E980.7
Dichloralphenazone	967.1	E852.0	E937.1	E950.2	E962.0	E980.2
Dichlorodifluo- romethane	987.4	E869.2	—	E952.8	E962.2	E982.8
Dichloroethane	982.3	E862.4	—	E950.9	E962.1	E980.9
Dichloroethylene	982.3	E862.4	—	E950.9	E962.1	E980.9
Dichloroethyl sulfide	987.8	E869.8	—	E952.8	E962.2	E982.8
Dichlorohydrin	982.3	E862.4	—	E950.9	E962.1	E980.9
Dichloromethane (solvent) (vapor)	982.3	E862.4	—	E950.9	E962.1	E980.9
Dichlorophen(e)	961.6	E857	E931.6	E950.4	E962.0	E980.4
Dichlorphenamide	974.2	E858.5	E944.2	E950.4	E962.0	E980.4
Dichlorvos	989.3	E863.1	—	E950.6	E962.1	E980.7
Diclofenac sodium	965.69	E850.6	E935.6	E950.0	E962.0	E980.0
Dicoumarin, dicumarol	964.2	E858.2	E934.2	E950.4	E962.0	E980.4
Dicyanogen (gas)	987.8	E869.8	—	E952.8	E962.2	E982.8
Dicyclomine	971.1	E855.4	E941.1	E950.4	E962.0	E980.4
Dieldrin (vapor)	989.2	E863.0	—	E950.6	E962.1	E980.7
Dienestrol	962.2	E858.0	E932.2	E950.4	E962.0	E980.4
Dietetics	977.0	E858.8	E947.0	E950.4	E962.0	E980.4
Diethazine	966.4	E855.0	E936.4	E950.4	E962.0	E980.4
Diethyl						
barbituric acid	967.0	E851	E937.0	E950.1	E962.0	E980.1
carbamazine	961.6	E857	E931.6	E950.4	E962.0	E980.4
carbinol	980.8	E860.8	—	E950.9	E962.1	E980.9
carbonate	982.8	E862.4	—	E950.9	E962.1	E980.9
dioxide	982.8	E862.4	—	E950.9	E962.1	E980.9
ether (vapor) — see Ether(s)						
glycol (monoacetate) (mo- noethyl ether)	982.8	E862.4	—	E950.9	E962.1	E980.9
propion	977.0	E858.8	E947.0	E950.4	E962.0	E980.4
stilbestrol	962.2	E858.0	E932.2	E950.4	E962.0	E980.4
Diethylene						
Diethylsulfone-diethyl- methane	967.8	E852.8	E937.8	E950.2	E962.0	E980.2
Difencloxazine	965.09	E850.2	E935.2	E950.0	E962.0	E980.0
Diffusin	963.4	E858.1	E933.4	E950.4	E962.0	E980.4
Diflos	971.0	E855.3	E941.0	E950.4	E962.0	E980.4
Digestants	973.4	E858.4	E943.4	E950.4	E962.0	E980.4
Digitalin(e)	972.1	E858.3	E942.1	E950.4	E962.0	E980.4
Digitalis glycosides	972.1	E858.3	E942.1	E950.4	E962.0	E980.4
Digitoxin	972.1	E858.3	E942.1	E950.4	E962.0	E980.4
Digoxin	972.1	E858.3	E942.1	E950.4	E962.0	E980.4
Dihydrocodeine	965.09	E850.2	E935.2	E950.0	E962.0	E980.0
Dihydrocodeinone	965.09	E850.2	E935.2	E950.0	E962.0	E980.0
Dihydroergocristine	972.9	E858.3	E942.9	E950.4	E962.0	E980.4
Dihydroergotamine	972.9	E858.3	E942.9	E950.4	E962.0	E980.4
Dihydroergotoxine	972.9	E858.3	E942.9	E950.4	E962.0	E980.4
Dihydrohydroxy- codeinone	965.09	E850.2	E935.2	E950.0	E962.0	E980.0
Dihydrohydroxymorphi- none	965.09	E850.2	E935.2	E950.0	E962.0	E980.0
Dihydroisocodeine	965.09	E850.2	E935.2	E950.0	E962.0	E980.0
Dihydromorphine	965.09	E850.2	E935.2	E950.0	E962.0	E980.0
Dihydromorphinone	965.09	E850.2	E935.2	E950.0	E962.0	E980.0
Dihydrostreptomycin	960.6	E856	E930.6	E950.4	E962.0	E980.4
Dihydrotachysterol	962.6	E858.0	E932.6	E950.4	E962.0	E980.4
Dihydroxyan- thraquinone	973.1	E858.4	E943.1	E950.4	E962.0	E980.4
Dihydroxycodeinone	965.09	E850.2	E935.2	E950.0	E962.0	E980.0

Index

Diiodohydroxyquin — Drug

	Poisoning	Accident	Therapeutic Use	Suicide Attempt	Assault	Undetermined
Diiodohydroxyquin	961.3	E857	E931.3	E950.4	E962.0	E980.4
topical	976.0	E858.7	E946.0	E950.4	E962.0	E980.4
Diiodohydroxyquinoline	961.3	E857	E931.3	E950.4	E962.0	E980.4
Dilantin	966.1	E855.0	E936.1	E950.4	E962.0	E980.4
Dilaudid	965.09	E850.2	E935.2	E950.0	E962.0	E980.0
Diloxanide	961.5	E857	E931.5	E950.4	E962.0	E980.4
Dimefline	970.0	E854.3	E940.0	E950.4	E962.0	E980.4
Dimenhydrinate	963.0	E858.1	E933.0	E950.4	E962.0	E980.4
Dimercaprol	963.8	E858.1	E933.8	E950.4	E962.0	E980.4
Dimercaptopropanol	963.8	E858.1	E933.8	E950.4	E962.0	E980.4
Dimetane	963.0	E858.1	E933.0	E950.4	E962.0	E980.4
Dimethicone	976.3	E858.7	E946.3	E950.4	E962.0	E980.4
Dimethindene	963.0	E858.1	E933.0	E950.4	E962.0	E980.4
Dimethisoquin	968.5	E855.2	E938.5	E950.4	E962.0	E980.4
Dimethisterone	962.2	E858.0	E932.2	E950.4	E962.0	E980.4
Dimethoxanate	975.4	E858.6	E945.4	E950.4	E962.0	E980.4
Dimethyl						
arsine, arsinic acid — see Arsenic						
carbinol	980.2	E860.3	—	E950.9	E962.1	E980.9
diguanide	962.3	E858.0	E932.3	E950.4	E962.0	E980.4
ketone	982.8	E862.4	—	E950.9	E962.1	E980.9
vapor	987.8	E869.8	—	E952.8	E962.2	E982.8
meperidine	965.09	E850.2	E935.2	E950.0	E962.0	E980.0
parathion	989.3	E863.1	—	E950.6	E962.1	E980.7
polysiloxane	973.8	E858.4	E943.8	E950.4	E962.0	E980.4
sulfate (fumes)	987.8	E869.8	—	E952.8	E962.2	E982.8
liquid	983.9	E864.3	—	E950.7	E962.1	E980.6
sulfoxide NEC	982.8	E862.4	—	E950.9	E962.1	E980.9
medicinal	976.4	E858.7	E946.4	E950.4	E962.0	E980.4
triptamine	969.6	E854.1	E939.6	E950.3	E962.0	E980.3
tubocurarine	975.2	E858.6	E945.2	E950.4	E962.0	E980.4
Dindevan	964.2	E858.2	E934.2	E950.4	E962.0	E980.4
Dinitrobenzene	983.0	E864.0	—	E950.7	E962.1	E980.6
vapor	987.8	E869.8	—	E952.8	E962.2	E982.8
Dinitro (-ortho-) cresol (herbicide) (spray)	989.4	E863.5	—	E950.6	E962.1	E980.7
insecticide	989.4	E863.4	—	E950.6	E962.1	E980.7
Dinitro-orthocresol (herbicide)	989.4	E863.5	—	E950.6	E962.1	E980.7
insecticide	989.4	E863.4	—	E950.6	E962.1	E980.7
Dinitrophenol (herbicide) (spray)	989.4	E863.5	—	E950.6	E962.1	E980.7
insecticide	989.4	E863.4	—	E950.6	E962.1	E980.7
Dinoprost	975.0	E858.6	E945.0	E950.4	E962.0	E980.4
Dioctyl sulfosuccinate (calcium) (sodium)	973.2	E858.4	E943.2	E950.4	E962.0	E980.4
Diodoquin	961.3	E857	E931.3	E950.4	E962.0	E980.4
Dione derivatives NEC	966.3	E855.0	E936.3	E950.4	E962.0	E980.4
Dionin	965.09	E850.2	E935.2	E950.0	E962.0	E980.0
Dioxane	982.8	E862.4	—	E950.9	E962.1	E980.9
Dioxin — see Herbicide						
Dioxyline	972.5	E858.3	E942.5	E950.4	E962.0	E980.4
Dipentene	982.8	E862.4	—	E950.9	E962.1	E980.9
Diphemanil	971.1	E855.4	E941.1	E950.4	E962.0	E980.4
Diphenadione	964.2	E858.2	E934.2	E950.4	E962.0	E980.4
Diphenhydramine	963.0	E858.1	E933.0	E950.4	E962.0	E980.4
Diphenidol	963.0	E858.1	E933.0	E950.4	E962.0	E980.4
Diphenoxylate	973.5	E858.4	E943.5	E950.4	E962.0	E980.4
Diphenylchloroarsine	985.1	E866.3	—	E950.8	E962.1	E980.8
Diphenylhydantoin (sodium)	966.1	E855.0	E936.1	E950.4	E962.0	E980.4
Diphenylpyraline	963.0	E858.1	E933.0	E950.4	E962.0	E980.4
Diphtheria						
antitoxin	979.9	E858.8	E949.9	E950.4	E962.0	E980.4
toxoid	978.5	E858.8	E948.5	E950.4	E962.0	E980.4
with tetanus toxoid	978.9	E858.8	E948.9	E950.4	E962.0	E980.4
with pertussis component	978.6	E858.8	E948.6	E950.4	E962.0	E980.4
vaccine	978.5	E858.8	E948.5	E950.4	E962.0	E980.4
Dipipanone	965.09	E850.2	E935.2	E950.0	E962.0	E980.0
Diplovax	979.5	E858.8	E949.5	E950.4	E962.0	E980.4
Diprophylline	975.1	E858.6	E945.1	E950.4	E962.0	E980.4
Dipyridamole	972.4	E858.3	E942.4	E950.4	E962.0	E980.4
Dipyrone	965.5	E850.5	E935.5	E950.0	E962.0	E980.0
Diquat	989.4	E863.5	—	E950.6	E962.1	E980.7
Disinfectant NEC	983.9	E861.4	—	E950.7	E962.1	E980.6
alkaline	983.2	E861.4	—	E950.7	E962.1	E980.6
aromatic	983.0	E861.4	—	E950.7	E962.1	E980.6
Disipal	966.4	E855.0	E936.4	E950.4	E962.0	E980.4
Disodium edetate	963.8	E858.1	E933.8	E950.4	E962.0	E980.4
Disulfamide	974.4	E858.5	E944.4	E950.4	E962.0	E980.4

	Poisoning	Accident	Therapeutic Use	Suicide Attempt	Assault	Undetermined
Disulfanilamide	961.0	E857	E931.0	E950.4	E962.0	E980.4
Disulfiram	977.3	E858.8	E947.3	E950.4	E962.0	E980.4
Dithiazanine	961.6	E857	E931.6	E950.4	E962.0	E980.4
Dithioglycerol	963.8	E858.1	E933.8	E950.4	E962.0	E980.4
Dithranol	976.4	E858.7	E946.4	E950.4	E962.0	E980.4
Diucardin	974.3	E858.5	E944.3	E950.4	E962.0	E980.4
Diupres	974.3	E858.5	E944.3	E950.4	E962.0	E980.4
Diuretics NEC	974.4	E858.5	E944.4	E950.4	E962.0	E980.4
carbonic acid anhydrase inhibitors	974.2	E858.5	E944.2	E950.4	E962.0	E980.4
mercurial	974.0	E858.5	E944.0	E950.4	E962.0	E980.4
osmotic	974.4	E858.5	E944.4	E950.4	E962.0	E980.4
purine derivatives	974.1	E858.5	E944.1	E950.4	E962.0	E980.4
saluretic	974.3	E858.5	E944.3	E950.4	E962.0	E980.4
Diuril	974.3	E858.5	E944.3	E950.4	E962.0	E980.4
Divinyl ether	968.2	E855.1	E938.2	E950.4	E962.0	E980.4
D-lysergic acid diethylamide	969.6	E854.1	E939.6	E950.3	E962.0	E980.3
DMCT	960.4	E856	E930.4	E950.4	E962.0	E980.4
DMSO	982.8	E862.4	—	E950.9	E962.1	E980.9
DMT	969.6	E854.1	E939.6	E950.3	E962.0	E980.3
DNOC	989.4	E863.5	—	E950.6	E962.1	E980.7
DOCA	962.0	E858.0	E932.0	E950.4	E962.0	E980.4
Dolophine	965.02	E850.1	E935.1	E950.0	E962.0	E980.0
Doloxene	965.8	E850.8	E935.8	E950.0	E962.0	E980.0
DOM	969.6	E854.1	E939.6	E950.3	E962.0	E980.3
Domestic gas — see Gas, utility						
Domiphen (bromide) (lozenges)	976.6	E858.7	E946.6	E950.4	E962.0	E980.4
Dopa (levo)	966.4	E855.0	E936.4	E950.4	E962.0	E980.4
Dopamine	971.2	E855.5	E941.2	E950.4	E962.0	E980.4
Doriden	967.5	E852.4	E937.5	E950.2	E962.0	E980.2
Dormiral	967.0	E851	E937.0	E950.1	E962.0	E980.1
Dormison	967.8	E852.8	E937.8	E950.2	E962.0	E980.2
Dornase	963.4	E858.1	E933.4	E950.4	E962.0	E980.4
Dorsacaine	968.5	E855.2	E938.5	E950.4	E962.0	E980.4
Dothiepin hydrochloride	969.05	E854.0	E939.0	E950.3	E962.0	E980.3
Doxapram	970.0	E854.3	E940.0	E950.4	E962.0	E980.4
Doxepin	969.05	E854.0	E939.0	E950.3	E962.0	E980.3
Doxorubicin	960.7	E856	E930.7	E950.4	E962.0	E980.4
Doxycycline	960.4	E856	E930.4	E950.4	E962.0	E980.4
Doxylamine	963.0	E858.1	E933.0	E950.4	E962.0	E980.4
Dramamine	963.0	E858.1	E933.0	E950.4	E962.0	E980.4
Drano (drain cleaner)	983.2	E864.2	—	E950.7	E962.1	E980.6
Dromoran	965.09	E850.2	E935.2	E950.0	E962.0	E980.0
Dromostanolone	962.1	E858.0	E932.1	E950.4	E962.0	E980.4
Droperidol	969.2	E853.1	E939.2	E950.3	E962.0	E980.3
Drotrecogin alfa	964.2	E858.2	E934.2	E950.4	E962.0	E980.4
Drug	977.9	E858.9	E947.9	E950.5	E962.0	E980.5
AHFS List						
4:00 antihistamine drugs	963.0	E858.1	E933.0	E950.4	E962.0	E980.4
8:04 amebacides	961.5	E857	E931.5	E950.4	E962.0	E980.4
arsenical anti-infectives	961.1	E857	E931.1	E950.4	E962.0	E980.4
quinoline derivatives	961.3	E857	E931.3	E950.4	E962.0	E980.4
8:08 anthelmintics	961.6	E857	E931.6	E950.4	E962.0	E980.4
quinoline derivatives	961.3	E857	E931.3	E950.4	E962.0	E980.4
8:12.04 antifungal antibiotics	960.1	E856	E930.1	E950.4	E962.0	E980.4
8:12.06 cephalosporins	960.5	E856	E930.5	E950.4	E962.0	E980.4
8:12.08 chloramphenicol	960.2	E856	E930.2	E950.4	E962.0	E980.4
8:12.12 erythromycins	960.3	E856	E930.3	E950.4	E962.0	E980.4
8:12.16 penicillins	960.0	E856	E930.0	E950.4	E962.0	E980.4
8:12.20 streptomycins	960.6	E856	E930.6	E950.4	E962.0	E980.4
8:12.24 tetracyclines	960.4	E856	E930.4	E950.4	E962.0	E980.4
8:12.28 other antibiotics	960.8	E856	E930.8	E950.4	E962.0	E980.4
antimycobacterial	960.6	E856	E930.6	E950.4	E962.0	E980.4
macrolides	960.3	E856	E930.3	E950.4	E962.0	E980.4
8:16 antituberculars	961.8	E857	E931.8	E950.4	E962.0	E980.4
antibiotics	960.6	E856	E930.6	E950.4	E962.0	E980.4
8:18 antivirals	961.7	E857	E931.7	E950.4	E962.0	E980.4
8:20 plasmodicides (antimalarials)	961.4	E857	E931.4	E950.4	E962.0	E980.4
8:24 sulfonamides	961.0	E857	E931.0	E950.4	E962.0	E980.4
8:26 sulfones	961.8	E857	E931.8	E950.4	E962.0	E980.4
8:28 treponemicides	961.2	E857	E931.2	E950.4	E962.0	E980.4
8:32 trichomonacides	961.5	E857	E931.5	E950.4	E962.0	E980.4
nitrofuran derivatives	961.9	E857	E931.9	E950.4	E962.0	E980.4
quinoline derivatives	961.3	E857	E931.3	E950.4	E962.0	E980.4
8:36 urinary germicides	961.9	E857	E931.9	E950.4	E962.0	E980.4
quinoline derivatives	961.3	E857	E931.3	E950.4	E962.0	E980.4
8:40 other anti-infectives	961.9	E857	E931.9	E950.4	E962.0	E980.4

Nontherapeutic use substance

▽ Subterms under main terms may continue to next column or page

Drug — continued	Poisoning	Accident	Therapeutic Use	Suicide Attempt	Assault	Undetermined
10:00 antineoplastic agents	963.1	E858.1	E933.1	E950.4	E962.0	E980.4
antibiotics	960.7	E856	E930.7	E950.4	E962.0	E980.4
progestogens	962.2	E858.0	E932.2	E950.4	E962.0	E980.4
12:04 parasympathomimetic (cholinergic) agents	971.0	E855.3	E941.0	E950.4	E962.0	E980.4
12:08 parasympatholytic (cholinergic-blocking) agents	971.1	E855.4	E941.1	E950.4	E962.0	E980.4
12:12 Sympathomimetic (adrenergic) agents	971.2	E855.5	E941.2	E950.4	E962.0	E980.4
12:16 sympatholytic (adrenergic-blocking) agents	971.3	E855.6	E941.3	E950.4	E962.0	E980.4
12:20 skeletal muscle relaxants						
central nervous system muscle-tone depressants	968.0	E855.1	E938.0	E950.4	E962.0	E980.4
myoneural blocking agents	975.2	E858.6	E945.2	E950.4	E962.0	E980.4
16:00 blood derivatives	964.7	E858.2	E934.7	E950.4	E962.0	E980.4
20:04.04 iron preparations	964.0	E858.2	E934.0	E950.4	E962.0	E980.4
20:04.08 liver and stomach preparations	964.1	E858.2	E934.1	E950.4	E962.0	E980.4
20:04 antianemia drugs	964.1	E858.2	E934.1	E950.4	E962.0	E980.4
20:12.04 anticoagulants	964.2	E858.2	E934.2	E950.4	E962.0	E980.4
20:12.08 antiheparin agents	964.5	E858.2	E934.5	E950.4	E962.0	E980.4
20:12.12 coagulants	964.5	E858.2	E934.5	E950.4	E962.0	E980.4
20:12.16 hemostatics NEC	964.5	E858.2	E934.5	E950.4	E962.0	E980.4
capillary active drugs	972.8	E858.3	E942.8	E950.4	E962.0	E980.4
24:04 cardiac drugs	972.9	E858.3	E942.9	E950.4	E962.0	E980.4
cardiotonic agents	972.1	E858.3	E942.1	E950.4	E962.0	E980.4
rhythm regulators	972.0	E858.3	E942.0	E950.4	E962.0	E980.4
24:06 antilipemic agents	972.2	E858.3	E942.2	E950.4	E962.0	E980.4
thyroid derivatives	962.7	E858.0	E932.7	E950.4	E962.0	E980.4
24:08 hypotensive agents	972.6	E858.3	E942.6	E950.4	E962.0	E980.4
adrenergic blocking agents	971.3	E855.6	E941.3	E950.4	E962.0	E980.4
ganglion blocking agents	972.3	E858.3	E942.3	E950.4	E962.0	E980.4
vasodilators	972.5	E858.3	E942.5	E950.4	E962.0	E980.4
24:12 vasodilating agents NEC	972.5	E858.3	E942.5	E950.4	E962.0	E980.4
coronary	972.4	E858.3	E942.4	E950.4	E962.0	E980.4
nicotinic acid derivatives	972.2	E858.3	E942.2	E950.4	E962.0	E980.4
24:16 sclerosing agents	972.7	E858.3	E942.7	E950.4	E962.0	E980.4
28:04 general anesthetics	968.4	E855.1	E938.4	E950.4	E962.0	E980.4
gaseous anesthetics	968.2	E855.1	E938.2	E950.4	E962.0	E980.4
halothane	968.1	E855.1	E938.1	E950.4	E962.0	E980.4
intravenous anesthetics	968.3	E855.1	E938.3	E950.4	E962.0	E980.4
28:08 analgesics and antipyretics	965.9	E850.9	E935.9	E950.0	E962.0	E980.0
antirheumatics	965.69	E850.6	E935.6	E950.0	E962.0	E980.0
aromatic analgesics	965.4	E850.4	E935.4	E950.0	E962.0	E980.0
non-narcotic NEC	965.7	E850.7	E935.7	E950.0	E962.0	E980.0
opium alkaloids	965.00	E850.2	E935.2	E950.0	E962.0	E980.0
heroin	965.01	E850.0	E935.0	E950.0	E962.0	E980.0
methadone	965.02	E850.1	E935.1	E950.0	E962.0	E980.0
specified type NEC	965.09	E850.2	E935.2	E950.0	E962.0	E980.0
pyrazole derivatives	965.5	E850.5	E935.5	E950.0	E962.0	E980.0
salicylates	965.1	E850.3	E935.3	E950.0	E962.0	E980.0
specified NEC	965.8	E850.8	E935.8	E950.0	E962.0	E980.0
28:10 narcotic antagonists	970.1	E854.3	E940.1	E950.4	E962.0	E980.4
28:12 anticonvulsants	966.3	E855.0	E936.3	E950.4	E962.0	E980.4
barbiturates	967.0	E851	E937.0	E950.1	E962.0	E980.1
benzodiazepine-based tranquilizers	969.4	E853.2	E939.4	E950.3	E962.0	E980.3
bromides	967.3	E852.2	E937.3	E950.2	E962.0	E980.2
hydantoin derivatives	966.1	E855.0	E936.1	E950.4	E962.0	E980.4
oxazolidine (derivatives)	966.0	E855.0	E936.0	E950.4	E962.0	E980.4
succinimides	966.2	E855.0	E936.2	E950.4	E962.0	E980.4
28:16.04 antidepressants	969.0	E854.0	E939.0	E950.3	E962.0	E980.3
28:16.08 tranquilizers	969.5	E853.9	E939.5	E950.3	E962.0	E980.3
benzodiazepine-based	969.4	E853.2	E939.4	E950.3	E962.0	E980.3

Drug — continued	Poisoning	Accident	Therapeutic Use	Suicide Attempt	Assault	Undetermined
28:16.08 tranquilizers — continued						
butyrophenone-based	969.2	E853.1	E939.2	E950.3	E962.0	E980.3
major NEC	969.3	E853.8	E939.3	E950.3	E962.0	E980.3
phenothiazine-based	969.1	E853.0	E939.1	E950.3	E962.0	E980.3
28:16.12 other psychotherapeutic agents	969.8	E855.8	E939.8	E950.3	E962.0	E980.3
28:20 respiratory and cerebral stimulants	970.9	E854.3	E940.9	E950.4	E962.0	E980.4
analeptics	970.0	E854.3	E940.0	E950.4	E962.0	E980.4
anorexigenic agents	977.0	E858.8	E947.0	E950.4	E962.0	E980.4
psychostimulants	969.70	E854.2	E939.7	E950.3	E962.0	E980.3
specified NEC	970.89 ▲	E854.3	E940.8	E950.4	E962.0	E980.4
28:24 sedatives and hypnotics	967.9	E852.9	E937.9	E950.2	E962.0	E980.2
barbiturates	967.0	E851	E937.0	E950.1	E962.0	E980.1
benzodiazepine-based tranquilizers	969.4	E853.2	E939.4	E950.3	E962.0	E980.3
chloral hydrate (group)	967.1	E852.0	E937.1	E950.2	E962.0	E980.2
glutethamide group	967.5	E852.4	E937.5	E950.2	E962.0	E980.2
intravenous anesthetics	968.3	E855.1	E938.3	E950.4	E962.0	E980.4
methaqualone (compounds)	967.4	E852.3	E937.4	E950.2	E962.0	E980.2
paraldehyde	967.2	E852.1	E937.2	E950.2	E962.0	E980.2
phenothiazine-based tranquilizers	969.1	E853.0	E939.1	E950.3	E962.0	E980.3
specified NEC	967.8	E852.8	E937.8	E950.2	E962.0	E980.2
thiobarbiturates	968.3	E855.1	E938.3	E950.4	E962.0	E980.4
tranquilizer NEC	969.5	E853.9	E939.5	E950.3	E962.0	E980.3
36:04 to 36:88 diagnostic agents	977.8	E858.8	E947.8	E950.4	E962.0	E980.4
40:00 electrolyte, caloric, and water balance agents NEC	974.5	E858.5	E944.5	E950.4	E962.0	E980.4
40:04 acidifying agents	963.2	E858.1	E933.2	E950.4	E962.0	E980.4
40:08 alkalinizing agents	963.3	E858.1	E933.3	E950.4	E962.0	E980.4
40:10 ammonia detoxicants	974.5	E858.5	E944.5	E950.4	E962.0	E980.4
40:12 replacement solutions	974.5	E858.5	E944.5	E950.4	E962.0	E980.4
plasma expanders	964.8	E858.2	E934.8	E950.4	E962.0	E980.4
40:16 sodium-removing resins	974.5	E858.5	E944.5	E950.4	E962.0	E980.4
40:18 potassium-removing resins	974.5	E858.5	E944.5	E950.4	E962.0	E980.4
40:20 caloric agents	974.5	E858.5	E944.5	E950.4	E962.0	E980.4
40:24 salt and sugar substitutes	974.5	E858.5	E944.5	E950.4	E962.0	E980.4
40:28 diuretics NEC	974.4	E858.5	E944.4	E950.4	E962.0	E980.4
carbonic acid anhydrase inhibitors	974.2	E858.5	E944.2	E950.4	E962.0	E980.4
mercurials	974.0	E858.5	E944.0	E950.4	E962.0	E980.4
purine derivatives	974.1	E858.5	E944.1	E950.4	E962.0	E980.4
saluretics	974.3	E858.5	E944.3	E950.4	E962.0	E980.4
thiazides	974.3	E858.5	E944.3	E950.4	E962.0	E980.4
40:36 irrigating solutions	974.5	E858.5	E944.5	E950.4	E962.0	E980.4
40:40 uricosuric agents	974.7	E858.5	E944.7	E950.4	E962.0	E980.4
44:00 enzymes	963.4	E858.1	E933.4	E950.4	E962.0	E980.4
fibrinolysis-affecting agents	964.4	E858.2	E934.4	E950.4	E962.0	E980.4
gastric agents	973.4	E858.4	E943.4	E950.4	E962.0	E980.4
48:00 expectorants and cough preparations						
antihistamine agents	963.0	E858.1	E933.0	E950.4	E962.0	E980.4
antitussives	975.4	E858.6	E945.4	E950.4	E962.0	E980.4
codeine derivatives	965.09	E850.2	E935.2	E950.0	E962.0	E980.0
expectorants	975.5	E858.6	E945.5	E950.4	E962.0	E980.4
narcotic agents NEC	965.09	E850.2	E935.2	E950.0	E962.0	E980.0
52:04.04 antibiotics (EENT)						
ENT agent	976.6	E858.7	E946.6	E950.4	E962.0	E980.4
ophthalmic preparation	976.5	E858.7	E946.5	E950.4	E962.0	E980.4
52:04.06 antivirals (EENT)						
ENT agent	976.6	E858.7	E946.6	E950.4	E962.0	E980.4
ophthalmic preparation	976.5	E858.7	E946.5	E950.4	E962.0	E980.4
52:04.08 sulfonamides (EENT)						
ENT agent	976.6	E858.7	E946.6	E950.4	E962.0	E980.4
ophthalmic preparation	976.5	E858.7	E946.5	E950.4	E962.0	E980.4
52:04.12 miscellaneous anti-infectives (EENT)						
ENT agent	976.6	E858.7	E946.6	E950.4	E962.0	E980.4
ophthalmic preparation	976.5	E858.7	E946.5	E950.4	E962.0	E980.4

Drug — continued	Poisoning	Accident	Therapeutic Use	Suicide Attempt	Assault	Undetermined
52:04 anti-infectives (EENT)						
ENT agent	976.6	E858.7	E946.6	E950.4	E962.0	E980.4
ophthalmic preparation	976.5	E858.7	E946.5	E950.4	E962.0	E980.4
52:08 anti-inflammatory agents (EENT)						
ENT agent	976.6	E858.7	E946.6	E950.4	E962.0	E980.4
ophthalmic preparation	976.5	E858.7	E946.5	E950.4	E962.0	E980.4
52:10 carbonic anhydrase inhibitors	974.2	E858.5	E944.2	E950.4	E962.0	E980.4
52:12 contact lens solutions	976.5	E858.7	E946.5	E950.4	E962.0	E980.4
52:16 local anesthetics (EENT)	968.5	E855.2	E938.5	E950.4	E962.0	E980.4
52:20 miotics	971.0	E855.3	E941.0	E950.4	E962.0	E980.4
52:24 mydriatics						
adrenergics	971.2	E855.5	E941.2	E950.4	E962.0	E980.4
anticholinergics	971.1	E855.4	E941.1	E950.4	E962.0	E980.4
antimuscarinics	971.1	E855.4	E941.1	E950.4	E962.0	E980.4
parasympatholytics	971.1	E855.4	E941.1	E950.4	E962.0	E980.4
spasmolytics	971.1	E855.4	E941.1	E950.4	E962.0	E980.4
sympathomimetics	971.2	E855.5	E941.2	E950.4	E962.0	E980.4
52:28 mouth washes and gargles	976.6	E858.7	E946.6	E950.4	E962.0	E980.4
52:32 vasoconstrictors (EENT)	971.2	E855.5	E941.2	E950.4	E962.0	E980.4
52:36 unclassified agents (EENT)						
ENT agent	976.6	E858.7	E946.6	E950.4	E962.0	E980.4
ophthalmic preparation	976.5	E858.7	E946.5	E950.4	E962.0	E980.4
56:04 antacids and adsorbents	973.0	E858.4	E943.0	E950.4	E962.0	E980.4
56:08 antidiarrhea agents	973.5	E858.4	E943.5	E950.4	E962.0	E980.4
56:10 antiflatulents	973.8	E858.4	E943.8	E950.4	E962.0	E980.4
56:12 cathartics NEC	973.3	E858.4	E943.3	E950.4	E962.0	E980.4
emollients	973.2	E858.4	E943.2	E950.4	E962.0	E980.4
irritants	973.1	E858.4	E943.1	E950.4	E962.0	E980.4
56:16 digestants	973.4	E858.4	E943.4	E950.4	E962.0	E980.4
56:20 emetics and antiemetics						
antiemetics	963.0	E858.1	E933.0	E950.4	E962.0	E980.4
emetics	973.6	E858.4	E943.6	E950.4	E962.0	E980.4
56:24 lipotropic agents	977.1	E858.8	E947.1	E950.4	E962.0	E980.4
56:40 miscellaneous G.I. drugs	973.8	E858.4	E943.8	E950.4	E962.0	E980.4
60:00 gold compounds	965.69	E850.6	E935.6	E950.0	E962.0	E980.0
64:00 heavy metal antagonists	963.8	E858.1	E933.8	E950.4	E962.0	E980.4
68:04 adrenals	962.0	E858.0	E932.0	E950.4	E962.0	E980.4
68:08 androgens	962.1	E858.0	E932.1	E950.4	E962.0	E980.4
68:12 contraceptives, oral	962.2	E858.0	E932.2	E950.4	E962.0	E980.4
68:16 estrogens	962.2	E858.0	E932.2	E950.4	E962.0	E980.4
68:18 gonadotropins	962.4	E858.0	E932.4	E950.4	E962.0	E980.4
68:20.08 insulins	962.3	E858.0	E932.3	E950.4	E962.0	E980.4
68:20 insulins and antidiabetic agents	962.3	E858.0	E932.3	E950.4	E962.0	E980.4
68:24 parathyroid	962.6	E858.0	E932.6	E950.4	E962.0	E980.4
68:28 pituitary (posterior)	962.5	E858.0	E932.5	E950.4	E962.0	E980.4
anterior	962.4	E858.0	E932.4	E950.4	E962.0	E980.4
68:32 progestogens	962.2	E858.0	E932.2	E950.4	E962.0	E980.4
68:34 other corpus luteum hormones NEC	962.2	E858.0	E932.2	E950.4	E962.0	E980.4
68:36 thyroid and antithyroid						
antithyroid	962.8	E858.0	E932.8	E950.4	E962.0	E980.4
thyroid (derivatives)	962.7	E858.0	E932.7	E950.4	E962.0	E980.4
72:00 local anesthetics						
NEC	968.9	E855.2	E938.9	E950.4	E962.0	E980.4
infiltration (intradermal) (subcutaneous) (submucosal)	968.5	E855.2	E938.5	E950.4	E962.0	E980.4
nerve blocking (peripheral) (plexus) (regional)	968.6	E855.2	E938.6	E950.4	E962.0	E980.4
spinal	968.7	E855.2	E938.7	E950.4	E962.0	E980.4
topical (surface)	968.5	E855.2	E938.5	E950.4	E962.0	E980.4
76:00 oxytocics	975.0	E858.6	E945.0	E950.4	E962.0	E980.4
78:00 radioactive agents	990	—	—	—	—	—
80:04 serums NEC	979.9	E858.8	E949.9	E950.4	E962.0	E980.4
immune gamma globulin (human)	964.6	E858.2	E934.6	E950.4	E962.0	E980.4
80:08 toxoids NEC	978.8	E858.8	E948.8	E950.4	E962.0	E980.4
diphtheria	978.5	E858.8	E948.5	E950.4	E962.0	E980.4

Drug — continued	Poisoning	Accident	Therapeutic Use	Suicide Attempt	Assault	Undetermined
80:08 toxoids — continued						
diphtheria — continued						
and diphtheria	978.9	E858.8	E948.9	E950.4	E962.0	E980.4
with pertussis component	978.6	E858.8	E948.6	E950.4	E962.0	E980.4
and tetanus	978.9	E858.8	E948.9	E950.4	E962.0	E980.4
with pertussis component	978.6	E858.8	E948.6	E950.4	E962.0	E980.4
tetanus	978.4	E858.8	E948.4	E950.4	E962.0	E980.4
80:12 vaccines	979.9	E858.8	E949.9	E950.4	E962.0	E980.4
bacterial NEC	978.8	E858.8	E948.8	E950.4	E962.0	E980.4
with						
other bacterial components	978.9	E858.8	E948.9	E950.4	E962.0	E980.4
pertussis component	978.6	E858.8	E948.6	E950.4	E962.0	E980.4
viral and rickettsial components	979.7	E858.8	E949.7	E950.4	E962.0	E980.4
rickettsial NEC	979.6	E858.8	E949.6	E950.4	E962.0	E980.4
with						
bacterial component	979.7	E858.8	E949.7	E950.4	E962.0	E980.4
pertussis component	978.6	E858.8	E948.6	E950.4	E962.0	E980.4
viral component	979.7	E858.8	E949.7	E950.4	E962.0	E980.4
viral NEC	979.6	E858.8	E949.6	E950.4	E962.0	E980.4
with						
bacterial component	979.7	E858.8	E949.7	E950.4	E962.0	E980.4
pertussis component	978.6	E858.8	E948.6	E950.4	E962.0	E980.4
rickettsial component	979.7	E858.8	E949.7	E950.4	E962.0	E980.4
84:04.04 antibiotics (skin and mucous membrane)	976.0	E858.7	E946.0	E950.4	E962.0	E980.4
84:04.08 fungicides (skin and mucous membrane)	976.0	E858.7	E946.0	E950.4	E962.0	E980.4
84:04.12 scabicides and pediculicides (skin and mucous membrane)	976.0	E858.7	E946.0	E950.4	E962.0	E980.4
84:04.16 miscellaneous local anti-infectives (skin and mucous membrane)	976.0	E858.7	E946.0	E950.4	E962.0	E980.4
84:06 anti-inflammatory agents (skin and mucous membrane)	976.0	E858.7	E946.0	E950.4	E962.0	E980.4
84:08 antipruritics and local anesthetics						
antipruritics	976.1	E858.7	E946.1	E950.4	E962.0	E980.4
local anesthetics	968.5	E855.2	E938.5	E950.4	E962.0	E980.4
84:12 astringents	976.2	E858.7	E946.2	E950.4	E962.0	E980.4
84:16 cell stimulants and proliferants	976.8	E858.7	E946.8	E950.4	E962.0	E980.4
84:20 detergents	976.2	E858.7	E946.2	E950.4	E962.0	E980.4
84:24 emollients, demulcents, and protectants	976.3	E858.7	E946.3	E950.4	E962.0	E980.4
84:28 keratolytic agents	976.4	E858.7	E946.4	E950.4	E962.0	E980.4
84:32 keratoplastic agents	976.4	E858.7	E946.4	E950.4	E962.0	E980.4
84:36 miscellaneous agents (skin and mucous membrane)	976.8	E858.7	E946.8	E950.4	E962.0	E980.4
86:00 spasmolytic agents	975.1	E858.6	E945.1	E950.4	E962.0	E980.4
antiasthmatics	975.7	E858.6	E945.7	E950.4	E962.0	E980.4
papaverine	972.5	E858.3	E942.5	E950.4	E962.0	E980.4
theophylline	974.1	E858.5	E944.1	E950.4	E962.0	E980.4
88:04 vitamin A	963.5	E858.1	E933.5	E950.4	E962.0	E980.4
88:08 vitamin B complex	963.5	E858.1	E933.5	E950.4	E962.0	E980.4
hematopoietic vitamin	964.1	E858.2	E934.1	E950.4	E962.0	E980.4
nicotinic acid derivatives	972.2	E858.3	E942.2	E950.4	E962.0	E980.4
88:12 vitamin C	963.5	E858.1	E933.5	E950.4	E962.0	E980.4
88:16 vitamin D	963.5	E858.1	E933.5	E950.4	E962.0	E980.4
88:20 vitamin E	963.5	E858.1	E933.5	E950.4	E962.0	E980.4
88:24 vitamin K activity	964.3	E858.2	E934.3	E950.4	E962.0	E980.4
88:28 multivitamin preparations	963.5	E858.1	E933.5	E950.4	E962.0	E980.4
92:00 unclassified therapeutic agents	977.8	E858.8	E947.8	E950.4	E962.0	E980.4
specified NEC	977.8	E858.8	E947.8	E950.4	E962.0	E980.4
Duboisine	971.1	E855.4	E941.1	E950.4	E962.0	E980.4

Substance	Poisoning	Accident	Therapeutic Use	Suicide Attempt	Assault	Undetermined
Dulcolax	973.1	E858.4	E943.1	E950.4	E962.0	E980.4
Duponol (C) (EP)	976.2	E858.7	E946.2	E950.4	E962.0	E980.4
Durabolin	962.1	E858.0	E932.1	E950.4	E962.0	E980.4
Dyclone	968.5	E855.2	E938.5	E950.4	E962.0	E980.4
Dyclonine	968.5	E855.2	E938.5	E950.4	E962.0	E980.4
Dydrogesterone	962.2	E858.0	E932.2	E950.4	E962.0	E980.4
Dyes NEC	989.89	E866.8	—	E950.9	E962.1	E980.9
diagnostic agents	977.8	E858.8	E947.8	E950.4	E962.0	E980.4
pharmaceutical NEC	977.4	E858.8	E947.4	E950.4	E962.0	E980.4
Dyfols	971.0	E855.3	E941.0	E950.4	E962.0	E980.4
Dymelor	962.3	E858.0	E932.3	E950.4	E962.0	E980.4
Dynamite	989.89	E866.8	—	E950.9	E962.1	E980.9
fumes	987.8	E869.8	—	E952.8	E962.2	E982.8
Dyphylline	975.1	E858.6	E945.1	E950.4	E962.0	E980.4
Ear preparations	976.6	E858.7	E946.6	E950.4	E962.0	E980.4
Echothiophate, ecothiopate	971.0	E855.3	E941.0	E950.4	E962.0	E980.4
Ecstasy	969.72	E854.2	E939.7	E950.3	E962.0	E980.3
Ectylurea	967.8	E852.8	E937.8	E950.2	E962.0	E980.2
Edathamil disodium	963.8	E858.1	E933.8	E950.4	E962.0	E980.4
Edecrin	974.4	E858.5	E944.4	E950.4	E962.0	E980.4
Edetate, disodium (calcium)	963.8	E858.1	E933.8	E950.4	E962.0	E980.4
Edrophonium	971.0	E855.3	E941.0	E950.4	E962.0	E980.4
Elase	976.8	E858.7	E946.8	E950.4	E962.0	E980.4
Elaterium	973.1	E858.4	E943.1	E950.4	E962.0	E980.4
Elder	988.2	E865.4	—	E950.9	E962.1	E980.9
berry (unripe)	988.2	E865.3	—	E950.9	E962.1	E980.9
Electrolytes NEC	974.5	E858.5	E944.5	E950.4	E962.0	E980.4
Electrolytic agent NEC	974.5	E858.5	E944.5	E950.4	E962.0	E980.4
Embramine	963.0	E858.1	E933.0	E950.4	E962.0	E980.4
Emetics	973.6	E858.4	E943.6	E950.4	E962.0	E980.4
Emetine (hydrochloride)	961.5	E857	E931.5	E950.4	E962.0	E980.4
Emollients	976.3	E858.7	E946.3	E950.4	E962.0	E980.4
Emylcamate	969.5	E853.8	E939.5	E950.3	E962.0	E980.3
Encyprate	969.09	E854.0	E939.0	E950.3	E962.0	E980.3
Endocaine	968.5	E855.2	E938.5	E950.4	E962.0	E980.4
Endrin	989.2	E863.0	—	E950.6	E962.1	E980.7
Enflurane	968.2	E855.1	E938.2	E950.4	E962.0	E980.4
Enovid	962.2	E858.0	E932.2	E950.4	E962.0	E980.4
ENT preparations (anti-infectives)	976.6	E858.7	E946.6	E950.4	E962.0	E980.4
Enzodase	963.4	E858.1	E933.4	E950.4	E962.0	E980.4
Enzymes NEC	963.4	E858.1	E933.4	E950.4	E962.0	E980.4
Epanutin	966.1	E855.0	E936.1	E950.4	E962.0	E980.4
Ephedra (tincture)	971.2	E855.5	E941.2	E950.4	E962.0	E980.4
Ephedrine	971.2	E855.5	E941.2	E950.4	E962.0	E980.4
Epiestriol	962.2	E858.0	E932.2	E950.4	E962.0	E980.4
Epilim — see Sodium valproate						
Epinephrine	971.2	E855.5	E941.2	E950.4	E962.0	E980.4
Epsom salt	973.3	E858.4	E943.3	E950.4	E962.0	E980.4
Equanil	969.5	E853.8	E939.5	E950.3	E962.0	E980.3
Equisetum (diuretic)	974.4	E858.5	E944.4	E950.4	E962.0	E980.4
Ergometrine	975.0	E858.6	E945.0	E950.4	E962.0	E980.4
Ergonovine	975.0	E858.6	E945.0	E950.4	E962.0	E980.4
Ergot NEC	988.2	E865.4	—	E950.9	E962.1	E980.9
medicinal (alkaloids)	975.0	E858.6	E945.0	E950.4	E962.0	E980.4
Ergotamine (tartrate) (for migraine) NEC	972.9	E858.3	E942.9	E950.4	E962.0	E980.4
Ergotrate	975.0	E858.6	E945.0	E950.4	E962.0	E980.4
Erythrityl tetranitrate	972.4	E858.3	E942.4	E950.4	E962.0	E980.4
Erythrol tetranitrate	972.4	E858.3	E942.4	E950.4	E962.0	E980.4
Erythromycin	960.3	E856	E930.3	E950.4	E962.0	E980.4
ophthalmic preparation	976.5	E858.7	E946.5	E950.4	E962.0	E980.4
topical NEC	976.0	E858.7	E946.0	E950.4	E962.0	E980.4
Eserine	971.0	E855.3	E941.0	E950.4	E962.0	E980.4
Eskabarb	967.0	E851	E937.0	E950.1	E962.0	E980.1
Eskalith	969.8	E855.8	E939.8	E950.3	E962.0	E980.3
Estradiol (cypionate) (dipropionate) (valerate)	962.2	E858.0	E932.2	E950.4	E962.0	E980.4
Estriol	962.2	E858.0	E932.2	E950.4	E962.0	E980.4
Estrogens (with progestogens)	962.2	E858.0	E932.2	E950.4	E962.0	E980.4
Estrone	962.2	E858.0	E932.2	E950.4	E962.0	E980.4
Etafedrine	971.2	E855.5	E941.2	E950.4	E962.0	E980.4
Ethacrynate sodium	974.4	E858.5	E944.4	E950.4	E962.0	E980.4
Ethacrynic acid	974.4	E858.5	E944.4	E950.4	E962.0	E980.4
Ethambutol	961.8	E857	E931.8	E950.4	E962.0	E980.4
Ethamide	974.2	E858.5	E944.2	E950.4	E962.0	E980.4
Ethamivan	970.0	E854.3	E940.0	E950.4	E962.0	E980.4
Ethamsylate	964.5	E858.2	E934.5	E950.4	E962.0	E980.4
Ethanol	980.0	E860.1	—	E950.9	E962.1	E980.9
beverage	980.0	E860.0	—	E950.9	E962.1	E980.9
Ethchlorvynol	967.8	E852.8	E937.8	E950.2	E962.0	E980.2
Ethebenecid	974.7	E858.5	E944.7	E950.4	E962.0	E980.4
Ether(s) (diethyl) (ethyl) (vapor)	987.8	E869.8	—	E952.8	E962.2	E982.8
anesthetic	968.2	E855.1	E938.2	E950.4	E962.0	E980.4
petroleum — see Ligroin						
solvent	982.8	E862.4	—	E950.9	E962.1	E980.9
Ethidine chloride (vapor)	987.8	E869.8	—	E952.8	E962.2	E982.8
liquid (solvent)	982.3	E862.4	—	E950.9	E962.1	E980.9
Ethinamate	967.8	E852.8	E937.8	E950.2	E962.0	E980.2
Ethinylestradiol	962.2	E858.0	E932.2	E950.4	E962.0	E980.4
Ethionamide	961.8	E857	E931.8	E950.4	E962.0	E980.4
Ethisterone	962.2	E858.0	E932.2	E950.4	E962.0	E980.4
Ethobral	967.0	E851	E937.0	E950.1	E962.0	E980.1
Ethocaine (infiltration) (topical)	968.5	E855.2	E938.5	E950.4	E962.0	E980.4
nerve block (peripheral) (plexus)	968.6	E855.2	E938.6	E950.4	E962.0	E980.4
spinal	968.7	E855.2	E938.7	E950.4	E962.0	E980.4
Ethoheptazine (citrate)	965.7	E850.7	E935.7	E950.0	E962.0	E980.0
Ethopropazine	966.4	E855.0	E936.4	E950.4	E962.0	E980.4
Ethosuximide	966.2	E855.0	E936.2	E950.4	E962.0	E980.4
Ethotoin	966.1	E855.0	E936.1	E950.4	E962.0	E980.4
Ethoxazene	961.9	E857	E931.9	E950.4	E962.0	E980.4
Ethoxzolamide	974.2	E858.5	E944.2	E950.4	E962.0	E980.4
Ethyl						
acetate (vapor)	982.8	E862.4	—	E950.9	E962.1	E980.9
alcohol	980.0	E860.1	—	E950.9	E962.1	E980.9
beverage	980.0	E860.0	—	E950.9	E962.1	E980.9
aldehyde (vapor)	987.8	E869.8	—	E952.8	E962.2	E982.8
liquid	989.89	E866.8	—	E950.9	E962.1	E980.9
aminobenzoate	968.5	E855.2	E938.5	E950.4	E962.0	E980.4
biscoumacetate	964.2	E858.2	E934.2	E950.4	E962.0	E980.4
bromide (anesthetic)	968.2	E855.1	E938.2	E950.4	E962.0	E980.4
carbamate (antineoplastic)	963.1	E858.1	E933.1	E950.4	E962.0	E980.4
carbinol	980.3	E860.4	—	E950.9	E962.1	E980.9
chaulmoograte	961.8	E857	E931.8	E950.4	E962.0	E980.4
chloride (vapor)	987.8	E869.8	—	E952.8	E962.2	E982.8
anesthetic (local)	968.5	E855.2	E938.5	E950.4	E962.0	E980.4
inhaled	968.2	E855.1	E938.2	E950.4	E962.0	E980.4
solvent	982.3	E862.4	—	E950.9	E962.1	E980.9
estranol	962.1	E858.0	E932.1	E950.4	E962.0	E980.4
ether — see Ether(s)						
formate (solvent) NEC	982.8	E862.4	—	E950.9	E962.1	E980.9
iodoacetate	987.5	E869.3	—	E952.8	E962.2	E982.8
lactate (solvent) NEC	982.8	E862.4	—	E950.9	E962.1	E980.9
methylcarbinol	980.8	E860.8	—	E950.9	E962.1	E980.9
morphine	965.09	E850.2	E935.2	E950.0	E962.0	E980.0
Ethylene (gas)	987.1	E869.8	—	E952.8	E962.2	E982.8
anesthetic (general)	968.2	E855.1	E938.2	E950.4	E962.0	E980.4
chlorohydrin (vapor)	982.3	E862.4	—	E950.9	E962.1	E980.9
dichloride (vapor)	982.3	E862.4	—	E950.9	E962.1	E980.9
glycol(s) (any) (vapor)	982.8	E862.4	—	E950.9	E962.1	E980.9
Ethylidene						
chloride NEC	982.3	E862.4	—	E950.9	E962.1	E980.9
diethyl ether	982.8	E862.4	—	E950.9	E962.1	E980.9
Ethynodiol	962.2	E858.0	E932.2	E950.4	E962.0	E980.4
Etidocaine	968.9	E855.2	E938.9	E950.4	E962.0	E980.4
infiltration (subcutaneous)	968.5	E855.2	E938.5	E950.4	E962.0	E980.4
nerve (peripheral) (plexus)	968.6	E855.2	E938.6	E950.4	E962.0	E980.4
Etilfen	967.0	E851	E937.0	E950.1	E962.0	E980.1
Etomide	965.7	E850.7	E935.7	E950.0	E962.0	E980.0
Etorphine	965.09	E850.2	E935.2	E950.0	E962.0	E980.0
Etoval	967.0	E851	E937.0	E950.1	E962.0	E980.1
Etryptamine	969.01	E854.0	E939.0	E950.3	E962.0	E980.3
Eucaine	968.5	E855.2	E938.5	E950.4	E962.0	E980.4
Eucalyptus (oil) NEC	975.5	E858.6	E945.5	E950.4	E962.0	E980.4
Eucatropine	971.1	E855.4	E941.1	E950.4	E962.0	E980.4
Eucodal	965.09	E850.2	E935.2	E950.0	E962.0	E980.0
Euneryl	967.0	E851	E937.0	E950.1	E962.0	E980.1
Euphthalmine	971.1	E855.4	E941.1	E950.4	E962.0	E980.4
Eurax	976.0	E858.7	E946.0	E950.4	E962.0	E980.4
Euresol	976.4	E858.7	E946.4	E950.4	E962.0	E980.4
Euthroid	962.7	E858.0	E932.7	E950.4	E962.0	E980.4
Evans blue	977.8	E858.8	E947.8	E950.4	E962.0	E980.4
Evipal	967.0	E851	E937.0	E950.1	E962.0	E980.1
sodium	968.3	E855.1	E938.3	E950.4	E962.0	E980.4

Nontherapeutic use substance

2011 ICD-9-CM

►◄ Revised Text ● New Line ▲ Revised Code

Subterms under main terms may continue to next column or page

Volume 2 — 311

Dulcolax — Evipal

	Poisoning	Accident	Therapeutic Use	Suicide Attempt	Assault	Undeter-mined
Evipan	967.0	E851	E937.0	E950.1	E962.0	E980.1
sodium	968.3	E855.1	E938.3	E950.4	E962.0	E980.4
Exalgin	965.4	E850.4	E935.4	E950.0	E962.0	E980.0
Excipients, pharmaceuti-cal	977.4	E858.8	E947.4	E950.4	E962.0	E980.4
Exhaust gas — *see* Carbon, monoxide						
Ex-Lax (phenolphthalein)	973.1	E858.4	E943.1	E950.4	E962.0	E980.4
Expectorants	975.5	E858.6	E945.5	E950.4	E962.0	E980.4
External medications (skin) (mucous membrane)	976.9	E858.7	E946.9	E950.4	E962.0	E980.4
dental agent	976.7	E858.7	E946.7	E950.4	E962.0	E980.4
ENT agent	976.6	E858.7	E946.6	E950.4	E962.0	E980.4
ophthalmic preparation	976.5	E858.7	E946.5	E950.4	E962.0	E980.4
specified NEC	976.8	E858.7	E946.8	E950.4	E962.0	E980.4
Eye agents (anti-infec-tive)	976.5	E858.7	E946.5	E950.4	E962.0	E980.4
Factor IX complex (hu-man)	964.5	E858.2	E934.5	E950.4	E962.0	E980.4
Fecal softeners	973.2	E858.4	E943.2	E950.4	E962.0	E980.4
Fenbutrazate	977.0	E858.8	E947.0	E950.4	E962.0	E980.4
Fencamfamin	970.89 ▲	E854.3	E940.8	E950.4	E962.0	E980.4
Fenfluramine	977.0	E858.8	E947.0	E950.4	E962.0	E980.4
Fenoprofen	965.61	E850.6	E935.6	E950.0	E962.0	E980.0
Fentanyl	965.09	E850.2	E935.2	E950.0	E962.0	E980.0
Fentazin	969.1	E853.0	E939.1	E950.3	E962.0	E980.3
Fenticlor, fentichlor	976.0	E858.7	E946.0	E950.4	E962.0	E980.4
Fer de lance (bite) (ven-om)	989.5	E905.0	—	E950.9	E962.1	E980.9
Ferric — *see* Iron						
Ferrocholinate	964.0	E858.2	E934.0	E950.4	E962.0	E980.4
Ferrous fumarate, gluconate, lactate, salt NEC, sulfate (medicinal)	964.0	E858.2	E934.0	E950.4	E962.0	E980.4
Ferrum — *see* Iron						
Fertilizers NEC	989.89	E866.5	—	E950.9	E962.1	E980.4
with herbicide mixture	989.4	E863.5	—	E950.6	E962.1	E980.7
Fibrinogen (human)	964.7	E858.2	E934.7	E950.4	E962.0	E980.4
Fibrinolysin	964.4	E858.2	E934.4	E950.4	E962.0	E980.4
Fibrinolysis-affecting agents	964.4	E858.2	E934.4	E950.4	E962.0	E980.4
Filix mas	961.6	E857	E931.6	E950.4	E962.0	E980.4
Fiorinal	965.1	E850.3	E935.3	E950.0	E962.0	E980.0
Fire damp	987.1	E869.8	—	E952.8	E962.2	E982.8
Fish, nonbacterial or nox-ious	988.0	E865.2	—	E950.9	E962.1	E980.9
shell	988.0	E865.1	—	E950.9	E962.1	E980.9
Flagyl	961.5	E857	E931.5	E950.4	E962.0	E980.4
Flavoxate	975.1	E858.6	E945.1	E950.4	E962.0	E980.4
Flaxedil	975.2	E858.6	E945.2	E950.4	E962.0	E980.4
Flaxseed (medicinal)	976.3	E858.7	E946.3	E950.4	E962.0	E980.4
Flomax	971.3	E855.6	E941.3	E950.4	E962.0	E980.4
Florantyrone	973.4	E858.4	E943.4	E950.4	E962.0	E980.4
Floraquin	961.3	E857	E931.3	E950.4	E962.0	E980.4
Florinef	962.0	E858.0	E932.0	E950.4	E962.0	E980.4
ENT agent	976.6	E858.7	E946.6	E950.4	E962.0	E980.4
ophthalmic preparation	976.5	E858.7	E946.5	E950.4	E962.0	E980.4
topical NEC	976.0	E858.7	E946.0	E950.4	E962.0	E980.4
Flowers of sulfur	976.4	E858.7	E946.4	E950.4	E962.0	E980.4
Floxuridine	963.1	E858.1	E933.1	E950.4	E962.0	E980.4
Flucytosine	961.9	E857	E931.9	E950.4	E962.0	E980.4
Fludrocortisone	962.0	E858.0	E932.0	E950.4	E962.0	E980.4
ENT agent	976.6	E858.7	E946.6	E950.4	E962.0	E980.4
ophthalmic preparation	976.5	E858.7	E946.5	E950.4	E962.0	E980.4
topical NEC	976.0	E858.7	E946.0	E950.4	E962.0	E980.4
Flumethasone	976.0	E858.7	E946.0	E950.4	E962.0	E980.4
Flumethiazide	974.3	E858.5	E944.3	E950.4	E962.0	E980.4
Flumidin	961.7	E857	E931.7	E950.4	E962.0	E980.4
Flunitrazepam	969.4	E853.2	E939.4	E950.3	E962.0	E980.3
Fluocinolone	976.0	E858.7	E946.0	E950.4	E962.0	E980.4
Fluocortolone	962.0	E858.0	E932.0	E950.4	E962.0	E980.4
Fluohydrocortisone	962.0	E858.0	E932.0	E950.4	E962.0	E980.4
ENT agent	976.6	E858.7	E946.6	E950.4	E962.0	E980.4
ophthalmic preparation	976.5	E858.7	E946.5	E950.4	E962.0	E980.4
topical NEC	976.0	E858.7	E946.0	E950.4	E962.0	E980.4
Fluonid	976.0	E858.7	E946.0	E950.4	E962.0	E980.4
Fluopromazine	969.1	E853.0	E939.1	E950.3	E962.0	E980.3
Fluoracetate	989.4	E863.7	—	E950.6	E962.1	E980.7
Fluorescein (sodium)	977.8	E858.8	E947.8	E950.4	E962.0	E980.4
Fluoride(s) (pesticides) (sodi-um) NEC	989.4	E863.4	—	E950.6	E962.1	E980.7

	Poisoning	Accident	Therapeutic Use	Suicide Attempt	Assault	Undeter-mined
Fluoride(s) (pesticides) (sodium) — *continued*						
hydrogen — see Hydrofluoric acid						
medicinal	976.7	E858.7	E946.7	E950.4	E962.0	E980.4
not pesticide NEC	983.9	E864.4	—	E950.7	E962.1	E980.6
stannous	976.7	E858.7	E946.7	E950.4	E962.0	E980.4
Fluorinated corticos-teroids	962.0	E858.0	E932.0	E950.4	E962.0	E980.4
Fluorine (compounds) (gas)	987.8	E869.8	—	E952.8	E962.2	E982.8
salt — see Fluoride(s)						
Fluoristan	976.7	E858.7	E946.7	E950.4	E962.0	E980.4
Fluoroacetate	989.4	E863.7	—	E950.6	E962.1	E980.7
Fluorodeoxyuridine	963.1	E858.1	E933.1	E950.4	E962.0	E980.4
Fluorometholone (topical) NEC	976.0	E858.7	E946.0	E950.4	E962.0	E980.4
ophthalmic preparation	976.5	E858.7	E946.5	E950.4	E962.0	E980.4
Fluorouracil	963.1	E858.1	E933.1	E950.4	E962.0	E980.4
Fluothane	968.1	E855.1	E938.1	E950.4	E962.0	E980.4
Fluoxetine hydrochlo-ride	969.03	E854.0	E939.0	E950.3	E962.0	E980.3
Fluoxymesterone	962.1	E858.0	E932.1	E950.4	E962.0	E980.4
Fluphenazine	969.1	E853.0	E939.1	E950.3	E962.0	E980.3
Fluprednisolone	962.0	E858.0	E932.0	E950.4	E962.0	E980.4
Flurandrenolide	976.0	E858.7	E946.0	E950.4	E962.0	E980.4
Flurazepam (hydrochlo-ride)	969.4	E853.2	E939.4	E950.3	E962.0	E980.3
Flurbiprofen	965.61	E850.6	E935.6	E950.0	E962.0	E980.0
Flurobate	976.0	E858.7	E946.0	E950.4	E962.0	E980.4
Flurothyl	969.8	E855.8	E939.8	E950.3	E962.0	E980.3
Fluroxene	968.2	E855.1	E938.2	E950.4	E962.0	E980.4
Folacin	964.1	E858.2	E934.1	E950.4	E962.0	E980.4
Folic acid	964.1	E858.2	E934.1	E950.4	E962.0	E980.4
Follicle stimulating hor-mone	962.4	E858.0	E932.4	E950.4	E962.0	E980.4
Food, foodstuffs, nonbacteri-al or noxious	988.9	E865.9	—	E950.9	E962.1	E980.9
berries, seeds	988.2	E865.3	—	E950.9	E962.1	E980.9
fish	988.0	E865.2	—	E950.9	E962.1	E980.9
mushrooms	988.1	E865.5	—	E950.9	E962.1	E980.9
plants	988.2	E865.9	—	E950.9	E962.1	E980.9
specified type NEC	988.2	E865.4	—	E950.9	E962.1	E980.9
shellfish	988.0	E865.1	—	E950.9	E962.1	E980.9
specified NEC	988.8	E865.8	—	E950.9	E962.1	E980.9
Fool's parsley	988.2	E865.4	—	E950.9	E962.1	E980.9
Formaldehyde (solution)	989.89	E861.4	—	E950.9	E962.1	E980.9
fungicide	989.4	E863.6	—	E950.6	E962.1	E980.7
gas or vapor	987.8	E869.8	—	E952.8	E962.2	E982.8
Formalin	989.89	E861.4	—	E950.9	E962.1	E980.9
fungicide	989.4	E863.6	—	E950.6	E962.1	E980.7
vapor	987.8	E869.8	—	E952.8	E962.2	E982.8
Formic acid	983.1	E864.1	—	E950.7	E962.1	E980.6
automobile	981	E862.1	—	E950.9	E962.1	E980.9
exhaust gas, not in tran-sit	986	E868.2	—	E952.0	E962.2	E982.0
vapor NEC	987.1	E869.8	—	E952.8	E962.2	E982.8
gas (domestic use) (*see also* Carbon, monoxide, fuel)						
utility	987.1	E868.1	—	E951.8	E962.2	E981.8
incomplete combustion of — see Carbon, monox-ide, fuel, utility						
in mobile container	987.0	E868.0	—	E951.1	E962.2	E981.1
piped (natural)	987.1	E867	—	E951.0	E962.2	E981.0
industrial, incomplete combus-tion	986	E868.3	—	E952.1	E962.2	E982.1
vapor	987.8	E869.8	—	E952.8	E962.2	E982.8
Fowler's solution	985.1	E866.3	—	E950.8	E962.1	E980.8
Foxglove	988.2	E865.4	—	E950.9	E962.1	E980.9
Fox green	977.8	E858.8	E947.8	E950.4	E962.0	E980.4
Framycetin	960.8	E856	E930.8	E950.4	E962.0	E980.4
Frangula (extract)	973.1	E858.4	E943.1	E950.4	E962.0	E980.4
Frei antigen	977.8	E858.8	E947.8	E950.4	E962.0	E980.4
Freons	987.4	E869.2	—	E952.8	E962.2	E982.8
Fructose	974.5	E858.5	E944.5	E950.4	E962.0	E980.4
Frusemide	974.4	E858.5	E944.4	E950.4	E962.0	E980.4
FSH	962.4	E858.0	E932.4	E950.4	E962.0	E980.4
Fuel						
Fugillin	960.8	E856	E930.8	E950.4	E962.0	E980.4
Fulminate of mercury	985.0	E866.1	—	E950.9	E962.1	E980.9
Fulvicin	960.1	E856	E930.1	E950.4	E962.0	E980.4

		External Cause (E-Code)				
	Poisoning	Accident	Therapeutic Use	Suicide Attempt	Assault	Undetermined
Fumadil	960.8	E856	E930.8	E950.4	E962.0	E980.4
Fumagillin	960.8	E856	E930.8	E950.4	E962.0	E980.4
Fumes (from)	987.9	E869.9	—	E952.9	E962.2	E982.9
carbon monoxide — see Carbon, monoxide						
charcoal (domestic use)	986	E868.3	—	E952.1	E962.2	E982.1
chloroform — see Chloroform						
coke (in domestic stoves, fireplaces)	986	E868.3	—	E952.1	E962.2	E982.1
corrosive NEC	987.8	E869.8	—	E952.8	E962.2	E982.8
ether — see Ether(s)						
freons	987.4	E869.2	—	E952.8	E962.2	E982.8
hydrocarbons	987.1	E869.8	—	E952.8	E962.2	E982.8
petroleum (liquefied)	987.0	E868.0	—	E951.1	E962.2	E981.1
distributed through pipes (pure or mixed with air)	987.0	E867	—	E951.0	E962.2	E981.0
lead — see Lead						
metals — see specified metal						
nitrogen dioxide	987.2	E869.0	—	E952.8	E962.2	E982.8
pesticides — see Pesticides						
petroleum (liquefied)	987.0	E868.0	—	E951.1	E962.2	E981.1
distributed through pipes (pure or mixed with air)	987.0	E867	—	E951.0	E962.2	E981.0
polyester	987.8	E869.8	—	E952.8	E962.2	E982.8
specified, source other (see also substance specified)	987.8	E869.8	—	E952.8	E962.2	E982.8
sulfur dioxide	987.3	E869.1	—	E952.8	E962.2	E982.8
Fumigants	989.4	E863.8	—	E950.6	E962.1	E980.7
Fungicides — see also Antifungals	989.4	E863.6	—	E950.6	E962.1	E980.7
Fungi, noxious, used as food	988.1	E865.5	—	E950.9	E962.1	E980.9
Fungizone	960.1	E856	E930.1	E950.4	E962.0	E980.4
topical	976.0	E858.7	E946.0	E950.4	E962.0	E980.4
Furacin	976.0	E858.7	E946.0	E950.4	E962.0	E980.4
Furadantin	961.9	E857	E931.9	E950.4	E962.0	E980.4
Furazolidone	961.9	E857	E931.9	E950.4	E962.0	E980.4
Furnace (coal burning) (domestic), gas from	986	E868.3	—	E952.1	E962.2	E982.1
industrial	986	E868.8	—	E952.1	E962.2	E982.1
Furniture polish	989.89	E861.2	—	E950.9	E962.1	E980.9
Furosemide	974.4	E858.5	E944.4	E950.4	E962.0	E980.4
Furoxone	961.9	E857	E931.9	E950.4	E962.0	E980.4
Fusel oil (amyl) (butyl) (propyl)	980.3	E860.4	—	E950.9	E962.1	E980.9
Fusidic acid	960.8	E856	E930.8	E950.4	E962.0	E980.4
Gallamine	975.2	E858.6	E945.2	E950.4	E962.0	E980.4
Gallotannic acid	976.2	E858.7	E946.2	E950.4	E962.0	E980.4
Gamboge	973.1	E858.4	E943.1	E950.4	E962.0	E980.4
Gamimune	964.6	E858.2	E934.6	E950.4	E962.0	E980.4
Gamma-benzene hexachloride (vapor)	989.2	E863.0	—	E950.6	E962.1	E980.7
Gamma globulin	964.6	E858.2	E934.6	E950.4	E962.0	E980.4
Gamma hydroxy butyrate (GHB)	968.4	E855.1	E938.4	E950.4	E962.0	E980.4
Gamulin	964.6	E858.2	E934.6	E950.4	E962.0	E980.4
Ganglionic blocking agents	972.3	E858.3	E942.3	E950.4	E962.0	E980.4
Ganja	969.6	E854.1	E939.6	E950.3	E962.0	E980.3
Garamycin	960.8	E856	E930.8	E950.4	E962.0	E980.4
ophthalmic preparation	976.5	E858.7	E946.5	E950.4	E962.0	E980.4
topical NEC	976.0	E858.7	E946.0	E950.4	E962.0	E980.4
Gardenal	967.0	E851	E937.0	E950.1	E962.0	E980.1
Gardepanyl	967.0	E851	E937.0	E950.1	E962.0	E980.1
Gas	987.9	E869.9	—	E952.9	E962.2	E982.9
acetylene	987.1	E868.1	—	E951.8	E962.2	E981.8
incomplete combustion of — see Carbon, monoxide, fuel, utility						
air contaminants, source or type not specified	987.9	E869.9	—	E952.9	E962.2	E982.9
anesthetic (general) NEC	968.2	E855.1	E938.2	E950.4	E962.0	E980.4
blast furnace	986	E868.8	—	E952.1	E962.2	E982.1
butane — see Butane						
carbon monoxide — see Carbon, monoxide						
chlorine	987.6	E869.8	—	E952.8	E962.2	E982.8

		External Cause (E-Code)				
	Poisoning	Accident	Therapeutic Use	Suicide Attempt	Assault	Undetermined
Gas — continued						
coal — see Carbon, monoxide, coal						
cyanide	987.7	E869.8	—	E952.8	E962.2	E982.8
dicyanogen	987.8	E869.8	—	E952.8	E962.2	E982.8
domestic — see Gas, utility						
exhaust — see Carbon, monoxide, exhaust gas						
from wood- or coal-burning stove or fireplace	986	E868.3	—	E952.1	E962.2	E982.1
fuel (domestic use) (see also Carbon, monoxide, fuel)						
industrial use	986	E868.8	—	E952.1	E962.2	E982.1
utility	987.1	E868.1	—	E951.8	E962.2	E981.8
incomplete combustion of — see Carbon, monoxide, fuel, utility						
in mobile container	987.0	E868.0	—	E951.1	E962.2	E981.1
piped (natural)	987.1	E867	—	E951.0	E962.2	E981.0
garage	986	E868.2	—	E952.0	E962.2	E982.0
hydrocarbon NEC	987.1	E869.8	—	E952.8	E962.2	E982.8
incomplete combustion of — see Carbon, monoxide, fuel, utility						
liquefied (mobile container)	987.0	E868.0	—	E951.1	E962.2	E981.1
piped	987.0	E867	—	E951.0	E962.2	E981.0
hydrocyanic acid	987.7	E869.8	—	E952.8	E962.2	E982.8
illuminating — see Gas, utility						
incomplete combustion, any — see Carbon, monoxide						
kiln	986	E868.8	—	E952.1	E962.2	E982.1
lacrimogenic	987.5	E869.3	—	E952.8	E962.2	E982.8
marsh	987.1	E869.8	—	E952.8	E962.2	E982.8
motor exhaust, not in transit	986	E868.8	—	E952.1	E962.2	E982.1
mustard — see Mustard, gas						
natural	987.1	E867	—	E951.0	E962.2	E981.0
nerve (war)	987.9	E869.9	—	E952.9	E962.2	E982.9
oils	981	E862.1	—	E950.9	E962.1	E980.9
petroleum (liquefied) (distributed in mobile containers)	987.0	E868.0	—	E951.1	E962.2	E981.1
piped (pure or mixed with air)	987.0	E867	—	E951.1	E962.2	E981.1
piped (manufactured) (natural) NEC	987.1	E867	—	E951.0	E962.2	E981.0
producer	986	E868.8	—	E952.1	E962.2	E982.1
propane — see Propane						
refrigerant (freon)	987.4	E869.2	—	E952.8	E962.2	E982.8
not freon	987.9	E869.9	—	E952.9	E962.2	E982.9
sewer	987.8	E869.8	—	E952.8	E962.2	E982.8
specified source NEC (see also substance specified)	987.8	E869.8	—	E952.8	E962.2	E982.8
stove — see Gas, utility						
tear	987.5	E869.3	—	E952.8	E962.2	E982.8
utility (for cooking, heating, or lighting) (piped) NEC	987.1	E868.1	—	E951.8	E962.2	E981.8
incomplete combustion of — see Carbon, monoxide, fuel, utility						
in mobile container	987.0	E868.0	—	E951.1	E962.2	E981.1
piped (natural)	987.1	E867	—	E951.0	E962.2	E981.0
water	987.1	E868.1	—	E951.8	E962.2	E981.8
incomplete combustion of — see Carbon, monoxide, fuel, utility						
Gaseous substance — see Gas						
Gasoline, gasolene	981	E862.1	—	E950.9	E962.1	E980.9
vapor	987.1	E869.8	—	E952.8	E962.2	E982.8
Gastric enzymes	973.4	E858.4	E943.4	E950.4	E962.0	E980.4
Gastrografin	977.8	E858.8	E947.8	E950.4	E962.0	E980.4
Gastrointestinal agents	973.9	E858.4	E943.9	E950.4	E962.0	E980.4
specified NEC	973.8	E858.4	E943.8	E950.4	E962.0	E980.4
Gaultheria procumbens	988.2	E865.4	—	E950.9	E962.1	E980.9
Gelatin (intravenous)	964.8	E858.2	E934.8	E950.4	E962.0	E980.4
absorbable (sponge)	964.5	E858.2	E934.5	E950.4	E962.0	E980.4
Gelfilm	976.8	E858.7	E946.8	E950.4	E962.0	E980.4
Gelfoam	964.5	E858.2	E934.5	E950.4	E962.0	E980.4
Gelsemine	970.89 ▲	E854.3	E940.8	E950.4	E962.0	E980.4

	Poisoning	Accident	Therapeutic Use	Suicide Attempt	Assault	Undetermined
External Cause (E-Code)						
Gelsemium (semper- virens)	988.2	E865.4	—	E950.9	E962.1	E980.9
Gemonil	967.0	E851	E937.0	E950.1	E962.0	E980.1
Gentamicin	960.8	E856	E930.8	E950.4	E962.0	E980.4
ophthalmic preparation	976.5	E858.7	E946.5	E950.4	E962.0	E980.4
topical NEC	976.0	E858.7	E946.0	E950.4	E962.0	E980.4
Gentian violet	976.0	E858.7	E946.0	E950.4	E962.0	E980.4
Gexane	976.0	E858.7	E946.0	E950.4	E962.0	E980.4
Gila monster (venom)	989.5	E905.0	—	E950.9	E962.1	E980.9
Ginger, Jamaica	989.89	E866.8	—	E950.9	E962.1	E980.9
Gitalin	972.1	E858.3	E942.1	E950.4	E962.0	E980.4
Gitoxin	972.1	E858.3	E942.1	E950.4	E962.0	E980.4
Glandular extract (medicinal) NEC	977.9	E858.9	E947.9	E950.5	E962.0	E980.5
Glaucarubin	961.5	E857	E931.5	E950.4	E962.0	E980.4
Globin zinc insulin	962.3	E858.0	E932.3	E950.4	E962.0	E980.4
Glucagon	962.3	E858.0	E932.3	E950.4	E962.0	E980.4
Glucochloral	967.1	E852.0	E937.1	E950.2	E962.0	E980.2
Glucocorticoids	962.0	E858.0	E932.0	E950.4	E962.0	E980.4
Glucose	974.5	E858.5	E944.5	E950.4	E962.0	E980.4
oxidase reagent	977.8	E858.8	E947.8	E950.4	E962.0	E980.4
Glucosulfone sodium	961.8	E857	E931.8	E950.4	E962.0	E980.4
Glue(s)	989.89	E866.6	—	E950.9	E962.1	E980.9
Glutamic acid (hydrochlo- ride)	973.4	E858.4	E943.4	E950.4	E962.0	E980.4
Glutaraldehyde	989.89	E861.4	—	E950.9	E962.1	E980.9
Glutathione	963.8	E858.1	E933.8	E950.4	E962.0	E980.4
Glutethimide (group)	967.5	E852.4	E937.5	E950.2	E962.0	E980.2
Glycerin (lotion)	976.3	E858.7	E946.3	E950.4	E962.0	E980.4
Glycerol (topical)	976.3	E858.7	E946.3	E950.4	E962.0	E980.4
Glyceryl						
guaiacolate	975.5	E858.6	E945.5	E950.4	E962.0	E980.4
triacetate (topical)	976.0	E858.7	E946.0	E950.4	E962.0	E980.4
trinitrate	972.4	E858.3	E942.4	E950.4	E962.0	E980.4
Glycine	974.5	E858.5	E944.5	E950.4	E962.0	E980.4
Glycobiarsol	961.1	E857	E931.1	E950.4	E962.0	E980.4
Glycols (ether)	982.8	E862.4	—	E950.9	E962.1	E980.9
Glycopyrrolate	971.1	E855.4	E941.1	E950.4	E962.0	E980.4
Glymidine	962.3	E858.0	E932.3	E950.4	E962.0	E980.4
Gold (compounds) (salts)	965.69	E850.6	E935.6	E950.0	E962.0	E980.0
Golden sulfide of antimo- ny	985.4	E866.2	—	E950.9	E962.1	E980.9
Goldylocks	988.2	E865.4	—	E950.9	E962.1	E980.9
Gonadal tissue extract	962.9	E858.0	E932.9	E950.4	E962.0	E980.4
female	962.2	E858.0	E932.2	E950.4	E962.0	E980.4
male	962.1	E858.0	E932.1	E950.4	E962.0	E980.4
Gonadotropin	962.4	E858.0	E932.4	E950.4	E962.0	E980.4
Grain alcohol	980.0	E860.1	—	E950.9	E962.1	E980.9
beverage	980.0	E860.0	—	E950.9	E962.1	E980.9
Gramicidin	960.8	E856	E930.8	E950.4	E962.0	E980.4
Gratiola officinalis	988.2	E865.4	—	E950.9	E962.1	E980.9
Grease	989.89	E866.8	—	E950.9	E962.1	E980.9
Green hellebore	988.2	E865.4	—	E950.9	E962.1	E980.9
Green soap	976.2	E858.7	E946.2	E950.4	E962.0	E980.4
Grifulvin	960.1	E856	E930.1	E950.4	E962.0	E980.4
Griseofulvin	960.1	E856	E930.1	E950.4	E962.0	E980.4
Growth hormone	962.4	E858.0	E932.4	E950.4	E962.0	E980.4
Guaiacol	975.5	E858.6	E945.5	E950.4	E962.0	E980.4
Guaiac reagent	977.8	E858.8	E947.8	E950.4	E962.0	E980.4
Guaifenesin	975.5	E858.6	E945.5	E950.4	E962.0	E980.4
Guaiphenesin	975.5	E858.6	E945.5	E950.4	E962.0	E980.4
Guanatol	961.4	E857	E931.4	E950.4	E962.0	E980.4
Guanethidine	972.6	E858.3	E942.6	E950.4	E962.0	E980.4
Guano	989.89	E866.5	—	E950.9	E962.1	E980.9
Guanochlor	972.6	E858.3	E942.6	E950.4	E962.0	E980.4
Guanoctine	972.6	E858.3	E942.6	E950.4	E962.0	E980.4
Guanoxan	972.6	E858.3	E942.6	E950.4	E962.0	E980.4
Hair treatment agent NEC	976.4	E858.7	E946.4	E950.4	E962.0	E980.4
Halcinonide	976.0	E858.7	E946.0	E950.4	E962.0	E980.4
Halethazole	976.0	E858.7	E946.0	E950.4	E962.0	E980.4
Hallucinogens	969.6	E854.1	E939.6	E950.3	E962.0	E980.3
Haloperidol	969.2	E853.1	E939.2	E950.3	E962.0	E980.3
Haloprogin	976.0	E858.7	E946.0	E950.4	E962.0	E980.4
Halotex	976.0	E858.7	E946.0	E950.4	E962.0	E980.4
Halothane	968.1	E855.1	E938.1	E950.4	E962.0	E980.4
Halquinols	976.0	E858.7	E946.0	E950.4	E962.0	E980.4
Hand sanitizer	976.0	E858.7	E946.0	E950.4	E962.0	E980.4
Harmonyl	972.6	E858.3	E942.6	E950.4	E962.0	E980.4
Hartmann's solution	974.5	E858.5	E944.5	E950.4	E962.0	E980.4
Hashish	969.6	E854.1	E939.6	E950.3	E962.0	E980.3

	Poisoning	Accident	Therapeutic Use	Suicide Attempt	Assault	Undetermined
External Cause (E-Code)						
Hawaiian wood rose seeds	969.6	E854.1	E939.6	E950.3	E962.0	E980.3
Headache cures, drugs, pow- ders NEC	977.9	E858.9	E947.9	E950.5	E962.0	E980.9
Heavenly Blue (morning glo- ry)	969.6	E854.1	E939.6	E950.3	E962.0	E980.3
Heavy metal antagonists	963.8	E858.1	E933.8	E950.4	E962.0	E980.4
anti-infectives	961.2	E857	E931.2	E950.4	E962.0	E980.4
Hedaquinium	976.0	E858.7	E946.0	E950.4	E962.0	E980.4
Hedge hyssop	988.2	E865.4	—	E950.9	E962.1	E980.9
Heet	976.8	E858.7	E946.8	E950.4	E962.0	E980.4
Helenin	961.6	E857	E931.6	E950.4	E962.0	E980.4
Hellebore (black) (green) (white)	988.2	E865.4	—	E950.9	E962.1	E980.9
Hemlock	988.2	E865.4	—	E950.9	E962.1	E980.9
Hemostatics	964.5	E858.2	E934.5	E950.4	E962.0	E980.4
capillary active drugs	972.8	E858.3	E942.8	E950.4	E962.0	E980.4
Henbane	988.2	E865.4	—	E950.9	E962.1	E980.9
Heparin (sodium)	964.2	E858.2	E934.2	E950.4	E962.0	E980.4
Heptabarbital, heptabarbi- tone	967.0	E851	E937.0	E950.1	E962.0	E980.1
Heptachlor	989.2	E863.0	—	E950.6	E962.1	E980.7
Heptalgin	965.09	E850.2	E935.2	E950.0	E962.0	E980.0
Herbicides	989.4	E863.5	—	E950.6	E962.1	E980.7
Heroin	965.01	E850.0	E935.0	E950.0	E962.0	E980.0
Herplex	976.5	E858.7	E946.5	E950.4	E962.0	E980.4
HES	964.8	E858.2	E934.8	E950.4	E962.0	E980.4
Hetastarch	964.8	E858.2	E934.8	E950.4	E962.0	E980.4
Hexachlorocyclohexane	989.2	E863.0	—	E950.6	E962.1	E980.7
Hexachlorophene	976.2	E858.7	E946.2	E950.4	E962.0	E980.4
Hexadimethrine (bro- mide)	964.5	E858.2	E934.5	E950.4	E962.0	E980.4
Hexafluorenium	975.2	E858.6	E945.2	E950.4	E962.0	E980.4
Hexa-germ	976.2	E858.7	E946.2	E950.4	E962.0	E980.4
Hexahydrophenol	980.8	E860.8	—	E950.9	E962.1	E980.9
Hexalin	980.8	E860.8	—	E950.9	E962.1	E980.9
Hexamethonium	972.3	E858.3	E942.3	E950.4	E962.0	E980.4
Hexamethyleneamine	961.9	E857	E931.9	E950.4	E962.0	E980.4
Hexamine	961.9	E857	E931.9	E950.4	E962.0	E980.4
Hexanone	982.8	E862.4	—	E950.9	E962.1	E980.9
Hexapropymate	967.8	E852.8	E937.8	E950.2	E962.0	E980.2
Hexestrol	962.2	E858.0	E932.2	E950.4	E962.0	E980.4
Hexethal (sodium)	967.0	E851	E937.0	E950.1	E962.0	E980.1
Hexetidine	976.0	E858.7	E946.0	E950.4	E962.0	E980.4
Hexobarbital, hexobarbi- tone	967.0	E851	E937.0	E950.1	E962.0	E980.1
sodium (anesthetic)	968.3	E855.1	E938.3	E950.4	E962.0	E980.4
soluble	968.3	E855.1	E938.3	E950.4	E962.0	E980.4
Hexocyclium	971.1	E855.4	E941.1	E950.4	E962.0	E980.4
Hexoestrol	962.2	E858.0	E932.2	E950.4	E962.0	E980.4
Hexone	982.8	E862.4	—	E950.9	E962.1	E980.9
Hexylcaine	968.5	E855.2	E938.5	E950.4	E962.0	E980.4
Hexylresorcinol	961.6	E857	E931.6	E950.4	E962.0	E980.4
Hinkle's pills	973.1	E858.4	E943.1	E950.4	E962.0	E980.4
Histalog	977.8	E858.8	E947.8	E950.4	E962.0	E980.4
Histamine (phosphate)	972.5	E858.3	E942.5	E950.4	E962.0	E980.4
Histoplasmin	977.8	E858.8	E947.8	E950.4	E962.0	E980.4
Holly berries	988.2	E865.3	—	E950.9	E962.1	E980.9
Homatropine	971.1	E855.4	E941.1	E950.4	E962.0	E980.4
Homo-tet	964.6	E858.2	E934.6	E950.4	E962.0	E980.4
Hormones (synthetic substi- tute) NEC	962.9	E858.0	E932.9	E950.4	E962.0	E980.4
adrenal cortical steroids	962.0	E858.0	E932.0	E950.4	E962.0	E980.4
antidiabetic agents	962.3	E858.0	E932.3	E950.4	E962.0	E980.4
follicle stimulating	962.4	E858.0	E932.4	E950.4	E962.0	E980.4
gonadotropic	962.4	E858.0	E932.4	E950.4	E962.0	E980.4
growth	962.4	E858.0	E932.4	E950.4	E962.0	E980.4
ovarian (substitutes)	962.2	E858.0	E932.2	E950.4	E962.0	E980.4
parathyroid (derivatives)	962.6	E858.0	E932.6	E950.4	E962.0	E980.4
pituitary (posterior)	962.5	E858.0	E932.5	E950.4	E962.0	E980.4
anterior	962.4	E858.0	E932.4	E950.4	E962.0	E980.4
thyroid (derivative)	962.7	E858.0	E932.7	E950.4	E962.0	E980.4
Hornet (sting)	989.5	E905.3	—	E950.9	E962.1	E980.9
Horticulture agent NEC	989.4	E863.9	—	E950.6	E962.1	E980.7
Hyaluronidase	963.4	E858.1	E933.4	E950.4	E962.0	E980.4
Hyazyme	963.4	E858.1	E933.4	E950.4	E962.0	E980.4
Hycodan	965.09	E850.2	E935.2	E950.0	E962.0	E980.0
Hydantoin derivatives	966.1	E855.0	E936.1	E950.4	E962.0	E980.4
Hydeltra	962.0	E858.0	E932.0	E950.4	E962.0	E980.4
Hydergine	971.3	E855.6	E941.3	E950.4	E962.0	E980.4
Hydrabamine penicillin	960.0	E856	E930.0	E950.4	E962.0	E980.4

Nontherapeutic use substance

Subterms under main terms may continue to next column or page

		External Cause (E-Code)							External Cause (E-Code)				
	Poisoning	Accident	Therapeutic Use	Suicide Attempt	Assault	Undeter-mined		Poisoning	Accident	Therapeutic Use	Suicide Attempt	Assault	Undeter-mined
Hydralazine, hydral-							**IDU**	976.5	E858.7	E946.5	E950.4	E962.0	E980.4
lazine	972.6	E858.3	E942.6	E950.4	E962.0	E980.4	**Iletin**	962.3	E858.0	E932.3	E950.4	E962.0	E980.4
Hydrargaphen	976.0	E858.7	E946.0	E950.4	E962.0	E980.4	**Ilex**	988.2	E865.4	—	E950.9	E962.1	E980.9
Hydrazine	983.9	E864.3	—	E950.7	E962.1	E980.6	**Illuminating gas** — see Gas,						
Hydriodic acid	975.5	E858.6	E945.5	E950.4	E962.0	E980.4	utility						
Hydrocarbon gas	987.1	E869.8	—	E952.8	E962.2	E982.8	**Ilopan**	963.5	E858.1	E933.5	E950.4	E962.0	E980.4
incomplete combustion of —							**Ilotycin**	960.3	E856	E930.3	E950.4	E962.0	E980.4
see Carbon, monoxide, fu-							ophthalmic preparation	976.5	E858.7	E946.5	E950.4	E962.0	E980.4
el, utility							topical NEC	976.0	E858.7	E946.0	E950.4	E962.0	E980.4
liquefied (mobile contain-							**Imipramine**	969.05	E854.0	E939.0	E950.3	E962.0	E980.3
er)	987.0	E868.0	—	E951.1	E962.2	E981.1	**Immu-G**	964.6	E858.2	E934.6	E950.4	E962.0	E980.4
piped (natural)	987.0	E867	—	E951.0	E962.2	E981.0	**Immuglobin**	964.6	E858.2	E934.6	E950.4	E962.0	E980.4
Hydrochloric acid (liquid)	983.1	E864.1	—	E950.7	E962.1	E980.6	**Immune serum globulin**	964.6	E858.2	E934.6	E950.4	E962.0	E980.4
medicinal	973.4	E858.4	E943.4	E950.4	E962.0	E980.4	**Immunosuppressive**						
vapor	987.8	E869.8	—	E952.8	E962.2	E982.8	agents	963.1	E858.1	E933.1	E950.4	E962.0	E980.4
Hydrochlorothiazide	974.3	E858.5	E944.3	E950.4	E962.0	E980.4	**Immu-tetanus**	964.6	E858.2	E934.6	E950.4	E962.0	E980.4
Hydrocodone	965.09	E850.2	E935.2	E950.0	E962.0	E980.0	**Indandione** (derivatives)	964.2	E858.2	E934.2	E950.4	E962.0	E980.4
Hydrocortisone	962.0	E858.0	E932.0	E950.4	E962.0	E980.4	**Inderal**	972.0	E858.3	E942.0	E950.4	E962.0	E980.4
ENT agent	976.6	E858.7	E946.6	E950.4	E962.0	E980.4	**Indian**						
ophthalmic preparation	976.5	E858.7	E946.5	E950.4	E962.0	E980.4	hemp	969.6	E854.1	E939.6	E950.3	E962.0	E980.3
topical NEC	976.0	E858.7	E946.0	E950.4	E962.0	E980.4	tobacco	988.2	E865.4	—	E950.9	E962.1	E980.9
Hydrocortone	962.0	E858.0	E932.0	E950.4	E962.0	E980.4	**Indigo carmine**	977.8	E858.8	E947.8	E950.4	E962.0	E980.4
ENT agent	976.6	E858.7	E946.6	E950.4	E962.0	E980.4	**Indocin**	965.69	E850.6	E935.6	E950.0	E962.0	E980.0
ophthalmic preparation	976.5	E858.7	E946.5	E950.4	E962.0	E980.4	**Indocyanine green**	977.8	E858.8	E947.8	E950.4	E962.0	E980.4
topical NEC	976.0	E858.7	E946.0	E950.4	E962.0	E980.4	**Indomethacin**	965.69	E850.6	E935.6	E950.0	E962.0	E980.0
Hydrocyanic acid — see							**Industrial**						
Cyanide(s)							alcohol	980.9	E860.9	—	E950.9	E962.1	E980.9
Hydroflumethiazide	974.3	E858.5	E944.3	E950.4	E962.0	E980.4	fumes	987.8	E869.8	—	E952.8	E962.2	E982.8
Hydrofluoric acid (liquid)	983.1	E864.1	—	E950.7	E962.1	E980.6	solvents (fumes) (vapors)	982.8	E862.9	—	E950.9	E962.1	E980.9
vapor	987.8	E869.8	—	E952.8	E962.2	E982.8	**Influenza vaccine**	979.6	E858.8	E949.6	E950.4	E962.0	E982.8
Hydrogen	987.8	E869.8	—	E952.8	E962.2	E982.8	**Ingested substances NEC**	989.9	E866.9	—	E950.9	E962.1	E980.9
arsenide	985.1	E866.3	—	E950.8	E962.1	E980.8	**INH** (isoniazid)	961.8	E857	E931.8	E950.4	E962.0	E980.4
arseniureted	985.1	E866.3	—	E950.8	E962.1	E980.8	**Inhalation, gas** (noxious) —						
cyanide (salts)	989.0	E866.8	—	E950.9	E962.1	E980.9	see Gas						
gas	987.7	E869.8	—	E952.8	E962.2	E982.8	**Ink**	989.89	E866.8	—	E950.9	E962.1	E980.9
fluoride (liquid)	983.1	E864.1	—	E950.7	E962.1	E980.6	**Innovar**	967.6	E852.5	E937.6	E950.2	E962.0	E980.2
vapor	987.8	E869.8	—	E952.8	E962.2	E982.8	**Inositol niacinate**	972.2	E858.3	E942.2	E950.4	E962.0	E980.4
peroxide (solution)	976.6	E858.7	E946.6	E950.4	E962.0	E980.4	**Inproquone**	963.1	E858.1	E933.1	E950.4	E962.0	E980.4
phosphureted	987.8	E869.8	—	E952.8	E962.2	E982.8	**Insecticides** — see also Pesti-						
sulfide (gas)	987.8	E869.8	—	E952.8	E962.2	E982.8	cides	989.4	E863.4	—	E950.6	E962.1	E980.7
arseniureted	985.1	E866.3	—	E950.8	E962.1	E980.8	chlorinated	989.2	E863.0	—	E950.6	E962.1	E980.7
sulfureted	987.8	E869.8	—	E952.8	E962.2	E982.8	mixtures	989.4	E863.3	—	E950.6	E962.1	E980.7
Hydromorphinol	965.09	E850.2	E935.2	E950.0	E962.0	E980.0	organochlorine (com-						
Hydromorphinone	965.09	E850.2	E935.2	E950.0	E962.0	E980.0	pounds)	989.2	E863.0	—	E950.6	E962.1	E980.7
Hydromorphone	965.09	E850.2	E935.2	E950.0	E962.0	E980.0	organophosphorus (com-						
Hydromox	974.3	E858.5	E944.3	E950.4	E962.0	E980.4	pounds)	989.3	E863.1	—	E950.6	E962.1	E980.7
Hydrophilic lotion	976.3	E858.7	E946.3	E950.4	E962.0	E980.4	**Insect (sting), venomous**	989.5	E905.5	—	E950.9	E962.1	E980.9
Hydroquinone	983.0	E864.0	—	E950.7	E962.1	E980.6	**Insular tissue extract**	962.3	E858.0	E932.3	E950.4	E962.0	E980.4
vapor	987.8	E869.8	—	E952.8	E962.2	E982.8	**Insulin** (amorphous) (globin)						
Hydrosulfuric acid (gas)	987.8	E869.8	—	E952.8	E962.2	E982.8	(isophane) (Lente) (NPH)						
Hydrous wool fat (lotion)	976.3	E858.7	E946.3	E950.4	E962.0	E980.4	(protamine) (Semilente) (Ul-						
Hydroxide, caustic	983.2	E864.2	—	E950.7	E962.1	E980.6	tralente) (zinc)	962.3	E858.0	E932.3	E950.4	E962.0	E980.4
Hydroxocobalamin	964.1	E858.2	E934.1	E950.4	E962.0	E980.4	**Intranarcon**	968.3	E855.1	E938.3	E950.4	E962.0	E980.4
Hydroxyamphetamine	971.2	E855.5	E941.2	E950.4	E962.0	E980.4	**Inulin**	977.8	E858.8	E947.8	E950.4	E962.0	E980.4
Hydroxychloroquine	961.4	E857	E931.4	E950.4	E962.0	E980.4	**Invert sugar**	974.5	E858.5	E944.5	E950.4	E962.0	E980.4
Hydroxydihy-							**Inza** — see Naproxen						
drocodeinone	965.09	E850.2	E935.2	E950.0	E962.0	E980.0	**Iodide NEC** — see also Io-						
Hydroxyethyl starch	964.8	E858.2	E934.8	E950.4	E962.0	E980.4	dine	976.0	E858.7	E946.0	E950.4	E962.0	E980.4
Hydroxyphenamate	969.5	E853.8	E939.5	E950.3	E962.0	E980.3	mercury (ointment)	976.0	E858.7	E946.0	E950.4	E962.0	E980.4
Hydroxyphenylbutazone	965.5	E850.5	E935.5	E950.0	E962.0	E980.0	methylate	976.0	E858.7	E946.0	E950.4	E962.0	E980.4
Hydroxyprogesterone	962.2	E858.0	E932.2	E950.4	E962.0	E980.4	potassium (expectorant)						
Hydroxyquinoline deriva-							NEC	975.5	E858.6	E945.5	E950.4	E962.0	E980.4
tives	961.3	E857	E931.3	E950.4	E962.0	E980.4	**Iodinated glycerol**	975.5	E858.6	E945.5	E950.4	E962.0	E980.4
Hydroxystilbamidine	961.5	E857	E931.5	E950.4	E962.0	E980.4	**Iodine** (antiseptic, external)						
Hydroxyurea	963.1	E858.1	E933.1	E950.4	E962.0	E980.4	(tincture) NEC	976.0	E858.7	E946.0	E950.4	E962.0	E980.4
Hydroxyzine	969.5	E853.8	E939.5	E950.3	E962.0	E980.3	diagnostic	977.8	E858.8	E947.8	E950.4	E962.0	E980.4
Hyoscine (hydrobromide)	971.1	E855.4	E941.1	E950.4	E962.0	E980.4	for thyroid conditions (antithy-						
Hyoscyamine	971.1	E855.4	E941.1	E950.4	E962.0	E980.4	roid)	962.8	E858.0	E932.8	E950.4	E962.0	E980.4
Hyoscyamus (albus)							vapor	987.8	E869.8	—	E952.8	E962.2	E982.8
(niger)	988.2	E865.4	—	E950.9	E962.1	E980.9	**Iodized oil**	977.8	E858.8	E947.8	E950.4	E962.0	E980.4
Hypaque	977.8	E858.8	E947.8	E950.4	E962.0	E980.4	**Iodobismitol**	961.2	E857	E931.2	E950.4	E962.0	E980.4
Hypertussis	964.6	E858.2	E934.6	E950.4	E962.0	E980.4	**Iodochlorhydroxyquin**	961.3	E857	E931.3	E950.4	E962.0	E980.4
Hypnotics NEC	967.9	E852.9	E937.9	E950.2	E962.0	E980.2	topical	976.0	E858.7	E946.0	E950.4	E962.0	E980.4
Hypochlorites — see Sodium,							**Iodoform**	976.0	E858.7	E946.0	E950.4	E962.0	E980.4
hypochlorite							**Iodopanoic acid**	977.8	E858.8	E947.8	E950.4	E962.0	E980.4
Hypotensive agents NEC	972.6	E858.3	E942.6	E950.4	E962.0	E980.4	**Iodophthalein**	977.8	E858.8	E947.8	E950.4	E962.0	E980.4
Ibufenac	965.69	E850.6	E935.6	E950.0	E962.0	E980.0	**Ion exchange resins**	974.5	E858.5	E944.5	E950.4	E962.0	E980.4
Ibuprofen	965.61	E850.6	E935.6	E950.0	E962.0	E980.0	**Iopanoic acid**	977.8	E858.8	E947.8	E950.4	E962.0	E980.4
ICG	977.8	E858.8	E947.8	E950.4	E962.0	E980.4	**Iophendylate**	977.8	E858.8	E947.8	E950.4	E962.0	E980.4
Ichthammol	976.4	E858.7	E946.4	E950.4	E962.0	E980.4	**Iothiouracil**	962.8	E858.0	E932.8	E950.4	E962.0	E980.4
Ichthyol	976.4	E858.7	E946.4	E950.4	E962.0	E980.4	**Ipecac**	973.6	E858.4	E943.6	E950.4	E962.0	E980.4
Idoxuridine	976.5	E858.7	E946.5	E950.4	E962.0	E980.4	**Ipecacuanha**	973.6	E858.4	E943.6	E950.4	E962.0	E980.4

Subterms under main terms may continue to next column or page

Substance	Poisoning	Accident	Therapeutic Use	Suicide Attempt	Assault	Undetermined
Ipodate	977.8	E858.8	E947.8	E950.4	E962.0	E980.4
Ipral	967.0	E851	E937.0	E950.1	E962.0	E980.1
Ipratropium	975.1	E858.6	E945.1	E950.4	E962.0	E980.4
Iproniazid	969.01	E854.0	E939.0	E950.3	E962.0	E980.3
Iron (compounds) (medicinal) (preparations)	964.0	E858.2	E934.0	E950.4	E962.0	E980.4
dextran	964.0	E858.2	E934.0	E950.4	E962.0	E980.4
nonmedicinal (dust) (fumes) NEC	985.8	E866.4	—	E950.9	E962.1	E980.9
Irritant drug	977.9	E858.9	E947.9	E950.5	E962.0	E980.5
Ismelin	972.6	E858.3	E942.6	E950.4	E962.0	E980.4
Isoamyl nitrite	972.4	E858.3	E942.4	E950.4	E962.0	E980.4
Isobutyl acetate	982.8	E862.4	—	E950.9	E962.1	E980.9
Isocarboxazid	969.01	E854.0	E939.0	E950.3	E962.0	E980.3
Isoephedrine	971.2	E855.5	E941.2	E950.4	E962.0	E980.4
Isoetharine	971.2	E855.5	E941.2	E950.4	E962.0	E980.4
Isofluorophate	971.0	E855.3	E941.0	E950.4	E962.0	E980.4
Isoniazid (INH)	961.8	E857	E931.8	E950.4	E962.0	E980.4
Isopentaquine	961.4	E857	E931.4	E950.4	E962.0	E980.4
Isophane insulin	962.3	E858.0	E932.3	E950.4	E962.0	E980.4
Isopregnenone	962.2	E858.0	E932.2	E950.4	E962.0	E980.4
Isoprenaline	971.2	E855.5	E941.2	E950.4	E962.0	E980.4
Isopropamide	971.1	E855.4	E941.1	E950.4	E962.0	E980.4
Isopropanol	980.2	E860.3	—	E950.9	E962.1	E980.9
topical (germicide)	976.0	E858.7	E946.0	E950.4	E962.0	E980.4
Isopropyl						
acetate	982.8	E862.4	—	E950.9	E962.1	E980.9
alcohol	980.2	E860.3	—	E950.9	E962.1	E980.9
topical (germicide)	976.0	E858.7	E946.0	E950.4	E962.0	E980.4
ether	982.8	E862.4	—	E950.9	E962.1	E980.9
Isoproterenol	971.2	E855.5	E941.2	E950.4	E962.0	E980.4
Isosorbide dinitrate	972.4	E858.3	E942.4	E950.4	E962.0	E980.4
Isothipendyl	963.0	E858.1	E933.0	E950.4	E962.0	E980.4
Isoxazolyl penicillin	960.0	E856	E930.0	E950.4	E962.0	E980.4
Isoxsuprine hydrochloride	972.5	E858.3	E942.5	E950.4	E962.0	E980.4
l-thyroxine sodium	962.7	E858.0	E932.7	E950.4	E962.0	E980.4
Jaborandi (pilocarpus) (extract)	971.0	E855.3	E941.0	E950.4	E962.0	E980.4
Jalap	973.1	E858.4	E943.1	E950.4	E962.0	E980.4
Jamaica						
dogwood (bark)	965.7	E850.7	E935.7	E950.0	E962.0	E980.0
ginger	989.89	E866.8	—	E950.9	E962.1	E980.9
Jatropha	988.2	E865.4	—	E950.9	E962.1	E980.9
curcas	988.2	E865.3	—	E950.9	E962.1	E980.9
Jectofer	964.0	E858.2	E934.0	E950.4	E962.0	E980.4
Jellyfish (sting)	989.5	E905.6	—	E950.9	E962.1	E980.9
Jequirity (bean)	988.2	E865.3	—	E950.9	E962.1	E980.9
Jimson weed	988.2	E865.4	—	E950.9	E962.1	E980.9
seeds	988.2	E865.3	—	E950.9	E962.1	E980.9
Juniper tar (oil) (ointment)	976.4	E858.7	E946.4	E950.4	E962.0	E980.4
Kallikrein	972.5	E858.3	E942.5	E950.4	E962.0	E980.4
Kanamycin	960.6	E856	E930.6	E950.4	E962.0	E980.4
Kantrex	960.6	E856	E930.6	E950.4	E962.0	E980.4
Kaolin	973.5	E858.4	E943.5	E950.4	E962.0	E980.4
Karaya (gum)	973.3	E858.4	E943.3	E950.4	E962.0	E980.4
Kemithal	968.3	E855.1	E938.3	E950.4	E962.0	E980.4
Kenacort	962.0	E858.0	E932.0	E950.4	E962.0	E980.4
Keratolytics	976.4	E858.7	E946.4	E950.4	E962.0	E980.4
Keratoplastics	976.4	E858.7	E946.4	E950.4	E962.0	E980.4
Kerosene, kerosine (fuel) (solvent) NEC	981	E862.1	—	E950.9	E962.1	E980.9
insecticide	981	E863.4	—	E950.6	E962.1	E980.7
vapor	987.1	E869.8	—	E952.8	E962.2	E982.8
Ketamine	968.3	E855.1	E938.3	E950.4	E962.0	E980.4
Ketobemidone	965.09	E850.2	E935.2	E950.0	E962.0	E980.0
Ketols	982.8	E862.4	—	E950.9	E962.1	E980.9
Ketone oils	982.8	E862.4	—	E950.9	E962.1	E980.9
Ketoprofen	965.61	E850.6	E935.6	E950.0	E962.0	E980.0
Kiln gas or vapor (carbon monoxide)	986	E868.8	—	E952.1	E962.2	E982.1
Konsyl	973.3	E858.4	E943.3	E950.4	E962.0	E980.4
Kosam seed	988.2	E865.3	—	E950.9	E962.1	E980.9
Krait (venom)	989.5	E905.0	—	E950.9	E962.1	E980.9
Kwell (insecticide)	989.2	E863.0	—	E950.6	E962.1	E980.7
anti-infective (topical)	976.0	E858.7	E946.0	E950.4	E962.0	E980.4
Laburnum (flowers)						
(seeds)	988.2	E865.3	—	E950.9	E962.1	E980.9
leaves	988.2	E865.4	—	E950.9	E962.1	E980.9
Lacquers	989.89	E861.6	—	E950.9	E962.1	E980.9
Lacrimogenic gas	987.5	E869.3	—	E952.8	E962.2	E982.8
Lactic acid	983.1	E864.1	—	E950.7	E962.1	E980.6
Lactobacillus acidophilus	973.5	E858.4	E943.5	E950.4	E962.0	E980.4
Lactoflavin	963.5	E858.1	E933.5	E950.4	E962.0	E980.4
Lactuca (virosa) (extract)	967.8	E852.8	E937.8	E950.2	E962.0	E980.2
Lactucarium	967.8	E852.8	E937.8	E950.2	E962.0	E980.2
Laevulose	974.5	E858.5	E944.5	E950.4	E962.0	E980.4
Lanatoside (C)	972.1	E858.3	E942.1	E950.4	E962.0	E980.4
Lanolin (lotion)	976.3	E858.7	E946.3	E950.4	E962.0	E980.4
Largactil	969.1	E853.0	E939.1	E950.3	E962.0	E980.3
Larkspur	988.2	E865.3	—	E950.9	E962.1	E980.9
Laroxyl	969.05	E854.0	E939.0	E950.3	E962.0	E980.3
Lasix	974.4	E858.5	E944.4	E950.4	E962.0	E980.4
Latex	989.82	E866.8	—	E950.9	E962.1	E980.9
Lathyrus (seed)	988.2	E865.3	—	E950.9	E962.1	E980.9
Laudanum	965.09	E850.2	E935.2	E950.0	E962.0	E980.0
Laudexium	975.2	E858.6	E945.2	E950.4	E962.0	E980.4
Laurel, black or cherry	988.2	E865.4	—	E950.9	E962.1	E980.9
Laurolinium	976.0	E858.7	E946.0	E950.4	E962.0	E980.4
Lauryl sulfoacetate	976.2	E858.7	E946.2	E950.4	E962.0	E980.4
Laxatives NEC	973.3	E858.4	E943.3	E950.4	E962.0	E980.4
emollient	973.2	E858.4	E943.2	E950.4	E962.0	E980.4
L-dopa	966.4	E855.0	E936.4	E950.4	E962.0	E980.4
Lead (dust) (fumes) (vapor) NEC	984.9	E866.0	—	E950.9	E962.1	E980.9
acetate (dust)	984.1	E866.0	—	E950.9	E962.1	E980.9
anti-infectives	961.2	E857	E931.2	E950.4	E962.0	E980.4
antiknock compound (tetraethyl)	984.1	E862.1	—	E950.9	E962.1	E980.9
arsenate, arsenite (dust) (insecticide) (vapor)	985.1	E863.4	—	E950.8	E962.1	E980.8
herbicide	985.1	E863.5	—	E950.8	E962.1	E980.8
carbonate	984.0	E866.0	—	E950.9	E962.1	E980.9
paint	984.0	E861.5	—	E950.9	E962.1	E980.9
chromate	984.0	E866.0	—	E950.9	E962.1	E980.9
paint	984.0	E861.5	—	E950.9	E962.1	E980.9
dioxide	984.0	E866.0	—	E950.9	E962.1	E980.9
inorganic (compound)	984.0	E866.0	—	E950.9	E962.1	E980.9
paint	984.0	E861.5	—	E950.9	E962.1	E980.9
iodide	984.0	E866.0	—	E950.9	E962.1	E980.9
pigment (paint)	984.0	E861.5	—	E950.9	E962.1	E980.9
monoxide (dust)	984.0	E866.0	—	E950.9	E962.1	E980.9
paint	984.0	E861.5	—	E950.9	E962.1	E980.9
organic	984.1	E866.0	—	E950.9	E962.1	E980.9
oxide	984.0	E866.0	—	E950.9	E962.1	E980.9
paint	984.0	E861.5	—	E950.9	E962.1	E980.9
paint	984.0	E861.5	—	E950.9	E962.1	E980.9
salts	984.0	E866.0	—	E950.9	E962.1	E980.9
specified compound NEC	984.8	E866.0	—	E950.9	E962.1	E980.9
tetra-ethyl	984.1	E862.1	—	E950.9	E962.1	E980.9
Lebanese red	969.6	E854.1	E939.6	E950.3	E962.0	E980.3
Lente Iletin (insulin)	962.3	E858.0	E932.3	E950.4	E962.0	E980.4
Leptazol	970.0	E854.3	E940.0	E950.4	E962.0	E980.4
Leritine	965.09	E850.2	E935.2	E950.0	E962.0	E980.0
Letter	962.7	E858.0	E932.7	E950.4	E962.0	E980.4
Lettuce opium	967.8	E852.8	E937.8	E950.2	E962.0	E980.2
Leucovorin (factor)	964.1	E858.2	E934.1	E950.4	E962.0	E980.4
Leukeran	963.1	E858.1	E933.1	E950.4	E962.0	E980.4
Levalbuterol	975.7	E858.6	E945.7	E950.4	E962.0	E980.4
Levallorphan	970.1	E854.3	E940.1	E950.4	E962.0	E980.4
Levanil	967.8	E852.8	E937.8	E950.2	E962.0	E980.2
Levarterenol	971.2	E855.5	E941.2	E950.4	E962.0	E980.4
Levodopa	966.4	E855.0	E936.4	E950.4	E962.0	E980.4
Levo-dromoran	965.09	E850.2	E935.2	E950.0	E962.0	E980.0
Levoid	962.7	E858.0	E932.7	E950.4	E962.0	E980.4
Levo-iso-methadone	965.02	E850.1	E935.1	E950.0	E962.0	E980.0
Levomepromazine	967.8	E852.8	E937.8	E950.2	E962.0	E980.2
Levoprome	967.8	E852.8	E937.8	E950.2	E962.0	E980.2
Levopropoxyphene	975.4	E858.6	E945.4	E950.4	E962.0	E980.4
Levorphan, levophanol	965.09	E850.2	E935.2	E950.0	E962.0	E980.0
Levothyroxine (sodium)	962.7	E858.0	E932.7	E950.4	E962.0	E980.4
Levsin	971.1	E855.4	E941.1	E950.4	E962.0	E980.4
Levulose	974.5	E858.5	E944.5	E950.4	E962.0	E980.4
Lewisite (gas)	985.1	E866.3	—	E950.8	E962.1	E980.8
Librium	969.4	E853.2	E939.4	E950.3	E962.0	E980.3
Lidex	976.0	E858.7	E946.0	E950.4	E962.0	E980.4
Lidocaine (infiltration) (topical)	968.5	E855.2	E938.5	E950.4	E962.0	E980.4
nerve block (peripheral) (plexus)	968.6	E855.2	E938.6	E950.4	E962.0	E980.4
spinal	968.7	E855.2	E938.7	E950.4	E962.0	E980.4
Lighter fluid	981	E862.1	—	E950.9	E962.1	E980.9

Nontherapeutic use substance

Subterms under main terms may continue to next column or page

	Poisoning	Accident	Therapeutic Use	Suicide Attempt	Assault	Undeter-mined
External Cause (E-Code)						
Lignocaine (infiltration) (topical)	968.5	E855.2	E938.5	E950.4	E962.0	E980.4
nerve block (peripheral) (plexus)	968.6	E855.2	E938.6	E950.4	E962.0	E980.4
spinal	968.7	E855.2	E938.7	E950.4	E962.0	E980.4
Ligroin(e) (solvent)	981	E862.0	—	E950.9	E962.1	E980.9
vapor	987.1	E869.8	—	E952.8	E962.2	E982.8
Ligustrum vulgare	988.2	E865.3	—	E950.9	E962.1	E980.9
Lily of the valley	988.2	E865.4	—	E950.9	E962.1	E980.9
Lime (chloride)	983.2	E864.2	—	E950.7	E962.1	E980.6
solution, sulferated	976.4	E858.7	E946.4	E950.4	E962.0	E980.4
Limonene	982.8	E862.4	—	E950.9	E962.1	E980.9
Lincomycin	960.8	E856	E930.8	E950.4	E962.0	E980.4
Lindane (insecticide) (vapor)	989.2	E863.0	—	E950.6	E962.1	E980.7
anti-infective (topical)	976.0	E858.7	E946.0	E950.4	E962.0	E980.4
Liniments NEC	976.9	E858.7	E946.9	E950.4	E962.0	E980.4
Linoleic acid	972.2	E858.3	E942.2	E950.4	E962.0	E980.4
Liothyronine	962.7	E858.0	E932.7	E950.4	E962.0	E980.4
Liotrix	962.7	E858.0	E932.7	E950.4	E962.0	E980.4
Lipancreatin	973.4	E858.4	E943.4	E950.4	E962.0	E980.4
Lipo-Lutin	962.2	E858.0	E932.2	E950.4	E962.0	E980.4
Lipotropic agents	977.1	E858.8	E947.1	E950.4	E962.0	E980.4
Liquefied petroleum gases	987.0	E868.0	—	E951.1	E962.2	E981.1
piped (pure or mixed with air)	987.0	E867	—	E951.0	E962.2	E981.0
Liquid petrolatum	973.2	E858.4	E943.2	E950.4	E962.0	E980.4
substance	989.9	E866.9	—	E950.9	E962.1	E980.9
specified NEC	989.89	E866.8	—	E950.9	E962.1	E980.9
Lirugen	979.4	E858.8	E949.4	E950.4	E962.0	E980.4
Lithane	969.8	E855.8	E939.8	E950.3	E962.0	E980.3
Lithium	985.8	E866.4	—	E950.9	E962.1	E980.9
carbonate	969.8	E855.8	E939.8	E950.3	E962.0	E980.3
Lithonate	969.8	E855.8	E939.8	E950.3	E962.0	E980.3
Liver (extract) (injection) (preparations)	964.1	E858.2	E934.1	E950.4	E962.0	E980.4
Lizard (bite) (venom)	989.5	E905.0	—	E950.9	E962.1	E980.9
LMD	964.8	E858.2	E934.8	E950.4	E962.0	E980.4
Lobelia	988.2	E865.4	—	E950.9	E962.1	E980.9
Lobeline	970.0	E854.3	E940.0	E950.4	E962.0	E980.4
Locorten	976.0	E858.7	E946.0	E950.4	E962.0	E980.4
Lolium temulentum	988.2	E865.3	—	E950.9	E962.1	E980.9
Lomotil	973.5	E858.4	E943.5	E950.4	E962.0	E980.4
Lomustine	963.1	E858.1	E933.1	E950.4	E962.0	E980.4
Lophophora williamsii	969.6	E854.1	E939.6	E950.3	E962.0	E980.3
Lorazepam	969.4	E853.2	E939.4	E950.3	E962.0	E980.3
Lotions NEC	976.9	E858.7	E946.9	E950.4	E962.0	E980.4
Lotronex	973.8	E858.4	E943.8	E950.4	E962.0	E980.4
Lotusate	967.0	E851	E937.0	E950.1	E962.0	E980.1
Lowila	976.2	E858.7	E946.2	E950.4	E962.0	E980.4
Loxapine	969.3	E853.8	E939.3	E950.3	E962.0	E980.3
Lozenges (throat)	976.6	E858.7	E946.6	E950.4	E962.0	E980.4
LSD (25)	969.6	E854.1	E939.6	E950.3	E962.0	E980.3
L-Tryptophan — see amino acid						
Lubricating oil NEC	981	E862.2	—	E950.9	E962.1	E980.9
Lucanthone	961.6	E857	E931.6	E950.4	E962.0	E980.4
Luminal	967.0	E851	E937.0	E950.1	E962.0	E980.1
Lung irritant (gas) NEC	987.9	E869.9	—	E952.9	E962.2	E982.9
Lutocylol	962.2	E858.0	E932.2	E950.4	E962.0	E980.4
Lutromone	962.2	E858.0	E932.2	E950.4	E962.0	E980.4
Lututrin	975.0	E858.6	E945.0	E950.4	E962.0	E980.4
Lye (concentrated)	983.2	E864.2	—	E950.7	E962.1	E980.6
Lygranum (skin test)	977.8	E858.8	E947.8	E950.4	E962.0	E980.4
Lymecycline	960.4	E856	E930.4	E950.4	E962.0	E980.4
Lymphogranuloma venereum antigen	977.8	E858.8	E947.8	E950.4	E962.0	E980.4
Lynestrenol	962.2	E858.0	E932.2	E950.4	E962.0	E980.4
Lyovac Sodium Edecrin	974.4	E858.5	E944.4	E950.4	E962.0	E980.4
Lypressin	962.5	E858.0	E932.5	E950.4	E962.0	E980.4
Lysergic acid (amide) (diethylamide)	969.6	E854.1	E939.6	E950.3	E962.0	E980.3
Lysergide	969.6	E854.1	E939.6	E950.3	E962.0	E980.3
Lysine vasopressin	962.5	E858.0	E932.5	E950.4	E962.0	E980.4
Lysol	983.0	E864.0	—	E950.7	E962.1	E980.6
Lytta (vitatta)	976.8	E858.7	E946.8	E950.4	E962.0	E980.4
Mace	987.5	E869.3	—	E952.8	E962.2	E982.8
Macrolides (antibiotics)	960.3	E856	E930.3	E950.4	E962.0	E980.4
Mafenide	976.0	E858.7	E946.0	E950.4	E962.0	E980.4
Magaldrate	973.0	E858.4	E943.0	E950.4	E962.0	E980.4
Magic mushroom	969.6	E854.1	E939.6	E950.3	E962.0	E980.3

	Poisoning	Accident	Therapeutic Use	Suicide Attempt	Assault	Undeter-mined
External Cause (E-Code)						
Magnamycin	960.8	E856	E930.8	E950.4	E962.0	E980.4
Magnesia magma	973.0	E858.4	E943.0	E950.4	E962.0	E980.4
Magnesium (compounds) (fumes) NEC	985.8	E866.4	—	E950.9	E962.1	E980.9
antacid	973.0	E858.4	E943.0	E950.4	E962.0	E980.4
carbonate	973.0	E858.4	E943.0	E950.4	E962.0	E980.4
cathartic	973.3	E858.4	E943.3	E950.4	E962.0	E980.4
citrate	973.3	E858.4	E943.3	E950.4	E962.0	E980.4
hydroxide	973.0	E858.4	E943.0	E950.4	E962.0	E980.4
oxide	973.0	E858.4	E943.0	E950.4	E962.0	E980.4
sulfate (oral)	973.3	E858.4	E943.3	E950.4	E962.0	E980.4
intravenous	966.3	E855.0	E936.3	E950.4	E962.0	E980.4
trisilicate	973.0	E858.4	E943.0	E950.4	E962.0	E980.4
Malathion (insecticide)	989.3	E863.1	—	E950.6	E962.1	E980.7
Male fern (oleoresin)	961.6	E857	E931.6	E950.4	E962.0	E980.4
Mandelic acid	961.9	E857	E931.9	E950.4	E962.0	E980.4
Manganese compounds (fumes) NEC	985.2	E866.4	—	E950.9	E962.1	E980.9
Mannitol (diuretic) (medicinal) NEC	974.4	E858.5	E944.4	E950.4	E962.0	E980.4
hexanitrate	972.4	E858.3	E942.4	E950.4	E962.0	E980.4
mustard	963.1	E858.1	E933.1	E950.4	E962.0	E980.4
Mannomustine	963.1	E858.1	E933.1	E950.4	E962.0	E980.4
MAO inhibitors	969.01	E854.0	E939.0	E950.3	E962.0	E980.3
Mapharsen	961.1	E857	E931.1	E950.4	E962.0	E980.4
Marcaine	968.9	E855.2	E938.9	E950.4	E962.0	E980.4
infiltration (subcutaneous)	968.5	E855.2	E938.5	E950.4	E962.0	E980.4
nerve block (peripheral) (plexus)	968.6	E855.2	E938.6	E950.4	E962.0	E980.4
Marezine	963.0	E858.1	E933.0	E950.4	E962.0	E980.4
Marihuana, marijuana (derivatives)	969.6	E854.1	E939.6	E950.3	E962.0	E980.3
Marine animals or plants (sting)	989.5	E905.6	—	E950.9	E962.1	E980.9
Marplan	969.01	E854.0	E939.0	E950.3	E962.0	E980.3
Marsh gas	987.1	E869.8	—	E952.8	E962.2	E982.8
Marsilid	969.01	E854.0	E939.0	E950.3	E962.0	E980.3
Matulane	963.1	E858.1	E933.1	E950.4	E962.0	E980.4
Mazindol	977.0	E858.8	E947.0	E950.4	E962.0	E980.4
MDMA	969.72	E854.2	E939.7	E950.3	E962.0	E980.3
Meadow saffron	988.2	E865.3	—	E950.9	E962.1	E980.9
Measles vaccine	979.4	E858.8	E949.4	E950.4	E962.0	E980.4
Meat, noxious or nonbacterial	988.8	E865.0	—	E950.9	E962.1	E980.9
Mebanazine	969.01	E854.0	E939.0	E950.3	E962.0	E980.3
Mebaral	967.0	E851	E937.0	E950.1	E962.0	E980.1
Mebendazole	961.6	E857	E931.6	E950.4	E962.0	E980.4
Mebeverine	975.1	E858.6	E945.1	E950.4	E962.0	E980.4
Mebhydroline	963.0	E858.1	E933.0	E950.4	E962.0	E980.4
Mebrophenhydramine	963.0	E858.1	E933.0	E950.4	E962.0	E980.4
Mebutamate	969.5	E853.8	E939.5	E950.3	E962.0	E980.3
Mecamylamine (chloride)	972.3	E858.3	E942.3	E950.4	E962.0	E980.4
Mechlorethamine hydrochloride	963.1	E858.1	E933.1	E950.4	E962.0	E980.4
Meclizene (hydrochloride)	963.0	E858.1	E933.0	E950.4	E962.0	E980.4
Meclofenoxate	970.0	E854.3	E940.0	E950.4	E962.0	E980.4
Meclozine (hydrochloride)	963.0	E858.1	E933.0	E950.4	E962.0	E980.4
Medazepam	969.4	E853.2	E939.4	E950.3	E962.0	E980.3
Medicine, medicinal substance	977.9	E858.9	E947.9	E950.5	E962.0	E980.5
specified NEC	977.8	E858.8	E947.8	E950.4	E962.0	E980.4
Medinal	967.0	E851	E937.0	E950.1	E962.0	E980.1
Medomin	967.0	E851	E937.0	E950.1	E962.0	E980.1
Medroxyprogesterone	962.2	E858.0	E932.2	E950.4	E962.0	E980.4
Medrysone	976.5	E858.7	E946.5	E950.4	E962.0	E980.4
Mefenamic acid	965.7	E850.7	E935.7	E950.0	E962.0	E980.0
Megahallucinogen	969.6	E854.1	E939.6	E950.3	E962.0	E980.3
Megestrol	962.2	E858.0	E932.2	E950.4	E962.0	E980.4
Meglumine	977.8	E858.8	E947.8	E950.4	E962.0	E980.4
Meladinin	976.3	E858.7	E946.3	E950.4	E962.0	E980.4
Melanizing agents	976.3	E858.7	E946.3	E950.4	E962.0	E980.4
Melarsoprol	961.1	E857	E931.1	E950.4	E962.0	E980.4
Melia azedarach	988.2	E865.3	—	E950.9	E962.1	E980.9
Mellaril	969.1	E853.0	E939.1	E950.3	E962.0	E980.3
Meloxine	976.3	E858.7	E946.3	E950.4	E962.0	E980.4
Melphalan	963.1	E858.1	E933.1	E950.4	E962.0	E980.4
Menadiol sodium diphosphate	964.3	E858.2	E934.3	E950.4	E962.0	E980.4
Menadione (sodium bisulfite)	964.3	E858.2	E934.3	E950.4	E962.0	E980.4
Menaphthone	964.3	E858.2	E934.3	E950.4	E962.0	E980.4

Nontherapeutic use substance

Subterms under main terms may continue to next column or page

Index

Meningococcal vaccine — Methyl

	Poisoning	Accident	Therapeutic Use	Suicide Attempt	Assault	Undetermined
Meningococcal vaccine	978.8	E858.8	E948.8	E950.4	E962.0	E980.4
Menningovax-C	978.8	E858.8	E948.8	E950.4	E962.0	E980.4
Menotropins	962.4	E858.0	E932.4	E950.4	E962.0	E980.4
Menthol NEC	976.1	E858.7	E946.1	E950.4	E962.0	E980.4
Mepacrine	961.3	E857	E931.3	E950.4	E962.0	E980.4
Meparfynol	967.8	E852.8	E937.8	E950.2	E962.0	E980.2
Mepazine	969.1	E853.0	E939.1	E950.3	E962.0	E980.3
Mepenzolate	971.1	E855.4	E941.1	E950.4	E962.0	E980.4
Meperidine	965.09	E850.2	E935.2	E950.0	E962.0	E980.0
Mephenamin(e)	966.4	E855.0	E936.4	E950.4	E962.0	E980.4
Mephenesin (carbamate)	968.0	E855.1	E938.0	E950.4	E962.0	E980.4
Mephenoxalone	969.5	E853.8	E939.5	E950.3	E962.0	E980.3
Mephentermine	971.2	E855.5	E941.2	E950.4	E962.0	E980.4
Mephenytoin	966.1	E855.0	E936.1	E950.4	E962.0	E980.4
Mephobarbital	967.0	E851	E937.0	E950.1	E962.0	E980.1
Mepiperphenidol	971.1	E855.4	E941.1	E950.4	E962.0	E980.4
Mepivacaine	968.9	E855.2	E938.9	E950.4	E962.0	E980.4
infiltration (subcutaneous)	968.5	E855.2	E938.5	E950.4	E962.0	E980.4
nerve block (peripheral) (plexus)	968.6	E855.2	E938.6	E950.4	E962.0	E980.4
topical (surface)	968.5	E855.2	E938.5	E950.4	E962.0	E980.4
Meprednisone	962.0	E858.0	E932.0	E950.4	E962.0	E980.4
Meprobam	969.5	E853.8	E939.5	E950.3	E962.0	E980.3
Meprobamate	969.5	E853.8	E939.5	E950.3	E962.0	E980.3
Mepyramine (maleate)	963.0	E858.1	E933.0	E950.4	E962.0	E980.4
Meralluride	974.0	E858.5	E944.0	E950.4	E962.0	E980.4
Merbaphen	974.0	E858.5	E944.0	E950.4	E962.0	E980.4
Merbromin	976.0	E858.7	E946.0	E950.4	E962.0	E980.4
Mercaptomerin	974.0	E858.5	E944.0	E950.4	E962.0	E980.4
Mercaptopurine	963.1	E858.1	E933.1	E950.4	E962.0	E980.4
Mercumatilin	974.0	E858.5	E944.0	E950.4	E962.0	E980.4
Mercuramide	974.0	E858.5	E944.0	E950.4	E962.0	E980.4
Mercuranin	976.0	E858.7	E946.0	E950.4	E962.0	E980.4
Mercurochrome	976.0	E858.7	E946.0	E950.4	E962.0	E980.4
Mercury, mercuric, mercurous (compounds) (cyanide) (fumes) (nonmedicinal) (vapor) NEC	985.0	E866.1	—	E950.9	E962.1	E980.9
ammoniated	976.0	E858.7	E946.0	E950.4	E962.0	E980.4
anti-infective	961.2	E857	E931.2	E950.4	E962.0	E980.4
topical	976.0	E858.7	E946.0	E950.4	E962.0	E980.4
chloride (antiseptic) NEC	976.0	E858.7	E946.0	E950.4	E962.0	E980.4
fungicide	985.0	E863.6	—	E950.6	E962.1	E980.7
diuretic compounds	974.0	E858.5	E944.0	E950.4	E962.0	E980.4
fungicide	985.0	E863.6	—	E950.6	E962.1	E980.7
organic (fungicide)	985.0	E863.6	—	E950.6	E962.1	E980.7
Merethoxylline	974.0	E858.5	E944.0	E950.4	E962.0	E980.4
Mersalyl	974.0	E858.5	E944.0	E950.4	E962.0	E980.4
Merthiolate (topical)	976.0	E858.7	E946.0	E950.4	E962.0	E980.4
ophthalmic preparation	976.5	E858.7	E946.5	E950.4	E962.0	E980.4
Meruvax	979.4	E858.8	E949.4	E950.4	E962.0	E980.4
Mescal buttons	969.6	E854.1	E939.6	E950.3	E962.0	E980.3
Mescaline (salts)	969.6	E854.1	E939.6	E950.3	E962.0	E980.3
Mesoridazine besylate	969.1	E853.0	E939.1	E950.3	E962.0	E980.3
Mestanolone	962.1	E858.0	E932.1	E950.4	E962.0	E980.4
Mestranol	962.2	E858.0	E932.2	E950.4	E962.0	E980.4
Metacresylacetate	976.0	E858.7	E946.0	E950.4	E962.0	E980.4
Metaldehyde (snail killer) NEC	989.4	E863.4	—	E950.6	E962.1	E980.7
Metals (heavy) (nonmedicinal) NEC	985.9	E866.4	—	E950.9	E962.1	E980.9
dust, fumes, or vapor NEC	985.9	E866.4	—	E950.9	E962.1	E980.9
light NEC	985.9	E866.4	—	E950.9	E962.1	E980.9
dust, fumes, or vapor NEC	985.9	E866.4	—	E950.9	E962.1	E980.9
pesticides (dust) (vapor)	985.9	E863.4	—	E950.6	E962.1	E980.7
Metamucil	973.3	E858.4	E943.3	E950.4	E962.0	E980.4
Metaphen	976.0	E858.7	E946.0	E950.4	E962.0	E980.4
Metaproterenol	975.1	E858.6	E945.1	E950.4	E962.0	E980.4
Metaraminol	972.8	E858.3	E942.8	E950.4	E962.0	E980.4
Metaxalone	968.0	E855.1	E938.0	E950.4	E962.0	E980.4
Metformin	962.3	E858.0	E932.3	E950.4	E962.0	E980.4
Methacycline	960.4	E856	E930.4	E950.4	E962.0	E980.4
Methadone	965.02	E850.1	E935.1	E950.0	E962.0	E980.0
Methallenestril	962.2	E858.0	E932.2	E950.4	E962.0	E980.4
Methamphetamine	969.72	E854.2	E939.7	E950.3	E962.0	E980.3
Methandienone	962.1	E858.0	E932.1	E950.4	E962.0	E980.4
Methandriol	962.1	E858.0	E932.1	E950.4	E962.0	E980.4
Methandrostenolone	962.1	E858.0	E932.1	E950.4	E962.0	E980.4
Methane gas	987.1	E869.8	—	E952.8	E962.2	E982.8

	Poisoning	Accident	Therapeutic Use	Suicide Attempt	Assault	Undetermined
Methanol	980.1	E860.2	—	E950.9	E962.1	E980.9
vapor	987.8	E869.8	—	E952.8	E962.2	E982.8
Methantheline	971.1	E855.4	E941.1	E950.4	E962.0	E980.4
Methaphenilene	963.0	E858.1	E933.0	E950.4	E962.0	E980.4
Methapyrilene	963.0	E858.1	E933.0	E950.4	E962.0	E980.4
Methaqualone (compounds)	967.4	E852.3	E937.4	E950.2	E962.0	E980.2
Metharbital, metharbitone	967.0	E851	E937.0	E950.1	E962.0	E980.1
Methazolamide	974.2	E858.5	E944.2	E950.4	E962.0	E980.4
Methdilazine	963.0	E858.1	E933.0	E950.4	E962.0	E980.4
Methedrine	969.72	E854.2	E939.7	E950.3	E962.0	E980.3
Methenamine (mandelate)	961.9	E857	E931.9	E950.4	E962.0	E980.4
Methenolone	962.1	E858.0	E932.1	E950.4	E962.0	E980.4
Methergine	975.0	E858.6	E945.0	E950.4	E962.0	E980.4
Methiacil	962.8	E858.0	E932.8	E950.4	E962.0	E980.4
Methicillin (sodium)	960.0	E856	E930.0	E950.4	E962.0	E980.4
Methimazole	962.8	E858.0	E932.8	E950.4	E962.0	E980.4
Methionine	977.1	E858.8	E947.1	E950.4	E962.0	E980.4
Methisazone	961.7	E857	E931.7	E950.4	E962.0	E980.4
Methitural	967.0	E851	E937.0	E950.1	E962.0	E980.1
Methixene	971.1	E855.4	E941.1	E950.4	E962.0	E980.4
Methobarbital, methobarbitone	967.0	E851	E937.0	E950.1	E962.0	E980.1
Methocarbamol	968.0	E855.1	E938.0	E950.4	E962.0	E980.4
Methohexital, methohexitone (sodium)	968.3	E855.1	E938.3	E950.4	E962.0	E980.4
Methoin	966.1	E855.0	E936.1	E950.4	E962.0	E980.4
Methopholine	965.7	E850.7	E935.7	E950.0	E962.0	E980.0
Methorate	975.4	E858.6	E945.4	E950.4	E962.0	E980.4
Methoserpidine	972.6	E858.3	E942.6	E950.4	E962.0	E980.4
Methotrexate	963.1	E858.1	E933.1	E950.4	E962.0	E980.4
Methotrimeprazine	967.8	E852.8	E937.8	E950.2	E962.0	E980.2
Methoxa-Dome	976.3	E858.7	E946.3	E950.4	E962.0	E980.4
Methoxamine	971.2	E855.5	E941.2	E950.4	E962.0	E980.4
Methoxsalen	976.3	E858.7	E946.3	E950.4	E962.0	E980.4
Methoxybenzyl penicillin	960.0	E856	E930.0	E950.4	E962.0	E980.4
Methoxychlor	989.2	E863.0	—	E950.6	E962.1	E980.7
Methoxyflurane	968.2	E855.1	E938.2	E950.4	E962.0	E980.4
Methoxyphenamine	971.2	E855.5	E941.2	E950.4	E962.0	E980.4
Methoxypromazine	969.1	E853.0	E939.1	E950.3	E962.0	E980.3
Methoxypsoralen	976.3	E858.7	E946.3	E950.4	E962.0	E980.4
Methscopolamine (bromide)	971.1	E855.4	E941.1	E950.4	E962.0	E980.4
Methsuximide	966.2	E855.0	E936.2	E950.4	E962.0	E980.4
Methyclothiazide	974.3	E858.5	E944.3	E950.4	E962.0	E980.4
Methyl						
acetate	982.8	E862.4	—	E950.9	E962.1	E980.9
acetone	982.8	E862.4	—	E950.9	E962.1	E980.9
alcohol	980.1	E860.2	—	E950.9	E962.1	E980.9
amphetamine	969.72	E854.2	E939.7	E950.3	E962.0	E980.3
androstanolone	962.1	E858.0	E932.1	E950.4	E962.0	E980.4
atropine	971.1	E855.4	E941.1	E950.4	E962.0	E980.4
benzene	982.0	E862.4	—	E950.9	E962.1	E980.9
bromide (gas)	987.8	E869.8	—	E952.8	E962.2	E982.8
fumigant	987.8	E863.8	—	E950.6	E962.2	E980.7
butanol	980.8	E860.8	—	E950.9	E962.1	E980.9
carbinol	980.1	E860.2	—	E950.9	E962.1	E980.9
cellosolve	982.8	E862.4	—	E950.9	E962.1	E980.9
cellulose	973.3	E858.4	E943.3	E950.4	E962.0	E980.4
chloride (gas)	987.8	E869.8	—	E952.8	E962.2	E982.8
cyclohexane	982.8	E862.4	—	E950.9	E962.1	E980.9
cyclohexanone	982.8	E862.4	—	E950.9	E962.1	E980.9
dihydromorphinone	965.09	E850.2	E935.2	E950.0	E962.0	E980.0
ergometrine	975.0	E858.6	E945.0	E950.4	E962.0	E980.4
ergonovine	975.0	E858.6	E945.0	E950.4	E962.0	E980.4
ethyl ketone	982.8	E862.4	—	E950.9	E962.1	E980.9
hydrazine	983.9	E864.3	—	E950.7	E962.1	E980.6
isobutyl ketone	982.8	E862.4	—	E950.9	E962.1	E980.9
morphine NEC	965.09	E850.2	E935.2	E950.0	E962.0	E980.0
parafynol	967.8	E852.8	E937.8	E950.2	E962.0	E980.2
parathion	989.3	E863.1	—	E950.6	E962.1	E980.7
pentynol NEC	967.8	E852.8	E937.8	E950.2	E962.0	E980.2
peridol	969.2	E853.1	E939.2	E950.3	E962.0	E980.3
phenidate	969.73	E854.2	E939.7	E950.3	E962.0	E980.3
prednisolone	962.0	E858.0	E932.0	E950.4	E962.0	E980.4
ENT agent	976.6	E858.7	E946.6	E950.4	E962.0	E980.4
ophthalmic preparation	976.5	E858.7	E946.5	E950.4	E962.0	E980.4
topical NEC	976.0	E858.7	E946.0	E950.4	E962.0	E980.4
propylcarbinol	980.8	E860.8	—	E950.9	E962.1	E980.9

Nontherapeutic use substance

▽ Subterms under main terms may continue to next column or page

▶◀ Revised Text　　● New Line　　▲ Revised Code　　2011 ICD-9-CM

External Cause (E-Code)

	Poisoning	Accident	Therapeutic Use	Suicide Attempt	Assault	Undetermined
Methyl — *continued*						
rosaniline NEC	976.0	E858.7	E946.0	E950.4	E962.0	E980.4
salicylate NEC	976.3	E858.7	E946.3	E950.4	E962.0	E980.4
sulfate (fumes)	987.8	E869.8	—	E952.8	E962.2	E982.8
liquid	983.9	E864.3	—	E950.7	E962.1	E980.6
sulfonal	967.8	E852.8	E937.8	E950.2	E962.0	E980.2
testosterone	962.1	E858.0	E932.1	E950.4	E962.0	E980.4
thiouracil	962.8	E858.0	E932.8	E950.4	E962.0	E980.4
Methylated spirit	980.0	E860.1	—	E950.9	E962.1	E980.9
Methyldopa	972.6	E858.3	E942.6	E950.4	E962.0	E980.4
Methylene						
blue	961.9	E857	E931.9	E950.4	E962.0	E980.4
chloride or dichloride (solvent)						
NEC	982.3	E862.4	—	E950.9	E962.1	E980.9
Methylhexabital	967.0	E851	E937.0	E950.1	E962.0	E980.1
Methylparaben (ophthalmic)	976.5	E858.7	E946.5	E950.4	E962.0	E980.4
Methyprylon	967.5	E852.4	E937.5	E950.2	E962.0	E980.2
Methysergide	971.3	E855.6	E941.3	E950.4	E962.0	E980.4
Metoclopramide	963.0	E858.1	E933.0	E950.4	E962.0	E980.4
Metofoline	965.7	E850.7	E935.7	E950.0	E962.0	E980.0
Metopon	965.09	E850.2	E935.2	E950.0	E962.0	E980.0
Metronidazole	961.5	E857	E931.5	E950.4	E962.0	E980.4
Metycaine	968.9	E855.2	E938.9	E950.4	E962.0	E980.4
infiltration (subcutaneous)	968.5	E855.2	E938.5	E950.4	E962.0	E980.4
nerve block (peripheral) (plexus)	968.6	E855.2	E938.6	E950.4	E962.0	E980.4
topical (surface)	968.5	E855.2	E938.5	E950.4	E962.0	E980.4
Metyrapone	977.8	E858.8	E947.8	E950.4	E962.0	E980.4
Mevinphos	989.3	E863.1	—	E950.6	E962.1	E980.7
Mezereon (berries)	988.2	E865.3	—	E950.9	E962.1	E980.9
Micatin	976.0	E858.7	E946.0	E950.4	E962.0	E980.4
Miconazole	976.0	E858.7	E946.0	E950.4	E962.0	E980.4
Midol	965.1	E850.3	E935.3	E950.0	E962.0	E980.0
Mifepristone	962.9	E858.0	E932.9	E950.4	E962.0	E980.4
Milk of magnesia	973.0	E858.4	E943.0	E950.4	E962.0	E980.4
Millipede (tropical) (venomous)	989.5	E905.4	—	E950.9	E962.1	E980.9
Miltown	969.5	E853.8	E939.5	E950.3	E962.0	E980.3
Mineral						
oil (medicinal)	973.2	E858.4	E943.2	E950.4	E962.0	E980.4
nonmedicinal	981	E862.1	—	E950.9	E962.1	E980.9
topical	976.3	E858.7	E946.3	E950.4	E962.0	E980.4
salts NEC	974.6	E858.5	E944.6	E950.4	E962.0	E980.4
spirits	981	E862.0	—	E950.9	E962.1	E980.9
Minocycline	960.4	E856	E930.4	E950.4	E962.0	E980.4
Mithramycin (antineoplastic)	960.7	E856	E930.7	E950.4	E962.0	E980.4
Mitobronitol	963.1	E858.1	E933.1	E950.4	E962.0	E980.4
Mitomycin (antineoplastic)	960.7	E856	E930.7	E950.4	E962.0	E980.4
Mitotane	963.1	E858.1	E933.1	E950.4	E962.0	E980.4
Moderil	972.6	E858.3	E942.6	E950.4	E962.0	E980.4
Mogadon — *see* Nitrazepam						
Molindone	969.3	E853.8	E939.3	E950.3	E962.0	E980.3
Monistat	976.0	E858.7	E946.0	E950.4	E962.0	E980.4
Monkshood	988.2	E865.4	—	E950.9	E962.1	E980.9
Monoamine oxidase inhibitors	969.01	E854.0	E939.0	E950.3	E962.0	E980.3
Monochlorobenzene	982.0	E862.4	—	E950.9	E962.1	E980.9
Monosodium glutamate	989.89	E866.8	—	E950.9	E962.1	E980.9
Monoxide, carbon — *see* Carbon, monoxide						
Moperone	969.2	E853.1	E939.2	E950.3	E962.0	E980.3
Morning glory seeds	969.6	E854.1	E939.6	E950.3	E962.0	E980.3
Moroxydine (hydrochloride)	961.7	E857	E931.7	E950.4	E962.0	E980.4
Morphazinamide	961.8	E857	E931.8	E950.4	E962.0	E980.4
Morphinans	965.09	E850.2	E935.2	E950.0	E962.0	E980.0
Morphine NEC	965.09	E850.2	E935.2	E950.0	E962.0	E980.0
antagonists	970.1	E854.3	E940.1	E950.4	E962.0	E980.4
Morpholinylethylmorphine	965.09	E850.2	E935.2	E950.0	E962.0	E980.0
Morrhuate sodium	972.7	E858.3	E942.7	E950.4	E962.0	E980.4
Moth balls — *see also* Pesticides	989.4	E863.4	—	E950.6	E962.1	E980.7
naphthalene	983.0	E863.4	—	E950.7	E962.1	E980.6
Motor exhaust gas — *see* Carbon, monoxide, exhaust gas						
Mouth wash	976.6	E858.7	E946.6	E950.4	E962.0	E980.4

External Cause (E-Code)

	Poisoning	Accident	Therapeutic Use	Suicide Attempt	Assault	Undetermined
Mucolytic agent	975.5	E858.6	E945.5	E950.4	E962.0	E980.4
Mucomyst	975.5	E858.6	E945.5	E950.4	E962.0	E980.4
Mucous membrane agents						
(external)	976.9	E858.7	E946.9	E950.4	E962.0	E980.4
specified NEC	976.8	E858.7	E946.8	E950.4	E962.0	E980.4
Mumps						
immune globulin (human)	964.6	E858.2	E934.6	E950.4	E962.0	E980.4
skin test antigen	977.8	E858.8	E947.8	E950.4	E962.0	E980.4
vaccine	979.6	E858.8	E949.6	E950.4	E962.0	E980.4
Mumpsvax	979.6	E858.8	E949.6	E950.4	E962.0	E980.4
Muriatic acid — *see* Hydrochloric acid						
Muscarine	971.0	E855.3	E941.0	E950.4	E962.0	E980.4
Muscle affecting agents						
NEC	975.3	E858.6	E945.3	E950.4	E962.0	E980.4
oxytocic	975.0	E858.6	E945.0	E950.4	E962.0	E980.4
relaxants	975.3	E858.6	E945.3	E950.4	E962.0	E980.4
central nervous system	968.0	E855.1	E938.0	E950.4	E962.0	E980.4
skeletal	975.2	E858.6	E945.2	E950.4	E962.0	E980.4
smooth	975.1	E858.6	E945.1	E950.4	E962.0	E980.4
Mushrooms, noxious	988.1	E865.5	—	E950.9	E962.1	E980.9
Mussel, noxious	988.0	E865.1	—	E950.9	E962.1	E980.9
Mustard (emetic)	973.6	E858.4	E943.6	E950.4	E962.0	E980.4
gas	987.8	E869.8	—	E952.8	E962.2	E982.8
nitrogen	963.1	E858.1	E933.1	E950.4	E962.0	E980.4
Mustine	963.1	E858.1	E933.1	E950.4	E962.0	E980.4
M-vac	979.4	E858.8	E949.4	E950.4	E962.0	E980.4
Mycifradin	960.8	E856	E930.8	E950.4	E962.0	E980.4
topical	976.0	E858.7	E946.0	E950.4	E962.0	E980.4
Mycitracin	960.8	E856	E930.8	E950.4	E962.0	E980.4
ophthalmic preparation	976.5	E858.7	E946.5	E950.4	E962.0	E980.4
Mycostatin	960.1	E856	E930.1	E950.4	E962.0	E980.4
topical	976.0	E858.7	E946.0	E950.4	E962.0	E980.4
Mydriacyl	971.1	E855.4	E941.1	E950.4	E962.0	E980.4
Myelobromal	963.1	E858.1	E933.1	E950.4	E962.0	E980.4
Myleran	963.1	E858.1	E933.1	E950.4	E962.0	E980.4
Myochrysin(e)	965.69	E850.6	E935.6	E950.0	E962.0	E980.0
Myoneural blocking agents	975.2	E858.6	E945.2	E950.4	E962.0	E980.4
Myristica fragrans	988.2	E865.3	—	E950.9	E962.1	E980.9
Myristicin	988.2	E865.3	—	E950.9	E962.1	E980.9
Mysoline	966.3	E855.0	E936.3	E950.4	E962.0	E980.4
Nafcillin (sodium)	960.0	E856	E930.0	E950.4	E962.0	E980.4
Nail polish remover	982.8	E862.4	—	E950.9	E962.1	E908.9
Nalidixic acid	961.9	E857	E931.9	E950.4	E962.0	E980.4
Nalorphine	970.1	E854.3	E940.1	E950.4	E962.0	E980.4
Naloxone	970.1	E854.3	E940.1	E950.4	E962.0	E980.4
Nandrolone (decanoate) (phenpropionate)	962.1	E858.0	E932.1	E950.4	E962.0	E980.4
Naphazoline	971.2	E855.5	E941.2	E950.4	E962.0	E980.4
Naphtha (painter's) (petroleum)	981	E862.0	—	E950.9	E962.1	E980.9
solvent	981	E862.0	—	E950.9	E962.1	E980.9
vapor	987.1	E869.8	—	E952.8	E962.2	E982.8
Naphthalene (chlorinated)	983.0	E864.0	—	E950.7	E962.1	E980.6
insecticide or moth repellent	983.0	E863.4	—	E950.7	E962.1	E980.6
vapor	987.8	E869.8	—	E952.8	E962.2	E982.8
Naphthol	983.0	E864.0	—	E950.7	E962.1	E980.6
Naphthylamine	983.0	E864.0	—	E950.7	E962.1	E980.6
Naprosyn — *see* Naproxen						
Naproxen	965.61	E850.6	E935.6	E950.0	E962.0	E980.0
Narcotic (drug)	967.9	E852.9	E937.9	E950.2	E962.0	E980.2
analgesic NEC	965.8	E850.8	E935.8	E950.0	E962.0	E980.0
antagonist	970.1	E854.3	E940.1	E950.4	E962.0	E980.4
specified NEC	967.8	E852.8	E937.8	E950.2	E962.0	E980.2
Narcotine	975.4	E858.6	E945.4	E950.4	E962.0	E980.4
Nardil	969.01	E854.0	E939.0	E950.3	E962.0	E980.3
Natrium cyanide — *see* Cyanide(s)						
Natural						
blood (product)	964.7	E858.2	E934.7	E950.4	E962.0	E980.4
gas (piped)	987.1	E867	—	E951.0	E962.2	E981.0
incomplete combustion	986	E867	—	E951.0	E962.2	E981.0
Nealbarbital, nealbarbitone	967.0	E851	E937.0	E950.1	E962.0	E980.1
Nectadon	975.4	E858.6	E945.4	E950.4	E962.0	E980.4
Nematocyst (sting)	989.5	E905.6	—	E950.9	E962.1	E980.9
Nembutal	967.0	E851	E937.0	E950.1	E962.0	E980.1
Neoarsphenamine	961.1	E857	E931.1	E950.4	E962.0	E980.4

	Poisoning	Accident	Therapeutic Use	Suicide Attempt	Assault	Undetermined
External Cause (E-Code)						
Neocinchophen	974.7	E858.5	E944.7	E950.4	E962.0	E980.4
Neomycin	960.8	E856	E930.8	E950.4	E962.0	E980.4
ENT agent	976.6	E858.7	E946.6	E950.4	E962.0	E980.4
ophthalmic preparation	976.5	E858.7	E946.5	E950.4	E962.0	E980.4
topical NEC	976.0	E858.7	E946.0	E950.4	E962.0	E980.4
Neonal	967.0	E851	E937.0	E950.1	E962.0	E980.1
Neoprontosil	961.0	E857	E931.0	E950.4	E962.0	E980.4
Neosalvarsan	961.1	E857	E931.1	E950.4	E962.0	E980.4
Neosilversalvarsan	961.1	E857	E931.1	E950.4	E962.0	E980.4
Neosporin	960.8	E856	E930.8	E950.4	E962.0	E980.4
ENT agent	976.6	E858.7	E946.6	E950.4	E962.0	E980.4
opthalmic preparation	976.5	E858.7	E946.5	E950.4	E962.0	E980.4
topical NEC	976.0	E858.7	E946.0	E950.4	E962.0	E980.4
Neostigmine	971.0	E855.3	E941.0	E950.4	E962.0	E980.4
Neraval	967.0	E851	E937.0	E950.1	E962.0	E980.1
Neravan	967.0	E851	E937.0	E950.1	E962.0	E980.1
Nerium oleander	988.2	E865.4	—	E950.9	E962.1	E980.9
Nerve gases (war)	987.9	E869.9	—	E952.9	E962.2	E982.9
Nesacaine	968.9	E855.2	E938.9	E950.4	E962.0	E980.4
infiltration (subcutaneous)	968.5	E855.2	E938.5	E950.4	E962.0	E980.4
nerve block (peripheral) (plexus)	968.6	E855.2	E938.6	E950.4	E962.0	E980.4
Neurobarb	967.0	E851	E937.0	E950.1	E962.0	E980.1
Neuroleptics NEC	969.3	E853.8	E939.3	E950.3	E962.0	E980.3
Neuroprotective agent	977.8	E858.8	E947.8	E950.4	E962.0	E980.4
Neutral spirits	980.0	E860.1	—	E950.9	E962.1	E980.9
beverage	980.0	E860.0	—	E950.9	E962.1	E980.9
Niacin, niacinamide	972.2	E858.3	E942.2	E950.4	E962.0	E980.4
Nialamide	969.01	E854.0	E939.0	E950.3	E962.0	E980.3
Nickle (carbonyl) (compounds) (fumes) (tetracarbonyl) (vapor)	985.8	E866.4	—	E950.9	E962.1	E980.9
Niclosamide	961.6	E857	E931.6	E950.4	E962.0	E980.4
Nicomorphine	965.09	E850.2	E935.2	E950.0	E962.0	E980.0
Nicotinamide	972.2	E858.3	E942.2	E950.4	E962.0	E980.4
Nicotine (insecticide) (spray) (sulfate) NEC	989.4	E863.4	—	E950.6	E962.1	E980.7
not insecticide	989.89	E866.8	—	E950.9	E962.1	E980.9
Nicotinic acid (derivatives)	972.2	E858.3	E942.2	E950.4	E962.0	E980.4
Nicotinyl alcohol	972.2	E858.3	E942.2	E950.4	E962.0	E980.4
Nicoumalone	964.2	E858.2	E934.2	E950.4	E962.0	E980.4
Nifenazone	965.5	E850.5	E935.5	E950.0	E962.0	E980.0
Nifuraldezone	961.9	E857	E931.9	E950.4	E962.0	E980.4
Nightshade (deadly)	988.2	E865.4	—	E950.9	E962.1	E980.9
Nikethamide	970.0	E854.3	E940.0	E950.4	E962.0	E980.4
Nilstat	960.1	E856	E930.1	E950.4	E962.0	E980.4
topical	976.0	E858.7	E946.0	E950.4	E962.0	E980.4
Nimodipine	977.8	E858.8	E947.8	E950.4	E962.0	E980.4
Niridazole	961.6	E857	E931.6	E950.4	E962.0	E980.4
Nisentil	965.09	E850.2	E935.2	E950.0	E962.0	E980.0
Nitrates	972.4	E858.3	E942.4	E950.4	E962.0	E980.4
Nitrazepam	969.4	E853.2	E939.4	E950.3	E962.0	E980.3
Nitric						
acid (liquid)	983.1	E864.1	—	E950.7	E962.1	E980.6
vapor	987.8	E869.8	—	E952.8	E962.2	E982.8
oxide (gas)	987.2	E869.0	—	E952.8	E962.2	E982.8
Nitrite, amyl (medicinal) (vapor)	972.4	E858.3	E942.4	E950.4	E962.0	E980.4
Nitroaniline	983.0	E864.0	—	E950.7	E962.1	E980.6
vapor	987.8	E869.8	—	E952.8	E962.2	E982.8
Nitrobenzene, nitrobenzol	983.0	E864.0	—	E950.7	E962.1	E980.6
vapor	987.8	E869.8	—	E952.8	E962.2	E982.8
Nitrocellulose	976.3	E858.7	E946.3	E950.4	E962.0	E980.4
Nitrofuran derivatives	961.9	E857	E931.9	E950.4	E962.0	E980.4
Nitrofurantoin	961.9	E857	E931.9	E950.4	E962.0	E980.4
Nitrofurazone	976.0	E858.7	E946.0	E950.4	E962.0	E980.4
Nitrogen (dioxide) (gas) (oxide)	987.2	E869.0	—	E952.8	E962.2	E982.8
mustard (antineoplastic)	963.1	E858.1	E933.1	E950.4	E962.0	E980.4
nonmedicinal	989.89	E866.8	—	E950.9	E962.1	E980.9
fumes	987.8	E869.0	—	E952.8	E962.2	E982.8
Nitroglycerin, nitroglycerol (medicinal)	972.4	E858.3	E942.4	E950.4	E962.0	E980.4
Nitrohydrochloric acid	983.1	E864.1	—	E950.7	E962.1	E980.6
Nitromersol	976.0	E858.7	E946.0	E950.4	E962.0	E980.4
Nitronaphthalene	983.0	E864.0	—	E950.7	E962.2	E980.6
Nitrophenol	983.0	E864.0	—	E950.7	E962.2	E980.6
Nitrothiazol	961.6	E857	E931.6	E950.4	E962.0	E980.4
Nitrotoluene, nitrotoluol	983.0	E864.0	—	E950.7	E962.1	E980.6

	Poisoning	Accident	Therapeutic Use	Suicide Attempt	Assault	Undetermined
External Cause (E-Code)						
Nitrotoluene, nitrotoluol — *continued*						
vapor	987.8	E869.8	—	E952.8	E962.2	E982.8
Nitrous	968.2	E855.1	E938.2	E950.4	E962.0	E980.4
acid (liquid)	983.1	E864.1	—	E950.7	E962.1	E980.6
fumes	987.2	E869.0	—	E952.8	E962.2	E982.8
oxide (anesthetic) NEC	968.2	E855.1	E938.2	E950.4	E962.0	E980.4
Nitrozone	976.0	E858.7	E946.0	E950.4	E962.0	E980.4
Noctec	967.1	E852.0	E937.1	E950.2	E962.0	E980.2
Noludar	967.5	E852.4	E937.5	E950.2	E962.0	E980.2
Noptil	967.0	E851	E937.0	E950.1	E962.0	E980.1
Noradrenalin	971.2	E855.5	E941.2	E950.4	E962.0	E980.4
Noramidopyrine	965.5	E850.5	E935.5	E950.0	E962.0	E980.0
Norepinephrine	971.2	E855.5	E941.2	E950.4	E962.0	E980.4
Norethandrolone	962.1	E858.0	E932.1	E950.4	E962.0	E980.4
Norethindrone	962.2	E858.0	E932.2	E950.4	E962.0	E980.4
Norethisterone	962.2	E858.0	E932.2	E950.4	E962.0	E980.4
Norethynodrel	962.2	E858.0	E932.2	E950.4	E962.0	E980.4
Norlestrin	962.2	E858.0	E932.2	E950.4	E962.0	E980.4
Norlutin	962.2	E858.0	E932.2	E950.4	E962.0	E980.4
Normison — see Benzodiazepines						
Normorphine	965.09	E850.2	E935.2	E950.0	E962.0	E980.0
Nortriptyline	969.05	E854.0	E939.0	E950.3	E962.0	E980.3
Noscapine	975.4	E858.6	E945.4	E950.4	E962.0	E980.4
Nose preparations	976.6	E858.7	E946.6	E950.4	E962.0	E980.4
Novobiocin	960.8	E856	E930.8	E950.4	E962.0	E980.4
Novocain (infiltration) (topical)	968.5	E855.2	E938.5	E950.4	E962.0	E980.4
nerve block (peripheral) (plexus)	968.6	E855.2	E938.6	E950.4	E962.0	E980.4
spinal	968.7	E855.2	E938.7	E950.4	E962.0	E980.4
Noxythiolin	961.9	E857	E931.9	E950.4	E962.0	E980.4
NPH Iletin (insulin)	962.3	E858.0	E932.3	E950.4	E962.0	E980.4
Numorphan	965.09	E850.2	E935.2	E950.0	E962.0	E980.0
Nunol	967.0	E851	E937.0	E950.1	E962.0	E980.1
Nupercaine (spinal anesthetic)	968.7	E855.2	E938.7	E950.4	E962.0	E980.4
topical (surface)	968.5	E855.2	E938.5	E950.4	E962.0	E980.4
Nutmeg oil (liniment)	976.3	E858.7	E946.3	E950.4	E962.0	E980.4
Nux vomica	989.1	E863.7	—	E950.6	E962.1	E980.7
Nydrazid	961.8	E857	E931.8	E950.4	E962.0	E980.4
Nylidrin	971.2	E855.5	E941.2	E950.4	E962.0	E980.4
Nystatin	960.1	E856	E930.1	E950.4	E962.0	E980.4
topical	976.0	E858.7	E946.0	E950.4	E962.0	E980.4
Nytol	963.0	E858.1	E933.0	E950.4	E962.0	E980.4
Oblivion	967.8	E852.8	E937.8	E950.2	E962.0	E980.2
Octyl nitrite	972.4	E858.3	E942.4	E950.4	E962.0	Chemical.4
Oestradiol (cypionate) (dipropionate) (valerate)	962.2	E858.0	E932.2	E950.4	E962.0	E980.4
Oestriol	962.2	E858.0	E932.2	E950.4	E962.0	E980.4
Oestrone	962.2	E858.0	E932.2	E950.4	E962.0	E980.4
Oil (of) NEC	989.89	E866.8	—	E950.9	E962.1	E980.9
bitter almond	989.0	E866.8	—	E950.9	E962.1	E980.9
camphor	976.1	E858.7	E946.1	E950.4	E962.0	E980.4
colors	989.89	E861.6	—	E950.9	E962.1	E980.9
fumes	987.8	E869.8	—	E952.8	E962.2	E982.8
lubricating	981	E862.2	—	E950.9	E962.1	E980.9
specified source, other — see substance specified						
vitriol (liquid)	983.1	E864.1	—	E950.7	E962.1	E980.6
fumes	987.8	E869.8	—	E952.8	E962.2	E982.8
wintergreen (bitter) NEC	976.3	E858.7	E946.3	E950.4	E962.0	E980.4
Ointments NEC	976.9	E858.7	E946.9	E950.4	E962.0	E980.4
Oleander	988.2	E865.4	—	E950.9	E962.1	E980.9
Oleandomycin	960.3	E856	E930.3	E950.4	E962.0	E980.4
Oleovitamin A	963.5	E858.1	E933.5	E950.4	E962.0	E980.4
Oleum ricini	973.1	E858.4	E943.1	E950.4	E962.0	E980.4
Olive oil (medicinal) NEC	973.2	E858.4	E943.2	E950.4	E962.0	E980.4
OMPA	989.3	E863.1	—	E950.6	E962.1	E980.7
Oncovin	963.1	E858.1	E933.1	E950.4	E962.0	E980.4
Ophthaine	968.5	E855.2	E938.5	E950.4	E962.0	E980.4
Ophthetic	968.5	E855.2	E938.5	E950.4	E962.0	E980.4
Opiates, opioids, opium NEC	965.00	E850.2	E935.2	E950.0	E962.0	E980.0
antagonists	970.1	E854.3	E940.1	E950.4	E962.0	E980.4
Oracon	962.2	E858.0	E932.2	E950.4	E962.0	E980.4
Oragrafin	977.8	E858.8	E947.8	E950.4	E962.0	E980.4
Oral contraceptives	962.2	E858.0	E932.2	E950.4	E962.0	E980.4
Orciprenaline	975.1	E858.6	E945.1	E950.4	E962.0	E980.4
Organidin	975.5	E858.6	E945.5	E950.4	E962.0	Chemical.4
Organophosphates	989.3	E863.1	—	E950.6	E962.1	E980.7

Subterms under main terms may continue to next column or page

	Poisoning	Accident	Therapeutic Use	Suicide Attempt	Assault	Undetermined
Orimune	979.5	E858.8	E949.5	E950.4	E962.0	E980.4
Orinase	962.3	E858.0	E932.3	E950.4	E962.0	E980.4
Orphenadrine	966.4	E855.0	E936.4	E950.4	E962.0	E980.4
Ortal (sodium)	967.0	E851	E937.0	E950.1	E962.0	E980.1
Orthoboric acid	976.0	E858.7	E946.0	E950.4	E962.0	E980.4
ENT agent	976.6	E858.7	E946.6	E950.4	E962.0	E980.4
ophthalmic preparation	976.5	E858.7	E946.5	E950.4	E962.0	E980.4
Orthocaine	968.5	E855.2	E938.5	E950.4	E962.0	E980.4
Ortho-Novum	962.2	E858.0	E932.2	E950.4	E962.0	E980.4
Orthotolidine (reagent)	977.8	E858.8	E947.8	E950.4	E962.0	E980.4
Osmic acid (liquid)	983.1	E864.1	—	E950.7	E962.1	E980.6
fumes	987.8	E869.8	—	E952.8	E962.2	E982.8
Osmotic diuretics	974.4	E858.5	E944.4	E950.4	E962.0	E980.4
Ouabain	972.1	E858.3	E942.1	E950.4	E962.0	E980.4
Ovarian hormones (synthetic substitutes)	962.2	E858.0	E932.2	E950.4	E962.0	E980.4
Ovral	962.2	E858.0	E932.2	E950.4	E962.0	E980.4
Ovulation suppressants	962.2	E858.0	E932.2	E950.4	E962.0	E980.4
Ovulen	962.2	E858.0	E932.2	E950.4	E962.0	E980.4
Oxacillin (sodium)	960.0	E856	E930.0	E950.4	E962.0	E980.4
Oxalic acid	983.1	E864.1	—	E950.7	E962.1	E980.6
Oxanamide	969.5	E853.8	E939.5	E950.3	E962.0	E980.3
Oxandrolone	962.1	E858.0	E932.1	E950.4	E962.0	E980.4
Oxaprozin	965.61	E850.6	E935.6	E950.0	E962.0	E980.0
Oxazepam	969.4	E853.2	E939.4	E950.3	E962.0	E980.3
Oxazolidine derivatives	966.0	E855.0	E936.0	E950.4	E962.0	E980.4
Ox bile extract	973.4	E858.4	E943.4	E950.4	E962.0	E980.4
Oxedrine	971.2	E855.5	E941.2	E950.4	E962.0	E980.4
Oxeladin	975.4	E858.6	E945.4	E950.4	E962.0	E980.4
Oxethazaine NEC	968.5	E855.2	E938.5	E950.4	E962.0	E980.4
Oxidizing agents NEC	983.9	E864.3	—	E950.7	E962.1	E980.6
Oxolinic acid	961.3	E857	E931.3	E950.4	E962.0	E980.4
Oxophenarsine	961.1	E857	E931.1	E950.4	E962.0	E980.4
Oxsoralen	976.3	E858.7	E946.3	E950.4	E962.0	E980.4
Oxtriphylline	975.7	E858.6	E945.7	E950.4	E962.0	E980.4
Oxybuprocaine	968.5	E855.2	E938.5	E950.4	E962.0	E980.4
Oxybutynin	975.1	E858.6	E945.1	E950.4	E962.0	E980.4
Oxycodone	965.09	E850.2	E935.2	E950.0	E962.0	E980.0
Oxygen	987.8	E869.8	—	E952.8	E962.2	E982.8
Oxylone	976.0	E858.7	E946.0	E950.4	E962.0	E980.4
ophthalmic preparation	976.5	E858.7	E946.5	E950.4	E962.0	E980.4
Oxymesterone	962.1	E858.0	E932.1	E950.4	E962.0	E980.4
Oxymetazoline	971.2	E855.5	E941.2	E950.4	E962.0	E980.4
Oxymetholone	962.1	E858.0	E932.1	E950.4	E962.0	E980.4
Oxymorphone	965.09	E850.2	E935.2	E950.0	E962.0	E980.0
Oxypertine	969.09	E854.0	E939.0	E950.3	E962.0	E980.3
Oxyphenbutazone	965.5	E850.5	E935.5	E950.0	E962.0	E980.0
Oxyphencyclimine	971.1	E855.4	E941.1	E950.4	E962.0	E980.4
Oxyphenisatin	973.1	E858.4	E943.1	E950.4	E962.0	E980.4
Oxyphenonium	971.1	E855.4	E941.1	E950.4	E962.0	E980.4
Oxyquinoline	961.3	E857	E931.3	E950.4	E962.0	E980.4
Oxytetracycline	960.4	E856	E930.4	E950.4	E962.0	E980.4
Oxytocics	975.0	E858.6	E945.0	E950.4	E962.0	E980.4
Oxytocin	975.0	E858.6	E945.0	E950.4	E962.0	E980.4
Ozone	987.8	E869.8	—	E952.8	E962.2	E982.8
PABA	976.3	E858.7	E946.3	E950.4	E962.0	E980.4
Packed red cells	964.7	E858.2	E934.7	E950.4	E962.0	E980.4
Paint NEC	989.89	E861.6	—	E950.9	E962.1	E980.9
cleaner	982.8	E862.9	—	E950.9	E962.1	E980.9
fumes NEC	987.8	E869.8	—	E952.8	E962.1	E982.8
lead (fumes)	984.0	E861.5	—	E950.9	E962.1	E980.9
solvent NEC	982.8	E862.9	—	E950.9	E962.1	E980.9
stripper	982.8	E862.9	—	E950.9	E962.1	E980.9
Palfium	965.09	E850.2	E935.2	E950.0	E962.0	E980.0
Palivizumab	979.9	E858.8	E949.6	E950.4	E962.0	E980.4
Paludrine	961.4	E857	E931.4	E950.4	E962.0	E980.4
PAM	977.2	E855.8	E947.2	E950.4	E962.0	E980.4
Pamaquine (naphthoate)	961.4	E857	E931.4	E950.4	E962.0	E980.4
Pamprin	965.1	E850.3	E935.3	E950.0	E962.0	E980.0
Panadol	965.4	E850.4	E935.4	E950.0	E962.0	E980.0
Pancreatic dornase (mucolytic)	963.4	E858.1	E933.4	E950.4	E962.0	E980.4
Pancreatin	973.4	E858.4	E943.4	E950.4	E962.0	E980.4
Pancrelipase	973.4	E858.4	E943.4	E950.4	E962.0	E980.4
Pangamic acid	963.5	E858.1	E933.5	E950.4	E962.0	E980.4
Panthenol	963.5	E858.1	E933.5	E950.4	E962.0	E980.4
topical	976.8	E858.7	E946.8	E950.4	E962.0	E980.4
Pantopaque	977.8	E858.8	E947.8	E950.4	E962.0	E980.4
Pantopon	965.00	E850.2	E935.2	E950.0	E962.0	E980.0
Pantothenic acid	963.5	E858.1	E933.5	E950.4	E962.0	E980.4
Panwarfin	964.2	E858.2	E934.2	E950.4	E962.0	E980.4
Papain	973.4	E858.4	E943.4	E950.4	E962.0	E980.4
Papaverine	972.5	E858.3	E942.5	E950.4	E962.0	E980.4
Para-aminobenzoic acid	976.3	E858.7	E946.3	E950.4	E962.0	E980.4
Para-aminophenol derivatives	965.4	E850.4	E935.4	E950.0	E962.0	E980.0
Para-aminosalicylic acid (derivatives)	961.8	E857	E931.8	E950.4	E962.0	E980.4
Paracetaldehyde (medicinal)	967.2	E852.1	E937.2	E950.2	E962.0	E980.2
Paracetamol	965.4	E850.4	E935.4	E950.0	E962.0	E980.0
Paracodin	965.09	E850.2	E935.2	E950.0	E962.0	E980.0
Paradione	966.0	E855.0	E936.0	E950.4	E962.0	E980.4
Paraffin(s) (wax)	981	E862.3	—	E950.9	E962.1	E980.9
liquid (medicinal)	973.2	E858.4	E943.2	E950.4	E962.0	E980.4
nonmedicinal (oil)	981	E962.1	—	E950.9	E962.1	E980.9
Paraldehyde (medicinal)	967.2	E852.1	E937.2	E950.2	E962.0	E980.2
Paramethadione	966.0	E855.0	E936.0	E950.4	E962.0	E980.4
Paramethasone	962.0	E858.0	E932.0	E950.4	E962.0	E980.4
Paraquat	989.4	E863.5	—	E950.6	E962.1	E980.7
Parasympatholytics	971.1	E855.4	E941.1	E950.4	E962.0	E980.4
Parasympathomimetics	971.0	E855.3	E941.0	E950.4	E962.0	E980.4
Parathion	989.3	E863.1	—	E950.6	E962.1	E980.7
Parathormone	962.6	E858.0	E932.6	E950.4	E962.0	E980.4
Parathyroid (derivatives)	962.6	E858.0	E932.6	E950.4	E962.0	E980.4
Paratyphoid vaccine	978.1	E858.8	E948.1	E950.4	E962.0	E980.4
Paredrine	971.2	E855.5	E941.2	E950.4	E962.0	E980.4
Paregoric	965.00	E850.2	E935.2	E950.0	E962.0	E980.0
Pargyline	972.3	E858.3	E942.3	E950.4	E962.0	E980.4
Paris green	985.1	E866.3	—	E950.8	E962.1	E980.8
insecticide	985.1	E863.4	—	E950.8	E962.1	E980.8
Parnate	969.01	E854.0	E939.0	E950.3	E962.0	E980.3
Paromomycin	960.8	E856	E930.8	E950.4	E962.0	E980.4
Paroxypropione	963.1	E858.1	E933.1	E950.4	E962.0	E980.4
Parzone	965.09	E850.2	E935.2	E950.0	E962.0	E980.0
PAS	961.8	E857	E931.8	E950.4	E962.0	E980.4
PCBs	981	E862.3	—	E950.9	E962.1	E980.9
PCP (pentachlorophenol)	989.4	E863.6	—	E950.6	E962.1	E980.7
herbicide	989.4	E863.5	—	E950.6	E962.1	E980.7
insecticide	989.4	E863.4	—	E950.6	E962.1	E980.7
phencyclidine	968.3	E855.1	E938.3	E950.4	E962.0	E980.4
Peach kernel oil (emulsion)	973.2	E858.4	E943.2	E950.4	E962.0	E980.4
Peanut oil (emulsion) NEC	973.2	E858.4	E943.2	E950.4	E962.0	E980.4
topical	976.3	E858.7	E946.3	E950.4	E962.0	E980.4
Pearly Gates (morning glory seeds)	969.6	E854.1	E939.6	E950.3	E962.0	E980.3
Pecazine	969.1	E853.0	E939.1	E950.3	E962.0	E980.3
Pecilocin	960.1	E856	E930.1	E950.4	E962.0	E980.4
Pectin (with kaolin) NEC	973.5	E858.4	E943.5	E950.4	E962.0	E980.4
Pelletierine tannate	961.6	E857	E931.6	E950.4	E962.0	E980.4
Pemoline	969.79	E854.2	E939.7	E950.3	E962.0	E980.3
Pempidine	972.3	E858.3	E942.3	E950.4	E962.0	E980.4
Penamecillin	960.0	E856	E930.0	E950.4	E962.0	E980.4
Penethamate hydriodide	960.0	E856	E930.0	E950.4	E962.0	E980.4
Penicillamine	963.8	E858.1	E933.8	E950.4	E962.0	E980.4
Penicillin (any type)	960.0	E856	E930.0	E950.4	E962.0	E980.4
Penicillinase	963.4	E858.1	E933.4	E950.4	E962.0	E980.4
Pentachlorophenol (fungicide)	989.4	E863.6	—	E950.6	E962.1	E980.7
herbicide	989.4	E863.5	—	E950.6	E962.1	E980.7
insecticide	989.4	E863.4	—	E950.6	E962.1	E980.7
Pentaerythritol	972.4	E858.3	E942.4	E950.4	E962.0	E980.4
chloral	967.1	E852.0	E937.1	E950.2	E962.0	E980.2
tetranitrate NEC	972.4	E858.3	E942.4	E950.4	E962.0	E980.4
Pentagastrin	977.8	E858.8	E947.8	E950.4	E962.0	E980.4
Pentalin	982.3	E862.4	—	E950.9	E962.1	E980.9
Pentamethonium (bromide)	972.3	E858.3	E942.3	E950.4	E962.0	E980.4
Pentamidine	961.5	E857	E931.5	E950.4	E962.0	E980.4
Pentanol	980.8	E860.8	—	E950.9	E962.1	E980.9
Pentaquine	961.4	E857	E931.4	E950.4	E962.0	E980.4
Pentazocine	965.8	E850.8	E935.8	E950.0	E962.0	E980.0
Penthienate	971.1	E855.4	E941.1	E950.4	E962.0	E980.4
Pentobarbital, pentobarbitone (sodium)	967.0	E851	E937.0	E950.1	E962.0	E980.1
Pentolinium (tartrate)	972.3	E858.3	E942.3	E950.4	E962.0	E980.4
Pentothal	968.3	E855.1	E938.3	E950.4	E962.0	E980.4
Pentylenetetrazol	970.0	E854.3	E940.0	E950.4	E962.0	E980.4
Pentylsalicylamide	961.8	E857	E931.8	E950.4	E962.0	E980.4
Pepsin	973.4	E858.4	E943.4	E950.4	E962.0	E980.4
Peptavlon	977.8	E858.8	E947.8	E950.4	E962.0	E980.4
Percaine (spinal)	968.7	E855.2	E938.7	E950.4	E962.0	E980.4

Nontherapeutic use substance

2011 ICD-9-CM

▶◀ Revised Text　　● New Line　　▲ Revised Code

Subterms under main terms may continue to next column or page

Volume 2 — 321

Orimune — Percaine

	Poisoning	Accident	Therapeutic Use	Suicide Attempt	Assault	Undetermined
Percaine — *continued*						
topical (surface)	968.5	E855.2	E938.5	E950.4	E962.0	E980.4
Perchloroethylene (vapor)	982.3	E862.4	—	E950.9	E962.1	E980.9
medicinal	961.6	E857	E931.6	E950.4	E962.0	E980.4
Percodan	965.09	E850.2	E935.2	E950.0	E962.0	E980.0
Percogesic	965.09	E850.2	E935.2	E950.0	E962.0	E980.0
Percorten	962.0	E858.0	E932.0	E950.4	E962.0	E980.4
Pergonal	962.4	E858.0	E932.4	E950.4	E962.0	E980.4
Perhexiline	972.4	E858.3	E942.4	E950.4	E962.0	E980.4
Periactin	963.0	E858.1	E933.0	E950.4	E962.0	E980.4
Periclor	967.1	E852.0	E937.1	E950.2	E962.0	E980.2
Pericyazine	969.1	E853.0	E939.1	E950.3	E962.0	E980.3
Peritrate	972.4	E858.3	E942.4	E950.4	E962.0	E980.4
Permanganates NEC	983.9	E864.3	—	E950.7	E962.1	E980.6
potassium (topical)	976.0	E858.7	E946.0	E950.4	E962.0	E980.4
Pernocton	967.0	E851	E937.0	E950.1	E962.0	E980.1
Pernoston	967.0	E851	E937.0	E950.1	E962.0	E980.1
Peronin(e)	965.09	E850.2	E935.2	E950.0	E962.0	E980.0
Perphenazine	969.1	E853.0	E939.1	E950.3	E962.0	E980.3
Pertofrane	969.05	E854.0	E939.0	E950.3	E962.0	E980.3
Pertussis						
immune serum (human)	964.6	E858.2	E934.6	E950.4	E962.0	E980.4
vaccine (with diphtheria toxoid) (with tetanus toxoid)	978.6	E858.8	E948.6	E950.4	E962.0	E980.4
Peruvian balsam	976.8	E858.7	E946.8	E950.4	E962.0	E980.4
Pesticides (dust) (fumes) (vapor)	989.4	E863.4	—	E950.6	E962.1	E980.7
arsenic	985.1	E863.4	—	E950.8	E962.1	E980.8
chlorinated	989.2	E863.0	—	E950.6	E962.1	E980.7
cyanide	989.0	E863.4	—	E950.6	E962.1	E980.7
kerosene	981	E863.4	—	E950.6	E962.1	E980.7
mixture (of compounds)	989.4	E863.3	—	E950.6	E962.1	E980.7
naphthalene	983.0	E863.4	—	E950.7	E962.1	E980.6
organochlorine (compounds)	989.2	E863.0	—	E950.6	E962.1	E980.7
petroleum (distillate) (products) NEC	981	E863.4	—	E950.6	E962.1	E980.7
specified ingredient NEC	989.4	E863.4	—	E950.6	E962.1	E980.7
strychnine	989.1	E863.4	—	E950.6	E962.1	E980.7
thallium	985.8	E863.7	—	E950.6	E962.1	E980.7
Pethidine (hydrochloride)	965.09	E850.2	E935.2	E950.0	E962.0	E980.0
Petrichloral	967.1	E852.0	E937.1	E950.2	E962.0	E980.2
Petrol	981	E862.1	—	E950.9	E962.1	E980.9
vapor	987.1	E869.8	—	E952.8	E962.2	E982.8
Petrolatum (jelly) (ointment)	976.3	E858.7	E946.3	E950.4	E962.0	E980.4
hydrophilic	976.3	E858.7	E946.3	E950.4	E962.0	E980.4
liquid	973.2	E858.4	E943.2	E950.4	E962.0	E980.4
topical	976.3	E858.7	E946.3	E950.4	E962.0	E980.4
nonmedicinal	981	E862.1	—	E950.9	E962.1	E980.9
Petroleum (cleaners) (fuels) (products) NEC	981	E862.1	—	E950.9	E962.1	E980.9
benzin(e) — see Ligroin						
ether — see Ligroin						
jelly — see Petrolatum						
naphtha — see Ligroin						
pesticide	981	E863.4	—	E950.6	E962.1	E980.7
solids	981	E862.3	—	E950.9	E962.1	E980.9
solvents	981	E862.0	—	E950.9	E962.1	E980.9
vapor	987.1	E869.8	—	E952.8	E962.2	E982.8
Peyote	969.6	E854.1	E939.6	E950.3	E962.0	E980.3
Phanodorm, phanodorn	967.0	E851	E937.0	E950.1	E962.0	E980.1
Phanquinone, phanquone	961.5	E857	E931.5	E950.4	E962.0	E980.4
Pharmaceutical excipient or adjunct	977.4	E858.8	E947.4	E950.4	E962.0	E980.4
Phenacemide	966.3	E855.0	E936.3	E950.4	E962.0	E980.4
Phenacetin	965.4	E850.4	E935.4	E950.0	E962.0	E980.0
Phenadoxone	965.09	E850.2	E935.2	E950.0	E962.0	E980.0
Phenaglycodol	969.5	E853.8	E939.5	E950.3	E962.0	E980.3
Phenantoin	966.1	E855.0	E936.1	E950.4	E962.0	E980.4
Phenaphthazine reagent	977.8	E858.8	E947.8	E950.4	E962.0	E980.4
Phenazocine	965.09	E850.2	E935.2	E950.0	E962.0	E980.0
Phenazone	965.5	E850.5	E935.5	E950.0	E962.0	E980.0
Phenazopyridine	976.1	E858.7	E946.1	E950.4	E962.0	E980.4
Phenbenicillin	960.0	E856	E930.0	E950.4	E962.0	E980.4
Phenbutrazate	977.0	E858.8	E947.0	E950.4	E962.0	E980.4
Phencyclidine	968.3	E855.1	E938.3	E950.4	E962.0	E980.4
Phendimetrazine	977.0	E858.8	E947.0	E950.4	E962.0	E980.4
Phenelzine	969.01	E854.0	E939.0	E950.3	E962.0	E980.3

	Poisoning	Accident	Therapeutic Use	Suicide Attempt	Assault	Undetermined
Phenergan	967.8	E852.8	E937.8	E950.2	E962.0	E980.2
Phenethicillin (potassium)	960.0	E856	E930.0	E950.4	E962.0	E980.4
Phenetsal	965.1	E850.3	E935.3	E950.0	E962.0	E980.0
Pheneturide	966.3	E855.0	E936.3	E950.4	E962.0	E980.4
Phenformin	962.3	E858.0	E932.3	E950.4	E962.0	E980.4
Phenglutarimide	971.1	E855.4	E941.1	E950.4	E962.0	E980.4
Phenicarbazide	965.8	E850.8	E935.8	E950.0	E962.0	E980.0
Phenindamine (tartrate)	963.0	E858.1	E933.0	E950.4	E962.0	E980.4
Phenindione	964.2	E858.2	E934.2	E950.4	E962.0	E980.4
Pheniprazine	969.01	E854.0	E939.0	E950.3	E962.0	E980.3
Pheniramine (maleate)	963.0	E858.1	E933.0	E950.4	E962.0	E980.4
Phenmetrazine	977.0	E858.8	E947.0	E950.4	E962.0	E980.4
Phenobal	967.0	E851	E937.0	E950.1	E962.0	E980.1
Phenobarbital	967.0	E851	E937.0	E950.1	E962.0	E980.1
Phenobarbitone	967.0	E851	E937.0	E950.1	E962.0	E980.1
Phenoctide	976.0	E858.7	E946.0	E950.4	E962.0	E980.4
Phenol (derivatives) NEC	983.0	E864.0	—	E950.7	E962.1	E980.6
disinfectant	983.0	E864.0	—	E950.7	E962.1	E980.6
pesticide	989.4	E863.4	—	E950.6	E962.1	E980.7
red	977.8	E858.8	E947.8	E950.4	E962.0	E980.4
Phenolphthalein	973.1	E858.4	E943.1	E950.4	E962.0	E980.4
Phenolsulfonphthalein	977.8	E858.8	E947.8	E950.4	E962.0	E980.4
Phenomorphan	965.09	E850.2	E935.2	E950.0	E962.0	E980.0
Phenonyl	967.0	E851	E937.0	E950.1	E962.0	E980.1
Phenoperidine	965.09	E850.2	E935.2	E950.0	E962.0	E980.0
Phenoquin	974.7	E858.5	E944.7	E950.4	E962.0	E980.4
Phenothiazines (tranquilizers) NEC	969.1	E853.0	E939.1	E950.3	E962.0	E980.3
insecticide	989.3	E863.4	—	E950.6	E962.1	E980.7
Phenoxybenzamine	971.3	E855.6	E941.3	E950.4	E962.0	E980.4
Phenoxymethyl penicillin	960.0	E856	E930.0	E950.4	E962.0	E980.4
Phenprocoumon	964.2	E858.2	E934.2	E950.4	E962.0	E980.4
Phensuximide	966.2	E855.0	E936.2	E950.4	E962.0	E980.4
Phentermine	977.0	E858.8	E947.0	E950.4	E962.0	E980.4
Phentolamine	971.3	E855.6	E941.3	E950.4	E962.0	E980.4
Phenyl						
butazone	965.5	E850.5	E935.5	E950.0	E962.0	E980.0
enediamine	983.0	E864.0	—	E950.7	E962.1	E980.6
hydrazine	983.0	E864.0	—	E950.7	E962.1	E980.6
antineoplastic	963.1	E858.1	E933.1	E950.4	E962.0	E980.4
mercuric compounds — see Mercury						
salicylate	976.3	E858.7	E946.3	E950.4	E962.0	E980.4
Phenylephrine	971.2	E855.5	E941.2	E950.4	E962.0	E980.4
Phenylethylbiguanide	962.3	E858.0	E932.3	E950.4	E962.0	E980.4
Phenylpropanolamine	971.2	E855.5	E941.2	E950.4	E962.0	E980.4
Phenylsulfthion	989.3	E863.1	—	E950.6	E962.1	E980.7
Phenyramidol, phenyramidon	965.7	E850.7	E935.7	E950.0	E962.0	E980.0
Phenytoin	966.1	E855.0	E936.1	E950.4	E962.0	E980.4
pHisoHex	976.2	E858.7	E946.2	E950.4	E962.0	E980.4
Pholcodine	965.09	E850.2	E935.2	E950.0	E962.0	E980.0
Phorate	989.3	E863.1	—	E950.6	E962.1	E980.7
Phosdrin	989.3	E863.1	—	E950.6	E962.1	E980.7
Phosgene (gas)	987.8	E869.8	—	E952.8	E962.2	E982.8
Phosphate (tricresyl)	989.89	E866.8	—	E950.9	E962.1	E980.9
organic	989.3	E863.1	—	E950.6	E962.1	E980.7
solvent	982.8	E862.4	—	E950.9	E926.1	E980.9
Phosphine	987.8	E869.8	—	E952.8	E962.2	E982.8
fumigant	987.8	E863.8	—	E950.6	E962.2	E980.7
Phospholine	971.0	E855.3	E941.0	E950.4	E962.0	E980.4
Phosphoric acid	983.1	E864.1	—	E950.7	E962.1	E980.6
Phosphorus (compounds) NEC	983.9	E864.3	—	E950.7	E962.1	E980.6
rodenticide	983.9	E863.7	—	E950.7	E962.1	E980.6
Phthalimidoglutarimide	967.8	E852.8	E937.8	E950.2	E962.0	E980.2
Phthalylsulfathiazole	961.0	E857	E931.0	E950.4	E962.0	E980.4
Phylloquinone	964.3	E858.2	E934.3	E950.4	E962.0	E980.4
Physeptone	965.02	E850.1	E935.1	E950.0	E962.0	E980.0
Physostigma venenosum	988.2	E865.4	—	E950.9	E962.1	E980.9
Physostigmine	971.0	E855.3	E941.0	E950.4	E962.0	E980.4
Phytolacca decandra	988.2	E865.4	—	E950.9	E962.1	E980.9
Phytomenadione	964.3	E858.2	E934.3	E950.4	E962.0	E980.4
Phytonadione	964.3	E858.2	E934.3	E950.4	E962.0	E980.4
Picric (acid)	983.0	E864.0	—	E950.7	E962.1	E980.6
Picrotoxin	970.0	E854.3	E940.0	E950.4	E962.0	E980.4
Pilocarpine	971.0	E855.3	E941.0	E950.4	E962.0	E980.4
Pilocarpus (jaborandi) extract	971.0	E855.3	E941.0	E950.4	E962.0	E980.4

Left margin (vertical): Index

Left margin (vertical): Percaine — Pilocarpus (jaborandi) extract

Substance	Poisoning	Accident	Therapeutic Use	Suicide Attempt	Assault	Undetermined
Pimaricin	960.1	E856	E930.1	E950.4	E962.0	E980.4
Piminodine	965.09	E850.2	E935.2	E950.0	E962.0	E980.0
Pine oil, pinesol (disinfectant)	983.9	E861.4	—	E950.7	E962.1	E980.6
Pinkroot	961.6	E857	E931.6	E950.4	E962.0	E980.4
Pipadone	965.09	E850.2	E935.2	E950.0	E962.0	E980.0
Pipamazine	963.0	E858.1	E933.0	E950.4	E962.0	E980.4
Pipazethate	975.4	E858.6	E945.4	E950.4	E962.0	E980.4
Pipenzolate	971.1	E855.4	E941.1	E950.4	E962.0	E980.4
Piperacetazine	969.1	E853.0	E939.1	E950.3	E962.0	E980.3
Piperazine NEC	961.6	E857	E931.6	E950.4	E962.0	E980.4
estrone sulfate	962.2	E858.0	E932.2	E950.4	E962.0	E980.4
Piper cubeba	988.2	E865.4	—	E950.9	E962.1	E980.9
Piperidione	975.4	E858.6	E945.4	E950.4	E962.0	E980.4
Piperidolate	971.1	E855.4	E941.1	E950.4	E962.0	E980.4
Piperocaine	968.9	E855.2	E938.9	E950.4	E962.0	E980.4
infiltration (subcutaneous)	968.5	E855.2	E938.5	E950.4	E962.0	E980.4
nerve block (peripheral) (plexus)	968.6	E855.2	E938.6	E950.4	E962.0	E980.4
topical (surface)	968.5	E855.2	E938.5	E950.4	E962.0	E980.4
Pipobroman	963.1	E858.1	E933.1	E950.4	E962.0	E980.4
Pipradrol	970.89 ▲	E854.3	E940.8	E950.4	E962.0	E980.4
Piscidia (bark) (erythrina)	965.7	E850.7	E935.7	E950.0	E962.0	E980.0
Pitch	983.0	E864.0	—	E950.7	E962.1	E980.6
Pitkin's solution	968.7	E855.2	E938.7	E950.4	E962.0	E980.4
Pitocin	975.0	E858.6	E945.0	E950.4	E962.0	E980.4
Pitressin (tannate)	962.5	E858.0	E932.5	E950.4	E962.0	E980.4
Pituitary extracts (posterior)	962.5	E858.0	E932.5	E950.4	E962.0	E980.4
anterior	962.4	E858.0	E932.4	E950.4	E962.0	E980.4
Pituitrin	962.5	E858.0	E932.5	E950.4	E962.0	E980.4
Placental extract	962.9	E858.0	E932.9	E950.4	E962.0	E980.4
Placidyl	967.8	E852.8	E937.8	E950.2	E962.0	E980.2
Plague vaccine	978.3	E858.8	E948.3	E950.4	E962.0	E980.4
Plant foods or fertilizers NEC	989.89	E866.5	—	E950.9	E962.1	E980.9
mixed with herbicides	989.4	E863.5	—	E950.6	E962.1	E980.7
Plants, noxious, used as food	988.2	E865.9	—	E950.9	E962.1	E980.9
berries and seeds	988.2	E865.3	—	E950.9	E962.1	E980.9
specified type NEC	988.2	E865.4	—	E950.9	E962.1	E980.9
Plasma (blood)	964.7	E858.2	E934.7	E950.4	E962.0	E980.4
expanders	964.8	E858.2	E934.8	E950.4	E962.0	E980.4
Plasmanate	964.7	E858.2	E934.7	E950.4	E962.0	E980.4
Plegicil	969.1	E853.0	E939.1	E950.3	E962.0	E980.3
Podophyllin	976.4	E858.7	E946.4	E950.4	E962.0	E980.4
Podophyllum resin	976.4	E858.7	E946.4	E950.4	E962.0	E980.4
Poison NEC	989.9	E866.9	—	E950.9	E962.1	E980.9
Poisonous berries	988.2	E865.3	—	E950.9	E962.1	E980.9
Pokeweed (any part)	988.2	E865.4	—	E950.9	E962.1	E980.9
Poldine	971.1	E855.4	E941.1	E950.4	E962.0	E980.4
Poliomyelitis vaccine	979.5	E858.8	E949.5	E950.4	E962.0	E980.4
Poliovirus vaccine	979.5	E858.8	E949.5	E950.4	E962.0	E980.4
Polish (car) (floor) (furniture) (metal) (silver)	989.89	E861.2	—	E950.9	E962.1	E980.9
abrasive	989.89	E861.3	—	E950.9	E962.1	E980.9
porcelain	989.89	E861.3	—	E950.9	E962.1	E980.9
Poloxalkol	973.2	E858.4	E943.2	E950.4	E962.0	E980.4
Polyaminostyrene resins	974.5	E858.5	E944.5	E950.4	E962.0	E980.4
Polychlorinated biphenyl — see PCBs						
Polycycline	960.4	E856	E930.4	E950.4	E962.0	E980.4
Polyester resin hardener	982.8	E862.4	—	E950.9	E962.1	E980.9
fumes	987.8	E869.8	—	E952.8	E962.2	E982.8
Polyestradiol (phosphate)	962.2	E858.0	E932.2	E950.4	E962.0	E980.4
Polyethanolamine alkyl sulfate	976.2	E858.7	E946.2	E950.4	E962.0	E980.4
Polyethylene glycol	976.3	E858.7	E946.3	E950.4	E962.0	E980.4
Polyferose	964.0	E858.2	E934.0	E950.4	E962.0	E980.4
Polymyxin B	960.8	E856	E930.8	E950.4	E962.0	E980.4
ENT agent	976.6	E858.7	E946.6	E950.4	E962.0	E980.4
ophthalmic preparation	976.5	E858.7	E946.5	E950.4	E962.0	E980.4
topical NEC	976.0	E858.7	E946.0	E950.4	E962.0	E980.4
Polynoxylin(e)	976.0	E858.7	E946.0	E950.4	E962.0	E980.4
Polyoxymethyleneurea	976.0	E858.7	E946.0	E950.4	E962.0	E980.4
Polytetrafluoroethylene (inhaled)	987.8	E869.8	—	E952.8	E962.2	E982.8
Polythiazide	974.3	E858.5	E944.3	E950.4	E962.0	E980.4
Polyvinylpyrrolidone	964.8	E858.2	E934.8	E950.4	E962.0	E980.4

Substance	Poisoning	Accident	Therapeutic Use	Suicide Attempt	Assault	Undetermined
Pontocaine (hydrochloride) (infiltration) (topical)	968.5	E855.2	E938.5	E950.4	E962.0	E980.4
nerve block (peripheral) (plexus)	968.6	E855.2	E938.6	E950.4	E962.0	E980.4
spinal	968.7	E855.2	E938.7	E950.4	E962.0	E980.4
Pot	969.6	E854.1	E939.6	E950.3	E962.0	E980.3
Potash (caustic)	983.2	E864.2	—	E950.7	E962.1	E980.6
Potassic saline injection (lactated)	974.5	E858.5	E944.5	E950.4	E962.0	E980.4
Potassium (salts) NEC	974.5	E858.5	E944.5	E950.4	E962.0	E980.4
aminosalicylate	961.8	E857	E931.8	E950.4	E962.0	E980.4
arsenite (solution)	985.1	E866.3	—	E950.8	E962.1	E980.8
bichromate	983.9	E864.3	—	E950.7	E962.1	E980.6
bisulfate	983.9	E864.3	—	E950.7	E962.1	E980.6
bromide (medicinal) NEC	967.3	E852.2	E937.3	E950.2	E962.0	E980.2
carbonate	983.2	E864.2	—	E950.7	E962.1	E980.6
chlorate NEC	983.9	E864.3	—	E950.7	E962.1	E980.6
cyanide — see Cyanide						
hydroxide	983.2	E864.2	—	E950.7	E962.1	E980.6
iodide (expectorant) NEC	975.5	E858.6	E945.5	E950.4	E962.0	E980.4
nitrate	989.89	E866.8	—	E950.9	E962.1	E980.9
oxalate	983.9	E864.3	—	E950.7	E962.1	E980.6
perchlorate NEC	977.8	E858.8	E947.8	E950.4	E962.0	E980.4
antithyroid	962.8	E858.0	E932.8	E950.4	E962.0	E980.4
permanganate	976.0	E858.7	E946.0	E950.4	E962.0	E980.4
nonmedicinal	983.9	E864.3	—	E950.7	E962.1	E980.6
Povidone-iodine (anti-infective) NEC	976.0	E858.7	E946.0	E950.4	E962.0	E980.4
Practolol	972.0	E858.3	E942.0	E950.4	E962.0	E980.4
Pralidoxime (chloride)	977.2	E858.8	E947.2	E950.4	E962.0	E980.4
Pramoxine	968.5	E855.2	E938.5	E950.4	E962.0	E980.4
Prazosin	972.6	E858.3	E942.6	E950.4	E962.0	E980.4
Prednisolone	962.0	E858.0	E932.0	E950.4	E962.0	E980.4
ENT agent	976.6	E858.7	E946.6	E950.4	E962.0	E980.4
ophthalmic preparation	976.5	E858.7	E946.5	E950.4	E962.0	E980.4
topical NEC	976.0	E858.7	E946.0	E950.4	E962.0	E980.4
Prednisone	962.0	E858.0	E932.0	E950.4	E962.0	E980.4
Pregnanediol	962.2	E858.0	E932.2	E950.4	E962.0	E980.4
Pregneninolone	962.2	E858.0	E932.2	E950.4	E962.0	E980.4
Preludin	977.0	E858.8	E947.0	E950.4	E962.0	E980.4
Premarin	962.2	E858.0	E932.2	E950.4	E962.0	E980.4
Prenylamine	972.4	E858.3	E942.4	E950.4	E962.0	E980.4
Preparation H	976.8	E858.7	E946.8	E950.4	E962.0	E980.4
Preservatives	989.89	E866.8	—	E950.9	E962.1	E980.9
Pride of China	988.2	E865.3	—	E950.9	E962.1	E980.9
Prilocaine	968.9	E855.2	E938.9	E950.4	E962.0	E980.4
infiltration (subcutaneous)	968.5	E855.2	E938.5	E950.4	E962.0	E980.4
nerve block (peripheral) (plexus)	968.6	E855.2	E938.6	E950.4	E962.0	E980.4
Primaquine	961.4	E857	E931.4	E950.4	E962.0	E980.4
Primidone	966.3	E855.0	E936.3	E950.4	E962.0	E980.4
Primula (veris)	988.2	E865.4	—	E950.9	E962.1	E980.9
Prinadol	965.09	E850.2	E935.2	E950.0	E962.0	E980.0
Priscol, Priscoline	971.3	E855.6	E941.3	E950.4	E962.0	E980.4
Privet	988.2	E865.4	—	E950.9	E962.1	E980.9
Privine	971.2	E855.5	E941.2	E950.4	E962.0	E980.4
Pro-Banthine	971.1	E855.4	E941.1	E950.4	E962.0	E980.4
Probarbital	967.0	E851	E937.0	E950.1	E962.0	E980.1
Probenecid	974.7	E858.5	E944.7	E950.4	E962.0	E980.4
Procainamide (hydrochloride)	972.0	E858.3	E942.0	E950.4	E962.0	E980.4
Procaine (hydrochloride) (infiltration) (topical)	968.5	E855.2	E938.5	E950.4	E962.0	E980.4
nerve block (peripheral) (plexus)	968.6	E855.2	E938.6	E950.4	E962.0	E980.4
penicillin G	960.0	E856	E930.0	E950.4	E962.0	E980.4
spinal	968.7	E855.2	E938.7	E950.4	E962.0	E980.4
Procalmidol	969.5	E853.8	E939.5	E950.3	E962.0	E980.3
Procarbazine	963.1	E858.1	E933.1	E950.4	E962.0	E980.4
Prochlorperazine	969.1	E853.0	E939.1	E950.3	E962.0	E980.3
Procyclidine	966.4	E855.0	E936.4	E950.4	E962.0	E980.4
Producer gas	986	E868.8	—	E952.1	E962.2	E982.1
Profenamine	966.4	E855.0	E936.4	E950.4	E962.0	E980.4
Profenil	975.1	E858.6	E945.1	E950.4	E962.0	E980.4
Progesterones	962.2	E858.0	E932.2	E950.4	E962.0	E980.4
Progestin	962.2	E858.0	E932.2	E950.4	E962.0	E980.4
Progestogens (with estrogens)	962.2	E858.0	E932.2	E950.4	E962.0	E980.4
Progestone	962.2	E858.0	E932.2	E950.4	E962.0	E980.4
Proguanil	961.4	E857	E931.4	E950.4	E962.0	E980.4
Prolactin	962.4	E858.0	E932.4	E950.4	E962.0	E980.4

Nontherapeutic use substance

▼ Subterms under main terms may continue to next column or page

2011 ICD-9-CM ▶◀ Revised Text ● New Line ▲ Revised Code October 2010 · Volume 2 — 323

	Poisoning	Accident	Therapeutic Use	Suicide Attempt	Assault	Undeter-mined
Proloid	962.7	E858.0	E932.7	E950.4	E962.0	E980.4
Proluton	962.2	E858.0	E932.2	E950.4	E962.0	E980.4
Promacetin	961.8	E857	E931.8	E950.4	E962.0	E980.4
Promazine	969.1	E853.0	E939.1	E950.3	E962.0	E980.3
Promedol	965.09	E850.2	E935.2	E950.0	E962.0	E980.0
Promethazine	967.8	E852.8	E937.8	E950.2	E962.0	E980.2
Promin	961.8	E857	E931.8	E950.4	E962.0	E980.4
Pronestyl (hydrochloride)	972.0	E858.3	E942.0	E950.4	E962.0	E980.4
Pronetalol, pronethalol	972.0	E858.3	E942.0	E950.4	E962.0	E980.4
Prontosil	961.0	E857	E931.0	E950.4	E962.0	E980.4
Propamidine isethionate	961.5	E857	E931.5	E950.4	E962.0	E980.4
Propanal (medicinal)	967.8	E852.8	E937.8	E950.2	E962.0	E980.2
Propane (gas) (distributed in mobile container)	987.0	E868.0	—	E951.1	E962.2	E981.1
distributed through pipes	987.0	E867		E951.0	E962.2	E981.0
incomplete combustion of — see Carbon monoxide, Propane						
Propanidid	968.3	E855.1	E938.3	E950.4	E962.0	E980.4
Propanol	980.3	E860.4	—	E950.9	E962.1	E980.9
Propantheline	971.1	E855.4	E941.1	E950.4	E962.0	E980.4
Proparacaine	968.5	E855.2	E938.5	E950.4	E962.0	E980.4
Propatyl nitrate	972.4	E858.3	E942.4	E950.4	E962.0	E980.4
Propicillin	960.0	E856	E930.0	E950.4	E962.0	E980.4
Propiolactone (vapor)	987.8	E869.8	—	E952.8	E962.2	E982.8
Propiomazine	967.8	E852.8	E937.8	E950.2	E962.0	E980.2
Propionaldehyde (medicinal)	967.8	E852.8	E937.8	E950.2	E962.0	E980.2
Propionate compound	976.0	E858.7	E946.0	E950.4	E962.0	E980.4
Propion gel	976.0	E858.7	E946.0	E950.4	E962.0	E980.4
Propitocaine	968.9	E855.2	E938.9	E950.4	E962.0	E980.4
infiltration (subcutaneous)	968.5	E855.2	E938.5	E950.4	E962.0	E980.4
nerve block (peripheral) (plexus)	968.6	E855.2	E938.6	E950.4	E962.0	E980.4
Propoxur	989.3	E863.2	—	E950.6	E962.1	E980.7
Propoxycaine	968.9	E855.2	E938.9	E950.4	E962.0	E980.4
infiltration (subcutaneous)	968.5	E855.2	E938.5	E950.4	E962.0	E980.4
nerve block (peripheral) (plexus)	968.6	E855.2	E938.6	E950.4	E962.0	E980.4
topical (surface)	968.5	E855.2	E938.5	E950.4	E962.0	E980.4
Propoxyphene (hydrochloride)	965.8	E850.8	E935.8	E950.0	E962.0	E980.0
Propranolol	972.0	E858.3	E942.0	E950.4	E962.0	E980.4
Propyl						
alcohol	980.3	E860.4	—	E950.9	E962.1	E980.9
carbinol	980.3	E860.4	—	E950.9	E962.1	E980.9
hexadrine	971.2	E855.5	E941.2	E950.4	E962.0	E980.4
iodone	977.8	E858.8	E947.8	E950.4	E962.0	E980.4
thiouracil	962.8	E858.0	E932.8	E950.4	E962.0	E980.4
Propylene	987.1	E869.8	—	E952.8	E962.2	E982.8
Propylparaben (ophthalmic)	976.5	E858.7	E946.5	E950.4	E962.0	E980.4
Proscillaridin	972.1	E858.3	E942.1	E950.4	E962.0	E980.4
Prostaglandins	975.0	E858.6	E945.0	E950.4	E962.0	E980.4
Prostigmin	971.0	E855.3	E941.0	E950.4	E962.0	E980.4
Protamine (sulfate)	964.5	E858.2	E934.5	E950.4	E962.0	E980.4
zinc insulin	962.3	E858.0	E932.3	E950.4	E962.0	E980.4
Protectants (topical)	976.3	E858.7	E946.3	E950.4	E962.0	E980.4
Protein hydrolysate	974.5	E858.5	E944.5	E950.4	E962.0	E980.4
Prothiaden — see Dothiepin hydrochloride						
Prothionamide	961.8	E857	E931.8	E950.4	E962.0	E980.4
Prothipendyl	969.5	E853.8	E939.5	E950.3	E962.0	E980.3
Protokylol	971.2	E855.5	E941.2	E950.4	E962.0	E980.4
Protopam	977.2	E858.8	E947.2	E950.4	E962.0	E980.4
Protoveratrine(s) (A) (B)	972.6	E858.3	E942.6	E950.4	E962.0	E980.4
Protriptyline	969.05	E854.0	E939.0	E950.3	E962.0	E980.3
Provera	962.2	E858.0	E932.2	E950.4	E962.0	E980.4
Provitamin A	963.5	E858.1	E933.5	E950.4	E962.0	E980.4
Proxymetacaine	968.5	E855.2	E938.5	E950.4	E962.0	E980.4
Proxyphylline	975.1	E858.6	E945.1	E950.4	E962.0	E980.4
Prozac — see Fluoxetine hydrochloride						
Prunus						
laurocerasus	988.2	E865.4	—	E950.9	E962.1	E980.9
virginiana	988.2	E865.4	—	E950.9	E962.1	E980.9
Prussic acid	989.0	E866.8	—	E950.9	E962.1	E980.9
vapor	987.7	E869.8	—	E952.8	E962.2	E982.8
Pseudoephedrine	971.2	E855.5	E941.2	E950.4	E962.0	E980.4

	Poisoning	Accident	Therapeutic Use	Suicide Attempt	Assault	Undeter-mined
Psilocin	969.6	E854.1	E939.6	E950.3	E962.0	E980.3
Psilocybin	969.6	E854.1	E939.6	E950.3	E962.0	E980.3
PSP	977.8	E858.8	E947.8	E950.4	E962.0	E980.4
Psychedelic agents	969.6	E854.1	E939.6	E950.3	E962.0	E980.3
Psychodysleptics	969.6	E854.1	E939.6	E950.3	E962.0	E980.3
Psychostimulants	969.70	E854.2	E939.7	E950.3	E962.0	E980.3
Psychotherapeutic agents	969.9	E855.9	E939.9	E950.3	E962.0	E980.3
antidepressants	969.00	E854.0	E939.0	E950.3	E962.0	E980.3
specified NEC	969.8	E855.8	E939.8	E950.3	E962.0	E980.3
tranquilizers NEC	969.5	E853.9	E939.5	E950.3	E962.0	E980.3
Psychotomimetic agents	969.6	E854.1	E939.6	E950.3	E962.0	E980.3
Psychotropic agents	969.9	E854.8	E939.9	E950.3	E962.0	E980.3
specified NEC	969.8	E854.8	E939.8	E950.3	E962.0	E980.3
Psyllium	973.3	E858.4	E943.3	E950.4	E962.0	E980.4
Pteroylglutamic acid	964.1	E858.2	E934.1	E950.4	E962.0	E980.4
Pteroyltriglutamate	963.1	E858.1	E933.1	E950.4	E962.0	E980.4
PTFE	987.8	E869.8	—	E952.8	E962.2	E982.8
Pulsatilla	988.2	E865.4	—	E950.9	E962.1	E980.9
Purex (bleach)	983.9	E864.3	—	E950.7	E962.1	E980.6
Purine diuretics	974.1	E858.5	E944.1	E950.4	E962.0	E980.4
Purinethol	963.1	E858.1	E933.1	E950.4	E962.0	E980.4
PVP	964.8	E858.2	E934.8	E950.4	E962.0	E980.4
Pyrabital	965.7	E850.7	E935.7	E950.0	E962.0	E980.0
Pyramidon	965.5	E850.5	E935.5	E950.0	E962.0	E980.0
Pyrantel (pamoate)	961.6	E857	E931.6	E950.4	E962.0	E980.4
Pyrathiazine	963.0	E858.1	E933.0	E950.4	E962.0	E980.4
Pyrazinamide	961.8	E857	E931.8	E950.4	E962.0	E980.4
Pyrazinoic acid (amide)	961.8	E857	E931.8	E950.4	E962.0	E980.4
Pyrazole (derivatives)	965.5	E850.5	E935.5	E950.0	E962.0	E980.0
Pyrazolone (analgesics)	965.5	E850.5	E935.5	E950.0	E962.0	E980.0
Pyrethrins, pyrethrum	989.4	E863.4	—	E950.6	E962.1	E980.7
Pyribenzamine	963.0	E858.1	E933.0	E950.4	E962.0	E980.4
Pyridine (liquid) (vapor)	982.0	E864.x	—	E950.9	E962.1	E980.9
aldoxime chloride	977.2	E858.8	E947.2	E950.4	E962.0	E980.4
Pyridium	976.1	E858.7	E946.1	E950.4	E962.0	E980.4
Pyridostigmine	971.0	E855.3	E941.0	E950.4	E962.0	E980.4
Pyridoxine	963.5	E858.1	E933.5	E950.4	E962.0	E980.4
Pyrilamine	963.0	E858.1	E933.0	E950.4	E962.0	E980.4
Pyrimethamine	961.4	E857	E931.4	E950.4	E962.0	E980.4
Pyrogallic acid	983.0	E864.0	—	E950.7	E962.1	E980.6
Pyroxylin	976.3	E858.7	E946.3	E950.4	E962.0	E980.4
Pyrrobutamine	963.0	E858.1	E933.0	E950.4	E962.0	E980.4
Pyrrocitine	968.5	E855.2	E938.5	E950.4	E962.0	E980.4
Pyrvinium (pamoate)	961.6	E857	E931.6	E950.4	E962.0	E980.4
PZI	962.3	E858.0	E932.3	E950.4	E962.0	E980.4
Quaalude	967.4	E852.3	E937.4	E950.2	E962.0	E980.2
Quaternary ammonium derivatives	971.1	E855.4	E941.1	E950.4	E962.0	E980.4
Quicklime	983.2	E864.2	—	E950.7	E962.1	E980.6
Quinacrine	961.3	E857	E931.3	E950.4	E962.0	E980.4
Quinaglute	972.0	E858.3	E942.0	E950.4	E962.0	E980.4
Quinalbarbitone	967.0	E851	E937.0	E950.1	E962.0	E980.1
Quinestradiol	962.2	E858.0	E932.2	E950.4	E962.0	E980.4
Quinethazone	974.3	E858.5	E944.3	E950.4	E962.0	E980.4
Quinidine (gluconate) (polygalacturonate) (salts) (sulfate)	972.0	E858.3	E942.0	E950.4	E962.0	E980.4
Quinine	961.4	E857	E931.4	E950.4	E962.0	E980.4
Quiniobine	961.3	E857	E931.3	E950.4	E962.0	E980.4
Quinolines	961.3	E857	E931.3	E950.4	E962.0	E980.4
Quotane	968.5	E855.2	E938.5	E950.4	E962.0	E980.4
Rabies						
immune globulin (human)	964.6	E858.2	E934.6	E950.4	E962.0	E980.4
vaccine	979.1	E858.8	E949.1	E950.4	E962.0	E980.4
Racemoramide	965.09	E850.2	E935.2	E950.0	E962.0	E980.0
Racemorphan	965.09	E850.2	E935.2	E950.0	E962.0	E980.0
Radiator alcohol	980.1	E860.2	—	E950.9	E962.1	E980.9
Radio-opaque (drugs) (materials)	977.8	E858.8	E947.8	E950.4	E962.0	E980.4
Ranunculus	988.2	E865.4	—	E950.9	E962.1	E980.9
Rat poison	989.4	E863.7	—	E950.6	E962.1	E980.7
Rattlesnake (venom)	989.5	E905.0	—	E950.9	E962.1	E980.9
Raudixin	972.6	E858.3	E942.6	E950.4	E962.0	E980.4
Rautensin	972.6	E858.3	E942.6	E950.4	E962.0	E980.4
Rautina	972.6	E858.3	E942.6	E950.4	E962.0	E980.4
Rautotal	972.6	E858.3	E942.6	E950.4	E962.0	E980.4
Rauwiloid	972.6	E858.3	E942.6	E950.4	E962.0	E980.4
Rauwolfia (alkaloids)	972.6	E858.3	E942.6	E950.4	E962.0	E980.4
Realgar	985.1	E866.3	—	E950.8	E962.1	E980.8

Nontherapeutic use substance

Subterms under main terms may continue to next column or page

		External Cause (E-Code)								External Cause (E-Code)				
	Poisoning	Accident	Therapeutic Use	Suicide Attempt	Assault	Undeter-mined		Poisoning	Accident	Therapeutic Use	Suicide Attempt	Assault	Undeter-mined
Red cells, packed	964.7	E858.2	E934.7	E950.4	E962.0	E980.4	Sambucus canadensis — continued						
Reducing agents, industrial							berry	988.2	E865.3	—	E950.9	E962.1	E980.9
NEC	983.9	E864.3	—	E950.7	E962.1	E980.6	Sandril	972.6	E858.3	E942.6	E950.4	E962.0	E980.4
Refrigerant gas (freon)	987.4	E869.2	—	E952.8	E962.2	E982.8	**Sanguinaria canadensis**	988.2	E865.4	—	E950.9	E962.1	E980.9
central nervous system	968.0	E855.1	E938.0	E950.4	E962.0	E980.4	**Saniflush** (cleaner)	983.9	E861.3	—	E950.7	E962.1	E980.6
not freon	987.9	E869.9	—	E952.9	E962.2	E982.9	Santonin	961.6	E857	E931.6	E950.4	E962.0	E980.4
Regroton	974.4	E858.5	E944.4	E950.4	E962.0	E980.4	Santyl	976.8	E858.7	E946.8	E950.4	E962.0	E980.4
Rela	968.0	E855.1	E938.0	E950.4	E962.0	E980.4	Sarkomycin	960.7	E856	E930.7	E950.4	E962.0	E980.4
Relaxants, skeletal muscle							Saroten	969.05	E854.0	E939.0	E950.3	E962.0	E980.3
(autonomic)	975.2	E858.6	E945.2	E950.4	E962.0	E980.4	Saturnine — see Lead						
Renese	974.3	E858.5	E944.3	E950.4	E962.0	E980.4	Savin (oil)	976.4	E858.7	E946.4	E950.4	E962.0	E980.4
Renografin	977.8	E858.8	E947.8	E950.4	E962.0	E980.4	Scammony	973.1	E858.4	E943.1	E950.4	E962.0	E980.4
Replacement solutions	974.5	E858.5	E944.5	E950.4	E962.0	E980.4	Scarlet red	976.8	E858.7	E946.8	E950.4	E962.0	E980.4
Rescinnamine	972.6	E858.3	E942.6	E950.4	E962.0	E980.4	**Scheele's green**	985.1	E866.3	—	E950.8	E962.1	E980.8
Reserpine	972.6	E858.3	E942.6	E950.4	E962.0	E980.4	insecticide	985.1	E863.4	—	E950.8	E962.1	E980.8
Resorcin, resorcinol	976.4	E858.7	E946.4	E950.4	E962.0	E980.4	**Schradan**	989.3	E863.1	—	E950.6	E962.1	E980.7
Respaire	975.5	E858.6	E945.5	E950.4	E962.0	E980.4	**Schweinfurt(h) green**	985.1	E866.3	—	E950.8	E962.1	E980.8
Respiratory agents NEC	975.8	E858.6	E945.8	E950.4	E962.0	E980.4	insecticide	985.1	E863.4	—	E950.8	E962.1	E980.8
Retinoic acid	976.8	E858.7	E946.8	E950.4	E962.0	E980.4	Scilla — see Squill						
Retinol	963.5	E858.1	E933.5	E950.4	E962.0	E980.4	**Sclerosing agents**	972.7	E858.3	E942.7	E950.4	F962.0	E980.4
Rh (D) immune globulin (hu-man)	964.6	E858.2	E934.6	E950.4	E962.0	E980.4	**Scopolamine**	971.1	E855.4	E941.1	E950.4	E962.0	E980.4
Rhodine	965.1	E850.3	E935.3	E950.0	E962.0	E980.0	**Scouring powder**	989.89	E861.3	—	E950.9	E962.1	E980.9
RhoGAM	964.6	E858.2	E934.6	E950.4	E962.0	E980.4	**Sea**						
Riboflavin	963.5	E858.1	E933.5	E950.4	E962.0	E980.4	anemone (sting)	989.5	E905.6	—	E950.9	E962.1	E980.9
Ricin	989.89	E866.8	—	E950.9	E962.1	E980.9	cucumber (sting)	989.5	E905.6	—	E950.9	E962.1	E980.9
Ricinus communis	988.2	E865.3	—	E950.9	E962.1	E980.9	snake (bite) (venom)	989.5	E905.0	—	E950.9	E962.1	E980.9
Rickettsial vaccine NEC	979.6	E858.8	E949.6	E950.4	E962.0	E980.4	urchin spine (puncture)	989.5	E905.6	—	E950.9	E962.1	E980.9
with viral and bacterial vac-cine	979.7	E858.8	E949.7	E950.4	E962.0	E980.4	Secbutabarbital	967.0	E851	E937.0	E950.1	E962.0	E980.1
Rifampin	960.6	E856	E930.6	E950.4	E962.0	E980.4	Secbutabarbitone	967.0	E851	E937.0	E950.1	E962.0	E980.1
Rimifon	961.8	E857	E931.8	E950.4	E962.0	E980.4	Secobarbital	967.0	E851	E937.0	E950.1	E962.0	E980.1
Ringer's injection (lactat-ed)	974.5	E858.5	E944.5	E950.4	E962.0	E980.4	Seconal	967.0	E851	E937.0	E950.1	E962.0	E980.1
Ristocetin	960.8	E856	E930.8	E950.4	E962.0	E980.4	Secretin	977.8	E858.8	E947.8	E950.4	E962.0	E980.4
Ritalin	969.73	E854.2	E939.7	E950.3	E962.0	E980.3	**Sedatives, nonbarbitu-rate**	967.9	E852.9	E937.9	E950.2	E962.0	E980.2
Roach killers — see Pesticides							specified NEC	967.8	E852.8	E937.8	E950.2	E962.0	E980.2
Rocky Mountain spotted fever vaccine	979.6	E858.8	E949.6	E950.4	E962.0	E980.4	Sedormid	967.8	E852.8	E937.8	E950.2	E962.0	E980.2
Rodenticides	989.4	E863.7	—	E950.6	E962.1	E980.7	**Seed** (plant)	988.2	E865.3	—	E950.9	E962.1	E980.9
Rohypnol	969.4	E853.2	E939.4	E950.3	E962.0	E980.3	disinfectant or dressing	989.89	E866.5	—	E950.9	E962.1	E980.9
Rolaids	973.0	E858.4	E943.0	E950.4	E962.0	E980.4	**Selective serotonin and norepinephrine reuptake inhibitors** (SSNRI)	969.02	E854.0	E939.0	E950.3	E962.0	E980.3
Rolitetracycline	960.4	E856	E930.4	E950.4	E962.0	E980.4	**Selective serotonin reuptake inhibitors** (SSRI)	969.03	E854.0	E939.0	E950.3	E962.0	E980.3
Romilar	975.4	E858.6	E945.4	E950.4	E962.0	E980.4	**Selenium** (fumes) NEC	985.8	E866.4	—	E950.9	E962.1	E980.9
Rose water ointment	976.3	E858.7	E946.3	E950.4	E962.0	E980.4	disulfide or sulfide	976.4	E858.7	E946.4	E950.4	E962.0	E980.4
Rosuvastatin calcium	972.1	E858.3	E942.2	E950.4	E962.0	E980.4	Selsun	976.4	E858.7	E946.4	E950.4	E962.0	E980.4
Rotenone	989.4	E863.7	—	E950.6	E962.1	E980.7	Senna	973.1	E858.4	E943.1	E950.4	E962.0	E980.4
Rotoxamine	963.0	E858.1	E933.0	E950.4	E962.0	E980.4	Septisol	976.2	E858.7	E946.2	E950.4	E962.0	E980.4
Rough-on-rats	989.4	E863.7	—	E950.6	E962.1	E980.7	Serax	969.4	E853.2	E939.4	E950.3	E962.0	E980.3
RU486	962.9	E858.0	E932.9	E950.4	E962.0	E980.4	Serenesil	967.8	E852.8	E937.8	E950.2	E962.0	E980.2
Rubbing alcohol	980.2	E860.3	—	E950.9	E962.1	E980.9	Serenium (hydrochloride)	961.9	E857	E931.9	E950.4	E962.0	E980.4
Rubella virus vaccine	979.4	E858.8	E949.4	E950.4	E962.0	E980.4	Serepax — see Oxazepam						
Rubelogen	979.4	E858.8	E949.4	E950.4	E962.0	E980.4	Sernyl	968.3	E855.1	E938.3	E950.4	E962.0	E980.4
Rubeovax	979.4	E858.8	E949.4	E950.4	E962.0	E980.4	Serotonin	977.8	E858.8	E947.8	E950.4	E962.0	E980.4
Rubidomycin	960.7	E856	E930.7	E950.4	E962.0	E980.4	Serpasil	972.6	E858.3	E942.6	E950.4	E962.0	E980.4
Rue	988.2	E865.4	—	E950.9	E962.1	E980.9	**Sewer gas**	987.8	E869.8	—	E952.8	E962.2	E982.8
Ruta	988.2	E865.4	—	E950.9	E962.1	E980.9	**Shampoo**	989.6	E861.0	—	E950.9	E962.1	E980.9
Sabadilla (medicinal)	976.0	E858.7	E946.0	E950.4	E962.0	E980.4	**Shellfish, nonbacterial or noxious**	988.0	E865.1	—	E950.9	E962.1	E980.9
pesticide	989.4	E863.4	—	E950.6	E962.1	E980.7	**Silicones NEC**	989.83	E866.8	E947.8	E950.9	E962.1	E980.9
Sabin oral vaccine	979.5	E858.8	E949.5	E950.4	E962.0	E980.4	**Silvadene**	976.0	E858.7	E946.0	E950.4	E962.0	E980.4
Saccharated iron oxide	964.0	E858.2	E934.0	E950.4	E962.0	E980.4	**Silver** (compound) (medici-nal) NEC	976.0	E858.7	E946.0	E950.4	E962.0	E980.4
Saccharin	974.5	E858.5	E944.5	E950.4	E962.0	E980.4	anti-infectives	976.0	E858.7	E946.0	E950.4	E962.0	E980.4
Safflower oil	972.2	E858.3	E942.2	E950.4	E962.0	E980.4	arsphenamine	961.1	E857	E931.1	E950.4	E962.0	E980.4
Salbutamol sulfate	975.7	E858.6	E945.7	E950.4	E962.0	E980.4	nitrate	976.0	E858.7	E946.0	E950.4	E962.0	E980.4
Salicylamide	965.1	E850.3	E935.3	E950.0	E962.0	E980.0	ophthalmic preparation	976.5	E858.7	E946.5	E950.4	E962.0	E980.4
Salicylate(s)	965.1	E850.3	E935.3	E950.0	E962.0	E980.0	toughened (keratolytic)	976.4	E858.7	E946.4	E950.4	E962.0	E980.4
methyl	976.3	E858.7	E946.3	E950.4	E962.0	E980.4	nonmedicinal (dust)	985.8	E866.4	—	E950.9	E962.1	E980.9
theobromine calcium	974.1	E858.5	E944.1	E950.4	E962.0	E980.4	protein (mild) (strong)	976.0	E858.7	E946.0	E950.4	E962.0	E980.4
Salicylazosulfapyridine	961.0	E857	E931.0	E950.4	E962.0	E980.4	salvarsan	961.1	E857	E931.1	E950.4	E962.0	E980.4
Salicylhydroxamic acid	976.0	E858.7	E946.0	E950.4	E962.0	E980.4	**Simethicone**	973.8	E858.4	E943.8	E950.4	E962.0	E980.4
Salicylic acid (keratolytic) NEC	976.4	E858.7	E946.4	E950.4	E962.0	E980.4	**Sinequan**	969.05	E854.0	E939.0	E950.3	E962.0	E980.3
congeners	965.1	E850.3	E935.3	E950.0	E962.0	E980.0	**Singoserp**	972.6	E858.3	E942.6	E950.4	E962.0	E980.4
salts	965.1	E850.3	E935.3	E950.0	E962.0	E980.0	**Sintrom**	964.2	E858.2	E934.2	E950.4	E962.0	E980.4
Saliniazid	961.8	E857	E931.8	E950.4	E962.0	E980.4	**Sitosterols**	972.2	E858.3	E942.2	E950.4	E962.0	E980.4
Salol	976.3	E858.7	E946.3	E950.4	E962.0	E980.4	**Skeletal muscle relax-ants**	975.2	E858.6	E945.2	E950.4	E962.0	E980.4
Salt (substitute) NEC	974.5	E858.5	E944.5	E950.4	E962.0	E980.4	**Skin**						
Saluretics	974.3	E858.5	E944.3	E950.4	E962.0	E980.4	agents (external)	976.9	E858.7	E946.9	E950.4	E962.0	E980.4
Saluron	974.3	E858.5	E944.3	E950.4	E962.0	E980.4	specified NEC	976.8	E858.7	E946.8	E950.4	E962.0	E980.4
Salvarsan 606 (neosilver) (sil-ver)	961.1	E857	E931.1	E950.4	E962.0	E980.4							
Sambucus canadensis	988.2	E865.4	—	E950.9	E962.1	E980.9							

Nontherapeutic use substance

▽ Subterms under main terms may continue to next column or page

	Poisoning	Accident	Therapeutic Use	Suicide Attempt	Assault	Undetermined
Skin — *continued*						
test antigen	977.8	E858.8	E947.8	E950.4	E962.0	E980.4
Sleep-eze	963.0	E858.1	E933.0	E950.4	E962.0	E980.4
Sleeping draught (drug) (pill)						
(tablet)	967.9	E852.9	E937.9	E950.2	E962.0	E980.2
Smallpox vaccine	979.0	E858.8	E949.0	E950.4	E962.0	E980.4
Smelter fumes NEC	985.9	E866.4	—	E950.9	E962.1	E980.9
Smog	987.3	E869.1	—	E952.8	E962.2	E982.8
Smoke NEC	987.9	E869.9	—	E952.9	E962.2	E982.9
Smooth muscle relaxant	975.1	E858.6	E945.1	E950.4	E962.0	E980.4
Snail killer	989.4	E863.4	—	E950.6	E962.1	E980.7
Snake (bite) (venom)	989.5	E905.0	—	E950.9	E962.1	E980.9
Snuff	989.89	E866.8	—	E950.9	E962.1	E980.9
Soap (powder) (product)	989.6	E861.1	—	E950.9	E962.1	E980.9
bicarb	963.3	E858.1	E933.3	E950.4	E962.0	E980.4
chlorinated — see Sodium, hypochlorite						
medicinal, soft	976.2	E858.7	E946.2	E950.4	E962.0	E980.4
Soda (caustic)	983.2	E864.2	—	E950.7	E962.1	E980.6
Sodium						
acetosulfone	961.8	E857	E931.8	E950.4	E962.0	E980.4
acetrizoate	977.8	E858.8	E947.8	E950.4	E962.0	E980.4
amytal	967.0	E851	E937.0	E950.1	E962.0	E980.1
arsenate — see Arsenic						
bicarbonate	963.3	E858.1	E933.3	E950.4	E962.0	E980.4
bichromate	983.9	E864.3	—	E950.7	E962.1	E980.6
biphosphate	963.2	E858.1	E933.2	E950.4	E962.0	E980.4
bisulfate	983.9	E864.3	—	E950.7	E962.1	E980.6
borate (cleanser)	989.6	E861.3	—	E950.9	E962.1	E980.9
bromide NEC	967.3	E852.2	E937.3	E950.2	E962.0	E980.2
cacodylate (nonmedicinal)						
NEC	978.8	E858.8	E948.8	E950.4	E962.0	E980.4
anti-infective	961.1	E857	E931.1	E950.4	E962.0	E980.4
herbicide	989.4	E863.5	—	E950.6	E962.1	E980.7
calcium edetate	963.8	E858.1	E933.8	E950.4	E962.0	E980.4
carbonate NEC	983.2	E864.2	—	E950.7	E962.1	E980.6
chlorate NEC	983.9	E864.3	—	E950.7	E962.1	E980.6
herbicide	983.9	E863.5	—	E950.7	E962.1	E980.6
chloride NEC	974.5	E858.5	E944.5	E950.4	E962.0	E980.4
chromate	983.9	E864.3	—	E950.7	E962.1	E980.6
citrate	963.3	E858.1	E933.3	E950.4	E962.0	E980.4
cyanide — see Cyanide(s)						
cyclamate	974.5	E858.5	E944.5	E950.4	E962.0	E980.4
diatrizoate	977.8	E858.8	E947.8	E950.4	E962.0	E980.4
dibunate	975.4	E858.6	E945.4	E950.4	E962.0	E980.4
dioctyl sulfosuccinate	973.2	E858.4	E943.2	E950.4	E962.0	E980.4
edetate	963.8	E858.1	E933.8	E950.4	E962.0	E980.4
ethacrynate	974.4	E858.5	E944.4	E950.4	E962.0	E980.4
fluoracetate (dust) (rodenticide)	989.4	E863.7	—	E950.6	E962.1	E980.7
fluoride — see Fluoride(s)						
free salt	974.5	E858.5	E944.5	E950.4	E962.0	E980.4
glucosulfone	961.8	E857	E931.8	E950.4	E962.0	E980.4
hydroxide	983.2	E864.2	—	E950.7	E962.1	E980.6
hypochlorite (bleach)						
NEC	983.9	E864.3	—	E950.7	E962.1	E980.6
disinfectant	983.9	E861.4	—	E950.7	E962.1	E980.6
medicinal (anti-infective) (external)	976.0	E858.7	E946.0	E950.4	E962.0	E980.4
vapor	987.8	E869.8	—	E952.8	E962.2	E982.8
hyposulfite	976.0	E858.7	E946.0	E950.4	E962.0	E980.4
indigotindisulfonate	977.8	E858.8	E947.8	E950.4	E962.0	E980.4
iodide	977.8	E858.8	E947.8	E950.4	E962.0	E980.4
iothalamate	977.8	E858.8	E947.8	E950.4	E962.0	E980.4
iron edetate	964.0	E858.2	E934.0	E950.4	E962.0	E980.4
lactate	963.3	E858.1	E933.3	E950.4	E962.0	E980.4
lauryl sulfate	976.2	E858.7	E946.2	E950.4	E962.0	E980.4
L-triiodothyronine	962.7	E858.0	E932.7	E950.4	E962.0	E980.4
metrizoate	977.8	E858.8	E947.8	E950.4	E962.0	E980.4
monofluoroacetate (dust) (rodenticide)	989.4	E863.7	—	E950.6	E962.1	E980.7
morrhuate	972.7	E858.3	E942.7	E950.4	E962.0	E980.4
nafcillin	960.0	E856	E930.0	E950.4	E962.0	E980.4
nitrate (oxidizing agent)	983.9	E864.3	—	E950.7	E962.1	E980.6
nitrite (medicinal)	972.4	E858.3	E942.4	E950.4	E962.0	E980.4
nitroferricyanide	972.6	E858.3	E942.6	E950.4	E962.0	E980.4
nitroprusside	972.6	E858.3	E942.6	E950.4	E962.0	E980.4
para-aminohippurate	977.8	E858.8	E947.8	E950.4	E962.0	E980.4
perborate (nonmedicinal)						
NEC	989.89	E866.8	—	E950.9	E962.1	E980.9
medicinal	976.6	E858.7	E946.6	E950.4	E962.0	E980.4
soap	989.6	E861.1	—	E950.9	E962.1	E980.9

	Poisoning	Accident	Therapeutic Use	Suicide Attempt	Assault	Undetermined
Sodium — *continued*						
percarbonate — see Sodium, perborate						
phosphate	973.3	E858.4	E943.3	E950.4	E962.0	E980.4
polystyrene sulfonate	974.5	E858.5	E944.5	E950.4	E962.0	E980.4
propionate	976.0	E858.7	E946.0	E950.4	E962.0	E980.4
psylliate	972.7	E858.3	E942.7	E950.4	E962.0	E980.4
removing resins	974.5	E858.5	E944.5	E950.4	E962.0	E980.4
salicylate	965.1	E850.3	E935.3	E950.0	E962.0	E980.0
sulfate	973.3	E858.4	E943.3	E950.4	E962.0	E980.4
sulfoxone	961.8	E857	E931.8	E950.4	E962.0	E980.4
tetradecyl sulfate	972.7	E858.3	E942.7	E950.4	E962.0	E980.4
thiopental	968.3	E855.1	E938.3	E950.4	E962.0	E980.4
thiosalicylate	965.1	E850.3	E935.3	E950.0	E962.0	E980.0
thiosulfate	976.0	E858.7	E946.0	E950.4	E962.0	E980.4
tolbutamide	977.8	E858.8	E947.8	E950.4	E962.0	E980.4
tyropanoate	977.8	E858.8	E947.8	E950.4	E962.0	E980.4
valproate	966.3	E855.0	E936.3	E950.4	E962.0	E980.4
Solanine	977.8	E858.8	E947.8	E950.4	E962.0	E980.4
Solanum dulcamara	988.2	E865.4	—	E950.9	E962.1	E980.9
Solapsone	961.8	E857	E931.8	E950.4	E962.0	E980.4
Solasulfone	961.8	E857	E931.8	E950.4	E962.0	E980.4
Soldering fluid	983.1	E864.1	—	E950.7	E962.1	E980.6
Solid substance	989.9	E866.9	—	E950.9	E962.1	E980.9
specified NEC	989.9	E866.8	—	E950.9	E962.1	E980.9
Solvents, industrial	982.8	E862.9	—	E950.9	E962.1	E980.9
naphtha	981	E862.0	—	E950.9	E962.1	E980.9
petroleum	981	E862.0	—	E950.9	E962.1	E980.9
specified NEC	982.8	E862.4	—	E950.9	E962.1	E980.9
Soma	968.0	E855.1	E938.0	E950.4	E962.0	E980.4
Somatotropin	962.4	E858.0	E932.4	E950.4	E962.0	E980.4
Sominex	963.0	E858.1	E933.0	E950.4	E962.0	E980.4
Somnos	967.1	E852.0	E937.1	E950.2	E962.0	E980.2
Somonal	967.0	E851	E937.0	E950.1	E962.0	E980.1
Soneryl	967.0	E851	E937.0	E950.1	E962.0	E980.1
Soothing syrup	977.9	E858.9	E947.9	E950.5	E962.0	E980.5
Sopor	967.4	E852.3	E937.4	E950.2	E962.0	E980.2
Soporific drug	967.9	E852.9	E937.9	E950.2	E962.0	E980.2
specified type NEC	967.8	E852.8	E937.8	E950.2	E962.0	E980.2
Sorbitol NEC	977.4	E858.8	E947.4	E950.4	E962.0	E980.4
Sotradecol	972.7	E858.3	E942.7	E950.4	E962.0	E980.4
Spacoline	975.1	E858.6	E945.1	E950.4	E962.0	E980.4
Spanish fly	976.8	E858.7	E946.8	E950.4	E962.0	E980.4
Sparine	969.1	E853.0	E939.1	E950.3	E962.0	E980.3
Sparteine	975.0	E858.6	E945.0	E950.4	E962.0	E980.4
Spasmolytics	975.1	E858.6	E945.1	E950.4	E962.0	E980.4
anticholinergics	971.1	E855.4	E941.1	E950.4	E962.0	E980.4
Spectinomycin	960.8	E856	E930.8	E950.4	E962.0	E980.4
Speed	969.72	E854.2	E939.7	E950.3	E962.0	E980.3
Spermicides	976.8	E858.7	E946.8	E950.4	E962.0	E980.4
Spider (bite) (venom)	989.5	E905.1	—	E950.9	E962.1	E980.9
antivenin	979.9	E858.8	E949.9	E950.4	E962.0	E980.4
Spigelia (root)	961.6	E857	E931.6	E950.4	E962.0	E980.4
Spiperone	969.2	E853.1	E939.2	E950.3	E962.0	E980.3
Spiramycin	960.3	E856	E930.3	E950.4	E962.0	E980.4
Spirilene	969.5	E853.8	E939.5	E950.3	E962.0	E980.3
Spirit(s) (neutral) NEC	980.0	E860.1	—	E950.9	E962.1	E980.9
beverage	980.0	E860.0	—	E950.9	E962.1	E980.9
industrial	980.9	E860.9	—	E950.9	E962.1	E980.9
mineral	981	E862.0	—	E950.9	E962.1	E980.9
of salt — see Hydrochloric acid						
surgical	980.9	E860.9	—	E950.9	E962.1	E980.9
Spironolactone	974.4	E858.5	E944.4	E950.4	E962.0	E980.4
Sponge, absorbable						
(gelatin)	964.5	E858.2	E934.5	E950.4	E962.0	E980.4
Sporostacin	976.0	E858.7	E946.0	E950.4	E962.0	E980.4
Sprays (aerosol)	989.89	E866.8	—	E950.9	E962.1	E980.9
cosmetic	989.89	E866.7	—	E950.9	E962.1	E980.9
medicinal NEC	977.9	E858.9	E947.9	E950.5	E962.0	E980.5
pesticides — see Pesticides						
specified content — see substance specified						
Spurge flax	988.2	E865.4	—	E950.9	E962.1	E980.9
Spurges	988.2	E865.4	—	E950.9	E962.1	E980.9
Squill (expectorant) NEC	975.5	E858.6	E945.5	E950.4	E962.0	E980.4
rat poison	989.4	E863.7	—	E950.6	E962.1	E980.7
Squirting cucumber (cathartic)	973.1	E858.4	E943.1	E950.4	E962.0	E980.4
SSNRI (selective serotonin and norepinephrine reuptake inhibitors)	969.02	E854.0	E939.0	E950.3	E962.0	E980.3

▽ Subterms under main terms may continue to next column or page

	Poisoning	Accident	Therapeutic Use	Suicide Attempt	Assault	Undetermined
SSRI (selective serotonin reuptake inhibitors)	969.03	E854.0	E939.0	E950.3	E962.0	E980.3
Stains	989.89	E866.8	—	E950.9	E962.1	E980.9
Stannous — see also Tin						
fluoride	976.7	E858.7	E946.7	E950.4	E962.0	E980.4
Stanolone	962.1	E858.0	E932.1	E950.4	E962.0	E980.4
Stanozolol	962.1	E858.0	E932.1	E950.4	E962.0	E980.4
Staphisagria or stavesacre						
(pediculicide)	976.0	E858.7	E946.0	E950.4	E962.0	E980.4
Stelazine	969.1	E853.0	E939.1	E950.3	E962.0	E980.3
Stemetil	969.1	E853.0	E939.1	E950.3	E962.0	E980.3
Sterculia (cathartic) (gum)	973.3	E858.4	E943.3	E950.4	E962.0	E980.4
Sternutator gas	987.8	E869.8	—	E952.8	E962.2	E982.8
Steroids NEC	962.0	E858.0	E932.0	E950.4	E962.0	E980.4
ENT agent	976.6	E858.7	E946.6	E950.4	E962.0	E980.4
ophthalmic preparation	976.5	E858.7	E946.5	E950.4	E962.0	E980.4
topical NEC	976.0	E858.7	E946.0	E950.4	E962.0	E980.4
Stibine	985.8	E866.4	—	E950.9	E962.1	E980.9
Stibophen	961.2	E857	E931.2	E950.4	E962.0	E980.4
Stilbamide, stilbamidine	961.5	E857	E931.5	E950.4	E962.0	E980.4
Stilbestrol	962.2	E858.0	E932.2	E950.4	E962.0	E980.4
Stimulants (central nervous						
system)	970.9	E854.3	E940.9	E950.4	E962.0	E980.4
analeptics	970.0	E854.3	E940.0	E950.4	E962.0	E980.4
opiate antagonist	970.1	E854.3	E940.1	E950.4	E962.0	E980.4
psychotherapeutic NEC	969.09	E854.0	E939.0	E950.3	E962.0	E980.3
specified NEC	970.89 ▲	E854.3	E940.8	E950.4	E962.0	E980.4
Storage batteries (acid)						
(cells)	983.1	E864.1	—	E950.7	E962.1	E980.6
Stovaine	968.9	E855.2	E938.9	E950.4	E962.0	E980.4
infiltration (subcutaneous)	968.5	E855.2	E938.5	E950.4	E962.0	E980.4
nerve block (peripheral) (plexus)	968.6	E855.2	E938.6	E950.4	E962.0	E980.4
spinal	968.7	E855.2	E938.7	E950.4	E962.0	E980.4
topical (surface)	968.5	E855.2	E938.5	E950.4	E962.0	E980.4
Stovarsal	961.1	E857	E931.1	E950.4	E962.0	E980.4
Stove gas — see Gas, utility						
Stoxil	976.5	E858.7	E946.5	E950.4	E962.0	E980.4
STP	969.6	E854.1	E939.6	E950.3	E962.0	E980.3
Stramonium (medicinal)						
NEC	971.1	E855.4	E941.1	E950.4	E962.0	E980.4
natural state	988.2	E865.4	—	E950.9	E962.1	E980.9
Streptodornase	964.4	E858.2	E934.4	E950.4	E962.0	E980.4
Streptoduocin	960.6	E856	E930.6	E950.4	E962.0	E980.4
Streptokinase	964.4	E858.2	E934.4	E950.4	E962.0	E980.4
Streptomycin	960.6	E856	E930.6	E950.4	E962.0	E980.4
Streptozocin	960.7	E856	E930.7	E950.4	E962.0	E980.4
Stripper (paint) (solvent)	982.8	E862.9	—	E950.9	E962.1	E980.9
Strobane	989.2	E863.0	—	E950.6	E962.1	E980.7
Strophanthin	972.1	E858.3	E942.1	E950.4	E962.0	E980.4
Strophanthus hispidus or kombe	988.2	E865.4	—	E950.9	E962.1	E980.9
Strychnine (rodenticide) (salts)	989.1	E863.7	—	E950.6	E962.1	E980.7
medicinal NEC	970.89 ▲	E854.3	E940.8	E950.4	E962.0	E980.4
Strychnos (ignatii) — see Strychnine						
Styramate	968.0	E855.1	E938.0	E950.4	E962.0	E980.4
Styrene	983.0	E864.0	—	E950.7	E962.1	E980.6
Succinimide (anticonvulsant)	966.2	E855.0	E936.2	E950.4	E962.0	E980.4
mercuric — see Mercury						
Succinylcholine	975.2	E858.6	E945.2	E950.4	E962.0	E980.4
Succinylsulfathiazole	961.0	E857	E931.0	E950.4	E962.0	E980.4
Sucrose	974.5	E858.5	E944.5	E950.4	E962.0	E980.4
Sulfacetamide	961.0	E857	E931.0	E950.4	E962.0	E980.4
ophthalmic preparation	976.5	E858.7	E946.5	E950.4	E962.0	E980.4
Sulfachlorpyridazine	961.0	E857	E931.0	E950.4	E962.0	E980.4
Sulfacytine	961.0	E857	E931.0	E950.4	E962.0	E980.4
Sulfadiazine	961.0	E857	E931.0	E950.4	E962.0	E980.4
silver (topical)	976.0	E858.7	E946.0	E950.4	E962.0	E980.4
Sulfadimethoxine	961.0	E857	E931.0	E950.4	E962.0	E980.4
Sulfadimidine	961.0	E857	E931.0	E950.4	E962.0	E980.4
Sulfaethidole	961.0	E857	E931.0	E950.4	E962.0	E980.4
Sulfafurazole	961.0	E857	E931.0	E950.4	E962.0	E980.4
Sulfaguanidine	961.0	E857	E931.0	E950.4	E962.0	E980.4
Sulfamerazine	961.0	E857	E931.0	E950.4	E962.0	E980.4
Sulfameter	961.0	E857	E931.0	E950.4	E962.0	E980.4
Sulfamethizole	961.0	E857	E931.0	E950.4	E962.0	E980.4
Sulfamethoxazole	961.0	E857	E931.0	E950.4	E962.0	E980.4
Sulfamethoxydiazine	961.0	E857	E931.0	E950.4	E962.0	E980.4
Sulfamethoxypyridazine	961.0	E857	E931.0	E950.4	E962.0	E980.4
Sulfamethylthiazole	961.0	E857	E931.0	E950.4	E962.0	E980.4
Sulfamylon	976.0	E858.7	E946.0	E950.4	E962.0	E980.4
Sulfan blue (diagnostic dye)	977.8	E858.8	E947.8	E950.4	E962.0	E980.4
Sulfanilamide	961.0	E857	E931.0	E950.4	E962.0	E980.4
Sulfanilylguanidine	961.0	E857	E931.0	E950.4	E962.0	E980.4
Sulfaphenazole	961.0	E857	E931.0	E950.4	E962.0	E980.4
Sulfaphenylthiazole	961.0	E857	E931.0	E950.4	E962.0	E980.4
Sulfaproxyline	961.0	E857	E931.0	E950.4	E962.0	E980.4
Sulfapyridine	961.0	E857	E931.0	E950.4	E962.0	E980.4
Sulfapyrimidine	961.0	E857	E931.0	E950.4	E962.0	E980.4
Sulfarsphenamine	961.1	E857	E931.1	E950.4	E962.0	E980.4
Sulfasalazine	961.0	E857	E931.0	E950.4	E962.0	E980.4
Sulfasomizole	961.0	E857	E931.0	E950.4	E962.0	E980.4
Sulfasuxidine	961.0	E857	E931.0	E950.4	E962.0	E980.4
Sulfinpyrazone	974.7	E858.5	E944.7	E950.4	E962.0	E980.4
Sulfisoxazole	961.0	E857	E931.0	E950.4	E962.0	E980.4
ophthalmic preparation	976.5	E858.7	E946.5	E950.4	E962.0	E980.4
Sulfomyxin	960.8	E856	E930.8	E950.4	E962.0	E980.4
Sulfonal	967.8	E852.8	E937.8	E950.2	E962.0	E980.2
Sulfonamides (mixtures)	961.0	E857	E931.0	E950.4	E962.0	E980.4
Sulfones	961.8	E857	E931.8	E950.4	E962.0	E980.4
Sulfonethylmethane	967.8	E852.8	E937.8	E950.2	E962.0	E980.2
Sulfonmethane	967.8	E852.8	E937.8	E950.2	E962.0	E980.2
Sulfonphthal, sulfonphthol	977.8	E858.8	E947.8	E950.4	E962.0	E980.4
Sulfonylurea derivatives, oral	962.3	E858.0	E932.3	E950.4	E962.0	E980.4
Sulfoxone	961.8	E857	E931.8	E950.4	E962.0	E980.4
Sulfur, sulfureted, sulfuric, sulfurous, sulfuryl (compounds) NEC	989.89	E866.8	—	E950.9	E962.1	E980.9
acid	983.1	E864.1	—	E950.7	E962.1	E980.6
dioxide	987.3	E869.1	—	E952.8	E962.2	E982.8
ether — see Ether(s)						
hydrogen	987.8	E869.8	—	E952.8	E962.2	E982.8
medicinal (keratolytic) (ointment) NEC	976.4	E858.7	E946.4	E950.4	E962.0	E980.4
pesticide (vapor)	989.4	E863.4	—	E950.6	E962.1	E980.7
vapor NEC	987.8	E869.8	—	E952.8	E962.2	E982.8
Sulkowitch's reagent	977.8	E858.8	E947.8	E950.4	E962.0	E980.4
Sulphadione	961.8	E857	E931.8	E950.4	E962.0	E980.4
Sulph — see also Sulf-						
Sulthiame, sultiame	966.3	E855.0	E936.3	E950.4	E962.0	E980.4
Superinone	975.5	E858.6	E945.5	E950.4	E962.0	E980.4
Suramin	961.5	E857	E931.5	E950.4	E962.0	E980.4
Surfacaine	968.5	E855.2	E938.5	E950.4	E962.0	E980.4
Surital	968.3	E855.1	E938.3	E950.4	E962.0	E980.4
Sutilains	976.8	E858.7	E946.8	E950.4	E962.0	E980.4
Suxamethonium (bromide) (chloride) (iodide)	975.2	E858.6	E945.2	E950.4	E962.0	E980.4
Suxethonium (bromide)	975.2	E858.6	E945.2	E950.4	E962.0	E980.4
Sweet oil (birch)	976.3	E858.7	E946.3	E950.4	E962.0	E980.4
Sym-dichloroethyl ether	982.3	E862.4	—	E950.9	E962.1	E980.9
Sympatholytics	971.3	E855.6	E941.3	E950.4	E962.0	E980.4
Sympathomimetics	971.2	E855.5	E941.2	E950.4	E962.0	E980.4
Synagis	979.6	E858.8	E949.6	E950.4	E962.0	E980.4
Synalar	976.0	E858.7	E946.0	E950.4	E962.0	E980.4
Synthroid	962.7	E858.0	E932.7	E950.4	E962.0	E980.4
Syntocinon	975.0	E858.6	E945.0	E950.4	E962.0	E950.4
Syrosingopine	972.6	E858.3	E942.6	E950.4	E962.0	E980.4
Systemic agents (primarily)	963.9	E858.1	E933.9	E950.4	E962.0	E980.4
specified NEC	963.8	E858.1	E933.8	E950.4	E962.0	E980.4
Tablets — see also specified substance	977.9	E858.9	E947.9	E950.5	E962.0	E980.5
Tace	962.2	E858.0	E932.2	E950.4	E962.0	E980.4
Tacrine	971.0	E855.3	E941.0	E950.4	E962.0	E980.4
Talbutal	967.0	E851	E937.0	E950.1	E962.0	E980.1
Talc	976.3	E858.7	E946.3	E950.4	E962.0	E980.4
Talcum	976.3	E858.7	E946.3	E950.4	E962.0	E980.4
Tamsulosin	971.3	E855.6	E941.3	E950.4	E962.0	E980.4
Tandearil, tanderil	965.5	E850.5	E935.5	E950.0	E962.0	E980.0
Tannic acid	983.1	E864.1	—	E950.7	E962.1	E980.6
medicinal (astringent)	976.2	E858.7	E946.2	E950.4	E962.0	E980.4
Tannin — see Tannic acid						
Tansy	988.2	E865.4	—	E950.9	E962.1	E980.9
TAO	960.3	E856	E930.3	E950.4	E962.0	E980.4
Tapazole	962.8	E858.0	E932.8	E950.4	E962.0	E980.4
Tar NEC	983.0	E864.0	—	E950.7	E962.1	E980.6
camphor — see Naphthalene						

SSRI — Tar NEC

		External Cause (E-Code)			
	Poisoning	Accident	Therapeutic Use	Suicide Attempt	Assault	Undetermined
---	---	---	---	---	---	---
Tar — *continued*						
fumes	987.8	E869.8	—	E952.8	E962.2	E982.8
Taractan	969.3	E853.8	E939.3	E950.3	E962.0	E980.3
Tarantula (venomous)	989.5	E905.1	—	E950.9	E962.1	E980.9
Tartar emetic (anti-infective)	961.2	E857	E931.2	E950.4	E962.0	E980.4
Tartaric acid	983.1	E864.1	—	E950.7	E962.1	E980.6
Tartrated antimony (anti-infective)	961.2	E857	E931.2	E950.4	E962.0	E980.4
TCA — *see* Trichloroacetic acid						
TDI	983.0	E864.0	—	E950.7	E962.1	E980.6
vapor	987.8	E869.8	—	E952.8	E962.2	E982.8
Tear gas	987.5	E869.3	—	E952.8	E962.2	E982.8
Teclothiazide	974.3	E858.5	E944.3	E950.4	E962.0	E980.4
Tegretol	966.3	E855.0	E936.3	E950.4	E962.0	E980.4
Telepaque	977.8	E858.8	E947.8	E950.4	E962.0	E980.4
Tellurium	985.8	E866.4	—	E950.9	E962.1	E980.9
fumes	985.8	E866.4	—	E950.9	E962.1	E980.9
TEM	963.1	E858.1	E933.1	E950.4	E962.0	E980.4
Temazepan — *see* Benzodiazepines						
TEPA	963.1	E858.1	E933.1	E950.4	E962.0	E980.4
TEPP	989.3	E863.1	—	E950.6	E962.1	E980.7
Terbutaline	971.2	E855.5	E941.2	E950.4	E962.0	E980.4
Teroxalene	961.6	E857	E931.6	E950.4	E962.0	E980.4
Terpin hydrate	975.5	E858.6	E945.5	E950.4	E962.0	E980.4
Terramycin	960.4	E856	E930.4	E950.4	E962.0	E980.4
Tessalon	975.4	E858.6	E945.4	E950.4	E962.0	E980.4
Testosterone	962.1	E858.0	E932.1	E950.4	E962.0	E980.4
Tetanus (vaccine)	978.4	E858.8	E948.4	E950.4	E962.0	E980.4
antitoxin	979.9	E858.8	E949.9	E950.4	E962.0	E980.4
immune globulin (human)	964.6	E858.2	E934.6	E950.4	E962.0	E980.4
toxoid	978.4	E858.8	E948.4	E950.4	E962.0	E980.4
with diphtheria toxoid	978.9	E858.8	E948.9	E950.4	E962.0	E980.4
with pertussis	978.6	E858.8	E948.6	E950.4	E962.0	E980.4
Tetrabenazine	969.5	E853.8	E939.5	E950.3	E962.0	E980.3
Tetracaine (infiltration) (topical)	968.5	E855.2	E938.5	E950.4	E962.0	E980.4
nerve block (peripheral) (plexus)	968.6	E855.2	E938.6	E950.4	E962.0	E980.4
spinal	968.7	E855.2	E938.7	E950.4	E962.0	E980.4
Tetrachlorethylene — *see* Tetrachloroethylene						
Tetrachlormethiazide	974.3	E858.5	E944.3	E950.4	E962.0	E980.4
Tetrachloroethane (liquid) (vapor)	982.3	E862.4	—	E950.9	E962.1	E980.9
paint or varnish	982.3	E861.6	—	E950.9	E962.1	E980.9
Tetrachloroethylene (liquid) (vapor)	982.3	E862.4	—	E950.9	E962.1	E980.9
medicinal	961.6	E857	E931.6	E950.4	E962.0	E980.4
Tetrachloromethane — *see* Carbon, tetrachloride						
Tetracycline	960.4	E856	E930.4	E950.4	E962.0	E980.4
ophthalmic preparation	976.5	E858.7	E946.5	E950.4	E962.0	E980.4
topical NEC	976.0	E858.7	E946.0	E950.4	E962.0	E980.4
Tetraethylammonium chloride	972.3	E858.3	E942.3	E950.4	E962.0	E980.4
Tetraethyl lead (antiknock compound)	984.1	E862.1	—	E950.9	E962.1	E980.9
Tetraethyl pyrophosphate	989.3	E863.1	—	E950.6	E962.1	E980.7
Tetraethylthiuram disulfide	977.3	E858.8	E947.3	E950.4	E962.0	E980.4
Tetrahydroaminoacridine	971.0	E855.3	E941.0	E950.4	E962.0	E980.4
Tetrahydrocannabinol	969.6	E854.1	E939.6	E950.3	E962.0	E980.3
Tetrahydronaphthalene	982.0	E862.4	—	E950.9	E962.1	E980.9
Tetrahydrozoline	971.2	E855.5	E941.2	E950.4	E962.0	E980.4
Tetralin	982.0	E862.4	—	E950.9	E962.1	E980.9
Tetramethylthiuram (disulfide) NEC	989.4	E863.6	—	E950.6	E962.1	E980.7
medicinal	976.2	E858.7	E946.2	E950.4	E962.0	E980.4
Tetronal	967.8	E852.8	E937.8	E950.2	E962.0	E980.2
Tetryl	983.0	E864.0	—	E950.7	E962.1	E980.6
Thalidomide	967.8	E852.8	E937.8	E950.2	E962.0	E980.2
Thallium (compounds) (dust) NEC	985.8	E866.4	—	E950.9	E962.1	E980.9
pesticide (rodenticide)	985.8	E863.7	—	E950.6	E962.1	E980.7
THC	969.6	E854.1	E939.6	E950.3	E962.0	E980.3
Thebacon	965.09	E850.2	E935.2	E950.0	E962.0	E980.0
Thebaine	965.09	E850.2	E935.2	E950.0	E962.0	E980.0

		External Cause (E-Code)			
	Poisoning	Accident	Therapeutic Use	Suicide Attempt	Assault	Undetermined
---	---	---	---	---	---	---
Theobromine (calcium salicylate)	974.1	E858.5	E944.1	E950.4	E962.0	E980.4
Theophylline (diuretic)	974.1	E858.5	E944.1	E950.4	E962.0	E980.4
ethylenediamine	975.7	E858.6	E945.7	E950.4	E962.0	E980.4
Thiabendazole	961.6	E857	E931.6	E950.4	E962.0	E980.4
Thialbarbital, thialbarbitone	968.3	E855.1	E938.3	E950.4	E962.0	E980.4
Thiamine	963.5	E858.1	E933.5	E950.4	E962.0	E980.4
Thiamylal (sodium)	968.3	E855.1	E938.3	E950.4	E962.0	E980.4
Thiazesim	969.09	E854.0	E939.0	E950.3	E962.0	E980.3
Thiazides (diuretics)	974.3	E858.5	E944.3	E950.4	E962.0	E980.4
Thiethylperazine	963.0	E858.1	E933.0	E950.4	E962.0	E980.4
Thimerosal (topical)	976.0	E858.7	E946.0	E950.4	E962.0	E980.4
ophthalmic preparation	976.5	E858.7	E946.5	E950.4	E962.0	E980.4
Thioacetazone	961.8	E857	E931.8	E950.4	E962.0	E980.4
Thiobarbiturates	968.3	E855.1	E938.3	E950.4	E962.0	E980.4
Thiobismol	961.2	E857	E931.2	E950.4	E962.0	E980.4
Thiocarbamide	962.8	E858.0	E932.8	E950.4	E962.0	E980.4
Thiocarbarsone	961.1	E857	E931.1	E950.4	E962.0	E980.4
Thiocarlide	961.8	E857	E931.8	E950.4	E962.0	E980.4
Thioguanine	963.1	E858.1	E933.1	E950.4	E962.0	E980.4
Thiomercaptomerin	974.0	E858.5	E944.0	E950.4	E962.0	E980.4
Thiomerin	974.0	E858.5	E944.0	E950.4	E962.0	E980.4
Thiopental, thiopentone (sodium)	968.3	E855.1	E938.3	E950.4	E962.0	E980.4
Thiopropazate	969.1	E853.0	E939.1	E950.3	E962.0	E980.3
Thioproperazine	969.1	E853.0	E939.1	E950.3	E962.0	E980.3
Thioridazine	969.1	E853.0	E939.1	E950.3	E962.0	E980.3
Thio-TEPA, thiotepa	963.1	E858.1	E933.1	E950.4	E962.0	E980.4
Thiothixene	969.3	E853.8	E939.3	E950.3	E962.0	E980.3
Thiouracil	962.8	E858.0	E932.8	E950.4	E962.0	E980.4
Thiourea	962.8	E858.0	E932.8	E950.4	E962.0	E980.4
Thiphenamil	971.1	E855.4	E941.1	E950.4	E962.0	E980.4
Thiram NEC	989.4	E863.6	—	E950.6	E962.1	E980.7
medicinal	976.2	E858.7	E946.2	E950.4	E962.0	E980.4
Thonzylamine	963.0	E858.1	E933.0	E950.4	E962.0	E980.4
Thorazine	969.1	E853.0	E939.1	E950.3	E962.0	E980.3
Thornapple	988.2	E865.4	—	E950.9	E962.1	E980.9
Throat preparation (lozenges) NEC	976.6	E858.7	E946.6	E950.4	E962.0	E980.4
Thrombin	964.5	E858.2	E934.5	E950.4	E962.0	E980.4
Thrombolysin	964.4	E858.2	E934.4	E950.4	E962.0	E980.4
Thymol	983.0	E864.0	—	E950.7	E962.1	E980.6
Thymus extract	962.9	E858.0	E932.9	E950.4	E962.0	E980.4
Thyroglobulin	962.7	E858.0	E932.7	E950.4	E962.0	E980.4
Thyroid (derivatives) (extract)	962.7	E858.0	E932.7	E950.4	E962.0	E980.4
Thyrolar	962.7	E858.0	E932.7	E950.4	E962.0	E980.4
Thyrothrophin, thyrotropin	977.8	E858.8	E947.8	E950.4	E962.0	E980.4
Thyroxin(e)	962.7	E858.0	E932.7	E950.4	E962.0	E980.4
Tigan	963.0	E858.1	E933.0	E950.4	E962.0	E980.4
Tigloidine	968.0	E855.1	E938.0	E950.4	E962.0	E980.4
Tin (chloride) (dust) (oxide) NEC	985.8	E866.4	—	E950.9	E962.1	E980.9
anti-infectives	961.2	E857	E931.2	E950.4	E962.0	E980.4
Tinactin	976.0	E858.7	E946.0	E950.4	E962.0	E980.4
Tincture, iodine — *see* Iodine						
Tindal	969.1	E853.0	E939.1	E950.3	E962.0	E980.3
Titanium (compounds) (vapor)	985.8	E866.4	—	E950.9	E962.1	E980.9
ointment	976.3	E858.7	E946.3	E950.4	E962.0	E980.4
Titroid	962.7	E858.0	E932.7	E950.4	E962.0	E980.4
TMTD — *see* Tetramethylthiuram disulfide						
TNT	989.89	E866.8	—	E950.9	E962.1	E980.9
fumes	987.8	E869.8	—	E952.8	E962.2	E982.8
Toadstool	988.1	E865.5	—	E950.9	E962.1	E980.9
Tobacco NEC	989.84	E866.8	—	E950.9	E962.1	E980.9
Indian	988.2	E865.4	—	E950.9	E962.1	E980.9
smoke, second-hand	987.8	E869.4	—	—	—	—
Tocopherol	963.5	E858.1	E933.5	E950.4	E962.0	E980.4
Tocosamine	975.0	E858.6	E945.0	E950.4	E962.0	E980.4
Tofranil	969.05	E854.0	E939.0	E950.3	E962.0	E980.3
Toilet deodorizer	989.89	E866.8	—	E950.9	E962.1	E980.9
Tolazamide	962.3	E858.0	E932.3	E950.4	E962.0	E980.4
Tolazoline	971.3	E855.6	E941.3	E950.4	E962.0	E980.4
Tolbutamide	962.3	E858.0	E932.3	E950.4	E962.0	E980.4
sodium	977.8	E858.8	E947.8	E950.4	E962.0	E980.4
Tolmetin	965.69	E850.6	E935.6	E950.0	E962.0	E980.0
Tolnaftate	976.0	E858.7	E946.0	E950.4	E962.0	E980.4
Tolpropamine	976.1	E858.7	E946.1	E950.4	E962.0	E980.4

		External Cause (E-Code)				
	Poisoning	Accident	Therapeutic Use	Suicide Attempt	Assault	Undetermined
Tolserol	968.0	E855.1	E938.0	E950.4	E962.0	E980.4
Toluene (liquid) (vapor)	982.0	E862.4	—	E950.9	E962.1	E980.9
diisocyanate	983.0	E864.0	—	E950.7	E962.1	E980.6
Toluidine	983.0	E864.0	—	E950.7	E962.1	E980.6
vapor	987.8	E869.8	—	E952.8	E962.2	E982.8
Toluol (liquid) (vapor)	982.0	E862.4	—	E950.9	E962.1	E980.9
Tolylene-2, 4-diiso-cyanate	983.0	E864.0	—	E950.7	E962.1	E980.6
Tonics, cardiac	972.1	E858.3	E942.1	E950.4	E962.0	E980.4
Toxaphene (dust) (spray)	989.2	E863.0	—	E950.6	E962.1	E980.7
Toxoids NEC	978.8	E858.8	E948.8	E950.4	E962.0	E980.4
Tractor fuel NEC	981	E862.1	—	E950.9	E962.1	E980.9
Tragacanth	973.3	E858.4	E943.3	E950.4	E962.0	E980.4
Tramazoline	971.2	E855.5	E941.2	E950.4	E962.0	E980.4
Tranquilizers	969.5	E853.9	E939.5	E950.3	E962.0	E980.3
benzodiazepine-based	969.4	E853.2	E939.4	E950.3	E962.0	E980.3
butyrophenone-based	969.2	E853.1	E939.2	E950.3	E962.0	E980.3
major NEC	969.3	E853.8	E939.3	E950.3	E962.0	E980.3
phenothiazine-based	969.1	E853.0	E939.1	E950.3	E962.0	E980.3
specified NEC	969.5	E853.8	E939.5	E950.3	E962.0	E980.3
Trantoin	961.9	E857	E931.9	E950.4	E962.0	E980.4
Tranxene	969.4	E853.2	E939.4	E950.3	E962.0	E980.3
Tranylcypromine (sulfate)	969.01	E854.0	E939.0	E950.3	E962.0	E980.3
Trasentine	975.1	E858.6	E945.1	E950.4	E962.0	E980.4
Travert	974.5	E858.5	E944.5	E950.4	E962.0	E980.4
Trecator	961.8	E857	E931.8	E950.4	E962.0	E980.4
Tretinoin	976.8	E858.7	E946.8	E950.4	E962.0	E980.4
Triacetin	976.0	E858.7	E946.0	E950.4	E962.0	E980.4
Triacetyloleandomycin	960.3	E856	E930.3	E950.4	E962.0	E980.4
Triamcinolone	962.0	E858.0	E932.0	E950.4	E962.0	E980.4
ENT agent	976.6	E858.7	E946.6	E950.4	E962.0	E980.4
medicinal (keratolytic)	976.4	E858.7	E946.4	E950.4	E962.0	E980.4
ophthalmic preparation	976.5	E858.7	E946.5	E950.4	E962.0	E980.4
topical NEC	976.0	E858.7	E946.0	E950.4	E962.0	E980.4
Triamterene	974.4	E858.5	E944.4	E950.4	E962.0	E980.4
Triaziquone	963.1	E858.1	E933.1	E950.4	E962.0	E980.4
Tribromacetaldehyde	967.3	E852.2	E937.3	E950.2	E962.0	E980.2
Tribromoethanol	968.2	E855.1	E938.2	E950.4	E962.0	E980.4
Tribromomethane	967.3	E852.2	E937.3	E950.2	E962.0	E980.2
Trichlorethane	982.3	E862.4	—	E950.9	E962.1	E980.9
Trichlormethiazide	974.3	E858.5	E944.3	E950.4	E962.0	E980.4
Trichloroacetic acid	983.1	E864.1	—	E950.7	E962.1	E980.6
Trichloroethanol	967.1	E852.0	E937.1	E950.2	E962.0	E980.2
Trichloroethylene (liquid) (vapor)	982.3	E862.4	—	E950.9	E962.1	E980.9
anesthetic (gas)	968.2	E855.1	E938.2	E950.4	E962.0	E980.4
Trichloroethyl phosphate	967.1	E852.0	E937.1	E950.2	E962.0	E980.2
Trichlorofluoromethane NEC	987.4	E869.2	—	E952.8	E962.2	E982.8
Trichlorotriethylamine	963.1	E858.1	E933.1	E950.4	E962.0	E980.4
Trichomonacides NEC	961.5	E857	E931.5	E950.4	E962.0	E980.4
Trichomycin	960.1	E856	E930.1	E950.4	E962.0	E980.4
Triclofos	967.1	E852.0	E937.1	E950.2	E962.0	E980.2
Tricresyl phosphate	989.89	E866.8	—	E950.9	E962.1	E980.9
solvent	982.8	E862.4	—	E950.9	E962.1	E980.9
Tricyclamol	966.4	E855.0	E936.4	E950.4	E962.0	E980.4
Tridesilon	976.0	E858.7	E946.0	E950.4	E962.0	E980.4
Tridihexethyl	971.1	E855.4	E941.1	E950.4	E962.0	E980.4
Tridione	966.0	E855.0	E936.0	E950.4	E962.0	E980.4
Triethanolamine NEC	983.2	E864.2	—	E950.7	E962.1	E980.6
detergent	983.2	E861.0	—	E950.7	E962.1	E980.6
trinitrate	972.4	E858.3	E942.4	E950.4	E962.0	E980.4
Triethanomelamine	963.1	E858.1	E933.1	E950.4	E962.0	E980.4
Triethylene melamine	963.1	E858.1	E933.1	E950.4	E962.0	E980.4
Triethylenephosphoramide	963.1	E858.1	E933.1	E950.4	E962.0	E980.4
Triethylenethiophosphoramide	963.1	E858.1	E933.1	E950.4	E962.0	E980.4
Trifluoperazine	969.1	E853.0	E939.1	E950.3	E962.0	E980.3
Trifluperidol	969.2	E853.1	E939.2	E950.3	E962.0	E980.3
Triflupromazine	969.1	E853.0	E939.1	E950.3	E962.0	E980.3
Trihexyphenidyl	971.1	E855.4	E941.1	E950.4	E962.0	E980.4
Triiodothyronine	962.7	E858.0	E932.7	E950.4	E962.0	E980.4
Trilene	968.2	E855.1	E938.2	E950.4	E962.0	E980.4
Trimeprazine	963.0	E858.1	E933.0	E950.4	E962.0	E980.4
Trimetazidine	972.4	E858.3	E942.4	E950.4	E962.0	E980.4
Trimethadione	966.0	E855.0	E936.0	E950.4	E962.0	E980.4
Trimethaphan	972.3	E858.3	E942.3	E950.4	E962.0	E980.4
Trimethidinium	972.3	E858.3	E942.3	E950.4	E962.0	E980.4
Trimethobenzamide	963.0	E858.1	E933.0	E950.4	E962.0	E980.4

		External Cause (E-Code)				
	Poisoning	Accident	Therapeutic Use	Suicide Attempt	Assault	Undetermined
Trimethylcarbinol	980.8	E860.8	—	E950.9	E962.1	E980.9
Trimethylpsoralen	976.3	E858.7	E946.3	E950.4	E962.0	E980.4
Trimeton	963.0	E858.1	E933.0	E950.4	E962.0	E980.4
Trimipramine	969.05	E854.0	E939.0	E950.3	E962.0	E980.3
Trimustine	963.1	E858.1	E933.1	E950.4	E962.0	E980.4
Trinitrin	972.4	E858.3	E942.4	E950.4	E962.0	E980.4
Trinitrophenol	983.0	E864.0	—	E950.7	E962.1	E980.6
Trinitrotoluene	989.89	E866.8	—	E950.9	E962.1	E980.9
fumes	987.8	E869.8	—	E952.8	E962.2	E982.8
Trional	967.8	E852.8	E937.8	E950.2	E962.0	E980.2
Trioxide of arsenic — see Arsenic						
Trioxsalen	976.3	E858.7	E946.3	E950.4	E962.0	E980.4
Tripelennamine	963.0	E858.1	E933.0	E950.4	E962.0	E980.4
Triperidol	969.2	E853.1	E939.2	E950.3	E962.0	E980.3
Triprolidine	963.0	E858.1	E933.0	E950.4	E962.0	E980.4
Trisoralen	976.3	E858.7	E946.3	E950.4	E962.0	E980.4
Troleandomycin	960.3	E856	E930.3	E950.4	E962.0	E980.4
Trolnitrate (phosphate)	972.4	E858.3	E942.4	E950.4	E962.0	E980.4
Trometamol	963.3	E858.1	E933.3	E950.4	E962.0	E980.4
Tromethamine	963.3	E858.1	E933.3	E950.4	E962.0	E980.4
Tronothane	968.5	E855.2	E938.5	E950.4	E962.0	E980.4
Tropicamide	971.1	E855.4	E941.1	E950.4	E962.0	E980.4
Troxidone	966.0	E855.0	E936.0	E950.4	E962.0	E980.4
Tryparsamide	961.1	E857	E931.1	E950.4	E962.0	E980.4
Trypsin	963.4	E858.1	E933.4	E950.4	E962.0	E980.4
Tryptizol	969.05	E854.0	E939.0	E950.3	E962.0	E980.3
Tuaminoheptane	971.2	E855.5	E941.2	E950.4	E962.0	E980.4
Tuberculin (old)	977.8	E858.8	E947.8	E950.4	E962.0	E980.4
Tubocurare	975.2	E858.6	E945.2	E950.4	E962.0	E980.4
Tubocurarine	975.2	E858.6	E945.2	E950.4	E962.0	E980.4
Turkish green	969.6	E854.1	E939.6	E950.3	E962.0	E980.3
Turpentine (spirits of) (liquid) (vapor)	982.8	E862.4	—	E950.9	E962.1	E980.9
Tybamate	969.5	E853.8	E939.5	E950.3	E962.0	E980.3
Tyloxapol	975.5	E858.6	E945.5	E950.4	E962.0	E980.4
Tymazoline	971.2	E855.5	E941.2	E950.4	E962.0	E980.4
Typhoid vaccine	978.1	E858.8	E948.1	E950.4	E962.0	E980.4
Typhus vaccine	979.2	E858.8	E949.2	E950.4	E962.0	E980.4
Tyrothricin	976.0	E858.7	E946.0	E950.4	E962.0	E980.4
ENT agent	976.6	E858.7	E946.6	E950.4	E962.0	E980.4
ophthalmic preparation	976.5	E858.7	E946.5	E950.4	E962.0	E980.4
Undecenoic acid	976.0	E858.7	E946.0	E950.4	E962.0	E980.4
Undecylenic acid	976.0	E858.7	E946.0	E950.4	E962.0	E980.4
Unna's boot	976.3	E858.7	E946.3	E950.4	E962.0	E980.4
Uracil mustard	963.1	E858.1	E933.1	E950.4	E962.0	E980.4
Uramustine	963.1	E858.1	E933.1	E950.4	E962.0	E980.4
Urari	975.2	E858.6	E945.2	E950.4	E962.0	E980.4
Urea	974.4	E858.5	E944.4	E950.4	E962.0	E980.4
topical	976.8	E858.7	E946.8	E950.4	E962.0	E980.4
Urethan(e) (antineoplastic)	963.1	E858.1	E933.1	E950.4	E962.0	E980.4
Urginea (maritima) (scilla) — see Squill						
Uric acid metabolism agents NEC	974.7	E858.5	E944.7	E950.4	E962.0	E980.4
Urokinase	964.4	E858.2	E934.4	E950.4	E962.0	E980.4
Urokon	977.8	E858.8	E947.8	E950.4	E962.0	E980.4
Urotropin	961.9	E857	E931.9	E950.4	E962.0	E980.4
Urtica	988.2	E865.4	—	E950.9	E962.1	E980.9
Utility gas — see Gas, utility						
Vaccine NEC	979.9	E858.8	E949.9	E950.4	E962.0	E980.4
bacterial NEC	978.8	E858.8	E948.8	E950.4	E962.0	E980.4
with						
other bacterial component	978.9	E858.8	E948.9	E950.4	E962.0	E980.4
pertussis component	978.6	E858.8	E948.6	E950.4	E962.0	E980.4
viral-rickettsial component	979.7	E858.8	E949.7	E950.4	E962.0	E980.4
mixed NEC	978.9	E858.8	E948.9	E950.4	E962.0	E980.4
BCG	978.0	E858.8	E948.0	E950.4	E962.0	E980.4
cholera	978.2	E858.8	E948.2	E950.4	E962.0	E980.4
diphtheria	978.5	E858.8	E948.5	E950.4	E962.0	E980.4
influenza	979.6	E858.8	E949.6	E950.4	E962.0	E980.4
measles	979.4	E858.8	E949.4	E950.4	E962.0	E980.4
meningococcal	978.8	E858.8	E948.8	E950.4	E962.0	E980.4
mumps	979.6	E858.8	E949.6	E950.4	E962.0	E980.4
paratyphoid	978.1	E858.8	E948.1	E950.4	E962.0	E980.4
pertussis (with diphtheria toxoid) (with tetanus toxoid)	978.6	E858.8	E948.6	E950.4	E962.0	E980.4
plague	978.3	E858.8	E948.3	E950.4	E962.0	E980.4

Nontherapeutic use substance

Subterms under main terms may continue to next column or page

Index | Vaccine NEC — Zinc

	Poisoning	Accident	Therapeutic Use	Suicide Attempt	Assault	Undetermined
Vaccine — *continued*						
poliomyelitis	979.5	E858.8	E949.5	E950.4	E962.0	E980.4
poliovirus	979.5	E858.8	E949.5	E950.4	E962.0	E980.4
rabies	979.1	E858.8	E949.1	E950.4	E962.0	E980.4
respiratory syncytial virus	979.6	E858.8	E949.6	E950.4	E962.0	E980.4
rickettsial NEC	979.6	E858.8	E949.6	E950.4	E962.0	E980.4
with						
bacterial component	979.7	E858.8	E949.7	E950.4	E962.0	E980.4
pertussis component	978.6	E858.8	E948.6	E950.4	E962.0	E980.4
viral component	979.7	E858.8	E949.7	E950.4	E962.0	E980.4
Rocky mountain spotted fever	979.6	E858.8	E949.6	E950.4	E962.0	E980.4
rotavirus	979.6	E858.8	E949.6	E950.4	E962.0	E980.4
rubella virus	979.4	E858.8	E949.4	E950.4	E962.0	E980.4
sabin oral	979.5	E858.8	E949.5	E950.4	E962.0	E980.4
smallpox	979.0	E858.8	E949.0	E950.4	E962.0	E980.4
tetanus	978.4	E858.8	E948.4	E950.4	E962.0	E980.4
typhoid	978.1	E858.8	E948.1	E950.4	E962.0	E980.4
typhus	979.2	E858.8	E949.2	E950.4	E962.0	E980.4
viral NEC	979.6	E858.8	E949.6	E950.4	E962.0	E980.4
with						
bacterial component	979.7	E858.8	E949.7	E950.4	E962.0	E980.4
pertussis component	978.6	E858.8	E948.6	E950.4	E962.0	E980.4
rickettsial component	979.7	E858.8	E949.7	E950.4	E962.0	E980.4
yellow fever	979.3	E858.8	E949.3	E950.4	E962.0	E980.4
Vaccinia immune globulin (human)	964.6	E858.2	E934.6	E950.4	E962.0	E980.4
Vaginal contraceptives	976.8	E858.7	E946.8	E950.4	E962.0	E980.4
Valethamate	971.1	E855.4	E941.1	E950.4	E962.0	E980.4
Valisone	976.0	E858.7	E946.0	E950.4	E962.0	E980.4
Valium	969.4	E853.2	E939.4	E950.3	E962.0	E980.3
Valmid	967.8	E852.8	E937.8	E950.2	E962.0	E980.2
Vanadium	985.8	E866.4	—	E950.9	E962.1	E980.9
Vancomycin	960.8	E856	E930.8	E950.4	E962.0	E980.4
Vapor — *see also* Gas	987.9	E869.9	—	E952.9	E962.2	E982.9
kiln (carbon monoxide)	986	E868.8	—	E952.1	E962.2	E982.1
lead — *see* Lead						
specified source NEC (see also specific substance)	987.8	E869.8	—	E952.8	E962.2	E982.8
Varidase	964.4	E858.2	E934.4	E950.4	E962.0	E980.4
Varnish	989.89	E861.6	—	E950.9	E962.1	E980.9
cleaner	982.8	E862.9	—	E950.9	E962.1	E980.9
Vaseline	976.3	E858.7	E946.3	E950.4	E962.0	E980.4
Vasodilan	972.5	E858.3	E942.5	E950.4	E962.0	E980.4
Vasodilators NEC	972.5	E858.3	E942.5	E950.4	E962.0	E980.4
coronary	972.4	E858.3	E942.4	E950.4	E962.0	E980.4
Vasopressin	962.5	E858.0	E932.5	E950.4	E962.0	E980.4
Vasopressor drugs	962.5	E858.0	E932.5	E950.4	E962.0	E980.4
Venom, venomous (bite) (sting)	989.5	E905.9	—	E950.9	E962.1	E980.9
arthropod NEC	989.5	E905.5	—	E950.9	E962.1	E980.9
bee	989.5	E905.3	—	E950.9	E962.1	E980.9
centipede	989.5	E905.4	—	E950.9	E962.1	E980.9
hornet	989.5	E905.3	—	E950.9	E962.1	E980.9
lizard	989.5	E905.0	—	E950.9	E962.1	E980.9
marine animals or plants	989.5	E905.6	—	E950.9	E962.1	E980.9
millipede (tropical)	989.5	E905.4	—	E950.9	E962.1	E980.9
plant NEC	989.5	E905.7	—	E950.9	E962.1	E980.9
marine	989.5	E905.6	—	E950.9	E962.1	E980.9
scorpion	989.5	E905.2	—	E950.9	E962.1	E980.9
snake	989.5	E905.0	—	E950.9	E962.1	E980.9
specified NEC	989.5	E905.8	—	E950.9	E962.1	E980.9
spider	989.5	E905.1	—	E950.9	E962.1	E980.9
wasp	989.5	E905.3	—	E950.9	E962.1	E980.9
Ventolin — *see* Salbutamol sulfate						
Veramon	967.0	E851	E937.0	E950.1	E962.0	E980.1
Veratrum						
album	988.2	E865.4	—	E950.9	E962.1	E980.9
alkaloids	972.6	E858.3	E942.6	E950.4	E962.0	E980.4
viride	988.2	E865.4	—	E950.9	E962.1	E980.9
Verdigris — *see also* Copper	985.8	E866.4	—	E950.9	E962.1	E980.9
Veronal	967.0	E851	E937.0	E950.1	E962.0	E980.1
Veroxil	961.6	E857	E931.6	E950.4	E962.0	E980.4
Versidyne	965.7	E850.7	E935.7	E950.0	E962.0	E980.0
Viagra	972.5	E858.3	E942.5	E950.4	E962.0	E980.4
Vienna						
green	985.1	E866.3	—	E950.8	E962.1	E980.8
insecticide	985.1	E863.4	—	E950.6	E962.1	E980.7
red	989.89	E866.8	—	E950.9	E962.1	E980.9
pharmaceutical dye	977.4	E858.8	E947.4	E950.4	E962.0	E980.4

	Poisoning	Accident	Therapeutic Use	Suicide Attempt	Assault	Undetermined
Vinbarbital, vinbarbitone	967.0	E851	E937.0	E950.1	E962.0	E980.1
Vinblastine	963.1	E858.1	E933.1	E950.4	E962.0	E980.4
Vincristine	963.1	E858.1	E933.1	E950.4	E962.0	E980.4
Vinesthene, vinethene	968.2	E855.1	E938.2	E950.4	E962.0	E980.4
Vinyl						
bital	967.0	E851	E937.0	E950.1	E962.0	E980.1
ether	968.2	E855.1	E938.2	E950.4	E962.0	E980.4
Vioform	961.3	E857	E931.3	E950.4	E962.0	E980.4
topical	976.0	E858.7	E946.0	E950.4	E962.0	E980.4
Viomycin	960.6	E856	E930.6	E950.4	E962.0	E980.4
Viosterol	963.5	E858.1	E933.5	E950.4	E962.0	E980.4
Viper (venom)	989.5	E905.0	—	E950.9	E962.1	E980.9
Viprynium (embonate)	961.6	E857	E931.6	E950.4	E962.0	E980.4
Virugon	961.7	E857	E931.7	E950.4	E962.0	E980.4
Visine	976.5	E858.7	E946.5	E950.4	E962.0	E980.4
Vitamins NEC	963.5	E858.1	E933.5	E950.4	E962.0	E980.4
B_{12}	964.1	E858.2	E934.1	E950.4	E962.0	E980.4
hematopoietic	964.1	E858.2	E934.1	E950.4	E962.0	E980.4
K	964.3	E858.2	E934.3	E950.4	E962.0	E980.4
Vleminckx's solution	976.4	E858.7	E946.4	E950.4	E962.0	E980.4
Voltaren — *see* Diclofenac sodium						
Warfarin (potassium) (sodium)	964.2	E858.2	E934.2	E950.4	E962.0	E980.4
rodenticide	989.4	E863.7	—	E950.6	E962.1	E980.7
Wasp (sting)	989.5	E905.3	—	E950.9	E962.1	E980.9
Water						
balance agents NEC	974.5	E858.5	E944.5	E950.4	E962.0	E980.4
gas	987.1	E868.1	—	E951.8	E962.2	E981.8
incomplete combustion of — *see* Carbon, monoxide, fuel, utility						
hemlock	988.2	E865.4	—	E950.9	E962.1	E980.9
moccasin (venom)	989.5	E905.0	—	E950.9	E962.1	E980.9
Wax (paraffin) (petroleum)	981	E862.3	—	E950.9	E962.1	E980.9
automobile	989.89	E861.2	—	E950.9	E962.1	E980.9
floor	981	E862.0	—	E950.9	E962.1	E980.9
Weed killers NEC	989.4	E863.5	—	E950.6	E962.1	E980.7
Welldorm	967.1	E852.0	E937.1	E950.2	E962.0	E980.2
White						
arsenic — *see* Arsenic						
hellebore	988.2	E865.4	—	E950.9	E962.1	E980.9
lotion (keratolytic)	976.4	E858.7	E946.4	E950.4	E962.0	E980.4
spirit	981	E862.0	—	E950.9	E962.1	E980.9
Whitewashes	989.89	E861.6	—	E950.9	E962.1	E980.9
Whole blood	964.7	E858.2	E934.7	E950.4	E962.0	E980.4
Wild						
black cherry	988.2	E865.4	—	E950.9	E962.1	E980.9
poisonous plants NEC	988.2	E865.4	—	E950.9	E962.1	E980.9
Window cleaning fluid	989.89	E861.3	—	E950.9	E962.1	E980.9
Wintergreen (oil)	976.3	E858.7	E946.3	E950.4	E962.0	E980.4
Witch hazel	976.2	E858.7	E946.2	E950.4	E962.0	E980.4
Wood						
alcohol	980.1	E860.2	—	E950.9	E962.1	E980.9
spirit	980.1	E860.2	—	E950.9	E962.1	E980.9
Woorali	975.2	E858.6	E945.2	E950.4	E962.0	E980.4
Wormseed, American	961.6	E857	E931.6	E950.4	E962.0	E980.4
Xanthine diuretics	974.1	E858.5	E944.1	E950.4	E962.0	E980.4
Xanthocillin	960.0	E856	E930.0	E950.4	E962.0	E980.4
Xanthotoxin	976.3	E858.7	E946.3	E950.4	E962.0	E980.4
Xigris	964.2	E858.2	E934.2	E950.4	E962.0	E980.4
Xylene (liquid) (vapor)	982.0	E862.4	—	E950.9	E962.1	E980.9
Xylocaine (infiltration) (topical)	968.5	E855.2	E938.5	E950.4	E962.0	E980.4
nerve block (peripheral) (plexus)	968.6	E855.2	E938.6	E950.4	E962.0	E980.4
spinal	968.7	E855.2	E938.7	E950.4	E962.0	E980.4
Xylol (liquid) (vapor)	982.0	E862.4	—	E950.9	E962.1	E980.9
Xylometazoline	971.2	E855.5	E941.2	E950.4	E962.0	E980.4
Yellow						
fever vaccine	979.3	E858.8	E949.3	E950.4	E962.0	E980.4
jasmine	988.2	E865.4	—	E950.9	E962.1	E980.9
Yew	988.2	E865.4	—	E950.9	E962.1	E980.9
Zactane	965.7	E850.7	E935.7	E950.0	E962.0	E980.0
Zaroxolyn	974.3	E858.5	E944.3	E950.4	E962.0	E980.4
Zephiran (topical)	976.0	E858.7	E946.0	E950.4	E962.0	E980.4
ophthalmic preparation	976.5	E858.7	E946.5	E950.4	E962.0	E980.4
Zerone	980.1	E860.2	—	E950.9	E962.1	E980.9
Zinc (compounds) (fumes) (salts) (vapor) NEC	985.8	E866.4	—	E950.9	E962.1	E980.9
anti-infectives	976.0	E858.7	E946.0	E950.4	E962.0	E980.4

Nontherapeutic use substance

▽ Subterms under main terms may continue to next column or page

▶◀ Revised Text   ● New Line   ▲ Revised Code

		External Cause (E-Code)				
	Poisoning	Accident	Therapeutic Use	Suicide Attempt	Assault	Undeter-mined
Zinc — *continued*						
antivaricose	972.7	E858.3	E942.7	E950.4	E962.0	E980.4
bacitracin	976.0	E858.7	E946.0	E950.4	E962.0	E980.4
chloride	976.2	E858.7	E946.2	E950.4	E962.0	E980.4
gelatin	976.3	E858.7	E946.3	E950.4	E962.0	E980.4
oxide	976.3	E858.7	E946.3	E950.4	E962.0	E980.4
peroxide	976.0	E858.7	E946.0	E950.4	E962.0	E980.4
pesticides	985.8	E863.4	—	E950.6	E962.1	E980.7
phosphide (rodenticide)	985.8	E863.7	—	E950.6	E962.1	E980.7
stearate	976.3	E858.7	E946.3	E950.4	E962.0	E980.4
sulfate (antivaricose)	972.7	E858.3	E942.7	E950.4	E962.0	E980.4
ENT agent	976.6	E858.7	E946.6	E950.4	E962.0	E980.4
ophthalmic solution	976.5	E858.7	E946.5	E950.4	E962.0	E980.4
topical NEC	976.0	E858.7	E946.0	E950.4	E962.0	E980.4
undecylenate	976.0	E858.7	E946.0	E950.4	E962.0	E980.4
Zovant	964.2	E858.2	E934.2	E950.4	E962.0	E980.4
Zoxazolamine	968.0	E855.1	E938.0	E950.4	E962.0	E980.4
Zygadenus (venenosus)	988.2	E865.4	—	E950.9	E962.1	E980.9
Zyprexa ●	969.3	E853.8	E939.3	E950.3	E962.0	E980.3

SECTION 3

Alphabetic Index to External Causes of Injury and Poisoning (E Code)

This section contains the index to the codes which classify environmental events, circumstances, and other conditions as the cause of injury and other adverse effects. Where a code from the section Supplementary Classification of External Causes of Injury and Poisoning (E800-E999) is applicable, it is intended that the E code shall be used in addition to a code from the main body of the classification, Chapters 1 to 17.

The alphabetic index to the E codes is organized by main terms which describe the accident, circumstance, event, or specific agent which caused the injury or other adverse effect.

Note — Transport accidents (E800-E848) include accidents involving:

- *aircraft and spacecraft (E840-E845)*
- *watercraft (E830-E838)*
- *motor vehicle (E810-E825)*
- *railway (E800-E807)*
- *other road vehicles (E826-E829)*

For definitions and examples related to transport accidents — see Volume 1 code categories E800-E848.

The fourth-digit subdivisions for use with categories E800-E848 to identify the injured person are found at the end of this section.

For identifying the place in which an accident or poisoning occurred (circumstances classifiable to categories E850-E869 and E880-E928) — see the listing in this section under "Accident, occurring."

See the Table of Drugs and Chemicals (Section 2 of this volume) for identifying the specific agent involved in drug overdose or a wrong substance given or taken in error, and for intoxication or poisoning by a drug or other chemical substance.

The specific adverse effect, reaction, or localized toxic effect to a correct drug or substance properly administered in therapeutic or prophylactic dosage should be classified according to the nature of the adverse effect (e.g., allergy, dermatitis, tachycardia) listed in Section 1 of this volume.

☑ **Additional Digit Required — Refer to the Tabular List for Digit Selection**   ⑫ **Subterms under main terms may continue to next column or page**

332 — Volume 2   ▶◀ **Revised Text**   ● **New Line**   ▲ **Revised Code**   **2011 ICD-9-CM**

A

Abandonment
 causing exposure to weather conditions —
  see Exposure
 child, with intent to injure or kill E968.4
 helpless person, infant, newborn E904.0
  with intent to injure or kill E968.4
Abortion, criminal, injury to child E968.8
Abuse (alleged) (suspected)
 adult
  by
   child E967.4
   ex-partner E967.3
   ex-spouse E967.3
   father E967.0
   grandchild E967.7
   grandparent E967.6
   mother E967.2
   non-related caregiver E967.8
   other relative E967.7
   other specified person E967.1
   partner E967.3
   sibling E967.5
   spouse E967.3
   stepfather E967.0
   stepmother E967.2
   unspecified person E967.9
 child
  by
   boyfriend of parent or guardian
    E967.0
   child E967.4
   father E967.0
   female partner of parent or guardian
    E967.2
   girlfriend of parent or guardian
    E967.2
   grandchild E967.7
   grandparent E967.6
   male partner of parent or guardian
    E967.0
   mother E967.2
   non-related caregiver E967.8
   other relative E967.7
   other specified person(s) E967.1
   sibling E967.5
   stepfather E967.0
   stepmother E967.2
   unspecified person E967.9
Accident (to) E928.9
 aircraft (in transit) (powered) E841 ☑
  at landing, take-off E840 ☑
  due to, caused by cataclysm — *see* categories E908 ☑, E909 ☑
  late effect of E929.1
  unpowered (*see also* Collision, aircraft,
   unpowered) E842 ☑
  while alighting, boarding E843 ☑
 amphibious vehicle
  on
   land — *see* Accident, motor vehicle
   water — *see* Accident, watercraft
 animal-drawn vehicle NEC E827 ☑
 animal, ridden NEC E828 ☑
 balloon (*see also* Collision, aircraft, unpowered) E842 ☑
 caused by, due to
  abrasive wheel (metalworking) E919.3
  animal NEC E906.9
   being ridden (in sport or transport)
    E828 ☑
  avalanche NEC E909.2
  band saw E919.4
  bench saw E919.4
  bore, earth-drilling or mining (land)
   (seabed) E919.1
  bulldozer E919.7
  cataclysmic
   earth surface movement or eruption
    E909.9
   storm E908.9
  chain
   hoist E919.2
    agricultural operations E919.0
    mining operations E919.1

Accident (to) — *continued*
caused by, due to — *continued*
 chain — *continued*
  saw E920.1
  circular saw E919.4
 cold (excessive) (*see also* Cold, exposure
  to) E901.9
 combine E919.0
 conflagration — *see* Conflagration
 corrosive liquid, substance NEC E924.1
 cotton gin E919.8
 crane E919.2
  agricultural operations E919.0
  mining operations E919.1
 cutting or piercing instrument (*see also*
  Cut) E920.9
 dairy equipment E919.8
 derrick E919.2
  agricultural operations E919.0
  mining operations E919.1
 drill E920.1
  earth (land) (seabed) E919.1
  hand (powered) E920.1
   not powered E920.4
  metalworking E919.3
  woodworking E919.4
 earth(-)
  drilling machine E919.1
  moving machine E919.7
  scraping machine E919.7
 electric
  current (*see also* Electric shock)
   E925.9
  motor (*see also* Accident, machine,
   by type of machine)
   current (of) — *see* Electric shock
 elevator (building) (grain) E919.2
  agricultural operations E919.0
  mining operations E919.1
 environmental factors NEC E928.9
 excavating machine E919.7
 explosive material (*see also* Explosion)
  E923.9
 farm machine E919.0
 firearm missile — *see* Shooting
 fire, flames (*see also* Fire)
  conflagration — *see* Conflagration
 forging (metalworking) machine E919.3
 forklift (truck) E919.2
  agricultural operations E919.0
  mining operations E919.1
 gas turbine E919.5
 harvester E919.0
 hay derrick, mower, or rake E919.0
 heat (excessive) (*see also* Heat) E900.9
 hoist (*see also* Accident, caused by, due
  to, lift) E919.2
  chain — *see* Accident, caused by, due
   to, chain
  shaft E919.1
 hot
  liquid E924.0
   caustic or corrosive E924.1
  object (not producing fire or flames)
   E924.8
  substance E924.9
   caustic or corrosive E924.1
   liquid (metal) NEC E924.0
   specified type NEC E924.8
 human bite E928.3
 ignition — *see* Ignition
 internal combustion engine E919.5
 landslide NEC E909.2
 lathe (metalworking) E919.3
  turnings E920.8
  woodworking E919.4
 lift, lifting (appliances) E919.2
  agricultural operations E919.0
  mining operations E919.1
  shaft E919.1
 lightning NEC E907
 machine, machinery (*see also* Accident,
  machine)
  drilling, metal E919.3
  manufacturing, for manufacture of
   beverages E919.8

Accident (to) — *continued*
caused by, due to — *continued*
 machine, machinery (*see also* Accident,
  machine) — *continued*
  manufacturing, for manufacture of
   — *continued*
   clothing E919.8
   foodstuffs E919.8
   paper E919.8
   textiles E919.8
  milling, metal E919.3
  moulding E919.4
  power press, metal E919.3
  printing E919.8
  rolling mill, metal E919.3
  sawing, metal E919.3
  specified type NEC E919.8
  spinning E919.8
  weaving E919.8
 natural factor NEC E928.9
 overhead plane E919.4
 plane E920.4
  overhead E919.4
 powered
  hand tool NEC E920.1
  saw E919.4
   hand E920.1
 printing machine E919.8
 pulley (block) E919.2
  agricultural operations E919.0
  mining operations E919.1
  transmission E919.6
 radial saw E919.4
 radiation — *see* Radiation
 reaper E919.0
 road scraper E919.7
  when in transport under its own
   power — *see* categories
   E810-E825 ☑
 roller coaster E919.8
 sander E919.4
 saw E920.4
  band E919.4
  bench E919.4
  chain E920.1
  circular E919.4
  hand E920.4
   powered E920.1
  powered, except hand E919.4
  radial E919.4
 sawing machine, metal E919.3
 shaft
  hoist E919.1
  lift E919.1
  transmission E919.6
 shears E920.4
  hand E920.4
   powered E920.1
  mechanical E919.3
 shovel E920.4
  steam E919.7
 spinning machine E919.8
 steam (*see also* Burning, steam)
  engine E919.5
  shovel E919.7
 thresher E919.0
 thunderbolt NEC E907
 tractor E919.0
  when in transport under its own
   power — *see* categories
   E810-E825 ☑
 transmission belt, cable, chain, gear,
  pinion, pulley, shaft E919.6
 turbine (gas) (water driven) E919.5
 under-cutter E919.1
 weaving machine E919.8
 winch E919.2
  agricultural operations E919.0
  mining operations E919.1
 diving E883.0
  with insufficient air supply E913.2
 glider (hang) (*see also* Collision, aircraft, unpowered) E842 ☑
 hovercraft
  on
   land — *see* Accident, motor vehicle

Accident (to) — *continued*
hovercraft — *continued*
 on — *continued*
  water — *see* Accident, watercraft
 ice yacht (*see also* Accident, vehicle NEC)
  E848
 in
  medical, surgical procedure
   as, or due to misadventure — *see*
    Misadventure
   causing an abnormal reaction or later
    complication without men-
    tion of misadventure — *see*
    Reaction, abnormal
 kite carrying a person (*see also* Collision, involving aircraft, unpowered) E842 ☑
 land yacht (*see also* Accident, vehicle NEC)
  E848
 late effect of — *see* Late effect
 launching pad E845 ☑
 machine, machinery (*see also* Accident,
  caused by, due to, by specific type of
  machine) E919.9
  agricultural including animal-powered
   E919.0
  earth-drilling E919.1
  earth moving or scraping E919.7
  excavating E919.7
  involving transport under own power
   on highway or transport vehicle
   — *see* categories
   E810-E825 ☑, E840-E845 ☑
  lifting (appliances) E919.2
  metalworking E919.3
  mining E919.1
  prime movers, except electric motors
   E919.5
   electric motors — *see* Accident, ma-
    chine, by specific type of ma-
    chine
  recreational E919.8
  specified type NEC E919.8
  transmission E919.6
  watercraft (deck) (engine room) (galley)
   (laundry) (loading) E836 ☑
  woodworking or forming E919.4
 motor vehicle (on public highway) (traffic)
  E819 ☑
  due to cataclysm — *see* categories
   E908 ☑, E909 ☑
  involving
   collision (*see also* Collision, motor
    vehicle) E812 ☑
   nontraffic, not on public highway — *see*
    categories E820-E825 ☑
   not involving collision — *see* categories
    E816-E819 ☑
 nonmotor vehicle NEC E829 ☑
  nonroad — *see* Accident, vehicle NEC
  road, except pedal cycle, animal-drawn
   vehicle, or animal being ridden
   E829 ☑
 nonroad vehicle NEC — *see* Accident, vehicle NEC
 not elsewhere classifiable involving
  cable car (not on rails) E847
   on rails E829 ☑
  coal car in mine E846
  hand truck — *see* Accident, vehicle NEC
  logging car E846
  sled(ge), meaning snow or ice vehicle
   E848
  tram, mine or quarry E846
  truck
   mine or quarry E846
   self-propelled, industrial E846
   station baggage E846
  tub, mine or quarry E846
  vehicle NEC E848
   snow and ice E848
   used only on industrial premises
    E846
  wheelbarrow E848
 occurring (at) (in)
  apartment E849.0
  baseball field, diamond E849.4

☑ Additional Digit Required — Refer to the Tabular List for Digit Selection   ⌄ Subterms under main terms may continue to next column or page

2011 ICD-9-CM   ▶◀ Revised Text   ● New Line   ▲ Revised Code   Volume 2 — 333

Accident (to) — *continued*
  occurring — *continued*
    construction site, any E849.3
    dock E849.8
      yard E849.3
    dormitory E849.7
    factory (building) (premises) E849.3
    farm E849.1
      buildings E849.1
      house E849.0
    football field E849.4
    forest E849.8
    garage (place of work) E849.3
      private (home) E849.0
    gravel pit E849.2
    gymnasium E849.4
    highway E849.5
    home (private) (residential) E849.0
      institutional E849.7
    hospital E849.7
    hotel E849.6
    house (private) (residential) E849.0
      movie E849.6
      public E849.6
    institution, residential E849.7
    jail E849.7
    mine E849.2
    motel E849.6
    movie house E849.6
    office (building) E849.6
    orphanage E849.7
    park (public) E849.4
      mobile home E849.8
      trailer E849.8
    parking lot or place E849.8
    place
      industrial NEC E849.3
      parking E849.8
      public E849.8
        specified place NEC E849.5
      recreational NEC E849.4
      sport NEC E849.4
    playground (park) (school) E849.4
    prison E849.6
    public building NEC E849.6
    quarry E849.2
    railway
      line NEC E849.8
      yard E849.3
    residence
      home (private) E849.0
    resort (beach) (lake) (mountain)
        (seashore) (vacation) E849.4
    restaurant E849.6
    sand pit E849.2
    school (building) (private) (public) (state)
        E849.6
      reform E849.7
      riding E849.4
    seashore E849.8
      resort E849.4
    shop (place of work) E849.3
      commercial E849.6
    skating rink E849.4
    sports palace E849.4
    stadium E849.4
    store E849.6
    street E849.5
    swimming pool (public) E849.4
      private home or garden E849.0
    tennis court, public E849.4
    theatre, theater E849.6
    trailer court E849.8
    tunnel E849.8
      under construction E849.2
    warehouse E849.3
    yard
      dock E849.3
      industrial E849.3
      private (home) E849.0
      railway E849.3
  off-road type motor vehicle (not on public
      highway) NEC E821 ☑
    on public highway — *see* categories
        E810-E819 ☑
  pedal cycle E826 ☑

Accident (to) — *continued*
  railway E807 ☑
    due to cataclysm — *see* categories
        E908 ☑, E909 ☑
    involving
      avalanche E909.2
      burning by engine, locomotive, train
          (*see also* Explosion, railway
          engine) E803 ☑
      collision (*see also* Collision, railway)
          E800 ☑
      derailment (*see also* Derailment, rail-
          way) E802 ☑
      explosion (*see also* Explosion, railway
          engine) E803 ☑
      fall (*see also* Fall, from, railway rolling
          stock) E804 ☑
      fire (*see also* Explosion, railway en-
          gine) E803 ☑
      hitting, being struck by
          object falling in, on, from, rolling
              stock, train, vehicle
              E806 ☑
          rolling stock, train, vehicle
              E805 ☑
      overturning, railway rolling stock,
          train, vehicle (*see also* Derail-
          ment, railway) E802 ☑
      running off rails, railway (*see also*
          Derailment, railway) E802 ☑
      specified circumstances NEC E806 ☑
      train or vehicle hit by
          avalanche E909.2
          falling object (earth, rock, tree)
              E806 ☑
              due to cataclysm — *see* cate-
                  gories
                  E908 ☑, E909 ☑
          landslide E909.2
  roller skate E885.1
  scooter (nonmotorized) E885.0
  skateboard E885.2
  ski(ing) E885.3
    jump E884.9
    lift or tow (with chair or gondola) E847
  snowboard E885.4
  snow vehicle, motor driven (not on public
      highway) E820 ☑
    on public highway — *see* categories
        E810-E819 ☑
  spacecraft E845 ☑
  specified cause NEC E928.8
  street car E829 ☑
  traffic NEC E819 ☑
  vehicle NEC (with pedestrian) E848
    battery powered
      airport passenger vehicle E846
      truck (baggage) (mail) E846
    powered commercial or industrial (with
        other vehicle or object within
        commercial or industrial premis-
        es) E846
  watercraft E838 ☑
    with
      drowning or submersion resulting
          from
          accident other than to watercraft
              E832 ☑
          accident to watercraft E830 ☑
      injury, except drowning or submer-
          sion, resulting from
          accident other than to watercraft
              — *see* categories
              E833-E838 ☑
          accident to watercraft E831 ☑
      due to, caused by cataclysm — *see* cate-
          gories E908 ☑, E909 ☑
    machinery E836 ☑
Acid throwing E961
Acosta syndrome E902.0
Activity (involving) E030
  aerobic and step exercise (class) E009.2
  alpine skiing E003.2
  animal care NEC E019.9
  arts and handcrafts NEC E012.9

Activity — *continued*
  athletics NEC E008.9
    played
      as a team or group NEC E007.9
      individually NEC E006.9
  baking E015.2
  ballet E005.0
  barbells E010.2
  baseball E007.3
  BASE (Building, Antenna, Span, Earth)
      jumping E004.2
  basketball E007.6
  bathing (personal) E013.0
  beach volleyball E007.7
  bike riding E006.4
  boogie boarding E002.7
  bowling E006.3
  boxing E008.0
  brass instrument playing E018.3
  building and construction E016.2
  bungee jumping E004.3
  calisthenics E009.1
  canoeing (in calm and turbulent water)
      E002.5
  capture the flag E007.8
  cardiorespiratory exercise NEC E009.9
  caregiving (providing) NEC E014.9
    bathing E014.0
    lifting E014.1
  cellular
    communication device E011.1
    telephone E011.1
  challenge course E009.4
  cheerleading E005.4
  circuit training E009.3
  cleaning
    floor E013.4
  climbing NEC E004.9
    mountain E004.0
    rock E004.0
    wall climbing E004.0
  combatives E008.4
  computer
    keyboarding E011.0
    technology NEC E011.9
  confidence course E009.4
  construction (building) E016.2
  cooking and baking E015.2
  cooking and grilling NEC E015.9
  cool down exercises E009.1
  cricket E007.9
  crocheting E012.0
  cross country skiing E003.3
  dancing (all types) E005.0
  digging
    dirt E016.0
  dirt digging E016.0
  dishwashing E015.0
  diving (platform) (springboard) E002.1
    underwater E002.4
  dodge ball E007.8
  downhill skiing E003.2
  drum playing E018.1
  dumbbells E010.2
  electronic
    devices NEC E011.9
      hand held interactive E011.1
    game playing (using) (with)
      interactive device E011.1
      keyboard or other stationary device
          E011.0
  elliptical machine E009.0
  exercise(s)
    machines (primarily for)
      cardiorespiratory conditioning
          E009.0
      muscle strengthening (non-machine)
          NEC E010.9
    external motion NEC E017.9
      roller coaster E017.0
  field hockey E007.4
  figure skating (pairs) (singles) E003.0
  flag football E007.1
  floor mopping and cleaning E013.4
  food preparation and clean up E015.0

Activity — *continued*
  football (American) NOS E007.0
    flag E007.1
    tackle E007.0
    touch E007.1
  four square E007.8
  free weights E010.2
  frisbee (ultimate) E008.3
  furniture
    building E012.2
    finishing E012.2
    repair E012.2
  game playing (electronic)
    using
      interactive device E011.1
      keyboard or other stationary device
          E011.0
  gardening E016.1
  golf E006.2
  grass drills E009.5
  grilling and smoking food E015.1
  grooming and shearing an animal E019.2
  guerilla drills E009.5
  gymnastics (rhythmic) E005.2
  handball E008.2
  handcrafts NEC E012.9
  hand held interactive electronic device
      E011.1
  hang gliding E004.4
  hiking (on level or elevated terrain) E001.0
  hockey (ice) E003.1
    field E007.4
  horseback riding E006.1
  household maintenance NEC E013.9
  ice NEC E003.9
    dancing E003.0
    hockey E003.1
    skating E003.0
  inline roller skating E006.0
  ironing E013.3
  judo E008.4
  jumping (off) NEC E004.9
    BASE (Building, Antenna, Span, Earth)
        E004.2
    bungee E004.3
    jacks E009.1
    rope E006.5
  jumping jacks E009.1
  jumping rope E006.5
  karate E008.4
  kayaking (in calm and turbulent water)
      E002.5
  keyboarding (computer) E011.0
  kickball E007.8
  knitting E012.0
  lacrosse E007.4
  land maintenance NEC E016.9
  landscaping E016.1
  laundry E013.1
  machines (exercise) primarily for cardiores-
      piratory conditioning E009.0
  maintenance
    building E016.9
    household NEC E013.9
    land E016.9
    property E016.9
  marching (on level or elevated terrain)
      E001.0
  martial arts E008.4
  microwave oven E015.2
  milking an animal E019.1
  mopping (floor) E013.4
  mountain climbing E004.0
  muscle strengthening
    exercises (non-machine) NEC E010.9
    machines E010.0
  musical keyboard (electronic) playing E018.0
  nordic skiing E003.3
  obstacle course E009.4
  oven (microwave) E015.2
  packing up and unpacking in moving to a
      new residence E013.5
  parasailing E002.9
  percussion instrument playing NEC E018.1
  personal
    bathing and showering E013.0

☑ **Additional Digit Required** — Refer to the Tabular List for Digit Selection   ▽ **Subterms under main terms may continue to next column or page**

334 — Volume 2   ▶◀ **Revised Text**   ● **New Line**   ▲ **Revised Code**   **2011 ICD-9-CM**

Bite — continued
  fer de lance E905.0
  gila monster E905.0
  human being
    accidental E928.3
    assault E968.7
  insect (nonvenomous) E906.4
    venomous — see Sting
  krait E905.0
  late effect of — see Late effect
  lizard E906.2
    venomous E905.0
  mamba E905.0
  marine animal
    nonvenomous E906.3
      snake E906.2
    venomous E905.6
      snake E905.0
  millipede E906.4
    venomous E905.4
  moray eel E906.3
  rat E906.1
  rattlesnake E905.0
  rodent, except rat E906.3
  serpent — see Bite, snake
  shark E906.3
  snake (venomous) E905.0
    nonvenomous E906.2
    sea E905.0
  spider E905.1
    nonvenomous E906.4
  tarantula (venomous) E905.1
  venomous NEC E905.9
    by specific animal — see category
      E905 ☑
  viper E905.0
  water moccasin E905.0
Blast (air)
  from nuclear explosion E996 ☑
  in
    terrorism E979.2
      from nuclear explosion E979.5
      underwater E979.0
    war operations E993.9
      from nuclear explosion ▶— see War
        operations, injury due to, nu-
        clear weapons◀
      underwater E992.9
Blizzard E908.3
Blow E928.9
  by law-enforcing agent, police (on duty)
    E975
    with blunt object (baton) (nightstick)
      (stave) (truncheon) E973
Blowing up — see also Explosion E923.9
Brawl (hand) (fists) (foot) E960.0
Breakage (accidental)
  cable of cable car not on rails E847
  ladder (causing fall) E881.0
  part (any) of
    animal-drawn vehicle E827 ☑
    ladder (causing fall) E881.0
    motor vehicle
      in motion (on public highway)
        E818 ☑
        not on public highway E825 ☑
    nonmotor road vehicle, except animal-
      drawn vehicle or pedal cycle
      E829 ☑
    off-road type motor vehicle (not on
      public highway) NEC E821 ☑
      on public highway E818 ☑
    pedal cycle E826 ☑
    scaffolding (causing fall) E881.1
    snow vehicle, motor-driven (not on
      public highway) E820 ☑
      on public highway E818 ☑
    vehicle NEC — see Accident, vehicle
Broken
  glass
    fall on E888.0
    injury by E920.8
  power line (causing electric shock) E925.1
Bumping against, into (accidentally)
  object (moving) E917.9
    caused by crowd E917.1

Bumping against, into — continued
  object — continued
    caused by crowd — continued
      with subsequent fall E917.6
    furniture E917.3
      with subsequent fall E917.7
    in
      running water E917.2
      sports E917.0
    stationary E917.4
      with subsequent fall E917.8
    person(s) E917.9
      with fall E886.9
        in sports E886.0
      as, or caused by, a crowd E917.1
        with subsequent fall E917.6
      in sports E917.0
        with fall E886.0
Burning, burns (accidental) (by) (from) (on)
  E899
  acid (any kind) E924.1
    swallowed — see Table of Drugs and
      Chemicals
  airgun E928.7
  bedclothes (see also Fire, specified NEC)
    E898.0
  blowlamp (see also Fire, specified NEC)
    E898.1
  blowtorch (see also Fire, specified NEC)
    E898.1
  boat, ship, watercraft — see categories
    E830 ☑, E831 ☑, E837 ☑
  bonfire (controlled) E897
    uncontrolled E892
  candle (see also Fire, specified NEC) E898.1
  caustic liquid, substance E924.1
    swallowed — see Table of Drugs and
      Chemicals
  chemical E924.1
    from swallowing caustic, corrosive sub-
      stance — see Table of Drugs and
      Chemicals
    in
      terrorism E979.7
      war operations E997.2
  cigar(s) or cigarette(s) (see also Fire, speci-
    fied NEC) E898.1
  clothes, clothing, nightdress — see Ignition,
    clothes
    with conflagration — see Conflagration
  conflagration — see Conflagration
  corrosive liquid, substance E924.1
    swallowed — see Table of Drugs and
      Chemicals
  electric current (see also Electric shock)
    E925.9
  firearm E928.7
  fire, flames (see also Fire) E899
  flare, Verey pistol E922.8
  heat
    from appliance (electrical) E924.8
    in local application, or packing during
      medical or surgical procedure
      E873.5
  homicide (attempt) (see also Assault, burn-
    ing) E968.0
  hot
    liquid E924.0
      caustic or corrosive E924.1
    object (not producing fire or flames)
      E924.8
    substance E924.9
      caustic or corrosive E924.1
      liquid (metal) NEC E924.0
      specified type NEC E924.8
    tap water E924.2
  ignition (see also Ignition)
    clothes, clothing, nightdress (see also
      Ignition, clothes)
      with conflagration — see Conflagra-
        tion
    highly inflammable material (benzine)
      (fat) (gasoline) (kerosene) (paraf-
      fin) (petrol) E894

Burning, burns — continued
  in
    terrorism E979.3
      from nuclear explosion E979.5
      petrol bomb E979.3
    war operations (from fire-producing de-
      vice or conventional weapon)
      E990.9
      from nuclear explosion (see also War
        operations, injury due to, nu-
        clear weapons) E996.2
      incendiary bomb E990.0
      petrol bomb E990.0
  inflicted by other person
    stated as
      homicidal, intentional (see also As-
        sault, burning) E968.0
      undetermined whether accidental or
        intentional (see also Burn,
        stated as undetermined
        whether accidental or inten-
        tional) E988.1
  internal, from swallowed caustic, corrosive
    liquid, substance — see Table of
    Drugs and Chemicals
  lamp (see also Fire, specified NEC) E898.1
  late effect of NEC E929.4
  lighter (cigar) (cigarette) (see also Fire,
    specified NEC) E898.1
  lightning E907
  liquid (boiling) (hot) (molten) E924.0
    caustic, corrosive E924.1
      swallowed — see Table of Drugs and
        Chemicals
  local application of externally applied sub-
    stance in medical or surgical care
    E873.5
  machinery — see Accident, machine
  matches (see also Fire, specified NEC) E898.1
  medicament, externally applied E873.5
  metal, molten E924.0
  object (hot) E924.8
    producing fire or flames — see Fire
  oven (electric) (gas) E924.8
  pipe (smoking) (see also Fire, specified NEC)
    E898.1
  radiation — see Radiation
  railway engine, locomotive, train (see also
    Explosion, railway engine) E803 ☑
  self-inflicted (unspecified whether acciden-
    tal or intentional) E988.1
    caustic or corrosive substance NEC
      E988.7
    stated as intentional, purposeful E958.1
      caustic or corrosive substance NEC
        E958.7
    stated as undetermined whether accidental
      or intentional E988.1
      caustic or corrosive substance NEC
        E988.7
  steam E924.0
    pipe E924.8
  substance (hot) E924.9
    boiling or molten E924.0
    caustic, corrosive (external) E924.1
      swallowed — see Table of Drugs and
        Chemicals
  suicidal (attempt) NEC E958.1
    caustic substance E958.7
    late effect of E959
  tanning bed E926.2
  therapeutic misadventure
    overdose of radiation E873.2
  torch, welding (see also Fire, specified NEC)
    E898.1
  trash fire (see also Burning, bonfire) E897
  vapor E924.0
  vitriol E924.1
  x-rays E926.3
    in medical, surgical procedure — see
      Misadventure, failure, in dosage,
      radiation
Butted by animal E906.8

C

Cachexia, lead or saturnine E866.0

Cachexia, lead or saturnine — continued
  from pesticide NEC (see also Table of Drugs
    and Chemicals) E863.4
Caisson disease E902.2
Capital punishment (any means) E978
Car sickness E903
Casualty (not due to war) NEC E928.9
  terrorism E979.8
  war (see also War operations) E995.9
Cat
  bite E906.3
  scratch E906.8
Cataclysmic (any injury)
  earth surface movement or eruption E909.9
    specified type NEC E909.8
  storm or flood resulting from storm E908.9
    specified type NEC E909.8
Catching fire — see Ignition
Caught
  between
    objects (moving) (stationary and mov-
      ing) E918
      and machinery — see Accident, ma-
        chine
  by cable car, not on rails E847
  in
    machinery (moving parts of) — see, Ac-
      cident, machine
    object E918
Cave-in (causing asphyxia, suffocation (by
  pressure) — see also Suffocation, due
  to, cave-in E913.3
  with injury other than asphyxia or suffoca-
    tion E916
    with asphyxia or suffocation (see also
      Suffocation, due to, cave-in)
      E913.3
  struck or crushed by E916
    with asphyxia or suffocation (see also
      Suffocation, due to, cave-in)
      E913.3
Change(s) in air pressure — see also Effects
  of, air pressure
  sudden, in aircraft (ascent) (descent) (caus-
    ing aeroneurosis or aviators' disease)
    E902.1
Chilblains E901.0
  due to manmade conditions E901.1
Choking (on) (any object except food or vomitus) E912
  apple E911
  bone E911
  food, any type (regurgitated) E911
  mucus or phlegm E912
  seed E911
Civil insurrection — see War operations
Cloudburst E908.8
Cold, exposure to (accidental) (excessive)
  (extreme) (place) E901.9
  causing chilblains or immersion foot E901.0
  due to
    manmade conditions E901.1
    specified cause NEC E901.8
    weather (conditions) E901.0
  late effect of NEC E929.5
  self-inflicted (undetermined whether acci-
    dental or intentional) E988.3
    suicidal E958.3
  suicidal E958.3
Colic, lead, painter's, or saturnine — see
  category E866 ☑
Collapse
  building E916
    burning (uncontrolled fire) E891.8
      in terrorism E979.3
      private E890.8
  dam E909.3
  due to heat — see Heat
  machinery — see Accident, machine or ve-
    hicle
  man-made structure E909.3
  postoperative NEC E878.9
  structure
    burning (uncontrolled fire) NEC E891.8
      in terrorism E979.3

☑ **Additional Digit Required** — Refer to the Tabular List for Digit Selection
▽ **Subterms under main terms may continue to next column or page**
336 — Volume 2 · October 2010
▶◀ Revised Text   ● New Line   ▲ Revised Code
2011 ICD-9-CM

Collision (accidental)

Note — In the case of collisions between different types of vehicles, persons and objects, priority in classification is in the following order:

    Aircraft

    Watercraft

    Motor vehicle

    Railway vehicle

    Pedal cycle

    Animal-drawn vehicle

    Animal being ridden

    Streetcar or other nonmotor road vehicle

    Other vehicle

    Pedestrian or person using pedestrian conveyance

    Object (except where falling from or set in motion by vehicle etc. listed above)

In the listing below, the combinations are listed only under the vehicle etc. having priority. For definitions, see Supplementary Classification of External Causes of Injury and Poisoning (E800-E999).

aircraft (with object or vehicle) (fixed) (movable) (moving) E841 ☑
  with
    person (while landing, taking off) (without accident to aircraft) E844 ☑
    powered (in transit) (with unpowered aircraft) E841 ☑
    while landing, taking off E840 ☑
    unpowered E842 ☑
    while landing, taking off E840 ☑
animal being ridden (in sport or transport) E828 ☑
  and
    animal (being ridden) (herded) (unattended) E828 ☑
    nonmotor road vehicle, except pedal cycle or animal-drawn vehicle E828 ☑
    object (fallen) (fixed) (movable) (moving) not falling from or set in motion by vehicle of higher priority E828 ☑
    pedestrian (conveyance or vehicle) E828 ☑
animal-drawn vehicle E827 ☑
  and
    animal (being ridden) (herded) (unattended) E827 ☑
    nonmotor road vehicle, except pedal cycle E827 ☑
    object (fallen) (fixed) (movable) (moving) not falling from or set in motion by vehicle of higher priority E827 ☑
    pedestrian (conveyance or vehicle) E827 ☑
    streetcar E827 ☑
motor vehicle (on public highway) (traffic accident) E812 ☑
  after leaving, running off, public highway (without antecedent collision) (without re-entry) E816 ☑
  with antecedent collision on public highway — see categories E810-E815
  with re-entrance collision with another motor vehicle E811 ☑
  and
    abutment (bridge) (overpass) E815 ☑
    animal (herded) (unattended) E815 ☑

Collision — continued

motor vehicle — continued
  and — continued
    animal — continued
      carrying person, property E813 ☑
    animal-drawn vehicle E813 ☑
    another motor vehicle (abandoned) (disabled) (parked) (stalled) (stopped) E812 ☑
      with, involving re-entrance (on same roadway) (across median strip) E811 ☑
    any object, person, or vehicle off the public highway resulting from a noncollision motor vehicle nontraffic accident E816 ☑
    avalanche, fallen or not moving E815 ☑
      falling E909.2
    boundary fence E815 ☑
    culvert E815 ☑
    fallen
      stone E815 ☑
      tree E815 ☑
    guard post or guard rail E815 ☑
    inter-highway divider E815 ☑
    landslide, fallen or not moving E815 ☑
      moving E909 ☑
    machinery (road) E815 ☑
    nonmotor road vehicle NEC E813 ☑
    object (any object, person, or vehicle off the public highway resulting from a noncollision motor vehicle nontraffic accident) E815 ☑
      off, normally not on, public highway resulting from a noncollision motor vehicle traffic accident E816 ☑
    pedal cycle E813 ☑
    pedestrian (conveyance) E814 ☑
    person (using pedestrian conveyance) E814 ☑
    post or pole (lamp) (light) (signal) (telephone) (utility) E815 ☑
    railway rolling stock, train, vehicle E810 ☑
    safety island E815 ☑
    street car E813 ☑
    traffic signal, sign, or marker (temporary) E815 ☑
    tree E815 ☑
    tricycle E813 ☑
    wall of cut made for road E815 ☑
  due to cataclysm — see categories E908 ☑, E909 ☑
  not on public highway, nontraffic accident E822 ☑
  and
    animal (carrying person, property) (herded) (unattended) E822 ☑
    animal-drawn vehicle E822 ☑
    another motor vehicle (moving), except off-road motor vehicle E822 ☑
      stationary E823 ☑
    avalanche, fallen, not moving E823 ☑
      moving E909.2
    landslide, fallen, not moving E823 ☑
      moving E909.2
    nonmotor vehicle (moving) E822 ☑
      stationary E823 ☑
    object (fallen) (normally) (fixed) (movable but not in motion) (stationary) E823 ☑
      moving, except when falling from, set in motion by, aircraft or cataclysm E822 ☑
    pedal cycle (moving) E822 ☑

Collision — continued

motor vehicle — continued
  not on public highway, nontraffic accident — continued
    and — continued
      pedal cycle — continued
        stationary E823 ☑
      pedestrian (conveyance) E822 ☑
      person (using pedestrian conveyance) E822 ☑
      railway rolling stock, train, vehicle (moving) E822 ☑
        stationary E823 ☑
      road vehicle (any) (moving) E822 ☑
        stationary E823 ☑
      tricycle (moving) E822 ☑
        stationary E823 ☑
  off-road type motor vehicle (not on public highway) E821 ☑
  and
    animal (being ridden) (-drawn vehicle) E821 ☑
    another off-road motor vehicle, except snow vehicle E821 ☑
    other motor vehicle, not on public highway E821 ☑
    other object or vehicle NEC, fixed or movable, not set in motion by aircraft, motor vehicle on highway, or snow vehicle, motor driven E821 ☑
    pedal cycle E821 ☑
    pedestrian (conveyance) E821 ☑
    railway train E821 ☑
  on public highway — see Collision, motor vehicle
pedal cycle E826 ☑
  and
    animal (carrying person, property) (herded) (unherded) E826 ☑
    animal-drawn vehicle E826 ☑
    another pedal cycle E826 ☑
    nonmotor road vehicle E826 ☑
    object (fallen) (fixed) (movable) (moving) not falling from or set in motion by aircraft, motor vehicle, or railway train NEC E826 ☑
    pedestrian (conveyance) E826 ☑
    person (using pedestrian conveyance) E826 ☑
    street car E826 ☑
pedestrian(s) (conveyance) E917.9
  with fall E886.9
  in sports E886.0
  and
    crowd, human stampede E917.1
      with subsequent fall E917.6
    furniture E917.3
      with subsequent fall E917.7
    machinery — see Accident, machine
    object (fallen) (moving) not falling from NEC, fixed or set in motion by any vehicle classifiable to E800-E848 ☑, E917.9
      with subsequent fall E917.6
      caused by a crowd E917.1
        with subsequent fall E917.6
      furniture E917.3
        with subsequent fall E917.7
    in
      running water E917.2
        with drowning or submersion — see Submersion
      sports E917.0
        with subsequent fall E917.5
      stationary E917.4
        with subsequent fall E917.8
    vehicle, nonmotor, nonroad E848
  in
    running water E917.2

Collision — continued

pedestrian(s) — continued
  in — continued
    running water — continued
      with drowning or submersion — see Submersion
    sports E917.0
      with fall E886.0
  person(s) (using pedestrian conveyance) (see also Collision, pedestrian) E917.9
railway (rolling stock) (train) (vehicle) (with (subsequent) derailment, explosion, fall or fire) E800 ☑
  with antecedent derailment E802 ☑
  and
    animal (carrying person) (herded) (unattended) E801 ☑
    another railway train or vehicle E800 ☑
    buffers E801 ☑
    fallen tree on railway E801 ☑
    farm machinery, nonmotor (in transport) (stationary) E801 ☑
    gates E801 ☑
    nonmotor vehicle E801 ☑
    object (fallen) (fixed) (movable) (moving) not falling from, set in motion by, aircraft or motor vehicle NEC E801 ☑
    pedal cycle E801 ☑
    pedestrian (conveyance) E805 ☑
    person (using pedestrian conveyance) E805 ☑
    platform E801 ☑
    rock on railway E801 ☑
    street car E801 ☑
snow vehicle, motor-driven (not on public highway) E820 ☑
  and
    animal (being ridden) (-drawn vehicle) E820 ☑
    another off-road motor vehicle E820 ☑
    other motor vehicle, not on public highway E820 ☑
    other object or vehicle NEC, fixed or movable, not set in motion by aircraft or motor vehicle on highway E820 ☑
    pedal cycle E820 ☑
    pedestrian (conveyance) E820 ☑
    railway train E820 ☑
  on public highway — see Collision, motor vehicle
street car(s) E829 ☑
  and
    animal, herded, not being ridden, unattended E829 ☑
    nonmotor road vehicle NEC E829 ☑
    object (fallen) (fixed) (movable) (moving) not falling from or set in motion by aircraft, animal-drawn vehicle, animal being ridden, motor vehicle, pedal cycle, or railway train E829 ☑
    pedestrian (conveyance) E829 ☑
    person (using pedestrian conveyance) E829 ☑
vehicle
  animal-drawn — see Collision, animal-drawn vehicle
  motor — see Collision, motor vehicle
  nonmotor
    nonroad E848
    and
      another nonmotor, nonroad vehicle E848

☑ Additional Digit Required — Refer to the Tabular List for Digit Selection   ⌐ Subterms under main terms may continue to next column or page

2011 ICD-9-CM   ▶◀ Revised Text   ● New Line   ▲ Revised Code   Volume 2 — 337

Collision — continued
  vehicle — continued
    nonmotor — continued
      nonroad — continued
        and — continued
          object (fallen) (fixed) (movable) (moving) not falling from or set in motion by aircraft, animal-drawn vehicle, animal being ridden, motor vehicle, nonmotor road vehicle, pedal cycle, railway train, or streetcar E848
      road, except animal being ridden, animal-drawn vehicle, or pedal cycle E829 ☑
      and
        animal, herded, not being ridden, unattended E829 ☑
        another nonmotor road vehicle, except animal being ridden, animal-drawn vehicle, or pedal cycle E829 ☑
        object (fallen) (fixed) (movable) (moving) not falling from or set in motion by, aircraft, animal-drawn vehicle, animal being ridden, motor vehicle, pedal cycle, or railway train E829 ☑
        pedestrian (conveyance) E829 ☑
        person (using pedestrian conveyance) E829 ☑
        vehicle, nonmotor, nonroad E829 ☑
  watercraft E838 ☑
    and
      person swimming or water skiing E838 ☑
    causing
      drowning, submersion E830 ☑
      injury except drowning, submersion E831 ☑
Combustion, spontaneous — see Ignition
Complication of medical or surgical procedure or treatment
  as an abnormal reaction — see Reaction, abnormal
  delayed, without mention of misadventure — see Reaction, abnormal
  due to misadventure — see Misadventure
Compression
  divers' squeeze E902.2
  trachea by
    food E911
    foreign body, except food E912
Conflagration
  building or structure, except private dwelling (barn) (church) (convalescent or residential home) (factory) (farm outbuilding) (hospital) (hotel) (institution) (educational) (domitory) (residential) (school) (shop) (store) (theater) E891.9
  with or causing (injury due to)
    accident or injury NEC E891.9
      specified circumstance NEC E891.8
    burns, burning E891.3
    carbon monoxide E891.2
    fumes E891.2
      polyvinylchloride (PVC) or similar material E891.1
    smoke E891.2
  causing explosion E891.0
  in terrorism E979.3
  not in building or structure E892

Conflagration — continued
  private dwelling (apartment) (boarding house) (camping place) (caravan) (farmhouse) (home (private)) (house) (lodging house) (private garage) (rooming house) (tenement) E890.9
  with or causing (injury due to)
    accident or injury NEC E890.9
      specified circumstance NEC E890.8
    burns, burning E890.3
    carbon monoxide E890.2
    fumes E890.2
      polyvinylchloride (PVC) or similar material E890.1
    smoke E890.2
  causing explosion E890.0
Constriction, external
  caused by
    hair E928.4
    other object E928.5
Contact with
  dry ice E901.1
  liquid air, hydrogen, nitrogen E901.1
Cramp(s)
  Heat — see Heat
  swimmers (see also category E910) E910.2
    not in recreation or sport E910.3
Cranking (car) (truck) (bus) (engine), injury by E917.9
Crash
  aircraft (in transit) (powered) E841 ☑
    at landing, take-off E840 ☑
    in
      terrorism E979.1
      war operations E994.9
    on runway NEC E840 ☑
    stated as
      homicidal E968.8
      suicidal E958.6
      undetermined whether accidental or intentional E988.6
    unpowered E842 ☑
  glider E842 ☑
  motor vehicle (see also Accident, motor vehicle)
    homicidal E968.5
    suicidal E958.5
    undetermined whether accidental or intentional E988.5
Crushed (accidentally) E928.9
  between
    boat(s), ship(s), watercraft (and dock or pier) (without accident to watercraft) E838 ☑
      after accident to, or collision, watercraft E831 ☑
    objects (moving) (stationary and moving) E918
  by
    avalanche NEC E909.2
    boat, ship, watercraft after accident to, collision, watercraft E831 ☑
    cave-in E916
      with asphyxiation or suffocation (see also Suffocation, due to, cave-in) E913.3
    crowd, human stampede E917.1
    falling
      aircraft (see also Accident, aircraft) E841 ☑
      in
        terrorism E979.1
        war operations E994.8
      earth, material E916
        with asphyxiation or suffocation (see also Suffocation, due to, cave-in) E913.3
      object E916
        on ship, watercraft E838 ☑
        while loading, unloading watercraft E838 ☑
    firearm E928.7
    landslide NEC E909.2
    lifeboat after abandoning ship E831 ☑
    machinery — see Accident, machine

Crushed — continued
  by — continued
    railway rolling stock, train, vehicle (part of) E805 ☑
    slide trigger mechanism, scope or other part of gun E928.7
    street car E829
    vehicle NEC — see Accident, vehicle NEC
  in
    machinery — see Accident, machine
    object E918
    transport accident — see categories E800-E848 ☑
  late effect of NEC E929.9
Cut, cutting (any part of body) (accidental) E920.9
  by
    arrow E920.8
    axe E920.4
    bayonet (see also Bayonet wound) E920.3
      in war operations E995.2
    blender E920.2
    broken glass E920.8
      following fall E888.0
    can opener E920.4
      powered E920.2
    chisel E920.4
    circular saw E919.4
    cutting or piercing instrument (see also category) E920 ☑
      following fall E888.0
      late effect of E929.8
    dagger E920.3
    dart E920.8
    drill — see Accident, caused by drill
    edge of stiff paper E920.8
    electric
      beater E920.2
      fan E920.2
      knife E920.2
      mixer E920.2
    firearm component E928.7
    fork E920.4
    garden fork E920.4
    hand saw or tool (not powered) E920.4
      powered E920.1
    hedge clipper E920.4
      powered E920.1
    hoe E920.4
    ice pick E920.4
    knife E920.3
      electric E920.2
      in war operations E995.2
    lathe turnings E920.8
    lawn mower E920.4
      powered E920.0
      riding E919.8
    machine — see Accident, machine
    meat
      grinder E919.8
      slicer E919.8
    nails E920.8
    needle E920.4
      hypodermic E920.5
    object, edged, pointed, sharp — see category E920 ☑
      following fall E888.0
    paper cutter E920.4
    piercing instrument (see also category) E920 ☑
      late effect of E929.8
    pitchfork E920.4
    powered
      can opener E920.2
      garden cultivator E920.1
        riding E919.8
      hand saw E920.1
      hand tool NEC E920.1
      hedge clipper E920.1
      household appliance or implement E920.2
      lawn mower (hand) E920.0
        riding E919.8
      rivet gun E920.1
      staple gun E920.1

Cut, cutting — continued
  by — continued
    rake E920.4
    saw
      circular E919.4
      hand E920.4
    scissors E920.4
    screwdriver E920.4
    sewing machine (electric) (powered) E920.2
      not powered E920.4
    shears E920.4
    shovel E920.4
    slide trigger mechanism, scope or other part of gun E928.7
    spade E920.4
    splinters E920.8
    sword E920.3
      in war operations E995.2
    tin can lid E920.8
    wood slivers E920.8
  homicide (attempt) E966
  inflicted by other person
    stated as
      intentional, homicidal E966
      undetermined whether accidental or intentional E986
  late effect of NEC E929.8
  legal
    execution E978
    intervention E974
  self-inflicted (unspecified whether accidental or intentional) E986
    stated as intentional, purposeful E956
  stated as undetermined whether accidental or intentional E986
  suicidal (attempt) E956
  terrorism E979.8
  war operations E995.2
Cyclone E908.1

Death due to injury occurring one year or more previous — see Late effect
Decapitation (accidental circumstances) NEC E928.9
  homicidal E966
  legal execution (by guillotine) E978
Deprivation — see also Privation
  homicidal intent E968.4
Derailment (accidental)
  railway (rolling stock) (train) (vehicle) (with subsequent collision) E802 ☑
    with
      collision (antecedent) (see also Collision, railway) E800 ☑
      explosion (subsequent) (without antecedent collision) E802 ☑
        antecedent collision E803 ☑
      fall (without collision (antecedent)) E802 ☑
      fire (without collision (antecedent)) E802 ☑
  street car E829 ☑
Descent
  parachute (voluntary) (without accident to aircraft) E844 ☑
    due to accident to aircraft — see categories E840-E842 ☑
Desertion
  child, with intent to injure or kill E968.4
  helpless person, infant, newborn E904.0
    with intent to injure or kill E968.4
Destitution — see Privation
Dirty bomb (see also War operations, injury due to, nuclear weapons) E996.9
Disability, late effect or sequela of injury — see Late effect
Disease
  Andes E902.0
  aviators' E902.1
  caisson E902.2
  range E902.0
Divers' disease, palsy, paralysis, squeeze E902.0

☑ Additional Digit Required — Refer to the Tabular List for Digit Selection   ⬚ Subterms under main terms may continue to next column or page

338 — Volume 2   ▶◀ Revised Text   ● New Line   ▲ Revised Code   2011 ICD-9-CM

Dog bite E906.0
Dragged by
   cable car (not on rails) E847
      on rails E829 ☑
   motor vehicle (on highway) E814 ☑
      not on highway, nontraffic accident
         E825 ☑
   street car E829 ☑
Drinking poison (accidental) — *see* Table of
   Drugs and Chemicals
Drowning — *see* Submersion
Dust in eye E914

E

Earth falling (on) (with asphyxia or suffocation
   (by pressure)) — *see also* Suffocation,
   due to, cave-in E913.3
   as, or due to, a cataclysm (involving any
      transport vehicle) — *see* categories
      E908 ☑, E909 ☑
   not due to cataclysmic action E913.3
      motor vehicle (in motion) (on public
         highway) E813 ☑
         not on public highway E825 ☑
      nonmotor road vehicle NEC E829 ☑
      pedal cycle E826 ☑
      railway rolling stock, train, vehicle
         E806 ☑
      street car E829 ☑
   struck or crushed by E916
      with asphyxiation or suffocation
         E913.3
      with injury other than asphyxia, suf-
         focation E916
Earthquake (any injury) E909.0
Effect(s) (adverse) of
   air pressure E902.9
      at high altitude E902.9
         in aircraft E902.1
         residence or prolonged visit (causing
            conditions classifiable to
            E902.0) E902.0
      due to
         diving E902.2
         specified cause NEC E902.8
      in aircraft E902.1
   cold, excessive (exposure to) (*see also* Cold,
      exposure to) E901.9
   heat (excessive) (*see also* Heat) E900.9
   hot
      place — *see* Heat
      weather E900.0
   insulation — *see* Heat
   late — *see* Late effect of
   motion E903
   nuclear explosion or weapon
      in
         terrorism E979.5
         war operations (*see also* War opera-
            tions, injury due to, nuclear
            weapons) E996.9
   radiation — *see* Radiation
   terrorism, secondary E979.9
   travel E903
Electric shock, electrocution (accidental)
   (from exposed wire, faulty appliance,
   high voltage cable, live rail, open socket)
   (by) (in) E925.9
   appliance or wiring
      domestic E925.0
      factory E925.2
      farm (building) E925.8
         house E925.0
      home E925.0
      industrial (conductor) (control appara-
         tus) (transformer) E925.2
      outdoors E925.8
      public building E925.8
      residential institution E925.8
      school E925.8
      specified place NEC E925.8
   caused by other person
      stated as
         intentional, homicidal E968.8

Electric shock, electrocution — *continued*
   caused by other person — *continued*
      stated as — *continued*
         undetermined whether accidental or
            intentional E988.4
   electric power generating plant, distribution
      station E925.1
   electroshock gun (taser) (stun gun) E925.8
      caused by other person E968.8
         legal intervention E975
         stated as accidental E925.8
         stated as intentional E968.8
      due to legal intervention E975
      stated as intentional self-harm (suicidal
         attempt) E958.4
      stated as undetermined whether acciden-
         tal or intentional E988.4
      suicide (attempt) E958.4
   homicidal (attempt) E968.8
   legal execution E978
   lightning E907
   machinery E925.9
      domestic E925.0
      factory E925.2
      farm E925.8
      home E925.0
   misadventure in medical or surgical proce-
      dure
      in electroshock therapy E873.4
   self-inflicted (undetermined whether acci-
      dental or intentional) E988.4
      stated as intentional E958.4
      stated as undetermined whether accidental
         or intentional E988.4
      suicidal (attempt) E958.4
   transmission line E925.1
Electrocution — *see* Electric shock
Embolism
   air (traumatic) NEC — *see* Air, embolism
Encephalitis
   lead or saturnine E866.0
      from pesticide NEC E863.4
Entanglement
   in
      bedclothes, causing suffocation E913.0
      wheel of pedal cycle E826 ☑
Entry of foreign body, material, any — *see*
   Foreign body
Execution, legal (any method) E978
Exertion, excessive physical, from pro-
   longed activity E927.2
Exhaustion
   cold — *see* Cold, exposure to
   due to excessive exertion E927.2 ▲
   heat — *see* Heat
Explosion (accidental) (in) (of) (on) E923.9
   acetylene E923.2
   aerosol can E921.8
   aircraft (in transit) (powered) E841 ☑
      at landing, take-off E840 ☑
      in
         terrorism E979.1
         war operations
            from
               enemy fire or explosive(s)
                  (device placed on air-
                  craft) E994.0
               own onboard explosives
                  E994.1
      unpowered E842 ☑
   air tank (compressed) (in machinery) E921.1
   anesthetic gas in operating theatre E923.2
   automobile tire NEC E921.8
      causing transport accident — *see* cate-
         gories E810-E825 ☑
   blasting (cap) (materials) E923.1
   boiler (machinery), not on transport vehicle
      E921.0
      steamship — *see* Explosion, watercraft
   bomb E923.8
      in
         terrorism E979.2
         war operations E993.8
           after cessation of hostilities
            E998.1

Explosion — *continued*
   bomb — *continued*
      in — *continued*
         war operations — *continued*
           atom, hydrogen or nuclear (*see*
            also War operations, injury
            due to, nuclear weapons)
            E996.9
           injury by fragments from E991.9
            antipersonnel bomb E991.3
   butane E923.2
   caused by
      other person
         stated as
           intentional, homicidal — *see* As-
            sault, explosive
           undetermined whether acciden-
            tal or homicidal E985.5
   coal gas E923.2
   detonator E923.1
   dynamite E923.1
   explosive (material) NEC E923.9
      gas(es) E923.2
      missile E923.8
         in
           terrorism E979.2
           war operations E993.1
            injury by fragments from
             E991.9
             antipersonnel bomb
              E991.3
      used in blasting operations E923.1
   fire-damp E923.2
   fireworks E923.0
   gas E923.2
      cylinder (in machinery) E921.1
      pressure tank (in machinery) E921.1
   gasoline (fumes) (tank) not in moving motor
      vehicle E923.2
   grain store (military) (munitions) E923.8
   grenade E923.8
      in
         terrorism E979.2
         war operations E993.8
           injury by fragments from E991.4
   homicide (attempt) — *see* Assault, explosive
   hot water heater, tank (in machinery) E921.0
   in mine (of explosive gases) NEC E923.2
   late effect of NEC E929.8
   machinery (*see also* Accident, machine)
      pressure vessel — *see* Explosion, pres-
         sure vessel
   methane E923.2
   missile E923.8
      in
         terrorism E979.2
         war operations E993.1
           injury by fragments from E991.4
   motor vehicle (part of)
      in motion (on public highway) E818 ☑
      not on public highway E825 ☑
   munitions (dump) (factory) E923.8
      in
         terrorism E979.2
         war operations E993.9
   of mine E923.8
      in
         terrorism
           at sea or in harbor E979.0
           land E979.2
           marine E979.0
         war operations
           after cessation of hostilities
            E998.0
           at sea or in harbor E992.2
           land E993.8
             after cessation of hostilities
               E998.0
             injury by fragments from
               E991.4
           marine E992.2
   own weapons
      in
         terrorism (*see also* Suicide) E979.2
         war operations E993.7
           injury by fragments from E991.9

Explosion — *continued*
   own weapons — *continued*
      in — *continued*
         war operations — *continued*
           injury by fragments from — *con-*
            tinued
            antipersonnel bomb E991.3
   pressure
      cooker E921.8
      gas tank (in machinery) E921.1
      vessel (in machinery) E921.9
         on transport vehicle — *see* cate-
            gories E800-E848 ☑
         specified type NEC E921.8
   propane E923.2
   railway engine, locomotive, train (boiler)
      (with subsequent collision, derail-
      ment, fall) E803 ☑
      with
         collision (antecedent) (*see also* Colli-
           sion, railway) E800 ☑
         derailment (antecedent) E802 ☑
         fire (without antecedent collision or
           derailment) E803 ☑
   secondary fire resulting from — *see* Fire
   self-inflicted (unspecified whether acciden-
      tal or intentional) E985.5
      stated as intentional, purposeful E955.5
   shell (artillery) E923.8
      in
         terrorism E979.2
         war operations E993.2
           injury by fragments from E991.4
   stated as undetermined whether caused
      accidentally or purposely inflicted
      E985.5
   steam or water lines (in machinery) E921.0
   suicide (attempted) E955.5
   terrorism — *see* Terrorism, explosion
   torpedo E923.8
      in
         terrorism E979.0
         war operations E992.0
   transport accident — *see* categories
      E800-E848 ☑
   war operations — *see* War operations, ex-
      plosion
   watercraft (boiler) E837 ☑
      causing drowning, submersion (after
         jumping from watercraft) E830 ☑
Exposure (weather) (conditions) (rain) (wind)
   E904.3
   with homicidal intent E968.4
   environmental
      to
         algae bloom E928.6
         blue-green algae bloom E928.6
         brown tide E928.6
         cyanobacteria bloom E928.6
         Florida red tide E928.6
         harmful alage
           and toxins E928.6
           bloom E928.6
         pfiesteria piscicida E928.6
         red tide E928.6
   excessive E904.3
      cold (*see also* Cold, exposure to) E901.9
         self-inflicted — *see* Cold, exposure
           to, self-inflicted
      heat (*see also* Heat) E900.9
   helpless person, infant, newborn due to
      abandonment or neglect E904.0
   noise E928.1
   prolonged in deep-freeze unit or refrigerator
      E901.1
   radiation — *see* Radiation
   resulting from transport accident — *see*
      categories E800-E848 ☑
   smoke from, due to
      fire — *see* Fire
      tobacco, second-hand E869.4
   vibration E928.2
External cause status E000.9
   child assisting in compensated work of   ●
      other family member E000.8   ●

☑ **Additional Digit Required** — Refer to the Tabular List for Digit Selection   ▽ **Subterms under main terms may continue to next column or page**

☑ Additional Digit Required — Refer to the Tabular List for Digit Selection   ✇ Subterms under main terms may continue to next column or page

340 — Volume 2 · October 2010   ▶◀ Revised Text   ● New Line   ▲ Revised Code   2011 ICD-9-CM

Fire, hot object or hot substance —
  continued
  controlled, normal (in brazier, fireplace,
      furnace, or stove) (charcoal) (coal)
      (coke) (electric) (gas) (wood)
    bonfire E897
    brazier, not in building or structure E897
    in building or structure, except private
        dwelling (barn) (church) (conva-
        lescent or residential home) (fac-
        tory) (farm outbuilding) (hospital)
        (hotel) (institution (educational)
        (dormitory) (residential)) (private
        garage) (school) (shop) (store)
        (theatre) E896
    in private dwelling (apartment) (board-
        ing house) (camping place) (cara-
        van) (farmhouse) (home (private))
        (house) (lodging house) (rooming
        house) (tenement) E895
    not in building or structure E897
    trash E897
  forest (uncontrolled) E892
  grass (uncontrolled) E892
  hay (uncontrolled) E892
  homicide (attempt) E968.0
    late effect of E969
  in, of, on, starting in E892
    aircraft (in transit) (powered) E841 ☑
      at landing, take-off E840 ☑
      stationary E892
      unpowered (balloon) (glider)
          E842 ☑
    balloon E842 ☑
    boat, ship, watercraft — *see* categories
        E830 ☑, E831 ☑, E837 ☑
    building or structure, except private
        dwelling (barn) (church) (conva-
        lescent or residential home) (fac-
        tory) (farm outbuilding) (hospital)
        (hotel) (institution (educational)
        (dormitory) (residential)) (school)
        (shop) (store) (theatre) (*see also*
        Conflagration, building or struc-
        ture, except private dwelling)
        E891.9
    forest (uncontrolled) E892
    glider E842 ☑
    grass (uncontrolled) E892
    hay (uncontrolled) E892
    lumber (uncontrolled) E892
    machinery — *see* Accident, machine
    mine (uncontrolled) E892
    motor vehicle (in motion) (on public
        highway) E818 ☑
      not on public highway E825 ☑
      stationary E892
    prairie (uncontrolled) E892
    private dwelling (apartment) (boarding
        house) (camping place) (caravan)
        (farmhouse) (home (private))
        (house) (lodging house) (private
        garage) (rooming house) (tene-
        ment) (*see also* Conflagration,
        private dwelling) E890.9
    railway rolling stock, train, vehicle (*see
        also* Explosion, railway engine)
        E803 ☑
      stationary E892
    room NEC E898.1
    street car (in motion) E829 ☑
      stationary E892
    terrorism (by fire-producing device)
        E979.3
      fittings or furniture (burning build-
          ing) (uncontrolled fire) E979.3
      from nuclear explosion E979.5
    transport vehicle, stationary NEC E892
    tunnel (uncontrolled) E892
    war operations (by fire-producing device
        or conventional weapon) E990.9
      from nuclear explosion (*see also* War
          operations, injury due to, nu-
          clear weapons) E996.2
      incendiary bomb E990.0
        petrol bomb E990.0

Fire, hot object or hot substance —
  continued
  late effect of NEC E929.4
  lumber (uncontrolled) E892
  mine (uncontrolled) E892
  prairie (uncontrolled) E892
  self-inflicted (unspecified whether acciden-
      tal or intentional) E988.1
    stated as intentional, purposeful E958.1
  specified NEC E898.1
    with
      conflagration — *see* Conflagration
      ignition (of)
        clothing — *see* Ignition, clothes
        highly inflammable material
            (benzine) (fat) (gasoline)
            (kerosene) (paraffin)
            (petrol) E894
    started by other person
      stated as
        with intent to injure or kill E968.0
        undetermined whether or not with
            intent to injure or kill E988.1
    suicide (attempted) E958.1
      late effect of E959
  tunnel (uncontrolled) E892
Fireball effects from nuclear explosion
  in
    terrorism E979.5
    war operations (*see also* War operations,
        injury due to, nuclear weapons)
        E996.2
Fireworks (explosion) E923.0
Flash burns from explosion — *see also* Explo-
    sion E923.9
Flood (any injury) (resulting from storm) E908.2
  caused by collapse of dam or manmade
      structure E909.3
Forced landing (aircraft) E840 ☑
Foreign body, object or material (entrance
    into) (accidental)
  air passage (causing injury) E915
    with asphyxia, obstruction, suffocation
        E912
      food or vomitus E911
    nose (with asphyxia, obstruction, suffo-
        cation) E912
      causing injury without asphyxia, ob-
          struction, suffocation E915
  alimentary canal (causing injury) (with ob-
      struction) E915
    with asphyxia, obstruction respiratory
        passage, suffocation E912
      food E911
    mouth E915
      with asphyxia, obstruction, suffoca-
          tion E912
        food E911
    pharynx E915
      with asphyxia, obstruction, suffoca-
          tion E912
        food E911
  aspiration (with asphyxia, obstruction respi-
      ratory passage, suffocation) E912
    causing injury without asphyxia, obstruc-
        tion respiratory passage, suffoca-
        tion E915
    food (regurgitated) (vomited) E911
      causing injury without asphyxia, ob-
          struction respiratory passage,
          suffocation E915
    mucus (not of newborn) E912
    phlegm E912
  bladder (causing injury or obstruction) E915
  bronchus, bronchi — *see* Foreign body, air
      passages
  conjunctival sac E914
  digestive system — *see* Foreign body, ali-
      mentary canal
  ear (causing injury or obstruction) E915
  esophagus (causing injury or obstruction)
      (*see also* Foreign body, alimentary
      canal) E915
  eye (any part) E914
  eyelid E914
  hairball (stomach) (with obstruction) E915

Foreign body, object or material —
  continued
  ingestion — *see* Foreign body, alimentary
      canal
  inhalation — *see* Foreign body, aspiration
  intestine (causing injury or obstruction)
      E915
  iris E914
  lacrimal apparatus E914
  larynx — *see* Foreign body, air passage
  late effect of NEC E929.8
  lung — *see* Foreign body, air passage
  mouth — *see* Foreign body, alimentary
      canal, mouth
  nasal passage — *see* Foreign body, air pas-
      sage, nose
  nose — *see* Foreign body, air passage, nose
  ocular muscle E914
  operation wound (left in) — *see* Misadven-
      ture, foreign object
  orbit E914
  pharynx — *see* Foreign body, alimentary
      canal, pharynx
  rectum (causing injury or obstruction) E915
  stomach (hairball) (causing injury or obstruc-
      tion) E915
  tear ducts or glands E914
  trachea — *see* Foreign body, air passage
  urethra (causing injury or obstruction) E915
  vagina (causing injury or obstruction) E915
Found dead, injured
  from exposure (to) — *see* Exposure
  on
    public highway E819 ☑
    railway right of way E807 ☑
Fracture (circumstances unknown or unspeci-
    fied) E887
  due to specified external means — *see*
      manner of accident
  late effect of NEC E929.3
  occurring in water transport NEC E835 ☑
Freezing — *see* Cold, exposure to
Frostbite E901.0
  due to manmade conditions E901.1
Frozen — *see* Cold, exposure to

G

Garrotting, homicidal (attempted) E963
Gored E906.8
Gunshot wound — *see also* Shooting E922.9

H

Hailstones, injury by E904.3
Hairball (stomach) (with obstruction) E915
Hanged himself — *see also* Hanging, self-in-
    flicted E983.0
Hang gliding E842 ☑
Hanging (accidental) E913.8
  caused by other person
    in accidental circumstances E913.8
    stated as
      intentional, homicidal E963
      undetermined whether accidental or
          intentional E983.0
  homicide (attempt) E963
  in bed or cradle E913.0
  legal execution E978
  self-inflicted (unspecified whether acciden-
      tal or intentional) E983.0
    in accidental circumstances E913.8
    stated as intentional, purposeful E953.0
  stated as undetermined whether accidental
      or intentional E983.0
  suicidal (attempt) E953.0
Heat (apoplexy) (collapse) (cramps) (effects of)
    (excessive) (exhaustion) (fever) (prostra-
    tion) (stroke) E900.9
  due to
    manmade conditions (as listed in E900.1,
        except boat, ship, watercraft)
        E900.1
    weather (conditions) E900.0
  from
    electric heating appartus causing burn-
        ing E924.8

Heat — *continued*
  from — *continued*
    nuclear explosion
      in
        terrorism E979.5
        war operations (*see also* War oper-
            ations, injury due to, nucle-
            ar weapons) E996.2
    generated in, boiler, engine, evaporator, fire
        room of boat, ship, watercraft
        E838 ☑
    inappropriate in local application or packing
        in medical or surgical procedure
        E873.5
  late effect of NEC E989
Hemorrhage
  delayed following medical or surgical
      treatment without mention of misad-
      venture — *see* Reaction, abnormal
  during medical or surgical treatment as
      misadventure — *see* Misadventure,
      cut
High
  altitude, effects E902.9
  level of radioactivity, effects — *see* Radia-
      tion
  pressure effects (*see also* Effects of, air pres-
      sure)
    from rapid descent in water (causing
        caisson or divers' disease, palsy,
        or paralysis) E902.2
  temperature, effects — *see* Heat
Hit, hitting (accidental) by
  aircraft (propeller) (without accident to air-
      craft) E844 ☑
    unpowered E842 ☑
  avalanche E909.2
  being thrown against object in or part of
      motor vehicle (in motion) (on public
      highway) E818 ☑
    not on public highway E825 ☑
    nonmotor road vehicle NEC E829 ☑
    street car E829 ☑
  boat, ship, watercraft
    after fall from watercraft E838 ☑
      damaged, involved in accident
          E831 ☑
    while swimming, water skiing E838 ☑
  bullet (*see also* Shooting) E922.9
    from air gun E922.4
    in
      terrorism E979.4
      war operations E991.2
        rubber E991.0
  flare, Verey pistol (*see also* Shooting) E922.8
  hailstones E904.3
  landslide E909.2
  law-enforcing agent (on duty) E975
    with blunt object (baton) (night stick)
        (stave) (truncheon) E973
  machine — *see* Accident, machine
  missile
    firearm (*see also* Shooting) E922.9
    in
      terrorism — *see* Terrorism, missile
      war operations — *see* War opera-
          tions, missile
  motor vehicle (on public highway) (traffic
      accident) E814 ☑
    not on public highway, nontraffic acci-
        dent E822 ☑
  nonmotor road vehicle NEC E829 ☑
  object
    falling E916
      from, in, on
        aircraft E844 ☑
          due to accident to aircraft —
              see categories
              E840–E842 ☑
            unpowered E842 ☑
          boat, ship, watercraft E838 ☑
            due to accident to watercraft
                E831 ☑
        building E916
          burning (uncontrolled fire)
              E891.8

Index

Hit, hitting — Injury, injured

Hit, hitting by — *continued*
  object — *continued*
    falling — *continued*
      from, in, on — *continued*
        building — *continued*
          burning — *continued*
            in terrorism E979.3
            private E890.8
        cataclysmic
          earth surface movement or
            eruption E909.9
          storm E908.9
        cave-in E916
          with asphyxiation or suffoca-
            tion (*see also* Suffoca-
            tion, due to, cave-in)
            E913.3
        earthquake E909.0
        motor vehicle (in motion) (on
          public highway) E818 ☑
          not on public highway
            E825 ☑
          stationary E916
        nonmotor road vehicle NEC
          E829 ☑
        pedal cycle E826 ☑
        railway rolling stock, train, vehicle
          E806 ☑
        street car E829 ☑
        structure, burning NEC E891.8
        vehicle, stationary E916
      moving NEC — *see* Striking against, ob-
        ject
      projected NEC — *see* Striking against,
        object
      set in motion by
        compressed air or gas, spring, strik-
          ing, throwing — *see* Striking
          against, object
        explosion — *see* Explosion
      thrown into, on, or towards
        motor vehicle (in motion) (on public
          highway) E818 ☑
          not on public highway E825 ☑
        nonmotor road vehicle NEC E829 ☑
        pedal cycle E826 ☑
        street car E829 ☑
      off-road type motor vehicle (not on public
        highway) E821 ☑
      on public highway E814 ☑
  other person(s) E917.9
    with blunt or thrown object E917.9
      in sports E917.0
        with subsequent fall E917.5
      intentionally, homicidal E968.2
    as, or caused by, a crowd E917.1
      with subsequent fall E917.6
      in sports E917.0
  pedal cycle E826 ☑
  police (on duty) E975
    with blunt object (baton) (nightstick)
      (stave) (truncheon) E973
  railway, rolling stock, train, vehicle (part of)
    E805 ☑
  shot — *see* Shooting
  snow vehicle, motor-driven (not on public
    highway) E820 ☑
    on public highway E814 ☑
  street car E829 ☑
  vehicle NEC — *see* Accident, vehicle NEC
Homicide, homicidal (attempt) (justifiable) —
  see also Assault E968.9
Hot
  liquid, object, substance, accident caused
    by (*see also* Accident, caused by, hot,
    by type of substance)
    late effect of E929.8
  place, effects — *see* Heat
  weather, effects E900.0
Humidity, causing problem E904.3
Hunger E904.1
  resulting from
    abandonment or neglect E904.0
    transport accident — *see* categories
      E800-E848 ☑
Hurricane (any injury) E908.0

Hypobarism, hypobaropathy — *see* Effects
  of, air pressure
Hypothermia — *see* Cold, exposure to

I

Ictus
  caloris — *see* Heat
  solaris E900.0
Ignition (accidental)
  anesthetic gas in operating theatre E923.2
  bedclothes
    with
      conflagration — *see* Conflagration
      ignition (of)
        clothing — *see* Ignition, clothes
        highly inflammable material
          (benzine) (fat) (gasoline)
          (kerosene) (paraffin)
          (petrol) E894
  benzine E894
  clothes, clothing (from controlled fire) (in
    building) E893.9
    with conflagration — *see* Conflagration
    from
      bonfire E893.2
      highly inflammable material E894
      sources or material as listed in E893.8
      trash fire E893.2
      uncontrolled fire — *see* Conflagra-
        tion
    in
      private dwelling E893.0
      specified building or structure, ex-
        cept private dwelling E893.1
    not in building or structure E893.2
  explosive material — *see* Explosion
  fat E894
  gasoline E894
  kerosene E894
  material
    explosive — *see* Explosion
    highly inflammable E894
      with conflagration — *see* Conflagra-
        tion
      with explosion E923.2
  nightdress — *see* Ignition, clothes
  paraffin E894
  petrol E894
Immersion — *see* Submersion
Implantation of quills of porcupine E906.8
Inanition (from) E904.9
  hunger — *see* Lack of, food
  resulting from homicidal intent E968.4
  thirst — *see* Lack of, water
Inattention after, at birth E904.0
  homicidal, infanticidal intent E968.4
Infanticide — *see also* Assault
Ingestion
  foreign body (causing injury) (with obstruc-
    tion) — *see* Foreign body, alimentary
    canal
  poisonous substance NEC — *see* Table of
    Drugs and Chemicals
Inhalation
  excessively cold substance, manmade
    E901.1
  foreign body — *see* Foreign body, aspiration
  liquid air, hydrogen, nitrogen E901.1
  mucus, not of newborn (with asphyxia, ob-
    struction respiratory passage, suffoca-
    tion) E912
  phlegm (with asphyxia, obstruction respira-
    tory passage, suffocation) E912
  poisonous gas — *see* Table of Drugs and
    Chemicals
  smoke from, due to
    fire — *see* Fire
    tobacco, second-hand E869.4
  vomitus (with asphyxia, obstruction respira-
    tory passage, suffocation) E911
Injury, injured (accidental(ly)) NEC E928.9
  by, caused by, from
    air rifle (BB gun) E922.4
    animal (not being ridden) NEC E906.9
      being ridden (in sport or transport)
        E828 ☑

Injury, injured — *continued*
  by, caused by, from — *continued*
    assault (*see also* Assault) E968.9
    avalanche E909.2
    bayonet (*see also* Bayonet wound)
      E920.3
    being thrown against some part of, or
      object in
      motor vehicle (in motion) (on public
        highway) E818 ☑
        not on public highway E825 ☑
      nonmotor road vehicle NEC E829 ☑
      off-road motor vehicle NEC E821 ☑
      railway train E806 ☑
      snow vehicle, motor-driven E820 ☑
      street car E829 ☑
    bending
      due to
        repetitive movement E927.3 ●
        sudden strenuous movement ●
          E927.0 ●
    bite, human E928.3
    broken glass E920.8
    bullet — *see* Shooting
    cave-in (*see also* Suffocation, due to,
      cave-in) E913.3
      without asphyxiation or suffocation
        E916
      earth surface movement or eruption
        E909.9
      storm E908.9
    cloudburst E908.8
    component of firearm or air gun E928.7
    cutting or piercing instrument (*see also*
      Cut) E920.9
    cyclone E908.1
    earthquake E909.0
    earth surface movement or eruption
      E909.9
    electric current (*see also* Electric shock)
      E925.9
    explosion (*see also* Explosion) E923.9
      of gun part E928.7
    fire — *see* Fire
    flare, Verey pistol E922.8
    flood E908.2
    foreign body — *see* Foreign body
    gun recoil E928.7
    hailstones E904.3
    hurricane E908.0
    landslide E909.2
    law-enforcing agent, police, in course of
      legal intervention — *see* Legal
      intervention
    lightning E907
    live rail or live wire — *see* Electric shock
    machinery (*see also* Accident, machine)
      aircraft, without accident to aircraft
        E844 ☑
      boat, ship, watercraft (deck) (engine
        room) (galley) (laundry)
        (loading) E836 ☑
    mechanism of firearm or air gun E928.7
    missile
      explosive E923.8
      firearm — *see* Shooting
      in
        terrorism — *see* Terrorism, mis-
          sile
        war operations — *see* War opera-
          tions, missile
    moving part of motor vehicle (in motion)
      (on public highway) E818 ☑
      not on public highway, nontraffic
        accident E825 ☑
      while alighting, boarding, entering,
        leaving — *see* Fall, from, mo-
        tor vehicle, while alighting,
        boarding
    nail E920.8
    needle (sewing) E920.4
      hypodermic E920.5
    noise E928.1

Injury, injured — *continued*
  by, caused by, from — *continued*
    object
      fallen on
        motor vehicle (in motion) (on
          public highway) E818 ☑
        not on public highway
          E825 ☑
      falling — *see* Hit by, object, falling
    paintball gun E922.5
    radiation — *see* Radiation
    railway rolling stock, train, vehicle (part
      of) E805 ☑
      door or window E806 ☑
    recoil of firearm E928.7
    rotating propeller, aircraft E844 ☑
    rough landing of off-road type motor
      vehicle (after leaving ground or
      rough terrain) E821 ☑
    snow vehicle E820 ☑
    saber (*see also* Wound, saber) E920.3
    shot — *see* Shooting
    sound waves E928.1
    splinter or sliver, wood E920.8
    straining
      due to
        repetitive movement E927.3 ●
        sudden strenuous movement ●
          E927.0 ●
    street car (door) E829 ☑
    suicide (attempt) E958.9
    sword E920.3
    terrorism — *see* Terrorism
    third rail — *see* Electric shock
    thunderbolt E907
    tidal wave E909.4
      caused by storm E908.0
    tornado E908.1
    torrential rain E908.2
    twisting
      due to
        repetitive movement E927.3 ●
        sudden strenuous movement ●
          E927.0 ●
    vehicle NEC — *see* Accident, vehicle NEC
    vibration E928.2
    volcanic eruption E909.1
    weapon burst, in war operations E993.9
    weightlessness (in spacecraft, real or
      simulated) E928.0
    wood splinter or sliver E920.8
  due to
    civil insurrection — *see* War operations
      occurring after cessation of hostilities
      E998.9
    terrorism — *see* Terrorism
    war operations — *see* War operations
      occurring after cessation of hostilities
      E998.9
    weapon of mass destruction [WMD]
      E997.3
  homicidal (*see also* Assault) E968.9
  inflicted (by)
    in course of arrest (attempted), suppres-
      sion of disturbance, maintenance
      of order, by law enforcing agents
      — *see* Legal intervention
    law-enforcing agent (on duty) — *see*
      Legal intervention
    other person
      stated as
        accidental E928.9
        homicidal, intentional — *see* As-
          sault
        undetermined whether acciden-
          tal or intentional — *see*
          Injury, stated as undeter-
          mined
    police (on duty) — *see* Legal interven-
      tion
  in, on
    civil insurrection — *see* War operations
    fight E960.0
    parachute descent (voluntary) (without
      accident to aircraft) E844 ☑

☑ **Additional Digit Required** — Refer to the Tabular List for Digit Selection   ▽ **Subterms under main terms may continue to next column or page**

Injury, injured — *continued*
in, on — *continued*
  parachute descent — *continued*
    with accident to aircraft — *see* categories E840–E842 ☑
    public highway E819 ☑
    railway right of way E807 ☑
    terrorism — *see* Terrorism
    war operations — *see* War operations
  late effect of E929.9
  purposely (inflicted) by other person(s) — *see* Assault
  self-inflicted (unspecified whether accidental or intentional) E988.9
  stated as
    accidental E928.9
    intentionally, purposely E958.9
  specified cause NEC E928.8
  stated as
    hanging E983.0
    knife E986
    late effect of E989
    puncture (any part of body) E986
    shooting — *see* Shooting, stated as undetermined whether accidental or intentional
    specified means NEC E988.8
    stab (any part of body) E986
    strangulation — *see* Suffocation, stated as undetermined whether accidental or intentional
    submersion E984
    suffocation — *see* Suffocation, stated as undetermined whether accidental or intentional
  undetermined whether accidentally or purposely inflicted (by) E988.9
    cut (any part of body) E986
    cutting or piercing instrument (classifiable to E920) E986
    drowning E984
    explosive(s) (missile) E985.5
    falling from high place E987.9
      manmade structure, except residential E987.1
    natural site E987.2
    residential premises E987.0
  to child due to criminal abortion E968.8
Insufficient nourishment — *see also* Lack of, food
homicidal intent E968.4
Insulation, effects — *see* Heat
Interruption of respiration by
  food lodged in esophagus E911
  foreign body, except food, in esophagus E912
Intervention, legal — *see* Legal intervention
Intoxication, drug or poison — *see* Table of Drugs and Chemicals
Irradiation — *see* Radiation

J

Jammed (accidentally)
  between objects (moving) (stationary and moving) E918
  in object E918
Jumped or fell from high place, so stated — *see* Jumping, from, high place, stated as in undetermined circumstances
Jumping
  before train, vehicle or other moving object (unspecified whether accidental or intentional) E988.0
  stated as
    intentional, purposeful E958.0
    suicidal (attempt) E958.0
  from
    aircraft
      by parachute (voluntarily) (without accident to aircraft) E844 ☑
      due to accident to aircraft — *see* categories E840–E842 ☑
    boat, ship, watercraft (into water)
      after accident to, fire on, watercraft E830 ☑

Jumping — *continued*
  from — *continued*
    boat, ship, watercraft — *continued*
      after accident to, fire on, watercraft — *continued*
        and subsequently struck by (part of) boat E831 ☑
      burning, crushed, sinking E830 ☑
        and subsequently struck by (part of) boat E831 ☑
      voluntarily, without accident (to boat) with injury other than drowning or submersion E883.0
    building (*see also* Jumping, from, high place)
    burning (uncontrolled fire) E891.8
      in terrorism E979.3
      private E890.8
    cable car (not on rails) E847
      on rails E829 ☑
    high place
      in accidental circumstances or in sport — *see* categories E880–E884 ☑
      stated as
        with intent to injure self E957.9
          man-made structures NEC E957.1
          natural sites E957.2
          residential premises E957.0
        in undetermined circumstances E987.9
          man-made structures NEC E987.1
          natural sites E987.2
          residential premises E987.0
        suicidal (attempt) E957.9
          man-made structures NEC E957.1
          natural sites E957.1
          residential premises E957.0
    motor vehicle (in motion) (on public highway) — *see* Fall, from, motor vehicle
    nonmotor road vehicle NEC E829 ☑
    street car E829 ☑
    structure (*see also* Jumping, from, high place)
      burning NEC (uncontrolled fire) E891.8
        in terrorism E979.3
  into water
    with injury other than drowning or submersion E883.0
    drowning or submersion — *see* Submersion
  from, off, watercraft — *see* Jumping, from, boat
Justifiable homicide — *see* Assault

K

Kicked by
  animal E906.8
  person(s) (accidentally) E917.9
    with intent to injure or kill E960.0
    as, or caused by a crowd E917.1
      with subsequent fall E917.6
    in fight E960.0
    in sports E917.0
      with subsequent fall E917.5
Kicking against
  object (moving) E917.9
    in sports E917.0
      with subsequent fall E917.5
    stationary E917.4
      with subsequent fall E917.8
  person — *see* Striking against, person
Killed, killing (accidentally) NEC — *see also* Injury E928.9
  in
    action — *see* War operations
    brawl, fight (hand) (fists) (foot) E960.0
      by weapon (*see also* Assault)
        cutting, piercing E966
        firearm — *see* Shooting, homicide

Killed, killing — *see also* Injury — *continued*
  self
    stated as
      accident E928.9
      suicide — *see* Suicide
    unspecified whether accidental or suicidal E988.9
Knocked down (accidentally) (by) NEC E928.9
  animal (not being ridden) E906.8
    being ridden (in sport or transport) E828 ☑
  blast from explosion (*see also* Explosion) E923.9
  crowd, human stampede E917.6
  late effect of — *see* Late effect
  person (accidentally) E917.9
    in brawl, fight E960.0
    in sports E917.5
  transport vehicle — *see* vehicle involved under Hit by
  while boxing E917.5

L

Laceration NEC E928.9
Lack of
  air (refrigerator or closed place), suffocation by E913.2
  care (helpless person) (infant) (newborn) E904.0
    homicidal intent E968.4
  food except as result of transport accident E904.1
    helpless person, infant, newborn due to abandonment or neglect E904.0
  water except as result of transport accident E904.2
    helpless person, infant, newborn due to abandonment or neglect E904.0
Landslide E909.2
  falling on, hitting
    motor vehicle (any) (in motion) (on or off public highway) E909.2
    railway rolling stock, train, vehicle E909.2
Late effect of
  accident NEC (accident classifiable to E928.9) E929.9
    specified NEC (accident classifiable to E910–E928.8) E929.8
  assault E969
  fall, accidental (accident classifiable to E880–E888) E929.3
  fire, accident caused by (accident classifiable to E890–E899) E929.4
  homicide, attempt (any means) E969
  injury due to terrorism E999.1
  injury undetermined whether accidentally or purposely inflicted (injury classifiable to E980–E988) E989
  legal intervention (injury classifiable to E970–E976) E977
  medical or surgical procedure, test or therapy
    as, or resulting in, or from
      abnormal or delayed reaction or complication — *see* Reaction, abnormal
      misadventure — *see* Misadventure
  motor vehicle accident (accident classifiable to E810–E825) E929.0
  natural or environmental factor, accident due to (accident classifiable to E900–E909) E929.5
  poisoning, accidental (accident classifiable to E850–E858, E860–E869) E929.2
  suicide, attempt (any means) E959
  transport accident NEC (accident classifiable to E800–E807, E826–E838, E840–E848) E929.1
  war operations, injury due to (injury classifiable to E990–E998) E999.0
Launching pad accident E845 ☑
Legal
  execution, any method E978
  intervention (by) (injury from) E976
    baton E973

Legal — *continued*
  intervention — *continued*
    bayonet E974
    blow E975
    blunt object (baton) (nightstick) (stave) (truncheon) E973
    cutting or piercing instrument E974
    dynamite E971
    execution, any method E973
    explosive(s) (shell) E971
    firearm(s) E970
    gas (asphyxiation) (poisoning) (tear) E972
    grenade E971
    late effect of E977
    machine gun E970
    manhandling E975
    mortar bomb E971
    nightstick E973
    revolver E970
    rifle E970
    specified means NEC E975
    stabbing E974
    stave E973
    truncheon E973
Lifting, injury
  due to ●
    repetitive movement E927.3 ●
    sudden strenuous movement E927.0 ●
Lightning (shock) (stroke) (struck by) E907
Liquid (noncorrosive) in eye E914
  corrosive E924.1
Loss of control
  motor vehicle (on public highway) (without antecedent collision) E816 ☑
    with
      antecedent collision on public highway — *see* Collision, motor vehicle
      involving any object, person or vehicle not on public highway E816 ☑
    not on public highway, nontraffic accident E825 ☑
      with antecedent collision — *see* Collision, motor vehicle, not on public highway
    on public highway — *see* Collision, motor vehicle
    off-road type motor vehicle (not on public highway) E821 ☑
      on public highway — *see* Loss of control, motor vehicle
    snow vehicle, motor-driven (not on public highway) E820 ☑
      on public highway — *see* Loss of control, motor vehicle
Lost at sea E832 ☑
  with accident to watercraft E830 ☑
  in war operations E995.8
Low
  pressure, effects — *see* Effects of, air pressure
  temperature, effects — *see* Cold, exposure to
Lying before train, vehicle or other moving object (unspecified whether accidental or intentional) E988.0
  stated as intentional, purposeful, suicidal (attempt) E958.0
Lynching — *see also* Assault E968.9

M

Malfunction, atomic power plant in water transport E838 ☑
Mangled (accidentally) NEC E928.9
Manhandling (in brawl, fight) E960.0
  legal intervention E975
Manslaughter (nonaccidental) — *see* Assault
Marble in nose E912
Mauled by animal E906.8
Medical procedure, complication of
  delayed or as an abnormal reaction
    without mention of misadventure — *see* Reaction, abnormal

☑ **Additional Digit Required** — Refer to the Tabular List for Digit Selection   🆆 **Subterms under main terms may continue to next column or page**

2011 ICD-9-CM   ▶◀ **Revised Text**   ● **New Line**   ▲ **Revised Code**   **October 2010 • Volume 2 — 343**

Medical procedure, complication of — *continued*
  due to or as a result of misadventure — *see* Misadventure
Melting of fittings and furniture in burning in terrorism E979.3
Minamata disease E865.2
Misadventure(s) to patient(s) during surgical or medical care E876.9
  contaminated blood, fluid, drug or biological substance (presence of agents and toxins as listed in E875) E875.9
    administered (by) NEC E875.9
      infusion E875.0
      injection E875.1
      specified means NEC E875.2
      transfusion E875.0
      vaccination E875.1
  cut, cutting, puncture, perforation or hemorrhage (accidental) (inadvertent) (inappropriate) (during) E870.9
    aspiration of fluid or tissue (by puncture or catheterization, except heart) E870.5
    biopsy E870.8
      needle (aspirating) E870.5
    blood sampling E870.5
    catheterization E870.5
      heart E870.6
    dialysis (kidney) E870.2
    endoscopic examination E870.4
    enema E870.7
    infusion E870.1
    injection E870.3
    lumbar puncture E870.5
    needle biopsy E870.5
    paracentesis, abdominal E870.5
    perfusion E870.2
    specified procedure NEC E870.8
    surgical operation E870.0
    thoracentesis E870.5
    transfusion E870.1
    vaccination E870.3
  excessive amount of blood or other fluid during transfusion or infusion E873.0
  failure
    in dosage E873.9
      electroshock therapy E873.4
      inappropriate temperature (too hot or too cold) in local application and packing E873.5
      infusion
        excessive amount of fluid E873.0
        incorrect dilution of fluid E873.1
      insulin-shock therapy E873.4
      nonadministration of necessary drug or medicinal E873.6
      overdose (*see also* Overdose)
        radiation, in therapy E873.2
      radiation
        inadvertent exposure of patient (receiving radiation for test or therapy) E873.3
          not receiving radiation for test or therapy — *see* Radiation
        overdose E873.2
      specified procedure NEC E873.8
      transfusion
        excessive amount of blood E873.0
    mechanical, of instrument or apparatus (during procedure) E874.9
      aspiration of fluid or tissue (by puncture or catheterization, except of heart) E874.4
      biopsy E874.8
        needle (aspirating) E874.4
      blood sampling E874.4
      catheterization E874.4
        heart E874.5
      dialysis (kidney) E874.2
      endoscopic examination E874.3
      enema E874.8
      infusion E874.1
      injection E874.8
      lumbar puncture E874.4

Misadventure(s) to patient(s) during surgical or medical care — *continued*
  failure — *continued*
    mechanical, of instrument or apparatus — *continued*
      needle biopsy E874.4
      paracentesis, abdominal E874.4
      perfusion E874.2
      specified procedure NEC E874.8
      surgical operation E874.0
      thoracentesis E874.4
      transfusion E874.1
      vaccination E874.8
    sterile precautions (during procedure) E872.9
      aspiration of fluid or tissue (by puncture or catheterization, except heart) E872.5
      biopsy E872.8
        needle (aspirating) E872.5
      blood sampling E872.5
      catheterization E872.5
        heart E872.6
      dialysis (kidney) E872.2
      endoscopic examination E872.4
      enema E872.8
      infusion E872.1
      injection E872.3
      lumbar puncture E872.5
      needle biopsy E872.5
      paracentesis, abdominal E872.5
      perfusion E872.2
      removal of catheter or packing E872.8
      specified procedure NEC E872.8
      surgical operation E872.0
      thoracentesis E872.5
      transfusion E872.1
      vaccination E872.3
    suture or ligature during surgical procedure E876.2
    to introduce or to remove tube or instrument E876.4
      foreign object left in body — *see* Misadventure, foreign object
  foreign object left in body (during procedure) E871.9
    aspiration of fluid or tissue (by puncture or catheterization, except heart) E871.5
    biopsy E871.8
      needle (aspirating) E871.5
    blood sampling E871.5
    catheterization E871.5
      heart E871.6
    dialysis (kidney) E871.2
    endoscopic examination E871.4
    enema E871.8
    infusion E871.1
    injection E871.3
    lumbar puncture E871.5
    needle biopsy E871.5
    paracentesis, abdominal E871.5
    perfusion E871.2
    removal of catheter or packing E871.7
    specified procedure NEC E871.8
    surgical operation E871.0
    thoracentesis E871.5
    transfusion E871.1
    vaccination E871.3
  hemorrhage — *see* Misadventure, cut
  inadvertent exposure of patient to radiation (being received for test or therapy) E873.3
  inappropriate
    temperature (too hot or too cold) in local application or packing E873.5
    infusion (*see also* Misadventure, by specific type, infusion)
      excessive amount of fluid E873.0
      incorrect dilution of fluid E873.1
      wrong fluid E876.1
    mismatched blood in transfusion E876.0
    nonadministration of necessary drug or medicinal E873.6
  overdose (*see also* Overdose)

Misadventure(s) to patient(s) during surgical or medical care — *continued*
  overdose (*see also* Overdose) — *continued*
    radiation, in therapy E873.2
  perforation — *see* Misadventure, cut
  performance of correct operation (procedure) on wrong
    body part E876.7
    side E876.7
    site E876.7
  performance of operation (procedure)
    intended for another patient E876.6
    on patient not scheduled for surgery E876.6
    on wrong patient E876.6
  performance of wrong operation on correct patient E876.5
  puncture — *see* Misadventure, cut
  specified type NEC E876.8
    failure
      suture or ligature during surgical operation E876.2
      to introduce or to remove tube or instrument E876.4
        foreign object left in body E871.9
    infusion of wrong fluid E876.1
    performance of inappropriate operation E876.5
    transfusion of mismatched blood E876.0
    wrong
      fluid in infusion E876.1
      placement of endotracheal tube during anesthetic procedure E876.3
  transfusion (*see also* Misadventure, by specific type, transfusion)
    excessive amount of blood E873.0
    mismatched blood E876.0
  wrong
    device implanted into correct surgical site E876.5
    drug given in error — *see* Table of Drugs and Chemicals
    fluid in infusion E876.1
    placement of endotracheal tube during anesthetic procedure E876.3
    procedure (operation) performed on the correct patient E876.5
Motion (effects) E903
  sickness E903
Mountain sickness E902.0
Mucus aspiration or inhalation, not of newborn (with asphyxia, obstruction respiratory passage, suffocation) E912
Mudslide of cataclysmic nature E909.2
Murder (attempt) — *see also* Assault E968.9

N

Nail, injury by E920.8
Needlestick (sewing needle) E920.4
  hypodermic E920.5
Neglect — *see also* Privation
  criminal E968.4
  homicidal intent E968.4
Noise (causing injury) (pollution) E928.1
Nuclear weapon — *see also* War operations, injury due to, nuclear weapons E996.9

O

Object
  falling
    from, in, on, hitting
      aircraft E844 ☑
        due to accident to aircraft — *see* categories E840-E842 ☑
      machinery (*see also* Accident, machine)
        not in operation E916
      motor vehicle (in motion) (on public highway) E818 ☑
        not on public highway E825 ☑
        stationary E916
      nonmotor road vehicle NEC E829 ☑

Object — *continued*
  falling — *continued*
    from, in, on, hitting — *continued*
      motor vehicle — *continued*
        pedal cycle E826 ☑
        person E916
        railway rolling stock, train, vehicle E806 ☑
        street car E829 ☑
        watercraft E838 ☑
          due to accident to watercraft E831 ☑
    set in motion by
      accidental explosion of pressure vessel — *see* category E921 ☑
      firearm — *see* category E922 ☑
      machine(ry) — *see* Accident, machine
      transport vehicle — *see* categories E800-E848 ☑
    thrown from, in, on, towards
      aircraft E844 ☑
      cable car (not on rails) E847
        on rails E829 ☑
      motor vehicle (in motion) (on public highway) E818 ☑
        not on public highway E825 ☑
      nonmotor road vehicle NEC E829 ☑
      pedal cycle E826 ☑
      street car E829 ☑
      vehicle NEC — *see* Accident, vehicle NEC
Obstruction
  air passages, larynx, respiratory passages by
      external means NEC — *see* Suffocation
      food, any type (regurgitated) (vomited) E911
      material or object, except food E912
      mucus E912
      phlegm E912
      vomitus E911
  digestive tract, except mouth or pharynx by
      food, any type E915
      foreign body (any) E915
  esophagus
    without asphyxia or obstruction of respiratory passage E915
    food E911
    foreign body, except food E912
  mouth or pharynx by
      food, any type E911
      material or object, except food E912
  respiration — *see* Obstruction, air passages
Oil in eye E914
Overdose
  anesthetic (drug) — *see* Table of Drugs and Chemicals
  drug — *see* Table of Drugs and Chemicals
Overexertion E927.9
  from
    lifting
      repetitive movement E927.3 ●
      sudden strenuous movement E927.0 ●
    maintaining prolonged positions E927.1
      holding E927.1
      sitting E927.1
      standing E927.1
    prolonged static position E927.1
    pulling
      repetitive movement E927.3 ●
      sudden strenuous movement E927.0 ●
    pushing
      repetitive movement E927.3 ●
      sudden strenuous movement E927.0 ●
    specified NEC E927.8 ●
    sudden strenuous movement E927.0
Overexposure (accidental) (to)
  cold (*see also* Cold, exposure to) E901.9
    due to manmade conditions E901.1
  heat (*see also* Heat) E900.9
  radiation — *see* Radiation

☑ **Additional Digit Required** — Refer to the Tabular List for Digit Selection   🖳 **Subterms under main terms may continue to next column or page**

2011 ICD-9-CM   ▶◀ **Revised Text**   ● **New Line**   ▲ **Revised Code**   **October 2010 • Volume 2 — 345**

Reaction, abnormal to or following — *continued*
  surgical operation (*see also* Reaction, abnormal, by specified type of operation) — *continued*
    restorative — *continued*
      with — *continued*
        transplant(ation) — *see* Reaction, abnormal, transplant
    specified operation NEC E878.8
  thoracentesis E879.4
  transfusion
    procedure E879.8
  transplant, transplantation (heart) (kidney) (liver) E878.0
    partial organ E878.4
  ureterostomy E878.3
  vaccination E879.8
Reduction in
  atmospheric pressure (*see also* Effects of, air pressure)
    while surfacing from
      deep water diving causing caisson or divers' disease, palsy or paralysis E902.2
      underground E902.8
Repetitive movements NEC E927.8 ●
Residual (effect) — *see* Late effect
Rock falling on or hitting (accidentally)
  motor vehicle (in motion) (on public highway) E818 ☑
    not on public highway E825 ☑
  nonmotor road vehicle NEC E829 ☑
  pedal cycle E826 ☑
  person E916
  railway rolling stock, train, vehicle E806 ☑
Running off, away
  animal (being ridden) (in sport or transport) E828 ☑
    not being ridden E906.8
  animal-drawn vehicle E827 ☑
  rails, railway (*see also* Derailment) E802 ☑
  roadway
    motor vehicle (without antecedent collision) E816 ☑
      with
        antecedent collision — *see* Collision motor vehicle
        subsequent collision
          involving any object, person or vehicle not on public highway E816 ☑
          on public highway E811 ☑
        nontraffic accident E825 ☑
          with antecedent collision — *see* Collision, motor vehicle, not on public highway
    nonmotor road vehicle NEC E829 ☑
    pedal cycle E826 ☑
Run over (accidentally) (by)
  animal (not being ridden) E906.8
    being ridden (in sport or transport) E828 ☑
  animal-drawn vehicle E827 ☑
  machinery — *see* Accident, machine
  motor vehicle (on public highway) — *see* Hit by, motor vehicle
  nonmotor road vehicle NEC E829 ☑
  railway train E805 ☑
  street car E829 ☑
  vehicle NEC E848

S

Saturnism E866.0
  from insecticide NEC E863.4
Scald, scalding (accidental) (by) (from) (in) E924.0
  acid — *see* Scald, caustic
  boiling tap water E924.2
  caustic or corrosive liquid, substance E924.1
    swallowed — *see* Table of Drugs and Chemicals
  homicide (attempt) — *see* Assault, burning

Scald, scalding — *continued*
  inflicted by other person
    stated as
      intentional or homicidal E968.3
      undetermined whether accidental or intentional E988.2
  late effect of NEC E929.8
  liquid (boiling) (hot) E924.0
  local application of externally applied substance in medical or surgical care E873.5
  molten metal E924.0
  self-inflicted (unspecified whether accidental or intentional) E988.2
    stated as intentional, purposeful E958.2
  stated as undetermined whether accidental or intentional E988.2
  steam E924.0
  tap water (boiling) E924.2
  transport accident — *see* categories E800-E848 ☑
  vapor E924.0
Scratch, cat E906.8
Sea
  sickness E903
Self-mutilation — *see* Suicide
Sequelae (of)
  in
    terrorism E999.1
    war operations E999.0
Shock
  anaphylactic (*see also* Table of Drugs and Chemicals) E947.9
    due to
      bite (venomous) — *see* Bite, venomous NEC
      sting — *see* Sting
  electric (*see also* Electric shock) E925.9
    from electric appliance or current (*see also* Electric shock) E925.9
Shooting, shot (accidental(ly)) E922.9
  air gun E922.4
  BB gun E922.4
  hand gun (pistol) (revolver) E922.0
  himself (*see also* Shooting, self-inflicted) E985.4
    hand gun (pistol) (revolver) E985.0
    military firearm, except hand gun E985.3
      hand gun (pistol) (revolver) E985.0
    rifle (hunting) E985.2
      military E985.3
    shotgun (automatic) E985.1
    specified firearm NEC E985.4
    Verey pistol E985.4
  homicide (attempt) E965.4
    air gun E968.6
    BB gun E968.6
    hand gun (pistol) (revolver) E965.0
    military firearm, except hand gun E965.3
      hand gun (pistol) (revolver) E965.0
    paintball gun E965.4
    rifle (hunting) E965.2
      military E965.3
    shotgun (automatic) E965.1
    specified firearm NEC E965.4
    Verey pistol E965.4
  in
    terrorism — *see* Terrorism, shooting
    war operations — *see* War operations, shooting
  inflicted by other person
    in accidental circumstances E922.9
      hand gun (pistol) (revolver) E922.0
      military firearm, except hand gun E922.3
        hand gun (pistol) (revolver) E922.0
      rifle (hunting) E922.2
        military E922.3
      shotgun (automatic) E922.1
      specified firearm NEC E922.8
      Verey pistol E922.8
    stated as
      intentional, homicidal E965.4
        hand gun (pistol) (revolver) E965.0

Shooting, shot — *continued*
  inflicted by other person — *continued*
    stated as — *continued*
      intentional, homicidal — *continued*
        military firearm, except hand gun E965.3
          hand gun (pistol) (revolver) E965.0
        paintball gun E965.4
        rifle (hunting) E965.2
          military E965.3
        shotgun (automatic) E965.1
        specified firearm NEC E965.4
        Verey pistol E965.4
      undetermined whether accidental or intentional E985.4
        air gun E985.6
        BB gun E985.6
        hand gun (pistol) (revolver) E985.0
        military firearm, except hand gun E985.3
          hand gun (pistol) (revolver) E985.0
        paintball gun E985.7
        rifle (hunting) E985.2
        shotgun (automatic) E985.1
        specified firearm NEC E985.4
        Verey pistol E985.4
  legal
    execution E978
    intervention E970
  military firearm, except hand gun E922.3
    hand gun (pistol) (revolver) E922.0
  paintball gun E922.5
  rifle (hunting) E922.2
    military E922.3
  self-inflicted (unspecified whether accidental or intentional) E985.4
    air gun E985.6
    BB gun E985.6
    hand gun (pistol) (revolver) E985.0
    military firearm, except hand gun E985.3
      hand gun (pistol) (revolver) E985.0
    paintball gun E985.7
    rifle (hunting) E985.2
      military E985.3
    shotgun (automatic) E985.1
    specified firearm NEC E985.4
    stated as
      accidental E922.9
        hand gun (pistol) (revolver) E922.0
        military firearm, except hand gun E922.3
          hand gun (pistol) (revolver) E922.0
        paintball gun E922.5
        rifle (hunting) E922.2
          military E922.3
        shotgun (automatic) E922.1
        specified firearm NEC E922.8
        Verey pistol E922.8
      intentional, purposeful E955.4
        hand gun (pistol) (revolver) E955.0
        military firearm, except hand gun E955.3
          hand gun (pistol) (revolver) E955.0
        paintball gun E955.7
        rifle (hunting) E955.2
          military E955.3
        shotgun (automatic) E955.1
        specified firearm NEC E955.4
        Verey pistol E955.4
  shotgun (automatic) E922.1
  specified firearm NEC E922.8
  stated as undetermined whether accidental or intentional E985.4
    hand gun (pistol) (revolver) E985.0
    military firearm, except hand gun E985.3
      hand gun (pistol) (revolver) E985.0
    paintball gun E985.7
    rifle (hunting) E985.2

Shooting, shot — *continued*
  stated as undetermined whether accidental or intentional — *continued*
    rifle — *continued*
      military E985.3
    shotgun (automatic) E985.1
    specified firearm NEC E985.4
    Verey pistol E985.4
  suicidal (attempt) E955.4
    air gun E955.6
    BB gun E955.6
    hand gun (pistol) (revolver) E955.0
    military firearm, except hand gun E955.3
      hand gun (pistol) (revolver) E955.0
    paintball gun E955.7
    rifle (hunting) E955.2
      military E955.3
    shotgun (automatic) E955.1
    specified firearm NEC E955.4
    Verey pistol E955.4
  Verey pistol E922.8
Shoving (accidentally) by other person — *see also* Pushing by other person E917.9
Sickness
  air E903
  alpine E902.0
  car E903
  motion E903
  mountain E902.0
  sea E903
  travel E903
Sinking (accidental)
  boat, ship, watercraft (causing drowning, submersion) E830 ☑
    causing injury except drowning, submersion E831 ☑
Siriasis E900.0
Skydiving E844 ☑
Slashed wrists — *see also* Cut, self-inflicted E986
Slipping (accidental)
  on
    deck (of boat, ship, watercraft) (icy) (oily) (wet) E835 ☑
    ice E885.9
    ladder of ship E833 ☑
      due to accident to watercraft E831 ☑
    mud E885.9
    oil E885.9
    snow E885.9
    stairs of ship E833 ☑
      due to accident to watercraft E831 ☑
    surface
      slippery E885 ☑
      wet E885 ☑
Sliver, wood, injury by E920.8
Smothering, smothered — *see also* Suffocation E913.9
Smouldering building or structure in terrorism E979.3
Sodomy (assault) E960.1
Solid substance in eye (any part) or adnexa E914
Sound waves (causing injury) E928.1
Splinter, injury by E920.8
Stab, stabbing E966
  accidental — *see* Cut
Starvation E904.1
  helpless person, infant, newborn — *see* Lack of food
  homicidal intent E968.4
  late effect of NEC E929.5
  resulting from accident connected with transport — *see* categories E800-E848 ☑
Stepped on
  by
    animal (not being ridden) E906.8
      being ridden (in sport or transport) E828 ☑
    crowd E917.1
    person E917.9
      in sports E917.0
  in sports E917.0

☑ Additional Digit Required — Refer to the Tabular List for Digit Selection   ⱳ Subterms under main terms may continue to next column or page

346 — Volume 2 · October 2010   ▶◀ Revised Text   ● New Line   ▲ Revised Code   2011 ICD-9-CM

Stepping on
object (moving) E917.9
in sports E917.0
with subsequent fall E917.5
stationary E917.4
with subsequent fall E917.8
person E917.9
as, or caused by a crowd E917.1
with subsequent fall E917.6
in sports E917.0
Sting E905.9
ant E905.5
bee E905.3
caterpillar E905.5
coral E905.6
hornet E905.3
insect NEC E905.5
jellyfish E905.6
marine animal or plant E905.6
nematocysts E905.6
scorpion E905.2
sea anemone E905.6
sea cucumber E905.6
wasp E905.3
yellow jacket E905.3
Storm E908.9
specified type NEC E908.8
Straining, injury
due to
repetitive movement E927.3
sudden strenuous movement E927.0
Strangling — see Suffocation
Strangulation — see Suffocation
Strenuous movements (in recreational or other activities) ▶NEC◀ E927.8
Striking against
bottom (when jumping or diving into water) E883.0
object (moving) E917.9
caused by crowd E917.1
with subsequent fall E917.6
furniture E917.3
with subsequent fall E917.7
in
running water E917.2
with drowning or submersion — see Submersion
sports E917.0
with subsequent fall E917.5
stationary E917.4
with subsequent fall E917.8
person(s) E917.9
with fall E886.9
in sports E886.0
as, or caused by, a crowd E917.1
with subsequent fall E917.6
in sports E917.0
with fall E886.0
Stroke
heat — see Heat
lightning E907
Struck by — see also Hit by
bullet
in
terrorism E979.4
war operations E991.2
rubber E991.0
lightning E907
missile
in terrorism — see Terrorism, missile
object
falling
from, in, on
building
burning (uncontrolled fire)
in terrorism E979.3
thunderbolt E907
Stumbling over animal, carpet, curb, rug or (small) object (with fall) E885.9
without fall — see Striking against, object
Submersion (accidental) E910.8
boat, ship, watercraft (causing drowning, submersion) E830
causing injury except drowning, submersion E831

Submersion (accidental) — continued
by other person
in accidental circumstances — see category E910
intentional, homicidal E964
stated as undetermined whether accidental or intentional E984
due to
accident
machinery — see Accident, machine to boat, ship, watercraft E830
transport — see categories E800-E848
avalanche E909.2
cataclysmic
earth surface movement or eruption E909.9
storm E908.9
cloudburst E908.8
cyclone E908.1
fall
from
boat, ship, watercraft (not involved in accident) E832
burning, crushed E830
involved in accident, collision E830
gangplank (into water) E832
overboard NEC E832
flood E908.2
hurricane E908.0
jumping into water E910.8
from boat, ship, watercraft
burning, crushed, sinking E830
involved in accident, collision E830
not involved in accident, for swim E910.2
in recreational activity (without diving equipment) E910.2
with or using diving equipment E910.1
to rescue another person E910.3
homicide (attempt) E964
in
bathtub E910.4
specified activity, not sport, transport or recreational E910.3
sport or recreational activity (without diving equipment) E910.2
with or using diving equipment E910.1
water skiing E910.0
swimming pool NEC E910.8
terrorism E979.8
war operations E995.4
intentional E995.3
water transport E832
due to accident to boat, ship, watercraft E830
landslide E909.2
overturning boat, ship, watercraft E909.2
sinking boat, ship, watercraft E909.2
submersion boat, ship, watercraft E909.2
tidal wave E909.4
caused by storm E908.0
torrential rain E908.2
late effect of NEC E929.8
quenching tank E910.8
self-inflicted (unspecified whether accidental or intentional) E984
in accidental circumstances — see category E910
stated as intentional, purposeful E954
stated as undetermined whether accidental or intentional E984
suicidal (attempted) E954
while
attempting rescue of another person E910.3
engaged in
marine salvage E910.3
underwater construction or repairs E910.3
fishing, not from boat E910.2

Submersion (accidental) — continued
while — continued
hunting, not from boat E910.2
ice skating E910.2
pearl diving E910.3
placing fishing nets E910.3
playing in water E910.2
scuba diving E910.1
nonrecreational E910.3
skin diving E910.1
snorkel diving E910.2
spear fishing underwater E910.1
surfboarding E910.2
swimming (swimming pool) E910.2
wading (in water) E910.2
water skiing E910.0
Sucked
into
jet (aircraft) E844
Suffocation (accidental) (by external means) (by pressure) (mechanical) E913.9
caused by other person
in accidental circumstances — see category E913
stated as
intentional, homicidal E963
undetermined whether accidental or intentional E983.9
by, in
hanging E983.0
plastic bag E983.1
specified means NEC E983.8
due to, by
avalanche E909.2
bedclothes E913.0
bib E913.0
blanket E913.0
cave-in E913.3
caused by cataclysmic earth surface movement or eruption E909.9
conflagration — see Conflagration
explosion — see Explosion
falling earth, other substance E913.3
fire — see Fire
food, any type (ingestion) (inhalation) (regurgitated) (vomited) E911
foreign body, except food (ingestion) (inhalation) E912
ignition — see Ignition
landslide E909.2
machine(ry) — see Accident, machine
material, object except food entering by nose or mouth, ingested, inhaled E912
mucus (aspiration) (inhalation), not of newborn E912
phlegm (aspiration) (inhalation) E912
pillow E913.0
plastic bag — see Suffocation, in, plastic bag
sheet (plastic) E913.0
specified means NEC E913.8
vomitus (aspiration) (inhalation) E911
homicidal (attempt) E963
in war operations E995.3
in
airtight enclosed place E913.2
baby carriage E913.0
bed E913.0
closed place E913.2
cot, cradle E913.0
perambulator E913.0
plastic bag (in accidental circumstances) E913.1
homicidal, purposely inflicted by other person E963
self-inflicted (unspecified whether accidental or intentional) E983.1
in accidental circumstances E913.1
intentional, suicidal E953.1
stated as undetermined whether accidentally or purposely inflicted E983.1

Suffocation — continued
in — continued
plastic bag — continued
suicidal, purposely self-inflicted E953.1
refrigerator E913.2
war operations E995.3
self-inflicted (see also Suffocation, stated as undetermined whether accidental or intentional) E953.9
in accidental circumstances — see category E913
stated as intentional, purposeful — see Suicide, suffocation
stated as undetermined whether accidental or intentional E983.9
by, in
hanging E983.0
plastic bag E983.1
specified means NEC E983.8
suicidal — see Suicide, suffocation
Suicide, suicidal (attempted) (by) E958.9
burning, burns E958.1
caustic substance E958.7
poisoning E950.7
swallowed E950.7
cold, extreme E958.3
cut (any part of body) E956
cutting or piercing instrument (classifiable to E920) E956
drowning E954
electrocution E958.4
explosive(s) (classifiable to E923) E955.5
fire E958.1
firearm (classifiable to E922) — see Shooting, suicidal
hanging E953.0
jumping
before moving object, train, vehicle E958.0
from high place — see Jumping, from, high place, stated as, suicidal
knife E956
late effect of E959
motor vehicle, crashing of E958.5
poisoning — see Table of Drugs and Chemicals
puncture (any part of body) E956
scald E958.2
shooting — see Shooting, suicidal
specified means NEC E958.8
stab (any part of body) E956
strangulation — see Suicide, suffocation
submersion E954
suffocation E953.9
by, in
hanging E953.0
plastic bag E953.1
specified means NEC E953.8
wound NEC E958.9
Sunburn E926.2
Sunstroke E900.0
Supersonic waves (causing injury) E928.1
Surgical procedure, complication of
delayed or as an abnormal reaction without mention of misadventure — see Reaction, abnormal
due to or as a result of misadventure — see Misadventure
Swallowed, swallowing
foreign body — see Foreign body, alimentary canal
poison — see Table of Drugs and Chemicals
substance
caustic — see Table of Drugs and Chemicals
corrosive — see Table of Drugs and Chemicals
poisonous — see Table of Drugs and Chemicals
Swimmers cramp — see also category E910 E910.2
not in recreation or sport E910.3
Syndrome, battered
baby or child — see Abuse, child
wife — see Assault

T

Tackle in sport E886.0
Terrorism (injury) (by) (in) E979.8
  air blast E979.2
  aircraft burned, destroyed, exploded, shot
    down E979.1
    used as a weapon E979.1
  anthrax E979.6
  asphyxia from
    chemical (weapons) E979.7
    fire, conflagration (caused by fire-produc-
      ing device) E979.3
      from nuclear explosion E979.5
    gas or fumes E979.7
  bayonet E979.8
  biological agents E979.6
  blast (air) (effects) E979.2
    from nuclear explosion E979.5
    underwater E979.0
  bomb (antipersonnel) (mortar) (explosion)
    (fragments) E979.2
  bullet(s) (from carbine, machine gun, pistol,
    rifle, shotgun) E979.4
  burn from
    chemical E979.7
    fire, conflagration (caused by fire-produc-
      ing device) E979.3
      from nuclear explosion E979.5
    gas E979.7
  burning aircraft E979.1
  chemical E979.7
  cholera E979.6
  conflagration E979.3
  crushed by falling aircraft E979.1
  depth-charge E979.0
  destruction of aircraft E979.1
  disability, as sequelae one year or more after
    injury E999.1
  drowning E979.8
  effect
    of nuclear weapon (direct) (secondary)
      E979.5
    secondary NEC E979.9
    sequelae E999.1
  explosion (artillery shell) (breech-block)
    (cannon block) E979.2
    aircraft E979.1
    bomb (antipersonnel) (mortar) E979.2
      nuclear (atom) (hydrogen) E979.5
    depth-charge E979.0
    grenade E979.2
    injury by fragments from E979.2
    land-mine E979.2
    marine weapon E979.0
    mine (land) E979.2
      at sea or in harbor E979.0
      marine E979.0
    missile (explosive) NEC E979.2
    munitions (dump) (factory) E979.2
    nuclear (weapon) E979.5
      other direct and secondary effects of
        E979.5
    sea-based artillery shell E979.0
    torpedo E979.0
  exposure to ionizing radiation from nuclear
    explosion E979.5
  falling aircraft E979.1
  firearms E979.4
  fireball effects from nuclear explosion
    E979.5
  fire or fire-producing device E979.3
  fragments from artillery shell, bomb NEC,
    grenade, guided missile, land-mine,
    rocket, shell, shrapnel E979.2
  gas or fumes E979.7
  grenade (explosion) (fragments) E979.2
  guided missile (explosion) (fragments)
    E979.2
    nuclear E979.5
  heat from nuclear explosion E979.5
  hot substances E979.3
  hydrogen cyanide E979.7
  land-mine (explosion) (fragments) E979.2
  laser(s) E979.8
  late effect of E999.1
  lewisite E979.7

Terrorism — continued
  lung irritant (chemical) (fumes) (gas) E979.7
  marine mine E979.0
  mine E979.2
    at sea E979.0
    in harbor E979.0
    land (explosion) (fragments) E979.2
    marine E979.0
  missile (explosion) (fragments) (guided)
    E979.2
    marine E979.0
    nuclear weapons E979.5
  mortar bomb (explosion) (fragments) E979.2
  mustard gas E979.7
  nerve gas E979.7
  nuclear weapons E979.5
  pellets (shotgun) E979.4
  petrol bomb E979.3
  phosgene E979.7
  piercing object E979.8
  poisoning (chemical) (fumes) (gas) E979.7
  radiation, ionizing from nuclear explosion
    E979.5
  rocket (explosion) (fragments) E979.2
  saber, sabre E979.8
  sarin E979.7
  screening smoke E979.7
  sequelae effect (of) E999.1
  shell (aircraft) (artillery) (cannon) (land-
    based) (explosion) (fragments)
    E979.2
    sea-based E979.0
  shooting E979.4
    bullet(s) E979.4
    pellet(s) (rifle) (shotgun) E979.4
  shrapnel E979.2
  smallpox E979.7
  stabbing object(s) E979.8
  submersion E979.8
  torpedo E979.0
  underwater blast E979.0
  vesicant (chemical) (fumes) (gas) E979.7
  weapon burst E979.2
Thermic fever E900.9
Thermoplegia E900.9
Thirst — see also Lack of water
  resulting from accident connected with
    transport — see categories
    E800-E848 ☑
Thrown (accidentally)
  against object in or part of vehicle
    by motion of vehicle
      aircraft E844 ☑
      boat, ship, watercraft E838 ☑
      motor vehicle (on public highway)
        E818 ☑
        not on public highway E825 ☑
        off-road type (not on public
          highway) E821 ☑
          on public highway E818 ☑
        snow vehicle E820 ☑
          on public highway
            E818 ☑
      nonmotor road vehicle NEC E829 ☑
      railway rolling stock, train, vehicle
        E806 ☑
      street car E829 ☑
  from
    animal (being ridden) (in sport or trans-
      port) E828 ☑
    high place, homicide (attempt) E968.1
    machinery — see Accident, machine
    vehicle NEC — see Accident, vehicle NEC
    off — see Thrown, from
    overboard (by motion of boat, ship, water-
      craft) E832 ☑
      by accident to boat, ship, watercraft
        E830 ☑
Thunderbolt NEC E907
Tidal wave (any injury) E909.4
  caused by storm E908.0
Took
  overdose of drug — see Table of Drugs and
    Chemicals
  poison — see Table of Drugs and Chemicals
Tornado (any injury) E908.1

Torrential rain (any injury) E908.2
Traffic accident NEC E819 ☑
Trampled by animal E906.8
  being ridden (in sport or transport) E828 ☑
Trapped (accidently)
  between
    objects (moving) (stationary and mov-
      ing) E918
  by
    door of
      elevator E918
      motor vehicle (on public highway)
        (while alighting, boarding) —
        see Fall, from, motor vehicle,
        while alighting
      railway train (underground) E806 ☑
      street car E829 ☑
      subway train E806 ☑
  in object E918
Trauma
  cumulative
    from
      repetitive
        impact E927.4
        motion or movements E927.3
    sudden from strenuous movement E927.0
Travel (effects) E903
  sickness E903
Tree
  falling on or hitting E916
    motor vehicle (in motion) (on public
      highway) E818 ☑
      not on public highway E825 ☑
    nonmotor road vehicle NEC E829 ☑
    pedal cycle E826 ☑
    person E916
    railway rolling stock, train, vehicle
      E806 ☑
    street car E829 ☑
Trench foot E901.0
Tripping over animal, carpet, curb, rug, or
    small object (with fall) E885 ☑
  without fall — see Striking against, object
Tsunami E909.4
Twisting, ▶injury◀
  due to   ●
    repetitive movement E927.3   ●
    sudden strenuous movement E927.0 ●

V

Violence, nonaccidental — see also Assault
  E968.9
Volcanic eruption (any injury) E909.1
Vomitus in air passages (with asphyxia, ob-
  struction or suffocation) E911

W

War operations (during hostilities) (injury) (by)
  (in) E995.9
  after cessation of hostilities, injury due to
    E998.9
  air blast E993.9
  aircraft burned, destroyed, exploded, shot
    down E994 ☑
  asphyxia from
    chemical E997.2
    fire, conflagration (caused by fire produc-
      ing device or conventional
      weapon) E990.9
      from nuclear explosion (see also War
        operations, injury due to, nu-
        clear weapons) E996.8
      incendiary bomb E990.0
      petrol bomb E990.0
    fumes E997.2
    gas E997.2
  baton (nightstick) E995.1
  battle wound NEC E995.8
  bayonet E995.2
  biological warfare agents E997.1
  blast (air) (effects) E993.9
    from nuclear explosion ▶— see War
      operations, injury due to, nuclear
      weapons◀
    underwater E992.9

War operations — continued
  bomb (mortar) (explosion) E993.2
    after cessation of hostilities E998.1
    fragments, injury by E991.4
      antipersonnel E991.3
  bullet(s) (from carbine, machine gun, pistol,
    rifle, shotgun) E991.2
    rubber E991.0
  burn from
    chemical E997.2
    fire, conflagration (caused by fire-produc-
      ing device or conventional
      weapon) E990.9
      from
        conventional weapon E990.3
        flamethrower E990.1
        incendiary bomb E990.0
        incendiary bullet E990.2
        nuclear explosion E996.2
        petrol bomb E990.0
    gas E997.2
  burning aircraft E994.3
  chemical E997.2
  chlorine E997.2
  conventional warfare, specified form NEC
    E995.8
  crushing by falling aircraft E994.8
  depth charge E992.1
  destruction of aircraft E994.9
  detonation of own munitions (ammunition)
    (artillery) (mortars), unintentional
    E993.6
  disability as sequela one year or more after
    injury E999.0
  discharge of own munitions launch device
    (autocannons) (automatic grenade
    launchers) (missile launchers) (small
    arms), unintentional E993.7
  drowning E995.4
  effect nuclear weapon (see also War opera-
    tions, injury due to, nuclear weapons)
    E996.9
  explosion (breech block) (cannon shell)
    E993.9
    after cessation of hostilities
      bomb placed in war E998.1
      mine placed in war E998.0
    aircraft E994.1
      due to
        enemy fire or explosives E994.0
        own onboard explosives E994.1
    artillery shell E993.2
    bomb (mortar) E993.2
      aerial E993.0
      atom (see also War operations, injury
        due to, nuclear weapons)
        E996.9
      hydrogen (see also War operations,
        injury due to, nuclear
        weapons) E996.9
      injury by fragments from E991.4
        antipersonnel E991.3
      nuclear (see also War operations, in-
        jury due to, nuclear weapons)
        E996.9
    depth charge E992.1
    injury by fragments from E991.4
      antipersonnel E991.3
    marine weapon NEC E992.8
    mine
      at sea or in harbor E992.2
      land E993.8
        injury by fragments from E991.4
      marine E992.2
    missile, guided E993.1
    mortar E993.2
    munitions (accidental) (being used in
      war) (dump) (factory) E993.9
      own E993.7
        ammunition (artillery) (mortars)
          E993.6
        launch device (autocannons)
          (automatic grenade
          launchers) (missile
          launchers) (small arms)
          E993.7

☑ Additional Digit Required — Refer to the Tabular List for Digit Selection   ☒ Subterms under main terms may continue to next column or page

348 — Volume 2 · October 2010   ▶◀ Revised Text   ● New Line   ▲ Revised Code   2011 ICD-9-CM

War operations — *continued*
  explosion — *continued*
    nuclear (weapon) (*see also* War operations, injury due to, nuclear weapons) E996.9
    own weapons (accidental) E993.7
      injury by fragments from E991.9
        antipersonnel E991.3
        sea-based artillery shell E992.3
        specified NEC E993.8
        torpedo E992.0
    exposure to ionizing radiation from nuclear explosion (*see also* War operations, injury due to, nuclear weapons) E996.3
    falling aircraft E994.8
    fireball effects from nuclear explosion E996.2
    fire or fire-producing device E990.9
      flamethrower E990.1
      incendiary bomb E990.0
      incendiary bullet E990.2
      indirectly caused from conventional weapon E990.3
      petrol bomb E990.0
    fragments from
      antipersonnel bomb E991.3
      artillery shell E991.4
      bomb NEC E991.4
      grenade E991.4
      guided missile E991.4
      land mine E991.4
      rocket E991.4
      shell E991.4
      shrapnel E991.9
    fumes E997.2
    gas E997.2
    grenade (explosion) E993.8
      fragments, injury by E991.4
    guided missile E993.1
      fragments, injury by E991.4
      nuclear (*see also* War operations, injury due to, nuclear weapons) E996.9
    heat from nuclear explosion E996.2
    injury due to
      aerial bomb E993.0
      air blast E993.9
      aircraft shot down E994.0
      artillery shell E993.2
      blast E993.9
        wave E993.9
        wind E993.9
      bomb E993.8
      but occurring after cessation of hostilities
        explosion of bombs E998.1
        explosion of mines E998.0
        specified NEC E998.8
      conventional warfare E995.9
        specified form NEC E995.8
      depth charge E992.1
      destruction of aircraft E994.9
        due to
          air to air missile E994.0
          collision with other aircraft E994.2
          enemy fire or explosives E994.0
          on board explosion (explosives) E994.1
          on board fire E994.3
          rocket propelled grenade [RPG] E994.0
          small arms fire E994.0
          surface to air missile E994.0
        specified NEC E994.8

War operations — *continued*
  injury due to — *continued*
    dirty bomb (*see also* War operations, injury due to, nuclear weapons) E996.9
    drowning E995.4
    explosion (direct pressure) (indirect pressure) (due to) E993.9
      depth charge E992.1
      improvised explosive device [IED]
        person borne E993.3
        roadside E993.5
        specified NEC E993.5
        transport vehicle (air) (land) (water) borne E993.4
        vehicle (air) (land) (water) borne E993.4
      marine mines (in harbor) (at sea) E992.2
      marine weapons E992.9
        specified NEC E992.8
      sea based artillery shell E992.3
      specified NEC E993.8
      torpedo E992.0
      unintentional (of own)
        autocannons E993.7
        automatic grenade launchers E993.7
        launch device discharge E993.7
        missile launchers E993.7
        munitions detonation (ammunition) (artillery) (mortars) E993.6
        small arms E993.7
    fragments (from) E991.9
      artillery E991.8
      artillery shells E991.4
      autocannons E991.8
      automatic grenade launchers [AGL] E991.8
      bombs E991.4
        antipersonnel E991.3
      detonation of unexploded ordnance [UXO] E991.4
      grenade E991.4
      guided missile E991.4
      improvised explosive device [IED]
        person borne E991.5
        roadside E991.7
        specified NEC E991.7
        transport vehicle (air) (land) (water) borne E991.6
        vehicle (air) (land) (water) borne E991.6
      land mine E991.4
      missile launchers E991.8
      mortars E991.8
      munitions (artillery shells) (bombs) (grenades) (rockets) (shells) E991.4
      rockets E991.4
      shells E991.4
      small arms E991.8
      specified NEC E991.9
      weapons (artillery) (autocannons) (mortars) (small arms) E991.8
    grenade E993.8
    guided missile E993.1
    hand to hand combat, unarmed E995.0
    improvised explosive device [IED]
      person borne E993.3
      roadside E993.5
      specified NEC E993.5
      transport vehicle (air) (land) (water) borne E993.4

War operations — *continued*
  injury due to — *continued*
    improvised explosive device [IED] — *continued*
      vehicle (air) (land) (water) borne E993.4
    inability to surface or obtain air E995.4
    land mine E993.8
    marine mines (in harbor) (at sea) E992.2
    marine weapons E992.9
      specified NEC E992.8
    mortar E993.2
    nuclear weapons E996.9
      beta burns E996.3
      blast debris E996.1
      blast pressure E996.0
      burns due to thermal radiation E996.2
      direct blast effect E996.0
      fallout exposure E996.3
      fireball effect E996.2
      flash burns E996.2
      heat effect E996.2
      indirect blast effect E996.1
      nuclear radiation effects E996.3
      radiation exposure (acute) E996.3
      radiation sickness E996.3
      secondary effects E996.3
      specified effects NEC E996.8
      thermal radiation effect E996.2
    piercing object E995.2
    restriction of airway, intentional E995.3
    sea based artillery shell E992.3
    shrapnel E991.9
    stave E995.1
    strangulation E995.3
    strike by blunt object (baton) (nightstick) (stave) E995.1
    submersion (accidental) (unintentional) E995.4
      intentional E995.3
    suffocation E995.3
      accidental E995.4
    torpedo E992.0
    underwater blast E992.9
    weapon of mass destruction [WMD] E997.3
  knife E995.2
  lacrimator (gas) (chemical) E997.2
  land mine (explosion) E993.8
    after cessation of hostilities E998.0
    fragments, injury by E991.4
  laser(s) E997.0
  late effect of E999.0
  lewisite E997.2
  lung irritant (chemical) (fumes) (gas) E997.2
  marine mine E992.2
  mine
    after cessation of hostilities E998.0
    at sea E992.2
    in harbor E992.2
    land (explosion) E993.8
      fragments, injury by E991.4
    marine E992.2
  missile (guided) (explosion) E993.1
    fragments, injury by E991.4
    marine E992.8
    nuclear (*see also* War operations, injury due to, nuclear weapons) E996.9
  mortar bomb (explosion) E993.2
    fragments, injury by E991.4
  mustard gas E997.2
  nerve gas E997.2
  phosgene E997.2
  piercing object E995.2

War operations — *continued*
  poisoning (chemical) (fumes) (gas) E997.2
  radiation, ionizing from nuclear explosion (*see also* War operations, injury due to, nuclear weapons) E996.3
  rocket (explosion) E993.8
    fragments, injury by E991.4
  saber, sabre E995.2
  screening smoke E997.8
  shell (aircraft) (artillery) (cannon) (land based) (explosion) E993.2
    fragments, injury by E991.4
    sea-based E992.3
  shooting E991.2
    after cessation of hostilities E998.8
    bullet(s) E991.2
      rubber E991.0
    pellet(s) (rifle) E991.1
    shrapnel E991.9
    submersion E995 ☑
    torpedo E992 ☑
  stave E995.2
  strike by blunt object (baton) (nightstick) (stave) E995.1
  submersion E995.4
    intentional E995.3
  sword E995.2
  torpedo E992.0
  unconventional warfare, except by nuclear weapon E997.9
    biological (warfare) E997.1
    gas, fumes, chemicals E997.2
    laser(s) E997.0
    specified type NEC E997.8
  underwater blast E992.9
  vesicant (chemical) (fumes) (gas) E997.2
  weapon burst E993.9
Washed
  away by flood — *see* Flood
  away by tidal wave — *see* Tidal wave
  off road by storm (transport vehicle) E908.9
  overboard E832 ☑
Weapon of mass destruction [WMD] E997.3
Weather exposure — *see also* Exposure
  cold E901.0
  hot E900.0
Weightlessness (causing injury) (effects of) (in spacecraft, real or simulated) E928.0
Wound (accidental) NEC — *see also* Injury E928.9
  battle (*see also* War operations) E995.9
  bayonet E920.3
    in
      legal intervention E974
      war operations E995.2
  gunshot — *see* Shooting
  incised — *see* Cut
  saber, sabre E920.3
    in war operations E995.2
Wrong
  body part, performance of correct operation (procedure) on E876.7
  device implanted into correct surgical site E876.5
  patient, performance of operation (procedure) on E876.6
  procedure (operation) performed on correct patient E876.5
  side, performance of correct operation (procedure) on E876.7
  site, performance of correct operation (procedure) on E876.7

☑ **Additional Digit Required** — Refer to the Tabular List for Digit Selection   ⟲ **Subterms under main terms may continue to next column or page**

2011 ICD-9-CM   ▶◀ Revised Text   ● New Line   ▲ Revised Code   Volume 2 — 349

War operations — Wrong

Railway Accidents (E800-E807)

The following fourth-digit subdivisions are for use with categories E800-E807 to identify the injured person:

.0 **Railway employee**
Any person who by virtue of his employment in connection with a railway, whether by the railway company or not, is at increased risk of involvement in a railway accident, such as:
  catering staff on train
    postal staff on train
    driver
    railway fireman
    guard
    shunter
    porter
    sleeping car attendant

.1 **Passenger on railway**
Any authorized person traveling on a train, except a railway employee
  EXCLUDES   intending passenger waiting at station (.8)
             unauthorized rider on railway vehicle (.8)

.2 **Pedestrian** See definition (r), E-Codes-2

.3 **Pedal cyclist** See definition (p), E-Codes-2

.8 **Other specified person** Intending passenger waiting at station
Unauthorized rider on railway vehicle

.9 **Unspecified person**

Motor Vehicle Traffic and Nontraffic Accidents (E810-E825)

The following fourth-digit subdivisions are for use with categories E810-E819 and E820-E825 to identify the injured person:

.0 **Driver of motor vehicle other than motorcycle** See definition (1), E-Codes-2

.1 **Passenger in motor vehicle other than motorcycle** See definition (1), E-Codes-2

.2 **Motorcyclist** See definition (1), E-Codes-2

.3 **Passenger on motorcycle** See definition (1), E-Codes-2

.4 **Occupant of streetcar**

.5 **Rider of animal; occupant of animal-drawn vehicle**

.6 **Pedal cyclist** See definition (p), E-Codes-2

.7 **Pedestrian** See definition (r), E-Codes-2

.8 **Other specified person**
Occupant of vehicle other than above
Person in railway train involved in accident
Unauthorized rider of motor vehicle

.9 **Unspecified person**

Other Road Vehicle Accidents (E826-E829)
(animal-drawn vehicle, streetcar, pedal cycle, and other nonmotor road vehicle accidents)

The following fourth-digit subdivisions are for use with categories E826-E829 to identify the injured person:

.0 **Pedestrian** See definition (r), E-Codes-2

.1 **Pedal cyclist** (does not apply to codes E827, E828, E829) See definition (p), E-Codes-2

.2 **Rider of animal** (does not apply to code E829)

.3 **Occupant of animal-drawn vehicle (does not apply to codes E828, E829)**

.4 **Occupant of streetcar**

.8 **Other specified person**

.9 **Unspecified person**

Water Transport Accidents (E830-E838)

The following fourth-digit subdivisions are for use with categories E830-E838 to identify the injured person:

.0 **Occupant of small boat, unpowered**

.1 **Occupant of small boat, powered** See definition (t), E-Codes-2
  EXCLUDES   water skier (.4)

.2 **Occupant of other watercraft — crew**
Persons:
  engaged in operation of watercraft
    providing passenger services [cabin attendants, ship's physician, catering personnel]
    working on ship during voyage in other capacity [musician in band, operators of shops and beauty parlors]

.3 **Occupant of other watercraft — other than crew**
Passenger
Occupant of lifeboat, other than crew, after abandoning ship

.4 **Water skier**

.5 **Swimmer**

.6 **Dockers, stevedores**
Longshoreman employed on the dock in loading and unloading ships

.8 **Other specified person**
Immigration and custom officials on board ship
Persons:
  accompanying passenger or member of crew visiting boat
Pilot (guiding ship into port)

.9 **Unspecified person**

Air and Space Transport Accidents (E840-E845)

The following fourth-digit subdivisions are for use with categories E840-E845 to identify the injured person:

.0 **Occupant of spacecraft**
  Crew
  Passenger (civilian)   in military aircraft [air force]
  (military)   [army] [national guard] [navy]
  Troops

.1 **Occupant of military aircraft, any**
  EXCLUDES   occupants of aircraft operated under jurisdiction of police departments (.5) parachutist (.7)

.2 **Crew of commercial aircraft (powered) in surface to surface transport**

.3 **Other occupant of commercial aircraft (powered) in surface to surface transport**
Flight personnel:
  not part of crew
    on familiarization flight Passenger on aircraft

.4 **Occupant of commercial aircraft (powered) in surface to air transport**
Occupant [crew] [passenger] of aircraft (powered) engaged in activities, such as:
  air drops of emergency supplies
    air drops of parachutists, except from military craft
    crop dusting
    lowering of construction material [bridge or telephone pole]
    sky writing

.5 **Occupant of other powered aircraft**
Occupant [crew] [passenger] of aircraft (powered) engaged in activities, such as:
  aerial spraying (crops)(fire retardants)
    aerobatic flying
    aircraft racing
    rescue operation
    storm surveillance
    traffic suveillance
Occupant of private plane NOS

.6 **Occupant of unpowered aircraft, except parachutist**
Occupant of aircraft classifiable to E842

.7 **Parachutist (military)(other)**
Person making voluntary descent
  person making descent after accident to aircraft (.1-.6)

.8 **Ground crew, airline employee**
Persons employed at airfields (civil)(military) or launching pads, not occupants of aircraft

.9 **Other person**

☑ **Additional Digit Required — Refer to the Tabular List for Digit Selection**   ▧ **Subterms under main terms may continue to next column or page**

350 — Volume 2   ▶◀ Revised Text   ● New Line   ▲ Revised Code   2011 ICD-9-CM

1. Infectious and Parasitic Diseases (001-139)

NOTE Categories for "late effects" of infectious and parasitic diseases are to be found at 137-139.

INCLUDES diseases generally recognized as communicable or transmissible as well as a few diseases of unknown but possibly infectious origin

EXCLUDES *acute respiratory infections (460-466)*
carrier or suspected carrier of infectious organism (V02.0-V02.9)
certain localized infections
influenza ▶(487.0-487.8, 488.01-488.19)◀

Intestinal Infectious Diseases (001-009)

EXCLUDES *helminthiases (120.0-129)*

✓4ᵗʰ 001 Cholera

DEF: An acute infectious enteritis caused by a potent enterotoxin produced by *Vibrio cholerae*; changes the permeability of the mucosa of the intestines and leads to diarrhea and dehydration.

001.0 Due to Vibrio cholerae

001.1 Due to Vibrio cholerae el tor

001.9 Cholera, unspecified

✓4ᵗʰ 002 Typhoid and paratyphoid fevers

DEF: Typhoid fever: an acute generalized illness caused by *Salmonella typhi*; clinical features are fever, headache, abdominal pain, cough, toxemia, leukopenia, abnormal pulse, rose spots on the skin, bacteremia, hyperplasia of intestinal lymph nodes, mesenteric lymphadenopathy, and Peyer's patches in the intestines.
DEF: Paratyphoid fever: a prolonged febrile illness, caused by salmonella serotypes other than *S. typhi*, especially *S. enteritidis* serotypes paratyphi A and B and *S. choleraesuis*.

002.0 Typhoid fever
Typhoid (fever) (infection) [any site]

002.1 Paratyphoid fever A

002.2 Paratyphoid fever B

002.3 Paratyphoid fever C

002.9 Paratyphoid fever, unspecified

✓4ᵗʰ 003 Other salmonella infections

INCLUDES infection or food poisoning by Salmonella [any serotype]
DEF: Infections caused by a genus of gram-negative, anaerobic bacteria of the family *Enterobacteriaceae*; major symptoms are enteric fevers, acute gastroenteritis and septicemia.

003.0 Salmonella gastroenteritis
Salmonellosis

003.1 Salmonella septicemia

✓5ᵗʰ 003.2 Localized salmonella infections

003.20 Localized salmonella infection, unspecified

003.21 Salmonella meningitis

003.22 Salmonella pneumonia

003.23 Salmonella arthritis

003.24 Salmonella osteomyelitis

003.29 Other

003.8 Other specified salmonella infections

003.9 Salmonella infection, unspecified

✓4ᵗʰ 004 Shigellosis

INCLUDES bacillary dysentery
DEF: Acute infectious dysentery caused by the genus *Shigella*, of the family *Enterobacteriaceae*; affecting the colon causing blood-stained stools, tenesmus, abdominal cramps and fever.

004.0 Shigella dysenteriae
Infection by group A Shigella (Schmitz) (Shiga)

004.1 Shigella flexneri
Infection by group B Shigella

004.2 Shigella boydii
Infection by group C Shigella

004.3 Shigella sonnei
Infection by group D Shigella

004.8 Other specified Shigella infections

004.9 Shigellosis, unspecified

✓4ᵗʰ 005 Other food poisoning (bacterial)

EXCLUDES *salmonella infections (003.0-003.9)*
toxic effect of:
food contaminants (989.7)
noxious foodstuffs (988.0-988.9)
DEF: Enteritis caused by ingesting contaminated foods and characterized by diarrhea, abdominal pain, vomiting; symptoms may be mild or life threatening.

005.0 Staphylococcal food poisoning
Staphylococcal toxemia specified as due to food

005.1 Botulism food poisoning
Botulism NOS
Food poisoning due to Clostridium botulinum
EXCLUDES *infant botulism (040.41)*
wound botulism (040.42)

005.2 Food poisoning due to Clostridium perfringens [C. welchii]
Enteritis necroticans

005.3 Food poisoning due to other Clostridia

005.4 Food poisoning due to Vibrio parahaemolyticus

✓5ᵗʰ 005.8 Other bacterial food poisoning

EXCLUDES *salmonella food poisoning (003.0-003.9)*

005.81 Food poisoning due to Vibrio vulnificus

005.89 Other bacterial food poisoning
Food poisoning due to Bacillus cereus

005.9 Food poisoning, unspecified

✓4ᵗʰ 006 Amebiasis

INCLUDES infection due to Entamoeba histolytica
EXCLUDES *amebiasis due to organisms other than Entamoeba histolytica (007.8)*
DEF: Infection of the large intestine caused by *Entamoeba histolytica*; usually asymptomatic but symptoms may range from mild diarrhea to profound life-threatening dysentery. Extraintestinal complications include hepatic abscess, which may rupture, causing life-threatening infections.

006.0 Acute amebic dysentery without mention of abscess
Acute amebiasis
DEF: Sudden, severe *Entamoeba histolytica* infection causing bloody stools.

006.1 Chronic intestinal amebiasis without mention of abscess
Chronic:
amebiasis
amebic dysentery

006.2 Amebic nondysenteric colitis
DEF: *Entamoeba histolytica* infection with inflamed colon but no dysentery.

006.3 Amebic liver abscess
Hepatic amebiasis

006.4 Amebic lung abscess
Amebic abscess of lung (and liver)

006.5 Amebic brain abscess
Amebic abscess of brain (and liver) (and lung)

006.6 Amebic skin ulceration
Cutaneous amebiasis

006.8 Amebic infection of other sites
Amebic: Ameboma
appendicitis
balanitis
EXCLUDES *specific infections by free-living amebae (136.21-136.29)*

006.9 Amebiasis, unspecified
Amebiasis NOS

✓4ᵗʰ
✓5ᵗʰ Additional Digit Required   Unspecified Code   Other Specified Code   Manifestation Code   ▶◀ Revised Text   ● New Code   ▲ Revised Code Title
2011 ICD-9-CM   **October 2010 • Volume 1 – 1**

Infectious and Parasitic Diseases

007–009.0

√4ᵗʰ **007 Other protozoal intestinal diseases**
   INCLUDES   protozoal:
        colitis
        diarrhea
        dysentery

007.0 Balantidiasis
    Infection by Balantidium coli

007.1 Giardiasis
    Infection by Giardia lamblia
    Lambliasis

007.2 Coccidiosis
    Infection by Isospora belli and Isospora hominis
    Isosporiasis

007.3 Intestinal trichomoniasis
    DEF: Colitis, diarrhea, or dysentery caused by the protozoa
    Trichomonas.

007.4 Cryptosporidiosis
    DEF: An intestinal infection by protozoan parasites causing
    intractable diarrhea in patients with AIDS and other
    immunosuppressed individuals.
    AHA: 4Q, '97, 30

007.5 Cyclosporiasis
    DEF: An infection of the small intestine by the protozoal organism,
    Cyclospora cayetenanesis, spread to humans through ingestion of
    contaminated water or food. Symptoms include watery diarrhea,
    loss of appetite, increased gas, stomach cramps, nausea, vomiting,
    muscle aches, low grade fever, and fatigue.
    AHA: 4Q, '00, 38

007.8 Other specified protozoal intestinal diseases
    Amebiasis due to organisms other than Entamoeba histolytica

007.9 Unspecified protozoal intestinal disease
    Flagellate diarrhea
    Protozoal dysentery NOS

√4ᵗʰ **008 Intestinal infections due to other organisms**
   INCLUDES   any condition classifiable to 009.0-009.3 with mention of
      the responsible organisms
   EXCLUDES   food poisoning by these organisms (005.0-005.9)

√5ᵗʰ **008.0 Escherichia coli [E. coli]**
    AHA: 4Q, '92, 17

008.00 E. coli, unspecified
    E. coli enteritis NOS

008.01 Enteropathogenic E. coli
    DEF: *E. coli* causing inflammation of intestines.

008.02 Enterotoxigenic E. coli
    DEF: A toxic reaction to *E. coli* of the intestinal mucosa,
    causing voluminous watery secretions.

008.03 Enteroinvasive E. coli
    DEF: *E. coli* infection penetrating intestinal mucosa.

008.04 Enterohemorrhagic E. coli
    DEF: E. coli infection penetrating the intestinal mucosa,
    producing microscopic ulceration and bleeding.

008.09 Other intestinal E. coli infections

008.1 Arizona group of paracolon bacilli

008.2 Aerobacter aerogenes
    Enterobacter aeogenes

008.3 Proteus (mirabilis) (morganii)

√5ᵗʰ **008.4 Other specified bacteria**
    AHA: 4Q, '92, 18

008.41 Staphylococcus
    Staphylococcal enterocolitis

008.42 Pseudomonas
    AHA: 2Q, '89, 10

008.43 Campylobacter

008.44 Yersinia enterocolitica

008.45 Clostridium difficile
    Pseudomembranous colitis
    DEF: An overgrowth of a species of bacterium that is a part
    of the normal colon flora in human infants and sometimes
    in adults; produces a toxin that causes pseudomembranous
    enterocolitis.; typically is seen in patients undergoing
    antibiotic therapy.
    A04.7 Enterocolitis due to clostridium difficile   I-10

008.46 Other anaerobes
    Anaerobic enteritis NOS
    Bacteroides (fragilis)
    Gram-negative anaerobes

008.47 Other gram-negative bacteria
    Gram-negative enteritis NOS
   EXCLUDES   gram-negative anaerobes (008.46)

008.49 Other
    AHA: 2Q, '89, 10; 1Q, '88, 6

008.5 Bacterial enteritis, unspecified

√5ᵗʰ **008.6 Enteritis due to specified virus**
    AHA: 4Q, '92, 18

008.61 Rotavirus

008.62 Adenovirus

008.63 Norwalk virus
    Norovirus
    Norwalk-like agent

008.64 Other small round viruses [SRVs]
    Small round virus NOS

008.65 Calicivirus
    DEF: Enteritis due to a subgroup of *Picornaviruses.*

008.66 Astrovirus

008.67 Enterovirus NEC
    Coxsackie virus
    Echovirus
   EXCLUDES   poliovirus (045.0-045.9)

008.69 Other viral enteritis
    Torovirus
    AHA: 1Q, '03, 10

008.8 Other organism, not elsewhere classified
    Viral:
      enteritis NOS
      gastroenteritis
   EXCLUDES   influenza with involvement of gastrointestinal tract
        ▶(487.8, 488.09, 488.19)◀
    A08.4 Viral intestinal infection unspecified   I-10

√4ᵗʰ **009 Ill-defined intestinal infections**
   EXCLUDES   diarrheal disease or intestinal infection due to specified
        organism (001.0-008.8)
      diarrhea following gastrointestinal surgery (564.4)
      intestinal malabsorption (579.0-579.9)
      ischemic enteritis (557.0-557.9)
      other noninfectious gastroenteritis and colitis (558.1-558.9)
      regional enteritis (555.0-555.9)
      ulcerative colitis (556)

009.0 Infectious colitis, enteritis, and gastroenteritis
    Colitis   ⎫
    Enteritis ⎬ septic
    Gastroenteritis ⎭
    Dysentery:
      NOS
      catarrhal
      hemorrhagic
    DEF: Colitis: An inflammation of mucous membranes of the colon.
    DEF: Enteritis: An inflammation of mucous membranes of the small
    intestine.
    DEF: Gastroenteritis: An inflammation of mucous membranes of
    stomach and intestines.
    AHA: 3Q, '99, 4
    A09 Infectious gastroenteritis and colitis unspec   I-10

   N Newborn Age: 0   P Pediatric Age: 0-17   M Maternity Age: 12-55   A Adult Age: 15-124

009.1 Colitis, enteritis, and gastroenteritis of presumed infectious origin
> EXCLUDES colitis NOS (558.9)
> enteritis NOS (558.9)
> gastroenteritis NOS (558.9)
> AHA: 3Q, '99, 6

009.2 Infectious diarrhea
Diarrhea:
  dysenteric
  epidemic
Infectious diarrheal disease NOS

009.3 Diarrhea of presumed infectious origin
> EXCLUDES diarrhea NOS (787.91)
> AHA: N-D, '87, 7

Tuberculosis (010-018)

INCLUDES infection by Mycobacterium tuberculosis (human)
(bovine)
EXCLUDES congenital tuberculosis (771.2)
late effects of tuberculosis (137.0-137.4)

The following fifth digit subclassification is for use with categories 010-018:
> 0 unspecified
> 1 bacteriological or histological examination not done
> 2 bacteriological or histological examination unknown (at present)
> 3 tubercle bacilli found (in sputum) by microscopy
> 4 tubercle bacilli not found (in sputum) by microscopy, but found by bacterial culture
> 5 tubercle bacilli not found by bacteriological examination, but tuberculosis confirmed histologically
> 6 tubercle bacilli not found by bacteriological or histological examination but tuberculosis confirmed by other methods [inoculation of animals]

DEF: An infection by *Mycobacterium tuberculosis* causing the formation of small, rounded nodules, called tubercles, that can disseminate throughout the body via lymph and blood vessels. Localized tuberculosis is most often seen in the lungs.

√4ᵗʰ **010 Primary tuberculous infection**
DEF: Tuberculosis of the lungs occurring when the patient is first infected.

§ √5ᵗʰ **010.0 Primary tuberculous infection**
[0-6] EXCLUDES nonspecific reaction to tuberculin skin test without active tuberculosis (795.5)
positive PPD (795.5)
positive tuberculin skin test without active tuberculosis (795.5)
DEF: Hilar or paratracheal lymph node enlargement in pulmonary tuberculosis.

§ √5ᵗʰ **010.1 Tuberculous pleurisy in primary progressive**
[0-6] **tuberculosis**
DEF: Inflammation and exudation in the lining of the tubercular lung.

§ √5ᵗʰ **010.8 Other primary progressive tuberculosis**
[0-6] EXCLUDES tuberculous erythema nodosum (017.1)

§ √5ᵗʰ **010.9 Primary tuberculous infection, unspecified**
[0-6]

√4ᵗʰ **011 Pulmonary tuberculosis**
Use additional code to identify any associated silicosis (502)

§ √5ᵗʰ **011.0 Tuberculosis of lung, infiltrative**
[0-6]

§ √5ᵗʰ **011.1 Tuberculosis of lung, nodular**
[0-6]

§ √5ᵗʰ **011.2 Tuberculosis of lung with cavitation**
[0-6]

§ √5ᵗʰ **011.3 Tuberculosis of bronchus**
[0-6] EXCLUDES isolated bronchial tuberculosis (012.2)

§ √5ᵗʰ **011.4 Tuberculous fibrosis of lung**
[0-6]

§ √5ᵗʰ **011.5 Tuberculous bronchiectasis**
[0-6]

§ √5ᵗʰ **011.6 Tuberculous pneumonia [any form]**
[0-6] DEF: Inflammatory pulmonary reaction to tuberculous cells.

§ √5ᵗʰ **011.7 Tuberculous pneumothorax**
[0-6] DEF: Spontaneous rupture of damaged tuberculous pulmonary tissue.

§ √5ᵗʰ **011.8 Other specified pulmonary tuberculosis**
[0-6]

§ √5ᵗʰ **011.9 Pulmonary tuberculosis, unspecified**
[0-6] Respiratory tuberculosis NOS
Tuberculosis of lung NOS

√4ᵗʰ **012 Other respiratory tuberculosis**
EXCLUDES respiratory tuberculosis, unspecified (011.9)

§ √5ᵗʰ **012.0 Tuberculous pleurisy**
[0-6] Tuberculosis of pleura
Tuberculous empyema
Tuberculous hydrothorax
EXCLUDES pleurisy with effusion without mention of cause (511.9)
tuberculous pleurisy in primary progressive tuberculosis (010.1)
DEF: Inflammation and exudation in the lining of the tubercular lung.

§ √5ᵗʰ **012.1 Tuberculosis of intrathoracic lymph nodes**
[0-6] Tuberculosis of lymph nodes:
hilar
mediastinal
tracheobronchial
Tuberculous tracheobronchial adenopathy
EXCLUDES that specified as primary (010.0-010.9)

§ √5ᵗʰ **012.2 Isolated tracheal or bronchial tuberculosis**
[0-6]

§ √5ᵗʰ **012.3 Tuberculous laryngitis**
[0-6] Tuberculosis of glottis

§ √5ᵗʰ **012.8 Other specified respiratory tuberculosis**
[0-6] Tuberculosis of:
mediastinum
nasopharynx
nose (septum)
sinus [any nasal]

√4ᵗʰ **013 Tuberculosis of meninges and central nervous system**

§ √5ᵗʰ **013.0 Tuberculous meningitis**
[0-6] Tuberculosis of meninges (cerebral) (spinal)
Tuberculous:
leptomeningitis
meningoencephalitis
EXCLUDES tuberculoma of meninges (013.1)

§ √5ᵗʰ **013.1 Tuberculoma of meninges**
[0-6]

§ √5ᵗʰ **013.2 Tuberculoma of brain**
[0-6] Tuberculosis of brain (current disease)

§ √5ᵗʰ **013.3 Tuberculous abscess of brain**
[0-6]

§ √5ᵗʰ **013.4 Tuberculoma of spinal cord**
[0-6]

§ √5ᵗʰ **013.5 Tuberculous abscess of spinal cord**
[0-6]

§ √5ᵗʰ **013.6 Tuberculous encephalitis or myelitis**
[0-6]

§ √5ᵗʰ **013.8 Other specified tuberculosis of central nervous system**
[0-6]

§ √5ᵗʰ **013.9 Unspecified tuberculosis of central nervous system**
[0-6] Tuberculosis of central nervous system NOS

√4ᵗʰ **014 Tuberculosis of intestines, peritoneum, and mesenteric glands**

§ √5ᵗʰ **014.0 Tuberculous peritonitis**
[0-6] Tuberculous ascites
DEF: Tuberculous inflammation of the membrane lining the abdomen.

§ Requires fifth digit. Valid digits are in [brackets] under each code. See beginning of section 010-018 for codes and definitions.

√4ᵗʰ
√5ᵗʰ Additional Digit Required   Unspecified Code   Other Specified Code   Manifestation Code   ▶◀ Revised Text   ● New Code   ▲ Revised Code Title

2011 ICD-9-CM   **Volume 1 – 3**

Infectious and Parasitic Diseases

014.8–018

§ ✓5ᵗʰ **014.8 Other**
[0-6]   Tuberculosis (of):
         anus
         intestine (large) (small)
         mesenteric glands
         rectum
         retroperitoneal (lymph nodes)
     Tuberculous enteritis

✓4ᵗʰ **015 Tuberculosis of bones and joints**
     Use additional code to identify manifestation, as:
     tuberculous:
         arthropathy (711.4)
         necrosis of bone (730.8)
         osteitis (730.8)
         osteomyelitis (730.8)
         synovitis (727.01)
         tenosynovitis (727.01)

§ ✓5ᵗʰ **015.0 Vertebral column**
[0-6]   Pott's disease
         Use additional code to identify manifestation, as:
             curvature of spine [Pott's] (737.4)
             kyphosis (737.4)
             spondylitis (720.81)

§ ✓5ᵗʰ **015.1 Hip**
[0-6]

§ ✓5ᵗʰ **015.2 Knee**
[0-6]

§ ✓5ᵗʰ **015.5 Limb bones**
[0-6]   Tuberculous dactylitis

§ ✓5ᵗʰ **015.6 Mastoid**
[0-6]   Tuberculous mastoiditis

§ ✓5ᵗʰ **015.7 Other specified bone**
[0-6]

§ ✓5ᵗʰ **015.8 Other specified joint**
[0-6]

§ ✓5ᵗʰ **015.9 Tuberculosis of unspecified bones and joints**
[0-6]

✓4ᵗʰ **016 Tuberculosis of genitourinary system**

§ ✓5ᵗʰ **016.0 Kidney**
[0-6]   Renal tuberculosis
         Use additional code to identify manifestation, as:
         tuberculous:
             nephropathy (583.81)
             pyelitis (590.81)
             pyelonephritis (590.81)

§ ✓5ᵗʰ **016.1 Bladder**
[0-6]

§ ✓5ᵗʰ **016.2 Ureter**
[0-6]

§ ✓5ᵗʰ **016.3 Other urinary organs**

§ ✓5ᵗʰ **016.4 Epididymis**   ♂
[0-6]

§ ✓5ᵗʰ **016.5 Other male genital organs**   ♂
[0-6]   Use additional code to identify manifestation, as:
         tuberculosis of:
             prostate (601.4)
             seminal vesicle (608.81)
             testis (608.81)

§ ✓5ᵗʰ **016.6 Tuberculous oophoritis and salpingitis**   ♀
[0-6]

§ ✓5ᵗʰ **016.7 Other female genital organs**   ♀
[0-6]   Tuberculous:
         cervicitis
         endometritis

§ ✓5ᵗʰ **016.9 Genitourinary tuberculosis, unspecified**
[0-6]

✓4ᵗʰ **017 Tuberculosis of other organs**

§ ✓5ᵗʰ **017.0 Skin and subcutaneous cellular tissue**
[0-6]   Lupus: Tuberculosis:
         exedens   colliquativa
         vulgaris   cutis
     Scrofuloderma   lichenoides
                        papulonecrotica
                        verrucosa cutis

     EXCLUDES *lupus erythematosus (695.4)*
             disseminated (710.0)
         lupus NOS (710.0)
         nonspecific reaction to tuberculin skin test without
             active tuberculosis (795.5)
         positive PPD (795.5)
         positive tuberculin skin test without active
             tuberculosis (795.5)

§ ✓5ᵗʰ **017.1 Erythema nodosum with hypersensitivity**
[0-6]   **reaction in tuberculosis**
     Bazin's disease
     Erythema:
         induratum
         nodosum, tuberculous
     Tuberculosis indurativa
     EXCLUDES *erythema nodosum NOS (695.2)*
     DEF: Tender, inflammatory, bilateral nodules appearing on the shins
     and thought to be an allergic reaction to tuberculotoxin.

§ ✓5ᵗʰ **017.2 Peripheral lymph nodes**
[0-6]   Scrofula
     Scrofulous abscess
     Tuberculous adenitis
     EXCLUDES *tuberculosis of lymph nodes:*
         bronchial and mediastinal (012.1)
         mesenteric and retroperitoneal (014.8)
         tuberculous tracheobronchial adenopathy (012.1)
     DEF: Scrofula: Old name for tuberculous cervical lymphadenitis.

§ ✓5ᵗʰ **017.3 Eye**
[0-6]   Use additional code to identify manifestation, as:
     tuberculous:
         chorioretinitis, disseminated (363.13)
         episcleritis (379.09)
         interstitial keratitis (370.59)
         iridocyclitis, chronic (364.11)
         keratoconjunctivitis (phlyctenular) (370.31)

§ ✓5ᵗʰ **017.4 Ear**
[0-6]   Tuberculosis of ear
     Tuberculous otitis media
     EXCLUDES *tuberculous mastoiditis (015.6)*

§ ✓5ᵗʰ **017.5 Thyroid gland**
[0-6]

§ ✓5ᵗʰ **017.6 Adrenal glands**
[0-6]   Addison's disease, tuberculous

§ ✓5ᵗʰ **017.7 Spleen**
[0-6]

§ ✓5ᵗʰ **017.8 Esophagus**
[0-6]

§ ✓5ᵗʰ **017.9 Other specified organs**
[0-6]   Use additional code to identify manifestation, as:
     tuberculosis of:
         endocardium [any valve] (424.91)
         myocardium (422.0)
         pericardium (420.0)

✓4ᵗʰ **018 Miliary tuberculosis**
     INCLUDES tuberculosis:
         disseminated
         generalized
         miliary, whether of a single specified site, multiple sites,
             or unspecified site
         polyserositis
     DEF: A form of tuberculosis caused by caseous material carried through the
     bloodstream planting seedlike tubercles in various body organs.

---

§   Requires fifth digit. Valid digits are in [brackets] under each code. See beginning of section 010-018 for codes and definitions.

Ⓝ Newborn Age: 0   Ⓟ Pediatric Age: 0-17   Ⓜ Maternity Age: 12-55   Ⓐ Adult Age: 15-124

§ ✓5ᵗʰ **018.0 Acute miliary tuberculosis**
[0-6]

§ ✓5ᵗʰ **018.8 Other specified miliary tuberculosis**
[0-6]

§ ✓5ᵗʰ **018.9 Miliary tuberculosis, unspecified**
[0-6]

Zoonotic Bacterial Diseases (020-027)

✓4ᵗʰ **020 Plague**
INCLUDES infection by Yersinia [Pasteurella] pestis

020.0 Bubonic
DEF: Most common acute and severe form of plague characterized by lymphadenopathy (buboes), chills, fever and headache.

020.1 Cellulocutaneous
DEF: Plague characterized by inflammation and necrosis of skin.

020.2 Septicemic
DEF: Plague characterized by massive infection in the bloodstream.

020.3 Primary pneumonic
DEF: Plague characterized by massive pulmonary Infection.

020.4 Secondary pneumonic
DEF: Lung infection as a secondary complication of plague.

020.5 Pneumonic, unspecified

020.8 Other specified types of plague
Abortive plague
Ambulatory plague
Pestis minor

020.9 Plague, unspecified

✓4ᵗʰ **021 Tularemia**
INCLUDES deerfly fever
infection by Francisella [Pasteurella] tularensis
rabbit fever
DEF: A febrile disease transmitted by the bites of deer flies, fleas and ticks, by inhalations of aerosolized *F. tularensis* or by ingestion of contaminated food or water; patients quickly develop fever, chills, weakness, headache, backache and malaise.

021.0 Ulceroglandular tularemia
DEF: Lesions occur at the site *Francisella tularensis* organism enters body, usually the fingers or hands.

021.1 Enteric tularemia
Tularemia:
cryptogenic
intestinal
typhoidal

021.2 Pulmonary tularemia
Bronchopneumonic tularemia

021.3 Oculoglandular tularemia
DEF: Painful conjunctival infection by *Francisella tularensis* organism with possible corneal, preauricular lymph, or lacrimal involvement.

021.8 Other specified tularemia
Tularemia:
generalized or disseminated
glandular

021.9 Unspecified tularemia

✓4ᵗʰ **022 Anthrax**
DEF: An bacterial disease usually transmitted by contact with infected animals or their discharges; primary routes of inoculation are cutaneous, gastrointestinal and by inhalation.
AHA: 4Q '02, 70

022.0 Cutaneous anthrax
Malignant pustule

022.1 Pulmonary anthrax
Respiratory anthrax
Wool-sorters' disease

022.2 Gastrointestinal anthrax

022.3 Anthrax septicemia

022.8 Other specified manifestations of anthrax

022.9 Anthrax, unspecified

✓4ᵗʰ **023 Brucellosis**
INCLUDES fever:
Malta
Mediterranean
undulant
DEF: An infectious disease caused by gram-negative, aerobic coccobacilli organisms transmitted to humans through contact with infected tissue or dairy products; fever, sweating, weakness and aching are symptoms.

023.0 Brucella melitensis
DEF: Infection from direct or indirect contact with infected sheep or goats.

023.1 Brucella abortus
DEF: Infection from direct or indirect contact with infected cattle.

023.2 Brucella suis
DEF: Infection from direct or indirect contact with infected swine.

023.3 Brucella canis
DEF: Infection from direct or indirect contact with infected dogs.

023.8 Other brucellosis
Infection by more than one organism

023.9 Brucellosis, unspecified

024 Glanders
Infection by:
Actinobacillus mallei
Malleomyces mallei
Pseudomonas mallei
Farcy
Malleus
DEF: Equine infection causing mucosal inflammation and skin ulcers in humans.

025 Melioidosis
Infection by:
Malleomyces pseudomallei
Pseudomonas pseudomallei
Whitmore's bacillus
Pseudoglanders
DEF: Rare infection caused by *Pseudomonas pseudomallei;* clinical symptoms range from localized infection to fatal septicemia.

✓4ᵗʰ **026 Rat-bite fever**

026.0 Spirillary fever
Rat-bite fever due to Spirillum minor [S. minus]
Sodoku

026.1 Streptobacillary fever
Epidemic arthritic erythema
Haverhill fever
Rat-bite fever due to Streptobacillus moniliformis

026.9 Unspecified rat-bite fever

✓4ᵗʰ **027 Other zoonotic bacterial diseases**

027.0 Listeriosis
Infection ⎫
Septicemia ⎬ by Listeria monocytogenes
Use additional code to identify manifestation, as meningitis (320.7)
EXCLUDES *congenital listeriosis (771.2)*

027.1 Erysipelothrix infection
Erysipeloid (of Rosenbach)
Infection ⎫ by Erysipelothrix insidiosa
Septicemia ⎬ [E. rhusiopathiae]
DEF: Usually associated with handling of fish, meat, or poultry; symptoms range from localized inflammation to septicemia.

027.2 Pasteurellosis
Pasteurella pseudotuberculosis infection
Mesenteric adenitis ⎫
Septic infection (cat bite) ⎬ by Pasteurella multocida
(dog bite) ⎭ [P. septica]
EXCLUDES *infection by:*
Francisella [Pasteurella] tularensis (021.0-021.9)
Yersinia [Pasteurella] pestis (020.0-020.9)
DEF: Swelling, abscesses, or septicemia from *Pasteurella multocida,* commonly transmitted to humans by a dog or cat scratch.

027.8 Other specified zoonotic bacterial diseases

---

§ Requires fifth digit. Valid digits are in [brackets] under each code. See beginning of section 010-018 for codes and definitions.

✓4ᵗʰ ✓5ᵗʰ Additional Digit Required   Unspecified Code   Other Specified Code   Manifestation Code   ▶◀ Revised Text   ● New Code   ▲ Revised Code Title

2011 ICD-9-CM   **Volume 1 – 5**

027.9 Unspecified zoonotic bacterial disease

Other Bacterial Diseases (030-041)

EXCLUDES   bacterial venereal diseases (098.0-099.9)
          bartonellosis (088.0)

√4ᵗʰ **030 Leprosy**
      INCLUDES   Hansen's disease
                infection by Mycobacterium leprae

030.0 Lepromatous [type L]
      Lepromatous leprosy (macular) (diffuse) (infiltrated) (nodular)
          (neuritic)
      DEF: Infectious, disseminated leprosy bacilli with lesions and
      deformities.

030.1 Tuberculoid [type T]
      Tuberculoid leprosy (macular) (maculoanesthetic) (major)
          (minor) (neuritic)
      DEF: Relatively benign, self-limiting leprosy with neuralgia and
      scales.

030.2 Indeterminate [group I]
      Indeterminate [uncharacteristic] leprosy (macular) (neuritic)
      DEF: Uncharacteristic leprosy, frequently an early manifestation.

030.3 Borderline [group B]
      Borderline or dimorphous leprosy (infiltrated) (neuritic)
      DEF: Transitional form of leprosy, neither lepromatous nor
      tuberculoid.

030.8 Other specified leprosy

030.9 Leprosy, unspecified

√4ᵗʰ **031 Diseases due to other mycobacteria**

031.0 Pulmonary
      Battey disease
      Infection by Mycobacterium:
          avium
          intracellulare [Battey bacillus]
          kansasii

031.1 Cutaneous
      Buruli ulcer
      Infection by Mycobacterium:
          marinum [M. balnei]
          ulcerans

031.2 Disseminated
      Disseminated mycobacterium avium-intracellulare complex
          (DMAC)
      Mycobacterium avium-intracellulare complex (MAC)
          bacteremia
      DEF: Disseminated mycobacterium avium-intracellulare complex
      (DMAC): A serious systemic form of MAC commonly observed in
      patients in the late course of AIDS.
      DEF: Mycobacterium avium-intracellulare complex (MAC) bacterium:
      Human pulmonary disease, lymphadenitis in children and systemic
      disease in immunocompromised individuals caused by a slow
      growing, gram-positive, aerobic organism.
      AHA: 4Q, '97, 31

031.8 Other specified mycobacterial diseases

031.9 Unspecified diseases due to mycobacteria
      Atypical mycobacterium infection NOS

√4ᵗʰ **032 Diphtheria**
      INCLUDES   infection by Corynebacterium diphtheriae

032.0 Faucial diphtheria
      Membranous angina, diphtheritic
      DEF: Diphtheria of the throat.

032.1 Nasopharyngeal diphtheria

032.2 Anterior nasal diphtheria

032.3 Laryngeal diphtheria
      Laryngotracheitis, diphtheritic

√5ᵗʰ **032.8 Other specified diphtheria**

032.81 Conjunctival diphtheria
      Pseudomembranous diphtheritic conjunctivitis

032.82 Diphtheritic myocarditis

032.83 Diphtheritic peritonitis

032.84 Diphtheritic cystitis

032.85 Cutaneous diphtheria

032.89 Other

032.9 Diphtheria, unspecified

√4ᵗʰ **033 Whooping cough**
      INCLUDES   pertussis
      Use additional code to identify any associated pneumonia (484.3)
      DEF: An acute, highly contagious respiratory tract infection caused by
      Bordetella pertussis and B. bronchiseptica; characteristic paroxysmal cough.

033.0 Bordetella pertussis [B. pertussis]

033.1 Bordetella parapertussis [B. parapertussis]

033.8 Whooping cough due to other specified organism
      Bordetella bronchiseptica [B. bronchiseptica]

033.9 Whooping cough, unspecified organism

√4ᵗʰ **034 Streptococcal sore throat and scarlet fever**

034.0 Streptococcal sore throat
      Septic: Streptococcal:
          angina   laryngitis
          sore throat   pharyngitis
      Streptococcal: tonsillitis
          angina
      J02.0 Streptococcal pharyngitis   I-10

034.1 Scarlet fever
      Scarlatina
      EXCLUDES   parascarlatina (057.8)
      DEF: Streptococcal infection and fever with red rash spreading from
      trunk.

035 Erysipelas
      EXCLUDES   postpartum or puerperal erysipelas (670.8)
      DEF: An acute superficial cellulitis involving the dermal lymphatics; it is often
      caused by group A streptococci.

√4ᵗʰ **036 Meningococcal infection**

036.0 Meningococcal meningitis
      Cerebrospinal fever (meningococcal)
      Meningitis:
          cerebrospinal
          epidemic

036.1 Meningococcal encephalitis

036.2 Meningococcemia
      Meningococcal septicemia

036.3 Waterhouse-Friderichsen syndrome, meningococcal
      Meningococcal hemorrhagic adrenalitis
      Meningococcic adrenal syndrome
      Waterhouse-Friderichsen syndrome NOS

√5ᵗʰ **036.4 Meningococcal carditis**

036.40 Meningococcal carditis, unspecified

036.41 Meningococcal pericarditis
      DEF: Meningococcal infection of the outer membrane of the
      heart.

036.42 Meningococcal endocarditis
      DEF: Meningococcal infection of the membranes lining the
      cavities of the heart.

036.43 Meningococcal myocarditis
      DEF: Meningococcal infection of the muscle of the heart.

√5ᵗʰ **036.8 Other specified meningococcal infections**

036.81 Meningococcal optic neuritis

036.82 Meningococcal arthropathy

036.89 Other

036.9 Meningococcal infection, unspecified
      Meningococcal infection NOS

Ⓝ Newborn Age: 0   Ⓟ Pediatric Age: 0-17   Ⓜ Maternity Age: 12-55   Ⓐ Adult Age: 15-124

037 Tetanus

EXCLUDES tetanus:
> complicating:
>> abortion (634-638 with .0, 639.0)
>> ectopic or molar pregnancy (639.0)
> neonatorum (771.3)
> puerperal (670.8)

DEF: An acute, often fatal, infectious disease caused by the anaerobic, spore-forming bacillus *Clostridium tetani;* the bacillus enters the body through a contaminated wound, burns, surgical wounds, or cutaneous ulcers. Symptoms: lockjaw, spasms, seizures, and paralysis.

✓4ᵗʰ 038 Septicemia

Use additional code for systemic inflammatory response syndrome (SIRS) (995.91-995.92)

EXCLUDES bacteremia (790.7)
> during labor (659.3)
> following ectopic or molar pregnancy (639.0)
> following infusion, injection, transfusion, or vaccination (999.3)
> postpartum, puerperal (670)
> septicemia (sepsis) of newborn (771.81)
> that complicating abortion (634-638 with .0, 639.0)

DEF: A systemic disease associated with the presence and persistence of pathogenic microorganisms or their toxins in the blood.
AHA: 2Q, '04, 16; 4Q, '88, 10; 3Q, '88, 12
TIP: Sequence any underlying cause (e.g., due to device or injury) first, before septicemia code.

038.0 Streptococcal septicemia
AHA: 4Q, '03, 79; 2Q, '96, 5

✓5ᵗʰ 038.1 Staphylococcal septicemia
AHA: 4Q, '97, 32

038.10 Staphylococcal septicemia, unspecified

038.11 Methicillin susceptible Staphylococcus aureus septicemia
MSSA septicemia
Staphylococcus aureus septicemia NOS
AHA: 4Q, '08, 69-70; 1Q, '05, 7; 2Q, '00, 5; 4Q, '98, 42
A41.0 Sepsis due to Staphylococcus aureus   `I-10`

038.12 Methicillin resistant Staphylococcus aureus septicemia
AHA: 4Q, '08, 69-73

038.19 Other staphylococcal septicemia
AHA: 2Q, '00, 5
A41.1 Sepsis due to other spec Staphylococcus   `I-10`

038.2 Pneumococcal septicemia [Streptococcus pneumoniae septicemia]
AHA: 2Q, '96, 5; 1Q, '91, 13

038.3 Septicemia due to anaerobes
Septicemia due to bacteroides
EXCLUDES gas gangrene (040.0)
> that due to anaerobic streptococci (038.0)

DEF: Infection of blood by microorganisms that thrive without oxygen.

✓5ᵗʰ 038.4 Septicemia due to other gram-negative organisms
DEF: Infection of blood by microorganisms categorized as gram-negative by Gram's method of staining for identification of bacteria.

038.40 Gram-negative organism, unspecified
Gram-negative septicemia NOS

038.41 Hemophilus influenzae [H. influenzae]

038.42 Escherichia coli [E. coli]
AHA: 4Q, '03, 73
A41.51 Sepsis due to Escherichia coli [E coli]   `I-10`

038.43 Pseudomonas

038.44 Serratia

038.49 Other
A41.59 Other Gram-negative sepsis   `I-10`

038.8 Other specified septicemias
EXCLUDES septicemia (due to):
> anthrax (022.3)
> gonococcal (098.89)
> herpetic (054.5)
> meningococcal (036.2)
> septicemic plague (020.2)

038.9 Unspecified septicemia
Septicemia NOS
EXCLUDES bacteremia NOS (790.7)
AHA: 4Q, '07, 97; 2Q, '05, 18-19; 2Q, '04, 16; 4Q, '03, 79; 2Q, '00, 3; 3Q, '99, 5, 9; 1Q, '98, 5; 3Q, '96, 16; 2Q, '96, 6
TIP: Ensure that documentation includes clinical evidence of systemic infection; do not code if documentation indicates "urosepsis" only.
A41.9 Sepsis unspecified   `I-10`

✓4ᵗʰ 039 Actinomycotic infections

INCLUDES actinomycotic mycetoma
> infection by Actinomycetales, such as species of Actinomyces, Actinomadura, Nocardia, Streptomyces
> maduromycosis (actinomycotic)
> schizomycetoma (actinomycotic)

DEF: Inflammatory lesions and abscesses at site of infection by *Actinomyces israelii.*

039.0 Cutaneous
Erythrasma
Trichomycosis axillaris

039.1 Pulmonary
Thoracic actinomycosis

039.2 Abdominal

039.3 Cervicofacial

039.4 Madura foot
EXCLUDES madura foot due to mycotic infection (117.4)

039.8 Of other specified sites

039.9 Of unspecified site
Actinomycosis NOS
Maduromycosis NOS
Nocardiosis NOS

✓4ᵗʰ 040 Other bacterial diseases

EXCLUDES bacteremia NOS (790.7)
> bacterial infection NOS (041.9)

040.0 Gas gangrene
Gas bacillus infection or gangrene
Infection by Clostridium:
> histolyticum
> oedematiens
> perfringens [welchii]
> septicum
> sordellii
Malignant edema
Myonecrosis, clostridial
Myositis, clostridial
AHA: 1Q, '95, 11

040.1 Rhinoscleroma
DEF: Growths on the nose and nasopharynx caused by *Klebsiella rhinoscleromatis.*

040.2 Whipple's disease
Intestinal lipodystrophy

040.3 Necrobacillosis
DEF: Infection with *Fusobacterium necrophorum* causing abscess or necrosis.
AHA: 4Q, '07, 85

 ✓4ᵗʰ / ✓5ᵗʰ Additional Digit Required   Unspecified Code   Other Specified Code   Manifestation Code   ▶◀ Revised Text   ● New Code   ▲ Revised Code Title

2011 ICD-9-CM   **Volume 1 – 7**

Infectious and Parasitic Diseases

040.4–042

√5ᵗʰ **040.4 Other specified botulism**

Non-foodborne intoxication due to toxins of Clostridium botulinum [C. botulinum]

> **EXCLUDES**   botulism NOS (005.1)
>   food poisoning due to toxins of Clostridium botulinum (005.1)

040.41 Infant botulism   P

> **DEF:** Colonization of Clostridium botulinum spores in the large intestine; release of neurotoxins results in constipation; may progress to neuromuscular paralysis; affects infants of less than six months.
> **AHA:** 4Q, '07, 60

040.42 Wound botulism

Non-foodborne botulism NOS

Use additional code to identify complicated open wound

> **AHA:** 4Q, '07, 60

√5ᵗʰ **040.8 Other specified bacterial diseases**

040.81 Tropical pyomyositis

040.82 Toxic shock syndrome

Use additional code to identify the organism

> **DEF:** Syndrome caused by staphylococcal exotoxin that may rapidly progress to severe and intractable shock; symptoms include sunburn-like rash with peeling of skin on palms and soles, sudden onset high fever, vomiting, diarrhea, myalgia, and hypotension.
> **AHA:** 4Q, '02, 44

040.89 Other

> **AHA:** N-D, '86, 7

√4ᵗʰ **041 Bacterial infection in conditions classified elsewhere and of unspecified site**

> **NOTE** This category is provided to be used as an additional code to identify the bacterial agent in diseases classified elsewhere. This category will also be used to classify bacterial infections of unspecified nature or site.
>
> **EXCLUDES**   septicemia (038.0-038.9)
>
> **AHA:** 2Q, '01, 12; J-A, '84, 19

√5ᵗʰ **041.0 Streptococcus**

041.00 Streptococcus, unspecified

041.01 Group A

> **AHA:** 1Q, '02, 3

041.02 Group B

> **B95.1** Streptococcus group B cause of dz class   I-10
> elsewhere

041.03 Group C

041.04 Group D [Enterococcus]

> **B95.2** Enterococcus as the cause of dz class elsewhere   I-10

041.05 Group G

041.09 Other Streptococcus

> **B95.4** Oth streptococcus cause of dz class elsewhere   I-10

√5ᵗʰ **041.1 Staphylococcus**

041.10 Staphylococcus, unspecified

> **AHA:** 2Q, '06, 15

041.11 Methicillin susceptible Staphylococcus aureus

MSSA

Staphylococcus aureus NOS

> **AHA:** 4Q, '08, 69-70; 2Q, '06, 16; 4Q, '03, 104, 106; 2Q, '01, 11; 4Q, '98, 42, 54; 4Q, '97, 32
> **B95.6** Staphylococcus aureus cause dz class   I-10
> elsewhere

041.12 Methicillin resistant Staphylococcus aureus

Methicillin-resistant staphylococcus aureus (MRSA)

> **AHA:** 4Q, '09, 98; 4Q, '08, 69-70, 73
> **TIP:** Do not assign if combination code (with localized infection) available, or if only colonization or carrier status documented.

041.19 Other Staphylococcus

> **AHA:** 2Q, '08, 3
> **B95.7** Other staphylococcus cause of dz class elsewhere   I-10

041.2 Pneumococcus

041.3 Klebsiella pneumoniae

> **AHA:** 4Q, '08, 149

041.4 Escherichia coli [E. coli]

> **B96.2** Escherichia coli cause of dz class elsewhere   I-10

041.5 Hemophilus influenzae [H. influenzae]

041.6 Proteus (mirabilis) (morganii)

041.7 Pseudomonas

> **AHA:** ▶1Q, '10, 9;◀ 4Q, '02, 45
> **B96.5** Pseudomonas as the cause of dz class elsewhere   I-10

√5ᵗʰ **041.8 Other specified bacterial infections**

041.81 Mycoplasma

Eaton's agent

Pleuropneumonia-like organisms [PPLO]

041.82 Bacteroides fragilis

> **DEF:** Anaerobic gram-negative bacilli of the gastrointestinal tract; frequently implicated in intra-abdominal infection; commonly resistant to antibiotics.

041.83 Clostridium perfringens

041.84 Other anaerobes

Gram-negative anaerobes

> **EXCLUDES**   Helicobacter pylori (041.86)

041.85 Other gram-negative organisms

Aerobacter aerogenes

Gram-negative bacteria NOS

Mima polymorpha

Serratia

> **EXCLUDES**   gram-negative anaerobes (041.84)
> **AHA:** 1Q, '95, 18

041.86 Helicobacter pylori [H. pylori]

> **AHA:** 4Q, '95, 60
> **B96.81** Helicobacter pylori cause of dz class elsewhere   I-10

041.89 Other specified bacteria

> **AHA:** 2Q, '06, 7; 2Q, '03, 7
> **A49.8** Other bacterial infections of unspec site   I-10

041.9 Bacterial infection, unspecified

> **AHA:** 2Q, '91, 9

Human Immunodeficiency Virus (HIV) Infection (042)

042 Human immunodeficiency virus [HIV] disease

Acquired immune deficiency syndrome

Acquired immunodeficiency syndrome

AIDS

AIDS-like syndrome

AIDS-related complex

ARC

HIV infection, symptomatic

Use additional code(s) to identify all manifestations of HIV

Use additional code to identify HIV-2 infection (079.53)

> **EXCLUDES**   asymptomatic HIV infection status (V08)
>   exposure to HIV virus (V01.79)
>   nonspecific serologic evidence of HIV (795.71)
>
> **AHA:** 4Q, '07, 63; 3Q, '06, 15; 1Q, '05, 7; 2Q, '04, 11; 1Q, '04, 5; 1Q, '03, 15; 1Q, '99, 14; 4Q, '97, 30, 31; 1Q, '93, 21; 2Q, '92, 11; 3Q, '90, 17; J-A, '87, 8
> **TIP:** Code only confirmed cases of HIV infection/illness; may be coded from provider's diagnostic statement.
> **B20** Human immunodeficiency virus [HIV] disease   I-10

N Newborn Age: 0   P Pediatric Age: 0-17   M Maternity Age: 12-55   A Adult Age: 15-124

Poliomyelitis and Other Non-Arthropod-Borne Viral Diseases and Prion Diseases of Central Nervous System (045-049)

✓4ᵗʰ **045 Acute poliomyelitis**

> EXCLUDES *late effects of acute poliomyelitis (138)*

> The following fifth-digit subclassification is for use with category 045:
>
> 0 **poliovirus, unspecified type**
> 1 **poliovirus type I**
> 2 **poliovirus type II**
> 3 **poliovirus type III**

§ ✓5ᵗʰ **045.0 Acute paralytic poliomyelitis specified as bulbar**

[0-3]   Infantile paralysis (acute) ⎱ specified as
      Poliomyelitis (acute) (anterior) ⎰   bulbar

      Polioencephalitis (acute) (bulbar)
      Polioencephalomyelitis (acute) (anterior) (bulbar)

> **DEF:** Acute paralytic infection occurring where the brain merges with the spinal cord; affecting breathing, swallowing, and heart rate.

§ ✓5ᵗʰ **045.1 Acute poliomyelitis with other paralysis**

[0-3]   Paralysis:
      acute atrophic, spinal
      infantile, paralytic
      Poliomyelitis (acute) ⎱
      anterior   ⎰ with paralysis except
      epidemic   bulbar

> **DEF:** Paralytic infection affecting peripheral or spinal nerves.

§ ✓5ᵗʰ **045.2 Acute nonparalytic poliomyelitis**

[0-3]   Poliomyelitis (acute) ⎱
      anterior   ⎰ specified as nonparalytic
      epidemic

> **DEF:** Nonparalytic infection causing pain, stiffness, and paresthesias.

§ ✓5ᵗʰ **045.9 Acute poliomyelitis, unspecified**

[0-3]   Infantile paralysis   ⎱
      Poliomyelitis (acute) ⎰ unspecified whether
      anterior   paralytic or
      epidemic   nonparalytic

✓4ᵗʰ **046 Slow virus infections and prion diseases of central nervous system**

046.0 Kuru

> **DEF:** A chronic, progressive, fatal nervous system disorder; clinical symptoms include cerebellar ataxia, trembling, spasticity and progressive dementia.

✓5ᵗʰ **046.1 Jakob-Creutzfeldt disease**

> Use additional code to identify dementia:
> with behavioral disturbance (294.11)
> without behavioral disturbance (294.10)

     046.11 Variant Creutzfeldt-Jakob disease
        vCJD
        AHA: 4Q, '08, 73-75

     046.19 Other and unspecified Creutzfeldt-Jacob disease
        CJD
        Familial Creutzfeldt-Jakob disease
        Iatrogenic Creutzfeldt-Jakob disease
        Jakob-Creutzfeldt disease, unspecified
        Sporadic Creutzfeldt-Jakob disease
        Subacute spongiform encephalopathy

>   EXCLUDES *variant Creutzfeldt-Jakob disease (vCJD) (046.11)*

>   **DEF:** Communicable, progressive spongiform encephalopathy thought to be caused by an infectious particle known as a "prion" (proteinaceous infection particle); a progressive, fatal disease manifested principally by mental deterioration.
>   **AHA:** 4Q, '08, 73-75

046.2 Subacute sclerosing panencephalitis

> Dawson's inclusion body encephalitis
> Van Bogaert's sclerosing leukoencephalitis

> **DEF:** Progressive viral infection causing cerebral dysfunction, blindness, dementia, and death (SSPE).

046.3 Progressive multifocal leukoencephalopathy

> Multifocal leukoencephalopathy NOS

> **DEF:** Infection affecting cerebral cortex in patients with weakened immune systems.

✓5ᵗʰ **046.7 Other specified prion diseases of central nervous system**

> EXCLUDES *Creutzfeldt-Jakob disease (046.11-046.19)*
> *Jakob-Creutzfeldt disease (046.11-046.19)*
> *kuru (046.0)*
> *variant Creutzfeldt-Jakob disease (vCJD) (046.11)*

     046.71 Gerstmann-Sträussler-Scheinker syndrome
        GSS syndrome
        AHA: 4Q, '08, 73-75

     046.72 Fatal familial insomnia
        FFI
        AHA: 4Q, '08, 73-75

     046.79 Other and unspecified prion disease of central nervous system

046.8 Other specified slow virus infection of central nervous system

046.9 Unspecified slow virus infection of central nervous system

✓4ᵗʰ **047 Meningitis due to enterovirus**

> INCLUDES meningitis:
>   abacterial
>   aseptic
>   viral

> EXCLUDES *meningitis due to:*
>   *adenovirus (049.1)*
>   *arthropod-borne virus (060.0-066.9)*
>   *leptospira (100.81)*
>   *virus of:*
>   *herpes simplex (054.72)*
>   *herpes zoster (053.0)*
>   *lymphocytic choriomeningitis (049.0)*
>   *mumps (072.1)*
>   *poliomyelitis (045.0-045.9)*
>   *any other infection specifically classified elsewhere*

> **AHA:** J-F, '87, 6

047.0 Coxsackie virus

047.1 ECHO virus

> Meningo-eruptive syndrome

047.8 Other specified viral meningitis

047.9 Unspecified viral meningitis

> Viral meningitis NOS
> A87.9 Viral meningitis unspecified   I-10

048 Other enterovirus diseases of central nervous system

> Boston exanthem

✓4ᵗʰ **049 Other non-arthropod-borne viral diseases of central nervous system**

> EXCLUDES *late effects of viral encephalitis (139.0)*

049.0 Lymphocytic choriomeningitis

> Lymphocytic:
>   meningitis (serous) (benign)
>   meningoencephalitis (serous) (benign)

049.1 Meningitis due to adenovirus

> **DEF:** Inflammation of lining of brain caused by Arenaviruses and usually occurring in adults in fall and winter months.

049.8 Other specified non-arthropod-borne viral diseases of central nervous system

> Encephalitis: Encephalitis:
>   acute: lethargica
>   inclusion body   Rio Bravo
>   necrotizing   von Economo's disease
>   epidemic

> EXCLUDES *human herpesvirus 6 encephalitis (058.21)*
> *other human herpesvirus encephalitis (058.29)*

049.9 Unspecified non-arthropod-borne viral diseases of central nervous system

> Viral encephalitis NOS

---

§   Requires fifth digit. Valid digits are in [brackets] under each code. See category 045 for codes and definitions.

✓4ᵗʰ
✓5ᵗʰ Additional Digit Required   Unspecified Code   Other Specified Code   Manifestation Code   ►◄ Revised Text   ● New Code   ▲ Revised Code Title

2011 ICD-9-CM   **Volume 1 – 9**

Infectious and Parasitic Diseases

050–054.6

Viral Diseases Generally Accompanied by Exanthem (050-059)

> **EXCLUDES** arthropod-borne viral diseases (060.0-066.9)
> Boston exanthem (048)

✓4ᵗʰ 050 Smallpox

050.0 Variola major
Hemorrhagic (pustular) smallpox
Malignant smallpox
Purpura variolosa
DEF: Form of smallpox known for its high mortality; exists only in laboratories.

050.1 Alastrim
Variola minor
DEF: Mild form of smallpox known for its low mortality rate.

050.2 Modified smallpox
Varioloid
DEF: Mild form occurring in patients with history of infection or vaccination.

050.9 Smallpox, unspecified

✓4ᵗʰ 051 Cowpox and paravaccinia

✓5ᵗʰ 051.0 Cowpox and vaccinia not from vaccination

051.01 Cowpox
DEF: A disease contracted by milking infected cows; vesicles usually appear on the fingers, hands and adjacent areas and usually disappear without scarring; other symptoms: local edema, lymphangitis, and regional lymphadenitis with or without fever.
AHA: 4Q, '08, 76-77

051.02 Vaccinia not from vaccination
EXCLUDES vaccinia (generalized) (from vaccination) (999.0)
AHA: 4Q, '08, 76-77

051.1 Pseudocowpox
Milkers' node
DEF: Hand lesions and mild fever in dairy workers caused by exposure to paravaccinia.

051.2 Contagious pustular dermatitis
Ecthyma contagiosum
Orf
DEF: Skin eruptions caused by exposure to poxvirus-infected sheep or goats.

051.9 Paravaccinia, unspecified

✓4ᵗʰ 052 Chickenpox

DEF: Contagious infection by *Varicella-zoster* virus causing rash with pustules and fever.

052.0 Postvaricella encephalitis
Postchickenpox encephalitis

052.1 Varicella (hemorrhagic) pneumonitis

052.2 Postvaricella myelitis
Postchickenpox myelitis
AHA: 4Q, '06, 58-63

052.7 With other specified complications
AHA: 1Q, '02, 3

052.8 With unspecified complication

052.9 Varicella without mention of complication
Chickenpox NOS   Varicella NOS

✓4ᵗʰ 053 Herpes zoster

INCLUDES shingles
zona
DEF: Self-limiting infection by *Varicella-zoster* virus causing unilateral eruptions and neuralgia along affected nerves.

053.0 With meningitis
DEF: *Varicella-zoster* virus infection causing inflammation of the lining of the brain and/or spinal cord.

✓5ᵗʰ 053.1 With other nervous system complications

053.10 With unspecified nervous system complication

053.11 Geniculate herpes zoster
Herpetic geniculate ganglionitis
DEF: Unilateral eruptions and neuralgia along the facial nerve geniculum affecting face and outer and middle ear.

053.12 Postherpetic trigeminal neuralgia
DEF: Severe oral or nasal pain following a herpes zoster infection.

053.13 Postherpetic polyneuropathy
DEF: Multiple areas of pain following a herpes zoster infection.

053.14 Herpes zoster myelitis
AHA: 4Q, '06, 58-63

053.19 Other

✓5ᵗʰ 053.2 With ophthalmic complications

053.20 Herpes zoster dermatitis of eyelid
Herpes zoster ophthalmicus

053.21 Herpes zoster keratoconjunctivitis

053.22 Herpes zoster iridocyclitis

053.29 Other

✓5ᵗʰ 053.7 With other specified complications

053.71 Otitis externa due to herpes zoster

053.79 Other

053.8 With unspecified complication

053.9 Herpes zoster without mention of complication
Herpes zoster NOS
B02.9 Zoster without complications   I-10

✓4ᵗʰ 054 Herpes simplex

EXCLUDES congenital herpes simplex (771.2)

054.0 Eczema herpeticum
Kaposi's varicelliform eruption
DEF: Herpes simplex virus invading site of preexisting skin inflammation.

✓5ᵗʰ 054.1 Genital herpes

AHA: J-F, '87, 15, 16

054.10 Genital herpes, unspecified
Herpes progenitalis
A60.00 Herpesviral infection urogenital system unspec   I-10

054.11 Herpetic vulvovaginitis   ♀

054.12 Herpetic ulceration of vulva   ♀

054.13 Herpetic infection of penis   ♂

054.19 Other

054.2 Herpetic gingivostomatitis

054.3 Herpetic meningoencephalitis
Herpes encephalitis   Simian B disease
EXCLUDES human herpesvirus 6 encephalitis (058.21)
other human herpesvirus encephalitis (058.29)
DEF: Inflammation of the brain and its lining, caused by infection of herpes simplex 1 in adults and simplex 2 in newborns.

✓5ᵗʰ 054.4 With ophthalmic complications

054.40 With unspecified ophthalmic complication

054.41 Herpes simplex dermatitis of eyelid

054.42 Dendritic keratitis

054.43 Herpes simplex disciform keratitis

054.44 Herpes simplex iridocyclitis

054.49 Other

054.5 Herpetic septicemia
AHA: 2Q, '00, 5

054.6 Herpetic whitlow
Herpetic felon
DEF: A primary infection of the terminal segment of a finger by herpes simplex; intense itching and pain start the disease, vesicles form, and tissue ultimately is destroyed.

N Newborn Age: 0   **P** Pediatric Age: 0-17   **M** Maternity Age: 12-55   **A** Adult Age: 15-124

✓5ᵗʰ 054.7 With other specified complications

    054.71 Visceral herpes simplex

    054.72 Herpes simplex meningitis

    054.73 Herpes simplex otitis externa

    054.74 Herpes simplex myelitis
        AHA: 4Q, '06, 58-63

    054.79 Other

054.8 With unspecified complication

054.9 Herpes simplex without mention of complication
    B00.9 Herpesviral infection unspecified   I-10

✓4ᵗʰ 055 Measles
    INCLUDES   morbilli
               rubeola

055.0 Postmeasles encephalitis

055.1 Postmeasles pneumonia

055.2 Postmeasles otitis media

✓6ᵗʰ 055.7 With other specified complications

    055.71 Measles keratoconjunctivitis
         Measles keratitis

    055.79 Other

055.8 With unspecified complication

055.9 Measles without mention of complication

✓4ᵗʰ 056 Rubella
    INCLUDES   German measles
    EXCLUDES   *congenital rubella (771.0)*
    DEF: Acute but usually benign togavirus infection causing fever, sore throat, and rash; associated with complications to fetus as a result of maternal infection.

✓6ᵗʰ 056.0 With neurological complications

    056.00 With unspecified neurological complication

    056.01 Encephalomyelitis due to rubella
         Encephalitis   ⎫
         Meningoencephalitis ⎬ due to rubella
                    ⎭

    056.09 Other

✓5ᵗʰ 056.7 With other specified complications

    056.71 Arthritis due to rubella

    056.79 Other

056.8 With unspecified complications

056.9 Rubella without mention of complication

✓4ᵗʰ 057 Other viral exanthemata
    DEF: Skin eruptions or rashes and fever caused by viruses, including poxviruses.

057.0 Erythema infectiosum [fifth disease]
    DEF: A moderately contagious, benign, epidemic disease, usually seen in children, of probable viral etiology; a red macular rash appears on face and may spread to the limbs and trunk.

057.8 Other specified viral exanthemata
     Dukes (-Filatow) disease
     Fourth disease
     Parascarlatina
     Pseudoscarlatina
    EXCLUDES   *exanthema subitum [sixth disease] (058.10-058.12)*
               roseola infantum (058.10-058.12)

057.9 Viral exanthem, unspecified

✓4ᵗʰ 058 Other human herpesvirus
    EXCLUDES   *congenital herpes (771.2)*
               cytomegalovirus (078.5)
               Epstein-Barr virus (075)
               herpes NOS (054.0-054.9)
               herpes simplex (054.0-054.9)
               herpes zoster (053.0-053.9)
               human herpesvirus NOS (054.0-054.9)
               human herpesvirus 1 (054.0-054.9)
               human herpesvirus 2 (054.0-054.9)
               human herpesvirus 3 (052.0-053.9)
               human herpesvirus 4 (075)
               human herpesvirus 5 (078.5)
               varicella (052.0-052.9)
               varicella-zoster virus (052.0-053.9)
    AHA: 4Q, '07, 61

✓5ᵗʰ 058.1 Roseola infantum
     Exanthema subitum [sixth disease]

    058.10 Roseola infantum, unspecified   P
         Exanthema subitum [sixth disease], unspecified
         AHA: 4Q, '07, 63

    058.11 Roseola infantum due to human herpesvirus 6   P
         Exanthema subitum [sixth disease] due to human herpesvirus 6

    058.12 Roseola infantum due to human herpesvirus 7   P
         Exanthema subitum [sixth disease] due to human herpesvirus 7

✓5ᵗʰ 058.2 Other human herpesvirus encephalitis
    EXCLUDES   *herpes encephalitis NOS (054.3)*
               herpes simplex encephalitis (054.3)
               human herpesvirus encephalitis NOS (054.3)
               simian B herpesvirus encephalitis (054.3)

    058.21 Human herpesvirus 6 encephalitis

    058.29 Other human herpesvirus encephalitis
         Human herpesvirus 7 encephalitis

✓5ᵗʰ 058.8 Other human herpesvirus infections

    058.81 Human herpesvirus 6 infection

    058.82 Human herpesvirus 7 infection

    058.89 Other human herpesvirus infection
         Human herpesvirus 8 infection
         Kaposi's sarcoma-associated herpesvirus infection
         AHA: 4Q, '07, 63

✓4ᵗʰ 059 Other poxvirus infections
    EXCLUDES   *contagious pustular dermatitis (051.2)*
               cowpox (051.01)
               ecthyma contagiosum (051.2)
               milker's nodule (051.1)
               orf (051.2)
               paravaccinia NOS (051.9)
               pseudocowpox (051.1)
               smallpox (050.0-050.9)
               vaccinia (generalized) (from vaccination) (999.0)
               vaccinia not from vaccination (051.02)
    AHA: 4Q, '08, 76-78

✓5ᵗʰ 059.0 Other orthopoxvirus infections

    059.00 Orthopoxvirus infection, unspecified

    059.01 Monkeypox

    059.09 Other orthopoxvirus infection

✓5ᵗʰ 059.1 Other parapoxvirus infections

    059.10 Parapoxvirus infection, unspecified

    059.11 Bovine stomatitis

    059.12 Sealpox

    059.19 Other parapoxvirus infections

✓5ᵗʰ 059.2 Yatapoxvirus infections

    059.20 Yatapoxvirus infection, unspecified

    059.21 Tanapox

    059.22 Yaba monkey tumor virus

✓4ᵗʰ / ✓5ᵗʰ Additional Digit Required   Unspecified Code   Other Specified Code   Manifestation Code   ►◄ Revised Text   ● New Code   ▲ Revised Code Title

2011 ICD-9-CM   **Volume 1 – 11**

Infectious and Parasitic Diseases

059.8–066.9

059.8 Other poxvirus infections

059.9 Poxvirus infections, unspecified

Arthropod-borne Viral Diseases (060-066)

Use additional code to identify any associated meningitis (321.2)

EXCLUDES late effects of viral encephalitis (139.0)

✓4ᵗʰ 060 Yellow fever

DEF: Fever and jaundice from infection by mosquito-borne virus of genus *Flavivirus*.

060.0 Sylvatic

Yellow fever: Yellow fever:
   jungle   sylvan

DEF: Yellow fever transmitted from animal to man, via mosquito.

060.1 Urban

DEF: Yellow fever transmitted from man to man, via mosquito.

060.9 Yellow fever, unspecified

061 Dengue

Breakbone fever

EXCLUDES hemorrhagic fever caused by dengue virus (065.4)

DEF: Acute, self-limiting infection by mosquito-borne virus characterized by fever and generalized aches.

✓4ᵗʰ 062 Mosquito-borne viral encephalitis

062.0 Japanese encephalitis

Japanese B encephalitis

DEF: Flavivirus causing inflammation of the brain, with a wide range of clinical manifestations.

062.1 Western equine encephalitis

DEF: Alphavirus WEE infection causing inflammation of the brain, found in areas west of the Mississippi; transmitted horse to mosquito to man.

062.2 Eastern equine encephalitis

EXCLUDES Venezuelan equine encephalitis (066.2)

DEF: Alphavirus EEE causing inflammation of the brain and spinal cord, found from Canada to South America and Mexico; transmitted horse to mosquito to man.

062.3 St. Louis encephalitis

DEF: Epidemic form caused by Flavivirus and transmitted by mosquito, and characterized by fever, difficulty in speech, and headache.

062.4 Australian encephalitis

Australian arboencephalitis
Australian X disease
Murray Valley encephalitis

DEF: Flavivirus causing inflammation of the brain, occurring in Australia and New Guinea.

062.5 California virus encephalitis

Encephalitis: Tahyna fever
   California
   La Crosse

DEF: Bunyamwere virus causing inflammation of the brain.

062.8 Other specified mosquito-borne viral encephalitis

Encephalitis by Ilheus virus

EXCLUDES West Nile virus (066.40-066.49)

062.9 Mosquito-borne viral encephalitis, unspecified

✓4ᵗʰ 063 Tick-borne viral encephalitis

INCLUDES diphasic meningoencephalitis

063.0 Russian spring-summer [taiga] encephalitis

063.1 Louping ill

DEF: Inflammation of brain caused by virus transmitted sheep to tick to man; incidence usually limited to British Isles.

063.2 Central European encephalitis

DEF: Inflammation of brain caused by virus transmitted by tick; limited to central Europe and presenting with two distinct phases.

063.8 Other specified tick-borne viral encephalitis

Langat encephalitis   Powassan encephalitis

063.9 Tick-borne viral encephalitis, unspecified

064 Viral encephalitis transmitted by other and unspecified arthropods

Arthropod-borne viral encephalitis, vector unknown
Negishi virus encephalitis

EXCLUDES viral encephalitis NOS (049.9)

✓4ᵗʰ 065 Arthropod-borne hemorrhagic fever

065.0 Crimean hemorrhagic fever [CHF Congo virus]

Central Asian hemorrhagic fever

065.1 Omsk hemorrhagic fever

065.2 Kyasanur Forest disease

065.3 Other tick-borne hemorrhagic fever

065.4 Mosquito-borne hemorrhagic fever

Chikungunya hemorrhagic fever
Dengue hemorrhagic fever

EXCLUDES Chikungunya fever (066.3)
dengue (061)
yellow fever (060.0-060.9)

065.8 Other specified arthropod-borne hemorrhagic fever

Mite-borne hemorrhagic fever

065.9 Arthropod-borne hemorrhagic fever, unspecified

Arbovirus hemorrhagic fever NOS

✓4ᵗʰ 066 Other arthropod-borne viral diseases

066.0 Phlebotomus fever

Changuinola fever   Sandfly fever

DEF: Sandfly-borne viral infection occurring in Asia, Mideast and South America.

066.1 Tick-borne fever

Nairobi sheep disease   Tick fever:
Tick fever: Kemerovo
   American mountain   Quaranfil
   Colorado

066.2 Venezuelan equine fever

Venezuelan equine encephalitis

DEF: Alphavirus VEE infection causing inflammation of the brain, usually limited to South America, Mexico, and Florida; transmitted horse to mosquito to man.

066.3 Other mosquito-borne fever

Fever (viral):   Fever (viral):
   Bunyamwera   Oropouche
   Bwamba   Pixuna
   Chikungunya   Rift valley
   Guama   Ross river
   Mayaro   Wesselsbron
   Mucambo   Zika
   O'Nyong-Nyong

EXCLUDES dengue (061)
yellow fever (060.0-060.9)

✓5ᵗʰ 066.4 West Nile fever

AHA: 4Q, '02, 44

DEF: Mosquito-borne fever causing fatal inflammation of the brain, the lining of the brain, or of the lining of the brain and spinal cord.

066.40 West Nile fever, unspecified

West Nile fever NOS
West Nile fever without complications
West Nile virus NOS

066.41 West Nile fever with encephalitis

West Nile encephalitis
West Nile encephalomyelitis

AHA: 4Q, '04, 51

066.42 West Nile fever with other neurologic manifestation

Use additional code to specify the neurologic manifestation

AHA: 4Q, '04, 51

066.49 West Nile fever with other complications

Use additional code to specify the other conditions

066.8 Other specified arthropod-borne viral diseases

Chandipura fever
Piry fever

066.9 Arthropod-borne viral disease, unspecified

Arbovirus infection NOS

Ⓝ Newborn Age: 0   Ⓟ Pediatric Age: 0-17   Ⓜ Maternity Age: 12-55   Ⓐ Adult Age: 15-124

Other Diseases Due to Viruses and Chlamydiae (070-079)

✓4ᵗʰ 070 Viral hepatitis

INCLUDES viral hepatitis (acute) (chronic)

EXCLUDES cytomegalic inclusion virus hepatitis (078.5)

The following fifth-digit subclassification is for use with categories 070.2 and 070.3:

0 acute or unspecified, without mention of hepatitis delta
1 acute or unspecified, with hepatitis delta
2 chronic, without mention of hepatitis delta
3 chronic, with hepatitis delta

DEF: Hepatitis A: HAV infection is self-limiting with flulike symptoms; transmission, fecal-oral.
DEF: Hepatitis B: HBV infection can be chronic and systemic; transmission, bodily fluids.
DEF: Hepatitis C: HCV infection can be chronic and systemic; transmission, blood transfusion and unidentified agents.
DEF: Hepatitis D (delta): HDV occurs only in the presence of hepatitis B virus.
DEF: Hepatitis E: HEV is epidemic form; transmission and nature under investigation.
AHA: 2Q,' 07, 5

070.0 Viral hepatitis A with hepatic coma

070.1 Viral hepatitis A without mention of hepatic coma
Infectious hepatitis

§ ✓5ᵗʰ 070.2 Viral hepatitis B with hepatic coma
[0-3] **AHA:** 4Q, '91, 28; **For code 070.20:** 2Q, '07, 6

§ ✓5ᵗʰ 070.3 Viral hepatitis B without mention of hepatic coma
[0-3] Serum hepatitis
AHA: 1Q, '93, 28; 4Q, '91, 28
B16.9 Acute hep B w/o delta-agent & w/o hepatic coma [I-10]

✓5ᵗʰ 070.4 Other specified viral hepatitis with hepatic coma
AHA: 4Q, '91, 28

070.41 Acute hepatitis C with hepatic coma

070.42 Hepatitis delta without mention of active hepatitis B disease with hepatic coma
Hepatitis delta with hepatitis B carrier state

070.43 Hepatitis E with hepatic coma

070.44 Chronic hepatitis C with hepatic coma
AHA: 2Q, '07, 5

070.49 Other specified viral hepatitis with hepatic coma

✓5ᵗʰ 070.5 Other specified viral hepatitis without mention of hepatic coma
AHA: 4Q, '91, 28

070.51 Acute hepatitis C without mention of hepatic coma

070.52 Hepatitis delta without mention of active hepatititis B disease or hepatic coma

070.53 Hepatitis E without mention of hepatic coma

070.54 Chronic hepatitis C without mention of hepatic coma
AHA: 4Q, '08, 120; 3Q, '07, 7; 2Q, '06, 13
B18.2 Chronic viral hepatitis C [I-10]

070.59 Other specified viral hepatitis without mention of hepatic coma

070.6 Unspecified viral hepatitis with hepatic coma
EXCLUDES unspecified viral hepatitis C with hepatic coma (070.71)

✓5ᵗʰ 070.7 Unspecified viral hepatitis C

070.70 Unspecified viral hepatitis C without hepatic coma
Unspecified viral hepatitis C NOS
AHA: 4Q, '04, 52
B19.20 Unspecified viral hepatis C w/o hepatic coma [I-10]

070.71 Unspecified viral hepatitis C with hepatic coma
AHA: 4Q, '04, 52

070.9 Unspecified viral hepatitis without mention of hepatic coma
Viral hepatitis NOS
EXCLUDES unspecified viral hepatitis C without hepatic coma (070.70)

071 Rabies
Hydrophobia
Lyssa
DEF: Acute infectious disease of the CNS caused by a rhabdovirus; usually spread by bites by infected animals; progresses from fever, restlessness, and extreme excitability, to hydrophobia, seizures, confusion and death.

✓4ᵗʰ 072 Mumps
DEF: Acute infectious disease caused by paramyxovirus; usually seen in children less than 15 years of age; salivary glands are typically enlarged, involves other organs, such as testes, pancreas and meninges.

072.0 Mumps orchitis ♂

072.1 Mumps meningitis

072.2 Mumps encephalitis
Mumps meningoencephalitis

072.3 Mumps pancreatitis

✓5ᵗʰ 072.7 Mumps with other specified complications

072.71 Mumps hepatitis

072.72 Mumps polyneuropathy

072.79 Other

072.8 Mumps with unspecified complication

072.9 Mumps without mention of complication
Epidemic parotitis
Infectious parotitis

✓4ᵗʰ 073 Ornithosis
INCLUDES parrot fever
psittacosis
DEF: Chlamydia psittaci infection often transmitted from birds to humans.

073.0 With pneumonia
Lobular pneumonitis due to ornithosis

073.7 With other specified complications

073.8 With unspecified complication

073.9 Ornithosis, unspecified

✓4ᵗʰ 074 Specific diseases due to Coxsackie virus
EXCLUDES Coxsackie virus:
infection NOS (079.2)
meningitis (047.0)

074.0 Herpangina
Vesicular pharyngitis
DEF: Acute infectious coxsackie virus infection causing throat lesions, fever, and vomiting; generally affects children in summer.

074.1 Epidemic pleurodynia
Bornholm disease
Devil's grip
Epidemic:
myalgia
myositis
DEF: Paroxysmal pain in chest, accompanied by fever and usually limited to children and young adults; caused by coxsackie virus.

✓5ᵗʰ 074.2 Coxsackie carditis

074.20 Coxsackie carditis, unspecified

074.21 Coxsackie pericarditis
DEF: Coxsackie infection of the outer lining of the heart.

074.22 Coxsackie endocarditis
DEF: Coxsackie infection within the heart's cavities.

074.23 Coxsackie myocarditis
Aseptic myocarditis of newborn
DEF: Coxsackie infection of the muscle of the heart.

074.3 Hand, foot, and mouth disease
Vesicular stomatitis and exanthem
DEF: Mild coxsackie infection causing lesions on hands, feet and oral mucosa, most commonly seen in preschool children.

§ Requires fifth digit. Valid digits are in [brackets] under each code. See category 070 for codes and definitions.

Infectious and Parasitic Diseases

074.8 Other specified diseases due to Coxsackie virus
Acute lymphonodular pharyngitis

075 Infectious mononucleosis
Glandular fever
Monocytic angina
Pfeiffer's disease
DEF: Acute infection by Epstein-Barr virus causing fever, sore throat, enlarged lymph glands and spleen, and fatigue; usually seen in teens and young adults.
AHA: 3Q, '01, 13; M-A, '87, 8

✓4ᵗʰ **076 Trachoma**
EXCLUDES late effect of trachoma (139.1)
DEF: A chronic infectious disease of the cornea and conjunctiva caused by a strain of the bacteria *Chlamydia trachomatis;* the infection can cause photophobia, pain, excessive tearing and sometimes blindness.

076.0 Initial stage
Trachoma dubium

076.1 Active stage
Granular conjunctivitis (trachomatous)
Trachomatous:
follicular conjunctivitis
pannus

076.9 Trachoma, unspecified
Trachoma NOS

✓4ᵗʰ **077 Other diseases of conjunctiva due to viruses and Chlamydiae**
EXCLUDES ophthalmic complications of viral diseases classified elsewhere

077.0 Inclusion conjunctivitis
Paratrachoma
Swimming pool conjunctivitis
EXCLUDES inclusion blennorrhea (neonatal) (771.6)
DEF: Pus in conjunctiva caused by *Chlamydiae trachomatis*.

077.1 Epidemic keratoconjunctivitis
Shipyard eye
DEF: Highly contagious corneal or conjunctival infection caused by adenovirus type 8; symptoms include inflammation and corneal infiltrates.

077.2 Pharyngoconjunctival fever
Viral pharyngoconjunctivitis

077.3 Other adenoviral conjunctivitis
Acute adenoviral follicular conjunctivitis

077.4 Epidemic hemorrhagic conjunctivitis
Apollo:
conjunctivitis
disease
Conjunctivitis due to enterovirus type 70
Hemorrhagic conjunctivitis (acute) (epidemic)

077.8 Other viral conjunctivitis
Newcastle conjunctivitis

✓5ᵗʰ **077.9 Unspecified diseases of conjunctiva due to viruses and Chlamydiae**

077.98 Due to Chlamydiae

077.99 Due to viruses
Viral conjunctivitis NOS

✓4ᵗʰ **078 Other diseases due to viruses and Chlamydiae**
EXCLUDES viral infection NOS (079.0-079.9)
viremia NOS (790.8)

078.0 Molluscum contagiosum
DEF: Benign poxvirus infection causing small bumps on the skin or conjunctiva; transmitted by close contact.

✓5ᵗʰ **078.1 Viral warts**
Viral warts due to human papilloma virus
DEF: A keratotic papilloma of the epidermis caused by the human papilloma virus; the superficial vegetative lesions last for varying durations and eventually regress spontaneously.
AHA: 2Q, '97, 9; 4Q, '93, 22

078.10 Viral warts, unspecified
Verruca:
NOS
Vulgaris
Warts (infectious)

078.11 Condyloma acuminatum
Condyloma NOS
Genital warts NOS
DEF: Clusters of mucosa or epidermal lesions on external genitalia; viral infection is sexually transmitted.

078.12 Plantar wart
Verruca plantaris
AHA: 4Q, '08, 78-79

078.19 Other specified viral warts
Common wart
Flat wart
Verruca plana

078.2 Sweating fever
Miliary fever
Sweating disease
DEF: A viral infection characterized by profuse sweating; various papular, vesicular and other eruptions cause the blockage of sweat glands.

078.3 Cat-scratch disease
Benign lymphoreticulosis (of inoculation)
Cat-scratch fever

078.4 Foot and mouth disease
Aphthous fever
Epizootic:
aphthae
stomatitis
DEF: Ulcers on oral mucosa, legs, and feet after exposure to infected animal.

078.5 Cytomegaloviral disease
Cytomegalic inclusion disease
Salivary gland virus disease
Use additional code to identify manifestation, as:
cytomegalic inclusion virus:
hepatitis (573.1)
pneumonia (484.1)
EXCLUDES congenital cytomegalovirus infection (771.1)
DEF: A herpesvirus associated with serious disease morbidity including fever, leukopenia, pneumonia, retinitis, hepatitis and organ transplant; often leads to hepatomegaly, splenomegaly and thrombocytopenia; a common post-transplant complication.
AHA: 1Q, '03, 10; 3Q, '98, 4; 2Q, '93, 11; 1Q, '89, 9

078.6 Hemorrhagic nephrosonephritis
Hemorrhagic fever:
epidemic
Korean
Russian
with renal syndrome
DEF: Viral infection causing kidney dysfunction and bleeding disorders.

078.7 Arenaviral hemorrhagic fever
Hemorrhagic fever: Hemorrhagic fever:
Argentine   Junin virus
Bolivian   Machupo virus

✓5ᵗʰ **078.8 Other specified diseases due to viruses and Chlamydiae**
EXCLUDES epidemic diarrhea (009.2)
lymphogranuloma venereum (099.1)

078.81 Epidemic vertigo

078.82 Epidemic vomiting syndrome
Winter vomiting disease

078.88 Other specified diseases due to Chlamydiae
AHA: 4Q, '96, 22

078.89 Other specified diseases due to viruses
Epidemic cervical myalgia
Marburg disease

✓4ᵗʰ **079 Viral and chlamydial infection in conditions classified elsewhere and of unspecified site**
NOTE This category is provided to be used as an additional code to identify the viral agent in diseases classifiable elsewhere. This category will also be used to classify virus infection of unspecified nature or site.

079.0 Adenovirus

N Newborn Age: 0   **P** Pediatric Age: 0-17   **M** Maternity Age: 12-55   **A** Adult Age: 15-124

079.1 ECHO virus

> **DEF:** An "orphan" enteric RNA virus, certain serotypes of which are associated with human disease, especially aseptic meningitis.

079.2 Coxsackie virus

> **DEF:** A heterogenous group of viruses associated with aseptic meningitis, myocarditis, pericarditis, and acute onset juvenile diabetes.

079.3 Rhinovirus

> **DEF:** Rhinoviruses affect primarily the upper respiratory tract. Over 100 distinct types infect humans.

079.4 Human papillomavirus

> **DEF:** Viral infection caused by the genus *Papillomavirus* causing cutaneous and genital warts, including verruca vulgaris and condyloma acuminatum; certain types are associated with cervical dysplasia, cancer and other genital malignancies.
> **AHA:** 2Q, '97, 9; 4Q, '93, 22
> **TIP:** Do not assign for viral warts; see instead subcategory 078.1.

√5ᵗʰ 079.5 Retrovirus

> **EXCLUDES** *human immunodeficiency virus, type 1 [HIV-1] (042)*
> *human T-cell lymphotrophic virus, type III [HTLV-III] (042)*
> *lymphadenopathy-associated virus [LAV] (042)*
> **DEF:** A large group of RNA viruses that carry reverse transcriptase and include the leukoviruses and lentiviruses.
> **AHA:** 4Q, '93, 22, 23

> **079.50 Retrovirus, unspecified**

> **079.51 Human T-cell lymphotrophic virus, type I [HTLV-I]**

> **079.52 Human T-cell lymphotrophic virus, type II [HTLV-II]**

> **079.53 Human immunodeficiency virus, type 2 [HIV-2]**

> **079.59 Other specified retrovirus**

079.6 Respiratory syncytial virus [RSV]

> **DEF:** The major respiratory pathogen of young children, causing severe bronchitis and bronchopneumonia, and minor infection in adults.
> **AHA:** 4Q, '96, 27, 28

√5ᵗʰ 079.8 Other specified viral and chlamydial infections

> **AHA:** 1Q, '88, 12

> **079.81 Hantavirus**

> > **DEF:** An infection caused by the Muerto Canyon virus whose primary rodent reservoir is the deer mouse Peromyscus maniculatus; commonly characterized by fever, myalgias, headache, cough.
> > **AHA:** 4Q, '95, 60

> **079.82 SARS-associated coronavirus**

> > **DEF:** A life-threatening respiratory disease, severe acute respiratory syndrome (SARS); etiology coronavirus; presenting symptoms may range from mild to severe forms of flu-like conditions; fever, chills, cough, headache, myalgia; diagnosis of SARS is based upon clinical, laboratory, and epidemiological criteria.
> > **AHA:** 4Q, '03, 46

> **079.83 Parvovirus B19**

> > Human parvovirus
> > Parvovirus NOS
> > **EXCLUDES** *erythema infectiosum [fifth disease] (057.0)*
> > **DEF:** The only known parvovirus to cause disease in humans; manifestation is erythema infectiosum; also associated with polyarthropathy, chronic anemia, red cell aplasia, and fetal hydrops.
> > **AHA:** 4Q, '07, 64

> **079.88 Other specified chlamydial infection**

> **079.89 Other specified viral infection**

√5ᵗʰ 079.9 Unspecified viral and chlamydial infections

> **EXCLUDES** *viremia NOS (790.8)*

> **079.98 Unspecified chlamydial infection**
> > Chlamydial infections NOS

> **079.99 Unspecified viral infection**
> > Viral infections NOS
> > **B97.8** Other viral agents cause of dz class elsewhere   **I-10**

Rickettsioses and Other Arthropod-borne Diseases (080-088)

> **EXCLUDES** *arthropod-borne viral diseases (060.0-066.9)*

080 Louse-borne [epidemic] typhus

> Typhus (fever):
>   classical
>   epidemic
>   exanthematic NOS
>   louse-borne
> **DEF:** *Rickettsia prowazekii;* causes severe headache, rash, high fever.

√4ᵗʰ 081 Other typhus

> **081.0 Murine [endemic] typhus**
> > Typhus (fever):
> >   endemic
> >   flea-borne
> > **DEF:** Milder typhus caused by *Rickettsia typhi (mooseri);* transmitted by rat flea.

> **081.1 Brill's disease**
> > Brill-Zinsser disease
> > Recrudescent typhus (fever)

> **081.2 Scrub typhus**
> > Japanese river fever
> > Kedani fever
> > Mite-borne typhus
> > Tsutsugamushi
> > **DEF:** Typhus caused by *Rickettsia tsutsugamushi* transmitted by chigger.

> **081.9 Typhus, unspecified**
> > Typhus (fever) NOS

√4ᵗʰ 082 Tick-borne rickettsioses

> **082.0 Spotted fevers**
> > Rocky mountain spotted fever
> > Sao Paulo fever

> **082.1 Boutonneuse fever**
> > African tick typhus
> > India tick typhus
> > Kenya tick typhus
> > Marseilles fever
> > Mediterranean tick fever

> **082.2 North Asian tick fever**
> > Siberian tick typhus

> **082.3 Queensland tick typhus**

> **√5ᵗʰ 082.4 Ehrlichiosis**
> > **AHA:** 3Q, '06, 11; 4Q, '00, 38

> > **082.40 Ehrlichiosis, unspecified**

> > **082.41 Ehrlichiosis chaffeensis [E. chaffeensis]**
> > > **DEF:** A febrile illness caused by bacterial infection, also called human monocytic ehrlichiosis (HME). Causal organism is *Ehrlichia chaffeensis*, transmitted by the Lone Star tick. Symptoms include fever, chills, myalgia, nausea, vomiting, diarrhea, confusion, and severe headache occurring one week after a tick bite. Clinical findings are lymphadenopathy, rash, thrombocytopenia, leukopenia, and abnormal liver function tests.

> > **082.49 Other ehrlichiosis**

> **082.8 Other specified tick-borne rickettsioses**
> > Lone star fever
> > **AHA:** 4Q, '99, 19

> **082.9 Tick-borne rickettsiosis, unspecified**
> > Tick-borne typhus NOS

√4ᵗʰ 083 Other rickettsioses

> **083.0 Q fever**
> > **DEF:** Infection of *Coxiella burnettii* usually acquired through airborne organisms.

> **083.1 Trench fever**
> > Quintan fever
> > Wolhynian fever

> **083.2 Rickettsialpox**
> > Vesicular rickettsiosis
> > **DEF:** Infection of *Rickettsia akari* usually acquired through a mite bite.

√4ᵗʰ / √5ᵗʰ Additional Digit Required   Unspecified Code   Other Specified Code   Manifestation Code   ►◄ Revised Text   ● New Code   ▲ Revised Code Title

2011 ICD-9-CM   **Volume 1 – 15**

083.8 Other specified rickettsioses

083.9 Rickettsiosis, unspecified

☑4ᵗʰ 084 Malaria

> **NOTE** Subcategories 084.0-084.6 exclude the listed conditions with mention of pernicious complications (084.8-084.9).
>
> **EXCLUDES** congenital malaria (771.2)
>
> **DEF:** Mosquito-borne disease causing high fever and prostration and cataloged by species of *Plasmodium: P. falciparum, P. malariae, P. ovale,* and *P. vivax.*

084.0 Falciparum malaria [malignant tertian]
    Malaria (fever):
        by Plasmodium falciparum
        subtertian

084.1 Vivax malaria [benign tertian]
    Malaria (fever) by Plasmodium vivax

084.2 Quartan malaria
    Malaria (fever) by Plasmodium malariae
    Malariae malaria

084.3 Ovale malaria
    Malaria (fever) by Plasmodium ovale

084.4 Other malaria
    Monkey malaria

084.5 Mixed malaria
    Malaria (fever) by more than one parasite

084.6 Malaria, unspecified
    Malaria (fever) NOS

084.7 Induced malaria
    Therapeutically induced malaria
    EXCLUDES accidental infection from syringe, blood transfusion, etc. (084.0-084.6, above, according to parasite species)
            transmission from mother to child during delivery (771.2)

084.8 Blackwater fever
    Hemoglobinuric:
        fever (bilious)
        malaria
    Malarial hemoglobinuria
    DEF: Severe hemic and renal complication of *Plasmodium falciparum* infection.

084.9 Other pernicious complications of malaria
    Algid malaria
    Cerebral malaria
    Use additional code to identify complication, as:
        malarial:
            hepatitis (573.2)
            nephrosis (581.81)

☑4ᵗʰ 085 Leishmaniasis

085.0 Visceral [kala-azar]
    Dumdum fever
    Infection by Leishmania:
        donovani
        infantum
    Leishmaniasis:
        dermal, post-kala-azar
        Mediterranean
        visceral (Indian)

085.1 Cutaneous, urban
    Aleppo boil
    Baghdad boil
    Delhi boil
    Infection by Leishmania tropica (minor)
    Leishmaniasis, cutaneous:
        dry form
        late
        recurrent
        ulcerating
    Oriental sore

085.2 Cutaneous, Asian desert
    Infection by Leishmania tropica major
    Leishmaniasis, cutaneous:
        acute necrotizing
        rural
        wet form
        zoonotic form

085.3 Cutaneous, Ethiopian
    Infection by Leishmania ethiopica
    Leishmaniasis, cutaneous:
        diffuse
        lepromatous

085.4 Cutaneous, American
    Chiclero ulcer
    Infection by Leishmania mexicana
    Leishmaniasis tegumentaria diffusa

085.5 Mucocutaneous (American)
    Espundia
    Infection by Leishmania braziliensis
    Uta

085.9 Leishmaniasis, unspecified

☑4ᵗʰ 086 Trypanosomiasis

> Use additional code to identify manifestations, as:
>   trypanosomiasis:
>   encephalitis (323.2)
>   meningitis (321.3)

086.0 Chagas' disease with heart involvement
    American trypanosomiasis   ⎫
    Infection by Trypanosoma cruzi ⎬ with heart involvement
    Any condition classifiable to 086.2 with heart involvement

086.1 Chagas' disease with other organ involvement
    American trypanosomiasis ⎫ with involvement of organ
    Infection by Trypanosoma cruzi ⎭   other than heart
    Any condition classifiable to 086.2 with involvement of organ other than heart

086.2 Chagas' disease without mention of organ involvement
    American trypanosomiasis
    Infection by Trypanosoma cruzi

086.3 Gambian trypanosomiasis
    Gambian sleeping sickness
    Infection by Trypanosoma gambiense

086.4 Rhodesian trypanosomiasis
    Infection by Trypanosoma rhodesiense
    Rhodesian sleeping sickness

086.5 African trypanosomiasis, unspecified
    Sleeping sickness NOS

086.9 Trypanosomiasis, unspecified

☑4ᵗʰ 087 Relapsing fever

> **INCLUDES** recurrent fever
>
> **DEF:** Infection of *Borrelia;* symptoms are episodic and include fever and arthralgia.

087.0 Louse-borne

087.1 Tick-borne

087.9 Relapsing fever, unspecified

☑4ᵗʰ 088 Other arthropod-borne diseases

088.0 Bartonellosis
    Carrión's disease   Verruga peruana
    Oroya fever

☑5ᵗʰ 088.8 Other specified arthropod-borne diseases

088.81 Lyme disease
    Erythema chronicum migrans
    DEF: A recurrent multisystem disorder caused by the spirochete *Borrelia burgdorferi* with the carrier being the tick; begins with lesions of erythema chronicum migrans; followed by arthritis of the large joints, myalgia, malaise, and neurological and cardiac manifestations.
    AHA: 4Q, '91, 15; 3Q, '90, 14; 2Q, '89, 10
    TIP: Do not assign if patient has been cured of Lyme disease but has residual chronic condition; refer instead to late-effect code 139.8.

Ⓝ Newborn Age: 0   Ⓟ Pediatric Age: 0-17   Ⓜ Maternity Age: 12-55   Ⓐ Adult Age: 15-124

088.82 Babesiosis
Babesiasis
DEF: A tick-borne disease caused by infection of *Babesia*, characterized by fever, malaise, listlessness, severe anemia and hemoglobinuria.
AHA: 4Q, '93, 23

088.89 Other

088.9 Arthropod-borne disease, unspecified

Syphilis and Other Venereal Diseases (090-099)

EXCLUDES nonvenereal endemic syphilis (104.0)
urogenital trichomoniasis (131.0)

√4ᵗʰ **090 Congenital syphilis**
DEF: Infection by spirochete*Treponema pallidum* acquired in utero from the infected mother.

090.0 Early congenital syphilis, symptomatic
Congenital syphilitic: Congenital syphilitic:
  choroiditis   splenomegaly
  coryza (chronic) Syphilitic (congenital):
  hepatomegaly   epiphysitis
  mucous patches osteochondritis
  periostitis   pemphigus
Any congenital syphilitic condition specified as early or manifest less than two years after birth

090.1 Early congenital syphilis, latent
Congenital syphilis without clinical manifestations, with positive serological reaction and negative spinal fluid test, less than two years after birth

090.2 Early congenital syphilis, unspecified
Congenital syphilis NOS, less than two years after birth

090.3 Syphilitic interstitial keratitis
Syphilitic keratitis:
  parenchymatous
  punctata profunda
EXCLUDES interstitial keratitis NOS (370.50)

√5ᵗʰ **090.4 Juvenile neurosyphilis**
Use additional code to identify any associated mental disorder
DEF: *Treponema pallidum* infection involving the nervous system.

090.40 Juvenile neurosyphilis, unspecified
Congenital neurosyphilis
Dementia paralytica juvenilis
Juvenile:
  general paresis
  tabes
  taboparesis

090.41 Congenital syphilitic encephalitis
DEF: Congenital *Treponema pallidum* infection involving the brain.

090.42 Congenital syphilitic meningitis
DEF: Congenital *Treponema pallidum* infection involving the lining of the brain and/or spinal cord.

090.49 Other

090.5 Other late congenital syphilis, symptomatic
Gumma due to congenital syphilis
Hutchinson's teeth
Syphilitic saddle nose
Any congenital syphilitic condition specified as late or manifest two years or more after birth

090.6 Late congenital syphilis, latent
Congenital syphilis without clinical manifestations, with positive serological reaction and negative spinal fluid test, two years or more after birth

090.7 Late congenital syphilis, unspecified
Congenital syphilis NOS, two years or more after birth

090.9 Congenital syphilis, unspecified

√4ᵗʰ **091 Early syphilis, symptomatic**
EXCLUDES early cardiovascular syphilis (093.0-093.9)
early neurosyphilis (094.0-094.9)

091.0 Genital syphilis (primary)
Genital chancre
DEF: Genital lesion at the site of initial infection by *Treponema pallidum.*

091.1 Primary anal syphilis
DEF: Anal lesion at the site of initial infection by *Treponema pallidum.*

091.2 Other primary syphilis
Primary syphilis of: Primary syphilis of:
  breast   lip
  fingers   tonsils
DEF: Lesion at the site of initial infection by *Treponema pallidum.*

091.3 Secondary syphilis of skin or mucous membranes
Condyloma latum   Secondary syphilis of:
Secondary syphilis of: skin
  anus   tonsils
  mouth   vulva
  pharynx
DEF: Transitory or chronic lesions following initial syphilis infection.

091.4 Adenopathy due to secondary syphilis
Syphilitic adenopathy (secondary)
Syphilitic lymphadenitis (secondary)

√5ᵗʰ **091.5 Uveitis due to secondary syphilis**

091.50 Syphilitic uveitis, unspecified

091.51 Syphilitic chorioretinitis (secondary)
DEF: Inflammation of choroid and retina as a secondary infection.

091.52 Syphilitic iridocyclitis (secondary)
DEF: Inflammation of iris and ciliary body as a secondary infection.

√5ᵗʰ **091.6 Secondary syphilis of viscera and bone**

091.61 Secondary syphilitic periostitis
DEF: Inflammation of outer layers of bone as a secondary infection.

091.62 Secondary syphilitic hepatitis
Secondary syphilis of liver

091.69 Other viscera

091.7 Secondary syphilis, relapse
Secondary syphilis, relapse (treated) (untreated)
DEF: Return of symptoms of syphilis following asymptomatic period.

√5ᵗʰ **091.8 Other forms of secondary syphilis**

091.81 Acute syphilitic meningitis (secondary)
DEF: Sudden, severe inflammation of the lining of the brain and/or spinal cord as a secondary infection.

091.82 Syphilitic alopecia
DEF: Hair loss following initial syphilis infection.

091.89 Other

091.9 Unspecified secondary syphilis

√4ᵗʰ **092 Early syphilis, latent**
INCLUDES syphilis (acquired) without clinical manifestations, with positive serological reaction and negative spinal fluid test, less than two years after infection

092.0 Early syphilis, latent, serological relapse after treatment

092.9 Early syphilis, latent, unspecified

√4ᵗʰ **093 Cardiovascular syphilis**

093.0 Aneurysm of aorta, specified as syphilitic
Dilatation of aorta, specified as syphilitic

093.1 Syphilitic aortitis
DEF: Inflammation of the aorta — the main artery leading from the heart.

√5ᵗʰ **093.2 Syphilitic endocarditis**
DEF: Inflammation of the tissues lining the cavities of the heart.

093.20 Valve, unspecified
Syphilitic ostial coronary disease

093.21 Mitral valve

093.22 Aortic valve
Syphilitic aortic incompetence or stenosis

093.23 Tricuspid valve

093.24 Pulmonary valve

√5ᵗʰ **093.8 Other specified cardiovascular syphilis**

093.81 Syphilitic pericarditis
DEF: Inflammation of the outer lining of the heart.

093.82 Syphilitic myocarditis
DEF: Inflammation of the muscle of the heart.

093.89 Other

093.9 Cardiovascular syphilis, unspecified

√4ᵗʰ **094 Neurosyphilis**
Use additional code to identify any associated mental disorder

094.0 Tabes dorsalis
Locomotor ataxia (progressive)
Posterior spinal sclerosis (syphilitic)
Tabetic neurosyphilis
Use additional code to identify manifestation, as:
neurogenic arthropathy [Charcot's joint disease] (713.5)
DEF: Progressive degeneration of nerves associated with long-term syphilis; causing pain, wasting away, incontinence, and ataxia.

094.1 General paresis
Dementia paralytica
General paralysis (of the insane) (progressive)
Paretic neurosyphilis
Taboparesis
DEF: Degeneration of brain associated with long-term syphilis, causing loss of brain function, progressive dementia, and paralysis.

094.2 Syphilitic meningitis
Meningovascular syphilis
EXCLUDES acute syphilitic meningitis (secondary) (091.81)
DEF: Inflammation of the lining of the brain and/or spinal cord.

094.3 Asymptomatic neurosyphilis

√5ᵗʰ **094.8 Other specified neurosyphilis**

094.81 Syphilitic encephalitis

094.82 Syphilitic Parkinsonism
DEF: Decreased motor function, tremors, and muscular rigidity.

094.83 Syphilitic disseminated retinochoroiditis
DEF: Inflammation of retina and choroid due to neurosyphilis.

094.84 Syphilitic optic atrophy
DEF: Degeneration of the eye and its nerves due to neurosyphilis.

094.85 Syphilitic retrobulbar neuritis
DEF: Inflammation of the posterior optic nerve due to neurosyphilis.

094.86 Syphilitic acoustic neuritis
DEF: Inflammation of acoustic nerve due to neurosyphilis.

094.87 Syphilitic ruptured cerebral aneurysm

094.89 Other

094.9 Neurosyphilis, unspecified
Gumma (syphilitic)   ⎫
Syphilis (early) (late)   ⎬ of central nervous system
Syphiloma   ⎭ NOS

095 Other forms of late syphilis, with symptoms
INCLUDES gumma (syphilitic)
syphilis, late, tertiary, or unspecified stage

095.0 Syphilitic episcleritis

095.1 Syphilis of lung

095.2 Syphilitic peritonitis

095.3 Syphilis of liver

095.4 Syphilis of kidney

095.5 Syphilis of bone

095.6 Syphilis of muscle
Syphilitic myositis

095.7 Syphilis of synovium, tendon, and bursa
Syphilitic:
bursitis
synovitis

095.8 Other specified forms of late symptomatic syphilis
EXCLUDES cardiovascular syphilis (093.0-093.9)
neurosyphilis (094.0-094.9)

095.9 Late symptomatic syphilis, unspecified

096 Late syphilis, latent
Syphilis (acquired) without clinical manifestations, with positive serological reaction and negative spinal fluid test, two years or more after infection

√4ᵗʰ **097 Other and unspecified syphilis**

097.0 Late syphilis, unspecified

097.1 Latent syphilis, unspecified
Positive serological reaction for syphilis

097.9 Syphilis, unspecified
Syphilis (acquired) NOS
EXCLUDES syphilis NOS causing death under two years of age (090.9)

√4ᵗʰ **098 Gonococcal infections**
DEF: Neisseria gonorrhoeae infection generally acquired in utero or in sexual congress.

098.0 Acute, of lower genitourinary tract
Gonococcal:
Bartholinitis (acute)
urethritis (acute)
vulvovaginitis (acute)
Gonorrhea (acute):
NOS
genitourinary (tract) NOS

√5ᵗʰ **098.1 Acute, of upper genitourinary tract**

098.10 Gonococcal infection (acute) of upper genitourinary tract, site unspecified

098.11 Gonococcal cystitis (acute) upper
Gonorrhea (acute) of bladder

098.12 Gonococcal prostatitis (acute) ♂

098.13 Gonococcal epididymo-orchitis (acute) ♂
Gonococcal orchitis (acute)
DEF: Acute inflammation of the testes.

098.14 Gonococcal seminal vesiculitis (acute) ♂
Gonorrhea (acute) of seminal vesicle

098.15 Gonococcal cervicitis (acute) ♀
Gonorrhea (acute) of cervix

098.16 Gonococcal endometritis (acute) ♀
Gonorrhea (acute) of uterus

098.17 Gonococcal salpingitis, specified as acute ♀
DEF: Acute inflammation of the fallopian tubes.

098.19 Other

098.2 Chronic, of lower genitourinary tract
Gonococcal:
Bartholinitis   ⎫
urethritis   ⎪ specified as chronic or with
vulvovaginitis   ⎬ duration of two months
Gonorrhea: ⎪ or more
NOS   ⎪
genitourinary (tract) ⎭
Any condition classifiable to 098.0 specified as chronic or with duration of two months or more

√5ᵗʰ **098.3 Chronic, of upper genitourinary tract**
INCLUDES any condition classifiable to 098.1 stated as chronic or with a duration of two months or more

098.30 Chronic gonococcal infection of upper genitourinary tract, site unspecified

098.31 Gonococcal cystitis, chronic
Gonorrhea of bladder, chronic
Any condition classifiable to 098.11, specified as chronic

098.32 Gonococcal prostatitis, chronic ♂
Any condition classifiable to 098.12, specified as chronic

098.33 Gonococcal epididymo-orchitis, chronic ♂
Chronic gonococcal orchitis
Any condition classifiable to 098.13, specified as chronic
DEF: Chronic inflammation of the testes.

098.34 Gonococcal seminal vesiculitis, chronic ♂
Gonorrhea of seminal vesicle, chronic
Any condition classifiable to 098.14, specified as chronic

098.35 Gonococcal cervicitis, chronic ♀
Gonorrhea of cervix, chronic
Any condition classifiable to 098.15, specified as chronic

098.36 Gonococcal endometritis, chronic ♀
Any condition classifiable to 098.16, specified as chronic
DEF: Chronic inflammation of the uterus.

098.37 Gonococcal salpingitis (chronic) ♀
DEF: Chronic inflammation of the fallopian tubes.

098.39 Other

√5ᵗʰ **098.4 Gonococcal infection of eye**

098.40 Gonococcal conjunctivitis (neonatorum)
Gonococcal ophthalmia (neonatorum)
DEF: Infection of conjunctiva present at birth.

098.41 Gonococcal iridocyclitis
DEF: Inflammation and infection of iris and ciliary body.

098.42 Gonococcal endophthalmia
DEF: Inflammation and infection of contents of eyeball.

098.43 Gonococcal keratitis
DEF: Inflammation and infection of the cornea.

098.49 Other

√5ᵗʰ **098.5 Gonococcal infection of joint**

098.50 Gonococcal arthritis
Gonococcal infection of joint NOS

098.51 Gonococcal synovitis and tenosynovitis

098.52 Gonococcal bursitis
DEF: Inflammation of the sac-like cavities in a joint.

098.53 Gonococcal spondylitis

098.59 Other
Gonococcal rheumatism

098.6 Gonococcal infection of pharynx

098.7 Gonococcal infection of anus and rectum
Gonococcal proctitis

√5ᵗʰ **098.8 Gonococcal infection of other specified sites**

098.81 Gonococcal keratosis (blennorrhagica)
DEF: Pustular skin lesions caused by *Neisseria gonorrhoeae*.

098.82 Gonococcal meningitis
DEF: Inflammation of lining of brain and/or spinal cord.

098.83 Gonococcal pericarditis
DEF: Inflammation of the outer lining of the heart.

098.84 Gonococcal endocarditis
DEF: Inflammation of tissues lining the cavities of heart.

098.85 Other gonococcal heart disease

098.86 Gonococcal peritonitis
DEF: Inflammation of the membrane lining the abdomen.

098.89 Other
Gonococcemia

√4ᵗʰ **099 Other venereal diseases**

099.0 Chancroid
Bubo (inguinal):
chancroidal
due to Hemophilus ducreyi
Chancre:
Ducrey's
simple
soft
Ulcus molle (cutis)(skin)
DEF: A sexually transmitted disease caused by *Haemophilus ducreyi*; identified by a painful primary ulcer at the site of inoculation (usually external genitalia) with related lymphadenitis.

099.1 Lymphogranuloma venereum
Climatic or tropical bubo
(Durand-) Nicolas-Favre disease
Esthiomene
Lymphogranuloma inguinale
DEF: Sexually transmitted infection of *Chlamydia trachomatis* causing skin lesions.

099.2 Granuloma inguinale
Donovanosis
Granuloma pudendi (ulcerating)
Granuloma venereum
Pudendal ulcer
DEF: Chronic, sexually transmitted infection of *Calymmatobacterium granulomatis* causing progressive, anogenital skin ulcers.

099.3 Reiter's disease
Reiter's syndrome
Use additional code for associated:
arthropathy (711.1)
conjunctivitis (372.33)
DEF: A symptom complex of unknown etiology consisting of urethritis, conjunctivitis, arthritis and myocutaneous lesions; occurs most commonly in young men and patients with HIV. Also a form of reactive arthritis.

√5ᵗʰ **099.4 Other nongonococcal urethritis [NGU]**

099.40 Unspecified
Nonspecific urethritis

099.41 Chlamydia trachomatis

099.49 Other specified organism

√5ᵗʰ **099.5 Other venereal diseases due to Chlamydia trachomatis**
EXCLUDES *Chlamydia trachomatis* infection of conjunctiva (076.0-076.9, 077.0, 077.9)
Lymphogranuloma venereum (099.1)
DEF: Venereal diseases caused by *Chlamydia trachomatis* at other sites besides the urethra (e.g., pharynx, anus and rectum, conjunctiva and peritoneum).

099.50 Unspecified site

099.51 Pharynx

099.52 Anus and rectum

099.53 Lower genitourinary sites
Use additional code to specify site of infection, such as:
bladder (595.4)
cervix (616.0)
vagina and vulva (616.11)
EXCLUDES *urethra (099.41)*

099.54 Other genitourinary sites
Use additional code to specify site of infection, such as:
pelvic inflammatory disease NOS (614.9)
testis and epididymis (604.91)

099.55 Unspecified genitourinary site

099.56 Peritoneum
Perihepatitis

099.59 Other specified site

099.8 Other specified venereal diseases

099.9 Venereal disease, unspecified

Infectious and Parasitic Diseases

100–110.2

Other Spirochetal Diseases (100-104)

✔4ᵗʰ 100   Leptospirosis
DEF: A blood infection of any spirochete of the genus Leptospire; transmitted to humans by exposure to contaminated animal tissues or water. Patients present with flulike symptoms, characteristic muscle aches involving the thighs and low back.

100.0   Leptospirosis icterohemorrhagica
Leptospiral or spirochetal jaundice (hemorrhagic)
Weil's disease

✔5ᵗʰ 100.8   Other specified leptospiral infections

100.81   Leptospiral meningitis (aseptic)

100.89   Other
Fever:
  Fort Bragg
  pretibial
  swamp
Infection by Leptospira:
  australis
  bataviae
  pyrogenes

100.9   Leptospirosis, unspecified

101   Vincent's angina
Acute necrotizing ulcerative:
  gingivitis
  stomatitis
Fusospirochetal pharyngitis
Spirochetal stomatitis
Trench mouth
Vincent's:
  gingivitis
  infection [any site]
DEF: Painful ulceration with edema and hypermic patches of the oropharyngeal and throat membranes; it is caused by spreading of acute ulcerative gingivitis.

✔4ᵗʰ 102   Yaws
INCLUDES   frambesia
              pian
DEF: An infectious, endemic, tropical disease caused by *Treponema pertenue;* usually affects persons 15 years old or younger; a primary cutaneous lesion develops, then a granulomatous skin eruption, and occasionally lesions that destroy skin and bone.

102.0   Initial lesions
Chancre of yaws
Frambesia, initial or primary
Initial frambesial ulcer
Mother yaw

102.1   Multiple papillomata and wet crab yaws
Butter yaws
Frambesioma
Pianoma
Plantar or palmar papilloma of yaws

102.2   Other early skin lesions
Cutaneous yaws, less than five years after infection
Early yaws (cutaneous) (macular) (papular) (maculopapular)
    (micropapular)
Frambeside of early yaws

102.3   Hyperkeratosis
Ghoul hand
Hyperkeratosis, palmar or plantar (early) (late) due to yaws
Worm-eaten soles
DEF: Overgrowth of skin of palm or bottoms of feet, due to yaws.

102.4   Gummata and ulcers
Gummatous frambeside
Nodular late yaws (ulcerated)
DEF: Rubbery lesions and areas of dead skin caused by yaws.

102.5   Gangosa
Rhinopharyngitis mutilans
DEF: Massive, mutilating lesions of the nose and oral cavity caused by yaws.

102.6   Bone and joint lesions
Goundou
Gumma, bone   } of yaws (late)
Gummatous osteitis or periostitis

Hydrarthrosis
Osteitis   } of yaws (early) (late)
Periostitis (hypertrophic)

102.7   Other manifestations
Juxta-articular nodules of yaws
Mucosal yaws

102.8   Latent yaws
Yaws without clinical manifestations, with positive serology

102.9   Yaws, unspecified

✔4ᵗʰ 103   Pinta
DEF: A chronic form of treponematosis, endemic in areas of tropical America; it is identified by the presence of red, violet, blue, coffee-colored or white spots on the skin.

103.0   Primary lesions
Chancre (primary)
Papule (primary)   } of pinta [carate]
Pintid

103.1   Intermediate lesions
Erythematous plaques
Hyperchronic lesions   } of pinta [carate]
Hyperkeratosis

103.2   Late lesions
Cardiovascular lesions
Skin lesions:
  achromic
  cicatricial   } of pinta [carate]
  dyschromic
Vitiligo

103.3   Mixed lesions
Achromic and hyperchromic skin lesions of pinta [carate]

103.9   Pinta, unspecified

✔4ᵗʰ 104   Other spirochetal infection

104.0   Nonvenereal endemic syphilis
Bejel
Njovera
DEF: *Treponema pallidum, T. pertenue, or T. caroteum* infection transmitted non-sexually, causing lesions on mucosa and skin.

104.8   Other specified spirochetal infections
EXCLUDES   relapsing fever (087.0-087.9)
               syphilis (090.0-097.9)

104.9   Spirochetal infection, unspecified

Mycoses (110-118)
Use additional code to identify manifestation as:
  arthropathy (711.6)
  meningitis (321.0-321.1)
  otitis externa (380.15)
EXCLUDES   infection by Actinomycetales, such as species of Actinomyces,
               Actinomadura, Nocardia, Streptomyces (039.0-039.9)

✔4ᵗʰ 110   Dermatophytosis
INCLUDES   infection by species of Epidermophyton, Microsporum,
               and Trichophyton
               tinea, any type except those in 111
DEF: Superficial infection of the skin caused by a parasitic fungus.

110.0   Of scalp and beard
Kerion
Sycosis, mycotic
Trichophytic tinea [black dot tinea], scalp

110.1   Of nail
Dermatophytic onychia
Onychomycosis
Tinea unguium
B35.1 Tinea unguium   I-10

110.2   Of hand
Tinea manuum

N Newborn Age: 0   **P** Pediatric Age: 0-17   **M** Maternity Age: 12-55   **A** Adult Age: 15-124

110.3 Of groin and perianal area
 Dhobie itch
 Eczema marginatum
 Tinea cruris

110.4 Of foot
 Athlete's foot
 Tinea pedis

110.5 Of the body
 Herpes circinatus
 Tinea imbricata [Tokelau]

110.6 Deep seated dermatophytosis
 Granuloma trichophyticum
 Majocchi's granuloma

110.8 Of other specified sites

110.9 Of unspecified site
 Favus NOS
 Microsporic tinea NOS
 Ringworm NOS

√4ᵗʰ **111 Dermatomycosis, other and unspecified**

111.0 Pityriasis versicolor
 Infection by Malassezia [Pityrosporum] furfur
 Tinea flava
 Tinea versicolor

111.1 Tinea nigra
 Infection by Cladosporium species
 Keratomycosis nigricans
 Microsporosis nigra
 Pityriasis nigra
 Tinea palmaris nigra

111.2 Tinea blanca
 Infection by Trichosporon (beigelii) cutaneum
 White piedra

111.3 Black piedra
 Infection by Piedraia hortai

111.8 Other specified dermatomycoses

111.9 Dermatomycosis, unspecified

√4ᵗʰ **112 Candidiasis**
 [INCLUDES] infection by Candida species
 moniliasis
 [EXCLUDES] *neonatal monilial infection (771.7)*
 DEF: Fungal infection caused by *Candida*; usually seen in mucous membranes or skin.

112.0 Of mouth
 Thrush (oral)
 B37.0 Candidal stomatitis   I-10

112.1 Of vulva and vagina   ♀
 Candidal vulvovaginitis
 Monilial vulvovaginitis
 B37.3 Candidiasis of vulva and vagina   I-10

112.2 Of other urogenital sites
 Candidal balanitis
 AHA: 4Q, '03, 105; 4Q, '96, 33

112.3 Of skin and nails
 Candidal intertrigo
 Candidal onychia
 Candidal perionyxis [paronychia]
 B37.2 Candidiasis of skin and nail   I-10

112.4 Of lung
 Candidal pneumonia
 AHA: 2Q, '98, 7

112.5 Disseminated
 Systemic candidiasis
 AHA: 2Q, '00, 5; 2Q, '89, 10

√5ᵗʰ **112.8 Of other specified sites**

112.81 Candidal endocarditis

112.82 Candidal otitis externa
 Otomycosis in moniliasis

112.83 Candidal meningitis

112.84 Candidal esophagitis
 AHA: 4Q, '92, 19
 B37.81 Candidal esophagitis   I-10

112.85 Candidal enteritis
 AHA: 4Q, '92, 19

112.89 Other
 AHA: 1Q, '92, 17; 3Q, '91, 20

112.9 Of unspecified site

√4ᵗʰ **114 Coccidioidomycosis**
 [INCLUDES] infection by Coccidioides (immitis)
 Posada-Wernicke disease
 DEF: A fungal disease caused by inhalation of dust particles containing arthrospores of *Coccidioides immitis;* a self-limited respiratory infection; the primary form is known as San Joaquin fever, desert fever or valley fever.
 AHA: 4Q, '93, 23

114.0 Primary coccidioidomycosis (pulmonary)
 Acute pulmonary coccidioidomycosis
 Coccidioidomycotic pneumonitis
 Desert rheumatism
 Pulmonary coccidioidomycosis
 San Joaquin Valley fever
 DEF: Acute, self-limiting *Coccidioides immitis* infection of the lung.
 B38.0 Acute pulmonary coccidioidomycosis   I-10

114.1 Primary extrapulmonary coccidioidomycosis
 Chancriform syndrome
 Primary cutaneous coccidioidomycosis
 DEF: Acute, self-limiting *Coccidioides immitis* infection in nonpulmonary site.

114.2 Coccidioidal meningitis
 DEF: *Coccidioides immitis* infection of the lining of the brain and/or spinal cord.

114.3 Other forms of progressive coccidioidomycosis
 Coccidioidal granuloma
 Disseminated coccidioidomycosis

114.4 Chronic pulmonary coccidioidomycosis

114.5 Pulmonary coccidioidomycosis, unspecified

114.9 Coccidioidomycosis, unspecified

√4ᵗʰ **115 Histoplasmosis**
 The following fifth-digit subclassification is for use with category 115:
 0 without mention of manifestation
 1 meningitis
 2 retinitis
 3 pericarditis
 4 endocarditis
 5 pneumonia
 9 other

§ √5ᵗʰ **115.0 Infection by Histoplasma capsulatum**
 [0-5, 9] American histoplasmosis
 Darling's disease
 Reticuloendothelial cytomycosis
 Small form histoplasmosis
 DEF: Infection resulting from inhalation of fungal spores, causing acute pneumonia, an influenza-like illness, or a disseminated disease of the reticuloendothelial system. In immunocompromised patients it can reactivate, affecting lungs, meninges, heart, peritoneum and adrenals.

§ √5ᵗʰ **115.1 Infection by Histoplasma duboisii**
 [0-5, 9] African histoplasmosis
 Large form histoplasmosis

§ √5ᵗʰ **115.9 Histoplasmosis, unspecified**
 [0-5, 9] Histoplasmosis NOS

√4ᵗʰ **116 Blastomycotic infection**

116.0 Blastomycosis
 Blastomycotic dermatitis
 Chicago disease
 Cutaneous blastomycosis
 Disseminated blastomycosis
 Gilchrist's disease
 Infection by Blastomyces [Ajellomyces] dermatitidis
 North American blastomycosis
 Primary pulmonary blastomycosis

---

§ Requires fifth digit. Valid digits are in [brackets] under each code. See category 115 for codes and definitions.

116.1 Paracoccidioidomycosis
Brazilian blastomycosis
Infection by Paracoccidioides [Blastomyces] brasiliensis
Lutz-Splendore-Almeida disease
Mucocutaneous-lymphangitic paracoccidioidomycosis
Pulmonary paracoccidioidomycosis
South American blastomycosis
Visceral paracoccidioidomycosis

116.2 Lobomycosis
Infections by Loboa [Blastomyces] loboi
Keloidal blastomycosis
Lobo's disease

√4ᵗʰ **117 Other mycoses**

117.0 Rhinosporidiosis
Infection by Rhinosporidium seeberi

117.1 Sporotrichosis
Cutaneous sporotrichosis
Disseminated sporotrichosis
Infection by Sporothrix [Sporotrichum] schenckii
Lymphocutaneous sporotrichosis
Pulmonary sporotrichosis
Sporotrichosis of the bones

117.2 Chromoblastomycosis
Chromomycosis
Infection by Cladosporidium carrionii, Fonsecaea compactum, Fonsecaea pedrosoi, Phialophora verrucosa

117.3 Aspergillosis
Infection by Aspergillus species, mainly A. fumigatus, A. flavus group, A. terreus group
AHA: 4Q, '97, 40

117.4 Mycotic mycetomas
Infection by various genera and species of Ascomycetes and Deuteromycetes, such as Acremonium [Cephalosporium] falciforme, Neotestudina rosatii, Madurella grisea, Madurella mycetomii, Pyrenochaeta romeroi, Zopfia [Leptosphaeria] senegalensis
Madura foot, mycotic
Maduromycosis, mycotic
EXCLUDES actinomycotic mycetomas (039.0-039.9)

117.5 Cryptococcosis
Busse-Buschke's disease
European cryptococcosis
Infection by Cryptococcus neoformans
Pulmonary cryptococcosis
Systemic cryptococcosis
Torula

117.6 Allescheriosis [Petriellidosis]
Infections by Allescheria [Petriellidium] boydii [Monosporium apiospermum]
EXCLUDES mycotic mycetoma (117.4)

117.7 Zygomycosis [Phycomycosis or Mucormycosis]
Infection by species of Absidia, Basidiobolus, Conidiobolus, Cunninghamella, Entomophthora, Mucor, Rhizopus, Saksenaea

117.8 Infection by dematiacious fungi, [Phaehyphomycosis]
Infection by dematiacious fungi, such as Cladosporium trichoides [bantianum], Dreschlera hawaiiensis, Phialophora gougerotii, Phialophora jeanselmi

117.9 Other and unspecified mycoses

118 Opportunistic mycoses
Infection of skin, subcutaneous tissues, and/or organs by a wide variety of fungi generally considered to be pathogenic to compromised hosts only (e.g., infection by species of Alternaria, Dreschlera, Fusarium)
Use additional code to identify manifestation, such as:
keratitis (370.8)

Helminthiases (120-129)

√4ᵗʰ **120 Schistosomiasis [bilharziasis]**
DEF: Infection caused by *Schistosoma*, a genus of flukes or trematode parasites.

120.0 Schistosoma haematobium
Vesical schistosomiasis NOS

120.1 Schistosoma mansoni
Intestinal schistosomiasis NOS

120.2 Schistosoma japonicum
Asiatic schistosomiasis NOS
Katayama disease or fever

120.3 Cutaneous
Cercarial dermatitis
Infection by cercariae of Schistosoma
Schistosome dermatitis
Swimmers' itch

120.8 Other specified schistosomiasis
Infection by Schistosoma:
bovis
intercalatum
mattheii
spindale
Schistosomiasis chestermani

120.9 Schistosomiasis, unspecified
Blood flukes NOS
Hemic distomiasis

√4ᵗʰ **121 Other trematode infections**

121.0 Opisthorchiasis
Infection by:
cat liver fluke
Opisthorchis (felineus) (tenuicollis) (viverrini)

121.1 Clonorchiasis
Biliary cirrhosis due to clonorchiasis
Chinese liver fluke disease
Hepatic distomiasis due to Clonorchis sinensis
Oriental liver fluke disease

121.2 Paragonimiasis
Infection by Paragonimus
Lung fluke disease (oriental)
Pulmonary distomiasis

121.3 Fascioliasis
Infection by Fasciola:
gigantica
hepatica
Liver flukes NOS
Sheep liver fluke infection

121.4 Fasciolopsiasis
Infection by Fasciolopsis (buski)
Intestinal distomiasis

121.5 Metagonimiasis
Infection by Metagonimus yokogawai

121.6 Heterophyiasis
Infection by:
Heterophyes heterophyes
Stellantchasmus falcatus

121.8 Other specified trematode infections
Infection by:
Dicrocoelium dendriticum
Echinostoma ilocanum
Gastrodiscoides hominis

121.9 Trematode infection, unspecified
Distomiasis NOS
Fluke disease NOS

√4ᵗʰ **122 Echinococcosis**
INCLUDES echinococciasis
hydatid disease
hydatidosis
DEF: Infection caused by larval forms of tapeworms of the genus *Echinococcus.*

122.0 Echinococcus granulosus infection of liver

| N Newborn Age: 0 | P Pediatric Age: 0-17 | M Maternity Age: 12-55 | A Adult Age: 15-124 |

2011 ICD-9-CM

122.1 Echinococcus granulosus infection of lung

122.2 Echinococcus granulosus infection of thyroid

122.3 Echinococcus granulosus infection, other

122.4 Echinococcus granulosus infection, unspecified

122.5 Echinococcus multilocularis infection of liver

122.6 Echinococcus multilocularis infection, other

122.7 Echinococcus multilocularis infection, unspecified

122.8 Echinococcosis, unspecified, of liver

122.9 Echinococcosis, other and unspecified

√4ᵗʰ **123 Other cestode infection**

123.0 Taenia solium infection, intestinal form
Pork tapeworm (adult) (infection)

123.1 Cysticercosis
Cysticerciasis
Infection by Cysticercus cellulosae [larval form of Taenia solium]
AHA: 2Q, '97, 8

123.2 Taenia saginata infection
Beef tapeworm (infection)
Infection by Taeniarhynchus saginatus

123.3 Taeniasis, unspecified

123.4 Diphyllobothriasis, intestinal
Diphyllobothrium (adult) (latum) (pacificum) infection
Fish tapeworm (infection)

123.5 Sparganosis [larval diphyllobothriasis]
Infection by:
Diphyllobothrium larvae
Sparganum (mansoni) (proliferum)
Spirometra larvae

123.6 Hymenolepiasis
Dwarf tapeworm (infection)
Hymenolepis (diminuta) (nana) infection
Rat tapeworm (infection)

123.8 Other specified cestode infection
Diplogonoporus (grandis) ⎫
Dipylidium (caninum)   ⎬ infection
Dog tapeworm (infection) ⎭

123.9 Cestode infection, unspecified
Tapeworm (infection) NOS

124 Trichinosis
Trichinella spiralis infection
Trichinellosis
Trichiniasis
DEF: Infection by *Trichinella spiralis,* the smallest of the parasitic nematodes.

√4ᵗʰ/√5ᵗʰ **125 Filarial infection and dracontiasis**

125.0 Bancroftian filariasis
Chyluria ⎫
Elephantiasis ⎪
Infection ⎬ due to Wuchereria bancrofti
Lymphadenitis ⎪
Lymphangitis ⎪
Wuchereriasis ⎭

125.1 Malayan filariasis
Brugia filariasis ⎫
Chyluria ⎪
Elephantiasis ⎬ due to Brugia [Wuchereria] malayi
Infection ⎪
Lymphadenitis ⎪
Lymphangitis ⎭

125.2 Loiasis
Eyeworm disease of Africa
Loa loa infection

125.3 Onchocerciasis
Onchocerca volvulus infection
Onchocercosis

125.4 Dipetalonemiasis
Infection by:
Acanthocheilonema perstans
Dipetalonema perstans

125.5 Mansonella ozzardi infection
Filariasis ozzardi

125.6 Other specified filariasis
Dirofilaria infection
Infection by:
Acanthocheilonema streptocerca
Dipetalonema streptocerca

125.7 Dracontiasis
Guinea-worm infection
Infection by Dracunculus medinensis

125.9 Unspecified filariasis

√4ᵗʰ **126 Ancylostomiasis and necatoriasis**
INCLUDES cutaneous larva migrans due to Ancylostoma
hookworm (disease) (infection)
uncinariasis

126.0 Ancylostoma duodenale

126.1 Necator americanus

126.2 Ancylostoma braziliense

126.3 Ancylostoma ceylanicum

126.8 Other specified Ancylostoma

126.9 Ancylostomiasis and necatoriasis, unspecified
Creeping eruption NOS
Cutaneous larva migrans NOS

√4ᵗʰ **127 Other intestinal helminthiases**

127.0 Ascariasis
Ascaridiasis
Infection by Ascaris lumbricoides
Roundworm infection

127.1 Anisakiasis
Infection by Anisakis larva

127.2 Strongyloidiasis
Infection by Strongyloides stercoralis
EXCLUDES *trichostrongyliasis (127.6)*

127.3 Trichuriasis
Infection by Trichuris trichiuria
Trichocephaliasis
Whipworm (disease) (infection)

127.4 Enterobiasis
Infection by Enterobius vermicularis
Oxyuriasis
Oxyuris vermicularis infection
Pinworm (disease) (infection)
Threadworm infection

127.5 Capillariasis
Infection by Capillaria philippinensis
EXCLUDES *infection by Capillaria hepatica (128.8)*

127.6 Trichostrongyliasis
Infection by Trichostrongylus species

127.7 Other specified intestinal helminthiasis
Infection by:
Oesophagostomum apiostomum and related species
Ternidens diminutus
other specified intestinal helminth
Physalopteriasis

127.8 Mixed intestinal helminthiasis
Infection by intestinal helminths classified to more than one
of the categories 120.0-127.7
Mixed helminthiasis NOS

127.9 Intestinal helminthiasis, unspecified

√4ᵗʰ **128 Other and unspecified helminthiases**

128.0 Toxocariasis
Larva migrans visceralis
Toxocara (canis) (cati) infection
Visceral larva migrans syndrome

128.1 Gnathostomiasis
Infection by Gnathostoma spinigerum and related species

128.8 Other specified helminthiasis
Infection by:
Angiostrongylus cantonensis
Capillaria hepatica
other specified helminth

128.9 Helminth infection, unspecified
Helminthiasis NOS
Worms NOS

129 Intestinal parasitism, unspecified

Other Infectious and Parasitic Diseases (130–136)

✓4ᵗʰ 130 Toxoplasmosis
INCLUDES infection by toxoplasma gondii
toxoplasmosis (acquired)
EXCLUDES *congenital toxoplasmosis (771.2)*

130.0 Meningoencephalitis due to toxoplasmosis
Encephalitis due to acquired toxoplasmosis

130.1 Conjunctivitis due to toxoplasmosis

130.2 Chorioretinitis due to toxoplasmosis
Focal retinochoroiditis due to acquired toxoplasmosis

130.3 Myocarditis due to toxoplasmosis

130.4 Pneumonitis due to toxoplasmosis

130.5 Hepatitis due to toxoplasmosis

130.7 Toxoplasmosis of other specified sites

130.8 Multisystemic disseminated toxoplasmosis
Toxoplasmosis of multiple sites

130.9 Toxoplasmosis, unspecified

131 Trichomoniasis
INCLUDES infection due to Trichomonas (vaginalis)

✓5ᵗʰ 131.0 Urogenital trichomoniasis

131.00 Urogenital trichomoniasis, unspecified
Fluor (vaginalis) ⎫ trichomonal or due to
Leukorrhea (vaginalis) ⎬ Trichomonas
⎭ (vaginalis)
DEF: *Trichomonas vaginalis* infection of reproductive and urinary organs, transmitted through coitus.

131.01 Trichomonal vulvovaginitis ♀
Vaginitis, trichomonal or due to Trichomonas (vaginalis)
DEF: *Trichomonas vaginalis* infection of vulva and vagina; often asymptomatic, transmitted through coitus.

131.02 Trichomonal urethritis
DEF: *Trichomonas vaginalis* infection of the urethra.

131.03 Trichomonal prostatitis ♂
DEF: *Trichomonas vaginalis* infection of the prostate.

131.09 Other

131.8 Other specified sites
EXCLUDES *intestinal (007.3)*

131.9 Trichomoniasis, unspecified

✓4ᵗʰ 132 Pediculosis and phthirus infestation

132.0 Pediculus capitis [head louse]

132.1 Pediculus corporis [body louse]

132.2 Phthirus pubis [pubic louse]
Pediculus pubis

132.3 Mixed infestation
Infestation classifiable to more than one of the categories 132.0-132.2

132.9 Pediculosis, unspecified

✓4ᵗʰ 133 Acariasis

133.0 Scabies
Infestation by Sarcoptes scabiei
Norwegian scabies
Sarcoptic itch

133.8 Other acariasis
Chiggers
Infestation by:
Demodex folliculorum
Trombicula

133.9 Acariasis, unspecified
Infestation by mites NOS

✓4ᵗʰ 134 Other infestation

134.0 Myiasis
Infestation by:
Dermatobia (hominis)
fly larvae
Gasterophilus (intestinalis)
maggots
Oestrus ovis

134.1 Other arthropod infestation
Infestation by: Jigger disease
chigoe   Scarabiasis
sand flea   Tungiasis
Tunga penetrans

134.2 Hirudiniasis
Hirudiniasis (external) (internal)
Leeches (aquatic) (land)

134.8 Other specified infestations

134.9 Infestation, unspecified
Infestation (skin) NOS   Skin parasites NOS

135 Sarcoidosis
Besnier-Boeck-Schaumann disease
Lupoid (miliary) of Boeck
Lupus pernio (Besnier)
Lymphogranulomatosis, benign (Schaumann's)
Sarcoid (any site):
NOS
Boeck
Darier-Roussy
Uveoparotid fever
DEF: A chronic, granulomatous reticulosis (abnormal increase in cells), affecting any organ or tissue; acute form has high rate of remission; chronic form is progressive.
D86.9 Sarcoidosis unspecified   I-10

✓4ᵗʰ 136 Other and unspecified infectious and parasitic diseases

136.0 Ainhum
Dactylolysis spontanea
DEF: A disease affecting the toes, especially the fifth digit, and the fingers, mostly seen in black adult males; characterized by a linear constriction around the affected digit leading to spontaneous amputation of the distal part of the digit.

136.1 Behçet's syndrome
DEF: A chronic inflammatory disorder of unknown etiology involving the small blood vessels; characterized by recurrent aphthous ulceration of the oral and pharyngeal mucous membranes and the genitalia, skin lesions, severe uveitis, retinal vascularitis and optic atrophy.

✓5ᵗʰ 136.2 Specific infections by free-living amebae
AHA: 4Q, '08, 79-81

136.21 Specific infection due to acanthamoeba
Use additional code to identify manifestation, such as:
keratitis (370.8)
AHA: 4Q, '08, 81

136.29 Other specific infections by free-living amebae
Meningoencephalitis due to Naegleria

136.3 Pneumocystosis
Pneumonia due to Pneumocystis carinii
Pneumonia due to Pneumocystis jiroveci
AHA: 1Q, '05, 7; 1Q, '03, 15; N-D, '87, 5-6
DEF: *Pneumocystis carinii* fungus causing pneumonia in immunocompromised patients; a leading cause of death among AIDS patients.

136.4 Psorospermiasis

136.5 Sarcosporidiosis
Infection by Sarcocystis lindemanni
DEF: *Sarcocystis* infection causing muscle cysts of intestinal inflammation.

Ⓝ Newborn Age: 0   Ⓟ Pediatric Age: 0-17   Ⓜ Maternity Age: 12-55   Ⓐ Adult Age: 15-124

136.8 Other specified infectious and parasitic diseases
Candiru infestation

136.9 Unspecified infectious and parasitic diseases
Infectious disease NOS
Parasitic disease NOS
AHA: 2Q, '91, 8

Late Effects of Infectious and Parasitic Diseases (137-139)

√4ᵗʰ **137 Late effects of tuberculosis**

NOTE This category is to be used to indicate conditions classifiable to 010-018 as the cause of late effects, which are themselves classified elsewhere. The "late effects" include those specified as such, as sequelae, or as due to old or inactive tuberculosis, without evidence of active disease.

137.0 Late effects of respiratory or unspecified tuberculosis

137.1 Late effects of central nervous system tuberculosis

137.2 Late effects of genitourinary tuberculosis

137.3 Late effects of tuberculosis of bones and joints

137.4 Late effects of tuberculosis of other specified organs

138 Late effects of acute poliomyelitis

NOTE This category is to be used to indicate conditions classifiable to 045 as the cause of late effects, which are themselves classified elsewhere. The "late effects" include conditions specified as such, or as sequelae, or as due to old or inactive poliomyelitis, without evidence of active disease.

B91 Sequelae of poliomyelitis   I-10

√4ᵗʰ **139 Late effects of other infectious and parasitic diseases**

NOTE This category is to be used to indicate conditions classifiable to categories 001-009, 020-041, 046-136 as the cause of late effects, which are themselves classified elsewhere. The "late effects" include conditions specified as such; they also include sequela of diseases classifiable to the above categories if there is evidence that the disease itself is no longer present.

139.0 Late effects of viral encephalitis
Late effects of conditions classifiable to 049.8-049.9, 062-064

139.1 Late effects of trachoma
Late effects of conditions classifiable to 076

139.8 Late effects of other and unspecified infectious and parasitic diseases
AHA: 2Q, '06, 17; 4Q, '91, 15; 3Q, '90, 14; M-A, '87, 8

2. Neoplasms (140-239)

NOTES

1. Content

This chapter contains the following broad groups:

140-195	Malignant neoplasms, stated or presumed to be primary, of specified sites, except of lymphatic and hematopoietic tissue
196-198	Malignant neoplasms, stated or presumed to be secondary, of specified sites
199	Malignant neoplasms, without specification of site
200-208	Malignant neoplasms, stated or presumed to be primary, of lymphatic and hematopoietic tissue
209	Neuroendocrine tumors
210-229	Benign neoplasms
230-234	Carcinoma in situ
235-238	Neoplasms of uncertain behavior [see Note, above category 235]
239	Neoplasms of unspecified nature

2. Functional activity

All neoplasms are classified in this chapter, whether or not functionally active. An additional code from Chapter 3 may be used to identify such functional activity associated with any neoplasm, e.g.:

> catecholamine-producing malignant pheochromocytoma of adrenal:
>> code 194.0, additional code 255.6
>
> basophil adenoma of pituitary with Cushing's syndrome:
>> code 227.3, additional code 255.0

3. Morphology [Histology]

For those wishing to identify the histological type of neoplasms, a comprehensive coded nomenclature, which comprises the morphology rubrics of the ICD-Oncology, is given in Appendix A.

4. Malignant neoplasms overlapping site boundaries

Categories 140-195 are for the classification of primary malignant neoplasms according to their point of origin. A malignant neoplasm that overlaps two or more subcategories within a three-digit rubric and whose point of origin cannot be determined should be classified to the subcategory .8 "Other."

For example, "carcinoma involving tip and ventral surface of tongue" should be assigned to 141.8. On the other hand, "carcinoma of tip of tongue, extending to involve the ventral surface" should be coded to 141.2, as the point of origin, the tip, is known. Three subcategories (149.8, 159.8, 165.8) have been provided for malignant neoplasms that overlap the boundaries of three-digit rubrics within certain systems.

Overlapping malignant neoplasms that cannot be classified as indicated above should be assigned to the appropriate subdivision of category 195 (Malignant neoplasm of other and ill-defined sites).

> **DEF:** An abnormal growth; morphology determines behavior, i.e., whether it will remain intact (benign) or spread to adjacent tissue (malignant). The term mass is not synonymous with neoplasm, as it is often used to describe cysts and thickenings such as those occurring with hematoma or infection.
> **AHA:** 2Q, '90, 7

Malignant Neoplasm of Lip, Oral Cavity, and Pharynx (140-149)

> **EXCLUDES** carcinoma in situ (230.0)

☑4ᵗʰ **140 Malignant neoplasm of lip**
> **EXCLUDES** skin of lip (173.0)

140.0 Upper lip, vermilion border
> Upper lip:
>> NOS
>> external
>> lipstick area

140.1 Lower lip, vermilion border
> Lower lip:
>> NOS
>> external
>> lipstick area

140.3 Upper lip, inner aspect
> Upper lip:
>> buccal aspect
>> frenulum
>> mucosa
>> oral aspect

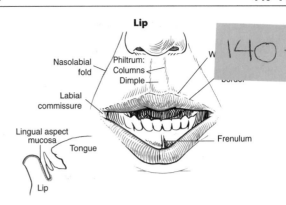

Lip

140.4 Lower lip, inner aspect
> Lower lip:
>> buccal aspect
>> frenulum
>> mucosa
>> oral aspect

140.5 Lip, unspecified, inner aspect
> Lip, not specified whether upper or lower:
>> buccal aspect
>> frenulum
>> mucosa
>> oral aspect

140.6 Commissure of lip
> Labial commissure

140.8 Other sites of lip
> Malignant neoplasm of contiguous or overlapping sites of lip whose point of origin cannot be determined

140.9 Lip, unspecified, vermilion border
> Lip, not specified as upper or lower:
>> NOS
>> external
>> lipstick area

☑4ᵗʰ **141 Malignant neoplasm of tongue**

141.0 Base of tongue
> Dorsal surface of base of tongue
> Fixed part of tongue NOS
> **AHA:** 4Q, '06, 90

141.1 Dorsal surface of tongue
> Anterior two-thirds of tongue, dorsal surface
> Dorsal tongue NOS
> Midline of tongue
> **EXCLUDES** dorsal surface of base of tongue (141.0)

141.2 Tip and lateral border of tongue

141.3 Ventral surface of tongue
> Anterior two-thirds of tongue, ventral surface
> Frenulum linguae

141.4 Anterior two-thirds of tongue, part unspecified
> Mobile part of tongue NOS

141.5 Junctional zone
> Border of tongue at junction of fixed and mobile parts at insertion of anterior tonsillar pillar

Tongue

☑4ᵗʰ ☑5ᵗʰ Additional Digit Required   Unspecified Code   Other Specified Code   Manifestation Code   ►◄ Revised Text   ● New Code   ▲ Revised Code Title

2011 ICD-9-CM   **Volume 1 – 27**

Main Salivary Glands

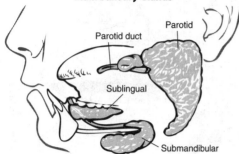

141.6 Lingual tonsil

141.8 Other sites of tongue
> Malignant neoplasm of contiguous or overlapping sites of tongue whose point of origin cannot be determined

141.9 Tongue, unspecified
> Tongue NOS

√4th **142 Malignant neoplasm of major salivary glands**
> INCLUDES salivary ducts
>
> EXCLUDES *malignant neoplasm of minor salivary glands:*
> *NOS (145.9)*
> *buccal mucosa (145.0)*
> *soft palate (145.3)*
> *tongue (141.0-141.9)*
> *tonsil, palatine (146.0)*

142.0 Parotid gland

142.1 Submandibular gland
> Submaxillary gland

142.2 Sublingual gland

142.8 Other major salivary glands
> Malignant neoplasm of contiguous or overlapping sites of salivary glands and ducts whose point of origin cannot be determined

142.9 Salivary gland, unspecified
> Salivary gland (major) NOS

√4th **143 Malignant neoplasm of gum**
> INCLUDES alveolar (ridge) mucosa
> gingiva (alveolar) (marginal)
> interdental papillae
>
> EXCLUDES *malignant odontogenic neoplasms (170.0-170.1)*

143.0 Upper gum

143.1 Lower gum

143.8 Other sites of gum
> Malignant neoplasm of contiguous or overlapping sites of gum whose point of origin cannot be determined

143.9 Gum, unspecified

√4th **144 Malignant neoplasm of floor of mouth**

144.0 Anterior portion
> Anterior to the premolar-canine junction

144.1 Lateral portion

144.8 Other sites of floor of mouth
> Malignant neoplasm of contiguous or overlapping sites of floor of mouth whose point of origin cannot be determined

144.9 Floor of mouth, part unspecified

√4th **145 Malignant neoplasm of other and unspecified parts of mouth**
> EXCLUDES *mucosa of lips (140.0-140.9)*

145.0 Cheek mucosa
> Buccal mucosa
> Cheek, inner aspect

145.1 Vestibule of mouth
> Buccal sulcus (upper) (lower)
> Labial sulcus (upper) (lower)

145.2 Hard palate

Mouth

Oropharynx

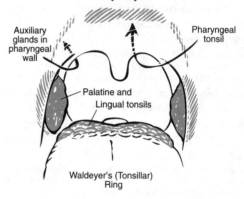

145.3 Soft palate
> EXCLUDES *nasopharyngeal [posterior] [superior] surface of soft palate (147.3)*

145.4 Uvula

145.5 Palate, unspecified
> Junction of hard and soft palate
> Roof of mouth

145.6 Retromolar area

145.8 Other specified parts of mouth
> Malignant neoplasm of contiguous or overlapping sites of mouth whose point of origin cannot be determined

145.9 Mouth, unspecified
> Buccal cavity NOS
> Minor salivary gland, unspecified site
> Oral cavity NOS

√4th **146 Malignant neoplasm of oropharynx**

146.0 Tonsil
> Tonsil:
> NOS
> faucial
> palatine
>
> EXCLUDES *lingual tonsil (141.6)*
> *pharyngeal tonsil (147.1)*
>
> AHA: S-O, '87, 8

146.1 Tonsillar fossa

146.2 Tonsillar pillars (anterior) (posterior)
> Faucial pillar
> Glossopalatine fold
> Palatoglossal arch
> Palatopharyngeal arch

146.3 Vallecula
> Anterior and medial surface of the pharyngoepiglottic fold

146.4 Anterior aspect of epiglottis
> Epiglottis, free border [margin]
> Glossoepiglottic fold(s)
>
> EXCLUDES *epiglottis:*
> *NOS (161.1)*
> *suprahyoid portion (161.1)*

N Newborn Age: 0   P Pediatric Age: 0-17   M Maternity Age: 12-55   A Adult Age: 15-124

Nasopharynx

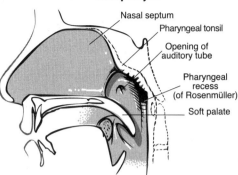

Nasal septum
Pharyngeal tonsil
Opening of auditory tube
Pharyngeal recess (of Rosenmüller)
Soft palate

146.5 Junctional region
Junction of the free margin of the epiglottis, the aryepiglottic fold, and the pharyngoepiglottic fold

146.6 Lateral wall of oropharynx

146.7 Posterior wall of oropharynx

146.8 Other specified sites of oropharynx
Branchial cleft
Malignant neoplasm of contiguous or overlapping sites of oropharynx whose point of origin cannot be determined

146.9 Oropharynx, unspecified
AHA: 2Q, '02, 6

√4ᵗʰ **147 Malignant neoplasm of nasopharynx**

147.0 Superior wall
Roof of nasopharynx

147.1 Posterior wall
Adenoid
Pharyngeal tonsil

147.2 Lateral wall
Fossa of Rosenmüller
Opening of auditory tube
Pharyngeal recess

147.3 Anterior wall
Floor of nasopharynx
Nasopharyngeal [posterior] [superior] surface of soft palate
Posterior margin of nasal septum and choanae

147.8 Other specified sites of nasopharynx
Malignant neoplasm of contiguous or overlapping sites of nasopharynx whose point of origin cannot be determined

147.9 Nasopharynx, unspecified
Nasopharyngeal wall NOS

√4ᵗʰ **148 Malignant neoplasm of hypopharynx**

148.0 Postcricoid region

148.1 Pyriform sinus
Pyriform fossa

Hypopharynx

Skull base from behind

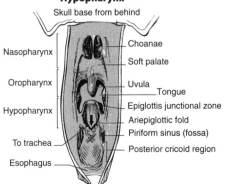

Nasopharynx
Oropharynx
Hypopharynx
To trachea
Esophagus

Choanae
Soft palate
Uvula
Tongue
Epiglottis junctional zone
Ariepiglottic fold
Piriform sinus (fossa)
Posterior cricoid region

148.2 Aryepiglottic fold, hypopharyngeal aspect
Aryepiglottic fold or interarytenoid fold:
NOS
marginal zone
EXCLUDES aryepiglottic fold or interarytenoid fold, laryngeal aspect (161.1)

148.3 Posterior hypopharyngeal wall

148.8 Other specified sites of hypopharynx
Malignant neoplasm of contiguous or overlapping sites of hypopharynx whose point of origin cannot be determined

148.9 Hypopharynx, unspecified
Hypopharyngeal wall NOS
Hypopharynx NOS

√4ᵗʰ **149 Malignant neoplasm of other and ill-defined sites within the lip, oral cavity, and pharynx**

149.0 Pharynx, unspecified

149.1 Waldeyer's ring

149.8 Other
Malignant neoplasms of lip, oral cavity, and pharynx whose point of origin cannot be assigned to any one of the categories 140-148
EXCLUDES "book leaf" neoplasm [ventral surface of tongue and floor of mouth] (145.8)

149.9 Ill-defined

Malignant Neoplasm of Digestive Organs and Peritoneum (150-159)

EXCLUDES carcinoma in situ (230.1-230.9)

√4ᵗʰ **150 Malignant neoplasm of esophagus**

150.0 Cervical esophagus

150.1 Thoracic esophagus

150.2 Abdominal esophagus
EXCLUDES adenocarcinoma (151.0)
cardio-esophageal junction (151.0)

150.3 Upper third of esophagus
Proximal third of esophagus

150.4 Middle third of esophagus

150.5 Lower third of esophagus
Distal third of esophagus
EXCLUDES adenocarcinoma (151.0)
cardio-esophageal junction (151.0)

150.8 Other specified part
Malignant neoplasm of contiguous or overlapping sites of esophagus whose point of origin cannot be determined

150.9 Esophagus, unspecified

√4ᵗʰ **151 Malignant neoplasm of stomach**
EXCLUDES benign carcinoid tumor of stomach (209.63)
malignant carcinoid tumor of stomach (209.23)

151.0 Cardia
Cardiac orifice
Cardio-esophageal junction
EXCLUDES squamous cell carcinoma (150.2, 150.5)

151.1 Pylorus
Prepylorus
Pyloric canal

151.2 Pyloric antrum
Antrum of stomach NOS

151.3 Fundus of stomach

151.4 Body of stomach

151.5 Lesser curvature, unspecified
Lesser curvature, not classifiable to 151.1-151.4

151.6 Greater curvature, unspecified
Greater curvature, not classifiable to 151.0-151.4

151.8 Other specified sites of stomach
Anterior wall, not classifiable to 151.0-151.4
Posterior wall, not classifiable to 151.0-151.4
Malignant neoplasm of contiguous or overlapping sites of
    stomach whose point of origin cannot be determined

151.9 Stomach, unspecified
Carcinoma ventriculi
Gastric cancer
AHA: 2Q, '01, 17

✓4th **152 Malignant neoplasm of small intestine, including duodenum**
EXCLUDES *benign carcinoid tumor of small intestine and duodenum*
    (209.40-209.43)
malignant carcinoid tumor of small intestine and duodenum
    (209.00-209.03)

152.0 Duodenum

152.1 Jejunum

152.2 Ileum
EXCLUDES *ileocecal valve (153.4)*

152.3 Meckel's diverticulum

152.8 Other specified sites of small intestine
Duodenojejunal junction
Malignant neoplasm of contiguous or overlapping sites of
    small intestine whose point of origin cannot be
    determined

152.9 Small intestine, unspecified

✓4th **153 Malignant neoplasm of colon**
EXCLUDES *benign carcinoid tumor of colon (209.50-209.56)*
malignant carcinoid tumor of colon (209.10-209.16)

153.0 Hepatic flexure

153.1 Transverse colon

153.2 Descending colon
Left colon

153.3 Sigmoid colon
Sigmoid (flexure)
EXCLUDES *rectosigmoid junction (154.0)*

153.4 Cecum
Ileocecal valve
C18.0 Malignant neoplasm of cecum   I-10

153.5 Appendix

153.6 Ascending colon
Right colon
C18.2 Malignant neoplasm of ascending colon   I-10

153.7 Splenic flexure

153.8 Other specified sites of large intestine
Malignant neoplasm of contiguous or overlapping sites of
    colon whose point of origin cannot be determined
EXCLUDES *ileocecal valve (153.4)*
rectosigmoid junction (154.0)

153.9 Colon, unspecified
Large intestine NOS
C18.9 Malignant neoplasm of colon unspecified   I-10

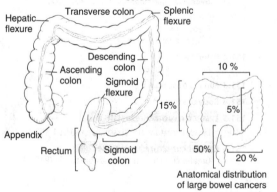

Colon

Transverse colon

Hepatic flexure   Splenic flexure

Descending colon

Ascending colon

Sigmoid flexure

Appendix

Rectum   Sigmoid colon

10 %
15%
5%
50%
20 %

Anatomical distribution
of large bowel cancers

✓4th **154 Malignant neoplasm of rectum, rectosigmoid junction, and anus**
EXCLUDES *benign carcinoid tumor of rectum (209.57)*
malignant carcinoid tumor of rectum (209.17)

154.0 Rectosigmoid junction
Colon with rectum
Rectosigmoid (colon)

154.1 Rectum
Rectal ampulla
C20 Malignant neoplasm of rectum   I-10

154.2 Anal canal
Anal sphincter
EXCLUDES *skin of anus (172.5, 173.5)*
AHA: 1Q, '01, 8

154.3 Anus, unspecified
EXCLUDES *anus:*
    margin (172.5, 173.5)
    skin (172.5, 173.5)
    perianal skin (172.5, 173.5)

154.8 Other
Anorectum
Cloacogenic zone
Malignant neoplasm of contiguous or overlapping sites of
    rectum, rectosigmoid junction, and anus whose point of
    origin cannot be determined

✓4th **155 Malignant neoplasm of liver and intrahepatic bile ducts**

155.0 Liver, primary
Carcinoma:
    hepatocellular
    liver cell
    liver, specified as primary
Hepatoblastoma
AHA: 4Q, '08, 82
C22.0 Liver cell carcinoma   I-10

155.1 Intrahepatic bile ducts
Canaliculi biliferi
Interlobular:
    bile ducts
    biliary canals
Intrahepatic:
    biliary passages
    canaliculi
    gall duct
EXCLUDES *hepatic duct (156.1)*

155.2 Liver, not specified as primary or secondary

✓4th **156 Malignant neoplasm of gallbladder and extrahepatic bile ducts**

156.0 Gallbladder

156.1 Extrahepatic bile ducts
Biliary duct or passage NOS
Common bile duct
Cystic duct
Hepatic duct
Sphincter of Oddi

156.2 Ampulla of Vater
DEF: Malignant neoplasm in the area of dilation at the juncture of the
common bile and pancreatic ducts near the opening into the lumen
of the duodenum.

156.8 Other specified sites of gallbladder and extrahepatic bile ducts
Malignant neoplasm of contiguous or overlapping sites of
    gallbladder and extrahepatic bile ducts whose point of
    origin cannot be determined

156.9 Biliary tract, part unspecified
Malignant neoplasm involving both intrahepatic and
    extrahepatic bile ducts

✓4th **157 Malignant neoplasm of pancreas**
AHA: 4Q, '07, 72

157.0 Head of pancreas
AHA: 2Q, '05, 9; 4Q, '00, 40

157.1 Body of pancreas

157.2 Tail of pancreas

N   Newborn Age: 0   P   Pediatric Age: 0-17   M   Maternity Age: 12-55   A   Adult Age: 15-124

Retroperitoneum and Peritoneum

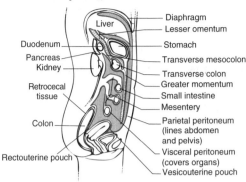

157.3 Pancreatic duct
Duct of:
    Santorini
    Wirsung

157.4 Islets of Langerhans
Islets of Langerhans, any part of pancreas
Use additional code to identify any functional activity
DEF: Malignant neoplasm within the structures of the pancreas that produce insulin, somatostatin and glucagon.

157.8 Other specified sites of pancreas
Ectopic pancreatic tissue
Malignant neoplasm of contiguous or overlapping sites of pancreas whose point of origin cannot be determined

157.9 Pancreas, part unspecified
AHA: 4Q, '89, 11
C25.9 Malignant neoplasm of pancreas unspecified   I-10

☑4ᵗʰ **158 Malignant neoplasm of retroperitoneum and peritoneum**

158.0 Retroperitoneum
Periadrenal tissue   Perirenal tissue
Perinephric tissue   Retrocecal tissue

158.8 Specified parts of peritoneum
Cul-de-sac (of Douglas)
Malignant neoplasm of contiguous or overlapping sites of retroperitoneum and peritoneum whose point of origin cannot be determined
Mesentery
Mesocolon
Omentum
Peritoneum:
    parietal
    pelvic
Rectouterine pouch

158.9 Peritoneum, unspecified

☑4ᵗʰ **159 Malignant neoplasm of other and ill-defined sites within the digestive organs and peritoneum**

159.0 Intestinal tract, part unspecified
Intestine NOS

159.1 Spleen, not elsewhere classified
Angiosarcoma ⎤ of spleen
Fibrosarcoma ⎦
EXCLUDES *Hodgkin's disease (201.0-201.9)*
lymphosarcoma (200.1)
reticulosarcoma (200.0)

159.8 Other sites of digestive system and intra-abdominal organs
Malignant neoplasm of digestive organs and peritoneum whose point of origin cannot be assigned to any one of the categories 150-158
EXCLUDES *anus and rectum (154.8)*
cardio-esophageal junction (151.0)
colon and rectum (154.0)

159.9 Ill-defined
Alimentary canal or tract NOS
Gastrointestinal tract NOS
EXCLUDES *abdominal NOS (195.2)*
intra-abdominal NOS (195.2)

Neoplasm of Respiratory and Intrathoracic Organs (160-165)

EXCLUDES *carcinoma in situ (231.0-231.9)*

☑4ᵗʰ **160 Malignant neoplasm of nasal cavities, middle ear, and accessory sinuses**

160.0 Nasal cavities
Cartilage of nose   Septum of nose
Conchae, nasal   Vestibule of nose
Internal nose
EXCLUDES *nasal bone (170.0)*
nose NOS (195.0)
olfactory bulb (192.0)
posterior margin of septum and choanae (147.3)
skin of nose (172.3, 173.3)
turbinates (170.0)

160.1 Auditory tube, middle ear, and mastoid air cells
Antrum tympanicum
Eustachian tube
Tympanic cavity
EXCLUDES *auditory canal (external) (172.2, 173.2)*
bone of ear (meatus) (170.0)
cartilage of ear (171.0)
ear (external) (skin) (172.2, 173.2)

160.2 Maxillary sinus
Antrum (Highmore) (maxillary)

160.3 Ethmoidal sinus

160.4 Frontal sinus

160.5 Sphenoidal sinus

160.8 Other
Malignant neoplasm of contiguous or overlapping sites of nasal cavities, middle ear, and accessory sinuses whose point of origin cannot be determined

160.9 Accessory sinus, unspecified

☑4ᵗʰ **161 Malignant neoplasm of larynx**

161.0 Glottis
Intrinsic larynx
Laryngeal commissure (anterior) (posterior)
True vocal cord
Vocal cord NOS

161.1 Supraglottis
Aryepiglottic fold or interarytenoid fold, laryngeal aspect
Epiglottis (suprahyoid portion) NOS
Extrinsic larynx
False vocal cords
Posterior (laryngeal) surface of epiglottis
Ventricular bands
EXCLUDES *anterior aspect of epiglottis (146.4)*
aryepiglottic fold or interarytenoid fold:
    NOS (148.2)
    hypopharyngeal aspect (148.2)
    marginal zone (148.2)

161.2 Subglottis

161.3 Laryngeal cartilages
Cartilage: Cartilage:
    arytenold   cuneiform
    cricoid   thyroid

161.8 Other specified sites of larynx
Malignant neoplasm of contiguous or overlapping sites of larynx whose point of origin cannot be determined
AHA: 3Q, '07, 7

161.9 Larynx, unspecified

☑4ᵗʰ **162 Malignant neoplasm of trachea, bronchus, and lung**
EXCLUDES *benign carcinoid tumor of bronchus (209.61)*
malignant carcinoid tumor of bronchus (209.21)

162.0 Trachea
Cartilage ⎤
Mucosa ⎦ of trachea

162.2 Main bronchus
Carina
Hilus of lung

☑4ᵗʰ / ☑5ᵗʰ Additional Digit Required   Unspecified Code   Other Specified Code   Manifestation Code   ►◄ Revised Text   ● New Code   ▲ Revised Code Title

2011 ICD-9-CM   **Volume 1 – 31**

162.3 Upper lobe, bronchus or lung

AHA: 1Q, '04, 4

C34.10 Malig neoplasm upper lobe bronchus/lung uns side   I-10

162.4 Middle lobe, bronchus or lung

162.5 Lower lobe, bronchus or lung

162.8 Other parts of bronchus or lung

Malignant neoplasm of contiguous or overlapping sites of bronchus or lung whose point of origin cannot be determined

AHA: 3Q, '06, 7

TIP: Assign when two separate tumors classifiable to category 162 are present, overlapping and no point of origin is determined.

162.9 Bronchus and lung, unspecified

AHA: 3Q, '06, 14-15; 2Q, '97, 3; 4Q, '96, 48

C34.90 Malig neoplas bronchus/lung unspec, unspec side   I-10

√4ᵗʰ **163 Malignant neoplasm of pleura**

163.0 Parietal pleura

163.1 Visceral pleura

163.8 Other specified sites of pleura

Malignant neoplasm of contiguous or overlapping sites of pleura whose point of origin cannot be determined

163.9 Pleura, unspecified

√4ᵗʰ **164 Malignant neoplasm of thymus, heart, and mediastinum**

164.0 Thymus

EXCLUDES *benign carcinoid tumor of the thymus (209.62)*
malignant carcinoid tumor of the thymus (209.22)

164.1 Heart

Endocardium   Myocardium
Epicardium   Pericardium

EXCLUDES *great vessels (171.4)*

164.2 Anterior mediastinum

164.3 Posterior mediastinum

164.8 Other

Malignant neoplasm of contiguous or overlapping sites of thymus, heart, and mediastinum whose point of origin cannot be determined

164.9 Mediastinum, part unspecified

√4ᵗʰ **165 Malignant neoplasm of other and ill-defined sites within the respiratory system and intrathoracic organs**

165.0 Upper respiratory tract, part unspecified

165.8 Other

Malignant neoplasm of respiratory and intrathoracic organs whose point of origin cannot be assigned to any one of the categories 160-164

165.9 Ill-defined sites within the respiratory system

Respiratory tract NOS

EXCLUDES *intrathoracic NOS (195.1)*
thoracic NOS (195.1)

Skull

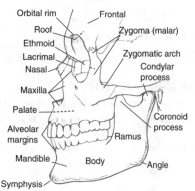

Orbital rim — Frontal
Roof — Zygoma (malar)
Ethmoid
Lacrimal — Zygomatic arch
Nasal — Condylar process
Maxilla
Palate — Coronoid process
Alveolar margins
Mandible — Body — Ramus — Angle
Symphysis

Malignant Neoplasm of Bone, Connective Tissue, Skin, and Breast (170-176)

EXCLUDES *carcinoma in situ:*
breast (233.0)
skin (232.0-232.9)

√4ᵗʰ **170 Malignant neoplasm of bone and articular cartilage**

INCLUDES cartilage (articular) (joint)
periosteum

EXCLUDES *bone marrow NOS (202.9)*
cartilage:
ear (171.0)
eyelid (171.0)
larynx (161.3)
nose (160.0)
synovia (171.0-171.9)

AHA: 4Q, '06, 103

TIP: Do not assign for bone metastasis; see instead code 198.5.

170.0 Bones of skull and face, except mandible

Bone: Bone:
  ethmoid   sphenoid
  frontal   temporal
  malar   zygomatic
  nasal   Maxilla (superior)
  occipital   Turbinate
  orbital   Upper jaw bone
  parietal   Vomer

EXCLUDES *carcinoma, any type except intraosseous or*
odontogenic:
maxilla, maxillary (sinus) (160.2)
upper jaw bone (143.0)
jaw bone (lower) (170.1)

170.1 Mandible

Inferior maxilla
Jaw bone NOS
Lower jaw bone

EXCLUDES *carcinoma, any type except intraosseous or*
odontogenic:
jaw bone NOS (143.9)
lower (143.1)
upper jaw bone (170.0)

170.2 Vertebral column, excluding sacrum and coccyx

Spinal column
Spine
Vertebra

EXCLUDES *sacrum and coccyx (170.6)*

170.3 Ribs, sternum, and clavicle

Costal cartilage
Costovertebral joint
Xiphoid process

170.4 Scapula and long bones of upper limb

Acromion
Bones NOS of upper limb
Humerus
Radius
Ulna

AHA: 2Q, '99, 9

170.5 Short bones of upper limb

Carpal   Scaphoid (of hand)
Cuneiform, wrist   Semilunar or lunate
Metacarpal   Trapezium
Navicular, of hand   Trapezoid
Phalanges of hand   Unciform
Pisiform

170.6 Pelvic bones, sacrum, and coccyx

Coccygeal vertebra
Ilium
Ischium
Pubic bone
Sacral vertebra

170.7 Long bones of lower limb

Bones NOS of lower limb
Femur
Fibula
Tibia

N Newborn Age: 0   P Pediatric Age: 0-17   M Maternity Age: 12-55   A Adult Age: 15-124

170.8 Short bones of lower limb
Astragalus [talus]   Navicular (of ankle)
Calcaneus   Patella
Cuboid   Phalanges of foot
Cuneiform, ankle   Tarsal
Metatarsal

170.9 Bone and articular cartilage, site unspecified

✓4th 171 Malignant neoplasm of connective and other soft tissue
INCLUDES blood vessel
bursa
fascia
fat
ligament, except uterine
muscle
peripheral, sympathetic, and parasympathetic nerves and
ganglia
synovia
tendon (sheath)
EXCLUDES *cartilage (of):*
articular (170.0-170.9)
larynx (161.3)
nose (160.0)
connective tissue:
breast (174.0-175.9)
internal organs — code to malignant neoplasm of the site
[e.g., leiomyosarcoma of stomach, 151.9]
heart (164.1)
uterine ligament (183.4)

171.0 Head, face, and neck
Cartilage of:
ear
eyelid
AHA: 2Q, '99, 6

171.2 Upper limb, including shoulder
Arm
Finger
Forearm
Hand

171.3 Lower limb, including hip
Foot
Leg
Popliteal space
Thigh
Toe

171.4 Thorax
Axilla
Diaphragm
Great vessels
EXCLUDES *heart (164.1)*
mediastinum (164.2-164.9)
thymus (164.0)

171.5 Abdomen
Abdominal wall
Hypochondrium
EXCLUDES *peritoneum (158.8)*
retroperitoneum (158.0)

171.6 Pelvis
Buttock
Groin
Inguinal region
Perineum
EXCLUDES *pelvic peritoneum (158.8)*
retroperitoneum (158.0)
uterine ligament, any (183.3-183.5)

171.7 Trunk, unspecified
Back NOS
Flank NOS

171.8 Other specified sites of connective and other soft tissue
Malignant neoplasm of contiguous or overlapping sites of
connective tissue whose point of origin cannot be
determined

171.9 Connective and other soft tissue, site unspecified

✓4th 172 Malignant melanoma of skin
INCLUDES melanocarcinoma
melanoma (skin) NOS
melanoma in situ of skin
EXCLUDES *skin of genital organs (184.0-184.9, 187.1-187.9)*
sites other than skin — code to malignant neoplasm of the
site
DEF: Malignant neoplasm of melanocytes; most common in skin, may
involve oral cavity, esophagus, anal canal, vagina, leptomeninges, or
conjunctiva.

172.0 Lip
EXCLUDES *vermilion border of lip (140.0-140.1, 140.9)*

172.1 Eyelid, including canthus

172.2 Ear and external auditory canal
Auricle (ear)
Auricular canal, external
External [acoustic] meatus
Pinna

172.3 Other and unspecified   parts of face
Cheek (external)
Chin
Eyebrow
Forehead
Nose, external
Temple

172.4 Scalp and neck

172.5 Trunk, except scrotum
Axilla   Perianal skin
Breast   Perineum
Buttock   Umbilicus
Groin
EXCLUDES *anal canal (154.2)*
anus NOS (154.3)
scrotum (187.7)

172.6 Upper limb, including shoulder
Arm   Forearm
Finger   Hand

172.7 Lower limb, including hip
Ankle   Leg
Foot   Popliteal area
Heel   Thigh
Knee   Toe

172.8 Other specified sites of skin
Malignant melanoma of contiguous or overlapping sites of
skin whose point of origin cannot be determined

172.9 Melanoma of skin, site unspecified

✓4th 173 Other malignant neoplasm of skin
INCLUDES malignant neoplasm of:
sebaceous glands
sudoriferous, sudoriparous glands
sweat glands
EXCLUDES *Kaposi's sarcoma (176.0-176.9)*
malignant melanoma of skin (172.0-172.9)
skin of genital organs (184.0-184.9, 187.1-187.9)
AHA: 1Q, '00, 18; 2Q, '96, 12
TIP: Do not assign for malignant neoplasm of skin documented as melanoma; see instead category 172.

173.0 Skin of lip
EXCLUDES *vermilion border of lip (140.0-140.1, 140.9)*

173.1 Eyelid, including canthus
EXCLUDES *cartilage of eyelid (171.0)*

173.2 Skin of ear and external auditory canal
Auricle (ear)
Auricular canal, external
External meatus
Pinna
EXCLUDES *cartilage of ear (171.0)*

173.3 Skin of other and unspecified parts of face
Cheek, external   Forehead
Chin   Nose, external
Eyebrow   Temple
AHA: 1Q, '00, 3

173.4 Scalp and skin of neck

173.5 Skin of trunk, except scrotum
Axillary fold
Perianal skin
Skin of:
    abdominal wall
    anus
    back
    breast
    buttock
    chest wall
    groin
    perineum
Umbilicus

> **EXCLUDES** *anal canal (154.2)*
> *anus NOS (154.3)*
> *skin of scrotum (187.7)*

AHA: 1Q, '01, 8

173.6 Skin of upper limb, including shoulder
Arm   Forearm
Finger   Hand

173.7 Skin of lower limb, including hip
Ankle   Leg
Foot   Popliteal area
Heel   Thigh
Knee   Toe

173.8 Other specified sites of skin
Malignant neoplasm of contiguous or overlapping sites of skin whose point of origin cannot be determined

173.9 Skin, site unspecified

√4ᵗʰ 174 Malignant neoplasm of female breast
Use additional code to identify estrogen receptor status (V86.0, V86.1)

> **INCLUDES** breast (female)
>   connective tissue
>   soft parts
> Paget's disease of:
>   breast
>   nipple

> **EXCLUDES** *skin of breast (172.5, 173.5)*

AHA: 3Q, '97, 8; 4Q, '89, 11
TIP: For bilateral breast malignancy, do not assign two codes unless documentation indicates separate sites (i.e., different fourth digits).

174.0 Nipple and areola ♀

174.1 Central portion ♀

174.2 Upper-inner quadrant ♀

174.3 Lower-inner quadrant ♀

174.4 Upper-outer quadrant ♀
AHA: 4Q, '08, 155; 1Q, '04, 3; 3Q, '97, 8

174.5 Lower-outer quadrant ♀

174.6 Axillary tail ♀

174.8 Other specified sites of female breast ♀
Ectopic sites
Inner breast
Lower breast
Midline of breast
Outer breast
Upper breast

Malignant neoplasm of contiguous or overlapping sites of breast whose point of origin cannot be determined

174.9 Breast (female), unspecified ♀
AHA: ▶3Q, '09, 3;◀ 3Q, '05, 11; 2Q, '94, 10; 4Q, '89, 11
C50.911 Malig neoplasm of uns site of rt female breast   I-10

√4ᵗʰ 175 Malignant neoplasm of male breast
Use additional code to identify estrogen receptor status (V86.0, V86.1)

> **EXCLUDES** *skin of breast (172.5, 173.5)*

175.0 Nipple and areola ♂

175.9 Other and unspecified sites of male breast ♂
Ectopic breast tissue, male

Female Breast

Upper outer quadrant — Upper inner quadrant — Midline — Areola — Nipple — Axillary tail — Mammary gland — Lower outer quadrant — Lower inner quadrant — Right Breast

√4ᵗʰ 176 Kaposi's sarcoma
AHA: 4Q, '91, 24

176.0 Skin
AHA: 4Q, '07, 63; 4Q, '94, 29; 4Q, '91, 24

176.1 Soft tissue
Blood vessel   Ligament
Connective tissue   Lymphatic(s) NEC
Fascia   Muscle

> **EXCLUDES** *lymph glands and nodes (176.5)*

176.2 Palate

176.3 Gastrointestinal sites

176.4 Lung

176.5 Lymph nodes

176.8 Other specified sites
Oral cavity NEC

176.9 Unspecified
Viscera NOS

Malignant Neoplasm of Genitourinary Organs (179-189)

> **EXCLUDES** *carcinoma in situ (233.1-233.9)*

179 Malignant neoplasm of uterus, part unspecified ♀

√4ᵗʰ 180 Malignant neoplasm of cervix uteri
> **INCLUDES** invasive malignancy [carcinoma]
> **EXCLUDES** *carcinoma in situ (233.1)*

180.0 Endocervix ♀
Cervical canal NOS
Endocervical canal
Endocervical gland

180.1 Exocervix ♀

180.8 Other specified sites of cervix ♀
Cervical stump
Squamocolumnar junction of cervix

Malignant neoplasm of contiguous or overlapping sites of cervix uteri whose point of origin cannot be determined

180.9 Cervix uteri, unspecified ♀

181 Malignant neoplasm of placenta ♀
Choriocarcinoma NOS
Chorioepithelioma NOS

> **EXCLUDES** *chorioadenoma (destruens) (236.1)*
> *hydatidiform mole (630)*
> *malignant (236.1)*
> *invasive mole (236.1)*
> *male choriocarcinoma NOS (186.0-186.9)*

√4ᵗʰ 182 Malignant neoplasm of body of uterus
> **EXCLUDES** *carcinoma in situ (233.2)*

182.0 Corpus uteri, except isthmus ♀
Cornu   Fundus
Endometrium   Myometrium
AHA: ▶3Q, '09, 5◀
C54.9 Malignant neoplasm of corpus uteri unspecified   I-10

182.1 Isthmus ♀
Lower uterine segment

N Newborn Age: 0   P Pediatric Age: 0-17   M Maternity Age: 12-55   A Adult Age: 15-124

182.8 Other specified sites of body of uterus ♀
Malignant neoplasm of contiguous or overlapping sites of body of uterus whose point of origin cannot be determined
EXCLUDES *uterus NOS (179)*

✓4ᵗʰ **183 Malignant neoplasm of ovary and other uterine adnexa**
EXCLUDES *Douglas' cul-de-sac (158.8)*

183.0 Ovary ♀
Use additional code to identify any functional activity
AHA: 4Q, '07, 96
C56.9 Malignant neoplasm of ovary unspecified side   I-10

183.2 Fallopian tube ♀
Oviduct
Uterine tube

183.3 Broad ligament ♀
Mesovarium
Parovarian region

183.4 Parametrium ♀
Uterine ligament NOS
Uterosacral ligament

183.5 Round ligament ♀
AHA: 3Q, '99, 5

183.8 Other specified sites of uterine adnexa ♀
Tubo-ovarian
Utero-ovarian
Malignant neoplasm of contiguous or overlapping sites of ovary and other uterine adnexa whose point of origin cannot be determined

183.9 Uterine adnexa, unspecified ♀

✓4ᵗʰ **184 Malignant neoplasm of other and unspecified female genital organs**
EXCLUDES *carcinoma in situ (233.30-233.39)*

184.0 Vagina ♀
Gartner's duct
Vaginal vault

184.1 Labia majora ♀
Greater vestibular [Bartholin's] gland

184.2 Labia minora ♀

184.3 Clitoris ♀

184.4 Vulva, unspecified ♀
External female genitalia NOS
Pudendum

184.8 Other specified sites of female genital ♀
Malignant neoplasm of contiguous or overlapping sites of female genital organs whose point of origin cannot be determined

184.9 Female genital organ, site unspecified ♀
Female genitourinary tract NOS

185 Malignant neoplasm of prostate ♂
EXCLUDES *seminal vesicles (187.8)*
AHA: 3Q, '03, 13; 3Q, '99, 5; 3Q, '92, 7
TIP: Assign as a secondary diagnosis if patient treated for BPH and incidental finding of carcinoma of the prostate is made.
C61 Malignant neoplasm of prostate   I-10

✓4ᵗʰ **186 Malignant neoplasm of testis**
Use additional code to identify any functional activity

186.0 Undescended testis ♂
Ectopic testis
Retained testis

186.9 Other and unspecified testis ♂
Testis:
NOS
descended
scrotal

✓4ᵗʰ **187 Malignant neoplasm of penis and other male genital organs**

187.1 Prepuce ♂
Foreskin

187.2 Glans penis ♂

187.3 Body of penis ♂
Corpus cavernosum

187.4 Penis, part unspecified ♂
Skin of penis NOS

187.5 Epididymis ♂

187.6 Spermatic cord ♂
Vas deferens

187.7 Scrotum ♂
Skin of scrotum

187.8 Other specified sites of male genital organs ♂
Seminal vesicle
Tunica vaginalis
Malignant neoplasm of contiguous or overlapping sites of penis and other male genital organs whose point of origin cannot be determined

187.9 Male genital organ, site unspecified ♂
Male genital organ or tract NOS

✓4ᵗʰ **188 Malignant neoplasm of bladder**
EXCLUDES *carcinoma in situ (233.7)*

188.0 Trigone of urinary bladder

188.1 Dome of urinary bladder

188.2 Lateral wall of urinary bladder

188.3 Anterior wall of urinary bladder

188.4 Posterior wall of urinary bladder

188.5 Bladder neck
Internal urethral orifice

188.6 Ureteric orifice

188.7 Urachus

188.8 Other specified sites of bladder
Malignant neoplasm of contiguous or overlapping sites of bladder whose point of origin cannot be determined

188.9 Bladder, part unspecified
Bladder wall NOS
AHA: 1Q, '00, 5
C67.9 Malignant neoplasm of bladder unspecified   I-10

✓4ᵗʰ **189 Malignant neoplasm of kidney and other and unspecified urinary organs**
EXCLUDES *benign carcinoid tumor of kidney (209.64)*
malignant carcinoid tumor of kidney (209.24)

189.0 Kidney, except pelvis
Kidney NOS
Kidney parenchyma
AHA: 2Q, '05, 4; 2Q, '04, 4
C64.9 Malig neoplasm kidney no renal pelvis uns side   I-10

189.1 Renal pelvis
Renal calyces
Ureteropelvic junction

189.2 Ureter
EXCLUDES *ureteric orifice of bladder (188.6)*

189.3 Urethra
EXCLUDES *urethral orifice of bladder (188.5)*

189.4 Paraurethral glands

189.8 Other specified sites of urinary organs
Malignant neoplasm of contiguous or overlapping sites of kidney and other urinary organs whose point of origin cannot be determined

189.9 Urinary organ, site unspecified
Urinary system NOS

✓4ᵗʰ/✓5ᵗʰ Additional Digit Required   Unspecified Code   Other Specified Code   Manifestation Code   ▶◀ Revised Text   ● New Code   ▲ Revised Code Title

Malignant Neoplasm of Other and Unspecified Sites (190-199)

EXCLUDES *carcinoma in situ (234.0-234.9)*

☑4ᵗʰ **190 Malignant neoplasm of eye**

EXCLUDES *carcinoma in situ (234.0)*
dark area on retina and choroid (239.81)
eyelid (skin) (172.1, 173.1)
    cartilage (171.0)
optic nerve (192.0)
orbital bone (170.0)
retinal freckle (239.81)

190.0 Eyeball, except conjunctiva, cornea, retina, and choroid
Ciliary body   Sclera
Crystalline lens   Uveal tract
Iris

190.1 Orbit
Connective tissue of orbit
Extraocular muscle
Retrobulbar
EXCLUDES *bone of orbit (170.0)*

190.2 Lacrimal gland

190.3 Conjunctiva

190.4 Cornea

190.5 Retina

190.6 Choroid

190.7 Lacrimal duct
Lacrimal sac
Nasolacrimal duct

190.8 Other specified sites of eye
Malignant neoplasm of contiguous or overlapping sites of eye whose point of origin cannot be determined

190.9 Eye, part unspecified

☑4ᵗʰ **191 Malignant neoplasm of brain**

EXCLUDES *cranial nerves (192.0)*
retrobulbar area (190.1)
AHA: 4Q, '07, 104

191.0 Cerebrum, except lobes and ventricles
Basal ganglia   Globus pallidus
Cerebral cortex   Hypothalamus
Corpus striatum   Thalamus

191.1 Frontal lobe
AHA: 4Q, '05, 118

191.2 Temporal lobe
Hippocampus
Uncus
AHA: ▶3Q, '09, 8;◀ 4Q, '06, 123

191.3 Parietal lobe

191.4 Occipital lobe

191.5 Ventricles
Choroid plexus
Floor of ventricle

191.6 Cerebellum NOS
Cerebellopontine angle

Brain and Meninges

Fourth ventricle
Cerebrum
Corpus callosum
Thalamus
Hypothalamus
Hypophysis
Pons
Cerebellum
Medulla oblongata
Midsagittal Section (between hemispheres)

191.7 Brain stem
Cerebral peduncle
Medulla oblongata
Midbrain
Pons

191.8 Other parts of brain
Corpus callosum
Tapetum
Malignant neoplasm of contiguous or overlapping sites of brain whose point of origin cannot be determined

191.9 Brain, unspecified
Cranial fossa NOS
AHA: ▶4Q, '09, 143◀

☑4ᵗʰ **192 Malignant neoplasm of other and unspecified parts of nervous system**

EXCLUDES *peripheral, sympathetic, and parasympathetic nerves and ganglia (171.0-171.9)*

192.0 Cranial nerves
Olfactory bulb

192.1 Cerebral meninges
Dura (mater)   Meninges NOS
Falx (cerebelli) (cerebri)   Tentorium

192.2 Spinal cord
Cauda equina

192.3 Spinal meninges

192.8 Other specified sites of nervous system
Malignant neoplasm of contiguous or overlapping sites of other parts of nervous system whose point of origin cannot be determined

192.9 Nervous system, part unspecified
Nervous system (central) NOS
EXCLUDES *meninges NOS (192.1)*

193 Malignant neoplasm of thyroid gland
Thyroglossal duct
Use additional code to identify any functional activity
C73 Malignant neoplasm of thyroid gland   ꟾ-10

☑4ᵗʰ **194 Malignant neoplasm of other endocrine glands and related structures**

EXCLUDES *islets of Langerhans (157.4)*
neuroendocrine tumors (209.00-209.69)
ovary (183.0)
testis (186.0-186.9)
thymus (164.0)

194.0 Adrenal gland
Adrenal cortex   Suprarenal gland
Adrenal medulla

194.1 Parathyroid gland

194.3 Pituitary gland and craniopharyngeal duct
Craniobuccal pouch   Rathke's pouch
Hypophysis   Sella turcica
AHA: J-A, '85, 9

194.4 Pineal gland

194.5 Carotid body

194.6 Aortic body and other paraganglia
Coccygeal body
Glomus jugulare
Para-aortic body

194.8 Other
Pluriglandular involvement NOS
NOTE If the sites of multiple involvements are known, they should be coded separately.

194.9 Endocrine gland, site unspecified

Ⓝ Newborn Age: 0   Ⓟ Pediatric Age: 0-17   Ⓜ Maternity Age: 12-55   Ⓐ Adult Age: 15-124

☑4ᵗʰ **195 Malignant neoplasm of other and ill-defined sites**

INCLUDES malignant neoplasms of contiguous sites, not elsewhere classified, whose point of origin cannot be determined

EXCLUDES malignant neoplasm:
lymphatic and hematopoietic tissue (200.0-208.9)
secondary sites (196.0-198.8)
unspecified site (199.0-199.1)

195.0 Head, face, and neck
Cheek NOS   Nose NOS
Jaw NOS   Supraclavicular region NOS
AHA: 4Q, '03, 107

195.1 Thorax
Axilla
Chest (wall) NOS
Intrathoracic NOS

195.2 Abdomen
Intra-abdominal NOS
AHA: 2Q, '97, 3

195.3 Pelvis
Groin
Inguinal region NOS
Presacral region
Sacrococcygeal region
Sites overlapping systems within pelvis, as:
rectovaginal (septum)
rectovesical (septum)

195.4 Upper limb

195.5 Lower limb

195.8 Other specified sites
Back NOS
Flank NOS
Trunk NOS

☑4ᵗʰ **196 Secondary and unspecified malignant neoplasm of lymph nodes**

EXCLUDES any malignant neoplasm of lymph nodes, specified as primary (200.0-202.9)
Hodgkin's disease (201.0-201.9)
lymphosarcoma (200.1)
other forms of lymphoma (202.0-202.9)
reticulosarcoma (200.0)
secondary neuroendocrine tumor of (distant) lymph nodes (209.71)
AHA: 2Q, '92, 3; M-J, '85, 3

196.0 Lymph nodes of head, face, and neck
Cervical   Scalene
Cervicofacial   Supraclavicular
AHA: 3Q, '07, 7
C77.0 Sec & uns malig neo lymph nodes head face & neck I-10

196.1 Intrathoracic lymph nodes
Bronchopulmonary   Mediastinal
Intercostal   Tracheobronchial
AHA: 3Q, '06, 7

196.2 Intra-abdominal lymph nodes
Intestinal   Retroperitoneal
Mesenteric
AHA: 4Q, '03, 111
C77.2 Sec & uns malig neoplasm intra-abd lymph nodes I-10

196.3 Lymph nodes of axilla and upper limb
Brachial   Infraclavicular
Epitrochlear   Pectoral

196.5 Lymph nodes of inguinal region and lower limb
Femoral   Popliteal
Groin   Tibial

196.6 Intrapelvic lymph nodes
Hypogastric   Obturator
Iliac   Parametrial

196.8 Lymph nodes of multiple sites

196.9 Site unspecified
Lymph nodes NOS

Lymph Nodes

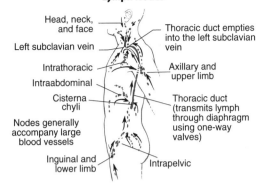

Head, neck, and face
Left subclavian vein
Intrathoracic
Intraabdominal
Cisterna chyli
Nodes generally accompany large blood vessels
Inguinal and lower limb
Thoracic duct empties into the left subclavian vein
Axillary and upper limb
Thoracic duct (transmits lymph through diaphragm using one-way valves)
Intrapelvic

☑4ᵗʰ **197 Secondary malignant neoplasm of respiratory and digestive systems**

EXCLUDES lymph node metastasis (196.0-196.9)
secondary neuroendocrine tumor of liver (209.72)
secondary neuroendocrine tumor of respiratory organs (209.79)
AHA: M-J, '85, 3

197.0 Lung
Bronchus
AHA: 1Q, '06, 4; 2Q, '99, 9
C78.00 Secondary malig neoplasm of lung unspec side I-10

197.1 Mediastinum
AHA: 3Q, '06, 7

197.2 Pleura
AHA: 1Q, '08, 16; 3Q, '07, 3; 4Q, '03, 110; 4Q, '89, 11
TIP: Do not assign for malignant pleural effusion; see instead code 511.81.
C78.2 Secondary malignant neoplasm of pleura I-10

197.3 Other respiratory organs
Trachea

197.4 Small intestine, including duodenum

197.5 Large intestine and rectum

197.6 Retroperitoneum and peritoneum
AHA: 2Q, '04, 4; 4Q, '89, 11
C78.6 Sec malignant neoplasm of retroperiton & periton I-10

197.7 Liver, specified as secondary
AHA: 1Q, '06, 4; 2Q, '05, 9
C78.7 Secondary malignant neoplasm of liver I-10

197.8 Other digestive organs and spleen
AHA: 2Q, '97, 3; 2Q, '92, 3

☑4ᵗʰ **198 Secondary malignant neoplasm of other specified sites**

EXCLUDES lymph node metastasis (196.0-196.9)
secondary neuroendocrine tumor of other specified sites (209.79)
AHA: M-J, '85, 3

198.0 Kidney

198.1 Other urinary organs

198.2 Skin
Skin of breast

198.3 Brain and spinal cord
AHA: 3Q, '07, 4; 3Q, '99, 7
C79.31 Secondary malignant neoplasm of brain I-10

198.4 Other parts of nervous system
Meninges (cerebral) (spinal)
AHA: J-F, '87, 7

198.5 Bone and bone marrow
AHA: 1Q, '07, 6; 4Q, '03, 110; 3Q, '99, 5; 2Q, '92, 3; 1Q, '91, 16; 4Q, '89, 10
C79.51 Secondary malignant neoplasm of bone I-10

198.6 Ovary ♀

198.7 Adrenal gland
Suprarenal gland
C79.70 Sec malignant neoplasm of adrenal gland uns side I-10

☑4ᵗʰ ☑5ᵗʰ Additional Digit Required   Unspecified Code   Other Specified Code   Manifestation Code   ►◄ Revised Text   ● New Code   ▲ Revised Code Title

2011 ICD-9-CM   **Volume 1 – 37**

✓5th **198.8 Other specified sites**

    198.81 Breast

        EXCLUDES *skin of breast (198.2)*

    198.82 Genital organs

    198.89 Other

        EXCLUDES *retroperitoneal lymph nodes (196.2)*

        AHA: 2Q, '05, 4; 2Q '97, 4

        TIP: Assign for intra-abdominal metastasis when no further specificity of site is documented.

        C79.89 Secondary malignant neoplasm of other spec sites   I-10

✓4th **199 Malignant neoplasm without specification of site**

    EXCLUDES *malignant carcinoid tumor of unknown primary site (209.20)*
        malignant (poorly differentiated) neuroendocrine carcinoma, any site (209.30)
        malignant (poorly differentiated) neuroendocrine tumor, any site (209.30)
        neuroendocrine carcinoma (high grade), any site (209.30)

  199.0 Disseminated

    Carcinomatosis
    Generalized:
      cancer   } unspecified site (primary)
      malignancy   }   (secondary)
    Multiple cancer

    AHA: 4Q, '89, 10

  199.1 Other

    Cancer   }
    Carcinoma   } unspecified site (primary)
    Malignancy   }   (secondary)

    AHA: 3Q, '06, 14-15; 1Q, '06, 4

    TIP: Assign if patient is assessed for a metastatic tumor but primary site is unknown.

    C80.1 Malignant neoplasm unspecified   I-10

  199.2 Malignant neoplasm associated with transplanted organ

    Code first complication of transplanted organ (996.80-996.89)
    Use additional code for specific malignancy

    AHA: 4Q, '08, 82-83

    TIP: Assign first the appropriate code from subcategory 996.8, Complications of transplanted organ; use additional code for the specific malignancy.

Malignant Neoplasm of Lymphatic and Hematopoietic Tissue (200-208)

  EXCLUDES *autoimmune lymphoproliferative syndrome (279.41)*
        secondary neoplasm of:
          bone marrow (198.5)
          spleen (197.8)
        secondary and unspecified neoplasm of lymph nodes (196.0-196.9)

The following fifth-digit subclassification is for use with categories 200-202:

  0 unspecified site, extranodal and solid organ sites
  1 lymph nodes of head, face, and neck
  2 intrathoracic lymph nodes
  3 intra-abdominal lymph nodes
  4 lymph nodes of axilla and upper limb
  5 lymph nodes of inguinal region and lower limb
  6 intrapelvic lymph nodes
  7 spleen
  8 lymph nodes of multiple sites

✓4th **200 Lymphosarcoma and reticulosarcoma and other specified malignant tumors of lymphatic tissue**

    AHA: 4Q, '07, 65; 2Q, '92, 3; N-D, '86, 5

§ ✓5th **200.0 Reticulosarcoma**

  [0-8]   Lymphoma (malignant):   Reticulum cell sarcoma:
        histiocytic (diffuse):   NOS
          nodular   pleomorphic cell type
          pleomorphic cell type
          reticulum cell type

    DEF: Malignant lymphoma of primarily histolytic cells; commonly originates in reticuloendothelium of lymph nodes.

    AHA: For Code 200.03: 3Q, '01, 12; **For Code 200.04:** ▶3Q, '09, 4◀

§ ✓5th **200.1 Lymphosarcoma**

  [0-8]   Lymphoblastoma (diffuse)
      Lymphoma (malignant):
        lymphoblastic (diffuse)
        lymphocytic (cell type) (diffuse)
        lymphosarcoma type
      Lymphosarcoma:
        NOS
        diffuse NOS
        lymphoblastic (diffuse)
        lymphocytic (diffuse)
        prolymphocytic

    EXCLUDES *lymphosarcoma:*
        follicular or nodular (202.0)
        mixed cell type (200.8)
        lymphosarcoma cell leukemia (207.8)

    DEF: Malignant lymphoma created from anaplastic lymphoid cells resembling lymphocytes or lymphoblasts.

§ ✓5th **200.2 Burkitt's tumor or lymphoma**

  [0-8]   Malignant lymphoma, Burkitt's type

    DEF: Large osteolytic lesion most common in jaw or as abdominal mass; usually found in central Africa but reported elsewhere.

§ ✓5th **200.3 Marginal zone lymphoma**

  [0-8]   Extranodal marginal zone B-cell lymphoma
      Mucosa associated lymphoid tissue [MALT]
      Nodal marginal zone B-cell lymphoma
      Splenic marginal zone B-cell lymphoma

    AHA: 4Q, '07, 65

§ ✓5th **200.4 Mantle cell lymphoma**

  [0-8]   **AHA:** 4Q, '07, 65

§ ✓5th **200.5 Primary central nervous system lymphoma**

  [0-8]   **AHA:** 4Q, '07, 66

§ ✓5th **200.6 Anaplastic large cell lymphoma**

  [0-8]   **AHA:** 4Q, '07, 66

§ ✓5th **200.7 Large cell lymphoma**

  [0-8]   **AHA:** 4Q, '07, 66

§ ✓5th **200.8 Other named variants**

  [0-8]   Lymphoma (malignant):
      lymphoplasmacytoid type
      mixed lymphocytic-histiocytic (diffuse)
    Lymphosarcoma, mixed cell type (diffuse)
    Reticulolymphosarcoma (diffuse)

✓4th **201 Hodgkin's disease**

    DEF: Painless, progressive enlargement of lymph nodes, spleen and general lymph tissue; symptoms include anorexia, lassitude, weight loss, fever, pruritis, night sweats, anemia.

    AHA: 2Q, '92, 3; N-D, '86, 5

§ ✓5th **201.0 Hodgkin's paragranuloma**

  [0-8]

§ ✓5th **201.1 Hodgkin's granuloma**

  [0-8]   **AHA:** 2Q, '99, 7

§ ✓5th **201.2 Hodgkin's sarcoma**

  [0-8]

§ ✓5th **201.4 Lymphocytic-histiocytic predominance**

  [0-8]

§ ✓5th **201.5 Nodular sclerosis**

  [0-8]   Hodgkin's disease, nodular sclerosis:
      NOS
      cellular phase

§ ✓5th **201.6 Mixed cellularity**

  [0-8]

§ ✓5th **201.7 Lymphocytic depletion**

  [0-8]   Hodgkin's disease, lymphocytic depletion:
      NOS
      diffuse fibrosis
      reticular type

§ ✓5th **201.9 Hodgkin's disease, unspecified**

  [0-8]   Hodgkin's: Malignant:
      disease NOS   lymphogranuloma
      lymphoma NOS   lymphogranulomatosis

§ Requires fifth digit. Valid digits are in [brackets] under each code. See beginning of section 200-208 for codes and definitions.

☑4th **202 Other malignant neoplasms of lymphoid and histiocytic tissue**
AHA: 2Q, '92, 3; N-D, '86, 5

§ ☑5th **202.0 Nodular lymphoma**
[0-8] Brill-Symmers disease
Lymphoma:
    follicular (giant) (large cell)
    lymphocytic, nodular
Lymphosarcoma:
    follicular (giant)
    nodular
DEF: Lymphomatous cells clustered into nodules within the lymph node; usually occurs in older adults and may involve all nodes and possibly extranodal sites.
AHA: For code 202.04: ▶3Q, '09, 4◀

§ ☑5th **202.1 Mycosis fungoides**
[0-8] **EXCLUDES** *peripheral T-cell lymphoma (202.7)*
DEF: Type of cutaneous T-cell lymphoma; may evolve into generalized lymphoma; formerly thought to be of fungoid origin.
AHA: 2Q, '92, 4

§ ☑5th **202.2 Sézary's disease**
[0-8] **DEF:** Type of cutaneous T-cell lymphoma with erythroderma, intense pruritus, peripheral lymphadenopathy, abnormal hyperchromatic mononuclear cells in skin, lymph nodes and peripheral blood.
AHA: 2Q, '99, 7

§ ☑5th **202.3 Malignant histiocytosis**
[0-8] Histiocytic medullary reticulosis
Malignant:
    reticuloendotheliosis
    reticulosis

§ ☑5th **202.4 Leukemic reticuloendotheliosis**
[0-8] Hairy-cell leukemia
DEF: Chronic leukemia with large, mononuclear cells with "hairy" appearance in marrow, spleen, liver, blood.

§ ☑5th **202.5 Letterer-Siwe disease**
[0-8] Acute:
    differentiated progressive histiocytosis
    histiocytosis X (progressive)
    infantile reticuloendotheliosis
    reticulosis of infancy
EXCLUDES *Hand-Schüller-Christian disease (277.89)*
histiocytosis (acute) (chronic) (277.89)
histiocytosis X (chronic) (277.89)
DEF: A recessive reticuloendotheliosis of early childhood, with a hemorrhagic tendency, eczema-like skin eruption, hepatosplenomegaly, lymph node enlargement, and progressive anemia; often a fatal disease with no established cause.

§ ☑5th **202.6 Malignant mast cell tumors**
[0-8] Malignant: Mast cell sarcoma
    mastocytoma   Systemic tissue mast
    mastocytosis   cell disease
EXCLUDES *mast cell leukemia (207.8)*

§ ☑5th **202.7 Peripheral T-cell lymphoma**
[0-8] **AHA:** 4Q, '07, 66

§ ☑5th **202.8 Other lymphomas**
[0-8] Lymphoma (malignant):
    NOS
    diffuse
EXCLUDES *benign lymphoma (229.0)*
AHA: 4Q, '06, 135; 2Q, '06, 20-21; 2Q, '92, 4; **For code 202.80:** 4Q, '08, 83; 1Q, '08, 16; 3Q, '07, 3
C85.70 Oth spec types non-Hodgkins lymphoma unspec site   [I-10]

§ ☑5th **202.9 Other and unspecified malignant neoplasms of**
[0-8] **lymphoid and histiocytic tissue**
Follicular dendritic cell sarcoma
Interdigitating dendritic cell sarcoma
Langerhans cell sarcoma
Malignant neoplasm of bone marrow NOS

☑4th **203 Multiple myeloma and immunoproliferative neoplasms**
AHA: 4Q, '08, 83-84; 4Q, '91, 26

The following fifth-digit subclassification is for use with category 203:
  0 without mention of having achieved remission
    Failed remission
  1 in remission
  2 in relapse

§ ☑5th **203.0 Multiple myeloma**
[0-2] Kahler's disease   Myelomatosis
EXCLUDES *solitary myeloma (238.6)*
AHA: 1Q, '96, 16; 4Q, '89, 10; **For code 203.00:** 2Q, '07, 8
For code 203.01: 4Q, '08, 91
C90.00 Multiple myeloma not in remission   [I-10]

§ ☑5th **203.1 Plasma cell leukemia**
[0-2] Plasmacytic leukemia
AHA: 4Q, '91, 26; S-0, '86, 12

§ ☑5th **203.8 Other immunoproliferative neoplasms**
[0-2] **AHA:** 4Q, '90, 26; S-O, '86, 12

☑4th **204 Lymphoid leukemia**
INCLUDES leukemia:
    lymphatic
    lymphoblastic
    lymphocytic
    lymphogenous
AHA: 4Q, '08, 83-84; 3Q, '93, 4

The following fifth-digit subclassification is for use with category 204:
  0 without mention of having achieved remission
    Failed remission
  1 in remission
  2 in relapse

§ ☑5th **204.0 Acute**
[0-2] **EXCLUDES** *acute exacerbation of chronic lymphoid leukemia (204.1)*
AHA: 3Q, '99, 6

§ ☑5th **204.1 Chronic**
[0-2] **C91.10** Chronic lymphocytic leukemia not in remission   [I-10]

§ ☑5th **204.2 Subacute**
[0-2]

§ ☑5th **204.8 Other lymphoid leukemia**
[0-2] Aleukemic leukemia: Aleukemic leukemia:
    lymphatic   lymphoid
    lymphocytic
AHA: ▶3Q, '09, 4◀
TIP: ▶Assign for T-cell large granular lymphocytic leukemia.◀

§ ☑5th **204.9 Unspecified lymphoid leukemia**
[0-2]

☑4th **205 Myeloid leukemia**
INCLUDES leukemia:
    granulocytic
    myeloblastic
    myelocytic
    myelogenous
    myelomonocytic
    myelosclerotic
    myelosis
AHA: 4Q, '08, 83-84; 3Q, '93, 3; 4Q, '91, 26; 4Q, '90, 3; M-J, '85, 18

The following fifth-digit subclassification is for use with category 205:
  0 without mention of having achieved remission
    Failed remission
  1 in remission
  2 in relapse

§ ☑5th **205.0 Acute**
[0-2] Acute promyelocytic leukemia
EXCLUDES *acute exacerbation of chronic myeloid leukemia (205.1)*
AHA: 2Q, '06, 20-2; **For code 205.00:** ▶4Q, '09, 79◀
C92.00 Acute myeloid leukemia not in remission   [I-10]

---

§   Requires fifth digit. Valid digits are in [brackets] under each code. See appropriate category for codes and definitions.

☑4th ☑5th Additional Digit Required   Unspecified Code   Other Specified Code   Manifestation Code   ▶◀ Revised Text   ● New Code   ▲ Revised Code Title

Neoplasms

205.1–209.29

§ ✓5ᵗʰ **205.1 Chronic**
[0-2]   Eosinophilic leukemia
      Neutrophilic leukemia
      AHA: 1Q, '00, 6; J-A, '85, 13 ; **For code 205.10:** 4Q, '08, 142

§ ✓5ᵗʰ **205.2 Subacute**
[0-2]

§ ✓5ᵗʰ **205.3 Myeloid sarcoma**
[0-2]   Chloroma
      Granulocytic sarcoma

§ ✓5ᵗʰ **205.8 Other myeloid leukemia**
[0-2]   Aleukemic leukemia: Aleukemic leukemia:
        granulocytic   myeloid
        myelogenous   Aleukemic myelosis

§ ✓5ᵗʰ **205.9 Unspecified myeloid leukemia**
[0-2]

✓4ᵗʰ **206 Monocytic leukemia**
  INCLUDES leukemia:
        histiocytic
        monoblastic
        monocytoid

AHA: 4Q, '08, 83-84

The following fifth-digit subclassification is for use with category 206:
  0 without mention of having achieved remission
      Failed remission
  1 in remission
  2 in relapse

§ ✓5ᵗʰ **206.0 Acute**
[0-2]   **EXCLUDES** *acute exacerbation of chronic monocytic leukemia*
        (206.1)

§ ✓5ᵗʰ **206.1 Chronic**
[0-2]

§ ✓5ᵗʰ **206.2 Subacute**
[0-2]

§ ✓5ᵗʰ **206.8 Other monocytic leukemia**
[0-2]   Aleukemic:
      monocytic leukemia
      monocytoid leukemia

§ ✓5ᵗʰ **206.9 Unspecified monocytic leukemia**
[0-2]

✓4ᵗʰ **207 Other specified leukemia**
  EXCLUDES *leukemic reticuloendotheliosis (202.4)*
        plasma cell leukemia (203.1)
  AHA: 4Q, '08, 83-85

The following fifth-digit subclassification is for use with category 207:
  0 without mention of having achieved remission
      Failed remission
  1 in remission
  2 in relapse

§ ✓5ᵗʰ **207.0 Acute erythremia and erythroleukemia**
[0-2]   Acute erythremic myelosis
      Di Guglielmo's disease
      Erythremic myelosis
      DEF: Erythremia: polycythemia vera.
      DEF: Erythroleukemia: a malignant blood dyscrasia (a
      myeloproliferative disorder).

§ ✓5ᵗʰ **207.1 Chronic erythremia**
[0-2]   Heilmeyer-Schöner disease

§ ✓5ᵗʰ **207.2 Megakaryocytic leukemia**
[0-2]   Megakaryocytic myelosis
      Thrombocytic leukemia

§ ✓5ᵗʰ **207.8 Other specified leukemia**
[0-2]   Lymphosarcoma cell leukemia

✓4ᵗʰ **208 Leukemia of unspecified cell type**
  AHA: 4Q, '08, 83-85

The following fifth-digit subclassification is for use with category 208:
  0 without mention of having achieved remission
      Failed remission
  1 in remission
  2 in relapse

§ ✓5ᵗʰ **208.0 Acute**
[0-2]   Acute leukemia NOS   Stem cell leukemia
      Blast cell leukemia
      EXCLUDES *acute exacerbation of chronic unspecified leukemia*
        (208.1)

§ ✓5ᵗʰ **208.1 Chronic**
[0-2]   Chronic leukemia NOS

§ ✓5ᵗʰ **208.2 Subacute**
[0-2]   Subacute leukemia NOS

§ ✓5ᵗʰ **208.8 Other leukemia of unspecified cell type**
[0-2]

§ ✓5ᵗʰ **208.9 Unspecified leukemia**
[0-2]   Leukemia NOS

Neuroendocrine Tumors (209)

✓4ᵗʰ **209 Neuroendocrine tumors**
  Code first any associated multiple endocrine neoplasia syndrome
      (258.01-258.03)
  Use additional code to identify associated endocrine syndrome, such
      as:
  carcinoid syndrome (259.2)
  EXCLUDES *benign pancreatic islet cell tumors (211.7)*
        malignant pancreatic islet cell tumors (157.4)
  AHA: ▶4Q, '09, 150;◀ 4Q, '08, 85-89

✓5ᵗʰ **209.0 Malignant carcinoid tumors of the small intestine**

  **209.00 Malignant carcinoid tumor of the small
       intestine, unspecified portion**

  209.01 Malignant carcinoid tumor of the duodenum

  209.02 Malignant carcinoid tumor of the jejunum

  209.03 Malignant carcinoid tumor of the ileum

✓5ᵗʰ **209.1 Malignant carcinoid tumors of the appendix, large
intestine, and rectum**

  **209.10 Malignant carcinoid tumor of the large
       intestine, unspecified portion**
       Malignant carcinoid tumor of the colon NOS

  209.11 Malignant carcinoid tumor of the appendix

  209.12 Malignant carcinoid tumor of the cecum

  209.13 Malignant carcinoid tumor of the ascending colon

  209.14 Malignant carcinoid tumor of the transverse colon

  209.15 Malignant carcinoid tumor of the descending colon

  209.16 Malignant carcinoid tumor of the sigmoid colon

  209.17 Malignant carcinoid tumor of the rectum

✓5ᵗʰ **209.2 Malignant carcinoid tumors of other and unspecified sites**

  209.20 Malignant carcinoid tumor of unknown primary site

  **209.21 Malignant carcinoid tumor of the bronchus and
       lung**

  209.22 Malignant carcinoid tumor of the thymus

  209.23 Malignant carcinoid tumor of the stomach
       AHA: 4Q, '08, 89

  209.24 Malignant carcinoid tumor of the kidney

  209.25 Malignant carcinoid tumor of the foregut NOS

  209.26 Malignant carcinoid tumor of the midgut NOS

  209.27 Malignant carcinoid tumor of the hindgut NOS

  209.29 Malignant carcinoid tumors of other sites

---

§ Requires fifth digit. Valid digits are in [brackets] under each code. See appropriate category for codes and definitions.

✓5ᵗʰ **209.3 Malignant poorly differentiated neuroendocrine tumors**
AHA: ▶4Q, '09, 73-74◀

209.30 Malignant poorly differentiated neuroendocrine carcinoma, any site
High grade neuroendocrine carcinoma, any site
Malignant poorly differentiated neuroendocrine tumor NOS
EXCLUDES *Merkel cell carcinoma (209.31-209.36)*

209.31 Merkel cell carcinoma of the face
Merkel cell carcinoma of the ear
Merkel cell carcinoma of the eyelid, including canthus
Merkel cell carcinoma of the lip

209.32 Merkel cell carcinoma of the scalp and neck

209.33 Merkel cell carcinoma of the upper limb

209.34 Merkel cell carcinoma of the lower limb

209.35 Merkel cell carcinoma of the trunk

209.36 Merkel cell carcinoma of other sites
Merkel cell carcinoma of the buttock
Merkel cell carcinoma of the genitals
Merkel cell carcinoma NOS
AHA: ▶4Q, '09, 74◀

✓5ᵗʰ **209.4 Benign carcinoid tumors of the small intestine**

209.40 Benign carcinoid tumor of the small intestine, unspecified portion

209.41 Benign carcinoid tumor of the duodenum

209.42 Benign carcinoid tumor of the jejunum

209.43 Benign carcinoid tumor of the ileum

✓5ᵗʰ **209.5 Benign carcinoid tumors of the appendix, large intestine, and rectum**

209.50 Benign carcinoid tumor of the large intestine, unspecified portion
Benign carcinoid tumor of the colon NOS

209.51 Benign carcinoid tumor of the appendix

209.52 Benign carcinoid tumor of the cecum

209.53 Benign carcinoid tumor of the ascending colon

209.54 Benign carcinoid tumor of the transverse colon

209.55 Benign carcinoid tumor of the descending colon

209.56 Benign carcinoid tumor of the sigmoid colon

209.57 Benign carcinoid tumor of the rectum

✓5ᵗʰ **209.6 Benign carcinoid tumors of other and unspecified sites**

209.60 Benign carcinoid tumor of unknown primary site
Carcinoid tumor NOS
Neuroendocrine tumor NOS

209.61 Benign carcinoid tumor of the bronchus and lung
AHA: ▶4Q, '09, 151◀

209.62 Benign carcinoid tumor of the thymus

209.63 Benign carcinoid tumor of the stomach

209.64 Benign carcinoid tumor of the kidney

209.65 Benign carcinoid tumor of the foregut NOS

209.66 Benign carcinoid tumor of the midgut NOS

209.67 Benign carcinoid tumor of the hindgut NOS

209.69 Benign carcinoid tumors of other sites

✓5ᵗʰ **209.7 Secondary neuroendocrine tumors**
Secondary carcinoid tumors
AHA: ▶4Q, '09, 74◀

209.70 Secondary neuroendocrine tumor, unspecified site

209.71 Secondary neuroendocrine tumor of distant lymph nodes
Mesentery metastasis of neuroendocrine tumor

209.72 Secondary neuroendocrine tumor of liver

209.73 Secondary neuroendocrine tumor of bone

209.74 Secondary neuroendocrine tumor of peritoneum
AHA: ▶4Q, '09, 150◀

209.75 Secondary Merkel cell carcinoma
Merkel cell carcinoma nodal presentation
Merkel cell carcinoma visceral metastatic presentation
Secondary Merkel cell carcinoma, any site

209.79 Secondary neuroendocrine tumor of other sites

Benign Neoplasms (210-229)

✓4ᵗʰ **210 Benign neoplasm of lip, oral cavity, and pharynx**
EXCLUDES *cyst (of):*
jaw (526.0-526.2, 526.89)
oral soft tissue (528.4)
radicular (522.8)

210.0 Lip
Frenulum labii
Lip (inner aspect) (mucosa) (vermilion border)
EXCLUDES *labial commissure (210.4)*
skin of lip (216.0)

210.1 Tongue
Lingual tonsil

210.2 Major salivary glands
Gland:
parotid
sublingual
submandibular
EXCLUDES *benign neoplasms of minor salivary glands:*
NOS (210.4)
buccal mucosa (210.4)
lips (210.0)
palate (hard) (soft) (210.4)
tongue (210.1)
tonsil, palatine (210.5)

210.3 Floor of mouth

210.4 Other and unspecified parts of mouth
Gingiva   Oral mucosa
Gum (upper) (lower)   Palate (hard) (soft)
Labial commissure   Uvula
Oral cavity NOS
EXCLUDES *benign odontogenic neoplasms of bone (213.0-213.1)*
developmental odontogenic cysts (526.0)
mucosa of lips (210.0)
nasopharyngeal [posterior] [superior] surface of soft palate (210.7)

210.5 Tonsil
Tonsil (faucial) (palatine)
EXCLUDES *lingual tonsil (210.1)*
pharyngeal tonsil (210.7)
tonsillar:
fossa (210.6)
pillars (210.6)

210.6 Other parts of oropharynx
Branchial cleft or vestiges
Epiglottis, anterior aspect
Fauces NOS
Mesopharynx NOS
Tonsillar:
fossa
pillars
Vallecula
EXCLUDES *epiglottis:*
NOS (212.1)
suprahyoid portion (212.1)

210.7 Nasopharynx
Adenoid tissue
Lymphadenoid tissue
Pharyngeal tonsil
Posterior nasal septum

210.8 Hypopharynx
Arytenoid fold
Laryngopharynx
Postcricoid region
Pyriform fossa

210.9 Pharynx, unspecified
Throat NOS

☑4ᵗʰ **211 Benign neoplasm of other parts of digestive system**
EXCLUDES *benign stromal tumors of digestive system (215.5)*

211.0 Esophagus

211.1 Stomach
Body
Cardia   ⎫
Fundus   ⎬ of stomach
Cardiac orifice
Pylorus
EXCLUDES *benign carcinoid tumors of the stomach (209.63)*
D13.1 Benign neoplasm of stomach   I-10

211.2 Duodenum, jejunum, and ileum
Small intestine NOS
EXCLUDES *ampulla of Vater (211.5)*
benign carcinoid tumors of the small intestine (209.40-209.43)
ileocecal valve (211.3)

211.3 Colon
Appendix
Cecum
Ileocecal valve
Large intestine NOS
EXCLUDES *benign carcinoid tumors of the large intestine (209.50-209.56)*
rectosigmoid junction (211.4)
AHA: 3Q, '05, 17; 2Q, '05, 16; 4Q, '01, 56
D12.6 Benign neoplasm of colon unspecified   I-10

211.4 Rectum and anal canal
Anal canal or sphincter
Anus NOS
Rectosigmoid junction
EXCLUDES *anus:*
margin (216.5)
skin (216.5)
benign carcinoid tumors of the rectum (209.57)
perianal skin (216.5)

211.5 Liver and biliary passages
Ampulla of Vater
Common bile duct
Cystic duct
Gallbladder
Hepatic duct
Sphincter of Oddi

211.6 Pancreas, except islets of Langerhans

211.7 Islets of Langerhans
Islet cell tumor
Use additional code to identify any functional activity

211.8 Retroperitoneum and peritoneum
Mesentery
Mesocolon
Omentum
Retroperitoneal tissue

211.9 Other and unspecified site
Alimentary tract NOS
Digestive system NOS
Gastrointestinal tract NOS
Intestinal tract NOS
Intestine NOS
Spleen, not elsewhere classified

☑4ᵗʰ **212 Benign neoplasm of respiratory and intrathoracic organs**

212.0 Nasal cavities, middle ear, and accessory sinuses
Cartilage of nose
Eustachian tube
Nares
Septum of nose
Sinus:
ethmoidal
frontal
maxillary
sphenoidal
EXCLUDES *auditory canal (external) (216.2)*
bone of:
ear (213.0)
nose [turbinates] (213.0)
cartilage of ear (215.0)
ear (external) (skin) (216.2)
nose NOS (229.8)
skin (216.3)
olfactory bulb (225.1)
polyp of:
accessory sinus (471.8)
ear (385.30-385.35)
nasal cavity (471.0)
posterior margin of septum and choanae (210.7)

212.1 Larynx
Cartilage: Epiglottis (suprahyoid portion) NOS
arytenoid   Glottis
cricoid   Vocal cords (false)(true)
cuneiform
thyroid
EXCLUDES *epiglottis, anterior aspect (210.6)*
polyp of vocal cord or larynx (478.4)

212.2 Trachea

212.3 Bronchus and lung
Carina
Hilus of lung
EXCLUDES *benign carcinoid tumors of bronchus and lung (209.61)*

212.4 Pleura

212.5 Mediastinum

212.6 Thymus
EXCLUDES *benign carcinoid tumors of thymus (209.62)*

212.7 Heart
EXCLUDES *great vessels (215.4)*

212.8 Other specified sites

212.9 Site unspecified
Respiratory organ NOS
Upper respiratory tract NOS
EXCLUDES *intrathoracic NOS (229.8)*
thoracic NOS (229.8)

☑4ᵗʰ **213 Benign neoplasm of bone and articular cartilage**
INCLUDES cartilage (articular) (joint)
periosteum
EXCLUDES *cartilage of:*
ear (215.0)
eyelid (215.0))
larynx (212.1)
nose (212.0)
exostosis NOS (726.91)
synovia (215.0-215.9)

213.0 Bones of skull and face
EXCLUDES *lower jaw bone (213.1)*

213.1 Lower jaw bone

213.2 Vertebral column, excluding sacrum and coccyx

213.3 Ribs, sternum, and clavicle

213.4 Scapula and long bones of upper limb

213.5 Short bones of upper limb

213.6 Pelvic bones, sacrum, and coccyx

213.7 Long bones of lower limb

213.8 Short bones of lower limb

213.9 Bone and articular cartilage, site unspecified

✓4ᵗʰ **214 Lipoma**

INCLUDES angiolipoma
fibrolipoma
hibernoma
lipoma (fetal) (infiltrating) (intramuscular)
myelolipoma
myxolipoma

DEF: Benign tumor frequently composed of mature fat cells; may occasionally be composed of fetal fat cells.

214.0 Skin and subcutaneous tissue of face

214.1 Other skin and subcutaneous tissue

214.2 Intrathoracic organs

214.3 Intra-abdominal organs

214.4 Spermatic cord   ♂

214.8 Other specified sites
AHA: 3Q, '94, 7

214.9 Lipoma, unspecified site

✓4ᵗʰ **215 Other benign neoplasm of connective and other soft tissue**

INCLUDES blood vessel
bursa
fascia
ligament
muscle
peripheral, sympathetic, and parasympathetic nerves and
ganglia
synovia
tendon (sheath)

EXCLUDES cartilage:
articular (213.0-213.9)
larynx (212.1)
nose (212.0)
connective tissue of:
breast (217)
internal organ, except lipoma and hemangioma — code
to benign neoplasm of the site
lipoma (214.0-214.9)

215.0 Head, face, and neck

215.2 Upper limb, including shoulder

215.3 Lower limb, including hip

215.4 Thorax
EXCLUDES *heart (212.7)*
mediastinum (212.5)
thymus (212.6)

215.5 Abdomen
Abdominal wall
Benign stromal tumors of abdomen
Hypochondrium

215.6 Pelvis
Buttock
Groin
Inguinal region
Perineum
EXCLUDES *uterine:*
leiomyoma (218.0-218.9)
ligament, any (221.0)

215.7 Trunk, unspecified
Back NOS
Flank NOS

215.8 Other specified sites

215.9 Site unspecified

✓4ᵗʰ **216 Benign neoplasm of skin**

INCLUDES blue nevus
dermatofibroma
hydrocystoma
pigmented nevus
syringoadenoma
syringoma

EXCLUDES *skin of genital organs (221.0-222.9)*
AHA: 1Q, '00, 21

216.0 Skin of lip
EXCLUDES *vermilion border of lip (210.0)*

216.1 Eyelid, including canthus
EXCLUDES *cartilage of eyelid (215.0)*

216.2 Ear and external auditory canal
Auricle (ear)
Auricular canal, external
External meatus
Pinna
EXCLUDES *cartilage of ear (215.0)*

216.3 Skin of other and unspecified parts of face
Cheek, external
Eyebrow
Nose, external
Temple

216.4 Scalp and skin of neck
AHA: 3Q, '91, 12

216.5 Skin of trunk, except scrotum

Axillary fold	Skin of:
Perianal skin	buttock
Skin of:	chest wall
abdominal wall	groin
anus	perineum
back	Umbilicus
breast	

EXCLUDES *anal canal (211.4)*
anus NOS (211.4)
skin of scrotum (222.4)

216.6 Skin of upper limb, including shoulder

216.7 Skin of lower limb, including hip

216.8 Other specified sites of skin

216.9 Skin, site unspecified

217 Benign neoplasm of breast
Breast (male) (female):
connective tissue
glandular tissue
soft parts
EXCLUDES *adenofibrosis (610.2)*
benign cyst of breast (610.0)
fibrocystic disease (610.1)
skin of breast (216.5)
AHA: 1Q, '00, 4

Types of Uterine Fibroids

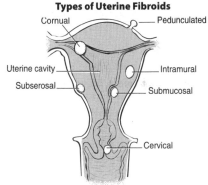

√4ᵗʰ **218 Uterine leiomyoma**

> **INCLUDES** fibroid (bleeding) (uterine)
> uterine:
>   fibromyoma
>   myoma

> **DEF:** Benign tumor primarily derived from uterine smooth muscle tissue; may contain fibrous, fatty, or epithelial tissue; also called uterine fibroid or myoma.

218.0 Submucous leiomyoma of uterus   ♀

218.1 Intramural leiomyoma of uterus   ♀
> Interstitial leiomyoma of uterus
> D25.1 Intramural leiomyoma of uterus   I-10

218.2 Subserous leiomyoma of uterus   ♀

218.9 Leiomyoma of uterus, unspecified   ♀
> **AHA:** 1Q, '03, 4
> D25.9 Leiomyoma of uterus unspecified   I-10

√4ᵗʰ **219 Other benign neoplasm of uterus**

219.0 Cervix uteri   ♀

219.1 Corpus uteri   ♀
> Endometrium
> Fundus
> Myometrium

219.8 Other specified parts of uterus   ♀

219.9 Uterus, part unspecified   ♀

220 Benign neoplasm of ovary   ♀
> Use additional code to identify any functional activity (256.0-256.1)
> **EXCLUDES** cyst:
>   corpus albicans (620.2)
>   corpus luteum (620.1)
>   endometrial (617.1)
>   follicular (atretic) (620.0)
>   graafian follicle (620.0)
>   ovarian NOS (620.2)
>   retention (620.2)
> D27.9 Benign neoplasm of ovary unspecified side   I-10

√4ᵗʰ **221 Benign neoplasm of other female genital organs**

> **INCLUDES** adenomatous polyp
> benign teratoma
> **EXCLUDES** cyst:
>   epoophoron (752.11)
>   fimbrial (752.11)
>   Gartner's duct (752.11)
>   parovarian (752.11)

221.0 Fallopian tube and uterine ligaments   ♀
> Oviduct
> Parametruim
> Uterine ligament (broad) (round) (uterosacral)
> Uterine tube

221.1 Vagina   ♀

221.2 Vulva   ♀
> Clitoris
> External female genitalia NOS
> Greater vestibular [Bartholin's] gland
> Labia (majora) (minora)
> Pudendum
> **EXCLUDES** Bartholin's (duct) (gland) cyst (616.2)

221.8 Other specified sites of female genital organs   ♀

221.9 Female genital organ, site unspecified   ♀
> Female genitourinary tract NOS

√4ᵗʰ **222 Benign neoplasm of male genital organs**

222.0 Testis   ♂
> Use additional code to identify any functional activity

222.1 Penis   ♂
> Corpus cavernosum
> Glans penis
> Prepuce

222.2 Prostate   ♂
> **EXCLUDES** adenomatous hyperplasia of prostate (600.20-600.21)
> prostatic:
>   adenoma (600.20-600.21)
>   enlargement (600.00-600.01)
>   hypertrophy (600.00-600.01)

222.3 Epididymis   ♂

222.4 Scrotum   ♂
> Skin of scrotum

222.8 Other specified sites of male genital organs   ♂
> Seminal vesicle
> Spermatic cord

222.9 Male genital organ, site unspecified   ♂
> Male genitourinary tract NOS

√4ᵗʰ **223 Benign neoplasm of kidney and other urinary organs**

223.0 Kidney, except pelvis
> Kidney NOS
> **EXCLUDES** benign carcinoid tumors of kidney (209.64)
> renal:
>   calyces (223.1)
>   pelvis (223.1)

223.1 Renal pelvis

223.2 Ureter
> **EXCLUDES** ureteric orifice of bladder (223.3)

223.3 Bladder

√5ᵗʰ **223.8 Other specified sites of urinary organs**

223.81 Urethra
> **EXCLUDES** urethral orifice of bladder (223.3)

223.89 Other
> Paraurethral glands

223.9 Urinary organ, site unspecified
> Urinary system NOS

√4ᵗʰ **224 Benign neoplasm of eye**
> **EXCLUDES** cartilage of eyelid (215.0)
> eyelid (skin) (216.1)
> optic nerve (225.1)
> orbital bone (213.0)

224.0 Eyeball, except conjunctiva, cornea, retina, and choroid
> Ciliary body
> Iris
> Sclera
> Uveal tract

224.1 Orbit
> **EXCLUDES** bone of orbit (213.0)

224.2 Lacrimal gland

224.3 Conjunctiva

224.4 Cornea

Eyeball

Posterior segment
Vitreous
Optic nerve
Optic disc
Choroid
Sclera
Retina
Pars plana
Lens
Iris
Conjunctiva
Sclera
Cornea
Anterior chamber

224.5 Retina
   EXCLUDES *hemangioma of retina (228.03)*

224.6 Choroid

224.7 Lacrimal duct
   Lacrimal sac
   Nasolacrimal duct

224.8 Other specified parts of eye

224.9 Eye, part unspecified

√4ᵗʰ **225 Benign neoplasm of brain and other parts of nervous system**
   EXCLUDES *hemangioma (228.02)*
   neurofibromatosis ▶(237.70-237.79)◀
   peripheral, sympathetic, and parasympathetic nerves and
   ganglia (215.0-215.9)
   retrobulbar (224.1)

225.0 Brain

225.1 Cranial nerves
   Acoustic neuroma
   AHA: 4Q, '04, 113

225.2 Cerebral meninges
   Meninges NOS
   Meningioma (cerebral)
   D32.9 Benign neoplasm of meninges unspecified   I-10

225.3 Spinal cord
   Cauda equina

225.4 Spinal meninges
   Spinal meningioma

225.8 Other specified sites of nervous system

225.9 Nervous system, part unspecified
   Nervous system (central) NOS
   EXCLUDES *meninges NOS (225.2)*

226 Benign neoplasm of thyroid glands
   Use additional code to identify any functional activity

√4ᵗʰ **227 Benign neoplasm of other endocrine glands and related structures**
   Use additional code to identify any functional activity
   EXCLUDES *ovary (220)*
   pancreas (211.6)
   testis (222.0)

227.0 Adrenal gland
   Suprarenal gland

227.1 Parathyroid gland

227.3 Pituitary gland and craniopharyngeal duct (pouch)
   Craniobuccal pouch
   Hypophysis
   Rathke's pouch
   Sella turcica

227.4 Pineal gland
   Pineal body

227.5 Carotid body

227.6 Aortic body and other paraganglia
   Coccygeal body
   Glomus jugulare
   Para-aortic body
   AHA: N-D, '84, 17

227.8 Other

227.9 Endocrine gland, site unspecified

√4ᵗʰ **228 Hemangioma and lymphangioma, any site**
   INCLUDES angioma (benign) (cavernous) (congenital) NOS
   cavernous nevus
   glomus tumor
   hemangioma (benign) (congenital)
   EXCLUDES *benign neoplasm of spleen, except hemangioma and*
   lymphangioma (211.9)
   glomus jugulare (227.6)
   nevus:
   NOS (216.0-216.9)
   blue or pigmented (216.0-216.9)
   vascular (757.32)
   AHA: 1Q, '00, 21

√5ᵗʰ **228.0 Hemangioma, any site**
   AHA: J-F, '85, 19
   DEF: A common benign tumor usually occurring in infancy;
   composed of newly formed blood vessels due to malformation of
   angioblastic tissue.

   228.00 Of unspecified site

   228.01 Of skin and subcutaneous tissue

   228.02 Of intracranial structures

   228.03 Of retina

   228.04 Of intra-abdominal structures
      Peritoneum
      Retroperitoneal tissue

   228.09 Of other sites
      Systemic angiomatosis
      AHA: 3Q, '91, 20

228.1 Lymphangioma, any site
   Congenital lymphangioma
   Lymphatic nevus

√4ᵗʰ **229 Benign neoplasm of other and unspecified sites**

229.0 Lymph nodes
   EXCLUDES *lymphangioma (228.1)*

229.8 Other specified sites
   Intrathoracic NOS
   Thoracic NOS

229.9 Site unspecified

Carcinoma In Situ (230-234)

   INCLUDES Bowen's disease
   erythroplasia
   Queyrat's erythroplasia
   EXCLUDES *leukoplakia — see Alphabetic Index*
   DEF: A neoplastic type; with tumor cells confined to epithelium of origin;
   without further invasion.

√4ᵗʰ **230 Carcinoma in situ of digestive organs**

230.0 Lip, oral cavity, and pharynx
   Gingiva
   Hypopharynx
   Mouth [any part]
   Nasopharynx
   Oropharynx
   Salivary gland or duct
   Tongue
   EXCLUDES *aryepiglottic fold or interarytenoid fold, laryngeal*
   aspect (231.0)
   epiglottis:
   NOS (231.0)
   suprahyoid portion (231.0)
   skin of lip (232.0)

230.1 Esophagus

230.2 Stomach
   Body ⎫
   Cardia ⎬ of stomach
   Fundus ⎭
   Cardiac orifice
   Pylorus

√4ᵗʰ
√5ᵗʰ Additional Digit Required   Unspecified Code   Other Specified Code   Manifestation Code   ▶◀ Revised Text   ● New Code   ▲ Revised Code Title

Neoplasms

230.3 Colon
Appendix
Cecum
Ileocecal valve
Large intestine NOS
> EXCLUDES rectosigmoid junction (230.4)

230.4 Rectum
Rectosigmoid junction

230.5 Anal canal
Anal sphincter

230.6 Anus, unspecified
> EXCLUDES anus:
> margin (232.5)
> skin (232.5)
> perianal skin (232.5)

230.7 Other and unspecified parts of intestine
Duodenum
Ileum
Jejunum
Small intestine NOS
> EXCLUDES ampulla of Vater (230.8)

230.8 Liver and biliary system
Ampulla of Vater
Common bile duct
Cystic duct
Gallbladder
Hepatic duct
Sphincter of Oddi

230.9 Other and unspecified digestive organs
Digestive organ NOS
Gastrointestinal tract NOS
Pancreas
Spleen

√4ᵗʰ **231 Carcinoma in situ of respiratory system**

231.0 Larynx
Cartilage:
  arytenoid
  cricoid
  cuneiform
  thyroid
Epiglottis:
  NOS
  posterior surface
  suprahyoid portion
Vocal cords (false)(true)
> EXCLUDES aryepiglottic fold or interarytenoid fold:
> NOS (230.0)
> hypopharyngeal aspect (230.0)
> marginal zone (230.0)

231.1 Trachea

231.2 Bronchus and lung
Carina
Hilus of lung

231.8 Other specified parts of respiratory system
Accessory sinuses
Middle ear
Nasal cavities
Pleura
> EXCLUDES ear (external) (skin) (232.2)
> nose NOS (234.8)
> skin (232.3)

231.9 Respiratory system, part unspecified
Respiratory organ NOS

√4ᵗʰ **232 Carcinoma in situ of skin**
> INCLUDES pigment cells
> EXCLUDES melanoma in situ of skin (172.0-172.9)

232.0 Skin of lip
> EXCLUDES vermilion border of lip (230.0)

232.1 Eyelid, including canthus

232.2 Ear and external auditory canal

232.3 Skin of other and unspecified parts of face

232.4 Scalp and skin of neck

232.5 Skin of trunk, except scrotum

Anus, margin	Skin of:
Axillary fold	breast
Perianal skin	buttock
Skin of:	chest wall
abdominal wall	groin
anus	perineum
back	Umbilicus

> EXCLUDES anal canal (230.5)
> anus NOS (230.6)
> skin of genital organs (233.30-233.39, 233.5-233.6)

232.6 Skin of upper limb, including shoulder

232.7 Skin of lower limb, including hip

232.8 Other specified sites of skin

232.9 Skin, site unspecified

√4ᵗʰ **233 Carcinoma in situ of breast and genitourinary system**
> TIP: For patients with carcinoma in situ found incidentally when admitted for treatment of another condition, sequence the 233 code as a secondary condition.

233.0 Breast
> EXCLUDES Paget's disease (174.0-174.9)
> skin of breast (232.5)
> TIP: Assign for tumors specified as intraductal carcinoma.

233.1 Cervix uteri ♀
Adenocarcinoma in situ of cervix
Cervical intraepithelial glandular neoplasia, grade III
Cervical intraepithelial neoplasia III [CIN III]
Severe dysplasia of cervix
> EXCLUDES cervical intraepithelial neoplasia II [CIN II] (622.12)
> cytologic evidence of malignancy without histologic confirmation (795.06)
> high grade squamous intraepithelial lesion (HGSIL) (795.04)
> moderate dysplasia of cervix (622.12)
> AHA: 3Q, '92, 7; 3Q, '92, 8; 1Q, '91, 11

233.2 Other and unspecified parts of uterus ♀

√5ᵗʰ **233.3 Other and unspecified female genital organs**
> AHA: 4Q, '07, 67

    233.30 Unspecified female genital organ ♀

    233.31 Vagina ♀
Severe dysplasia of vagina
Vaginal intraepithelial neoplasia III [VAIN III]

    233.32 Vulva ♀
Severe dysplasia of vulva
Vulvar intraepithelial neoplasia III [VIN III]

    233.39 Other female genital organ ♀

233.4 Prostate ♂

233.5 Penis ♂

233.6 Other and unspecified male genital organs ♂

233.7 Bladder

233.9 Other and unspecified urinary organs

√4ᵗʰ **234 Carcinoma in situ of other and unspecified sites**

234.0 Eye
> EXCLUDES cartilage of eyelid (234.8)
> eyelid (skin) (232.1)
> optic nerve (234.8)
> orbital bone (234.8)

234.8 Other specified sites
Endocrine gland [any]

234.9 Site unspecified
Carcinoma in situ NOS

N Newborn Age: 0   P Pediatric Age: 0-17   M Maternity Age: 12-55   A Adult Age: 15-124

Neoplasms of Uncertain Behavior (235-238)

NOTE Categories 235–238 classify by site certain histomorphologically well-defined neoplasms, the subsequent behavior of which cannot be predicted from the present appearance.

TIP: Typically assigned for cases in which the tumor is in transition and may be undergoing malignant transformation, but continued study is required for accurate classification.

√4th **235 Neoplasm of uncertain behavior of digestive and respiratory systems**

> **EXCLUDES** *stromal tumors of uncertain behavior of digestive system (238.1)*

235.0 Major salivary glands
Gland:
  parotid
  sublingual
  submandibular
> **EXCLUDES** *minor salivary glands (235.1)*

235.1 Lip, oral cavity, and pharynx
Gingiva
Hypopharynx
Minor salivary glands
Mouth
Nasopharynx
Oropharynx
Tongue
> **EXCLUDES** *aryepiglottic fold or interarytenoid fold, laryngeal aspect (235.6)*
> *epiglottis:*
>   *NOS (235.6)*
>   *suprahyoid portion (235.6)*
> *skin of lip (238.2)*

235.2 Stomach, intestines, and rectum

235.3 Liver and biliary passages
Ampulla of Vater
Bile ducts [any]
Gallbladder
Liver

235.4 Retroperitoneum and peritoneum

235.5 Other and unspecified digestive organs
Anal:
  canal
  sphincter
Anus NOS
Esophagus
Pancreas
Spleen
> **EXCLUDES** *anus:*
>   *margin (238.2)*
>   *skin (238.2)*
> *perianal skin (238.2)*

235.6 Larynx
> **EXCLUDES** *aryepiglottic fold or interarytenoid fold:*
>   *NOS (235.1)*
>   *hypopharyngeal aspect (235.1)*
>   *marginal zone (235.1)*

235.7 Trachea, bronchus, and lung

235.8 Pleura, thymus, and mediastinum

235.9 Other and unspecified respiratory organs
Accessory sinuses
Middle ear
Nasal cavities
Respiratory organ NOS
> **EXCLUDES** *ear (external) (skin) (238.2)*
> *nose (238.8)*
> *skin (238.2)*

√4th **236 Neoplasm of uncertain behavior of genitourinary organs**

236.0 Uterus ♀

236.1 Placenta ♀
Chorioadenoma (destruens)
Invasive mole
Malignant hydatid(iform) mole

236.2 Ovary ♀
> Use additional code to identify any functional activity

236.3 Other and unspecified female genital organs ♀

236.4 Testis ♂
> Use additional code to identify any functional activity

236.5 Prostate ♂

236.6 Other and unspecified male genital organs ♂

236.7 Bladder

√5th **236.9 Other and unspecified urinary organs**

> **236.90 Urinary organ, unspecified**

> **236.91 Kidney and ureter**

> **236.99 Other**

√4th **237 Neoplasm of uncertain behavior of endocrine glands and nervous system**

237.0 Pituitary gland and craniopharyngeal duct
> Use additional code to identify any functional activity

237.1 Pineal gland

237.2 Adrenal gland
Suprarenal gland
> Use additional code to identify any functional activity

237.3 Paraganglia
Aortic body
Carotid body
Coccygeal body
Glomus jugulare
AHA: N-D, '84, 17

237.4 Other and unspecified endocrine glands
Parathyroid gland
Thyroid gland

237.5 Brain and spinal cord

237.6 Meninges
Meninges:
  NOS
  cerebral
  spinal

√5th **237.7 Neurofibromatosis**
> **DEF:** An inherited condition with developmental changes in the nervous system, muscles, bones and skin; multiple soft tumors (neurofibromas) distributed over the entire body.

> **237.70 Neurofibromatosis, unspecified**

> **237.71 Neurofibromatosis, type 1 [von Recklinghausen's disease]**

> **237.72 Neurofibromatosis, type 2 [acoustic neurofibromatosis]**
>> **DEF:** Inherited condition with cutaneous lesions, benign tumors of peripheral nerves and bilateral 8th nerve masses.

> ● **237.73 Schwannomatosis**
> ● **237.79 Other neurofibromatosis**

237.9 Other and unspecified parts of nervous system
Cranial nerves
> **EXCLUDES** *peripheral, sympathetic, and parasympathetic nerves and ganglia (238.1)*

√4th **238 Neoplasm of uncertain behavior of other and unspecified sites and tissues**

238.0 Bone and articular cartilage
> **EXCLUDES** *cartilage:*
>   *ear (238.1)*
>   *eyelid (238.1)*
>   *larynx (235.6)*
>   *nose (235.9)*
>   *synovia (238.1)*
> **AHA:** 4Q, '04, 128

238.1 Connective and other soft tissue
Peripheral, sympathetic, and parasympathetic nerves and ganglia
Stromal tumors of digestive system
> EXCLUDES *cartilage (of):*
> *articular (238.0)*
> *larynx (235.6)*
> *nose (235.9)*
> *connective tissue of breast (238.3)*

238.2 Skin
> EXCLUDES *anus NOS (235.5)*
> *skin of genital organs (236.3, 236.6)*
> *vermilion border of lip (235.1)*
> **TIP:** Assign when documentation indicates keratoacanthoma only.

238.3 Breast
> EXCLUDES *skin of breast (238.2)*

238.4 Polycythemia vera
> **DEF:** Abnormal proliferation of all bone marrow elements, increased red cell mass and total blood volume; unknown etiology, frequently associated with splenomegaly, leukocytosis, and thrombocythemia.
> **D45** Polycythemia vera   [I-10]

238.5 Histiocytic and mast cells
Mast cell tumor NOS
Mastocytoma NOS

238.6 Plasma cells
Plasmacytoma NOS
Solitary myeloma

☑5ᵗʰ **238.7 Other lymphatic and hematopoietic tissues**
> EXCLUDES *acute myelogenous leukemia (205.0)*
> *chronic myelomonocytic leukemia (205.1)*
> *myelosclerosis NOS (289.89)*
> *myelosis:*
> *NOS (205.9)*
> *megakaryocytic (207.2)*
> **AHA:** 3Q, '01, 13; 1Q, '97, 5; 2Q, '89, 8

238.71 Essential thrombocythemia
Essential hemorrhagic thrombocythemia
Essential thrombocytosis
Idiopathic (hemorrhagic) thrombocythemia
Primary thrombocytosis
> **AHA:** 4Q, '06, 63-66
> **D47.3** Essential (hemorrhagic) thrombocythemia   [I-10]

238.72 Low grade myelodysplastic syndrome lesions
Refractory anemia (RA)
Refractory anemia with excess blasts-1 (RAEB-1)
Refractory anemia with ringed sideroblasts (RARS)
Refractory cytopenia with multilineage dysplasia (RCMD)
Refractory cytopenia with multilineage dysplasia and ringed sideroblasts (RCMD-RS)
> **DEF:** Refractory anemia (RA): Form of bone marrow disorder (myelodysplastic syndrome) that interferes with red blood cell production in the bone marrow; unresponsive to hematinics; characteristic normal or hypercellular marrow with abnormal erythrocyte development and reticulocytopenia.
> **AHA:** 4Q, '06, 63-66

238.73 High grade myelodysplastic syndrome lesions
Refractory anemia with excess blasts-2 (RAEB-2)
> **AHA:** 4Q, '06, 63-66

238.74 Myelodysplastic syndrome with 5q deletion
5q minus syndrome NOS
> EXCLUDES *constitutional 5q deletion (758.39)*
> *high grade myelodysplastic syndrome with 5q deletion (238.73)*
> **AHA:** 4Q, '06, 63-66

238.75 Myelodysplastic syndrome, unspecified
> **AHA:** 4Q, '06, 63-66
> **D46.9** Myelodysplastic syndrome unspecified   [I-10]

238.76 Myelofibrosis with myeloid metaplasia
Agnogenic myeloid metaplasia
Idiopathic myelofibrosis (chronic)
Myelosclerosis with myeloid metaplasia
Primary myelofibrosis
> EXCLUDES *myelofibrosis NOS (289.83)*
> *myelophthisic anemia (284.2)*
> *myelophthisis (284.2)*
> *secondary myelofibrosis (289.83)*
> **AHA:** 4Q, '06, 63-66

238.77 Post-transplant lymphoproliferative disorder [PTLD]
Code first complications of transplant (996.80-996.89)
> **DEF:** Excessive proliferation of B-cell lymphocytes following Epstein-Barr virus infection in organ transplant patients; may progress to non-Hodgkins lymphoma.
> **AHA:** 4Q, '08, 90-91

238.79 Other lymphatic and hematopoietic tissues
Lymphoproliferative disease (chronic) NOS
Megakaryocytic myelosclerosis
Myeloproliferative disease (chronic) NOS
Panmyelosis (acute)
> **AHA:** 4Q, '06, 63-66

238.8 Other specified sites
Eye   Heart
> EXCLUDES *eyelid (skin) (238.2)*
> *cartilage (238.1)*

238.9 Site unspecified

Neoplasms of Unspecified Nature (239)

☑4ᵗʰ **239 Neoplasms of unspecified nature**
> **NOTE** Category 239 classifies by site neoplasms of unspecified morphology and behavior. The term "mass," unless otherwise stated, is not to be regarded as a neoplastic growth.
> **INCLUDES** "growth" NOS
> neoplasm NOS
> new growth NOS
> tumor NOS
> **TIP:** Do not assign for inpatient cases; more information should be available.

239.0 Digestive system
> EXCLUDES *anus:*
> *margin (239.2)*
> *skin (239.2)*
> *perianal skin (239.2)*

239.1 Respiratory system

239.2 Bone, soft tissue, and skin
> EXCLUDES *anal canal (239.0)*
> *anus NOS (239.0)*
> *bone marrow (202.9)*
> *cartilage:*
> *larynx (239.1)*
> *nose (239.1)*
> *connective tissue of breast (239.3)*
> *skin of genital organs (239.5)*
> *vermilion border of lip (239.0)*

239.3 Breast
> EXCLUDES *skin of breast (239.2)*

239.4 Bladder

239.5 Other genitourinary organs

239.6 Brain
> EXCLUDES *cerebral meninges (239.7)*
> *cranial nerves (239.7)*

239.7 Endocrine glands and other parts of nervous system
> EXCLUDES *peripheral, sympathetic, and parasympathetic nerves and ganglia (239.2)*

☑5ᵗʰ **239.8 Other specified sites**

EXCLUDES *eyelid (skin) (239.2)*
cartilage (239.2)
great vessels (239.2)
optic nerve (239.7)

AHA: ▶4Q, '09, 75◀

239.81 Retina and choroid
Dark area on retina
Retinal freckle

TIP: ▶Assign for documentation of retinal "freckles" or spots that may be indicative of malignant melanoma. Histologic confirmation is not required.◀

239.89 Other specified sites

239.9 Site unspecified

☑4ᵗʰ
☑5ᵗʰ Additional Digit Required   Unspecified Code   Other Specified Code   Manifestation Code   ▶◀ Revised Text   ● New Code   ▲ Revised Code Title

2011 ICD-9-CM   **February 2010 • Volume 1 – 49**

Endocrine, Nutritional and Metabolic Diseases, and Immunity

240–244.8

3. Endocrine, Nutritional and Metabolic Diseases, and Immunity Disorders (240-279)

EXCLUDES *endocrine and metabolic disturbances specific to the fetus and newborn (775.0-775.9)*

NOTE All neoplasms, whether functionally active or not, are classified in Chapter 2. Codes in Chapter 3 (i.e., 242.8, 246.0, 251-253, 255-259) may be used to identify such functional activity associated with any neoplasm, or by ectopic endocrine tissue.

Disorders of Thyroid Gland (240-246)

✓4th **240 Simple and unspecified goiter**

> **DEF:** An enlarged thyroid gland often caused by an inadequate dietary intake of iodine.

240.0 Goiter, specified as simple
Any condition classifiable to 240.9, specified as simple

240.9 Goiter, unspecified
Enlargement of thyroid
Goiter or struma:
  NOS
  diffuse colloid
  endemic
  hyperplastic
  nontoxic (diffuse)
  parenchymatous
  sporadic
  EXCLUDES *congenital (dyshormonogenic) goiter (246.1)*

✓4th **241 Nontoxic nodular goiter**

> **EXCLUDES** *adenoma of thyroid (226)*
> *cystadenoma of thyroid (226)*

241.0 Nontoxic uninodular goiter
Thyroid nodule
Uninodular goiter (nontoxic)
> **DEF:** Enlarged thyroid, commonly due to decreased thyroid production, with single nodule; no clinical hypothyroidism.
> E04.1 Nontoxic single thyroid nodule I-10

241.1 Nontoxic multinodular goiter
Multinodular goiter (nontoxic)
> **DEF:** Enlarged thyroid, commonly due to decreased thyroid production with multiple nodules; no clinical hypothyroidism.

241.9 Unspecified nontoxic nodular goiter
Adenomatous goiter
Nodular goiter (nontoxic) NOS
Struma nodosa (simplex)

✓4th **242 Thyrotoxicosis with or without goiter**

> **EXCLUDES** *neonatal thyrotoxicosis (775.3)*

> **DEF:** A condition caused by excess quantities of thyroid hormones being introduced into the tissues

The following fifth-digit subclassification is for use with categories 242:
  0 **without mention of thyrotoxic crisis or storm**
  1 **with mention of thyrotoxic crisis or storm**

§ ✓5th **242.0 Toxic diffuse goiter**
[0-1] Basedow's disease
Exophthalmic or toxic goiter NOS
Graves' disease
Primary thyroid hyperplasia
> **DEF:** Diffuse thyroid enlargement accompanied by hyperthyroidism, bulging eyes, and dermopathy.

§ ✓5th **242.1 Toxic uninodular goiter**
[0-1] Thyroid nodule ⎫ toxic or with hyperthyroidism
Uninodular goiter ⎭
> **DEF:** Symptomatic hyperthyroidism with a single nodule on the enlarged thyroid gland. Abrupt onset of symptoms; including extreme nervousness, insomnia, weight loss, tremors, and psychosis or coma.

§ ✓5th **242.2 Toxic multinodular goiter**
[0-1] Secondary thyroid hyperplasia
> **DEF:** Symptomatic hyperthyroidism with multiple nodules on the enlarged thyroid gland. Abrupt onset of symptoms; including extreme nervousness, insomnia, weight loss, tremors, and psychosis or coma.

The Endocrine System

§ ✓5th **242.3 Toxic nodular goiter, unspecified**
[0-1] Adenomatous goiter ⎫
Nodular goiter ⎬ toxic or with hyperthyroidism
Struma nodosa ⎭

Any condition classifiable to 241.9 specified as toxic or with hyperthyroidism

§ ✓5th **242.4 Thyrotoxicosis from ectopic thyroid nodule**
[0-1]

§ ✓5th **242.8 Thyrotoxicosis of other specified origin**
[0-1] Overproduction of thyroid-stimulating hormone [TSH]
Thyrotoxicosis:
  factitia from ingestion of excessive thyroid material
Use additional E code to identify cause, if drug-induced

§ ✓5th **242.9 Thyrotoxicosis without mention of goiter or other**
[0-1] **cause**
Hyperthyroidism NOS
Thyrotoxicosis NOS
E05.90 Thyrotoxicosis uns w/o thyrotoxic crisis or storm I-10

243 Congenital hypothyroidism
Congenital thyroid insufficiency
Cretinism (athyrotic) (endemic)
Use additional code to identify associated mental retardation
> **EXCLUDES** *congenital (dyshormonogenic) goiter (246.1)*
> **DEF:** Underproduction of thyroid hormone present from birth.

✓4th **244 Acquired hypothyroidism**

> **INCLUDES** athyroidism (acquired)
> hypothyroidism (acquired)
> myxedema (adult) (juvenile)
> thyroid (gland) insufficiency (acquired)

244.0 Postsurgical hypothyroidism
> **DEF:** Underproduction of thyroid hormone due to surgical removal of all or part of the thyroid gland.
> E89.0 Postprocedural hypothyroidism I-10

244.1 Other postablative hypothyroidism
Hypothyroidism following therapy, such as irradiation

244.2 Iodine hypothyroidism
Hypothyroidism resulting from administration or ingestion of iodide
> **EXCLUDES** ►*hypothyroidism resulting from administration of radioactive iodine (244.1)*◄
> Use additional E code to identify drug

244.3 Other iatrogenic hypothyroidism
Hypothyroidism resulting from:
  P-aminosalicylic acid [PAS]
  Phenylbutazone
  Resorcinol
Iatrogenic hypothyroidism NOS
Use additional E code to identify drug

244.8 Other specified acquired hypothyroidism
Secondary hypothyroidism NEC
AHA: J-A, '85, 9

---

§ Requires fifth digit. Valid digits are in [brackets] under each code. See category 242 for codes and definitions.

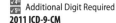

244.9 Unspecified hypothyroidism

Hypothyroidism }
Myxedema   } primary or NOS

AHA: 3Q, '99, 19; 4Q, '96, 29

E03.9 Hypothyroidism unspecified   I-10

✓4ᵗʰ 245 Thyroiditis

245.0 Acute thyroiditis

Abscess of thyroid
Thyroiditis:
    nonsuppurative, acute
    pyogenic
    suppurative

Use additional code to identify organism

DEF: Inflamed thyroid caused by infection, with abscess and liquid puris.

245.1 Subacute thyroiditis

Thyroiditis: Thyroiditis:
   de Quervain's   granulomatous
   giant cell   viral

DEF: Inflammation of the thyroid, characterized by fever and painful enlargement of the thyroid gland, with granulomas in the gland.

245.2 Chronic lymphocytic thyroiditis

Hashimoto's disease   Thyroiditis:
Struma lymphomatosa   autoimmune
                  lymphocytic (chronic)

DEF: Autoimmune disease of thyroid; lymphocytes infiltrate the gland and thyroid antibodies are produced; women more often affected.

245.3 Chronic fibrous thyroiditis

Struma fibrosa
Thyroiditis:
   invasive (fibrous)
   ligneous
   Riedel's

DEF: Persistent fibrosing inflammation of thyroid with adhesions to nearby structures; rare condition

245.4 Iatrogenic thyroiditis

Use additional code to identify cause

DEF: Thyroiditis resulting from treatment or intervention by physician or in a patient intervention setting.

245.8 Other and unspecified chronic thyroiditis

Chronic thyroiditis: Chronicthyroiditis:
   NOS   nonspecific

245.9 Thyroiditis, unspecified

Thyroiditis NOS

✓4ᵗʰ 246 Other disorders of thyroid

246.0 Disorders of thyrocalcitonin secretion

Hypersecretion of calcitonin or thyrocalcitonin

246.1 Dyshormonogenic goiter

Congenital (dyshormonogenic) goiter
Goiter due to enzyme defect in synthesis of thyroid hormone
Goitrous cretinism (sporadic)

246.2 Cyst of thyroid

EXCLUDES cystadenoma of thyroid (226)

246.3 Hemorrhage and infarction of thyroid

246.8 Other specified disorders of thyroid

Abnormality of thyroid-binding globulin
Atrophy of thyroid
Hyper-TBG-nemia
Hypo-TBG-nemia

AHA: 2Q, '06, 5

246.9 Unspecified disorder of thyroid

E07.9 Disorder of thyroid unspecified   I-10

Diseases of Other Endocrine Glands (249-259)

✓4ᵗʰ 249 Secondary diabetes mellitus

INCLUDES diabetes mellitus (due to) (in) (secondary) (with):
     drug-induced or chemical induced infection

Use additional code to identify any associated insulin use (V58.67)

EXCLUDES gestational diabetes (648.8)
    hyperglycemia NOS (790.29)
    neonatal diabetes mellitus (775.1)
    nonclinical diabetes (790.29)
    Type I diabetes — see category 250
    Type II diabetes — see category 250

The following fifth-digit subclassification is for use with category 249:
   0 not stated as uncontrolled, or unspecified
   1 uncontrolled

AHA: 4Q, '08, 91-95

TIP: If the secondary DM is due to pancreatectomy, code first 251.3 Postsurgical hypoinsulinemia; also assign a code from category 249 and any manifestations, and code V88.1x Acquired absence of pancreas.

§ ✓5ᵗʰ **249.0 Secondary diabetes mellitus without mention**
[0-1]   **of complication**

Secondary diabetes mellitus without mention of complication or manifestation classifiable to 249.1-249.9
Secondary diabetes mellitus NOS

E09.9 Drug/chemical induced diabetes mellitus w/o comp   I-10

§ ✓5ᵗʰ **249.1 Secondary diabetes mellitus with ketoacidosis**
[0-1]   Secondary diabetes mellitus with diabetic acidosis without mention of coma
Secondary diabetes mellitus with diabetic ketosis without mention of coma

§ ✓5ᵗʰ **249.2 Secondary diabetes mellitus with hyperosmolarity**
[0-1]   Secondary diabetes mellitus with hyperosmolar (nonketotic) coma

§ ✓5ᵗʰ **249.3 Secondary diabetes mellitus with other coma**
[0-1]   Secondary diabetes mellitus with diabetic coma (with ketoacidosis)
Secondary diabetes mellitus with diabetic hypoglycemic coma
Secondary diabetes mellitus with insulin coma NOS

EXCLUDES secondary diabetes mellitus with hyperosmolar coma (249.2)

§ ✓5ᵗʰ **249.4 Secondary diabetes mellitus with renal manifestations**
[0-1]   Use additional code to identify manifestation, as:
    chronic kidney disease (585.1-585.9)
    diabetic nephropathy NOS (583.81)
    diabetic nephrosis (581.81)
    intercapillary glomerulosclerosis (581.81)
    Kimmelstiel-Wilson syndrome (581.81)

§ ✓5ᵗʰ **249.5 Secondary diabetes mellitus with ophthalmic**
[0-1]   **manifestations**

Use additional code to identify manifestation, as:
    diabetic blindness (369.00-369.9)
    diabetic cataract (366.41)
    diabetic glaucoma (365.44)
    diabetic macular edema (362.07)
    diabetic retinal edema (362.07)
    diabetic retinopathy (362.01-362.07)

§ ✓5ᵗʰ **249.6 Secondary diabetes mellitus with neurological**
[0-1]   **manifestations**

Use additional code to identify manifestation, as:
    diabetic amyotrophy (353.5)
    diabetic gastroparalysis (536.3)
    diabetic gastroparesis (536.3)
    diabetic mononeuropathy (354.0-355.9)
    diabetic neurogenic arthropathy (713.5)
    diabetic peripheral autonomic neuropathy (337.1)
    diabetic polyneuropathy (357.2)

AHA: For code 249.60: 4Q, '08, 94

§ ✓5ᵗʰ **249.7 Secondary diabetes mellitus with peripheral**
[0-1]   **circulatory disorders**

Use additional code to identify manifestation, as:
    diabetic gangrene (785.4)
    diabetic peripheral angiopathy (443.81)

---

§   Requires fifth digit. Valid digits are in [brackets] under each code. See category 249 for codes and definitions.

    N Newborn Age: 0   **P** Pediatric Age: 0-17   **M** Maternity Age: 12-55   **A** Adult Age: 15-124

§ ✓5ᵗʰ **249.8 Secondary diabetes mellitus with other specified**
[0-1] **manifestations**
    Secondary diabetic hypoglycemia in diabetes mellitus
    Secondary hypoglycemic shock in diabetes mellitus

    Use additional code to identify manifestation, as:
      any associated ulceration (707.10-707.9)
      diabetic bone changes (731.8)

§ ✓5ᵗʰ **249.9 Secondary diabetes mellitus with unspecified**
[0-1] **complication**

✓4ᵗʰ **250 Diabetes mellitus**

    EXCLUDES *gestational diabetes (648.8)*
      hyperglycemia NOS (790.29)
      neonatal diabetes mellitus (775.1)
      nonclinical diabetes (790.29)
      secondary diabetes (249.0-249.9)

    The following fifth-digit subclassification is for use with category 250:
    0 type II or unspecified type, not state as uncontrolled
      Fifth-digit 0 is for use for type II patients, even if the patient
       requires insulin
      Use additional code, if applicable, for associated long-term
       (current) insulin use V58.67
    1 type I [juvenile type], not stated as uncontrolled
    2 type II or unspecified type, uncontrolled
      Fifth-digit 2 is for use for type II patients, even if the patient
       requires insulin
      Use additional code, if applicable, for associated long-term
       (current) insulin use V58.67
    3 type I [juvenile type], uncontrolled

    DEF: Diabetes mellitus: Inability to metabolize carbohydrates, proteins, and fats due to insufficient secretion of insulin. Symptoms may be unremarkable, with long-term complications, involving kidneys, nerves, blood vessels, and eyes.
    DEF: Uncontrolled diabetes: A nonspecific term indicating that the current treatment regimen does not keep the blood sugar level of a patient within acceptable levels.
    AHA: 4Q, '04, 56; 2Q, '04, 17; 2Q, '02, 13; 2Q,'01, 16; 2Q,'98, 15; 4Q, '97, 32; 2Q, '97, 14; 3Q, '96, 5; 4Q, '93, 19; 2Q, '92, 5; 3Q, '91, 3; 2Q, '90, 22; N-D, '85, 11
    TIP: Use of insulin does not ensure type I DM; if patient is on routine insulin, assign also V58.67 Long-term (current) use of insulin.

§ ✓5ᵗʰ **250.0 Diabetes mellitus without mention of complication**
[0-3]   Diabetes mellitus without mention of complication or
      manifestation classifiable to 250.1-250.9
    Diabetes (mellitus) NOS
    AHA: 1Q, '06, 14; 4Q, '97, 32; 3Q, '91, 3, 12; N-D, '85, 11; **For code 250.00:** ▶4Q, '09, 77;◀1Q, '05, 15; 4Q, '04, 55; 4Q, '03, 105, 108; 2Q, '03, 16; 1Q, '02, 7, 11; **For code 250.01:** 4Q, '04, 55; 4Q, '03, 110; 2Q, '03, 6; **For code 250.02:** 1Q, '03, 5
    E11.9 Type 2 diabetes mellitus w/o complications   I-10

§ ✓5ᵗʰ **250.1 Diabetes with ketoacidosis**
[0-3]   Diabetic:
    acidosis   }
    ketosis   } without mention of coma
    DEF: Diabetic hyperglycemic crisis causing ketone presence in body fluids.
    AHA: 3Q, '91, 6; **For code 250.11:** 4Q, '03, 82; **For code 250.13:** 2Q, '06, 19-20
    E10.10 Type 1 diabetes mellitus w/ketoacidosis w/o coma   I-10

§ ✓5ᵗʰ **250.2 Diabetes with hyperosmolarity**
[0-3]   Hyperosmolar (nonketotic) coma
    AHA: 4Q, '93, 19; 3Q, '91, 7

§ ✓5ᵗʰ **250.3 Diabetes with other coma**
[0-3]   Diabetic coma (with ketoacidosis)
    Diabetic hypoglycemic coma
    Insulin coma NOS
    EXCLUDES *diabetes with hyperosmolar coma (250.2)*
    DEF: Coma (not hyperosmolar) caused by hyperglycemia or hypoglycemia as complication of diabetes.
    AHA: 3Q, '91, 7, 12

---

§ ✓5ᵗʰ **250.4 Diabetes with renal manifestations**
[0-3]   Use additional code to identify manifestation, as:
    chronic kidney disease (585.1-585.9)
    diabetic:
      nephropathy NOS (583.81)
      nephrosis (581.81)
    intercapillary glomerulosclerosis (581.81)
    Kimmelstiel-Wilson syndrome (581.81)
    AHA: 3Q, '91, 8, 12; S-O, '87, 9; S-O, '84, 3; **For code 250.40:** 1Q, '03, 20
    E11.22 Type 2 diabetes mellitus w/diabetic CKD   I-10

§ ✓5ᵗʰ **250.5 Diabetes with ophthalmic manifestations**
[0-3]   Use additional code to identify manifestation, as:
    diabetic:
      blindness (369.00-369.9)
      cataract (366.41)
      glaucoma (365.44)
      macular edema (362.07)
      retinal edema (362.07)
      retinopathy (362.01-362.07)
    AHA: 4Q, '05, 65; 3Q, '91, 8; S-O, '85, 11; **For code 250.50:** 4Q, '05, 67
    E10.36 Type 1 diabetes mellitus with diabetic cataract   I-10

§ ✓5ᵗʰ **250.6 Diabetes with neurological manifestations**
[0-3]   Use additional code to identify manifestation, as:
    diabetic:
      amyotrophy (353.5)
      gastroparalysis (536.3)
      gastroparesis (536.3)
      mononeuropathy (354.0-355.9)
      neurogenic arthropathy (713.5)
      peripheral autonomic neuropathy (337.1)
      polyneuropathy (357.2)
    AHA: ▶4Q, '09, 151;◀ 2Q, '09, 13, 15; 3Q, '08, 5; 2Q, '93, 6; 2Q, '92, 15; 3Q, '91, 9; N-D, '84, 9; **For code 250.60:** 4Q, '03, 105; **For code 250.61:** 2Q, '04, 7
    E11.40 Type 2 diabetes mellitus w/diab neuropathy uns   I-10

§ ✓5ᵗʰ **250.7 Diabetes with peripheral circulatory disorders**
[0-3]   Use additional code to identify manifestation, as:
    diabetic:
      gangrene (785.4)
      peripheral angiopathy (443.81)
    DEF: Blood vessel damage or disease, usually in the feet, legs, or hands, as a complication of diabetes.
    AHA: 1Q, '96, 10; 3Q, '94, 5; 2Q, '94, 17; 3Q, '91, 10, 12; 3Q, '90, 15; **For code 250.70:** 1Q, '04, 14
    E10.51 Type 1 DM w/diab periph angiopathy w/o gangrene   I-10

§ ✓5ᵗʰ **250.8 Diabetes with other specified manifestations**
[0-3]   Diabetic hypoglycemia NOS
    Hypoglycemic shock NOS

    Use additional code to identify manifestation, as:
      any associated ulceration (707.10-707.9)
      diabetic bone changes (731.8)
    AHA: 4Q, '00, 44; 4Q, '97, 43; 2Q, '97, 16; 4Q, '93, 20; 3Q, '91, 10; **For code 250.80:** 1Q, '04, 14
    TIP: Assign for diabetic osteomyelitis, along with code 731.8 and the appropriate code from category 730.
    E11.610 Type 2 DM with diabetic neuropathic arthropathy   I-10

§ ✓5ᵗʰ **250.9 Diabetes with unspecified complication**
[0-3]   **AHA:** 2Q, '92, 15; 3Q, '91, 7, 12
    TIP: Do not assign with any other code in category 250.
    E10.8 Type 1 diabetes mellitus with unspecified comp   I-10

✓4ᵗʰ **251 Other disorders of pancreatic internal secretion**

251.0 Hypoglycemic coma
    Iatrogenic hyperinsulinism
    Non-diabetic insulin coma

    Use additional E code to identify cause, if drug-induced
    EXCLUDES *hypoglycemic coma in diabetes mellitus (249.3, 250.3)*
    DEF: Coma induced by low blood sugar in non-diabetic patient.
    AHA: M-A, '85, 8

---

§ Requires fifth digit. Valid digits are in [brackets] under each code. See appropriate category for codes and definitions.

✓4ᵗʰ / ✓5ᵗʰ Additional Digit Required   Unspecified Code   Other Specified Code   Manifestation Code   ▶◀ Revised Text   ● New Code   ▲ Revised Code Title

251.1 Other specified hypoglycemia

Hyperinsulinism: Hyperplasia of pancreatic
   NOS   islet beta cells NOS
   ectopic
   functional

Use additional E code to identify cause, if drug-induced

EXCLUDES hypoglycemia:
     in diabetes mellitus (249.8, 250.8)
     in infant of diabetic mother (775.0)
    hypoglycemic coma (251.0)
    neonatal hypoglycemia (775.6)

DEF: Excessive production of insulin by the pancreas; associated with obesity and insulin-producing tumors.

AHA: 1Q, '03, 10

251.2 Hypoglycemia, unspecified

Hypoglycemia: Hypoglycemia:
   NOS   spontaneous
   reactive

EXCLUDES hypoglycemia:
     with coma (251.0)
     in diabetes mellitus (249.8, 250.8)
    leucine-induced (270.3)

AHA: M-A, '85, 8

E16.2 Hypoglycemia unspecified   I-10

251.3 Postsurgical hypoinsulinemia

Hypoinsulinemia following complete or partial
     pancreatectomy
Postpancreatectomy hyperglycemia

Use additional code to identify (any associated):
    acquired absence of pancreas ►(V88.11-V88.12)◄
    insulin use (V58.67)
    secondary diabetes mellitus (249.00-249.91)

EXCLUDES transient hyperglycemia post procedure (790.29)
            transient hypoglycemia post procedure (251.2)

AHA: 3Q, '91, 6

251.4 Abnormality of secretion of glucagon

Hyperplasia of pancreatic islet alpha cells with glucagon
     excess

DEF: Production malfunction of a pancreatic hormone secreted by cells of the islets of Langerhans.

251.5 Abnormality of secretion of gastrin

Hyperplasia of pancreatic alpha cells with gastrin excess
Zollinger-Ellison syndrome

251.8 Other specified disorders of pancreatic internal secretion

AHA: 2Q, '98, 15; 3Q, '91, 6

E16.8 Oth spec d/o of pancreatic internal secretion   I-10

251.9 Unspecified disorder of pancreatic internal secretion

Islet cell hyperplasia NOS

√4ᵗʰ **252 Disorders of parathyroid gland**

EXCLUDES hungry bone syndrome (275.5)

√5ᵗʰ **252.0 Hyperparathyroidism**

EXCLUDES ectopic hyperparathyroidism (259.3)

DEF: Abnormally high secretion of parathyroid hormones causing bone deterioration, reduced renal function, kidney stones.

252.00 Hyperparathyroidism, unspecified

E21.3 Hyperparathyroidism unspecified   I-10

Dorsal View of Parathyroid Glands

252.01 Primary hyperparathyroidism

Hyperplasia of parathyroid

DEF: Parathyroid dysfunction commonly caused by hyperplasia of two or more glands; characteristic hypercalcemia and increased parathyroid hormone levels.

252.02 Secondary hyperparathyroidism, non-renal

EXCLUDES secondary hyperparathyroidism (of renal
           origin) (588.81)

DEF: Underlying disease of nonrenal origin decreases blood levels of calcium causing the parathyroid to release increased levels of parathyroid hormone; parathyroid hormone levels return to normal once underlying condition is treated and blood calcium levels are normal.

AHA: 4Q, '04, 57-59

252.08 Other hyperparathyroidism

Tertiary hyperparathyroidism

DEF: Tertiary hyperparathyroidism: chronic secondary hyperparathyroidism with adenomatous parathyroid causing irreversible abnormal production of parathyroid hormone (PTH); PTH remains high after the serum calcium levels are brought under control.

252.1 Hypoparathyroidism

Parathyroiditis (autoimmune)
Tetany:
   parathyroid
   parathyroprival

EXCLUDES pseudohypoparathyroidism (275.4)
            pseudopseudohypoparathyroidism (275.4)
            tetany NOS (781.7)
            transitory neonatal hypoparathyroidism (775.4)

DEF: Abnormally low secretion of parathyroid hormones which causes decreased calcium and increased phosphorus in the blood, resulting in muscle cramps, tetany, urinary frequency and cataracts.

252.8 Other specified disorders of parathyroid gland

Cyst   } of parathyroid
Hemorrhage

252.9 Unspecified disorder of parathyroid gland

√4ᵗʰ **253 Disorders of the pituitary gland and its hypothalamic control**

INCLUDES the listed conditions whether the disorder is in the
           pituitary or the hypothalamus

EXCLUDES Cushing's syndrome (255.0)

253.0 Acromegaly and gigantism

Overproduction of growth hormone

DEF: Acromegaly: chronic, middle age condition; caused by hypersecretion of the pituitary growth hormone; enlarged parts of skeleton, especially the nose, ears, jaws, fingers and toes.

DEF: Gigantism: pituitary gigantism caused by excess growth of short flat bones; men may grow 78 to 80 inches tall.

253.1 Other and unspecified anterior pituitary hyperfunction

Forbes-Albright syndrome

EXCLUDES overproduction of:
     ACTH (255.3)
     thyroid-stimulating hormone [TSH] (242.8)

DEF: Spontaneous galactorrhea-amenorrhea syndrome unrelated to pregnancy; usually related to presence of pituitary tumor.

AHA: J-A, '85, 9

253.2 Panhypopituitarism

Cachexia, pituitary   Sheehan's syndrome
Necrosis of pituitary (postpartum)   Simmonds' disease
Pituitary insufficiency NOS

EXCLUDES iatrogenic hypopituitarism (253.7)

DEF: Damage to or absence of pituitary gland leading to impaired sexual function, weight loss, fatigue, bradycardia, hypotension, pallor, depression, and impaired growth in children; called Simmonds' disease if cachexia is prominent.

253.3 Pituitary dwarfism

Isolated deficiency of (human) growth hormone [HGH]
Lorain-Levi dwarfism

DEF: Dwarfism with infantile physical characteristics due to abnormally low secretion of growth hormone and gonadotropin deficiency.

253.4 Other anterior pituitary disorders

Isolated or partial deficiency of an anterior pituitary hormone,
     other than growth hormone
Prolactin deficiency

AHA: J-A, '85, 9

253.5 Diabetes insipidus
Vasopressin deficiency
EXCLUDES *nephrogenic diabetes insipidus (588.1)*
DEF: Metabolic disorder causing insufficient antidiuretic hormone release; symptoms include frequent urination, thirst, ravenous hunger, loss of weight, fatigue.

253.6 Other disorders of neurohypophysis
Syndrome of inappropriate secretion of antidiuretic hormone [ADH]
EXCLUDES *ectopic antidiuretic hormone secretion (259.3)*
E22.2 Synd inappropriate secrectn antiduretic hormone   I-10

253.7 Iatrogenic pituitary disorders
Hypopituitarism:
  hormone-induced
  hypophysectomy-induced
  postablative
  radiotherapy-induced
Use additional E code to identify cause
DEF: Pituitary dysfunction that results from drug therapy, radiation therapy, or surgery, causing mild to severe symptoms.

253.8 Other disorders of the pituitary and other syndromes of diencephalohypophyseal origin
Abscess of pituitary   Cyst of Rathke's pouch
Adiposogenital dystrophy   Fröhlich's syndrome
EXCLUDES *craniopharyngioma (237.0)*

253.9 Unspecified
Dyspituitarism

✓4ᵗʰ 254 Diseases of thymus gland
EXCLUDES *aplasia or dysplasia with immunodeficiency (279.2)*
hypoplasia with immunodeficiency (279.2)
myasthenia gravis (358.00-358.01)

254.0 Persistent hyperplasia of thymus
Hypertrophy of thymus
DEF: Continued abnormal growth of the twin lymphoid lobes that produce T lymphocytes.

254.1 Abscess of thymus

254.8 Other specified diseases of thymus gland
Astrophy ⎫
Cyst ⎬ of thymus
EXCLUDES *thymoma (212.6)*

254.9 Unspecified disease of thymus gland

✓4ᵗʰ 255 Disorders of adrenal glands
INCLUDES the listed conditions whether the basic disorder is in the adrenals or is pituitary-induced

255.0 Cushing's syndrome
Adrenal hyperplasia due to excess ACTH
Cushing's syndrome:
  NOS
  iatrogenic
  idiopathic
  pituitary-dependent
Ectopic ACTH syndrome
Iatrogenic syndrome of excess cortisol
Overproduction of cortisol
Use additional E code to identify cause, if drug-induced
EXCLUDES *congenital adrenal hyperplasia (255.2)*
DEF: Due to adrenal cortisol oversecretion or glucocorticoid medications; may cause excess fatty tissue of the face, neck and body; osteoporosis and curvature of spine, hypertension, diabetes mellitus, female genitourinary problems, male impotence, degeneration of muscle tissues, weakness.

✓5ᵗʰ 255.1 Hyperaldosteronism
DEF: Oversecretion of aldosterone causing fluid retention, hypertension.
AHA: 4Q, '03, 48

255.10 Hyperaldosteronism, unspecified
Aldosteronism NOS
Primary aldosteronism, unspecified
EXCLUDES *Conn's syndrome (255.12)*

255.11 Glucocorticoid-remediable aldosteronism
Familial aldosteronism type I
EXCLUDES *Conn's syndrome (255.12)*
DEF: Rare autosomal dominant familial form of primary aldosteronism in which the secretion of aldosterone is under the influence of adrenocortiotrophic hormone (ACTH) rather than the renin-angiotensin mechanism; moderate hypersecretion of aldosterone and suppressed plasma renin activity rapidly reversed by administration of glucosteroids; symptoms include hypertension and mild hypokalemia.

255.12 Conn's syndrome
DEF: A type of primary aldosteronism caused by an adenoma of the glomerulosa cells in the adrenal cortex; presence of hypertension.

255.13 Bartter's syndrome
DEF: A cluster of symptoms caused by a defect in the ability of the kidney to reabsorb potassium; signs include alkalosis (hypokalemic alkalosis), increased aldosterone, increased plasma renin, and normal blood pressure; symptoms include muscle cramping, weakness, constipation, frequency of urination, and failure to grow; also known as urinary potassium wasting or juxtaglomerular cell hyperplasia.

255.14 Other secondary aldosteronism
AHA: 3Q, '06, 24

255.2 Adrenogenital disorders
Achard-Thiers syndrome
Adrenogenital syndromes, virilizing or feminizing, whether acquired or associated with congenital adrenal hyperplasia consequent on inborn enzyme defects in hormone synthesis
Congenital adrenal hyperplasia
Female adrenal pseudohermaphroditism
Male:
  macrogenitosomia praecox
  sexual precocity with adrenal hyperplasia
Virilization (female) (suprarenal)
EXCLUDES *adrenal hyperplasia due to excess ACTH (255.0)*
isosexual virilization (256.4)

255.3 Other corticoadrenal overactivity
Acquired benign adrenal androgenic overactivity
Overproduction of ACTH

✓5ᵗʰ 255.4 Corticoadrenal insufficiency
EXCLUDES *tuberculous Addison's disease (017.6)*
DEF: Underproduction of adrenal hormones causing low blood pressure.
AHA: 4Q, '07, 68; 3Q, '06, 24

255.41 Glucocorticoid deficiency
Addisonian crisis
Addison's disease NOS
Adrenal atrophy (autoimmune)
Adrenal calcification
Adrenal crisis
Adrenal hemorrhage
Adrenal infarction
Adrenal insufficiency NOS
Combined glucocorticoid and mineralocorticoid deficiency
Corticoadrenal insufficiency NOS
DEF: Decreased function of the adrenal cortex resulting in insufficient production of glucocorticoid, the hormone regulating carbohydrate, fat, and protein metabolism; manifestations: hyponatremia, hyperpigmentation, orthostatic hypotension, anemia, loss of appetite, and malaise.
AHA: 4Q, '07, 68, 69
E27.1 Primary adrenocortical insufficiency   I-10

255.42 Mineralocorticoid deficiency
Hypoaldosteronism
EXCLUDES *combined glucocorticoid and mineralocorticoid deficiency (255.41)*
DEF: Decreased function of the adrenal cortex resulting in insufficient production of mineralocorticoid, which regulates electrolyte and water balance; manifestations: hyponatremia, hyperkalemia, and mild acidosis.

Endocrine, Nutritional and Metabolic Diseases, and Immunity   255.5–259.8

255.5 Other adrenal hypofunction
Adrenal medullary insufficiency
> EXCLUDES   *Waterhouse-Friderichsen syndrome (meningococcal) (036.3)*

255.6 Medulloadrenal hyperfunction
Catecholamine secretion by pheochromocytoma

255.8 Other specified disorders of adrenal glands
Abnormality of cortisol-binding globulin

255.9 Unspecified disorder of adrenal glands

√4th **256 Ovarian dysfunction**
AHA: 4Q, '00, 51

256.0 Hyperestrogenism   ♀
> DEF: Excess secretion of estrogen by the ovaries; characterized by ovaries containing multiple follicular cysts filled with serous fluid.

256.1 Other ovarian hyperfunction   ♀
Hypersecretion of ovarian androgens
AHA: 3Q, '95, 15

256.2 Postablative ovarian failure   ♀
Ovarian failure:
  iatrogenic
  postirradiation
  postsurgical
Use additional code for states associated with artificial menopause (627.4)
> EXCLUDES   *acquired absence of ovary (V45.77)*
> *asymptomatic age-related (natural) postmenopausal status (V49.81)*
> DEF: Failed ovarian function after medical or surgical intervention.
AHA: 2Q, '02, 12

√5th **256.3 Other ovarian failure**
Use additional code for states associated with natural menopause (627.2)
> EXCLUDES   *asymptomatic age-related (natural) postmenopausal status (V49.81)*
AHA: 4Q, '01, 41

  256.31 Premature menopause   A ♀
> DEF: Permanent cessation of ovarian function before the age of 40 occuring naturally of unknown cause.

  256.39 Other ovarian failure   ♀
  Delayed menarche
  Ovarian hypofunction
  Primary ovarian failure NOS

256.4 Polycystic ovaries   ♀
Isosexual virilization
Stein-Leventhal syndrome
> DEF: Multiple serous filled cysts of ovary; symptoms of infertility, hirsutism, oligomenorrhea or amenorrhea.
E28.2 Polycystic ovarian syndrome   I-10

256.8 Other ovarian dysfunction   ♀

256.9 Unspecified ovarian dysfunction   ♀

√4th **257 Testicular dysfunction**

257.0 Testicular hyperfunction   ♂
Hypersecretion of testicular hormones

257.1 Postablative testicular hypofunction   ♂
Testicular hypofunction:
  iatrogenic
  postirradiation
  postsurgical

257.2 Other testicular hypofunction
Defective biosynthesis of testicular androgen
Eunuchoidism:
  NOS
  hypogonadotropic
Failure:
  Leydig's cell, adult
  seminiferous tubule, adult
Testicular hypogonadism
> EXCLUDES   *azoospermia (606.0)*

257.8 Other testicular dysfunction
> EXCLUDES   *androgen insensitivity syndromes (259.50-259.52)*

257.9 Unspecified testicular dysfunction   ♂

√4th **258 Polyglandular dysfunction and related disorders**

√5th **258.0 Polyglandular activity in multiple endocrine adenomatosis**
Multiple endocrine neoplasia [MEN] syndromes
Use additional codes to identify any malignancies and other conditions associated with the syndromes
AHA: ▶4Q, '09, 150;◀ 4Q, '07, 70

  258.01 Multiple endocrine neoplasia [MEN] type I
  Wermer's syndrome
> DEF: Wermer's syndrome: A rare hereditary condition characterized by the presence of adenomas or hyperplasia in more than one endocrine gland causing premature aging.
AHA: 4Q, '08, 86, 89; 4Q, '07, 70, 72

  258.02 Multiple endocrine neoplasia [MEN] type IIA
  Sipple's syndrome
> DEF: Sipple's syndrome: A hereditary disorder caused by a defect in the RET gene causing overactivity of the thyroid, adrenal, and parathyroid glands, resulting in adrenal pheochromocytoma and thyroid medullary carcinoma.

  258.03 Multiple endocrine neoplasia [MEN] type IIB

258.1 Other combinations of endocrine dysfunction
Lloyd's syndrome
Schmidt's syndrome

258.8 Other specified polyglandular dysfunction

258.9 Polyglandular dysfunction, unspecified

√4th **259 Other endocrine disorders**

259.0 Delay in sexual development and puberty, not elsewhere classified
Delayed puberty

259.1 Precocious sexual development and puberty, not elsewhere classified   P
Sexual precocity: Sexual precocity:
  NOS   cryptogenic
  constitutional   idiopathic

259.2 Carcinoid syndrome
Hormone secretion by carcinoid tumors
> DEF: Presence of carcinoid tumors that spread to liver; characterized by cyanotic flushing of skin, diarrhea, bronchospasm, acquired tricuspid and pulmonary stenosis, sudden drops in blood pressure, edema, ascites.
AHA: 4Q, '08, 85-86, 89

259.3 Ectopic hormone secretion, not elsewhere classified
Ectopic:
  antidiuretic hormone secretion [ADH]
  hyperparathyroidism
> EXCLUDES   *ectopic ACTH syndrome (255.0)*
AHA: N-D, '85, 4

259.4 Dwarfism, not elsewhere classified
Dwarfism: Dwarfism:
  NOS   constitutional
> EXCLUDES   *dwarfism:*
> *achondroplastic (756.4)*
> *intrauterine (759.7)*
> *nutritional (263.2)*
> *pituitary (253.3)*
> *renal (588.0)*
> *progeria (259.8)*

√5th **259.5 Androgen insensitivity syndrome**
> DEF: X chromosome abnormality that prohibits the body from recognizing androgen; XY genotype with ambiguous genitalia.
AHA: 4Q, '08, 95-96; 4Q, '05, 53

  259.50 Androgen insensitivity, unspecified

  259.51 Androgen insensitivity syndrome
  Complete androgen insensitivity
  de Quervain's syndrome
  Goldberg-Maxwell Syndrome

  259.52 Partial androgen insensitivity
  Partial androgen insensitivity syndrome
  Reifenstein syndrome

259.8 Other specified endocrine disorders
Pineal gland dysfunction   Werner's syndrome
Progeria

259.9 Unspecified endocrine disorder
Disturbance:
   endocrine NOS
   hormone NOS
   Infantilism NOS

Nutritional Deficiencies (260-269)

EXCLUDES *deficiency anemias (280.0-281.9)*

TIP: Assign first a code for the underlying condition (e.g., anorexia nervosa) if specified.

260 Kwashiorkor
Nutritional edema with dyspigmentation of skin and hair

DEF: Syndrome, particulary of children; excessive carbohydrate with inadequate protein intake, inhibited growth potential, anomalies in skin and hair pigmentation, edema and liver disease.

AHA: ▶3Q, '09, 6◀

TIP: ▶Do not assign when documentation indicates "mild or moderate protein malnutrition" only. Kwashiorkor is a rare severe protein deficiency.◀

E40 Kwashiorkor   I-10

261 Nutritional marasmus
Nutritional atrophy   Severe malnutrition NOS
Severe calorie deficiency

DEF: Protein-calorie malabsorption or malnutrition in children; characterized by tissue wasting, dehydration, and subcutaneous fat depletion; may occur with infectious disease; also called infantile atrophy.

AHA: 4Q, '07, 97; 3Q, '06, 14; 2Q, '06, 12

E41 Nutritional marasmus   I-10

262 Other severe, protein-calorie malnutrition
Nutritional edema without mention of dyspigmentation of skin and hair

AHA: 4Q, '92, 24; J-A, '85, 12

✓4ᵗʰ 263 Other and unspecified protein-calorie malnutrition
AHA: 4Q, '92, 24

263.0 Malnutrition of moderate degree
DEF: Malnutrition characterized by biochemical changes in electrolytes, lipids, blood plasma.
AHA: ▶3Q, '09, 6;◀ J-A, '85, 1

263.1 Malnutrition of mild degree
AHA: J-A, '85, 1

263.2 Arrested development following protein-calorie malnutrition
Nutritional dwarfism
Physical retardation due to malnutrition

263.8 Other protein-calorie malnutrition

263.9 Unspecified protein-calorie malnutrition
Dystrophy due to malnutrition
Malnutrition (calorie) NOS
EXCLUDES *nutritional deficiency NOS (269.9)*
AHA: 4Q, '03, 109; N-D, '84, 19
E46 Unspecified protein-calorie malnutrition   I-10

✓4ᵗʰ 264 Vitamin A deficiency

264.0 With conjunctival xerosis
DEF: Vitamin A deficiency with conjunctival dryness.

264.1 With conjunctival xerosis and Bitot's spot
Bitot's spot in the young child
DEF: Vitamin A deficiency with conjunctival dryness, superficial spots of keratinized epithelium.

264.2 With corneal xerosis
DEF: Vitamin A deficiency with corneal dryness.

264.3 With corneal ulceration and xerosis
DEF: Vitamin A deficiency with corneal dryness, epithelial ulceration.

264.4 With keratomalacia
DEF: Vitamin A deficiency creating corneal dryness; progresses to corneal insensitivity, softness, necrosis; usually bilateral.

264.5 With night blindness
DEF: Vitamin A deficiency causing vision failure in dim light.

264.6 With xerophthalmic scars of cornea
DEF: Vitamin A deficiency with corneal scars from dryness.

264.7 Other ocular manifestations of vitamin A deficiency
Xerophthalmia due to vitamin A deficiency

264.8 Other manifestations of vitamin A deficiency
Follicular keratosis ⎫
Xeroderma   ⎬ due to vitamin A deficiency

264.9 Unspecified vitamin A deficiency
Hypovitaminosis A NOS

✓4ᵗʰ 265 Thiamine and niacin deficiency states

265.0 Beriberi
DEF: Inadequate vitamin B_1 (thiamine) intake, affects heart and peripheral nerves; individual may become edematous and develop cardiac disease due to the excess fluid; affects alcoholics and people with a diet of excessive polished rice.

265.1 Other and unspecified manifestations of thiamine deficiency
Other vitamin B_1 deficiency states

265.2 Pellagra
Deficiency:
   niacin (-tryptophan)
   nicotinamide
   nicotinic acid
   vitamin PP
Pellagra (alcoholic)
DEF: Niacin deficiency causing dermatitis, inflammation of mucous membranes, diarrhea, and psychic disturbances.

✓4ᵗʰ 266 Deficiency of B-complex components

266.0 Ariboflavinosis
Riboflavin [vitamin B_2] deficiency
DEF: Vitamin B_2 (riboflavin) deficiency marked by swollen lips and tongue fissures, corneal vascularization, scaling lesions, and anemia.
AHA: S-O, '86, 10

266.1 Vitamin B_6 deficiency
Deficiency:
   pyridoxal
   pyridoxamine
   pyridoxine
Vitamin B_6 deficiency syndrome
EXCLUDES *vitamin B_6-responsive sideroblastic anemia (285.0)*
DEF: Vitamin B_6 deficiency causing skin, lip, and tongue disturbances, peripheral neuropathy; and convulsions in infants.

266.2 Other B-complex deficiencies
Deficiency:
   cyanocobalamin
   folic acid
   vitamin B_{12}
EXCLUDES *combined system disease with anemia (281.0-281.1)*
deficiency anemias (281.0-281.9)
subacute degeneration of spinal cord with anemia (281.0-281.1)
E53.8 Deficiency of other specified B group vitamins   I-10

266.9 Unspecified vitamin B deficiency

267 Ascorbic acid deficiency
Deficiency of vitamin C
Scurvy
EXCLUDES *scorbutic anemia (281.8)*
DEF: Vitamin C deficiency causing swollen gums, myalgia, weight loss, and weakness.

✓4ᵗʰ 268 Vitamin D deficiency
EXCLUDES *vitamin D-resistant:*
osteomalacia (275.3)
rickets (275.3)

268.0 Rickets, active
EXCLUDES *celiac rickets (579.0)*
renal rickets (588.0)
DEF: Inadequate vitamin D intake, usually in pediatrics, that affects bones most involved with muscular action; may cause nodules on ends and sides of bones; delayed closure of fontanels in infants; symptoms may include muscle soreness, and profuse sweating.

268.1 Rickets, late effect
Any condition specified as due to rickets and stated to be a late effect or sequela of rickets
Code first the nature of late effect
DEF: Distorted or demineralized bones as a result of vitamin D deficiency.

Endocrine, Nutritional and Metabolic Diseases, and Immunity

268.2–271.3

268.2 Osteomalacia, unspecified

DEF: Softening of bones due to decrease in calcium; marked by pain, tenderness, muscular weakness, anorexia, and weight loss.

268.9 Unspecified vitamin D deficiency

Avitaminosis D

√4ᵗʰ **269 Other nutritional deficiencies**

269.0 Deficiency of vitamin K

EXCLUDES deficiency of coagulation factor due to vitamin K deficiency (286.7)
vitamin K deficiency of newborn (776.0)

269.1 Deficiency of other vitamins

Deficiency:
vitamin E
vitamin P

269.2 Unspecified vitamin deficiency

Multiple vitamin deficiency NOS

269.3 Mineral deficiency, not elsewhere classified

Deficiency:
calcium, dietary
iodine

EXCLUDES deficiency:
calcium NOS (275.4)
potassium (276.8)
sodium (276.1)

269.8 Other nutritional deficiency

EXCLUDES adult failure to thrive (783.7)
failure to thrive in childhood (783.41)
feeding problems (783.3)
newborn (779.31-779.34)

269.9 Unspecified nutritional deficiency

Other Metabolic and Immunity Disorders (270-279)

Use additional code to identify any associated mental retardation

√4ᵗʰ **270 Disorders of amino-acid transport and metabolism**

EXCLUDES abnormal findings without manifest disease (790.0-796.9)
disorders of purine and pyrimidine metabolism (277.1-277.2)
gout (274.00-274.9)

270.0 Disturbances of amino-acid transport

Cystinosis
Cystinuria
Fanconi (-de Toni) (-Debré) syndrome
Glycinuria (renal)
Hartnup disease

270.1 Phenylketonuria [PKU]

Hyperphenylalaninemia

DEF: Inherited metabolic condition causing excess phenylpyruvic and other acids in urine; results in mental retardation, neurological manifestations, including spasticity and tremors, light pigmentation, eczema, and mousy odor.

270.2 Other disturbances of aromatic amino-acid metabolism

Albinism
Alkaptonuria
Alkaptonuric ochronosis
Disturbances of metabolism of tyrosine and tryptophan
Homogentisic acid defects
Hydroxykynureninuria
Hypertyrosinemia
Indicanuria
Kynureninase defects
Oasthouse urine disease
Ochronosis
Tyrosinosis
Tyrosinuria
Waardenburg syndrome

EXCLUDES vitamin B₆-deficiency syndrome (266.1)

AHA: 3Q, '99, 20

270.3 Disturbances of branched-chain amino-acid metabolism

Disturbances of metabolism of leucine, isoleucine, and valine
Hypervalinemia
Intermittent branched-chain ketonuria
Leucine-induced hypoglycemia
Leucinosis
Maple syrup urine disease

AHA: 3Q, '00, 8

270.4 Disturbances of sulphur-bearing amino-acid metabolism

Cystathioninemia
Cystathioninuria
Disturbances of metabolism of methionine, homocystine, and cystathionine
Homocystinuria
Hypermethioninemia
Methioninemia

AHA: 2Q, '07, 7;1Q, '04, 6

270.5 Disturbances of histidine metabolism

Carnosinemia
Histidinemia
Hyperhistidinemia
Imidazole aminoaciduria

270.6 Disorders of urea cycle metabolism

Argininosuccinic aciduria
Citrullinemia
Disorders of metabolism of ornithine, citrulline, argininosuccinic acid, arginine, and ammonia
Hyperammonemia
Hyperomithinemia

270.7 Other disturbances of straight-chain amino-acid metabolism

Glucoglycinuria
Glycinemia (with methyl-malonic acidemia)
Hyperglycinemia
Hyperlysinemia
Other disturbances of metabolism of glycine, threonine, serine, glutamine, and lysine
Pipecolic acidemia
Saccharopinuria

AHA: 3Q, '00, 8

270.8 Other specified disorders of amino-acid metabolism

Alaninemia   Iminoacidopathy
Ethanolaminuria   Prolinemia
Glycoprolinuria   Prolinuria
Hydroxyprolinemia   Sarcosinemia
Hyperprolinemia

270.9 Unspecified disorder of amino-acid metabolism

√4ᵗʰ **271 Disorders of carbohydrate transport and metabolism**

EXCLUDES abnormality of secretion of glucagon (251.4)
diabetes mellitus (249.0-249.9, 250.0-250.9)
hypoglycemia NOS (251.2)
mucopolysaccharidosis (277.5)

271.0 Glycogenosis

Amylopectinosis
Glucose-6-phosphatase deficiency
Glycogen storage disease
McArdle's disease
Pompe's disease
von Gierke's disease

DEF: Excess glycogen storage; rare inherited trait affects liver, kidneys; causes various symptoms depending on type, though often weakness and muscle cramps.

AHA: 1Q, '98, 5

271.1 Galactosemia

Galactose-1-phosphate uridyl transferase deficiency
Galactosuria

DEF: Any of three genetic disorders due to defective galactose metabolism; symptoms include failure to thrive in infancy, jaundice, liver and spleen damage, cataracts, and mental retardation.

271.2 Hereditary fructose intolerance

Essential benign fructosuria
Fructosemia

DEF: Chromosome recessive disorder of carbohydrate metabolism; in infants, occurs after dietary sugar introduced; characterized by enlarged spleen, yellowish cast to skin, and progressive inability to thrive.

271.3 Intestinal disaccharidase deficiencies and disaccharide malabsorption

Intolerance or malabsorption (congenital) (of):
glucose-galactose
lactose
sucrose-isomaltose

E73.9 Lactose intolerance unspecified   **I-10**

271.4 Renal glycosuria
Renal diabetes
DEF: Persistent abnormal levels of glucose in urine, with normal blood glucose levels; caused by failure of the renal tubules to reabsorb glucose.

271.8 Other specified disorders of carbohydrate transport and metabolism
Essential benign pentosuria
Fucosidosis
Glycolic aciduria
Hyperoxaluria (primary)
Mannosidosis
Oxalosis
Xylosuria
Xylulosuria

271.9 Unspecified disorder of carbohydrate transport and metabolism

✓4ᵗʰ **272 Disorders of lipoid metabolism**
EXCLUDES localized cerebral lipidoses (330.1)

272.0 Pure hypercholesterolemia
Familial hypercholesterolemia
Fredrickson Type IIa hyperlipoproteinemia
Hyperbetalipoproteinemia
Hyperlipidemia, Group A
Low-density-lipoid-type [LDL] hyperlipoproteinemia
AHA: 4Q, '05, 71
E78.0 Pure hypercholesterolemia   I-10

272.1 Pure hyperglyceridemia
Endogenous hyperglyceridemia
Fredrickson Type IV hyperlipoproteinemia
Hyperlipidemia, Group B
Hyperprebetalipoproteinemia
Hypertriglyceridemia, essential
Very-low-density-lipoid-type [VLDL] hyperlipoproteinemia

272.2 Mixed hyperlipidemia
Broad- or floating-betalipoproteinemia
Combined hyperlipidemia
Elevated cholesterol with elevated triglycerides NEC
Fredrickson Type IIb or III hyperlipoproteinemia
Hypercholesterolemia with endogenous hyperglyceridemia
Hyperbetalipoproteinemia with prebetalipoproteinemia
Tubo-eruptive xanthoma
Xanthoma tuberosum
DEF: Elevated levels of lipoprotein, a complex of fats and proteins, in blood due to inherited metabolic disorder.

272.3 Hyperchylomicronemia
Bürger-Grütz syndrome
Fredrickson type I or V hyperlipoproteinemia
Hyperlipidemia, Group D
Mixed hyperglyceridemia

272.4 Other and unspecified hyperlipidemia
Alpha-lipoproteinemia
Hyperlipidemia NOS
Hyperlipoproteinemia NOS
DEF: Hyperlipoproteinemia: elevated levels of transient chylomicrons in the blood which are a form of lipoproteins that transport dietary cholesterol and triglycerides from the small intestine to the blood.
AHA: 1Q, '05, 17
E78.4 Other hyperlipidemia   I-10

272.5 Lipoprotein deficiencies
Abetalipoproteinemia
Bassen-Kornzweig syndrome
High-density lipoid deficiency
Hypoalphalipoproteinemia
Hypobetalipoproteinemia (familial)
DEF: Abnormally low levels of lipoprotein, a complex of fats and protein, in the blood.

272.6 Lipodystrophy
Barraquer-Simons disease
Progressive lipodystrophy
Use additional E code to identify cause, if iatrogenic
EXCLUDES intestinal lipodystrophy (040.2)
DEF: Disturbance of fat metabolism resulting in loss of fatty tissue in some areas of the body.

Lipid Metabolism

272.7 Lipidoses
Chemically-induced lipidosis
Disease:
Anderson's
Fabry's
Gaucher's
I cell [mucolipidosis I]
lipoid storage NOS
Niemann-Pick
pseudo-Hurler's or mucolipdosis III
triglyceride storage, Type I or II
Wolman's or triglyceride storage, Type III
Mucolipidosis II
Primary familial xanthomatosis
EXCLUDES cerebral lipidoses (330.1)
Tay-Sachs disease (330.1)
DEF: Lysosomal storage diseases marked by an abnormal amount of lipids in reticuloendothelial cells.

272.8 Other disorders of lipoid metabolism
Hoffa's disease or liposynovitis prepatellaris
Launois-Bensaude's lipomatosis
Lipoid dermatoarthritis

272.9 Unspecified disorder of lipoid metabolism

✓4ᵗʰ **273 Disorders of plasma protein metabolism**
EXCLUDES agammaglobulinemia and hypogammaglobulinemia (279.0-279.2)
coagulation defects (286.0-286.9)
hereditary hemolytic anemias (282.0-282.9)

273.0 Polyclonal hypergammaglobulinemia
Hypergammaglobulinemic purpura:
benign primary
Waldenström's
DEF: Elevated blood levels of gamma globulins, frequently found in patients with chronic infectious diseases.

273.1 Monoclonal paraproteinemia
Benign monoclonal hypergammaglobulinemia [BMH]
Monoclonal gammopathy:
NOS
associated with lymphoplasmacytic dyscrasias
benign
Paraproteinemia:
benign (familial)
secondary to malignant or inflammatory disease

273.2 Other paraproteinemias
Cryoglobulinemic:
purpura
vasculitis
Mixed cryoglobulinemia
AHA: 2Q, '08, 17

273.3 Macroglobulinemia
Macroglobulinemia (idiopathic) (primary)
Waldenström's macroglobulinemia
DEF: Elevated blood levels of macroglobulins (plasma globulins of high weight); characterized by malignant neoplasms of bone marrow, spleen, liver, or lymph nodes; symptoms include weakness, fatigue, bleeding disorders, and vision problems.

Endocrine, Nutritional and Metabolic Diseases, and Immunity

273.4–276.1

273.4 Alpha-1-antitrypsin deficiency
AAT deficiency
DEF: Disorder of plasma protein metabolism that results in a deficiency of Alpha-1-antitrypsin, an acute-phase reactive protein, released into the blood in response to infection or injury to protect tissue against the harmful effect of enzymes.

273.8 Other disorders of plasma protein metabolism
Abnormality of transport protein
Bisalbuminemia
AHA: 2Q, '98, 11
E88.09 Oth disorders of plasma-protein metablolis NEC   I-10

273.9 Unspecified disorder of plasma protein metabolism

274 Gout
EXCLUDES   *lead gout (984.0-984.9)*
DEF: Purine and pyrimidine metabolic disorders; manifested by hyperuricemia and recurrent acute inflammatory arthritis; monosodium urate or monohydrate crystals may be deposited in and around the joints, leading to joint destruction, and severe crippling.
AHA: 2Q, '95, 4

274.0 Gouty arthropathy
AHA: 4Q, '09, 76-77

274.00 Gouty arthropathy, unspecified
M10.00 Idiopathic gout unspecified site   I-10

274.01 Acute gouty arthropathy
Acute gout
Gout attack
Gout flare
Podagra

274.02 Chronic gouty arthropathy without mention of tophus (tophi)
Chronic gout

274.03 Chronic gouty arthropathy with tophus (tophi)
Chronic tophaceous gout
Gout with tophi NOS
AHA: 4Q, '09, 77

274.1 Gouty nephropathy

274.10 Gouty nephropathy, unspecified
AHA: N-D, '85, 15

274.11 Uric acid nephrolithiasis
DEF: Sodium urate stones in the kidney.

274.19 Other

274.8 Gout with other specified manifestations

274.81 Gouty tophi of ear
DEF: Chalky sodium urate deposit in the ear due to gout; produces chronic inflammation of external ear.

274.82 Gouty tophi of other sites
Gouty tophi of heart
EXCLUDES   *gout with tophi NOS (274.03)*
    gouty arthropathy with tophi (274.03)

274.89 Other
Use additional code to identify manifestations, as:
  gouty:
    iritis (364.11)
    neuritis (357.4)

274.9 Gout, unspecified
M10.9 Gout unspecified   I-10

275 Disorders of mineral metabolism
EXCLUDES   *abnormal findings without manifest disease (790.0-796.9)*

275.0 Disorders of iron metabolism
EXCLUDES   *anemia:*
     iron deficiency (280.0-280.9)
     sideroblastic (285.0)
AHA: 2Q, '97, 11

275.01 Hereditary hemochromatosis
Bronzed diabetes
Pigmentary cirrhosis (of liver)
Primary (hereditary) hemochromatosis

275.02 Hemochromatosis due to repeated red blood cell transfusions
Iron overload due to repeated red blood cell transfusions
Transfusion (red blood cell) associated hemochromatosis

275.03 Other hemochromatosis
Hemochromatosis NOS
E83.11 Hematochromatosis   I-10

275.09 Other disorders of iron metabolism
E83.10 Disorder of iron-metabolism unspecified   I-10

275.1 Disorders of copper metabolism
Hepatolenticular degeneration
Wilson's disease

275.2 Disorders of magnesium metabolism
HypermagnesemiaHypomagnesemia
AHA: ▶1Q, '10, 14;◀ 3Q, '09, 21
E83.40 Disorders of magnesium metabolism unspec   I-10

275.3 Disorders of phosphorus metabolism
Familial hypophosphatemia
Hypophosphatasia
Vitamin D-resistant:
  osteomalacia
  rickets

275.4 Disorders of calcium metabolism
EXCLUDES   *hungry bone syndrome (275.5)*
     parathyroid disorders (252.00-252.9)
     vitamin D deficiency (268.0-268.9)
AHA: 4Q, '97, 33

275.40 Unspecified disorder of calcium metabolism

275.41 Hypocalcemia
DEF: Abnormally decreased blood calcium level; symptoms include hyperactive deep tendon reflexes, muscle, abdominal cramps, and carpopedal spasm.
AHA: 3Q, '07, 5
E83.51 Hypocalcemia   I-10

275.42 Hypercalcemia
DEF: Abnormally increased blood calcium level; symptoms include muscle weakness, fatigue, nausea, depression, and constipation.
AHA: 4Q, '03, 110

275.49 Other disorders of calcium metabolism
Nephrocalcinosis
Pseudohypoparathyroidism
Pseudopseudohypoparathyroidism
DEF: Nephrocalcinosis: calcium phosphate deposits in the tubules of the kidney with resultant renal insufficiency.
DEF: Pseudohypoparathyroidism: inherited hypoparathyroidismdisorder; caused by inadequate response to parathyroid hormone, not hormonal deficiency; includes muscle cramps, tetany, urinary frequency, blurred vision due to cataracts, and dry scaly skin.
DEF: Pseudopseudohypoparathyroidism: clinical manifestations of hypoparathyroidism without affecting blood calcium levels.

275.5 Hungry bone syndrome
DEF: Marked and prolonged hypocalcemia; usually involves an extended history of elevated levels of parathyroid hormone, related bone demineralization causing the bone to sequester calcium.
AHA: 4Q, 08, 96-97

275.8 Other specified disorders of mineral metabolism

275.9 Unspecified disorder of mineral metabolism

276 Disorders of fluid, electrolyte, and acid-base balance
EXCLUDES   *diabetes insipidus (253.5)*
     familial periodic paralysis (359.3)

276.0 Hyperosmolality and/or hypernatremia
Sodium [Na] excess
Sodium [Na] overload

276.1 Hyposmolality and/or hyponatremia
Sodium [Na] deficiency
E87.1 Hypo-osmolality and hyponatremia   I-10

N Newborn Age: 0   P Pediatric Age: 0-17   M Maternity Age: 12-55   A Adult Age: 15-124

276.2 Acidosis

Acidosis:	Acidosis:
NOS	metabolic
lactic	respiratory

EXCLUDES *diabetic acidosis (249.1, 250.1)*

DEF: Disorder involves decrease of pH (hydrogen ion) concentration in blood and cellular tissues; caused by increase in acid and decrease in bicarbonate.

AHA: J-F, '87, 15

E87.2 Acidosis　　　　I-10

276.3 Alkalosis

Alkalosis:	Alkalosis:
NOS	respiratory
metabolic	

DEF: Increased blood alkalinity (base) without relative loss of base in body fluids; caused by increased arterial plasma bicarbonate concentration or loss of carbon dioxide due to hyperventilation.

276.4 Mixed acid-base balance disorder

Hypercapnia with mixed acid-base disorder

√5ᵗʰ **276.5 Volume depletion**

EXCLUDES *hypovolemic shock:*
postoperative (998.0)
traumatic (958.4)

AHA: 4Q, '05, 54; 2Q, '05, 9; 1Q, '03, 5, 22; 3Q, '02, 21; 4Q, '97, 30; 2Q, '88, 9

276.50 Volume depletion, unspecified

DEF: Depletion of total body water (dehydration) and/or contraction of total intravascular plasma (hypovolemia).

E86.9 Volume depletion unspecified　　　　I-10

276.51 Dehydration

DEF: Depletion of total body water; blood volume may be normal while fluid is pulled from other tissues.

AHA: 1Q, '08, 10

E86.0 Dehydration　　　　I-10

276.52 Hypovolemia

Depletion of volume of plasma

DEF: Depletion of volume plasma; depletion of total blood volume.

√5ᵗʰ **276.6 Fluid overload**

EXCLUDES *ascites (789.51-789.59)*
localized edema (782.3)

AHA: 3Q, '07, 9; 4Q, '06, 136

● **276.61 Transfusion associated circulatory overload**

Fluid overload due to transfusion (blood) (blood components)

TACO

● **276.69 Other fluid overload**

Fluid retention

E87.7 Fluid overload　　　　I-10

276.7 Hyperpotassemia

Hyperkalemia	Potassium [K]:
Potassium [K]:	intoxication
excess	overload

DEF: Elevated blood levels of potassium; symptoms include abnormal EKG readings, weakness; related to defective renal excretion.

AHA: 1Q, '05, 9; 2Q,'01, 12

E87.5 Hyperkalemia　　　　I-10

276.8 Hypopotassemia

Hypokalemia

Potassium [K] deficiency

DEF: Decreased blood levels of potassium; symptoms include neuromuscular disorders.

E87.6 Hypokalemia　　　　I-10

276.9 Electrolyte and fluid disorders not elsewhere classified

Electrolyte imbalance

Hyperchloremia

Hypochloremia

EXCLUDES *electrolyte imbalance:*
associated with hyperemesis gravidarum (643.1)
complicating labor and delivery (669.0)
following abortion and ectopic or molar pregnancy (634-638 with .4, 639.4)

AHA: J-F, '87, 15

E87.8 Oth disorders of electrolyte & fluid balance NEC　　　　I-10

√4ᵗʰ **277 Other and unspecified disorders of metabolism**

√5ᵗʰ **277.0 Cystic fibrosis**

Fibrocystic disease of the pancreas

Mucoviscidosis

DEF: Genetic disorder of infants, children, and young adults marked by exocrine gland dysfunction; characterized by chronic pulmonary disease with excess mucus production, pancreatic deficiency, and high levels of electrolytes in the sweat.

AHA: 4Q, '90, 16; 3Q, '90, 18

TIP: Sequencing of CF is determined by circumstances of admission. If a patient is admitted for CF, sequence the CF first. If admitted for a complication of CF (e.g., pneumothorax, acute bronchitis, or acute cor pulmonale), sequence the complication first.

277.00 Without mention of meconium ileus

Cystic fibrosis NOS

AHA: 2Q, '03, 12

E84.9 Cystic fibrosis unspecified　　　　I-10

277.01 With meconium ileus　　　　N

Meconium:
ileus (of newborn)
obstruction of intestine in mucoviscidosis

277.02 With pulmonary manifestations

Cystic fibrosis with pulmonary exacerbation

Use additional code to identify any infectious organism present, such as:
pseudomonas (041.7)

277.03 With gastrointestinal manifestations

EXCLUDES *with meconium ileus (277.01)*

AHA: 4Q, '02, 45

277.09 With other manifestations

277.1 Disorders of porphyrin metabolism

Hematoporphyria

Hematoporphyrinuria

Hereditary coproporphyria

Porphyria

Porphyrinuria

Protocoproporphyria

Protoporphyria

Pyrroloporphyria

277.2 Other disorders of purine and pyrimidine metabolism

Hypoxanthine-guanine-phosphoribosyltransferase deficiency [HG-PRT deficiency]

Lesch-Nyhan syndrome

Xanthinuria

EXCLUDES *gout (274.00-274.9)*
orotic aciduric anemia (281.4)

√5ᵗʰ **277.3 Amyloidosis**

DEF: Conditions of diverse etiologies characterized by the accumulation of insoluble fibrillar proteins (amyloid) in various organs and tissues of the body, compromising vital functions.

AHA: 1Q, '96, 16

277.30 Amyloidosis, unspecified

Amyloidosis NOS

AHA: 4Q, '06, 66

277.31 Familial Mediterranean fever

Benign paroxysmal peritonitis

Hereditary amyloid nephropathy

Periodic familial polyserositis

Recurrent polyserositis

DEF: Early-life onset of recurrent attacks characterized by high fevers with pain and inflammation of chest and abdominal cavities, skin and joints, also rash or vasculitis. Etiology unknown, possibly genetic, but may be precipitated by stress, trauma or exertion.

AHA: 4Q, '06, 66

277.39 Other amyloidosis

Hereditary cardiac amyloidosis

Inherited systemic amyloidosis

Neuropathic (Portuguese) (Swiss) amyloidosis

Secondary amyloidosis

AHA: 1Q, '09, 9; 2Q, '08, 8; 4Q, '06, 66

√4ᵗʰ √5ᵗʰ Additional Digit Required	Unspecified Code	Other Specified Code	Manifestation Code	▶◀ Revised Text	● New Code	▲ Revised Code Title

277.4 Disorders of bilirubin excretion

Hyperbilirubinemia:
   congenital
   constitutional
Syndrome:
   Crigler-Najjar
   Dubin-Johnson
   Gilbert's
   Rotor's

   EXCLUDES *hyperbilirubinemias specific to the perinatal period (774.0-774.7)*

277.5 Mucopolysaccharidosis

Gargoylism
Hunter's syndrome
Hurler's syndrome
Lipochondrodystrophy
Maroteaux-Lamy syndrome
Morquio-Brailsford disease
Osteochondrodystrophy
Sanfilippo's syndrome
Scheie's syndrome

DEF: Metabolic disorders evidenced by excretion of various mucopolysaccharides in urine and infiltration of these substances into connective tissue, with resulting defects of bone, cartilage and connective tissue.

277.6 Other deficiencies of circulating enzymes

Hereditary angioedema

277.7 Dysmetabolic syndrome X

Use additional code for associated manifestation, such as:
   cardiovascular disease (414.00-414.07)
   obesity ▶(278.00-278.03)◀

DEF: A specific group of metabolic disorders that are related to the state of insulin resistance (decreased cellular response to insulin) without elevated blood sugars; often related to elevated cholesterol and triglycerides, obesity, cardiovascular disease, and high blood pressure.
AHA: 4Q, '01, 42

✓5ᵗʰ 277.8 Other specified disorders of metabolism

AHA: 4Q, '03, 50; 2Q, '01, 18; S-O, '87, 9

277.81 Primary carnitine deficiency

277.82 Carnitine deficiency due to inborn errors of metabolism

277.83 Iatrogenic carnitine deficiency

Carnitine deficiency due to:
   hemodialysis
   valproic acid therapy

277.84 Other secondary carnitine deficiency

277.85 Disorders of fatty acid oxidation

Carnitine palmitoyltransferase deficiencies (CPT1, CPT2)
Glutaric aciduria type II (type IIA, IIB, IIC)
Long chain 3-hydroxyacyl CoA dehydrogenase deficiency (LCHAD)
Long chain/very long chain acyl CoA dehydrogenase deficiency (LCAD, VLCAD)
Medium chain acyl CoA dehydrogenase deficiency (MCAD)
Short chain acyl CoA dehydrogenase deficiency (SCAD)

   EXCLUDES *primary carnitine deficiency (277.81)*

277.86 Peroxisomal disorders

Adrenomyeloneuropathy
Neonatal adrenoleukodystrophy
Rhizomelic chrondrodysplasia punctata
X-linked adrenoleukodystrophy
Zellweger syndrome

   EXCLUDES *infantile Refsum disease (356.3)*

277.87 Disorders of mitochondrial metabolism

Kearns-Sayre syndrome
Mitochondrial Encephalopathy, Lactic Acidosis and Stroke-like episodes (MELAS syndrome)
Mitochondrial Neurogastrointestinal Encephalopathy syndrome (MNGIE)
Myoclonus with Epilepsy and with Ragged Red Fibers (MERRF syndrome)
Neuropathy, Ataxia and Retinitis Pigmentosa (NARP syndrome)

Use additional code for associated conditions

   EXCLUDES *disorders of pyruvate metabolism (271.8)*
     Leber's optic atrophy (377.16)
     Leigh's subacute necrotizing encephalopathy (330.8)
     Reye's syndrome (331.81)
AHA: 4Q, '04, 62

277.88 Tumor lysis syndrome

Spontaneous tumor lysis syndrome
Tumor lysis syndrome following antineoplastic drug therapy

Use additional E code to identify cause, if drug-induced

DEF: A potentially fatal metabolic complication of tumor necrosis caused by either spontaneous or treatment-related accumulation of byproducts from dying cancer cells; symptoms include hyperkalemia, hyperphosphatemia, hypocalcemia, hyperuricemia, and hyperuricosuria.
AHA: 4Q, '09, 78-79

277.89 Other specified disorders of metabolism

Hand-Schüller-Christian disease
Histiocytosis (acute) (chronic)
Histiocytosis X (chronic)

   EXCLUDES *histiocytosis:*
     acute differentiated progressive (202.5)
     X, acute (progressive) (202.5)

277.9 Unspecified disorder of metabolism

Enzymopathy NOS

✓4ᵗʰ 278 Overweight, obesity and other hyperalimentation

   EXCLUDES *hyperalimentation NOS (783.6)*
     poisoning by vitamins NOS (963.5)
     polyphagia (783.6)

✓5ᵗʰ 278.0 Overweight and obesity

Use additional code to identify Body Mass Index (BMI), if known (V85.0-V85.54)

   EXCLUDES *adiposogenital dystrophy (253.8)*
     obesity of endocrine origin NOS (259.9)
AHA: 4Q, '05, 97

278.00 Obesity, unspecified

Obesity NOS
DEF: BMI (body mass index) between 30.0 and 39.9.
AHA: 4Q, '01, 42; 1Q, '99, 5, 6

278.01 Morbid obesity

Severe obesity
DEF: BMI (body mass index) 40 or greater.
AHA: 2Q, '09, 11; 2Q, '06, 5-6; 3Q, '03, 6-8
E66.01 Morbid (severe) obesity due to excess calories   `I-10`

278.02 Overweight

DEF: BMI (body mass index) between 25 and 29.9.
AHA: 4Q, '05, 55
E66.3 Overweight   `I-10`

278.03 Obesity hypoventilation syndrome

Pickwickian syndrome
E66.2 Morbid obesity w/alveolar hyperventilation   `I-10`

278.1 Localized adiposity

Fat pad
AHA: 2Q, '06, 10

278.2 Hypervitaminosis A

278.3 Hypercarotinemia

DEF: Elevated blood carotene level due to ingesting excess carotenoids or the inability to convert carotenoids to vitamin A.

   Ⓝ Newborn Age: 0   Ⓟ Pediatric Age: 0-17   Ⓜ Maternity Age: 12-55   Ⓐ Adult Age: 15-124

278.4 Hypervitaminosis D

> **DEF:** Weakness, fatigue, loss of weight, and other symptoms resulting from ingesting excessive amounts of vitamin D.

278.8 Other hyperalimentation

> **AHA:** 2Q, '09, 11

√4th 279 Disorders involving the immune mechanism

> ►Use additional code for associated manifestations◄

√5th 279.0 Deficiency of humoral immunity

> **DEF:** Inadequate immune response to bacterial infections with potential reinfection by viruses due to lack of circulating immunoglobulins (acquired antibodies).

279.00 Hypogammaglobulinemia, unspecified
Agammaglobulinemia NOS

279.01 Selective IgA immunodeficiency

279.02 Selective IgM immunodeficiency

279.03 Other selective immunoglobulin deficiencies
Selective deficiency of IgG

279.04 Congenital hypogammaglobulinemia
Agammaglobulinemia:
Bruton's type
X-linked

279.05 Immunodeficiency with increased IgM
Immunodeficiency with hyper-IgM:
autosomal recessive
X-linked

279.06 Common variable immunodeficiency
Dysgammaglobulinemia (acquired) (congenital) (primary)
Hypogammaglobulinemia:
acquired primary
congenital non-sex-linked
sporadic

279.09 Other
Transient hypogammaglobulinemia of infancy

√5th 279.1 Deficiency of cell-mediated immunity

279.10 Immunodeficiency with predominant T-cell defect, unspecified

> **AHA:** S-O, '87, 10

279.11 DiGeorge's syndrome
Pharyngeal pouch syndrome
Thymic hypoplasia

> **DEF:** Congenital hypoplasia or aplasia of the thymus, parathyroid glands; related heart defects, anomalies of the great vessels, esophageal atresia, and abnormalities of facial structures.

279.12 Wiskott-Aldrich syndrome

> **DEF:** A disease characterized by chronic conditions, such as eczema, suppurative otitis media and anemia; results from an X-linked recessive gene and is classified as an immune deficiency syndrome.

279.13 Nezelof's syndrome
Cellular immunodeficiency with abnormal immunoglobulin deficiency

> **DEF:** Immune system disorder characterized by a pathological deficiency in cellular immunity and humoral antibodies resulting in inability to fight infectious diseases.

279.19 Other

> **EXCLUDES** ataxia-telangiectasia (334.8)

279.2 Combined immunity deficiency
Agammaglobulinemia:
autosomal recessive
Swiss-type
x-linked recessive
Severe combined immunodeficiency [SCID]
Thymic:
alymphoplasia
aplasia or dysplasia with immunodeficiency

> **EXCLUDES** thymic hypoplasia (279.11)

> **DEF:** Agammaglobulinemia: No immunoglobulins in the blood.
> **DEF:** Thymic alymphoplasia: Severe combined immunodeficiency; result of failed lymphoid tissue development.

279.3 Unspecified immunity deficiency

√5th 279.4 Autoimmune disease, not elsewhere classified

> **EXCLUDES** transplant failure or rejection (996.80-996.89)
> **AHA:** 4Q, '09, 80; 3Q, 08, 5

279.41 Autoimmune lymphoproliferative syndrome
ALPS

> **DEF:** Rare genetic alteration of the Fas protein; impairs normal cellular apoptosis (normal cell death), causing abnormal accumulation of lymphocytes in the lymph glands, liver, and spleen; symptoms include neutropenia, anemia, and thrombocytopenia.

279.49 Autoimmune disease, not elsewhere classified
Autoimmune disease NOS

√5th 279.5 Graft-versus-host disease
Code first underlying cause, such as:
complication of blood transfusion (999.89)
complication of transplanted organ (996.80-996.89)
Use additional code to identify associated manifestations, such as:
desquamative dermatitis (695.89)
diarrhea (787.91)
elevated bilirubin (782.4)
hair loss (704.09)

> **DEF:** A complication of transplantation, most commonly bone marrow; may involve skin, GI tract, liver and cause increased susceptibility to infection; results when donor cells responsible for immune response attack the cells of the transplant recipient.
> **AHA:** 4Q, 08, 97-99, 154

279.50 Graft-versus-host disease, unspecified

> **AHA:** 4Q, 08, 99

279.51 Acute graft-versus-host disease

> **AHA:** 4Q, 08, 99

279.52 Chronic graft-versus-host disease

279.53 Acute on chronic graft-versus-host disease

279.8 Other specified disorders involving the immune mechanism
Single complement [C_1-C_9] deficiency or dysfunction

279.9 Unspecified disorder of immune mechanism

> **AHA:** 3Q, '92, 13

√4th √5th Additional Digit Required   Unspecified Code   Other Specified Code   Manifestation Code   ►◄ Revised Text   ● New Code   ▲ Revised Code Title

2011 ICD-9-CM   **October 2010 • Volume 1 – 63**

4. Diseases of the Blood and Blood-Forming Organs (280-289)

> **EXCLUDES** anemia complicating pregnancy or the puerperium (648.2)

☑4th **280 Iron deficiency anemias**

> **INCLUDES** anemia:
> asiderotic
> hypochromic-microcytic
> sideropenic

> **EXCLUDES** familial microcytic anemia (282.49)

280.0 Secondary to blood loss (chronic)

Normocytic anemia due to blood loss

> **EXCLUDES** acute posthemorrhagic anemia (285.1)

AHA: 4Q, '93, 34

280.1 Secondary to inadequate dietary iron intake

280.8 Other specified iron deficiency anemias

Paterson-Kelly syndrome
Plummer-Vinson syndrome
Sideropenic dysphagia

280.9 Iron deficiency anemia, unspecified

Anemia:	Anemia:
achlorhydric	idiopathic hypochromic
chlorotic	iron [Fe] deficiency NOS

☑4th **281 Other deficiency anemias**

281.0 Pernicious anemia

Anemia:
Addison's
Biermer's
congenital pernicious
Congenital intrinsic factor [Castle's] deficiency

> **EXCLUDES** combined system disease without mention of anemia (266.2)
> subacute degeneration of spinal cord without mention of anemia (266.2)

DEF: Chronic progressive anemia due to Vitamin B12 malabsorption; caused by lack of a secretion of intrinsic factor, which is produced by the gastric mucosa of the stomach.

AHA: N-D, '84, 1; S-O, '84, 16

281.1 Other vitamin B$_{12}$ deficiency anemia

Anemia:
vegan's
vitamin B$_{12}$ deficiency (dietary)
due to selective vitamin B$_{12}$ malabsorption with proteinuria
Syndrome:
Imerslund's
Imerslund-Gräsbeck

> **EXCLUDES** combined system disease without mention of anemia (266.2)
> subacute degeneration of spinal cord without mention of anemia (266.2)

281.2 Folate-deficiency anemia

Congenital folate malabsorption
Folate or folic acid deficiency anemia:
NOS
dietary
drug-induced
Goat's milk anemia
Nutritional megaloblastic anemia (of infancy)

Use additional E code to identify drug

DEF: Macrocytic anemia resembles pernicious anemia but without absence of hydrochloric acid secretions; responsive to folic acid therapy.

281.3 Other specified megaloblastic anemias not elsewhere classified

Combined B$_{12}$ and folate-deficiency anemia
Refractory megaloblastic anemia

DEF: Megaloblasts predominant in bone marrow with few normoblasts; rare familial type associated with proteinuria and genitourinary tract anomalies.

281.4 Protein-deficiency anemia

Amino-acid-deficiency anemia

281.8 Anemia associated with other specified nutritional deficiency

Scorbutic anemia

281.9 Unspecified deficiency anemia

Anemia:
dimorphic
macrocytic
megaloblastic NOS
nutritional NOS
simple chronic

☑4th **282 Hereditary hemolytic anemias**

DEF: Escalated rate of erythrocyte destruction; similar to all anemias, occurs when imbalance exists between blood loss and blood production.

282.0 Hereditary spherocytosis

Acholuric (familial) jaundice
Congenital hemolytic anemia (spherocytic)
Congenital spherocytosis
Minkowski-Chauffard syndrome
Spherocytosis (familial)

> **EXCLUDES** hemolytic anemia of newborn (773.0-773.5)

DEF: Hereditary, chronic illness marked by abnormal red blood cell membrane; symptoms include enlarged spleen, jaundice; and anemia in severe cases.

282.1 Hereditary elliptocytosis

Elliptocytosis (congenital)
Ovalocytosis (congenital) (hereditary)

DEF: Genetic hemolytic anemia characterized by malformed, elliptical erythrocytes; there is increased destruction of red cells with resulting anemia.

282.2 Anemias due to disorders of glutathione metabolism

Anemia:
6-phosphogluconic dehydrogenase deficiency
enzyme deficiency, drug-induced
erythrocytic glutathione deficiency
glucose-6-phosphate dehydrogenase [G-6-PD] deficiency
glutathione-reductase deficiency
hemolytic nonspherocytic (hereditary), type I
Disorder of pentose phosphate pathway
Favism

282.3 Other hemolytic anemias due to enzyme deficiency

Anemia:
hemolytic nonspherocytic (hereditary), type II
hexokinase deficiency
pyruvate kinase [PK] deficiency
triosephosphate isomerase deficiency

☑5th **282.4 Thalassemias**

> **EXCLUDES** sickle-cell:
> disease (282.60-282.69)
> trait (282.5)

DEF: Inherited hemolytic disorders characterized by decreased production of at least one polypeptide globin chain results in defective hemoglobin synthesis; symptoms include severe anemia, expanded marrow spaces, transfusional and absorptive iron overload, impaired growth rate, thickened cranial bones, and pathologic fractures.

AHA: 4Q, '03, 51

282.41 Sickle-cell thalassemia without crisis

Sickle-cell thalassemia NOS
Thalassemia Hb-S disease without crisis

282.42 Sickle-cell thalassemia with crisis

Sickle-cell thalassemia with vaso-occlusive pain
Thalassemia Hb-S disease with crisis

Use additional code for type of crisis, such as:
acute chest syndrome (517.3)
splenic sequestration (289.52)

282.49 Other thalassemia

Cooley's anemia
Hb-Bart's disease
Hereditary leptocytosis
Mediterranean anemia (with other hemoglobinopathy)
Microdrepanocytosis
Thalassemia (alpha) (beta) (intermedia) (major) (minima) (minor) (mixed) (trait) (with other hemoglobinopathy)
Thalassemia NOS

☑4th ☑5th Additional Digit Required   Unspecified Code   Other Specified Code   Manifestation Code   ▶◀ Revised Text   ● New Code   ▲ Revised Code Title

2011 ICD-9-CM   **Volume 1 – 65**

Diseases of the Blood and Blood-Forming Organs

282.5–284.1

282.5 Sickle-cell trait
Hb-AS genotype
Hemoglobin S [Hb-S] trait

Heterozygous:
  hemoglobin S
  Hb-S

> **EXCLUDES**   *that with other hemoglobinopathy (282.60-282.69)*
> *that with thalassemia (282.49)*

DEF: Heterozygous genetic makeup characterized by one gene for normal hemoglobin and one for sickle-cell hemoglobin; clinical disease rarely present.

TIP: Do not assign along with another code for sickle-cell disease or thalassemia.

√5ᵗʰ 282.6 Sickle-cell disease
Sickle-cell anemia

> **EXCLUDES**   *sickle-cell thalassemia (282.41-282.42)*
> *sickle-cell trait (282.5)*

DEF: Inherited blood disorder; sickle-shaped red blood cells are hard and pointed, clogging blood flow; anemia characterized by periodic episodes of pain, acute abdominal discomfort, skin ulcerations of the legs, increased infections.

282.60 Sickle-cell disease, unspecified
Sickle-cell anemia NOS
AHA: 2Q, '97, 11

282.61 Hb-SS disease without crisis

282.62 Hb-SS disease with crisis
Hb-SS disease with vaso-occlusive pain
Sickle-cell crisis NOS

Use additional code for type of crisis, such as:
  acute chest syndrome (517.3)
  splenic sequestration (289.52)
AHA: 4Q, '03, 56; 2Q, '98, 8; 2Q, '91, 15

282.63 Sickle-cell/Hb-C disease without crisis
Hb-S/Hb-C disease without crisis

282.64 Sickle-cell/Hb-C disease with crisis
Hb-S/Hb-C disease with crisis
Sickle-cell/Hb-C disease with vaso-occlusive pain

Use additional code for type of crisis, such as:
  acute chest syndrome (517.3)
  splenic sequestration (289.52)
AHA: 4Q, '03, 51

282.68 Other sickle-cell disease without crisis
Hb-S/Hb-D
Hb-S/Hb-E
Sickle-cell/Hb-D   } diseases without
Sickle-cell/Hb-E   crisis
AHA: 4Q, '03, 51

282.69 Other sickle-cell disease with crisis
Hb-S/Hb-D
Hb-S/Hb-E
Sickle-cell/Hb-D   } diseases with crisis
Sickle-cell/Hb-E

Other sickle-cell disease with vaso-occlusive pain

Use additional code for type of crisis, such as:
  acute chest syndrome (517.3)
  splenic sequestration (289.52)

282.7 Other hemoglobinopathies
Abnormal hemoglobin NOS
Congenital Heinz-body anemia
Disease:
  hemoglobin C [Hb-C]
  hemoglobin D [Hb-D]
  hemoglobin E [Hb-E]
  hemoglobin Zurich [Hb-Zurich]
Hemoglobinopathy NOS
Hereditary persistence of fetal hemoglobin [HPFH]
Unstable hemoglobin hemolytic disease

> **EXCLUDES**   *familial polycythemia (289.6)*
> *hemoglobin M [Hb-M] disease (289.7)*
> *high-oxygen-affinity hemoglobin (289.0)*

DEF: Any disorder of hemoglobin due to alteration of molecular structure; may include overt anemia.

282.8 Other specified hereditary hemolytic anemias
Stomatocytosis

282.9 Hereditary hemolytic anemia, unspecified
Hereditary hemolytic anemia NOS

√4ᵗʰ 283 Acquired hemolytic anemias
DEF: Non-hereditary anemia characterized by premature destruction of red blood cells; caused by infectious organisms, poisons, and physical agents.
AHA: N-D, '84, 1

283.0 Autoimmune hemolytic anemias
Autoimmune hemolytic disease (cold type) (warm type)
Chronic cold hemagglutinin disease
Cold agglutinin disease or hemoglobinuria
Hemolytic anemia:
  cold type (secondary) (symptomatic)
  drug-induced
  warm type (secondary) (symptomatic)

Use additional E code to identify cause, if drug-induced

> **EXCLUDES**   *Evans' syndrome (287.32)*
> *hemolytic disease of newborn (773.0-773.5)*

AHA: 3Q, '08, 5

√5ᵗʰ 283.1 Non-autoimmune hemolytic anemias
Use additional E code to identify cause
DEF: Hemolytic anemia and thrombocytopenia with acute renal failure; relatively rare condition; 50 percent of patients require renal dialysis.
AHA: 4Q, '93, 25

283.10 Non-autoimmune hemolytic anemia, unspecified

283.11 Hemolytic-uremic syndrome

283.19 Other non-autoimmune hemolytic anemias
Hemolytic anemia:
  mechanical
  microangiopathic
  toxic

283.2 Hemoglobinuria due to hemolysis from external causes
Acute intravascular hemolysis
Hemoglobinuria:
  from exertion
  march
  paroxysmal (cold) (nocturnal)
  due to other hemolysis
Marchiafava-Micheli syndrome

Use additional E code to identify cause

283.9 Acquired hemolytic anemia, unspecified
Acquired hemolytic anemia NOS
Chronic idiopathic hemolytic anemia

√4ᵗʰ 284 Aplastic anemia and other bone marrow failure syndromes
DEF: Bone marrow failure to produce the normal amount of blood components; generally non-responsive to usual therapy.
AHA: 1Q, '91, 14; N-D, '84, 1; S-O, '84, 16

√5ᵗʰ 284.0 Constitutional aplastic anemia
AHA: 1Q, '91, 14

284.01 Constitutional red blood cell aplasia
Aplasia, (pure) red cell:
  congenital
  of infants
  primary
Blackfan-Diamond syndrome
Familial hypoplastic anemia
AHA: 4Q, '06, 67-69

284.09 Other constitutional aplastic anemia
Fanconi's anemia
Pancytopenia with malformations
AHA: 4Q, '06, 67-69

284.1 Pancytopenia

> **EXCLUDES**   *pancytopenia (due to) (with):*
> *aplastic anemia NOS (284.9)*
> *bone marrow infiltration (284.2)*
> *constitutional red blood cell aplasia (284.01)*
> *drug induced (284.89)*
> *hairy cell leukemia (202.4)*
> *human immunodeficiency virus disease (042)*
> *leukoerythroblastic anemia (284.2)*
> *malformations (284.09)*
> *myelodysplastic syndromes (238.72-238.75)*
> *myeloproliferative disease (238.79)*
> *other constitutional aplastic anemia (284.09)*

AHA: 4Q, '06, 67-69

Ⓝ Newborn Age: 0   Ⓟ Pediatric Age: 0-17   Ⓜ Maternity Age: 12-55   Ⓐ Adult Age: 15-124

284.2 **Myelophthisis**
Leukoerythroblastic anemia
Myelophthisic anemia

Code first the underlying disorder, such as:
malignant neoplasm of breast (174.0-174.9, 175.0-175.9)
tuberculosis (015.0-015.9)

EXCLUDES *idiopathic myelofibrosis (238.76)*
myelofibrosis NOS (289.83)
myelofibrosis with myeloid metaplasia (238.76)
primary myelofibrosis (238.76)
secondary myelofibrosis (289.83)

DEF: A secondary disease process involving replacement of normal hematopoeitic tissue in the bone marrow with abnormal tissue, such as fibrous tissue or tumors. Occurs with advanced-stage neoplasms, granulomatous diseases such as miliary tuberculosis, and other inflammatory diseases.
AHA: 4Q, '06, 67-69

√5ᵗʰ **284.8 Other specified aplastic anemias**
AHA: 4Q, '07, 72; 3Q, '05, 11; 1Q, '97, 5; 1Q, '92, 15; 1Q, '91, 14

284.81 Red cell aplasia (acquired) (adult) (with thymoma)
Red cell aplasia NOS

284.89 Other specified aplastic anemias
Aplastic anemia (due to):
chronic systemic disease
drugs
infection
radiation
toxic (paralytic)
Use additional E code to identify cause
AHA: 1Q, '09, 20; 2Q, '08, 6

284.9 Aplastic anemia, unspecified
Anemia:
aplastic (idiopathic) NOS
aregenerative
hypoplastic NOS

Anemia:
nonregenerative
Medullary hypoplasia

EXCLUDES *refractory anemia (238.72)*

√4ᵗʰ **285 Other and unspecified anemias**
AHA: 1Q, '91, 14; N-D, '84, 1

285.0 Sideroblastic anemia
Anemia:
hypochromic with iron loading
sideroachrestic
sideroblastic:
acquired
congenital
hereditary
primary
secondary (drug-induced) (due to disease)
sex-linked hypochromic
vitamin B6-responsive
Pyridoxine-responsive (hypochromic) anemia
Use additional E code to identify cause, if drug induced

EXCLUDES *refractory sideroblastic anemia (238.72)*

DEF: Characterized by a disruption of final heme synthesis; results in iron overload of reticuloendothelial tissues.

285.1 Acute posthemorrhagic anemia
Anemia due to acute blood loss

EXCLUDES *anemia due to chronic blood loss (280.0)*
blood loss anemia NOS (280.0)

AHA: 1Q, '07, 19; 2Q, '92, 15

√4ᵗʰ **285.2 Anemia of chronic disease**
Anemia in (due to) (with) chronic illness
AHA: 4Q, '00, 39

285.21 Anemia in chronic kidney disease
Anemia in end stage renal disease
Erythropoietin-resistant anemia (EPO resistant anemia)
TIP: Assign also a code for the chronic kidney disease (585.X).

285.22 Anemia in neoplastic disease
EXCLUDES *anemia due to antineoplastic chemotherapy (285.3)*
▶*aplastic anemia due to antineoplastic chemotherapy (284.89)*◀

AHA: 4Q, '09, 81
TIP: Assign also a code for the neoplasm causing the anemia. Do not assign if anemia is caused by chemotherapy drugs, which is instead reported with 285.3.
D63.0 Anemia in neoplastic disease   I-10

285.29 Anemia of other chronic disease
Anemia in other chronic illness

285.3 Antineoplastic chemotherapy induced anemia
Anemia due to antineoplastic chemotherapy
EXCLUDES *anemia due to drug NEC — code to type of anemia*
anemia in neoplastic disease (285.22)
aplastic anemia due to antineoplastic chemotherapy (284.89)

DEF: Reversible adverse effect of chemotherapy, causing inhibition of bone marrow production; decrease in red blood cell production prevents adequate oxygenation of the tissues and organs causing fatique, SOB, and exacerbation of other medical conditions.
AHA: 4Q, '09, 80-82

285.8 Other specified anemias
Anemia:
dyserythropoietic (congenital)
dyshematopoietic (congenital)
von Jaksch's
Infantile pseudoleukemia
AHA: 1Q, '91, 16

285.9 Anemia, unspecified
Anemia:
NOS
essential
normocytic, not due
to blood loss

Anemia:
profound
progressive
secondary
Oligocythemia

EXCLUDES *anemia (due to):*
blood loss:
acute (285.1)
chronic or unspecified (280.0)
iron deficiency (280.0-280.9)

AHA: 1Q, '09, 17, 20; 1Q, '07, 19; 1Q, '02, 14; 2Q, '92, 16; M-A, '85, 13; N-D, '84, 1
TIP: Assign for "postoperative anemia" if there is no mention of blood loss.

√4ᵗʰ **286 Coagulation defects**
AHA: 2Q, '06, 17

286.0 Congenital factor VIII disorder
Antihemophilic globulin [AHG] deficiency
Factor VIII (functional) deficiency
Hemophilia:
NOS
A
classical
familial
hereditary
Subhemophilia

EXCLUDES *factor VIII deficiency with vascular defect (286.4)*

DEF: Hereditary, sex-linked, results in missing antihemophilic globulin (AHG) (factor VIII); causes abnormal coagulation characterized by increased bleeding, large bruises of skin, bleeding in mouth, nose, gastrointestinal tract; hemorrhages into joints, resulting in swelling and impaired function.

286.1 Congenital factor IX disorder
Christmas disease
Deficiency:
factor IX (functional)
plasma thromboplastin component [PTC]
Hemophilia B

DEF: Deficiency of plasma thromboplastin component (PTC) (factor IX) and plasma thromboplastin antecedent (PTA); PTC deficiency clinically indistinguishable from classical hemophilia.

286.2 Congenital factor XI deficiency
Hemophilia C
Plasma thromboplastin antecedent [PTA] deficiency
Rosenthal's disease

√4ᵗʰ √5ᵗʰ Additional Digit Required   Unspecified Code   Other Specified Code   Manifestation Code   ▶◀ Revised Text   ● New Code   ▲ Revised Code Title

2011 ICD-9-CM   October 2010 • Volume 1 – **67**

Diseases of the Blood and Blood-Forming Organs

286.3 – 287.39

286.3 Congenital deficiency of other clotting factors
Congenital afibrinogenemia
Deficiency:
  AC globulin factor:
    I [fibrinogen]
    II [prothrombin]
    V [labile]
    VII [stable]
    X [Stuart-Prower]
    XII [Hageman]
    XIII [fibrin stabilizing]
  Laki-Lorand factor
  proaccelerin
Disease:
  Owren's
  Stuart-Prower
Dysfibrinogenemia (congenital)
Dysprothrombinemia (constitutional)
Hypoproconvertinemia
Hypoprothrombinemia (hereditary)
Parahemophilia

286.4 von Willebrand's disease
Angiohemophilia (A) (B)
Constitutional thrombopathy
Factor VIII deficiency with vascular defect
Pseudohemophilia type B
Vascular hemophilia
von Willebrand's (-Jürgens') disease

> **EXCLUDES** *factor VIII deficiency:*
>   *NOS (286.0)*
>   *with functional defect (286.0)*
>   *hereditary capillary fragility (287.8)*

DEF: Abnormal blood coagulation caused by deficient blood Factor VII; congenital; symptoms include excess or prolonged bleeding.

286.5 Hemorrhagic disorder due to intrinsic circulating anticoagulants
Antithrombinemia
Antithromboplastinemia
Antithromboplastino-
  genemia
Hyperheparinemia
Increase in:
  anti-VIIIa
  anti-IXa
  anti-Xa
Increase in:
  anti-XIa
  antithrombin
Secondary hemophilia
Systemic lupus erythematosus
  [SLE] inhibitor

AHA: 3Q, '04, 7; No.5, '93, 16; 3Q, '92, 15; 3Q, '90, 14

TIP: Do not assign for Coumadin/warfarin toxicity, poisoning or adverse effect. Follow coding guidelines for poisoning and adverse reactions.

286.6 Defibrination syndrome
Afibrinogenemia, acquired
Consumption coagulopathy
Diffuse or disseminated intravascular coagulation [DIC syndrome]
Fibrinolytic hemorrhage, acquired
Hemorrhagic fibrinogenolysis
Pathologic fibrinolysis
Purpura:
  fibrinolytic
  fulminans

> **EXCLUDES** *that complicating:*
>   *abortion (634-638 with .1, 639.1)*
>   *pregnancy or the puerperium (641.3, 666.3)*
>   *disseminated intravascular coagulation in newborn (776.2)*

DEF: Characterized by destruction of circulating fibrinogen; often precipitated by other conditions, such as injury, causing release of thromboplastic particles in blood stream.

AHA: 4Q, '93, 29

286.7 Acquired coagulation factor deficiency
Deficiency of coagulation factor due to:
  liver disease
  vitamin K deficiency
Hypoprothrombinemia, acquired

Use additional E code to identify cause, if drug induced

> **EXCLUDES** *vitamin K deficiency of newborn (776.0)*

AHA: 4Q, '93, 29

286.9 Other and unspecified coagulation defects
Defective coagulation NOS
Deficiency, coagulation factor NOS
Delay, coagulation
Disorder:
  coagulation
  hemostasis

> **EXCLUDES** *abnormal coagulation profile (790.92)*
>   *hemorrhagic disease of newborn (776.0)*
>   *that complicating:*
>   *abortion (634-638 with .1, 639.1)*
>   *pregnancy or the puerperium (641.3, 666.3)*

AHA: 4Q, '99, 22; 4Q, '93, 29

✓4ᵗʰ 287 Purpura and other hemorrhagic conditions

> **EXCLUDES** *hemorrhagic thrombocythemia (238.79)*
>   *purpura fulminans (286.6)*

AHA: 1Q, '91, 14

287.0 Allergic purpura
Peliosis rheumatica
Purpura:
  anaphylactoid
  autoimmune
  Henoch's
  nonthrombocytopenic:
    hemorrhagic
    idiopathic
Purpura:
  rheumatica
  Schönlein-Henoch
  vascular
Vasculitis, allergic

> **EXCLUDES** *hemorrhagic purpura (287.39)*
>   *purpura annularis telangiectodes (709.1)*

DEF: Any hemorrhagic condition, thrombocytic or nonthrombocytopenic in origin, caused by a presumed allergic reaction.

287.1 Qualitative platelet defects
Thrombasthenia (hemorrhagic) (hereditary)
Thrombocytasthenia
Thrombocytopathy (dystrophic)
Thrombopathy (Bernard-Soulier)

> **EXCLUDES** *von Willebrand's disease (286.4)*

287.2 Other nonthrombocytopenic purpuras
Purpura:
  NOS
  senile
Purpura;
  simplex

✓5ᵗʰ 287.3 Primary thrombocytopenia

> **EXCLUDES** *thrombotic thrombocytopenic purpura (446.6)*
>   *transient thrombocytopenia of newborn (776.1)*

DEF: Decrease in number of blood platelets in circulating blood and purpural skin hemorrhages.

AHA: 4Q, '05, 56

287.30 Primary thrombocytopenia, unspecified
Megakaryocytic hypoplasia

287.31 Immune thrombocytopenic purpura
Idiopathic thrombocytopenic purpura
Tidal platelet dysgenesis

DEF: Tidal platelet dysgenesis: Platelet counts fluctuate from normal to very low within periods of 20 to 40 days and may involve autoimmune platelet destruction.

AHA: 4Q, '05, 57

287.32 Evans' syndrome
DEF: Combination of immunohemolytic anemia and autoimmune hemolytic anemia, sometimes with neutropenia.

287.33 Congenital and hereditary thrombocytopenic purpura
Congenital and hereditary thrombocytopenia
Thrombocytopenia with absent radii (TAR) syndrome

> **EXCLUDES** *Wiskott-Aldrich syndrome (279.12)*

DEF: Thrombocytopenia with absent radii (TAR) syndrome: autosomal recessive syndrome characterized by thrombocytopenia and bilateral radial aplasia; manifestations include skeletal, gastrointestinal, hematologic, and cardiac system abnormalities.

287.39 Other primary thrombocytopenia

☑5ᵗʰ **287.4 Secondary thrombocytopenia**
    Use additional E code to identify cause
    EXCLUDES *heparin-induced thrombocytopenia (HIT) (289.84)*
        transient thrombocytopenia of newborn (776.1)
    AHA: M-A, '85, 14

●   **287.41 Posttransfusion purpura**
    Posttransfusion purpura from whole blood (fresh) or
      blood products
    PTP

●   **287.49 Other secondary thrombocytopenia**
    Thrombocytopenia (due to):
      dilutional
      drugs
      extracorporeal circulation of blood
      massive blood transfusion
      platelet alloimmunization
      secondary NOS
    DEF: Reduced number of platelets in circulating blood as
    consequence of an underlying disease or condition.

287.5 Thrombocytopenia, unspecified

287.8 Other specified hemorrhagic conditions
    Capillary fragility (hereditary)
    Vascular pseudohemophilia

287.9 Unspecified hemorrhagic conditions
    Hemorrhagic diathesis (familial)

☑4ᵗʰ **288 Diseases of white blood cells**
    EXCLUDES *leukemia (204.0-208.9)*
    AHA: 4Q, '06, 69; 1Q, '91, 14

☑5ᵗʰ **288.0 Neutropenia**
    Decreased absolute neutrophil count [ANC]
    Use additional code for any associated:
      fever (780.61)
      mucositis (478.11, 528.00-528.09, 538, 616.81)
    EXCLUDES *neutropenic splenomegaly (289.53)*
        transitory neonatal neutropenia (776.7)
    DEF: Sudden, severe condition characterized by reduced number of
    white blood cells; results in sores in the throat, stomach or skin;
    symptoms include chills, fever.
    AHA: 4Q, '06, 69-73; 3Q, '05, 11; 3Q, '99, 6; 2Q, '99, 9; 3Q, '96, 16;
    2Q, '96, 6

  288.00 Neutropenia, unspecified
    AHA: 4Q, '06, 69-73

  288.01 Congenital neutropenia
    Congenital agranulocytosis
    Infantile genetic agranulocytosis
    Kostmann's syndrome
    AHA: 4Q, '06, 69-73

  288.02 Cyclic neutropenia
    Cyclic hematopoiesis Periodic neutropenia
    AHA: 4Q, '06, 69-73

  288.03 Drug induced neutropenia
    Use additional E code to identify drug
    AHA: 4Q, '06, 69-73
    TIP: Assign for neutropenic fever due to chemotherapy
    drugs, along with codes for the fever, adverse effect, and
    the underlying malignancy.

  288.04 Neutropenia due to infection
    AHA: 4Q, '06, 69-73

  288.09 Other neutropenia
    Agranulocytosis
    Neutropenia:
      immune
      toxic
    AHA: 4Q, '06, 69-73

**288.1 Functional disorders of polymorphonuclear
neutrophils**
    Chronic (childhood) granulomatous disease
    Congenital dysphagocytosis
    Job's syndrome
    Lipochrome histiocytosis (familial)
    Progressive septic granulomatosis

288.2 Genetic anomalies of leukocytes
    Anomaly (granulation) (granulocyte) or syndrome:
      Alder's (-Reilly)
      Chédiak-Steinbrinck (-Higashi)
      Jordan's
      May-Hegglin
      Pelger-Huet
    Hereditary:
      hypersegmentation
      hyposegmentation
      leukomelanopathy

288.3 Eosinophilia
    Eosinophilia: Eosinophilia:
      allergic   secondary
      hereditary   Eosinophilic leukocytosis
      idiopathic
    EXCLUDES *Löffler's syndrome (518.3)*
        pulmonary eosinophilia (518.3)
    DEF: Elevated number of eosinophils in the blood; characteristic of
    allergic states and various parasitic infections.
    AHA: 3Q, '00, 11

288.4 Hemophagocytic syndromes
    Familial hemophagocytic lymphohistiocytosis
    Familial hemophagocytic reticulosis
    Hemophagocytic syndrome, infection-associated
    Histiocytic syndromes
    Macrophage activation syndrome
    AHA: 4Q, '06, 69-73

☑5ᵗʰ **288.5 Decreased white blood cell count**
    EXCLUDES *neutropenia (288.01-288.09)*

  288.50 Leukocytopenia, unspecified
    Decreased leukocytes, unspecified
    Decreased white blood cell count, unspecified
    Leukopenia NOS
    AHA: 4Q, '06, 69-73

  288.51 Lymphocytopenia
    Decreased lymphocytes
    AHA: 4Q, '06, 69-73

  288.59 Other decreased white blood cell count
    Basophilic leukopenia   Monocytopenia
    Eosinophilic leukopenia Plasmacytopenia
    AHA: 4Q, '06, 69-73

☑5ᵗʰ **288.6 Elevated white blood cell count**
    EXCLUDES *eosinophilia (288.3)*

  288.60 Leukocytosis, unspecified
    Elevated leukocytes, unspecified
    Elevated white blood cell count, unspecified
    AHA: 4Q, '06, 69-73

  288.61 Lymphocytosis (symptomatic)
    Elevated lymphocytes
    AHA: 4Q, '06, 69-73

  288.62 Leukemoid reaction
    Basophilic leukemoid reaction
    Lymphocytic leukemoid reaction
    Monocytic leukemoid reaction
    Myelocytic leukemoid reaction
    Neutrophilic leukemoid reaction
    AHA: 4Q, '06, 69-73

  288.63 Monocytosis (symptomatic)
    EXCLUDES *infectious mononucleosis (075)*
    AHA: 4Q, '06, 69-73

  288.64 Plasmacytosis
    AHA: 4Q, '06, 69-73

  288.65 Basophilia
    AHA: 4Q, '06, 69-73

288.66 Bandemia
Bandemia without diagnosis of specific infection

EXCLUDES confirmed infection — code to infection leukemia (204.00-208.9)

DEF: Increase in early neutrophil cells, called band cells; may indicate infection.

AHA: 4Q, '07, 73

TIP: Do not assign based on lab values alone; physician must substantiate bandemia without evidence of corresponding infection.

288.69 Other elevated white blood cell count
AHA: 4Q, '06, 69-73

288.8 Other specified disease of white blood cells
EXCLUDES decreased white blood cell counts (288.50-288.59)
elevated white blood cell counts (288.60-288.69)
immunity disorders (279.0-279.9)

AHA: M-A, '87, 12

288.9 Unspecified disease of white blood cells

✓4ᵗʰ 289 Other diseases of blood and blood-forming organs

289.0 Polycythemia, secondary
High-oxygen-affinity hemoglobin

Polycythemia:
acquired
benign
due to:
fall in plasma volume
high altitude
emotional
erythropoietin
hypoxemic
nephrogenous
relative
spurious
stress

EXCLUDES polycythemia:
neonatal (776.4)
primary (238.4)
vera (238.4)

DEF: Elevated number of red blood cells in circulating blood as result of reduced oxygen supply to the tissues.

D75.1 Secondary polycythemia   I-10

289.1 Chronic lymphadenitis
Chronic:
adenitis } any lymph node, except
lymphadenitis } mesenteric

EXCLUDES acute lymphadenitis (683)
mesenteric (289.2)
enlarged glands NOS (785.6)

DEF: Persistent inflammation of lymph node tissue; origin of infection is usually elsewhere.

I88.1 Chronic lymphadenitis except mesenteric   I-10

289.2 Nonspecific mesenteric lymphadenitis
Mesenteric lymphadenitis (acute) (chronic)

DEF: Inflammation of the lymph nodes in peritoneal fold that encases abdominal organs; disease resembles acute appendicitis; unknown etiology.

I88.0 Nonspecific mesenteric lymphadenitis   I-10

289.3 Lymphadenitis, unspecified, except mesenteric
AHA: 2Q, '92, 8

I88.9 Nonspecific lymphadenitis unspecified   I-10

289.4 Hypersplenism
"Big spleen" syndromeHypersplenia
Dyssplenism

EXCLUDES primary splenic neutropenia (289.53)

DEF: An overactive spleen causing a deficiency of the peripheral blood components, an increase in bone marrow cells and sometimes a notable increase in the size of the spleen.

D73.1 Hypersplenism   I-10

✓4ᵗʰ 289.5 Other diseases of spleen

289.50 Disease of spleen, unspecified
D73.9 Disease of spleen unspecified   I-10

289.51 Chronic congestive splenomegaly
D73.2 Chronic congestive splenomegaly   I-10

289.52 Splenic sequestration
Code first sickle-cell disease in crisis (282.42, 282.62, 282.64, 282.69)

DEF: Blood is entrapped in the spleen due to vessel occlusion; most often associated with sickle-cell disease; spleen becomes enlarged and there is a sharp drop in hemoglobin.

AHA: 4Q, '03, 51

289.53 Neutropenic splenomegaly
AHA: 4Q, '06, 73

D73.81 Neutropenic splenomegaly   I-10

289.59 Other
Lien migrans   Splenic:
Perisplenitis   fibrosis
Splenic: infarction
abscess   rupture, nontraumatic
atrophy   Splenitis
cyst   Wandering spleen

EXCLUDES bilharzial splenic fibrosis (120.0-120.9)
hepatolienal fibrosis (571.5)
splenomegaly NOS (789.2)

D73.89 Other diseases of spleen   I-10

289.6 Familial polycythemia
Familial:
benign polycythemia
erythrocytosis

DEF: Elevated number of red blood cells.

289.7 Methemoglobinemia
Congenital NADH [DPNH]-methemoglobin- reductase deficiency
Hemoglobin M [Hb-M] disease
Methemoglobinemia:
NOS
acquired (with sulfhemoglobinemia)
hereditary
toxic
Stokvis' disease
Sulfhemoglobinemia

Use additional E code to identify cause

DEF: Presence of blood methemoglobin, a chemically altered form of hemoglobin; causes cyanosis, headache, ataxia, dyspnea, tachycardia, nausea, stupor, and coma.

D74.0 Congenital methemoglobinemia   I-10

Ⓝ Newborn Age: 0   Ⓟ Pediatric Age: 0-17   Ⓜ Maternity Age: 12-55   Ⓐ Adult Age: 15-124

√5ᵗʰ **289.8 Other specified diseases of blood and blood-forming organs**

DEF: Hypercoagulable states: a group of inherited or acquired abnormalities of specific proteins and anticoagulant factors; also called thromboembolic states or thrombotic disorders, result in abnormal development of blood clots.

AHA: 4Q, '03, 56; 1Q, '02, 16; 2Q, '89, 8; M-A, '87, 12

289.81 Primary hypercoagulable state

Activated protein C resistance
Antithrombin III deficiency
Factor V Leiden mutation
Lupus anticoagulant
Protein C deficiency
Protein S deficiency
Prothrombin gene mutation

DEF: Activated protein C resistance: decreased effectiveness of protein C to degrade factor V, necessary to inhibit clotting cascade; also called Factor V Leiden mutation.

DEF: Antithrombin III, deficiency: deficiency in plasma antithrombin III, one of six naturally occurring antithrombins that limit coagulation.

DEF: Factor V Leiden mutation: also called activated protein C resistance.

DEF: Lupus anticoagulant: autoimmune deficiency in a circulating anticoagulant that inhibits the conversion of prothrombin into thrombin; also called anti-phospholipid syndrome.

DEF: Protein C deficiency: deficiency of activated protein C which functions to bring the blood-clotting process into balance; same outcome as factor V Leiden mutation.

DEF: Protein S deficiency: similar to protein C deficiency; protein S is a vitamin K dependent cofactor in the activation of protein C.

DEF: Prothrombin gene mutation: increased levels of prothrombin, or factor II, a plasma protein that is converted to thrombin, which acts upon fibrinogen to form the fibrin.

D68.59 Other primary thrombophilia   I-10

289.82 Secondary hypercoagulable state

EXCLUDES *heparin-induced thrombocytopenia (HIT) (289.84)*

D68.69 Other thrombophilia   I-10

289.83 **Myelofibrosis**

Myelofibrosis NOS   Secondary myelofibrosis

Code first the underlying disorder, such as:
malignant neoplasm of breast (174.0-174.9, 175.0-175.9)

Use additional code for associated therapy-related myelodysplastic syndrome, if applicable (238.72, 238.73)

Use additional external cause code if due to antineoplastic chemotherapy (E933.1)

EXCLUDES *idiopathic myelofibrosis (238.76)*
leukoerythroblastic anemia (284.2)
myelofibrosis with myeloid metaplasia (238.76)
myelophthisic anemia (284.2)
myelophthisis (284.2)
primary myelofibrosis (238.76)

DEF: A progressive bone marrow disease characterized by the replacement of bone marrow with the overgrowth of neoplastic stem cells and fibrotic tissue, also progressive anemia and enlarged spleen.

AHA: 4Q, '06, 73

D75.81 Myelofibrosis   I-10

289.84 Heparin-induced thrombocytopenia [HIT]

DEF: Immune-mediated reaction to heparin therapy causing an abrupt fall in platelet count and serious complications such as pulmonary embolism, stroke, AMI or DVT.

AHA: 4Q, '08, 100-101

289.89 Other specified diseases of blood and blood-forming organs

Hypergammaglobulinemia
Pseudocholinesterase deficiency

D75.89 Oth specified dz of blood & blood-forming organs   I-10

289.9 Unspecified diseases of blood and blood-forming organs

Blood dyscrasia NOS   Erythroid hyperplasia

AHA: M-A, '85, 14

D75.9 Disease of blood and blood-forming organs unspecified   I-10

√4ᵗʰ
√5ᵗʰ Additional Digit Required   Unspecified Code   Other Specified Code   Manifestation Code   ►◄ Revised Text   ● New Code   ▲ Revised Code Title
2011 ICD-9-CM   **Volume 1 – 71**

5. Mental Disorders (290-319)

Psychoses (290-299)

EXCLUDES *mental retardation (317-319)*

Organic Psychotic Conditions (290-294)

INCLUDES psychotic organic brain syndrome
EXCLUDES *nonpsychotic syndromes of organic etiology (310.0-310.9)*
psychoses classifiable to 295-298 and without impairment of orientation, comprehension, calculation, learning capacity, and judgment, but associated with physical disease, injury, or condition affecting the brain [eg., following childbirth] (295.0-298.8)

✓4ᵗʰ **290 Dementias**
Code first the associated neurological condition
EXCLUDES *dementia due to alcohol (291.0-291.2)*
dementia due to drugs (292.82)
dementia not classified as senile, presenile, or arteriosclerotic (294.10-294.11)
psychoses classifiable to 295-298 occurring in the senium without dementia or delirium (295.0-298.8)
senility with mental changes of nonpsychotic severity (310.1)
transient organic psychotic conditions (293.0-293.9)

290.0 Senile dementia, uncomplicated   A
Senile dementia:
NOS
simple type
EXCLUDES *mild memory disturbances, not amounting to dementia, associated with senile brain disease (310.8)*
senile dementia with:
delirium or confusion (290.3)
delusional [paranoid] features (290.20)
depressive features (290.21)
AHA: 4Q, '99, 4
F03 Unspecified dementia   I-10

✓5ᵗʰ **290.1 Presenile dementia**
Brain syndrome with presenile brain disease
EXCLUDES *arteriosclerotic dementia (290.40-290.43)*
dementia associated with other cerebral conditions (294.10-294.11)
AHA: N-D, '84, 20

290.10 Presenile dementia, uncomplicated   A
Presenile dementia:
NOS
simple type

290.11 Presenile dementia with delirium   A
Presenile dementia with acute confusional state
AHA: 1Q, '88, 3

290.12 Presenile dementia with delusional features   A
Presenile dementia, paranoid type

290.13 Presenile dementia with depressive features   A
Presenile dementia, depressed type

✓5ᵗʰ **290.2 Senile dementia with delusional or depressive features**
EXCLUDES *senile dementia:*
NOS (290.0)
with delirium and/or confusion (290.3)

290.20 Senile dementia with delusional features   A
Senile dementia, paranoid type
Senile psychosis NOS

290.21 Senile dementia with depressive features   A

290.3 Senile dementia with delirium   A
Senile dementia with acute confusional state
EXCLUDES *senile:*
dementia NOS (290.0)
psychosis NOS (290.20)
AHA: ▶3Q, '09, 11◀

✓5ᵗʰ **290.4 Vascular dementia**
Multi-infarct dementia or psychosis
Use additional code to identify cerebral atherosclerosis (437.0)
EXCLUDES *suspected cases with no clear evidence of arteriosclerosis (290.9)*
AHA: 1Q, '88, 3

290.40 Vascular dementia, uncomplicated   A
Arteriosclerotic dementia:
NOS
simple type
F01.50 Vascular dementia without behavioral disturbance   I-10

290.41 Vascular dementia with delirium   A
Arteriosclerotic dementia with acute confusional state

290.42 Vascular dementia with delusions   A
Arteriosclerotic dementia, paranoid type

290.43 Vascular dementia with depressed mood   A
Arteriosclerotic dementia, depressed type

290.8 Other specified senile psychotic conditions
Presbyophrenic psychosis

290.9 Unspecified senile psychotic condition   A

✓4ᵗʰ **291 Alcohol induced mental disorders**
EXCLUDES *alcoholism without psychosis (303.0-303.9)*
AHA: 1Q, '88, 3; S-O, '86, 3

291.0 Alcohol withdrawal delirium
Alcoholic delirium
Delirium tremens
EXCLUDES *alcohol withdrawal (291.81)*
AHA: 2Q, '91, 11
F10.921 Alcohol use unspecified w/intoxication delirium   I-10

291.1 Alcohol induced persisting amnestic disorder
Alcoholic polyneuritic psychosis
Korsakoff's psychosis, alcoholic
Wernicke-Korsakoff syndrome (alcoholic)
DEF: Prominent and lasting reduced memory span, disordered time appreciation and confabulation, occurring in alcoholics, as sequel to acute alcoholic psychosis.
AHA: 1Q, '88, 3

291.2 Alcohol induced persisting dementia
Alcoholic dementia NOS
Alcoholism associated with dementia NOS
Chronic alcoholic brain syndrome
F10.27 Alcohol depend alcohol-induced persist dementia   I-10

291.3 Alcohol induced psychotic disorder with hallucinations
Alcoholic:
hallucinosis (acute)
psychosis with hallucinosis
EXCLUDES *alcohol withdrawal with delirium (291.0)*
schizophrenia (295.0-295.9) and paranoid states (297.0-297.9) taking the form of chronic hallucinosis with clear consciousness in an alcoholic
DEF: Psychosis lasting less than six months with slight or no clouding of consciousness in which auditory hallucinations predominate.
AHA: 2Q, '91, 11

291.4 Idiosyncratic alcohol intoxication
Pathologic:
alcohol intoxication
drunkenness
EXCLUDES *acute alcohol intoxication (305.0)*
in alcoholism (303.0)
simple drunkenness (305.0)
DEF: Unique behavioral patterns, like belligerence, after intake of relatively small amounts of alcohol; behavior not due to excess consumption.

Mental Disorders

291.5 Alcohol induced psychotic disorder with delusions
Alcoholic:
  paranoia
  psychosis, paranoid type
> EXCLUDES *nonalcoholic paranoid states (297.0-297.9)*
>   *schizophrenia, paranoid type (295.3)*

√5ᵗʰ **291.8 Other specified alcohol induced mental disorders**
AHA: 3Q, '94, 13; J-A, '85, 10

291.81 Alcohol withdrawal
Alcohol:
  abstinence syndrome or symptoms
  withdrawal syndrome or symptoms
> EXCLUDES *alcohol withdrawal:*
>   *delirium (291.0)*
>   *hallucinosis (291.3)*
>   *delirium tremens (291.0)*

AHA: 4Q, '96, 28; 2Q, '91, 11
F10.239 Alcohol dependence with withdrawal   I-10
unspecified

291.82 Alcohol induced sleep disorders
Alcohol induced circadian rhythm sleep disorders
Alcohol induced hypersomnia
Alcohol induced insomnia
Alcohol induced parasomnia

291.89 Other
Alcohol induced anxiety disorder
Alcohol induced mood disorder
Alcohol induced sexual dysfunction

291.9 Unspecified alcohol induced mental disorders
Alcoholic:
  mania NOS
  psychosis NOS
Alcoholism (chronic) with psychosis
Alcohol related disorder NOS

√4ᵗʰ **292 Drug induced mental disorders**
> INCLUDES organic brain syndrome associated with consumption of
>   drugs

Use additional code for any associated drug dependence
(304.0-304.9)
Use additional E code to identify drug
AHA: 3Q, '04, 8; 2Q, '91, 11; S-O, '86, 3

292.0 Drug withdrawal
Drug:
  abstinence syndrome or symptoms
  withdrawal syndrome or symptoms
AHA: 1Q, '97, 12; 1Q, '88, 3
TIP: Assign only for patients who suffer mental or behavioral
disturbances due to drug withdrawal, regardless of the
circumstances.
F19.939 Oth psychoactive sbstnc use uns w/withdraw uns   I-10

√5ᵗʰ **292.1 Drug induced psychotic disorders**

292.11 Drug induced psychotic disorder with delusions
Paranoid state induced by drugs

292.12 Drug induced psychotic disorder with hallucinations
Hallucinatory state induced by drugs
> EXCLUDES *states following LSD or other hallucinogens,*
>   *lasting only a few days or less ["bad*
>   *trips"] (305.3)*

292.2 Pathological drug intoxication
Drug reaction:
  NOS   } resulting in brief psychotic
  idiosyncratic   states
  pathologic
> EXCLUDES *expected brief psychotic reactions to hallucinogens*
>   *["bad trips"] (305.3)*
>   *physiological side-effects of drugs (e.g., dystonias)*

√5ᵗʰ **292.8 Other specified drug induced mental disorders**

292.81 Drug induced delirium
AHA: 1Q, '88, 3
F19.921 Oth psychoactv sbstnc use uns   I-10
intoxcat delirium

292.82 Drug induced persisting dementia

292.83 Drug induced persisting amnestic disorder

292.84 Drug induced mood disorder
Depressive state induced by drugs

292.85 Drug induced sleep disorders
Drug induced circadian rhythm sleep disorder
Drug induced hypersomnia
Drug induced insomnia
Drug induced parasomnia

292.89 Other
Drug induced anxiety disorder
Drug induced organic personality syndrome
Drug induced sexual dysfunction
Drug intoxication

292.9 Unspecified drug induced mental disorder
Drug related disorder NOS
Organic psychosis NOS due to or associated with drugs

√4ᵗʰ **293 Transient mental disorders due to conditions classified elsewhere**
> INCLUDES transient organic mental disorders not associated with
>   alcohol or drugs

Code first the associated physical or neurological condition
> EXCLUDES *confusional state or delirium superimposed on senile*
>   *dementia (290.3)*
>   *dementia due to:*
>   *alcohol (291.0-291.9)*
>   *arteriosclerosis (290.40-290.43)*
>   *drugs (292.82)*
>   *senility (290.0)*

293.0 Delirium due to conditions classified elsewhere
Acute:
  confusional state
  infective psychosis
  organic reaction
  posttraumatic organic psychosis
  psycho-organic syndrome
Acute psychosis associated with endocrine, metabolic, or
  cerebrovascular disorder
Epileptic:
  confusional state
  twilight state
AHA: 1Q, '88, 3
F05 Delirium due to known physiological condition   I-10

293.1 Subacute delirium
Subacute:
  confusional state
  infective psychosis
  organic reaction
  posttraumatic organic psychosis
  psycho-organic syndrome
  psychosis associated with endocrine or metabolic disorder

√5ᵗʰ **293.8 Other specified transient mental disorders due to conditions classified elsewhere**

293.81 Psychotic disorder with delusions in conditions classified elsewhere
Transient organic psychotic condition, paranoid type

293.82 Psychotic disorder with hallucinations in conditions classified elsewhere
Transient organic psychotic condition, hallucinatory type

293.83 Mood disorder in conditions classified elsewhere
Transient organic psychotic condition, depressive type

293.84 Anxiety disorder in conditions classified elsewhere
AHA: 4Q, '96, 29

293.89 Other
Catatonic disorder in conditions classified elsewhere

N Newborn Age: 0   P Pediatric Age: 0-17   M Maternity Age: 12-55   A Adult Age: 15-124

293.9 Unspecified transient mental disorder in conditions classified elsewhere
Organic psychosis:
infective NOS
posttraumatic NOS
transient NOS
Psycho-organic syndrome

☑4ᵗʰ 294 Persistent mental disorders due to conditions classified elsewhere
INCLUDES organic psychotic brain syndromes (chronic), not elsewhere classified
AHA: M-A, '85, 12

294.0 Amnestic disorder in conditions classified elsewhere
Korsakoff's psychosis or syndrome (nonalcoholic)
Code first underlying condition
EXCLUDES alcoholic:
amnestic syndrome (291.1)
Korsakoff's psychosis (291.1)

☑5ᵗʰ 294.1 Dementia in conditions classified elsewhere
Dementia of the Alzheimer's type
Code first any underlying physical condition, as:
dementia in:
Alzheimer's disease (331.0)
cerebral lipidoses (330.1)
dementia with Lewy bodies (331.82)
dementia with Parkinsonism (331.82)
epilepsy (345.0-345.9)
frontal dementia (331.19)
frontotemporal dementia (331.19)
general paresis [syphilis] (094.1)
hepatolenticular degeneration (275.1)
Huntington's chorea (333.4)
Jakob-Creutzfeldt disease (046.11-046.19)
multiple sclerosis (340)
Pick's disease of the brain (331.11)
polyarteritis nodosa (446.0)
syphilis (094.1)
EXCLUDES dementia:
arteriosclerotic (290.40-290.43)
presenile (290.10-290.13)
senile (290.0)
epileptic psychosis NOS (294.8)
AHA: 4Q, '00, 40; 1Q, '99, 14; N-D, '85, 5

294.10 *Dementia in conditions classified elsewhere without behavioral disturbance*
Dementia in conditions classified elsewhere NOS
F02.80 Dementia in oth dz class elsw w/o behavrl distur ⏹I-10

294.11 *Dementia in conditions classified elsewhere with behavioral disturbance*
Aggressive behavior
Combative behavior
Violent behavior
Wandering off
AHA: 4Q, '00, 41
TIP: Review entire medical record for documentation of behavioral disturbance (aggressive, combative, violent behavior, wandering off); requires physician substantiation.

294.8 Other persistent mental disorders due to conditions classified elsewhere
Amnestic disorder NOS
Dementia NOS
Epileptic psychosis NOS
Mixed paranoid and affective organic psychotic states
Use additional code for associated epilepsy (345.0-345.9)
EXCLUDES mild memory disturbances, not amounting to dementia (310.8)
AHA: ▶3Q, '09, 11;◀ 3Q, '03, 14; 1Q, '88, 5
F06.8 Oth spec mental disord d/t known physiol cond ⏹I-10

294.9 Unspecified persistent mental disorders due to conditions classified elsewhere
Cognitive disorder NOS
Organic psychosis (chronic)
AHA: 2Q, '07, 4

Other Psychoses (295-299)

Use additional code to identify any associated physical disease, injury, or condition affecting the brain with psychoses classifiable to 295-298

☑4ᵗʰ 295 Schizophrenic disorders
INCLUDES schizophrenia of the types described in 295.0-295.9 occurring in children
EXCLUDES *childhood type schizophrenia (299.9)*
infantile autism (299.0)

The following fifth-digit subclassification is for use with category 295:
0 unspecified
1 subchronic
2 chronic
3 subchronic with acute exacerbation
4 chronic with acute exacerbation
5 in remission

DEF: Group of disorders with disturbances in thought (delusions, hallucinations), mood (blunted, flattened, inappropriate affect), sense of self; also bizarre, purposeless behavior, repetitious activity, or inactivity.

§ ☑5ᵗʰ 295.0 Simple type
[0-5] Schizophrenia simplex
EXCLUDES *latent schizophrenia (295.5)*

§ ☑5ᵗʰ 295.1 Disorganized type
[0-5] Hebephrenia
Hebephrenic type schizophrenia
DEF: Inappropriate behavior; results in extreme incoherence and disorganization of time, place and sense of social appropriateness; withdrawal from routine social interaction may occur.

§ ☑5ᵗʰ 295.2 Catatonic type
[0-5] Catatonic (schizophrenia):
agitation
excitation
excited type
stupor
withdrawn type
Schizophrenic:
catalepsy
catatonia
flexibilitas cerea
DEF: Extreme changes in motor activity; one extreme is decreased response or reaction to the environment and the other is spontaneous activity.

§ ☑5ᵗʰ 295.3 Paranoid type
[0-5] Paraphrenic schizophrenia
EXCLUDES *involutional paranoid state (297.2)*
paranoia (297.1)
paraphrenia (297.2)
DEF: Preoccupied with delusional suspicions and auditory hallucinations related to single theme; usually hostile, grandiose, overly religious, occasionally hypochondriacal.
F20.0 Paranoid schizophrenia ⏹I-10

§ ☑5ᵗʰ 295.4 Schizophreniform disorder
[0-5] Oneirophrenia
Schizophreniform:
attack
psychosis, confusional type
EXCLUDES *acute forms of schizophrenia of:*
catatonic type (295.2)
hebephrenic type (295.1)
paranoid type (295.3)
simple type (295.0)
undifferentiated type (295.8)

§ ☑5ᵗʰ 295.5 Latent schizophrenia
[0-5] Latent schizophrenic reaction
Schizophrenia:
borderline
incipient
prepsychotic
prodromal
pseudoneurotic
pseudopsychopathic
EXCLUDES *schizoid personality (301.20-301.22)*
AHA: For code 295.50: 1Q, '06, 10

---

§   Requires fifth digit. Valid digits are in [brackets] under each code. See category 295 for codes and definitions.

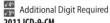
☑4ᵗʰ
☑5ᵗʰ Additional Digit Required   Unspecified Code   Other Specified Code   Manifestation Code   ▶◀ Revised Text   ● New Code   ▲ Revised Code Title
2011 ICD-9-CM   **February 2010 · Volume 1 – 75**

Mental Disorders

295.6–296.90

§ ✓5ᵗʰ **295.6 Residual type**
[0-5]   Chronic undifferentiated schizophrenia
     Restzustand (schizophrenic)
     Schizophrenic residual state
     AHA: For code 295.62: 4Q, '06, 78

§ ✓5ᵗʰ **295.7 Schizoaffective disorder**
[0-5]   Cyclic schizophrenia
     Mixed schizophrenic and affective psychosis
     Schizo-affective psychosis
     Schizophreniform psychosis, affective type
     F25.9 Schizoaffective disorder unspecified   I-10

§ ✓5ᵗʰ **295.8 Other specified types of schizophrenia**
[0-5]   Acute (undifferentiated) schizophrenia
     Atypical schizophrenia
     Cenesthopathic schizophrenia
     EXCLUDES *infantile autism (299.0)*

§ ✓5ᵗʰ **295.9 Unspecified schizophrenia**
[0-5]   Schizophrenia:
       NOS
       mixed NOS
       undifferentiated NOS
       undifferentiated type
     Schizophrenic reaction NOS
     Schizophreniform psychosis NOS
     AHA: 3Q, '95, 6
     F20.9 Schizophrenia unspecified   I-10

✓4ᵗʰ **296 Episodic mood disorders**
     INCLUDES episodic affective disorders
     EXCLUDES *neurotic depression (300.4)*
         reactive depressive psychosis (298.0)
         reactive excitation (298.1)

     The following fifth-digit subclassification is for use with categories 296.0-296.6:

     0 unspecified
     1 mild
     2 moderate
     3 severe, without mention of psychotic behavior
     4 severe, specified as with psychotic behavior
     5 in partial or unspecified remission
     6 in full remission

     AHA: M-A, '85, 14

§ ✓5ᵗʰ **296.0 Bipolar I disorder, single manic episode**
[0-6]   Hypomania (mild) NOS
     Hypomanic psychosis
     Mania (monopolar) NOS
     Manic-depressive psychosis or reaction: } single episode or unspecified
       hypomanic
       manic

     EXCLUDES *circular type, if there was a previous attack of depression (296.4)*
     DEF: Mood disorder identified by hyperactivity; may show extreme agitation or exaggerated excitability; speech and thought processes may be accelerated.

§ ✓5ᵗʰ **296.1 Manic disorder, recurrent episode**
[0-6]   Any condition classifiable to 296.0, stated to be recurrent
     EXCLUDES *circular type, if there was a previous attack of depression (296.4)*

§ ✓5ᵗʰ **296.2 Major depressive disorder, single episode**
[0-6]   Depressive psychosis
     Endogenous depression
     Involutional melancholia
     Manic-depressive psychosis or reaction, depressed type   } single episode or unspecified
     Monopolar depression
     Psychotic depression

     EXCLUDES *circular type, if previous attack was of manic type (296.5)*
         depression NOS (311)
         reactive depression (neurotic) (300.4)
         psychotic (298.0)
     DEF: Mood disorder that produces depression; may exhibit as sadness, low self-esteem, or guilt feelings; other manifestations may be withdrawal from friends and family; interrupted sleep.
     AHA: For code 296.20: ▶3Q, '09, 18◀
     F32.9 Major depressive disorder single episode uns   I-10

§ ✓5ᵗʰ **296.3 Major depressive disorder, recurrent episode**
[0-6]   Any condition classifiable to 296.2, stated to be recurrent
     EXCLUDES *circular type, if previous attack was of manic type (296.5)*
         depression NOS (311)
         reactive depression (neurotic) (300.4)
         psychotic (298.0)
     F33.2 Maj dprsv disord recur sev w/o psychot features   I-10

§ ✓5ᵗʰ **296.4 Bipolar I disorder, most recent episode (or current) manic**
[0-6]   Bipolar disorder, now manic
     Manic-depressive psychosis, circular type but currently manic
     EXCLUDES *brief compensatory or rebound mood swings (296.99)*
     F31.2 Bipolar d/o currnt epis mnic sev w/psychotc ftur   I-10

§ ✓5ᵗʰ **296.5 Bipolar I disorder, most recent episode (or current) depressed**
[0-6]   Bipolar disorder, now depressed
     Manic-depressive psychosis, circular type but currently depressed
     EXCLUDES *brief compensatory or rebound mood swings (296.99)*
     F31.30 Bipol disord currnt epis dprsd mild/mod sev uns   I-10

§ ✓5ᵗʰ **296.6 Bipolar I disorder, most recent episode (or current) mixed**
[0-6]   Manic-depressive psychosis, circular type, mixed

296.7 Bipolar I disorder, most recent episode (or current) unspecified
     Atypical bipolar affective disorder NOS
     Manic-depressive psychosis, circular type, current condition not specified as either manic or depressive
     DEF: Manic-depressive disorder referred to as bipolar because of the mood range from manic to depressive.

✓5ᵗʰ **296.8 Other and unspecified bipolar disorders**

296.80 Bipolar disorder, unspecified
     Bipolar disorder NOS
     Manic-depressive:
       reaction NOS
       syndrome NOS
     F31.9 Bipolar disorder unspecified   I-10

296.81 Atypical manic disorder

296.82 Atypical depressive disorder

296.89 Other
     Bipolar II disorder
     Manic-depressive psychosis, mixed type
     F31.81 Bipolar II disorder   I-10

✓5ᵗʰ **296.9 Other and unspecified episodic mood disorder**
     EXCLUDES *psychogenic affective psychoses (298.0-298.8)*

296.90 Unspecified episodic mood disorder
     Affective psychosis NOS
     Melancholia NOS
     Mood disorder NOS
     AHA: M-A, '85, 14
     F39 Unspecified mood [affective] disorder   I-10

---

§   Requires fifth digit. Valid digits are in [brackets] under each code. See appropriate category for codes and definitions

N Newborn Age: 0   P Pediatric Age: 0-17   M Maternity Age: 12-55   A Adult Age: 15-124

296.99 **Other specified episodic mood disorder**
    Mood swings:
        brief compensatory
        rebound

☑4ᵗʰ **297 Delusional disorders**
    INCLUDES paranoid disorders
    EXCLUDES *acute paranoid reaction (298.3)*
        alcoholic jealousy or paranoid state (291.5)
        paranoid schizophrenia (295.3)

297.0 **Paranoid state, simple**

297.1 **Delusional disorder**
    Chronic paranoid psychosis
    Sander's disease
    Systematized delusions
    EXCLUDES *paranoid personality disorder (301.0)*
    F22 Delusional disorders   I-10

297.2 **Paraphrenia**
    Involutional paranoid state
    Late paraphrenia
    Paraphrenia (involutional)
    DEF: Paranoid schizophrenic disorder that persists over a prolonged
    period but does not distort personality despite persistent delusions.

297.3 **Shared psychotic disorder**
    Folie à deux
    Induced psychosis or paranoid disorder
    DEF: Mental disorder two people share; first person with the
    delusional disorder convinces second person because of a close
    relationship and shared experiences to accept the delusions.

297.8 **Other specified paranoid states**
    Paranoia querulans
    Sensitiver Beziehungswahn
    EXCLUDES *acute paranoid reaction or state (298.3)*
        senile paranoid state (290.20)

297.9 **Unspecified paranoid state**
    Paranoid:
        disorder NOS
        psychosis NOS
        reaction NOS
        state NOS
    AHA: J-A, '85, 9

☑4ᵗʰ **298 Other nonorganic psychoses**
    INCLUDES psychotic conditions due to or provoked by:
        emotional stress
        environmental factors as major part of etiology

298.0 **Depressive type psychosis**
    Psychogenic depressive psychosis
    Psychotic reactive depression
    Reactive depressive psychosis
    EXCLUDES *manic-depressive psychosis, depressed type*
        (296.2-296.3)
        neurotic depression (300.4)
        reactive depression NOS (300.4)

298.1 **Excitative type psychosis**
    Acute hysterical psychosis
    Psychogenic excitation
    Reactive excitation
    EXCLUDES *manic-depressive psychosis, manic type*
        (296.0-296.1)
    DEF: Affective disorder similar to manic-depressive psychosis, in the
    manic phase, seemingly brought on by stress.

298.2 **Reactive confusion**
    Psychogenic confusion
    Psychogenic twilight state
    EXCLUDES *acute confusional state (293.0)*
    DEF: Confusion, disorientation, cloudiness in consciousness; brought
    on by severe emotional upheaval.

298.3 **Acute paranoid reaction**
    Acute psychogenic paranoid psychosis
    Bouffée délirante
    EXCLUDES *paranoid states (297.0-297.9)*

298.4 **Psychogenic paranoid psychosis**
    Protracted reactive paranoid psychosis

298.8 **Other and unspecified reactive psychosis**
    Brief psychotic disorder
    Brief reactive psychosis NOS
    Hysterical psychosis
    Psychogenic psychosis NOS
    Psychogenic stupor
    EXCLUDES *acute hysterical psychosis (298.1)*

298.9 **Unspecified psychosis**
    Atypical psychosis
    Psychosis NOS
    Psychotic disorder NOS
    AHA: 3Q, '06, 22
    F28 Oth psych d/o not d/t sbstnc/knwn physiolog cond   I-10

☑4ᵗʰ **299 Pervasive developmental disorders**
    EXCLUDES *adult type psychoses occurring in childhood, as:*
        affective disorders (296.0-296.9)
        manic-depressive disorders (296.0-296.9)
        schizophrenia (295.0-295.9)

    The following fifth-digit subclassification is for use with category 299:
        0 current or active state
        1 residual state

§ ☑5ᵗʰ **299.0 Autistic disorder**
    [0-1]   Childhood autism
        Infantile psychosis
        Kanner's syndrome
        EXCLUDES *disintegrative psychosis (299.1)*
            Heller's syndrome (299.1)
            schizophrenic syndrome of childhood (299.9)
        DEF: Severe mental disorder of children, results in impaired social
        behavior; abnormal development of communicative skills, appears
        to be unaware of the need for emotional support and little
        emotional response to family members.

§ ☑5ᵗʰ **299.1 Childhood disintegrative disorder**
    [0-1]   Heller's syndrome
        Use additional code to identify any associated neurological
            disorder
        EXCLUDES *infantile autism (299.0)*
            schizophrenic syndrome of childhood (299.9)
        DEF: Mental disease of children identified by impaired development
        of reciprocal social skills, verbal and nonverbal communication skills,
        imaginative play.

§ ☑5ᵗʰ **299.8 Other specified pervasive developmental disorders**
    [0-1]   Asperger's disorder
        Atypical childhood psychosis
        Borderline psychosis of childhood
        EXCLUDES *simple stereotypes without psychotic disturbance*
            (307.3)

§ ☑5ᵗʰ **299.9 Unspecified pervasive developmental disorder**
    [0-1]   Child psychosis NOS
        Pervasive developmental disorder NOS
        Schizophrenia, childhood type NOS
        Schizophrenic syndrome of childhood NOS
        EXCLUDES *schizophrenia of adult type occurring in childhood*
            (295.0-295.9)

---

§   Requires fifth digit. Valid digits are in [brackets] under each code. See category 299 for codes and definitions.

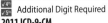 Additional Digit Required   Unspecified Code   Other Specified Code   Manifestation Code   ▶◀ Revised Text   ● New Code   ▲ Revised Code Title

Mental Disorders

300–300.4

Neurotic Disorders, Personality Disorders, and Other Nonpsychotic Mental Disorders (300-316)

✓4ᵗʰ 300 Anxiety, dissociative and somatoform disorders

✓5ᵗʰ 300.0 Anxiety states

> **EXCLUDES** anxiety in:
>> acute stress reaction (308.0)
>> transient adjustment reaction (309.24)
>> neurasthenia (300.5)
>> psychophysiological disorders (306.0-306.9)
>> separation anxiety (309.21)

> **DEF:** Mental disorder characterized by anxiety and avoidance behavior not particularly related to any specific situation or stimulus; symptoms include emotional instability, apprehension, fatigue.

300.00 Anxiety state, unspecified
> Anxiety:
>> neurosis
>> reaction
>> state (neurotic)
> Atypical anxiety disorder
> **AHA:** 1Q, '02, 6
> **TIP:** For chest pain due to anxiety, assign chest pain code first, because chest pain is not integral to the diagnosis of anxiety.
> **F41.9** Anxiety disorder unspecified   I-10

300.01 Panic disorder without agoraphobia
> Panic:
>> attack
>> state
> **EXCLUDES** panic disorder with agoraphobia (300.21)
> **DEF:** Neurotic disorder characterized by recurrent panic or anxiety, apprehension, fear or terror; symptoms include shortness of breath, palpitations, dizziness, shakiness; fear of dying may persist.
> **F41.0** Panic d/o [epis paroxysmal anxiety] w/o agoraphobia   I-10

300.02 Generalized anxiety disorder

300.09 Other

✓5ᵗʰ 300.1 Dissociative, conversion and factitious disorders

> **EXCLUDES** adjustment reaction (309.0-309.9)
>> anorexia nervosa (307.1)
>> gross stress reaction (308.0-308.9)
>> hysterical personality (301.50-301.59)
>> psychophysiologic disorders (306.0-306.9)

300.10 Hysteria, unspecified

300.11 Conversion disorder
> Astasia-abasia, hysterical
> Conversion hysteria or reaction
> Hysterical:
>> blindness
>> deafness
>> paralysis
> **DEF:** Mental disorder that impairs physical functions with no physiological basis; sensory motor symptoms include seizures, paralysis, temporary blindness; increase in stress or avoidance of unpleasant responsibilities may precipitate onset of symptoms.
> **AHA:** N-D, '85, 15

300.12 Dissociative amnesia
> Hysterical amnesia

300.13 Dissociative fugue
> Hysterical fugue
> **DEF:** Dissociative hysteria; identified by loss of memory, flight from familiar surroundings; conscious activity is not associated with perception of surroundings, no later memory of episode.

300.14 Dissociative identity disorder

300.15 Dissociative disorder or reaction, unspecified
> **DEF:** Hysterical neurotic episode; sudden but temporary changes in perceived identity, memory, consciousness, segregated memory patterns exist separate from dominant personality.

300.16 Factitious disorder with predominantly psychological signs and symptoms
> Compensation neurosis
> Ganser's syndrome, hysterical
> **DEF:** A disorder characterized by the purposeful assumption of mental illness symptoms; which are acted out more often when another person is present.

300.19 Other and unspecified factitious illness
> Factitious disorder (with combined psychological and physical signs and symptoms) (with predominantly physical signs and symptoms) NOS
> **EXCLUDES** multiple operations or hospital addiction syndrome (301.51)

✓5ᵗʰ 300.2 Phobic disorders

> **EXCLUDES** anxiety state not associated with a specific situation or object (300.00-300.09)
>> obsessional phobias (300.3)

300.20 Phobia, unspecified
> Anxiety-hysteria NOS
> Phobia NOS

300.21 Agoraphobia with panic disorder
> Fear of:
>> open spaces
>> streets   } with panic attacks
>> travel
> Panic disorder with agoraphobia
> **EXCLUDES** agoraphobia without panic disorder (300.22)
>> panic disorder without agoraphobia (300.01)

300.22 Agoraphobia without mention of panic attacks
> Any condition classifiable to 300.21 without mention of panic attacks

300.23 Social phobia
> Fear of:
>> eating in public
>> public speaking
>> washing in public

300.29 Other isolated or specific phobias
> Acrophobia   Claustrophobia
> Animal phobias   Fear of crowds

300.3 Obsessive-compulsive disorders
> Anancastic neurosis
> Compulsive neurosis
> Obsessional phobia [any]
> **EXCLUDES** obsessive-compulsive symptoms occurring in:
>> endogenous depression (296.2-296.3)
>> organic states (eg., encephalitis)
>> schizophrenia (295.0-295.9)

300.4 Dysthymic disorder
> Anxiety depression
> Depression with anxiety
> Depressive reaction
> Neurotic depressive state
> Reactive depression
> **EXCLUDES** adjustment reaction with depressive symptoms (309.0-309.1)
>> depression NOS (311)
>> manic-depressive psychosis, depressed type (296.2-296.3)
>> reactive depressive psychosis (298.0)
> **DEF:** Depression without psychosis; less severe depression related to personal change or unexpected circumstances; also referred to as "reactional depression."
> **F34.1** Dysthymic disorder   I-10

Ⓝ Newborn Age: 0   Ⓟ Pediatric Age: 0-17   Ⓜ Maternity Age: 12-55   Ⓐ Adult Age: 15-124

300.5 Neurasthenia
Fatigue neurosis
Nervous debility
Psychogenic:
   asthenia
   general fatigue
Use additional code to identify any associated physical
   disorder

> **EXCLUDES** *anxiety state (300.00-300.09)*
> *neurotic depression (300.4)*
> *psychophysiological disorders (306.0-306.9)*
> *specific nonpsychotic mental disorders following*
> * organic brain damage (310.0-310.9)*

DEF: Physical and mental symptoms caused primarily by what is
known as mental exhaustion; symptoms include chronic weakness,
fatigue.

300.6 Depersonalization disorder
Derealization (neurotic)
Neurotic state with depersonalization episode

> **EXCLUDES** *depersonalization associated with:*
> *anxiety (300.00-300.09)*
> *depression (300.4)*
> *manic-depressive disorder or psychosis*
> * (296.0-296.9)*
> *schizophrenia (295.0-295.9)*

DEF: Dissociative disorder characterized by feelings of strangeness
about self or body image; symptoms include dizziness, anxiety, fear
of insanity, loss of reality of surroundings.

300.7 Hypochondriasis
Body dysmorphic disorder

> **EXCLUDES** *hypochondriasis in:*
> *hysteria (300.10-300.19)*
> *manic-depressive psychosis, depressed type*
> * (296.2-296.3)*
> *neurasthenia (300.5)*
> *obsessional disorder (300.3)*
> *schizophrenia (295.0-295.9)*

√5ᵗʰ **300.8 Somatoform disorders**

    300.81 Somatization disorder
       Briquet's disorder
       Severe somatoform disorder

    300.82 Undifferentiated somatoform disorder
       Atypical somatoform disorder
       Somatoform disorder NOS

       DEF: Disorders in which patients have symptoms that
       suggest an organic disease but no evidence of physical
       disorder after repeated testing.
       AHA: 4Q, '96, 29

    300.89 Other somatoform disorders
       Occupational neurosis, including writers' cramp
       Psychasthenia
       Psychasthenic neurosis

300.9 Unspecified nonpsychotic mental disorder
Psychoneurosis NOS

√4ᵗʰ **301 Personality disorders**
> **INCLUDES** character neurosis

Use additional code to identify any associated neurosis or psychosis,
or physical condition

> **EXCLUDES** *nonpsychotic personality disorder associated with organic*
> * brain syndromes (310.0-310.9)*

301.0 Paranoid personality disorder
Fanatic personality
Paranoid personality (disorder)
Paranoid traits

> **EXCLUDES** *acute paranoid reaction (298.3)*
> *alcoholic paranoia (291.5)*
> *paranoid schizophrenia (295.3)*
> *paranoid states (297.0-297.9)*

AHA: J-A, '85, 9

√5ᵗʰ **301.1 Affective personality disorder**
> **EXCLUDES** *affective psychotic disorders (296.0-296.9)*
> *neurasthenia (300.5)*
> *neurotic depression (300.4)*

    301.10 Affective personality disorder, unspecified

    301.11 Chronic hypomanic personality disorder
       Chronic hypomanic disorder
       Hypomanic personality

    301.12 Chronic depressive personality disorder
       Chronic depressive disorder
       Depressive character or personality

    301.13 Cyclothymic disorder
       Cycloid personality
       Cyclothymia
       Cyclothymic personality

√5ᵗʰ **301.2 Schizoid personality disorder**
> **EXCLUDES** *schizophrenia (295.0-295.9)*

    301.20 Schizoid personality disorder, unspecified

    301.21 Introverted personality

    301.22 Schizotypal personality disorder

301.3 Explosive personality disorder
Aggressive:
   personality
   reaction
Aggressiveness
Emotional instability (excessive)
Pathological emotionality
Quarrelsomeness

> **EXCLUDES** *dyssocial personality (301.7)*
> *hysterical neurosis (300.10-300.19)*

301.4 Obsessive-compulsive personality disorder
Anancastic personality
Obsessional personality

> **EXCLUDES** *obsessive-compulsive disorder (300.3)*
> *phobic state (300.20-300.29)*

√5ᵗʰ **301.5 Histrionic personality disorder**
> **EXCLUDES** *hysterical neurosis (300.10-300.19)*

DEF: Extreme emotional behavior, often theatrical; often concerned
about own appeal; may demand attention, exhibit seductive
behavior.

    301.50 Histrionic personality disorder, unspecified
       Hysterical personality NOS

    301.51 Chronic factitious illness with physical symptoms
       Hospital addiction syndrome
       Multiple operations syndrome
       Munchausen syndrome

    301.59 Other histrionic personality disorder
       Personality:
          emotionally unstable
          labile
          psychoinfantile

301.6 Dependent personality disorder
Asthenic personality
Inadequate personality
Passive personality

> **EXCLUDES** *neurasthenia (300.5)*
> *passive-aggressive personality (301.84)*

DEF: Overwhelming feeling of helplessness; fears of abandonment
may persist; difficulty in making personal decisions without
confirmation by others; low self-esteem due to irrational sensitivity
to criticism.

301.7 Antisocial personality disorder
Amoral personality
Asocial personality
Dyssocial personality
Personality disorder with predominantly sociopathic or
  asocial manifestation

> **EXCLUDES** *disturbance of conduct without specifiable*
> * personality disorder (312.0-312.9)*
> *explosive personality (301.3)*

DEF: Continuous antisocial behavior that violates rights of others;
social traits include extreme aggression, total disregard for
traditional social rules.
AHA: S-O, '84, 16

√4ᵗʰ
√5ᵗʰ Additional Digit Required   Unspecified Code   Other Specified Code   Manifestation Code   ▶◀ Revised Text   ● New Code   ▲ Revised Code Title
2011 ICD-9-CM   **Volume 1 – 79**

Mental Disorders

301.8–302.9

√5ᵗʰ **301.8 Other personality disorders**

301.81 Narcissistic personality disorder
DEF: Grandiose fantasy or behavior, lack of social empathy, hypersensitive to the lack of others' judgment, exploits others; need for continual admiration.

301.82 Avoidant personality disorder
DEF: Personality disorder marked by feelings of social inferiority; sensitivity to criticism, emotionally restrained due to fear of rejection.

301.83 Borderline personality disorder
DEF: Personality disorder characterized by unstable moods, self-image, and interpersonal relationships; uncontrolled anger, impulsive and self-destructive acts, fears of abandonment, feelings of emptiness and boredom, recurrent suicide threats or self-mutilation.
F60.3 Borderline personality disorder   I-10

301.84 Passive-aggressive personality
DEF: Pattern of procrastination and refusal to meet standards; introduce own obstacles to success and exploit failure.

301.89 Other
Personality: Personality:
   eccentric   masochistic
   "haltlose" type   psychoneurotic
   immature
EXCLUDES psychoinfantile personality (301.59)

301.9 Unspecified personality disorder
Pathological personality NOS
Personality disorder NOS
Psychopathic:
   constitutional state
   personality (disorder)

√4ᵗʰ **302 Sexual and gender identity disorders**
EXCLUDES sexual disorder manifest in:
   organic brain syndrome (290.0-294.9, 310.0-310.9)
   psychosis (295.0-298.9)

302.0 Ego-dystonic sexual orientation
Ego-dystonic lesbianism
Sexual orientation conflict disorder
EXCLUDES homosexual pedophilia (302.2)

302.1 Zoophilia
Bestiality
DEF: A sociodeviant disorder marked by engaging in sexual intercourse with animals.

302.2 Pedophilia
DEF: A sociodeviant condition of adults characterized by sexual activity with children.

302.3 Transvestic fetishism
EXCLUDES trans-sexualism (302.5)
DEF: The desire to dress in clothing of opposite sex.

302.4 Exhibitionism
DEF: Sexual deviant behavior; exposure of genitals to strangers; behavior prompted by intense sexual urges and fantasies.

√5ᵗʰ **302.5 Trans-sexualism**
Sex reassignment surgery status
EXCLUDES transvestism (302.3)
DEF: Gender identity disturbance; overwhelming desire to change anatomic sex, due to belief that individual is a member of the opposite sex.

302.50 With unspecified sexual history

302.51 With asexual history

302.52 With homosexual history

302.53 With heterosexual history

302.6 Gender identity disorder in children
Feminism in boys
Gender identity disorder NOS
EXCLUDES gender identity disorder in adult (302.85)
   trans-sexualism (302.50-302.53)
   transvestism (302.3)

√5ᵗʰ **302.7 Psychosexual dysfunction**
EXCLUDES impotence of organic origin (607.84)
   normal transient symptoms from ruptured hymen
   transient or occasional failures of erection due to
     fatigue, anxiety, alcohol, or drugs

302.70 Psychosexual dysfunction, unspecified
Sexual dysfunction NOS

302.71 Hypoactive sexual desire disorder
EXCLUDES decreased sexual desire NOS (799.81)

302.72 With inhibited sexual excitement
Female sexual arousal disorder
Frigidity
Impotence
Male erectile disorder

302.73 Female orgasmic disorder   ♀

302.74 Male orgasmic disorder   ♂

302.75 Premature ejaculation   ♂

302.76 Dyspareunia, psychogenic   ♀
DEF: Difficult or painful sex due to psychosomatic state.

302.79 With other specified psychosexual dysfunctions
Sexual aversion disorder

√5ᵗʰ **302.8 Other specified psychosexual disorders**

302.81 Fetishism
DEF: Psychosexual disorder noted for intense sexual urges and arousal precipitated by fantasies; use of inanimate objects, such as clothing, to stimulate sexual arousal, orgasm.

302.82 Voyeurism
DEF: Psychosexual disorder characterized by uncontrollable impulse to observe others, without their knowledge, who are nude or engaged in sexual activity.

302.83 Sexual masochism
DEF: Psychosexual disorder noted for need to achieve sexual gratification through humiliating or hurtful acts inflicted on self.

302.84 Sexual sadism
DEF: Psychosexual disorder noted for need to achieve sexual gratification through humiliating or hurtful acts inflicted on someone else.

302.85 Gender identity disorder in adolescents or adults
Use additional code to identify sex reassignment surgery status (302.5)
EXCLUDES gender identity disorder NOS (302.6)
   gender identity disorder in children (302.6)

302.89 Other
Frotteurism
Nymphomania
Satyriasis

302.9 Unspecified psychosexual disorder
Paraphilia NOS
Pathologic sexuality NOS
Sexual deviation NOS
Sexual disorder NOS

N Newborn Age: 0   P Pediatric Age: 0-17   M Maternity Age: 12-55   A Adult Age: 15-124

☑4ᵗʰ **303 Alcohol dependence syndrome**

Use additional code to identify any associated condition, as:
alcoholic psychoses (291.0-291.9)
drug dependence (304.0-304.9)
physical complications of alcohol, such as:
cerebral degeneration (331.7)
cirrhosis of liver (571.2)
epilepsy (345.0-345.9)
gastritis (535.3)
hepatitis (571.1)
liver damage NOS (571.3)

EXCLUDES *drunkenness NOS (305.0)*

The following fifth-digit subclassification is for use with category 303:
0 unspecified
1 continuous
2 episodic
3 in remission

AHA: ▶1Q, '10, 20-21;◀ 3Q, '95, 6; 2Q, '91, 9; 4Q, '88, 8; S-O, '86, 3
TIP: The patient has become physically addicted to alcohol and often experiences withdrawal symptoms when not drinking. Do not assign both 303.0X and 303.9X on the same encounter.

§ ☑5ᵗʰ **303.0 Acute alcoholic intoxication**
[0-3] Acute drunkenness in alcoholism

§ ☑5ᵗʰ **303.9 Other and unspecified alcohol dependence**
[0-3] Chronic alcoholism
Dipsomania
AHA: 2Q, '02, 4; 2Q, '89, 9; **For code 303.90:** 2Q, '07, 6
F10.20 Alcohol dependence uncomplicated   I-10
F10.21 Alcohol dependence in remission   I-10

☑4ᵗʰ **304 Drug dependence**
EXCLUDES *nondependent abuse of drugs (305.1-305.9)*

The following fifth-digit subclassification is for use with category 304:
0 unspecified
1 continuous
2 episodic
3 in remission

AHA: ▶1Q, '10, 20-21;◀ 2Q, '91, 10; 4Q, '88, 8; S-O, '86, 3

§ ☑5ᵗʰ **304.0 Opioid type dependence**
[0-3] Heroin
Meperidine
Methadone
Morphine
Opium
Opium alkaloids and their derivatives
Synthetics with morphine-like effects
AHA: 2Q, '06, 7

§ ☑5ᵗʰ **304.1 Sedative, hypnotic or anxiolytic dependence**
[0-3] Barbiturates
Nonbarbiturate sedatives and tranquilizers with a similar
effect:
chlordiazepoxide
diazepam
glutethimide
meprobamate
methaqualone

§ ☑5ᵗʰ **304.2 Cocaine dependence**
[0-3] Coca leaves and derivatives
F14.20 Cocaine dependence uncomplicated   I-10

§ ☑5ᵗʰ **304.3 Cannabis dependence**
[0-3] Hashish
Hemp
Marihuana

§ ☑5ᵗʰ **304.4 Amphetamine and other psychostimulant dependence**
[0-3] Methylphenidate
Phenmetrazine

§ ☑5ᵗʰ **304.5 Hallucinogen dependence**
[0-3] Dimethyltryptamine [DMT]
Lysergic acid diethylamide [LSD] and derivatives
Mescaline
Psilocybin

§ ☑5ᵗʰ **304.6 Other specified drug dependence**
[0-3] Absinthe addiction
Glue sniffing
Inhalant dependence
Phencyclidine dependence
EXCLUDES *tobacco dependence (305.1)*

§ ☑5ᵗʰ **304.7 Combinations of opioid type drug with any other**
[0-3] **AHA:** M-A, '86, 12

§ ☑5ᵗʰ **304.8 Combinations of drug dependence excluding**
[0-3] **opioid type drug**
AHA: M-A, '86, 12

§ ☑5ᵗʰ **304.9 Unspecified drug dependence**
[0-3] Drug addiction NOS
Drug dependence NOS
AHA: For code 304.90: 4Q, '03, 103

☑4ᵗʰ **305 Nondependent abuse of drugs**
NOTE Includes cases where a person, for whom no other diagnosis is possible, has come under medical care because of the maladaptive effect of a drug on which he is not dependent and that he has taken on his own initiative to the detriment of his health or social functioning.

EXCLUDES *alcohol dependence syndrome (303.0-303.9)*
drug dependence (304.0-304.9)
drug withdrawal syndrome (292.0)
poisoning by drugs or medicinal substances (960.0-979.9)

The following fifth-digit subclassification is for use with codes 305.0, 305.2-305.9:
0 unspecified
1 continuous
2 episodic
3 in remission

AHA: ▶1Q, '10, 20-21;◀ 2Q, '91, 10; 4Q, '88, 8; S-O, '86, 3

§ ☑5ᵗʰ **305.0 Alcohol abuse**
[0-3] Drunkenness NOS
Excessive drinking of alcohol NOS
"Hangover" (alcohol)
Inebriety NOS
EXCLUDES *acute alcohol intoxication in alcoholism (303.0)*
alcoholic psychoses (291.0-291.9)
AHA: 3Q, '96, 16; **For code 305.00:** 4Q, '09, 112
F10.10 Alcohol abuse uncomplicated   I-10

305.1 Tobacco use disorder
Tobacco dependence
EXCLUDES *history of tobacco use (V15.82)*
smoking complicating pregnancy (649.0)
tobacco use disorder complicating pregnancy (649.0)
AHA: 1Q, '09, 16; 2Q, '96, 10; N-D, '84, 12
F17.210 Nicotine dependence cigarettes uncomplicated   I-10

§ ☑5ᵗʰ **305.2 Cannabis abuse**
[0-3] **F12.10** Cannabis abuse uncomplicated   I-10

§ ☑5ᵗʰ **305.3 Hallucinogen abuse**
[0-3] Acute intoxication from hallucinogens ["bad trips"]
LSD reaction

§ ☑5ᵗʰ **305.4 Sedative, hypnotic or anxiolytic abuse**
[0-3]

§ ☑5ᵗʰ **305.5 Opioid abuse**
[0-3]

§ ☑5ᵗʰ **305.6 Cocaine abuse**
[0-3] **AHA:** 1Q, '93, 25; **For code 305.60:** 1Q, '05, 6
F14.10 Cocaine abuse uncomplicated   I-10

§ ☑5ᵗʰ **305.7 Amphetamine or related acting sympathomimetic**
[0-3] **abuse**
AHA: For code 305.70: 2Q, '03, 10-11

§ ☑5ᵗʰ **305.8 Antidepressant type abuse**
[0-3]

---

§ Requires fifth digit. Valid digits are in [brackets] under each code. See appropriate category for codes and definitions.

Mental Disorders

305.9–307.23

§ ✓5ᵗʰ **305.9 Other, mixed, or unspecified drug abuse**
[0-3]   Caffeine intoxication
     Inhalant abuse
     "Laxative habit"
     Misuse of drugs NOS
     Nonprescribed use of drugs or patent medicinals
     Phencyclidine abuse
     AHA: 3Q, '99, 20

✓4ᵗʰ **306 Physiological malfunction arising from mental factors**
   INCLUDES   psychogenic:
       physical symptoms
       physiological   } not involving tissue
       manifestations   damage

   EXCLUDES   hysteria (300.11-300.19)
      physical symptoms secondary to a psychiatric disorder
       classified elsewhere
      psychic factors associated with physical conditions involving
       tissue damage classified elsewhere (316)
      specific nonpsychotic mental disorders following organic
       brain damage (310.0-310.9)

   DEF: Functional disturbances or interruptions due to mental or psychological causes; no tissue damage sustained in these conditions.

306.0 Musculoskeletal
   Psychogenic paralysis   Psychogenic torticollis
   EXCLUDES   Gilles de la Tourette's syndrome (307.23)
      paralysis as hysterical or conversion reaction (300.11)
      tics (307.20-307.22)

306.1 Respiratory
   Psychogenic: Psychogenic:
     air hunger   hyperventilation
     cough   yawning
     hiccough
   EXCLUDES   psychogenic asthma (316 and 493.9)

306.2 Cardiovascular
   Cardiac neurosis
   Cardiovascular neurosis
   Neurocirculatory asthenia
   Psychogenic cardiovascular disorder
   EXCLUDES   psychogenic paroxysmal tachycardia (316 and 427.2)
   DEF: Neurocirculatory asthenia: functional nervous and circulatory irregularities with palpitations, dyspnea, fatigue, rapid pulse, precordial pain, fear of effort, discomfort during exercise, anxiety; also called DaCosta's syndrome, Effort syndrome, Irritable or Soldier's Heart.
   AHA: J-A, '85, 14

306.3 Skin
   Psychogenic pruritus
   EXCLUDES   psychogenic:
      alopecia (316 and 704.00)
      dermatitis (316 and 692.9)
      eczema (316 and 691.8 or 692.9)
      urticaria (316 and 708.0-708.9)

306.4 Gastrointestinal
   Aerophagy
   Cyclical vomiting, psychogenic
   Diarrhea, psychogenic
   Nervous gastritis
   Psychogenic dyspepsia
   EXCLUDES   cyclical vomiting NOS (536.2)
      associated with migraine (346.2)
      globus hystericus (300.11)
      mucous colitis (316 and 564.9)
      psychogenic:
       cardiospasm (316 and 530.0)
       duodenal ulcer (316 and 532.0-532.9)
       gastric ulcer (316 and 531.0-531.9)
       peptic ulcer NOS (316 and 533.0-533.9)
       vomiting NOS (307.54)
   DEF: Aerophagy: excess swallowing of air, usually unconscious; related to anxiety; results in distended abdomen or belching, often interpreted by the patient as a physical disorder.
   AHA: 2Q, '89, 11

✓5ᵗʰ **306.5 Genitourinary**
   EXCLUDES   enuresis, psychogenic (307.6)
      frigidity (302.72)
      impotence (302.72)
      psychogenic dyspareunia (302.76)

306.50 Psychogenic genitourinary malfunction, unspecified

306.51 Psychogenic vaginismus   ♀
   Functional vaginismus
   DEF: Psychogenic response resulting in painful contractions of vaginal canal muscles; can be severe enough to prevent sexual intercourse.

306.52 Psychogenic dysmenorrhea   ♀

306.53 Psychogenic dysuria

306.59 Other
   AHA: M-A, '87, 11

306.6 Endocrine

306.7 Organs of special sense
   EXCLUDES   hysterical blindness or deafness (300.11)
      psychophysical visual disturbances (368.16)

306.8 Other specified psychophysiological malfunction
   Bruxism
   Teeth grinding

306.9 Unspecified psychophysiological malfunction
   Psychophysiologic disorder NOS
   Psychosomatic disorder NOS

✓4ᵗʰ **307 Special symptoms or syndromes, not elsewhere classified**
   NOTE This category is intended for use if the psychopathology is manifested by a single specific symptom or group of symptoms which is not part of an organic illness or other mental disorder classifiable elsewhere.
   EXCLUDES   those due to mental disorders classified elsewhere
      those of organic origin

▲ **307.0 Adult onset fluency disorder**
   EXCLUDES   ►childhood onset fluency disorder (315.35)◄
      dysphasia (784.59)
      ►fluency disorder due to late effect of cerebrovascular
       accident (438.14)
      fluency disorder in conditions classified elsewhere
       (784.52)◄
      lisping or lalling (307.9)
      retarded development of speech (315.31-315.39)

307.1 Anorexia nervosa
   EXCLUDES   eating disturbance NOS (307.50)
      feeding problem (783.3)
       of nonorganic origin (307.59)
      loss of appetite (783.0)
       of nonorganic origin (307.59)
   AHA: 2Q, '06, 12; 4Q, '89, 11
   TIP: Assign an additional code for any associated malnutrition.

✓5ᵗʰ **307.2 Tics**
   EXCLUDES   nail-biting or thumb-sucking (307.9)
      stereotypes occurring in isolation (307.3)
      tics of organic origin (333.3)
   DEF: Involuntary muscle response usually confined to the face, shoulders.

307.20 Tic disorder, unspecified
   Tic disorder NOS

307.21 Transient tic disorder

307.22 Chronic motor or vocal tic disorder

307.23 Tourette's disorder
   Motor-verbal tic disorder
   DEF: Syndrome of facial and vocal tics in childhood; progresses to spontaneous or involuntary jerking, obscene utterances, other uncontrollable actions considered inappropriate.

---

§   Requires fifth digit. Valid digits are in [brackets] under each code. See category 305 for codes and definitions.

N Newborn Age: 0   P Pediatric Age: 0-17   M Maternity Age: 12-55   A Adult Age: 15-124

307.3 Stereotypic movement disorder
Body-rocking
Head banging
Spasmus nutans
Stereotypes NOS
EXCLUDES tics (307.20-307.23)
of organic origin (333.3)

√5ᵗʰ **307.4 Specific disorders of sleep of nonorganic origin**
EXCLUDES narcolepsy (347.00-347.11)
organic hypersomnia (327.10-327.19)
organic insomnia (327.00-327.09)
those of unspecified cause (780.50-780.59)

307.40 Nonorganic sleep disorder, unspecified

307.41 Transient disorder of initiating or maintaining sleep
Adjustment insomnia
Hyposomnia ⎤ associated with intermittent
Insomnia ⎥ emotional reactions
Sleeplessness ⎦ or conflicts

307.42 Persistent disorder of initiating or maintaining sleep
Hyposomnia, Insomnia, or sleeplessness associated with:
anxiety
conditioned arousal
depression (major) (minor)
psychosis
Idiopathic insomnia
Paradoxical insomnia
Primary insomnia
Psychophysiological insomnia

307.43 Transient disorder of initiating or maintaining wakefulness
Hypersomnia associated with acute or intermittent emotional reactions or conflicts

307.44 Persistent disorder of initiating or maintaining wakefulness
Hypersomnia associated with depression (major) (minor)
Insufficient sleep syndrome
Primary hypersomnia
EXCLUDES sleep deprivation (V69.4)

307.45 Circadian rhythm sleep disorder of nonorganic origin

307.46 Sleep arousal disorder
Night terror disorder
Night terrors
Sleep terror disorder
Sleepwalking
Somnambulism
DEF: Sleepwalking marked by extreme terror, panic, screaming, confusion; no recall of event upon arousal; term may refer to simply the act of sleepwalking.

307.47 Other dysfunctions of sleep stages or arousal from sleep
Nightmare disorder
Nightmares:
NOS
REM-sleep type
Sleep drunkenness

307.48 Repetitive intrusions of sleep
Repetitive intrusion of sleep with:
atypical polysomnographic features
environmental disturbances
repeated REM-sleep interruptions

307.49 Other
"Short-sleeper"
Subjective insomnia complaint

√5ᵗʰ **307.5 Other and unspecified disorders of eating**
EXCLUDES anorexia:
nervosa (307.1)
of unspecified cause (783.0)
overeating, of unspecified cause (783.6)
vomiting:
NOS (787.03)
cyclical (536.2)
associated with migraine (346.2)
psychogenic (306.4)

307.50 Eating disorder, unspecified
Eating disorder NOS

307.51 Bulimia nervosa
Overeating of nonorganic origin
DEF: Mental disorder commonly characterized by binge eating followed by self-induced vomiting; perceptions of being fat; and fear the inability to stop eating voluntarily.

307.52 Pica
Perverted appetite of nonorganic origin
DEF: Compulsive eating disorder characterized by craving for substances other than food, such as paint chips or dirt.

307.53 Rumination disorder
Regurgitation, of nonorganic origin, of food with reswallowing
EXCLUDES obsessional rumination (300.3)

307.54 Psychogenic vomiting

307.59 Other
Feeding disorder of infancy or early childhood of nonorganic origin
Infantile feeding disturbances ⎤ of nonorganic
Loss of appetite ⎦ origin

307.6 Enuresis
Enuresis (primary) (secondary) of nonorganic origin
EXCLUDES enuresis of unspecified cause (788.3)
DEF: Involuntary urination past age of normal control; also called bedwetting; no trace to biological problem; focus on psychological issues.

307.7 Encopresis
Encopresis (continuous) (discontinuous) of nonorganic origin
EXCLUDES encopresis of unspecified cause ▶(787.60-787.63)◄
DEF: Inability to control bowel movements; cause traced to psychological, not biological, problems.

√5ᵗʰ **307.8 Pain disorders related to psychological factors**

307.80 Psychogenic pain, site unspecified

307.81 Tension headache
EXCLUDES headache:
NOS (784.0)
migraine (346.0-346.9)
syndromes (339.00-339.89)
tension type (339.10-339.12)
AHA: 4Q, '08, 103; N-D, '85, 16

307.89 Other
Code first to type or site of pain
EXCLUDES pain disorder exclusively attributed to psychological factors (307.80)
psychogenic pain (307.80)

307.9 Other and unspecified special symptoms or syndromes, not elsewhere classified
Communication disorder NOS
Hair plucking
Lalling
Lisping
Masturbation
Nail-biting
Thumb-sucking

√4ᵗʰ√5ᵗʰ Additional Digit Required   Unspecified Code   Other Specified Code   Manifestation Code   ▶◄ Revised Text   ● New Code   ▲ Revised Code Title

2011 ICD-9-CM   **October 2010 • Volume 1 – 83**

Mental Disorders

308–310.9

✓4ᵗʰ **308   Acute reaction to stress**

> **INCLUDES** ▸combat and operational stress reaction◂
>
> **EXCLUDES** *adjustment reaction or disorder (309.0-309.9)*
> *chronic stress reaction (309.1-309.9)*

308.0   Predominant disturbance of emotions

> Anxiety
> Emotional crisis   } as acute reaction to exceptional
> Panic state   } [gross] stress

308.1   Predominant disturbance of consciousness

> Fugues as acute reaction to exceptional [gross] stress

308.2   Predominant psychomotor disturbance

> Agitation states   } as acute reaction to exceptional
> Stupor   } [gross] stress

308.3   Other acute reactions to stress

> Acute situational disturbance
> Acute stress disorder
>
> **EXCLUDES** *prolonged posttraumatic emotional disturbance*
> *(309.81)*

308.4   Mixed disorders as reaction to stress

308.9   Unspecified acute reaction to stress

✓4ᵗʰ **309   Adjustment reaction**

> **INCLUDES** adjustment disorders
> reaction (adjustment) to chronic stress
>
> **EXCLUDES** *acute reaction to major stress (308.0-308.9)*
> *neurotic disorders (300.0-300.9)*

309.0   Adjustment disorder with depressed mood

> Grief reaction
>
> **EXCLUDES** *affective psychoses (296.0-296.9)*
> *neurotic depression (300.4)*
> *prolonged depressive reaction (309.1)*
> *psychogenic depressive psychosis (298.0)*
>
> **F43.21** Adjustment disorder with depressed mood   I-10

309.1   Prolonged depressive reaction

> **EXCLUDES** *affective psychoses (296.0-296.9)*
> *brief depressive reaction (309.0)*
> *neurotic depression (300.4)*
> *psychogenic depressive psychosis (298.0)*

✓5ᵗʰ **309.2   With predominant disturbance of other emotions**

309.21   Separation anxiety disorder

> **DEF:** Abnormal apprehension by a child when physically
> separated from support environment; byproduct of
> abnormal symbiotic child-parent relationship.

309.22   Emancipation disorder of adolescence and early adult life

> **DEF:** Adjustment reaction of late adolescence; conflict over
> independence from parental supervision; symptoms
> include difficulty in making decisions, increased reliance on
> parental advice, deliberate adoption of values in
> opposition of parents.

309.23   Specific academic or work inhibition

309.24   Adjustment disorder with anxiety

309.28   Adjustment disorder with mixed anxiety and depressed mood

> Adjustment reaction with anxiety and depression
> **F43.23** Adjustment d/o w/mixed anxiety & depressed   I-10
> mood

309.29   Other

> Culture shock

309.3   Adjustment disorder with disturbance of conduct

> Conduct disturbance   } as adjustment reaction
> Destructiveness   }
>
> **EXCLUDES** *destructiveness in child (312.9)*
> *disturbance of conduct NOS (312.9)*
> *dyssocial behavior without manifest psychiatric*
> *disorder (V71.01-V71.02)*
> *personality disorder with predominantly sociopathic*
> *or asocial manifestations (301.7)*

309.4   Adjustment disorder with mixed disturbance of emotions and conduct

✓5ᵗʰ **309.8   Other specified adjustment reactions**

309.81   Posttraumatic stress disorder

> Chronic posttraumatic stress disorder
> Concentration camp syndrome
> Posttraumatic stress disorder NOS
> Post-traumatic stress disorder (PTSD)
>
> **EXCLUDES** *acute stress disorder (308.3)*
> *posttraumatic brain syndrome:*
> *nonpsychotic (310.2)*
> *psychotic (293.0-293.9)*
>
> **DEF:** Preoccupation with traumatic events beyond normal
> experience; i.e., rape, personal assault, etc,; also recurring
> flashbacks of trauma; symptoms include difficulty
> remembering, sleeping, or concentrating, and guilt feelings
> for surviving.

309.82   Adjustment reaction with physical symptoms

309.83   Adjustment reaction with withdrawal

> Elective mutism as adjustment reaction
> Hospitalism (in children) NOS

309.89   Other

309.9   Unspecified adjustment reaction

> Adaptation reaction NOS
> Adjustment reaction NOS

✓4ᵗʰ **310   Specific nonpsychotic mental disorders due to brain damage**

> **EXCLUDES** *neuroses, personality disorders, or other nonpsychotic*
> *conditions occurring in a form similar to that seen with*
> *functional disorders but in association with a physical*
> *condition (300.0-300.9, 301.0-301.9)*

310.0   Frontal lobe syndrome

> Lobotomy syndrome
> Postleucotomy syndrome [state]
>
> **EXCLUDES** *postcontusion syndrome (310.2)*

310.1   Personality change due to conditions classified elsewhere

> Cognitive or personality change of other type, of
> nonpsychotic severity
> Organic psychosyndrome of nonpsychotic severity
> Presbyophrenia NOS
> Senility with mental changes of nonpsychotic severity
>
> **EXCLUDES** *mild cognitive impairment (331.83)*
> *postconcussion syndrome (310.2)*
> *signs and symptoms involving emotional state*
> *(799.21-799.29)*
>
> **DEF:** Personality disorder caused by organic factors, such as brain
> lesions, head trauma, or cerebrovascular accident (CVA).
> **AHA:** 2Q, '05, 6

310.2   Postconcussion syndrome

> Postcontusion syndrome or encephalopathy
> Posttraumatic brain syndrome, nonpsychotic
> Status postcommotio cerebri
>
> Use additional code to identify associated post-traumatic
> headache, if applicable (339.20-339.22)
>
> **EXCLUDES** *frontal lobe syndrome (310.0)*
> *postencephalitic syndrome (310.8)*
> *any organic psychotic conditions following head*
> *injury (293.0-294.0)*
>
> **DEF:** Nonpsychotic disorder due to brain trauma, causes symptoms
> unrelated to any disease process; symptoms include amnesia, serial
> headaches, rapid heartbeat, fatigue, disrupted sleep patterns,
> inability to concentrate.
> **AHA:** 4Q, '90, 24
> **TIP:** For treatment within 24 to 48 hours of the concussion, clarify
> with physician whether the concussion is still in the acute phase; if
> so, assign instead a code from 850.X subcategory.

310.8   Other specified nonpsychotic mental disorders following organic brain damage

> Mild memory disturbance
> Postencephalitic syndrome
> Other focal (partial) organic psychosyndromes
>
> **EXCLUDES** *memory loss of unknown cause (780.93)*

310.9   Unspecified nonpsychotic mental disorder following organic brain damage

> **AHA:** 4Q, '03, 103

N Newborn Age: 0   P Pediatric Age: 0-17   M Maternity Age: 12-55   A Adult Age: 15-124

311 Depressive disorder, not elsewhere classified
Depressive disorder NOS
Depressive state NOS
Depression NOS
    EXCLUDES *acute reaction to major stress with depressive symptoms*
(308.0)
affective personality disorder (301.10-301.13)
affective psychoses (296.0-296.9)
brief depressive reaction (309.0)
depressive states associated with stressful events
(309.0-309.1)
disturbance of emotions specific to childhood and
adolescence, with misery and unhappiness (313.1)
mixed adjustment reaction with depressive symptoms
(309.4)
neurotic depression (300.4)
prolonged depressive adjustment reaction (309.1)
psychogenic depressive psychosis (298.0)
    AHA: 4Q, '03, 75

√4ᵗʰ 312 Disturbance of conduct, not elsewhere classified
    EXCLUDES *adjustment reaction with disturbance of conduct (309.3)*
drug dependence (304.0-304.9)
dyssocial behavior without manifest psychiatric disorder
(V71.01-V71.02)
personality disorder with predominantly sociopathic or
asocial manifestations (301.7)
sexual deviations (302.0-302.9)

The following fifth-digit subclassification is for use with categories
312.0-312.2
  0 unspecified
  1 mild
  2 moderate
  3 severe

§ **√5ᵗʰ 312.0 Undersocialized conduct disorder, aggressive type**
  [0-3]   Aggressive outburst
Anger reaction
Unsocialized aggressive disorder
DEF: Mental condition identified by behaviors disrespectful of others'
rights and of age-appropriate social norms or rules; symptoms
include bullying, vandalism, verbal and physical abusiveness, lying,
stealing, defiance.

§ **√5ᵗʰ 312.1 Undersocialized conduct disorder, unaggressive type**
  [0-3]   Childhood truancy, unsocialized
Solitary stealing
Tantrums

§ **√5ᵗʰ 312.2 Socialized conduct disorder**
  [0-3]   Childhood truancy, socialized
Group delinquency
    EXCLUDES *gang activity without manifest psychiatric disorder*
(V71.01)

√5ᵗʰ 312.3 Disorders of impulse control, not elsewhere classified
  312.30 Impulse control disorder, unspecified
  312.31 Pathological gambling
  312.32 Kleptomania
  312.33 Pyromania
  312.34 Intermittent explosive disorder
  312.35 Isolated explosive disorder
  312.39 Other
      Trichotillomania

312.4 Mixed disturbance of conduct and emotions
Neurotic delinquency
    EXCLUDES *compulsive conduct disorder (312.3)*

**√5ᵗʰ 312.8 Other specified disturbances of conduct, not elsewhere
classified**
  312.81 Conduct disorder, childhood onset type
  312.82 Conduct disorder, adolescent onset type
  312.89 Other conduct disorder
      Conduct disorder of unspecified onset

312.9 Unspecified disturbance of conduct
Delinquency (juvenile)
Disruptive behavior disorder NOS

√4ᵗʰ 313 Disturbance of emotions specific to childhood and adolescence
    EXCLUDES *adjustment reaction (309.0-309.9)*
emotional disorder of neurotic type (300.0-300.9)
masturbation, nail-biting, thumbsucking, and other isolated
symptoms (307.0-307.9)

313.0 Overanxious disorder
Anxiety and fearfulness ⎫ of childhood and
Overanxious disorder   ⎬ adolescence
    EXCLUDES *abnormal separation anxiety (309.21)*
anxiety states (300.00-300.09)
hospitalism in children (309.83)
phobic state (300.20-300.29)

313.1 Misery and unhappiness disorder
    EXCLUDES *depressive neurosis (300.4)*

√5ᵗʰ 313.2 Sensitivity, shyness, and social withdrawal disorder
    EXCLUDES *infantile autism (299.0)*
schizoid personality (301.20-301.22)
schizophrenia (295.0-295.9)

  313.21 Shyness disorder of childhood
      Sensitivity reaction of childhood or adolescence

  313.22 Introverted disorder of childhood
      Social withdrawal ⎫ of childhood and
      Withdrawal reaction ⎬ adolescence

  313.23 Selective mutism
      EXCLUDES *elective mutism as adjustment reaction*
(309.83)

313.3 Relationship problems
Sibling jealousy
    EXCLUDES *relationship problems associated with aggression,*
destruction, or other forms of conduct
disturbance (312.0-312.9)

**√5ᵗʰ 313.8 Other or mixed emotional disturbances of childhood or
adolescence**
  313.81 Oppositional defiant disorder
      DEF: Mental disorder of children noted for pervasive
opposition, defiance of authority.

  313.82 Identity disorder
      Identity problem
      DEF: Distress of adolescents caused by inability to form
acceptable self-identity; uncertainty about career choice,
sexual orientation, moral values.

  313.83 Academic underachievement disorder

  313.89 Other   **P**
      Reactive attachment disorder of infancy or early
childhood

  313.9 Unspecified emotional disturbance of   **P**
  childhood or adolescence
      Mental disorder of infancy, childhood or adolescence NOS

√4ᵗʰ 314 Hyperkinetic syndrome of childhood
    EXCLUDES *hyperkinesis as symptom of underlying disorder — code the*
underlying disorder

√5ᵗʰ 314.0 Attention deficit disorder
Adult
Child
    DEF: A behavioral disorder usually diagnosed at an early age;
characterized by the inability to focus attention for a normal period
of time.
    TIP: These codes may be assigned for patients of any age.

  314.00 Without mention of hyperactivity
      Predominantly inattentive type
      AHA: 1Q, '97, 8

---

§ Requires fifth digit. Valid digits are in [brackets] under each code. See category 312 for codes and definitions.

314.01 With hyperactivity
Combined type
Overactivity NOS
Predominantly hyperactive/impulsive type
Simple disturbance of attention with overactivity
AHA: 1Q, '97, 8
F90.1 ADHD predominantly hyperactive type `I-10`

314.1 Hyperkinesis with developmental delay
Developmental disorder of hyperkinesis
Use additional code to identify any associated neurological disorder

314.2 Hyperkinetic conduct disorder
Hyperkinetic conduct disorder without developmental delay
EXCLUDES hyperkinesis with significant delays in specific skills (314.1)

314.8 Other specified manifestations of hyperkinetic syndrome

314.9 Unspecified hyperkinetic syndrome
Hyperkinetic reaction of childhood or adolescence NOS
Hyperkinetic syndrome NOS

√4ᵗʰ **315 Specific delays in development**
EXCLUDES that due to a neurological disorder (320.0-389.9)

√5ᵗʰ **315.0 Specific reading disorder**

315.00 Reading disorder, unspecified

315.01 Alexia
DEF: Lack of ability to understand written language; manifestation of aphasia.

315.02 Developmental dyslexia
DEF: Serious impairment of reading skills unexplained in relation to general intelligence and teaching processes.

315.09 Other
Specific spelling difficulty

315.1 Mathematics disorder
Dyscalculia

315.2 Other specific learning difficulties
Disorder of written expression
EXCLUDES specific arithmetical disorder (315.1)
specific reading disorder (315.00-315.09)

√5ᵗʰ **315.3 Developmental speech or language disorder**

315.31 Expressive language disorder
Developmental aphasia
Word deafness
EXCLUDES acquired aphasia (784.3)
elective mutism (309.83, 313.0, 313.23)

315.32 Mixed receptive-expressive language disorder
Central auditory processing disorder
EXCLUDES acquired auditory processing disorder (388.45)

315.34 Speech and language developmental delay due to hearing loss
AHA: 4Q, '07, 80, 81

315.35 Childhood onset fluency disorder
Cluttering NOS
Stuttering NOS
EXCLUDES adult onset fluency disorder (307.0)
fluency disorder due to late effect of cerebrovascular accident (438.14)
fluency disorder in conditions classified elsewhere (784.52)
F98.5 Stuttering [stammering] `I-10`

315.39 Other
Developmental articulation disorder
Dyslalia
Phonological disorder
EXCLUDES lisping and lalling (307.9)
AHA: 3Q, '07, 7

315.4 Developmental coordination disorder
Clumsiness syndrome
Dyspraxia syndrome
Specific motor development disorder

315.5 Mixed development disorder
AHA: 2Q, '02, 11

315.8 Other specified delays in development
F88 Other disorders of psychological development `I-10`

315.9 Unspecified delay in development
Developmental disorder NOS
Learning disorder NOS

316 Psychic factors associated with diseases classified elsewhere
Psychologic factors in physical conditions classified elsewhere
Use additional code to identify the associated physical condition, as:
psychogenic:
asthma (493.9)
dermatitis (692.9)
duodenal ulcer (532.0-532.9)
eczema (691.8, 692.9)
gastric ulcer (531.0-531.9)
mucous colitis (564.9)
paroxysmal tachycardia (427.2)
ulcerative colitis (556)
urticaria (708.0-708.9)
psychosocial dwarfism (259.4)
EXCLUDES physical symptoms and physiological malfunctions, not involving tissue damage, of mental origin (306.0-306.9)

Mental Retardation (317-319)

Use additional code(s) to identify any associated psychiatric or physical condition(s)

317 Mild mental retardation
High-grade defect
IQ 50-70
Mild mental subnormality
F70 Mild mental retardation `I-10`

√4ᵗʰ **318 Other specified mental retardation**

318.0 Moderate mental retardation
IQ 35-49
Moderate mental subnormality

318.1 Severe mental retardation
IQ 20-34
Severe mental subnormality

318.2 Profound mental retardation
IQ under 20
Profound mental subnormality

319 Unspecified mental retardation
Mental deficiency NOS
Mental subnormality NOS
F79 Unspecified mental reatardation `I-10`

N Newborn Age: 0   P Pediatric Age: 0-17   M Maternity Age: 12-55   A Adult Age: 15-124

6. Diseases of the Nervous System and Sense Organs (320-389)

Inflammatory Diseases of the Central Nervous System (320-326)

✓4ᵗʰ **320 Bacterial meningitis**

> INCLUDES   arachnoiditis
> leptomeningitis
> meningitis   } bacterial
> meningoencephalitis
> meningomyelitis
> pachymeningitis

> **DEF:** Bacterial infection causing inflammation of the lining of the brain and/or spinal cord.
> **AHA:** J-F, '87, 6

320.0 Hemophilus meningitis
> Meningitis due to Hemophilus influenzae [H. influenzae]

320.1 Pneumococcal meningitis

320.2 Streptococcal meningitis

320.3 Staphylococcal meningitis

320.7 Meningitis in other bacterial diseases classified elsewhere

> Code first underlying disease, as:
> actinomycosis (039.8)
> listeriosis (027.0)
> typhoid fever (002.0)
> whooping cough (033.0-033.9)

> > EXCLUDES   meningitis (in):
> > epidemic (036.0)
> > gonococcal (098.82)
> > meningococcal (036.0)
> > salmonellosis (003.21)
> > syphilis:
> > NOS (094.2)
> > congenital (090.42)
> > meningovascular (094.2)
> > secondary (091.81)
> > tuberculous (013.0)

✓5ᵗʰ **320.8 Meningitis due to other specified bacteria**

320.81 Anaerobic meningitis
> Bacteroides (fragilis)
> Gram-negative anaerobes

320.82 Meningitis due to gram-negative bacteria, not elsewhere classified

> Aerobacter aerogenes   Klebsiella
> pneumoniae   Proteus morganii
> Escherichia coli [E. coli]   Pseudomonas
> Friedländer bacillus

> > EXCLUDES   gram-negative anaerobes (320.81)

320.89 Meningitis due to other specified bacteria
> Bacillus pyocyaneus

320.9 Meningitis due to unspecified bacterium
> Meningitis: Meningitis:
> bacterial NOS   pyogenic NOS
> purulent NOS   suppurative NOS

✓4ᵗʰ **321 Meningitis due to other organisms**

> INCLUDES   arachnoiditis
> leptomeningitis   } due to organisms other
> meningitis   than bacterial
> pachymeningitis

> **DEF:** Infection causing inflammation of the lining of the brain and/or spinal cord, due to organisms other than bacteria.
> **AHA:** J-F, '87, 6

321.0 Cryptococcal meningitis
> Code first underlying disease (117.5)

321.1 Meningitis in other fungal diseases
> Code first underlying disease (110.0-118)

> > EXCLUDES   meningitis in:
> > candidiasis (112.83)
> > coccidioidomycosis (114.2)
> > histoplasmosis (115.01, 115.11, 115.91)

321.2 Meningitis due to viruses not elsewhere classified

> Code first underlying disease, as:
> meningitis due to arbovirus (060.0-066.9)

> > EXCLUDES   meningitis (due to):
> > abacterial (047.0-047.9)
> > adenovirus (049.1)
> > aseptic NOS (047.9)
> > Coxsackie (virus)(047.0)
> > ECHO virus (047.1)
> > enterovirus (047.0-047.9)
> > herpes simplex virus (054.72)
> > herpes zoster virus (053.0)
> > lymphocytic choriomeningitis virus (049.0)
> > mumps (072.1)
> > viral NOS (047.9)
> > meningo-eruptive syndrome (047.1)

> **AHA:** 4Q, '04, 51

321.3 Meningitis due to trypanosomiasis
> Code first underlying disease (086.0-086.9)

321.4 Meningitis in sarcoidosis
> Code first underlying disease (135)

321.8 Meningitis due to other nonbacterial organisms classified elsewhere
> Code first underlying disease

> > EXCLUDES   leptospiral meningitis (100.81)

✓4ᵗʰ **322 Meningitis of unspecified cause**

> INCLUDES   arachnoiditis
> leptomeningitis   } with no organism
> meningitis   specified as cause
> pachymeningitis

> **DEF:** Infection causing inflammation of the lining of the brain and/or spinal cord, due to unspecified cause.
> **AHA:** J-F, '87, 6

322.0 Nonpyogenic meningitis
> Meningitis with clear cerebrospinal fluid

322.1 Eosinophilic meningitis

322.2 Chronic meningitis

322.9 Meningitis, unspecified

✓4ᵗʰ **323 Encephalitis, myelitis, and encephalomyelitis**

> INCLUDES   acute disseminated encephalomyelitis
> meningoencephalitis, except bacterial
> meningomyelitis, except bacterial
> myelitis:
> ascending
> transverse

> > EXCLUDES   acute transverse myelitis NOS (341.20)
> > acute transverse myelitis in conditions classified elsewhere (341.21)
> > bacterial:
> > meningoencephalitis (320.0-320.9)
> > meningomyelitis (320.0-320.9)
> > idiopathic transverse myelitis (341.22)

> **DEF:** Encephalitis: inflammation of brain tissues.
> **DEF:** Myelitis: inflammation of the spinal cord.
> **DEF:** Encephalomyelitis: inflammation of brain and spinal cord.

✓4ᵗʰ
✓5ᵗʰ Additional Digit Required   Unspecified Code   Other Specified Code   Manifestation Code   ▶◀ Revised Text   ● New Code   ▲ Revised Code Title

2011 ICD-9-CM   **Volume 1 – 87**

Diseases of the Nervous System and Sense Organs

323.0–324.9

√5ᵗʰ **323.0 Encephalitis, myelitis, and encephalomyelitis in viral diseases classified elsewhere**

Code first underlying disease, as:
cat-scratch disease (078.3)
infectious mononucleosis (075)
ornithosis (073.7)

323.01 Encephalitis and encephalomyelitis in viral diseases classified elsewhere

EXCLUDES *encephalitis (in):*
arthropod-borne viral (062.0-064)
herpes simplex (054.3)
mumps (072.2)
other viral diseases of central nervous system (049.8-049.9)
poliomyelitis (045.0-045.9)
rubella (056.01)
slow virus infections of central nervous system (046.0-046.9)
viral NOS (049.9)
West Nile (066.41)

AHA: 4Q, '06, 58-63

323.02 Myelitis in viral diseases classified elsewhere

EXCLUDES *myelitis (in):*
herpes simplex (054.74)
herpes zoster (053.14)
poliomyelitis (045.0-045.9)
rubella (056.01)
other viral diseases of central nervous system (049.8-049.9)

AHA: 4Q, '06, 58-63

323.1 Encephalitis, myelitis, and encephalomyelitis in rickettsial diseases classified elsewhere

Code first underlying disease (080-083.9)

DEF: Inflammation of the brain caused by rickettsial disease carried by louse, tick, or mite.

323.2 Encephalitis, myelitis, and encephalomyelitis in protozoal diseases classified elsewhere

Code first underlying disease, as:
malaria (084.0-084.9)
trypanosomiasis (086.0-086.9)

DEF: Inflammation of the brain caused by protozoal disease carried by mosquitoes and flies.

√5ᵗʰ **323.4 Other encephalitis, myelitis, and encephalomyelitis due to infection classified elsewhere**

Code first underlying disease

323.41 Other encephalitis and encephalomyelitis due to infection classified elsewhere

EXCLUDES *encephalitis (in):*
meningococcal (036.1)
syphilis:
NOS (094.81)
congenital (090.41)
toxoplasmosis (130.0)
tuberculosis (013.6)
meningoencephalitis due to free-living ameba [Naegleria] (136.29)

AHA: 4Q, '06, 58-63

323.42 Other myelitis due to infection classified elsewhere

EXCLUDES *myelitis (in):*
syphilis (094.89)
tuberculosis (013.6)

AHA: 4Q, '06, 58-63

√5ᵗʰ **323.5 Encephalitis, myelitis, and encephalomyelitis following immunization procedures**

Use additional E code to identify vaccine

323.51 Encephalitis and encephalomyelitis following immunization procedures

Encephalitis postimmunization or postvaccinal
Encephalomyelitis postimmunization or postvaccinal
AHA: 4Q, '06, 58-63

323.52 Myelitis following immunization procedures

Myelitis postimmunization or postvaccinal
AHA: 4Q, '06, 58-63

√5ᵗʰ **323.6 Postinfectious encephalitis, myelitis, and encephalomyelitis**

Code first underlying disease

DEF: Infection, inflammation of brain several weeks following the outbreak of a systemic infection.

323.61 Infectious acute disseminated encephalomyelitis [ADEM]

Acute necrotizing hemorrhagic encephalopathy

EXCLUDES *noninfectious acute disseminated encephalomyelitis (ADEM) (323.81)*

AHA: 4Q, '06, 58-63

323.62 Other postinfectious encephalitis and encephalomyelitis

EXCLUDES *encephalitis:*
postchickenpox (052.0)
postmeasles (055.0)

AHA: 4Q, '06, 58-63

323.63 Postinfectious myelitis

EXCLUDES *postchickenpox myelitis (052.2)*
herpes simplex myelitis (054.74)
herpes zoster myelitis (053.14)

AHA: 4Q, '06, 58-63

√5ᵗʰ **323.7 Toxic encephalitis, myelitis, and encephalomyelitis**

Code first underlying cause, as:
carbon tetrachloride (982.1)
hydroxyquinoline derivatives (961.3)
lead (984.0-984.9)
mercury (985.0)
thallium (985.8)

AHA: 2Q, '97, 8

323.71 Toxic encephalitis and encephalomyelitis

AHA: 4Q, '06, 58-63

323.72 Toxic myelitis

AHA: 4Q, '06, 58-63

√5ᵗʰ **323.8 Other causes of encephalitis, myelitis, and encephalomyelitis**

323.81 Other causes of encephalitis and encephalomyelitis

Noninfectious acute disseminated encephalomyelitis (ADEM)
AHA: 4Q, '06, 58-63

323.82 Other causes of myelitis

Transverse myelitis NOS
AHA: 4Q, '06, 58-63

323.9 Unspecified cause of encephalitis, myelitis, and encephalomyelitis

√4ᵗʰ **324 Intracranial and intraspinal abscess**

324.0 Intracranial abscess

Abscess (embolic):
cerebellar
cerebral
Abscess (embolic) of brain [any part]:
epidural
extradural
otogenic
subdural

EXCLUDES *tuberculous (013.3)*

324.1 Intraspinal abscess

Abscess (embolic) of spinal cord [any part]:
epidural
extradural
subdural

EXCLUDES *tuberculous (013.5)*

324.9 Of unspecified site

Extradural or subdural abscess NOS

Ⓝ Newborn Age: 0   Ⓟ Pediatric Age: 0-17   Ⓜ Maternity Age: 12-55   Ⓐ Adult Age: 15-124

325 Phlebitis and thrombophlebitis of intracranial venous sinuses

Embolism
Endophlebitis
Phlebitis, septic or suppurative
Thrombophlebitis
Thrombosis

} of cavernous, lateral or other intracranial or unspecified intracranial venous sinus

> **EXCLUDES** that specified as:
>   complicating pregnancy, childbirth, or the puerperium (671.5)
>   of nonpyogenic origin (437.6)

> **DEF:** Inflammation and formation of blood clot in a vein within the brain or its lining.

326 Late effects of intracranial abscess or pyogenic infection

> **NOTE** This category is to be used to indicate conditions whose primary classification is to 320-325 [excluding 320.7, 321.0-321.8, 323.01-323.42, 323.6-323.7] as the cause of late effects, themselves classifiable elsewhere. The "late effects" include conditions specified as such, or as sequelae, which may occur at any time after the resolution of the causal condition.

> Use additional code to identify condition, as:
>   hydrocephalus (331.4)
>   paralysis (342.0-342.9, 344.0-344.9)

Organic sleep disorders (327)

> **TIP:** If the sleep disorder is not documented with the etiology related to an organic disease process, see instead subcategory 307.4.

✓4ᵗʰ 327 Organic sleep disorders

> AHA: 4Q, '05, 59-64

✓5ᵗʰ 327.0 Organic disorders of initiating and maintaining sleep [Organic insomnia]

> **EXCLUDES** insomnia NOS (780.52)
>   insomnia not due to a substance or known physiological condition (307.41-307.42)
>   insomnia with sleep apnea NOS (780.51)

327.00 Organic insomnia, unspecified

327.01 Insomnia due to medical condition classified elsewhere

> Code first underlying condition
> **EXCLUDES** insomnia due to mental disorder (327.02)

327.02 Insomnia due to mental disorder

> Code first mental disorder
> **EXCLUDES** alcohol induced insomnia (291.82)
>   drug induced insomnia (292.85)

327.09 Other organic insomnia

✓5ᵗʰ 327.1 Organic disorder of excessive somnolence [Organic hypersomnia]

> **EXCLUDES** hypersomnia NOS (780.54)
>   hypersomnia not due to a substance or known physiological condition (307.43-307.44)
>   hypersomnia with sleep apnea NOS (780.53)

327.10 Organic hypersomnia, unspecified

327.11 Idiopathic hypersomnia with long sleep time

327.12 Idiopathic hypersomnia without long sleep time

327.13 Recurrent hypersomnia

> Kleine-Levin syndrome
> Menstrual related hypersomnia

327.14 Hypersomnia due to medical condition classified elsewhere

> Code first underlying condition
> **EXCLUDES** hypersomnia due to mental disorder (327.15)

327.15 Hypersomnia due to mental disorder

> Code first mental disorder
> **EXCLUDES** alcohol induced hypersomnia (291.82)
>   drug induced hypersomnia (292.85)

327.19 Other organic hypersomnia

✓5ᵗʰ 327.2 Organic sleep apnea

> **EXCLUDES** Cheyne-Stokes breathing (786.04)
>   hypersomnia with sleep apnea NOS (780.53)
>   insomnia with sleep apnea NOS (780.51)
>   sleep apnea in newborn (770.81-770.82)
>   sleep apnea NOS (780.57)

327.20 Organic sleep apnea, unspecified

327.21 Primary central sleep apnea

327.22 High altitude periodic breathing

327.23 Obstructive sleep apnea (adult) (pediatric)

> **G47.33** Obstructive sleep apnea (adult) (pediatric)   **I-10**

327.24 Idiopathic sleep related nonobstructive alveolar hypoventilation

> Sleep related hypoxia

327.25 Congenital central alveolar hypoventilation syndrome

327.26 Sleep related hypoventilation/ hypoxemia in conditions classifiable elsewhere

> Code first underlying condition

327.27 Central sleep apnea in conditions classified elsewhere

> Code first underlying condition

327.29 Other organic sleep apnea

✓4ᵗʰ 327.3 Circadian rhythm sleep disorder

> Organic disorder of sleep wake cycle
> Organic disorder of sleep wake schedule
> **EXCLUDES** alcohol induced circadian rhythm sleep disorder (291.82)
>   circadian rhythm sleep disorder of nonorganic origin (307.45)
>   disruption of 24 hour sleep wake cycle NOS (780.55)
>   drug induced circadian rhythm sleep disorder (292.85)

327.30 Circadian rhythm sleep disorder, unspecified

327.31 Circadian rhythm sleep disorder, delayed sleep phase type

327.32 Circadian rhythm sleep disorder, advanced sleep phase type

327.33 Circadian rhythm sleep disorder, irregular sleep-wake type

327.34 Circadian rhythm sleep disorder, free-running type

327.35 Circadian rhythm sleep disorder, jet lag type

327.36 Circadian rhythm sleep disorder, shift work type

327.37 Circadian rhythm sleep disorder in conditions classified elsewhere

> Code first underlying condition

327.39 Other circadian rhythm sleep disorder

✓5ᵗʰ 327.4 Organic parasomnia

> **EXCLUDES** alcohol induced parasomnia (291.82)
>   drug induced parasomnia (292.85)
>   parasomnia not due to a known physiological condition (307.47)

327.40 Organic parasomnia, unspecified

327.41 Confusional arousals

327.42 REM sleep behavior disorder

327.43 Recurrent isolated sleep paralysis

327.44 Parasomnia in conditions classified elsewhere

> Code first underlying condition

327.49 Other organic parasomnia

✓5ᵗʰ 327.5 Organic sleep related movement disorders

> **EXCLUDES** restless legs syndrome (333.94)
>   sleep related movement disorder NOS (780.58)

327.51 Periodic limb movement disorder

> Periodic limb movement sleep disorder

327.52 Sleep related leg cramps

✓4ᵗʰ ✓5ᵗʰ Additional Digit Required   Unspecified Code   Other Specified Code   Manifestation Code   ▶◀ Revised Text   ● New Code   ▲ Revised Code Title

2011 ICD-9-CM   **Volume 1 – 89**

327.53 Sleep related bruxism

327.59 Other organic sleep related movement disorders

327.8 Other organic sleep disorders
AHA: 2Q, '07, 6

Hereditary and Degenerative Diseases of the Central Nervous System (330-337)

EXCLUDES *hepatolenticular degeneration (275.1)*
multiple sclerosis (340)
other demyelinating diseases of central nervous system (341.0-341.9)

√4ᵗʰ **330 Cerebral degenerations usually manifest in childhood**
Use additional code to identify associated mental retardation

330.0 Leukodystrophy
Krabbe's disease   Pelizaeus-Merzbacher disease
Leukodystrophy: Sulfatide lipidosis
  NOS
  globoid cell
  metachromatic
  sudanophilic
DEF: Hereditary disease of arylsulfatase or cerebroside sulfatase; characterized by a diffuse loss of myelin in CNS; infantile form causes blindness, motor disturbances, rigidity, mental deterioration and, occasionally, convulsions.

330.1 Cerebral lipidoses
Amaurotic (familial) idiocy
Disease:
  Batten
  Jansky-Bielschowsky
  Kufs'
  Spielmeyer-Vogt
  Tay-Sachs
Gangliosidosis
DEF: Genetic disorder causing abnormal lipid accumulation in the reticuloendothelial cells of the brain.

330.2 Cerebral degeneration in generalized lipidoses
Code first underlying disease, as:
  Fabry's disease (272.7)
  Gaucher's disease (272.7)
  Niemann-Pick disease (272.7)
  sphingolipidosis (272.7)

330.3 Cerebral degeneration of childhood in other diseases classified elsewhere
Code first underlying disease, as:
  Hunter's disease (277.5)
  mucopolysaccharidosis (277.5)

330.8 Other specified cerebral degenerations in childhood
Alpers' disease or gray-matter degeneration
Infantile necrotizing encephalomyelopathy
Leigh's disease
Subacute necrotizing encephalopathy or
  encephalomyelopathy
AHA: N-D, '85, 5

330.9 Unspecified cerebral degeneration in childhood

√4ᵗʰ **331 Other cerebral degenerations**
Use additional code, where applicable, to identify dementia:
  with behavioral disturbance (294.11)
  without behavioral disturbance (294.10)

331.0 Alzheimer's disease
DEF: Diffuse atrophy of cerebral cortex; causing a progressive decline in intellectual and physical functions, including memory loss, personality changes and profound dementia.
AHA: 4Q, '00, 41; 4Q, '99, 7; N-D, '84, 20
G30.9 Alzheimer's disease unspecified   I-10

√5ᵗʰ **331.1 Frontotemporal dementia**
DEF: Rare, progressive degenerative brain disease, similar to Alzheimer's; cortical atrophy affects the frontal and temporal lobes.
AHA: 4Q, '03, 57

331.11 Pick's disease
DEF: A progressive frontotemporal dementia with asymmetrical atrophy of the frontal and temporal regions of the cerebral cortex, abnormal rounded brain cells called Pick cells with the presence of abnormal staining of protein (called tau); symptoms include prominent apathy, behavioral changes such as disinhibition and restlessness, echolalia, impairment of language, memory, and intellect, increased carelessness, poor personal hygiene, and decreased attention span.

331.19 Other frontotemporal dementia
Frontal dementia

331.2 Senile degeneration of brain
EXCLUDES *senility NOS (797)*

331.3 Communicating hydrocephalus
Secondary normal pressure hydrocephalus
EXCLUDES *congenital hydrocephalus (742.3)*
idiopathic normal pressure hydrocephalus (331.5)
normal pressure hydrocephalus (331.5)
spina bifida with hydrocephalus (741.0)
DEF: Subarachnoid hemorrhage and meningitis causing excess buildup of cerebrospinal fluid in cavities due to nonabsorption of fluid back through fluid pathways.
AHA: S-O, '85, 12

331.4 Obstructive hydrocephalus
Acquired hydrocephalus NOS
EXCLUDES *congenital hydrocephalus (742.3)*
idiopathic normal pressure hydrocephalus (331.5)
normal pressure hydrocephalus (331.5)
spina bifida with hydrocephalus (741.0)
DEF: Obstruction of cerebrospinal fluid passage from brain into spinal canal.
AHA: 4Q, '03, 106; 1Q, '99, 9
G91.1 Obstructive hydrocephalus   I-10

331.5 Idiopathic normal pressure hydrocephalus [INPH]
Normal pressure hydrocephalus NOS
EXCLUDES *congenital hydrocephalus (742.3)*
secondary normal pressure hydrocephalus (331.3)
spina bifida with hydrocephalus (741.0)
DEF: Abnormal increase of cerebrospinal fluid in the brain's ventricles; results in dementia, progressive mental impairment, gait disturbance, and impaired bladder control.
AHA: 4Q, '07, 74

331.7 Cerebral degeneration in diseases classified elsewhere
Code first underlying disease, as:
  alcoholism (303.0-303.9)
  beriberi (265.0)
  cerebrovascular disease (430-438)
  congenital hydrocephalus (741.0, 742.3)
  myxedema (244.0-244.9)
  neoplastic disease (140.0-239.9)
  vitamin B12 deficiency (266.2)
EXCLUDES *cerebral degeneration in:*
Jakob-Creutzfeldt disease (046.11-046.19)
progressive multifocal leukoencephalopathy (046.3)
subacute spongiform encephalopathy (046.1)

√5ᵗʰ **331.8 Other cerebral degeneration**

331.81 Reye's syndrome   P
DEF: Rare childhood illness, often developed after a viral upper respiratory infection; characterized by vomiting, elevated serum transaminase, changes in liver and other viscera; brain swelling, disturbances of consciousness and seizures; can be fatal.

331.82 Dementia with Lewy bodies
Dementia with Parkinsonism
Lewy body dementia
Lewy body disease
DEF: A cerebral dementia with neurophysiologic changes, increased hippocampal volume, hypoperfusion in the occipital lobes, and beta amyloid deposits with neurofibrillarity tangles, atrophy of cortex and brainstem, hallmark neuropsychologic characteristics are fluctuating cognition with pronounced variation in attention and alertness; recurrent hallucinations; and parkinsonism.
AHA: 4Q, '03, 57
G31.83 Dementia with Lewy bodies   I-10

331.83 Mild cognitive impairment, so stated
> *EXCLUDES*   altered mental status (780.97)
> cerebral degeneration (331.0-331.9)
> change in mental status (780.97)
> cognitive deficits following (late effects of) cerebral hemorr- hage or infarction (438.0)
> cognitive impairment due to intracranial or head injury (850-854, 959.01)
> cognitive impairment due to late effect of intracranial injury (907.0)
> cognitive impairment due to skull fracture (800-801, 803-804)
> dementia (290.0-290.43, 294.8)
> mild memory disturbance (310.8)
> neurologic neglect syndrome (781.8)
> personality change, nonpsychotic (310.1)

AHA: 4Q, '06, 75

331.89 Other
Cerebral ataxia

331.9 Cerebral degeneration, unspecified

✓4ᵗʰ 332 Parkinson's disease
> *EXCLUDES*   dementia with Parkinsonism (331.82)

332.0 Paralysis agitans
Parkinsonism or Parkinson's disease:
NOS
idiopathic
primary
DEF: Form of progessive parkinsonism, characterized by masklike facial expressions, in ability to stand or walk smoothly, muscle weakness, and involuntary trembling movement.
AHA: M-A, '87, 7
G20 Parkinson's disease   I-10

332.1 Secondary Parkinsonism
Neuroleptic-induced Parkinsonism
Parkinsonism due to drugs
Use additional E code to identify drug, if drug-induced
> *EXCLUDES*   Parkinsonism (in):
> Huntington's disease (333.4)
> progressive supranuclear palsy (333.0)
> Shy-Drager syndrome (333.0)
> syphilitic (094.82)

✓4ᵗʰ 333 Other extrapyramidal disease and abnormal movement disorders
> *INCLUDES*   other forms of extrapyramidal, basal ganglia, or striatopallidal disease
> *EXCLUDES*   abnormal movements of head NOS (781.0)
> sleep related movement disorders (327.51-327.59)

333.0 Other degenerative diseases of the basal ganglia
Atrophy or degeneration:
olivopontocerebellar [Déjérine-Thomas syndrome]
pigmentary pallidal [Hallervorden-Spatz disease]
striatonigral
Parkinsonian syndrome associated with:
idiopathic orthostatic hypotension
symptomatic orthostatic hypotension
Progressive supranuclear ophthalmoplegia
Shy-Drager syndrome
AHA: 3Q, '96, 8

333.1 Essential and other specified forms of tremor
Benign essential tremor
Familial tremor
Medication-induced postural tremor
Use additional E code to identify drug, if drug-induced
> *EXCLUDES*   tremor NOS (781.0)

333.2 Myoclonus
Familial essential myoclonus
Palatal myoclonus
> *EXCLUDES*   progressive myoclonic epilepsy (345.1)
> Unverricht-Lundborg disease (345.1)

Use additional E code to identify drug, if drug-induced
DEF: Spontaneous movements or contractions of muscles.
AHA: 3Q, '97, 4; M-A, '87, 12

333.3 Tics of organic origin
Use additional E code to identify drug, if drug-induced
> *EXCLUDES*   Gilles de la Tourette's syndrome (307.23)
> habit spasm (307.22)
> tic NOS (307.20)

333.4 Huntington's chorea
DEF: Genetic disease characterized by chronic progressive mental deterioration; dementia and death within 15 years of onset.

333.5 Other choreas
Hemiballism(us)
Paroxysmal choreo-athetosis
Use additional E code to identify drug, if drug-induced
> *EXCLUDES*   Sydenham's or rheumatic chorea (392.0-392.9)

333.6 Genetic torsion dystonia
Dystonia:
deformans progressiva
musculorum deformans
(Schwalbe-) Ziehen-Oppenheim disease
DEF: Sustained muscular contractions, causing twisting and repetitive movements that result in abnormal postures of trunk and limbs; etiology unknown.

✓5ᵗʰ 333.7 Acquired torsion dystonia

333.71 Athetoid cerebral palsy
Double athetosis (syndrome)
Vogt's disease
> *EXCLUDES*   infantile cerebral palsy (343.0-343.9)
AHA: 4Q, '06, 76-78

333.72 Acute dystonia due to drugs
Acute dystonic reaction due to drugs
Neuroleptic induced acute dystonia
Use additional E code to identify drug
> *EXCLUDES*   blepharospasm due to drugs (333.85)
> orofacial dyskinesia due to drugs (333.85)
> secondary Parkinsonism (332.1)
> subacute dyskinesia due to drugs (333.85)
> tardive dyskinesia (333.85)
AHA: 4Q, '06, 76-78

333.79 Other acquired torsion dystonia
AHA: 4Q, '06, 76-78

✓6ᵗʰ 333.8 Fragments of torsion dystonia
Use additional E code to identify drug, if drug-induced

333.81 Blepharospasm
> *EXCLUDES*   blepharospasm due to drugs (333.85)
DEF: Uncontrolled winking or blinking due to orbicularis oculi muscle spasm.

333.82 Orofacial dyskinesia
> *EXCLUDES*   orofacial dyskinesia due to drugs (333.85)
DEF: Uncontrolled movement of mouth or facial muscles.

333.83 Spasmodic torticollis
> *EXCLUDES*   torticollis:
> NOS (723.5)
> hysterical (300.11)
> psychogenic (306.0)
DEF: Uncontrolled movement of head due to spasms of neck muscle.

333.84 Organic writers' cramp
> *EXCLUDES*   pychogenic (300.89)

333.85 Subacute dyskinesia due to drugs
Blepharospasm due to drugs
Orofacial dyskinesia due to drugs
Tardive dyskinesia
Use additional E code to identify drug
> *EXCLUDES*   *acute dystonia due to drugs (333.72)*
> *acute dystonic reaction due to drugs (333.72)*
> *secondary Parkinsonism (332.1)*
> **AHA:** 4Q, '06, 76-78

333.89 Other

√5ᵗʰ **333.9 Other and unspecified extrapyramidal diseases and abnormal movement disorders**

333.90 Unspecified extrapyramidal disease and abnormal movement disorder
Medication-induced movement disorders NOS
Use additional E code to identify drug, if drug-induced

333.91 Stiff-man syndrome

333.92 Neuroleptic malignant syndrome
Use additional E code to identify drug
> *EXCLUDES*   *neuroleptic induced Parkinsonism (332.1)*
> **AHA:** 4Q, '94, 37

333.93 Benign shuddering attacks
> **AHA:** 4Q, '94, 37

333.94 Restless legs syndrome [RLS]
> **DEF:** Neurological disorder of unknown etiology with an irresistible urge to move the legs, which may temporarily relieve the symptoms, is accompanied by motor restlessness and sensations of pain, burning, prickling, or tingling.
> **AHA:** 4Q, '06, 79
> **TIP:** Assign an additional code if the underlying cause of the RLS is specified (e.g., iron deficiency anemia).
> **G25.81** Restless legs syndrome   I•10

333.99 Other
Neuroleptic-induced acute akathisia
Use additional E code to identify drug, if drug-induced
> **AHA:** 4Q, '04, 95; 2Q, '04, 12; 4Q, '94, 37

√4ᵗʰ **334 Spinocerebellar disease**
> *EXCLUDES*   *olivopontocerebellar degeneration (333.0)*
> *peroneal muscular atrophy (356.1)*

334.0 Friedreich's ataxia
> **DEF:** Genetic recessive disease of children; sclerosis of dorsal, lateral spinal cord columns; characterized by ataxia, speech impairment, swaying and irregular movements, with muscle paralysis, especially of lower limbs.

334.1 Hereditary spastic paraplegia

334.2 Primary cerebellar degeneration
Cerebellar ataxia:
  Marie's
  Sanger-Brown
Dyssynergia cerebellaris myoclonica
Primary cerebellar degeneration:
  NOS
  hereditary
  sporadic
> **AHA:** M-A, '87, 9

334.3 Other cerebellar ataxia
Cerebellar ataxia NOS
Use additional E code to identify drug, if drug-induced

334.4 Cerebellar ataxia in diseases classified elsewhere
Code first underlying disease, as:
  alcoholism (303.0-303.9)
  myxedema (244.0-244.9)
  neoplastic disease (140.0-239.9)

334.8 Other spinocerebellar diseases
Ataxia-telangiectasia [Louis-Bar syndrome]
Corticostriatal-spinal degeneration

334.9 Spinocerebellar disease, unspecified

√4ᵗʰ **335 Anterior horn cell disease**

335.0 Werdnig-Hoffmann disease
Infantile spinal muscular atrophy
Progressive muscular atrophy of infancy
> **DEF:** Spinal muscle atrophy manifested in prenatal period or shortly after birth; symptoms include hypotonia, atrophy of skeletal muscle; death occurs in infancy.

√5ᵗʰ **335.1 Spinal muscular atrophy**

335.10 Spinal muscular atrophy, unspecified

335.11 Kugelberg-Welander disease
Spinal muscular atrophy:
  familial
  juvenile
> **DEF:** Hereditary; juvenile muscle atrophy; appears during first two decades of life; due to lesions of anterior horns of spinal cord; includes wasting, diminution of lower body muscles and twitching.

335.19 Other
Adult spinal muscular atrophy

√5ᵗʰ **335.2 Motor neuron disease**

335.20 Amyotrophic lateral sclerosis   A
Motor neuron disease (bulbar) (mixed type)
> **AHA:** 4Q, '95, 81

335.21 Progressive muscular atrophy
Duchenne-Aran muscular atrophy
Progressive muscular atrophy (pure)

335.22 Progressive bulbar palsy

335.23 Pseudobulbar palsy

335.24 Primary lateral sclerosis

335.29 Other

335.8 Other anterior horn cell diseases

335.9 Anterior horn cell disease, unspecified

√4ᵗʰ **336 Other diseases of spinal cord**

336.0 Syringomyelia and syringobulbia
> **AHA:** 1Q, '89, 10

336.1 Vascular myelopathies
Acute infarction of spinal cord (embolic) (nonembolic)
Arterial thrombosis of spinal cord
Edema of spinal cord
Hematomyelia
Subacute necrotic myelopathy

336.2 Subacute combined degeneration of spinal cord in diseases classified elsewhere
Code first underlying disease, as:
  pernicious anemia (281.0)
  other vitamin B12 deficiency anemia (281.1)
  vitamin B12 deficiency (266.2)

336.3 Myelopathy in other diseases classified elsewhere
Code first underlying disease, as:
  myelopathy in neoplastic disease (140.0-239.9)
> *EXCLUDES*   *myelopathy in:*
> *intervertebral disc disorder (722.70-722.73)*
> *spondylosis (721.1, 721.41-721.42, 721.91)*
> **AHA:** 3Q, '99, 5

336.8 Other myelopathy
Myelopathy:
  drug-induced
  radiation-induced
Use additonal E code to identify cause

336.9 Unspecified disease of spinal cord
Cord compression NOS
Myelopathy NOS
> *EXCLUDES*   *myelitis (323.02, 323.1, 323.2, 323.42, 323.52, 323.63, 323.72, 323.82, 323.9)*
> *spinal (canal) stenosis (723.0, 724.00-724.09)*

N   Newborn Age: 0   P   Pediatric Age: 0-17   M   Maternity Age: 12-55   A   Adult Age: 15-124

☑4ᵗʰ **337 Disorders of the autonomic nervous system**

INCLUDES disorders of peripheral autonomic, sympathetic, parasympathetic, or vegetative system

EXCLUDES familial dysautonomia [Riley-Day syndrome] (742.8)

☑5ᵗʰ **337.0 Idiopathic peripheral autonomic neuropathy**

337.00 Idiopathic peripheral autonomic neuropathy, unspecified

337.01 Carotid sinus syndrome
Carotid sinus syncope
DEF: Vagal activation caused by pressure on the carotid sinus baroreceptors; sympathetic nerve impulses may cause sinus arrest or AV block.
AHA: 4Q, '08, 101-102

337.09 Other idiopathic peripheral autonomic neuropathy
Cervical sympathetic dystrophy or paralysis

337.1 Peripheral autonomic neuropathy in disorders classified elsewhere
Code first underlying disease, as:
amyloidosis (277.30-277.39)
diabetes (249.6, 250.6)
AHA: 2Q, '09, 13; 2Q, '93, 6; 3Q, '91, 9; N-D, '84, 9

☑5ᵗʰ **337.2 Reflex sympathetic dystrophy**
DEF: Disturbance of the sympathetic nervous system evidenced by sweating, pain, pallor and edema following injury to nerves or blood vessels.
AHA: 4Q, '93, 24

337.20 Reflex sympathetic dystrophy, unspecified
Complex regional pain syndrome type I, unspecified

337.21 Reflex sympathetic dystrophy of the upper limb
Complex regional pain syndrome type I of the upper limb

337.22 Reflex sympathetic dystrophy of the lower limb
Complex regional pain syndrome type I of the lower limb

337.29 Reflex sympathetic dystrophy of other specified site
Complex regional pain syndrome type I of other specified site

337.3 Autonomic dysreflexia
Use additional code to identify the cause, such as:
fecal impaction ▶(560.32)◀
pressure ulcer (707.00-707.09)
urinary tract infection (599.0)
DEF: Noxious stimuli evokes paroxysmal hypertension, bradycardia, excess sweating, headache, pilomotor responses, facial flushing, and nasal congestion due to uncontrolled parasympathetic nerve response; occurs in patients with spinal cord injury above sympathetic outflow tract (T₆).
AHA: 4Q, '98, 37

337.9 Unspecified disorder of autonomic nervous system

Pain (338)

☑4ᵗʰ **338 Pain, not elsewhere classified**
Use additional code to identify:
pain associated with psychological factors (307.89)
EXCLUDES generalized pain (780.96)
headache syndromes (339.00-339.89)
localized pain, unspecified type — code to pain by site
migraines (346.0-346.9)
pain disorder exclusively attributed to psychological factors (307.80)
vulvar vestibulitis (625.71)
vulvodynia (625.70-625.79)
AHA: 2Q, '07, 12
TIP: Do not assign a 338 code if the pain is not specified as acute or chronic, unless post-thoracotomy, postoperative, neoplasm related or central pain syndrome.

338.0 Central pain syndrome
Déjérine-Roussy syndrome
Myelopathic pain syndrome
Thalamic pain syndrome (hyperesthetic)
AHA: 4Q, '06, 79-81

☑5ᵗʰ **338.1 Acute pain**

338.11 Acute pain due to trauma
AHA: 1Q, '07, 7; 4Q, '06, 79-81

338.12 Acute post-thoracotomy pain
Post-thoracotomy pain NOS
AHA: 4Q, '06, 79-81

338.18 Other acute postoperative pain
Postoperative pain NOS
AHA: 2Q, '07, 11; 4Q, '06, 79-81
G89.18 Other acute postprocedural pain   I-10

338.19 Other acute pain
EXCLUDES neoplasm related acute pain (338.3)
AHA: 2Q, '07, 11; 4Q, '06, 79-81

☑5ᵗʰ **338.2 Chronic pain**
EXCLUDES causalgia (355.9)
lower limb (355.71)
upper limb (354.4)
chronic pain syndrome (338.4)
myofascial pain syndrome (729.1)
neoplasm related chronic pain (338.3)
reflex sympathetic dystrophy (337.20-337.29)

338.21 Chronic pain due to trauma
AHA: 4Q, '06, 79-81

338.22 Chronic post-thoracotomy pain
AHA: 4Q, '06, 79-81

338.28 Other chronic postoperative pain
AHA: 4Q, '06, 79-81
G89.28 Other chronic postprocedural pain   I-10

338.29 Other chronic pain
AHA: 4Q, '06, 79-81

338.3 Neoplasm related pain (acute) (chronic)
Cancer associated pain
Pain due to malignancy (primary) (secondary)
Tumor associated pain
AHA: 2Q, '07, 11; 4Q, '06, 79-81
G89.3 Neoplasm related pain (acute) (chronic)   I-10

338.4 Chronic pain syndrome
Chronic pain associated with significant psychosocial dysfunction
AHA: 2Q, '07, 11; 4Q, '06, 79-81
G89.4 Chronic pain syndrome   I-10

Other Headache Syndromes (339)

☑4ᵗʰ **339 Other headache syndromes**
EXCLUDES headache:
NOS (784.0)
due to lumbar puncture (349.0)
migraine (346.0-346.9)
AHA: 4Q, '08, 102-105

☑5ᵗʰ **339.0 Cluster headaches and other trigeminal autonomic cephalgias**
TACS

339.00 Cluster headache syndrome, unspecified
Ciliary neuralgia
Cluster headache NOS
Histamine cephalgia
Lower half migraine
Migrainous neuralgia

339.01 Episodic cluster headache

339.02 Chronic cluster headache

339.03 Episodic paroxysmal hemicrania
Paroxysmal hemicrania NOS

339.04 Chronic paroxysmal hemicrania

339.05 Short lasting unilateral neuralgiform headache with conjunctival injection and tearing
SUNCT

339.09 Other trigeminal autonomic cephalgias

Diseases of the Nervous System and Sense Organs

339.1–343.9

√5ᵗʰ **339.1 Tension type headache**

> EXCLUDES   tension headache NOS (307.81)
> tension headache related to psychological factors (307.81)
>
> AHA: 4Q, '08, 103

339.10 Tension type headache, unspecified

339.11 Episodic tension type headache

339.12 Chronic tension type headache

√5ᵗʰ **339.2 Post-traumatic headache**

> TIP: Do not assign during the acute phase of the trauma (e.g., head injury). When assigning 339.2X, report also a late effect code (e.g., 907.0 for intracranial injury).

339.20 Post-traumatic headache, unspecified

> AHA: 4Q, '08, 108

339.21 Acute post-traumatic headache

339.22 Chronic post-traumatic headache

339.3 Drug induced headache, not elsewhere classified
> Medication overuse headache
> Rebound headache

√5ᵗʰ **339.4 Complicated headache syndromes**

339.41 Hemicrania continua

339.42 New daily persistent headache
> NDPH

339.43 Primary thunderclap headache

339.44 Other complicated headache syndrome

√5ᵗʰ **339.8 Other specified headache syndromes**

339.81 Hypnic headache

339.82 Headache associated with sexual activity
> Orgasmic headache
> Preorgasmic headache

339.83 Primary cough headache

339.84 Primary exertional headache

339.85 Primary stabbing headache

339.89 Other specified headache syndromes

Other Disorders of the Central Nervous System (340-349)

340 Multiple sclerosis
> Disseminated or multiple sclerosis:
> NOS
> brain stem
> cord
> generalized
>
> G35 Multiple sclerosis   I-10

√4ᵗʰ **341 Other demyelinating diseases of central nervous system**

341.0 Neuromyelitis optica

341.1 Schilder's disease
> Baló's concentric sclerosis
> Encephalitis periaxialis:
> concentrica [Baló's]
> diffusa [Schilder's]
>
> DEF: Chronic leukoencephalopathy of children and adolescents; symptoms include blindness, deafness, bilateral spasticity and progressive mental deterioration.

√5ᵗʰ **341.2 Acute (transverse) myelitis**

> EXCLUDES   acute (transverse) myelitis (in) (due to):
> following immunization procedures (323.52)
> infection classified elsewhere (323.42)
> postinfectious (323.63)
> protozoal diseases classified elsewhere (323.2)
> rickettsial diseases classified elsewhere (323.1)
> toxic (323.72)
> viral diseases classified elsewhere (323.02)
> transverse myelitis NOS (323.82)

341.20 Acute (transverse) myelitis NOS
> AHA: 4Q, '06, 58-63

341.21 Acute (transverse) myelitis in conditions classified elsewhere

> Code first underlying condition
> AHA: 4Q, '06, 58-63

341.22 Idiopathic transverse myelitis
> AHA: 4Q, '06, 58-63

341.8 Other demyelinating diseases of central nervous system
> Central demyelination of corpus callosum
> Central pontine myelinosis
> Marchiafava (-Bignami) disease
>
> AHA: N-D, '87, 6

341.9 Demyelinating disease of central nervous system, unspecified

√4ᵗʰ **342 Hemiplegia and hemiparesis**

> NOTE This category is to be used when hemiplegia (complete) (incomplete) is reported without further specification, or is stated to be old or long-standing but of unspecified cause. The category is also for use in multiple coding to identify these types of hemiplegia resulting from any cause.
>
> EXCLUDES   congenital (343.1)
> hemiplegia due to late effect of cerebrovascular accident (438.20-438.22)
> infantile NOS (343.4)

> The following fifth-digits are for use with codes 342.0-342.9:
> 0 affecting unspecified side
> 1 affecting dominant side
> 2 affecting nondominant side

> AHA: 4Q, '94, 38

§ √5ᵗʰ **342.0 Flaccid hemiplegia**
[0-2]

§ √5ᵗʰ **342.1 Spastic hemiplegia**
[0-2]

§ √5ᵗʰ **342.8 Other specified hemiplegia**
[0-2]

§ √5ᵗʰ **342.9 Hemiplegia, unspecified**
[0-2]   AHA: 3Q, '06, 5; 4Q, '98, 87
> G81.90 Hemiplegia unspecified affect unspecified side   I-10

√4ᵗʰ **343 Infantile cerebral palsy**

> INCLUDES   cerebral:
> palsy NOS
> spastic infantile paralysis
> congenital spastic paralysis (cerebral)
> Little's disease
> paralysis (spastic) due to birth injury:
> intracranial
> spinal
>
> EXCLUDES   athetoid cerebral palsy (333.71)
> hereditary cerebral paralysis, such as:
> hereditary spastic paraplegia (334.1)
> Vogt's disease (333.71)
> spastic paralysis specified as noncongenital or noninfantile (344.0-344.9)

343.0 Diplegic
> Congenital diplegia
> Congenital paraplegia
> DEF: Paralysis affecting both sides of the body simultaneously.

343.1 Hemiplegic
> Congenital hemiplegia
> EXCLUDES   infantile hemiplegia NOS (343.4)

343.2 Quadriplegic
> Tetraplegic

343.3 Monoplegic

343.4 Infantile hemiplegia
> Infantile hemiplegia (postnatal) NOS

343.8 Other specified infantile cerebral palsy

343.9 Infantile cerebral palsy, unspecified
> Cerebral palsy NOS
> AHA: 4Q, '05, 89
> G80.9 Cerebral palsy unspecified   I-10

---

§   Requires fifth digit. Valid digits are in [brackets] under each code. See category 342 for codes and definitions.

N Newborn Age: 0   P Pediatric Age: 0-17   M Maternity Age: 12-55   A Adult Age: 15-124

☑4ᵗʰ **344　Other paralytic syndromes**

NOTE This category is to be used when the listed conditions are reported without further specification or are stated to be old or long-standing but of unspecified cause. The category is also for use in multiple coding to identify these conditions resulting from any cause.

INCLUDES paralysis (complete) (incomplete), except as classifiable to 342 and 343

EXCLUDES congenital or infantile cerebral palsy (343.0-343.9)
hemiplegia (342.0-342.9)
congenital or infantile (343.1, 343.4)

☑5ᵗʰ **344.0　Quadriplegia and quadriparesis**
TIP: Assign also a code from subcategory 438.5 if late effect of CVA.

344.00　Quadriplegia unspecified
AHA: 4Q, '03, 103; 4Q, '98, 38
G82.50 Quadriplegia unspecified　　　　I-10

344.01　C$_1$-C$_4$ complete

344.02　C$_1$-C$_4$ incomplete

344.03　C$_5$-C$_7$ complete

344.04　C$_5$-C$_7$ incomplete

344.09　Other
AHA: 1Q, '01, 12; 4Q, '98, 39

344.1　Paraplegia
Paralysis of both lower limbs
Paraplegia (lower)
AHA: 4Q, '03, 110; M-A, '87, 10
G82.20 Paraplegia unspecified　　　　I-10

344.2　Diplegia of upper limbs
Diplegia (upper)
Paralysis of both upper limbs

☑5ᵗʰ **344.3　Monoplegia of lower limb**
Paralysis of lower limb
EXCLUDES monoplegia of lower limb due to late effect of cerebrovascular accident (438.40-438.42)

344.30　Affecting unspecified side

344.31　Affecting dominant side

344.32　Affecting nondominant side

☑5ᵗʰ **344.4　Monoplegia of upper limb**
Paralysis of upper limb
EXCLUDES monoplegia of upper limb due to late effect of cerebrovascular accident (438.30-438.32)

344.40　Affecting unspecified side

344.41　Affecting dominant side

344.42　Affecting nondominant side

344.5　Unspecified monoplegia

☑5ᵗʰ **344.6　Cauda equina syndrome**
DEF: Dull pain and paresthesias in sacrum, perineum and bladder due to compression of spinal nerve roots; pain radiates down buttocks, back of thigh, calf of leg and into foot with prickling, burning sensations.

344.60　Without mention of neurogenic bladder

344.61　With neurogenic bladder
Acontractile bladder
Autonomic hyperreflexia of bladder
Cord bladder
Detrusor hyperreflexia
AHA: M-J, '87, 12; M-A, '87, 10

☑5ᵗʰ **344.8　Other specified paralytic syndromes**

344.81　Locked-in state
DEF: State of consciousness where patients are paralyzed and unable to respond to environmental stimuli; patients have eye movements, and stimuli can enter the brain but patients unable to respond.
AHA: 4Q, '93, 24

344.89　Other specified paralytic syndrome
AHA: 2Q, '99, 4

344.9　Paralysis, unspecified

☑4ᵗʰ **345　Epilepsy and recurrent seizures**

The following fifth-digit subclassification is for use with categories 345.0, .1, .4-.9:
0　without mention of intractable epilepsy
1　with intractable epilepsy
pharmacoresistant (pharmacologically resistant)
poorly controlled
refractory (medically)
treatment resistant

EXCLUDES hippocampal sclerosis (348.81)
mesial temporal sclerosis (348.81)
temporal sclerosis (348.81)

DEF: Brain disorder characterized by electrical-like disturbances; may include occasional impairment or loss of consciousness, abnormal motor phenomena and psychic or sensory disturbances.
AHA: ▶4Q, '09, 82;◀ 1Q, '93, 24; 2Q, '92, 8; 4Q, '92, 23

§ ☑5ᵗʰ **345.0　Generalized nonconvulsive epilepsy**
[0-1]　Absences:　　Pykno-epilepsy
atonic　　　Seizures:
typical　　akinetic
Minor epilepsy　atonic
Petit mal
AHA: For code 345.00: 1Q, '04, 18

§ ☑5ᵗʰ **345.1　Generalized convulsive epilepsy**
[0-1]　Epileptic seizures:　Grand mal
clonic　　　Major epilepsy
myoclonic　　Progressive myoclonic epilepsy
tonic　　　Unverricht-Lundborg disease
tonic-clonic
EXCLUDES convulsions:
NOS (780.39)
infantile (780.39)
newborn (779.0)
infantile spasms (345.6)
DEF: Convulsive seizures with tension of limbs (tonic) or rhythmic contractions (clonic).
AHA: 3Q, '97, 4

345.2　Petit mal status
Epileptic absence status
DEF: Minor myoclonic spasms and sudden momentary loss of consciousness in epilepsy.

345.3　Grand mal status
Status epilepticus NOS
EXCLUDES epilepsia partialis continua (345.7)
status:
psychomotor (345.7)
temporal lobe (345.7)
DEF: Sudden loss of consciousness followed by generalized convulsions in epilepsy.
AHA: 3Q, '05, 12
G40.301 Gen idiopath epilep&epi syn not intractabl w/se　　　　I-10

§ ☑5ᵗʰ **345.4　Localization-related (focal) (partial) epilepsy and**
[0-1]　**epileptic syndromes with complex partial seizures**
Epilepsy:
limbic system
partial:
secondarily generalized
with impairment of consciousness
with memory and ideational disturbances
psychomotor
psychosensory
temporal lobe
Epileptic automatism
AHA: For code 345.41 ▶4Q, '09, 83◀

§ ☑5ᵗʰ **345.5　Localization-related (focal) (partial) epilepsy and**
[0-1]　**epileptic syndromes with simple partial seizures**
Epilepsy:　　　　Epilepsy:
Bravais-Jacksonian NOS　somatomotor
focal (motor) NOS　　somatosensory
Jacksonian NOS　　visceral
motor partial　　visual
partial NOS:
without impairment of consciousness
sensory-induced

---

§　Requires fifth digit. Valid digits are in [brackets] under each code. See category 345 for codes and definitions.

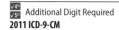

☑4ᵗʰ
☑5ᵗʰ　Additional Digit Required　　Unspecified Code　　Other Specified Code　　Manifestation Code　　▶◀ Revised Text　　● New Code　　▲ Revised Code Title

§ ✓5th **345.6 Infantile spasms**
[0-1]   Hypsarrhythmia   Lightning spasms
Salaam attacks
EXCLUDES *salaam tic (781.0)*
AHA: N-D, '84, 12

§ ✓5th **345.7 Epilepsia partialis continua**
[0-1]   Kojevnikov's epilepsy
DEF: Continuous muscle contractions and relaxation; result of abnormal neural discharge.

§ ✓5th **345.8 Other forms of epilepsy and recurrent seizures**
[0-1]   Epilepsy:
cursive [running]
gelastic

§ ✓5th **345.9 Epilepsy, unspecified**
[0-1]   Epileptic convulsions, fits, or seizures NOS
Recurrent seizures NOS
Seizure disorder NOS
EXCLUDES *convulsion (convulsive) disorder (780.39)*
convulsive seizure or fit NOS (780.39)
recurrent convulsions (780.39)
AHA: 1Q, '08, 17; N-D, '87, 12; For code 345.90: 2Q, '09, 10
G40.909 Epilepsy uns not intractbl w/o status epilepticus   I-10

✓4th **346 Migraine**
EXCLUDES *headache:*
NOS (784.0)
syndromes (339.00-339.89)
AHA: 4Q, '08, 103, 105-107

The following fifth-digit subclassification is for use with category 346:
0 **without mention of intractable migraine without mention of status migrainosus**
1 **with intractable migraine, so stated without mention of status migrainosus**
2 **without mention of intractable migraine with status migrainosus**
3 **with intractable migraine, so stated, with status migrainosus**

DEF: Benign vascular headache of extreme pain; commonly associated with irritability, nausea, vomiting and often photophobia; premonitory visual hallucination of a crescent in the visual field (scotoma).

§ ✓5th **346.0 Migraine with aura**
[0-3]   Basilar migraine
Classic migraine
Migraine preceded or accompanied by transient focal neurological phenomena
Migraine triggered seizures
Migraine with acute-onset aura
Migraine with aura without headache (migraine equivalents)
Migraine with prolonged aura
Migraine with typical aura
Retinal migraine
EXCLUDES *persistent migraine aura (346.5, 346.6)*

§ ✓5th **346.1 Migraine without aura**
[0-3]   Common migraine

§ ✓5th **346.2 Variants of migraine, not elsewhere classified**
[0-3]   Abdominal migraine
Cyclical vomiting associated with migraine
Ophthalmoplegic migraine
Periodic headache syndromes in child or adolescent
EXCLUDES *cyclical vomiting NOS (536.2)*
psychogenic cyclical vomiting (306.4)

§ ✓5th **346.3 Hemiplegic migraine**
[0-3]   Familial migraine   Sporadic migraine

§ ✓5th **346.4 Menstrual migraine**   ♀
[0-3]   Menstrual headache   Premenstrual migraine
Menstrually related migraine Pure menstrual migraine
Premenstrual headache

§ ✓5th **346.5 Persistent migraine aura without cerebral infarction**
[0-3]   Persistent migraine aura NOS

§ ✓5th **346.6 Persistent migraine aura with cerebral infarction**
[0-3]   AHA: For code 346.60: 4Q, '08, 108
TIP: Assign also a code for the specific type of cerebral infarction.

§ ✓5th **346.7 Chronic migraine without aura**
[0-3]   Transformed migraine without aura

§ ✓5th **346.8 Other forms of migraine**
[0-3]

§ ✓5th **346.9 Migraine, unspecified**
[0-3]   AHA: N-D, '85, 16
G43.90 Migraine unspecified not intractable   I-10

✓4th **347 Cataplexy and narcolepsy**
DEF: Cataplexy: Sudden onset of muscle weakness with loss of tone and strength; caused by aggressive or passionate emotions.
DEF: Narcolepsy: Brief, recurrent, uncontrollable episodes of sound sleep.

✓5th **347.0 Narcolepsy**

347.00 Without cataplexy
Narcolepsy NOS

347.01 With cataplexy

✓5th **347.1 Narcolepsy in conditions classified elsewhere**
Code first underlying condition

347.10 Without cataplexy

347.11 With cataplexy

✓4th **348 Other conditions of brain**

348.0 Cerebral cysts
Arachnoid cyst   Porencephaly, acquired
Porencephalic cyst   Pseudoporencephaly
EXCLUDES *porencephaly (congenital) (742.4)*

348.1 Anoxic brain damage
Use additional E code to identify cause
EXCLUDES *that occurring in:*
abortion (634-638 with .7, 639.8)
ectopic or molar pregnancy (639.8)
labor or delivery (668.2, 669.4)
that of newborn (767.0, 768.0-768.9, 772.1-772.2)
DEF: Brain injury due to lack of oxygen, other than birth trauma.
G93.1 Anoxic brain damage not elsewhere classified   I-10

348.2 Benign intracranial hypertension
Pseudotumor cerebri
EXCLUDES *hypertensive encephalopathy (437.2)*
DEF: Elevated pressure in brain due to fluid retention in brain cavities.

✓5th **348.3 Encephalopathy, not elsewhere classified**
AHA: 4Q, '03, 58; 3Q, '97, 4

348.30 Encephalopathy, unspecified
G93.40 Encephalopathy unspecified   I-10

348.31 Metabolic encephalopathy
Septic encephalopathy
EXCLUDES *toxic metabolic encephalopathy (349.82)*
TIP: Physician documentation may include "acute confusional state," usually denoting delirium secondary to the encephalopathy.

348.39 Other encephalopathy
EXCLUDES *encephalopathy:*
alcoholic (291.2)
hepatic (572.2)
hypertensive (437.2)
toxic (349.82)

348.4 Compression of brain
Compression
Herniation } brain (stem)
Posterior fossa compression syndrome
DEF: Elevated pressure in brain due to blood clot, tumor, fracture, abscess, other condition.
AHA: 4Q, '94, 37
TIP: Assign for Arnold-Chiari syndrome, Type I. For Type II, III, or IV, refer to categories 741 and 742.

348.5 Cerebral edema
DEF: Elevated pressure in the brain due to fluid retention in brain tissues.
AHA: ▶1Q, '10, 8;◄ 3Q, '09, 8
G93.6 Cerebral edema   I-10

---

§ Requires fifth digit. Valid digits are in [brackets] under each code. See appropriate category for codes and definitions.

√5th **348.8 Other conditions of brain**
AHA: S-O, '87, 9

348.81 Temporal sclerosis
Hippocampal sclerosis
Mesial temporal sclerosis
DEF: ▶Abnormal hardening or scarring of frontal lobe tissues due to injury, tumor, congenital anomaly, or hypoxia, resulting in loss of functional neurons; commonly associated with temporal lobe epilepsy.◀
AHA: ▶4Q, '09, 83◀

348.89 Other conditions of brain
Cerebral: Cerebral:
    calcification   fungus

348.9 Unspecified condition of brain

√4th **349 Other and unspecified disorders of the nervous system**
AHA: 4Q, '08, 109

349.0 Reaction to spinal or lumbar puncture
Headache following lumbar puncture
AHA: 2Q, '99, 9; 3Q, '90, 18
G97.1 Other reaction to spinal and lumbar puncture   I-10

349.1 Nervous system complications from surgically implanted device
EXCLUDES immediate postoperative complications (997.00-997.09)
mechanical complications of nervous system device (996.2)

349.2 Disorders of meninges, not elsewhere classified
Adhesions, meningeal (cerebral) (spinal)
Cyst, spinal meninges
Meningocele, acquired
Pseudomeningocele, acquired
AHA: 1Q, '06, 15; 2Q, '98, 18; 3Q, '94, 4

√5th **349.3 Dural tear**

349.31 Accidental puncture or laceration of dura during a procedure
Incidental (inadvertent) durotomy
AHA: 4Q, '08, 109-110
TIP: Do not assign code 998.2 Accidental puncture or laceration during a procedure, for an incidental dural tear.

349.39 Other dural tear

√5th **349.8 Other specified disorders of nervous system**

349.81 Cerebrospinal fluid rhinorrhea
EXCLUDES cerebrospinal fluid otorrhea (388.61)
DEF: Cerebrospinal fluid discharging from the nose; caused by fracture of frontal bone with tearing of dura mater and arachnoid.

349.82 Toxic encephalopathy
Toxic metabolic encephalopathy
Use additional E code to identify cause
DEF: Brain tissue degeneration due to toxic substance.
AHA: 4Q, '93, 29
G92 Toxic encephalopathy   I-10

349.89 Other

349.9 Unspecified disorders of nervous system
Disorder of nervous system (central) NOS

Cranial Nerves

Olfactory bulb (I)
Optic nerve (II)
Oculomotor nerve (III)
Trochlear nerve (IV)
Trigeminal nerve (V)
Abducens nerve (VI)
Pons
Facial nerve (VII)
Vestibulocochlear nerve (VIII)
Glossopharyngeal nerve (IX)
Vagus nerve (X)
Accessory nerve (XI)
Hypoglossal nerve (XII)

Trigeminal and Facial Nerve Branches

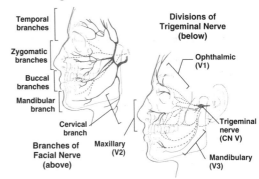

Temporal branches
Zygomatic branches
Buccal branches
Mandibular branch
Cervical branch
Branches of Facial Nerve (above)
Maxillary (V2)
Divisions of Trigeminal Nerve (below)
Ophthalmic (V1)
Trigeminal nerve (CN V)
Mandibulary (V3)

Disorders of the Peripheral Nervous System (350-359)

EXCLUDES diseases of:
acoustic [8th] nerve (388.5)
oculomotor [3rd, 4th, 6th] nerves (378.0-378.9)
optic [2nd] nerve (377.0-377.9)
peripheral autonomic nerves (337.0-337.9)
neuralgia
neuritis   } NOS or "rheumatic" (729.2)
radiculitis
peripheral neuritis in pregnancy (646.4)

√4th **350 Trigeminal nerve disorders**
INCLUDES disorders of 5th cranial nerve

350.1 Trigeminal neuralgia
Tic douloureux   Trigeminal neuralgia NOS
Trifacial neuralgia
EXCLUDES postherpetic (053.12)
G50.0 Trigeminal neuralgia   I-10

350.2 Atypical face pain

350.8 Other specified trigeminal nerve disorders

350.9 Trigeminal nerve disorder, unspecified

√4th **351 Facial nerve disorders**
INCLUDES disorders of 7th cranial nerve
EXCLUDES that in newborn (767.5)

351.0 Bell's palsy
Facial palsy
DEF: Unilateral paralysis of face due to lesion on facial nerve; produces facial distortion.
G51.0 Bell's palsy   I-10

351.1 Geniculate ganglionitis
Geniculate ganglionitis NOS
EXCLUDES herpetic (053.11)
DEF: Inflammation of tissue at bend in facial nerve.

351.8 Other facial nerve disorders
Facial myokymia
Melkersson's syndrome
AHA: 3Q, '02, 13

351.9 Facial nerve disorder, unspecified

√4th **352 Disorders of other cranial nerves**

352.0 Disorders of olfactory [lst] nerve

352.1 Glossopharyngeal neuralgia
DEF: Pain between throat and ear along petrosal and jugular ganglia.
AHA: 2Q, '02, 8

352.2 Other disorders of glossopharyngeal [9th] nerve

352.3 Disorders of pneumogastric [10th] nerve
Disorders of vagal nerve
EXCLUDES paralysis of vocal cords or larynx (478.30-478.34)
DEF: Nerve disorder affecting ear, tongue, pharynx, larynx, esophagus, viscera and thorax.

352.4 Disorders of accessory [11th] nerve
DEF: Nerve disorder affecting palate, pharynx, larynx, thoracic viscera, sternocleidomastoid and trapezius muscles.

352.5 Disorders of hypoglossal [12th] nerve
DEF: Nerve disorder affecting tongue muscles.

√4th √5th Additional Digit Required   Unspecified Code   Other Specified Code   Manifestation Code   ▶◀ Revised Text   ● New Code   ▲ Revised Code Title

352.6 Multiple cranial nerve palsies
Collet-Sicard syndrome
Polyneuritis cranialis

352.9 Unspecified disorder of cranial nerves

✓4ᵗʰ **353 Nerve root and plexus disorders**
EXCLUDES conditions due to:
    intervertebral disc disorders (722.0-722.9)
    spondylosis (720.0-721.9)
    vertebrogenic disorders (723.0-724.9)

353.0 Brachial plexus lesions
Cervical rib syndrome
Costoclavicular syndrome
Scalenus anticus syndrome
Thoracic outlet syndrome
EXCLUDES *brachial neuritis or radiculitis NOS (723.4)*
    that in newborn (767.6)
DEF: Acquired disorder in tissue along nerves in shoulder; causes corresponding motor and sensory dysfunction.
AHA: 3Q, '06, 12

353.1 Lumbosacral plexus lesions
DEF: Acquired disorder in tissue along nerves in lower back; causes corresponding motor and sensory dysfunction.

353.2 Cervical root lesions, not elsewhere classified

353.3 Thoracic root lesions, not elsewhere classified

353.4 Lumbosacral root lesions, not elsewhere classified

Peripheral Nervous System

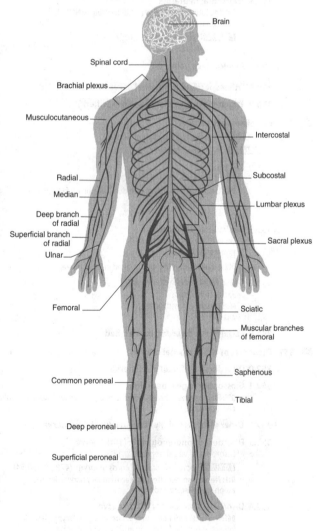

Brain
Spinal cord
Brachial plexus
Musculocutaneous
Intercostal
Radial
Subcostal
Median
Lumbar plexus
Deep branch of radial
Superficial branch of radial
Sacral plexus
Ulnar
Femoral
Sciatic
Muscular branches of femoral
Saphenous
Common peroneal
Tibial
Deep peroneal
Superficial peroneal

353.5 Neuralgic amyotrophy
Parsonage-Aldren-Turner syndrome
Code first any associated underlying disease, such as:
    diabetes mellitus (249.6, 250.6)

353.6 Phantom limb (syndrome)
DEF: Abnormal tingling or a burning sensation, transient aches, and intermittent or continuous pain perceived as originating in the absent limb.

353.8 Other nerve root and plexus disorders

353.9 Unspecified nerve root and plexus disorder

✓4ᵗʰ **354 Mononeuritis of upper limb and mononeuritis multiplex**
DEF: Inflammation of a single nerve; known as mononeuritis multiplex when several nerves in unrelated body areas are affected.

354.0 Carpal tunnel syndrome
Median nerve entrapment
Partial thenar atrophy
DEF: Compression of median nerve by tendons; causes pain, tingling, numbness and burning sensation in hand.
G56.00 Carpal tunnel syndrome unspecified side   `I-10`

354.1 Other lesion of median nerve
Median nerve neuritis

354.2 Lesion of ulnar nerve
Cubital tunnel syndrome
Tardy ulnar nerve palsy

354.3 Lesion of radial nerve
Acute radial nerve palsy
AHA: N-D, '87, 6

354.4 Causalgia of upper limb
Complex regional pain syndrome type II of the upper limb
EXCLUDES *causalgia:*
    NOS (355.9)
    lower limb (355.71)
    complex regional pain syndrome type II of the lower limb (355.71)
DEF: Peripheral nerve damage, upper limb; usually due to injury; causes burning sensation and trophic skin changes.

354.5 Mononeuritis multiplex
Combinations of single conditions classifiable to 354 or 355

354.8 Other mononeuritis of upper limb

354.9 Mononeuritis of upper limb, unspecified

✓4ᵗʰ **355 Mononeuritis of lower limb**
355.0 Lesion of sciatic nerve
EXCLUDES *sciatica NOS (724.3)*
DEF: Acquired disorder of sciatic nerve; causes motor and sensory dysfunction in back, buttock and leg.
AHA: 2Q, '89, 12

355.1 Meralgia paresthetica
Lateral cutaneous femoral nerve of thigh compression or syndrome
DEF: Inguinal ligament entraps lateral femoral cutaneous nerve; causes tingling, pain and numbness along outer thigh.

355.2 Other lesion of femoral nerve

355.3 Lesion of lateral popliteal nerve
Lesion of common peroneal nerve

355.4 Lesion of medial popliteal nerve

355.5 Tarsal tunnel syndrome
DEF: Compressed, entrapped posterior tibial nerve; causes tingling, pain and numbness in sole of foot.

355.6 Lesion of plantar nerve
Morton's metatarsalgia, neuralgia, or neuroma

✓5ᵗʰ **355.7 Other mononeuritis of lower limb**
355.71 Causalgia of lower limb
EXCLUDES *causalgia:*
    NOS (355.9)
    upper limb (354.4)
    complex regional pain syndrome type II of upper limb (354.4)
DEF: Dysfunction of lower limb peripheral nerve, usually due to injury; causes burning pain and trophic skin changes.

Ⓝ Newborn Age: 0   Ⓟ Pediatric Age: 0-17   Ⓜ Maternity Age: 12-55   Ⓐ Adult Age: 15-124

355.79 Other mononeuritis of lower limb

355.8 Mononeuritis of lower limb, unspecified

355.9 Mononeuritis of unspecified site
Causalgia NOS
Complex regional pain syndrome NOS

> **EXCLUDES** causalgia:
> lower limb (355.71)
> upper limb (354.4)
> complex regional pain syndrome:
> lower limb (355.71)
> upper limb (354.4)
>
> G58.9 Mononeuropathy unspecified   [I-10]

356 Hereditary and idiopathic peripheral neuropathy

356.0 Hereditary peripheral neuropathy
Déjérine-Sottas disease

356.1 Peroneal muscular atrophy
Charcôt-Marie-Tooth disease
Neuropathic muscular atrophy
DEF: Genetic disorder, in muscles innervated by peroneal nerves; symptoms include muscle wasting in lower limbs and locomotor difficulties.

356.2 Hereditary sensory neuropathy
DEF: Inherited disorder in dorsal root ganglia, optic nerve, and cerebellum, causing sensory losses, shooting pains, and foot ulcers.

356.3 Refsum's disease
Heredopathia atactica polyneuritiformis
DEF: Genetic disorder of lipid metabolism; causes persistent, painful inflammation of nerves and retinitis pigmentosa.

356.4 Idiopathic progressive polyneuropathy

356.8 Other specified idiopathic peripheral neuropathy
Supranuclear paralysis

356.9 Unspecified
G60.9 Hereditary & idiopathic neuropathy unspecified   [I-10]

357 Inflammatory and toxic neuropathy

357.0 Acute infective polyneuritis
Guillain-Barré syndrome   Postinfectious polyneuritis
DEF: Guillain-Barré syndrome: acute demyelinating polyneuropathy preceded by viral illness (i.e., herpes, cytomegalovirus [CMV], Epstein-Barr virus [EBV]) or a bacterial illness; areflexic motor paralysis with mild sensory disturbance and acellular rise in spinal fluid protein.
AHA: 2Q, '98, 12

357.1 Polyneuropathy in collagen vascular disease
Code first underlying disease, as:
disseminated lupus erythematosus (710.0)
polyarteritis nodosa (446.0)
rheumatoid arthritis (714.0)

357.2 Polyneuropathy in diabetes
Code first underlying disease (249.6, 250.6)
AHA: ▶4Q, '09, 151;◀ 2Q, '09, 13, 15; 3Q, '08, 5; 4Q, '03, 105; 2Q, '92, 15; 3Q, '91, 9

357.3 Polyneuropathy in malignant disease
Code first underlying disease (140.0-208.9)

357.4 Polyneuropathy in other diseases classified elsewhere
Code first underlying disease, as:
amyloidosis (277.30-277.39)
beriberi (265.0)
chronic uremia (585.9)
deficiency of B vitamins (266.0-266.9)
diphtheria (032.0-032.9)
hypoglycemia (251.2)
pellagra (265.2)
porphyria (277.1)
sarcoidosis (135)
uremia NOS (586)

> **EXCLUDES** polyneuropathy in:
> herpes zoster (053.13)
> mumps (072.72)
>
> **AHA:** 2Q, '08, 8; 2Q, '98, 15
> G63 Polyneuropathy in dz classified elsewhere   [I-10]

357.5 Alcoholic polyneuropathy

357.6 Polyneuropathy due to drugs
Use additional E code to identify drug

357.7 Polyneuropathy due to other toxic agents
Use additional E code to identify toxic agent

357.8 Other
AHA: 4Q, '02, 47; 2Q, '98, 12

357.81 Chronic inflammatory demyelinating polyneuritis
DEF: Inflammation of peripheral nerves resulting in destruction of myelin sheath; associated with diabetes mellitus, dysproteinemias, renal failure and malnutrition; symptoms include tingling, numbness, burning pain, diminished tendon reflexes, weakness of lower extremities.

357.82 Critical illness polyneuropathy
Acute motor neuropathy
DEF: An acute axonal neuropathy, both sensory and motor, that is associated with Systemic Inflammatory Response Syndrome (SIRS).
AHA: 4Q, '03, 111

357.89 Other inflammatory and toxic neuropathy

357.9 Unspecified

358 Myoneural disorders

358.0 Myasthenia gravis
DEF: Autoimmune disorder of acetylcholine at neuromuscular junction; causing fatigue of voluntary muscles.
AHA: 4Q, '03, 59

358.00 Myasthenia gravis without (acute) exacerbation
Myasthenia gravis NOS
G70.00 Myasthenia gravis w/o (acute) exacerbation   [I-10]

358.01 Myasthenia gravis with (acute) exacerbation
Myasthenia gravis in crisis
AHA: 4Q, '07, 109; 1Q, '05, 4; 4Q, '04, 139

358.1 Myasthenic syndromes in diseases classified elsewhere
Eaton-Lambert syndrome from stated cause classified elsewhere
Code first underlying disease, as:
botulism (005.1, 040.41-040.42)
hypothyroidism (244.0-244.9)
malignant neoplasm (140.0-208.9)
pernicious anemia (281.0)
thyrotoxicosis (242.0-242.9)

358.2 Toxic myoneural disorders
Use additional E code to identify toxic agent

358.8 Other specified myoneural disorders

358.9 Myoneural disorders, unspecified
AHA: 2Q, '02, 16

359 Muscular dystrophies and other myopathies
> **EXCLUDES** idiopathic polymyositis (710.4)

359.0 Congenital hereditary muscular dystrophy
Benign congenital myopathy   Myotubular myopathy
Central core disease   Nemaline body disease
Centronuclear myopathy

> **EXCLUDES** arthrogryposis multiplex congenita (754.89)
>
> **DEF:** Genetic disorder; causing progressive or nonprogressive muscle weakness.

359.1 Hereditary progressive muscular dystrophy
Muscular dystrophy: Muscular dystrophy:
NOS   Gower's
distal   Landouzy-Déjérine
Duchenne   limb-girdle
Erb's   ocular
fascioscapulohumeral   oculopharyngeal
DEF: Genetic degenerative, muscle disease; causes progressive weakness, wasting of muscle with no nerve involvement.

√5ᵗʰ **359.2 Myotonic disorders**

> **EXCLUDES** *periodic paralysis (359.3)*
> **DEF:** Impaired movement due to spasmatic, rigid muscles.
> **AHA:** 4Q, '07, 75

359.21 Myotonic muscular dystrophy
> Dystrophia myotonica
> Myotonia atrophica
> Myotonic dystrophy
> Proximal myotonic myopathy [PROMM]
> Steinert's disease

359.22 Myotonia congenita
> Acetazolamide responsive myotonia congenita
> Dominant form [Thomsen's disease]
> Myotonia levior
> Recessive form [Becker's disease]

359.23 Myotonic chondrodystrophy
> Congenital myotonic chondrodystrophy
> Schwartz-Jampel disease

359.24 Drug induced myotonia
> Use additional E code to identify drug

359.29 Other specified myotonic disorder
> Myotonia fluctuans
> Myotonia permanens
> Paramyotonia congenita (of von Eulenburg)

359.3 Periodic paralysis
> Familial periodic paralysis
> Hypokalemic familial periodic paralysis
> Hyperkalemic periodic paralysis
> Hypokalemic periodic paralysis
> Potassium sensitive periodic paralysis
> **EXCLUDES** *paramyotonia congenita (of von Eulenburg) (359.29)*
> **DEF:** Genetic disorder; characterized by rapidly progressive flaccid paralysis; attacks often occur after exercise or exposure to cold or dietary changes.

359.4 Toxic myopathy
> Use additional E code to identify toxic agent
> **DEF:** Muscle disorder caused by toxic agent.
> **AHA:** 1Q, '88, 5

359.5 Myopathy in endocrine diseases classified elsewhere
> *Code first underlying disease, as:*
>   Addison's disease (255.41)
>   Cushing's syndrome (255.0)
>   hypopituitarism (253.2)
>   myxedema (244.0-244.9)
>   thyrotoxicosis (242.0-242.9)
> **DEF:** Muscle disorder secondary to dysfunction in hormone secretion.

359.6 Symptomatic inflammatory myopathy in diseases classified elsewhere
> *Code first underlying disease, as:*
>   amyloidosis (277.30-277.39)
>   disseminated lupus erythematosus (710.0)
>   malignant neoplasm (140.0-208.9)
>   polyarteritis nodosa (446.0)
>   rheumatoid arthritis (714.0)
>   sarcoidosis (135)
>   scleroderma (710.1)
>   Sjögren's disease (710.2)

√5ᵗʰ **359.7 Inflammatory and immune myopathies, NEC**

359.71 Inclusion body myositis
> IBM
> **DEF:** ▶Progressive, debilitating inflammatory muscle disease characterized by dysphagia, chronic muscle swelling, weakness, and atrophy (wasting); impairs fine motor functions.◀
> **AHA:** ▶4Q, '09, 84◀

359.79 Other inflammatory and immune myopathies, NEC
> Inflammatory myopathy NOS

√5ᵗʰ **359.8 Other myopathies**
> **AHA:** 4Q, '02, 47; 3Q, '90, 17

359.81 Critical illness myopathy
> Acute necrotizing myopathy
> Acute quadriplegic myopathy
> Intensive care (ICU) myopathy
> Myopathy of critical illness

359.89 Other myopathies

359.9 Myopathy, unspecified

Disorders of the Eye and Adnexa (360-379)

> Use additional external cause code, if applicable, to identify the cause of the eye condition

√4ᵗʰ **360 Disorders of the globe**
> **INCLUDES** disorders affecting multiple structures of eye

√5ᵗʰ **360.0 Purulent endophthalmitis**
> **EXCLUDES** *bleb associated endophthalmitis (379.63)*

360.00 Purulent endophthalmitis, unspecified

360.01 Acute endophthalmitis

360.02 Panophthalmitis

360.03 Chronic endophthalmitis

360.04 Vitreous abscess

√5ᵗʰ **360.1 Other endophthalmitis**
> **EXCLUDES** *bleb associated endophthalmitis (379.63)*

360.11 Sympathetic uveitis
> **DEF:** Inflammation of vascular layer of uninjured eye; follows injury to other eye.

360.12 Panuveitis
> **DEF:** Inflammation of entire vascular layer of eye, including choroid, iris and ciliary body.

360.13 Parasitic endophthalmitis NOS
> **DEF:** Parasitic infection causing inflammation of the entire eye.

360.14 Ophthalmia nodosa
> **DEF:** Conjunctival inflammation caused by embedded hairs.

360.19 Other
> Phacoanaphylactic endophthalmitis

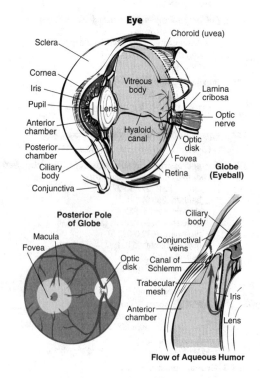

Eye

Globe (Eyeball)

Posterior Pole of Globe

Flow of Aqueous Humor

Adnexa

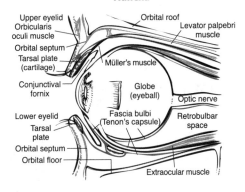

Upper eyelid
Orbicularis oculi muscle
Orbital septum
Tarsal plate (cartilage)
Conjunctival fornix
Lower eyelid
Tarsal plate
Orbital septum
Orbital floor
Orbital roof
Levator palpebri muscle
Müller's muscle
Globe (eyeball)
Fascia bulbi (Tenon's capsule)
Optic nerve
Retrobulbar space
Extraocular muscle

✓5th **360.2 Degenerative disorders of globe**
AHA: 3Q, '91, 3

360.20 Degenerative disorder of globe, unspecified

360.21 Progressive high (degenerative) myopia
Malignant myopia
DEF: Severe, progressive nearsightedness in adults, complicated by serious disease of the choroid; leads to retinal detachment and blindness.

360.23 Siderosis
DEF: Iron pigment deposits within tissue of eyeball; caused by high iron content of blood.

360.24 Other metallosis
Chalcosis
DEF: Metal deposits, other than iron, within eyeball tissues.

360.29 Other
EXCLUDES xerophthalmia (264.7)

✓5th **360.3 Hypotony of eye**

360.30 Hypotony, unspecified
DEF: Low osmotic pressure causing lack of tone, tension and strength.

360.31 Primary hypotony

360.32 Ocular fistula causing hypotony
DEF: Low intraocular pressure due to leak through abnormal passage.

360.33 Hypotony associated with other ocular disorders

360.34 Flat anterior chamber
DEF: Low pressure behind cornea, causing compression.

✓5th **360.4 Degenerated conditions of globe**

360.40 Degenerated globe or eye, unspecified

360.41 Blind hypotensive eye
Atrophy of globe
Phthisis bulbi
DEF: Vision loss due to extremely low intraocular pressure.

360.42 Blind hypertensive eye
Absolute glaucoma
DEF: Vision loss due to painful, high intraocular pressure.

360.43 Hemophthalmos, except current injury
EXCLUDES traumatic (871.0-871.9, 921.0-921.9)
DEF: Pool of blood within eyeball, not from current injury.

360.44 Leucocoria
DEF: Whitish mass or reflex in the pupil behind lens; also called cat's eye reflex; often indicative of retinoblastoma.

✓5th **360.5 Retained (old) intraocular foreign body, magnetic**
►Use additional code to identify foreign body (V90.11)◄
EXCLUDES current penetrating injury with magnetic foreign body (871.5)
retained (old) foreign body of orbit (376.6)

360.50 Foreign body, magnetic, intraocular, unspecified

360.51 Foreign body, magnetic, in anterior chamber

360.52 Foreign body, magnetic, in iris or ciliary body

360.53 Foreign body, magnetic, in lens

360.54 Foreign body, magnetic, in vitreous

360.55 Foreign body, magnetic, in posterior wall

360.59 Foreign body, magnetic, in other or multiple sites

✓5th **360.6 Retained (old) intraocular foreign body, nonmagnetic**
Retained (old) foreign body:
NOS
nonmagnetic
►Use additional code to identify foreign body (V90.01-V90.10, V90.12, V90.2-V90.9)◄
EXCLUDES current penetrating injury with (nonmagnetic) foreign body (871.6)
retained (old) foreign body in orbit (376.6)

360.60 Foreign body, intraocular, unspecified

360.61 Foreign body in anterior chamber

360.62 Foreign body in iris or ciliary body

360.63 Foreign body in lens

360.64 Foreign body in vitreous

360.65 Foreign body in posterior wall

360.69 Foreign body in other or multiple sites

✓5th **360.8 Other disorders of globe**

360.81 Luxation of globe
DEF: Displacement of eyeball.

360.89 Other

360.9 Unspecified disorder of globe

✓4th **361 Retinal detachments and defects**
DEF: Disorders of light-sensitive layer at back of eye, which separates from blood supply, disrupting vision.

✓5th **361.0 Retinal detachment with retinal defect**
Rhegmatogenous retinal detachment
EXCLUDES detachment of retinal pigment epithelium (362.42-362.43)
retinal detachment (serous) (without defect) (361.2)

361.00 Retinal detachment with retinal defect, unspecified

361.01 Recent detachment, partial, with single defect

361.02 Recent detachment, partial, with multiple defects

361.03 Recent detachment, partial, with giant tear

361.04 Recent detachment, partial, with retinal dialysis
Dialysis (juvenile) of retina (with detachment)

361.05 Recent detachment, total or subtotal

361.06 Old detachment, partial
Delimited old retinal detachment

361.07 Old detachment, total or subtotal

✓5th **361.1 Retinoschisis and retinal cysts**
EXCLUDES juvenile retinoschisis (362.73)
microcystoid degeneration of retina (362.62)
parasitic cyst of retina (360.13)

361.10 Retinoschisis, unspecified
DEF: Separation of retina due to degenerative process of aging; should not be confused with acute retinal detachment.

361.11 Flat retinoschisis
DEF: Slow, progressive split of retinal sensory layers.

361.12 Bullous retinoschisis
DEF: Fluid retention between split retinal sensory layers.

361.13 Primary retinal cysts

361.14 Secondary retinal cysts

361.19 Other
Pseudocyst of retina

361.2 Serous retinal detachment
Retinal detachment without retinal defect
> **EXCLUDES** *central serous retinopathy (362.41)*
> *retinal pigment epithelium detachment*
> *(362.42-362.43)*

√5ᵗʰ **361.3 Retinal defects without detachment**
> **EXCLUDES** *chorioretinal scars after surgery for detachment*
> *(363.30-363.35)*
> *peripheral retinal degeneration without defect*
> *(362.60-362.66)*

361.30 Retinal defect, unspecified
Retinal break(s) NOS

361.31 Round hole of retina without detachment

361.32 Horseshoe tear of retina without detachment
Operculum of retina without mention of detachment

361.33 Multiple defects of retina without detachment

√5ᵗʰ **361.8 Other forms of retinal detachment**

361.81 Traction detachment of retina
Traction detachment with vitreoretinal organization

361.89 Other
AHA: 3Q, '99, 12

361.9 Unspecified retinal detachment
AHA: N-D, '87, 10

√4ᵗʰ **362 Other retinal disorders**
> **EXCLUDES** *chorioretinal scars (363.30-363.35)*
> *chorioretinitis (363.0-363.2)*

√5ᵗʰ **362.0 Diabetic retinopathy**
Code first diabetes (249.5, 250.5)
DEF: Retinal changes in diabetes of long duration; causes hemorrhages, microaneurysms, waxy deposits and proliferative noninflammatory degenerative disease of retina.
AHA: 4Q, '05, 65; 3Q, '91, 8

362.01 Background diabetic retinopathy
Diabetic retinal microaneurysms
Diabetic retinopathy NOS

362.02 Proliferative diabetic retinopathy
DEF: Occurrence of the ischemic effects of vessel blockages result in neovascularization; new blood vessels begin to form to compensate for restricted blood flow; multiple areas of the retina and inner vitreous may be affected.
AHA: 3Q, '96, 5

362.03 Nonproliferative diabetic retinopathy NOS

362.04 Mild nonproliferative diabetic retinopathy
DEF: Early stages of degenerative condition of the retina due to diabetes; microaneurysm formation; small balloon-like swelling of the retinal vessels.

362.05 Moderate nonproliferative diabetic retinopathy
DEF: Stage of degenerative condition of the retina due to diabetes with pronounced microaneurysms; vessel blockages can occur.

362.06 Severe nonproliferative diabetic retinopathy
DEF: Stage of degenerative condition of the retina due to diabetes in which vascular breakdown in the retina results in multiple vascular blockages, or "beadings," with intraretinal hemorrhages.
AHA: 4Q, '05, 67

362.07 Diabetic macular edema
NOTE Code 362.07 must be used with a code for diabetic retinopathy (362.01-362.06)
Diabetic retinal edema
DEF: Leakage from retinal blood vessels causes swelling of the macula and impaired vision; exudates or plaques may develop in the posterior pole of the retina due to the breakdown of retinal vasculature.

√5ᵗʰ **362.1 Other background retinopathy and retinal vascular changes**

362.10 Background retinopathy, unspecified
AHA: 1Q, '06, 12

362.11 Hypertensive retinopathy
DEF: Retinal irregularities caused by systemic hypertension.
AHA: 3Q, '90, 3

362.12 Exudative retinopathy
Coats' syndrome
AHA: 3Q, '99, 12

362.13 Changes in vascular appearance
Vascular sheathing of retina
Use additional code for any associated atherosclerosis (440.8)

362.14 Retinal microaneurysms NOS
DEF: Microscopic dilation of retinal vessels in nondiabetic.

362.15 Retinal telangiectasia
DEF: Dilation of blood vessels of the retina.

362.16 Retinal neovascularization NOS
Neovascularization:	Neovascularization:
choroidal	subretinal

DEF: New and abnormal vascular growth in the retina.

362.17 Other intraretinal microvascular abnormalities
Retinal sclerosis
Retinal varices

362.18 Retinal vasculitis
Eales' disease	Retinal:
Retinal:	perivasculitis
arteritis	phlebitis
endarteritis	

DEF: Inflammation of retinal blood vessels.

√5ᵗʰ **362.2 Other proliferative retinopathy**
AHA: 4Q, '08, 110-111

362.20 Retinopathy of prematurity, unspecified
Retinopathy of prematurity NOS

362.21 Retrolental fibroplasia
Cicatricial retinopathy of prematurity
DEF: Fibrous tissue in vitreous, from retina to lens, causing blindness; associated with premature infants requiring high amounts of oxygen.

362.22 Retinopathy of prematurity, stage 0

362.23 Retinopathy of prematurity, stage 1

362.24 Retinopathy of prematurity, stage 2

362.25 Retinopathy of prematurity, stage 3

362.26 Retinopathy of prematurity, stage 4

362.27 Retinopathy of prematurity, stage 5

362.29 Other nondiabetic proliferative retinopathy
AHA: 3Q, '96, 5

√5ᵗʰ **362.3 Retinal vascular occlusion**
DEF: Obstructed blood flow to and from retina.

362.30 Retinal vascular occlusion, unspecified

362.31 Central retinal artery occlusion

362.32 Arterial branch occlusion

362.33 Partial arterial occlusion
Hollenhorst plaque
Retinal microembolism

362.34 Transient arterial occlusion
Amaurosis fugax
AHA: 1Q, '00, 16

362.35 Central retinal vein occlusion
AHA: 2Q, '93, 6

362.36 Venous tributary (branch) occlusion

362.37 Venous engorgement
Occlusion:
incipient } of retinal vein
partial

√5ᵗʰ **362.4 Separation of retinal layers**
> **EXCLUDES** *retinal detachment (serous) (361.2)*
> *rhegmatogenous (361.00-361.07)*

362.40 Retinal layer separation, unspecified

362.41 Central serous retinopathy
DEF: Serous-filled blister causing detachment of retina from pigment epithelium.

N Newborn Age: 0   P Pediatric Age: 0-17   M Maternity Age: 12-55   A Adult Age: 15-124

362.42 Serous detachment of retinal pigment epithelium
Exudative detachment of retinal pigment epithelium
DEF: Blister of fatty fluid causing detachment of retina from pigment epithelium.

362.43 Hemorrhagic detachment of retinal pigment epithelium
DEF: Blood-filled blister causing detachment of retina from pigment epithelium.

√5ᵗʰ **362.5 Degeneration of macula and posterior pole**
EXCLUDES degeneration of optic disc (377.21-377.24)
hereditary retinal degeneration [dystrophy] (362.70-362.77)

362.50 Macular degeneration (senile), unspecified

362.51 Nonexudative senile macular degeneration
Senile macular degeneration:
atrophic
dry

362.52 Exudative senile macular degeneration
Kuhnt-Junius degeneration
Senile macular degeneration:
disciform
wet
DEF: Leakage in macular blood vessels with loss of visual acuity.

362.53 Cystoid macular degeneration
Cystoid macular edema
DEF: Retinal swelling and cyst formation in macula.

362.54 Macular cyst, hole, or pseudohole

362.55 Toxic maculopathy
Use additional E code to identify drug, if drug induced

362.56 Macular puckering
Preretinal fibrosis

362.57 Drusen (degenerative)
DEF: White, hyaline deposits on Bruch's membrane (lamina basalis choroideae).

√5ᵗʰ **362.6 Peripheral retinal degenerations**
EXCLUDES hereditary retinal degeneration [dystrophy] (362.70-362.77)
retinal degeneration with retinal defect (361.00-361.07)

362.60 Peripheral retinal degeneration, unspecified

362.61 Paving stone degeneration
DEF: Degeneration of peripheral retina; causes thinning through which choroid is visible.

362.62 Microcystoid degeneration
Blessig's cysts   Iwanoff's cysts

362.63 Lattice degeneration
Palisade degeneration of retina
DEF: Degeneration of retina; often bilateral, usually benign; characterized by lines intersecting at irregular intervals in peripheral retina; retinal thinning and retinal holes may occur.

362.64 Senile reticular degeneration
DEF: Net-like appearance of retina; sign of degeneration.

362.65 Secondary pigmentary degeneration
Pseudoretinitis pigmentosa

362.66 Secondary vitreoretinal degenerations

√5ᵗʰ **362.7 Hereditary retinal dystrophies**
DEF: Genetically induced progressive changes in retina.

362.70 Hereditary retinal dystrophy, unspecified

362.71 Retinal dystrophy in systemic or cerebroretinal lipidoses
Code first underlying disease, as:
cerebroretinal lipidoses (330.1)
systemic lipidoses (272.7)

362.72 Retinal dystrophy in other systemic disorders and syndromes
Code first underlying disease, as:
Bassen-Kornzweig syndrome (272.5)
Refsum's disease (356.3)

362.73 Vitreoretinal dystrophies
Juvenile retinoschisis

362.74 Pigmentary retinal dystrophy
Retinal dystrophy, albipunctate
Retinitis pigmentosa

362.75 Other dystrophies primarily involving the sensory retina
Progressive cone(-rod) dystrophy
Stargardt's disease

362.76 Dystrophies primarily involving the retinal pigment epithelium
Fundus flavimaculatus
Vitelliform dystrophy

362.77 Dystrophies primarily involving Bruch's membrane
Dystrophy:
hyaline
pseudoinflammatory foveal
Hereditary drusen

√5ᵗʰ **362.8 Other retinal disorders**
EXCLUDES chorioretinal inflammations (363.0-363.2)
chorioretinal scars (363.30-363.35)

362.81 Retinal hemorrhage
Hemorrhage:
preretinal
retinal (deep) (superficial)
subretinal
AHA: 4Q, '96, 43

362.82 Retinal exudates and deposits

362.83 Retinal edema
Retinal:
cotton wool spots
edema (localized) (macular) (peripheral)
DEF: Retinal swelling due to fluid accumulation.

362.84 Retinal ischemia
DEF: Reduced retinal blood supply.

362.85 Retinal nerve fiber bundle defects

362.89 Other retinal disorders

362.9 Unspecified retinal disorder

√4ᵗʰ **363 Chorioretinal inflammations, scars, and other disorders of choroid**

√5ᵗʰ **363.0 Focal chorioretinitis and focal retinochoroiditis**
EXCLUDES focal chorioretinitis or retinochoroiditis in:
histoplasmosis (115.02, 115.12, 115.92)
toxoplasmosis (130.2)
congenital infection (771.2)

363.00 Focal chorioretinitis, unspecified
Focal:
choroiditis or chorioretinitis NOS
retinitis or retinochoroiditis NOS

363.01 Focal choroiditis and chorioretinitis, juxtapapillary

363.03 Focal choroiditis and chorioretinitis of other posterior pole

363.04 Focal choroiditis and chorioretinitis, peripheral

363.05 Focal retinitis and retinochoroiditis, juxtapapillary
Neuroretinitis

363.06 Focal retinitis and retinochoroiditis, macular or paramacular

363.07 Focal retinitis and retinochoroiditis of other posterior pole

363.08 Focal retinitis and retinochoroiditis, peripheral

√5ᵗʰ **363.1 Disseminated chorioretinitis and disseminated retinochoroiditis**
EXCLUDES disseminated choroiditis or chorioretinitis in secondary syphilis (091.51)
neurosyphilitic disseminated retinitis or retinochoroiditis (094.83)
retinal (peri)vasculitis (362.18)

363.10 Disseminated chorioretinitis, unspecified
Disseminated:
choroiditis or chorioretinitis NOS
retinitis or retinochoroiditis NOS

363.11 Disseminated choroiditis and, chorioretinitis posterior pole

363.12 Disseminated choroiditis and chorioretinitis, peripheral

363.13 Disseminated choroiditis and chorioretinitis, generalized
Code first any underlying disease, as:
tuberculosis (017.3)

363.14 Disseminated retinitis and retinochoroiditis, metastatic

363.15 Disseminated retinitis and retinochoroiditis, pigment epitheliopathy
Acute posterior multifocal placoid pigment epitheliopathy
DEF: Widespread inflammation of retina and choroid; characterized by pigmented epithelium involvement.

√5ᵗʰ **363.2 Other and unspecified forms of chorioretinitis and retinochoroiditis**
EXCLUDES panophthalmitis (360.02)
sympathetic uveitis (360.11)
uveitis NOS (364.3)

363.20 Chorioretinitis, unspecified
Choroiditis NOS   Uveitis, posterior NOS
Retinitis NOS

363.21 Pars planitis
Posterior cyclitis
DEF: Inflammation of peripheral retina and ciliary body; characterized by bands of white cells.

363.22 Harada's disease
DEF: Retinal detachment and bilateral widespread exudative choroiditis; symptoms include headache, vomiting, increased lymphocytes in cerebrospinal fluid; with temporary or permanent deafness.

√5ᵗʰ **363.3 Chorioretinal scars**
Scar (postinflammatory) (postsurgical) (posttraumatic):
choroid
retina

363.30 Chorioretinal scar, unspecified

363.31 Solar retinopathy
DEF: Retinal scarring caused by solar radiation.

363.32 Other macular scars

363.33 Other scars of posterior pole

363.34 Peripheral scars

363.35 Disseminated scars

√5ᵗʰ **363.4 Choroidal degenerations**

363.40 Choroidal degeneration, unspecified
Choroidal sclerosis NOS

363.41 Senile atrophy of choroid
DEF: Wasting away of choroid; due to aging.

363.42 Diffuse secondary atrophy of choroid
DEF: Wasting away of choroid in systemic disease.

363.43 Angioid streaks of choroid
DEF: Degeneration of choroid; characterized by dark brown streaks radiating from optic disc; occurs with pseudoxanthoma, elasticum or Paget's disease.

√5ᵗʰ **363.5 Hereditary choroidal dystrophies**
Hereditary choroidal atrophy:
partial [choriocapillaris]
total [all vessels]

363.50 Hereditary choroidal dystrophy or atrophy, unspecified

363.51 Circumpapillary dystrophy of choroid, partial

363.52 Circumpapillary dystrophy of choroid, total
Helicoid dystrophy of choroid

363.53 Central dystrophy of choroid, partial
Dystrophy, choroidal:
central areolar
circinate

363.54 Central choroidal atrophy, total
Dystrophy, choroidal:
central gyrate
serpiginous

363.55 Choroideremia
DEF: Hereditary choroid degeneration, occurs in first decade; characterized by constricted visual field and ultimately blindness in males; less debilitating in females.

363.56 Other diffuse or generalized dystrophy, partial
Diffuse choroidal sclerosis

363.57 Other diffuse or generalized dystrophy, total
Generalized gyrate atrophy, choroid

√5ᵗʰ **363.6 Choroidal hemorrhage and rupture**

363.61 Choroidal hemorrhage, unspecified

363.62 Expulsive choroidal hemorrhage

363.63 Choroidal rupture

√5ᵗʰ **363.7 Choroidal detachment**

363.70 Choroidal detachment, unspecified

363.71 Serous choroidal detachment
DEF: Detachment of choroid from sclera; due to blister of serous fluid.

363.72 Hemorrhagic choroidal detachment
DEF: Detachment of choroid from sclera; due to blood-filled blister.

363.8 Other disorders of choroid

363.9 Unspecified disorder of choroid

√4ᵗʰ **364 Disorders of iris and ciliary body**

√5ᵗʰ **364.0 Acute and subacute iridocyclitis**
Anterior uveitis
Cylitis
Iridocyclitis } acute, subacute
Iritis

EXCLUDES gonococcal (098.41)
herpes simplex (054.44)
herpes zoster (053.22)

364.00 Acute and subacute iridocyclitis, unspecified

364.01 Primary iridocyclitis

364.02 Recurrent iridocyclitis

364.03 Secondary iridocyclitis, infectious

364.04 Secondary iridocyclitis, noninfectious
Aqueous: Aqueous:
cells   flare
fibrin

364.05 Hypopyon
DEF: Accumulation of white blood cells between cornea and lens.

√5ᵗʰ **364.1 Chronic iridocyclitis**
EXCLUDES posterior cyclitis (363.21)

364.10 Chronic iridocyclitis, unspecified

364.11 Chronic iridocyclitis in diseases classified elsewhere

Code first underlying disease, as:
sarcoidosis (135)
tuberculosis (017.3)
EXCLUDES syphilitic iridocyclitis (091.52)
DEF: Persistent inflammation of iris and ciliary body; due to underlying disease or condition.

Ⓝ Newborn Age: 0   Ⓟ Pediatric Age: 0-17   Ⓜ Maternity Age: 12-55   Ⓐ Adult Age: 15-124

√5ᵗʰ **364.2 Certain types of iridocyclitis**
  EXCLUDES *posterior cyclitis (363.21)*
       sympathetic uveitis (360.11)

  364.21 Fuchs' heterochromic cyclitis
    DEF: Chronic cyclitis characterized by differences in the color of the two irises; the lighter iris appears in the inflamed eye.

  364.22 Glaucomatocyclitic crises
    DEF: An uncommon inflammatory unilateral eye condition, characteristic recurrent episodes of high intraocular pressure accompanied by mild inflammation.

  364.23 Lens-induced iridocyclitis
    DEF: Inflammation of iris; due to immune reaction to proteins in lens following trauma or other lens abnormality.

  364.24 Vogt-Koyanagi syndrome
    DEF: Uveomeningitis with exudative iridocyclitis and choroiditis; causes depigmentation of hair and skin, detached retina; tinnitus and loss of hearing.

364.3 Unspecified iridocyclitis
  Uveitis NOS

√5ᵗʰ **364.4 Vascular disorders of iris and ciliary body**

  364.41 Hyphema
    Hemorrhage of iris or ciliary body
    DEF: Hemorrhage in anterior chamber; also called hyphemia or "blood shot" eyes.

  364.42 Rubeosis iridis
    Neovascularization of iris or ciliary body
    DEF: Blood vessel and connective tissue formation on surface of iris; symptomatic of diabetic retinopathy, central retinal vein occlusion and retinal detachment.

√5ᵗʰ **364.5 Degenerations of iris and ciliary body**

  364.51 Essential or progressive iris atrophy

  364.52 Iridoschisis
    DEF: Splitting of the iris into two layers.

  364.53 Pigmentary iris degeneration
    Acquired heterochromia
    Pigment dispersion syndrome } of iris
    Translucency

  364.54 Degeneration of pupillary margin
    Atrophy of sphincter } of iris
    Ectropion of pigment epithelium

  364.55 Miotic cysts of pupillary margin
    DEF: Serous-filled sacs in pupillary margin of iris.

  364.56 Degenerative changes of chamber angle

  364.57 Degenerative changes of ciliary body

  364.59 Other iris atrophy
    Iris atrophy (generalized) (sector shaped)

√5ᵗʰ **364.6 Cysts of iris, ciliary body, and anterior chamber**
  EXCLUDES *miotic pupillary cyst (364.55)*
       parasitic cyst (360.13)

  364.60 Idiopathic cysts
    DEF: Fluid-filled sacs in iris or ciliary body; unknown etiology.

  364.61 Implantation cysts
    Epithelial down-growth, anterior chamber
    Implantation cysts (surgical) (traumatic)

  364.62 Exudative cysts of iris or anterior chamber

  364.63 Primary cyst of pars plana
    DEF: Fluid-filled sacs of outermost ciliary ring.

  364.64 Exudative cyst of pars plana
    DEF: Protein, fatty-filled sacs of outermost ciliary ring; due to fluid leak from blood vessels.

√5ᵗʰ **364.7 Adhesions and disruptions of iris and ciliary body**
  EXCLUDES *flat anterior chamber (360.34)*

  364.70 Adhesions of iris, unspecified
    Synechiae (iris) NOS

  364.71 Posterior synechiae
    DEF: Adhesion binding iris to lens.

  364.72 Anterior synechiae
    DEF: Adhesion binding the iris to cornea.

  364.73 Goniosynechiae
    Peripheral anterior synechiae
    DEF: Adhesion binding the iris to cornea at the angle of the anterior chamber.

  364.74 Pupillary membranes
    Iris bombé
    Pupillary:
      occlusion
      seclusion
    DEF: Membrane traversing the pupil and blocking vision.

  364.75 Pupillary abnormalities
    Deformed pupil
    Ectopic pupil
    Rupture of sphincter, pupil

  364.76 Iridodialysis
    DEF: Separation of the iris from the ciliary body base; due to trauma or surgical accident.

  364.77 Recession of chamber angle
    DEF: Receding of anterior chamber angle of the eye, restricts vision.

√5ᵗʰ **364.8 Other disorders of iris and ciliary body**
  AHA: 2Q, '07, 9

  364.81 Floppy iris syndrome
    Intraoperative floppy iris syndrome [IFIS]
    Use additional E code to identify cause, such as:
      sympatholytics [antiadrenergics] causing adverse effect in therapeutic use (E941.3)
    DEF: Condition complicating cataract surgery for patients who have received alpha blocker treatment for urinary retention problems; iris dilator muscle fails to dilate, and the iris may billow or flap.
    AHA: 4Q, '07, 77, 79

  364.82 Plateau iris syndrome
    DEF: A postoperative chronic angle-closure glaucoma characterized by closing of the anterior chamber angle secondary to a large or anteriorly positioned ciliary body that impairs the normal flow of aqueous fluid.
    AHA: 4Q, '08, 112

  364.89 Other disorders of iris and ciliary body
    Prolapse of iris NOS
    EXCLUDES *prolapse of iris in recent wound (871.1)*

364.9 Unspecified disorder of iris and ciliary body

√4ᵗʰ **365 Glaucoma**
  EXCLUDES *blind hypertensive eye [absolute glaucoma] (360.42)*
       congenital glaucoma (743.20-743.22)
  DEF: Rise in intraocular pressure restricting blood flow; multiple causes.

√5ᵗʰ **365.0 Borderline glaucoma [glaucoma suspect]**
  AHA: 1Q, '90, 8

  365.00 Preglaucoma, unspecified

  365.01 Open angle with borderline findings
    Open angle with:
      borderline intraocular pressure
      cupping of optic discs
    DEF: Minor block of aqueous outflow from eye.

  365.02 Anatomical narrow angle

  365.03 Steroid responders

  365.04 Ocular hypertension
    DEF: High fluid pressure within eye; no clear cause.

√5ᵗʰ **365.1 Open-angle glaucoma**

  365.10 Open-angle glaucoma, unspecified
    Wide-angle glaucoma NOS

  365.11 Primary open angle glaucoma
    Chronic simple glaucoma
    DEF: High intraocular pressure, despite free flow of aqueous.

Plateau Iris Syndrome

Normal Aqueous Flow

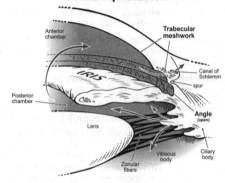

365.12 Low tension glaucoma

365.13 Pigmentary glaucoma

> **DEF:** High intraocular pressure; due to iris pigment granules blocking aqueous flow.

365.14 Glaucoma of childhood
Infantile or juvenile glaucoma

365.15 Residual stage of open angle glaucoma

☑5ᵗʰ **365.2 Primary angle-closure glaucoma**

> **DEF:** Glaucoma caused by a shift in the position of the iris of the eye that blocks the surface of the trabecular meshwork causing impairment of the normal flow of aqueous fluid.

365.20 Primary angle-closure glaucoma, unspecified

365.21 Intermittent angle-closure glaucoma
Angle-closure glaucoma:
interval
subacute

> **DEF:** Recurring attacks of high intraocular pressure; due to blocked aqueous flow.

365.22 Acute angle-closure glaucoma

> **DEF:** Sudden, severe rise in intraocular pressure due to blockage in aqueous drainage.

365.23 Chronic angle-closure glaucoma

> **AHA:** 2Q, '98, 16

365.24 Residual stage of angle-closure glaucoma

☑5ᵗʰ **365.3 Corticosteroid-induced glaucoma**

> **DEF:** Elevated intraocular pressure; due to long-term corticosteroid therapy.

365.31 Glaucomatous stage

365.32 Residual stage

☑5ᵗʰ **365.4 Glaucoma associated with congenital anomalies, dystrophies, and systemic syndromes**

365.41 Glaucoma associated with chamber angle anomalies

365.42 Glaucoma associated with anomalies of iris

365.43 Glaucoma associated with other anterior segment anomalies

Angle Closure Glaucoma

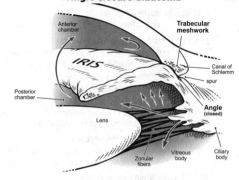

365.44 Glaucoma associated with systemic syndromes

> *Code first associated disease, as*
> neurofibromatosis ▶(237.70-237.79)◀
> Sturge-Weber (-Dimitri) syndrome (759.6)

☑5ᵗʰ **365.5 Glaucoma associated with disorders of the lens**

365.51 Phacolytic glaucoma

> **DEF:** Elevated intraocular pressure; due to lens protein blocking aqueous flow.

365.52 Pseudoexfoliation glaucoma

> **DEF:** Glaucoma characterized by small grayish particles deposited on the lens.

365.59 Glaucoma associated with other lens disorders

☑5ᵗʰ **365.6 Glaucoma associated with other ocular disorders**

365.60 Glaucoma associated with unspecified ocular disorder

365.61 Glaucoma associated with pupillary block

> **DEF:** Acute, open-angle glaucoma caused by mature cataract; aqueous flow is blocked by lens material and macrophages.

365.62 Glaucoma associated with ocular inflammations

365.63 Glaucoma associated with vascular disorders

365.64 Glaucoma associated with tumors or cysts

365.65 Glaucoma associated with ocular trauma

☑5ᵗʰ **365.8 Other specified forms of glaucoma**

365.81 Hypersecretion glaucoma

365.82 Glaucoma with increased episcleral venous pressure

365.83 Aqueous misdirection
Malignant glaucoma

> **DEF:** A form of secondary angle-closure glaucoma that occurs when aqueous humor flows into the posterior chamber of the eye (vitreous) rather than through the normal recycling channels.
> **AHA:** 4Q, '02, 48

365.89 Other specified glaucoma

> **AHA:** 2Q, '98, 16

365.9 Unspecified glaucoma

> **AHA:** 3Q, '03, 14; 2Q, '01, 16
> H40.9 Unspecified glaucoma   I-10

☑4ᵗʰ **366 Cataract**

> **EXCLUDES** congenital cataract (743.30-743.34)
> **DEF:** A variety of conditions that create a cloudy, or calcified lens that obstructs vision.

☑5ᵗʰ **366.0 Infantile, juvenile, and presenile cataract**

366.00 Nonsenile cataract, unspecified

366.01 Anterior subcapsular polar cataract

> **DEF:** Defect within the front, center lens surface.

366.02 Posterior subcapsular polar cataract

> **DEF:** Defect within the rear, center lens surface.

366.03 Cortical, lamellar, or zonular cataract

> **DEF:** Opacities radiating from center to edge of lens; appear as thin, concentric layers of lens.

N Newborn Age: 0   P Pediatric Age: 0-17   M Maternity Age: 12-55   A Adult Age: 15-124

Cataract

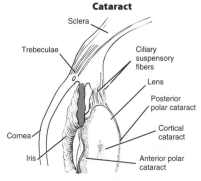

Sclera
Trebeculae
Ciliary suspensory fibers
Lens
Posterior polar cataract
Cortical cataract
Cornea
Iris
Anterior polar cataract

366.04 Nuclear cataract

366.09 Other and combined forms of nonsenile cataract

√5ᵗʰ **366.1 Senile cataract**
AHA: 3Q, '91, 9; S-0, '85, 10

366.10 Senile cataract, unspecified   Ⓐ
AHA: 1Q, '03, 5

366.11 Pseudoexfoliation of lens capsule   Ⓐ

366.12 Incipient cataract   Ⓐ
Cataract: Cataract:
coronary   punctate
immature NOS   Water clefts
DEF: Minor disorders of lens not affecting vision; due to aging.

366.13 Anterior subcapsular polar senile cataract   Ⓐ

366.14 Posterior subcapsular polar senile cataract   Ⓐ

366.15 Cortical senile cataract   Ⓐ

366.16 Nuclear sclerosis   Ⓐ
Cataracta brunescens
Nuclear cataract
AHA: 4Q, '07, 79

366.17 Total or mature cataract   Ⓐ

366.18 Hypermature cataract   Ⓐ
Morgagni cataract

366.19 Other and combined forms of senile cataract   Ⓐ

√5ᵗʰ **366.2 Traumatic cataract**

366.20 Traumatic cataract, unspecified

366.21 Localized traumatic opacities
Vossius' ring

366.22 Total traumatic cataract

366.23 Partially resolved traumatic cataract

√5ᵗʰ **366.3 Cataract secondary to ocular disorders**

366.30 Cataracta complicata, unspecified

366.31 Glaucomatous flecks (subcapsular)
Code first underlying glaucoma (365.0-365.9)

366.32 Cataract in inflammatory disorders
Code first underlying condition, as:
chronic choroiditis (363.0-363.2)

366.33 Cataract with neovascularization
Code first underlying condition, as:
chronic iridocyclitis (364.10)

366.34 Cataract in degenerative disorders
Sunflower cataract
Code first underlying condition, as:
chalcosis (360.24)
degenerative myopia (360.21)
pigmentary retinal dystrophy (362.74)

√5ᵗʰ **366.4 Cataract associated with other disorders**

366.41 Diabetic cataract
Code first diabetes (249.5, 250.5)
AHA: 3Q, '91, 9; S-O, '85, 11

366.42 Tetanic cataract
Code first underlying disease, as:
calcinosis (275.4)
hypoparathyroidism (252.1)

366.43 Myotonic cataract
Code first underlying disorder (359.21, 359.23)

366.44 Cataract associated with other syndromes
Code first underlying condition, as:
craniofacial dysostosis (756.0)
galactosemia (271.1)

366.45 Toxic cataract
Drug-induced cataract
Use additional E code to identify drug or other toxic substance

366.46 Cataract associated with radiation and other physical influences
Use additional E code to identify cause

√5ᵗʰ **366.5 After-cataract**

366.50 After-cataract, unspecified
Secondary cataract NOS

366.51 Soemmering's ring
DEF: A donut-shaped lens remnant and a capsule behind the pupil as a result of cataract surgery or trauma.

366.52 Other after-cataract, not obscuring vision

366.53 After-cataract, obscuring vision

366.8 Other cataract
Calcification of lens

366.9 Unspecified cataract
AHA: ▶4Q, '09, 131◀
H26.9 Unspecified cataract   I-10

√4ᵗʰ **367 Disorders of refraction and accommodation**

367.0 Hypermetropia
Far-sightedness
Hyperopia
DEF: Refraction error, called also hyperopia, focal point is posterior to retina; abnormally short anteroposterior diameter or subnormal refractive power; causes farsightedness.

367.1 Myopia
Near-sightedness
DEF: Refraction error, focal point is anterior to retina; causes near-sightedness.

√5ᵗʰ **367.2 Astigmatism**

367.20 Astigmatism, unspecified

367.21 Regular astigmatism

367.22 Irregular astigmatism

√5ᵗʰ **367.3 Anisometropia and aniseikonia**

367.31 Anisometropia
DEF: Eyes with refractive powers that differ by at least one diopter.

367.32 Aniseikonia
DEF: Eyes with unequal retinal imaging; usually due to refractive error.

367.4 Presbyopia
DEF: Loss of crystalline lens elasticity; causes errors of accommodation; due to aging.

√5ᵗʰ **367.5 Disorders of accommodation**

367.51 Paresis of accommodation
Cycloplegia
DEF: Partial paralysis of ciliary muscle, causing focus problems.

367.52 Total or complete internal ophthalmoplegia
DEF: Total paralysis of ciliary muscle; large pupil incapable of focus.

367.53 Spasm of accommodation
DEF: Abnormal contraction of ciliary muscle; causes focus problems.

✓5ᵗʰ **367.8 Other disorders of refraction and accommodation**

367.81 Transient refractive change

367.89 Other
Drug-induced } disorders of refraction and
Toxic } accommodation

367.9 Unspecified disorder of refraction and accommodation

✓4ᵗʰ **368 Visual disturbances**
EXCLUDES electrophysiological disturbances (794.11-794.14)

✓5ᵗʰ **368.0 Amblyopia ex anopsia**
DEF: Vision impaired due to disuse; esotropia often cause.

368.00 Amblyopia, unspecified

368.01 Strabismic amblyopia
Suppression amblyopia

368.02 Deprivation amblyopia
DEF: Decreased vision associated with suppressed retinal image of one eye.

368.03 Refractive amblyopia

✓5ᵗʰ **368.1 Subjective visual disturbances**

368.10 Subjective visual disturbance, unspecified

368.11 Sudden visual loss

368.12 Transient visual loss
Concentric fading
Scintillating scotoma

368.13 Visual discomfort
Asthenopia   Photophobia
Eye strain

368.14 Visual distortions of shape and size
Macropsia   Micropsia
Metamorphopsia

368.15 Other visual distortions and entoptic phenomena
Photopsia   Refractive:
Refractive: polyopia
   diplopia   Visual halos

368.16 Psychophysical visual disturbances
Prosopagnosia
Visual:
   agnosia
   disorientation syndrome
   hallucinations
   object agnosia

368.2 Diplopia
Double vision
H53.2 Diplopia   I-10

✓5ᵗʰ **368.3 Other disorders of binocular vision**

368.30 Binocular vision disorder, unspecified

368.31 Suppression of binocular vision

368.32 Simultaneous visual perception without fusion

368.33 Fusion with defective stereopsis
DEF: Faulty depth perception though normal ability to focus.

368.34 Abnormal retinal correspondence

✓5ᵗʰ **368.4 Visual field defects**

368.40 Visual field defect, unspecified

368.41 Scotoma involving central area
Scotoma: Scotoma:
   central   paracentral
   centrocecal
DEF: Vision loss (blind spot) in central five degrees of visual field.

368.42 Scotoma of blind spot area
Enlarged: Paracecal scotoma
   angioscotoma
   blind spot

368.43 Sector or arcuate defects
Scotoma: Scotoma:
   arcuate   Seidel
   Bjerrum
DEF: Arc-shaped blind spot caused by retinal nerve damage.

368.44 Other localized visual field defect
Scotoma: Visual field defect:
   NOS   nasal step
   ring   peripheral

368.45 Generalized contraction or constriction

368.46 Homonymous bilateral field defects
Hemianopsia (altitudinal) (homonymous)
Quadrant anopia
DEF: Disorders found in the corresponding vertical halves of the visual fields of both eyes.

368.47 Heteronymous bilateral field defects
Hemianopsia: Hemianopsia:
   binasal   bitemporal
DEF: Disorders in the opposite halves of the visual fields of both eyes.

✓5ᵗʰ **368.5 Color vision deficiencies**
Color blindness

368.51 Protan defect
Protanomaly
Protanopia
DEF: Mild difficulty distinguishing green and red hues with shortened spectrum; sex-linked affecting one percent of males.

368.52 Deutan defect
Deuteranomaly
Deuteranopia
DEF: Male-only disorder; difficulty in distinguishing green and red, no shortened spectrum.

368.53 Tritan defect
Tritanomaly
Tritanopia
DEF: Difficulty in distinguishing blue and yellow; occurs often due to drugs, retinal detachment and central nervous system diseases.

368.54 Achromatopsia
Monochromatism (cone) (rod)
DEF: Complete color blindness; caused by disease, injury to retina, optic nerve or pathway.

368.55 Acquired color vision deficiencies

368.59 Other color vision deficiencies

✓5ᵗʰ **368.6 Night blindness**
Nyctalopia
DEF: Nyctalopia: disorder of vision in dim light or night blindness.

368.60 Night blindness, unspecified

368.61 Congenital night blindness
Hereditary night blindness
Oguchi's disease

368.62 Acquired night blindness
EXCLUDES that due to vitamin A deficiency (264.5)

368.63 Abnormal dark adaptation curve
Abnormal threshold } of cones or rods
Delayed adaptation }

368.69 Other night blindness

368.8 Other specified visual disturbances
Blurred vision NOS
AHA: 4Q, '02, 56

368.9 Unspecified visual disturbance
AHA: 3Q, '06, 22; 1Q, '04, 15

Ⓝ Newborn Age: 0   Ⓟ Pediatric Age: 0-17   Ⓜ Maternity Age: 12-55   Ⓐ Adult Age: 15-124

√4ᵗʰ **369 Blindness and low vision**

> **NOTE** Visual impairment refers to a functional limitation of the eye (e.g., limited visual acuity or visual field). It should be distinguished from visual disability, indicating a limitation of the abilities of the individual (e.g., limited reading skills, vocational skills), and from visual handicap, indicating a limitation of personal and socioeconomic independence (e.g., limited mobility, limited employability).
>
> The levels of impairment defined in the table on this page are based on the recommendations of the WHO Study Group on Prevention of Blindness (Geneva, November 6-10, 1972; WHO Technical Report Series 518), and of the International Council of Ophthalmology (1976).
>
> Note that definitions of blindness vary in different settings.
>
> For international reporting WHO defines blindness as profound impairment. This definition can be applied to blindness of one eye (369.1, 369.6) and to blindness of the individual (369.0).
>
> For determination of benefits in the U.S.A., the definition of legal blindness as severe impairment is often used. This definition applies to blindness of the individual only.
>
> **EXCLUDES** correctable impaired vision due to refractive errors (367.0-367.9)

√5ᵗʰ **369.0 Profound impairment, both eyes**

    369.00 Impairment level not further specified
       Blindness:
         NOS according to WHO definition
         both eyes

    369.01 Better eye: total impairment; lesser eye: total impairment

    369.02 Better eye: near-total impairment; lesser eye: not further specified

    369.03 Better eye: near-total impairment; lesser eye: total impairment

    369.04 Better eye: near-total impairment; lesser eye: near-total impairment

    369.05 Better eye: profound impairment; lesser eye: not further specified

    369.06 Better eye: profound impairment; lesser eye: total impairment

    369.07 Better eye: profound impairment; lesser eye: near-total impairment

    369.08 Better eye: profound impairment; lesser eye: profound impairment

√4ᵗʰ **369.1 Moderate or severe impairment, better eye, profound impairment lesser eye**

    369.10 Impairment level not further specified
       Blindness, one eye, low vision other eye

    369.11 Better eye: severe impairment; lesser eye: blind, not further specified

    369.12 Better eye: severe impairment; lesser eye: total impairment

    369.13 Better eye: severe impairment; lesser eye: near-total impairment

    369.14 Better eye: severe impairment; lesser eye: profound impairment

    369.15 Better eye: moderate impairment; lesser eye: blind, not further specified

    369.16 Better eye: moderate impairment; lesser eye: total impairment

    369.17 Better eye: moderate impairment; lesser eye: near-total impairment

    369.18 Better eye: moderate impairment; lesser eye: profound impairment

√5ᵗʰ **369.2 Moderate or severe impairment, both eyes**

    369.20 Impairment level not further specified
       Low vision, both eyes NOS

    369.21 Better eye: severe impairment; lesser eye: not further specified

    369.22 Better eye: severe impairment; lesser eye: severe impairment

    369.23 Better eye: moderate impairment; lesser eye: not further specified

    369.24 Better eye: moderate impairment; lesser eye: severe impairment

    369.25 Better eye: moderate impairment; lesser eye: moderate impairment

   369.3 Unqualified visual loss, both eyes
      EXCLUDES blindness NOS:
         legal [U.S.A. definition] (369.4)
         WHO definition (369.00)

   369.4 Legal blindness, as defined in U.S.A.
      Blindness NOS according to U.S.A. definition
      EXCLUDES legal blindness with specification of impairment level (369.01-369.08, 369.11-369.14, 369.21-369.22)
      H54.8 Legal blindness as defined in USA   I-10

√5ᵗʰ **369.6 Profound impairment, one eye**

    369.60 Impairment level not further specified
       Blindness, one eye

    369.61 One eye: total impairment; other eye: not specified

    369.62 One eye: total impairment; other eye: near normal vision

    369.63 One eye: total impairment; other eye: normal vision

    369.64 One eye: near-total impairment; other eye: not specified

    369.65 One eye: near-total impairment; other eye: near-normal vision

    369.66 One eye: near-total impairment; other eye: normal vision

    369.67 One eye: profound impairment; other eye: not specified

Classification		LEVELS OF VISUAL IMPAIRMENT		Additional descriptors which may be encountered
"legal"	WHO	Visual acuity and/or visual field limitation (whichever is worse)		
(NEAR-) NORMAL VISION		RANGE OF NORMAL VISION 20/10 20/13 20/16 20/20 20/25 2.0 1.6 1.25 1.0 0.8		
		NEAR-NORMAL VISION 20/30 20/40 20/50 20/60 0.7 0.6 0.5 0.4 0.3		
LOW VISION		MODERATE VISUAL IMPAIRMENT 20/70 20/80 20/100 20/125 20/160 0.25 0.20 0.16 0.12		Moderate low vision
		SEVERE VISUAL IMPAIRMENT 20/200 20/250 20/320 20/400 0.10 0.08 0.06 0.05 Visual field: 20 degrees or less		Severe low vision, "Legal" blindness
LEGAL BLINDNESS (U.S.A.) both eyes	BLINDNESS (WHO) one or both eyes	PROFOUND VISUAL IMPAIRMENT 20/500 20/630 20/800 20/1000 0.04 0.03 0.025 0.02 Count fingers at: less than 3m (10 ft.) Visual field: 10 degrees or less		Profound low vision, Moderate blindness
		NEAR-TOTAL VISUAL IMPAIRMENT Visual acuity: less than 0.02 (20/1000) Count fingers at: 1m (3 ft.) or less Hand movements: 5m (15 ft.) or less Light projection, light perception Visual field: 5 degrees or less		Severe blindness, Near-total blindness
		TOTAL VISUAL IMPAIRMENT No light perception (NLP)		Total blindness

Visual acuity refers to best achievable acuity with correction.
Non-listed Snellen fractions may be classified by converting to the nearest decimal equivalent, e.g. 10/200 = 0.05, 6/30 = 0.20.
CF (count fingers) without designation of distance, may be classified to profound impairment.
HM (hand motion) without designation of distance, may be classified to near-total impairment.
Visual field measurements refer to the largest field diameter for a 1/100 white test object.

√4ᵗʰ √5ᵗʰ Additional Digit Required   Unspecified Code   Other Specified Code   Manifestation Code   ▶◀ Revised Text   ● New Code   ▲ Revised Code Title

2011 ICD-9-CM   **Volume 1 – 109**

369.68 One eye: profound impairment; other eye: near-normal vision

369.69 One eye: profound impairment; other eye: normal vision

√5ᵗʰ **369.7 Moderate or severe impairment, one eye**

369.70 Impairment level not further specified
Low vision, one eye

369.71 One eye: severe impairment; other eye: not specified

369.72 One eye: severe impairment; other eye: near-normal vision

369.73 One eye: severe impairment; other eye: normal vision

369.74 One eye: moderate impairment; other eye: not specified

369.75 One eye: moderate impairment; other eye: near-normal vision

369.76 One eye: moderate impairment; other eye: normal vision

369.8 Unqualified visual loss, one eye

369.9 Unspecified visual loss
AHA: 4Q, '02, 114; 3Q, '02, 20

√4ᵗʰ **370 Keratitis**

√5ᵗʰ **370.0 Corneal ulcer**
EXCLUDES *that due to vitamin A deficiency (264.3)*

370.00 Corneal ulcer, unspecified

370.01 Marginal corneal ulcer

370.02 Ring corneal ulcer

370.03 Central corneal ulcer

370.04 Hypopyon ulcer
Serpiginous ulcer
DEF: Corneal ulcer with an accumulation of pus in the eye's anterior chamber.

370.05 Mycotic corneal ulcer
DEF: Fungal infection causing corneal tissue loss.

370.06 Perforated corneal ulcer
DEF: Tissue loss through all layers of cornea.

370.07 Mooren's ulcer
DEF: Tissue loss, with chronic inflammation, at junction of cornea and sclera; seen in elderly.

√5ᵗʰ **370.2 Superficial keratitis without conjunctivitis**
EXCLUDES *dendritic [herpes simplex] keratitis (054.42)*

370.20 Superficial keratitis, unspecified

370.21 Punctate keratitis
Thygeson's superficial punctate keratitis
DEF: Formation of cellular and fibrinous deposits (keratic precipitates) on posterior surface; deposits develop after injury or iridocyclitis.

370.22 Macular keratitis
Keratitis: Keratitis:
areolar   stellate
nummular   striate

370.23 Filamentary keratitis
DEF: Keratitis characterized by twisted filaments of mucoid material on the cornea's surface.

370.24 Photokeratitis
Snow blindness   Welders' keratitis
DEF: Painful, inflamed cornea; due to extended exposure to ultraviolet light.
AHA: 3Q, '96, 6

√5ᵗʰ **370.3 Certain types of keratoconjunctivitis**

370.31 Phlyctenular keratoconjunctivitis
Phlyctenulosis
Use additional code for any associated tuberculosis (017.3)
DEF: Miniature blister on conjunctiva or cornea; associated with tuberculosis and malnutrition disorders.

370.32 Limbar and corneal involvement in vernal conjunctivitis
Use additional code for vernal conjunctivitis (372.13)
DEF: Corneal itching and inflammation in conjunctivitis; often limited to lining of eyelids.

370.33 Keratoconjunctivitis sicca, not specified as Sjögren's
EXCLUDES *Sjögren's syndrome (710.2)*
DEF: Inflammation of conjunctiva and cornea; characterized by "horny" looking tissue and excess blood in these areas; decreased flow of lacrimal (tear) is a contributing factor.

370.34 Exposure keratoconjunctivitis
DEF: Incomplete closure of eyelid causing dry, inflamed eye.

370.35 Neurotrophic keratoconjunctivitis

√5ᵗʰ **370.4 Other and unspecified keratoconjunctivitis**

370.40 Keratoconjunctivitis, unspecified
Superficial keratitis with conjunctivitis NOS

370.44 Keratitis or keratoconjunctivitis in exanthema
Code first underlying condition (050.0-052.9)
EXCLUDES *herpes simplex (054.43)*
herpes zoster (053.21)
measles (055.71)

370.49 Other
EXCLUDES *epidemic keratoconjunctivitis (077.1)*

√5ᵗʰ **370.5 Interstitial and deep keratitis**

370.50 Interstitial keratitis, unspecified

370.52 Diffuse interstitial keratitis
Cogan's syndrome
DEF: Inflammation of cornea; with deposits in middle corneal layers; may obscure vision.

370.54 Sclerosing keratitis
DEF: Chronic corneal inflammation leading to opaque scarring.

370.55 Corneal abscess
DEF: Pocket of pus and inflammation on the cornea.

370.59 Other
EXCLUDES *disciform herpes simplex keratitis (054.43)*
syphilitic keratitis (090.3)

√5ᵗʰ **370.6 Corneal neovascularization**

370.60 Corneal neovascularization, unspecified

370.61 Localized vascularization of cornea
DEF: Limited infiltration of cornea by new blood vessels.

370.62 Pannus (corneal)
DEF: Buildup of superficial vascularization and granulated tissue under epithelium of cornea.
AHA: 3Q, '02, 20

370.63 Deep vascularization of cornea
DEF: Deep infiltration of cornea by new blood vessels.

370.64 Ghost vessels (corneal)

370.8 Other forms of keratitis
Code first underlying condition, such as:
Acanthamoeba (136.21)
Fusarium (118)
AHA: 4Q, '08, 80-81; 3Q, '94, 5

370.9 Unspecified keratitis

√4ᵗʰ **371 Corneal opacity and other disorders of cornea**

√5ᵗʰ **371.0 Corneal scars and opacities**
EXCLUDES *that due to vitamin A deficiency (264.6)*

371.00 Corneal opacity, unspecified
Corneal scar NOS

371.01 Minor opacity of cornea
Corneal nebula

371.02 Peripheral opacity of cornea
Corneal macula not interfering with central vision

N Newborn Age: 0   P Pediatric Age: 0-17   M Maternity Age: 12-55   A Adult Age: 15-124

371.03 Central opacity of cornea
Corneal:
leucoma
macula } interfering with central vision

371.04 Adherent leucoma
DEF: Dense, opaque corneal growth adhering to the iris; also spelled as leukoma.

371.05 Phthisical cornea
Code first underlying tuberculosis (017.3)

√5ᵗʰ **371.1 Corneal pigmentations and deposits**

371.10 Corneal deposit, unspecified

371.11 Anterior pigmentations
Stähli's lines

371.12 Stromal pigmentations
Hematocornea

371.13 Posterior pigmentations
Krukenberg spindle

371.14 Kayser-Fleischer ring
DEF: Copper deposits forming ring at outer edge of cornea; seen in Wilson's disease and other liver disorders.

371.15 Other deposits associated with metabolic disorders

371.16 Argentous deposits
DEF: Silver deposits in cornea.

√5ᵗʰ **371.2 Corneal edema**

371.20 Corneal edema, unspecified

371.21 Idiopathic corneal edema
DEF: Corneal swelling and fluid retention of unknown cause.

371.22 Secondary corneal edema
DEF: Corneal swelling and fluid retention caused by an underlying disease, injury, or condition.

371.23 Bullous keratopathy
DEF: Corneal degeneration; characterized by recurring, rupturing epithelial "blisters;" ruptured blebs expose corneal nerves; occurs in glaucoma, iridocyclitis and Fuchs' epithelial dystrophy.

371.24 Corneal edema due to wearing of contact lenses

√5ᵗʰ **371.3 Changes of corneal membranes**

371.30 Corneal membrane change, unspecified

371.31 Folds and rupture of Bowman's membrane

371.32 Folds in Descemet's membrane

371.33 Rupture in Descemet's membrane

√5ᵗʰ **371.4 Corneal degenerations**

371.40 Corneal degeneration, unspecified

371.41 Senile corneal changes
Arcus senilis　　Hassall-Henle bodies

371.42 Recurrent erosion of cornea
EXCLUDES Mooren's ulcer (370.07)

371.43 Band-shaped keratopathy
DEF: Horizontal bands of superficial corneal calcium deposits.

371.44 Other calcerous degenerations of cornea

371.45 Keratomalacia NOS
EXCLUDES that due to vitamin A deficiency (264.4)
DEF: Destruction of the cornea by keratinization of the epithelium with ulceration and perforation of the cornea; seen in cases of vitamin A deficiency.

371.46 Nodular degeneration of cornea
Salzmann's nodular dystrophy

371.48 Peripheral degenerations of cornea
Marginal degeneration of cornea [Terrien's]

371.49 Other
Discrete colliquative keratopathy

√5ᵗʰ **371.5 Hereditary corneal dystrophies**
DEF: Genetic disorder; leads to opacities, edema or lesions of cornea.

371.50 Corneal dystrophy, unspecified

371.51 Juvenile epithelial corneal dystrophy

371.52 Other anterior corneal dystrophies
Corneal dystrophy:　　Corneal dystrophy:
microscopic cystic　　ring-like

371.53 Granular corneal dystrophy

371.54 Lattice corneal dystrophy

371.55 Macular corneal dystrophy

371.56 Other stromal corneal dystrophies
Crystalline corneal dystrophy

371.57 Endothelial corneal dystrophy
Combined corneal dystrophy
Cornea guttata
Fuchs' endothelial dystrophy

371.58 Other posterior corneal dystrophies
Polymorphous corneal dystrophy

√5ᵗʰ **371.6 Keratoconus**
DEF: Bilateral bulging protrusion of anterior cornea; often due to noninflammatory thinning.

371.60 Keratoconus, unspecified

371.61 Keratoconus, stable condition

371.62 Keratoconus, acute hydrops

√5ᵗʰ **371.7 Other corneal deformities**

371.70 Corneal deformity, unspecified

371.71 Corneal ectasia
DEF: Bulging protrusion of thinned, scarred cornea.

371.72 Descemetocele
DEF: Protrusion of Descemet's membrane into cornea.

371.73 Corneal staphyloma
DEF: Protrusion of cornea into adjacent tissue.

√5ᵗʰ **371.8 Other corneal disorders**

371.81 Corneal anesthesia and hypoesthesia
DEF: Decreased or absent sensitivity of cornea.

371.82 Corneal disorder due to contact lens
EXCLUDES corneal edema due to contact lens (371.24)
DEF: Contact lens wear causing cornea disorder, excluding swelling.

371.89 Other
AHA: 3Q, '99, 12

371.9 Unspecified corneal disorder

√4ᵗʰ **372 Disorders of conjunctiva**
EXCLUDES keratoconjunctivitis (370.3-370.4)

√5ᵗʰ **372.0 Acute conjunctivitis**

372.00 Acute conjunctivitis, unspecified

372.01 Serous conjunctivitis, except viral
EXCLUDES viral conjunctivitis NOS (077.9)
AHA: 3Q, '08, 6

372.02 Acute follicular conjunctivitis
Conjunctival folliculosis NOS
EXCLUDES conjunctivitis:
adenoviral (acute follicular) (077.3)
epidemic hemorrhagic (077.4)
inclusion (077.0)
Newcastle (077.8)
epidemic keratoconjunctivitis (077.1)
pharyngoconjunctival fever (077.2)
DEF: Severe conjunctival inflammation with dense infiltrations of lymphoid tissues of inner eyelids; may be traced to a viral or chlamydial etiology.

√4ᵗʰ
√5ᵗʰ Additional Digit Required　　Unspecified Code　　Other Specified Code　　Manifestation Code　　▶◀ Revised Text　　● New Code　　▲ Revised Code Title

Diseases of the Nervous System and Sense Organs

372.03–373.11

372.03 Other mucopurulent conjunctivitis
Catarrhal conjunctivitis
EXCLUDES   *blennorrhea neonatorum (gonococcal)*
(098.40)
neonatal conjunctivitis(771.6)
ophthalmia neonatorum NOS (771.6)

372.04 Pseudomembranous conjunctivitis
Membranous conjunctivitis
EXCLUDES   *diphtheritic conjunctivitis (032.81)*
DEF: Severe inflammation of conjunctiva; false membrane
develops on inner surface of eyelid; membrane can be
removed without harming epithelium, due to bacterial
infections, toxic and allergic factors, and viral infections.

372.05 Acute atopic conjunctivitis
DEF: Sudden, severe conjunctivitis due to allergens.

372.06 Acute chemical conjunctivitis
Acute toxic conjunctivitis
Use additional E code to identify the chemical or toxic
agent
EXCLUDES   *burn of eye and adnexa (940.0-940.9)*
chemical corrosion injury of eye
(940.2-940.3)
AHA: ▶4Q, '09, 85◀

✓5ᵗʰ 372.1 Chronic conjunctivitis

372.10 Chronic conjunctivitis, unspecified

372.11 Simple chronic conjunctivitis

372.12 Chronic follicular conjunctivitis
DEF: Persistent conjunctival inflammation with dense,
localized infiltrations of lymphoid tissues of inner eyelids.

372.13 Vernal conjunctivitis
AHA: 3Q, '96, 8

372.14 Other chronic allergic conjunctivitis
AHA: 3Q, '96, 8

372.15 Parasitic conjunctivitis
Code first underlying disease, as:
filariasis (125.0-125.9)
mucocutaneous leishmaniasis (085.5)

✓5ᵗʰ 372.2 Blepharoconjunctivitis

372.20 Blepharoconjunctivitis, unspecified

372.21 Angular blepharoconjunctivitis
DEF: Inflammation at junction of upper and lower eyelids;
may block lacrimal secretions.

372.22 Contact blepharoconjunctivitis

✓5ᵗʰ 372.3 Other and unspecified conjunctivitis

372.30 Conjunctivitis, unspecified
H10.9 Unspecified conjunctivitis   I-10

372.31 Rosacea conjunctivitis
Code first underlying rosacea dermatitis (695.3)

372.33 Conjunctivitis in mucocutaneous disease
Code first underlying disease, as:
erythema multiforme (695.10-695.19)
Reiter's disease (099.3)
EXCLUDES   *ocular pemphigoid (694.61)*

372.34 Pingueculitis
EXCLUDES   *pinguecula (372.51)*
AHA: 4Q, '08, 112-113

372.39 Other
AHA: 2Q, '07, 9

✓5ᵗʰ 372.4 Pterygium
EXCLUDES   *pseudopterygium (372.52)*
DEF: Wedge-shaped, conjunctival thickening that advances from the
inner corner of the eye toward the cornea.

372.40 Pterygium, unspecified

372.41 Peripheral pterygium, stationary

372.42 Peripheral pterygium, progressive

372.43 Central pterygium

372.44 Double pterygium

372.45 Recurrent pterygium

✓5ᵗʰ 372.5 Conjunctival degenerations and deposits

372.50 Conjunctival degeneration, unspecified

372.51 Pinguecula
EXCLUDES   *pingueculitis (372.34)*
DEF: Proliferative spot on the bulbar conjunctiva located
near the sclerocorneal junction, usually on the nasal side; it
is seen in elderly people.

372.52 Pseudopterygium
DEF: Conjunctival scar joined to the cornea; it looks like a
pterygium but is not attached to the tissue.

372.53 Conjunctival xerosis
EXCLUDES   *conjunctival xerosis due to vitamin A*
deficiency (264.0, 264.1, 264.7)
DEF: Dry conjunctiva due to vitamin A deficiency; related to
Bitot's spots; may develop into xerophthalmia and
keratomalacia.

372.54 Conjunctival concretions
DEF: Calculus or deposit on conjunctiva.

372.55 Conjunctival pigmentations
Conjunctival argyrosis
DEF: Color deposits in conjunctiva.

372.56 Conjunctival deposits

✓5ᵗʰ 372.6 Conjunctival scars

372.61 Granuloma of conjunctiva

372.62 Localized adhesions and strands of conjunctiva
DEF: Abnormal fibrous connections in conjunctiva.

372.63 Symblepharon
Extensive adhesions of conjunctiva
DEF: Adhesion of the eyelids to the eyeball.

372.64 Scarring of conjunctiva
Contraction of eye socket (after enucleation)

✓5ᵗʰ 372.7 Conjunctival vascular disorders and cysts

372.71 Hyperemia of conjunctiva
DEF: Conjunctival blood vessel congestion causing eye
redness.

372.72 Conjunctival hemorrhage
Hyposphagma Subconjunctival hemorrhage

372.73 Conjunctival edema
Chemosis of conjunctiva
Subconjunctival edema
DEF: Fluid retention and swelling in conjunctival tissue.

372.74 Vascular abnormalities of conjunctiva
Aneurysm(ata) of conjunctiva

372.75 Conjunctival cysts
DEF: Abnormal sacs of fluid in conjunctiva.

✓5ᵗʰ 372.8 Other disorders of conjunctiva

372.81 Conjunctivochalasis
DEF: Bilateral condition of redundant conjunctival tissue
between globe and lower eyelid margin; may cover lower
punctum, interfering with normal tearing.
AHA: 4Q, '00, 41

372.89 Other disorders of conjunctiva

372.9 Unspecified disorder of conjunctiva

✓4ᵗʰ 373 Inflammation of eyelids

✓5ᵗʰ 373.0 Blepharitis
EXCLUDES   *blepharoconjunctivitis (372.20-372.22)*

373.00 Blepharitis, unspecified

373.01 Ulcerative blepharitis

373.02 Squamous blepharitis

✓5ᵗʰ 373.1 Hordeolum and other deep inflammation of eyelid
DEF: Purulent, localized, staphylococcal infection in sebaceous
glands of eyelids.

373.11 Hordeolum externum
Hordeolum NOS   Stye
DEF: Infection of the oil glands in the eyelash follicles.

Ⓝ Newborn Age: 0   Ⓟ Pediatric Age: 0-17   Ⓜ Maternity Age: 12-55   Ⓐ Adult Age: 15-124

373.12 Hordeolum internum
  Infection of meibomian gland
  DEF: Infection of the oil gland of the eyelid margin.

373.13 Abscess of eyelid
  Furuncle of eyelid
  DEF: Inflamed pocket of pus on the eyelid.

373.2 Chalazion
  Meibomian (gland) cyst
  EXCLUDES *infected meibomian gland (373.12)*
  DEF: Chronic inflammation of the meibomian gland, causing an eyelid mass.

√5ᵗʰ **373.3 Noninfectious dermatoses of eyelid**

  373.31 Eczematous dermatitis of eyelid

  373.32 Contact and allergic dermatitis of eyelid

  373.33 Xeroderma of eyelid

  373.34 Discoid lupus erythematosus of eyelid

373.4 *Infective dermatitis of eyelid of types resulting in deformity*
  Code first underlying disease, as:
  leprosy (030.0-030.9)
  lupus vulgaris (tuberculous) (017.0)
  yaws (102.0-102.9)

373.5 *Other infective dermatitis of eyelid*
  Code first underlying disease, as:
  actinomycosis (039.3)
  impetigo (684)
  mycotic dermatitis (110.0-111.9)
  vaccinia (051.0)
    postvaccination (999.0)
  EXCLUDES *herpes:*
      simplex (054.41)
      zoster (053.20)

373.6 *Parasitic infestation of eyelid*
  Code first underlying disease, as:
  leishmaniasis (085.0-085.9)
  loiasis (125.2)
  onchocerciasis (125.3)
  pediculosis (132.0)

373.8 Other inflammations of eyelids

373.9 Unspecified inflammation of eyelid

√4ᵗʰ **374 Other disorders of eyelids**

√5ᵗʰ **374.0 Entropion and trichiasis of eyelid**
  DEF: Entropion: turning inward of eyelid edge toward eyeball.
  DEF: Trichiasis: ingrowing eyelashes marked by irritation with possible distortion of sight.

  374.00 Entropion, unspecified

  374.01 Senile entropion   Ⓐ

  374.02 Mechanical entropion

  374.03 Spastic entropion

  374.04 Cicatricial entropion

  374.05 Trichiasis without entropion

√5ᵗʰ **374.1 Ectropion**
  DEF: Turning outward (eversion) of eyelid edge; exposes palpebral conjunctiva; dryness irritation result.

  374.10 Ectropion, unspecified

  374.11 Senile ectropion   Ⓐ

  374.12 Mechanical ectropion

  374.13 Spastic ectropion

  374.14 Cicatricial ectropion

√5ᵗʰ **374.2 Lagophthalmos**
  DEF: Incomplete closure of eyes; causes dry eye and other complications.

  374.20 Lagophthalmos, unspecified

  374.21 Paralytic lagophthalmos

  374.22 Mechanical lagophthalmos

  374.23 Cicatricial lagophthalmos

Entropion and Ectropion

Normal eyelashes   Entropion   Ectropion

√5ᵗʰ **374.3 Ptosis of eyelid**

  374.30 Ptosis of eyelid, unspecified
    AHA: 2Q, '96, 11

  374.31 Paralytic ptosis
    DEF: Drooping of upper eyelid due to nerve disorder.

  374.32 Myogenic ptosis
    DEF: Drooping of upper eyelid due to muscle disorder.

  374.33 Mechanical ptosis
    DEF: Outside force causes drooping of upper eyelid.

  374.34 Blepharochalasis
    Pseudoptosis
    DEF: Loss of elasticity, thickened or indurated skin of eyelids associated with recurrent episodes of idiopathic edema causing intracellular tissue atrophy.

√5ᵗʰ **374.4 Other disorders affecting eyelid function**
  EXCLUDES *blepharoclonus (333.81)*
      blepharospasm (333.81)
      facial nerve palsy (351.0)
      third nerve palsy or paralysis (378.51-378.52)
      tic (psychogenic) (307.20-307.23)
        organic (333.3)

  374.41 Lid retraction or lag

  374.43 Abnormal innervation syndrome
    Jaw-blinking
    Paradoxical facial movements

  374.44 Sensory disorders

  374.45 Other sensorimotor disorders
    Deficient blink reflex

  374.46 Blepharophimosis
    Ankyloblepharon
    DEF: Narrowing of palpebral fissure horizontally; caused by laterally displaced inner canthi; either acquired or congenital.

√5ᵗʰ **374.5 Degenerative disorders of eyelid and periocular area**

  374.50 Degenerative disorder of eyelid, unspecified

  *374.51 **Xanthelasma***
    Xanthoma (planum) (tuberosum) of eyelid
    Code first underlying condition (272.0-272.9)
    DEF: Fatty tumors of the eyelid linked to high fat content of blood.

  374.52 Hyperpigmentation of eyelid
    Chloasma
    Dyspigmentation
    DEF: Excess pigment of eyelid.

  374.53 Hypopigmentation of eyelid
    Vitiligo of eyelid
    DEF: Lack of color pigment of the eyelid.

  374.54 Hypertrichosis of eyelid
    DEF: Excessive eyelash growth.

  374.55 Hypotrichosis of eyelid
    Madarosis of eyelid
    DEF: Less than normal, or absent, eyelashes.

  374.56 Other degenerative disorders of skin affecting eyelid

Diseases of the Nervous System and Sense Organs

374.8–376.12

✓5ᵗʰ **374.8 Other disorders of eyelid**

374.81 Hemorrhage of eyelid
EXCLUDES *black eye (921.0)*

374.82 Edema of eyelid
Hyperemia of eyelid
DEF: Swelling and fluid retention in eyelid.
AHA: 4Q, '08, 131

374.83 Elephantiasis of eyelid
DEF: Filarial disease causing dermatitis and enlargement of eyelid.

374.84 Cysts of eyelids
Sebaceous cyst of eyelid

374.85 Vascular anomalies of eyelid

374.86 Retained foreign body of eyelid
▶Use additional code to identify foreign body (V90.01-V90.9)◀

374.87 Dermatochalasis
DEF: Acquired form of connective tissue disorder associated with decreased elastic tissue and abnormal elastin formation resulting in loss of elasticity of the skin of the eyelid, generally associated with aging.

374.89 Other disorders of eyelid

374.9 Unspecified disorder of eyelid

✓4ᵗʰ **375 Disorders of lacrimal system**

✓5ᵗʰ **375.0 Dacryoadenitis**

375.00 Dacryoadenitis, unspecified

375.01 Acute dacryoadenitis
DEF: Severe, sudden inflammation of the lacrimal gland.

375.02 Chronic dacryoadenitis
DEF: Persistent inflammation of the lacrimal gland.

375.03 Chronic enlargement of lacrimal gland

✓5ᵗʰ **375.1 Other disorders of lacrimal gland**

375.11 Dacryops
DEF: Overproduction and constant flow of tears; may cause distended lacrimal duct.

375.12 Other lacrimal cysts and cystic degeneration

375.13 Primary lacrimal atrophy

375.14 Secondary lacrimal atrophy
DEF: Wasting away of the lacrimal gland due to another disease.

375.15 Tear film insufficiency, unspecified
Dry eye syndrome
AHA: 3Q, '96, 6
DEF: Eye dryness and irritation from insufficient tear production.

375.16 Dislocation of lacrimal gland

✓5ᵗʰ **375.2 Epiphora**
DEF: Abnormal development of tears due to stricture of lacrimal passages.

375.20 Epiphora, unspecified as to cause

375.21 Epiphora due to excess lacrimation
DEF: Tear overflow due to overproduction.

375.22 Epiphora due to insufficient drainage
DEF: Tear overflow due to blocked drainage.

✓5ᵗʰ **375.3 Acute and unspecified inflammation of lacrimal passages**
EXCLUDES *neonatal dacryocystitis (771.6)*

375.30 Dacryocystitis, unspecified

375.31 Acute canaliculitis, lacrimal

375.32 Acute dacryocystitis
Acute pericdacryocystitis

375.33 Phlegmonous dacryocystitis
DEF: Infection of the tear sac with pockets of pus.

Lacrimal System

Superior and inferior lobes of lacrimal gland
Medial angle
Lacrimal ducts
Lacrimal canaliculi
Nasolacrimal sac
Lacrimal caruncle
Superior, inferior lacrimal puncta
Left eye

✓5ᵗʰ **375.4 Chronic inflammation of lacrimal passages**

375.41 Chronic canaliculitis

375.42 Chronic dacryocystitis

375.43 Lacrimal mucocele

✓5ᵗʰ **375.5 Stenosis and insufficiency of lacrimal passages**

375.51 Eversion of lacrimal punctum
DEF: Abnormal turning outward of the tear duct.

375.52 Stenosis of lacrimal punctum
DEF: Abnormal narrowing of the tear duct.

375.53 Stenosis of lacrimal canaliculi

375.54 Stenosis of lacrimal sac
DEF: Abnormal narrowing of the tear sac.

375.55 Obstruction of nasolacrimal duct, neonatal
EXCLUDES *congenital anomaly of nasola- crimal duct (743.65)*
DEF: Acquired, abnormal obstruction of tear drainage system from the eye to the nose; in an infant.

375.56 Stenosis of nasolacrimal duct, acquired

375.57 Dacryolith
DEF: Concretion or stone anywhere in lacrimal system.

✓5ᵗʰ **375.6 Other changes of lacrimal passages**

375.61 Lacrimal fistula
DEF: Abnormal communication from the lacrimal system.

375.69 Other

✓5ᵗʰ **375.8 Other disorders of lacrimal system**

375.81 Granuloma of lacrimal passages
DEF: Abnormal nodules within lacrimal system.

375.89 Other

375.9 Unspecified disorder of lacrimal system

✓4ᵗʰ **376 Disorders of the orbit**

✓5ᵗʰ **376.0 Acute inflammation of orbit**

376.00 Acute inflammation of orbit, unspecified

376.01 Orbital cellulitis
Abscess of orbit
DEF: Infection of tissue between the orbital bone and eyeball.

376.02 Orbital periostitis
DEF: Inflammation of connective tissue covering the orbital bone.

376.03 Orbital osteomyelitis
DEF: Inflammation of the orbital bone.

376.04 Tenonitis

✓5ᵗʰ **376.1 Chronic inflammatory disorders of orbit**

376.10 Chronic inflammation of orbit, unspecified

376.11 Orbital granuloma
Pseudotumor (inflammatory) of orbit
DEF: Abnormal nodule between orbital bone and eyeball.

376.12 Orbital myositis
DEF: Painful inflammation of the muscles of the eye.

376.13 *Parasitic infestation of orbit*
  Code first underlying disease, as:
    hydatid infestation of orbit (122.3, 122.6, 122.9)
    myiasis of orbit (134.0)

✓5ᵗʰ **376.2 Endocrine exophthalmos**
  Code first underlying thyroid disorder (242.0-242.9)

  376.21 *Thyrotoxic exophthalmos*
    DEF: Painful inflammation of eye muscles.

  376.22 *Exophthalmic ophthalmoplegia*
    DEF: Inability to rotate eye as a result of bulging eyes.

✓5ᵗʰ **376.3 Other exophthalmic conditions**

  376.30 **Exophthalmos, unspecified**
    DEF: Abnormal protrusion of eyeball.

  376.31 **Constant exophthalmos**
    DEF: Continuous, abnormal protrusion or bulging of eyeball.

  376.32 **Orbital hemorrhage**
    DEF: Bleeding behind the eyeball, causing it to bulge forward.

  376.33 **Orbital edema or congestion**
    DEF: Fluid retention behind eyeball, causing forward bulge.

  376.34 **Intermittent exophthalmos**

  376.35 **Pulsating exophthalmos**
    DEF: Bulge or protrusion; associated with a carotid-cavernous fistula.

  376.36 **Lateral displacement of globe**
    DEF: Abnormal displacement of the eyeball away from nose, toward temple.

✓5ᵗʰ **376.4 Deformity of orbit**

  376.40 **Deformity of orbit, unspecified**

  376.41 **Hypertelorism of orbit**
    DEF: Abnormal increase in interorbital distance; associated with congenital facial deformities; may be accompanied by mental deficiency.

  376.42 **Exostosis of orbit**
    DEF: Abnormal bony growth of orbit.

  376.43 **Local deformities due to bone disease**
    DEF: Acquired abnormalities of orbit; due to bone disease.

  376.44 **Orbital deformities associated with craniofacial deformities**

  376.45 **Atrophy of orbit**
    DEF: Wasting away of bone tissue of orbit.

  376.46 **Enlargement of orbit**

  376.47 **Deformity due to trauma or surgery**

✓5ᵗʰ **376.5 Enophthalmos**
  DEF: Recession of eyeball deep into eye socket.

  376.50 **Enophthalmos, unspecified as to cause**

  376.51 **Enophthalmos due to atrophy of orbital tissue**

  376.52 **Enophthalmos due to trauma or surgery**

376.6 **Retained (old) foreign body following penetrating wound of orbit**
  Retrobulbar foreign body
  ▶Use additional code to identify foreign body (V90.01-V90.9)◀

✓5ᵗʰ **376.8 Other orbital disorders**

  376.81 **Orbital cysts**
    Encephalocele of orbit
    AHA: 3Q, '99, 13

  376.82 **Myopathy of extraocular muscles**
    DEF: Disease in the muscles that control eyeball movement.

  376.89 **Other**

376.9 **Unspecified disorder of orbit**

✓4ᵗʰ **377 Disorders of optic nerve and visual pathways**

✓5ᵗʰ **377.0 Papilledema**

  377.00 **Papilledema, unspecified**

  377.01 **Papilledema associated with increased intracranial pressure**

  377.02 **Papilledema associated with decreased ocular pressure**

  377.03 **Papilledema associated with retinal disorder**

  377.04 **Foster-Kennedy syndrome**
    DEF: Retrobulbar optic neuritis, central scotoma and optic atrophy; caused by tumors in frontal lobe of brain that press downward.

✓5ᵗʰ **377.1 Optic atrophy**

  377.10 **Optic atrophy, unspecified**

  377.11 **Primary optic atrophy**
    EXCLUDES *neurosyphilitic optic atrophy (094.84)*

  377.12 **Postinflammatory optic atrophy**
    DEF: Adverse effect of inflammation causing wasting away of eye.

  377.13 **Optic atrophy associated with retinal dystrophies**
    DEF: Progressive changes in retinal tissue due to metabolic disorder causing wasting away of eye.

  377.14 **Glaucomatous atrophy [cupping] of optic disc**

  377.15 **Partial optic atrophy**
    Temporal pallor of optic disc

  377.16 **Hereditary optic atrophy**
    Optic atrophy:
      dominant hereditary
      Leber's

✓5ᵗʰ **377.2 Other disorders of optic disc**

  377.21 **Drusen of optic disc**

  377.22 **Crater-like holes of optic disc**

  377.23 **Coloboma of optic disc**
    DEF: Ocular malformation caused by the failure of fetal fissure of optic stalk to close.

  377.24 **Pseudopapilledema**

✓5ᵗʰ **377.3 Optic neuritis**
  EXCLUDES *meningococcal optic neuritis (036.81)*

  377.30 **Optic neuritis, unspecified**

  377.31 **Optic papillitis**
    DEF: Swelling and inflammation of the optic disc.

  377.32 **Retrobulbar neuritis (acute)**
    EXCLUDES *syphilitic retrobulbar neuritis (094.85)*
    DEF: Inflammation of optic nerve immediately behind the eyeball.

  377.33 **Nutritional optic neuropathy**
    DEF: Malnutrition causing optic nerve disorder.

  377.34 **Toxic optic neuropathy**
    Toxic amblyopia
    DEF: Toxic substance causing optic nerve disorder.

  377.39 **Other**
    EXCLUDES *ischemic optic neuropathy (377.41)*

✓5ᵗʰ **377.4 Other disorders of optic nerve**

  377.41 **Ischemic optic neuropathy**
    DEF: Decreased blood flow affecting optic nerve.

  377.42 **Hemorrhage in optic nerve sheaths**
    DEF: Bleeding in meningeal lining of optic nerve.

  377.43 **Optic nerve hypoplasia**
    AHA: 4Q, '06, 81

  377.49 **Other**
    Compression of optic nerve

✓5ᵗʰ **377.5 Disorders of optic chiasm**

  377.51 **Associated with pituitary neoplasms and disorders**
    DEF: Abnormal pituitary growth causing disruption in nerve chain from retina to brain.

  377.52 **Associated with other neoplasms**
    DEF: Abnormal growth, other than pituitary, causing disruption in nerve chain from retina to brain.

  377.53 **Associated with vascular disorders**
    DEF: Vascular disorder causing disruption in nerve chain from retina to brain.

✓4ᵗʰ
✓5ᵗʰ Additional Digit Required   Unspecified Code   Other Specified Code   Manifestation Code   ▶◀ Revised Text   ● New Code   ▲ Revised Code Title

Diseases of the Nervous System and Sense Organs

377.54–378.61

377.54 Associated with inflammatory disorders
DEF: Inflammatory disease causing disruption in nerve chain from retina to brain.

√5th **377.6 Disorders of other visual pathways**

377.61 Associated with neoplasms

377.62 Associated with vascular disorders

377.63 Associated with inflammatory disorders

√5th **377.7 Disorders of visual cortex**
EXCLUDES visual:
agnosia (368.16)
hallucinations (368.16)
halos (368.15)

377.71 Associated with neoplasms

377.72 Associated with vascular disorders

377.73 Associated with inflammatory

377.75 Cortical blindness
DEF: Blindness due to brain disorder, rather than eye disorder.

377.9 Unspecified disorder of optic nerve and visual pathways

√4th **378 Strabismus and other disorders of binocular eye movements**
EXCLUDES nystagmus and other irregular eye movements (379.50-379.59)
DEF: Misalignment of the eyes due to imbalance in extraocular muscles.

√5th **378.0 Esotropia**
Convergent concomitant strabismus
EXCLUDES intermittent esotropia (378.20-378.22)
DEF: Visual axis deviation created by one eye fixing upon an image and the other eye deviating inward.

378.00 Esotropia, unspecified

378.01 Monocular esotropia

378.02 Monocular esotropia with A pattern

378.03 Monocular esotropia with V pattern

378.04 Monocular esotropia with other noncomitancies
Monocular esotropia with X or Y pattern

378.05 Alternating esotropia

378.06 Alternating esotropia with A pattern

378.07 Alternating esotropia with V pattern

378.08 Alternating esotropia with other noncomitancies
Alternating esotropia with X or Y pattern

√5th **378.1 Exotropia**
Divergent concomitant strabismus
EXCLUDES intermittent exotropia (378.20, 378.23-378.24)
DEF: Visual axis deviation created by one eye fixing upon an image and the other eye deviating outward.

378.10 Exotropia, unspecified

378.11 Monocular exotropia

378.12 Monocular exotropia with A pattern

378.13 Monocular exotropia with V pattern

378.14 Monocular exotropia with other noncomitancies
Monocular exotropia with X or Y pattern

378.15 Alternating exotropia

378.16 Alternating exotropia with A pattern

378.17 Alternating exotropia with V pattern

378.18 Alternating exotropia with other noncomitancies
Alternating exotropia with X or Y pattern

Eye Musculature

Superior rectus
Superior oblique
Lateral rectus
Medial rectus
Inferior oblique
Inferior rectus
Muscles and actions (right eye)

R.   L.
Monocular (one eye only) esotropia (inward)

Monocular exotropia (outward)

Monocular hypertropia (upward)

√5th **378.2 Intermittent heterotropia**
EXCLUDES vertical heterotropia (intermittent) (378.31)
DEF: Deviation of eyes seen only at intervals; it is also called strabismus.

378.20 Intermittent heterotropia, unspecified
Intermittent: Intermittent:
esotropia NOS   exotropia NOS

378.21 Intermittent esotropia, monocular

378.22 Intermittent esotropia, alternating

378.23 Intermittent exotropia, monocular

378.24 Intermittent exotropia, alternating

√5th **378.3 Other and unspecified heterotropia**

378.30 Heterotropia, unspecified

378.31 Hypertropia
Vertical heterotropia (constant) (intermittent)

378.32 Hypotropia

378.33 Cyclotropia

378.34 Monofixation syndrome
Microtropia

378.35 Accommodative component in esotropia

√5th **378.4 Heterophoria**
DEF: Deviation occurring only when the other eye is covered.

378.40 Heterophoria, unspecified

378.41 Esophoria

378.42 Exophoria

378.43 Vertical heterophoria

378.44 Cyclophoria

378.45 Alternating hyperphoria

√5th **378.5 Paralytic strabismus**
DEF: Deviation of the eye due to nerve paralysis affecting muscle.

378.50 Paralytic strabismus, unspecified

378.51 Third or oculomotor nerve palsy, partial
AHA: 3Q, '91, 9

378.52 Third or oculomotor nerve palsy, total
AHA: 2Q, '89, 12

378.53 Fourth or trochlear nerve palsy
AHA: 2Q, '01, 21

378.54 Sixth or abducens nerve palsy
AHA: 2Q, '89, 12

378.55 External ophthalmoplegia

378.56 Total ophthalmoplegia

√5th **378.6 Mechanical strabismus**
DEF: Deviation of the eye due to an outside force upon the extraocular muscles.

378.60 Mechanical strabismus, unspecified

378.61 Brown's (tendon) sheath syndrome
DEF: Congenital or acquired shortening of the anterior sheath of superior oblique muscle; eye is unable to move upward and inward; usually unilateral.

N Newborn Age: 0   P Pediatric Age: 0-17   M Maternity Age: 12-55   A Adult Age: 15-124

378.62 Mechanical strabismus from other musculofascial disorders

378.63 Limited duction associated with other conditions

√5ᵗʰ **378.7 Other specified strabismus**

  378.71 Duane's syndrome
DEF: Congenital, affects one eye; due to abnormal fibrous bands attached to rectus muscle; inability to abduct affected eye with retraction of globe.

  378.72 Progressive external ophthalmoplegia
DEF: Paralysis progressing from one eye muscle to another.

  378.73 Strabismus in other neuromuscular disorders

√5ᵗʰ **378.8 Other disorders of binocular eye movements**
EXCLUDES nystagmus (379.50-379.56)

  378.81 Palsy of conjugate gaze
DEF: Paralysis progressing from one eye muscle to another.

  378.82 Spasm of conjugate gaze
DEF: Muscle contractions impairing parallel movement of eye.

  378.83 Convergence insufficiency or palsy

  378.84 Convergence excess or spasm

  378.85 Anomalies of divergence

  378.86 Internuclear ophthalmoplegia
DEF: Eye movement anomaly due to brainstem lesion.

  378.87 Other dissociated deviation of eye movements
Skew deviation

378.9 Unspecified disorder of eye movements
Ophthalmoplegia NOS
Strabismus NOS
AHA: 2Q, '01, 21

√4ᵗʰ **379 Other disorders of eye**

√5ᵗʰ **379.0 Scleritis and episcleritis**
EXCLUDES syphilitic episcleritis (095.0)

  379.00 Scleritis, unspecified
Episcleritis NOS

  379.01 Episcleritis periodica fugax
DEF: Hyperemia (engorgement) of the sclera and overlying conjunctiva characterized by a sudden onset and short duration.

  379.02 Nodular episcleritis
DEF: Inflammation of the outermost layer of the sclera, with formation of nodules.

  379.03 Anterior scleritis

  379.04 Scleromalacia perforans
DEF: Scleral thinning, softening and degeneration; seen with rheumatoid arthritis.

  379.05 Scleritis with corneal involvement
Scleroperikeratitis

  379.06 Brawny scleritis
DEF: Severe scleral inflammation with thickening corneal margins.

  379.07 Posterior scleritis
Sclerotenonitis

  379.09 Other
Scleral abscess

√5ᵗʰ **379.1 Other disorders of sclera**
EXCLUDES blue sclera (743.47)

  379.11 Scleral ectasia
Scleral staphyloma NOS
DEF: Protrusion of the contents of the eyeball where the sclera has thinned.

  379.12 Staphyloma posticum
DEF: Ring-shaped protrusion or bulging of sclera and uveal tissue at posterior pole of eye.

  379.13 Equatorial staphyloma
DEF: Ring-shaped protrusion or bulging of sclera and uveal tissue midway between front and back of eye.

  379.14 Anterior staphyloma, localized

  379.15 Ring staphyloma

  379.16 Other degenerative disorders of sclera

  379.19 Other

√5ᵗʰ **379.2 Disorders of vitreous body**
DEF: Disorder of clear gel that fills space between retina and lens.

  379.21 Vitreous degeneration
Vitreous:
cavitation
detachment
liquefaction

  379.22 Crystalline deposits in vitreous
Asteroid hyalitis
Synchysis scintillans

  379.23 Vitreous hemorrhage
AHA: 3Q, '91, 15

  379.24 Other vitreous opacities
Vitreous floaters

  379.25 Vitreous membranes and strands

  379.26 Vitreous prolapse
DEF: Slipping of vitreous from normal position.

  379.29 Other disorders of vitreous
EXCLUDES vitreous abscess (360.04)
AHA: 1Q, '99, 11

√5ᵗʰ **379.3 Aphakia and other disorders of lens**
EXCLUDES after-cataract (366.50-366.53)

  379.31 Aphakia
EXCLUDES cataract extraction status (V45.61)
DEF: Absence of eye's crystalline lens.

  379.32 Subluxation of lens

  379.33 Anterior dislocation of lens
DEF: Lens displaced toward iris.

  379.34 Posterior dislocation of lens
DEF: Lens displaced backward toward vitreous.

  379.39 Other disorders of lens

√5ᵗʰ **379.4 Anomalies of pupillary function**

  379.40 Abnormal pupillary function, unspecified

  379.41 Anisocoria
DEF: Unequal pupil diameter.

  379.42 Miosis (persistent), not due to miotics
DEF: Abnormal contraction of pupil less than 2 mil.

  379.43 Mydriasis (persistent), not due to mydriatics
DEF: Morbid dilation of pupil.

  379.45 Argyll Robertson pupil, atypical
Argyll Robertson phenomenon or pupil, nonsyphilitic
EXCLUDES Argyll Robertson pupil (syphilitic) (094.89)
DEF: Failure of pupil to respond to light; affects both eyes; may be caused by diseases such as syphilis of the central nervous system or miosis.

  379.46 Tonic pupillary reaction
Adie's pupil or syndrome

  379.49 Other
Hippus   Pupillary paralysis

√5ᵗʰ **379.5 Nystagmus and other irregular eye movements**

  379.50 Nystagmus, unspecified
DEF: Involuntary, rapid, rhythmic movement of eyeball; vertical, horizontal, rotatory or mixed; cause may be congenital, acquired, physiological, neurological, myopathic, or due to ocular diseases.
AHA: 4Q, '02, 68; 2Q, '01, 21

  379.51 Congenital nystagmus

  379.52 Latent nystagmus

  379.53 Visual deprivation nystagmus

  379.54 Nystagmus associated with disorders of the vestibular system

  379.55 Dissociated nystagmus

379.56 Other forms of nystagmus

379.57 Deficiencies of saccadic eye movements
Abnormal optokinetic response
DEF: Saccadic eye movements; small, rapid, involuntary movements by both eyes simultaneously, due to changing point of fixation on visualized object.

379.58 Deficiencies of smooth pursuit movements

379.59 Other irregularities of eye movements
Opsoclonus

√5ᵗʰ **379.6 Inflammation (infection) of postprocedural bleb**
Postprocedural blebitis

379.60 Inflammation (infection) of postprocedural bleb, unspecified
AHA: 4Q, '06, 82

379.61 Inflammation (infection) of postprocedural bleb, stage 1
AHA: 4Q, '06, 82

379.62 Inflammation (infection) of postprocedural bleb, stage 2
AHA: 4Q, '06, 82

379.63 Inflammation (infection) of postprocedural bleb, stage 3
Bleb associated endophthalmitis
AHA: 4Q, '06, 82

379.8 Other specified disorders of eye and adnexa

√5ᵗʰ **379.9 Unspecified disorder of eye and adnexa**

379.90 Disorder of eye, unspecified

379.91 Pain in or around eye

379.92 Swelling or mass of eye

379.93 Redness or discharge of eye

379.99 Other ill-defined disorders of eye
EXCLUDES *blurred vision NOS (368.8)*

Diseases of the Ear and Mastoid Process (380-389)

Use additional external cause code, if applicable, to identify the cause of the ear condition

√4ᵗʰ **380 Disorders of external ear**

√5ᵗʰ **380.0 Perichondritis and chondritis of pinna**
Chondritis of auricle   Perichondritis of auricle

380.00 Perichondritis of pinna, unspecified

380.01 Acute perichondritis of pinna

380.02 Chronic perichondritis of pinna

380.03 Chondritis of pinna
DEF: Infection that has progressed into the cartilage; presents as indurated and edematous skin over the pinna; vascular compromise occurs with tissue necrosis and deformity.
AHA: 4Q, '04, 76

√5ᵗʰ **380.1 Infective otitis externa**

380.10 Infective otitis externa, unspecified
Otitis externa (acute):
    NOS
    circumscribed
    diffuse
    hemorrhagica
    infective NOS

380.11 Acute infection of pinna
EXCLUDES *furuncular otitis externa (680.0)*

380.12 Acute swimmers' ear
Beach ear
Tank ear
DEF: Otitis externa due to swimming.

Ear and Mastoid Process

Helix, Antihelix, Concha, Mastoid process, External auditory meatus, Tragus, Antitragus

380.13 Other acute infections of external ear
Code first underlying disease, as:
    erysipelas (035)
    impetigo (684)
    seborrheic dermatitis (690.10-690.18)
EXCLUDES *herpes simplex (054.73)*
      herpes zoster (053.71)

380.14 Malignant otitis externa
DEF: Severe necrotic otitis externa; due to bacteria.

380.15 Chronic mycotic otitis externa
Code first underlying disease, as:
    aspergillosis (117.3)
    otomycosis NOS (111.9)
EXCLUDES *candidal otitis externa (112.82)*

380.16 Other chronic infective otitis externa
Chronic infective otitis externa NOS

√5ᵗʰ **380.2 Other otitis externa**

380.21 Cholesteatoma of external ear
Keratosis obturans of external ear (canal)
EXCLUDES *cholesteatoma NOS (385.30-385.35)*
      postmastoidectomy (383.32)
DEF: Cystlike mass filled with debris, including cholesterol; rare, congenital condition.

380.22 Other acute otitis externa
Acute otitis externa:
    actinic
    chemical
    contact
    eczematoid
    reactive

380.23 Other chronic otitis externa
Chronic otitis externa NOS

√5ᵗʰ **380.3 Noninfectious disorders of pinna**

380.30 Disorder of pinna, unspecified

380.31 Hematoma of auricle or pinna

380.32 Acquired deformities of auricle or pinna
EXCLUDES *cauliflower ear (738.7)*
AHA: 3Q, '03, 12

380.39 Other
EXCLUDES *gouty tophi of ear (274.81)*

380.4 Impacted cerumen
Wax in ear

√5ᵗʰ **380.5 Acquired stenosis of external ear canal**
Collapse of external ear canal

380.50 Acquired stenosis of external ear canal, unspecified as to cause

380.51 Secondary to trauma
DEF: Narrowing of the external ear canal; due to trauma.

380.52 Secondary to surgery
DEF: Postsurgical narrowing of the external ear canal.

380.53 Secondary to inflammation
DEF: Narrowing of the external ear canal; due to chronic inflammation.

√5ᵗʰ **380.8 Other disorders of external ear**

380.81 Exostosis of external ear canal

Diseases of the Nervous System and Sense Organs

380.89 Other

380.9 Unspecified disorder of external ear

√4ᵗʰ **381** Nonsuppurative otitis media and Eustachian tube disorders

√5ᵗʰ **381.0** Acute nonsuppurative otitis media
Acute tubotympanic catarrh
Otitis media, acute or subacute:
catarrhal
exudative
transudative
with effusion
EXCLUDES otitic barotrauma (993.0)

381.00 Acute nonsuppurative otitis media, unspecified

381.01 Acute serous otitis media
Acute or subacute secretory otitis media
DEF: Sudden, severe infection of the middle ear.

381.02 Acute mucoid otitis media
Acute or subacute seromucinous otitis media
Blue drum syndrome
DEF: Sudden, severe infection of the middle ear, with mucous.

381.03 Acute sanguinous otitis media
DEF: Sudden, severe infection of the middle ear, with blood.

381.04 Acute allergic serous otitis media

381.05 Acute allergic mucoid otitis media

381.06 Acute allergic sanguinous otitis media

√5ᵗʰ **381.1** Chronic serous otitis media
Chronic tubotympanic catarrh

381.10 Chronic serous otitis media, simple or unspecified
DEF: Persistent infection of the middle ear, without pus.

381.19 Other
Serosanguinous chronic otitis media

√5ᵗʰ **381.2** Chronic mucoid otitis media
Glue ear
EXCLUDES adhesive middle ear disease (385.10-385.19)
DEF: Chronic condition; characterized by viscous fluid in middle ear; due to obstructed Eustachian tube.

381.20 Chronic mucoid otitis media, simple or unspecified

381.29 Other
Mucosanguinous chronic otitis media

381.3 Other and unspecified chronic nonsuppurative otitis media
Otitis media, chronic: Otitis media, chronic:
allergic   seromucinous
exudative   transudative
secretory   with effusion

381.4 Nonsuppurative otitis media, not specified as acute or chronic
Otitis media: Otitis media:
allergic   secretory
catarrhal   seromucinous
exudative   serous
mucoid   transudative
with effusion

√5ᵗʰ **381.5** Eustachian salpingitis

381.50 Eustachian salpingitis, unspecified

381.51 Acute Eustachian salpingitis
DEF: Sudden, severe inflammation of the Eustachian tube.

381.52 Chronic Eustachian salpingitis
DEF: Persistent inflammation of the Eustachian tube.

√5ᵗʰ **381.6** Obstruction of Eustachian tube
Stenosis ⎫
Stricture ⎭ of Eustachian tube

381.60 Obstruction of Eustachian tube, unspecified

381.61 Osseous obstruction of Eustachian tube
Obstruction of Eustachian tube from cholesteatoma, polyp, or other osseous lesion

381.62 Intrinsic cartilaginous obstruction of Eustachian tube
DEF: Blockage of Eustachian tube; due to cartilage overgrowth.

381.63 Extrinsic cartilaginous obstruction of Eustachian tube
Compression of Eustachian tube

381.7 Patulous Eustachian tube
DEF: Distended, oversized Eustachian tube.

√5ᵗʰ **381.8** Other disorders of Eustachian tube

381.81 Dysfunction of Eustachian tube

381.89 Other

381.9 Unspecified Eustachian tube disorder

√4ᵗʰ **382** Suppurative and unspecified otitis media

√5ᵗʰ **382.0** Acute suppurative otitis media
Otitis media, acute: Otitis media, acute:
necrotizing NOS   purulent

382.00 Acute suppurative otitis media without spontaneous rupture of ear drum
DEF: Sudden, severe inflammation of middle ear, with pus.

382.01 Acute suppurative otitis media with spontaneous rupture of ear drum
DEF: Sudden, severe inflammation of middle ear, with pressure tearing ear drum tissue.

382.02 *Acute suppurative otitis media in diseases classified elsewhere*
Code first underlying disease, as:
influenza ▶(487.8, 488.09, 488.19)◀
scarlet fever (034.1)
EXCLUDES postmeasles otitis (055.2)

382.1 Chronic tubotympanic suppurative otitis media
Benign chronic suppurative   ⎫
ottis media   ⎬ (with anterior perforation
Chronic tubotympanic disease ⎭   of ear drum)
DEF: Inflammation of tympanic cavity and auditory tube; with pus formation.

382.2 Chronic atticoantral suppurative otitis media
Chronic atticoantral disease ⎫ (with posterior or superior
Persistent mucosal disease   ⎬   maginal perforation
                                           ⎭   of ear drum)
DEF: Inflammation of upper tympanic membrane and mastoid antrum with pus formation.

382.3 Unspecified chronic suppurative otitis media
Chronic purulent otitis media
EXCLUDES tuberculous otitis media (017.4)

382.4 Unspecified suppurative otitis media
Purulent otitis media NOS

382.9 Unspecified otitis media
Otitis media: Otitis media:
NOS   chronic NOS
acute NOS
AHA: N-D, '84, 16
H66.93 Otitis media unspecified bilateral   I-10

√4ᵗʰ **383** Mastoiditis and related conditions

√5ᵗʰ **383.0** Acute mastoiditis
Abscess of mastoid
Empyema of mastoid

383.00 Acute mastoiditis without complications
DEF: Sudden, severe inflammation of mastoid air cells.

383.01 Subperiosteal abscess of mastoid
DEF: Pocket of pus within the mastoid bone.

383.02 Acute mastoiditis with other complications
Gradenigo's syndrome

383.1 Chronic mastoiditis
Caries of mastoid   Fistula of mastoid
EXCLUDES tuberculous mastoiditis (015.6)
DEF: Persistent inflammation of the mastoid air cells.

380.89–383.1

√4ᵗʰ
√5ᵗʰ Additional Digit Required   Unspecified Code   Other Specified Code   Manifestation Code   ▶◀ Revised Text   ● New Code   ▲ Revised Code Title

Diseases of the Nervous System and Sense Organs

383.2–385.32

✓5ᵗʰ **383.2 Petrositis**

Coalescing osteitis
Inflammation } of petrous bone
Osteomyelitis

383.20 Petrositis, unspecified

383.21 Acute petrositis
DEF: Sudden, severe inflammation of dense bone behind the ear.

383.22 Chronic petrositis
DEF: Persistent inflammation of dense bone behind the ear.

✓5ᵗʰ **383.3 Complications following mastoidectomy**

383.30 Postmastoidectomy complication, unspecified

383.31 Mucosal cyst of postmastoidectomy cavity
DEF: Mucous-lined cyst cavity following removal of mastoid bone.

383.32 Recurrent cholesteatoma of postmastoidectomy cavity
DEF: Cystlike mass of cell debris in cavity following removal of mastoid bone.

383.33 Granulations of postmastoidectomy cavity
Chronic inflammation of postmastoidectomy cavity
DEF: Granular tissue in cavity following removal of mastoid bone.

✓5ᵗʰ **383.8 Other disorders of mastoid**

383.81 Postauricular fistula
DEF: Abnormal passage behind mastoid cavity.

383.89 Other

383.9 Unspecified mastoiditis

✓4ᵗʰ **384 Other disorders of tympanic membrane**

✓5ᵗʰ **384.0 Acute myringitis without mention of otitis media**

384.00 Acute myringitis, unspecified
Acute tympanitis NOS
DEF: Sudden, severe inflammation of ear drum.

384.01 Bullous myringitis
Myringitis bullosa hemorrhagica
DEF: Type of viral otitis media characterized by the appearance of serous or hemorrhagic blebs on the tympanic membrane.

384.09 Other

384.1 Chronic myringitis without mention of otitis media
Chronic tympanitis
DEF: Persistent inflammation of ear drum; with no evidence of middle ear infection.

✓5ᵗʰ **384.2 Perforation of tympanic membrane**
Perforation of ear drum:
NOS
persistent posttraumatic
postinflammatory
EXCLUDES otitis media with perforation of tympanic membrane (382.00-382.9)
traumatic perforation [current injury] (872.61)

384.20 Perforation of tympanic membrane, unspecified

384.21 Central perforation of tympanic membrane

384.22 Attic perforation of tympanic membrane
Pars flaccida

384.23 Other marginal perforation of tympanic membrane

384.24 Multiple perforations of tympanic membrane

384.25 Total perforation of tympanic membrane

✓5ᵗʰ **384.8 Other specified disorders of tympanic membrane**

384.81 Atrophic flaccid tympanic membrane
Healed perforation of ear drum

384.82 Atrophic nonflaccid tympanic membrane

384.9 Unspecified disorder of tympanic membrane

Middle and Inner Ear

Osseous labyrinth
Semicircular canals
Auditory ossicles:
Stapes
Incus
Malleus
Utricle and saccule
CN VIII
Cochlea in bone
External auditory canal
Cochlea (round window)
Eustachian tube
Pharynx

Exposed view of middle and inner ear

✓4ᵗʰ **385 Other disorders of middle ear and mastoid**
EXCLUDES mastoiditis (383.0-383.9)

✓5ᵗʰ **385.0 Tympanosclerosis**

385.00 Tympanosclerosis, unspecified as to involvement

385.01 Tympanosclerosis involving tympanic membrane only
DEF: Tough, fibrous tissue impeding functions of ear drum.

385.02 Tympanosclerosis involving tympanic membrane and ear ossicles
DEF: Tough, fibrous tissue impeding functions of middle ear bones (stapes, malleus, incus).

385.03 Tympanosclerosis involving tympanic membrane, ear ossicles, and middle ear
DEF: Tough, fibrous tissue impeding functions of ear drum, middle ear bones and middle ear canal.

385.09 Tympanosclerosis involving other combination of structures

✓5ᵗʰ **385.1 Adhesive middle ear disease**
Adhesive otitis
Otitis media:
chronic adhesive
fibrotic
EXCLUDES glue ear (381.20-381.29)
DEF: Adhesions of middle ear structures.

385.10 Adhesive middle ear disease, unspecified as to involvement

385.11 Adhesions of drum head to incus

385.12 Adhesions of drum head to stapes

385.13 Adhesions of drum head to promontorium

385.19 Other adhesions and combinations

✓5ᵗʰ **385.2 Other acquired abnormality of ear ossicles**

385.21 Impaired mobility of malleus
Ankylosis of malleus

385.22 Impaired mobility of other ear ossicles
Ankylosis of ear ossicles, except malleus

385.23 Discontinuity or dislocation of ear ossicles
DEF: Disruption in auditory chain; created by malleus, incus and stapes.

385.24 Partial loss or necrosis of ear ossicles
DEF: Tissue loss in malleus, incus and stapes.

✓5ᵗʰ **385.3 Cholesteatoma of middle ear and mastoid**
Cholesterosis
Epidermosis } of (middle) ear
Keratosis
Polyp
EXCLUDES cholesteatoma:
external ear canal (380.21)
recurrent of postmastoidectomy cavity (383.32)
DEF: Cystlike mass of middle ear and mastoid antrum filled with debris, including cholesterol.

385.30 Cholesteatoma, unspecified

385.31 Cholesteatoma of attic

385.32 Cholesteatoma of middle ear

Cholesteatoma

Middle ear chamber

Cholesteatoma sac   Ear drum

385.33 Cholesteatoma of middle ear and mastoid
DEF: Cystlike mass of cell debris in middle ear and mastoid air cells behind ear.
AHA: 3Q, '00, 10

385.35 Diffuse cholesteatosis

√5ᵗʰ **385.8 Other disorders of middle ear and mastoid**

385.82 Cholesterin granuloma
DEF: Granuloma formed of fibrotic tissue; contains cholesterol crystals surrounded by foreign-body cells; found in the middle ear and mastoid area.

385.83 Retained foreign body of middle ear
▶Use additional code to identify foreign body (V90.01-V90.9)◀
AHA: 3Q, '94, 7; N-D, '87, 9

385.89 Other

385.9 Unspecified disorder of middle ear and mastoid

√4ᵗʰ **386 Vertiginous syndromes and other disorders of vestibular system**
EXCLUDES vertigo NOS (780.4)
AHA: M-A, '85, 12

√5ᵗʰ **386.0 Ménière's disease**
Endolymphatic hydrops
Lermoyez's syndrome
Ménière's syndrome or vertigo
DEF: Distended membranous labyrinth of middle ear from endolymphatic hydrops; causes ischemia, failure of nerve function; hearing and balance dysfunction; symptoms include fluctuating deafness, ringing in ears and dizziness.

386.00 Ménière's disease, unspecified
Ménière's disease (active)
H81.03 Ménière's disease bilateral   I-10

386.01 Active Ménière's disease, cochleovestibular

386.02 Active Ménière's disease, cochlear

386.03 Active Ménière's disease, vestibular

386.04 Inactive Ménière's disease
Ménière's disease in remission

√5ᵗʰ **386.1 Other and unspecified peripheral vertigo**
EXCLUDES epidemic vertigo (078.81)

386.10 Peripheral vertigo, unspecified

386.11 Benign paroxysmal positional vertigo
Benign paroxysmal positional nystagmus

386.12 Vestibular neuronitis
Acute (and recurrent) peripheral vestibulopathy
DEF: Transient benign vertigo, unknown cause; characterized by response to caloric stimulation on one side, nystagmus with rhythmic movement of eyes; normal auditory function present.

386.19 Other
Aural vertigo   Otogenic vertigo

386.2 Vertigo of central origin
Central positional nystagmus
Malignant positional vertigo

√5ᵗʰ **386.3 Labyrinthitis**

386.30 Labyrinthitis, unspecified

386.31 Serous labyrinthitis
Diffuse labyrinthitis
DEF: Inflammation of labyrinth; with fluid buildup.

386.32 Circumscribed labyrinthitis
Focal labyrinthitis

386.33 Suppurative labyrinthitis
Purulent labyrinthitis
DEF: Inflammation of labyrinth; with pus.

386.34 Toxic labyrinthitis
DEF: Inflammation of labyrinth; due to toxic reaction.

386.35 Viral labyrinthitis

√5ᵗʰ **386.4 Labyrinthine fistula**

386.40 Labyrinthine fistula, unspecified

386.41 Round window fistula

386.42 Oval window fistula

386.43 Semicircular canal fistula

386.48 Labyrinthine fistula of combined sites

√5ᵗʰ **386.5 Labyrinthine dysfunction**

386.50 Labyrinthine dysfunction, unspecified

386.51 Hyperactive labyrinth, unilateral
DEF: Abnormal increased sensitivity of labyrinth to stimuli such as sound, pressure or gravitational change, affecting one ear.

386.52 Hyperactive labyrinth, bilateral
DEF: Abnormal increased sensitivity of labyrinth to stimuli such as sound, pressure or gravitational change, affecting both ears.

386.53 Hypoactive labyrinth, unilateral
DEF: Abnormal decreased sensitivity of labyrinth to stimuli such as sound, pressure or gravitational change, affecting one ear.

386.54 Hypoactive labyrinth, bilateral
DEF: Abnormal decreased sensitivity of labyrinth to stimuli such as sound, pressure or gravitational change, affecting both ears.

386.55 Loss of labyrinthine reactivity, unilateral
DEF: Decreased function of the labyrinth sensors, affecting one ear

386.56 Loss of labyrinthine reactivity, bilateral
DEF: Decreased function of the labyrinth sensors, affecting both ears

386.58 Other forms and combinations

386.8 Other disorders of labyrinth

386.9 Unspecified vertiginous syndromes and labyrinthine disorders

√4ᵗʰ **387 Otosclerosis**
INCLUDES otospongiosis
DEF: Synonym for otospongiosis, spongy bone formation in the labyrinth bones of the ear; it causes progressive hearing impairment.

387.0 Otosclerosis involving oval window, nonobliterative
DEF: Tough, fibrous tissue impeding functions of oval window.

387.1 Otosclerosis involving oval window, obliterative
DEF: Tough, fibrous tissue blocking oval window.

387.2 Cochlear otosclerosis
Otosclerosis involving:
otic capsule
round window
DEF: Tough, fibrous tissue impeding functions of cochlea.

387.8 Other otosclerosis

387.9 Otosclerosis, unspecified

√4ᵗʰ **388 Other disorders of ear**

√5ᵗʰ **388.0 Degenerative and vascular disorders of ear**

388.00 Degenerative and vascular disorders, unspecified

388.01 Presbyacusis
DEF: Progressive, bilateral perceptive hearing loss caused by advancing age; it is also known as presbycusis.

√4ᵗʰ√5ᵗʰ Additional Digit Required   Unspecified Code   Other Specified Code   Manifestation Code   ▶◀ Revised Text   ● New Code   ▲ Revised Code Title

388.02 Transient ischemic deafness
DEF: Restricted blood flow to auditory organs causing temporary hearing loss.

√5ᵗʰ **388.1 Noise effects on inner ear**

388.10 Noise effects on inner ear, unspecified

388.11 Acoustic trauma (explosive) to ear
Otitic blast injury

388.12 Noise-induced hearing loss

388.2 Sudden hearing loss, unspecified

√5ᵗʰ **388.3 Tinnitus**
DEF: Abnormal noises in ear; may be heard by others beside the affected individual; noises include ringing, clicking, roaring and buzzing.

388.30 Tinnitus, unspecified

388.31 Subjective tinnitus

388.32 Objective tinnitus

√5ᵗʰ **388.4 Other abnormal auditory perception**

388.40 Abnormal auditory perception, unspecified

388.41 Diplacusis
DEF: Perception of a single auditory sound as two sounds at two different levels of intensity.

388.42 Hyperacusis
DEF: Exceptionally acute sense of hearing caused by such conditions as Bell's palsy; this term may also refer to painful sensitivity to sounds.

388.43 Impairment of auditory discrimination
DEF: Impaired ability to distinguish tone of sound.

388.44 Recruitment
DEF: Perception of abnormally increased loudness caused by a slight increase in sound intensity; it is a term used in audiology.

388.45 Acquired auditory processing disorder
Auditory processing disorder NOS
EXCLUDES central auditory processing disorder (315.32)
DEF: Difficulty in recognizing and interpreting sounds; a failure of the brain to process auditory information; due to neurological problems due to injury, infection, and degenerative conditions.
AHA: 4Q, '07, 79

388.5 Disorders of acoustic nerve
Acoustic neuritis
Degeneration } of acoustic or eighth nerve
Disorder
EXCLUDES acoustic neuroma (225.1)
syphilitic acoustic neuritis (094.86)
AHA: M-A, '87, 8

√5ᵗʰ **388.6 Otorrhea**

388.60 Otorrhea, unspecified
Discharging ear NOS

388.61 Cerebrospinal fluid otorrhea
EXCLUDES cerebrospinal fluid rhinorrhea (349.81)
DEF: Spinal fluid leakage from ear.

388.69 Other
Otorrhagia

√5ᵗʰ **388.7 Otalgia**

388.70 Otalgia, unspecified
Earache NOS

388.71 Otogenic pain

388.72 Referred pain

388.8 Other disorders of ear

388.9 Unspecified disorder of ear

√4ᵗʰ **389 Hearing loss**

√5ᵗʰ **389.0 Conductive hearing loss**
Conductive deafness
EXCLUDES mixed conductive and sensorineural hearing loss (389.20-389.22)
DEF: Dysfunction in sound-conducting structures of external or middle ear causing hearing loss.
AHA: 4Q, '07, 80; 4Q, '89, 5

389.00 Conductive hearing loss, unspecified

389.01 Conductive hearing loss, external ear

389.02 Conductive hearing loss, tympanic membrane

389.03 Conductive hearing loss, middle ear

389.04 Conductive hearing loss, inner ear

389.05 Conductive hearing loss, unilateral

389.06 Conductive hearing loss, bilateral
AHA: 4Q, '07, 81

389.08 Conductive hearing loss of combined types

√5ᵗʰ **389.1 Sensorineural hearing loss**
Perceptive hearing loss or deafness
EXCLUDES abnormal auditory perception (388.40-388.44)
mixed conductive and sensorineural hearing loss (389.20-389.22)
psychogenic deafness (306.7)
DEF: Nerve conduction causing hearing loss.
AHA: 4Q, '07, 80; 4Q, '89, 5

389.10 Sensorineural hearing loss, unspecified
AHA: 1Q, '93, 29

389.11 Sensory hearing loss, bilateral

389.12 Neural hearing loss, bilateral

389.13 Neural hearing loss, unilateral

389.14 Central hearing loss

389.15 Sensorineural hearing loss, unilateral
AHA: 4Q, '06, 84

389.16 Sensorineural hearing loss, asymmetrical
AHA: 4Q, '06, 84

389.17 Sensory hearing loss, unilateral

389.18 Sensorineural hearing loss, bilateral
AHA: 4Q, '06, 84

√5ᵗʰ **389.2 Mixed conductive and sensorineural hearing loss**
Deafness or hearing loss of type classifiable to 389.00-389.08 with type classifiable to 389.10-389.18
AHA: 4Q, '07, 80

389.20 Mixed hearing loss, unspecified

389.21 Mixed hearing loss, unilateral

389.22 Mixed hearing loss, bilateral

389.7 Deaf, non-speaking, not elsewhere classifiable

389.8 Other specified forms of hearing loss

389.9 Unspecified hearing loss
Deafness NOS
AHA: 1Q, '04, 15
H91.93 Unspecified hearing loss bilateral   I-10

7. Diseases of the Circulatory System (390-459)

Acute Rheumatic Fever (390-392)

DEF: Febrile disease occurs mainly in children or young adults following throat infection by group A streptococci; symptoms include fever, joint pain, lesions of heart, blood vessels and joint connective tissue, abdominal pain, skin changes, and chorea.

390 Rheumatic fever without mention of heart involvement

Arthritis, rheumatic, acute or subacute
Rheumatic fever (active) (acute)
Rheumatism, articular, acute or subacute

EXCLUDES *that with heart involvement (391.0-391.9)*

✓4ᵗʰ 391 Rheumatic fever with heart involvement

EXCLUDES *chronic heart diseases of rheumatic origin (393-398.99) unless rheumatic fever is also present or there is evidence of recrudescence or activity of the rheumatic process*

391.0 Acute rheumatic pericarditis

Rheumatic:
  fever (active) (acute) with pericarditis
  pericarditis (acute)

Any condition classifiable to 390 with pericarditis

EXCLUDES *that not specified as rheumatic (420.0-420.9)*

DEF: Sudden, severe inflammation of heart lining due to rheumatic fever.

391.1 Acute rheumatic endocarditis

Rheumatic:
  endocarditis, acute
  fever (active) (acute) with endocarditis or valvulitis
  valvulitis acute

Any condition classifiable to 390 with endocarditis or valvulitis

DEF: Sudden, severe inflammation of heart cavities due to rheumatic fever.

391.2 Acute rheumatic myocarditis

Rheumatic fever (active) (acute) with myocarditis

Any condition classifiable to 390 with myocarditis

DEF: Sudden, severe inflammation of heart muscles due to rheumatic fever.

391.8 Other acute rheumatic heart disease

Rheumatic:
  fever (active) (acute) with other or multiple types of heart involvement
  pancarditis, acute

Any condition classifiable to 390 with other or multiple types of heart involvement

391.9 Acute rheumatic heart disease, unspecified

Rheumatic:
  carditis, acute
  fever (active) (acute) with unspecified type of heart involvement
  heart disease, active or acute

Any condition classifiable to 390 with unspecified type of heart involvement

Sections of Heart Muscle

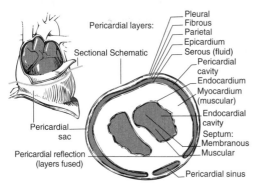

Pericardial layers:
Sectional Schematic

Pleural
Fibrous
Parietal
Epicardium
Serous (fluid)
Pericardial cavity
Endocardium
Myocardium (muscular)
Endocardial cavity
Septum:
Membranous
Muscular

Pericardial sac
Pericardial reflection (layers fused)
Pericardial sinus

✓4ᵗʰ 392 Rheumatic chorea

INCLUDES Sydenham's chorea

EXCLUDES *chorea:*
  NOS (333.5)
  Huntington's (333.4)

DEF: Childhood disease linked with rheumatic fever and streptococcal infections; symptoms include spasmodic, involuntary movements of limbs or facial muscles, psychic symptoms, and irritability.

392.0 With heart involvement

Rheumatic chorea with heart involvement of any type classifiable to 391

392.9 Without mention of heart involvement

Chronic Rheumatic Heart Disease (393-398)

393 Chronic rheumatic pericarditis

Adherent pericardium, rheumatic
Chronic rheumatic:
  mediastinopericarditis
  myopericarditis

EXCLUDES *pericarditis NOS or not specified as rheumatic (423.0-423.9)*

DEF: Persistent inflammation of heart lining due to rheumatic heart disease.

✓4ᵗʰ 394 Diseases of mitral valve

EXCLUDES *that with aortic valve involvement (396.0-396.9)*

394.0 Mitral stenosis

Mitral (valve):
  obstruction (rheumatic)
  stenosis NOS

DEF: Narrowing, of mitral valve between left atrium and left ventricle; due to rheumatic heart disease.

TIP: ▶Assign when documentation indicates mitral valve stenosis or obstruction with no further specification of cause.◀

394.1 Rheumatic mitral insufficiency

Rheumatic mitral:
  incompetence
  regurgitation

EXCLUDES *that not specified as rheumatic (424.0)*

DEF: Malfunction of mitral valve between left atrium and left ventricle; due to rheumatic heart disease.

AHA: 2Q, '05, 14

394.2 Mitral stenosis with insufficiency

Mitral stenosis with incompetence or regurgitation

DEF: A narrowing or stricture of the mitral valve situated between the left atrium and left ventricle; valve does not completely close, is insufficient (inadequate) in preventing regurgitation into the atrium; also called incompetence.

AHA: 1Q, '07, 11

394.9 Other and unspecified mitral valve diseases

Mitral (valve):
  disease (chronic)
  failure

✓4ᵗʰ 395 Diseases of aortic valve

EXCLUDES *that not specified as rheumatic (424.1)*
  that with mitral valve involvement (396.0-396.9)

395.0 Rheumatic aortic stenosis

Rheumatic aortic (valve) obstruction

DEF: Narrowing of the aortic valve; results in backflow into ventricle; due to rheumatic heart disease.

AHA: 4Q, '88, 8

395.1 Rheumatic aortic insufficiency

Rheumatic aortic:
  incompetence
  regurgitation

DEF: Malfunction of the aortic valve; results in backflow into left ventricle; due to rheumatic heart disease.

395.2 Rheumatic aortic stenosis with insufficiency

Rheumatic aortic stenosis with incompetence or regurgitation

DEF: Malfunction and narrowing, of the aortic valve; results in backflow into left ventricle; due to rheumatic heart disease.

395.9 Other and unspecified rheumatic aortic diseases

Rheumatic aortic (valve) disease

| ✓4ᵗʰ ✓5ᵗʰ Additional Digit Required | Unspecified Code | Other Specified Code | Manifestation Code | ▶◀ Revised Text | ● New Code | ▲ Revised Code Title |

2011 ICD-9-CM | **February 2010 • Volume 1 – 123**

Diseases of the Circulatory System

396–402.91

√4ᵗʰ **396 Diseases of mitral and aortic valves**

INCLUDES involvement of both mitral and aortic valves, whether specified as rheumatic or not

AHA: N-D, '87, 8

396.0 Mitral valve stenosis and aortic valve stenosis
Atypical aortic (valve) stenosis
Mitral and aortic (valve) obstruction (rheumatic)

396.1 Mitral valve stenosis and aortic valve insufficiency

396.2 Mitral valve insufficiency and aortic valve stenosis
AHA: 2Q, '09, 17; 1Q, '09, 18; 2Q, '00, 16

396.3 Mitral valve insufficiency and aortic valve insufficiency
Mitral and aortic (valve):
incompetence
regurgitation
I08.0 Rheumatic d/o of both mitral & aortic valves   I-10

396.8 Multiple involvement of mitral and aortic valves
Stenosis and insufficiency of mitral or aortic valve with stenosis or insufficiency, or both, of the other valve

396.9 Mitral and aortic valve diseases, unspecified

√4ᵗʰ **397 Diseases of other endocardial structures**

397.0 Diseases of tricuspid valve
Tricuspid (valve) (rheumatic):
disease
insufficiency
obstruction
regurgitation
stenosis
DEF: Malfunction of the valve between right atrium and right ventricle; due to rheumatic heart disease.
AHA: 3Q, '06, 7; 2Q, '00, 16
I07.2 Rheumatic tricuspid stenosis and insufficiency   I-10

397.1 Rheumatic diseases of pulmonary valve
EXCLUDES that not specified as rheumatic (424.3)

397.9 Rheumatic diseases of endocardium, valve unspecified
Rheumatic:
endocarditis (chronic)
valvulitis (chronic)
EXCLUDES that not specified as rheumatic (424.90-424.99)

√4ᵗʰ **398 Other rheumatic heart disease**

398.0 Rheumatic myocarditis
Rheumatic degeneration of myocardium
EXCLUDES myocarditis not specified as rheumatic (429.0)
DEF: Chronic inflammation of heart muscle; due to rheumatic heart disease.

√5ᵗʰ **398.9 Other and unspecified rheumatic heart diseases**

398.90 Rheumatic heart disease, unspecified
Rheumatic:
carditis
heart disease NOS
EXCLUDES carditis not specified as rheumatic (429.89)
heart disease NOS not specified as rheumatic (429.9)

398.91 Rheumatic heart failure (congestive)
Rheumatic left ventricular failure
DEF: Decreased cardiac output, edema and hypertension; due to rheumatic heart disease.
AHA: 2Q, '05, 14; 1Q, '95, 6; 3Q, '88, 3
I09.81 Rheumatic heart failure   I-10

398.99 Other

Hypertensive Disease (401-405)

EXCLUDES that complicating pregnancy, childbirth, or the puerperium (642.0-642.9)
that involving coronary vessels (410.00-414.9)
AHA: 3Q, '90, 3; 2Q, '89, 12; S-O, '87, 9; J-A, '84, 11

√4ᵗʰ **401 Essential hypertension**

INCLUDES high blood pressure
hyperpiesia
hyperpiesis
hypertension (arterial) (essential) (primary) (systemic)
hypertensive vascular:
degeneration
disease

EXCLUDES elevated blood pressure without diagnosis of hypertension (796.2)
pulmonary hypertension (416.0-416.9)
that involving vessels of:
brain (430-438)
eye (362.11)
DEF: Hypertension that occurs without apparent organic cause; idiopathic.
AHA: 2Q, '92, 5

401.0 Malignant
DEF: Severe high arterial blood pressure; results in necrosis in kidney, retina, etc.; hemorrhages occur and death commonly due to uremia or rupture of cerebral vessel.
AHA: M-J, '85, 19

401.1 Benign
DEF: Mildly elevated arterial blood pressure.

401.9 Unspecified
AHA: ▶4Q, '09, 77, 129;◀ 1Q, '09, 18; 2Q, '08, 16; 4Q, '05, 71; 3Q, '05, 8; 4Q, '04, 78; 4Q, '03, 105, 108, 111; 3Q, '03, 14; 2Q, '03, 16; 4Q, '97, 37
I10 Essential (primary) hypertension   I-10

√4ᵗʰ **402 Hypertensive heart disease**

INCLUDES hypertensive:
cardiomegaly
cardiopathy
cardiovascular disease
heart (disease) (failure)
any condition classifiable to 429.0-429.3, 429.8, 429.9 due to hypertension
Use additional code to specify type of heart failure (428.0-428.43), if known
AHA: 4Q, '02, 49; 2Q, '93, 9; N-D, '84, 18
TIP: Assign when a cardiac condition is stated (due to hypertension) or implied (hypertensive).

√5ᵗʰ **402.0 Malignant**

402.00 Without heart failure

402.01 With heart failure
AHA: 4Q, '08, 180

√5ᵗʰ **402.1 Benign**

402.10 Without heart failure

402.11 With heart failure

√5ᵗʰ **402.9 Unspecified**

402.90 Without heart failure
I11.9 Hypertensive heart disease without heart failure   I-10

402.91 With heart failure
AHA: 4Q, '02, 52; 1Q, '93, 19; 2Q, '89, 12

N Newborn Age: 0   P Pediatric Age: 0-17   M Maternity Age: 12-55   A Adult Age: 15-124

√4ᵗʰ **403 Hypertensive chronic kidney disease**

INCLUDES arteriolar nephritis
arteriosclerosis of:
   kidney
   renal arterioles
arteriosclerotic nephritis (chronic) (interstitial)
hypertensive:
   nephropathy
   renal failure
   uremia (chronic)
nephrosclerosis
renal sclerosis with hypertension

any condition classifiable to 585 ►and 587◄ with any condition classifiable to 401

EXCLUDES *acute kidney failure (584.5-584.9)*
renal disease stated as not due to hypertension
renovascular hypertension (405.0-405.9 with fifth-digit 1)

The following fifth-digit subclassification is for use with category 403:
  0 with chronic kidney disease stage I through stage IV, or unspecified
    Use additional code to identify the stage of chronic kidney disease (585.1-585.4, 585.9)
  1 with chronic kidney disease stage V or end stage renal disease
    Use additional code to identify the stage of chronic kidney disease (585.5, 585.6)

AHA: 4Q, '06, 84-86; 4Q, '05, 68; 4Q, '92, 22; 2Q, '92, 5
TIP: Assign whenever a patient has both chronic kidney disease and hypertension (presumed cause-and-effect relationship).

§ √5ᵗʰ **403.0 Malignant**
  [0-1]

§ √5ᵗʰ **403.1 Benign**
  [0-1]

§ √5ᵗʰ **403.9 Unspecified**
  [0-1]   **AHA: For code 403.90:** 1Q, '08, 10 ;2Q, '07, 3; 4Q, '06, 86; **For code 403.91:** 1Q ,'08, 7; 4Q, '05, 69; 1Q, '04, 14; 1Q, '03, 20; 2Q, '01, 11; 3Q, '91, 8
    I12.9 HTN CKD w/stage I thru IV CKD/UNS CKD   I-10

√4ᵗʰ **404 Hypertensive heart and chronic kidney disease**

INCLUDES disease:
   cardiorenal
   cardiovascular renal
any condition classifiable to 402 with any condition classifiable to 403

Use additional code to specify type of heart failure (428.0-428.43), if known

The following fifth-digit subclassification is for use with category 404:
  0 without heart failure and with chronic kidney disease stage I through stage IV, or unspecified
    Use additional code to identify the stage of chronic kidney disease (585.1-585.4, 585.9)
  1 with heart failure and with chronic kidney disease stage I through stage IV, or unspecified
    Use additional code to identify the stage of chronic kidney disease (585.1-585.4, 585.9)
  2 without heart failure and with chronic kidney disease stage V or end stage renal disease
    Use additional code to identify the stage of chronic kidney disease (585.5, 585.6)
  3 with heart failure and chronic kidney disease stage V or end stage renal disease
    Use additional code to identify the stage of chronic kidney disease (585.5, 585.6)

AHA: 4Q, '06, 84-86; 4Q, '05, 68; 4Q, '02, 49; 3Q, '90, 3; J-A, '84, 14

§ √5ᵗʰ **404.0 Malignant**
  [0-3]

§ √5ᵗʰ **404.1 Benign**
  [0-3]

§ √5ᵗʰ **404.9 Unspecified**
  [0-3]   **I13.0** HTN heart & CKD HF & stage I thru IV CKD/UNS CKD   I-10

√4ᵗʰ **405 Secondary hypertension**

DEF: High arterial blood pressure due to or with a variety of primary diseases, such as renal disorders, CNS disorders, endocrine, and vascular diseases.
AHA: 3Q, '90, 3; S-O, '87, 9, 11; J-A, '84, 14

√5ᵗʰ **405.0 Malignant**

    405.01 Renovascular

    405.09 Other

√5ᵗʰ **405.1 Benign**

    405.11 Renovascular

    405.19 Other

√5ᵗʰ **405.9 Unspecified**

    405.91 Renovascular

    405.99 Other
      AHA: 3Q, '00, 4

Ischemic Heart Disease (410-414)

INCLUDES that with mention of hypertension
Use additional code to identify presence of hypertension (401.0-405.9)
AHA: 3Q, '91, 10; J-A, '84, 5

√4ᵗʰ **410 Acute myocardial infarction**

INCLUDES cardiac infarction
coronary (artery):
   embolism
   occlusion
   rupture
   thrombosis
infarction of heart, myocardium, or ventricle
rupture of heart, myocardium, or ventricle
ST elevation (STEMI) and non-ST elevation (NSTEMI) myocardial infarction
any condition classifiable to 414.1-414.9 specified as acute or with a stated duration of 8 weeks or less

The following fifth-digit subclassification is for use with category 410:
  0 episode of care unspecified
    Use when the source document does not contain sufficient information for the assigment of fifth-digit 1 or 2.
  1 initial episode of care
    Use fifth-digit 1 to designate the first episode of care (regardless of facility site) for a newly diagnosed myocardial infarction. The fifth-digit 1 is assigned regardless of the number of times a patient may be transferred during the initial episode of care.
  2 subsequent episode of care
    Use fifth-digit 2 to designate an episode of care following the initial episode when the patient is admitted for further observation, evaluation or treatment for a myocardial infarction that has received initial treatment, but is still less than 8 weeks old.

DEF: A sudden insufficiency of blood supply to an area of the heart muscle; usually due to a coronary artery occlusion.
AHA: 2Q, '06, 9; 4Q, '05, 69; 3Q, '01, 21; 3Q, '98, 15; 4Q, '97, 37; 3Q, '95, 9; 4Q, 92, 24; 1Q, '92, 10; 3Q, '91, 18; 1Q, '91, 14; 3Q, '89, 3
TIP: Assign an acute MI code with a fifth digit of "1," initial episode of care, for all care provided before the AMI has resolved, regardless of type or number of transfers between facilities.

§ √5ᵗʰ **410.0 Of anterolateral wall**
  [0-2]   ST elevation myocardial infarction (STEMI) of anterolateral wall
      AHA: For code 410.01: 4Q, '09, 129; 4Q, '08, 72

§ √5ᵗʰ **410.1 Of other anterior wall**
  [0-2]   Infarction:
      anterior (wall) NOS ⎫ (with contiguous portion of
      anteroapical   ⎬ intraventricular
      anteroseptal   ⎭ septum)
    ST elevation myocardial infarction (STEMI) of other anterior wall
      AHA: For code 410.11: 3Q, '03, 10

§ √5ᵗʰ **410.2 Of inferolateral wall**
  [0-2]   ST elevation myocardial infarction (STEMI) of inferolateral wall

---

§ Requires fifth digit. Valid digits are in [brackets] under each code. See appropriate category for codes and definitions.

√4ᵗʰ/√5ᵗʰ Additional Digit Required   Unspecified Code   Other Specified Code   Manifestation Code   ►◄ Revised Text   ● New Code   ▲ Revised Code Title

Acute Myocardial Infarction

Anatomic Sites

- Anterolateral 410.0
- Other lateral 410.5
- Posterobasal 410.6
- Postero-lateral 410.5
- Anteroseptal 410.1
- Inferoposterior 410.3
- Atrium only 410.8
- Septum only 410.8
- Apical 410.1
- Other and septum 410.4
- Papillary muscle

§ √5ᵗʰ **410.3 Of inferoposterior wall**
[0-2]　ST elevation myocardial infarction (STEMI) of inferoposterior wall

§ √5ᵗʰ **410.4 Of other inferior wall**
[0-2]　Infarction:
　　diaphragmatic wall NOS ⎤ (with contiguous portion of
　　inferior (wall) NOS ⎦ intraventricular septum)
　　ST elevation myocardial infarction (STEMI) of other inferior wall
AHA: 1Q, '00, 7, 26; 4Q, '99, 9; 3Q, '97, 10; **For code 410.41:** ▶3Q, '09, 10;◀ 2Q, '01, 8, 9
I21.19 STEMI invlv oth coronary artery of inferior wall　I-10

§ √5ᵗʰ **410.5 Of other lateral wall**
[0-2]　Infarction:
　　apical-lateral
　　basal-lateral
　　high lateral
　　posterolateral
　　ST elevation myocardial infarction (STEMI) of other lateral wall
AHA: For code 410.51: ▶3Q, '09, 9◀

§ √5ᵗʰ **410.6 True posterior wall infarction**
[0-2]　Infarction:
　　posterobasal
　　strictly posterior
　　ST elevation myocardial infarction (STEMI) of true posterior wall

§ √5ᵗʰ **410.7 Subendocardial infarction**
[0-2]　Non-ST elevation myocardial infarction (NSTEMI)
　　Nontransmural infarction
AHA: 1Q, '00, 7; **For code 410.71:** 4Q, '05, 71; 2Q, '05, 19
I21.4 Non-ST elevation (NSTEMI) myocardial infarction　I-10

§ √5ᵗʰ **410.8 Of other specified sites**
[0-2]　Infarction of:
　　atrium
　　papillary muscle
　　septum alone
　　ST elevation myocardial infarction (STEMI) of other specified sites

§ √5ᵗʰ **410.9 Unspecified site**
[0-2]　Acute myocardial infarction NOS
　　Coronary occlusion NOS
　　Myocardial infarction NOS
AHA: 1Q, '96, 17; 1Q, '92, 9; **For code 410.91:** 2Q, '05, 18; 3Q, '02, 5
I21.3 ST elevation myocardial infarction of uns site　I-10

√4ᵗʰ **411 Other acute and subacute forms of ischemic heart disease**
AHA: 4Q, '94, 55; 3Q, '91, 24

411.0 Postmyocardial infarction syndrome
　　Dressler's syndrome
DEF: Complication developing several days/weeks after myocardial infarction; symptoms include fever, leukocytosis, chest pain, pericarditis, pleurisy, and pneumonitis; tendency to recur.

411.1 Intermediate coronary syndrome
　　Impending infarction　　Preinfarction syndrome
　　Preinfarction angina　　Unstable angina
EXCLUDES angina (pectoris) (413.9)
　　　　decubitus (413.0)
DEF: A condition representing an intermediate stage between angina of effort and acute myocardial infarction. It is often documented by the physician as "unstable angina."
AHA: 3Q, '07, 9; 4Q, '05, 105; 2Q, '04, 3; 1Q, '03, 12; 3Q, '01, 15; 2Q, '01, 7, 9; 4Q, '98, 86; 2Q, '96, 10; 3Q, '91, 24; 1Q, '91, 14; 3Q, '90, 6; 4Q, '89, 10
TIP: Do not assign code 411.1 on the same episode of care as an acute myocardial infarction (category 410). Assign 411.1 for accelerated angina.
I20.0 Unstable angina　I-10

√5ᵗʰ **411.8 Other**
AHA: 3Q, '91, 18; 3Q, '89, 4

411.81 Acute coronary occlusion without myocardial infarction
　　Acute coronary (artery):
　　　embolism ⎤
　　　obstruction ⎥ without or not resulting
　　　occlusion ⎥ in myocardial
　　　thrombosis ⎦ infarction
EXCLUDES obstruction without infarction due to atherosclerosis (414.00-414.07)
　　　　occlusion without infarction due to atherosclerosis (414.00-414.07)
DEF: Interrupted blood flow to a portion of the heart; without tissue death.
AHA: 3Q, '91, 24; 1Q, '91, 14

411.89 Other
　　Coronary insufficiency (acute)
　　Subendocardial ischemia
AHA: 3Q, '01, 14; 1Q, '92, 9

412 Old myocardial infarction
　　Healed myocardial infarction
　　Past myocardial infarction diagnosed on ECG [EKG] or other special investigation, but currently presenting no symptoms
AHA: 2Q, '03, 10; 2Q, '01, 9; 3Q, '98, 15; 2Q, '91, 22; 3Q, '90, 7
TIP: Assign for any acute myocardial infarction stated to be older than 8 weeks.
I25.2 Old myocardial infarction　I-10

√4ᵗʰ **413 Angina pectoris**
DEF: Severe constricting pain in the chest, often radiating from the precordium to the left shoulder and down the arm, due to ischemia of the heart muscle; usually caused by coronary disease; pain is often precipitated by effort or excitement.

413.0 Angina decubitus
　　Nocturnal angina
DEF: Angina occurring only in the recumbent position.

413.1 Prinzmetal angina
　　Variant angina pectoris
DEF: Angina occurring when patient is recumbent; associated with ST-segment elevations.
AHA: 3Q, '06, 23

413.9 Other and unspecified angina pectoris
　　Angina:　　　　Anginal syndrome
　　　NOS　　　　Status anginosus
　　　cardiac　　　Stenocardia
　　　equivalent　　Syncope anginosa
　　　of effort
　　Use additional code(s) for symptoms associated with angina equivalent
EXCLUDES preinfarction angina (411.1)
AHA: 2Q, '08, 16; 3Q, '02, 4; 3Q, '91, 16; 3Q, '90, 6
TIP: For patients with both angina and coronary artery disease, sequence the CAD (subcategory 414.0) code first.
I20.9 Angina pectoris unspecified　I-10

---

§　Requires fifth digit. Valid digits are in [brackets] under each code. See category 410 for codes and definitions.

Ⓝ Newborn Age: 0　　Ⓟ Pediatric Age: 0-17　　Ⓜ Maternity Age: 12-55　　Ⓐ Adult Age: 15-124

√4ᵗʰ **414 Other forms of chronic ischemic heart disease**

> **EXCLUDES** *arteriosclerotic cardiovascular disease [ASCVD] (429.2)*
> *cardiovascular:*
> *arteriosclerosis or sclerosis (429.2)*
> *degeneration or disease (429.2)*

√5ᵗʰ **414.0 Coronary atherosclerosis**

Arteriosclerotic heart disease [ASHD] Coronary (artery): arteritis or endarteritis
Atherosclerotic heart disease atheroma
Coronary (artery): sclerosis
arteriosclerosis stricture

Use additional code, if applicable, to identify chronic total occlusion of coronary artery (414.2)

> **EXCLUDES** *embolism of graft (996.72)*
> *occlusion NOS of graft (996.72)*
> *thrombus of graft (996.72)*

DEF: A chronic condition marked by thickening and loss of elasticity of the coronary artery; caused by deposits of plaque containing cholesterol, lipoid material and lipophages.
AHA: 2Q, '97, 13; 2Q, '95, 17; 4Q, '94, 49; 2Q, '94, 13; 1Q, '94, 6; 3Q, '90, 7

414.00 Of unspecified type of vessel, native or graft ▣A
AHA: 1Q, '04, 24; 2Q, '03, 16; 3Q, '01, 15; 4Q, '99, 4; 3Q, '97, 15; 4Q, '96, 31

414.01 Of native coronary artery ▣A
DEF: Plaque deposits in natural heart vessels.
AHA: ►3Q, '09, 9, 10;◄ 3Q, '08, 10; 2Q, '08, 16; 3Q, '06, 25; 4Q, '05, 71; 2Q, '04, 3; 4Q, '03, 108; 3Q, '03, 9, 14; 3Q, '02, 4-9; 3Q, '01, 15; 2Q, '01, 8, 9; 3Q, '97, 15; 2Q, '96, 10; 4Q, '96, 31
TIP: Assign for documentation of CAD NOS in a patient with no history of coronary artery bypass procedure.
I25.10 ASHD of native cor artery w/o angina pectoris ▣I-10

414.02 Of autologous vein bypass graft ▣A
DEF: Plaque deposit in grafted vein originating within patient.

414.03 Of nonautologous biological bypass graft ▣A
DEF: Plaque deposits in grafted vessel originating outside patient.

414.04 Of artery bypass graft ▣A
Internal mammary artery
DEF: Plaque deposits in grafted artery originating within patient.
AHA: 4Q, '96, 31

414.05 Of unspecified type of bypass graft ▣A
Bypass graft NOS
AHA: 3Q, '97, 15; 4Q, '96, 31

414.06 Of native coronary artery of transplanted heart
AHA: 4Q, '03, 60; 4Q, '02, 53

414.07 Of bypass graft (artery) (vein) of transplanted heart ▣A

√5ᵗʰ **414.1 Aneurysm and dissection of heart**
AHA: 4Q, '02, 54

414.10 Aneurysm of heart (wall)
Aneurysm (arteriovenous):
mural
ventricular

Arteries of the Heart

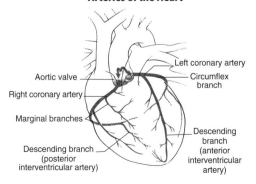

Aortic valve
Right coronary artery
Marginal branches
Descending branch (posterior interventricular artery)
Left coronary artery
Circumflex branch
Descending branch (anterior interventricular artery)

414.11 Aneurysm of coronary vessels
Aneurysm (arteriovenous) of coronary vessels
DEF: Dilatation of all three-vessel wall layers forming a sac filled with blood.
AHA: 3Q, '03, 10; 1Q, '99, 17

414.12 Dissection of coronary artery
DEF: A tear in the intimal arterial wall of a coronary artery resulting in the sudden intrusion of blood within the layers of the wall.

414.19 Other aneurysm of heart
Arteriovenous fistula, acquired, of heart

414.2 Chronic total occlusion of coronary artery
Complete occlusion of coronary artery
Total occlusion of coronary artery
Code first coronary atherosclerosis (414.00-414.07)
> **EXCLUDES** *acute coronary occlusion with myo- cardial infarction (410.00-410.92)*
> *acute coronary occlusion without myocardial infarction (411.81)*
DEF: Complete blockage of coronary artery due to plaque accumulation over an extended period of time; results in substantial reduction of blood flow.
AHA: 4Q, '07, 82

414.3 Coronary atherosclerosis due to lipid rich plaque ▣A
Code first coronary atherosclerosis (414.00-414.07)
AHA: 4Q, '08, 113

414.8 Other specified forms of chronic ischemic heart disease
Chronic coronary insufficiency
Ischemia, myocardial (chronic)
Any condition classifiable to 410 specified as chronic, or presenting with symptoms after 8 weeks from date of infarction
> **EXCLUDES** *coronary insufficiency (acute) (411.89)*
AHA: 3Q, '01, 15; 1Q, '92, 10; 3Q, '90, 7, 15; 2Q, '90, 19
I25.89 Other forms of chronic ischemic heart disease ▣I-10

414.9 Chronic ischemic heart disease, unspecified
Ischemic heart disease NOS

Diseases of Pulmonary Circulation (415-417)

√4ᵗʰ **415 Acute pulmonary heart disease**

415.0 Acute cor pulmonale
> **EXCLUDES** *cor pulmonale NOS (416.9)*
DEF: A heart-lung disease marked by dilation and failure of the right side of heart; due to pulmonary embolism; ventilatory function is impaired and pulmonary hypertension results.

√5ᵗʰ **415.1 Pulmonary embolism and infarction**
Pulmonary (artery) (vein): Pulmonary (artery) (vein):
apoplexy infarction (hemorrhagic)
embolism thrombosis
> **EXCLUDES** *chronic pulmonary embolism (416.2)*
> *personal history of pulmonary embolism (V12.51)*
> *that complicating:*
> *abortion (634-638 with .6, 639.6)*
> *ectopic or molar pregnancy (639.6)*
> *pregnancy, childbirth, or the puerperium (673.0-673.8)*
DEF: Embolism: Closure of the pulmonary artery or branch; due to thrombosis (blood clot).
DEF: Infarction: Necrosis of lung tissue; due to obstructed arterial blood supply, most often by pulmonary embolism.
AHA: 4Q, '90, 25

415.11 Iatrogenic pulmonary embolism and infarction
Use additional code for associated septic pulmonary embolism, if applicable, 415.12
AHA: 4Q, '95, 58
TIP: Do not assign additional code of 997.39 Other respiratory complications, with code 415.11.

415.12 Septic pulmonary embolism
Septic embolism NOS
Code first underlying infection, such as:
septicemia (038.0-038.9)
> **EXCLUDES** *septic arterial embolism (449)*
AHA: 4Q, '07, 84-86

Diseases of the Circulatory System

415.19–421.0

415.19 Other
4Q, '09, 86
I26.99 Other pulmonary embolism w/o acute
cor pulmonale `I-10`

✔4ᵗʰ 416 Chronic pulmonary heart disease

416.0 Primary pulmonary hypertension
Idiopathic pulmonary arteriosclerosis
Pulmonary hypertension (essential) (idiopathic) (primary)

EXCLUDES ▶pulmonary hypertension NOS (416.8)
secondary pulmonary hypertension (416.8)◀

DEF: A rare increase in pulmonary circulation, often resulting in right
ventricular failure or fatal syncope.
I27.0 Primary pulmonary hypertension `I-10`

416.1 Kyphoscoliotic heart disease
DEF: High blood pressure within the lungs as a result of curvature of
the spine.

416.2 Chronic pulmonary embolism
Use additional code, if applicable, for associated long-term
(current) use of anticoagulants (V58.61)

EXCLUDES personal history of pulmonary embolism (V12.51)
DEF: A long-standing condition commonly associated with
pulmonary hypertension in which small blood clots travel to the
lungs repeatedly over many weeks, months, or years, requiring
continuation of established anticoagulant or thrombolytic therapy.
AHA: 4Q, '09, 85-86

416.8 Other chronic pulmonary heart diseases
▶Pulmonary hypertension NOS◀
Pulmonary hypertension, secondary
I27.89 Other specified pulmonary heart diseases `I-10`

416.9 Chronic pulmonary heart disease, unspecified
Chronic cardiopulmonary disease
Cor pulmonale (chronic) NOS

✔4ᵗʰ 417 Other diseases of pulmonary circulation

417.0 Arteriovenous fistula of pulmonary vessels
EXCLUDES congenital arteriovenous fistula (747.3)
DEF: Abnormal communication between blood vessels within lung.

417.1 Aneurysm of pulmonary artery
EXCLUDES congenital aneurysm (747.3)

417.8 Other specified diseases of pulmonary circulation
Pulmonary:
arteritis
endarteritis
Rupture } of pulmonary vessel
Stricture

417.9 Unspecified disease of pulmonary circulation

Other Forms of Heart Disease (420-429)

✔4ᵗʰ 420 Acute pericarditis
INCLUDES acute:
mediastinopericarditis
myopericarditis
pericardial effusion
pleuropericarditis
pneumopericarditis

EXCLUDES acute rheumatic pericarditis (391.0)
postmyocardial infarction syndrome [Dressler's] (411.0)
DEF: Inflammation of the pericardium (heart sac); pericardial friction rub
results from this inflammation and is heard as a scratchy or leathery sound.

420.0 Acute pericarditis in diseases classified elsewhere
Code first underlying disease, as:
actinomycosis (039.8)
amebiasis (006.8)
chronic uremia (585.9)
nocardiosis (039.8)
tuberculosis (017.9)
uremia NOS (586)

EXCLUDES pericarditis (acute) (in):
Coxsackie (virus) (074.21)
gonococcal (098.83)
histoplasmosis (115.0-115.9 with
fifth-digit 3)
meningococcal infection (036.41)
syphilitic (093.81)

Anatomy

Blood Flow

✔5ᵗʰ 420.9 Other and unspecified acute pericarditis

420.90 Acute pericarditis, unspecified
Pericarditis (acute):   Periocarditis (acute):
NOS   sicca
infective NOS
AHA: 2Q, '89, 12

420.91 Acute idiopathic pericarditis
Pericarditis, acute: Periocarditis (acute):
benign   viral
nonspecific

420.99 Other
Pericarditis (acute):   Pericarditis (acute):
pneumococcal   suppurative
purulent   Pneumopyopericardium
staphylococcal   Pyopericardium
streptococcal

EXCLUDES pericarditis in diseases classified elsewhere
(420.0)

✔4ᵗʰ 421 Acute and subacute endocarditis
DEF: Bacterial inflammation of the endocardium (intracardiac area); major
symptoms include fever, fatigue, heart murmurs, splenomegaly, embolic
episodes and areas of infarction.

421.0 Acute and subacute bacterial endocarditis
Endocarditis (acute)(chronic) (subacute):
bacterial
infective NOS
lenta
malignant
purulent
septic
ulcerative
vegetative
Infective aneurysm
Subacute bacterial endocarditis [SBE]

Use additional code to identify infectious organism [e.g.,
Streptococcus 041.0, Staphylococcus 041.1]
AHA: 4Q, '08, 73; 1Q, '99, 12; 1Q, '91, 15
I33.0 Acute and subacute infective endocarditis `I-10`

421.1 **Acute and subacute infective endocarditis in diseases classified elsewhere**

Code first underlying disease, as:
blastomycosis (116.0)
Q fever (083.0)
typhoid (fever) (002.0)

EXCLUDES   *endocarditis (in):*
    Coxsackie (virus) (074.22)
    gonococcal (098.84)
    histoplasmosis (115.0-115.9 with fifth-digit 4)
    meningococcal infection (036.42)
    monilial (112.81)

421.9 Acute endocarditis, unspecified

Endocarditis
Myoendocarditis ⎫ acute or subacute
Periendocarditis ⎭

EXCLUDES   *acute rheumatic endocarditis (391.1)*

422 Acute myocarditis

EXCLUDES   *acute rheumatic myocarditis (391.2)*

DEF: Acute inflammation of the muscular walls of the heart (myocardium).

422.0 **Acute myocarditis in diseases classified elsewhere**

Code first underlying disease, as:
myocarditis (acute):
  influenzal ▶(487.8, 488.09, 488.19)◀
  tuberculous (017.9)

EXCLUDES   *myocarditis (acute) (due to):*
    aseptic, of newborn (074.23)
    Coxsackie (virus) (074.23)
    diphtheritic (032.82)
    meningococcal infection (036.43)
    syphilitic (093.82)
    toxoplasmosis (130.3)

422.9 Other and unspecified acute myocarditis

422.90 Acute myocarditis, unspecified

Acute or subacute (interstitial) myocarditis

422.91 Idiopathic myocarditis

Myocarditis (acute or subacute):
  Fiedler's
  giant cell
  isolated (diffuse) (granulomatous)
  nonspecific granulomatous

422.92 Septic myocarditis

Myocarditis, acute or subacute:
  pneumococcal
  staphylococcal

Use additional code to identify infectious organism
[e.g., Staphylococcus 041.1]

EXCLUDES   *myocarditis, acute or subacute:*
    in bacterial diseases classified elsewhere (422.0)
    streptococcal (391.2)

422.93 Toxic myocarditis

DEF: Inflammation of the heart muscle due to an adverse reaction to certain drugs or chemicals reaching the heart through the bloodstream.

422.99 Other

Cardiac Tamponade

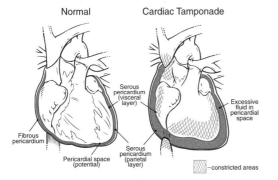

Normal   Cardiac Tamponade

Serous pericardium (visceral layer)
Excessive fluid in pericardial space
Fibrous pericardium
Pericardial space (potential)
Serous pericardium (parietal layer)
▨ --constricted areas

---

423 Other diseases of pericardium

EXCLUDES   *that specified as rheumatic (393)*

423.0 Hemopericardium

DEF: Blood in the pericardial sac (pericardium).

423.1 Adhesive pericarditis

Adherent pericardium   Pericarditis:
Fibrosis of pericardium   adhesive
Milk spots   obliterative
                    Soldiers' patches

DEF: Two layers of serous pericardium adhere to each other by fibrous adhesions.

423.2 Constrictive pericarditis

Concato's disease
Pick's disease of heart (and liver)

DEF: Inflammation identified by a rigid, thickened and sometimes calcified pericardium; ventricles of the heart not adequately filled; congestive heart failure may result.

423.3 Cardiac tamponade

Code first the underlying cause

DEF: Life-threatening condition in which fluid or blood accumulates between the muscle of the heart (myocardium) and the outer sac (pericardium), resulting in compression of the heart, which decreases cardiac output.

AHA: 4Q, '07, 86, 87

423.8 Other specified diseases of pericardium

Calcification ⎫ of pericardium
Fistula   ⎭

AHA: 2Q, '89, 12

423.9 Unspecified disease of pericardium

AHA: 1Q, '07, 11

424 Other diseases of endocardium

EXCLUDES   *bacterial endocarditis (421.0-421.9)*
    rheumatic endocarditis (391.1, 394.0-397.9)
    syphilitic endocarditis (093.20-093.24)

424.0 Mitral valve disorders

Mitral (valve):
  incompetence ⎫ NOS of specified cause,
  insufficiency   ⎬ except rheumatic
  regurgitation ⎭

EXCLUDES   *mitral (valve):*
    disease (394.9)
    failure (394.9)
    stenosis (394.0)
    the listed conditions:
      specified as rheumatic (394.1)
      unspecified as to cause but with mention of:
        diseases of aortic valve (396.0-396.9)
        mitral stenosis or obstruction (394.2)

AHA: 3Q, '06, 7; 2Q, '00, 16; 3Q, '98, 11; N-D, '87, 8; N-D, '84, 8

I34.8 Other nonrheumatic mitral valve disorders   I-10

424.1 Aortic valve disorders

Aortic (valve):
  incompetence ⎫
  insufficiency   ⎬ NOS of specified cause,
  regurgitation   ⎪ except rheumatic
  stenosis   ⎭

EXCLUDES   *hypertrophic subaortic stenosis (425.1)*
    that specified as rheumatic (395.0-395.9)
    that of unspecified cause but with mention of diseases of mitral valve (396.0-396.9)

AHA: 4Q, '08, 179; 4Q, '88, 8; N-D, '87, 8

424.2 Tricuspid valve disorders, specified as nonrheumatic

Tricuspid valve:
  incompetence ⎫
  insufficiency   ⎬ of specified cause, except
  regurgitation   ⎪ rheumatic
  stenosis   ⎭

EXCLUDES   *rheumatic or of unspecified cause (397.0)*

424.3 Pulmonary valve disorders

Pulmonic: Pulmonic:
  incompetence NOS   regurgitation NOS
  insufficiency NOS   stenosis NOS

EXCLUDES   *that specified as rheumatic (397.1)*

Additional Digit Required   Unspecified Code   Other Specified Code   Manifestation Code   ▶◀ Revised Text   ● New Code   ▲ Revised Code Title

2011 ICD-9-CM   **October 2010 · Volume 1 – 129**

Heart Valve Disorders

Valve stenosis
(trouble opening)

Incompetent valve
(trouble closing)

causes regurgitation
(backflow of blood)

Insufficient valve
(unable to close completely)

Shortened, fused
chorda tendinae

Ventricular hypertrophy

Normal Heart Valve Function

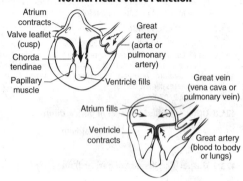

Atrium
contracts

Valve leaflet
(cusp)

Chorda
tendinae

Papillary
muscle

Great
artery
(aorta or
pulmonary
artery)

Ventricle fills

Great vein
(vena cava or
pulmonary vein)

Atrium fills

Ventricle
contracts

Great artery
(blood to body
or lungs)

√5ᵗʰ **424.9 Endocarditis, valve unspecified**

424.90 Endocarditis, valve unspecified, unspecified cause
Endocarditis (chronic):
NOS
nonbacterial thrombotic
Valvular:
incompetence
insufficiency ⎤
regurgitation ⎬ of unspecified valve,
stenosis ⎦ unspecified cause
Valvulitis (chronic)
I38 Endocarditis valve unspecified   I-10

424.91 Endocarditis in diseases classified elsewhere
Code first underlying disease as:
atypical verrucous endocarditis [Libman-Sacks]
(710.0)
disseminated lupus erythematosus (710.0)
tuberculosis (017.9)
EXCLUDES syphilitic (093.20-093.24)

424.99 Other
Any condition classifiable to 424.90 with specified
cause, except rheumatic
EXCLUDES endocardial fibroelastosis (425.3)
that specified as rheumatic (397.9)

√4ᵗʰ **425 Cardiomyopathy**
INCLUDES myocardiopathy
AHA: J-A, '85, 15

425.0 Endomyocardial fibrosis

425.1 Hypertrophic obstructive cardiomyopathy
Hypertrophic subaortic stenosis (idiopathic)
DEF: Cardiomyopathy marked by left ventricle hypertrophy, enlarged
septum; results in obstructed blood flow.

425.2 Obscure cardiomyopathy of Africa
Becker's disease
Idiopathic mural endomyocardial disease

425.3 Endocardial fibroelastosis
Elastomyofibrosis
DEF: A condition marked by left ventricle hypertrophy and
conversion of the endocardium into a thick fibroelastic coat; capacity
of the ventricle may be reduced, but is often increased.

425.4 Other primary cardiomyopathies
Cardiomyopathy: Cardiomyopathy:
NOS   idiopathic
congestive   nonobstructive
constrictive   obstructive
familial   restrictive
hypertrophic   Cardiovascular collagenosis
AHA: ▶4Q, '09, 141;◀ 1Q, '07, 20; 2Q, '05, 14; 1Q, '00, 22; 4Q, '97, 55;
2Q, '90, 19
TIP: For congestive cardiomyopathy, assign first a code for the CHF
(category 428) if the treatment is directed toward the CHF.
I42.8 Other cardiomyopathies   I-10

425.5 Alcoholic cardiomyopathy
DEF: Heart disease as result of excess alcohol consumption.
AHA: S-O, '85, 15

425.7 Nutritional and metabolic cardiomyopathy
Code first underlying disease, as:
amyloidosis (277.30-277.39)
beriberi (265.0)
cardiac glycogenosis (271.0)
mucopolysaccharidosis (277.5)
thyrotoxicosis (242.0-242.9)
EXCLUDES gouty tophi of heart (274.82)

425.8 Cardiomyopathy in other diseases classified elsewhere
Code first underlying disease, as:
Friedreich's ataxia (334.0)
myotonia atrophica (359.21)
progressive muscular dystrophy (359.1)
sarcoidosis (135)
EXCLUDES cardiomyopathy in Chagas' disease (086.0)
AHA: 2Q, '93, 9
I43 Cardiomyopathy in diseases classified elsewhere   I-10

425.9 Secondary cardiomyopathy, unspecified

√4ᵗʰ **426 Conduction disorders**
DEF: Disruption or disturbance in the electrical impulses that regulate
heartbeats.

426.0 Atrioventricular block, complete
Third degree atrioventricular block
AHA: 2Q, '06, 14
TIP: Assign if documentation indicates intermittent complete heart
block.

√5ᵗʰ **426.1 Atrioventricular block, other and unspecified**
AHA: 2Q, '06, 14
TIP: Assign separate codes for each type of AV block documented.

426.10 Atrioventricular block, unspecified
Atrioventricular [AV] block (incomplete) (partial)

426.11 First degree atrioventricular block
Incomplete atrioventricular block, first degree
Prolonged P-R interval NOS
AHA: 2Q, '06, 14
I44.0 Atrioventricular block first degree   I-10

426.12 Mobitz (type) II atrioventricular block
Incomplete atrioventricular block:
Mobitz (type) II
second degree, Mobitz (type) II
DEF: Impaired conduction of excitatory impulse from
cardiac atrium to ventricle through AV node.
AHA: 2Q, '06, 14

Nerve Conduction of the Heart

Sinoatrial node
(pacemaker)

Internodal tracts:
Anterior
Middle
Posterior

Atrioventricular
node

Common bundle
(of His)

Atrioventricular block

Accessory bundle
(of Kent)

Right bundle branch

Right bundle branch block

Moderator band

Bachmann's bundle

Left bundle branch block

Left bundle branch:
Anterior fascicle
Posterior fascicle

Left bundle branch
hemiblock

Purkinje fibers

Ⓝ Newborn Age: 0   Ⓟ Pediatric Age: 0-17   Ⓜ Maternity Age: 12-55   Ⓐ Adult Age: 15-124

426.13 Other second degree atrioventricular block
Incomplete atrioventricular block:
Mobitz (type) I [Wenckebach's]
second degree:
NOS
Mobitz (type) I
with 2:1 atrioventricular response [block]
Wenckebach's phenomenon
DEF: Wenckebach's phenomenon: impulses generated at constant rate to sinus node, P-R interval lengthens; results in cycle of ventricular inadequacy and shortened P-R interval; second-degree A-V block commonly called "Mobitz type 1."

426.2 Left bundle branch hemiblock
Block: Block:
left anterior fascicular   left posterior fascicular

426.3 Other left bundle branch block
Left bundle branch block:
NOS
anterior fascicular with posterior fascicular
complete
main stem
I44.7 Left bundle-branch block unspecified   `I-10`

426.4 Right bundle branch block
AHA: 3Q, '00, 3
I45.10 Unspecified right bundle-branch block   `I-10`

`√5ᵗʰ` **426.5 Bundle branch block, other and unspecified**

426.50 Bundle branch block, unspecified

426.51 Right bundle branch block and left posterior fascicular block

426.52 Right bundle branch block and left anterior fascicular block

426.53 Other bilateral bundle branch block
Bifascicular block NOS
Bilateral bundle branch block NOS
Right bundle branch with left bundle branch block (incomplete) (main stem)

426.54 Trifascicular block

426.6 Other heart block
Intraventricular block:
NOS
diffuse
myofibrillar
Sinoatrial block
Sinoauricular block

426.7 Anomalous atrioventricular excitation
Atrioventricular conduction:
accelerated
accessory
pre-excitation
Ventricular pre-excitation
Wolff-Parkinson-White syndrome
DEF: Wolff-Parkinson-White: normal conduction pathway is bypassed; results in short P-R interval on EKG; tendency to supraventricular tachycardia.

`√6ᵗʰ` **426.8 Other specified conduction disorders**

426.81 Lown-Ganong-Levine syndrome
Syndrome of short P-R interval, normal QRS complexes, and supraventricular tachycardias

426.82 Long QT syndrome
DEF: Condition characterized by recurrent syncope, malignant arrhythmias, and sudden death; characteristic prolonged Q-T interval on electrocardiogram.
AHA: 4Q, '05, 72

426.89 Other
Dissociation:
atrioventricular [AV]
interference
isorhythmic
Nonparoxysmal AV nodal tachycardia

426.9 Conduction disorder, unspecified
Heart block NOS
Stokes-Adams syndrome

Normal and Long QT Electrocardiogram

`√4ᵗʰ` **427 Cardiac dysrhythmias**
EXCLUDES *that complicating:*
abortion (634-638 with .7, 639.8)
ectopic or molar pregnancy (639.8)
labor or delivery (668.1, 669.4)
DEF: Disruption or disturbance in the rhythm of heartbeats.
AHA: J-A, '85, 15

427.0 Paroxysmal supraventricular tachycardia
Paroxysmal tachycardia: Paroxysmal tachycardia:
atrial [PAT]   junctional
atrioventricular [AV]   nodal
DEF: Rapid atrial rhythm.

427.1 Paroxysmal ventricular tachycardia
Ventricular tachycardia (paroxysmal)
DEF: Rapid ventricular rhythm.
AHA: 2Q, '09, 14; 1Q, '08, 14; 2Q, '06, 15-16; 3Q, '95, 9; M-A, '86, 11
TIP: If a ventricular tachycardia is documented as sustained or nonsustained but is induced during an EP study, assign 427.1.
I47.2 Ventricular tachycardia   `I-10`

427.2 Paroxysmal tachycardia, unspecified
Bouveret-Hoffmann syndrome
Paroxysmal tachycardia:
NOS
essential

`√5ᵗʰ` **427.3 Atrial fibrillation and flutter**
TIP: Assign V58.61 Long-term (current) use of anticoagulants, as a secondary diagnosis if the patient is maintained on Coumadin.

427.31 Atrial fibrillation
DEF: Irregular, rapid atrial contractions.
AHA: 4Q, '08, 135; 3Q, '05, 8; 4Q, '04, 78, 121; 3Q, '04, 7; 4Q, '03, 95, 105; 1Q, '03, 8; 2Q, '99, 17; 3Q, '95, 8
I48.0 Atrial fibrillation   `I-10`

427.32 Atrial flutter
DEF: Regular, rapid atrial contractions.
AHA: 4Q, '03, 94
I48.1 Atrial flutter   `I-10`

`√5ᵗʰ` **427.4 Ventricular fibrillation and flutter**

427.41 Ventricular fibrillation
DEF: Irregular, rapid ventricular contractions.
AHA: 2Q, '09, 14-15; 3Q, '02, 5

427.42 Ventricular flutter
DEF: Regular, rapid, ventricular contractions.

427.5 Cardiac arrest
Cardiorespiratory arrest
AHA: 3Q, '02, 5; 2Q, '00, 12; 3Q, '95, 8; 2Q, '88, 8
I46.9 Cardiac arrest cause unspecified   `I-10`

`√5ᵗʰ` **427.6 Premature beats**

427.60 Premature beats, unspecified
Ectopic beats
Extrasystoles
Extrasystolic arrhythmia
Premature contractions or systoles NOS

427.61 Supraventricular premature beats
Atrial premature beats, contractions, or systoles

427.69 Other
Ventricular premature beats, contractions, or systoles
AHA: 4Q, '93, 42

Diseases of the Circulatory System

427.8–429.1

✓5ᵗʰ 427.8 Other specified cardiac dysrhythmias

427.81 Sinoatrial node dysfunction

Sinus bradycardia: Syndrome:
- persistent   sick sinus
- severe   tachycardia-bradycardia

EXCLUDES *sinus bradycardia NOS (427.89)*

DEF: Complex cardiac arrhythmia; appears as severe sinus bradycardia, sinus bradycardia with tachycardia, or sinus bradycardia with atrioventricular block.

AHA: 3Q, '00, 8

I49.5 Sick sinus syndrome   `I-10`

427.89 Other

Rhythm disorder:
- coronary sinus
- ectopic
- nodal

Wandering (atrial) pacemaker

EXCLUDES *carotid sinus syncope (337.0)*
neonatal bradycardia (779.81)
neonatal tachycardia (779.82)
reflex bradycardia (337.0)
tachycardia NOS (785.0)

I49.8 Other specified cardiac arrhythmias   `I-10`

427.9 Cardiac dysrhythmia, unspecified

Arrhythmia (cardiac) NOS

AHA: 2Q, '89, 10

✓4ᵗʰ 428 Heart failure

Code, if applicable, heart failure due to hypertension first (402.0-402.9, with fifth-digit 1 or 404.0-404.9 with fifth-digit 1 or 3)

EXCLUDES *following cardiac surgery (429.4)*
rheumatic (398.91)
that complicating:
    abortion (634-638 with .7, 639.8)
    ectopic or molar pregnancy (639.8)
    labor or delivery (668.1, 669.4)

AHA: 4Q, '02, 49; 3Q, '98, 5; 2Q, '90, 16; 2Q, '90, 19; 2Q, '89, 10; 3Q, '88, 3

428.0 Congestive heart failure, unspecified

Congestive heart disease
Right heart failure (secondary to left heart failure)

EXCLUDES *fluid overload NOS ▶(276.69)◀*

DEF: Mechanical inadequacy; caused by inability of heart to pump and circulate blood; results in fluid collection in lungs, hypertension, congestion and edema of tissue.

AHA: 4Q, '09, 141; 1Q, '09, 8, 18; 4Q, '08, 72, 180, 182; 3Q, '08, 12; 3Q, '07, 9; 1Q, '07, 20; 3Q, '06, 7; 4Q, '05, 120; 3Q, '05, 8; 1Q, '05, 5, 9; 1Q, '05, 5, 9; 4Q, '04, 140; 3Q, '04, 7; 4Q, '03, 109; 1Q, '03, 9; 4Q, '02, 52; 2Q, '01, 13; 4Q, '00, 48; 2Q, '00, 16; 1Q, '00, 22; 4Q, '99, 4; 1Q, '99, 11; 4Q, '97, 55; 3Q, '97, 10; 3Q, '96, 9; 3Q, '91, 18; 3Q, '91, 19; 2Q, '89, 12

TIP: Assign additional code(s) from subcategory 428.2, 428.3, or 428.4 to specify the type of heart failure.

I50.9 Heart failure unspecified   `I-10`

428.1 Left heart failure

Acute edema of lung   ⎫ with heart disease NOS or
Acute pulmonary edema ⎬ heart failure
Cardiac asthma   ⎭
Left ventricular failure

DEF: Mechanical inadequacy of left ventricle; causing fluid in lungs.

✓5ᵗʰ 428.2 Systolic heart failure

EXCLUDES *combined systolic and diastolic heart failure (428.40-428.43)*

DEF: Heart failure due to a defect in expulsion of blood caused by an abnormality in systolic function, or ventricular contractile dysfunction.

428.20 Unspecified

I50.20 Unspecified systolic congestive heart failure   `I-10`

428.21 Acute

I50.21 Acute systolic congestive heart failure   `I-10`

428.22 Chronic

AHA: 4Q, '05, 120

428.23 Acute on chronic

AHA: 1Q, '09, 8, 18; 1Q, '03, 9

Echocardiography of Heart Failure

Four-chamber echocardiograms, two-dimensional views.
LV: Left ventricle
RV: Right ventricle
RA: Right atrium
LA: Left atrium

Systolic dysfunction with dilated LV

Diastolic dysfunction with LV hypertrophy

✓5ᵗʰ 428.3 Diastolic heart failure

EXCLUDES *combined systolic and diastolic heart failure (428.40-428.43)*

DEF: Heart failure due to resistance to ventricular filling caused by an abnormality in the diastolic function.

428.30 Unspecified

AHA: 4Q, '02, 52

I50.30 Unspecified diastolic congestive heart failure   `I-10`

428.31 Acute

428.32 Chronic

AHA: 3Q, '08, 12

I50.32 Chronic diastolic congestive heart failure   `I-10`

428.33 Acute on chronic

AHA: 4Q, '09, 141; 3Q, '08, 12; 1Q, '07, 20

I50.33 Acute on chronic diastolic heart failure   `I-10`

✓5ᵗʰ 428.4 Combined systolic and diastolic heart failure

428.40 Unspecified

428.41 Acute

AHA: 4Q, '04, 140

428.42 Chronic

428.43 Acute on chronic

AHA: 3Q, '06, 7; 4Q, '02, 52

428.9 Heart failure, unspecified

Cardiac failure NOS   Myocardial failure NOS
Heart failure NOS   Weak heart

AHA: 2Q, '89, 10; N-D, '85, 14

✓4ᵗʰ 429 Ill-defined descriptions and complications of heart disease

429.0 Myocarditis, unspecified

Myocarditis   ⎫
  NOS   ⎪
  chronic (interstitial) ⎬ (with mention of
  fibroid   ⎪ arteriosclerosis)
  senile   ⎭

Use additional code to identify presence of arteriosclerosis

EXCLUDES *acute or subacute (422.0-422.9)*
rheumatic (398.0)
  acute (391.2)
that due to hypertension (402.0-402.9)

429.1 Myocardial degeneration

Degeneration of heart or ⎫
  myocardium: ⎪
  fatty   ⎪
  mural   ⎬ (with mention of
  muscular   ⎪ arteriosclerosis)
Myocardial: ⎪
  degeneration   ⎪
  disease   ⎭

Use additional code to identify presence of arteriosclerosis

EXCLUDES *that due to hypertension (402.0-402.9)*

N Newborn Age: 0   **P** Pediatric Age: 0-17   **M** Maternity Age: 12-55   **A** Adult Age: 15-124

429.2 Cardiovascular disease, unspecified
Arteriosclerotic cardiovascular disease [ASCVD]
Cardiovascular arteriosclerosis
Cardiovascular:
   degeneration   ⎫
   disease   ⎬ (with mention of arteriosclerosis)
   sclerosis   ⎭
Use additional code to identify presence of arteriosclerosis
EXCLUDES *that due to hypertension (402.0-402.9)*

429.3 Cardiomegaly
Cardiac: Ventricular dilatation
   dilatation
   hypertrophy
EXCLUDES *that due to hypertension (402.0-402.9)*
I51.7 Cardiomegaly   I-10

429.4 Functional disturbances following cardiac surgery
Cardiac insufficiency ⎫ following cardiac surgery or
Heart failure   ⎬ due to prosthesis
Postcardiotomy syndrome
Postvalvulotomy syndrome
EXCLUDES *cardiac failure in the immediate postoperative period (997.1)*
AHA: 2Q, '02, 12; N-D, '85, 6

429.5 Rupture of chordae tendineae
DEF: Torn tissue, between heart valves and papillary muscles.

429.6 Rupture of papillary muscle
DEF: Torn muscle, between chordae tendineae and heart wall.

√5ᵗʰ **429.7 Certain sequelae of myocardial infarction, not elsewhere classified**
Use additional code to identify the associated myocardial infarction:
   with onset of 8 weeks or less (410.00-410.92)
   with onset of more than 8 weeks (414.8)
EXCLUDES *congenital defects of heart (745, 746)*
coronary aneurysm (414.11)
disorders of papillary muscle (429.6, 429.81)
postmyocardial infarction syndrome (411.0)
rupture of chordae tendineae (429.5)
AHA: 3Q, '89, 5

  429.71 Acquired cardiac septal defect   A
      EXCLUDES *acute septal infarction (410.00-410.92)*
      DEF: Abnormal communication, between opposite heart chambers; due to defect of septum; not present at birth.

  429.79 Other   A
      Mural thrombus (atrial) (ventricular), acquired, following myocardial infarction
      AHA: 1Q, '92, 10

√5ᵗʰ **429.8 Other ill-defined heart diseases**

  429.81 Other disorders of papillary muscle
      Papillary muscle: Papillary muscle:
         atrophy   incompetence
         degeneration   incoordination
         dysfunction   scarring

  429.82 Hyperkinetic heart disease
      DEF: Condition of unknown origin in young adults; marked by increased cardiac output at rest, increased rate of ventricular ejection; may lead to heart failure.

  429.83 Takotsubo syndrome
      Broken heart syndrome
      Reversible left ventricular dysfunction following sudden emotional stress
      Stress induced cardiomyopathy
      Transient left ventricular apical ballooning syndrome
      AHA: 4Q, '06, 87

  429.89 Other
      Carditis
      EXCLUDES *that due to hypertension (402.0-402.9)*
      AHA: 2Q, '06, 18; 3Q, '05, 14; 1Q, '92, 10

Berry Aneurysms

429.9 Heart disease, unspecified
Heart disease (organic) NOS
Morbus cordis NOS
EXCLUDES *that due to hypertension (402.0-402.9)*
AHA: 1Q, '09, 7; 1Q, '93, 19
I51.9 Heart disease unspecified   I-10

Cerebrovascular Disease (430-438)

INCLUDES with mention of hypertension (conditions classifiable to 401-405)
Use additional code to identify presence of hypertension
EXCLUDES *any condition classifiable to 430-434, 436, 437 occurring during pregnancy, childbirth, or the puerperium, or specified as puerperal (674.0)*
iatrogenic cerebrovascular infarction or hemorrhage (997.02)
AHA: 1Q, '93, 27; 3Q, '91, 10; 3Q, '90, 3; 2Q, '89, 8; M-A, '85, 6

430 Subarachnoid hemorrhage
Meningeal hemorrhage
Ruptured:
   berry aneurysm
   (congenital) cerebral aneurysm NOS
   EXCLUDES *syphilitic ruptured cerebral aneurysm (094.87)*
AHA: 4Q, '04, 77
DEF: Bleeding in space between brain and lining.

431 Intracerebral hemorrhage
Hemorrhage (of):   Hemorrhage (of):
  basilar   internal capsule
  bulbar   intrapontine
  cerebellar   pontine
  cerebral   subcortical
  cerebromeningeal ventricular
  corticalRupture of blood vessel in brain
DEF: Bleeding within the brain.
AHA: ▶1Q, '10, 8;◀ 3Q, '07, 4; 4Q, '04, 77
I61.9 Nontraumatic intracerebral hemorrhage unspec   I-10

√4ᵗʰ **432 Other and unspecified intracranial hemorrhage**
AHA: 4Q, '04, 7

  432.0 Nontraumatic extradural hemorrhage
      Nontraumatic epidural hemorrhage
      DEF: Bleeding, nontraumatic, between skull and brain lining.

  432.1 Subdural hemorrhage
      Subdural hematoma, nontraumatic
      DEF: Bleeding, between outermost and other layers of brain lining.

  432.9 Unspecified intracranial hemorrhage
      Intracranial hemorrhage NOS

Cerebrovascular Arteries

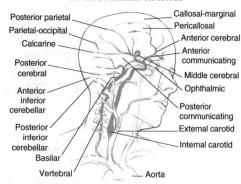

✓4th 433 Occlusion and stenosis of precerebral arteries

> INCLUDES   embolism
> narrowing   of basilar, carotid, and vertebral
> obstruction   arteries
> thrombosis

Use additional code, if applicable, to identify status post administration of tPA (rtPA) in a different facility within the last 24 hours prior to admission to current facility (V45.88)

> EXCLUDES   insufficiency NOS of precerebral arteries (435.0–435.9)

The following fifth-digit subclassification is for use with category 433:
> **0 without mention of cerebral infarction**
> **1 with cerebral infarction**

> **DEF:** Blockage, stricture, arteries branching into brain.
> **AHA:** 2Q, '95, 14; 3Q, '90, 16

§ ✓5th **433.0 Basilar artery**
[0-1]

§ ✓5th **433.1 Carotid artery**
[0-1]   **AHA:** 1Q, '00, 16; **For code 433.10:** 1Q, '06, 17; 1Q, '02, 7, 10
> I65.29 Occlusion and stenosis of unspec carotid artery   `I-10`
> I63.239 Cerbral infarct d/t usp occ/stenosis of uns carotid art   `I-10`
> I63.449 Cerbral infarct d/t embo of uns cerebellar art   `I-10`

§ ✓5th **433.2 Vertebral artery**
[0-1]

§ ✓5th **433.3 Multiple and bilateral**
[0-1]   **AHA:** 2Q, '02, 19

§ ✓5th **433.8 Other specified precerebral artery**
[0-1]

§ ✓5th **433.9 Unspecified precerebral artery**
[0-1]   Precerebral artery NOS

✓4th 434 Occlusion of cerebral arteries

Use additional code, if applicable, to identify status post administration of tPA (rtPA) in a different facility within the last 24 hours prior to admission to current facility (V45.88)

The following fifth-digit subclassification is for use with category 434:
> **0 without mention of cerebral infarction**
> **1 with cerebral infarction**

> **AHA:** 2Q, '95, 14

§ ✓5th **434.0 Cerebral thrombosis**
[0-1]   Thrombosis of cerebral arteries
> **AHA: For code 434.01:** 4Q, '04, 77

§ ✓5th **434.1 Cerebral embolism**
[0-1]   **AHA: For code 434.11:** 4Q, '04, 77; 3Q, '97, 11
> I63.449 Cerbral infarct d/t embo of uns cerebellar art   `I-10`

§ ✓5th **434.9 Cerebral artery occlusion, unspecified**
[0-1]   **AHA: For code 434.91:** 4Q, '08, 108; 3Q, '07, 9; 1Q, '07, 23; 4Q, '04, 77-78; 4Q, '98, 87

✓4th 435 Transient cerebral ischemia

> INCLUDES   cerebrovascular insufficiency (acute) with transient focal neurological signs and symptoms
> insufficiency of basilar, carotid, and vertebral arteries
> spasm of cerebral arteries

> EXCLUDES   acute cerebrovascular insufficiency NOS (437.1)
> that due to any condition classifiable to 433 (433.0–433.9)

> **DEF:** Temporary restriction of blood flow to arteries branching into brain.

435.0 Basilar artery syndrome

435.1 Vertebral artery syndrome

435.2 Subclavian steal syndrome
> **DEF:** Cerebrovascular insufficiency, due to occluded subclavian artery; symptoms include pain in mastoid and posterior head regions, flaccid paralysis of arm and diminished or absent radial pulse on affected side.

435.3 Vertebrobasilar artery syndrome
> **DEF:** Transient ischemic attack; due to brainstem dysfunction; symptoms include confusion, vertigo, binocular blindness, diplopia, unilateral or bilateral weakness and paresthesis of extremities.
> **AHA:** 4Q, '95, 60

435.8 Other specified transient cerebral ischemias

435.9 Unspecified transient cerebral ischemia
> Impending cerebrovascular accident
> Intermittent cerebral ischemia
> Transient ischemic attack [TIA]
> **AHA:** N-D, '85, 12
> G45.9 Transient cerebral ischemic attack unspecified   `I-10`

436 Acute, but ill-defined, cerebrovascular disease

Apoplexy, apoplectic: Apoplexy, apoplectic:
NOS   seizure
attack   Cerebral seizure
cerebral

> EXCLUDES   any condition classifiable to categories 430-435
> cerebrovascular accident (434.91)
> CVA (ischemic) (434.91)
> embolic (434.11)
> hemorrhagic (430, 431, 432.0-432.9)
> thrombotic (434.01)
> postoperative cerebrovascular accident (997.02)
> stroke (ischemic) (434.91)
> embolic (434.11)
> hemorrhagic (430, 431, 432.0-432.9)
> thrombotic (434.01)

> **AHA:** 4Q, '04, 77; 4Q, '99, 3
> **TIP:** Do not assign when documentation indicates "CVA, stroke, or cerebral infarction." See instead default code 434.91.

✓4th 437 Other and ill-defined cerebrovascular disease

437.0 Cerebral atherosclerosis   `A`
> Atheroma of cerebral arteries
> Cerebral arteriosclerosis
> I67.2 Cerebral atherosclerosis   `I-10`

437.1 Other generalized ischemic cerebrovascular disease
> Acute cerebrovascular insufficiency NOS
> Cerebral ischemia (chronic)
> **AHA:** 1Q, '09, 8

437.2 Hypertensive encephalopathy
> **DEF:** Cerebral manifestations (such as visual disturbances and headache) due to high blood pressure.
> **AHA:** J-A, '84, 14

437.3 Cerebral aneurysm, nonruptured
> Internal carotid artery, intracranial portion
> Internal carotid artery NOS
> EXCLUDES   congenital cerebral aneurysm, nonruptured (747.81)
> internal carotid artery, extracranial portion (442.81)
> **AHA:** 2Q, '09, 12

437.4 Cerebral arteritis
> **DEF:** Inflammation of a cerebral artery or arteries.
> **AHA:** 4Q, '99, 21

437.5 Moyamoya disease
> **DEF:** Cerebrovascular ischemia; vessels occlude and rupture causing tiny hemorrhages at base of brain; predominantly affects Japanese.

---

§   Requires fifth digit. Valid digits are in [brackets] under each code. See appropriate category for codes and definitions.

   N Newborn Age: 0   P Pediatric Age: 0-17   M Maternity Age: 12-55   A Adult Age: 15-124

437.6 Nonpyogenic thrombosis of intracranial venous sinus

> **EXCLUDES** *pyogenic (325)*

437.7 Transient global amnesia

> **DEF:** Episode of short-term memory loss, not often recurrent; pathogenesis unknown; with no signs or symptoms of neurological disorder.
>
> **AHA:** 4Q, '92, 20

437.8 Other

437.9 Unspecified

> Cerebrovascular disease or lesion NOS
>
> **AHA:** 1Q, '09, 9

√4th **438 Late effects of cerebrovascular disease**

> **NOTE** This category is to be used to indicate conditions in 430-437 as the cause of late effects. The "late effects" include conditions specified as such, as sequelae, which may occur at any time after the onset of the causal condition.
>
> **EXCLUDES** *personal history of:*
> *cerebral infarction without residual deficits (V12.54)*
> *PRIND [Prolonged reversible ischemic neurologic deficit] (V12.54)*
> *RIND [Reversible ischemic neurological deficit] (V12.54)*
> *transient ischemic attack [TIA] (V12.54)*
>
> **AHA:** 3Q, '06, 3-4, 6; 4Q, '99, 4, 6, 7; 4Q, '98, 39, 88; 4Q, '97, 35, 37; 4Q, '92, 21;N-D,'86, 12; M-A, '86, 7
>
> **TIP:** Assign instead code V12.54 TIA and cerebral infarction without residual effects, if no residual deficits are present.

438.0 Cognitive deficits

√5th **438.1 Speech and language deficits**

> **438.10 Speech and language deficit, unspecified**
>
> **438.11 Aphasia**
> > **DEF:** Impairment or absence of the ability to communicate by speech, writing or signs or to comprehend the spoken or written language due to disease or injury to the brain.
> > **AHA:** 4Q, '03, 105; 4Q, '97, 36
>
> **438.12 Dysphasia**
> > **DEF:** Impaired speech; marked by inability to sequence language.
> > **AHA:** 4Q, '99, 3, 9
>
> **438.13 Dysarthria**
> > **DEF:** Speech disorder caused by paralysis, spasticity, or other nerve damage resulting in difficulty expressing words or sounds; characterized by slurring, interrupted rhythm of speech, or distorted vowel sounds.
> > **AHA:** 4Q, '09, 87-88
> > **TIP:** If dysarthria or other speech disturbances are not due to underlying cerebrovascular disease, see subcategory 784.5 codes.
>
> **438.14 Fluency disorder**
> > ►Stuttering due to late effect of cerebrovascular accident◄
> > **DEF:** Interruption in the flow of speech that significantly interferes with communication; characterized by primary sound and syllable repetitions, articulatory fixations, and abnormal prolongation of speech sounds.
> > **AHA:** 4Q, '09, 87-88
>
> **438.19 Other speech and language deficits**

√5th **438.2 Hemiplegia/hemiparesis**

> **DEF:** Paralysis of one side of the body.
> **AHA:** ►1Q, '10, 5◄
>
> **438.20 Hemiplegia affecting unspecified side**
> > **AHA:** 4Q, '07, 94; 4Q, '03, 105; 4Q, '99, 3, 9
> > I69.959 Hempl & hemiparesis flw uns CVD affect uns side   I-10
>
> **438.21 Hemiplegia affecting dominant side**
>
> **438.22 Hemiplegia affecting nondominant side**
> > **AHA:** 4Q, '03, 105; 1Q, '02, 16

√5th **438.3 Monoplegia of upper limb**

> **DEF:** Paralysis of one limb or one muscle group.
>
> **438.30 Monoplegia of upper limb affecting unspecified side**
>
> **438.31 Monoplegia of upper limb affecting dominant side**
>
> **438.32 Monoplegia of upper limb affecting nondominant side**

√5th **438.4 Monoplegia of lower limb**

> **438.40 Monoplegia of lower limb affecting unspecified side**
>
> **438.41 Monoplegia of lower limb affecting dominant side**
>
> **438.42 Monoplegia of lower limb affecting nondominant side**

√5th **438.5 Other paralytic syndrome**

> Use additional code to identify type of paralytic syndrome, such as:
> locked-in state (344.81)
> quadriplegia (344.00-344.09)
>
> **EXCLUDES** *late effects of cerebrovascular accident with:*
> *hemiplegia/hemiparesis (438.20-438.22)*
> *monoplegia of lower limb (438.40-438.42)*
> *monoplegia of upper limb (438.30-438.32)*
>
> **438.50 Other paralytic syndrome affecting unspecified side**
>
> **438.51 Other paralytic syndrome affecting dominant side**
>
> **438.52 Other paralytic syndrome affecting nondominant side**
>
> **438.53 Other paralytic syndrome, bilateral**
> > **AHA:** 4Q, '98, 39

438.6 Alterations of sensations

> Use additional code to identify the altered sensation

438.7 Disturbances of vision

> Use additional code to identify the visual disturbance
> **AHA:** 4Q, '02, 56

√5th **438.8 Other late effects of cerebrovascular disease**

> **438.81 Apraxia**
> > **DEF:** Inability to activate learned movements; no known sensory or motor impairment.
>
> **438.82 Dysphagia**
> > Use additional code to identify the type of dysphagia, if known (787.20-787.29)
> > **DEF:** Inability or difficulty in swallowing.
> > **AHA:** 4Q, '07, 94
> > I69.991 Dysphagia following uns cerebrovascular dis   I-10
>
> **438.83 Facial weakness**
> > Facial droop
>
> **438.84 Ataxia**
> > **AHA:** 4Q, '02, 56
>
> **438.85 Vertigo**
>
> **438.89 Other late effects of cerebrovascular disease**
> > Use additional code to identify the late effect
> > **AHA:** 2Q, '09, 10; 1Q, '05, 13; 4Q, '98, 39
> > **TIP:** Assign 438.89 and 728.87 Muscle weakness, for residual weakness secondary to late effect of CVA.
> > I69.998 Other sequelae flw uns cerebrovascular disease   I-10

438.9 Unspecified late effects of cerebrovascular disease

Diseases of the Circulatory System

440–440.22

Map of Major Arteries

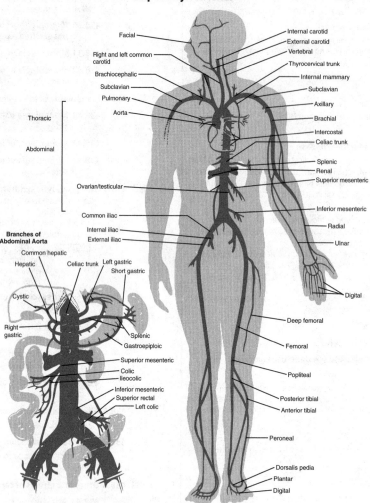

Diseases of Arteries, Arterioles, and Capillaries (440-449)

☑4ᵗʰ 440 Atherosclerosis

INCLUDES arteriolosclerosis
arteriosclerosis (obliterans) (senile)
arteriosclerotic vascular disease
atheroma
degeneration:
   arterial
   arteriovascular
   vascular
endarteritis deformans or obliterans
senile:
   arteritis
   endarteritis

EXCLUDES atheroembolism (445.01-445.89)
atherosclerosis of bypass graft of the extremities
(440.30-440.32)

DEF: Stricture and reduced elasticity of artery; due to plaque deposits.

440.0 Of aorta   A

    AHA: 2Q, '93, 7; 2Q, '93, 8; 4Q, '88, 8

440.1 Of renal artery   A

    EXCLUDES atherosclerosis of renal arterioles (403.00-403.91)

☑5ᵗʰ 440.2 Of native arteries of the extremities

Use additional code, if applicable, to identify chronic total
occlusion of artery of the extremities (440.4)

    EXCLUDES atherosclerosis of bypass graft of the extremities
(440.30-440.32)

AHA: 4Q, '94, 49; 4Q, '93, 27; 4Q, '92, 25; 3Q, '90, 15; M-A, '87, 6
TIP: Codes are listed in order of increasing severity; all patients who
have gangrene (regardless of whether ulceration, rest pain, and/or
intermittent claudication are present) are coded to 440.24. Patients
without gangrene, but with ulceration (regardless of whether they
also suffer from rest pain or intermittent claudication) are coded to
440.23.

440.20 Atherosclerosis of the extremities, unspecified   A

    I70.209 Uns atherosclero natv art of extrem uns extrem   I-10

440.21 Atherosclerosis of the extremities with intermittent claudication   A

    DEF: Atherosclerosis; marked by pain, tension and weakness
after walking; no symptoms while at rest.

    I70.219 Atherosclerosis native arteries ext   I-10
interm claud uns ext

440.22 Atherosclerosis of the extremities with rest pain   A

    INCLUDES any condition classifiable to 440.21

    DEF: Atherosclerosis, marked by pain, tension and weakness
while at rest.

☑N Newborn Age: 0   ☑P Pediatric Age: 0-17   ☑M Maternity Age: 12-55   ☑A Adult Age: 15-124

440.23 Atherosclerosis of the extremities with ulceration 　A

> INCLUDES any condition classifiable to 440.21 and 440.22

Use additional code for any associated ulceration (707.10-707.9)

AHA: 4Q, '00, 44

I70.249 Atherosclero natv art lt leg ulceration uns site 　I-10

440.24 Atherosclerosis of the extremities with gangrene

> INCLUDES any condition classifiable to 440.21, 440.22, and 440.23 with ischemic gangrene 785.4

Use additional code for any associated ulceration (707.10-707.9)

> EXCLUDES gas gangrene (040.0)

AHA: 4Q, '03, 109; 3Q, '03, 14; 4Q, '95, 54; 1Q, '95, 11

440.29 Other 　A

√5ʰ **440.3 Of bypass graft of extremities**

> EXCLUDES atherosclerosis of native arteries of the extremities (440.21-440.24)
> embolism [occlusion NOS] [thrombus] of graft (996.74)

AHA: 4Q, '94, 49

440.30 Of unspecified graft 　A

440.31 Of autologous vein bypass graft 　A

440.32 Of nonautologous biological bypass graft 　A

440.4 Chronic total occlusion of artery of the extremities
Complete occlusion of artery of the extremities
Total occlusion of artery of the extremities

Code first atherosclerosis of arteries of the extremities (440.20-440.29, 440.30-440.32)

> EXCLUDES acute occlusion of artery of extremity (444.21-444.22)

AHA: 4Q, '07, 82

440.8 Of other specified arteries 　A

> EXCLUDES basilar (433.0)
> carotid (433.1)
> cerebral (437.0)
> coronary (414.00-414.07)
> mesenteric (557.1)
> precerebral (433.0-433.9)
> pulmonary (416.0)
> vertebral (433.2)

AHA: 3Q, '09, 9

TIP: Assign for arteriosclerosis of the iliac artery.

440.9 Generalized and unspecified atherosclerosis 　A
Arteriosclerotic vascular disease NOS

> EXCLUDES arteriosclerotic cardiovascular disease [ASCVD] (429.2)

I70.91 Generalized atherosclerosis 　I-10

√4ʰ **441 Aortic aneurysm and dissection**

> EXCLUDES ►aortic ectasia (447.70-447.73)◄
> syphilitic aortic aneurysm (093.0)
> traumatic aortic aneurysm (901.0, 902.0)

√5ʰ **441.0 Dissection of aorta**

DEF: Dissection or splitting of wall of the aorta; due to blood entering through intimal tear or interstitial hemorrhage.

AHA: 4Q, '89, 10

441.00 Unspecified site

441.01 Thoracic
AHA: 1Q, '09, 16; 4Q, '07, 87

441.02 Abdominal

441.03 Thoracoabdominal

441.1 Thoracic aneurysm, ruptured

441.2 Thoracic aneurysm without mention of rupture
AHA: 3Q, '92, 10
I71.2 Thoracic aortic aneurysm without rupture 　I-10

441.3 Abdominal aneurysm, ruptured

Thoracic and Abdominal Aortic Aneurysm

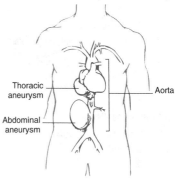

Thoracic aneurysm
Abdominal aneurysm
Aorta

441.4 Abdominal aneurysm without mention of rupture
AHA: 4Q, '00, 64; 1Q, '99, 15, 16, 17; 3Q, '92, 10
I71.4 Abdominal aortic aneurysm without rupture 　I-10

441.5 Aortic aneurysm of unspecified site, ruptured
Rupture of aorta NOS

441.6 Thoracoabdominal aneurysm, ruptured

441.7 Thoracoabdominal aneurysm, without mention of rupture
AHA: 2Q, '06, 16

441.9 Aortic aneurysm of unspecified site without mention of rupture
Aneurysm
Dilatation 　} of aorta
Hyaline necrosis

√4ʰ **442 Other aneurysm**

> INCLUDES aneurysm (ruptured) (cirsoid) (false) (varicose)
> aneurysmal varix

> EXCLUDES arteriovenous aneurysm or fistula:
> acquired (447.0)
> congenital (747.60-747.69)
> traumatic (900.0-904.9)

DEF: Dissection or splitting of arterial wall; due to blood entering through intimal tear or interstitial hemorrhage.

442.0 Of artery of upper extremity

442.1 Of renal artery

442.2 Of iliac artery
AHA: 1Q, '99, 16, 17

442.3 Of artery of lower extremity
Aneurysm: 　　　Aneurysm:
femoral artery 　　popliteal artery
AHA: 2Q, '08, 13; 3Q, '02, 24-26; 1Q, '99, 16

√5ʰ **442.8 Of other specified artery**

442.81 Artery of neck
Aneurysm of carotid artery (common) (external) (internal, extracranial portion)

> EXCLUDES internal carotid artery, intra-cranial portion (437.3)

442.82 Subclavian artery

442.83 Splenic artery

442.84 Other visceral artery
Aneurysm:
celiac
gastroduodenal
gastroepiploic
hepatic 　　　} artery
pancreaticoduodenal
superior mesenteric

√4ʰ
√5ʰ Additional Digit Required　　Unspecified Code　　Other Specified Code　　Manifestation Code　　►◄ Revised Text　　● New Code　　▲ Revised Code Title

2011 ICD-9-CM　　　　　　　　　　　　　　　　　　　　　　　　　　　　　　**October 2010 • Volume 1 – 137**

442.89 Other

Aneurysm:
 mediastinal artery
 spinal artery

EXCLUDES   *cerebral (nonruptured) (437.3)*
 congenital (747.81)
 ruptured (430)
 coronary (414.11)
 heart (414.10)
 pulmonary (417.1)

442.9 Of unspecified site

√4th 443 Other peripheral vascular disease

443.0 Raynaud's syndrome

Raynaud's:
 disease
 phenomenon (secondary)

Use additional code to identify gangrene (785.4)

DEF: Constriction of the arteries, due to cold or stress; bilateral ischemic attacks of fingers, toes, nose or ears; symptoms include pallor, paresthesia and pain.

I73.00 Raynaud's syndrome without gangrene   I-10

443.1 Thromboangiitis obliterans [Buerger's disease]

Presenile gangrene

DEF: Inflammatory disease of extremity blood vessels, mainly the lower; occurs primarily in young men and leads to tissue ischemia and gangrene.

√5th 443.2 Other arterial dissection

EXCLUDES   *dissection of aorta (441.00-441.03)*
 dissection of coronary arteries (414.12)

AHA: 4Q, '02, 54

443.21 Dissection of carotid artery

443.22 Dissection of iliac artery

443.23 Dissection of renal artery

443.24 Dissection of vertebral artery

443.29 Dissection of other artery

√5th 443.8 Other specified peripheral vascular diseases

443.81 Peripheral angiopathy in diseases classified elsewhere

Code first underlying disease, as:
 diabetes mellitus (249.7, 250.7)

AHA: 1Q, '04, 14; 3Q, '91, 10

I79.8 Oth d/o art arterioles & cap in dz clas elsw   I-10

443.82 Erythromelalgia

DEF: Rare syndrome of paroxysmal vasodilation; maldistribution of blood flow causes redness, pain, increased skin temperature, and burning sensations in various parts of the body.

AHA: 4Q, '05, 73

443.89 Other

Acrocyanosis
Acroparesthesia:
 simple [Schultze's type]
 vasomotor [Nothnagel's type]
Erythrocyanosis

EXCLUDES   *chilblains (991.5)*
 frostbite (991.0-991.3)
 immersion foot (991.4)

AHA: 4Q, '07, 124

I73.89 Other specified peripheral vascular dz   I-10

443.9 Peripheral vascular disease, unspecified

Intermittent claudication NOS
Peripheral:
 angiopathy NOS
 vascular disease NOS
Spasm of artery

EXCLUDES   *atherosclerosis of the arteries of the extremities (440.20-440.22)*
 spasm of cerebral artery (435.0-435.9)

AHA: 4Q, '92, 25; 3Q, '91, 10

I73.9 Peripheral vascular disease unspecified   I-10

Arterial Diseases and Disorders

Lipids
Calcium deposits

Intimal proliferation

Atherosclerosis narrowing lumen

Thrombus (clot) forming in lumen

Organization of thrombus and recanalization

Embolus (from elsewhere) occluding lumen

Aneurysm bypasses lumen or...

...bulges from arterial wall

Arteriovenous fistula

√4th 444 Arterial embolism and thrombosis

INCLUDES   infarction:
 embolic
 thrombotic
 occlusion

EXCLUDES   *atheroembolism (445.01-445.89)*
 that complicating:
 abortion (634-638 with .6, 639.6)
 ectopic or molar pregnancy (639.6)
 pregnancy, childbirth, or the pueperium (673.0-673.8)
 septic arterial embolism (449)

AHA: 2Q, '92, 11; 4Q, '90, 27

444.0 Of abdominal aorta

Aortic bifurcation syndrome
Aortoiliac obstruction
Leriche's syndrome
Saddle embolus

AHA: 2Q, '93, 7; 4Q, '90, 27

444.1 Of thoracic aorta

Embolism or thrombosis of aorta (thoracic)

√5th 444.2 Of arteries of the extremities

AHA: M-A, '87, 6

444.21 Upper extremity

444.22 Lower extremity

Arterial embolism or thrombosis:
 femoral
 peripheral NOS
 popliteal

EXCLUDES   *iliofemoral (444.81)*

AHA: 4Q, '07, 85; 3Q, '03, 10; 1Q, '03, 17; 3Q, '90, 16

I74.3 Embo & thromb of arteries of the low extremities   I-10

√5th 444.8 Of other specified artery

444.81 Iliac artery

AHA: 1Q, '03, 16

444.89 Other

EXCLUDES   *basilar (433.0)*
 carotid (433.1)
 cerebral (434.0-434.9)
 coronary (410.00-410.92)
 mesenteric (557.0)
 ophthalmic (362.30-362.34)
 precerebral (433.0-433.9)
 pulmonary (415.19)
 renal (593.81)
 retinal (362.30-362.34)
 vertebral (433.2)

444.9 Of unspecified artery

√4th 445 Atheroembolism

INCLUDES   atherothrombotic microembolism
 cholesterol embolism

AHA: 4Q, '02, 57

√5th 445.0 Of extremities

445.01 Upper extremity

445.02 Lower extremity

N   Newborn Age: 0   P   Pediatric Age: 0-17   M   Maternity Age: 12-55   A   Adult Age: 15-124

√5ᵗʰ **445.8 Of other sites**

445.81 Kidney

Use additional code for any associated acute kidney failure or chronic kidney disease (584, 585)

445.89 Other site

√4ᵗʰ **446 Polyarteritis nodosa and allied conditions**

446.0 Polyarteritis nodosa
Disseminated necrotizing periarteritis
Necrotizing angiitis
Panarteritis (nodosa)
Periarteritis (nodosa)
DEF: Inflammation of small and mid-size arteries; symptoms related to involved arteries in kidneys, muscles, gastrointestinal tract and heart; results in tissue death.

446.1 Acute febrile mucocutaneous lymph node syndrome [MCLS]
Kawasaki disease
DEF: Acute febrile disease of children; marked by erythema of conjunctiva and mucous membranes of upper respiratory tract, skin eruptions and edema.

√5ᵗʰ **446.2 Hypersensitivity angiitis**

EXCLUDES *antiglomerular basement membrane disease without pulmonary hemorrhage (583.89)*

446.20 Hypersensitivity angiitis, unspecified

446.21 Goodpasture's syndrome
Antiglomerular basement membrane antibody-mediated nephritis with pulmonary hemorrhage
Use additional code to identify renal disease (583.81)
DEF: Glomerulonephritis associated with hematuria, progresses rapidly; results in death from renal failure.

446.29 Other specified hypersensitivity angiitis
AHA: 1Q, '95, 3

446.3 Lethal midline granuloma
Malignant granuloma of face
DEF: Granulomatous lesion; in nose or paranasal sinuses; often fatal; occurs chiefly in males.
AHA: 3Q, '00, 11

446.4 Wegener's granulomatosis
Necrotizing respiratory granulomatosis
Wegener's syndrome
DEF: A disease occurring mainly in men; marked by necrotizing granulomas and ulceration of the upper respiratory tract; cause is a vasculitis affecting small vessels due to an immune disorder.
AHA: 3Q, '00, 11

446.5 Giant cell arteritis
Bagratuni's syndrome   Horton's disease
Cranial arteritis   Temporal arteritis
DEF: Inflammation of arteries; due to giant cells affecting carotid artery branches, resulting in occlusion; symptoms include fever, headache and neurological problems.
M31.6 Other giant cell arteritis   I-10

446.6 Thrombotic microangiopathy
Moschcowitz's syndrome
Thrombotic thrombocytopenic purpura
DEF: Blockage of small blood vessels; due to hyaline deposits; symptoms include purpura, CNS disorders; results in protracted disease or rapid death.

446.7 Takayasu's disease
Aortic arch arteritis
Pulseless disease
DEF: Progressive obliterative arteritis of brachiocephalic trunk, left subclavian, and left common carotid arteries above aortic arch; results in ischemia in brain, heart and arm.

√4ᵗʰ **447 Other disorders of arteries and arterioles**

447.0 Arteriovenous fistula, acquired
Arteriovenous aneurysm, acquired
EXCLUDES *cerebrovascular (437.3)*
coronary (414.19)
pulmonary (417.0)
surgically created arteriovenous shunt or fistula:
complication (996.1, 996.61-996.62)
status or presence (V45.11)
traumatic (900.0-904.9)
DEF: Communication between an artery and vein caused by error in healing.

447.1 Stricture of artery
AHA: 2Q, '93, 8; M-A, '87, 6
I77.1 Stricture of artery   I-10

447.2 Rupture of artery
Erosion
Fistula, except
    arteriovenous } of artery
Ulcer
EXCLUDES *traumatic rupture of artery (900.0-904.9)*

447.3 Hyperplasia of renal artery
Fibromuscular hyperplasia of renal artery
DEF: Overgrowth of cells in muscular lining of renal artery.

447.4 Celiac artery compression syndrome
Celiac axis syndrome
Marable's syndrome

447.5 Necrosis of artery

447.6 Arteritis, unspecified
Aortitis NOS   Endarteritis NOS
EXCLUDES *arteritis, endarteritis:*
aortic arch (446.7)
cerebral (437.4)
coronary (414.00-414.07)
deformans (440.0-440.9)
obliterans (440.0-440.9)
pulmonary (417.8)
senile (440.0-440.9)
polyarteritis NOS (446.0)
syphilitic aortitis (093.1)
AHA: 1Q, '95, 3

● √5ᵗʰ **447.7 Aortic ectasia**
Ectasis aorta
EXCLUDES *aortic aneurysm and dissection (441.00-441.9)*

● **447.70 Aortic ectasia, unspecified site**

● **447.71 Thoracic aortic ectasia**

● **447.72 Abdominal aortic ectasia**

● **447.73 Thoracoabdominal aortic ectasia**

447.8 Other specified disorders of arteries and arterioles
Fibromuscular hyperplasia of arteries, except renal

447.9 Unspecified disorders of arteries and arterioles

√4ᵗʰ **448 Disease of capillaries**

448.0 Hereditary hemorrhagic telangiectasia
Rendu-Osler-Weber disease
DEF: Genetic disease with onset after puberty; results in multiple telangiectases, dilated venules on skin and mucous membranes; recurrent bleeding may occur.

448.1 Nevus, non-neoplastic
Nevus: Nevus:
  araneus   spider
  senile   stellar
EXCLUDES *neoplastic (216.0-216.9)*
port wine (757.32)
strawberry (757.32)
DEF: Enlarged or malformed blood vessels of skin; results in reddish swelling, skin patch, or birthmark.

448.9 Other and unspecified capillary diseases
Capillary:
  hemorrhage
  hyperpermeability
  thrombosis
EXCLUDES *capillary fragility (hereditary) (287.8)*

Diseases of the Circulatory System

449–453.71

449   Septic arterial embolism

Code first underlying infection, such as:
    infective endocarditis (421.0)
    lung abscess (513.0)
Use additional code to identify the site of the embolism (433.0-433.9, 444.0-444.9)

EXCLUDES   septic pulmonary embolism (415.12)
AHA: 4Q, '07, 84-85

Diseases of Veins and Lymphatics, and Other Diseases of Circulatory System (451-459)

✓4ᵗʰ 451   Phlebitis and thrombophlebitis

INCLUDES   endophlebitis
    inflammation, vein
    periphlebitis
    suppurative phlebitis

Use additional E code to identify drug, if drug-induced

EXCLUDES   that complicating:
    abortion (634-638 with .7, 639.8)
    ectopic or molar pregnancy (639.8)
    pregnancy, childbirth, or the puerperium (671.0-671.9)
    that due to or following:
      implant or catheter device (996.61-996.62)
      infusion, perfusion, or transfusion (999.2)

DEF: Inflammation of a vein (phlebitis) with formation of a thrombus (thrombophlebitis).
AHA: 1Q, '92, 16
TIP: Do not assign an additional code from category 453 for thrombosis; if both conditions are present, assign only a code from category 451.

451.0   Of superficial vessels of lower extremities
Saphenous vein (greater) (lesser)
AHA: 3Q, '91, 16

✓5ᵗʰ 451.1   Of deep vessels of lower extremities
AHA: 3Q, '91, 16

451.11   Femoral vein (deep) (superficial)

451.19   Other
Femoropopliteal vein
Popliteal vein
Tibial vein

451.2   Of lower extremities, unspecified
AHA: 4Q, '04, 80

✓5ᵗʰ 451.8   Of other sites
EXCLUDES   intracranial venous sinus (325)
    nonpyogenic (437.6)
    portal (vein) (572.1)

451.81   Iliac vein

451.82   Of superficial veins of upper extremities
Antecubital vein
Basilic vein
Cephalic vein

451.83   Of deep veins of upper extremities
Brachial vein
Radial vein
Ulnar vein

451.84   Of upper extremities, unspecified

451.89   Other
Axillary vein
Jugular vein
Subclavian vein
Thrombophlebitis of breast (Mondor's disease)

451.9   Of unspecified site

452   Portal vein thrombosis
Portal (vein) obstruction
EXCLUDES   hepatic vein thrombosis (453.0)
    phlebitis of portal vein (572.1)
DEF: Formation of a blood clot in main vein of liver.

✓4ᵗʰ 453   Other venous embolism and thrombosis
EXCLUDES   that complicating:
    abortion (634-638 with .7, 639.8)
    ectopic or molar pregnancy (639.8)
    pregnancy, childbirth, or the puerperium (671.0-671.9)
AHA: 1Q, '92, 16

453.0   Budd-Chiari syndrome
Hepatic vein thrombosis
DEF: Thrombosis or other obstruction of hepatic vein; symptoms include enlarged liver, extensive collateral vessels, intractable ascites and severe portal hypertension.

453.1   Thrombophlebitis migrans
DEF: Slow, advancing thrombophlebitis; appearing first in one vein then another.

453.2   Of inferior vena cava

453.3   Of renal vein

✓5ᵗʰ 453.4   Acute venous embolism and thrombosis of deep vessels of lower extremity
AHA: 4Q, '09, 88-92; 3Q, '08,16

453.40   Acute venous embolism and thrombosis of unspecified deep vessels of lower extremity
Deep vein thrombosis NOS
DVT NOS
I82.40 Embo & thrombo of uns deep veins   **I-10**
of lower extrem

453.41   Acute venous embolism and thrombosis of deep vessels of proximal lower extremity
Femoral   Thigh
Iliac   Upper leg NOS
Popliteal
AHA: 4Q, '04, 79

453.42   Acute venous embolism and thrombosis of deep vessels of distal lower extremity
Calf   Peroneal
Lower leg NOS   Tibial

✓5ᵗʰ 453.5   Chronic venous embolism and thrombosis of deep vessels of lower extremity
Use additional code, if applicable, for associated long-term (current) use of anticoagulants (V58.61)
EXCLUDES   personal history of venous thrombosis and embolism (V12.51)
AHA: 4Q, '09, 88-92

453.50   Chronic venous embolism and thrombosis of unspecified deep vessels of lower

453.51   Chronic venous embolism and thrombosis of deep vessels of proximal lower extremity
▶Femoral
Iliac
Popliteal
Thigh
Upper leg NOS◀

453.52   Chronic venous embolism and thrombosis of deep vessels of distal lower extremity
▶Calf
Lower leg NOS
Peroneal
Tibial◀

453.6   Venous embolism and thrombosis of superficial vessels of lower extremity
Saphenous vein (greater) (lesser)
▶Use additional code, if applicable, for associated long-term (current) use of anticoagulants (V58.61)◀
AHA: 4Q, '09, 88-92

✓5ᵗʰ 453.7   Chronic venous embolism and thrombosis of other specified vessels
Use additional code, if applicable, for associated long-term (current) use of anticoagulants (V58.61)
EXCLUDES   personal history of venous thrombosis and embolism (V12.51)
AHA: 4Q, '09, 88-92

453.71   Chronic venous embolism and thrombosis of superficial veins of upper extremity
Antecubital vein   Cephalic vein
Basilic vein

Map of Major Veins

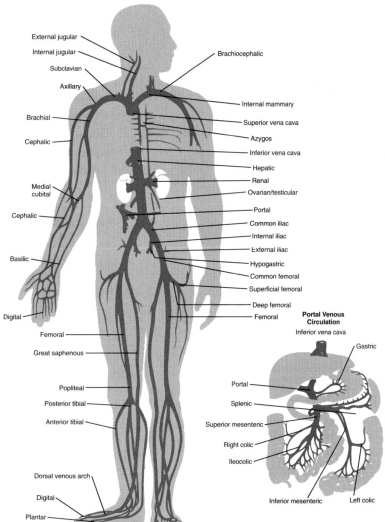

Portal Venous Circulation

453.72 Chronic venous embolism and thrombosis of deep veins of upper extremity
Brachial vein   Ulnar vein
Radial vein

453.73 Chronic venous embolism and thrombosis of upper extremity, unspecified

453.74 Chronic venous embolism and thrombosis of axillary veins

453.75 Chronic venous embolism and thrombosis of subclavian veins

453.76 Chronic venous embolism and thrombosis of internal jugular veins

453.77 Chronic venous embolism and thrombosis of other thoracic veins
Brachiocephalic (innominate)
Superior vena cava

453.79 Chronic venous embolism and thrombosis of other specified veins

√5ᵗʰ **453.8 Acute venous embolism and thrombosis of other specified veins**

EXCLUDES cerebral (434.0-434.9)
coronary (410.00-410.92)
intracranial venous sinus (325)
    nonpyogenic (437.6)
mesenteric (557.0)
portal (452)
precerebral (433.0-433.9)
pulmonary (415.19)

AHA: ▶4Q, '09, 88-92;◀3Q, '91, 16; M-A, '87, 6

453.81 Acute venous embolism and thrombosis of superficial veins of upper extremity
Antecubital vein
Basilic vein
Cephalic vein

453.82 Acute venous embolism and thrombosis of deep veins of upper extremity
Brachial vein   Ulnar vein
Radial vein

453.83 Acute venous embolism and thrombosis of upper extremity, unspecified

453.84 Acute venous embolism and thrombosis of axillary veins

453.85 Acute venous embolism and thrombosis of subclavian veins

453.86 Acute venous embolism and thrombosis of internal jugular veins

453.87 Acute venous embolism and thrombosis of other thoracic veins
Brachiocephalic (innominate)
Superior vena cava

453.89 Acute venous embolism and thrombosis of other specified veins
I82.89 Embolism and thrombosis of other   I-10
specified veins

453.9 Of unspecified site
Embolism of vein   Thrombosis (vein)

☑4ᵗʰ **454 Varicose veins of lower extremities**

EXCLUDES *that complicating pregnancy, childbirth, or the puerperium (671.0)*

DEF: Dilated leg veins; due to incompetent vein valves that allow reversed blood flow and cause tissue erosion or weakness of wall; may be painful.

AHA: 2Q, '91, 20

454.0 With ulcer Ⓐ

Varicose ulcer (lower extremity, any part)

Varicose veins with ulcer of lower extremity [any part] or of unspecified site

Any condition classifiable to 454.9 with ulcer or specified as ulcerated

AHA: 4Q, '99, 18

454.1 With inflammation Ⓐ

Stasis dermatitis

Varicose veins with inflammation of lower extremity [any part] or of unspecified site

Any condition classifiable to 454.9 with inflammation or specified as inflamed

454.2 With ulcer and inflammation Ⓐ

Varicose veins with ulcer and inflammation of lower extremity [any part] or of unspecified site

Any condition classifiable to 454.9 with ulcer and inflammation

454.8 With other complications

Edema   Swelling

Pain

AHA: 4Q, '02, 58

454.9 Asymptomatic varicose veins Ⓐ

Phlebectasia

Varicose veins } of lower extremity [any part] or of unspecified site

Varix

Varicose veins NOS

AHA: 4Q, '02, 58

TIP: Do not assign if patient seen for surgical treatment of varicose veins; query physician for specific symptom (inflammation, pain, edema, swelling).

☑4ᵗʰ **455 Hemorrhoids**

INCLUDES hemorrhoids (anus) (rectum)

piles

varicose veins, anus or rectum

EXCLUDES *that complicating pregnancy, childbirth, or the puerperium (671.8)*

DEF: Varicose condition of external hemorrhoidal veins causing painful swellings at the anus.

455.0 Internal hemorrhoids without mention of complication

AHA: 3Q, '05, 17

I84.21 Internal hemorrhoids without complication I-10

455.1 Internal thrombosed hemorrhoids

455.2 Internal hemorrhoids with other complication

Internal hemorrhoids: Internal hemorrhoids:

bleeding   strangulated

prolapsed   ulcerated

AHA: 3Q, '05, 17; 1Q, '03, 8

I84.111 Internal bleeding hemorrhoids I-10

455.3 External hemorrhoids without mention of complication

AHA: 1Q, '07, 13; 3Q, '05, 17

I84.22 External hemorrhoids without complicaton I-10

455.4 External thrombosed hemorrhoids

455.5 External hemorrhoids with other complication

External hemorrhoids: External hemorrhoids:

bleeding   strangulated

prolapsed   ulcerated

AHA: 3Q, '05, 17; 1Q, '03, 8

455.6 Unspecified hemorrhoids without mention of complication

Hemorrhoids NOS

455.7 Unspecified thrombosed hemorrhoids

Thrombosed hemorrhoids, unspecified whether internal or external

455.8 Unspecified hemorrhoids with other complication

Hemorrhoids, unspecified whether internal or external:

bleeding

prolapsed

strangulated

ulcerated

455.9 Residual hemorrhoidal skin tags

Skin tags, anus or rectum

☑4ᵗʰ **456 Varicose veins of other sites**

456.0 Esophageal varices with bleeding

DEF: Distended, tortuous, veins of lower esophagus, usually due to portal hypertension.

456.1 Esophageal varices without mention of bleeding

☑5ᵗʰ **456.2 Esophageal varices in diseases classified elsewhere**

Code first underlying cause, as:

cirrhosis of liver (571.0-571.9)

portal hypertension (572.3)

456.20 With bleeding

AHA: N-D, '85, 14

I85.11 Secondary esophageal varices with bleeding I-10

456.21 Without mention of bleeding

AHA: 3Q, '05, 15; 2Q, '02, 4

456.3 Sublingual varices

DEF: Distended, tortuous veins beneath tongue.

456.4 Scrotal varices ♂

Varicocele

456.5 Pelvic varices

Varices of broad ligament

456.6 Vulval varices ♀

Varices of perineum

EXCLUDES *that complicating pregnancy, childbirth, or the puerperium (671.1)*

456.8 Varices of other sites

Varicose veins of nasal septum (with ulcer)

EXCLUDES *placental varices (656.7)*

retinal varices (362.17)

varicose ulcer of unspecified site (454.0)

varicose veins of unspecified site (454.9)

AHA: 2Q, '02, 4

☑4ᵗʰ **457 Noninfectious disorders of lymphatic channels**

457.0 Postmastectomy lymphedema syndrome Ⓐ

Elephantiasis

Obliteration of lymphatic } due to mastectomy

vessel

DEF: Reduced lymphatic circulation following mastectomy; symptoms include swelling of the arm on the operative side.

AHA: 2Q, '02, 12

457.1 Other lymphedema

Elephantiasis (nonfilarial) NOS   Lymphedema:

Lymphangiectasis   secondary

Lymphedema: Obliteration, lymphatic

acquired (chronic)   vessel

praecox

EXCLUDES *elephantiasis (nonfilarial):*

congenital (757.0)

eyelid (374.83)

vulva (624.8)

DEF: Fluid retention due to reduced lymphatic circulation; due to other than mastectomy.

AHA: 3Q, '04, 5

I89.0 Lymphedema not elsewhere classified I-10

457.2 Lymphangitis

Lymphangitis: Lymphangitis:

NOS   subacute

chronic

EXCLUDES *acute lymphangitis (682.0-682.9)*

Ⓝ Newborn Age: 0   Ⓟ Pediatric Age: 0-17   Ⓜ Maternity Age: 12-55   Ⓐ Adult Age: 15-124

457.8 Other noninfectious disorders of lymphatic channels
Chylocele (nonfilarial)
Chylous:
  ascites
  cyst
Lymph node or vessel:
  fistula
  infarction
  rupture
> *EXCLUDES* *chylocele:*
> *filarial (125.0-125.9)*
> *tunica vaginalis (nonfilarial) (608.84)*

AHA: 1Q, '04, 5; 3Q, '03, 17

457.9 Unspecified noninfectious disorder of lymphatic channels

✓4ᵗʰ 458 Hypotension
> *INCLUDES* hypopiesis
> *EXCLUDES* *cardiovascular collapse (785.50)*
> *maternal hypotension syndrome (669.2)*
> *shock (785.50-785.59)*
> *Shy-Drager syndrome (333.0)*

458.0 Orthostatic hypotension
Hypotension: Hypotension:
  orthostatic (chronic)   postural
DEF: Low blood pressure; occurs when standing.
AHA: 3Q, '00, 8; 3Q, '91, 9
I95.1 Orthostatic hypotension   I-10

458.1 Chronic hypotension
Permanent idiopathic hypotension
DEF: Persistent low blood pressure.

✓5ᵗʰ 458.2 Iatrogenic hypotension
DEF: Abnormally low blood pressure; due to medical treatment.
AHA: 4Q, '03, 60; 3Q, '02, 12; 4Q, '95, 57

458.21 Hypotension of hemodialysis
Intra-dialytic hypotension
AHA: 4Q, '03, 61

458.29 Other iatrogenic hypotension
Postoperative hypotension
I95.81 Postprocedural hypotension   I-10

458.8 Other specified hypotension
AHA: 4Q, '97, 37

458.9 Hypotension, unspecified
Hypotension (arterial) NOS
I95.9 Hypotension unspecified   I-10

✓4ᵗʰ 459 Other disorders of circulatory system

459.0 Hemorrhage, unspecified
Rupture of blood vessel NOS
Spontaneous hemorrhage NEC
> *EXCLUDES* *hemorrhage:*
> *gastrointestinal NOS (578.9)*
> *in newborn NOS (772.9)*
> *secondary or recurrent following trauma (958.2)*
> *traumatic rupture of blood vessel (900.0-904.9)*
> *nontraumatic hematoma of soft tissue (729.92)*

AHA: 4Q, '90, 26
R58 Hemorrhage not elsewhere classified   I-10

✓5ᵗʰ 459.1 Postphlebitic syndrome
Chronic venous hypertension due to deep vein thrombosis
> *EXCLUDES* *chronic venous hypertension without deep vein*
> *thrombosis (459.30-459.39)*

DEF: Various conditions following deep vein thrombosis; including edema, pain, stasis dermatitis, cellulitis, varicose veins and ulceration of the lower leg.
AHA: 4Q, '02, 58; 2Q, '91, 20

459.10 Postphlebitic syndrome without complications
Asymptomatic postphlebitic syndrome
Postphlebitic syndrome NOS

459.11 Postphlebitic syndrome with ulcer

459.12 Postphlebitic syndrome with inflammation

459.13 Postphlebitic syndrome with ulcer and inflammation

459.19 Postphlebitic syndrome with other complication

459.2 Compression of vein
Stricture of vein
Vena cava syndrome (inferior) (superior)

✓5ᵗʰ 459.3 Chronic venous hypertension (idiopathic)
Stasis edema
> *EXCLUDES* *chronic venous hypertension due to deep vein*
> *thrombosis (459.10-459.9)*
> *varicose veins (454.0-454.9)*

AHA: 4Q, '02, 59

459.30 Chronic venous hypertension without complications
Asymptomatic chronic venous hypertension
Chronic venous hypertension NOS

459.31 Chronic venous hypertension with ulcer
AHA: 4Q, '02, 43

459.32 Chronic venous hypertension with inflammation

459.33 Chronic venous hypertension with ulcer and inflammation

459.39 Chronic venous hypertension with other complication

✓5ᵗʰ 459.8 Other specified disorders of circulatory system

459.81 Venous (peripheral) insufficiency, unspecified
Chronic venous insufficiency NOS
Use additional code for any associated ulceration (707.10-707.9)
DEF: Insufficient drainage, venous blood, any part of body, results in edema or dermatosis.
AHA: 3Q, '04, 5; 2Q, '91, 20; M-A, '87, 6
TIP: Assign for stasis dermatitis without varicose veins or past DVT.
I87.2 Venous insufficiency (chronic) (peripheral)   I-10

459.89 Other
Collateral circulation (venous), any site
Phlebosclerosis
Venofibrosis

459.9 Unspecified circulatory system disorder

---

8. Diseases of the Respiratory System (460-519)

Use additional code to identify infectious organism

Acute Respiratory Infections (460-466)

EXCLUDES *pneumonia and influenza ▶(480.0-488.19)◀*

460 Acute nasopharyngitis [common cold]

Coryza (acute)	Rhinitis:
Nasal catarrh, acute	acute
Nasopharyngitis:	infective
NOS	
acute	
infective NOS	

EXCLUDES *nasopharyngitis, chronic (472.2)*
pharyngitis:
acute or unspecified (462)
chronic (472.1)
rhinitis:
allergic (477.0-477.9)
chronic or unspecified (472.0)
sore throat:
acute or unspecified (462)
chronic (472.1)

DEF: Acute inflammation of mucous membranes; extends from nares to pharynx.
AHA: 1Q, '88, 12

✓4ᵗʰ 461 Acute sinusitis

INCLUDES abscess
empyema
infection   acute, of sinus
inflammation   (accessory) (nasal)
suppuration

EXCLUDES *chronic or unspecified sinusitis (473.0-473.9)*

461.0 Maxillary
Acute antritis

461.1 Frontal

461.2 Ethmoidal

461.3 Sphenoidal

461.8 Other acute sinusitis
Acute pansinusitis

461.9 Acute sinusitis, unspecified
Acute sinusitis NOS
J01.90 Acute sinusitis unspecified   `I-10`

462 Acute pharyngitis
Acute sore throat NOS
Pharyngitis (acute):
NOS
gangrenous
infective
phlegmonous
pneumococcal
staphylococca
suppurative
ulcerative
Sore throat (viral) NOS
Viral pharyngitis

EXCLUDES *abscess:*
peritonsillar [quinsy] (475)
pharyngeal NOS (478.29)
retropharyngeal (478.24)
chronic pharyngitis (472.1)
infectious mononucleosis (075)
that specified as (due to):
Coxsackie (virus) (074.0)
gonococcus (098.6)
herpes simplex (054.79)
influenza ▶(487.1, 488.02, 488.12)◀
septic (034.0)
streptococcal (034.0)

AHA: 4Q, '99, 26; S-O, '85, 8
J02.9 Acute pharyngitis unspecified   `I-10`

Respiratory System

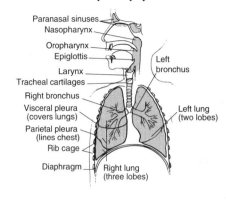

463 Acute tonsillitis

Tonsillitis (acute):	Tonsillitis (acute):
NOS	septic
follicular	staphylococcal
gangrenous	suppurative
infective	ulcerative
pneumococcal	viral

EXCLUDES *chronic tonsillitis (474.0)*
hypertrophy of tonsils (474.1)
peritonsillar abscess [quinsy] (475)
sore throat:
acute or NOS (462)
septic (034.0)
streptococcal tonsillitis (034.0)

AHA: N-D, '84, 16

✓4ᵗʰ 464 Acute laryngitis and tracheitis

EXCLUDES *that associated with influenza ▶(487.1, 488.02, 488.12)◀*
that due to Streptococcus (034.0)

✓5ᵗʰ 464.0 Acute laryngitis
Laryngitis (acute):
NOS
edematous
Hemophilus influenzae [H. influenzae]
pneumococcal
septic
suppurative
ulcerative

EXCLUDES *chronic laryngitis (476.0-476.1)*
influenzal laryngitis ▶(487.1, 488.02, 488.12)◀

AHA: 4Q, '01, 42

464.00 Without mention of obstruction

464.01 With obstruction

✓5ᵗʰ 464.1 Acute tracheitis
Tracheitis (acute):
NOS
catarrhal
viral

EXCLUDES *chronic tracheitis (491.8)*

464.10 Without mention of obstruction

464.11 With obstruction

✓5ᵗʰ 464.2 Acute laryngotracheitis
Laryngotracheitis (acute)
Tracheitis (acute) with laryngitis (acute)

EXCLUDES *chronic laryngotracheitis (476.1)*

464.20 Without mention of obstruction

464.21 With obstruction

✓5ᵗʰ 464.3 Acute epiglottitis
Viral epiglottitis

EXCLUDES *epiglottitis, chronic (476.1)*

464.30 Without mention of obstruction

464.31 With obstruction

Diseases of the Respiratory System   464.4–473.9

Upper Respiratory System

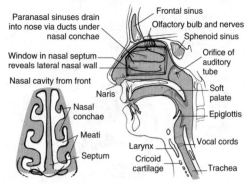

Paranasal sinuses drain into nose via ducts under nasal conchae

Window in nasal septum reveals lateral nasal wall

Nasal cavity from front

Frontal sinus
Olfactory bulb and nerves
Sphenoid sinus
Orifice of auditory tube
Soft palate
Epiglottis
Vocal cords
Trachea

Naris
Nasal conchae
Meati
Septum
Larynx
Cricoid cartilage

464.4 Croup
Croup syndrome

DEF: Acute laryngeal obstruction due to allergy, foreign body or infection; symptoms include barking cough, hoarseness and harsh, persistent high-pitched respiratory sound.

J05.0 Acute obstructive laryngitis [croup]   I-10

✓5ᵗʰ 464.5 Supraglottitis, unspecified

DEF: A rapidly advancing generalized upper respiratory infection of the lingual tonsillar area, epiglottic folds, false vocal cords, and the epiglottis.

AHA: 4Q, '01, 42

464.50 Without mention of obstruction
AHA: 4Q, '01, 43

464.51 With obstruction

✓4ᵗʰ 465 Acute upper respiratory infections of multiple or unspecified sites

EXCLUDES upper respiratory infection due to:
influenza ▶(487.1, 488.02, 488.12)◀
Streptococcus (034.0)

465.0 Acute laryngopharyngitis
DEF: Acute infection of the vocal cords and pharynx.

465.8 Other multiple sites
Multiple URI
AHA: 4Q, '07, 85

465.9 Unspecified site
Acute URI NOS
Upper respiratory infection (acute)
J06.9 Acute upper respiratory infection unspecified   I-10

✓4ᵗʰ 466 Acute bronchitis and bronchiolitis

INCLUDES that with:
bronchospasm
obstruction

466.0 Acute bronchitis
Bronchitis, acute or subacute:
fibrinous
membranous
pneumococcal
purulent
septic
viral
with tracheitis
Croupous bronchitis
Tracheobronchitis, acute

EXCLUDES acute bronchitis with chronic obstructive pulmonary disease (491.22)

DEF: Acute inflammation of main branches of bronchial tree due to infectious or irritant agents; symptoms include cough with a varied production of sputum, fever, substernal soreness, and lung rales.

AHA: 4Q, '04, 137; 1Q, '04, 3; 4Q, '02, 46; 4Q, '96, 28; 4Q, '91, 24; 1Q, '88, 12

TIP: If documented with COPD, assign only 491.22 Obstructive chronic bronchitis with acute bronchitis.

J20.9 Acute bronchitis unspecified   I-10

✓5ᵗʰ 466.1 Acute bronchiolitis
Bronchiolitis (acute)
Capillary pneumonia

DEF: Acute inflammation of smallest branches of bronchial tree due to infectious or irritant agents; symptoms include cough, tachycardia, and lung crackles.

466.11 Acute bronchiolitis due to respiratory syncytial virus (RSV)
AHA: 1Q, '05, 10; 4Q, '96, 27
J21.0 Acute bronchiolitis d/t resp syncytial virus   I-10

466.19 Acute bronchiolitis due to other infectious organisms
Use additional code to identify organism
J21.8 Acute bronchiolitis d/t oth specified organisms   I-10

Other Diseases of the Upper Respiratory Tract (470-478)

470 Deviated nasal septum
Deflected septum (nasal) (acquired)
EXCLUDES congenital (754.0)

✓4ᵗʰ 471 Nasal polyps
EXCLUDES adenomatous polyps (212.0)

471.0 Polyp of nasal cavity
Polyp: Polyp:
choanal   nasopharyngeal

471.1 Polypoid sinus degeneration
Woakes' syndrome or ethmoiditis

471.8 Other polyp of sinus
Polyp of sinus:
accessory
ethmoidal
maxillary
sphenoidal

471.9 Unspecified nasal polyp
Nasal polyp NOS

✓4ᵗʰ 472 Chronic pharyngitis and nasopharyngitis

472.0 Chronic rhinitis
Ozena   Rhinitis:
Rhinitis: hypertrophic
NOS   obstructive
atrophic   purulent
granulomatous   ulcerative

EXCLUDES allergic rhinitis (477.0-477.9)
DEF: Persistent inflammation of mucous membranes of nose.

472.1 Chronic pharyngitis
Chronic sore throat   Pharyngitis:
Pharyngitis: granular (chronic)
atrophic   hypertrophic

472.2 Chronic nasopharyngitis
EXCLUDES acute or unspecified nasopharyngitis (460)
DEF: Persistent inflammation of mucous membranes extending from nares to pharynx.

✓4ᵗʰ 473 Chronic sinusitis
INCLUDES abscess
empyema
infection   (chronic) of sinus (accessory) (nasal)
suppuration

EXCLUDES acute sinusitis (461.0-461.9)

473.0 Maxillary
Antritis (chronic)
J32.0 Chronic maxillary sinusitis   I-10

473.1 Frontal

473.2 Ethmoidal
EXCLUDES Woakes' ethmoiditis (471.1)

473.3 Sphenoidal

473.8 Other chronic sinusitis
Pansinusitis (chronic)

473.9 Unspecified sinusitis (chronic)
Sinusitis (chronic) NOS
J32.9 Chronic sinusitis unspecified   I-10

N Newborn Age: 0   **P** Pediatric Age: 0-17   **M** Maternity Age: 12-55   **A** Adult Age: 15-124

Paranasal Sinuses

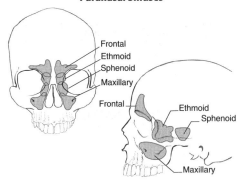

Frontal
Ethmoid
Sphenoid
Maxillary

Frontal
Ethmoid
Sphenoid
Maxillary

√4ᵗʰ 474 Chronic disease of tonsils and adenoids

√5ᵗʰ 474.0 Chronic tonsillitis and adenoiditis
> *EXCLUDES* *acute or unspecified tonsillitis (463)*
> AHA: 4Q, '97, 38

474.00 Chronic tonsillitis

474.01 Chronic adenoiditis

474.02 Chronic tonsillitis and adenoiditis

√5ᵗʰ 474.1 Hypertrophy of tonsils and adenoids
> Enlargement
> Hyperplasia } of tonsils or adenoids
> Hypertrophy
>
> *EXCLUDES* *that with:*
> > *adenoiditis (474.01)*
> > *adenoiditis and tonsillitis (474.02)*
> > *tonsillitis (474.00)*

474.10 Tonsils with adenoids
> AHA: 2Q, '05, 16

474.11 Tonsils alone

474.12 Adenoids alone

474.2 Adenoid vegetations
> DEF: Fungus-like growth of lymph tissue between the nares and pharynx.

474.8 Other chronic disease of tonsils and adenoids
> Amygdalolith
> Calculus, tonsil
> Cicatrix of tonsil (and adenoid)
> Tonsillar tag
> Ulcer, tonsil

474.9 Unspecified chronic disease of tonsils and adenoids
> Disease (chronic) of tonsils (and adenoids)

475 Peritonsillar abscess
> Abscess of tonsil   Quinsy
> Peritonsillar cellulitis
> *EXCLUDES* *tonsillitis:*
> > *acute or NOS (463)*
> > *chronic (474.0)*
> J36 Peritonsillar abscess   I-10

√4ᵗʰ 476 Chronic laryngitis and laryngotracheitis

476.0 Chronic laryngitis
> Laryngitis: Laryngitis:
> > catarrhal   sicca
> > hypertrophic

476.1 Chronic laryngotracheitis
> Laryngitis, chronic, with tracheitis (chronic)
> Tracheitis, chronic, with laryngitis
> *EXCLUDES* *chronic tracheitis (491.8)*
> > *laryngitis and tracheitis, acute or unspecified*
> > *(464.00-464.51)*

√4ᵗʰ 477 Allergic rhinitis
> *INCLUDES* allergic rhinitis (nonseasonal) (seasonal)
> hay fever
> spasmodic rhinorrhea
> *EXCLUDES* *allergic rhinitis with asthma (bronchial) (493.0)*
> DEF: True immunoglobulin E (IgE)-mediated allergic reaction of nasal mucosa; seasonal (typical hay fever) or perennial (year-round allergens: dust, food, dander).

477.0 Due to pollen
> Pollinosis

477.1 Due to food
> AHA: 4Q, '00, 42

477.2 Due to animal (cat) (dog) hair and dander

477.8 Due to other allergen

477.9 Cause unspecified
> AHA: 2Q, '97, 9
> J30.9 Allergic rhinitis unspecified   I-10

√4ᵗʰ 478 Other diseases of upper respiratory tract

478.0 Hypertrophy of nasal turbinates
> DEF: Overgrowth, enlargement of shell-shaped bones in nasal cavity.

√5ᵗʰ 478.1 Other diseases of nasal cavity and sinuses
> *EXCLUDES* *varicose ulcer of nasal septum (456.8)*

478.11 Nasal mucositis (ulcerative)
> Use additional E code to identify adverse effects of therapy, such as:
> > antineoplastic and immunosuppressive drugs
> > (E930.7, E933.1)
> > radiation therapy (E879.2)
> AHA: 4Q, '06, 88-90

478.19 Other diseases of nasal cavity and sinuses
> Abscess
> Necrosis } of nose (septum)
> Ulcer
> Cyst or mucocele of sinus (nasal)
> Rhinolith
> AHA: 4Q, '06, 88-90
> J34.1 Cyst and mucocele of nose and nasal sinus   I-10

√5ᵗʰ 478.2 Other diseases of pharynx, not elsewhere classified

478.20 Unspecified disease of pharynx

478.21 Cellulitis of pharynx or nasopharynx

478.22 Parapharyngeal abscess

478.24 Retropharyngeal abscess
> DEF: Purulent infection, behind pharynx and front of precerebral fascia.

478.25 Edema of pharynx or nasopharynx

478.26 Cyst of pharynx or nasopharynx

478.29 Other
> Abscess of pharynx or nasopharynx
> *EXCLUDES* *ulcerative pharyngitis (462)*

√5ᵗʰ 478.3 Paralysis of vocal cords or larynx
> DEF: Loss of motor ability of vocal cords or larynx; due to nerve or muscle damage.

478.30 Paralysis, unspecified
> Laryngoplegia
> Paralysis of glottis

478.31 Unilateral, partial

478.32 Unilateral, complete

478.33 Bilateral, partial

478.34 Bilateral, complete

478.4 Polyp of vocal cord or larynx
> *EXCLUDES* *adenomatous polyps (212.1)*

√4ᵗʰ
√5ᵗʰ Additional Digit Required   Unspecified Code   Other Specified Code   Manifestation Code   ►◄ Revised Text   ● New Code   ▲ Revised Code Title

2011 ICD-9-CM   **Volume 1 – 147**

478.5 Other diseases of vocal cords

Abscess
Cellulitis } of vocal cords
Granuloma
Leukoplakia

Chorditis (fibrinous) (nodosa) (tuberosa)
Singers' nodes

478.6 Edema of larynx

Edema (of):   Edema (of):
  glottis   supraglottic
  subglottic

☑5ᵗʰ **478.7 Other diseases of larynx, not elsewhere classified**

478.70 Unspecified disease of larynx

478.71 Cellulitis and perichondritis of larynx

DEF: Inflammation of deep soft tissues or lining of bone of the larynx.

478.74 Stenosis of larynx

478.75 Laryngeal spasm

Laryngismus (stridulus)

DEF: Involuntary muscle contraction of the larynx.

478.79 Other

Abscess
Necrosis
Obstruction } of larynx
Pachyderma
Ulcer

EXCLUDES ulcerative laryngitis (464.00-464.01)
AHA:3Q, '91, 20

478.8 Upper respiratory tract hypersensitivity reaction, site unspecified

EXCLUDES hypersensitivity reaction of lower respiratory tract, as:
extrinsic allergic alveolitis (495.0-495.9)
pneumoconiosis (500-505)

478.9 Other and unspecified diseases of upper respiratory tract

Abscess } of trachea
Cicatrix

Pneumonia and Influenza (480-488)

EXCLUDES pneumonia:
allergic or eosinophilic (518.3)
aspiration:
NOS (507.0)
newborn (770.18)
solids and liquids (507.0-507.8)
congenital (770.0)
lipoid (507.1)
passive (514)
rheumatic (390)
ventilator-associated (997.31)

☑4ᵗʰ **480 Viral pneumonia**

480.0 Pneumonia due to adenovirus

480.1 Pneumonia due to respiratory syncytial virus

AHA: 4Q, '96, 28; 1Q, '88, 12

480.2 Pneumonia due to parainfluenza virus

480.3 Pneumonia due to SARS-associated coronavirus

DEF: A severe adult respiratory syndrome caused by the coronavirus, specified as inflammation of the lungs with consolidation.
AHA: 4Q, '03, 46-47

480.8 Pneumonia due to other virus not elsewhere classified

EXCLUDES congenital rubella pneumonitis (771.0)
pneumonia complicating viral diseases classified
elsewhere (484.1-484.8)

480.9 Viral pneumonia, unspecified

AHA: 3Q, '98, 5

481 Pneumococcal pneumonia [Streptococcus pneumoniae pneumonia]

Lobar pneumonia, organism unspecified
AHA: 2Q, '98, 7; 4Q, '92, 19; 1Q, '92, 18; 1Q, '91, 13; 1Q, '88, 13; M-A, '85, 6

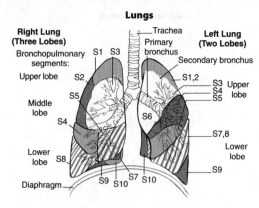

Lungs

Right Lung
(Three Lobes)
Trachea
Primary
bronchus
Left Lung
(Two Lobes)
Bronchopulmonary
segments:
Upper lobe
S1 S3
Secondary bronchus
S2
S1,2
S3 Upper
S4 lobe
S5
Middle
lobe
S5
S6
S4
S7,8
Lower
lobe
S8
Lower
lobe
S9
Diaphragm
S9 S10
S7 S10

☑4ᵗʰ **482 Other bacterial pneumonia**

AHA: 4Q, '93, 39

482.0 Pneumonia due to Klebsiella pneumoniae

482.1 Pneumonia due to Pseudomonas

482.2 Pneumonia due to Hemophilus influenzae [H. influenzae]

AHA: 2Q, '05, 19

☑5ᵗʰ **482.3 Pneumonia due to Streptococcus**

EXCLUDES Streptococcus pneumoniae (481)
AHA: 1Q, '88, 13

482.30 Streptococcus, unspecified

482.31 Group A

482.32 Group B

482.39 Other Streptococcus

☑5ᵗʰ **482.4 Pneumonia due to Staphylococcus**

AHA: 3Q, '91, 16

482.40 Pneumonia due to Staphylococcus, unspecified

482.41 Methicillin susceptible pneumonia due to Staphylococcus aureus

MSSA pneumonia
Pneumonia due to Staphylococcus aureus NOS
J15.21 Pneumonia due to staphylococcus aureus   I-10

482.42 Methicillin resistant pneumonia due to Staphylococcus aureus

AHA: 4Q, '08, 69, 71, 72

482.49 Other Staphylococcus pneumonia

☑5ᵗʰ **482.8 Pneumonia due to other specified bacteria**

EXCLUDES pneumonia, complicating infectious disease
classified elsewhere (484.1-484.8)
AHA: 3Q, '88, 11

482.81 Anaerobes

Bacteroides (melaninogenicus)
Gram-negative anaerobes

482.82 Escherichia coli [E. coli]

482.83 Other gram-negative bacteria

Gram-negative pneumonia NOS
Proteus
Serratia marcescens

EXCLUDES gram-negative anaerobes (482.81)
Legionnaires' disease (482.84)
AHA: 2Q, '98, 5; 3Q, '94, 9
TIP: Do not assign based solely on laboratory findings of gram-negative bacteria on gram-stain. Physician substantiation is required.
J15.6 Pneumonia d/t oth aerobic Gram-negative   I-10
bacteria

482.84 Legionnaires' disease

DEF: Severe and often fatal infection by Legionella pneumophilia; symptoms include high fever, gastrointestinal pain, headache, myalgia, dry cough, and pneumonia; usually transmitted airborne via air conditioning systems.
AHA: 4Q, '97, 38

N Newborn Age: 0   P Pediatric Age: 0-17   M Maternity Age: 12-55   A Adult Age: 15-124

482.89 Other specified bacteria
AHA: 2Q, '97, 6
TIP: Do not assign based on documentation of "mixed bacterial pneumonia" or "gram-positive pneumonia." See instead 482.9.

482.9 Bacterial pneumonia unspecified
AHA: 2Q, '98, 6; 2Q, '97, 6; 1Q, '94, 17
J15.9 Unspecified bacterial pneumonia   `I-10`

√4th 483 Pneumonia due to other specified organism
AHA: N-D, '87, 5
TIP: Do not assign if pneumonia due to candidiasis; see code 112.4.

483.0 Mycoplasma pneumoniae
Eaton's agent
Pleuropneumonia-like organism [PPLO]

483.1 Chlamydia
AHA: 4Q, '96, 31

483.8 Other specified organism

√4th 484 Pneumonia in infectious diseases classified elsewhere

484.1 *Pneumonia in cytomegalic inclusion disease*
Code first underlying disease (078.5)

484.3 *Pneumonia in whooping cough*
Code first underlying disease (033.0-033.9)

484.5 *Pneumonia in anthrax*
Code first underlying disease (022.1)

484.6 *Pneumonia in aspergillosis*
Code first underlying disease (117.3)
AHA: 4Q, '97, 40

484.7 *Pneumonia in other systemic mycoses*
Code first underlying disease
EXCLUDES *pneumonia in:*
candidiasis (112.4)
coccidioidomycosis (114.0)
histoplasmosis (115.0-115.9 with fifth-digit 5)

484.8 *Pneumonia in other infectious diseases classified elsewhere*
Code first underlying disease, as:
Q fever (083.0)
typhoid fever (002.0)
EXCLUDES *pneumonia in:*
actinomycosis (039.1)
measles (055.1)
nocardiosis (039.1)
ornithosis (073.0)
Pneumocystis carinii (136.3)
salmonellosis (003.22)
toxoplasmosis (130.4)
tuberculosis (011.6)
tularemia (021.2)
varicella (052.1)

485 Bronchopneumonia, organism unspecified
Bronchopneumonia: Pneumonia:
hemorrhagic   lobular
terminal   segmental
Pleurobronchopneumonia
EXCLUDES *bronchiolitis (acute) (466.11-466.19)*
chronic (491.8)
lipoid pneumonia (507.1)

486 Pneumonia, organism unspecified
EXCLUDES *hypostatic or passive pneumonia (514)*
inhalation or aspiration pneumonia due to foreign materials (507.0-507.8)
pneumonitis due to fumes and vapors (506.0)
AHA: ▶1Q, '10, 3, 12;◀ 3Q, '09, 16; 4Q, '08, 142; 4Q, '99, 6; 3Q, '99, 9; 3Q, '98, 7; 2Q, '98, 4, 5; 1Q, '98, 8; 3Q, '97, 9; 3Q, '94, 10; 3Q, '88, 11
TIP: Never assume a causal organism based on laboratory or radiology findings alone.
J18.9 Pneumonia unspecified organism   `I-10`

√4th 487 Influenza
Influenza caused by unspecified influenza virus
EXCLUDES *Hemophilus influenzae [H. influenzae]:*
infection NOS (041.5)
influenza due to identified avian influenza virus
▶(488.01-488.09)◀
influenza due to identified novel H1N1 influenza virus
▶(488.11-488.19)◀
influenza due to novel 2009 H1N1 [swine] influenza virus
▶(488.11-488.19)◀
laryngitis (464.00-464.01)
meningitis (320.0)

487.0 With pneumonia
Influenza with pneumonia, any form
Influenzal:
bronchopneumonia
pneumonia
Use additional code to identify the type of pneumonia (480.0-480.9, 481, 482.0-482.9, 483.0-483.8, 485)
AHA: 1Q, '06, 18; 2Q, '05, 18

487.1 With other respiratory manifestations
▶Influenza NEC◀   Influenzal:
Influenza NOS   pharyngitis
Influenzal: respiratory infection (upper)(acute)
laryngitis
AHA: ▶1Q, '10, 4;◀ 1Q, '06, 18; 2Q, '05, 18; 4Q, '99, 26
TIP: Selection of the principal diagnosis will be dependent on the circumstances of admission
J10.1 Influenza d/t oth influenza virus w/resp manifst   `I-10`

487.8 With other manifestations
Encephalopathy due to influenza
Influenza with involvement of gastrointestinal tract
EXCLUDES *"intestinal flu" [viral gastroenteritis] (008.8)*

√4th 488 Influenza due to certain identified influenza viruses
EXCLUDES *influenza caused by unspecified influenza viruses (487.0-487.8)*
AHA: 4Q, '09, 92-93
TIP: Do not assign a code from this category unless the specified influenza virus is confirmed.

√5th 488.0 Influenza due to identified avian influenza virus
Avian influenza
Bird flu
Influenza A/H5N1
DEF: Infection caused by contact with bird influenza viruses; results in flu-like symptoms that may progress to other severe and life-threatening complications.
AHA: 4Q, '07, 87

● **488.01 Influenza due to identified avian influenza virus with pneumonia**
Avian influenzal:
bronchopneumonia
pneumonia
Influenza due to identified avian influenza virus with pneumonia, any form
Use additional code to identify the type of pneumonia (480.0- 480.9, 481, 482.0-482.9, 483.0-483.8, 485)

● **488.02 Influenza due to identified avian influenza virus with other respiratory manifestations**
Avian influenzal:
laryngitis
pharyngitis
respiratory infection (acute) (upper)
Identified avian influenza NOS

● **488.09 Influenza due to identified avian influenza virus with other manifestations**
Avian influenza with involvement of gastrointestinal tract
Encephalopathy due to identified avian influenza
EXCLUDES *"intestinal flu" [viral gastroenteritis] (008.8)*

Bronchioli and Alveoli

√5ᵗʰ **488.1 Influenza due to identified novel H1N1 influenza virus**
2009 H1N1 [swine] influenza virus
Novel 2009 influenza H1N1
Novel H1N1 influenza
Novel influenza A/H1N1
Swine flu
AHA: ▶1Q, '10, 3-4◀

● **488.11 Influenza due to identified novel H1N1 influenza virus with pneumonia**
Novel H1N1 influenzal:
bronchopneumonia
pneumonia
Influenza due to identified novel H1N1 with pneumonia, any form
Use additional code to identify the type of pneumonia (480.0- 480.9, 481, 482.0-482.9, 483.0-483.8, 485)

● **488.12 Influenza due to identified novel H1N1 influenza virus with other respiratory manifestations**
Novel H1N1 influenza NOS
Novel H1N1 influenzal:
laryngitis
pharyngitis
respiratory infection (acute) (upper)

● **488.19 Influenza due to identified novel H1N1 influenza virus with other manifestations**
Encephalopathy due to identified novel H1N1 influenza
Novel H1N1 influenza with involvement of gastrointestinal tract
EXCLUDES *"intestinal flu" [viral gastroenteritis] (008.8)*

Chronic Obstructive Pulmonary Disease and Allied Conditions (490-496)
AHA: 3Q, '88, 5
TIP: Due to the overlapping nature of conditions that make up COPD, it's essential that the coder review all instructional notes carefully.

490 Bronchitis, not specified as acute or chronic
Bronchitis NOS: Tracheobronchitis NOS
catarrhal
with tracheitis NOS
EXCLUDES *bronchitis:*
allergic NOS (493.9)
asthmatic NOS (493.9)
due to fumes and vapors (506.0)
J40 Bronchitis not specified as acute or chronic   I-10

√4ᵗʰ **491 Chronic bronchitis**
EXCLUDES *chronic obstructive asthma (493.2)*

491.0 Simple chronic bronchitis
Catarrhal bronchitis, chronic   Smokers' cough
J41.0 Simple chronic bronchitis   I-10

491.1 Mucopurulent chronic bronchitis
Bronchitis (chronic) (recurrent):
fetid
mucopurulent
purulent
DEF: Chronic bronchial infection characterized by both mucus and pus secretions in the bronchial tree; recurs after asymptomatic periods; signs are coughing, expectoration and secondary changes in the lung.
AHA: 3Q, '88, 12

√5ᵗʰ **491.2 Obstructive chronic bronchitis**
Bronchitis:
emphysematous
obstructive (chronic) (diffuse)
Bronchitis with:
chronic airway obstruction
emphysema
EXCLUDES *asthmatic bronchitis (acute) NOS (493.9)*
chronic obstructive asthma (493.2)
AHA: 3Q, '97, 9; 4Q, '91, 25; 2Q, '91, 21

491.20 Without exacerbation
Emphysema with chronic bronchitis
AHA: 3Q, '97, 9

491.21 With (acute) exacerbation
Acute exacerbation of chronic obstructive pulmonary disease [COPD]
Decompensated chronic obstructive pulmonary disease [COPD]
Decompensated chronic obstructive pulmonary disease [COPD] with exacerbation
EXCLUDES *chronic obstructive asthma with acute exacerbation (493.22)*
AHA: ▶1Q, '10, 12;◀ 1Q, '04, 3; 3Q, '02, 18, 19; 4Q, '01, 43; 2Q, '96, 10
J44.1 Chronic obst pulmonary disease w/exacerbation I-10

491.22 With acute bronchitis
AHA: 3Q, '06, 20; 4Q, '04, 82
J44.0 Chronic obst pulm dz acute lower respiratory inf I-10

491.8 Other chronic bronchitis
Chronic:
tracheitis
tracheobronchitis

491.9 Unspecified chronic bronchitis
J42 Unspecified chronic bronchitis   I-10

√4ᵗʰ **492 Emphysema**
AHA: 2Q, '91, 21

492.0 Emphysematous bleb
Giant bullous emphysema
Ruptured emphysematous bleb
Tension pneumatocele
Vanishing lung
DEF: Formation of vesicle or bulla in emphysematous lung, more than one millimeter; contains serum or blood.
AHA: 2Q, '93, 3

Interrelationship Between Chronic Airway Obstruction, Chronic Bronchitis, and Emphysema

Diseases of the Respiratory System

492.8–496

492.8 Other emphysema
Emphysema (lung or pulmonary):
NOS
centriacinar
centrilobular
obstructive
panacinar
panlobular
unilateral
vesicular
MacLeod's syndrome
Swyer-James syndrome
Unilateral hyperlucent lung
EXCLUDES *emphysema:*
with chronic bronchitis (491.20-491.22)
compensatory (518.2)
due to fumes and vapors (506.4)
interstitial (518.1)
newborn (770.2)
mediastinal (518.1)
surgical (subcutaneous) (998.81)
traumatic (958.7)
AHA: 4Q, '08, 175; 1Q, '05, 4; 4Q, '93, 41; J-A, '84, 17
J43.9 Emphysema unspecified   I-10

√4ᵗʰ **493 Asthma**
EXCLUDES *wheezing NOS (786.07)*

The following fifth-digit subclassification is for use with codes
493.0-493.2, 493.9:
  0 unspecified
  1 with status asthmaticus
  2 with (acute) exacerbation

DEF: Status asthmaticus: severe, intractable episode of asthma unresponsive
to normal therapeutic measures.
AHA: 4Q, '04, 137; 4Q, '03, 62; 4Q, '01, 43; 4Q, '00, 42; 1Q, '91, 13; 3Q, '88, 9; J-A,
'85, 8; N-D, '84, 17
TIP: If documentation indicates both exacerbation and status asthmaticus,
assign only the code for status asthmaticus.

§ √5ᵗʰ **493.0 Extrinsic asthma**
[0-2]   Asthma:
allergic with stated cause
atopic
childhood
hay
platinum
Hay fever with asthma
EXCLUDES *asthma:*
allergic NOS (493.9)
detergent (507.8)
miners' (500)
wood (495.8)
DEF: Transient stricture of airway diameters of bronchi; due to
environmental factor; also called allergic (bronchial) asthma.
J45.20 Mild intermittent asthma uncomplicated   I-10

§ √5ᵗʰ **493.1 Intrinsic asthma**
[0-2]   Late-onset asthma
DEF: Transient stricture of airway diameters of bronchi; due to
pathophysiological disturbances.
AHA: 3Q, '88, 9; M-A, '85, 7

§ √5ᵗʰ **493.2 Chronic obstructive asthma**
[0-2]   Asthma with chronic obstructive pulmonary disease [COPD]
Chronic asthmatic bronchitis
EXCLUDES *acute bronchitis (466.0)*
chronic obstructive bronchitis (491.20-491.22)
DEF: Persistent narrowing of airway diameters in the bronchial tree,
restricting airflow and causing constant labored breathing.
AHA: 2Q, '91, 21; 2Q, '90, 20; For code 493.20: 4Q, '03, 108; For code
493.22: 1Q, '09, 17; 3Q, '06, 20

√5ᵗʰ **493.8 Other forms of asthma**
AHA: 4Q, '03, 62

    493.81 Exercise induced bronchospasm

    493.82 Cough variant asthma

§ √5ᵗʰ **493.9 Asthma, unspecified**
[0-2]   Asthma (bronchial) (allergic NOS)
Bronchitis:
allergic
asthmatic
AHA: 4Q, '97, 40, For code 493.90: 4Q, '04, 137; 4Q, '03, 108; 4Q, '99, 25;
1Q, '97, 7; For code 493.91: 1Q, '05, 5; For code 493.92: 1Q, '03, 9
J45.909 Unspecified asthma uncomplicated   I-10
J45.901 Unspecified asthma with acute exacerbation   I-10

√4ᵗʰ **494 Bronchiectasis**
Bronchiectasis (fusiform) (postinfectious) (recurrent)
Bronchiolectasis
EXCLUDES *congenital (748.61)*
tuberculous bronchiectasis (current disease) (011.5)
DEF: Dilation of bronchi; due to infection or chronic conditions; causes
decreased lung capacity and recurrent infections of lungs.
AHA: 4Q, '00, 42

    494.0 Bronchiectasis without acute exacerbation
      J47.9 Bronchiectasis uncomplicated   I-10

    494.1 Bronchiectasis with acute exacerbation

√4ᵗʰ **495 Extrinsic allergic alveolitis**
INCLUDES allergic alveolitis and pneumonitis due to inhaled organic
dust particles of fungal, thermophilic actinomycete,
or other origin
DEF: Pneumonitis due to particles inhaled into lung, often at workplace;
symptoms include cough, chills, fever, increased heart and respiratory rates;
develops within hours of exposure.

    495.0 Farmers' lung

    495.1 Bagassosis

    495.2 Bird-fanciers' lung
Budgerigar-fanciers' disease or lung
Pigeon-fanciers' disease or lung

    495.3 Suberosis
Cork-handlers' disease or lung

    495.4 Malt workers' lung
Alveolitis due to Aspergillus clavatus

    495.5 Mushroom workers' lung

    495.6 Maple bark-strippers' lung
Alveolitis due to Cryptostroma corticale

    495.7 "Ventilation" pneumonitis
Allergic alveolitis due to fungal, thermophilic actinomycete,
and other organisms growing in ventilation [air
conditioning] systems

    495.8 Other specified allergic alveolitis and pneumonitis

Cheese-washers' lung	Grain-handlers' disease or lung
Coffee workers' lung	Pituitary snuff-takers' disease
Fish-meal workers' lung	Sequoiosis or red-cedar asthma
Furriers' lung	Wood asthma

    495.9 Unspecified allergic alveolitis and pneumonitis
Alveolitis, allergic (extrinsic)
Hypersensitivity pneumonitis

    496 Chronic airway obstruction, not elsewhere classified
NOTE This code is not to be used with any code from categories
491-493
Chronic:
nonspecific lung disease
obstructive lung disease
obstructive pulmonary disease [COPD] NOS
EXCLUDES *chronic obstructive lung disease [COPD] specified (as) (with):*
allergic alveolitis (495.0-495.9)
asthma (493.20-493.22)
bronchiectasis (494.0-494.1)
bronchitis (491.20-491.22)
with emphysema (491.20-491.22)
decompensated (491.21)
emphysema (492.0-492.8)
AHA: ▶◄1Q, '10, 5, 18;◄ 1Q, '09, 16; 3Q, '07, 10; 4Q, '03, 109; 2Q, '00, 15; 2Q, '92,
16; 2Q, '91, 21; 3Q, '88, 56
TIP: COPD is a nonspecific term that encompasses many different respiratory
conditions; review medical record and query physician for more specific documentation of emphysema, bronchitis, asthma, etc.
J44.9 Chronic obstructive pulmonary disease unspec   I-10

---

§   Requires fifth digit. Valid digits are in [brackets] under each code. See category 493 for codes and definitions.

Diseases of the Respiratory System

500–511.89

Pneumoconioses and Other Lung Diseases Due to External Agents (500-508)

DEF: Permanent deposits of particulate matter, within lungs; due to occupational or environmental exposure; results in chronic induration and fibrosis. (See specific listings in 500-508 code range).

500   Coal workers' pneumoconiosis   A
     Anthracosilicosis   Coal workers' lung
     Anthracosis   Miner's asthma
     Black lung disease

501   Asbestosis   A

502   Pneumoconiosis due to other silica or silicates
     Pneumoconiosis due to talc
     Silicotic fibrosis (massive) of lung
     Silicosis (simple) (complicated)

503   Pneumoconiosis due to other inorganic dust
     Aluminosis (of lung)   Graphite fibrosis (of lung)
     Baritosis   Siderosis
     Bauxite fibrosis (of lung)   Stannosis
     Berylliosis

504   Pneumonopathy due to inhalation of other dust
     Byssinosis
     Cannabinosis
     Flax-dressers' disease
     EXCLUDES   *allergic alveolitis (495.0-495.9)*
          asbestosis (501)
          bagassosis (495.1)
          farmers' lung (495.0)

505   Pneumoconiosis, unspecified

√4ᵗʰ 506   Respiratory conditions due to chemical fumes and vapors
     Use additional E code to identify cause

     506.0   Bronchitis and pneumonitis due to fumes and vapors
         Chemical bronchitis (acute)
         AHA: 3Q, '08, 7

     506.1   Acute pulmonary edema due to fumes and vapors
         Chemical pulmonary edema (acute)
         EXCLUDES   *acute pulmonary edema NOS (518.4)*
               chronic or unspecified pulmonary edema (514)
         AHA: 3Q, '88, 4

     506.2   Upper respiratory inflammation due to fumes and vapors
         AHA: 3Q, '05, 10

     506.3   Other acute and subacute respiratory conditions due to fumes and vapors

     506.4   Chronic respiratory conditions due to fumes and vapors
         Emphysema (diffuse) (chronic) ⎫ due to inhalation
         Obliterative bronchiolitis   ⎬ of chemical
            (chronic) (subacute)   fumes and
         Pulmonary fibrosis (chronic) ⎭ vapors

     506.9   Unspecified respiratory conditions due to fumes and vapors
         Silo-fillers' disease

√4ᵗʰ 507   Pneumonitis due to solids and liquids
     EXCLUDES   *fetal aspiration pneumonitis (770.18)*
     AHA: 3Q, '91, 16

     507.0   Due to inhalation of food or vomitus
         Aspiration pneumonia (due to):
           NOS
           food (regurgitated)
           gastric secretions
           milk
           saliva
           vomitus
         AHA: 1Q, '08, 18; 1Q, '89,10
         TIP: Assign an additional code for pneumonia due to a specific organism if that documentation is provided in addition to aspiration pneumonia.
         J69.0 Pneumonitis due to inhalation of food and vomit   I-10

     507.1   Due to inhalation of oils and essences
         Lipoid pneumonia (exogenous)
         EXCLUDES   *endogenous lipoid pneumonia (516.8)*

     507.8   Due to other solids and liquids
         Detergent asthma

√4ᵗʰ 508   Respiratory conditions due to other and unspecified external agents
     Use additional E code to identify cause

     508.0   Acute pulmonary manifestations due to radiation
         Radiation pneumonitis
         AHA: 2Q, '88, 4

     508.1   Chronic and other pulmonary manifestations due to radiation
         Fibrosis of lung following radiation

     508.8   Respiratory conditions due to other specified external agents

     508.9   Respiratory conditions due to unspecified external agent

Other Diseases of Respiratory System (510-519)

√4ᵗʰ 510   Empyema
     Use additional code to identify infectious organism (041.0-041.9)
     EXCLUDES   *abscess of lung (513.0)*
     DEF: Purulent infection within pleural space.

     510.0   With fistula
         Fistula: Fistula:
           bronchocutaneous   mediastinal
           bronchopleural   pleural
           hepatopleural   thoracic

         Any condition classifiable to 510.9 with fistula
         DEF: Purulent infection of respiratory cavity, with communication from cavity to another structure.

     510.9   Without mention of fistula
         Abscess: Pleurisy:
           pleura   purulent
           thorax   septic
         Empyema (chest) (lung)   seropurulent
           (pleura)   suppurative
         Fibrinopurulent pleurisy   Pyopneumothorax
                                       Pyothorax
         AHA: 4Q, '07, 113; 3Q, '94, 6
         J86.9 Pyothorax without fistula   I-10

√4ᵗʰ 511   Pleurisy
     EXCLUDES   *pleurisy with mention of tuberculosis, current disease (012.0)*
     DEF: Inflammation of serous membrane of lungs and lining of thoracic cavity; causes exudation in cavity or membrane surface.

     511.0   Without mention of effusion or current tuberculosis
         Adhesion, lung or pleura   Pleurisy:
         Calcification of pleura   NOS
         Pleurisy (acute) (sterile):   pneumococcal
           diaphragmatic   staphylococcal
           fibrinous   streptococcal
           interlobar   Thickening of pleura
         AHA: 3Q, '94, 5

     511.1   With effusion, with mention of a bacterial cause other than tuberculosis
         Pleurisy with effusion (exudative) (serous):
           pneumococcal
           staphylococcal
           streptococcal
           other specified nontuberculous bacterial cause

     √5ᵗʰ 511.8   Other specified forms of effusion, except tuberculous
         EXCLUDES   *traumatic (860.2-860.5, 862.29, 862.39)*
         AHA: 4Q, '08, 113-114; 1Q, '97, 10

         511.81   Malignant pleural effusion
            Code first malignant neoplasm, if known
            J91.0 Malignant pleural effusion   I-10

         511.89   Other specified forms of effusion, except tuberculous
            Encysted pleurisy   Hydropneumothorax
            Hemopneumothorax   Hydrothorax
            Hemothorax

N   Newborn Age: 0   P   Pediatric Age: 0-17   M   Maternity Age: 12-55   A   Adult Age: 15-124

511.9 Unspecified pleural effusion

Pleural effusion NOS   Pleurisy:
Pleurisy: serous
    exudative   with effusion NOS
    serofibrinous

AHA: 2Q, '03, 7; 3Q, '91, 19; 4Q, '89, 11

TIP: Do not assign when the pleural effusion is a symptom of CHF and no therapeutic treatment (e.g., thoracentesis) is directed towards the pleural effusion.

J90 Pleural effusion not elsewhere classified   `I-10`

✓4ᵗʰ 512 Pneumothorax

DEF: Collapsed lung; due to gas or air in pleural space.

512.0 Spontaneous tension pneumothorax

DEF: Leaking air from lung into lining causing collapse.

AHA: 3Q, '94, 5

512.1 Iatrogenic pneumothorax

Postoperative pneumothorax

DEF: Air trapped in the lining of the lung following surgery.

AHA: 4Q, '94, 40

TIP: Pneumothorax is a known risk associated with most thoracic surgery; do not assign based on radiology findings alone, without physician substantiation.

J95.81 Postprocedural pneumothorax   `I-10`

512.8 Other spontaneous pneumothorax

Pneumothorax: Pneumothorax:
    NOS   chronic
    acute

EXCLUDES *pneumothorax:*
    congenital (770.2)
    traumatic (860.0-860.1, 860.4-860.5)
    tuberculous, current disease (011.7)

AHA: 2Q, '93, 3

J93.9 Pneumothorax unspecified   `I-10`

✓4ᵗʰ 513 Abscess of lung and mediastinum

513.0 Abscess of lung

Abscess (multiple) of lung
Gangrenous or necrotic pneumonia
Pulmonary gangrene or necrosis

AHA: 4Q, '07, 85; 2Q, '98, 7

513.1 Abscess of mediastinum

514 Pulmonary congestion and hypostasis

Hypostatic:
    bronchopneumonia
    pneumonia
Passive pneumonia
Pulmonary congestion (chronic) (passive)
Pulmonary edema:
    NOS
    chronic

EXCLUDES *acute pulmonary edema:*
    NOS (518.4)
    with mention of heart disease or failure (428.1)
hypostatic pneumonia due to or specified as a specific type of pneumonia — code to the type of pneumonia ▶*(480.0-480.9, 481, 482.0-482.9, 483.0-483.8, 485, 486, 487.0, 488.01, 488.11)*◀

DEF: Excessive retention of interstitial fluid in the lungs and pulmonary vessels; due to poor circulation.

AHA: 2Q, '98, 6; 3Q, '88, 5

J81.1 Chronic pulmonary edema   `I-10`

515 Postinflammatory pulmonary fibrosis

Cirrhosis of lung
Fibrosis of lung (atrophic) (confluent) (massive) (perialveolar) (peribronchial) } chronic or unspecified
Induration of lung

DEF: Fibrosis and scarring of the lungs due to inflammatory reaction.

J84.1 Other interstitial pulmonary diseases w/fibrosis   `I-10`

✓4ᵗʰ 516 Other alveolar and parietoalveolar pneumonopathy

516.0 Pulmonary alveolar proteinosis

DEF: Reduced ventilation; due to proteinaceous deposits on alveoli; symptoms include dyspnea, cough, chest pain, weakness, weight loss, and hemoptysis.

516.1 *Idiopathic pulmonary hemosiderosis*

Code first underlying disease ▶*(275.01-275.09)*◀
Essential brown induration of lung

EXCLUDES ▶*acute idiopathic pulmonary hemorrhage in infants [AIPHI] (786.31)*◀

DEF: Fibrosis of alveolar walls; marked by abnormal amounts hemosiderin in lungs; primarily affects children; symptoms include anemia, fluid in lungs, and blood in sputum; etiology unknown.

516.2 Pulmonary alveolar microlithiasis

DEF: Small calculi in pulmonary alveoli resembling sand-like particles on x-ray.

516.3 Idiopathic fibrosing alveolitis

Alveolar capillary block
Diffuse (idiopathic) (interstitial) pulmonary fibrosis
Hamman-Rich syndrome

516.8 Other specified alveolar and parietoalveolar pneumonopathies

Endogenous lipoid pneumonia
Interstitial pneumonia (desquamative) (lymphoid)

EXCLUDES *lipoid pneumonia, exogenous or unspecified (507.1)*

AHA: ▶1Q, '10, 6;◀ 2Q, '06, 20; 1Q, '92, 12

516.9 Unspecified alveolar and parietoalveolar pneumonopathy

✓4ᵗʰ 517 Lung involvement in conditions classified elsewhere

EXCLUDES *rheumatoid lung (714.81)*

517.1 *Rheumatic pneumonia*

Code first underlying disease (390)

517.2 *Lung involvement in systemic sclerosis*

Code first underlying disease (710.1)

517.3 *Acute chest syndrome*

Code first sickle-cell disease in crisis (282.42, 282.62, 282.64, 282.69)

AHA: 4Q, '03, 51, 56

517.8 *Lung involvement in other diseases classified elsewhere*

Code first underlying disease, as:
    amyloidosis (277.30-277.39)
    polymyositis (710.4)
    sarcoidosis (135)
    Sjögren's disease (710.2)
    systemic lupus erythematosus (710.0)

EXCLUDES *syphilis (095.1)*

AHA: 2Q, '03, 7

✓4ᵗʰ 518 Other diseases of lung

518.0 Pulmonary collapse

Atelectasis   Middle lobe syndrome
Collapse of lung

EXCLUDES *atelectasis:*
    congenital (partial) (770.5)
    primary (770.4)
    tuberculous, current disease (011.8)

AHA: 4Q, '90, 25

J98.11 Atelectasis   `I-10`

518.1 Interstitial emphysema

Mediastinal emphysema

EXCLUDES *surgical (subcutaneous) emphysema (998.81)*
    that in fetus or newborn (770.2)
    traumatic emphysema (958.7)

DEF: Escaped air from the alveoli trapped in the interstices of the lung; trauma or cough may cause the disease.

518.2 Compensatory emphysema

DEF: Distention of all or part of the lung caused by disease processes or surgical intervention that decreased volume in another part of the lung; overcompensation reaction to the loss of capacity in another part of the lung.

518.3 Pulmonary eosinophilia

Eosinophilic asthma   Tropical eosinophilia
Löffler's syndrome
Pneumonia:
    allergic
    eosinophilic

DEF: Infiltration into pulmonary parenchyma of eosinophils; results in cough, fever, and dyspnea.

✓4ᵗʰ / ✓5ᵗʰ Additional Digit Required   Unspecified Code   Other Specified Code   Manifestation Code   ▶◀ Revised Text   ● New Code   ▲ Revised Code Title

Diseases of the Respiratory System

518.4–519.9

518.4 Acute edema of lung, unspecified
Acute pulmonary edema NOS
Pulmonary edema, postoperative

EXCLUDES pulmonary edema:
    acute, with mention of heart disease or failure
      (428.1)
    chronic or unspecified (514)
    due to external agents (506.0-508.9)

DEF: Severe, sudden fluid retention within lung tissues.

TIP: Do not assign separately if associated with CHF or heart disease; it is incorporated into those codes.

518.5 Pulmonary insufficiency following trauma and surgery
Adult respiratory distress syndrome
Pulmonary insufficiency following:
    shock
    surgery
    trauma
Shock lung

EXCLUDES adult respiratory distress syndrome associated with
    other conditions (518.82)
    pneumonia:
      aspiration (507.0)
      hypostatic (514)
    respiratory failure in other conditions (518.81,
      518.83-518.84)

AHA: 4Q, '04, 139; 3Q, '88, 3; 3Q, '88, 7; S-O, '87, 1

J95.82 Postprocedural respiratory failure   I-10

518.6 Allergic bronchopulmonary aspergillosis
DEF: Noninvasive hypersensitive reaction; due to allergic reaction to *Aspergillus fumigatus* (mold).
AHA: 4Q, '97, 39

518.7 Transfusion related acute lung injury [TRALI]
DEF: A relatively rare, but serious pulmonary complication of blood transfusion, with acute respiratory distress, noncardiogenic pulmonary edema, cyanosis, hypoxemia, hypotension, fever and chills.
AHA: 4Q, '06, 91

√5ᵗʰ 518.8 Other diseases of lung

518.81 Acute respiratory failure
Respiratory failure NOS

EXCLUDES acute and chronic respiratory failure (518.84)
    acute respiratory distress (518.82)
    chronic respiratory failure (518.83)
    respiratory arrest (799.1)
    respiratory failure, newborn (770.84)

AHA: ▶1Q, '10, 18-19;◄ 3Q, '09, 14; 2Q, '09, 11; 1Q, '08, 18; 3Q, '07, 6; 2Q, '06, 25; 4Q, '05, 96; 2Q, '05, 19; 1Q, '05, 3-8; 1Q, '05, 3-8; 4Q, '04, 139; 1Q, '03, 15; 4Q, '98, 41; 3Q, '91, 14; 2Q, '91, 3; 4Q, '90, 25; 2Q, '90, 20; 3Q, '88, 7; 3Q, '88, 10; S-O, '87, 1

TIP: If both respiratory failure and another acute condition are responsible for admission, either may be sequenced as principal diagnosis.

J96.0 Acute respiratory failure   I-10

518.82 Other pulmonary insufficiency, not elsewhere classified
Acute respiratory distress
Acute respiratory insufficiency
Adult respiratory distress syndrome NEC

EXCLUDES adult respiratory distress syndrome
    associated with trauma and surgery
    (518.5)
    pulmonary insufficiency following trauma
      and surgery (518.5)
    respiratory distress:
      NOS (786.09)
      newborn (770.89)
      syndrome, newborn (769)
    shock lung (518.5)

AHA: 4Q, '03, 105; 2Q, '91, 21; 3Q, '88, 7

J80 Acute respiratory distress syndrome   I-10

518.83 Chronic respiratory failure
AHA: 4Q, '05, 96; 4Q, '03, 103, 111
J96.1 Chronic respiratory failure   I-10

518.84 Acute and chronic respiratory failure
Acute on chronic respiratory failure
J96.2 Acute and chronic respiratory failure   I-10

518.89 Other diseases of lung, not elsewhere classified
Broncholithiasis   Lung disease NOS
Calcification of lung   Pulmolithiasis

DEF: Broncholithiasis: calculi in lumen of transbronchial tree.
DEF: Pulmolithiasis: calculi in lung.
AHA: 3Q, '90, 18; 4Q, '88, 6
J98.4 Other disorders of lung   I-10

√4ᵗʰ 519 Other diseases of respiratory system

√5ᵗʰ 519.0 Tracheostomy complications

519.00 Tracheostomy complication, unspecified

519.01 Infection of tracheostomy
Use additional code to identify type of infection, such as:
    abscess or cellulitis of neck (682.1)
    septicemia (038.0-038.9)
Use additional code to identify organism
    (041.00-041.9)
AHA: 4Q, '98, 41

519.02 Mechanical complication of tracheostomy
Tracheal stenosis due to tracheostomy

519.09 Other tracheostomy complications
Hemorrhage due to tracheostomy
Tracheoesophageal fistula due to tracheostomy

√5ᵗʰ 519.1 Other diseases of trachea and bronchus, not elsewhere classified
AHA: 3Q, '02, 18; 3Q, '88, 6

519.11 Acute bronchospasm
Bronchospasm NOS

EXCLUDES acute bronchitis with bronchospasm (466.0)
    asthma (493.00-493.92)
    exercise induced bronchospasm (493.81)

AHA: 4Q, '06, 92

519.19 Other diseases of trachea and bronchus
Calcification ⎫
Stenosis   ⎬ of bronchus or trachea
Ulcer   ⎭

AHA: 4Q, '06, 92

519.2 Mediastinitis
DEF: Inflammation of tissue between organs behind sternum.

519.3 Other diseases of mediastinum, not elsewhere classified
Fibrosis ⎫
Hernia   ⎬ of mediastinum
Retraction ⎭

519.4 Disorders of diaphragm
Diaphragmitis   Relaxation of diaphragm
Paralysis of diaphragm

EXCLUDES congenital defect of diaphragm (756.6)
    diaphragmatic hernia (551-553 with .3)
    congenital (756.6)

519.8 Other diseases of respiratory system, not elsewhere classified
AHA: 4Q, '89, 12

519.9 Unspecified disease of respiratory system
Respiratory disease (chronic) NOS

N Newborn Age: 0   **P** Pediatric Age: 0-17   **M** Maternity Age: 12-55   **A** Adult Age: 15-124

9. Diseases of the Digestive System (520-579)

Diseases of Oral Cavity, Salivary Glands, and Jaws (520-529)

☑4ᵗʰ **520 Disorders of tooth development and eruption**

520.0 Anodontia
Absence of teeth (complete) (congenital) (partial)
Hypodontia
Oligodontia
> **EXCLUDES** *acquired absence of teeth (525.10-525.19)*

520.1 Supernumerary teeth
Distomolar
Fourth molar
Mesiodens
Paramolar
Supplemental teeth
> **EXCLUDES** *supernumerary roots (520.2)*

520.2 Abnormalities of size and form
Concrescence ⎫
Fusion   ⎬ of teeth
Gemination ⎭

Dens evaginatus
Dens in dente
Dens invaginatus
Enamel pearls
Macrodontia
Microdontia
Peg-shaped [conical] teeth
Supernumerary roots
Taurodontism
Tuberculum paramolare
> **EXCLUDES** *that due to congenital syphilis (090.5)*
> *tuberculum Carabelli, which is regarded as a normal variation*

520.3 Mottled teeth
Mottling of enamel
Dental fluorosis
Nonfluoride enamel opacities

Digestive System

The Oral Cavity

Teeth

Maxillary view

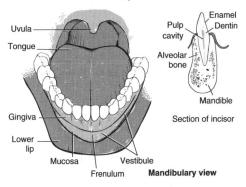

Mandibulary view

520.4 Disturbances of tooth formation
Aplasia and hypoplasia of cementum
Dilaceration of tooth
Enamel hypoplasia (neonatal) (postnatal) (prenatal)
Horner's teeth
Hypocalcification of teeth
Regional odontodysplasia
Turner's tooth
> **EXCLUDES** *Hutchinson's teeth and mulberry molars in congenital syphilis (090.5)*
> *mottled teeth (520.3)*

520.5 Hereditary disturbances in tooth structure, not elsewhere classified
Amelogensis   ⎫
Dentinogenesis ⎬ imperfecta
Odontogenesis   ⎭

Dentinal dysplasia
Shell teeth

520.6 Disturbances in tooth eruption
Teeth:
  embedded
  impacted
  natal
  neonatal
  prenatal
  primary [deciduous]:
    persistent
    shedding, premature
Tooth eruption:
  late
  obstructed
  premature
> **EXCLUDES** *exfoliation of teeth (attributable to disease of surrounding tissues) (525.0-525.19)*
> **AHA:** 1Q, '06, 18; 2Q, '05, 15

520.7 Teething syndrome

520.8 Other specified disorders of tooth development and eruption
Color changes during tooth formation
Pre-eruptive color changes
> **EXCLUDES** *posteruptive color changes (521.7)*

520.9 Unspecified disorder of tooth development and eruption

☑4ᵗʰ
☑5ᵗʰ Additional Digit Required   Unspecified Code   Other Specified Code   Manifestation Code   ▶◀ Revised Text   ● New Code   ▲ Revised Code Title
2011 ICD-9-CM   **Volume 1 – 155**

✓4th **521 Diseases of hard tissues of teeth**

✓5th **521.0 Dental caries**
AHA: 4Q, '01, 44

521.00 Dental caries, unspecified

521.01 Dental caries limited to enamel
Initial caries
White spot lesion

521.02 Dental caries extending into dentine

521.03 Dental caries extending into pulp

521.04 Arrested dental caries

521.05 Odontoclasia
Infantile melanodontia
Melanodontoclasia
EXCLUDES *internal and external resorption of teeth (521.40-521.49)*
DEF: A pathological dental condition described as stained areas, loss of tooth substance, and hypoplasia linked to nutritional deficiencies during tooth development and to cariogenic oral conditions.

521.06 Dental caries pit and fissure
Primary dental caries, pit and fissure origin

521.07 Dental caries of smooth surface
Primary dental caries, smooth surface origin

521.08 Dental caries of root surface
Primary dental caries, root surface

521.09 Other dental caries
AHA: 3Q, '02, 14

✓5th **521.1 Excessive attrition (approximal wear) (occlusal wear)**

521.10 Excessive attrition, unspecified

521.11 Excessive attrition, limited to enamel

521.12 Excessive attrition, extending into dentine

521.13 Excessive attrition, extending into pulp

521.14 Excessive attrition, localized

521.15 Excessive attrition, generalized

✓5th **521.2 Abrasion**
Abrasion:
dentifrice
habitual
occupational } of teeth
ritual
traditional
Wedge defect NOS

521.20 Abrasion, unspecified

521.21 Abrasion, limited to enamel

521.22 Abrasion, extending into dentine

521.23 Abrasion, extending into pulp

521.24 Abrasion, localized

521.25 Abrasion, generalized

✓5th **521.3 Erosion**
Erosion of teeth:
NOS
due to:
medicine
persistent vomiting
idiopathic
occupational

521.30 Erosion, unspecified

521.31 Erosion, limited to enamel

521.32 Erosion, extending into dentine

521.33 Erosion, extending into pulp

521.34 Erosion, localized

521.35 Erosion, generalized

✓5th **521.4 Pathological resorption**
DEF: Loss of dentin and cementum due to disease process.

521.40 Pathological resorption, unspecified

521.41 Pathological resorption, internal

521.42 Pathological resorption, external

521.49 Other pathological resorption
Internal granuloma of pulp

521.5 Hypercementosis
Cementation hyperplasia
DEF: Excess deposits of cementum, on tooth root.

521.6 Ankylosis of teeth
DEF: Adhesion of tooth to surrounding bone.

521.7 Intrinsic posteruptive color changes
Staining [discoloration] of teeth:
NOS
due to:
drugs
metals
pulpal bleeding
EXCLUDES *accretions [deposits] on teeth (523.6)*
extrinsic color changes (523.6)
pre-eruptive color changes (520.8)

✓5th **521.8 Other specified diseases of hard tissues of teeth**

521.81 Cracked tooth
EXCLUDES *asymptomatic craze lines in enamel — omit code*
broken tooth due to trauma (873.63, 873.73)
fractured tooth due to trauma (873.63, 873.73)

521.89 Other specified diseases of hard tissues of teeth
Irradiated enamel
Sensitive dentin

521.9 Unspecified disease of hard tissues of teeth

✓4th **522 Diseases of pulp and periapical tissues**

522.0 Pulpitis
Pulpal:
abscess
polyp
Pulpitis:
acute
chronic (hyperplastic) (ulcerative)
suppurative

522.1 Necrosis of the pulp
Pulp gangrene
DEF: Death of pulp tissue.

522.2 Pulp degeneration
Denticles
Pulp calcifications
Pulp stones

522.3 Abnormal hard tissue formation in pulp
Secondary or irregular dentin

522.4 Acute apical periodontitis of pulpal origin
DEF: Severe inflammation of periodontal ligament due to pulpal inflammation or necrosis.

522.5 Periapical abscess without sinus
Abscess:
dental
dentoalveolar
EXCLUDES *periapical abscess with sinus (522.7)*

522.6 Chronic apical periodontitis
Apical or periapical granuloma
Apical periodontitis NOS

522.7 Periapical abscess with sinus
Fistula:
alveolar process
dental

522.8 Radicular cyst
Cyst:
apical (periodontal)
periapical
radiculodental
residual radicular
DEF: Cyst in tissue around tooth apex due to chronic infection of granuloma around root.

522.9 Other and unspecified diseases of pulp and periapical tissues

√4ᵗʰ **523 Gingival and periodontal diseases**

√5ᵗʰ **523.0 Acute gingivitis**
EXCLUDES *acute necrotizing ulcerative gingivitis (101)*
herpetic gingivostomatitis (054.2)

523.00 Acute gingivitis, plaque induced
Acute gingivitis NOS

523.01 Acute gingivitis, non-plaque induced

√5ᵗʰ **523.1 Chronic gingivitis**
Gingivitis (chronic):
desquamative
hyperplastic
simple marginal
ulcerative
EXCLUDES *herpetic gingivostomatitis (054.2)*

523.10 Chronic gingivitis, plaque induced
Chronic gingivitis NOS
Gingivitis NOS

523.11 Chronic gingivitis, non-plaque induced

√5ᵗʰ **523.2 Gingival recession**
Gingival recession (postinfective) (postoperative)

523.20 Gingival recession, unspecified

523.21 Gingival recession, minimal

523.22 Gingival recession, moderate

523.23 Gingival recession, severe

523.24 Gingival recession, localized

523.25 Gingival recession, generalized

√5ᵗʰ **523.3 Aggressive and acute periodontitis**
Acute:
pericementitis
pericoronitis
EXCLUDES *acute apical periodontitis (522.4)*
periapical abscess (522.5, 522.7)
DEF: Severe inflammation of tissues supporting teeth.

523.30 Aggressive periodontitis, unspecified

523.31 Aggressive periodontitis, localized
Periodontal abscess

523.32 Aggressive periodontitis, generalized

523.33 Acute periodontitis

√5ᵗʰ **523.4 Chronic periodontitis**
Chronic pericoronitis
Pericementitis (chronic)
Periodontitis:
NOS
complex
simplex
EXCLUDES *chronic apical periodontitis (522.6)*

523.40 Chronic periodontitis, unspecified

523.41 Chronic periodontitis, localized

523.42 Chronic periodontitis, generalized

523.5 Periodontosis

523.6 Accretions on teeth
Dental calculus:
subgingival
supragingival
Deposits on teeth:
betel
materia alba
soft
tartar
tobacco
Extrinsic discoloration of teeth
EXCLUDES *intrinsic discoloration of teeth (521.7)*
DEF: Foreign material on tooth surface, usually plaque or calculus.

523.8 Other specified periodontal diseases
Giant cell:
epulis
peripheral granuloma
Gingival:
cysts
enlargement NOS
fibromatosis
Gingival polyp
Periodontal lesions due to traumatic occlusion
Peripheral giant cell granuloma
EXCLUDES *leukoplakia of gingiva (528.6)*

523.9 Unspecified gingival and periodontal disease
AHA: 3Q, '02, 14

√4ᵗʰ **524 Dentofacial anomalies, including malocclusion**

√5ᵗʰ **524.0 Major anomalies of jaw size**
EXCLUDES *hemifacial atrophy or hypertrophy (754.0)*
unilateral condylar hyperplasia or hypoplasia of mandible (526.89)

524.00 Unspecified anomaly
DEF: Unspecified deformity of jaw size.

524.01 Maxillary hyperplasia
DEF: Overgrowth or over development of upper jaw bone.

524.02 Mandibular hyperplasia
DEF: Overgrowth or over development of lower jaw bone.

524.03 Maxillary hypoplasia
DEF: Incomplete or underdeveloped upper jaw bone.

524.04 Mandibular hypoplasia
DEF: Incomplete or underdeveloped lower jaw bone.

524.05 Macrogenia
DEF: Enlarged jaw, especially chin; affects bone, soft tissue, or both.

524.06 Microgenia
DEF: Underdeveloped mandible, characterized by an extremely small chin.

524.07 Excessive tuberosity of jaw
Entire maxillary tuberosity

524.09 Other specified anomaly

√5ᵗʰ **524.1 Anomalies of relationship of jaw to cranial base**

524.10 Unspecified anomaly
Prognathism
Retrognathism
DEF: Prognathism: protrusion of lower jaw.
DEF: Retrognathism: jaw is located posteriorly to a normally positioned jaw; backward position of mandible.

524.11 Maxillary asymmetry
DEF: Absence of symmetry of maxilla.

524.12 Other jaw asymmetry

524.19 Other specified anomaly

Diseases of the Digestive System

524.2–524.9

Angle's Classification of Malocclusion

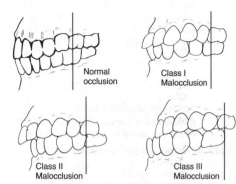

Normal occlusion

Class I Malocclusion

Class II Malocclusion

Class III Malocclusion

√5ᵗʰ **524.2 Anomalies of dental arch relationship**
Anomaly of dental arch
EXCLUDES hemifacial atrophy or hypertrophy (754.0)
soft tissue impingement (524.81-524.82)
unilateral condylar hyperplasia or hypoplasia of
mandible (526.89)

524.20 Unspecified anomaly of dental arch relationship

524.21 Malocclusion, Angle's class I
Neutro-occlusion

524.22 Malocclusion, Angle's class II
Disto-occlusion Division I
Disto-occlusion Division II

524.23 Malocclusion, Angle's class III
Mesio-occlusion

524.24 Open anterior occlusal relationship
Anterior open bite

524.25 Open posterior occlusal relationship
Posterior open bite

524.26 Excessive horizontal overlap
Excessive horizontal overjet

524.27 Reverse articulation
Anterior articulation
Crossbite
Posterior articulation

524.28 Anomalies of interarch distance
Excessive interarch distance
Inadequate interarch distance

524.29 Other anomalies of dental arch relationship
Other anomalies of dental arch

√5ᵗʰ **524.3 Anomalies of tooth position of fully erupted teeth**
EXCLUDES impacted or embedded teeth with abnormal position
of such teeth or adjacent teeth (520.6)

524.30 Unspecified anomaly of tooth position
Diastema of teeth NOS
Displacement of teeth NOS
Transposition of teeth NOS

524.31 Crowding of teeth

524.32 Excessive spacing of teeth

524.33 Horizontal displacement of teeth
Tipped teeth
Tipping of teeth

524.34 Vertical displacement of teeth
Extruded tooth
Infraeruption of teeth
Intruded tooth
Supraeruption of teeth

524.35 Rotation of tooth/teeth

524.36 Insufficient interocclusal distance of teeth (ridge)
Lack of adequate intermaxillary vertical dimension

524.37 Excessive interocclusal distance of teeth
Excessive intermaxillary vertical dimension
Loss of occlusal vertical dimension

524.39 Other anomalies of tooth position

524.4 Malocclusion, unspecified
DEF: Malposition of top and bottom teeth; interferes with chewing.

√5ᵗʰ **524.5 Dentofacial functional abnormalities**

524.50 Dentofacial functional abnormality, unspecified

524.51 Abnormal jaw closure

524.52 Limited mandibular range of motion

524.53 Deviation in opening and closing of the mandible

524.54 Insufficient anterior guidance
Insufficient anterior occlusal guidance

524.55 Centric occlusion maximum intercuspation discrepancy
Centric occlusion of teeth discrepancy

524.56 Non-working side interference
Balancing side interference

524.57 Lack of posterior occlusal support

524.59 Other dentofacial functional abnormalities
Abnormal swallowing
Mouth breathing
Sleep postures
Tongue, lip, or finger habits

√5ᵗʰ **524.6 Temporomandibular joint disorders**
EXCLUDES current temporomandibular joint:
dislocation (830.0-830.1)
strain (848.1)

524.60 Temporomandibular joint disorders, unspecified
Temporomandibular joint-pain-dysfunction
syndrome [TMJ]

524.61 Adhesions and ankylosis (bony or fibrous)
DEF: Stiffening or union of temporomandibular joint due to
bony or fibrous union across joint.

524.62 Arthralgia of temporomandibular joint
DEF: Pain in temporomandibular joint; not inflammatory in
nature.

524.63 Articular disc disorder (reducing or non-reducing)

524.64 Temporomandibular joint sounds on opening and/or closing the jaw

524.69 Other specified temporomandibular joint disorders

√5ᵗʰ **524.7 Dental alveolar anomalies**

524.70 Unspecified alveolar anomaly

524.71 Alveolar maxillary hyperplasia
DEF: Excessive tissue formation in the dental alveoli of
upper jaw.

524.72 Alveolar mandibular hyperplasia
DEF: Excessive tissue formation in the dental alveoli of lower
jaw.

524.73 Alveolar maxillary hypoplasia
DEF: Incomplete or underdeveloped alveolar tissue of upper
jaw.

524.74 Alveolar mandibular hypoplasia
DEF: Incomplete or underdeveloped alveolar tissue of lower
jaw.

524.75 Vertical displacement of alveolus and teeth
Extrusion of alveolus and teeth

524.76 Occlusal plane deviation

524.79 Other specified alveolar anomaly

√5ᵗʰ **524.8 Other specified dentofacial anomalies**

524.81 Anterior soft tissue impingement

524.82 Posterior soft tissue impingement

524.89 Other specified dentofacial anomalies

524.9 Unspecified dentofacial anomalies

Ⓝ Newborn Age: 0   Ⓟ Pediatric Age: 0-17   Ⓜ Maternity Age: 12-55   Ⓐ Adult Age: 15-124

Diseases of the Digestive System

525–525.9

☑4ᵗʰ **525 Other diseases and conditions of the teeth and supporting structures**

525.0 Exfoliation of teeth due to systemic causes
DEF: Deterioration of teeth and surrounding structures due to systemic disease.

☑5ᵗʰ **525.1 Loss of teeth due to trauma, extraction, or periodontal disease**
Code first class of edentulism (525.40-525.44, 525.50-525.54)
AHA: 4Q, '05, 74; 4Q, '01, 44

525.10 Acquired absence of teeth, unspecified
Tooth extraction status, NOS

525.11 Loss of teeth due to trauma

525.12 Loss of teeth due to periodontal disease

525.13 Loss of teeth due to caries

525.19 Other loss of teeth

☑5ᵗʰ **525.2 Atrophy of edentulous alveolar ridge**

525.20 Unspecified atrophy of edentulous alveolar ridge
Atrophy of the mandible NOS
Atrophy of the maxilla NOS

525.21 Minimal atrophy of the mandible

525.22 Moderate atrophy of the mandible

525.23 Severe atrophy of the mandible

525.24 Minimal atrophy of the maxilla

525.25 Moderate atrophy of the maxilla

525.26 Severe atrophy of the maxilla

525.3 Retained dental root

☑5ᵗʰ **525.4 Complete edentulism**
Use additional code to identify cause of edentulism (525.10-525.19)
AHA: 4Q, '05, 74

525.40 Complete edentulism, unspecified
Edentulism NOS

525.41 Complete edentulism, class I

525.42 Complete edentulism, class II

525.43 Complete edentulism, class III

525.44 Complete edentulism, class IV

☑5ᵗʰ **525.5 Partial edentulism**
Use additional code to identify cause of edentulism (525.10-525.19)
AHA: 4Q, '05, 74

525.50 Partial edentulism, unspecified

525.51 Partial edentulism, class I

525.52 Partial edentulism, class II

525.53 Partial edentulism, class III

525.54 Partial edentulism, class IV

☑5ᵗʰ **525.6 Unsatisfactory restoration of tooth**
Defective bridge, crown, fillings
Defective dental restoration
EXCLUDES dental restoration status (V45.84)
unsatisfactory endodontic treatment (526.61-526.69)

525.60 Unspecified unsatisfactory restoration of tooth
Unspecified defective dental restoration

525.61 Open restoration margins
Dental restoration failure of marginal integrity
Open margin on tooth restoration

525.62 Unrepairable overhanging of dental restorative materials
Overhanging of tooth restoration

525.63 Fractured dental restorative material without loss of material
EXCLUDES cracked tooth (521.81)
fractured tooth (873.63, 873.73)

525.64 Fractured dental restorative material with loss of material
EXCLUDES cracked tooth (521.81)
fractured tooth (873.63, 873.73)

525.65 Contour of existing restoration of tooth biologically incompatible with oral health
Dental restoration failure of periodontal anatomical integrity
Unacceptable contours of existing restoration
Unacceptable morphology of existing restoration

525.66 Allergy to existing dental restorative material
Use additional code to identify the specific type of allergy

525.67 Poor aesthetics of existing restoration
Dental restoration aesthetically inadequate or displeasing

525.69 Other unsatisfactory restoration of existing tooth

☑5ᵗʰ **525.7 Endosseous dental implant failure**

525.71 Osseointegration failure of dental implant
Failure of dental implant due to infection
Failure of dental implant due to unintentional loading
Failure of dental implant osseointegration due to premature loading
Failure of dental implant to osseointegrate prior to intentional prosthetic loading
Hemorrhagic complications of dental implant placement
Iatrogenic osseointegration failure of dental implant
Osseointegration failure of dental implant due to complications of systemic disease
Osseointegration failure of dental implant due to poor bone quality
Pre-integration failure of dental implant NOS
Pre-osseointegration failure of dental implant

525.72 Post-osseointegration biological failure of dental implant
Failure of dental implant due to lack of attached gingiva
Failure of dental implant due to occlusal trauma (caused by poor prosthetic design)
Failure of dental implant due to parafunctional habits
Failure of dental implant due to periodontal infection (peri-implantitis)
Failure of dental implant due to poor oral hygiene
Failure of dental implant to osseointegrate following intentional prosthetic loading
Iatrogenic post-osseointegration failure of dental implant
Post-osseointegration failure of dental implant due to complications of systemic disease

525.73 Post-osseointegration mechanic failure of dental implant
Failure of dental prosthesis causing loss of dental implant
Fracture of dental implant
Mechanical failure of dental implant NOS
EXCLUDES cracked tooth (521.81)
fractured dental restorative material with loss of material (525.64)
fractured dental restorative material without loss of material (525.63)
fractured tooth (873.63, 873.73)

525.79 Other endosseous dental implant failure
Dental implant failure NOS

525.8 Other specified disorders of the teeth and supporting structures
Enlargement of alveolar ridge NOS
Irregular alveolar process

525.9 Unspecified disorder of the teeth and supporting structures

Diseases of the Digestive System

526–528.09

✓4ᵗʰ **526 Diseases of the jaws**

526.0 Developmental odontogenic cysts
Cyst:
dentigerous
eruption
follicular
lateral developmental
lateral periodontal
primordial
Keratocyst
EXCLUDES *radicular cyst (522.8)*

526.1 Fissural cysts of jaw
Cyst:
globulomaxillary
incisor canal
median anterior maxillary
median palatal
nasopalatine
palatine of papilla
EXCLUDES *cysts of oral soft tissues (528.4)*

526.2 Other cysts of jaws
Cyst of jaw:
NOS
aneurysmal
hemorrhagic
traumatic

526.3 Central giant cell (reparative) granuloma
EXCLUDES *peripheral giant cell granuloma (523.8)*

526.4 Inflammatory conditions
Abscess
Osteitis } of jaw (acute) (chronic)
Osteomyelitis (neonatal) } (suppurative)
Periostitis

Sequestrum of jaw bone
EXCLUDES *alveolar osteitis (526.5)*
osteonecrosis of jaw (733.45)

526.5 Alveolitis of jaw
Alveolar osteitis
Dry socket
DEF: Inflammation of alveoli or tooth socket.

✓5ᵗʰ **526.6 Periradicular pathology associated with previous endodontic treatment**

526.61 Perforation of root canal space

526.62 Endodontic overfill

526.63 Endodontic underfill

526.69 Other periradicular pathology associated with previous endodontic treatment

✓5ᵗʰ **526.8 Other specified diseases of the jaws**

526.81 Exostosis of jaw
Torus mandibularis
Torus palatinus
DEF: Spur or bony outgrowth on the jaw.

526.89 Other
Cherubism
Fibrous dysplasia } of jaw(s)
Latent bone cyst }
Osteoradionecrosis

Unilateral condylar hyperplasia or hypoplasia of mandible

526.9 Unspecified disease of the jaws

✓4ᵗʰ **527 Diseases of the salivary glands**

527.0 Atrophy
DEF: Wasting away, necrosis of salivary gland tissue.

527.1 Hypertrophy
DEF: Overgrowth or overdeveloped salivary gland tissue.

527.2 Sialoadenitis
Parotitis:
NOS
allergic
toxic
Sialoangitis
Sialodochitis
EXCLUDES *epidemic or infectious parotitis (072.0-072.9)*
uveoparotid fever (135)
DEF: Inflammation of salivary gland.

527.3 Abscess

527.4 Fistula
EXCLUDES *congenital fistula of salivary gland (750.24)*

527.5 Sialolithiasis
Calculus } of salivary gland or duct
Stone }
Sialodocholithiasis

527.6 Mucocele
Mucous:
extravasation cyst of salivary gland
retention cyst of salivary gland
Ranula
DEF: Dilated salivary gland cavity filled with mucous.

527.7 Disturbance of salivary secretion
Hyposecretion
Ptyalism
Sialorrhea
Xerostomia

527.8 Other specified diseases of the salivary glands
Benign lymphoepithelial lesion of salivary gland
Sialectasia
Sialosis
Stenosis } of salivary duct
Stricture }

527.9 Unspecified disease of the salivary glands

✓4ᵗʰ **528 Diseases of the oral soft tissues, excluding lesions specific for gingiva and tongue**

✓5ᵗʰ **528.0 Stomatitis and mucositis (ulcerative)**
EXCLUDES *cellulitis and abscess of mouth (528.3)*
diphtheritic stomatitis (032.0)
epizootic stomatitis (078.4)
gingivitis (523.0-523.1)
oral thrush (112.0)
Stevens-Johnson syndrome (695.13)
stomatitis:
acute necrotizing ulcerative (101)
aphthous (528.2)
gangrenous (528.1)
herpetic (054.2)
Vincent's (101)
DEF: Stomatitis: Inflammation of oral mucosa; labial and buccal mucosa, tongue, palate, floor of the mouth, and gingivae.
AHA: 2Q, '99, 9
TIP: Do not assign if documented as fungal oral thrush, or as due to candidiasis. See instead 112.0.

528.00 Stomatitis and mucositis, unspecified
Mucositis NOS
Ulcerative mucositis NOS
Ulcerative stomatitis NOS
Vesicular stomatitis NOS
AHA: 4Q, '06, 88-90

528.01 Mucositis (ulcerative) due to antineoplastic therapy
Use additional E code to identify adverse effects of therapy, such as:
antineoplastic and immunosuppressive drugs (E930.7, E933.1)
radiation therapy (E879.2)
AHA: 4Q, '06, 88-90

528.02 Mucositis (ulcerative) due to other drugs
Use additional E code to identify drug
AHA: 4Q, '06, 88-90

528.09 Other stomatitis and mucositis (ulcerative)
AHA: 4Q, '06, 88-90

Ⓝ Newborn Age: 0   Ⓟ Pediatric Age: 0-17   Ⓜ Maternity Age: 12-55   Ⓐ Adult Age: 15-124

528.1 Cancrum oris
Gangrenous stomatitis
Noma
DEF: A severely gangrenous lesion of mouth due to fusospirochetal infection; destroys buccal, labial and facial tissues; can be fatal; found primarily in debilitated and malnourished children.

528.2 Oral aphthae
Aphthous stomatitis
Canker sore
Periadenitis mucosa necrotica recurrens
Recurrent aphthous ulcer
Stomatitis herpetiformis
EXCLUDES *herpetic stomatitis (054.2)*
DEF: Small oval or round ulcers of the mouth marked by a grayish exudate and a red halo effect.

528.3 Cellulitis and abscess
Cellulitis of mouth (floor)
Ludwig's angina
Oral fistula
EXCLUDES *abscess of tongue (529.0)*
cellulitis or abscess of lip (528.5)
fistula (of):
dental (522.7)
lip (528.5)
gingivitis (523.00-523.11)

528.4 Cysts
Dermoid cyst
Epidermoid cyst
Epstein's pearl   } of mouth
Lymphoepithelial cyst
Nasoalveolar cyst
Nasolabial cyst
EXCLUDES *cyst:*
gingiva (523.8)
tongue (529.8)

528.5 Diseases of lips
Abscess
Cellulitis   } of lips
Fistula
Hypertrophy
Cheilitis:
NOS
angular
Cheilodynia
Cheilosis
EXCLUDES *actinic cheilitis (692.79)*
congenital fistula of lip (750.25)
leukoplakia of lips (528.6)
AHA: S-O, '86, 10

528.6 Leukoplakia of oral mucosa, including tongue
Leukokeratosis of oral mucosa
Leukoplakia of:
gingiva
lips
tongue
EXCLUDES *carcinoma in situ (230.0, 232.0)*
leukokeratosis nicotina palati (528.79)
DEF: Thickened white patches of epithelium on mucous membranes of mouth.

√5ᵗʰ 528.7 Other disturbances of oral epithelium, including tongue
EXCLUDES *carcinoma in situ (230.0, 232.0)*
leukokeratosis NOS (702.8)

528.71 Minimal keratinized residual ridge mucosa
Minimal keratinization of alveolar ridge mucosa

528.72 Excessive keratinized residual ridge mucosa
Excessive keratinization of alveolar ridge mucosa

528.79 Other disturbances of oral epithelium, including tongue
Erythroplakia of mouth or tongue
Focal epithelial hyperplasia of mouth or tongue
Leukoedema of mouth or tongue
Leukokeratosis nicotina palate
Other oral epithelium disturbances

528.8 Oral submucosal fibrosis, including of tongue

528.9 Other and unspecified diseases of the oral soft tissues
Cheek and lip biting
Denture sore mouth
Denture stomatitis
Melanoplakia
Papillary hyperplasia of palate
Eosinophilic granuloma
Irritative hyperplasisa   } of oral mucosa
Pyogenic granuloma
Ulcer (traumatic)

√4ᵗʰ 529 Diseases and other conditions of the tongue

529.0 Glossitis
Abscess   } of tongue
Ulceration (traumatic)
EXCLUDES *glossitis:*
benign migratory (529.1)
Hunter's (529.4)
median rhomboid (529.2)
Moeller's (529.4)

529.1 Geographic tongue
Benign migratory glossitis
Glossitis areata exfoliativa
DEF: Chronic glossitis; marked by filiform papillae atrophy and inflammation; no known etiology.

529.2 Median rhomboid glossitis
DEF: A noninflammatory, congenital disease characterized by rhomboid-like lesions at the middle third of the tongue's dorsal surface.

529.3 Hypertrophy of tongue papillae
Black hairy tongue
Coated tongue
Hypertrophy of foliate papillae
Lingua villosa nigra

529.4 Atrophy of tongue papillae
Bald tongue
Glazed tongue
Glossitis:
Hunter's
Moeller's
Glossodynia exfoliativa
Smooth atrophic tongue

529.5 Plicated tongue
Fissured
Furrowed   } tongue
Scrotal
EXCLUDES *fissure of tongue, congenital (750.13)*
DEF: Cracks, fissures or furrows, on dorsal surface of tongue.

529.6 Glossodynia
Glossopyrosis
Painful tongue
EXCLUDES *glossodynia exfoliativa (529.4)*

529.8 Other specified conditions of the tongue
Atrophy
Crenated   } (of) tongue
Enlargement
Hypertrophy
Glossocele
Glossoptosis
EXCLUDES *erythroplasia of tongue (528.79)*
leukoplakia of tongue (528.6)
macroglossia (congenital) (750.15)
microglossia (congenital) (750.16)
oral submucosal fibrosis (528.8)

529.9 Unspecified condition of the tongue

Diseases of the Digestive System

530–530.9

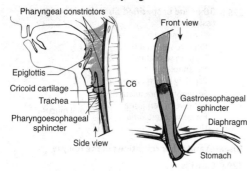

Esophagus

Pharyngeal constrictors

Front view

Epiglottis
Cricoid cartilage
Trachea

C6

Gastroesophageal sphincter

Pharyngoesophageal sphincter

Diaphragm

Side view

Stomach

Diseases of Esophagus, Stomach, and Duodenum (530-538)

√4ᵗʰ **530 Diseases of esophagus**
> **EXCLUDES** *esophageal varices (456.0-456.2)*

530.0 Achalasia and cardiospasm
Achalasia (of cardia)
Aperistalsis of esophagus
Megaesophagus
> **EXCLUDES** *congenital cardiospasm (750.7)*

DEF: Failure of smooth muscle fibers to relax at gastrointestinal junctures, such as esophagogastric sphincter when swallowing.

√5ᵗʰ ### 530.1 Esophagitis
Esophagitis: Esphagitis:
  chemical   postoperative
  peptic   regurgitant

Use additional E code to identify cause, if induced by chemical
> **EXCLUDES** *tuberculous esophagitis (017.8)*

AHA: 4Q, '93, 27; 1Q, '92, 17; 3Q, '91, 20

TIP: Do not assign if esophagitis due to candidiasis; see instead code 112.84.

530.10 Esophagitis, unspecified
Esophagitis NOS
AHA: 3Q, '05, 17

530.11 Reflux esophagitis
DEF: Inflammation of lower esophagus; due to regurgitated gastric acid.
AHA: 4Q, '95, 82
K21.0 Gastro-esophageal reflux disease w/esophagitis   I-10

530.12 Acute esophagitis
DEF: An acute inflammation of the mucous lining or submucosal coat of the esophagus.
AHA: 4Q, '01, 45

530.13 Eosinophilic esophagitis
AHA: 4Q, '08, 115-116

530.19 Other esophagitis
Abscess of esophagus
AHA: 3Q, '01, 10
K20 Esophagitis   I-10

√5ᵗʰ ### 530.2 Ulcer of esophagus
Ulcer of esophagus:
  fungal
  peptic
Ulcer of esophagus due to ingestion of:
  aspirin
  chemicals
  medicines
Use additional E code to identify cause, if induced by chemical or drug
AHA: 4Q, '03, 63

530.20 Ulcer of esophagus without bleeding
Ulcer of esophagus NOS

530.21 Ulcer of esophagus with bleeding
> **EXCLUDES** *bleeding esophageal varices (456.0, 456.20)*

530.3 Stricture and stenosis of esophagus
Compression of esophagus
Obstruction of esophagus
> **EXCLUDES** *congenital stricture of esophagus (750.3)*

AHA: 2Q, '01, 4; 2Q, '97, 3; 1Q, '88, 13

TIP: If esophageal obstruction is due to impacted foreign body, such as meat or other substance, assign instead code 935.1.
K22.2 Esophageal obstruction   I-10

530.4 Perforation of esophagus
Rupture of esophagus
> **EXCLUDES** *traumatic perforation of esophagus (862.22, 862.32, 874.4-874.5)*

530.5 Dyskinesia of esophagus
Corkscrew esophagus
Curling esophagus
Esophagospasm
Spasm of esophagus
> **EXCLUDES** *cardiospasm (530.0)*

DEF: Difficulty performing voluntary esophageal movements.
AHA: 1Q, '88, 13; N-D, '84, 19

530.6 Diverticulum of esophagus, acquired
Diverticulum, acquired:
  epiphrenic
  pharyngoesophageal
  pulsion
  subdiaphragmatic
  traction
  Zenker's (hypopharyngeal)
Esophageal pouch, acquired
Esophagocele, acquired
> **EXCLUDES** *congenital diverticulum of esophagus (750.4)*

AHA: J-F, '85, 3

530.7 Gastroesophageal laceration-hemorrhage syndrome
Mallory-Weiss syndrome
DEF: Laceration of distal esophagus and proximal stomach due to vomiting, hiccups or other sustained activity.

√5ᵗʰ ### 530.8 Other specified disorders of esophagus

530.81 Esophageal reflux
Gastroesophageal reflux
> **EXCLUDES** *reflux esophagitis (530.11)*

DEF: Regurgitation of the gastric contents into esophagus and possibly pharynx.
AHA: 2Q, '01, 4; 1Q, '95, 7; 4Q, '92, 27
K21.9 Gastro-esophageal reflux dz w/o esophagitis   I-10

530.82 Esophageal hemorrhage
> **EXCLUDES** *hemorrhage due to esophageal varices (456.0-456.2)*

AHA: 1Q, '05, 17

530.83 Esophageal leukoplakia

530.84 Tracheoesophageal fistula
> **EXCLUDES** *congenital tracheoesophageal fistula (750.3)*

530.85 Barrett's esophagus
DEF: A metaplastic disorder in which specialized columnar epithelial cells replace the normal squamous epithelial cells; secondary to chronic gastroesophageal reflux damage to the mucosa; increases risk of developing adenocarcinoma.
AHA: 4Q, '03, 63
K22.7 Barrett's esophagus   I-10

530.86 Infection of esophagostomy
Use additional code to specify infection

530.87 Mechanical complication of esophagostomy
Malfunction of esophagostomy

530.89 Other
> **EXCLUDES** *Paterson-Kelly syndrome (280.8)*

530.9 Unspecified disorder of esophagus

Stomach

Esophagus

Diaphragm

Cardiac portion — Stomach

Pylorus — Fundus

Greater curvature

Pancreas

Sphincter of Oddi

Pancreatic duct

Common bile duct

Proximal duodenum

☑4ᵗʰ **531 Gastric ulcer**

INCLUDES ulcer (peptic):
  prepyloric
  pylorus
  stomach

Use additional E code to identify drug, if drug-induced

EXCLUDES *peptic ulcer NOS (533.0-533.9)*

The following fifth-digit subclassification is for use with category 531:
  0 **without mention of obstruction**
  1 **with obstruction**

DEF: Destruction of tissue in lumen of stomach due to action of gastric acid and pepsin on gastric mucosa decreasing resistance to ulcers.
AHA: 1Q, '91, 15; 4Q, '90, 27

§ ☑5ᵗʰ **531.0 Acute with hemorrhage**
[0-1]   AHA: N-D, '84, 15

§ ☑5ᵗʰ **531.1 Acute with perforation**
[0-1]

§ ☑5ᵗʰ **531.2 Acute with hemorrhage and perforation**
[0-1]

§ ☑5ᵗʰ **531.3 Acute without mention of hemorrhage or perforation**
[0-1]

§ ☑5ᵗʰ **531.4 Chronic or unspecified with hemorrhage**
[0-1]   AHA: 4Q, '90, 22
       K25.4 Chronic/unspec gastric ulcer w/hemorrhage   I-10

§ ☑5ᵗʰ **531.5 Chronic or unspecified with perforation**
[0-1]

§ ☑5ᵗʰ **531.6 Chronic or unspecified with hemorrhage and**
[0-1]   **perforation**

§ ☑5ᵗʰ **531.7 Chronic without mention of hemorrhage or**
[0-1]   **perforation**

§ ☑5ᵗʰ **531.9 Unspecified as acute or chronic, without mention**
[0-1]   **of hemorrhage or perforation**
       K25.9 Gastric ulcer uns acute/chronic w/o hem/perf   I-10

☑4ᵗʰ **532 Duodenal ulcer**

INCLUDES erosion (acute) of duodenum
  ulcer (peptic):
  duodenum
  postpyloric

Use additional E code to identify drug, if drug-induced

EXCLUDES *peptic ulcer NOS (533.0-533.9)*

The following fifth-digit subclassification is for use with category 532:
  0 **without mention of obstruction**
  1 **with obstruction**

DEF: Ulcers in duodenum due to action of gastric acid and pepsin on mucosa decreasing resistance to ulcers.
AHA: 4Q, '90, 27; 1Q, '91, 15

§ ☑5ᵗʰ **532.0 Acute with hemorrhage**
[0-1]   AHA: 4Q, '90, 22

§ ☑5ᵗʰ **532.1 Acute with perforation**
[0-1]

§ ☑5ᵗʰ **532.2 Acute with hemorrhage and perforation**
[0-1]

§ ☑5ᵗʰ **532.3 Acute without mention of hemorrhage or perforation**
[0-1]

§ ☑5ᵗʰ **532.4 Chronic or unspecified with hemorrhage**
[0-1]   K26.4 Chronic/unspecified duodenal ulcer w/hemorrhage   I-10

§ ☑5ᵗʰ **532.5 Chronic or unspecified with perforation**
[0-1]

§ ☑5ᵗʰ **532.6 Chronic or unspecified with hemorrhage and**
[0-1]   **perforation**

§ ☑5ᵗʰ **532.7 Chronic without mention of hemorrhage or**
[0-1]   **perforation**

§ ☑5ᵗʰ **532.9 Unspecified as acute or chronic, without mention**
[0-1]   **of hemorrhage or perfortaion**
       K26.9 Duodenal ulcer uns acute/chronic w/o hem/perf   I-10

☑4ᵗʰ **533 Peptic ulcer, site unspecified**

INCLUDES gastroduodenal ulcer NOS
  peptic ulcer NOS
  stress ulcer NOS

Use additional E code to identify drug, if drug-induced

EXCLUDES *peptic ulcer:*
  duodenal (532.0-532.9)
  gastric (531.0-531.9)

The following fifth-digit subclassification is for use with category 533:
  0 **without mention of obstruction**
  1 **with obstruction**

DEF: Ulcer of mucous membrane of esophagus, stomach or duodenum due to gastric acid secretion.
AHA: 1Q, '91, 15; 4Q, '90, 27

§ ☑5ᵗʰ **533.0 Acute with hemorrhage**
[0-1]

§ ☑5ᵗʰ **533.1 Acute with perforation**
[0-1]

§ ☑5ᵗʰ **533.2 Acute with hemorrhage and perforation**
[0-1]

§ ☑5ᵗʰ **533.3 Acute without mention of hemorrhage and**
[0-1]   **perforation**

§ ☑5ᵗʰ **533.4 Chronic or unspecified with hemorrhage**
[0-1]

§ ☑5ᵗʰ **533.5 Chronic or unspecified with perforation**
[0-1]

§ ☑5ᵗʰ **533.6 Chronic or unspecified with hemorrhage and**
[0-1]   **perforation**

§ ☑5ᵗʰ **533.7 Chronic without mention of hemorrhage or**
[0-1]   **perforation**
       AHA: 2Q, '89, 16

§ ☑5ᵗʰ **533.9 Unspecified as acute or chronic, without**
[0-1]   **mention of hemorrhage or perforation**

☑4ᵗʰ **534 Gastrojejunal ulcer**

INCLUDES ulcer (peptic) or erosion:
  anastomotic
  gastrocolic
  gastrointestinal
  gastrojejunal
  jejunal
  marginal
  stomal

EXCLUDES *primary ulcer of small intestine (569.82)*

The following fifth-digit subclassification is for use with category 534:
  0 **without mention of obstruction**
  1 **with obstruction**

AHA: 1Q, '91, 15; 4Q, '90, 27

§ ☑5ᵗʰ **534.0 Acute with hemorrhage**
[0-1]

§ ☑5ᵗʰ **534.1 Acute with perforation**
[0-1]

§ ☑5ᵗʰ **534.2 Acute with hemorrhage and perforation**
[0-1]

---

§ Requires fifth digit. Valid digits are in [brackets] under each code. See appropriate category for codes and definitions.

☑4ᵗʰ ☑5ᵗʰ Additional Digit Required   Unspecified Code   Other Specified Code   Manifestation Code   ▶◀ Revised Text   ● New Code   ▲ Revised Code Title

2011 ICD-9-CM   **Volume 1 – 163**

Diseases of the Digestive System

534.3–537.6

§ ✓5ᵗʰ **534.3 Acute without mention of hemorrhage or perforation**
[0-1]

§ ✓5ᵗʰ **534.4 Chronic or unspecified with hemorrhage**
[0-1]

§ ✓5ᵗʰ **534.5 Chronic or unspecified with perforation**
[0-1]

§ ✓5ᵗʰ **534.6 Chronic or unspecified with hemorrhage and perforation**
[0-1]

§ ✓5ᵗʰ **534.7 Chronic without mention of hemorrhage or perforation**
[0-1]

§ ✓5ᵗʰ **534.9 Unspecified as acute or chronic, without mention**
[0-1]   **of hemorrhage or perforation**

✓4ᵗʰ **535 Gastritis and duodenitis**

The following fifth-digit subclassification is for use with category 535:
0 without mention of hemorrhage
1 with hemorrhage

AHA: 2Q, '92, 9; 4Q, '91, 25

§ ✓5ᵗʰ **535.0 Acute gastritis**
[0-1]   **AHA:** 2Q, '92, 8; N-D, '86, 9

§ ✓5ᵗʰ **535.1 Atrophic gastritis**
[0-1]   Gastritis:
     atrophic-hyperplastic
     chronic (atrophic)
   DEF: Inflammation of stomach, with mucous membrane atrophy and peptic gland destruction.
   AHA: 1Q, '94, 18
   K29.50 Unspecified chronic gastritis without bleeding   I-10

§ ✓5ᵗʰ **535.2 Gastric mucosal hypertrophy**
[0-1]   Hypertrophic gastritis

§ ✓5ᵗʰ **535.3 Alcoholic gastritis**
[0-1]

§ ✓5ᵗʰ **535.4 Other specified gastritis**
[0-1]   Gastritis: Gastritis:
     allergic   superficial
     bile induced   toxic
     irritant
   EXCLUDES *eosinophilic gastritis (535.7)*
   AHA: 4Q, '90, 27

§ ✓5ᵗʰ **535.5 Unspecified gastritis and gastroduodenitis**
[0-1]   **AHA: For code 535.50:** 3Q, '05, 17; 4Q, '99, 25

§ ✓5ᵗʰ **535.6 Duodenitis**
[0-1]   **DEF:** Inflammation of intestine, between pylorus and jejunum.
   AHA: For code 535.60: 3Q, '05, 17
   K29.80 Duodenitis without bleeding   I-10

§ ✓5ᵗʰ **535.7 Eosinophilic gastritis**
[0-1]   **AHA:** 4Q, '08, 115-116

✓4ᵗʰ **536 Disorders of function of stomach**
   EXCLUDES *functional disorders of stomach specified as psychogenic (306.4)*

536.0 Achlorhydria
   DEF: Absence of gastric acid due to gastric mucosa atrophy; unresponsive to histamines; also known as gastric anacidity.

536.1 Acute dilatation of stomach
   Acute distention of stomach

536.2 Persistent vomiting
   Cyclical vomiting
   Habit vomiting
   Persistent vomiting [not of pregnancy]
   Uncontrollable vomiting
   EXCLUDES *bilious emesis (vomiting) (787.04)*
       excessive vomiting in pregnancy (643.0-643.9)
       vomiting NOS (787.03)
         cyclical, associated with migraine (346.2)
       vomiting of fecal matter (569.87)

536.3 Gastroparesis
   Gastroparalysis
   Code first underlying disease, such as: diabetes mellitus (249.6, 250.6)
   DEF: Slight degree of paralysis within muscular coat of stomach.
   AHA: 4Q, '08, 94; 2Q, '04, 7; 2Q, '01, 4; 4Q, '94, 42

✓5ᵗʰ **536.4 Gastrostomy complications**
   AHA: 4Q, '98, 42
   TIP: Do not assign code 997.4 Digestive system complications, for any gastrostomy complications.

536.40 Gastrostomy complication, unspecified

536.41 Infection of gastrostomy
   Use additional code to specify type of infection, such as:
     abscess or cellulitis of abdomen (682.2)
     septicemia (038.0-038.9)
   Use additional code to identify organism (041.00-041.9)
   AHA: 4Q, '98, 42

536.42 Mechanical complication of gastrostomy

536.49 Other gastrostomy complications
   AHA: 4Q, '98, 42

536.8 Dyspepsia and other specified disorders of function of stomach
   Achylia gastrica
   Hourglass contraction of stomach
   Hyperacidity
   Hyperchlorhydria
   Hypochlorhydria
   Indigestion
   Tachygastria
   EXCLUDES *achlorhydria (536.0)*
       heartburn (787.1)
   AHA: 2Q, '93, 6; 2Q, '89, 16; N-D, '84, 9
   K30 Dyspepsia   I-10

536.9 Unspecified functional disorder of stomach
   Functional gastrointestinal:
     disorder
     disturbance
     irritation

✓4ᵗʰ **537 Other disorders of stomach and duodenum**

537.0 Acquired hypertrophic pyloric stenosis
   Constriction ⎫
   Obstruction ⎬ of pylorus, acquired or adult
   Stricture ⎭
   EXCLUDES *congenital or infantile pyloric stenosis (750.5)*
   AHA: 2Q, '01, 4; J-F, '85, 14

537.1 Gastric diverticulum
   EXCLUDES *congenital diverticulum of stomach (750.7)*
   DEF: Herniated sac or pouch within stomach or duodenum.
   AHA: J-F, '85, 4

537.2 Chronic duodenal ileus
   DEF: Persistent obstruction between pylorus and jejunum.

537.3 Other obstruction of duodenum
   Cicatrix ⎫
   Stenosis ⎬
   Stricture } of duodenum
   Volvulus ⎭
   EXCLUDES *congenital obstruction of duodenum (751.1)*

537.4 Fistula of stomach or duodenum
   Gastrocolic fistula
   Gastrojejunocolic fistula

537.5 Gastroptosis
   DEF: Downward displacement of stomach.

537.6 Hourglass stricture or stenosis of stomach
   Cascade stomach
   EXCLUDES *congenital hourglass stomach (750.7)*
       hourglass contraction of stomach (536.8)

---

§ Requires fifth digit. Valid digits are in [brackets] under each code. See appropriate category for codes and definitions.

Duodenum

- Common bile duct
- Bulb of duodenum
- Stomach
- Ligament of Trietz
- Jejunum
- Duodenal papilla of Vater
- Pancreas

Appendix

- Appendicular artery
- Mesoappendix
- Cecum
- Vermiform appendix

✓5ᵗʰ **537.8 Other specified disorders of stomach and duodenum**
AHA: 4Q, '91, 25

537.81 Pylorospasm
EXCLUDES *congenital pylorospasm (750.5)*
DEF: Spasm of the pyloric sphincter.

537.82 Angiodysplasia of stomach and duodenum (without mention of hemorrhage)
AHA: 2Q, '07, 7; 3Q, '96, 10; 4Q, '90, 4

537.83 Angiodysplasia of stomach and duodenum with hemorrhage
DEF: Bleeding of stomach and duodenum due to vascular abnormalities.
AHA: 2Q, '07, 7

537.84 Dieulafoy lesion (hemorrhagic) of stomach and duodenum
DEF: An abnormally large and convoluted submucosal artery protruding through a defect in the mucosa in the stomach or intestines that can erode the epithelium causing hemorrhaging.
AHA: 4Q, '02, 60

537.89 Other
Gastric or duodenal:
  prolapse
  rupture
Intestinal metaplasia of gastric mucosa
Passive congestion of stomach
EXCLUDES *diverticula of duodenum (562.00-562.01)*
        gastrointestinal hemorrhage (578.0-578.9)
AHA: 3Q, '05, 15; N-D, '84, 7
TIP: Assign for congestive portal gastropathy or portal hypertensive gastropathy.

537.9 Unspecified disorder of stomach and duodenum

538 Gastrointestinal mucositis (ulcerative)
Use additional E code to identify adverse effects of therapy, such as:
  antineoplastic and immunosuppressive drugs (E930.7, E933.1)
  radiation therapy (E879.2)
EXCLUDES *mucositis (ulcerative) of mouth and oral soft tissue (528.00-528.09)*
AHA: 4Q, '06, 88-90

Appendicitis (540-543)

✓4ᵗʰ **540 Acute appendicitis**
DEF: Inflammation of vermiform appendix due to fecal obstruction, neoplasm or foreign body of appendiceal lumen; causes infection, edema and infarction of appendiceal wall; may result in mural necrosis, and perforation.
AHA: N-D, '84, 19

540.0 With generalized peritonitis
Appendicitis (acute) with: { perforation / peritonitis (generalized) / rupture } { fulminating / gangrenous / obstructive }
Cecitis (acute) with perforation, peritonitis (generalized), rupture
Rupture of appendix
EXCLUDES *acute appendicitis with peritoneal abscess (540.1)*
K35.0 Acute appendicitis w/generalized peritonitis   I-10

540.1 With peritoneal abscess
Abscess of appendix
With generalized peritonitis
AHA: N-D, '84, 19

540.9 Without mention of peritonitis
Acute appendicitis without mention of perforation, peritonitis, or rupture:
  fulminating
  gangrenous
  inflamed
  obstructive
Acute cecitis without mention of perforation, peritonitis, or rupture
AHA: 1Q, '01, 15; 4Q, '97, 52
K35.9 Acute appendicitis unspecified   I-10

541 Appendicitis, unqualified
AHA: 2Q, '90, 26
TIP: Do not assign for normal appendix found at appendectomy. Assign instead symptom code (e.g., abdominal pain).

542 Other appendicitis
Appendicitis:
  chronic
  recurrent
Appendicitis:
  relapsing
  subacute
EXCLUDES *hyperplasia (lymphoid) of appendix (543.0)*
AHA: 1Q, '01, 15

✓4ᵗʰ **543 Other diseases of appendix**
543.0 Hyperplasia of appendix (lymphoid)
DEF: Proliferation of cells in appendix tissue.

Inguinal Hernias

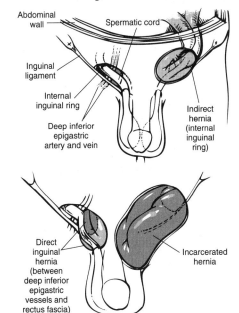

- Abdominal wall
- Spermatic cord
- Inguinal ligament
- Internal inguinal ring
- Deep inferior epigastric artery and vein
- Indirect hernia (internal inguinal ring)
- Direct inguinal hernia (between deep inferior epigastric vessels and rectus fascia)
- Incarcerated hernia

543.9 Other and unspecified diseases of appendix

Appendicular or appendiceal:
  colic
  concretion
  fistula

Diverticulum ⎫
Fecalith   ⎪
Intussusception ⎬ of appendix
Mucocele   ⎪
Stercolith ⎭

Hernia of Abdominal Cavity (550-553)

INCLUDES hernia:
  acquired
  congenital, except diaphragmatic or hiatal

√4ᵗʰ **550 Inguinal hernia**

INCLUDES bubonocele
  inguinal hernia (direct) (double) (indirect) (oblique)
    (sliding)
  scrotal hernia

The following fifth-digit subclassification is for use with category 550:
  0 unilateral or unspecified (not specified as recurrent)
    Unilateral NOS
  1 unilateral or unspecified, recurrent
  2 bilateral (not specified as recurrent)
    Bilateral NOS
  3 bilateral, recurrent

DEF: Hernia protrusion of an abdominal organ or tissue through inguinal canal.
DEF: Indirect inguinal hernia: (external or oblique) leaves abdomen through deep inguinal ring, passes through inguinal canal lateral to the inferior epigastric artery.
DEF: Direct inguinal hernia: (internal) emerges between inferior epigastric artery and rectus muscle edge.
AHA: N-D, '85, 12

§ √5ᵗʰ **550.0 Inguinal hernia, with gangrene**
  [0-3]   Inguinal hernia with gangrene (and obstruction)

§ √5ᵗʰ **550.1 Inguinal hernia, with obstruction, without mention**
  [0-3]   **of gangrene**
    Inguinal hernia with mention of incarceration, irreducibility, or strangulation

§ √5ᵗʰ **550.9 Inguinal hernia, without mention of obstruction**
  [0-3]   **or gangrene**
    Inguinal hernia NOS
    AHA: For code 550.91: 3Q, '03, 10; 1Q, '03, 4
    K40.90 Uni ingin hernia w/o obst/gangrene not spec recur [I-10]

√4ᵗʰ **551 Other hernia of abdominal cavity, with gangrene**
  INCLUDES that with gangrene (and obstruction)

  √5ᵗʰ **551.0 Femoral hernia with gangrene**

    551.00 Unilateral or unspecified (not specified as recurrent)
      Femoral hernia NOS with gangrene

    551.01 Unilateral or unspecified, recurrent

    551.02 Bilateral (not specified as recurrent)

    551.03 Bilateral, recurrent

Hernias of Abdominal Cavity

Femoral Hernia

Diaphragmatic Hernias

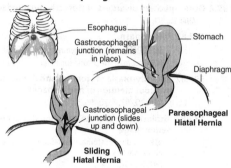

551.1 Umbilical hernia with gangrene
  Parumbilical hernia specified as gangrenous

√5ᵗʰ **551.2 Ventral hernia with gangrene**

  551.20 Ventral, unspecified, with gangrene

  551.21 Incisional, with gangrene
    Hernia:
      postoperative ⎫ specified as
      recurrent, ventral ⎬ gangrenous

  551.29 Other
    Epigastric hernia specified as gangrenous

551.3 Diaphragmatic hernia with gangrene
  Hernia:
    hiatal (esophageal) (sliding) ⎫ specified as
    paraesophageal   ⎬ gangrenous
    Thoracic stomach   ⎭
    EXCLUDES congenital diaphragmatic hernia (756.6)

551.8 Hernia of other specified sites, with gangrene
  Any condition classifiable to 553.8 if specified as gangrenous

551.9 Hernia of unspecified site, with gangrene
  Any condition classifiable to 553.9 if specified as gangrenous

√4ᵗʰ **552 Other hernia of abdominal cavity, with obstruction, but without mention of gangrene**
  EXCLUDES that with mention of gangrene (551.0-551.9)

  √5ᵗʰ **552.0 Femoral hernia with obstruction**
    Femoral hernia specified as incarcerated, irreducible, strangulated, or causing obstruction

    552.00 Unilateral or unspecified (not specified as recurrent)

    552.01 Unilateral or unspecified, recurrent

    552.02 Bilateral (not specified as recurrent)

    552.03 Bilateral, recurrent

  552.1 Umbilical hernia with obstruction
    Parumbilical hernia specified as incarcerated, irreducible, strangulated, or causing obstruction

  √5ᵗʰ **552.2 Ventral hernia with obstruction**
    Ventral hernia specified as incarcerated, irreducible, strangulated, or causing obstruction

    552.20 Ventral, unspecified, with obstruction

§ Requires fifth digit. Valid digits are in [brackets] under each code. See category 550 for codes and definitions.

N Newborn Age: 0   P Pediatric Age: 0-17   M Maternity Age: 12-55   A Adult Age: 15-124

552.21 Incisional, with obstruction

Hernia:
postoperative
recurrent,   } specified as incarcerated,
ventral   irreducible, strangulated,
                  or causing obstruction

AHA: 3Q, '03, 11

552.29 Other

Epigastric hernia specified as incarcerated,
irreducible, strangulated, or causing
obstruction

552.3 Diaphragmatic hernia with obstruction

Hernia:
hiatal (esophageal)   } specified as caracerated,
(sliding)   irreducible,
paraesophageal   strangulated, or
Thoracic stomach   causing obstruction

EXCLUDES congenital diaphragmatic hernia (756.6)

552.8 Hernia of other specified sites, with obstruction

Any condition classifiable to 553.8 if specified as incarcerated,
irreducible, strangulated, or causing obstruction

AHA: 1Q, '04, 10

552.9 Hernia of unspecified site, with obstruction

Any condition classifiable to 553.9 if specified as incarcerated,
irreducible, strangulated, or causing obstruction

√4ᵗʰ **553 Other hernia of abdominal cavity without mention of obstruction or gangrene**

EXCLUDES the listed conditions with mention of:
gangrene (and obstruction) (551.0-551.9)
obstruction (552.0-552.9)

√5ᵗʰ **553.0 Femoral hernia**

553.00 Unilateral or unspecified (not specified as recurrent)
Femoral hernia NOS

553.01 Unilateral or unspecified, recurrent

553.02 Bilateral (not specified as recurrent)

553.03 Bilateral, recurrent

553.1 Umbilical hernia
Parumbilical hernia
K42.9 Umbilical hernia without obstruction/gangrene   I-10

√5ᵗʰ **553.2 Ventral hernia**

553.20 Ventral, unspecified
AHA: 2Q, '06, 10; 3Q, '03, 6

553.21 Incisional
Hernia:
postoperative
recurrent, ventral
AHA: 3Q, '03, 6
K43.91 Incisional hernia w/o obstruction or gangrene   I-10

553.29 Other
Hernia:
epigastric
spigelian

553.3 Diaphragmatic hernia
Hernia:
hiatal (esophageal) (sliding)
paraesophageal
Thoracic stomach
EXCLUDES congenital:
diaphragmatic hernia (756.6)
hiatal hernia (750.6)
esophagocele (530.6)
AHA: 2Q, '01, 6; 1Q, '00, 6
K44.9 Diaphragmatic hernia w/o obstruction/gangrene   I-10

553.8 Hernia of other specified sites
Hernia:
ischiatic
ischiorectal
lumbar
obturator
pudendal
retroperitoneal
sciatic
Other abdominal hernia of specified site
EXCLUDES vaginal enterocele (618.6)

553.9 Hernia of unspecified site
Enterocele   Hernia:
Epiplocele   intestinal
Hernia: intra-abdominal
NOS   Rupture (nontraumatic)
interstitial   Sarcoepiplocele

Noninfectious Enteritis and Colitis (555-558)

√4ᵗʰ **555 Regional enteritis**

INCLUDES Crohn's disease
Granulomatous enteritis

EXCLUDES ulcerative colitis (556)

DEF: Inflammation of intestine; classified to site.
TIP: Assign separate code for fistula, if present. Sequence 555 code as
first-listed/principal diagnosis (if underlying cause of fistula).

555.0 Small intestine
Ileitis: Regional enteritis or Crohn's disease of:
regional   duodenum
segmental   ileum
terminal   jejunum

555.1 Large intestine
Colitis:
granulmatous
regional
transmural
Regional enteritis or Crohn's disease of:
colon
large bowel
rectum
AHA: 3Q, '99, 8

555.2 Small intestine with large intestine
Regional ileocolitis
AHA: 1Q, '03, 18

555.9 Unspecified site
Crohn's disease NOS
Regional enteritis NOS
AHA: 1Q, '09, 5; 2Q, '05, 11; 3Q, '99, 8; 4Q, '97, 42; 2Q, '97, 3
K50.90 Crohns disease unspecified w/o complications   I-10

√4ᵗʰ **556 Ulcerative colitis**
DEF: Chronic inflammation of mucosal lining of intestinal tract; may be single
area or entire colon.
AHA: 3Q, '99, 8

556.0 Ulcerative (chronic) enterocolitis

556.1 Ulcerative (chronic) ileocolitis

556.2 Ulcerative (chronic) proctitis

556.3 Ulcerative (chronic) proctosigmoiditis

556.4 Pseudopolyposis of colon

Large Intestine

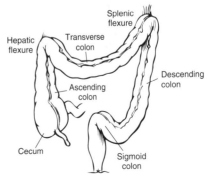

√4ᵗʰ
√5ᵗʰ   Additional Digit Required   Unspecified Code   Other Specified Code   Manifestation Code   ►◄ Revised Text   ● New Code   ▲ Revised Code Title

2011 ICD-9-CM   Volume 1 – 167

Diseases of the Digestive System

556.5 Left-sided ulcerative (chronic) colitis

556.6 Universal ulcerative (chronic) colitis
Pancolitis

556.8 Other ulcerative colitis

556.9 Ulcerative colitis, unspecified
Ulcerative enteritis NOS
AHA: 1Q, '03, 10
K51.90 Ulcerative colitis unspecified w/o complications   I-10

✓4ᵗʰ **557 Vascular insufficiency of intestine**
EXCLUDES *necrotizing enterocolitis of the newborn (777.50-777.53)*
DEF: Inadequacy of intestinal vessels.

557.0 Acute vascular insufficiency of intestine
Acute:
hemorrhagic enterocolitis
ischemic colitis, enteritis, or enterocolitis
massive necrosis of intestine
Bowel infarction
Embolism of mesenteric artery
Fulminant enterocolitis
Hemorrhagic necrosis of intestine
Infarction of appendices epiploicae
Intestinal gangrene
Intestinal infarction (acute) (agnogenic) (hemorrhagic)
    (nonocclusive)
Mesenteric infarction (embolic) (thrombotic)
Necrosis of intestine
Terminal hemorrhagic enteropathy
Thrombosis of mesenteric artery
AHA: 2Q, '08, 15; 4Q, '01, 53
TIP: Do not assign an additional code for GI bleeding; it is inherent in 557.0.
K55.0 Acute vascular disorders of intestine   I-10

557.1 Chronic vascular insufficiency of intestine
Angina, abdominal
Chronic ischemic colitis, enteritis, or enterocolitis
Ischemic stricture of intestine
Mesenteric:
angina
artery syndrome (superior)
vascular insufficiency
AHA: 3Q, '96, 9; 4Q, '90, 4; N-D, '86, 11; N-D, '84, 7

557.9 Unspecified vascular insufficiency of intestine
Alimentary pain due to vascular insufficiency
Ischemic colitis, enteritis, or enterocolitis NOS
K55.9 Vascular disorder of intestine unspecified   I-10

✓4ᵗʰ **558 Other and unspecified noninfectious gastroenteritis and colitis**
EXCLUDES *infectious:*
colitis, enteritis, or gastroenteritis (009.0-009.1)
diarrhea (009.2-009.3)

558.1 Gastroenteritis and colitis due to radiation
Radiation enterocolitis

558.2 Toxic gastroenteritis and colitis
Use additional E code to identify cause

558.3 Allergic gastroenteritis and colitis
Use additional code to identify type of food allergy
   (V15.01-V15.05)
DEF: True immunoglobulin E (IgE)-mediated allergic reaction of the lining of the stomach, intestines, or colon to food proteins; causes nausea, vomiting, diarrhea, and abdominal cramping.
AHA: 4Q, '08, 116; 1Q, '03, 12; 4Q, '00, 42

✓5ᵗʰ **558.4 Eosinophilic gastroenteritis and colitis**
AHA: 4Q, '08, 116

558.41 Eosinophilic gastroenteritis
Eosinophilic enteritis
AHA: 4Q, '08, 116

558.42 Eosinophilic colitis
AHA: 4Q, '08, 115-116

558.9 Other and unspecified noninfectious gastroenteritis and colitis
Colitis
Enteritis
Gastroenteritis } NOS, dietetic, or
Ileitis   noninfectious
Jejunitis
Sigmoiditis
AHA: 2Q, '08, 10; 1Q, '08, 10; 3Q, '99, 4, 6; N-D, '87, 7
K52.9 Noninfective gastroenteritis & colitis unspec   I-10

Other Diseases of Intestines and Peritoneum (560-569)

✓4ᵗʰ **560 Intestinal obstruction without mention of hernia**
EXCLUDES *duodenum (537.2-537.3)*
inguinal hernia with obstruction (550.1)
intestinal obstruction complicating hernia (552.0-552.9)
mesenteric:
embolism (557.0)
infarction (557.0)
thrombosis (557.0)
neonatal intestinal obstruction (277.01, 777.1-777.2, 777.4)
TIP: If intestinal obstruction is due to abdominal carcinomatosis or Crohn's disease, sequence that condition first.

560.0 Intussusception
Intussusception (colon) (intestine) (rectum)
Invagination of intestine or colon
EXCLUDES *intussusception of appendix (543.9)*
DEF: Prolapse of a bowel section into adjacent section; occurs primarily in children; symptoms include paroxysmal pain, vomiting, presence of blood, and mucous passage from rectum.
AHA: 4Q, '98, 82

560.1 Paralytic ileus
Adynamic ileus
Ileus (of intestine) (of bowel) (of colon)
Paralysis of intestine or colon
EXCLUDES *gallstone ileus (560.31)*
DEF: Obstruction of ileus due to inhibited bowel motility.
AHA: J-F, '87, 13
K56.0 Paralytic ileus   I-10

560.2 Volvulus
Knotting
Strangulation } if intestine, bowel, or colon
Torsion
Twist
DEF: Entanglement of bowel; causes obstruction; may compromise bowel circulation.

✓5ᵗʰ **560.3 Impaction of intestine**

560.30 Impaction of intestine, unspecified
Impaction of colon

560.31 Gallstone ileus
Obstruction of intestine by gallstone

560.32 Fecal impaction
EXCLUDES *constipation (564.00-564.09)*
incomplete defecation (787.61)
K56.4 Other impaction of intestine   I-10

560.39 Other
Concretion of intestine
Enterolith
AHA: 4Q, '98, 38
K56.4 Other impaction of intestine   I-10

✓5ᵗʰ **560.8 Other specified intestinal obstruction**

560.81 Intestinal or peritoneal adhesions with obstruction (postoperative) (postinfection)
EXCLUDES *adhesions without obstruction (568.0)*
DEF: Obstruction of peritoneum or intestine due to abnormal union of tissues.
AHA: ▶1Q, '10, 11;◄ 4Q, '95, 55; 3Q, '95, 6; N-D, '87, 9
TIP: Do not assign additional code 997.4 Digestive system complications.
K56.5 Intestinal adhes [bands] w/obst (postproc) (postinfec)   I-10

Volvulus and Diverticulitis

Knotted intestine (volvulus)

Diverticulum

560.89 Other
Acute pseudo-obstruction of intestine
Mural thickening causing obstruction
> **EXCLUDES** *ischemic stricture of intestine (557.1)*
AHA: 2Q, '97, 3; 1Q, '88, 6

560.9 Unspecified intestinal obstruction
Enterostenosis
Obstruction
Occlusion   } of intestine or colon
Stenosis
Stricture
> **EXCLUDES** *congenital stricture or stenosis of intestine (751.1-751.2)*
K56.60 Unspecified intestinal obstruction ⬚I-10

✓4ᵗʰ **562 Diverticula of intestine**
Use additional code to identify any associated:
peritonitis (567.0-567.9)
> **EXCLUDES** *congenital diverticulum of colon (751.5)*
> *diverticulum of appendix (543.9)*
> *Meckel's diverticulum (751.0)*
AHA: 4Q, '91, 25; J-F, '85, 1

✓5ᵗʰ **562.0 Small intestine**

562.00 Diverticulosis of small intestine (without mention of hemorrhage)
Diverticulosis:
duodenum
ileum   } without mention of diverticulitis
jejunum
> **DEF:** Saclike herniations of mucous lining of small intestine.

562.01 Diverticulitis of small intestine (without mention of hemorrhage)
Diverticulitis (with diverticulosis):
duodenum
ileum
jejunum
small intestine
> **DEF:** Inflamed saclike herniations of mucous lining of small intestine

562.02 Diverticulosis of small intestine with hemorrhage

562.03 Diverticulitis of small intestine with hemorrhage

✓5ᵗʰ **562.1 Colon**

562.10 Diverticulosis of colon (without mention of hemorrhage)
Diverticulosis:
NOS   } without metion of
intestine (large) diverticulitis
Diverticular disease (colon)
> **DEF:** Saclike herniations of mucous lining of large intestine.
AHA: 3Q, '05, 17; 3Q, '02, 15; 4Q, '90, 21; J-F, '85, 5
K57.90 Divrticulos intest part uns w/o perf/absc w/o bldg ⬚I-10

562.11 Diverticulitis of colon (without mention of hemorrhage)
Diverticulitis (with diverticulosis):
NOS
colon
intestine (large)
> **DEF:** Inflamed saclike herniations of mucosal lining of large intestine.
AHA: 1Q, '96, 14; J-F, '85, 5
K57.92 Divrticulit intest part uns w/o perf/absc w/o bldg ⬚I-10

562.12 Diverticulosis of colon with hemorrhage

562.13 Diverticulitis of colon with hemorrhage

✓4ᵗʰ **564 Functional digestive disorders, not elsewhere classified**
> **EXCLUDES** *functional disorders of stomach (536.0-536.9)*
> *those specified as psychogenic (306.4)*

✓5ᵗʰ **564.0 Constipation**
> **EXCLUDES** ▸*fecal impaction (560.32)*
> *incomplete defecation (787.61)*◂
AHA: 4Q, '01, 45

564.00 Constipation, unspecified
K59.00 Constipation unspecified ⬚I-10

564.01 Slow transit constipation
> **DEF:** Delay in the transit of fecal material through the colon secondary to smooth muscle dysfunction or decreased peristaltic contractions along the colon: also called colonic inertia or delayed transit.

564.02 Outlet dysfunction constipation
> **DEF:** Failure to relax the paradoxical contractions of the striated pelvic floor muscles during the attempted defecation.

564.09 Other constipation

564.1 Irritable bowel syndrome
Irritable colon
Spastic colon
> **DEF:** Functional gastrointestinal disorder (FGID); symptoms include diarrhea, constipation, abdominal pain, gas, distended abdomen, nausea, vomiting, emotional distress, and depression.
AHA: 1Q, '88, 6
K58.9 Irritable bowel syndrome without diarrhea ⬚I-10

564.2 Postgastric surgery syndromes
Dumping syndrome
Jejunal syndrome
Postgastrectomy syndrome
Postvagotomy syndrome
> **EXCLUDES** *malnutrition following gastrointestinal surgery (579.3)*
> *postgastrojejunostomy ulcer (534.0-534.9)*
AHA: 1Q, '95, 11

564.3 Vomiting following gastrointestinal surgery
Vomiting (bilious) following gastrointestinal surgery

564.4 Other postoperative functional disorders
Diarrhea following gastrointestinal surgery
> **EXCLUDES** *colostomy and enterostomy complications (569.60-569.69)*

Anal Fistula and Abscess

Urethra
Fistula
Bladder
Abscess
Rectum

564.5 Functional diarrhea
EXCLUDES diarrhea:
NOS (787.91)
psychogenic (306.4)
DEF: Diarrhea with no detectable organic cause.

564.6 Anal spasm
Proctalgia fugax

564.7 Megacolon, other than Hirschsprung's
Dilatation of colon
EXCLUDES megacolon:
congenital [Hirschsprung's] (751.3)
toxic (556)
DEF: Enlarged colon; congenital or acquired; can occur acutely or become chronic.

√5ᵗʰ 564.8 Other specified functional disorders of intestine
EXCLUDES malabsorption (579.0-579.9)
AHA: 1Q, '88, 6

564.81 Neurogenic bowel
DEF: Disorder of bowel due to spinal cord lesion above conus medullaris; symptoms include precipitous micturition, nocturia, headache, sweating, nasal obstruction and spastic contractions.
AHA: 1Q, '01, 12; 4Q, '98, 45

564.89 Other functional disorders of intestine
Atony of colon
DEF: Absence of normal bowel tone or strength.

564.9 Unspecified functional disorder of intestine

√4ᵗʰ 565 Anal fissure and fistula

565.0 Anal fissure
EXCLUDES anal sphincter tear (healed) (non-traumatic) (old) (569.43)
traumatic (863.89, 863.99)
DEF: Ulceration of cleft at anal mucosa; causes pain, itching, bleeding, infection, and sphincter spasm; may occur with hemorrhoids.

565.1 Anal fistula
Fistula:
anorectal
rectal
rectum to skin
EXCLUDES fistula of rectum to internal organs — see Alphabetic Index
ischiorectal fistula (566)
rectovaginal fistula (619.1)
DEF: Abnormal opening on cutaneous surface near anus; may lack connection with rectum.
AHA: 1Q, '07, 13

566 Abscess of anal and rectal regions
Abscess:
ischiorectal
perianal
perirectal
Cellulitis:
anal
perirectal
rectal
Ischiorectal fistula

Psoas Muscle Abscess

√4ᵗʰ 567 Peritonitis and retroperitoneal infections
EXCLUDES peritonitis:
benign paroxysmal (277.31)
pelvic, female (614.5, 614.7)
periodic familial (277.31)
puerperal (670.8)
with or following:
abortion (634-638 with .0, 639.0)
appendicitis (540.0-540.1)
ectopic or molar pregnancy (639.0)
DEF: Inflammation of the peritoneal cavity.

567.0 Peritonitis in infectious diseases classified elsewhere
Code first underlying disease
EXCLUDES peritonitis:
gonococcal (098.86)
syphilitic (095.2)
tuberculous (014.0)

567.1 Pneumococcal peritonitis

√5ᵗʰ 567.2 Other suppurative peritonitis
AHA: 4Q, '05, 74; 2Q, '01, 11, 12; 3Q, '99, 9; 2Q, '98, 19

567.21 Peritonitis (acute) generalized
Pelvic peritonitis, male
TIP: For pelvic peritonitis in a female patient, refer to code 614.5.

567.22 Peritoneal abscess
Abscess (of):
abdominopelvic
mesenteric
omentum
peritoneum
retrocecal
subdiaphragmatic
subhepatic
subphrenic
K65.1 Peritoneal abscess　　I-10

567.23 Spontaneous bacterial peritonitis
EXCLUDES bacterial peritonitis NOS (567.29)

567.29 Other suppurative peritonitis
Subphrenic peritonitis

√5ᵗʰ 567.3 Retroperitoneal infections
AHA: 4Q, '05, 74

567.31 Psoas muscle abscess
DEF: Infection that extends into or around the psoas muscle that connects the lumbar vertebrae to the femur.

567.38 Other retroperitoneal abscess
AHA: 4Q, '05, 77

567.39 Other retroperitoneal infections

√5ᵗʰ 567.8 Other specified peritonitis
AHA: 4Q, '05, 74

567.81 Choleperitonitis
Peritonitis due to bile
DEF: Inflammation or infection due to presence of bile in the peritoneum resulting from rupture of the bile passages or gallbladder.

567.82 Sclerosing mesenteritis
Fat necrosis of peritoneum
(Idiopathic) sclerosing mesenteric fibrosis
Mesenteric lipodystrophy
Mesenteric panniculitis
Retractile mesenteritis
DEF: Inflammatory processes involving the mesenteric fat; progresses to fibrosis and necrosis of tissue.
AHA: 4Q, '05, 77

567.89 Other specified peritonitis
Chronic proliferative peritonitis
Mesenteric saponification
Peritonitis due to urine

567.9 Unspecified peritonitis
Peritonitis NOS
Peritonitis of unspecified cause
AHA: 1Q, '04, 10

N Newborn Age: 0　　　**P** Pediatric Age: 0-17　　　**M** Maternity Age: 12-55　　　**A** Adult Age: 15-124

☑4ᵗʰ **568 Other disorders of peritoneum**

568.0 Peritoneal adhesions (postoperative) (postinfection)
Adhesions (of):
abdominal (wall)
diaphragm
intestine
male pelvis
mesenteric
omentum
stomach
Adhesive bands

EXCLUDES   adhesions:
pelvic, female (614.6)
with obstruction:
duodenum (537.3)
intestine (560.81)

DEF: Abnormal union of tissues in peritoneum.
AHA: 3Q, '03, 7, 11; 4Q, '95, 55; 3Q, '95, 7; S-O, '85, 11
TIP: Do not assign additional code 997.4 Digestive system complications.
K66.0 Peritoneal adhesns (postprocedural) (postinfection)   I-10

☑5ᵗʰ **568.8 Other specified disorders of peritoneum**

568.81 Hemoperitoneum (nontraumatic)

568.82 Peritoneal effusion (chronic)
EXCLUDES   *ascites NOS (789.51-789.59)*
DEF: Persistent leakage of fluid within peritoneal cavity.

568.89 Other
Peritoneal:
cyst
granuloma

568.9 Unspecified disorder of peritoneum

☑4ᵗʰ **569 Other disorders of intestine**

569.0 Anal and rectal polyp
Anal and rectal polyp NOS
EXCLUDES   *adenomatous anal and rectal polyp (211.4)*

569.1 Rectal prolapse
Procidentia: Prolapse:
anus (sphincter)   anal canal
rectum (sphincter)   rectal mucosa
Proctoptosis
EXCLUDES   *prolapsed hemorrhoids (455.2, 455.5)*

569.2 Stenosis of rectum and anus
Stricture of anus (sphincter)

569.3 Hemorrhage of rectum and anus
EXCLUDES   *gastrointestinal bleeding NOS (578.9)*
melena (578.1)
AHA: 3Q, '05, 17
K62.5 Hemorrhage of anus and rectum   I-10

☑5ᵗʰ **569.4 Other specified disorders of rectum and anus**

569.41 Ulcer of anus and rectum
Solitary ulcer   } of anus (sphincter) or
Stercoral ulcer   }   rectum (sphincter)

569.42 Anal or rectal pain
AHA: 1Q, '03, 8; 1Q, '96, 13

Rectum and Anus

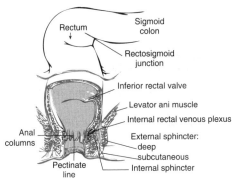

Sigmoid colon
Rectum
Rectosigmoid junction
Inferior rectal valve
Levator ani muscle
Internal rectal venous plexus
Anal columns
External sphincter:
deep
subcutaneous
Pectinate line
Internal sphincter

569.43 Anal sphincter tear (healed) (old)
Tear of anus, nontraumatic
Use additional code for any associated fecal incontinence ▶(787.60-787.63)◀
EXCLUDES   *anal fissure (565.0)*
anal sphincter tear (healed) (old)
complicating delivery (654.8)
AHA: 4Q, '07, 88

569.44 Dysplasia of anus
Anal intraepithelial neoplasia I and II (AIN I and II) (histologically confirmed)
Dysplasia of anus NOS
Mild and moderate dysplasia of anus (histologically confirmed)
EXCLUDES   *abnormal results from anal cytologic examination without histologic confirmation (796.70-796.79)*
anal intraepithelial neoplasia III (230.5, 230.6)
carcinoma in situ of anus (230.5, 230.6)
HGSIL of anus (796.74)
severe dysplasia of anus (230.5, 230.6)
AHA: 4Q, '08, 117

569.49 Other
Granuloma   } of rectum (sphincter)
Rupture   }
Hypertrophy of anal papillae
Proctitis NOS
▶Use additional code for associated fecal incontinence (787.60-787.63)◀
EXCLUDES   *fistula of rectum to:*
internal organs — see Alphabetic Index
skin (565.1)
hemorrhoids (455.0-455.9)

569.5 Abscess of intestine
EXCLUDES   *appendiceal abscess (540.1)*
K63.0 Abscess of intestine   I-10

☑5ᵗʰ **569.6 Colostomy and enterostomy complications**
DEF: Complication in a surgically created opening, from intestine to surface skin.
AHA: 4Q, '95, 58
TIP: Do not assign additional code 997.4 Digestive system complications.

569.60 Colostomy and enterostomy complication, unspecified

569.61 Infection of colostomy or enterostomy
Use additional code to identify organism (041.00-041.9)
Use additional code to specify type of infection, such as:
abscess or cellulitis of abdomen (682.2)
septicemia (038.0-038.9)

569.62 Mechanical complication of colostomy and enterostomy
Malfunction of colostomy and enterostomy
AHA: 2Q, '05, 11 ; 1Q, '03, 10; 4Q, '98, 44

569.69 Other complication
Fistula   Prolapse
Hernia
AHA: 3Q, '98, 16

☑5ᵗʰ **569.7 Complications of intestinal pouch**
TIP: Do not assign code 997.4 Digestive system complications in addition to a code from this subcategory.

569.71 Pouchitis
Inflammation of internal ileoanal pouch
DEF: Inflammatory complication of an existing surgically created ileoanal pouch, resulting in multiple GI complaints, including diarrhea, abdominal pain, rectal bleeding, fecal urgency, or incontinence.
AHA: 4Q, '09, 94

569.79 Other complications of intestinal pouch

☑4ᵗʰ
☑5ᵗʰ Additional Digit Required   Unspecified Code   Other Specified Code   Manifestation Code   ▶◀ Revised Text   ● New Code   ▲ Revised Code Title
2011 ICD-9-CM   **October 2010 · Volume 1 – 171**

☑5ᵗʰ 569.8 Other specified disorders of intestine
> AHA: 4Q, '91, 25

569.81 Fistula of intestine, excluding rectum and anus
> Fistula: Fistula:
> abdominal wall   enteroenteric
> enterocolic   ileorectal
>> *EXCLUDES* *fistula of intestine to internal organs — see*
>> *Alphabetic Index*
>> *persistent postoperative fistula (998.6)*
> AHA: 3Q, '99, 8

569.82 Ulceration of intestine
> Primary ulcer of intestine
> Ulceration of colon
>> *EXCLUDES* *that with perforation (569.83)*

569.83 Perforation of intestine

569.84 Angiodysplasia of intestine (without mention of hemorrhage)
> DEF: Small vascular abnormalities of the intestinal tract without bleeding problems.
> AHA: 3Q, '96, 10; 4Q, '90, 4; 4Q, '90, 21
> TIP: Assign code 569.84 or 569.85 for documentation of either intestinal arteriovenous (AV) malformation or angiodysplasia.

569.85 Angiodysplasia of intestine with hemorrhage
> DEF: Small vascular abnormalities of the intestinal tract with bleeding problems.
> AHA: 3Q, '96, 9

569.86 Dieulafoy lesion (hemorrhagic) of intestine
> AHA: 4Q, '02, 60-61

569.87 Vomiting of fecal matter
> DEF: ▶Spasmodic expulsion of partially digested substance with similar odor to fecal matter; often suggestive of bowel obstruction or other underlying causal pathology.◀
> AHA: ▶4Q, '09, 105◀

569.89 Other
> Enteroptosis
> Granuloma ⎫
> Prolapse ⎬ of intestine
> ⎭
> Pericolitis
> Perisigmoiditis
> Visceroptosis
>> *EXCLUDES* *gangrene of intestine, mesentery, or*
>> *omentum (557.0)*
>> *hemorrhage of intestine NOS (578.9)*
>> *obstruction of intestine (560.0-560.9)*
> AHA: 3Q, '96, 9

569.9 Unspecified disorder of intestine

Other Diseases of Digestive System (570-579)

570 Acute and subacute necrosis of liver
> Acute hepatic failure
> Acute or subacute hepatitis, not specified as infective
> Necrosis of liver (acute) (diffuse) (massive) (subacute)
> Parenchymatous degeneration of liver
> Yellow atrophy (liver) (acute) (subacute)
>> *EXCLUDES* *icterus gravis of newborn (773.0-773.2)*
>> *serum hepatitis (070.2-070.3)*
>> *that with:*
>> *abortion (634-638 with .7, 639.8)*
>> *ectopic or molar pregnancy (639.8)*
>> *pregnancy, childbirth, or the puerperium (646.7)*
>> *viral hepatitis (070.0-070.9)*
> AHA: 2Q, '05, 9; 1Q, '00, 22
> K72.00 Acute and subacute hepatic failure without coma   [I-10]

☑4ᵗʰ 571 Chronic liver disease and cirrhosis

571.0 Alcoholic fatty liver   [A]

571.1 Acute alcoholic hepatitis   [A]
> Acute alcoholic liver disease
> AHA: 2Q, '02, 4

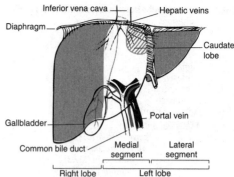

Liver

571.2 Alcoholic cirrhosis of liver   [A]
> Florid cirrhosis
> Laennec's cirrhosis (alcoholic)
> DEF: Fibrosis and dysfunction of liver due to alcoholic liver disease.
> AHA: 3Q, '07, 7; 2Q, '07, 6; 2Q, '02, 4; 1Q, '02, 3; N-D, '85, 14
> TIP: For a patient admitted for bleeding esophageal varices due to alcoholic liver cirrhosis, sequence the liver cirrhosis first.
> K70.30 Alcoholic cirrhosis of liver without ascites   [I-10]

571.3 Alcoholic liver damage, unspecified   [A]

☑5ᵗʰ 571.4 Chronic hepatitis
>> *EXCLUDES* *viral hepatitis (acute) (chronic) (070.0-070.9)*

571.40 Chronic hepatitis, unspecified

571.41 Chronic persistent hepatitis

571.42 Autoimmune hepatitis
> AHA: 4Q, '08, 120

571.49 Other
> Chronic hepatitis:
> active
> aggressive
> Recurrent hepatitis
> AHA: 3Q, '99, 19; N-D, '85, 14

571.5 Cirrhosis of liver without mention of alcohol
> Cirrhosis of liver:
> NOS
> cryptogenic
> macronodular
> micronodular
> posthepatitic
> postnecrotic
> Healed yellow atrophy (liver)
> Portal cirrhosis
> Code first, if applicable, viral hepatitis (acute) (chronic) (070.0-070.9)
> DEF: Fibrosis and dysfunction of liver; not alcohol related.
> AHA: 3Q, '07, 7; 2Q, '07, 5
> TIP: For a patient admitted for bleeding esophageal varices due to liver cirrhosis, sequence the liver cirrhosis first.

571.6 Biliary cirrhosis
> Chronic nonsuppurative destructive cholangitis
> Cirrhosis:
> cholangitic
> cholestatic

571.8 Other chronic nonalcoholic liver disease
> Chronic yellow atrophy (liver)
> Fatty liver, without mention of alcohol
> AHA: 2Q, '96, 12

571.9 Unspecified chronic liver disease without mention of alcohol

☑4ᵗʰ 572 Liver abscess and sequelae of chronic liver disease

572.0 Abscess of liver
>> *EXCLUDES* *amebic liver abscess (006.3)*

[N] Newborn Age: 0   [P] Pediatric Age: 0-17   [M] Maternity Age: 12-55   [A] Adult Age: 15-124

572.1 Portal pyemia

Phlebitis of portal vein　　　Pylephlebitis
Portal thrombophlebitis　　　Pylethrombophlebitis

DEF: Inflammation of portal vein or branches; may be due to intestinal disease; symptoms include fever, chills, jaundice, sweating, and abscess in various body parts.

572.2 Hepatic encephalopathy

Hepatic coma
Hepatocerebral intoxication
Portal-systemic encephalopathy

EXCLUDES *hepatic coma associated with viral hepatitis — see category 070*

AHA: 2Q, '07, 5; 2Q, '05, 9; 1Q, '02, 3; 3Q, '95, 14

TIP: Do not assign if hepatic coma is documented with viral hepatitis; see category 070 with fourth digit indicating hepatic coma.

K72.91 Hepatic failure unspecified with coma ⌐I-10⌐

572.3 Portal hypertension

▶Use additional code for any associated complications, such as: portal hypertensive gastropathy (537.89)◀

DEF: Abnormally high blood pressure in the portal vein.

AHA: 3Q, '05, 15

K76.6 Portal hypertension ⌐I-10⌐

572.4 Hepatorenal syndrome

EXCLUDES *that following delivery (674.8)*

DEF: Hepatic and renal failure characterized by cirrhosis with ascites or obstructive jaundice, oliguria, and low sodium concentration.

AHA: 3Q, '93, 15

572.8 Other sequelae of chronic liver disease

✓4ᵗʰ 573 Other disorders of liver

EXCLUDES *amyloid or lardaceous degeneration of liver (277.39)*
congenital cystic disease of liver (751.62)
glycogen infiltration of liver (271.0)
hepatomegaly NOS (789.1)
portal vein obstruction (452)

573.0 Chronic passive congestion of liver

DEF: Blood accumulation in liver tissue.

573.1 Hepatitis in viral diseases classified elsewhere

Code first underlying disease as:
Coxsackie virus disease (074.8)
cytomegalic inclusion virus disease (078.5)
infectious mononucleosis (075)

EXCLUDES *hepatitis (in):*
mumps (072.71)
viral (070.0-070.9)
yellow fever (060.0-060.9)

573.2 Hepatitis in other infectious diseases classified elsewhere

Code first underlying disease, as:
malaria (084.9)

EXCLUDES *hepatitis in:*
late syphilis (095.3)
secondary syphilis (091.62)
toxoplasmosis (130.5)

573.3 Hepatitis, unspecified

Toxic (noninfectious) hepatitis
Use additional E code to identify cause

AHA: 3Q, '98, 3, 4; 4Q, '90, 26

K75.9 Inflammatory liver disease unspecified ⌐I-10⌐

573.4 Hepatic infarction

573.8 Other specified disorders of liver

Hepatoptosis

573.9 Unspecified disorder of liver

Gallbladder and Bile Ducts

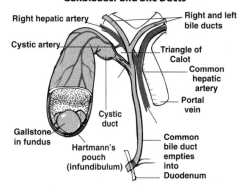

✓4ᵗʰ 574 Cholelithiasis

The following fifth-digit subclassification is for use with category 574:

0　without mention of obstruction
1　with obstruction

§ ✓5ᵗʰ 574.0 Calculus of gallbladder with acute cholecystitis
[0-1]

Billary calculus
Calculus of cystic duct ⎫ with acute cholecystitis
Cholelithiasis ⎭

Any condition classifiable to 574.2 with acute cholecystitis

AHA: 4Q, '96, 32

K80.00 Calculus of GB w/acute cholecystitis w/o obst ⌐I-10⌐

§ ✓5ᵗʰ 574.1 Calculus of gallbladder with other cholecystitis
[0-1]

Billary calculus
Calculus of cystic duct ⎫ with cholecystitis
Cholelithiasis ⎭

Cholecystitis with cholelithiasis NOS

Any condition classifiable to 574.2 with cholecystitis (chronic)

AHA: 3Q, '99, 9; 4Q, '96, 32, 69; 2Q, '96, 13; **For code 574.10:** 1Q, '03, 5

K80.10 Calculus of GB w/chronic cholecystitis w/o obst ⌐I-10⌐

§ ✓5ᵗʰ 574.2 Calculus of gallbladder without mention of cholecystitis
[0-1]

Biliary:
calculus NOS
colic NOS
Calculus of cystic duct
Cholelithiasis NOS
Colic (recurrent) of gallbladder
Gallstone (impacted)

AHA: For code 574.20: 1Q, '88, 14

K80.20 Calculus of GB w/o cholecystitis w/o obst ⌐I-10⌐

§ ✓5ᵗʰ 574.3 Calculus of bile duct with acute cholecystitis
[0-1]

Calculus of bile duct (any) ⎫ with acute cholecystitis
Choledocholithiasis ⎭

Any condition classifiable to 574.5 with acute cholecystitis

§ ✓5ᵗʰ 574.4 Calculus of bile duct with other cholecystitis
[0-1]

Calculus of bile duct
(any) ⎫ with cholecystitis (chronic)
Choledocholithiasis ⎭

Any condition classifiable to 574.5 with cholecystitis (chronic)

§ ✓5ᵗʰ 574.5 Calculus of bile duct without mention of cholecystitis
[0-1]

Calculus of:
bile duct [any]
common duct
hepatic duct
Choledocholithiasis
Hepatic:
colic (recurrent)
lithiasis

AHA: 3Q, '94, 11

§ ✓5ᵗʰ 574.6 Calculus of gallbladder and bile duct with acute cholecystitis
[0-1]

Any condition classifiable to 574.0 and 574.3

AHA: 4Q, '96, 32

§ ✓5ᵗʰ 574.7 Calculus of gallbladder and bile duct with other cholecytitis
[0-1]

Any condition classifiable to 574.1 and 574.4

AHA: 4Q, '96, 32

---

§ Requires fifth digit. Valid digits are in [brackets] under each code. See category 574 for codes and definitions.

✓4ᵗʰ
✓5ᵗʰ　Additional Digit Required　　　Unspecified Code　　　Other Specified Code　　　Manifestation Code　　　▶◀ Revised Text　　　● New Code　　　▲ Revised Code Title

2011 ICD-9-CM　　　　　　**October 2010 • Volume 1 – 173**

Diseases of the Digestive System

574.8–577.0

§ ✓5th **574.8 Calculus of gallbladder and bile duct with acute**
[0-1]   **and chronic cholcystitis**
      Any condition classifiable to 574.6 and 574.7
      AHA: 4Q, '96, 32

§ ✓5th **574.9 Calculus of gallbladder and bile duct without cholecystitis**
[0-1]   Any condition classifiable to 574.2 and 574.5
      AHA: 4Q, '96, 32

✓4th **575 Other disorders of gallbladder**

    575.0 Acute cholecystitis

        Abscess of gallbladder
        Angiocholecystitis
        Cholecystitis:
          emphysematous (acute)   } without mention of
          gangrenous   calculus
          suppurative
        Empyema of gallbladder
        Gangrene of gallbladder

        EXCLUDES *that with:*
            acute and chronic cholecystitis (575.12)
            choledocholithiasis (574.3)
            choledocholithiasis and cholelithiasis (574.6)
            cholelithiasis (574.0)

        AHA: 3Q, '91, 17
        TIP: Do not assign a separate cholecystitis code from category 575 with a code from category 574; cholecystitis is inherent.
        K81.0 Acute cholecystitis   I-10

   ✓5th **575.1 Other cholecystitis**

        Cholecystitis:
          NOS   } without mention of calculus
          chronic

        EXCLUDES *that with:*
            choledocholithiasis (574.4)
            choledocholithiasis and cholelithiasis (574.8)
            cholelithiasis (574.1)

        AHA: 4Q, '96, 32

        575.10 Cholecystitis, unspecified
            Cholecystitis NOS

        575.11 Chronic cholecystitis
            K81.1 Chronic cholecystitis   I-10

        575.12 Acute and chronic cholecystitis
            AHA: 4Q, '97, 52; 4Q, '96, 32

    575.2 Obstruction of gallbladder

        Occlusion   } of cystic duct or gallbladder without
        Stenosis   mention of calculus
        Stricture

        EXCLUDES *that with calculus (574.0-574.2 with fifth-digit 1)*

    575.3 Hydrops of gallbladder
        Mucocele of gallbladder
        DEF: Serous fluid accumulation in bladder.
        AHA: 2Q, '89, 13

    575.4 Perforation of gallbladder
        Rupture of cystic duct or gallbladder

    575.5 Fistula of gallbladder
        Fistula:
          cholecystoduodenal
          cholecystoenteric

    575.6 Cholesterolosis of gallbladder
        Strawberry gallbladder
        DEF: Cholesterol deposits in gallbladder tissue.
        AHA: 4Q, '90, 17

    575.8 Other specified disorders of gallbladder

        Adhesions
        Atrophy
        Cyst   }
        Hypertrophy   } of cystic duct or gallbladder
        Nonfunctioning
        Ulcer

        Biliary dyskinesia

        EXCLUDES *Hartmann's pouch of intestine (V44.3)*
            nonvisualization of gallbladder (793.3)

        AHA: 4Q, '90, 26; 2Q, '89, 13

    575.9 Unspecified disorder of gallbladder

✓4th **576 Other disorders of biliary tract**

    EXCLUDES *that involving the:*
        cystic duct (575.0-575.9)
        gallbladder (575.0-575.9)

    576.0 Postcholecystectomy syndrome
        DEF: Jaundice or abdominal pain following cholecystectomy.
        AHA: 1Q, '88, 10
        TIP: Do not assign additional code 997.4 Digestive system complications.

    576.1 Cholangitis
        Cholangitis: Cholangitis:
          NOS   recurrent
          acute   sclerosing
          ascending   secondary
          chronic   stenosing
          primary   suppurative
        AHA: 2Q, '99, 13
        K83.0 Cholangitis   I-10

    576.2 Obstruction of bile duct
        Occlusion   } of bile duct, except cystic duct, without
        Stenosis   mention of calculus
        Stricture

        EXCLUDES *congenital (751.61)*
            that with calculus (574.3-574.5 with fifth-digit 1)

        AHA: 3Q, '03, 17-18; 1Q, '01, 8; 2Q, '99, 13
        K83.1 Obstruction of bile duct   I-10

    576.3 Perforation of bile duct
        Rupture of bile duct, except cystic duct

    576.4 Fistula of bile duct
        Choledochoduodenal fistula

    576.5 Spasm of sphincter of Oddi

    576.8 Other specified disorders of biliary tract

        Adhesions
        Atrophy
        Cyst   }
        Hypertrophy   } of bile duct (any)
        Nonfunctioning
        Ulcer

        EXCLUDES *congenital choledochal cyst (751.69)*
        AHA: 3Q, '03, 17; 2Q, '99, 14

    576.9 Unspecified disorder of biliary tract

✓4th **577 Diseases of pancreas**

    577.0 Acute pancreatitis
        Abscess of pancreas
        Necrosis of pancreas:
          acute
          infective
        Pancreatitis:
          NOS
          acute (recurrent)
          apoplectic
          hemorrhagic
          subacute
          suppurative

        EXCLUDES *mumps pancreatitis (072.3)*
        AHA: 3Q, '99, 9; 2Q, '98, 19; 2Q, '96, 13; 2Q, '89, 9
        K85.0 Idiopathic acute pancreatitis   I-10

---

§ Requires fifth digit. Valid digits are in [brackets] under each code. See category 574 for codes and definitions.

Pancreas

Head   Neck   Body   Tail

Common
bile duct

Spleen

Accesory
pancreatic
duct

Pancreatic
duct (of Wirsung)

Uncinate
process

Duodenum

Superior
mesenteric
artery
and vein

577.1 Chronic pancreatitis
Chronic pancreatitis:
- NOS
- infectious
- interstitial

Pancreatitis:
- painless
- recurrent
- relapsing

AHA: 1Q, '01, 8; 2Q, '96, 13; 3Q, '94, 11

K86.1 Other chronic pancreatitis   `I-10`

577.2 Cyst and pseudocyst of pancreas
K86.2 Cyst of pancreas   `I-10`

577.8 Other specified diseases of pancreas
Atrophy ⎫
Calculus ⎬ of pancreas
Cirrhosis ⎮
Fibrosis ⎭

Pancreatic:
- infantilism
- necrosis:
  - NOS
  - aseptic
  - fat

Pancreatolithiasis

EXCLUDES *fibrocystic disease of pancreas (277.00-277.09)*
islet cell tumor of pancreas (211.7)
pancreatic steatorrhea (579.4)

AHA: 1Q, '01, 8

577.9 Unspecified disease of pancreas

578 Gastrointestinal hemorrhage
EXCLUDES *that with mention of:*
angiodysplasia of stomach and duodenum (537.83)
angiodysplasia of intestine (569.85)
diverticulitis, intestine:
  large (562.13)
  small (562.03)
diverticulosis, intestine:
  large (562.12)
  small (562.02)
gastritis and duodenitis (535.0-535.6)
ulcer:
  duodenal, gastric, gastrojejuunal or peptic
    (531.00-534.91)

AHA: 2Q, '92, 9; 4Q, '90, 20

578.0 Hematemesis
Vomiting of blood

AHA: 2Q, '02, 4

578.1 Blood in stool
Melena

EXCLUDES *melena of the newborn (772.4, 777.3)*
occult blood (792.1)

AHA: 2Q, '06, 17; 2Q, '92, 8

K92.1 Melena   `I-10`

578.9 Hemorrhage of gastrointestinal tract, unspecified
Gastric hemorrhage
Intestinal hemorrhage

AHA: 4Q, '06, 91; 3Q, '05, 17; N-D, '86, 9

TIP: Assign 578.9 if the physician does not establish a causal link between GI bleeding and any possible causes found on endoscopy.

K92.2 Gastrointestinal hemorrhage unspecified   `I-10`

579 Intestinal malabsorption

579.0 Celiac disease
Celiac: Gee (-Herter) disease
  crisis   Gluten enteropathy
  infantilism   Idiopathic steatorrhea
  rickets   Nontropical sprue

DEF: Malabsorption syndrome due to gluten consumption; symptoms include fetid, bulky, frothy, oily stools, distended abdomen, gas, asthenia, electrolyte depletion and vitamin B, D and K deficiency.

579.1 Tropical sprue
Sprue:
- NOS
- tropical

Tropical steatorrhea

DEF: Diarrhea, occurs in tropics; may be due to enteric infection and malnutrition.

579.2 Blind loop syndrome
Postoperative blind loop syndrome

DEF: Obstruction or impaired passage in small intestine due to alterations, from strictures or surgery; causes stasis, abnormal bacterial flora, diarrhea, weight loss, multiple vitamin deficiency, and megaloblastic anemia.

TIP: Do not assign additional code 997.4 Digestive system complications.

579.3 Other and unspecified postsurgical nonabsorption
Hypoglycemia ⎫ following gastrointestinal
Malnutrition ⎬ surgery

AHA: 4Q, '03, 104

579.4 Pancreatic steatorrhea
DEF: Excess fat in feces due to absence of pancreatic secretions in intestine.

579.8 Other specified intestinal malabsorption
Enteropathy:
- exudative
- protein-losing

Steatorrhea (chronic)

AHA: 1Q, '88, 6

579.9 Unspecified intestinal malabsorption
Malabsorption syndrome NOS

AHA: 4Q, '04, 59

`√4th` `√5th` Additional Digit Required   Unspecified Code   Other Specified Code   Manifestation Code   ▶◀ Revised Text   ● New Code   ▲ Revised Code Title

2011 ICD-9-CM   **Volume 1 – 175**

10. Diseases of the Genitourinary System (580-629)

Nephritis, Nephrotic Syndrome, and Nephrosis (580-589)

EXCLUDES *hypertensive chronic kidney disease (403.00-403.91, 404.00-404.93)*

✓4ᵗʰ 580 Acute glomerulonephritis

INCLUDES acute nephritis

DEF: Acute, severe inflammation in tuft of capillaries that filter the kidneys.

580.0 With lesion of proliferative glomerulonephritis
Acute (diffuse) proliferative glomerulonephritis
Acute poststreptococcal glomerulonephritis

580.4 With lesion of rapidly progressive glomerulonephritis
Acute nephritis with lesion of necrotizing glomerulitis

DEF: Acute glomerulonephritis; progresses to ESRD with diffuse epithelial proliferation.

✓5ᵗʰ 580.8 With other specified pathological lesion in kidney

580.81 *Acute glomerulonephritis in diseases classified elsewhere*

Code first underlying disease, as:
infectious hepatitis (070.0-070.9)
mumps (072.79)
subacute bacterial endocarditis (421.0)
typhoid fever (002.0)

580.89 Other
Glomerulonephritis, acute, with lesion of:
exudative nephritis
interstitial (diffuse) (focal) nephritis

580.9 Acute glomerulonephritis with unspecified pathological lesion in kidney
Glomerulonephritis
NOS
hemorrhagic ⎫
Nephritis   ⎬ specified as acute
Nephropathy ⎭

✓4ᵗʰ 581 Nephrotic syndrome

DEF: Disease process marked by symptoms such as extensive edema, notable proteinuria, hypoalbuminemia, and susceptibility to intercurrent infections.

581.0 With lesion of proliferative glomerulonephritis

581.1 With lesion of membranous glomerulonephritis
Epimembranous nephritis
Idiopathic membranous glomerular disease
Nephrotic syndrome with lesion of:
focal glomerulosclerosis
sclerosing membranous glomerulonephritis
segmental hyalinosis

581.2 With lesion of membranoproliferative glomerulonephritis
Nephrotic syndrome with lesion (of):
endothelial ⎫
hypocomplementemic persistent ⎪
lobular ⎬ glomerulonephritis
mesangiocapillary ⎪
mixed membranous and ⎪
proliferative ⎭

DEF: Glomerulonephritis combined with clinical features of nephrotic syndrome; characterized by uneven thickening of glomerular capillary walls and mesangial cell increase; slowly progresses to ESRD.

581.3 With lesion of minimal change glomerulonephritis
Foot process disease
Lipoid nephrosis
Minimal change:
glomerular disease
glomerulitis
nephrotic syndrome

AHA: 1Q, '07, 23

Kidney

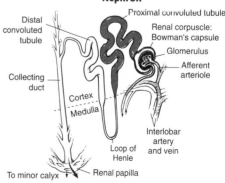

✓5ᵗʰ 581.8 With other specified pathological lesion in kidney

581.81 *Nephrotic syndrome in diseases classified elsewhere*

Code first underlying disease, as:
amyloidosis (277.30-277.39)
diabetes mellitus (249.4, 250.4)
tes mellitus (250.4)
malaria (084.9)
polyarteritis (446.0)
systemic lupus erythematosus (710.0)

EXCLUDES *nephrosis in epidemic hemorrhagic fever (078.6)*

AHA: 3Q, '91, 8, 12; S-O, '85, 3

581.89 Other
Glomerulonephritis with edema and lesion of:
exudative nephritis
interstitial (diffuse) (focal) nephritis

581.9 Nephrotic syndrome with unspecified pathological lesion in kidney
Glomerulonephritis with edema NOS
Nephritis:
nephrotic NOS
with edema NOS
Nephrosis NOS
Renal disease with edema NOS

✓4ᵗʰ 582 Chronic glomerulonephritis

INCLUDES chronic nephritis

DEF: Slow progressive type of nephritis characterized by inflammation of the capillary loops in the glomeruli of the kidney, which leads to renal failure.

582.0 With lesion of proliferative glomerulonephritis
Chronic (diffuse) proliferative glomerulonephritis

582.1 With lesion of membranous glomerulonephritis
Chronic glomerulonephritis:
membranous
sclerosing
Focal glomerulosclerosis
Segmental hyalinosis

AHA: S-O, '84, 16

Nephron

✓4ᵗʰ
✓5ᵗʰ Additional Digit Required   Unspecified Code   Other Specified Code   Manifestation Code   ▶◀ Revised Text   ● New Code   ▲ Revised Code Title

Diseases of the Genitourinary System

582.2–584.9

582.2 With lesion of membranoproliferative glomerulonephritis
Chronic glomerulonephritis:
endothelial
hypocomplementemic persistent
lobular
membranoproliferative
mesangiocapillary
mixed membranous and proliferative
DEF: Chronic glomerulonephritis with mesangial cell proliferation.

582.4 With lesion of rapidly progressive glomerulonephritis
Chronic nephritis with lesion of necrotizing glomerulitis
DEF: Chronic glomerulonephritis rapidly progresses to ESRD; marked by diffuse epithelial proliferation.

√5ᵗʰ **582.8 With other specified pathological lesion in kidney**

582.81 Chronic glomerulonephritis in diseases classified elsewhere
Code first underlying disease, as:
amyloidosis (277.30-277.39)
systemic lupus erythematosus (710.0)

582.89 Other
Chronic glomerulonephritis with lesion of:
exudative nephritis
interstitial (diffuse) (focal) nephritis

582.9 Chronic glomerulonephritis with unspecified pathological lesion in kidney
Glomerulonephritis:
NOS
hemorrhagic   } specified as chronic
Nephritis
Nephropathy
AHA: 2Q, '01, 12

√4ᵗʰ **583 Nephritis and nephropathy, not specified as acute or chronic**
INCLUDES "renal disease" so stated, not specified as acute or chronic but with stated pathology or cause

583.0 With lesion of proliferative glomerulonephritis
Proliferative:
glomerulonephritis (diffuse) NOS
nephritis NOS
nephropathy NOS

583.1 With lesion of membranous glomerulonephritis
Membranous:
glomerulonephritis NOS
nephritis NOS
Membranous nephropathy NOS
DEF: Kidney inflammation or dysfunction with deposits on glomerular capillary basement membranes.
N05.2 Uns nephritic syndr w/ diffuse membranous gln   I-10

583.2 With lesion of membranoproliferative glomerulonephritis
Membranoproliferative:
glomerulonephritis NOS
nephritis NOS
nephropathy NOS
Nephritis NOS, with lesion of:
hypocomplementemic persistant
lobular
mesangiocapillary   } glomerulonephritis
mixed membranous and
   proliferative
DEF: Kidney inflammation or dysfunction with mesangial cell proliferation.

583.4 With lesion of rapidly progressive glomerulonephritis
Necrotizing or rapidly progressive:
glomerulitis NOS
glomerulonephritis NOS
nephritis NOS
nephropathy NOS
Nephritis, unspecified, with lesion of necrotizing glomerulitis
DEF: Kidney inflammation or dysfunction; rapidly progresses to ESRD marked by diffuse epithelial proliferation.

583.6 With lesion of renal cortical necrosis
Nephritis, NOS   } with (renal) cortical necrosis
Nephropathy NOS
Renal cortical necrosis NOS

583.7 With lesion of renal medullary necrosis
Nephritis, NOS   } with (renal) medullary
Nephropathy NOS   } [papillary] necrosis

√5ᵗʰ **583.8 With other specified pathological lesion in kidney**

583.81 Nephritis and nephropathy, not specified as acute or chronic, in diseases classified elsewhere
Code first underlying disease, as:
amyloidosis (277.30-277.39)
diabetes mellitus (249.4, 250.4)
gonococcal infection (098.19)
Goodpasture's syndrome (446.21)
systemic lupus erythematosus (710.0)
tuberculosis (016.0)
EXCLUDES gouty nephropathy (274.10)
syphilitic nephritis (095.4)
AHA: 2Q, '03, 7; 3Q, '91, 8; S-O, '85, 3

583.89 Other
Glomerulitis
Glomerulonephritis   } with lesions of:
Nephritis   } exudative nephritis
Nephropathy   } interstitial nephritis
Renal disease

583.9 With unspecified pathological lesion in kidney
Glomerulitis
Glomerulonephritis   } NOS
Nephritis
Nephropathy
EXCLUDES nephropathy complicating pregnancy, labor, or the puerperium (642.0-642.9, 646.2)
renal disease NOS with no stated cause (593.9)

√4ᵗʰ **584 Acute kidney failure**
INCLUDES acute renal failure
EXCLUDES following labor and delivery (669.3)
posttraumatic (958.5)
that complicating:
abortion (634-638 with .3, 639.3)
ectopic or molar pregnancy (639.3)
DEF: State resulting from increasing urea and related substances from the blood (azotemia), often with urine output of less than 500 ml per day.
AHA: 1Q, '93, 18; 2Q, '92, 5; 4Q, '92, 22
TIP: Do not assign combination code for hypertensive renal disease unless chronic kidney disease is also present.

584.5 Acute kidney failure with lesion of tubular necrosis
Lower nephron nephrosis
Renal failure with (acute) tubular necrosis
Tubular necrosis:
NOS
acute
DEF: Acute decline in kidney efficiency with destruction of tubules.
N17.0 Acute renal failure with tubular necrosis   I-10

584.6 Acute kidney failure with lesion of renal cortical necrosis
DEF: Acute decline in kidney efficiency with destruction of renal tissues that filter blood.

584.7 Acute kidney failure with lesion of renal medullary [papillary] necrosis
Necrotizing renal papillitis
DEF: Acute decline in kidney efficiency with destruction of renal tissues that collect urine.

584.8 Acute kidney failure with other specified pathological lesion in kidney
AHA: N-D, '85, 1

584.9 Acute kidney failure, unspecified
Acute kidney injury (nontraumatic)
EXCLUDES traumatic kidney injury (866.00-866.13)
AHA: ▶4Q, '09, 98;◀ 4Q, '08, 192; 4Q, '07, 97; 2Q, '05, 18; 2Q, '03, 7; 1Q, '03, 22; 3Q, '02, 21, 28; 2Q, '01, 14; 1Q, '00, 22; 3Q, '96, 9; 4Q, '88, 1
N17.9 Acute renal failure unspecified   I-10

☑4ᵗʰ 585　Chronic kidney disease [CKD]
Chronic uremia

Code first hypertensive chronic kidney disease, if applicable, (403.00-403.91, 404.00-404.93)

Use additional code to identify kidney transplant status, if applicable (V42.0)

Use additional code to identify manifestation as:
uremic:
　neuropathy (357.4)
　pericarditis (420.0)

AHA: 4Q, '06, 84-86; 4Q, '05, 68, 77; 1Q, '04, 5; 4Q, '03, 61, 111; 2Q, '03, 7; 2Q, '01, 12, 13; 1Q, '01, 3; 4Q, '98, 55; 3Q, '98, 6, 7; 2Q, '98, 20; 3Q, '96, 9; 1Q, '93, 18; 3Q, '91, 8; 4Q, '89, 1; N-D, '85, 15; S-O, '84, 3

585.1　Chronic kidney disease, Stage I
DEF: Some kidney damage; normal or slightly increased GFR (> 90).

585.2　Chronic kidney disease, Stage II (mild)
DEF: Kidney damage with mild decrease in GFR (60–89).

585.3　Chronic kidney disease, Stage III (moderate)
AHA: 4Q, '05, 69
DEF: Kidney damage with moderate decrease in GFR (30–59).
N18.3 Chronic kidney disease stage III moderate　`I-10`

585.4　Chronic kidney disease, Stage IV (severe)
DEF: Kidney damage with severe decrease in GFR (15–29).
N18.4 Chronic kidney disease stage IV severe　`I-10`

585.5　Chronic kidney disease, Stage V
EXCLUDES　*chronic kidney disease, stage V requiring chronic dialysis (585.6)*
DEF: Kidney failure with GFR value of less than 15.

585.6　End stage renal disease
Chronic kidney disease requiring chronic dialysis
DEF: Federal government indicator of a stage V CKD patient undergoing treatment by dialysis or transplantation.
AHA: 4Q, '08, 193; 1Q, '08, 7; 4Q, '07, 86; 3Q, '07, 5, 9; 4Q, '06, 136; 4Q, '05, 79
N18.6 End stage renal disease　`I-10`

585.9　Chronic kidney disease, unspecified
Chronic renal disease
Chronic renal failure NOS
Chronic renal insufficiency
AHA: 1Q, '08, 10; 2Q, '07, 3; 4Q, '06, 86; 4Q, '05, 79
N18.9 Chronic kidney disease unspecified　`I-10`

586　Renal failure, unspecified
Uremia NOS
EXCLUDES　*following labor and delivery (669.3)*
posttraumatic renal failure (958.5)
that complicating:
　abortion (634-638 with .3, 639.3)
　ectopic or molar pregnancy (639.3)
uremia:
　extrarenal (788.9)
　prenal (788.9)
DEF: Renal failure: kidney functions cease; malfunction may be due to inability to excrete metabolized substances or retain level of electrolytes.
DEF: Uremia: excess urea, creatinine and other nitrogenous products of protein and amino acid metabolism in blood due to reduced excretory function in bilateral kidney disease; also called azotemia.
AHA: 3Q, '98, 6; 1Q, '93, 18; 1Q, '88, 3
N19 Unspecified renal failure　`I-10`

Genitourinary System

Inferior vena cava
Aorta
Right kidney
Left kidney
Ureter
Anterior division of internal iliac artery
Ovarian or testicular artery and vein
Superior and Inferior vesicular arteries
Urinary bladder
Ureteral orifice
Urethra
Urogenital diaphragm

587　Renal sclerosis, unspecified
Atrophy of kidney
Contracted kidney
Renal:
　cirrhosis
　fibrosis

☑4ᵗʰ 588　Disorders resulting from impaired renal function

588.0　Renal osteodystrophy
Azotemic osteodystrophy
Phosphate-losing tubular disorders
Renal:
　dwarfism
　infantilism
　rickets
DEF: Condition resulting from chronic renal failure results in osteomalacia, osteoporosis or osteosclerosis; an abnormal level of phosphorus in the blood and impaired stimulation of the parathyroid.

588.1　Nephrogenic diabetes insipidus
EXCLUDES　*diabetes insipidus NOS (253.5)*
DEF: Type of diabetes due to renal tubules inability to reabsorb water; not responsive to vasopressin; may develop into chronic renal insufficiency.

☑5ᵗʰ 588.8　Other specified disorders resulting from impaired renal function
EXCLUDES　*secondary hypertension (405.0-405.9)*

588.81　Secondary hyperparathyroidism (of renal origin)
Secondary hyperparathyroidism NOS
DEF: Parathyroid dysfunction caused by chronic renal failure; phosphate clearance is impaired, phosphate is released from bone, vitamin D is not produced, intestinal calcium absorption is low, and blood levels of calcium are lowered causing excessive production of parathyroid hormone.
AHA: 4Q, '04, 58-59
N25.81 Secondary hyperparathyroidism of renal origin　`I-10`

588.89　Other specified disorders resulting from impaired renal function
Hypokalemic nephropathy

588.9　Unspecified disorder resulting from impaired renal function

☑4ᵗʰ 589　Small kidney of unknown cause

589.0　Unilateral small kidney

589.1　Bilateral small kidneys

589.9　Small kidney, unspecified

Other Diseases of Urinary System (590-599)

☑4ᵗʰ 590　Infections of kidney
Use additional code to identify organism, such as Escherichia coli [E. coli] (041.4)

☑5ᵗʰ 590.0　Chronic pyelonephritis
Chronic pyelitis
Chronic pyonephrosis
Code if applicable, any casual condition first

590.00　Without lesion of renal medullary necrosis

590.01　With lesion of renal medullary necrosis

☑5ᵗʰ 590.1　Acute pyelonephritis
Acute pyelitis
Acute pyonephrosis

590.10　Without lesion of renal medullary necrosis

590.11　With lesion of renal medullary necrosis

590.2　Renal and perinephric abscess
Abscess:
　kidney
　nephritic
　perirenal
Carbuncle of kidney

☑4ᵗʰ ☑5ᵗʰ Additional Digit Required　　Unspecified Code　　Other Specified Code　　Manifestation Code　　▶◀ Revised Text　　● New Code　　▲ Revised Code Title

2011 ICD-9-CM　　　　　　　　　　　　　　　　　　　　　　　　　　　　**Volume 1 – 179**

590.3 Pyeloureteritis cystica
Infection of renal pelvis and ureter
Ureteritis cystica
DEF: Inflammation and formation of submucosal cysts in the kidney, pelvis, and ureter.

√5ᵗʰ **590.8 Other pyelonephritis or pyonephrosis, not specified as acute or chronic**

590.80 Pyelonephritis, unspecified
Pyelitis NOS
Pyelonephritis NOS
AHA: 1Q, '98, 10; 4Q, '97, 40
N11.9 Chronic tubulo-interstitial nephritis uns   I-10

590.81 Pyelitis or pyelonephritis in diseases classified elsewhere
Code first underlying disease, as:
tuberculosis (016.0)

590.9 Infection of kidney, unspecified
EXCLUDES urinary tract infection NOS (599.0)

591 Hydronephrosis
Hydrocalycosis
Hydronephrosis
Hydroureteronephrosis
EXCLUDES congenital hydronephrosis (753.29)
hydroureter (593.5)
DEF: Distention of kidney and pelvis, with urine build-up due to ureteral obstruction; pyonephrosis may result.
AHA: 2Q, '98, 9
TIP: Hydronephrosis is not inherent in urinary obstructions and should be coded separately.
N13.30 Unspecified hydronephrosis   I-10

√4ᵗʰ **592 Calculus of kidney and ureter**
EXCLUDES nephrocalcinosis (275.4)

592.0 Calculus of kidney
Nephrolithiasis NOS
Renal calculus or stone
Staghorn calculus
Stone in kidney
EXCLUDES uric acid nephrolithiasis (274.11)
AHA: 1Q, '00, 4
N20.0 Calculus of kidney   I-10

592.1 Calculus of ureter
Ureteric stone
Ureterolithiasis
AHA: 2Q, '98, 9; 1Q, '98, 10; 1Q, '91, 11
N20.1 Calculus of ureter   I-10

592.9 Urinary calculus, unspecified
AHA: 1Q, '98, 10; 4Q, '97, 40

√4ᵗʰ **593 Other disorders of kidney and ureter**

593.0 Nephroptosis
Floating kidney
Mobile kidney

593.1 Hypertrophy of kidney

593.2 Cyst of kidney, acquired
Cyst (multiple) (solitary) of kidney, not congenital
Peripelvic (lymphatic) cyst
EXCLUDES calyceal or pyelogenic cyst of kidney (591)
congenital cyst of kidney (753.1)
polycystic (disease of) kidney (753.1)
DEF: Abnormal, fluid-filled sac in the kidney, not present at birth.
AHA: 4Q, '90, 3
N28.1 Cyst of kidney acquired   I-10

593.3 Stricture or kinking of ureter
Angulation ⎫
Constriction ⎬ of ureter (post-operative)
Stricture of pelviureteric junction
DEF: Stricture or knot in tube connecting kidney to bladder.
AHA: 2Q, '98, 9

593.4 Other ureteric obstruction
Idiopathic retroperitoneal fibrosis
Occlusion NOS of ureter
EXCLUDES that due to calculus (592.1)
AHA: ▶1Q, '10, 9;◄ 2Q, '97, 4

593.5 Hydroureter
EXCLUDES congenital hydroureter (753.22)
hydroureteronephrosis (591)

593.6 Postural proteinuria
Benign postural proteinuria
Orthostatic proteinuria
EXCLUDES proteinuria NOS (791.0)
DEF: Excessive amounts of serum protein in the urine caused by the body position, e.g., orthostatic and lordotic.

√5ᵗʰ **593.7 Vesicoureteral reflux**
DEF: Backflow of urine, from bladder into ureter due to obstructed bladder neck.
AHA: 4Q, '94, 42

593.70 Unspecified or without reflux nephropathy

593.71 With reflux nephropathy, unilateral

593.72 With reflux nephropathy, bilateral

593.73 With reflux nephropathy NOS

√5ᵗʰ **593.8 Other specified disorders of kidney and ureter**

593.81 Vascular disorders of kidney
Renal (artery):
embolism
hemorrhage
thrombosis
Renal infarction

593.82 Ureteral fistula
Intestinoureteral fistula
EXCLUDES fistula between ureter and female genital tract (619.0)
DEF: Abnormal communication, between tube connecting kidney to bladder and another structure.

593.89 Other
Adhesions, kidney or ureter
Periureteritis
Polyp of ureter
Pyelectasia
Ureterocele
EXCLUDES tuberculosis of ureter (016.2)
ureteritis cystica (590.3)

593.9 Unspecified disorder of kidney and ureter
Acute renal disease
Acute renal insufficiency
Renal disease NOS
Salt-losing nephritis or syndrome
EXCLUDES chronic renal insufficiency (585.9)
cystic kidney disease (753.1)
nephropathy, so stated (583.0-583.9)
renal disease:
arising in pregnancy or the puerperium (642.1-642.2, 642.4-642.7, 646.2)
not specified as acute or chronic, but with stated pathology or cause (583.0-583.9)
AHA: 4Q, '05, 79; 1Q, '93, 17
N28.9 Disorder of kidney and ureter unspecified   I-10

√4ᵗʰ **594 Calculus of lower urinary tract**

594.0 Calculus in diverticulum of bladder
DEF: Stone or mineral deposit in abnormal sac on the bladder wall.

594.1 Other calculus in bladder
Urinary bladder stone
EXCLUDES staghorn calculus (592.0)
DEF: Stone or mineral deposit in bladder.

594.2 Calculus in urethra
DEF: Stone or mineral deposit in tube that empties urine from bladder.

594.8 Other lower urinary tract calculus
AHA: J-F, '85, 16

594.9 Calculus of lower urinary tract, unspecified
EXCLUDES calculus of urinary tract NOS (592.9)

N Newborn Age: 0   P Pediatric Age: 0-17   M Maternity Age: 12-55   A Adult Age: 15-124

Bladder

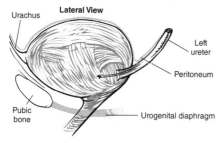

Anterior View

Fundus · Left ureter · Right ureter · Lateral wall · Ureteral orifice · Trigone · Uvula of bladder · Urethra

Lateral View

Urachus · Left ureter · Peritoneum · Pubic bone · Urogenital diaphragm

√4ᵗʰ 595 Cystitis

EXCLUDES *prostatocystitis (601.3)*

Use additional code to identify organism, such as Escherichia coli [E. coli] (041.4)

595.0 Acute cystitis
EXCLUDES *trigonitis (595.3)*
DEF: Acute inflammation of bladder.
AHA: 2Q, '99, 15
N30.00 Acute cystitis without hematuria   I-10

595.1 Chronic interstitial cystitis
Hunner's ulcer
Panmural fibrosis of bladder
Submucous cystitis
DEF: Inflamed lesion affecting bladder wall; symptoms include urinary frequency, pain on bladder filling, nocturia, and distended bladder.

595.2 Other chronic cystitis
Chronic cystitis NOS
Subacute cystitis
EXCLUDES *trigonitis (595.3)*
DEF: Persistent inflammation of bladder.

595.3 Trigonitis
Follicular cystitis
Trigonitis (acute) (chronic)
Urethrotrigonitis
DEF: Inflammation of the triangular area of the bladder called the trigonum vesicae.

595.4 Cystitis in diseases classified elsewhere
Code first underlying disease, as:
actinomycosis (039.8)
amebiasis (006.8)
bilharziasis (120.0-120.9)
Echinococcus infestation (122.3, 122.6)
EXCLUDES *cystitis:*
diphtheritic (032.84)
gonococcal (098.11, 098.31)
monilial (112.2)
trichomonal (131.09)
tuberculous (016.1)

√5ᵗʰ 595.8 Other specified types of cystitis

595.81 Cystitis cystica
DEF: Inflammation of the bladder characterized by formation of multiple cysts.

595.82 Irradiation cystitis
Use additional E code to identify cause
DEF: Inflammation of the bladder due to effects of radiation.

595.89 Other
Abscess of bladder:
Cystitis:
bullous
emphysematous
glandularis

595.9 Cystitis, unspecified

√4ᵗʰ 596 Other disorders of bladder
Use additional code to identify urinary incontinence (625.6, 788.30-788.39)
AHA: M-A, '87, 10

596.0 Bladder neck obstruction
Contracture (acquired)
Obstruction (acquired) } of bladder neck or vesicourethral
Stenosis (acquired)   orifice
EXCLUDES *congenital (753.6)*
DEF: Bladder outlet and vesicourethral obstruction; occurs as a consequence of benign prostatic hypertrophy or prostatic cancer; may also occur in either sex due to strictures, following radiation, cystoscopy, catheterization, injury, infection, blood clots, bladder cancer, impaction or disease compressing bladder neck.
AHA: 3Q, '02, 28; 2Q, '01, 14; N-D, '86, 10
N32.0 Bladder-neck obstruction   I-10

596.1 Intestinovesical fistula
Fistula:
enterovesical
vesicocolic
vesicoenteric
vesicorectal
DEF: Abnormal communication, between intestine and bladder.

596.2 Vesical fistula, not elsewhere classified
Fistula:
bladder NOS
urethrovesical
vesicocutaneous
vesicoperineal
EXCLUDES *fistula between bladder and female genital tract (619.0)*
DEF: Abnormal communication between bladder and another structure.

596.3 Diverticulum of bladder
Diverticulitis
Diverticulum (acquired) (false) } of bladder
EXCLUDES *that with calculus in diverticulum of bladder (594.0)*
DEF: Abnormal pouch in bladder wall.

596.4 Atony of bladder
High compliance bladder
Hypotonicity
Inertia } of bladder
EXCLUDES *neurogenic bladder (596.54)*
DEF: Distended, bladder with loss of expulsive force; linked to CNS disease.

√5ᵗʰ 596.5 Other functional disorders of bladder
EXCLUDES *cauda equina syndrome with neurogenic bladder (344.61)*

596.51 Hypertonicity of bladder
Hyperactivity
Overactive bladder
DEF: Abnormal tension of muscular wall of bladder; may appear after surgery of voluntary nerve.
N32.81 Overactive bladder   I-10

596.52 Low bladder compliance
DEF: Low bladder capacity; causes increased pressure and frequent urination.

596.53 Paralysis of bladder
DEF: Impaired bladder motor function due to nerve or muscle damage.

596.54 Neurogenic bladder NOS
DEF: Unspecified dysfunctional bladder due to lesion of central, peripheral nervous system; may result in incontinence, residual urine retention, urinary infection, stones and renal failure.
AHA: 1Q, '01, 12
N31.9 Neuromuscular dysfunction of   I-10
bladder unspecified

Diseases of the Genitourinary System

595–596.54

Diseases of the Genitourinary System

596.55–599.83

596.55 Detrusor sphincter dyssynergia
DEF: Instability of the urinary bladder sphincter muscle associated with urinary incontinence.

596.59 Other functional disorder of bladder
Detrusor instability
DEF: Detrusor instability: instability of bladder; marked by uninhibited contractions often leading to incontinence.

596.6 Rupture of bladder, nontraumatic

596.7 Hemorrhage into bladder wall
Hyperemia of bladder
EXCLUDES acute hemorrhagic cystitis (595.0)

596.8 Other specified disorders of bladder
Bladder: Bladder:
calcified   hemorrhage
contracted   hypertrophy
EXCLUDES cystocele, female (618.01-618.02, 618.09, 618.2-618.4)
hernia or prolapse of bladder, female (618.01-618.02, 618.09, 618.2-618.4)
AHA: J-F, '85, 8

596.9 Unspecified disorder of bladder
AHA: J-F, '85, 8

√4ᵗʰ **597 Urethritis, not sexually transmitted, and urethral syndrome**
EXCLUDES nonspecific urethritis, so stated (099.4)

597.0 Urethral abscess
Abscess: Abscess of:
periurethral   Cowper's gland
urethral (gland)   Littré's gland
Abscess of: Periurethral cellulitis
bulbourethral gland
EXCLUDES urethral caruncle (599.3)
DEF: Pocket of pus in tube that empties urine from the bladder.

√5ᵗʰ **597.8 Other urethritis**

597.80 Urethritis, unspecified

597.81 Urethral syndrome NOS

597.89 Other
Adenitis, Skene's glands
Cowperitis
Meatitis, urethral
Ulcer, urethra (meatus)
Verumontanitis
EXCLUDES trichomonal (131.02)

√4ᵗʰ **598 Urethral stricture**
Use additional code to identify urinary incontinence (625.6, 788.30-788.39)
INCLUDES pinhole meatus
stricture of urinary meatus
EXCLUDES congenital stricture of urethra and urinary meatus (753.6)
DEF: Narrowing of tube that empties urine from bladder.

√5ᵗʰ **598.0 Urethral stricture due to infection**

598.00 Due to unspecified infection

598.01 Due to infective diseases classified elsewhere
Code first underlying disease, as:
gonococcal infection (098.2)
schistosomiasis (120.0-120.9)
syphilis (095.8)

598.1 Traumatic urethral stricture
Stricture of urethra:
late effect of injury
postobstetric
EXCLUDES postoperative following surgery on genitourinary tract (598.2)

598.2 Postoperative urethral stricture
Postcatheterization stricture of urethra
AHA: 3Q, '97, 6

598.8 Other specified causes of urethral stricture
AHA: N-D, '84, 9

598.9 Urethral stricture, unspecified

√4ᵗʰ **599 Other disorders of urethra and urinary tract**

599.0 Urinary tract infection, site not specified
EXCLUDES candidiasis of urinary tract (112.2)
urinary tract infection of newborn (771.82)
Use additional code to identify organism, such as Escherichia coli [E. coli] (041.4)
AHA: ▶1Q, '10, 9;◀ 3Q, '09, 10-11; 3Q, '05, 12; 2Q, '04, 13; 4Q, '03, 79; 4Q, '99, 6; 2Q, '99, 15;1Q, '98, 5; 2Q, '96, 7; 4Q, '96, 33; 2Q, '95, 7; 1Q, '92, 13
TIP: Do not assign if UTI due to candidiasis; see code 112.2.
N39.0 Urinary tract infection site not specified   I-10

599.1 Urethral fistula
Fistula: Urinary fistula NOS
urethroperineal
urethrorectal
EXCLUDES fistula:
urethroscrotal (608.89)
urethrovaginal (619.0)
urethrovesicovaginal (619.0)
AHA: 3Q, '97, 6

599.2 Urethral diverticulum
DEF: Abnormal pouch in urethral wall.

599.3 Urethral caruncle
Polyp of urethra

599.4 Urethral false passage
DEF: Abnormal opening in urethra due to surgery; trauma or disease.

599.5 Prolapsed urethral mucosa
Prolapse of urethra   Urethrocele
EXCLUDES urethrocele, female (618.03, 618.09, 618.2-618.4)

√5ᵗʰ **599.6 Urinary obstruction**
Use additional code to identify urinary incontinence (625.6, 788.30-788.39)
EXCLUDES obstructive nephropathy NOS (593.89)
AHA: 4Q, '05, 80

599.60 Urinary obstruction, unspecified
Obstructive uropathy NOS
Urinary (tract) obstruction NOS
N13.9 Obstructive and reflux uropathy unspec   I-10

599.69 Urinary obstruction, not elsewhere classified
Code, if applicable, any causal condition first, such as:
hyperplasia of prostate (600.0-600.9 with fifth-digit 1)
AHA: 4Q, '06, 93

√5ᵗʰ **599.7 Hematuria**
Hematuria (benign) (essential)
EXCLUDES hemoglobinuria (791.2)
AHA: 4Q, '08, 121; 1Q, '00, 5; 3Q, '95, 8

599.70 Hematuria, unspecified
R31.9 Hematuria unspecified   I-10

599.71 Gross hematuria

599.72 Microscopic hematuria

√5ᵗʰ **599.8 Other specified disorders of urethra and urinary tract**
Use additional code to identify urinary incontinence (625.6, 788.30-788.39), if present
EXCLUDES symptoms and other conditions classifiable to 788.0-788.2, 788.4-788.9, 791.0-791.9

599.81 Urethral hypermobility
DEF: Hyperactive urethra.

599.82 Intrinsic (urethral) sphincter deficiency [ISD]
DEF: Malfunctioning urethral sphincter.
AHA: 2Q, '96, 15

599.83 Urethral instability
DEF: Inconsistent functioning of urethra.

N Newborn Age: 0   P Pediatric Age: 0-17   M Maternity Age: 12-55   A Adult Age: 15-124

599.84 Other specified disorders of urethra
Rupture of urethra (nontraumatic)
Urethral:
  cyst
  granuloma
DEF: Rupture of urethra due to herniation or breaking down of tissue; not due to trauma.
DEF: Urethral cyst: abnormal sac in urethra; usually fluid filled.
DEF: Granuloma: inflammatory cells forming small nodules in urethra.
AHA: 1Q, '09, 15

599.89 Other specified disorders of urinary tract

599.9 Unspecified disorder of urethra and urinary tract

Diseases of Male Genital Organs (600-608)

√4ᵗʰ 600 Hyperplasia of prostate
INCLUDES enlarged prostate
DEF: Fibrostromal proliferation in periurethral glands, causes blood in urine; etiology unknown.
AHA: 3Q, '05, 20; 4Q, '00, 43; 3Q, '94, 12; 3Q, '92, 7; N-D, '86, 10

√5ᵗʰ 600.0 Hypertrophy (benign) of prostate
Benign prostatic hypertrophy   Soft enlarged prostate
Enlargement of prostate
Smooth enlarged prostate
AHA: 4Q, '06, 93-95; 3Q, '05, 20; 4Q, '03, 63; 1Q, '03, 6; 3Q, '02, 28; 2Q, '01, 14

600.00 Hypertrophy (benign) of prostate without urinary obstruction and other lower urinary tract symptoms [LUTS] A ♂
Hypertrophy (benign) of prostate NOS
N40.0 Enlarged prostate without LUTS   I-10

600.01 Hypertrophy (benign) of prostate with urinary obstruction and other lower urinary tract symptoms [LUTS] A ♂
Hypertrophy (benign) of prostate with urinary retention
Use additional code to identify symptoms:
  incomplete bladder emptying (788.21)
  nocturia (788.43)
  straining on urination (788.65)
  urinary frequency (788.41)
  urinary hesitancy (788.64)
  urinary incontinence (788.30-788.39)
  urinary obstruction (599.69)
  urinary retention (788.20)
  urinary urgency (788.63)
  weak urinary stream (788.62)
AHA: 4Q, '06, 93-95; 4Q, '03, 64

√5ᵗʰ 600.1 Nodular prostate
Hard, firm prostate
Multinodular prostate
EXCLUDES malignant neoplasm of prostate (185)
DEF: Hard, firm nodule in prostate.
AHA: 4Q, '03, 63

600.10 Nodular prostate without urinary obstruction A ♂
Nodular prostate NOS

600.11 Nodular prostate with urinary obstruction A ♂
Nodular prostate with urinary retention

Male Pelvic Organs

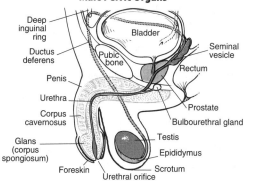

Deep inguinal ring
Ductus deferens
Penis
Urethra
Corpus cavernosus
Glans (corpus spongiosum)
Foreskin
Bladder
Pubic bone
Seminal vesicle
Rectum
Prostate
Bulbourethral gland
Testis
Epididymus
Scrotum
Urethral orifice

√5ᵗʰ 600.2 Benign localized hyperplasia of prostate
Adenofibromatous hypertrophy of prostate
Adenoma of prostate
Fibroadenoma of prostate
Fibroma of prostate
Myoma of prostate
Polyp of prostate
EXCLUDES benign neoplasms of prostate (222.2)
hypertrophy of prostate (600.00-600.01)
malignant neoplasm of prostate (185)
DEF: Benign localized hyperplasia clearly defined epithelial tumor.
AHA: 4Q, '06, 93-95; 4Q, '03, 63

600.20 Benign localized hyperplasia of prostate without urinary obstruction and other lower urinary tract symptoms [LUTS] A ♂
Benign localized hyperplasia of prostate NOS

600.21 Benign localized hyperplasia of prostate with urinary obstruction and other lower urinary tract symptoms [LUTS] A ♂
Benign localized hyperplasia of prostate with urinary retention
Use additional code to identify symptoms:
  incomplete bladder emptying (788.21)
  nocturia (788.43)
  straining on urination (788.65)
  urinary frequency (788.41)
  urinary hesitancy (788.64)
  urinary incontinence (788.30-788.39)
  urinary obstruction (599.69)
  urinary retention (788.20)
  urinary urgency (788.63)
  weak urinary stream (788.62)

600.3 Cyst of prostate A ♂
DEF: Sacs of fluid, which differentiate this from either nodular or adenomatous tumors.

√5ᵗʰ 600.9 Hyperplasia of prostate, unspecified
Median bar
Prostatic obstruction NOS
AHA: 4Q, '06, 93-95; 4Q, '03, 63

600.90 Hyperplasia of prostate, unspecified, without urinary obstruction and other lower urinary tract symptoms [LUTS] A ♂
Hyperplasia of prostate NOS

600.91 Hyperplasia of prostate, unspecified with urinary obstruction and other lower urinary tract symptoms [LUTS] A ♂
Hyperplasia of prostate, unspecified, with urinary retention
Use additional code to identify symptoms:
  incomplete bladder emptying (788.21)
  nocturia (788.43)
  straining on urination (788.65)
  urinary frequency (788.41)
  urinary hesitancy (788.64)
  urinary incontinence (788.30-788.39)
  urinary obstruction (599.69)
  urinary retention (788.20)
  urinary urgency (788.63)
  weak urinary stream (788.62)

√4ᵗʰ 601 Inflammatory diseases of prostate
Use additional code to identify organism, such as Staphylococcus (041.1), or Streptococcus (041.0)

601.0 Acute prostatitis A ♂

601.1 Chronic prostatitis A ♂

601.2 Abscess of prostate A ♂

601.3 Prostatocystitis A ♂

601.4 *Prostatitis in diseases classified elsewhere* 🅰 ♂

Code first underlying disease, as:
actinomycosis (039.8)
blastomycosis (116.0)
syphilis (095.8)
tuberculosis (016.5)
EXCLUDES *prostatitis:*
gonococcal (098.12, 098.32)
monilial (112.2)
trichomonal (131.03)

601.8 **Other specified inflammatory diseases of prostate** 🅰 ♂

Prostatitis:
cavitary
diverticular
granulomatous

601.9 **Prostatitis, unspecified** 🅰 ♂

Prostatitis NOS

✓4ᵗʰ 602 **Other disorders of prostate**

602.0 **Calculus of prostate** 🅰 ♂

Prostatic stone
DEF: Stone or mineral deposit in prostate.

602.1 **Congestion or hemorrhage of prostate** 🅰 ♂

DEF: Bleeding or fluid collection in prostate.

602.2 **Atrophy of prostate** 🅰 ♂

602.3 **Dysplasia of prostate** ♂

Prostatic intraepithelial neoplasia I (PIN I)
Prostatic intraepithelial neoplasia II (PIN II)
EXCLUDES *prostatic intraepithelial neoplasia III (PIN III) (233.4)*
DEF: Abnormality of shape and size of the intraepithelial tissues of the prostate; premalignant condition characterized by stalks and absence of a basilar cell layer; synonyms are intraductal dysplasia, large acinar atypical hyperplasia, atypical primary hyperplasia, hyperplasia with malignant changes, marked atypia, or duct-acinar dysplasia.
AHA: 4Q, '01, 46

602.8 **Other specified disorders of prostate** 🅰 ♂

Fistula ⎫
Infarction ⎬ of prostate
Stricture ⎭
Periprostatic adhesions

602.9 **Unspecified disorder of prostate** 🅰 ♂

✓4ᵗʰ 603 **Hydrocele**

INCLUDES hydrocele of spermatic cord, testis or tunica vaginalis
EXCLUDES *congenital (778.6)*
DEF: Circumscribed collection of fluid in tunica vaginalis, spermatic cord or testis.

603.0 **Encysted hydrocele** ♂

603.1 **Infected hydrocele** ♂

Use additional code to identify organism

603.8 **Other specified types of hydrocele** ♂

603.9 **Hydrocele, unspecified** ♂

✓4ᵗʰ 604 **Orchitis and epididymitis**

Use additional code to identify organism, such as Escherichia coli [E. coli] (041.4), Staphylococcus (041.1), or Streptococcus (041.0)

604.0 **Orchitis, epididymitis, and epididymo-orchitis, with abscess** ♂

Abscess of epididymis or testis

✓5ᵗʰ 604.9 **Other orchitis, epididymitis, and epididymo-orchitis, without mention of abscess**

604.90 **Orchitis and epididymitis, unspecified** ♂

604.91 *Orchitis and epididymitis in diseases classified elsewhere* ♂

Code first underlying disease, as:
diphtheria (032.89)
filariasis (125.0-125.9)
syphilis (095.8)
EXCLUDES *orchitis:*
gonococcal (098.13, 098.33)
mumps (072.0)
tuberculous (016.5)
tuberculous epididymitis (016.4)

604.99 **Other** ♂

605 **Redundant prepuce and phimosis** ♂

Adherent prepuce
Paraphimosis
Phimosis (congenital)
Tight foreskin
DEF: Constriction of preputial orifice causing inability of the prepuce to be drawn back over the glans; it may be congenital or caused by infection.
AHA: 3Q, '08, 9

✓4ᵗʰ 606 **Infertility, male**

AHA: 2Q, '96, 9

606.0 **Azoospermia** 🅰 ♂

Absolute infertility
Infertility due to:
germinal (cell) aplasia
spermatogenic arrest (complete)
DEF: Absence of spermatozoa in the semen or inability to produce spermatozoa.

606.1 **Oligospermia** 🅰 ♂

Infertility due to:
germinal cell desquamation
hypospermatogenesis
incomplete spermatogenic arrest
DEF: Insufficient number of sperm in semen.

606.8 **Infertility due to extratesticular causes** 🅰 ♂

Infertility due to:
drug therapy
infection
obstruction of efferent ducts
radiation
systemic disease

606.9 **Male infertility, unspecified** 🅰 ♂

✓4ᵗʰ 607 **Disorders of penis**

EXCLUDES *phimosis (605)*

607.0 **Leukoplakia of penis** ♂

Kraurosis of penis
EXCLUDES *carcinoma in situ of penis (233.5)*
erythroplasia of Queyrat (233.5)
DEF: White, thickened patches on glans penis.

607.1 **Balanoposthitis** ♂

Balanitis
Use additional code to identify organism
DEF: Inflammation of glans penis and prepuce.

607.2 **Other inflammatory disorders of penis** ♂

Abscess ⎫
Boil ⎬ of corpus cavernosum or
Carbuncle ⎥ penis
Cellulitis ⎭
Cavernitis (penis)
Use additional code to identify organism
EXCLUDES *herpetic infection (054.13)*

Common Inguinal Canal Anomalies

Peritoneal cavity
Normal anatomy
Vas deferens
Obliterated process vaginalis
Tunica vaginalis
Testis
Scrotal hernia
Inguinal hernia
Hydrocele of the cord
Communicating hydrocele
Hydrocele of tunica vaginalis

607.3 Priapism ♂

Painful erection

DEF: Prolonged penile erection without sexual stimulation.

√5th 607.8 Other specified disorders of penis

607.81 Balanitis xerotica obliterans ♂

Induratio penis plastica

DEF: Inflammation of the glans penis, caused by stricture of the opening of the prepuce.

607.82 Vascular disorders of penis ♂

Embolisim

Hematoma

(nontraumatic) } of corpus cavernosum

Hemorrhage or penis

Thrombosis

607.83 Edema of penis ♂

DEF: Fluid retention within penile tissues.

607.84 Impotence of organic origin A ♂

EXCLUDES nonorganic (302.72)

DEF: Physiological cause interfering with erection.

AHA: 3Q, '91, 11

TIP: If impotence is a result of previous radical prostatectomy, assign also 997.99.

607.85 Peyronie's disease ♂

DEF: A severe curvature of the erect penis due to fibrosis of the cavernous sheaths.

AHA: 4Q, '03, 64

607.89 Other ♂

Atrophy

Fibrosis } of corpus cavernosum or

Hypertrophy penis

Ulcer (chronic)

607.9 Unspecified disorder of penis ♂

√4th 608 Other disorders of male genital organs

608.0 Seminal vesiculitis ♂

Abscess

Cellulitis } of seminal vesicle

Vesiculitis (seminal)

Use additional code to identify organism

EXCLUDES gonococcal infection (098.14, 098.34)

DEF: Inflammation of seminal vesicle.

608.1 Spermatocele ♂

DEF: Cystic enlargement of the epididymis or the testis; the cysts contain spermatozoa.

√5th 608.2 Torsion of testis

DEF: Twisted or rotated testis; may compromise blood flow.

608.20 Torsion of testis, unspecified ♂

AHA: 4Q, '06, 95

608.21 Extravaginal torsion of spermatic cord ♂

DEF: Torsion of the spermatic cord just below the tunica vaginalis attachments.

AHA: 4Q, '06, 95

608.22 Intravaginal torsion of spermatic cord ♂

Torsion of spermatic cord NOS

DEF: Torsion within the tunica vaginalis also called the "bell-clapper" anomaly. It usually occurs in older children.

AHA: 4Q, '06, 95

Torsion of the Testis

608.23 Torsion of appendix testis ♂

DEF: Torsion of small solid projection of tissue on the upper outer surface of the testis (hydatid of Morgagni); a remnant of the embryologic Müllerian duct.

AHA: 4Q, '06, 95

608.24 Torsion of appendix epididymis ♂

DEF: Torsion of small stalked appendage of the head of the epididymis (pedunculated hydatid); a detached embryologic efferent duct.

AHA: 4Q, '06, 95

608.3 Atrophy of testis ♂

608.4 Other inflammatory disorders of male genital organs ♂

Abscess

Boil } of scrotum, spermatic cord, testis

Carbuncle [except abscess], tunica

Cellulitis vaginalis, or vas deferens

Vasitis

Use additional code to identify organism

EXCLUDES abscess of testis (604.0)

√5th 608.8 Other specified disorders of male genital organs

608.81 Disorders of male genital organs in diseases classified elsewhere ♂

Code first underlying disease, as:

filariasis (125.0-125.9)

tuberculosis (016.5)

608.82 Hematospermia ♂

DEF: Presence of blood in the ejaculate; relatively common, affecting men of any age after puberty; cause is often the result of a viral or bacterial infection and inflammation.

AHA: 4Q, '01, 46

608.83 Vascular disorders ♂

Hematoma (non-

traumatic) } of seminal vessel, spermatic

cord, testis, scrotum,

Hemorrhage tunica vaginalis, or vas

Thrombosis deferens

Hematocele NOS, male

AHA: 4Q, '03, 110

TIP: Assign for Fournier's gangrene, which is a result of an infection in the genital area.

608.84 Chylocele of tunica vaginalis ♂

DEF: Chylous effusion into tunica vaginalis; due to infusion of lymphatic fluids.

608.85 Stricture ♂

Stricture of:

spermatic cord

tunica vaginalis

vas deferens

608.86 Edema ♂

608.87 Retrograde ejaculation ♂

DEF: Condition where the semen travels to the bladder rather than out through the urethra due to damaged nerves causing the bladder neck to remain open during ejaculation.

AHA: 4Q, '01, 46

608.89 Other ♂

Atrophy } of seminal vessel, spermatic

Fibrosis cord, testis, scrotum,

Hypertrophy tunica vaginalis, or vas

Ulcer deferens

EXCLUDES atrophy of testis (608.3)

608.9 Unspecified disorder of male genital organs ♂

√4th
√5th Additional Digit Required   Unspecified Code   Other Specified Code   Manifestation Code   ►◄ Revised Text   ● New Code   ▲ Revised Code Title

2011 ICD-9-CM   **Volume 1 – 185**

Diseases of the Genitourinary System

610–614.0

Disorders of Breast (610-612)

✓4ᵗʰ **610 Benign mammary dysplasias**

610.0 Solitary cyst of breast
Cyst (solitary) of breast

610.1 Diffuse cystic mastopathy   A
Chronic cystic mastitis
Cystic breast
Fibrocystic disease of
breast
DEF: Extensive formation of nodular cysts in breast tissue; symptoms include tenderness, change in size and hyperplasia of ductal epithelium.
AHA: 2Q, '06, 10
TIP: Assign in addition to screening mammography V code; is a normal variant, commonly found in normal breasts and not a pathological condition.

610.2 Fibroadenosis of breast
Fibroadenosis of breast:
NOS
chronic
cystic
diffuse
periodic
segmental
DEF: Non-neoplastic nodular condition of breast.

610.3 Fibrosclerosis of breast
DEF: Fibrous tissue in breast.

610.4 Mammary duct ectasia
Comedomastitis
Duct ectasia
Mastitis:
periductal
plasma cell
DEF: Atrophy of duct epithelium; causes distended collecting ducts of mammary gland, drying up of breast secretion, intraductal inflammation and periductal and interstitial chronic inflammatory reaction.

610.8 Other specified benign mammary dysplasias
Mazoplasia
Sebaceous cyst of breast
AHA: 2Q, '09, 9

610.9 Benign mammary dysplasia, unspecified

✓4ᵗʰ **611 Other disorders of breast**
EXCLUDES *that associated with lactation or the puerperium (675.0-676.9)*

611.0 Inflammatory disease of breast
Abscess (acute) (chronic) (nonpuerperal) of:
areola
breast
Mammillary fistula
Mastitis (acute) (subacute) (nonpuerperal):
NOS
infective
retromammary
submammary
EXCLUDES *carbuncle of breast (680.2)*
chronic cystic mastitis (610.1)
neonatal infective mastitis (771.5)
thrombophlebitis of breast [Mondor's disease] (451.89)

611.1 Hypertrophy of breast
Gynecomastia
Hypertrophy of breast:
NOS
massive pubertal
EXCLUDES *breast engorgement in newborn (778.7)*
disproportion of reconstructed breast (612.1)

611.2 Fissure of nipple

611.3 Fat necrosis of breast
Fat necrosis (segmental) of breast
Code first breast necrosis due to breast graft (996.79)
DEF: Splitting of neutral fats in adipose tissue cells as a result of trauma; a firm circumscribed mass is then formed in the breast.

611.4 Atrophy of breast

611.5 Galactocele
DEF: Milk-filled cyst in breast due to blocked duct.

611.6 Galactorrhea not associated with childbirth
DEF: Flow of milk not associated with childbirth or pregnancy.

✓5ᵗʰ **611.7 Signs and symptoms in breast**

611.71 Mastodynia
Pain in breast

611.72 Lump or mass in breast
AHA: ▶4Q, '09, 106;◀ 2Q, '03, 4-5
TIP: Do not assign if the underlying cause of the breast lump or mass is determined and documented during the episode of care.

611.79 Other
Induration of breast
Inversion of nipple
Nipple discharge
Retraction of nipple

✓5ᵗʰ **611.8 Other specified disorders of breast**
AHA: 4Q, '08, 121-122

611.81 Ptosis of breast   A
EXCLUDES *ptosis of native breast in relation to reconstructed breast (612.1)*

611.82 Hypoplasia of breast   A
Micromastia
EXCLUDES *congenital absence of breast (757.6)*
hypoplasia of native breast in relation to reconstructed breast (612.1)

611.83 Capsular contracture of breast implant   A
TIP: Do not assign additional code from category 996 Complications peculiar to certain specified procedures.

611.89 Other specified disorders of breast
Hematoma (nontraumatic) of breast
Infarction of breast
Occlusion of breast duct
Subinvolution of breast (postlactational) (postpartum)

611.9 Unspecified breast disorder

✓4ᵗʰ **612 Deformity and disproportion of reconstructed breast**
AHA: 4Q, '08, 123

612.0 Deformity of reconstructed breast   A
Contour irregularity in reconstructed breast
Excess tissue in reconstructed breast
Misshapen reconstructed breast

612.1 Disproportion of reconstructed breast   A
Breast asymmetry between native breast and reconstructed breast
Disproportion between native breast and reconstructed breast

Inflammatory Disease of Female Pelvic Organs (614-616)

Use additional code to identify organism, such as Staphylococcus (041.1), or Streptococcus (041.0)
EXCLUDES *that associated with pregnancy, abortion, childbirth, or the puerperium (630-676.9)*

✓4ᵗʰ **614 Inflammatory disease of ovary, fallopian tube, pelvic cellular tissue, and peritoneum**
EXCLUDES *endometritis (615.0-615.9)*
major infection following delivery (670.0-670.8)
that complicating:
abortion (634-638 with .0, 639.0)
ectopic or molar pregnancy (639.0)
pregnancy or labor (646.6)

614.0 Acute salpingitis and oophoritis   ♀
Any condition classifiable to 614.2, specified as acute or subacute
DEF: Acute inflammation of ovary and fallopian tube.

N Newborn Age: 0   P Pediatric Age: 0-17   M Maternity Age: 12-55   A Adult Age: 15-124

614.1 Chronic salpingitis and oophoritis ♀
   Hydrosalpinx
   Salpingitis:
      follicularis
      isthmica nodosa
   Any condition classifiable to 614.2, specified as chronic
   DEF: Persistent inflammation of ovary and fallopian tube.

614.2 Salpingitis and oophoritis not specified as acute, subacute, or chronic ♀
   Abscess (of):
      fallopian tube
      ovary
      tubo-ovarian
   Oophoritis
   Perioophoritis
   Perisalpingitis
   Pyosalpinx
   Salpingitis
   Salpingo-oophoritis
   Tubo-ovarian inflammatory disease
   EXCLUDES *gonococcal infection (chronic) (098.37)*
      acute (098.17)
      tuberculous (016.6)
   AHA: 2Q, '91, 5

614.3 Acute parametritis and pelvic cellulitis ♀
   Acute inflammatory pelvic disease
   Any condition classifiable to 614.4, specified as acute
   DEF: Parametritis: inflammation of the parametrium; pelvic cellulitis is a synonym for parametritis.

614.4 Chronic or unspecified parametritis and pelvic cellulitis ♀
   Abscess (of):
      broad ligament
      parametrium   ⎫
      pelvis, femal   ⎬ chronic or NOS
      pouch of Douglas   ⎭
   Chronic inflammatory pelvic disease
   Pelvic cellulitis, female
   EXCLUDES *tuberculous (016.7)*

614.5 Acute or unspecified pelvic peritonitis, female ♀
   AHA: 4Q, '05, 74
   TIP: For pelvic peritonitis in a male patient, refer to code 567.21.

614.6 Pelvic peritoneal adhesions, female (postoperative) (postinfection) ♀
   Adhesions:
      peritubal
      tubo-ovarian
   Use additional code to identify any associated infertility (628.2)
   DEF: Fibrous scarring abnormally joining structures within abdomen.
   AHA: 3Q, '03, 6; 1Q, '03, 4; 3Q, '95, 7; 3Q, '94, 12
   N73.6 Female pelvic peritoneal adhesions (postinfective) `I-10`

614.7 Other chronic pelvic peritonitis, female ♀
   EXCLUDES *tuberculous (016.7)*

614.8 Other specified inflammatory disease of female pelvic organs and tissues ♀

614.9 Unspecified inflammatory disease of female pelvic organs and tissues ♀
   Pelvic infection or inflammation, female NOS
   Pelvic inflammatory disease [PID]

`√4ᵗʰ` **615 Inflammatory diseases of uterus, except cervix**
   EXCLUDES *following delivery (670.0-670.8)*
      hyperplastic endometritis (621.30-621.35)
      that complicating:
         abortion (634-638 with .0, 639.0)
         ectopic or molar pregnancy (639.0)
         pregnancy or labor (646.6)

615.0 Acute ♀
   Any condition classifiable to 615.9, specified as acute or subacute

615.1 Chronic ♀
   Any condition classifiable to 615.9, specified as chronic

615.9 Unspecified inflammatory disease of uterus ♀
   Endometritis   Myometritis
   Endomyometritis   Perimetritis
   Intrauterine infection   Pyometra
   Metritis   Uterine abscess
   N71.9 Inflammatory disease of uterus unspecified `I-10`

`√4ᵗʰ` **616 Inflammatory disease of cervix, vagina, and vulva**
   EXCLUDES *that complicating:*
      abortion (634-638 with .0, 639.0)
      ectopic or molar pregnancy (639.0)
      pregnancy, childbirth, or the puerperium (646.6)

616.0 Cervicitis and endocervicitis ♀
   Cervicitis   ⎫ with or without mention of
   Endocervicitis   ⎬   erosion or ectropion
   Nabothian (gland) cyst or follicle
   EXCLUDES *erosion or ectropion without mention of cervicitis (622.0)*
   N72 Inflammatory disease of cervix uteri `I-10`

`√5ᵗʰ` **616.1 Vaginitis and vulvovaginitis**
   EXCLUDES *vulvar vestibulitis (625.71)*
   DEF: Inflammation or infection of vagina or external female genitalia.

   616.10 Vaginitis and vulvovaginitis, unspecified ♀
      Vaginitis:
         NOS
         postirradiation
      Vulvitis NOS
      Vulvovaginitis NOS
      Use additional code to identify organism, such as Escherichia coli [E. coli] (041.4), Staphylococcus (041.1), or Streptococcus (041.0)
      EXCLUDES *noninfective leukorrhea (623.5)*
         postmenopausal or senile vaginitis (627.3)

   616.11 Vaginitis and vulvovaginitis in diseases classified elsewhere ♀
      Code first underlying disease, as:
         pinworm vaginitis (127.4)
      EXCLUDES *herpetic vulvovaginitis (054.11)*
         monilial vulvovaginitis (112.1)
         trichomonal vaginitis or vulvovaginitis (131.01)

616.2 Cyst of Bartholin's gland ♀
   Bartholin's duct cyst
   DEF: Fluid-filled sac within gland of vaginal orifice.

616.3 Abscess of Bartholin's gland ♀
   Vulvovaginal gland abscess

616.4 Other abscess of vulva ♀
   Abscess   ⎫
   Carbuncle ⎬ of vulva
   Furuncle   ⎭

`√5ᵗʰ` **616.5 Ulceration of vulva**

   616.50 Ulceration of vulva, unspecified ♀
      Ulcer NOS of vulva

   616.51 Ulceration of vulva in diseases classified elsewhere ♀
      Code first underlying disease, as:
         Behçet's syndrome (136.1)
         tuberculosis (016.7)
      EXCLUDES *vulvar ulcer (in):*
         gonococcal (098.0)
         herpes simplex (054.12)
         syphilitic (091.0)

Diseases of the Genitourinary System

616.8–618.1

✓5ᵗʰ **616.8 Other specified inflammatory diseases of cervix, vagina, and vulva**

> **EXCLUDES** *noninflammatory disorders of:*
> *cervix (622.0-622.9)*
> *vagina (623.0-623.9)*
> *vulva (624.0-624.9)*

616.81 Mucositis (ulcerative) of cervix, vagina, and vulva ♀

> Use additional E code to identify adverse effects of therapy, such as:
> antineoplastic and immunosuppressive drugs (E930.7, E933.1)
> radiation therapy (E879.2)
> **AHA:** 4Q, '06, 88-90

616.89 Other inflammatory disease of cervix, vagina and vulva ♀

> Caruncle, vagina or labium
> Ulcer, vagina
> **AHA:** 4Q, '06, 88-90

616.9 Unspecified inflammatory disease of cervix, vagina, and vulva ♀

Other Disorders of Female Genital Tract (617-629)

✓4ᵗʰ **617 Endometriosis**

617.0 Endometriosis of uterus ♀

> Adenomyosis
> Endometriosis:
>> cervix
>> internal
>> myometrium
>
> **EXCLUDES** *stromal endometriosis (236.0)*
> **DEF:** Aberrant uterine mucosal tissue; creating products of menses and inflamed uterine tissues.
> **AHA:** 3Q, '92, 7
> **N80.0** Endometriosis of uterus   `I-10`

617.1 Endometriosis of ovary ♀

> Chocolate cyst of ovary
> Endometrial cystoma of ovary
> **DEF:** Aberrant uterine tissue; creating products of menses and inflamed ovarian tissues.
> **N80.1** Endometriosis of ovary   `I-10`

617.2 Endometriosis of fallopian tube ♀

> **DEF:** Aberrant uterine tissue; creating products of menses and inflamed tissues of fallopian tubes.

617.3 Endometriosis of pelvic peritoneum ♀

> Endometriosis:
>> broad ligament
>> cul-de-sac (Douglas')
>> parametrium
>> round ligament
>
> **DEF:** Aberrant uterine tissue; creating products of menses and inflamed peritoneum tissues.

617.4 Endometriosis of rectovaginal septum and vagina ♀

> **DEF:** Aberrant uterine tissue; creating products of menses and inflamed tissues in and behind vagina.

617.5 Endometriosis of intestine ♀

> Endometriosis: Endometriosis:
>> appendix   rectum
>> colon
>
> **DEF:** Aberrant uterine tissue; creating products of menses and inflamed intestinal tissues.

617.6 Endometriosis in scar of skin ♀

617.8 Endometriosis of other specified sites ♀

> Endometriosis: Endometriosis:
>> bladder   umbilicus
>> lung   vulva

617.9 Endometriosis, site unspecified ♀

Female Genitourinary System

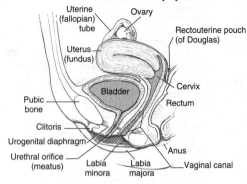

Common Sites of Endometriosis

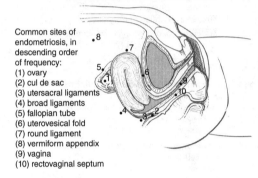

Common sites of endometriosis, in descending order of frequency:
(1) ovary
(2) cul de sac
(3) utersacral ligaments
(4) broad ligaments
(5) fallopian tube
(6) uterovesical fold
(7) round ligament
(8) vermiform appendix
(9) vagina
(10) rectovaginal septum

✓4ᵗʰ **618 Genital prolapse**

> Use additional code to identify urinary incontinence (625.6, 788.31, 788.33-788.39)
> **EXCLUDES** *that complicating pregnancy, labor, or delivery (654.4)*

✓5ᵗʰ **618.0 Prolapse of vaginal walls without mention of uterine prolapse**

> **EXCLUDES** *that with uterine prolapse (618.2-618.4)*
> *enterocele (618.6)*
> *vaginal vault prolapse following hysterectomy (618.5)*

618.00 Unspecified prolapse of vaginal walls ♀

> Vaginal prolapse NOS

618.01 Cystocele, midline ♀

> Cystocele NOS
> **DEF:** Defect in the pubocervical fascia, the supportive layer of the bladder, causing bladder drop and herniated into the vagina along the midline.
> **N81.11** Cystocele midline   `I-10`

618.02 Cystocele, lateral ♀

> Paravaginal
> **DEF:** Loss of support of the lateral attachment of the vagina at the arcus tendinous results in bladder drop; bladder herniates into the vagina laterally.

618.03 Urethrocele ♀

618.04 Rectocele ♀

> Proctocele
> ▶Use additional code for associated fecal incontinence (787.60-787.63)◀
> **N81.6** Rectocele   `I-10`

618.05 Perineocele ♀

618.09 Other prolapse of vaginal walls without mention of uterine prolapse ♀

> Cystourethrocele

618.1 Uterine prolapse without mention of vaginal wall prolapse ♀

> Descensus uteri   Uterine prolapse:
> Uterine prolapse: first degree
>> NOS   second degree
>> complete   third degree
>
> **EXCLUDES** *that with mention of cystocele, urethrocele, or rectocele (618.2-618.4)*

Ⓝ Newborn Age: 0   Ⓟ Pediatric Age: 0-17   Ⓜ Maternity Age: 12-55   Ⓐ Adult Age: 15-124

Vaginal Midline Cystocele

Vaginal Lateral Cystocele

Types of Vaginal Hernias

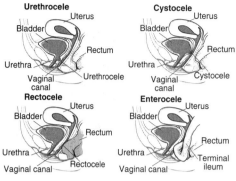

618.2 Uterovaginal prolapse, incomplete   ♀
  DEF: Downward displacement of uterus downward into vagina.
  N81.2 Incomplete uterovaginal prolapse   I-10

618.3 Uterovaginal prolapse, complete   ♀
  DEF: Downward displacement of uterus exposed within external genitalia.

618.4 Uterovaginal prolapse, unspecified   ♀
  N81.4 Uterovaginal prolapse unspecified   I-10

618.5 Prolapse of vaginal vault after hysterectomy   ♀
  N99.3 Prolapse of vaginal vault after hysterectomy   I-10

618.6 Vaginal enterocele, congenital or acquired   ♀
  Pelvic enterocele, congenital or acquired
  DEF: Vaginal vault hernia formed by the loop of the small intestine protruding into the rectal vaginal pouch; can also accompany uterine prolapse or follow hysterectomy.
  N81.5 Vaginal enterocele   I-10

618.7 Old laceration of muscles of pelvic floor   ♀

✓5ᵗʰ **618.8 Other specified genital prolapse**

  618.81 Incompetence or weakening of pubocervical tissue   ♀

  618.82 Incompetence or weakening of rectovaginal tissue   ♀

  618.83 Pelvic muscle wasting   ♀
    Disuse atrophy of pelvic muscles and anal sphincter

  618.84 Cervical stump prolapse   ♀
    AHA: 4Q, '06, 97

  618.89 Other specified genital prolapse   ♀

618.9 Unspecified genital prolapse   ♀

✓4ᵗʰ **619 Fistula involving female genital tract**
  EXCLUDES vesicorectal and intestinovesical fistula (596.1)

  619.0 Urinary-genital tract fistula, female   ♀
    Fistula: Fistula:
      cervicovesical   uteroureteric
      ureterovaginal   uterovesical
      urethrovaginal   vesicocervicovaginal
      urethrovesicovaginal   vesicovaginal

  619.1 Digestive-genital tract fistula, female   ♀
    Fistula: Fistula:
      intestinouterine   rectovulval
      intestinovaginal   sigmoidovaginal
      rectovaginal   uterorectal

  619.2 Genital tract-skin fistula, female   ♀
    Fistula:
      uterus to abdominal wall
      vaginoperineal

  619.8 Other specified fistulas involving female genital tract   ♀
    Fistula:
      cervix
      cul-de-sac (Douglas')
      uterus
      vagina
    DEF: Abnormal communication between female reproductive tract and skin.

  619.9 Unspecified fistula involving female genital tract   ♀

✓4ᵗʰ **620 Noninflammatory disorders of ovary, fallopian tube, and broad ligament**
  EXCLUDES hydrosalpinx (614.1)

  620.0 Follicular cyst of ovary   ♀
    Cyst of graafian follicle
    DEF: Fluid-filled, encapsulated cyst due to occluded follicle duct that secretes hormones into ovaries.
    N83.0 Follicular cyst of ovary   I-10

  620.1 Corpus luteum cyst or hematoma   ♀
    Corpus luteum hemorrhage or rupture
    Lutein cyst
    DEF: Fluid-filled cyst due to serous developing from corpus luteum or clotted blood.
    N83.1 Corpus luteum cyst   I-10

  620.2 Other and unspecified ovarian cyst   ♀
    Cyst:
      NOS
      corpus albicans
      retention NOS   } of ovary
      serous
      theca-lutein
    Simple cystoma of ovary
    EXCLUDES cystadenoma (benign) (serous) (220)
                developmental cysts (752.0)
                neoplastic cysts (220)
                polycystic ovaries (256.4)
                Stein-Leventhal syndrome (256.4)
    N83.20 Unspecified ovarian cysts   I-10

  620.3 Acquired atrophy of ovary and fallopian tube   ♀
    Senile involution of ovary

  620.4 Prolapse or hernia of ovary and fallopian tube   ♀
    Displacement of ovary and fallopian tube
    Salpingocele

  620.5 Torsion of ovary, ovarian pedicle, or fallopian tube   ♀
    Torsion:
      accessory tube
      hydatid of Morgagni

  620.6 Broad ligament laceration syndrome   ♀
    Masters-Allen syndrome

  620.7 Hematoma of broad ligament   ♀
    Hematocele, broad ligament
    DEF: Blood within peritoneal fold that supports uterus.

Diseases of the Genitourinary System

620.8–622.2

Uterus and Ovaries

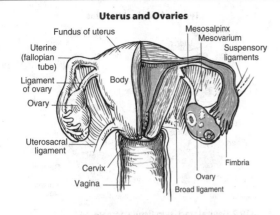

620.8 Other noninflammatory disorders of ovary, fallopian tube, and broad ligament ♀

Cyst   } of broad ligament or
Polyp   }   fallopian tube

Infarction   } of ovary or fallopian tube
Rupture   }
Hematosalpinx

EXCLUDES *hematosalpinx in ectopic pregnancy (639.2)*
peritubal adhesions (614.6)
torsion of ovary, ovarian pedicle, or fallopian tube (620.5)

620.9 Unspecified noninflammatory disorder of ovary, fallopian tube, and broad ligament ♀

✓4ᵗʰ 621 Disorders of uterus, not elsewhere classified

621.0 Polyp of corpus uteri ♀

Polyp:
  endometrium
  uterus NOS

EXCLUDES *cervical polyp NOS (622.7)*

N84.0 Polyp of corpus uteri   **I-10**

621.1 Chronic subinvolution of uterus ♀

EXCLUDES *puerperal (674.8)*

DEF: Abnormal size of uterus after delivery; the uterus does not return to its normal size after the birth of a child.

AHA: 1Q, '91, 11

621.2 Hypertrophy of uterus ♀

Bulky or enlarged uterus

EXCLUDES *puerperal (674.8)*

✓5ᵗʰ 621.3 Endometrial hyperplasia

DEF: Abnormal cystic overgrowth of endometrial tissue.

621.30 Endometrial hyperplasia, unspecified ♀

Endometrial hyperplasia NOS
Hyperplasia (adenomatous) (cystic) (glandular) of endometrium
Hyperplastic endometritis

621.31 Simple endometrial hyperplasia without atypia ♀

EXCLUDES *benign endometrial hyperplasia (621.34)*

621.32 Complex endometrial hyperplasia without atypia ♀

EXCLUDES *benign endometrial hyperplasia (621.34)*

621.33 Endometrial hyperplasia with atypia ♀

EXCLUDES *endometrial intraepithelial neoplasia [EIN] (621.35)*

621.34 Benign endometrial hyperplasia ♀

DEF: Excessive cell growth of the endometrium due to primary hormonal changes (menopause) that result in secondary effects to the endometrial stroma and associated structures.

AHA: 4Q, '09, 95-96

621.35 Endometrial intraepithelial neoplasia [EIN] ♀

EXCLUDES *malignant neoplasm of endometrium with endometrial intraepithelial neoplasia [EIN] (182.0)*

DEF: Abnormal premalignant neoplastic changes of the endometrial glands prone to malignant transformation.

AHA: 4Q, '09, 95-96

TIP: Do not confuse (EIN) with unrelated serous intraepithelial carcinoma (serous EIC), which is an early phase of (Type II) papillary serous adenocarcinoma of the endometrium.

621.4 Hematometra ♀

Hemometra

EXCLUDES *that in congenital anomaly ▶(752.2-752.39)◀*

DEF: Accumulated blood in uterus.

621.5 Intrauterine synechiae ♀

Adhesions of uterus   Band(s) of uterus

621.6 Malposition of uterus ♀

Anteversion
Retroflexion   } of uterus
Retroversion

EXCLUDES *malposition complicating pregnancy, labor, or delivery (654.3-654.4)*
prolapse of uterus (618.1-618.4)

621.7 Chronic inversion of uterus ♀

EXCLUDES *current obstetrical trauma (665.2)*
prolapse of uterus (618.1-618.4)

621.8 Other specified disorders of uterus, not elsewhere classified ♀

Atrophy, acquired
Cyst
Fibrosis NOS   } of uterus
Old laceration (postpartum)
Ulcer

EXCLUDES *bilharzial fibrosis (120.0-120.9)*
endometriosis (617.0)
fistulas (619.0-619.8)
inflammatory diseases (615.0-615.9)

621.9 Unspecified disorder of uterus ♀

✓4ᵗʰ 622 Noninflammatory disorders of cervix

EXCLUDES *abnormality of cervix complicating pregnancy, labor, or delivery (654.5-654.6)*
fistula (619.0-619.8)

622.0 Erosion and ectropion of cervix ♀

Eversion   } of cervix
Ulcer   }

EXCLUDES *that in chronic cervicitis (616.0)*

DEF: Ulceration or turning outward of uterine cervix.

✓5ᵗʰ 622.1 Dysplasia of cervix (uteri)

EXCLUDES *abnormal results from cervical cytologic examination without histologic confirmation (795.00-795.09)*
carcinoma in situ of cervix (233.1)
cervical intraepithelial neoplasia III [CIN III] (233.1)
HGSIL of cervix (795.04)

DEF: Abnormal cell structures in portal between uterus and vagina.

AHA: 1Q, '91, 11

622.10 Dysplasia of cervix, unspecified ♀

Anaplasia of cervix   Cervical dysplasia NOS
Cervical atypism

622.11 Mild dysplasia of cervix ♀

Cervical intraepithelial neoplasia I [CIN I]

622.12 Moderate dysplasia of cervix ♀

Cervical intraepithelial neoplasia II [CIN II]

EXCLUDES *carcinoma in situ of cervix (233.1)*
cervical intraepithelial neoplasia III [CIN III] (233.1)
severe dysplasia (233.1)

622.2 Leukoplakia of cervix (uteri) ♀

EXCLUDES *carcinoma in situ of cervix (233.1)*

DEF: Thickened, white patches on portal between uterus and vagina.

622.3 Old laceration of cervix ♀
Adhesions
Band(s)   } of cervix
Cicatrix (postpartum)
EXCLUDES *current obstetrical trauma (665.3)*
DEF: Scarring or other evidence of old wound on cervix.

622.4 Stricture and stenosis of cervix ♀
Atresia (acquired)
Contracture   } of cervix
Occlusion
Pinpoint os uteri
EXCLUDES *congenital (752.49)*
that complicating labor (654.6)

622.5 Incompetence of cervix ♀
EXCLUDES *complicating pregnancy (654.5)*
that affecting fetus or newborn (761.0)
DEF: Inadequate functioning of cervix; marked by abnormal widening during pregnancy; causing miscarriage.

622.6 Hypertrophic elongation of cervix ♀
DEF: Overgrowth of cervix tissues extending down into vagina.

622.7 Mucous polyp of cervix ♀
Polyp NOS of cervix
EXCLUDES *adenomatous polyp of cervix (219.0)*

622.8 Other specified noninflammatory disorders of cervix ♀
Atrophy (senile)
Cyst   } of cervix
Fibrosis
Hemorrhage
EXCLUDES *endometriosis (617.0)*
fistula (619.0-619.8)
inflammatory diseases (616.0)

622.9 Unspecified noninflammatory disorder of cervix ♀

√4ᵗʰ **623 Noninflammatory disorders of vagina**
EXCLUDES *abnormality of vagina complicating pregnancy, labor, or delivery (654.7)*
congenital absence of vagina (752.49)
congenital diaphragm or bands (752.49)
fistulas involving vagina (619.0-619.8)

623.0 Dysplasia of vagina ♀
Mild and moderate dysplasia of vagina
Vaginal intraepithelial neoplasia I and II [VAIN I and II]
EXCLUDES *abnormal results from vaginal cytological examination without histologic confirmation (795.10-795.19)*
carcinoma in situ of vagina (233.31)
HGSIL of vagina (795.14)
severe dysplasia of vagina (233.31)
vaginal intraepithelial neoplasia III [VAIN III] (233.31)

623.1 Leukoplakia of vagina ♀
DEF: Thickened white patches on vaginal canal.

623.2 Stricture or atresia of vagina ♀
Adhesions (postoperative) (postradiation) of vagina
Occlusion of vagina
Stenosis, vagina
Use additional E code to identify any external cause
EXCLUDES *congenital atresia or stricture (752.49)*

623.3 Tight hymenal ring ♀
Rigid hymen
Tight hymenal ring } acquired or congenital
Tight introitus
EXCLUDES *imperforate hymen (752.42)*

623.4 Old vaginal laceration ♀
EXCLUDES *old laceration involving muscles of pelvic floor (618.7)*
DEF: Scarring or other evidence of old wound on vagina.

623.5 Leukorrhea, not specified as infective ♀
Leukorrhea NOS of vagina
Vaginal discharge NOS
EXCLUDES *trichomonal (131.00)*
DEF: Viscid whitish discharge from vagina.

623.6 Vaginal hematoma ♀
EXCLUDES *current obstetrical trauma (665.7)*

623.7 Polyp of vagina ♀

623.8 Other specified noninflammatory disorders of vagina ♀
Cyst   } of vagina
Hemorrhage

623.9 Unspecified noninflammatory disorder of vagina ♀

√4ᵗʰ **624 Noninflammatory disorders of vulva and perineum**
EXCLUDES *abnormality of vulva and perineum complicating pregnancy, labor, or delivery (654.8)*
condyloma acuminatum (078.11)
fistulas involving:
perineum — see Alphabetic Index
vulva (619.0-619.8)
vulval varices (456.6)
vulvar involvement in skin conditions (690-709.9)

√5ᵗʰ **624.0 Dystrophy of vulva**
EXCLUDES *carcinoma in situ of vulva (233.32)*
severe dysplasia of vulva (233.32)
vulvar intraepithelial neoplasia III [VIN III] (233.32)
AHA: 4Q, '07, 90

624.01 Vulvar intraepithelial neoplasia I [VIN I] ♀
Mild dysplasia of vulva

624.02 Vulvar intraepithelial neoplasia II [VIN II] ♀
Moderate dysplasia of vulva
AHA: 4Q, '07, 91

624.09 Other dystrophy of vulva ♀
Kraurosis of vulva
Leukoplakia of vulva

624.1 Atrophy of vulva ♀

624.2 Hypertrophy of clitoris ♀
EXCLUDES *that in endocrine disorders (255.2, 256.1)*

624.3 Hypertrophy of labia ♀
Hypertrophy of vulva NOS
DEF: Overgrowth of fleshy folds on either side of vagina.

624.4 Old laceration or scarring of vulva ♀
DEF: Scarring or other evidence of old wound on external female genitalia.

624.5 Hematoma of vulva ♀
EXCLUDES *that complicating delivery (664.5)*
DEF: Blood in tissue of external genitalia.

624.6 Polyp of labia and vulva ♀

624.8 Other specified noninflammatory disorders of vulva and perineum ♀
Cyst
Edema   } of vulva
Stricture
AHA: 1Q, '03, 13; 1Q, '95, 8

624.9 Unspecified noninflammatory disorder of vulva and perineum ♀

√4ᵗʰ **625 Pain and other symptoms associated with female genital organs**

625.0 Dyspareunia ♀
EXCLUDES *psychogenic dyspareunia (302.76)*
DEF: Difficult or painful sexual intercourse.

625.1 Vaginismus ♀
Colpospasm
Vulvismus
EXCLUDES *psychogenic vaginismus (306.51)*
DEF: Vaginal spasms; due to involuntary contraction of musculature; prevents intercourse.

625.2 Mittelschmerz ♀
Intermenstrual pain
Ovulation pain
DEF: Pain occurring between menstrual periods.

625.3 Dysmenorrhea ♀
Painful menstruation
EXCLUDES *psychogenic dysmenorrhea (306.52)*
AHA: 2Q, '94, 12
N94.6 Dysmenorrhea unspecified   I-10

Diseases of the Genitourinary System

622.3–625.3

625.4 Premenstrual tension syndromes ♀
Menstrual molimen
Premenstrual dysphoric disorder
Premenstrual syndrome
Premenstrual tension NOS
　　EXCLUDES *menstrual migraine (346.4)*
　　AHA: 4Q, '03, 116

625.5 Pelvic congestion syndrome ♀
Congestion-fibrosis syndrome
Taylor's syndrome
　　DEF: Excessive accumulation of blood in vessels of pelvis; may occur
　　after orgasm; causes abnormal menstruation, lower back pain and
　　vaginal discharge.

625.6 Stress incontinence, female ♀
　　EXCLUDES *mixed incontinence (788.33)*
　　　　　　stress incontinence, male (788.32)
　　DEF: Involuntary leakage of urine due to insufficient sphincter
　　control; occurs upon sneezing, laughing, coughing, sudden
　　movement or lifting.
　　N39.3 Stress incontinence(female) (male)　　I-10

√5ᵗʰ **625.7 Vulvodynia**
　　DEF: Vulvar pain without an identifiable cause that persists for three
　　months or longer.
　　AHA: 4Q, '08, 124

　　625.70 Vulvodynia, unspecified ♀
　　　　Vulvodynia NOS

　　625.71 Vulvar vestibulitis ♀

　　625.79 Other vulvodynia ♀

625.8 Other specified symptoms associated with ♀
female genital organs
　　AHA: N-D, '85, 16

625.9 Unspecified symptom associated with female ♀
genital organs
　　AHA: 4Q, '06, 110
　　R39.8 Oth symptoms & signs involv genitourinary system　　I-10

√4ᵗʰ **626 Disorders of menstruation and other abnormal bleeding from**
female genital tract
　　EXCLUDES *menopausal and premenopausal bleeding (627.0)*
　　　　　　pain and other symptoms associated with menstrual cycle
　　　　　　(625.2-625.4)
　　　　　　postmenopausal bleeding (627.1)
　　　　　　▶*precocious puberty (259.1)*◄

626.0 Absence of menstruation ♀
　　Amenorrhea (primary) (secondary)

626.1 Scanty or infrequent menstruation ♀
　　Hypomenorrhea　Oligomenorrhea

626.2 Excessive or frequent menstruation ♀
　　Heavy periods　　　　Menorrhagia
　　Menometrorrhagia　　Plymenorrhea
　　EXCLUDES *premenopausal (627.0)*
　　　　　　that in puberty (626.3)
　　N92.0 Excess & frequent menstruation w/regular cycle　　I-10

626.3 Puberty bleeding ♀
　　Excessive bleeding associated with onset of menstrual
　　　　periods
　　Pubertal menorrhagia

626.4 Irregular menstrual cycle ♀
　　Irregular:　　　　Irregular:
　　　bleeding NOS　　　periods
　　　menstruation

626.5 Ovulation bleeding ♀
　　Regular intermenstrual bleeding

626.6 Metrorrhagia ♀
　　Bleeding unrelated to menstrual cycle
　　Irregular intermenstrual bleeding

626.7 Postcoital bleeding ♀
　　DEF: Bleeding from vagina after sexual intercourse.

626.8 Other ♀
　　Dysfunctional or functional uterine hemorrhage NOS
　　Menstruation:
　　　retained
　　　suppression of
　　N92.5 Other specified irregular menstruation　　I-10

626.9 Unspecified ♀

√4ᵗʰ **627 Menopausal and postmenopausal disorders**
　　EXCLUDES *asymptomatic age-related (natural) postmenopausal status*
　　　　　　(V49.81)

627.0 Premenopausal menorrhagia ♀
　　Excessive bleeding associated with onset of menopause
　　Menorrhagia:
　　　climacteric
　　　menopausal
　　　preclimacteric

627.1 Postmenopausal bleeding ♀
　　N95.0 Postmenopausal bleeding　　I-10

627.2 Symptomatic menopausal or female climacteric states ♀
　　Symptoms, such as flushing, sleeplessness, headache, lack
　　　of concentration, associated with the menopause

627.3 Postmenopausal atrophic vaginitis ♀
　　Senile (atrophic) vaginitis

627.4 Symptomatic states associated with artificial ♀
menopause
　　Postartificial menopause syndromes
　　Any condition classifiable to 627.1, 627.2, or 627.3 which
　　　follows induced menopause
　　DEF: Conditions arising after hysterectomy.

627.8 Other specified menopausal and postmenopausal ♀
disorders
　　EXCLUDES *premature menopause NOS (256.31)*

627.9 Unspecified menopausal and postmenopausal ♀
disorder

√4ᵗʰ **628 Infertility, female**
　　INCLUDES primary and secondary sterility
　　DEF: Infertility: inability to conceive for at least one year with regular
　　intercourse.
　　DEF: Primary infertility: occurring in patients who have never conceived.
　　DEF: Secondary infertility: occurring in patients who have previously
　　conceived.
　　AHA: 2Q, '96, 9; 1Q, '95, 7

628.0 Associated with anovulation ♀
　　Anovulatory cycle
　　Use additional code for any associated Stein-Leventhal
　　　syndrome (256.4)

628.1 Of pituitary-hypothalamic origin ♀
　　Code first underlying cause, as:
　　　adiposogenital dystrophy (253.8)
　　　anterior pituitary disorder (253.0-253.4)

628.2 Of tubal origin ♀
　　Infertility associated with congenital anomaly of tube
　　Tubal:
　　　block
　　　occlusion
　　　stenosis
　　Use additional code for any associated peritubal adhesions
　　　(614.6)

628.3 Of uterine origin ♀
　　Infertility associated with congenital anomaly of uterus
　　Nonimplantation
　　Use additional code for any associated tuberculous
　　　endometritis (016.7)

628.4 Of cervical or vaginal origin ♀
　　Infertility associated with:
　　　anomaly of cervical mucus
　　　congenital structural anomaly
　　　dysmucorrhea

628.8 Of other specified origin ♀

628.9 Of unspecified origin ♀

N Newborn Age: 0　　P Pediatric Age: 0-17　　M Maternity Age: 12-55　　A Adult Age: 15-124

☑4ᵗʰ **629 Other disorders of female genital organs**

629.0 Hematocele, female, not elsewhere classified   ♀

  EXCLUDES *hematocele or hematoma:*
        broad ligament (620.7)
        fallopian tube (620.8)
        that associated with ectopic pregnancy
            (633.00-633.91)
        uterus (621.4)
        vagina (623.6)
        vulva (624.5)

629.1 Hydrocele, canal of Nuck   ♀
    Cyst of canal of Nuck (acquired)
      EXCLUDES *congenital (752.41)*

☑5ᵗʰ **629.2 Female genital mutilation status**
    Female circumcision status
    Female genital cutting
    AHA: 4Q, '04, 88

  629.20 Female genital mutilation status, unspecified   ♀
      Female genital cutting status, unspecified
      Female genital mutilation status NOS

  629.21 Female genital mutilation Type I status   ♀
      Clitorectomy status
      Female genital cutting Type I status
      DEF: Female genital mutilation involving clitorectomy, with
      part or all of the clitoris removed.

  629.22 Female genital mutilation Type II status   ♀
      Clitorectomy with excision of labia
            minora status
      Female genital cutting Type II status
      DEF: Female genital mutilation involving clitoris and the
      labia minora amputation.
      AHA: 4Q, '04, 90

  629.23 Female genital mutilation Type III status   ♀
      Female genital cutting Type III status
      Infibulation status
      DEF: Female genital mutilation involving removal, most or
      all of the labia minora excised, labia majora incised which is
      then made into a hood of skin over the urethral and vaginal
      opening.
      AHA: 4Q, '04, 90

  629.29 Other female genital mutilation status   ♀
      Female genital cutting Type IV status
      Female genital mutilation Type IV status
      Other female genital cutting status
      AHA: 4Q, '06, 97

☑5ᵗʰ **629.8 Other specified disorders of female genital organs**

  ▲ **629.81 Recurrent pregnancy loss without current**   ♀
            pregnancy
      EXCLUDES ▶*recurrent pregnancy loss with current*
                  pregnancy (646.3)◀
      AHA: 4Q, '06, 98

  629.89 Other specified disorders of female   ♀
            genital organs
      AHA: 4Q, '06, 98

629.9 Unspecified disorder of female genital organs   ♀

11. Complications of Pregnancy, Childbirth, and the Puerperium (630-679)

Ectopic and Molar Pregnancy (630-633)

Use additional code from category 639 to identify any complications

630 Hydatidiform mole   M♀
Trophoblastic disease NOS
Vesicular mole

EXCLUDES   chorioadenoma (destruens) (236.1)
chorionepithelioma (181)
malignant hydatidiform mole (236.1)

DEF: Abnormal product of pregnancy; marked by mass of cysts resembling bunch of grapes due to chorionic villi proliferation, and dissolution; must be surgically removed.

631 Other abnormal product of conception   M♀
Blighted ovum
Mole:
   NOS
   carneous
   fleshy
   stone

632 Missed abortion   M♀
Early fetal death before completion of 22 weeks' gestation with retention of dead fetus
Retained products of conception, not following spontaneous or induced abortion or delivery

EXCLUDES   failed induced abortion (638.0-638.9)
fetal death (intrauterine) (late) (656.4)
missed delivery (656.4)
that with abnormal product of conception (630, 631)

AHA: 1Q, '01, 5
002.1 Missed abortion   I-10

✓4ᵗʰ 633 Ectopic pregnancy
INCLUDES   ruptured ectopic pregnancy
DEF: Fertilized egg develops outside uterus.
AHA: 4Q, '02, 61

✓5ᵗʰ 633.0 Abdominal pregnancy
Intraperitoneal pregnancy

633.00 Abdominal pregnancy without intrauterine pregnancy   M♀

633.01 Abdominal pregnancy with intrauterine pregnancy   M♀

✓5ᵗʰ 633.1 Tubal pregnancy
Fallopian pregnancy
Rupture of (fallopian) tube due to pregnancy
Tubal abortion
AHA: 2Q, '90, 27

633.10 Tubal pregnancy without intrauterine pregnancy   M♀
    000.1 Tubal pregnancy   I-10

633.11 Tubal pregnancy with intrauterine pregnancy   M♀

✓5ᵗʰ 633.2 Ovarian pregnancy

633.20 Ovarian pregnancy without intrauterine pregnancy   M♀

633.21 Ovarian pregnancy with intrauterine pregnancy   M♀

✓5ᵗʰ 633.8 Other ectopic pregnancy
Pregnancy:
   cervical
   combined
   cornual
   intraligamentous
   mesometric
   mural

633.80 Other ectopic pregnancy without intrauterine pregnancy   M♀

633.81 Other ectopic pregnancy with intrauterine pregnancy   M♀

✓5ᵗʰ 633.9 Unspecified ectopic pregnancy

633.90 Unspecified ectopic pregnancy without intrauterine pregnancy   M♀

633.91 Unspecified ectopic pregnancy with intrauterine pregnancy   M♀

Other Pregnancy with Abortive Outcome (634-639)

The following fourth-digit subdivisions are for use with categories 634-638:

.0 Complicated by genital tract and pelvic infection
Endometritis
Salpingo-oophoritis
Sepsis NOS
Septicemia NOS
Any condition classifiable to 639.0 with condition classifiable to 634-638
   EXCLUDES   urinary tract infection (634-638 with .7)

.1 Complicated by delayed or excessive hemorrhage
Afibrinogenemia
Defibrination syndrome
Intravascular hemolysis
Any condition classifiable to 639.1 with condition classifiable to 634-638

.2 Complicated by damage to pelvic organs and tissues
Laceration, perforation, or tear of:
   bladder
   uterus
Any condition classifiable to 639.2 with condition classifiable to 634-638

.3 Complicated by renal failure
Oliguria
Uremia
Any condition classifiable to 639.3, with condition classifiable to 634-638

.4 Complicated by metabolic disorder
Electrolyte imbalance with conditions classfiable to 634-638

.5 Complicated by shock
Circulatory collapse
Shock (postoperative) (septic)
Any condition classifiable to 639.5 with condition classifiable to 634-638

.6 Complicated by embolism
Embolism:
   NOS
   amniotic fluid
   pulmonary
Any condition classifiable to 639.6, with condition classifiable to 634-638

.7 With other specified complications
Cardiac arrest or failure
Urinary tract infection
Any condition classiable to 639.8 with condition classifiable to 634-638

.8 With unspecified complication
.9 Without mention of complication

§ ✓4ᵗʰ 634 Spontaneous abortion

Requires fifth-digit to identify stage:
   0 unspecified
   1 incomplete
   2 complete

INCLUDES   miscarriage
        spontaneous abortion
DEF: Spontaneous premature expulsion of the products of conception from the uterus.
AHA: 2Q, '91, 16

§§ ✓5ᵗʰ 634.0 Complicated by genital tract and pelvic infection   M♀
[0-2]

§§ ✓5ᵗʰ 634.1 Complicated by delayed or excessive hemorrhage   M♀
[0-2]   **AHA:** For Code 634.11: 1Q, '03, 6

§§ ✓5ᵗʰ 634.2 Complicated by damage to pelvic organs or tissues   M♀
[0-2]

§§ ✓5ᵗʰ 634.3 Complicated by renal failure   M♀
[0-2]

§§ ✓5ᵗʰ 634.4 Complicated by metabolic disorder   M♀
[0-2]

§§ ✓5ᵗʰ 634.5 Complicated by shock   M♀
[0-2]

§§ ✓5ᵗʰ 634.6 Complicated by embolism   M♀
[0-2]

---

§   See beginning of section 634-639 for fourth-digit definitions.
§§   Requires fifth digit. Valid digits are in [brackets] under each code. See appropriate category for codes and definitions.

✓4ᵗʰ ✓5ᵗʰ Additional Digit Required   Unspecified Code   Other Specified Code   Manifestation Code   ▶◀ Revised Text   ● New Code   ▲ Revised Code Title

Ectopic Pregnancy Sites

§§ √5ᵗʰ **634.7 With other specified complications** Ⓜ♀
[0-2]

§§ √5ᵗʰ **634.8 With unspecified complication** Ⓜ♀
[0-2]

§§ √5ᵗʰ **634.9 Without mention of complication** Ⓜ♀
[0-2]

§ √4ᵗʰ **635 Legally induced abortion**

Requires fifth-digit to identify stage:
  0 unspecified
  1 incomplete
  2 complete

INCLUDES abortion or termination of pregnancy:
  elective
  legal
  therapeutic

EXCLUDES *menstrual extraction or regulation (V25.3)*

DEF: Intentional expulsion of products of conception from uterus performed by medical professionals inside boundaries of law.
AHA: 2Q, '94, 14

§§ √5ᵗʰ **635.0 Complicated by genital tract and pelvic infection** Ⓜ♀
[0-2]

§§ √5ᵗʰ **635.1 Complicated by delayed or excessive hemorrhage** Ⓜ♀
[0-2]

§§ √5ᵗʰ **635.2 Complicated by damage to pelvic organs or tissues** Ⓜ♀
[0-2]

§§ √5ᵗʰ **635.3 Complicated by renal failure** Ⓜ♀
[0-2]

§§ √5ᵗʰ **635.4 Complicated by metabolic disorder** Ⓜ♀
[0-2]

§§ √5ᵗʰ **635.5 Complicated by shock** Ⓜ♀
[0-2]

§§ √5ᵗʰ **635.6 Complicated by embolism** Ⓜ♀
[0-2]

§§ √5ᵗʰ **635.7 With other specified complications** Ⓜ♀
[0-2]

§§ √5ᵗʰ **635.8 With unspecified complication** Ⓜ♀
[0-2]

§§ √5ᵗʰ **635.9 Without mention of complication** Ⓜ♀
[0-2]   AHA: For code 635.92: 2Q, '94, 14

§ √4ᵗʰ **636 Illegally induced abortion**

Requires fifth-digit to identify stage:
  0 unspecified
  1 incomplete
  2 complete

INCLUDES abortion:
  criminal
  illegal
  self-induced

DEF: Intentional expulsion of products of conception from uterus; outside boundaries of law.

§§ √5ᵗʰ **636.0 Complicated by genital tract and pelvic infection** Ⓜ♀
[0-2]

§§ √5ᵗʰ **636.1 Complicated by delayed or excessive hemorrhage** Ⓜ♀
[0-2]

§§ √5ᵗʰ **636.2 Complicated by damage to pelvic organs or tissues** Ⓜ♀
[0-2]

§§ √5ᵗʰ **636.3 Complicated by renal failure** Ⓜ♀
[0-2]

§§ √5ᵗʰ **636.4 Complicated by metabolic disorder** Ⓜ♀
[0-2]

§§ √5ᵗʰ **636.5 Complicated by shock** Ⓜ♀
[0-2]

§§ √5ᵗʰ **636.6 Complicated by embolism** Ⓜ♀
[0-2]

§§ √5ᵗʰ **636.7 With other specified complications** Ⓜ♀
[0-2]

§§ √5ᵗʰ **636.8 With unspecified complication** Ⓜ♀
[0-2]

§§ √5ᵗʰ **636.9 Without mention of complication** Ⓜ♀
[0-2]

§ √4ᵗʰ **637 Unspecified abortion**

Requires fifth-digit to identify stage:
  0 unspecified
  1 incomplete
  2 complete

INCLUDES abortion NOS
  retained products of conception following abortion, not classifiable elsewhere

§§ √5ᵗʰ **637.0 Complicated by genital tract and pelvic infection** Ⓜ♀
[0-2]

§§ √5ᵗʰ **637.1 Complicated by delayed or excessive hemorrhage** Ⓜ♀
[0-2]

§§ √5ᵗʰ **637.2 Complicated by damage to pelvic organs or tissues** Ⓜ♀
[0-2]

§§ √5ᵗʰ **637.3 Complicated by renal failure** Ⓜ♀
[0-2]

§§ √5ᵗʰ **637.4 Complicated by metabolic disorder** Ⓜ♀
[0-2]

§§ √5ᵗʰ **637.5 Complicated by shock** Ⓜ♀
[0-2]

§§ √5ᵗʰ **637.6 Complicated by embolism** Ⓜ♀
[0-2]

§§ √5ᵗʰ **637.7 With other specified complications** Ⓜ♀
[0-2]

§§ √5ᵗʰ **637.8 With unspecified complication** Ⓜ♀
[0-2]

§§ √5ᵗʰ **637.9 Without mention of complication** Ⓜ♀
[0-2]

§ √4ᵗʰ **638 Failed attempted abortion**

INCLUDES failure of attempted induction of (legal) abortion
EXCLUDES *incomplete abortion (634.0-637.9)*
DEF: Continued pregnancy despite an attempted legal abortion.

638.0 Complicated by genital tract and pelvic infection Ⓜ♀

638.1 Complicated by delayed or excessive hemorrhage Ⓜ♀

638.2 Complicated by damage to pelvic organs or tissues Ⓜ♀

638.3 Complicated by renal failure Ⓜ♀

638.4 Complicated by metabolic disorder Ⓜ♀

638.5 Complicated by shock Ⓜ♀

638.6 Complicated by embolism Ⓜ♀

638.7 With other specified complications Ⓜ♀

638.8 With unspecified complication Ⓜ♀

638.9 Without mention of complication Ⓜ♀

§ See beginning of section 634-639 for fourth-digit definitions.
§§ Requires fifth digit. Valid digits are in [brackets] under each code. See appropriate category for codes and definitions.

Ⓝ Newborn Age: 0   Ⓟ Pediatric Age: 0-17   Ⓜ Maternity Age: 12-55   Ⓐ Adult Age: 15-124

☑4ᵗʰ **639 Complications following abortion and ectopic and molar pregnancies**

NOTE This category is provided for use when it is required to classify separately the complications classifiable to the fourth-digit level in categories 634-638; for example:

a) when the complication itself was responsible for an episode of medical care, the abortion, ectopic or molar pregnancy itself having been dealt with at a previous episode

b) when these conditions are immediate complications of ectopic or molar pregnancies classifiable to 630-633 where they cannot be identified at fourth-digit level.

639.0 Genital tract and pelvic infection   Ⓜ♀

Endometritis
Parametritis
Pelvic peritonitis
Salpingitis   } following conditions classifiable to 630-638
Salpingo-oophoritis
Sepsis NOS
Septicemia NOS

EXCLUDES urinary tract infection (639.8)

639.1 Delayed or excessive hemorrhage   Ⓜ♀

Afibrinogenemia   } following conditions
Defibrination syndrome   classfiable to
Intravascular   630-638

639.2 Damage to pelvic organs and tissues   Ⓜ♀
Laceration, perforation, or tear of:

bladder
bowel
broad ligament
cervix   } following conditions classifiable to 630-638
periurethral tissue
uterus
vagina

639.3 Kidney failure   Ⓜ♀

Oliguria
Renal (kidney):
  failure (acute)   } following conditions
  shutdown   classifiable to
  tubular necrosis   630-638
Uremia

639.4 Metabolic disorders   Ⓜ♀
Electrolyte imbalance following conditions classifiable to 630-638

639.5 Shock   Ⓜ♀

Circulatory collapse   } following conditions
Shock (postoperative)   classifiable to
  (septic)   630-638

639.6 Embolism   Ⓜ♀
Embolism:

NOS
air
amniotic fluid
blood-clot
fat   } following conditions classifiable to 630-638
pulmonary
pyemic
septic
soap

639.8 Other specified complications following abortion or ectopic and molar pregnancy   Ⓜ♀

Acute yellow atrophy
  or necrosis of
  liver   } following conditons classifiable to 630-638
Cardiac arrest or failure
Cerebral anoxia
Urinary tract infection

639.9 Unspecified complication following abortion or ectopic and molar pregnancy   Ⓜ♀

Complication(s) not further specified following conditions classifiable to 630-638

Complications Mainly Related to Pregnancy (640-649)

INCLUDES the listed conditions even if they arose or were present during labor, delivery, or the puerperium

AHA: 2Q, '90, 11

The following fifth-digit subclassification is for use with categories 640-649 to denote the current episode of care. Valid fifth-digits are in [brackets] under each code.

0 unspecified as to episode of care or not applicable

1 delivered, with or without mention of antepartum condition
Antepartum condition with delivery
Delivery NOS (with mention of antepartum complication during current episode of care)
Intrapartum obstetric condition (with mention of antepartum complication during current episode of care)
Pregnancy, delivered (with mention of antepartum complication during current episode of care)

2 delivered, with mention of postpartum complication
Delivery with mention of puerperal complication during current episode of care

3 antepartum condition or complication
Antepartum obstetric condtion, not delivered during the current episode of care

4 postpartum condition of complication
Postpartum or puerperal obstetric condition or complication following delivery that occurred:
during previous episode of care
outside hospital, with subsequent admission for observation or care

☑4ᵗʰ **640 Hemorrhage in early pregnancy**

INCLUDES hemorrhage before completion of 22 weeks' gestation

§ ☑5ᵗʰ **640.0 Threatened abortion**   Ⓜ♀
[0,1,3]   **DEF:** Bloody discharge during pregnancy; cervix may be dilated and pregnancy is threatened, but the pregnancy is not terminated.

§ ☑5ᵗʰ **640.8 Other specified hemorrhage in early pregnancy**   Ⓜ♀
[0,1,3]

§ ☑5ᵗʰ **640.9 Unspecified hemorrhage in early pregnancy**   Ⓜ♀
[0,1,3]

☑4ᵗʰ **641 Antepartum hemorrhage, abruptio placentae, and placenta previa**

§ ☑5ᵗʰ **641.0 Placenta previa without hemorrhage**   Ⓜ♀
[0,1,3]
Low impantation of placenta
Placenta previa noted: } without
  during pregnancy   hemorrhage
  before labor (and delivered
  by caesarean delivery)

DEF: Placenta implanted in lower segment of uterus; commonly causes hemorrhage in the last trimester of pregnancy.

Placenta Previa

Low (marginal) implantation   Partial placenta previa   Total placenta previa

Abruptio Placentae

Partial separation (concealed bleeding)   Partial separation (apparent hemorrhage)   Complete separation (concealed hemorrhage)

---

§ Requires fifth digit. Valid digits are in [brackets] under each code. See beginning of section 640-649 for codes and definitions.

☑4ᵗʰ / ☑5ᵗʰ Additional Digit Required   Unspecified Code   Other Specified Code   Manifestation Code   ▶◀ Revised Text   ● New Code   ▲ Revised Code Title

2011 ICD-9-CM   **Volume 1 – 197**

Complications of Pregnancy, Childbirth, and the Puerperium   641.1–643.9

§ √5ᵗʰ **641.1 Hemorrhage from placenta previa** Ⓜ♀
[0,1,3]
    Low-lying placenta ⎫
    Placenta previa ⎪
      incomplete   ⎬ NOS or with hemorrhage
      marginal   ⎪   (intrapartum)
      partial   ⎪
      total   ⎭

    EXCLUDES *hemorrhage from vasa previa (663.5)*

§ √5ᵗʰ **641.2 Premature separation of placenta** Ⓜ♀
[0,1,3]
    Ablatio placentae
    Abruptio placentae
    Accidental antepartum hemorrhage
    Couvelaire uterus
    Detachment of placenta (premature)
    Premature separation of normally implanted placenta
    DEF: Abruptio placentae: premature detachment of the placenta, characterized by shock, oliguria and decreased fibrinogen.
    045.90 Premature sep of placenta unspec, uns trimester   I-10

§ √5ᵗʰ **641.3 Antepartum hemorrhage associated** Ⓜ♀
[0,1,3] **with coagulation defects**
    Antepartum or intrapartum hemorrhage associated with:
      afibrinogenemia
      hyperfibrinolysis
      hypofibrinogenemia
    EXCLUDES *coagulation defects not associated with antepartum hemorrhage (649.3)*
    DEF: Uterine hemorrhage prior to delivery.

§ √5ᵗʰ **641.8 Other antepartum hemorrhage** Ⓜ♀
[0,1,3]
    Antepartum or intrapartum hemorrhage associated with:
      trauma
      uterine leiomyoma

§ √5ᵗʰ **641.9 Unspecified antepartum hemorrhage** Ⓜ♀
[0,1,3]
    Hemorrhage:
      antepartum NOS
      intrapartum NOS
      of pregnancy NOS

√4ᵗʰ **642 Hypertension complicating pregnancy, childbirth, and the puerperium**

§ √5ᵗʰ **642.0 Benign essential hypertension complicating** Ⓜ♀
[0-4] **pregnancy, childbirth, and the puerperium**
    Hypertension   ⎫ specified as complicating, or
      benign essential ⎪   as reason for obstetric
      chronic NOS   ⎬   care during pregnancy,
      essential   ⎪   childbirth, or the
      pre-existing NOS ⎭   puerperium
    010.02 Pre-exist essential hypertension comp childbirth   I-10

§ √5ᵗʰ **642.1 Hypertension secondary to renal disease,** Ⓜ♀
[0-4] **complicating pregnancy, childbirth, and the puerperium**
    Hypertension secondary to renal disease, specified as complicating, or as a reason for obstetric care during pregnancy, childbirth, or the puerperium

§ √5ᵗʰ **642.2 Other pre-existing hypertension complicating** Ⓜ♀
[0-4] **pregnancy, childbirth, and the puerperium**
    Hypertensive   ⎫ specified as complicating,
      chronic kidney disease ⎪   or as a reason for
      heart and chronic   ⎪   obstetric care
        kidney disease   ⎬   during pregnancy,
      heart disease   ⎪   childbirth, or the
      Malignant hypertension ⎭   puerperium

§ √5ᵗʰ **642.3 Transient hypertension of pregnancy** Ⓜ♀
[0-4]
    Gestational hypertension
    Transient hypertension, so described, in pregnancy, childbirth, or the puerperium
    AHA: 3Q, '90, 4
    013.9 Gestatnl pg-inducd HTN w/o sig protnuria uns tri   I-10

§ √5ᵗʰ **642.4 Mild or unspecified pre-eclampsia** Ⓜ♀
[0-4]
    Hypertension in pregnancy, childbirth, or the puerperium, not specified as pre-existing, with either albuminuria or edema, or both; mild or unspecified
    Pre-eclampsia:
      NOS
      mild
    Toxemia (pre-eclamptic):
      NOS
      mild
    EXCLUDES *albuminuria in pregnancy, without mention of hypertension (646.2)*
                edema in pregnancy, without mention of hypertension (646.1)
    AHA: For code 642.41: ▶4Q, '09, 153◀
    014.00 Mild pre-eclampsia unspecified trimester   I-10

§ √5ᵗʰ **642.5 Severe pre-eclampsia** Ⓜ♀
[0-4]
    Hypertension in pregnancy, childbirth, or the puerperium, not specified as pre-existing, with either albuminuria or edema, or both; specified as severe
    Pre-eclampsia, severe
    Toxemia (pre-eclamptic), severe
    AHA: N-D, '85, 3

§ √5ᵗʰ **642.6 Eclampsia** Ⓜ♀
[0-4]
    Toxemia:
      eclamptic
      with convulsions

§ √5ᵗʰ **642.7 Pre-eclampsia or eclampsia superimposed** Ⓜ♀
[0-4] **on pre-existing hypertension**
    Conditions classifiable to 642.4-642.6, with conditions classifiable to 642.0-642.2

§ √5ᵗʰ **642.9 Unspecified hypertension complicating** Ⓜ♀
[0-4] **pregnancy, childbirth, or the puerperium**
    Hypertension NOS, without mention of albuminuria or edema, complicating pregnancy, childbirth, or the puerperium
    AHA: For code 642.94: 1Q, '09, 17

√4ᵗʰ **643 Excessive vomiting in pregnancy**
    INCLUDES hyperemesis ⎫
      vomiting: ⎬ arising during pregnancy
        persistent   ⎪
        vicious   ⎭
    hyperemesis gravidarum

§ √5ᵗʰ **643.0 Mild hyperemesis gravidarum** Ⓜ♀
[0,1,3]
    Hyperemesis gravidarum, mild or unspecified, starting before the end of the 22nd week of gestation
    DEF: Detrimental vomiting and nausea.

§ √5ᵗʰ **643.1 Hyperemesis gravidarum with metabolic** Ⓜ♀
[0,1,3] **disturbance**
    Hyperemesis gravidarum, starting before the end of the 22nd week of gestation, with metabolic disturbance, such as:
      carbohydrate depletion
      dehydration
      electrolyte imbalance

§ √5ᵗʰ **643.2 Late vomiting of pregnancy** Ⓜ♀
[0,1,3]
    Excessive vomiting starting after 22 completed weeks of gestation

§ √5ᵗʰ **643.8 Other vomiting complicating pregnancy** Ⓜ♀
[0,1,3]
    Vomiting due to organic disease or other cause, specified as complicating pregnancy, or as a reason for obstetric care during pregnancy
    Use additional code to specify cause

§ √5ᵗʰ **643.9 Unspecified vomiting of pregnancy** Ⓜ♀
[0,1,3]
    Vomiting as a reason for care during pregnancy, length of gestation unspecified

---

§   Requires fifth digit. Valid digits are in [brackets] under each code. See beginning of section 640-649 for codes and definitions.

Ⓝ Newborn Age: 0   Ⓟ Pediatric Age: 0-17   Ⓜ Maternity Age: 12-55   Ⓐ Adult Age: 15-124

✓4ᵗʰ **644** **Early or threatened labor**

§ ✓5ᵗʰ **644.0** **Threatened premature labor** Ⓜ♀
[0,3]   Premature labor after 22 weeks, but before 37 completed weeks of gestation without delivery
EXCLUDES *that occurring before 22 completed weeks of gestation (640.0)*
060.00 Preterm labor without delivery unspec trimester [I-10]

§ ✓5ᵗʰ **644.1** **Other threatened labor** Ⓜ♀
[0,3]   False labor:
NOS ⎫
after 37 completed weeks ⎬ without delivery
of gestation ⎪
Threatened labor NOS ⎭

§ ✓5ᵗʰ **644.2** **Early onset of delivery** Ⓜ♀
[0,1]   Onset (spontaneous) of delivery ⎫ before 37 completed
Premature labor with onset of ⎬ weeks of
delivery ⎭ gestation
AHA: 2Q, '91, 16
TIP: Assign if an attempted termination of pregnancy results in a liveborn fetus.
060.14x0 Pt labor 3rd tri w/pt del 3rd tri not applic/uns [I-10]

✓4ᵗʰ **645** **Late pregnancy**
AHA: 4Q, '00, 43; 4Q, '91, 26

§ ✓5ᵗʰ **645.1** **Post term pregnancy** Ⓜ♀
[0,1,3]   Pregnancy over 40 completed weeks to 42 completed weeks gestation
048.0 Post-term pregnancy [I-10]

§ ✓5ᵗʰ **645.2** **Prolonged pregnancy** Ⓜ♀
[0,1,3]   Pregnancy which has advanced beyond 42 completed weeks gestation

✓4ᵗʰ **646** **Other complications of pregnancy, not elsewhere classified**
Use additional code(s) to further specify complication
AHA: 4Q, '95, 59

§ ✓5ᵗʰ **646.0** **Papyraceous fetus** Ⓜ♀
[0,1,3]   **DEF:** Fetus that dies in the second trimester of pregnancy and is retained in the uterus, with subsequent atrophy and mummification; commonly occurs in twin pregnancy, nonviable fetus becomes compressed by growth of living twin.

§ ✓5ᵗʰ **646.1** **Edema or excessive weight gain in** Ⓜ♀
[0-4] **pregnancy, without mention of hypertension**
Gestational edema
Maternal obesity syndrome
EXCLUDES *that with mention of hypertension (642.0-642.9)*

§ ✓5ᵗʰ **646.2** **Unspecified renal disease in pregnancy,** Ⓜ♀
[0-4] **without mention of hypertension**
Albuminuria ⎫ in pregnancy or the
Nephropathy NOS ⎬ puerperium, without
Renal disease NOS ⎪ mention of
Uremia ⎭ hypertension
Gestational proteinuria
EXCLUDES *that with mention of hypertension (642.0-642.9)*

▲ § ✓5ᵗʰ **646.3** **Recurrent pregnancy loss** Ⓜ♀
[0,1,3]   **EXCLUDES** *with current abortion (634.0-634.9)*
without current pregnancy (629.81)
DEF: Three or more consecutive spontaneous abortions.

§ ✓5ᵗʰ **646.4** **Peripheral neuritis in pregnancy** Ⓜ♀
[0-4]

§ ✓5ᵗʰ **646.5** **Asymptomatic bacteriuria in pregnancy** Ⓜ♀
[0-4]

§ ✓5ᵗʰ **646.6** **Infections of genitourinary tract in pregnancy** Ⓜ♀
[0-4]   Conditions classifiable to 590, 595, 597, 599.0, 616 complicating pregnancy, childbirth, or the puerperium
Conditions classifiable to 614.0-614.5, 614.7-614.9, 615 complicating pregnancy or labor
EXCLUDES *major puerperal infection (670.0-670.8)*
AHA: For code 646.63: 4Q, '04, 90
023.90 Unspec GU tract infection in pregnancy uns tri [I-10]

§ ✓5ᵗʰ **646.7** **Liver disorders in pregnancy** Ⓜ♀
[0,1,3]   Acute yellow atrophy of liver ⎫
(obstetric) (true) ⎬ of pregnancy
Icterus gravis ⎪
Necrosis of liver ⎭
EXCLUDES *hepatorenal syndrome following delivery (674.8)*
viral hepatitis (647.6)

§ ✓5ᵗʰ **646.8** **Other specified complications of pregnancy** Ⓜ♀
[0-4]   Fatigue during pregnancy
Herpes gestationis
Insufficient weight gain of pregnancy
AHA: 3Q, '98, 16; J-F, '85, 15

§ ✓5ᵗʰ **646.9** **Unspecified complication of pregnancy** Ⓜ♀
[0,1,3]

✓4ᵗʰ **647** **Infectious and parasitic conditions in the mother classifiable elsewhere, but complicating pregnancy, childbirth, or the puerperium**
INCLUDES the listed conditions when complicating the pregnant state, aggravated by the pregnancy, or when a main reason for obstetric care
Use additional code(s) to further specify complication
EXCLUDES *those conditions in the mother known or suspected to have affected the fetus (655.0-655.9)*

§ ✓5ᵗʰ **647.0** **Syphilis** Ⓜ♀
[0-4]   Conditions classifiable to 090-097

§ ✓5ᵗʰ **647.1** **Gonorrhea** Ⓜ♀
[0-4]   Conditions classifiable to 098

§ ✓5ᵗʰ **647.2** **Other venereal diseases** Ⓜ♀
[0-4]   Conditions classifiable to 099

§ ✓5ᵗʰ **647.3** **Tuberculosis** Ⓜ♀
[0-4]   Conditions classifiable to 010-018

§ ✓5ᵗʰ **647.4** **Malaria** Ⓜ♀
[0-4]   Conditions classifiable to 084

§ ✓5ᵗʰ **647.5** **Rubella** Ⓜ♀
[0-4]   Conditions classifiable to 056

§ ✓5ᵗʰ **647.6** **Other viral diseases** Ⓜ♀
[0-4]   Conditions classifiable to 042, 050-055, 057-079, 795.05, 795.15, 796.75
AHA: J-F, '85, 15
TIP: Assign when pregnant patient has any HIV-related condition or is stated to have an asymptomatic HIV infection.
098.52 Other viral diseases complicating childbirth [I-10]

§ ✓5ᵗʰ **647.8** **Other specified infectious and parasitic** Ⓜ♀
[0-4] **diseases**

§ ✓5ᵗʰ **647.9** **Unspecified infection or infestation** Ⓜ♀
[0-4]

✓4ᵗʰ **648** **Other current conditions in the mother classifiable elsewhere, but complicating pregnancy, childbirth, or the puerperium**
INCLUDES the listed conditions when complicating the pregnant state, aggravated by the pregnancy, or when a main reason for obstetric care
Use additional code(s) to identify the condition
EXCLUDES *those conditions in the mother known or suspected to have affected the fetus (655.0-655.9)*

§ ✓5ᵗʰ **648.0** **Diabetes mellitus** Ⓜ♀
[0-4]   Conditions classifiable to 249, 250
EXCLUDES *gestational diabetes (648.8)*
AHA: 3Q, '91, 5, 11
024.32 Uns pre-existing diabetes mellitus in childbirth [I-10]

§ ✓5ᵗʰ **648.1** **Thyroid dysfunction** Ⓜ♀
[0-4]   Conditions classifiable to 240-246

§ ✓5ᵗʰ **648.2** **Anemia** Ⓜ♀
[0-4]   Conditions classifiable to 280-285
AHA: For Code 648.22: 1Q, '02, 14; For code 648.24: 1Q, '09, 17
TIP: Assign with fifth digit 2 for postpartum anemia.
099.013 Anemia complicating pregnancy third trimester [I-10]

---

§   Requires fifth digit. Valid digits are in [brackets] under each code. See beginning of section 640-649 for codes and definitions.

✓4ᵗʰ / ✓5ᵗʰ Additional Digit Required   Unspecified Code   Other Specified Code   Manifestation Code   ▶◀ Revised Text   ● New Code   ▲ Revised Code Title

§ ✓5ᵗʰ **648.3 Drug dependence**   Ⓜ♀
[0-4]   Conditions classifiable to 304
> AHA: 2Q, '98, 13; 4Q, '88, 8

§ ✓5ᵗʰ **648.4 Mental disorders**   Ⓜ♀
[0-4]   Conditions classifiable to 290-303, 305.0, 305.2-305.9,
     306-316, 317-319
> AHA: 2Q, '98, 13; 4Q, '95, 63

> 099.314 Alcohol use complicating childbirth   I-10

§ ✓5ᵗʰ **648.5 Congenital cardiovascular disorders**   Ⓜ♀
[0-4]   Conditions classifiable to 745-747

§ ✓5ᵗʰ **648.6 Other cardiovascular diseases**   Ⓜ♀
[0-4]   Conditions classifiable to 390-398, 410-429
> **EXCLUDES** *cerebrovascular disorders in the puerperium (674.0)*
> *peripartum cardiomyopathy (674.5)*
> *venous complications (671.0-671.9)*

> AHA: 3Q, '98, 11

§ ✓5ᵗʰ **648.7 Bone and joint disorders of back, pelvis, and**   Ⓜ♀
[0-4]   **lower limbs**
     Conditions classifiable to 720-724, and those classifiable to
     711-719 or 725-738, specified as affecting the lower
     limbs

§ ✓5ᵗʰ **648.8 Abnormal glucose tolerance**   Ⓜ♀
[0-4]   Conditions classifiable to 790.21-790.29
     Gestational diabetes
     Use additional code, if applicable, for associated long-term
     (current) insulin use (V58.67)
> **DEF:** Glucose intolerance arising in pregnancy, resolving at end of
> pregnancy.

> AHA: 3Q, '91, 5; **For code 648.83:** 4Q, '04, 56

> **TIP:** Do not assign if patient was diabetic before becoming pregnant;
> should never be assigned in combination with code 648.0X.

> 024.429 Gestational diab mellitus childbirth uns cntrl   I-10

§ ✓5ᵗʰ **648.9 Other current conditions classifiable elsewhere**   Ⓜ♀
[0-4]   Conditions classifiable to 440-459, 795.01-795.04, 795.06,
     795.10-795.14, 795.16, 796.70-796.74, 796.76
     Nutritional deficiencies [conditions classifiable to 260-269]
> AHA: 3Q, '06, 14; 4Q, '04, 88; N-D, '87, 10; **For code 648.91:** 1Q, '02, 14;
> **For code 648.93:** 4Q, '04, 90; **For code 648.94:** 1Q, '09, 17

> **TIP:** Assign for group B streptococcus carrier patients, along with
> code V02.51 Carrier or suspected carrier of infectious diseases.

✓4ᵗʰ **649 Other conditions or status of the mother complicating**
     pregnancy, childbirth, or the puerperium
> AHA: 4Q, '06, 99

§ ✓5ᵗʰ **649.0 Tobacco use disorder complicating pregnancy,**   Ⓜ♀
[0-4]   **childbirth, or the puerperium**
     Smoking complicating pregnancy, childbirth, or the
     puerperium
> AHA: 4Q, '06, 99

> 099.334 Smoking tobacco complicating childbirth   I-10

§ ✓5ᵗʰ **649.1 Obesity complicating pregnancy, childbirth,**   Ⓜ♀
[0-4]   **or the puerperium**
     Use additional code to identify the obesity ▶(278.00-
     278.03)◀
> AHA: 4Q, '06, 99

> 099.214 Obesity complicating childbirth   I-10

§ ✓5ᵗʰ **649.2 Bariatric surgery status complicating**   Ⓜ♀
[0-4]   **pregnancy, childbirth, or the puerperium**
     Gastric banding status complicating pregnancy, childbirth, or
     the puerperium
     Gastric bypass status for obesity complicating pregnancy,
     childbirth, or the puerperium
     Obesity surgery status complicating pregnancy, childbirth, or
     the puerperium
> AHA: 4Q, '06, 99, 118

§ ✓5ᵗʰ **649.3 Coagulation defects complicating pregnancy,**   Ⓜ♀
[0-4]   **childbirth, or the puerperium**
     Conditions classifiable to 286, 287, 289
     Use additional code to identify the specific coagulation defect
     (286.0-286.9, 287.0-287.9, 289.0-289.9)
> **EXCLUDES** *coagulation defects causing antepartum*
> *hemorrhage (641.3)*
> *postpartum coagulation defects (666.3)*

> AHA: 4Q, '06, 99

§ ✓5ᵗʰ **649.4 Epilepsy complicating pregnancy, childbirth,**   Ⓜ♀
[0-4]   **or the puerperium**
     Conditions classifiable to 345
     Use additional code to identify the specific type of epilepsy
     (345.00-345.91)
> **EXCLUDES** *eclampsia (642.6)*

> AHA: 4Q, '06, 99

§ ✓5ᵗʰ **649.5 Spotting complicating pregnancy**   Ⓜ♀
[0,1,3]   **EXCLUDES** *antepartum hemorrhage (641.0-641.9)*
> *hemorrhage in early pregnancy (640.0-640.9)*

> AHA: 4Q, '06, 99

§ ✓5ᵗʰ **649.6 Uterine size date discrepancy**   Ⓜ♀
[0-4]   **EXCLUDES** *suspected problem with fetal growth not found*
> *(V89.04)*

> AHA: 4Q, '06, 99

§ ✓5ᵗʰ **649.7 Cervical shortening**   Ⓜ♀
[0,1,3]   **EXCLUDES** *suspected cervical shortening not found (V89.05)*
> **DEF:** A cervix that has shortened to < 25 mm in length by the 16th
> week of pregnancy; warning sign for impending premature delivery;
> treated by cervical cerclage placement or progesterone.

> AHA: 4Q, '08, 124-125; **For code 649.73:** 4Q, '08, 125

Normal Delivery, and Other Indications for Care in Pregnancy, Labor, and Delivery (650-659)

The following fifth-digit subclassification is for use with categories 651-659 to
denote the current episode of care. Valid fifth-digits are in [brackets] under each
code.

   0 unspecified as to episode of care or not applicable
   1 delivered, with or without mention of antepartum condition
   2 delivered, with mention of postpartum complication
   3 antepartum condition or complication
   4 postpartum condition or complication

650 Normal delivery   Ⓜ♀
> **NOTE** Delivery requiring minimal or no assistance, with or without
> episiotomy, without fetal manipulation [e.g., rotation version]
> or instrumentation [forceps] of spontaneous, cephalic, vaginal,
> full-term, single, live-born infant. This code is for use as a single
> diagnosis code and is not to be used with any other code in the
> range 630-676.

Use additional code to indicate outcome of delivery (V27.0)
> **EXCLUDES** *breech delivery (assisted) (spontaneous) NOS (652.2)*
> *delivery by vacuum extractor, forceps, cesarean section, or*
> *breech extraction, without specified complication*
> *(669.5-669.7)*

> AHA: 2Q, '02, 10; 3Q, '01, 12; 3Q, '00, 5; 4Q, '95, 28, 59

> **TIP:** Code 650 is to be assigned only for the episode of care during which the
> patient delivers and may be assigned if the patient is admitted for induction
> of labor.

> 080 Encounter for full-term uncomplicated delivery   I-10

✓4ᵗʰ **651 Multiple gestation**
   ▶Use additional code to specify placenta status (V91.00-V91.99)◀

§ ✓5ᵗʰ **651.0 Twin pregnancy**   Ⓜ♀
[0,1,3]   **EXCLUDES** *fetal conjoined twins (678.1)*
> AHA: 3Q, '06, 16

> 030.009 Twin pregnancy unspecified, unspecified trimester   I-10

§ ✓5ᵗʰ **651.1 Triplet pregnancy**   Ⓜ♀
[0,1,3]

§ ✓5ᵗʰ **651.2 Quadruplet pregnancy**   Ⓜ♀
[0,1,3]

§ ✓5ᵗʰ **651.3 Twin pregnancy with fetal loss and retention of one**   Ⓜ♀
[0,1,3] **fetus**
     Vanishing twin syndrome (651.33)

---

§   Requires fifth digit. Valid digits are in [brackets] under each code. See beginning of section 640-649 for codes and definitions.

Ⓝ Newborn Age: 0   Ⓟ Pediatric Age: 0-17   Ⓜ Maternity Age: 12-55   Ⓐ Adult Age: 15-124

Malposition and Malpresentation

Breech

Mother's pelvis

Shoulder (arm prolapse)

Compound (extremity together with head)

Face (mentum)

Oblique

Cephalopelvic Disproportion

Pubic symphysis

Cephalopelvic disproportion due to: Contraction of pelvic inlet, or large fetus, or hydrocephalus

Ischial tuberosity

Contraction of pelvic outlet (from below)

Pubic symphysis

Pelvic inlet from above

§ ✓5ᵗʰ **651.4 Triplet pregnancy with fetal loss and retention of one** Ⓜ♀
[0,1,3] **or more fetus(es)**

§ ✓5ᵗʰ **651.5 Quadruplet pregnancy with fetal loss and retention** Ⓜ♀
[0,1,3] **of one or more fetus(es)**

§ ✓5ᵗʰ **651.6 Other multiple pregnancy with fetal loss and** Ⓜ♀
[0,1,3] **retention of one or more fetus(es)**

§ ✓5ᵗʰ **651.7 Multiple gestation following (elective)** Ⓜ♀
[0,1,3] **fetal reduction**
Fetal reduction of multiple fetuses reduced to single fetus
AHA: 3Q, '06, 18; **For code 651.71:** 4Q, '05, 81

§ ✓5ᵗʰ **651.8 Other specified multiple gestation** Ⓜ♀
[0,1,3]

§ ✓5ᵗʰ **651.9 Unspecified multiple gestation** Ⓜ♀
[0,1,3]

✓4ᵗʰ **652 Malposition and malpresentation of fetus**
Code first any associated obstructed labor (660.0)

§ ✓5ᵗʰ **652.0 Unstable lie** Ⓜ♀
[0,1,3] **DEF:** Changing fetal position.

§ ✓5ᵗʰ **652.1 Breech or other malpresentation successfully** Ⓜ♀
[0,1,3] **converted to cephalic presentation**
Cephalic version NOS

§ ✓5ᵗʰ **652.2 Breech presentation without mention of version** Ⓜ♀
[0,1,3] Breech delivery (assisted) (spontaneous) NOS
Buttocks presentation
Complete breech
Frank breech
EXCLUDES *footling presentation (652.8)*
incomplete breech (652.8)
DEF: Fetal presentation of buttocks or feet at birth canal.
032.1xx0 Maternal care breech presentation not applic/uns 【I-10】

§ ✓5ᵗʰ **652.3 Transverse or oblique presentation** Ⓜ♀
[0,1,3] Oblique lie　　　　Transverse lie
EXCLUDES *transverse arrest of fetal head (660.3)*
DEF: Delivery of fetus, shoulder first.

§ ✓5ᵗʰ **652.4 Face or brow presentation** Ⓜ♀
[0,1,3] Mentum presentation

§ ✓5ᵗʰ **652.5 High head at term** Ⓜ♀
[0,1,3] Failure of head to enter pelvic brim
032.4xx0 Maternal care high head at term not applic/uns 【I-10】

§ ✓5ᵗʰ **652.6 Multiple gestation with malpresentation** Ⓜ♀
[0,1,3] **of one fetus or more**

§ ✓5ᵗʰ **652.7 Prolapsed arm** Ⓜ♀
[0,1,3]

§ ✓5ᵗʰ **652.8 Other specified malposition or malpresentation** Ⓜ♀
[0,1,3] Compound presentation

§ ✓5ᵗʰ **652.9 Unspecified malposition or malpresentation** Ⓜ♀
[0,1,3]

✓4ᵗʰ **653 Disproportion**
Code first any associated obstructed labor (660.1)

§ ✓5ᵗʰ **653.0 Major abnormality of bony pelvis, not** Ⓜ♀
[0,1,3] **further specified**
Pelvic deformity NOS

§ ✓5ᵗʰ **653.1 Generally contracted pelvis** Ⓜ♀
[0,1,3] Contracted pelvis NOS

§ ✓5ᵗʰ **653.2 Inlet contraction of pelvis** Ⓜ♀
[0,1,3] Inlet contraction (pelvis)

§ ✓5ᵗʰ **653.3 Outlet contraction of pelvis** Ⓜ♀
[0,1,3] Outlet contraction (pelvis)

§ ✓5ᵗʰ **653.4 Fetopelvic disproportion** Ⓜ♀
[0,1,3] Cephalopelvic disproportion NOS
Disproportion of mixed maternal and fetal origin, with normally formed fetus
033.4xx0 Mtrn care dispropor mtrn & fetal orig not applic 【I-10】

§ ✓5ᵗʰ **653.5 Unusually large fetus causing disproportion** Ⓜ♀
[0,1,3] Disproportion of fetal origin with normally formed fetus
Fetal disproportion NOS
EXCLUDES *that when the reason for medical care was concern for the fetus (656.6)*

§ ✓5ᵗʰ **653.6 Hydrocephalic fetus causing disproportion** Ⓜ♀
[0,1,3] **EXCLUDES** *that when the reason for medical care was concern for the fetus (655.0)*

§ ✓5ᵗʰ **653.7 Other fetal abnormality causing disproportion** Ⓜ♀
[0,1,3] Fetal:
ascites
hydrops
myelomeningocele
sacral teratoma
tumor
EXCLUDES *conjoined twins causing disproportion (678.1)*

§ ✓5ᵗʰ **653.8 Disproportion of other origin** Ⓜ♀
[0,1,3] **EXCLUDES** *shoulder (girdle) dystocia (660.4)*

§ ✓5ᵗʰ **653.9 Unspecified disproportion** Ⓜ♀
[0,1,3]

✓4ᵗʰ **654 Abnormality of organs and soft tissues of pelvis**
INCLUDES the listed conditions during pregnancy, childbirth, or the puerperium
Code first any associated obstructed labor (660.2)
EXCLUDES *trauma to perineum and vulva complicating current delivery (664.0-664.9)*

§ ✓5ᵗʰ **654.0 Congenital abnormalities of uterus** Ⓜ♀
[0-4] Double uterus
Uterus bicornis

§ ✓5ᵗʰ **654.1 Tumors of body of uterus** Ⓜ♀
[0-4] Uterine fibroids

§ ✓5ᵗʰ **654.2 Previous cesarean delivery** Ⓜ♀
[0,1,3] Uterine scar from previous cesarean delivery
AHA: 1Q, '92, 8
034.21 Maternal care for scar from prev cesarean del 【I-10】

---

§ Requires fifth digit. Valid digits are in [brackets] under each code. See beginning of section 640-649 for codes and definitions.

✓4ᵗʰ /✓5ᵗʰ Additional Digit Required　　Unspecified Code　　Other Specified Code　　Manifestation Code　　▶◀ Revised Text　　● New Code　　▲ Revised Code Title

2011 ICD-9-CM　　　　　　　　　　　　　　　　　　　　　　　　　　　**Volume 1 – 201**

§ √5ᵗʰ **654.3 Retroverted and incarcerated gravid uterus** Ⓜ♀
[0-4]   **DEF:** Retroverted: tilted back uterus; no change in angle of longitudinal axis.
     DEF: Incarcerated: immobile, fixed uterus.

§ √5ᵗʰ **654.4 Other abnormalities in shape or position of** Ⓜ♀
[0-4]   **gravid uterus and of neighboring structures**
     Cystocele
     Pelvic floor repair
     Pendulous abdomen
     Prolapse of gravid uterus
     Rectocele
     Rigid pelvic floor

§ √5ᵗʰ **654.5 Cervical incompetence** Ⓜ♀
[0-4]   Presence of Shirodkar suture with or without mention of cervical incompetence
     DEF: Abnormal cervix; tendency to dilate in second trimester; causes premature fetal expulsion.
     DEF: Shirodkar suture: purse-string suture used to artificially close incompetent cervix.

§ √5ᵗʰ **654.6 Other congenital or acquired abnormality of cervix** Ⓜ♀
[0-4]   Cicatricial cervix
     Polyp of cervix
     Previous surgery to cervix
     Rigid cervix (uteri)
     Stenosis or stricture of cervix
     Tumor of cervix

§ √5ᵗʰ **654.7 Congenital or acquired abnormality of vagina** Ⓜ♀
[0-4]   Previous surgery to vagina
     Septate vagina
     Stenosis of vagina (acquired) (congenital)
     Stricture of vagina
     Tumor of vagina

§ √5ᵗʰ **654.8 Congenital or acquired abnormality of vulva** Ⓜ♀
[0-4]   Anal sphincter tear (healed) (old) complicating delivery
     Fibrosis of perineum
     Persistent hymen
     Previous surgery to perineum or vulva
     Rigid perineum
     Tumor of vulva
     EXCLUDES *anal sphincter tear (healed) (old) not associated with delivery (569.43)*
       varicose veins of vulva (671.1)
     AHA: 1Q, '03, 14

§ √5ᵗʰ **654.9 Other and unspecified** Ⓜ♀
[0-4]   Uterine scar NEC

√4ᵗʰ **655 Known or suspected fetal abnormality affecting management of mother**
     INCLUDES the listed conditions in the fetus as a reason for observation or obstetrical care of the mother, or for termination of pregnancy
     AHA: 3Q, '90, 4
     TIP: Only assign when the fetal condition affects the management of the mother. Assign on mother's chart when in utero procedures are performed on the fetus.

§ √5ᵗʰ **655.0 Central nervous system malformation in fetus** Ⓜ♀
[0,1,3]   Fetal or suspected fetal:
     anencephaly
     hydrocephalus
     spina bifida (with myelomeningocele)

§ √5ᵗʰ **655.1 Chromosomal abnormality in fetus** Ⓜ♀
[0,1,3]

§ √5ᵗʰ **655.2 Hereditary disease in family possibly** Ⓜ♀
[0,1,3] **affecting fetus**

§ √5ᵗʰ **655.3 Suspected damage to fetus from viral disease** Ⓜ♀
[0,1,3] **in the mother**
     Suspected damage to fetus from maternal rubella

§ √5ᵗʰ **655.4 Suspected damage to fetus from other disease in** Ⓜ♀
[0,1,3] **the mother**
     Suspected damage to fetus from maternal:
     alcohol addiction
     listeriosis
     toxoplasmosis

§ √5ᵗʰ **655.5 Suspected damage to fetus from drugs** Ⓜ♀
[0,1,3]

§ √5ᵗʰ **655.6 Suspected damage to fetus from radiation** Ⓜ♀
[0,1,3]

§ √5ᵗʰ **655.7 Decreased fetal movements** Ⓜ♀
[0,1,3]   **AHA:** 4Q, '97, 41

§ √5ᵗʰ **655.8 Other known or suspected fetal abnormality, not** Ⓜ♀
[0,1,3] **elsewhere classified**
     Suspected damage to fetus from:
     environmental toxins
     intrauterine contraceptive device
     AHA: 3Q, '06, 16, 18

§ √5ᵗʰ **655.9 Unspecified** Ⓜ♀
[0,1,3]

√4ᵗʰ **656 Other known or suspected fetal and placental problems affecting management of mother**
     EXCLUDES *fetal hematologic conditions (678.0)*
       suspected placental problems not found (V89.02)

§ √5ᵗʰ **656.0 Fetal-maternal hemorrhage** Ⓜ♀
[0,1,3]   Leakage (microscopic) of fetal blood into maternal circulation

§ √5ᵗʰ **656.1 Rhesus isoimmunization** Ⓜ♀
[0,1,3]   Anti-D [Rh] antibodies
     Rh incompatibility
     DEF: Antibodies developing against Rh factor; mother with Rh negative develops antibodies against Rh positive fetus.
     036.0190 Mtrn care anti-D Rh antibds uns tri not applic   I-10

§ √5ᵗʰ **656.2 Isoimmunization from other and unspecified** Ⓜ♀
[0,1,3] **blood-group incompatibility**
     ABO isoimmunization
     AHA: 4Q, '06, 135

§ √5ᵗʰ **656.3 Fetal distress** Ⓜ♀
[0,1,3]   Fetal metabolic acidemia
     EXCLUDES *abnormal fetal acid-base balance (656.8)*
       abnormality in fetal heart rate or rhythm (659.7)
       fetal bradycardia (659.7)
       fetal tachycardia (659.7)
       meconium in liquor (656.8)
     DEF: Life-threatening disorder; fetal anoxia, hemolytic disease and other miscellaneous diseases cause fetal distress.
     AHA: N-D, '86, 4

§ √5ᵗʰ **656.4 Intrauterine death** Ⓜ♀
[0,1,3]   Fetal death:
     NOS
     after completion of 22 weeks' gestation
     late
     Missed delivery
     EXCLUDES *missed abortion (632)*

§ √5ᵗʰ **656.5 Poor fetal growth** Ⓜ♀
[0,1,3]   "Light-for-dates"
     "Placental insufficiency"
     "Small-for-dates"
     036.5190 Mtrn care known/spct placental insuff uns tri   I-10

§ √5ᵗʰ **656.6 Excessive fetal growth** Ⓜ♀
[0,1,3]   "Large-for-dates"
     036.60x0 Mtrn care excess fetl grwth uns tri not applic   I-10

§ √5ᵗʰ **656.7 Other placental conditions** Ⓜ♀
[0,1,3]   Abnormal placenta
     Placental infarct
     EXCLUDES *placental polyp (674.4)*
       placentitis (658.4)

§ √5ᵗʰ **656.8 Other specified fetal and placental problems** Ⓜ♀
[0,1,3]   Abnormal acid-base balance
     Intrauterine acidosis
     Lithopedian
     Meconium in liquor
     Subchorionic hematoma
     DEF: Lithopedion: Calcified fetus; not expelled by mother.
     036.20x0 Mtrn care hydrops fetalis uns tri not applic/uns   I-10

§ √5ᵗʰ **656.9 Unspecified fetal and placental problem** Ⓜ♀
[0,1,3]

---

§ Requires fifth digit. Valid digits are in [brackets] under each code. See beginning of section 640-649 for codes and definitions.

Ⓝ Newborn Age: 0   Ⓟ Pediatric Age: 0-17   Ⓜ Maternity Age: 12-55   Ⓐ Adult Age: 15-124

√4ᵗʰ **657 Polyhydramnios**   Ⓜ♀
    [0,1,3]

   § √5ᵗʰ   Use 0 as fourth-digit for this category

      Hydramnios

      EXCLUDES *suspected polyhydramnios not found (V89.01)*

      DEF: Excess amniotic fluid.

      AHA: 3Q, '06, 16; 4Q, '91, 26

      040.9xx0 Polyhydraminos uns trimester not applicable/uns   I-10

√4ᵗʰ **658 Other problems associated with amniotic cavity and membranes**

      EXCLUDES *amniotic fluid embolism (673.1)*
                    suspected problems with amniotic cavity and membranes
                    not found (V89.01)

   § √5ᵗʰ **658.0 Oligohydramnios**   Ⓜ♀
     [0,1,3]   Oligohydramnios without mention of rupture of membranes

      DEF: Deficient amount of amniotic fluid.

      AHA: 3Q, '06, 16

      041.00x0 Oligohydraminos uns trimester not applicable/uns   I-10

   § √5ᵗʰ **658.1 Premature rupture of membranes**   Ⓜ♀
     [0,1,3]   Rupture of amniotic sac less than 24 hours prior
             to the onset of labor

      AHA: For code 658.13: 1Q, '01, 5; 4Q, '98, 77

      042.00 Prmat rom ool w/in 24 hrs of rup uns wks gestatn   I-10

   § √5ᵗʰ **658.2 Delayed delivery after spontaneous or**   Ⓜ♀
     [0,1,3] **unspecified rupture of membranes**
      Prolonged rupture of membranes NOS
      Rupture of amniotic sac 24 hours or more prior to the
             onset of labor

   § √5ᵗʰ **658.3 Delayed delivery after artificial rupture**   Ⓜ♀
     [0,1,3] **of membranes**

   § √5ᵗʰ **658.4 Infection of amniotic cavity**   Ⓜ♀
     [0,1,3]   Amnionitis
      Chorioamnionitis
      Membranitis
      Placentitis

      041.1090 Inf amniotic sac & memb uns, uns tri not applic/uns   I-10

   § √5ᵗʰ **658.8 Other**   Ⓜ♀
     [0,1,3]   Amnion nodosum
      Amniotic cyst

   § √5ᵗʰ **658.9 Unspecified**   Ⓜ♀
     [0,1,3]

√4ᵗʰ **659 Other indications for care or intervention related to labor and delivery, not elsewhere classified**

   § √5ᵗʰ **659.0 Failed mechanical induction**   Ⓜ♀
     [0,1,3]   Failure of induction of labor by surgical or other
             instrumental methods

   § √5ᵗʰ **659.1 Failed medical or unspecified induction**   Ⓜ♀
     [0,1,3]   Failed induction NOS
      Failure of induction of labor by medical methods,
             such as oxytocic drugs

      061.9 Failed induction of labor unspecified   I-10

   § √5ᵗʰ **659.2 Maternal pyrexia during labor, unspecified**   Ⓜ♀
     [0,1,3]   **DEF:** Fever during labor.

      075.2 Pyrexia during labor not elsewhere classified   I-10

   § √5ᵗʰ **659.3 Generalized infection during labor**   Ⓜ♀
     [0,1,3]   Septicemia during labor

   § √5ᵗʰ **659.4 Grand multiparity**   Ⓜ♀
     [0,1,3]   **EXCLUDES** *supervision only, in pregnancy (V23.3)*
                   without current pregnancy (V61.5)

      DEF: Having borne six or more children previously.

   § √5ᵗʰ **659.5 Elderly primigravida**   Ⓜ♀
     [0,1,3]   First pregnancy in a woman who will be 35 years of age or
             older at expected date of delivery

      EXCLUDES *supervision only, in pregnancy (V23.81)*

      AHA: 3Q, '01, 12

      009.519 Supervisn of elderly primigravida uns trimester   I-10

---

   § √5ᵗʰ **659.6 Elderly multigravida**   Ⓜ♀
     [0,1,3]   Second or more pregnancy in a woman who will be 35 years
             of age or older at expected date of delivery

      EXCLUDES *elderly primigravida 659.5*
                   supervision only, in pregnancy (V23.82)

      AHA: 3Q, '01, 12

      009.529 Supervisn of elderly multigravida uns trimester   I-10

   § √5ᵗʰ **659.7 Abnormality in fetal heart rate or rhythm**   Ⓜ♀
     [0,1,3]   Depressed fetal heart tones
      Fetal:
        bradycardia
        tachycardia
      Fetal heart rate decelerations
      Non-reassuring fetal heart rate or rhythm

      AHA: 4Q, '98, 48

      076 Abn in fetal heart rate & rhythm comp L&D   I-10

   § √5ᵗʰ **659.8 Other specified indications for care or**   Ⓜ♀
     [0,1,3] **intervention related to labor and delivery**
      Pregnancy in a female less than 16 years
             old at expected date of delivery
      Very young maternal age

      AHA: 3Q, '01, 12

   § √5ᵗʰ **659.9 Unspecified indication for care or intervention**   Ⓜ♀
     [0,1,3] **related to labor and delivery**

Complications Occurring Mainly in the Course of Labor and Delivery (660-669)

The following fifth-digit subclassification is for use with categories 660-669 to denote the current episode of care. Valid fifth-digits are in [brackets] under each code.
   0   **unspecified as to episode of care or not applicable**
   1   **delivered, with or without mention of antepartum condition**
   2   **delivered, with mention of postpartum complication**
   3   **antepartum condition or complication**
   4   **postpartum condition or complication**

√4ᵗʰ **660 Obstructed labor**

      AHA: 3Q, '95, 10

   § √5ᵗʰ **660.0 Obstruction caused by malposition of fetus at**   Ⓜ♀
     [0,1,3] **onset of labor**

      Any condition classifiable to 652, causing obstruction during
         labor

      Use additional code from 652.0-652.9 to identify condition

   § √5ᵗʰ **660.1 Obstruction by bony pelvis**   Ⓜ♀
     [0,1,3]   Any condition classifiable to 653, causing obstruction during
         labor

      Use additional code from 653.0-653.9 to identify condition

   § √5ᵗʰ **660.2 Obstruction by abnormal pelvic soft tissues**   Ⓜ♀
     [0,1,3]   Prolapse of anterior lip of cervix
      Any condition classifiable to 654, causing obstruction during
         labor

      Use additional code from 654.0-654.9 to identify condition

   § √5ᵗʰ **660.3 Deep transverse arrest and persistent**   Ⓜ♀
     [0,1,3] **occipitoposterior position**

      064.0xx0 Obst labor incpl rotat of fetal head not applic   I-10

   § √5ᵗʰ **660.4 Shoulder (girdle) dystocia**   Ⓜ♀
     [0,1,3]   Impacted shoulders

      DEF: Obstructed labor due to impacted fetal shoulders.

      066.0 Obstructed labor due to shoulder dystocia   I-10

   § √5ᵗʰ **660.5 Locked twins**   Ⓜ♀
     [0,1,3]

   § √5ᵗʰ **660.6 Failed trial of labor, unspecified**   Ⓜ♀
     [0,1,3]   Failed trial of labor, without mention of
             condition or suspected condition

   § √5ᵗʰ **660.7 Failed forceps or vacuum extractor,**   Ⓜ♀
     [0,1,3] **unspecified**

      Application of ventouse or forceps, without mention of
         condition

   § √5ᵗʰ **660.8 Other causes of obstructed labor**   Ⓜ♀
     [0,1,3]   Use additional code to identify condition

      AHA: 4Q, '04, 88

---

§   Requires fifth digit. Valid digits are in [brackets] under each code. See beginning of section 640-649 for codes and definitions.

√4ᵗʰ √5ᵗʰ **Additional Digit Required**   Unspecified Code   Other Specified Code   Manifestation Code   ►◄ Revised Text   ● New Code   ▲ Revised Code Title

2011 ICD-9-CM   **Volume 1 – 203**

§ ✓5ᵗʰ **660.9 Unspecified obstructed labor**   Ⓜ♀
[0,1,3]   Dystocia:
     NOS
     fetal NOS
     maternal NOS

✓4ᵗʰ **661 Abnormality of forces of labor**

§ ✓5ᵗʰ **661.0 Primary uterine inertia**   Ⓜ♀
[0,1,3]   Failure of cervical dilation
     Hypotonic uterine dysfunction, primary
     Prolonged latent phase of labor
     DEF: Lack of efficient contractions during labor causing prolonged labor.
     062.0 Primary inadequate contractions   I-10

§ ✓5ᵗʰ **661.1 Secondary uterine inertia**   Ⓜ♀
[0,1,3]   Arrested active phase of labor
     Hypotonic uterine dysfunction, secondary
     062.1 Secondary uterine inertia   I-10

§ ✓5ᵗʰ **661.2 Other and unspecified uterine inertia**   Ⓜ♀
[0,1,3]   Atony of uterus without hemorrhage
     Desultory labor
     Irregular labor
     Poor contractions
     Slow slope active phase of labor
     EXCLUDES *atony of uterus with hemorrhage (666.1)*
       postpartum atony of uterus without hemorrhage (669.8)

§ ✓5ᵗʰ **661.3 Precipitate labor**   Ⓜ♀
[0,1,3]   **DEF:** Rapid labor and delivery.

§ ✓5ᵗʰ **661.4 Hypertonic, incoordinate, or prolonged**   Ⓜ♀
[0,1,3] **uterine contractions**
     Cervical spasm
     Contraction ring (dystocia)
     Dyscoordinate labor
     Hourglass contraction of uterus
     Hypertonic uterine dysfunction
     Incoordinate uterine action
     Retraction ring (Bandl's) (pathological)
     Tetanic contractions
     Uterine dystocia NOS
     Uterine spasm

§ ✓5ᵗʰ **661.9 Unspecified abnormality of labor**   Ⓜ♀
[0,1,3]

✓4ᵗʰ **662 Long labor**

§ ✓5ᵗʰ **662.0 Prolonged first stage**   Ⓜ♀
[0,1,3]

§ ✓5ᵗʰ **662.1 Prolonged labor, unspecified**   Ⓜ♀
[0,1,3]

§ ✓5ᵗʰ **662.2 Prolonged second stage**   Ⓜ♀
[0,1,3]

§ ✓5ᵗʰ **662.3 Delayed delivery of second twin, triplet, etc.**   Ⓜ♀
[0,1,3]

✓4ᵗʰ **663 Umbilical cord complications**

§ ✓5ᵗʰ **663.0 Prolapse of cord**   Ⓜ♀
[0,1,3]   Presentation of cord
     DEF: Abnormal presentation of fetus; marked by protruding umbilical cord during labor; can cause fetal death.

§ ✓5ᵗʰ **663.1 Cord around neck, with compression**   Ⓜ♀
[0,1,3]   Cord tightly around neck
     069.1xx0 L&D comp by cord arnd neck w comprs not applic/uns   I-10

§ ✓5ᵗʰ **663.2 Other and unspecified cord entanglement,**   Ⓜ♀
[0,1,3] **with compression**
     Entanglement of cords of twins in mono-amniotic sac
     Knot in cord (with compression)

§ ✓5ᵗʰ **663.3 Other and unspecified cord entanglement,**   Ⓜ♀
[0,1,3] **without mention of compression**
     AHA: For code 663.31: 2Q, '03, 9
     069.2xx0 L&D comp by oth cord entanglement not applic/uns   I-10

§ ✓5ᵗʰ **663.4 Short cord**   Ⓜ♀
[0,1,3]

§ ✓5ᵗʰ **663.5 Vasa previa**   Ⓜ♀
[0,1,3]   **DEF:** Abnormal presentation of fetus marked by blood vessels of umbilical cord in front of fetal head.

§ ✓5ᵗʰ **663.6 Vascular lesions of cord**   Ⓜ♀
[0,1,3]   Bruising of cord
     Hematoma of cord
     Thrombosis of vessels of cord

§ ✓5ᵗʰ **663.8 Other umbilical cord complications**   Ⓜ♀
[0,1,3]   Velamentous insertion of umbilical cord

§ ✓5ᵗʰ **663.9 Unspecified umbilical cord complication**   Ⓜ♀
[0,1,3]

✓4ᵗʰ **664 Trauma to perineum and vulva during delivery**
     INCLUDES damage from instruments
       that from extension of episiotomy
     AHA: 1Q, '92, 11; N-D, '84, 10

§ ✓5ᵗʰ **664.0 First-degree perineal laceration**   Ⓜ♀
[0,1,4]   Perineal laceration, rupture, or tear involving:
     fourchette
     hymen
     labia
     skin
     vagina
     vulva
     070.0 First degree perineal laceration during delivery   I-10

§ ✓5ᵗʰ **664.1 Second-degree perineal laceration**   Ⓜ♀
[0,1,4]   Perineal laceration, rupture, or tear (following episiotomy) involving:
     pelvic floor
     perineal muscles
     vaginal muscles
     EXCLUDES *that involving anal sphincter (664.2)*
     AHA: For code 664.11: 4Q, '08, 192
     070.1 Second degree perineal laceration dur delivery   I-10

§ ✓5ᵗʰ **664.2 Third-degree perineal laceration**   Ⓜ♀
[0,1,4]   Perineal laceration, rupture, or tear (following episiotomy) involving:
     anal sphincter
     rectovaginal septum
     sphincter NOS
     EXCLUDES *anal sphincter tear during delivery not associated with third-degree perineal laceration (664.6)*
       that with anal or rectal mucosal laceration (664.3)
     070.2 Third degree perineal laceration during delivery   I-10

§ ✓5ᵗʰ **664.3 Fourth-degree perineal laceration**   Ⓜ♀
[0,1,4]   Perineal laceration, rupture, or tear as classifiable to 664.2 and involving also:
     anal mucosa
     rectal mucosa

§ ✓5ᵗʰ **664.4 Unspecified perineal laceration**   Ⓜ♀
[0,1,4]   Central laceration
     AHA: 1Q, '92, 8

§ ✓5ᵗʰ **664.5 Vulval and perineal hematoma**   Ⓜ♀
[0,1,4]   **AHA:** N-D, '84, 10

§ ✓5ᵗʰ **664.6 Anal sphincter tear complicating delivery,**   Ⓜ♀
[0,1,4] **not associated with third-degree perineal laceration**
     EXCLUDES *third-degree perineal laceration (664.2)*
     AHA: For code 664.61: 4Q, '07, 88, 90

§ ✓5ᵗʰ **664.8 Other specified trauma to perineum and vulva**   Ⓜ♀
[0,1,4] ▶Periurethral trauma◀
     AHA: For code 664.81: 4Q, '07, 125
     TIP: Assign when documentation indicates periurethral laceration only.

§ ✓5ᵗʰ **664.9 Unspecified trauma to perineum and vulva**   Ⓜ♀
[0,1,4]

---

§ Requires fifth digit. Valid digits are in [brackets] under each code. See beginning of section 640-649 for codes and definitions.

Ⓝ Newborn Age: 0   Ⓟ Pediatric Age: 0-17   Ⓜ Maternity Age: 12-55   Ⓐ Adult Age: 15-124

Perineal Lacerations

First degree
Second degree
Anus
Third degree
Fourth degree

§ ✓4ᵗʰ **665 Other obstetrical trauma**
  [INCLUDES] damage from instruments

§ ✓5ᵗʰ **665.0 Rupture of uterus before onset of labor** Ⓜ♀
  [0,1,3]

§ ✓5ᵗʰ **665.1 Rupture of uterus during labor** Ⓜ♀
  [0,1] Rupture of uterus NOS

§ ✓5ᵗʰ **665.2 Inversion of uterus** Ⓜ♀
  [0,2,4]

§ ✓5ᵗʰ **665.3 Laceration of cervix** Ⓜ♀
  [0,1,4]

§ ✓5ᵗʰ **665.4 High vaginal laceration** Ⓜ♀
  [0,1,4] Laceration of vaginal wall or sulcus without mention of perineal laceration
  071.4 Obstetric high vaginal laceration alone ⏐I-10⏐

§ ✓5ᵗʰ **665.5 Other injury to pelvic organs** Ⓜ♀
  [0,1,4] [EXCLUDES] ▶periurethral trauma (664.8)◀
  Injury to:
    bladder
    urethra
  AHA: M-A, '87, 10
  071.5 Other obstetric injury to pelvic organs ⏐I-10⏐

§ ✓5ᵗʰ **665.6 Damage to pelvic joints and ligaments** Ⓜ♀
  [0,1,4] Avulsion of inner symphyseal cartilage
  Damage to coccyx
  Separation of symphysis (pubis)
  AHA: N-D, '84, 12

§ ✓5ᵗʰ **665.7 Pelvic hematoma** Ⓜ♀
  [0,1,2,4] Hematoma of vagina

§ ✓5ᵗʰ **665.8 Other specified obstetrical trauma** Ⓜ♀
  [0-4]

§ ✓5ᵗʰ **665.9 Unspecified obstetrical trauma** Ⓜ♀
  [0-4]

✓4ᵗʰ **666 Postpartum hemorrhage**
  AHA: 1Q, '88, 14

§ ✓5ᵗʰ **666.0 Third-stage hemorrhage** ♀
  [0,2,4] Hemorrhage associated with retained, trapped, or adherent placenta
  Retained placenta NOS

§ ✓5ᵗʰ **666.1 Other immediate postpartum hemorrhage** Ⓜ♀
  [0,2,4] Atony of uterus with hemorrhage
  Hemorrhage within the first 24 hours following delivery of placenta
  Postpartum atony of uterus with hemorrhage
  Postpartum hemorrhage (atonic) NOS
  [EXCLUDES] atony of uterus without hemorrhage (661.2)
    postpartum atony of uterus without hemorrhage (669.8)
  072.1 Other immediate postpartum hemorrhage ⏐I-10⏐

§ ✓5ᵗʰ **666.2 Delayed and secondary postpartum hemorrhage** Ⓜ♀
  [0,2,4] Hemorrhage:
    after the first 24 hours following delivery
    associated with retained portions of placenta or membranes
  Postpartum hemorrhage specified as delayed or secondary
  Retained products of conception NOS, following delivery

§ ✓5ᵗʰ **666.3 Postpartum coagulation defects** Ⓜ♀
  [0,2,4] Postpartum:
    afibrinogenemia
    fibrinolysis

✓4ᵗʰ **667 Retained placenta or membranes, without hemorrhage**
  [NOTE] Requires fifth digit; valid digits are in [brackets] under each code. See beginning of section 660-669 for definitions.
  DEF: Postpartum condition resulting from failure to expel placental membrane tissues due to failed contractions of uterine wall.
  AHA: 1Q, '88, 14
  TIP: A retained placenta is one that has not separated or been expelled within one hour after completion of the second stage of labor (birth of the fetus).

§ ✓5ᵗʰ **667.0 Retained placenta without hemorrhage** Ⓜ♀
  [0,2,4] Placenta accreta
  Retained placenta:
    NOS   } without hemorrhage
    total
  073.0 Retained placenta without hemorrhage ⏐I-10⏐

§ ✓5ᵗʰ **667.1 Retained portions of placenta or** Ⓜ♀
  [0,2,4] **membranes, without hemorrhage**
  Retained products of conception following delivery, without hemorrhage

✓4ᵗʰ **668 Complications of the administration of anesthetic or other sedation in labor and delivery**
  [INCLUDES] complications arising from the administration of a general or local anesthetic, analgesic, or other sedation in labor and delivery
  [EXCLUDES] reaction to spinal or lumbar puncture (349.0)
    spinal headache (349.0)
  Use additional code(s) to further specify complication

§ ✓5ᵗʰ **668.0 Pulmonary complications** Ⓜ♀
  [0-4] Inhalation (aspiration) of
    stomach contents or
    secretions   } following anesthesia or other sedation in labor or delivery
  Mendelson's syndrome
  Pressure collapse of lung

§ ✓5ᵗʰ **668.1 Cardiac complications** Ⓜ♀
  [0-4] Cardiac arrest or failure following anesthesia or other sedation in labor and delivery

§ ✓5ᵗʰ **668.2 Central nervous system complications** Ⓜ♀
  [0-4] Cerebral anoxia following anesthesia or other sedation in labor and delivery

§ ✓5ᵗʰ **668.8 Other complications of anesthesia or** Ⓜ♀
  [0-4] **other sedation in labor and delivery**
  AHA: 2Q, '99, 9

§ ✓5ᵗʰ **668.9 Unspecified complication of anesthesia** Ⓜ♀
  [0-4] **and other sedation**

✓4ᵗʰ **669 Other complications of labor and delivery, not elsewhere classified**

§ ✓5ᵗʰ **669.0 Maternal distress** Ⓜ♀
  [0-4] Metabolic disturbance in labor and delivery

§ ✓5ᵗʰ **669.1 Shock during or following labor and delivery** Ⓜ♀
  [0-4] Obstetric shock

§ ✓5ᵗʰ **669.2 Maternal hypotension syndrome** Ⓜ♀
  [0-4] DEF: Low arterial blood pressure in mother during labor and delivery.

§ ✓5ᵗʰ **669.3 Acute kidney failure following labor and delivery** Ⓜ♀
  [0,2,4]

---

§ Requires fifth digit. Valid digits are in [brackets] under each code. See beginning of section 640-649 for codes and definitions.

✓4ᵗʰ
✓5ᵗʰ Additional Digit Required | Unspecified Code | Other Specified Code | Manifestation Code | ▶◀ Revised Text | ● New Code | ▲ Revised Code Title

Complications of Pregnancy, Childbirth, and the Puerperium

669.4–673.8

§ ✓5ᵗʰ **669.4 Other complications of obstetrical surgery and procedures** Ⓜ♀
[0-4]
Cardiac:
arrest   ⎫ following cesarean or other obstetrical
failure   ⎬ surgery or procedure, including
Cerebral anoxia ⎭ delivery NOS
EXCLUDES complications of obstetrical surgical wounds (674.1-674.3)

§ ✓5ᵗʰ **669.5 Forceps or vacuum extractor delivery without mention of indication** Ⓜ♀
[0,1]
Delivery by ventouse, without mention of indication

§ ✓5ᵗʰ **669.6 Breech extraction, without mention of indication** Ⓜ♀
[0,1]
EXCLUDES breech delivery NOS (652.2)

§ ✓5ᵗʰ **669.7 Cesarean delivery, without mention of indication** Ⓜ♀
[0,1]
AHA: For code 669.71: 1Q, '01, 11
082 Encounter for cesarean delivery w/o indication   I-10

§ ✓5ᵗʰ **669.8 Other complications of labor and delivery** Ⓜ♀
[0-4]
AHA: 4Q, '06, 135

§ ✓5ᵗʰ **669.9 Unspecified complication of labor and delivery** Ⓜ♀
[0-4]

Complications of the Puerperium (670-677)

NOTE Categories 671 and 673-676 include the listed conditions even if they occur during pregnancy or childbirth.

The following fifth-digit subclassification is for use with categories 670-676 to denote the current episode of care. Valid fifth-digits are in [brackets] under each code.

0   unspecified as to episode of care or not applicable
1   delivered, with or without mention of antepartum condition
2   delivered, with mention of postpartum complication
3   antepartum condition or complication
4   postpartum condition or complication

✓4ᵗʰ **670 Major puerperal infection**
EXCLUDES infection following abortion (639.0)
minor genital tract infection following delivery (646.6)
puerperal pyrexia NOS (672)
puerperal fever NOS (672)
puerperal pyrexia of unknown origin (672)
urinary tract infection following delivery (646.6)
DEF: Infection and inflammation following childbirth.
AHA: 4Q, '91, 26; 2Q, '91, 7

§ ✓5ᵗʰ **670.0 Major puerperal infection, unspecified** Ⓜ♀
[0,2,4]   **AHA:** For code 670.02: 3Q, '07, 8

§ ✓5ᵗʰ **670.1 Puerperal endometritis** Ⓜ♀
[0,2,4]

§ ✓5ᵗʰ **670.2 Puerperal sepsis** Ⓜ♀
[0,2,4]
Puerperal pyemia
▶Use additional code to identify severe sepsis (995.92) and any associated acute organ dysfunction, if applicable◀
AHA: For code 670.24: 4Q, '09, 98
TIP: Do not assign a code from category 038 or 995.91 Sepsis, along with a code from this subcategory. If applicable, assign additional codes to indicate severe sepsis (995.92), and any associated acute organ dysfunction.

§ ✓5ᵗʰ **670.3 Puerperal septic thrombophlebitis** Ⓜ♀
[0,2,4]

§ ✓5ᵗʰ **670.8 Other major puerperal infection** Ⓜ♀
[0,2,4]
Puerperal: Puerperal:
pelvic cellulitis   salpingitis
peritonitis

✓4ᵗʰ **671 Venous complications in pregnancy and the puerperium**
EXCLUDES personal history of venous complications prior to pregnancy, such as:
thrombophlebitis (V12.52)
thrombosis and embolism (V12.51)

§ ✓5ᵗʰ **671.0 Varicose veins of legs** Ⓜ♀
[0-4]
Varicose veins NOS
DEF: Distended, tortuous veins on legs associated with pregnancy.

§ ✓5ᵗʰ **671.1 Varicose veins of vulva and perineum** Ⓜ♀
[0-4]
DEF: Distended, tortuous veins on external female genitalia associated with pregnancy.

§ ✓5ᵗʰ **671.2 Superficial thrombophlebitis** Ⓜ♀
[0-4]
Phlebitis NOS
Thrombophlebitis (superficial)
Thrombosis NOS
▶Use additional code to identify the superficial thrombophlebitis (453.6, 453.71, 453.81)◀

§ ✓5ᵗʰ **671.3 Deep phlebothrombosis, antepartum** Ⓜ♀
[0,1,3]
Deep vein thrombosis antepartum
Use additional code to identify the deep vein thrombosis (453.40-453.42, 453.50-453.52, 453.72-453.79, 453.82-453.89)
Use additional code for long term (current) use of anticoagulants, if applicable (V58.61)

§ ✓5ᵗʰ **671.4 Deep phlebothrombosis, postpartum** Ⓜ♀
[0,2,4]
Deep-vein thrombosis, postpartum
Pelvic thrombophlebitis, postpartum
Phlegmasia alba dolens (puerperal)
Use additional code to identify the deep vein thrombosis (453.40-453.42, 453.50-453.52, 453.72-453.79, 453.82-453.89)
Use additional code for long term (current) use of anticoagulants, if applicable (V58.61)

§ ✓5ᵗʰ **671.5 Other phlebitis and thrombosis** Ⓜ♀
[0-4]
Cerebral venous thrombosis
Thrombosis of intracranial venous sinus

§ ✓5ᵗʰ **671.8 Other venous complications** Ⓜ♀
[0-4]
Hemorrhoids

§ ✓5ᵗʰ **671.9 Unspecified venous complication** Ⓜ♀
[0-4]

✓4ᵗʰ **672 Pyrexia of unknown origin during the puerperium** Ⓜ♀
[0,2,4]

§ ✓5ᵗʰ   Use 0 as fourth-digit for this category
Postpartum fever NOS
Puerperal fever NOS
Puerperal pyrexia NOS
DEF: Fever of unknown origin experienced by the mother after childbirth.
AHA: 4Q, '91, 26
086.4 Pyrexia of unknown origin following delivery   I-10

✓4ᵗʰ **673 Obstetrical pulmonary embolism**
INCLUDES pulmonary emboli in pregnancy, childbirth, or the puerperium, or specified as puerperal
EXCLUDES embolism following abortion (639.6)

§ ✓5ᵗʰ **673.0 Obstetrical air embolism** Ⓜ♀
[0-4]
DEF: Sudden blocking of pulmonary artery with air or nitrogen bubbles during pregnancy.

§ ✓5ᵗʰ **673.1 Amniotic fluid embolism** Ⓜ♀
[0-4]
DEF: Sudden onset of pulmonary artery blockage from amniotic fluid entering the mother's circulation near the end of pregnancy due to strong uterine contractions.

§ ✓5ᵗʰ **673.2 Obstetrical blood-clot embolism** Ⓜ♀
[0-4]
Puerperal pulmonary embolism NOS
AHA: For code 673.24: 1Q, '05, 6
DEF: Blood clot blocking artery in the lung; associated with pregnancy.
TIP: If a pregnant or postpartum patient develops a pulmonary embolism that progresses to acute respiratory failure, the code for the pregnancy/delivery complication (673.2X) should be sequenced first.

§ ✓5ᵗʰ **673.3 Obstetrical pyemic and septic embolism** Ⓜ♀
[0-4]

§ ✓5ᵗʰ **673.8 Other pulmonary embolism** Ⓜ♀
[0-4]
Fat embolism

---

§   Requires fifth digit. Valid digits are in [brackets] under each code. See beginning of section 640-649 for codes and definitions.

Ⓝ Newborn Age: 0   Ⓟ Pediatric Age: 0-17   Ⓜ Maternity Age: 12-55   Ⓐ Adult Age: 15-124

✓4ᵗʰ **674 Other and unspecified complications of the puerperium, not elsewhere classified**

§ ✓5ᵗʰ **674.0 Cerebrovascular disorders in the puerperium** Ⓜ♀
[0-4]   Any condition classifiable to 430-434, 436-437 occurring during pregnancy, childbirth, or the puerperium, or specified as puerperal
EXCLUDES *intracranial venous sinus thrombosis (671.5)*

§ ✓5ᵗʰ **674.1 Disruption of cesarean wound** Ⓜ♀
[0,2,4]   Dehiscence or disruption of uterine wound
EXCLUDES *uterine rupture before onset of labor (665.0)*
uterine rupture during labor (665.1)

§ ✓5ᵗʰ **674.2 Disruption of perineal wound** Ⓜ♀
[0,2,4]   Breakdown of perineum
Disruption of wound of:
   episiotomy
   perineal laceration
Secondary perineal tear
AHA: For code 674.24: 1Q, '97, 9

§ ✓5ᵗʰ **674.3 Other complications of obstetrical surgical** Ⓜ♀
[0,2,4] **wounds**
Hematoma ⎫
Hemorrhage ⎬ of cesarean section or
Infection ⎭   perineal wound
EXCLUDES *damage from instruments in delivery (664.0-665.9)*
AHA: For code 674.32: 2Q, '91, 7; For code 674.34: ▶4Q, '09, 98◀

§ ✓5ᵗʰ **674.4 Placental polyp** Ⓜ♀
[0,2,4]

§ ✓5ᵗʰ **674.5 Peripartum cardiomyopathy** Ⓜ♀
[0-4]   Postpartum cardiomyopathy
DEF: Any structural or functional abnormality of the ventricular myocardium, non-inflammatory disease of obscure or unknown etiology with onset during the postpartum period.
AHA: 4Q, '03, 65

§ ✓5ᵗʰ **674.8 Other** Ⓜ♀
[0,2,4]   Hepatorenal syndrome, following delivery
Postpartum:
   subinvolution of uterus
   uterine hypertrophy
AHA: 3Q, '98, 16

§ ✓5ᵗʰ **674.9 Unspecified** Ⓜ♀
[0,2,4]   Sudden death of unknown cause during the puerperium

✓4ᵗʰ **675 Infections of the breast and nipple associated with childbirth**
INCLUDES the listed conditions during pregnancy, childbirth, or the puerperium

§ ✓5ᵗʰ **675.0 Infections of nipple** Ⓜ♀
[0-4]   Abscess of nipple

§ ✓5ᵗʰ **675.1 Abscess of breast** Ⓜ♀
[0-4]   Abscess: Abscess:
     mammary   purulent
     subareolar   retromammary
     submammary   submammary

§ ✓5ᵗʰ **675.2 Nonpurulent mastitis** Ⓜ♀
[0-4]   Lymphangitis of breast
Mastitis:
   NOS
   interstitial
   parenchymatous

§ ✓5ᵗʰ **675.8 Other specified infections of the breast and** Ⓜ♀
[0-4] **nipple**

§ ✓5ᵗʰ **675.9 Unspecified infection of the breast and nipple** Ⓜ♀
[0-4]

✓4ᵗʰ **676 Other disorders of the breast associated with childbirth and disorders of lactation**
INCLUDES the listed conditions during pregnancy, the puerperium, or lactation

§ ✓5ᵗʰ **676.0 Retracted nipple** Ⓜ♀
[0-4]

§ ✓5ᵗʰ **676.1 Cracked nipple** Ⓜ♀
[0-4]   Fissure of nipple

Lactation Process: Ejection Reflex Arc

§ ✓5ᵗʰ **676.2 Engorgement of breasts** Ⓜ♀
[0-4]   **DEF:** Abnormal accumulation of milk in ducts of breast.

§ ✓5ᵗʰ **676.3 Other and unspecified   disorder of breast** Ⓜ♀
[0-4]

§ ✓5ᵗʰ **676.4 Failure of lactation** Ⓜ♀
[0-4]   Agalactia
DEF: Abrupt ceasing of milk secretion by breast.

§ ✓5ᵗʰ **676.5 Suppressed lactation** Ⓜ♀
[0-4]

§ ✓5ᵗʰ **676.6 Galactorrhea** Ⓜ♀
[0-4]   **EXCLUDES** *galactorrhea not associated with childbirth (611.6)*
DEF: Excessive or persistent milk secretion by breast; may be in absence of nursing.

§ ✓5ᵗʰ **676.8 Other disorders of lactation** Ⓜ♀
[0-4]   Galactocele
DEF: Galactocele: Obstructed mammary gland, creating retention cyst, results in milk-filled cysts enlarging mammary gland.

§ ✓5ᵗʰ **676.9 Unspecified disorder of lactation** Ⓜ♀
[0-4]

677 Late effect of complication of pregnancy, childbirth, and the puerperium ♀
NOTE This category is to be used to indicate conditions in 632-648.9 and 651-676.9 as the cause of the late effect, themselves classifiable elsewhere. The "late effects" include conditions specified as such, or as sequelae, which may occur at any time after puerperium.
Code first any sequelae
AHA: 1Q, '97, 9; 4Q, '94, 42
TIP: Sequence as a secondary diagnosis, after the code for the late effect complication. May be assigned at any time after the initial postpartum period (six weeks following delivery).

Other Maternal and Fetal Complications (678-679)

The following fifth-digit subclassification is for use with categories 678-679 to denote the current episode of care. Valid fifth-digits are in [brackets] under each code.
   0   unspecified as to episode of care or not applicable
   1   delivered, with or without mention of antepartum condition
   2   delivered, with mention of postpartum complication
   3   antepartum condition or complication
   4   postpartum condition or complication

✓4ᵗʰ **678 Other fetal conditions**

§ ✓5ᵗʰ **678.0 Fetal hematologic conditions** Ⓜ♀
[0,1,3]   Fetal anemia
Fetal thrombocytopenia
Fetal twin to twin transfusion
EXCLUDES *fetal and neonatal hemorrhage (772.0-772.9)*
fetal hematologic disorders affecting newborn (776.0-776.9)
fetal-maternal hemorrhage (656.00-656.03)
isoimmunization incompatibility (656.10-656.13, 656.20-656.23)
AHA: 4Q, '08, 125-127

§ ✓5ᵗʰ **678.1 Fetal conjoined twins** Ⓜ♀
[0,1,3]   **AHA:** 4Q, '08, 125-127

---

§ Requires fifth digit. Valid digits are in [brackets] under each code. See beginning of section 640-649 for codes and definitions.

✓4ᵗʰ / ✓5ᵗʰ Additional Digit Required   Unspecified Code   Other Specified Code   Manifestation Code   ▶◀ Revised Text   ● New Code   ▲ Revised Code Title

√4ᵗʰ **679 Complications of in utero procedures**
     AHA: 4Q, '08, 127-128, 158

§ √5ᵗʰ **679.0 Maternal complications from in utero procedure** Ⓜ♀
[0-4]   **EXCLUDES** *maternal history of in utero procedure during*
                previous pregnancy (V23.86)

§ √5ᵗʰ **679.1 Fetal complications from in utero procedure** Ⓜ♀
[0-4]   Fetal complications from amniocentesis
     EXCLUDES *newborn affected by in utero procedure*
                (760.61-760.64)
     TIP: Assign only on the mother's record. Although there is a fetal
     complication, it affects the mother's pregnancy.

---

§   Requires fifth digit. Valid digits are in [brackets] under each code. See beginning of section 640-649 for codes and definitions.

Ⓝ Newborn Age: 0   Ⓟ Pediatric Age: 0-17   Ⓜ Maternity Age: 12-55   Ⓐ Adult Age: 15-124

12. Diseases of the Skin and Subcutaneous Tissue (680-709)

Infections of Skin and Subcutaneous Tissue (680-686)

EXCLUDES *certain infections of skin classified under "Infectious and Parasitic Diseases," such as:*
erysipelas (035)
erysipeloid of Rosenbach (027.1)
herpes:
  simplex (054.0-054.9)
  zoster (053.0-053.9)
molluscum contagiosum (078.0)
viral warts (078.10-078.19)

✓4ᵗʰ 680 Carbuncle and furuncle

INCLUDES boil
furunculosis

DEF: Carbuncle: necrotic boils in skin and subcutaneous tissue of neck or back mainly due to staphylococcal infection.
DEF: Furuncle: circumscribed inflammation of corium and subcutaneous tissue due to staphylococcal infection.

680.0 Face
Ear [any part]
Face [any part, except eye]
Nose (septum)
Temple (region)
EXCLUDES *eyelid (373.13)*
lacrimal apparatus (375.31)
orbit (376.01)

680.1 Neck

680.2 Trunk
Abdominal wall
Back [any part, except buttocks]
Breast
Chest wall
Flank
Groin
Pectoral region
Perineum
Umbilicus
EXCLUDES *buttocks (680.5)*
external genital organs:
  female (616.4)
  male (607.2, 608.4)

680.3 Upper arm and forearm
Arm [any part, except hand]
Axilla
Shoulder

680.4 Hand
Finger [any]
Thumb
Wrist

680.5 Buttock
Anus
Gluteal region

680.6 Leg, except foot
Ankle
Hip
Knee
Thigh

680.7 Foot
Heel
Toe

680.8 Other specified sites
Head [any part, except face]
Scalp
EXCLUDES *external genital organs:*
  female (616.4)
  male (607.2, 608.4)

680.9 Unspecified site
Boil NOS
Carbuncle NOS
Furuncle NOS

Skin and Subcutaneous Layer

Hair follicle
Epidermis
Dermis
Hypodermis (subcutaneous layer)
Bulb
Sebaceous gland
Arrector pili muscle
Thick-skin epidermis
Hair shaft
Pacinian corpuscle
Hair matrix
Sweat (eccrine gland)
Sensory nerve
Blood vessels

✓4ᵗʰ 681 Cellulitis and abscess of finger and toe

INCLUDES that with lymphangitis

Use additional code to identify organism, such as Staphylococcus (041.1)

DEF: Acute suppurative inflammation and edema in subcutaneous tissue or muscle of finger or toe.
AHA: 2Q, '91, 5; J-F, '87, 12
TIP: Coding of cellulitis due to superficial injury, burn, or frostbite requires two codes, one for the injury and one for the cellulitis. Sequencing depends on the circumstances of the admission.

✓5ᵗʰ 681.0 Finger

681.00 Cellulitis and abscess, unspecified
L03.019 Cellulitis of unspecified finger   I-10

681.01 Felon
Pulp abscess
Whitlow
EXCLUDES *herpetic whitlow (054.6)*
DEF: Painful abscess of fingertips caused by infection in the closed space of terminal phalanx.

681.02 Onychia and paronychia of finger
Panaritium ⎫
Perionychia ⎬ of finger
DEF: Onychia: inflammation of nail matrix; causes nail loss.
DEF: Paronychia: inflammation of tissue folds around nail.

✓5ᵗʰ 681.1 Toe

681.10 Cellulitis and abscess, unspecified
AHA: 1Q, '05, 14
L03.039 Cellulitis of unspecified toe   I-10

681.11 Onychia and paronychia of toe
Panaritium ⎫
Perionychia ⎬ of toe

681.9 Cellulitis and abscess of unspecified digit
Infection of nail NOS

✓4ᵗʰ 682 Other cellulitis and abscess

INCLUDES abscess (acute) ⎫
cellulitis (diffuse) ⎬ (with lymphangitis) except
lymphangitis, acute ⎭ of finger or toe

Use additional code to identify organism, such as Staphylococcus (041.1)

EXCLUDES *lymphangitis (chronic) (subacute) (457.2)*

DEF: Cellulitis: Acute suppurative inflammation of deep subcutaneous tissue and sometimes muscle due to infection of wound, burn or other lesion.
AHA: 2Q, '91, 5; J-F, '87, 12; S-O, '85, 10
TIP: Coding of cellulitis due to superficial injury, burn, or frostbite requires two codes, one for the injury and one for the cellulitis. Sequencing depends on the circumstances of the admission.

682.0 Face
Cheek, external   Nose, external
Chin   Submandibular
Forehead   Temple (region)
EXCLUDES *ear [any part] (380.10-380.16)*
eyelid (373.13)
lacrimal apparatus (375.31)
lip (528.5)
mouth (528.3)
nose (internal) (478.1)
orbit (376.01)
L03.211 Cellulitis of face   I-10

✓4ᵗʰ ✓5ᵗʰ Additional Digit Required   Unspecified Code   Other Specified Code   Manifestation Code   ▶◀ Revised Text   ● New Code   ▲ Revised Code Title

2011 ICD-9-CM   **Volume 1 – 209**

Diseases of the Skin and Subcutaneous Tissue

682.1–686.1

682.1 Neck
L03.221 Cellulitis of neck   I-10

682.2 Trunk
Abdominal wall
Back [any part, except buttock]
Chest wall
Flank
Groin
Pectoral region
Perineum
Umbilicus, except newborn
> **EXCLUDES** *anal and rectal regions (566)*
> *breast:*
>   *NOS (611.0)*
>   *puerperal (675.1)*
> *external genital organs:*
>   *female (616.3-616.4)*
>   *male (604.0, 607.2, 608.4)*
> *umbilicus, newborn (771.4)*

AHA: 4Q, '98, 42
L03.319 Cellulitis of trunk unspecified   I-10

682.3 Upper arm and forearm
Arm [any part, except hand]
Axilla
Shoulder
> **EXCLUDES** *hand (682.4)*

AHA: 2Q, '03, 7
L03.113 Cellulitis of right upper limb   I-10

682.4 Hand, except fingers and thumb
Wrist
> **EXCLUDES** *finger and thumb (681.00-681.02)*

682.5 Buttock
Gluteal region
> **EXCLUDES** *anal and rectal regions (566)*
L03.317 Cellulitis of buttock   I-10

682.6 Leg, except foot
Ankle
Hip
Knee
Thigh
AHA: 1Q, '09, 10; 3Q, '04, 5; 4Q, '03, 108
L03.115 Cellulitis of right lower limb   I-10

682.7 Foot, except toes
Heel
> **EXCLUDES** *toe (681.10-681.11)*

682.8 Other specified sites
Head [except face]
Scalp
> **EXCLUDES** *face (682.0)*

682.9 Unspecified site
Abscess NOS
Cellulitis NOS
Lymphangitis, acute NOS
> **EXCLUDES** *lymphangitis NOS (457.2)*

683 Acute lymphadenitis
Abscess (acute)
Adenitis, acute   } lymph gland or node,
Lymphadenitis, acute   except mesenteric
Use additional code to identify organism, such as Staphylococcus (041.1)
> **EXCLUDES** *enlarged glands NOS (785.6)*
> *lymphadenitis:*
>   *chronic or subacute, except mesenteric (289.1)*
>   *mesenteric (acute) (chronic) (subacute) (289.2)*
>   *unspecified (289.3)*

DEF: Acute inflammation of lymph nodes due to primary infection located elsewhere in the body.

Lymphatic System of Head and Neck

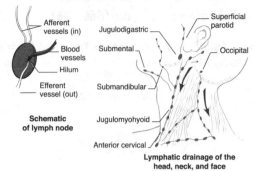

Schematic of lymph node

Lymphatic drainage of the head, neck, and face

684 Impetigo
Impetiginization of other dermatoses
Impetigo (contagiosa) [any site] [any organism]:
    bullous
    circinate
    neonatorum
    simplex
Pemphigus neonatorum
> **EXCLUDES** *impetigo herpetiformis (694.3)*

DEF: Infectious skin disease commonly occurring in children; caused by group A streptococci or *Staphylococcus aureus*; skin lesions usually appear on the face and consist of subcorneal vesicles and bullae that burst and form yellow crusts.

✓4ᵗʰ **685 Pilonidal cyst**
> **INCLUDES** fistula   } coccygeal or pilonidal
>   sinus

DEF: Hair-containing cyst or sinus in the tissues of the sacrococcygeal area; often drains through opening at the postanal dimple.

685.0 With abscess

685.1 Without mention of abscess

✓4ᵗʰ **686 Other local infections of skin and subcutaneous tissue**
Use additional code to identify any infectious organism (041.0-041.8)

✓5ᵗʰ **686.0 Pyoderma**
Dermatitis:
    purulent
    septic
    suppurative
DEF: Nonspecific purulent skin disease related most to furuncles, pustules, or possibly carbuncles.

686.00 Pyoderma, unspecified

686.01 Pyoderma gangrenosum
DEF: Persistent debilitating skin disease characterized by irregular, boggy, blue-red ulcerations, with central healing and undermined edges.
AHA: 4Q, '97, 42

686.09 Other pyoderma

686.1 Pyogenic granuloma
Granuloma: Granuloma:
    septic   telangiectaticum
    suppurative
> **EXCLUDES** *pyogenic granuloma of oral mucosa (528.9)*

DEF: Solitary polypoid capillary hemangioma often associated with local irritation, trauma, and superimposed inflammation; located on the skin and gingival or oral mucosa.

Stages of Pilonidal Disease

686.8 Other specified local infections of skin and subcutaneous tissue
Bacterid (pustular)
Dermatitis vegetans
Ecthyma
Perlèche

EXCLUDES dermatitis infectiosa eczematoides (690.8)
panniculitis (729.30-729.39)

686.9 Unspecified local infection of skin and subcutaneous tissue
Fistula of skin NOS
Skin infection NOS

EXCLUDES fistula to skin from internal organs — see Alphabetic Index

Other Inflammatory Conditions of Skin and Subcutaneous Tissue (690-698)

EXCLUDES panniculitis (729.30-729.39)

√4th **690 Erythematosquamous dermatosis**

EXCLUDES eczematous dermatitis of eyelid (373.31)
parakeratosis variegata (696.2)
psoriasis (696.0-696.1)
seborrheic keratosis (702.11-702.19)

√5th **690.1 Seborrheic dermatitis**
AHA: 4Q, '95, 58

690.10 Seborrheic dermatitis, unspecified
Seborrheic dermatitis NOS
L21.9 Seborrheic dermatitis unspecified   I-10

690.11 Seborrhea capitis   P
Cradle cap

690.12 Seborrheic infantile dermatitis   P

690.18 Other seborrheic dermatitis

690.8 Other erythematosquamous dermatosis

√4th **691 Atopic dermatitis and related conditions**
DEF: Atopic dermatitis: chronic, pruritic, inflammatory skin disorder found on the face and antecubital and popliteal fossae; often accompanied by allergic rhinitis, hay fever, asthma, and extreme itching; also called allergic dermatitis, or disseminated neurodermatitis.

691.0 Diaper or napkin rash
Ammonia dermatitis
Diaper or napkin:
dermatitis
erythema
rash
Psoriasiform napkin eruption

691.8 Other atopic dermatitis and related conditions
Atopic dermatitis
Besnier's prurigo
Eczema:
atopic
flexural
intrinsic (allergic)
Neurodermatitis:
atopic
diffuse (of Brocq)

√4th **692 Contact dermatitis and other eczema**

INCLUDES dermatitis:
NOS
contact
occupational
venenata
eczema (acute) (chronic):
NOS
allergic
erythematous
occupational

EXCLUDES allergy NOS (995.3)
contact dermatitis of eyelids (373.32)
dermatitis due to substances taken internally (693.0-693.9)
eczema of external ear (380.22)
perioral dermatitis (695.3)
urticarial reactions (708.0-708.9, 995.1)

DEF: Contact dermatitis: acute or chronic dermatitis caused by initial irritant effect of a substance, or by prior sensitization to a substance coming once again in contact with skin.

692.0 Due to detergents

692.1 Due to oils and greases

692.2 Due to solvents
Dermatitis due to solvents of:
chlorocompound
cyclohexane
ester
glycol } group
hydrocarbon
ketone

692.3 Due to drugs and medicines in contact with skin
Dermatitis (allergic) (contact) due to:
arnica
fungicides
iodine
keratolytics
mercurials
neomycin
pediculocides
phenols
scabicides
any drug applied to skin
Dermatitis medicamentosa due to drug applied to skin

Use additional E code to identify drug

EXCLUDES allergy NOS due to drugs (995.27)
dermatitis due to ingested drugs (693.0)
dermatitis medicamentosa NOS (693.0)

692.4 Due to other chemical products
Dermatitis due to:
acids
adhesive plaster
alkalis
caustics
dichromate
insecticide
nylon
plastic
rubber
AHA: 3Q, '08, 6-7; 2Q, '89, 16

692.5 Due to food in contact with skin
Dermatitis, contact, due to:
cereals
fish
flour
fruit
meat
milk

EXCLUDES dermatitis due to:
dyes (692.89)
ingested foods (693.1)
preservatives (692.89)

Diseases of the Skin and Subcutaneous Tissue

692.6–693.9

692.6 Due to plants [except food]
Dermatitis due to:
lacquer tree [Rhus verniciflua]
poison:
ivy [Rhus toxicodendron]
oak [Rhus diversiloba]
sumac [Rhus venenata]
vine [Rhus radicans]
primrose [Primula]
ragweed [Senecio jacobae]
other plants in contact with the skin
EXCLUDES allergy NOS due to pollen (477.0)
nettle rash (708.8)

√5ᵗʰ 692.7 Due to solar radiation
EXCLUDES sunburn due to other ultraviolet radiation exposure
(692.82)

692.70 Unspecified dermatitis due to sun

692.71 Sunburn
First degree sunburn
Sunburn NOS
AHA: 4Q, '01, 47
TIP: Do not assign if sunburn is due to tanning bed use; see instead code 692.82.

692.72 Acute dermatitis due to solar radiation
Acute solar skin damage NOS
Berlogue dermatitis
Photoallergic response
Phototoxic response
Polymorphus light eruption
Use additional E code to identify drug, if drug induced
EXCLUDES sunburn (692.71, 692.76-692.77)
DEF: Berloque dermatitis: Phytophotodermatitis due to sun exposure after use of a product containing bergamot oil; causes red patches, that turn brown.
DEF: Photoallergic response: Dermatitis due to hypersensitivity to the sun; causes papulovesicular, eczematous or exudative eruptions.
DEF: Phototoxic response: Chemically induced sensitivity to sun causes burn-like reaction, occasionally vesiculation and subsequent hyperpigmentation.
DEF: Polymorphous light eruption: Inflammatory skin eruptions due to sunlight exposure; eruptions differ in size and shape.
DEF: Acute solar skin damage (NOS): Rapid, unspecified injury to skin from sun.

692.73 Actinic reticuloid and actinic granuloma
DEF: Actinic reticuloid: Dermatosis aggravated by light, causes chronic eczema-like eruption on exposed skin which extends to other unexposed surfaces; occurs in the elderly.
DEF: Actinic granuloma: Inflammatory response of skin to sun causing small nodule of microphages.

692.74 Other chronic dermatitis due to solar radiation
Chronic solar skin damage NOS
Solar elastosis
EXCLUDES actinic [solar] keratosis (702.0)
DEF: Solar elastosis: Premature aging of skin of light-skinned people; causes inelasticity, thinning or thickening, wrinkling, dryness, scaling and hyperpigmentation.
DEF: Chronic solar skin damage (NOS): Chronic skin impairment due to exposure to the sun, not otherwise specified.

692.75 Disseminated superficial actinic porokeratosis [DSAP]
DEF: Autosomal dominant skin condition occurring in skin that has been overexposed to the sun; characterized by superficial annular, keratotic, brownish-red spots or thickenings with depressed centers and sharp, ridged borders, may evolve into squamous cell carcinoma.
AHA: 4Q, '00, 43

692.76 Sunburn of second degree
AHA: 4Q, '01, 47
TIP: Do not assign if sunburn is due to tanning bed use; see instead code 692.82.

692.77 Sunburn of third degree
AHA: 4Q, '01, 47
TIP: Do not assign if sunburn is due to tanning bed use; see instead code 692.82.

692.79 Other dermatitis due to solar radiation
Hydroa aestivale
Photodermatitis
Photosensitiveness } (due to sun)
Solar skin damage NOS

√5ᵗʰ 692.8 Due to other specified agents

692.81 Dermatitis due to cosmetics

692.82 Dermatitis due to other radiation
Infrared rays
Light, except from sun
Radiation NOS
Tanning bed
Ultraviolet rays, except from sun
X-rays
EXCLUDES solar radiation (692.70-692.79)
AHA: 4Q, '01, 47; 3Q, '00, 5

692.83 Dermatitis due to metals
Jewelry

692.84 Due to animal (cat) (dog) dander
Due to animal (cat) (dog) hair

692.89 Other
Dermatitis due to:
cold weather
dyes
hot weather
preservatives
EXCLUDES allergy (NOS) (rhinitis) due to animal hair or dander (477.2)
allergy to dust (477.8)
sunburn (692.71, 692.76-692.77)

692.9 Unspecified cause
Dermatitis:
NOS
contact NOS
venenata NOS
Eczema NOS
L23.9 Allergic contact dermatitis unspecified cause [I-10]

√4ᵗʰ 693 Dermatitis due to substances taken internally
EXCLUDES adverse effect NOS of drugs and medicines (995.20)
allergy NOS (995.3)
contact dermatitis (692.0-692.9)
urticarial reactions (708.0-708.9, 995.1)
DEF: Inflammation of skin due to ingested substance.

693.0 Due to drugs and medicines
Dermatitis medicamentosa NOS
Use additional E code to identify drug
EXCLUDES that due to drugs in contact with skin (692.3)
AHA: 2Q, '07, 8
TIP: Assign for palmar plantar erythrodysesthesia (PPE) or hand-foot syndrome due to chemotherapy drugs.
L27.0 Gen skin eruption d/t Rx & med taken internally [I-10]

693.1 Due to food

693.8 Due to other specified substances taken internally

693.9 Due to unspecified substance taken internally
EXCLUDES dermatitis NOS (692.9)

✓4ᵗʰ 694 Bullous dermatoses

694.0 Dermatitis herpetiformis
  Dermatosis herpetiformis
  Duhring's disease
  Hydroa herpetiformis

  EXCLUDES *herpes gestationis (646.8)*
      dermatitis herpetiformis:
        juvenile (694.2)
        senile (694.5)

  DEF: Chronic, multisystem disease manifested most in the cutaneous system; seen as an extremely pruritic eruption of various lesions that frequently heal leaving hyperpigmentation or hypopigmentation and occasionally scarring; usually associated with an asymptomatic gluten-sensitive enteropathy, and immunogenic factors.

694.1 Subcorneal pustular dermatosis
  Sneddon-Wilkinson disease or syndrome

  DEF: Chronic relapses of sterile pustular blebs beneath the horny skin layer of the trunk and skin folds; resembles dermatitis herpetiformis.

694.2 Juvenile dermatitis herpetiformis
  Juvenile pemphigoid

694.3 Impetigo herpetiformis

  DEF: Rare dermatosis associated with pregnancy; marked by itching pustules in third trimester, hypocalcemia, tetany, fever and lethargy; may result in maternal or fetal death.

694.4 Pemphigus
  Pemphigus:
    NOS
    erythematosus
    foliaceus
    malignant
    vegetans
    vulgaris

  EXCLUDES *pemphigus neonatorum (684)*

  DEF: Chronic, relapsing, sometimes fatal skin diseases; causes vesicles, bullae; autoantibodies against intracellular connections cause acantholysis.

694.5 Pemphigoid
  Benign pemphigus NOS
  Bullous pemphigoid
  Herpes circinatus bullosus
  Senile dermatitis herpetiformis

✓5ᵗʰ 694.6 Benign mucous membrane pemphigoid
  Cicatricial pemphigoid
  Mucosynechial atrophic bullous dermatitis

  694.60 Without mention of ocular involvement

  694.61 With ocular involvement
    Ocular pemphigus

    DEF: Mild self-limiting, subepidermal blistering of mucosa including the conjunctiva, seen predominantly in the elderly, produces adhesions and scarring.

694.8 Other specified bullous dermatoses
  EXCLUDES *herpes gestationis (646.8)*

694.9 Unspecified bullous dermatoses

✓4ᵗʰ 695 Erythematous conditions

695.0 Toxic erythema
  Erythema venenatum

✓5ᵗʰ 695.1 Erythema multiforme
  Use additional code to identify associated manifestations, such as:
    arthropathy associated with dermatological disorders (713.3)
    conjunctival edema (372.73)
    conjunctivitis (372.04, 372.33)
    corneal scars and opacities (371.00-371.05)
    corneal ulcer (370.00-370.07)
    edema of eyelid (374.82)
    inflammation of eyelid (373.8)
    keratoconjunctivitis sicca (370.33)
    mechanical lagophthalmos (374.22)
    mucositis (478.11, 528.00, 538, 616.81)
    stomatitis (528.00)
    symblepharon (372.63)
  Use additional E-code to identify drug, if drug-induced
  Use additional code to identify percentage of skin exfoliation (695.50-695.59)

  EXCLUDES *(Staphylococcal) scalded skin syndrome (695.81)*

  DEF: Symptom complex with varied skin eruption pattern of macular, bullous, papular, nodose, or vesicular lesions on the neck, face, and legs; gastritis and rheumatic pains; secondary to number of factors, including infections, ingestants, physical agents, malignancy and pregnancy.

  AHA: 4Q, '08, 128-130

  695.10 Erythema multiforme, unspecified
    Erythema iris
    Herpes iris

  695.11 Erythema multiforme minor

  695.12 Erythema multiforme major

  695.13 Stevens-Johnson syndrome

  695.14 Stevens-Johnson syndrome-toxic epidermal necrolysis overlap syndrome
    SJS-TEN overlap syndrome
    AHA: 4Q, '08, 131

  695.15 Toxic epidermal necrolysis
    Lyell's syndrome

  695.19 Other erythema multiforme

695.2 Erythema nodosum
  EXCLUDES *tuberculous erythema nodosum (017.1)*

  DEF: Panniculitis (an inflammatory reaction of the subcutaneous fat) of women, usually seen as a hypersensitivity reaction to infections, drugs, sarcoidosis, and specific enteropathies; the acute stage associated with fever, malaise, and arthralgia; the lesions are pink to blue in color as tender nodules and are found on the front of the legs below the knees.

695.3 Rosacea
  Acne:
    erythematosa
    rosacea
  Perioral dermatitis
  Rhinophyma

  DEF: Chronic skin disease, usually of the face, characterized by persistent erythema and telangiectasis with acute episodes of edema, engorgement papules, and pustules.

695.4 Lupus erythematosus
  Lupus:
    erythematodes (discoid)
    erythematosus (discoid), not disseminated

  EXCLUDES *lupus (vulgaris) NOS (017.0)*
      systemic [disseminated] lupus erythematosus (710.0)

  DEF: Group of connective tissue disorders occurring as various cutaneous diseases of unknown origin; it primarily affects women between the ages of 20 and 40.

✓4ᵗʰ ✓5ᵗʰ Additional Digit Required   Unspecified Code   Other Specified Code   Manifestation Code   ▶◀ Revised Text   ● New Code   ▲ Revised Code Title

2011 ICD-9-CM   **Volume 1 – 213**

Diseases of the Skin and Subcutaneous Tissue

695.5–698.2

√5ᵗʰ **695.5 Exfoliation due to erythematous conditions according to extent of body surface involved**
> Code first erythematous condition causing exfoliation, such as:
>> Ritter's disease (695.81)
>> (Staphylococcal) scalded skin syndrome (695.81)
>> Stevens-Johnson syndrome (695.13)
>> Stevens-Johnson syndrome-toxic epidermal necrolysis overlap syndrome (695.14)
>> toxic epidermal necrolysis (695.15)
> **AHA:** 4Q, '08, 128-131

695.50 Exfoliation due to erythematous condition involving less than 10 percent of body surface
> Exfoliation due to erythematous condition NOS

695.51 Exfoliation due to erythematous condition involving 10-19 percent of body surface

695.52 Exfoliation due to erythematous condition involving 20-29 percent of body surface

695.53 Exfoliation due to erythematous condition involving 30-39 percent of body surface
> **AHA:** 4Q, '08, 131

695.54 Exfoliation due to erythematous condition involving 40-49 percent of body surface

695.55 Exfoliation due to erythematous condition involving 50-59 percent of body surface

695.56 Exfoliation due to erythematous condition involving 60-69 percent of body surface

695.57 Exfoliation due to erythematous condition involving 70-79 percent of body surface

695.58 Exfoliation due to erythematous condition involving 80-89 percent of body surface

695.59 Exfoliation due to erythematous condition involving 90 percent or more of body surface

√5ᵗʰ **695.8 Other specified erythematous conditions**

695.81 Ritter's disease
> Dermatitis exfoliativa neonatorum
> (Staphylococcal) Scalded skin syndrome
> Use additional code to identify percentage of skin exfoliation (695.50-695.59)
> **DEF:** Infectious skin disease of young children marked by eruptions ranging from a localized bullous to widespread of easily ruptured fine vesicles and bullae; results in exfoliation of large planes of skin and leaves raw areas.

695.89 Other
> Erythema intertrigo
> Intertrigo
> Pityriasis rubra (Hebra)
> **EXCLUDES** mycotic intertrigo (111.0-111.9)
> **AHA:** S-O, '86, 10

695.9 Unspecified erythematous condition
> Erythema NOS
> Erythroderma (secondary)

√4ᵗʰ **696 Psoriasis and similar disorders**

696.0 Psoriatic arthropathy
> **DEF:** Psoriasis associated with inflammatory arthritis; often involves interphalangeal joints.

696.1 Other psoriasis
> Acrodermatitis continua
> Dermatitis repens
> Psoriasis:
>> NOS
>> any type, except arthropathic
> **EXCLUDES** psoriatic arthropathy (696.0)
> **L40.9** Psoriasis unspecified   I-10

696.2 Parapsoriasis
> Parakeratosis variegata
> Parapsoriasis lichenoides chronica
> Pityriasis lichenoides et varioliformis
> **DEF:** Erythrodermas similar to lichen, planus and psoriasis; symptoms include redness and itching; resistant to treatment.

696.3 Pityriasis rosea
> Pityriasis circinata (et maculata)
> **DEF:** Common, self-limited rash of unknown etiology marked by a solitary erythematous, salmon or fawn-colored herald plaque on the trunk, arms or thighs; followed by development of papular or macular lesions that tend to peel and form a scaly collarette.

696.4 Pityriasis rubra pilaris
> Devergie's disease
> Lichen ruber acuminatus
> **EXCLUDES** pityriasis rubra (Hebra) (695.89)
> **DEF:** Inflammatory disease of hair follicles; marked by firm, red lesions topped by horny plugs; may form patches; occurs on fingers elbows, knees.

696.5 Other and unspecified pityriasis
> Pityriasis:
>> NOS
>> alba
>> streptogenes
> **EXCLUDES** pityriasis:
>> simplex (690.18)
>> versicolor (111.0)

696.8 Other

√4ᵗʰ **697 Lichen**
> **EXCLUDES** lichen:
>> obtusus corneus (698.3)
>> pilaris (congenital) (757.39)
>> ruber acuminatus (696.4)
>> sclerosus et atrophicus (701.0)
>> scrofulosus (017.0)
>> simplex chronicus (698.3)
>> spinulosus (congenital) (757.39)
>> urticatus (698.2)

697.0 Lichen planus
> Lichen: Lichen:
>> planopilaris   ruber planus
> **DEF:** Inflammatory, pruritic skin disease; marked by angular, flat-top, violet-colored papules; may be acute and widespread or chronic and localized.

697.1 Lichen nitidus
> Pinkus' disease
> **DEF:** Chronic, inflammatory, asymptomatic skin disorder, characterized by numerous glistening, flat-topped, discrete, skin-colored micropapules most often on penis, lower abdomen, inner thighs, wrists, forearms, breasts and buttocks.

697.8 Other lichen, not elsewhere classified
> Lichen:
>> ruber moniliforme
>> striata

697.9 Lichen, unspecified

√4ᵗʰ **698 Pruritus and related conditions**
> **EXCLUDES** pruritus specified as psychogenic (306.3)
> **DEF:** Pruritus: Intense, persistent itching due to irritation of sensory nerve endings from organic or psychogenic causes.

698.0 Pruritus ani
> Perianal itch

698.1 Pruritus of genital organs

698.2 Prurigo
> Lichen urticatus
> Prurigo:
>> NOS
>> Hebra's
>> mitis
>> simplex
> Urticaria papulosa (Hebra)
> **EXCLUDES** prurigo nodularis (698.3)

698.3 Lichenification and lichen simplex chronicus
Hyde's disease
Neurodermatitis (circumscripta) (local)
Prurigo nodularis
EXCLUDES *neurodermatitis, diffuse (of Brocq) (691.8)*
DEF: Lichenification: thickening of skin due to prolonged rubbing or scratching.
DEF: Lichen simplex chronicus: eczematous dermatitis, of face, neck, extremities, scrotum, vulva, and perianal region due to repeated itching, rubbing and scratching; spontaneous or evolves with other dermatoses.

698.4 Dermatitis factitia [artefacta]
Dermatitis ficta
Neurotic excoriation
Use additional code to identify any associated mental disorder
DEF: Various types of self-inflicted skin lesions characterized in appearance as an erythema to a gangrene.

698.8 Other specified pruritic conditions
Pruritus:
hiemalis
senilis
Winter itch

698.9 Unspecified pruritic disorder
Itch NOS
Pruritus NOS
L29.9 Pruritus unspecified   I-10

Other Diseases of Skin and Subcutaneous Tissue (700-709)

EXCLUDES *conditions confined to eyelids (373.0-374.9)*
congenital conditions of skin, hair, and nails (757.0-757.9)

700 Corns and callosities
Callus
Clavus
DEF: Corns: Conical or horny thickening of skin on toes, due to friction, pressure from shoes and hosiery; pain and inflammation may develop.
DEF: Callosities: Localized overgrowth (hyperplasia) of the horny epidermal layer due to pressure or friction.

√4ᵗʰ 701 Other hypertrophic and atrophic conditions of skin
EXCLUDES *dermatomyositis (710.3)*
hereditary edema of legs (757.0)
scleroderma (generalized) (710.1)

701.0 Circumscribed scleroderma
Addison's keloid
Dermatosclerosis, localized
Lichen sclerosus et atrophicus
Morphea
Scleroderma, circumscribed or localized
DEF: Thickened, hardened, skin and subcutaneous tissue; may involve musculoskeletal system.

701.1 Keratoderma, acquired
Acquired:
ichthyosis
keratoderma palmaris et plantaris
Elastosis perforans serpiginosa
Hyperkeratosis:
NOS
follicularis in cutem penetrans
palmoplantaris climacterica
Keratoderma:
climactericum
tylodes, progressive
Keratosis (blennorrhagica)
EXCLUDES *Darier's disease [keratosis follicularis] (congenital) (757.39)*
keratosis:
arsenical (692.4)
gonococcal (098.81)
AHA:4Q, '94, 48

701.2 Acquired acanthosis nigricans
Keratosis nigricans
DEF: Diffuse velvety hyperplasia of the spinous skin layer of the axilla and other body folds marked by gray, brown, or black pigmentation; in adult form often associated with malignant acanthosis nigricans in a benign, nevoid form relatively generalized.

701.3 Striae atrophicae
Atrophic spots of skin
Atrophoderma maculatum
Atrophy blanche (of Milian)
Degenerative colloid atrophy
Senile degenerative atrophy
Striae distensae
DEF: Bands of atrophic, depressed, wrinkled skin associated with stretching of skin from pregnancy, obesity, or rapid growth during puberty.

701.4 Keloid scar
Cheloid
Hypertrophic scar
Keloid
DEF: Overgrowth of scar tissue due to excess amounts of collagen during connective tissue repair; occurs mainly on upper trunk, face.

701.5 Other abnormal granulation tissue
Excessive granulation

701.8 Other specified hypertrophic and atrophic conditions of skin
Acrodermatitis atrophicans chronica
Atrophia cutis senilis
Atrophoderma neuriticum
Confluent and reticulate papillomatosis
Cutis laxa senilis
Elastosis senilis
Folliculitis ulerythematosa reticulata
Gougerot-Carteaud syndrome or disease
AHA: 1Q, '08, 7
TIP: Assign for nephrogenic fibrosing dermopathy (NFD) or nephrogenic systemic dermopathy (NSD), a systemic condition occurring only in patients with kidney disease.

701.9 Unspecified hypertrophic and atrophic conditions of skin
Atrophoderma
Skin tag

√4ᵗʰ 702 Other dermatoses
EXCLUDES *carcinoma in situ (232.0-232.9)*

702.0 Actinic keratosis
DEF: Wart-like growth, red or skin-colored; may form a cutaneous horn.
AHA: 1Q, '92, 18

√5ᵗʰ 702.1 Seborrheic keratosis
DEF: Common, benign, lightly pigmented, warty growth composed of basaloid cells.

702.11 Inflamed seborrheic keratosis
AHA: 4Q, '94, 48

702.19 Other seborrheic keratosis
Seborrheic keratosis NOS

702.8 Other specified dermatoses

√4ᵗʰ 703 Diseases of nail
EXCLUDES *congenital anomalies (757.5)*
onychia and paronychia (681.02, 681.11)

703.0 Ingrowing nail
Ingrowing nail with infection
Unguis incarnatus
EXCLUDES *infection, nail NOS (681.9)*

703.8 Other specified diseases of nail
Dystrophia unguium
Hypertrophy of nail
Koilonychia
Leukonychia (punctata) (striata)
Onychauxis
Onychogryposis
Onycholysis

703.9 Unspecified disease of nail

Diseases of the Skin and Subcutaneous Tissue

704–706.1

√4ᵗʰ **704　Diseases of hair and hair follicles**
  EXCLUDES *congenital anomalies (757.4)*

√5ᵗʰ **704.0　Alopecia**
  EXCLUDES *madarosis (374.55)*
  　　　syphilitic alopecia (091.82)
  DEF: Lack of hair, especially on scalp; often called baldness; may be partial or total; occurs at any age.

  704.00　Alopecia, unspecified
  　　Baldness
  　　Loss of hair

  704.01　Alopecia areata
  　　Ophiasis
  　　DEF: Alopecia areata: usually reversible, inflammatory, patchy hair loss found in beard or scalp.
  　　DEF: Ophiasis: alopecia areata of children; marked by band around temporal and occipital scalp margins.

  704.02　Telogen effluvium
  　　DEF: Shedding of hair from premature telogen development in follicles due to stress, including shock, childbirth, surgery, drugs or weight loss.

  704.09　Other
  　　Folliculitis decalvans
  　　Hypotrichosis:
  　　　NOS
  　　　postinfectional NOS
  　　Pseudopelade

704.1　Hirsutism
  　Hypertrichosis:
  　　NOS
  　　lanuginosa, acquired
  　Polytrichia
  　EXCLUDES *hypertrichosis of eyelid (374.54)*
  　DEF: Excess hair growth; often in unexpected places and amounts.

704.2　Abnormalities of the hair
  　Atrophic hair
  　Clastothrix
  　Fragilitas crinium
  　Trichiasis:
  　　NOS
  　　cicatrical
  　Trichorrhexis (nodosa)
  　EXCLUDES *trichiasis of eyelid (374.05)*

704.3　Variations in hair color
  　Canities (premature)
  　Grayness, hair (premature)
  　Heterochromia of hair
  　Poliosis:
  　　NOS
  　　circumscripta, acquired

704.8　Other specified diseases of hair and hair follicles
  　Folliculitis:
  　　NOS
  　　abscedens et suffodiens
  　　pustular
  　Perifolliculitis:
  　　NOS
  　　capitis abscedens et suffodiens
  　　scalp
  　Sycosis:
  　　NOS
  　　barbae [not parasitic]
  　　lupoid
  　　vulgaris

704.9　Unspecified disease of hair and hair follicles

√4ᵗʰ **705　Disorders of sweat glands**

705.0　Anhidrosis
  　Hypohidrosis
  　Oligohidrosis
  　DEF: Lack or deficiency of ability to sweat.

705.1　Prickly heat
  　Heat rash
  　Miliaria rubra (tropicalis)
  　Sudamina

√5ᵗʰ **705.2　Focal hyperhidrosis**
  EXCLUDES *generalized (secondary) hyperhidrosis (780.8)*

  705.21　Primary focal hyperhidrosis
  　　Focal hyperhidrosis NOS
  　　Hyperhidrosis NOS
  　　Hyperhidrosis of:
  　　　axilla
  　　　face
  　　　palms
  　　　soles
  　　DEF: A rare disorder of the sweat glands resulting in excessive production of sweat; occurs in the absence of any underlying condition, almost always focal, confined to one or more specific areas of the body.
  　　AHA: 4Q, '04, 91

  705.22　Secondary focal hyperhidrosis
  　　Frey's syndrome
  　　DEF: Secondary focal hyperhidrosis: a symptom of an underlying disease process resulting in excessive sweating beyond what the body requires to maintain thermal control, confined to one or more specific areas of the body.
  　　DEF: Frey's syndrome: an auriculotemporal syndrome due to lesion on the parotid gland; characteristic redness and excessive sweating on the cheek in connection with eating.
  　　AHA: 4Q, '04, 91

√5ᵗʰ **705.8　Other specified disorders of sweat glands**

  705.81　Dyshidrosis
  　　Cheiropompholyx
  　　Pompholyx
  　　DEF: Vesicular eruption, on hands, feet causing itching and burning.

  705.82　Fox-Fordyce disease
  　　DEF: Chronic, usually pruritic disease evidenced by small follicular papular eruptions, especially in the axillary and pubic areas; develops from the closure and rupture of the affected apocrine glands' intraepidermal portion of the ducts.

  705.83　Hidradenitis
  　　Hidradenitis suppurativa
  　　DEF: Inflamed sweat glands.

  705.89　Other
  　　Bromhidrosis
  　　Chromhidrosis
  　　Granulosis rubra nasi
  　　Urhidrosis
  　　EXCLUDES *generalized hyperhidrosis (780.8)*
  　　　hidrocystoma (216.0-216.9)
  　　DEF: Bromhidrosis: foul-smelling axillary sweat due to decomposed bacteria.
  　　DEF: Chromhidrosis: secretion of colored sweat.
  　　DEF: Granulosis rubra nasi: idiopathic condition of children; causes redness, sweating around nose, face and chin; tends to end by puberty.
  　　DEF: Urhidrosis: urinous substance, such as uric acid, in sweat; occurs in uremia.

705.9　Unspecified disorder of sweat glands
  　Disorder of sweat glands NOS

√4ᵗʰ **706　Diseases of sebaceous glands**

706.0　Acne varioliformis
  　Acne:
  　　frontalis
  　　necrotica
  　DEF: Rare form of acne characterized by persistent brown papulo-pustules usually on the brow and temporoparietal part of the scalp.

706.1　Other acne
  　Acne:　　　　　　　　Acne:
  　　NOS　　　　　　　　vulgaris
  　　conglobata　　　　Blackhead
  　　cystic　　　　　　　Comedo
  　　pustular
  　EXCLUDES *acne rosacea (695.3)*

Ⓝ Newborn Age: 0　　　Ⓟ Pediatric Age: 0-17　　　Ⓜ Maternity Age: 12-55　　　Ⓐ Adult Age: 15-124

706.2 Sebaceous cyst
Atheroma, skin
Keratin cyst
Wen

DEF: Benign epidermal cyst, contains sebum and keratin; presents as firm, circumscribed nodule.

706.3 Seborrhea

EXCLUDES seborrhea:
    capitis (690.11)
    sicca (690.18)
  seborrheic
    dermatitis (690.10)
    keratosis (702.11-702.19)

DEF: Seborrheic dermatitis marked by excessive secretion of sebum; the sebum forms an oily coating, crusts, or scales on the skin; it is also called hypersteatosis.

706.8 Other specified diseases of sebaceous glands
Asteatosis (cutis)
Xerosis cutis

706.9 Unspecified disease of sebaceous glands

√4ᵗʰ 707 Chronic ulcer of skin

INCLUDES non-infected sinus of skin
             non-healing ulcer

EXCLUDES varicose ulcer (454.0, 454.2)

AHA: 4Q, '04, 92

√5ᵗʰ 707.0 Pressure ulcer
Bed sore
Decubitus ulcer
Plaster ulcer

Use additional code to identify pressure ulcer stage (707.20-707.25)

AHA: 4Q, '08, 132-133; 1Q, '04, 14; 4Q, '03, 110; 4Q, '99, 20; 1Q, '96, 15; 3Q, '90, 15; N-D, '87, 9

707.00 Unspecified site

707.01 Elbow

707.02 Upper back
Shoulder blades

707.03 Lower back
Coccyx
Sacrum
AHA: 3Q, '08, 17; 1Q, '05, 16
L89.159 Pressure ulcer of sacral region uns stage   I-10

707.04 Hip
L89.209 Pressure ulcer of unspecified hip uns stage   I-10

707.05 Buttock
L89.309 Pressure ulcer of unspecified buttock uns stage   I-10

707.06 Ankle

707.07 Heel
AHA: ▶4Q, '09, 150;◀ 1Q, '05, 16
L89.609 Pressure ulcer of unspecified heel uns stage   I-10

707.09 Other site
Head
L89.899 Pressure ulcer of other site unspecified stage   I-10

Four Stages of Pressure Ulcers

First Stage
Persistent focal erythema

Second Stage
Partial thickness skin loss involving epidermis, dermis, or both

Third Stage
Full thickness skin loss extending through subcutaneous tissue

Fourth Stage
Necrosis of soft tissue extending to muscle and bone

Cutaneous Lesions

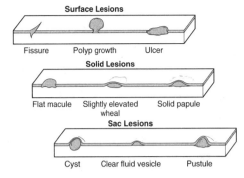

Surface Lesions
Fissure   Polyp growth   Ulcer

Solid Lesions
Flat macule   Slightly elevated wheal   Solid papule

Sac Lesions
Cyst   Clear fluid vesicle   Pustule

√5ᵗʰ 707.1 Ulcer of lower limbs, except pressure ulcer
Ulcer, chronic:
  neurogenic ⎱
  trophic   ⎰ of lower limb

Code, if applicable, any causal condition first:
  atherosclerosis of the extremities with ulceration (440.23)
  chronic venous hypertension with ulcer (459.31)
  chronic venous hypertension with ulcer and inflammation (459.33)
  diabetes mellitus (249.80-249.81, 250.80-250.83)
  postphlebitic syndrome with ulcer (459.11)
  postphlebitic syndrome with ulcer and inflammation (459.13)

AHA: 4Q, '00, 44; 4Q, '99, 15

707.10 Ulcer of lower limb, unspecified
AHA: 3Q, '04, 5; 4Q, '02, 43
L97.901 Non-prss chr ulcr uns part uns lw leg brkdwn skn   I-10

707.11 Ulcer of thigh

707.12 Ulcer of calf
L97.229 Non-press chronic ulcer left calf w/uns severity   I-10

707.13 Ulcer of ankle
L97.309 Non-press chronic ulcer uns ankle uns severity   I-10

707.14 Ulcer of heel and midfoot
Plantar surface of midfoot
L97.409 Non-press chr ulcer uns heel & midft uns sevrity   I-10

707.15 Ulcer of other part of foot
Toes
L97.509 Non-press chr ulcer oth part uns ft uns severity   I-10

707.19 Ulcer of other part of lower limb
L97.819 Non-press chr ulcer oth part rt low leg uns sevr   I-10

√5ᵗʰ 707.2 Pressure ulcer stages
Code first site of pressure ulcer (707.00-707.09)
AHA: 4Q, '08, 132-134
TIP: If a pressure ulcer progresses during an admission from one stage to another, assign only the code for the higher stage.

707.20 Pressure ulcer, unspecified stage
Healing pressure ulcer NOS
Healing pressure ulcer, unspecified stage

707.21 Pressure ulcer stage I
Healing pressure ulcer, stage I
Pressure pre-ulcer skin changes limited to persistent focal erythema

707.22 Pressure ulcer stage II
Healing pressure ulcer, stage II
Pressure ulcer with abrasion, blister, partial thickness skin loss involving epidermis and/or dermis

707.23 Pressure ulcer stage III
Healing pressure ulcer, stage III
Pressure ulcer with full thickness skin loss involving damage or necrosis of subcutaneous tissue
AHA: ▶4Q, '09, 150◀

√4ᵗʰ / √5ᵗʰ Additional Digit Required   Unspecified Code   Other Specified Code   Manifestation Code   ▶◀ Revised Text   ● New Code   ▲ Revised Code Title

707.24 Pressure ulcer stage IV
Healing pressure ulcer, stage IV
Pressure ulcer with necrosis of soft tissues through to underlying muscle, tendon, or bone

707.25 Pressure ulcer, unstageable
TIP: Assign only if ulcer is covered by eschar, has been treated with skin or other graft, or is documented as a deep tissue injury but not documented as due to trauma.

707.8 Chronic ulcer of other specified sites
Ulcer, chronic:
neurogenic
trophic   } of other specified sites

L98.499 Non-press chr ulcer skin oth sites uns severity   [I-10]

707.9 Chronic ulcer of unspecified site
Chronic ulcer NOS   Tropical ulcer NOS
Trophic ulcer NOS   Ulcer of skin NOS

√4ᵗʰ 708 Urticaria
EXCLUDES edema:
    angioneurotic (995.1)
    Quincke's (995.1)
    hereditary angioedema (277.6)
    urticaria:
      giant (995.1)
      papulosa (Hebra) (698.2)
      pigmentosa (juvenile) (congenital) (757.33)

DEF: Skin disorder marked by raised edematous patches of skin or mucous membrane with intense itching; also called hives.

708.0 Allergic urticaria

708.1 Idiopathic urticaria

708.2 Urticaria due to cold and heat
Thermal urticaria

708.3 Dermatographic urticaria
Dermatographia
Factitial urticaria

708.4 Vibratory urticaria

708.5 Cholinergic urticaria

708.8 Other specified urticaria
Nettle rash
Urticaria:
    chronic
    recurrent periodic

708.9 Urticaria, unspecified
Hives NOS

√4ᵗʰ 709 Other disorders of skin and subcutaneous tissue

√5ᵗʰ 709.0 Dyschromia
EXCLUDES albinism (270.2)
    pigmented nevus (216.0-216.9)
    that of eyelid (374.52-374.53)
DEF: Pigment disorder of skin or hair.

709.00 Dyschromia, unspecified

709.01 Vitiligo
DEF: Persistent, progressive development of nonpigmented white patches on otherwise normal skin.

709.09 Other

709.1 Vascular disorders of skin
Angioma serpiginosum
Purpura (primary)annularis telangiectodes

709.2 Scar conditions and fibrosis of skin
Adherent scar (skin)
Cicatrix
Disfigurement (due to scar)
Fibrosis, skin NOS
Scar NOS
EXCLUDES keloid scar (701.4)
AHA: N-D, '84, 19

709.3 Degenerative skin disorders
Calcinosis: Degeneration, skin
  circumscripta   Deposits, skin
  cutis   Senile dermatosis NOS
Colloid milium   Subcutaneous calcification

709.4 Foreign body granuloma of skin and subcutaneous tissue
►Use additional code to identify foreign body (V90.01-V90.9)◄
EXCLUDES residual foreign body without granuloma of skin and subcutaneous tissue (729.6)
    that of muscle (728.82)

709.8 Other specified disorders of skin
Epithelial hyperplasia
Menstrual dermatosis
Vesicular eruption
DEF: Epithelial hyperplasia: increased number of epithelial cells.
DEF: Vesicular eruption: liquid-filled structures appearing through skin.
AHA: 4Q, '08, 99; N-D, '87, 6
L98.8 Other spec disorders skin & subcutaneous tissue   [I-10]

709.9 Unspecified disorder of skin and subcutaneous tissue
Dermatosis NOS

---

13. Diseases of the Musculoskeletal System and Connective Tissue (710-739)

Use additional external cause code, if applicable, to identify the cause of the musculoskeletal condition

The following fifth-digit subclassification is for use with categories 711-712, 715-716, 718-719, and 730:

0 site unspecified
1 shoulder region
   Acromioclavicular joint(s)
   Clavicle
   Glenohumeral joint(s)
   Scapula
   Sternoclavicular joint(s)
2 upper arm
   Elbow joint
   Humerus
3 forearm
   Radius
   Ulna
   Wrist joint
4 hand
   Carpus
   Metacarpus
   Phalanges [fingers]
5 pelvic region and thigh
   Buttock
   Femur
   Hip (joint)

6 lower leg
   Fibula
   Knee joint
   Patella
   Tibia
7 ankle and foot
   Ankle joint
   Digits [toes]
   Metatarsus
   Phalanges, foot
   Tarsus
   Other joints in foot
8 other specified sites
   Head
   Neck
   Ribs
   Skull
   Trunk
   Vertebral column
9 multiple sites

Arthropathies and Related Disorders (710-719)

    EXCLUDES *disorders of spine (720.0-724.9)*

✓4ᵗʰ **710 Diffuse diseases of connective tissue**
    INCLUDES all collagen diseases whose effects are not mainly confined to a single system
    EXCLUDES *those affecting mainly the cardiovascular system, i.e., polyarteritis nodosa and allied conditions (446.0-446.7)*

710.0 Systemic lupus erythematosus
   Disseminated lupus erythematosus
   Libman-Sacks disease
   Use additional code to identify manifestation, as:
      endocarditis (424.91)
      nephritis (583.81)
        chronic (582.81)
      nephrotic syndrome (581.81)
     EXCLUDES *lupus erythematosus (discoid) NOS (695.4)*
   DEF: A chronic multisystemic inflammatory disease affecting connective tissue; marked by anemia, leukopenia, muscle and joint pains, fever, rash of a butterfly pattern around cheeks and forehead area; of unknown etiology.
   AHA: 2Q, '03, 7-8; 2Q, '97, 8
   M32.9 Systemic lupus erythematosus unspecified [I-10]

710.1 Systemic sclerosis
   Acrosclerosis
   CRST syndrome
   Progressive systemic sclerosis
   Scleroderma
   Use additional code to identify manifestation, as:
      lung involvement (517.2)
      myopathy (359.6)
     EXCLUDES *circumscribed scleroderma (701.0)*
   DEF: Systemic disease, involving excess fibrotic collagen build-up; symptoms include thickened skin, fibrotic degenerative changes in various organs, and vascular abnormalities; condition occurs more often in females.
   AHA: 1Q, '88, 6

710.2 Sicca syndrome
   Keratoconjunctivitis sicca
   Sjögren's disease
   DEF: Autoimmune disease; associated with keratoconjunctivitis, laryngopharyngitis, rhinitis, dry mouth, enlarged parotid gland, and chronic polyarthritis.

710.3 Dermatomyositis
   Poikilodermatomyositis
   Polymyositis with skin involvement
   DEF: Polymyositis characterized by flat-top purple papules on knuckles; upper eyelid rash, edema of eyelids and orbit area, red rash on forehead, neck, shoulders, trunk and arms; symptoms include fever, weight loss aching muscles; visceral cancer.

710.4 Polymyositis
   DEF: Chronic, progressive, inflammatory skeletal muscle disease; causes weakness of limb girdles, neck, pharynx; may precede or follow scleroderma, Sjogren's disease, systemic lupus erythematosus, arthritis, or malignancy.

710.5 Eosinophilia myalgia syndrome
   Toxic oil syndrome
   Use additional E code to identify drug, if drug induced
   DEF: Eosinophilia myalgia syndrome (EMS): inflammatory, multisystem fibrosis; associated with ingesting elementary L-tryptophan; symptoms include myalgia, weak limbs and bulbar muscles, distal sensory loss, areflexia, arthralgia, cough, fever, fatigue, skin rashes, myopathy, and eosinophil counts greater than 1000/microliter.
   DEF: Toxic oil syndrome: syndrome similar to EMS due to ingesting contaminated cooking oil
   AHA: 4Q, '92, 21

710.8 Other specified diffuse diseases of connective tissue
   Multifocal fibrosclerosis (idiopathic) NEC
   Systemic fibrosclerosing syndrome
   AHA: M-A, '87, 12

710.9 Unspecified diffuse connective tissue disease
   Collagen disease NOS

✓4ᵗʰ **711 Arthropathy associated with infections**
    INCLUDES arthritis
          arthropathy } associated with conditions
          polyarthritis   classifiable below
          polyarthropathy }

    EXCLUDES *rheumatic fever (390)*

The following fifth-digit subclassification is for use with category 711; valid digits are in [brackets] under each code. See list at beginning of chapter for definitions.
   0 site unspecified
   1 shoulder region
   2 upper arm
   3 forearm
   4 hand
   5 pelvic region and thigh
   6 lower leg
   7 ankle and foot
   8 other specified sites
   9 multiple sites
   AHA: 1Q, '92, 17

§ ✓5ᵗʰ **711.0 Pyogenic arthritis**
  [0-9]   Arthritis or polyarthritis (due to):
       coliform [Escherichia coli]
       Hemophilus influenzae [H. influenzae]
       pneumococcal
       Pseudomonas
       staphylococcal
       streptococcal
   Pyarthrosis
   Use additional code to identify infectious organism (041.0-041.8)
   DEF: Infectious arthritis caused by various bacteria; marked by inflamed synovial membranes, and purulent effusion in joints.
   AHA: 1Q, '92, 16; 1Q, '91, 15
   M00.869 Arthritis due to other bacteria unspecified knee [I-10]

§ ✓5ᵗʰ ***711.1 Arthropathy associated with Reiter's disease and***
  [0-9]   ***nonspecific urethritis***
   Code first underlying disease as:
      nonspecific urethritis (099.4)
      Reiter's disease (099.3)
   DEF: Reiter's disease: joint disease marked by diarrhea, urethritis, conjunctivitis, keratosis and arthritis; of unknown etiology; affects young males.
   DEF: Urethritis: inflamed urethra.

---

§ Requires fifth digit. Valid digits are in [brackets] under each code. See beginning of section 710-739 for codes and defintions.

✓4ᵗʰ✓5ᵗʰ Additional Digit Required   Unspecified Code   Other Specified Code   Manifestation Code   ►◄ Revised Text   ● New Code   ▲ Revised Code Title

Joint Structures

Muscle
Periosteum (covers bone)
Cortical bone
Medullary bone
Fascia over Muscle
Sesamoid bone
Bursa (with synovial fluid)
Tendon (muscle to bone)
Muscle insertion into bone (crosses one or more joints)
Retinaculum
Tendon sheath around
Tendon
Synovium lines
Joint capsule around
Synovial cavity (with fluid)
Articular cartilage
Ligament (bone to bone)
Bursa
Bone covered with periosteum

§ √5ᵗʰ **711.2 Arthropathy in Behçet's syndrome**
[0-9] *Code first underlying disease (136.1)*
DEF: Behçet's syndrome: Chronic inflammatory disorder, of unknown etiology; affects small blood vessels; causes ulcers of oral and pharyngeal mucous membranes and genitalia, skin lesions, retinal vasculitis, optic atrophy and severe uveitis.

§ √5ᵗʰ **711.3 Postdysenteric arthropathy**
[0-9] *Code first underlying disease as:*
dysentery (009.0)
enteritis, infectious (008.0-009.3)
paratyphoid fever (002.1-002.9)
typhoid fever (002.0)
EXCLUDES *salmonella arthritis (003.23)*

§ √5ᵗʰ **711.4 Arthropathy associated with other bacterial diseases**
[0-9] *Code first underlying disease as:*
diseases classifiable to 010-040, 090-099, except as in 711.1, 711.3, and 713.5
leprosy (030.0-030.9)
tuberculosis (015.0-015.9)
EXCLUDES *gonococcal arthritis (098.50)*
meningococcal arthritis (036.82)

§ √5ᵗʰ **711.5 Arthropathy associated with other viral diseases**
[0-9] *Code first underlying disease as:*
diseases classifiable to 045-049, 050-079, 480, 487
O'nyong nyong (066.3)
EXCLUDES *that due to rubella (056.71)*

§ √5ᵗʰ **711.6 Arthropathy associated with mycoses**
[0-9] *Code first underlying disease (110.0-118)*

§ √5ᵗʰ **711.7 Arthropathy associated with helminthiasis**
[0-9] *Code first underlying disease as:*
filariasis (125.0-125.9)

§ √5ᵗʰ **711.8 Arthropathy associated with other infectious and parasitic diseases**
[0-9]
Code first underlying disease as:
diseases classifiable to 080-088, 100-104, 130-136
EXCLUDES *arthropathy associated with sarcoidosis (713.7)*
AHA: 4Q, '91, 15; 3Q, '90, 14

§ √5ᵗʰ **711.9 Unspecified infective arthritis**
[0-9] Infective arthritis or polyarthritis (acute) (chronic) (subacute) NOS

√4ᵗʰ **712 Crystal arthropathies**
INCLUDES crystal-induced arthritis and synovitis
EXCLUDES *gouty arthropathy (274.00-274.03)*
DEF: Joint disease due to urate crystal deposit in joints or synovial membranes.

The following fifth-digit subclassification is for use with category 712; valid digits are in [brackets] under each code. See list at beginning of chapter for definitions.
0 **site unspecified**
1 **shoulder region**
2 **upper arm**
3 **forearm**
4 **hand**
5 **pelvic region and thigh**
6 **lower leg**
7 **ankle and foot**
8 **other specified sites**
9 **multiple sites**

§ √5ᵗʰ **712.1 Chondrocalcinosis due to dicalcium phosphate**
[0-9] **crystals**
Chondrocalcinosis due to dicalcium phosphate crystals (with other crystals)
Code first underlying disease (275.4)

§ √5ᵗʰ **712.2 Chondrocalcinosis due to pyrophosphate crystals**
[0-9] *Code first underlying disease (275.4)*

§ √5ᵗʰ **712.3 Chondrocalcinosis, unspecified**
[0-9] *Code first underlying disease (275.4)*

§ √5ᵗʰ **712.8 Other specified crystal arthropathies**
[0-9]

§ √5ᵗʰ **712.9 Unspecified crystal arthropathy**
[0-9]

√4ᵗʰ **713 Arthropathy associated with other disorders classified elsewhere**
INCLUDES arthritis   associated with
arthropathy   conditions
polyarthritis   classifiable
polyarthropathy   below

713.0 Arthropathy associated with other endocrine and metabolic disorders
Code first underlying disease as:
acromegaly (253.0)
hemochromatosis ▶(275.01-275.09)◀
hyperparathyroidism (252.00-252.08)
hypogammaglobulinemia (279.00-279.09)
hypothyroidism (243-244.9)
lipoid metabolism disorder (272.0-272.9)
ochronosis (270.2)
EXCLUDES *arthropathy associated with:*
amyloidosis (713.7)
crystal deposition disorders, except gout (712.1-712.9)
diabetic neuropathy (713.5)
gout (274.00-274.03)

713.1 Arthropathy associated with gastrointestinal conditions other than infections
Code first underlying disease as:
regional enteritis (555.0-555.9)
ulcerative colitis (556)

713.2 Arthropathy associated with hematological disorders
Code first underlying disease as:
hemoglobinopathy (282.4-282.7)
hemophilia (286.0-286.2)
leukemia (204.0-208.9)
malignant reticulosis (202.3)
multiple myelomatosis (203.0)
EXCLUDES *arthropathy associated with Henoch-Schönlein purpura (713.6)*

713.3 Arthropathy associated with dermatological disorders
Code first underlying disease as:
erythema multiforme (695.10-695.19)
erythema nodosum (695.2)
EXCLUDES *psoriatic arthropathy (696.0)*

---

§ Requires fifth digit. Valid digits are in [brackets] under each code. See beginning of section 710-739 for codes and defintions.

713.4 **Arthropathy associated with respiratory disorders**

Code first underlying disease as:
diseases classifiable to 490-519

EXCLUDES arthropathy associated with respiratory infections (711.0, 711.4-711.8)

713.5 **Arthropathy associated with neurological disorders**

Charcôt's arthropathy ⎫ associated with diseases
Neuropathic arthritis ⎬ classifiable elsewhere

Code first underlying disease as:
neuropathic joint disease [Charcôt's joints]:
NOS (094.0)
diabetic (249.6, 250.6)
syringomyelic (336.0)
tabetic [syphilitic] (094.0)

713.6 **Arthropathy associated with hypersensitivity reaction**

Code first underlying disease as:
Henoch (-Schönlein) purpura (287.0)
serum sickness (999.5)

EXCLUDES allergic arthritis NOS (716.2)

713.7 **Other general diseases with articular involvement**

Code first underlying disease as:
amyloidosis (277.30-277.39)
familial Mediterranean fever (277.31)
sarcoidosis (135)

AHA: 2Q, '97, 12

713.8 **Arthropathy associated with other condition classifiable elsewhere**

Code first underlying disease as:
conditions classifiable elsewhere except as in 711.1-711.8, 712, and 713.0-713.7

✓4ᵗʰ **714 Rheumatoid arthritis and other inflammatory polyarthropathies**

EXCLUDES rheumatic fever (390)
rheumatoid arthritis of spine NOS (720.0)

AHA: 2Q, '95, 3

714.0 Rheumatoid arthritis
Arthritis or polyarthritis:
atrophic
rheumatic (chronic)
Use additional code to identify manifestation, as:
myopathy (359.6)
polyneuropathy (357.1)

EXCLUDES juvenile rheumatoid arthritis NOS (714.30)

DEF: Chronic systemic disease principally of joints, manifested by inflammatory changes in articular structures and synovial membranes, atrophy, and loss in bone density.

AHA: 2Q, '06, 20; 1Q, '90, 5

M06.9 Rheumatoid arthritis unspecified   I-10

714.1 Felty's syndrome
Rheumatoid arthritis with splenoadenomegaly and leukopenia

DEF: Syndrome marked by rheumatoid arthritis, splenomegaly, leukopenia, pigmented spots on lower extremity skin, anemia, and thrombocytopenia.

714.2 Other rheumatoid arthritis with visceral or systemic involvement
Rheumatoid carditis

✓5ᵗʰ **714.3 Juvenile chronic polyarthritis**
DEF: Rheumatoid arthritis of more than one joint; lasts longer than six weeks in age 17 or younger; symptoms include fever, erythematous rash, weight loss, lymphadenopathy, hepatosplenomegaly and pericarditis.

714.30 Polyarticular juvenile rheumatoid arthritis, chronic or unspecified
Juvenile rheumatoid arthritis NOS
Still's disease

714.31 Polyarticular juvenile rheumatoid arthritis, acute

714.32 Pauciarticular juvenile rheumatoid arthritis

714.33 Monoarticular juvenile rheumatoid arthritis

714.4 Chronic postrheumatic arthropathy
Chronic rheumatoid nodular fibrositis
Jaccoud's syndrome

DEF: Persistent joint disorder; follows previous rheumatic infection.

✓5ᵗʰ **714.8 Other specified inflammatory polyarthropathies**

714.81 Rheumatoid lung
Caplan's syndrome
Diffuse interstitial rheumatoid disease of lung
Fibrosing alveolitis, rheumatoid

DEF: Lung disorders associated with rheumatoid arthritis.

714.89 Other

714.9 Unspecified inflammatory polyarthropathy
Inflammatory polyarthropathy or polyarthritis NOS

EXCLUDES polyarthropathy NOS (716.5)

✓4ᵗʰ **715 Osteoarthrosis and allied disorders**

NOTE Localized, in the subcategories below, includes bilateral involvement of the same site.

INCLUDES arthritis or polyarthritis:
degenerative
hypertrophic
degenerative joint disease
osteoarthritis

EXCLUDES Marie-Strümpell spondylitis (720.0)
osteoarthrosis [osteoarthritis] of spine (721.0-721.9)

The following fifth-digit subclassification is for use with category 715; valid digits are in [brackets] under each code. See list at beginning of chapter for definitions.
0 site unspecified
1 shoulder region
2 upper arm
3 forearm
4 hand
5 pelvic region and thigh
6 lower leg
7 ankle and foot
8 other specified sites
9 multiple sites

§ ✓5ᵗʰ **715.0 Osteoarthrosis, generalized**
[0,4,9] Degenerative joint disease, involving multiple joints
Primary generalized hypertrophic osteoarthrosis

DEF: Chronic noninflammatory arthritis; marked by degenerated articular cartilage and enlarged bone; symptoms include pain and stiffness with activity.

§ ✓5ᵗʰ **715.1 Osteoarthrosis, localized, primary**
[0-8] Localized osteoarthropathy, idiopathic
M17.0 Bilateral primary osteoarthritis of knee   I-10

§ ✓5ᵗʰ **715.2 Osteoarthrosis, localized, secondary**
[0-8] Coxae malum senilis

§ ✓5ᵗʰ **715.3 Osteoarthrosis, localized, not specified whether**
[0-8] **primary or secondary**
Otto's pelvis

AHA: For code 715.35: 3Q, '04, 12; 2Q, '04, 15; For code 715.36: 4Q, '03, 118; 2Q, '95, 5

M16.9 Osteoarthritis of hip unspecified   I-10

§ ✓5ᵗʰ **715.8 Osteoarthrosis involving, or with mention of**
[0,9] **more than one site, but not specified as generalized**

§ ✓5ᵗʰ **715.9 Osteoarthrosis, unspecified whether**
[0-8] **generalized or localized**

AHA: For code 715.90: 2Q, '97, 12

M19.90 Unspecified osteoarthritis unspecified site   I-10
M17.9 Osteoarthritis of knee unspecified   I-10

---

§ Requires fifth digit. Valid digits are in [brackets] under each code. See beginning of section 710-739 for codes and defintions.

✓4ᵗʰ
✓5ᵗʰ Additional Digit Required   Unspecified Code   Other Specified Code   Manifestation Code   ▶◀ Revised Text   ● New Code   ▲ Revised Code Title
2011 ICD-9-CM   **Volume 1 – 221**

√4ᵗʰ **716 Other and unspecified arthropathies**

EXCLUDES *cricoarytenoid arthropathy (478.79)*

The following fifth-digit subclassification is for use with category 716; valid digits are in [brackets] under each code. See list at beginning of chapter for definitions.
- 0 site unspecified
- 1 shoulder region
- 2 upper arm
- 3 forearm
- 4 hand
- 5 pelvic region and thigh
- 6 lower leg
- 7 ankle and foot
- 8 other specified sites
- 9 multiple sites

AHA: 2Q, '95, 3

§ √5ᵗʰ **716.0 Kaschin-Beck disease**
[0-9]   Endemic polyarthritis
DEF: Chronic degenerative disease of spine and peripheral joints; occurs in eastern Siberian, northern Chinese, and Korean youth; may be a mycotoxicosis caused by eating cereals infected with fungus.

§ √5ᵗʰ **716.1 Traumatic arthropathy**
[0-9]   AHA: For Code 716.11: 1Q, '02, 9; For code 716.15: 2Q, '09, 11

§ √5ᵗʰ **716.2 Allergic arthritis**
[0-9]   EXCLUDES *arthritis associated with Henoch-Schönlein purpura or serum sickness (713.6)*

§ √5ᵗʰ **716.3 Climacteric arthritis**   ♀
[0-9]   Menopausal arthritis
DEF: Ovarian hormone deficiency; causes pain in small joints, shoulders, elbows or knees; affects females at menopause; also called arthropathia ovaripriva.

§ √5ᵗʰ **716.4 Transient arthropathy**
[0-9]   EXCLUDES *palindromic rheumatism (719.3)*

§ √5ᵗʰ **716.5 Unspecified polyarthropathy or polyarthritis**
[0-9]

§ √5ᵗʰ **716.6 Unspecified monoarthritis**
[0-8]   Coxitis

§ √5ᵗʰ **716.8 Other specified arthropathy**
[0-9]

§ √5ᵗʰ **716.9 Arthropathy, unspecified**
[0-9]   Arthritis
     Arthropathy } (acute) (chronic) (subacute)
     Articular rheumatism (chronic)
     Inflammation of joint NOS
     M12.9 Arthropathy unspecified   I-10

√4ᵗʰ **717 Internal derangement of knee**

INCLUDES degeneration
     rupture, old } of articular cartilage or
     tear, old   meniscus of knee

EXCLUDES *acute derangement of knee (836.0-836.6)*
     ankylosis (718.5)
     contracture (718.4)
     current injury (836.0-836.6)
     deformity (736.4-736.6)
     recurrent dislocation (718.3)

717.0 Old bucket handle tear of medial meniscus
     Old bucket handle tear of unspecified cartilage

717.1 Derangement of anterior horn of medial meniscus

717.2 Derangement of posterior horn of medial meniscus

717.3 Other and unspecified derangement of medial meniscus
     Degeneration of internal semilunar cartilage

Disruption and Tears of Meniscus

Bucket-handle   Flap-type   Peripheral   Radial

Horizontal cleavage   Vertical   Congenital discoid meniscus

Internal Derangements of Knee

Disruptions of Cruciate Ligament — Anterior — Posterior

Chondromalacia of Patella

"Kissing" lesion of femur

√5ᵗʰ **717.4 Derangement of lateral meniscus**

     717.40 Derangement of lateral meniscus, unspecified

     717.41 Bucket handle tear of lateral meniscus

     717.42 Derangement of anterior horn of lateral meniscus

     717.43 Derangement of posterior horn of lateral meniscus

     717.49 Other

717.5 Derangement of meniscus, not elsewhere classified
     Congenital discoid meniscus
     Cyst of semilunar cartilage
     Derangement of semilunar cartilage NOS

717.6 Loose body in knee
     Joint mice, knee
     Rice bodies, knee (joint)
DEF: The presence in the joint synovial area of a small, frequently calcified, loose body created from synovial membrane, organized fibrin fragments of articular cartilage or arthritis osteophytes.

717.7 Chondromalacia of patella
     Chondromalacia patellae
     Degeneration [softening] of articular cartilage of patella
DEF: Softened patella cartilage.
AHA: M-A, '85, 14; N-D, '84, 9

√5ᵗʰ **717.8 Other internal derangement of knee**

     717.81 Old disruption of lateral collateral ligament

     717.82 Old disruption of medial collateral ligament

     717.83 Old disruption of anterior cruciate ligament

     717.84 Old disruption of posterior cruciate ligament

     717.85 Old disruption of other ligaments of knee
         Capsular ligament of knee

     717.89 Other
         Old disruption of ligaments NOS

717.9 Unspecified internal derangement of knee
     Derangement NOS of knee

---

§   Requires fifth digit. Valid digits are in [brackets] under each code. See beginning of section 710-739 for codes and definitions.

Ⓝ Newborn Age: 0   Ⓟ Pediatric Age: 0-17   Ⓜ Maternity Age: 12-55   Ⓐ Adult Age: 15-124

☑4ᵗʰ **718 Other derangement of joint**

    EXCLUDES *current injury (830.0-848.9)*
          jaw (524.60-524.69)

The following fifth-digit subclassification is for use with category 718; valid digits are in [brackets] under each code. See list at beginning of chapter for definitions.

    0 **site unspecified**
    1 **shoulder region**
    2 **upper arm**
    3 **forearm**
    4 **hand**
    5 **pelvic region and thigh**
    6 **lower leg**
    7 **ankle and foot**
    8 **other specified sites**
    9 **multiple sites**

§ ☑5ᵗʰ **718.0 Articular cartilage disorder**
  [0-5,7-9] Meniscus:
        disorder
        rupture, old
        tear, old
      Old rupture of ligament(s) of joint NOS
      EXCLUDES *articular cartilage disorder:*
          in ochronosis (270.2)
          knee (717.0-717.9)
          chondrocalcinosis (275.4)
          metastatic calcification (275.4)

§ ☑5ᵗʰ **718.1 Loose body in joint**
  [0-5,7-9] Joint mice
      EXCLUDES *knee (717.6)*
      DEF: Calcified loose bodies in synovial fluid; due to arthritic osteophytes.
      AHA: For code 718.17: 2Q, '01, 15

§ ☑5ᵗʰ **718.2 Pathological dislocation**
  [0-9]   Dislocation or displacement of joint, not recurrent and not current injury
           Spontaneous dislocation (joint)

§ ☑5ᵗʰ **718.3 Recurrent dislocation of joint**
  [0-9]   **AHA:** N-D, '87, 7

§ ☑5ᵗʰ **718.4 Contracture of joint**
  [0-9]   **AHA:** 4Q, '98, 40
      TIP: Assign an additional code from category 438 if the contracture is a result of a CVA.

§ ☑5ᵗʰ **718.5 Ankylosis of joint**
  [0-9]   Ankylosis of joint (fibrous) (osseous)
      EXCLUDES *spine (724.9)*
          stiffness of joint without mention of ankylosis (719.5)
      DEF: Immobility and solidification of joint; due to disease, injury or surgical procedure.

§ ☑5ᵗʰ **718.6 Unspecified intrapelvic protrusion of acetabulum**
  [0,5]   Protrusio acetabuli, unspecified
      DEF: Sinking of the floor of acetabulum, causing femoral head to protrude, limits hip movement; of unknown etiology.

§ ☑5ᵗʰ **718.7 Developmental dislocation of joint**
  [0-9]   **EXCLUDES** *congenital dislocation of joint (754.0-755.8)*
              traumatic dislocation of joint (830-839)
      AHA: 4Q, '01, 48

Joint Derangements and Disorders

Loose body in joint   Dislocation of joint

Joint contracture   Ankylosis of joint   Synovial effusion (fluid)   Hemarthrosis (blood)

§ ☑5ᵗʰ **718.8 Other joint derangement, not elsewhere classified**
  [0-9]   Flail joint (paralytic)   Instability of joint
      EXCLUDES *deformities classifiable to 736 (736.0-736.9)*
      AHA: For code 718.81: 2Q, '00, 14
      TIP: Assign 718.81 for multidirectional shoulder instability.

§ ☑5ᵗʰ **718.9 Unspecified derangement of joint**
  [0-5,7-9] **EXCLUDES** *knee (717.9)*

☑4ᵗʰ **719 Other and unspecified disorders of joint**
    EXCLUDES *jaw (524.60-524.69)*

The following fifth-digit subclassification is for use with codes 719.0-719.6, 719.8-719.9; valid digits are in [brackets] under each code. See list at beginning of chapter for definitions.

    0 **site unspecified**
    1 **shoulder region**
    2 **upper arm**
    3 **forearm**
    4 **hand**
    5 **pelvic region and thigh**
    6 **lower leg**
    7 **ankle and foot**
    8 **other specified sites**
    9 **multiple sites**

§ ☑5ᵗʰ **719.0 Effusion of joint**
  [0-9]   Hydrarthrosis
         Swelling of joint, with or without pain
      EXCLUDES *intermittent hydrarthrosis (719.3)*
      M25.469 Effusion unspecified knee   I-10

§ ☑5ᵗʰ **719.1 Hemarthrosis**
  [0-9]   **EXCLUDES** *current injury (840.0-848.9)*

§ ☑5ᵗʰ **719.2 Villonodular synovitis**
  [0-9]   **DEF:** Overgrowth of synovial tissue, especially at knee joint; due to macrophage infiltration of giant cells in synovial villi and fibrous nodules.

§ ☑5ᵗʰ **719.3 Palindromic rheumatism**
  [0-9]   Hench-Rosenberg syndrome
         Intermittent hydrarthrosis
      DEF: Recurrent episodes of afebrile arthritis and periarthritis marked by their complete disappearance after a few days or hours; causes swelling, redness, and disability usually affecting only one joint; no known cause.

§ ☑5ᵗʰ **719.4 Pain in joint**
  [0-9]   Arthralgia
      AHA: For code 719.46: 1Q, '01, 3
      TIP: Assign 719.46 for patellofemoral syndrome, a chronic knee pain common among athletes.
      M25.519 Pain in unspecified shoulder   I-10
      M25.552 Pain in left hip   I-10

§ ☑5ᵗʰ **719.5 Stiffness of joint, not elsewhere classified**
  [0-9]

§ ☑5ᵗʰ **719.6 Other symptoms referable to joint**
  [0-9]   Joint crepitus
         Snapping hip
      AHA: 1Q, '94, 15; **For code 719.66:** 2Q, '07, 6
      TIP: Assign 719.66 for patellar clunk syndrome, which is a fibrous reaction caused by chronic pressure on the patella, S/P knee replacement surgery.

719.7 Difficulty in walking
      EXCLUDES *abnormality of gait (781.2)*
      AHA: 2Q, '04, 15; 4Q, '03, 66
      R26.2 Difficulty in walking not elsewhere classified   I-10

§ ☑5ᵗʰ **719.8 Other specified disorders of joint**
  [0-9]   Calcification of joint
         Fistula of joint
      EXCLUDES *temporomandibular joint-pain-dysfunction syndrome [Costen's syndrome] (524.60)*

§ ☑5ᵗʰ **719.9 Unspecified disorder of joint**
  [0-9]

---

§   Requires fifth digit. Valid digits are in [brackets] under each code. See beginning of section 710-739 for codes and defintions.

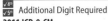

☑4ᵗʰ / ☑5ᵗʰ   Additional Digit Required   Unspecified Code   Other Specified Code   Manifestation Code   ▶◀ Revised Text   ● New Code   ▲ Revised Code Title

Dorsopathies (720–724)

EXCLUDES *curvature of spine (737.0-737.9)*
osteochondrosis of spine (juvenile) (732.0)
adult (732.8)

✓4ᵗʰ 720 Ankylosing spondylitis and other inflammatory spondylopathies

720.0 Ankylosing spondylitis
Rheumatoid arthritis of spine NOS
Spondylitis:
    Marie-Strümpell
    rheumatoid
DEF: Rheumatoid arthritis of spine and sacroiliac joints; fusion and deformity in spine follows; affects mainly males; cause unknown.

720.1 Spinal enthesopathy
Disorder of peripheral ligamentous or muscular attachments of spine
Romanus lesion
DEF: Tendinous or muscular vertebral bone attachment abnormality.

720.2 Sacroiliitis, not elsewhere classified
Inflammation of sacroiliac joint NOS
DEF: Pain due to inflammation in joint, at juncture of sacrum and hip.

✓5ᵗʰ 720.8 Other inflammatory spondylopathies

720.81 Inflammatory spondylopathies in diseases classified elsewhere

Code first underlying disease as:
    tuberculosis (015.0)

720.89 Other

720.9 Unspecified inflammatory spondylopathy
Spondylitis NOS

✓4ᵗʰ 721 Spondylosis and allied disorders
DEF: Degenerative changes in spinal joint.
AHA: 2Q, '89, 14

721.0 Cervical spondylosis without myelopathy
Cervical or cervicodorsal:
    arthritis
    osteoarthritis
    spondylarthritis

721.1 Cervical spondylosis with myelopathy
Anterior spinal artery compression syndrome
Spondylogenic compression of cervical spinal cord
Vertebral artery compression syndrome
M47.12 Other spondylosis w/myelopathy cervical region   I-10

721.2 Thoracic spondylosis without myelopathy
Thoracic:
    arthritis
    osteoarthritis
    spondylarthritis

721.3 Lumbosacral spondylosis without myelopathy
Lumbar or lumbosacral:
    arthritis
    osteoarthritis
    spondylarthritis
AHA: 4Q, '02, 107
M47.817 Spondylosis w/o myelopath/radiculopath lumboscrl   I-10

✓5ᵗʰ 721.4 Thoracic or lumbar spondylosis with myelopathy

721.41 Thoracic region
Spondylogenic compression of thoracic spinal cord

721.42 Lumbar region

721.5 Kissing spine
Baastrup's syndrome
DEF: Compression of spinous processes of adjacent vertebrae; due to mutual contact.

721.6 Ankylosing vertebral hyperostosis

721.7 Traumatic spondylopathy
Kümmell's disease or spondylitis

721.8 Other allied disorders of spine

✓5ᵗʰ 721.9 Spondylosis of unspecified site

721.90 Without mention of myelopathy
Spinal:
    arthritis (deformans) (degenerative) (hypertrophic)
    osteoarthritis NOS
    Spondylarthrosis NOS

721.91 With myelopathy
Spondylogenic compression of spinal cord NOS

✓4ᵗʰ 722 Intervertebral disc disorders
AHA: 1Q, '88, 10

722.0 Displacement of cervical intervertebral disc without myelopathy
Neuritis (brachial) or radiculitis due to displacement or rupture of cervical intervertebral disc
Any condition classifiable to 722.2 of the cervical or cervicothoracic intervertebral disc
M50.20 Other cerv disc displacement uns cerv region   I-10

✓5ᵗʰ 722.1 Displacement of thoracic or lumbar intervertebral disc without myelopathy

722.10 Lumbar intervertebral disc without myelopathy
Lumbago or sciatica due to displacement of intervertebral disc
Neuritis or radiculitis due to displacement or rupture of lumbar intervertebral disc
Any condition classifiable to 722.2 of the lumbar or lumbosacral intervertebral disc
AHA: 4Q, '08, 184; 1Q, '07, 9; 3Q, '03, 12; 1Q, '03, 7; 4Q, '02, 107
M51.26 Oth intervertebral disc displcmnt lumbar region   I-10

722.11 Thoracic intervertebral disc without myelopathy
Any condition classifiable to 722.2 of thoracic intervertebral disc

722.2 Displacement of intervertebral disc, site unspecified, without myelopathy
Discogenic syndrome NOS
Herniation of nucleus pulposus NOS
Intervertebral disc NOS:
    extrusion
    prolapse
    protrusion
    rupture
Neuritis or radiculitis due to displacement or rupture of intervertebral disc

✓5ᵗʰ 722.3 Schmorl's nodes
DEF: Irregular bone defect in the margin of the vertebral body; causes herniation into end plate of vertebral body.

722.30 Unspecified region

722.31 Thoracic region

722.32 Lumbar region

722.39 Other

Normal Anatomy of Vertebral Disc

Lamina
Ligamentum flavum
Disk annulus
Nucleus pulposus
Normal Top View

Spinal canal
Spinal cord in dural sac
Intervertebral disk
Annulus
Nucleus pulposus
Vertebral body
Spinal nerve
Lamina
Normal Side View

Derangement of Vertebral Disc

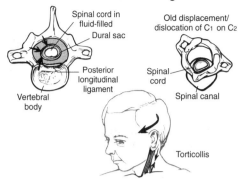

Stenosis in Cervical Region

722.4 Degeneration of cervical intervertebral disc
Degeneration of cervicothoracic intervertebral disc
M50.30 Other cerv disc degeneration uns cerv region   I-10

√5ᵗʰ **722.5 Degeneration of thoracic or lumbar intervertebral disc**

722.51 Thoracic or thoracolumbar intervertebral disc

722.52 Lumbar or lumbosacral intervertebral disc
AHA: 2Q, '06, 18; 4Q, '04, 133
M51.37 Oth intervertebral disc degen lumbosacral region   I-10

722.6 Degeneration of intervertebral disc, site unspecified
Degenerative disc disease NOS
Narrowing of intervertebral disc or space NOS

√5ᵗʰ **722.7 Intervertebral disc disorder with myelopathy**

722.70 Unspecified region

722.71 Cervical region

722.72 Thoracic region

722.73 Lumbar region

√5ᵗʰ **722.8 Postlaminectomy syndrome**
DEF: Spinal disorder due to spinal laminectomy surgery.
AHA: J-F, '87, 7
TIP: Assign if documentation indicates that scar tissue has formed following disc surgery.

722.80 Unspecified region

722.81 Cervical region

722.82 Thoracic region

722.83 Lumbar region
AHA: 2Q, '97, 15
M96.1 Postlaminectomy syndrome NEC   I-10

√5ᵗʰ **722.9 Other and unspecified disc disorder**
Calcification of intervertebral cartilage or disc
Discitis

722.90 Unspecified region
AHA: N-D, '84, 19

722.91 Cervical region

722.92 Thoracic region

722.93 Lumbar region
M51.86 Other intervertebral disc disorder lumbar region   I-10

√4ᵗʰ **723 Other disorders of cervical region**
EXCLUDES conditions due to:
intervertebral disc disorders (722.0-722.9)
spondylosis (721.0-721.9)
AHA: 3Q, '94, 14; 2Q, '89, 14

723.0 Spinal stenosis in cervical region
AHA: 4Q, '03, 101
M48.02 Spinal stenosis cervical region   I-10

723.1 Cervicalgia
Pain in neck
DEF: Pain in cervical spine or neck region.
M54.2 Cervicalgia   I-10

723.2 Cervicocranial syndrome
Barré-Liéou syndrome
Posterior cervical sympathetic syndrome
DEF: Neurologic disorder of upper cervical spine and nerve roots.

723.3 Cervicobrachial syndrome (diffuse)
DEF: Complex of symptoms due to scalenus anterior muscle compressing the brachial plexus; pain radiates from shoulder to arm or back of neck.
AHA: N-D, '85, 12

723.4 Brachial neuritis or radiculitis NOS
Cervical radiculitis
Radicular syndrome of upper limbs

723.5 Torticollis, unspecified
Contracture of neck
EXCLUDES congenital (754.1)
due to birth injury (767.8)
hysterical (300.11)
ocular torticollis (781.93)
psychogenic (306.0)
spasmodic (333.83)
traumatic, current (847.0)
DEF: Abnormally positioned neck relative to head due to cervical muscle or fascia contractions; also called wryneck.
AHA: 2Q, '01, 21; 1Q, '95, 7

723.6 Panniculitis specified as affecting neck
DEF: Inflammation of the panniculus adiposus (subcutaneous fat) in the neck.

723.7 Ossification of posterior longitudinal ligament in cervical region

723.8 Other syndromes affecting cervical region
Cervical syndrome NEC
Klippel's disease
Occipital neuralgia
AHA: 1Q, '00, 7

723.9 Unspecified musculoskeletal disorders and symptoms referable to neck
Cervical (region) disorder NOS

√4ᵗʰ **724 Other and unspecified disorders of back**
EXCLUDES collapsed vertebra (code to cause, e.g., osteoporosis, 733.00-733.09)
conditions due to:
intervertebral disc disorders (722.0-722.9)
spondylosis (721.0-721.9)
AHA: 2Q, '89, 14

√5ᵗʰ **724.0 Spinal stenosis, other than cervical**

724.00 Spinal stenosis, unspecified region
M48.00 Spinal stenosis site unspecified   I-10

724.01 Thoracic region

▲ **724.02 Lumbar region, without neurogenic claudication**
►Lumbar region NOS◄
AHA: 4Q, '08, 109; 4Q, '07, 120; 1Q, '07, 10, 20; 4Q, '99, 13
M48.06 Spinal stenosis lumbar region   I-10

● **724.03 Lumbar region, with neurogenic claudication**

724.09 Other

724.1 Pain in thoracic spine

Diseases of the Musculoskeletal System and Connective Tissue

724.2–727.00

724.2 Lumbago
Low back pain
Low back syndrome
Lumbalgia
AHA: 2Q, '07, 11; N-D, '85, 12
M54.5 Low back pain [I-10]

724.3 Sciatica
Neuralgia or neuritis of sciatic nerve
EXCLUDES *specified lesion of sciatic nerve (355.0)*
AHA: 2Q, '89, 12
M54.30 Sciatica unspecified side [I-10]

724.4 Thoracic or lumbosacral neuritis or radiculitis, unspecified
Radicular syndrome of lower limbs
AHA: 2Q, '99, 3
M51.14 Intervertebral disc d/o w/radiculopathy thoracic [I-10]

724.5 Backache, unspecified
Vertebrogenic (pain) syndrome NOS
M54.9 Dorsalgia unspecified [I-10]

724.6 Disorders of sacrum
Ankylosis
Instability } lumbosacral or sacroiliac (joint)

724.7 Disorders of coccyx [✓5th]

724.70 Unspecified disorder of coccyx

724.71 Hypermobility of coccyx

724.79 Other
Coccygodynia

724.8 Other symptoms referable to back
Ossification of posterior longitudinal ligament NOS
Panniculitis specified as sacral or affecting back

724.9 Other unspecified back disorders
Ankylosis of spine NOS
Compression of spinal nerve root NEC
Spinal disorder NOS
EXCLUDES *sacroiliitis (720.2)*

Rheumatism, Excluding the Back (725-729)

INCLUDES disorders of muscles and tendons and their attachments, and of other soft tissues

725 Polymyalgia rheumatica
DEF: Joint and muscle pain, pelvis, and shoulder girdle stiffness, high sedimentation rate and temporal arteritis; occurs in elderly.
M35.3 Polymyalgia rheumatica [I-10]

726 Peripheral enthesopathies and allied syndromes [✓4th]
NOTE Enthesopathies are disorders of peripheral ligamentous or muscular attachments.
EXCLUDES *spinal enthesopathy (720.1)*

726.0 Adhesive capsulitis of shoulder

726.1 Rotator cuff syndrome of shoulder and allied disorders [✓5th]

726.10 Disorders of bursae and tendons in shoulder region, unspecified
Rotator cuff syndrome NOS
Supraspinatus syndrome NOS
AHA: 2Q, '01, 11
M75.11 Rotator cuff syndrome right shoulder [I-10]

726.11 Calcifying tendinitis of shoulder

726.12 Bicipital tenosynovitis

726.19 Other specified disorders
EXCLUDES *complete rupture of rotator cuff, nontraumatic (727.61)*

726.2 Other affections of shoulder region, not elsewhere classified
Periarthritis of shoulder
Scapulohumeral fibrositis

726.3 Enthesopathy of elbow region [✓5th]

726.30 Enthesopathy of elbow, unspecified

726.31 Medial epicondylitis

726.32 Lateral epicondylitis
Epicondylitis NOS
Golfers' elbow
Tennis elbow

726.33 Olecranon bursitis
Bursitis of elbow

726.39 Other

726.4 Enthesopathy of wrist and carpus
Bursitis of hand or wrist
Periarthritis of wrist

726.5 Enthesopathy of hip region
Bursitis of hip
Gluteal tendinitis
Iliac crest spur
Psoas tendinitis
Trochanteric tendinitis

726.6 Enthesopathy of knee [✓5th]

726.60 Enthesopathy of knee, unspecified
Bursitis of knee NOS

726.61 Pes anserinus tendinitis or bursitis
DEF: Inflamed tendons of sartorius, gracilis and semitendinosus muscles of medial aspect of knee.

726.62 Tibial collateral ligament bursitis
Pellegrini-Stieda syndrome

726.63 Fibular collateral ligament bursitis

726.64 Patellar tendinitis

726.65 Prepatellar bursitis
AHA: 2Q, '06, 15

726.69 Other
Bursitis:
infrapatellar
subpatellar

726.7 Enthesopathy of ankle and tarsus [✓5th]

726.70 Enthesopathy of ankle and tarsus, unspecified
Metatarsalgia NOS
EXCLUDES *Morton's metatarsalgia (355.6)*

726.71 Achilles bursitis or tendinitis

726.72 Tibialis tendinitis
Tibialis (anterior) (posterior) tendinitis

726.73 Calcaneal spur
DEF: Overgrowth of calcaneus bone; causes pain on walking; due to chronic avulsion injury of plantar fascia from calcaneus.

726.79 Other
Peroneal tendinitis

726.8 Other peripheral enthesopathies

726.9 Unspecified enthesopathy [✓5th]

726.90 Enthesopathy of unspecified site
Capsulitis NOS
Periarthritis NOS
Tendinitis NOS

726.91 Exostosis of unspecified site
Bone spur NOS
AHA: 2Q, '01, 15

727 Other disorders of synovium, tendon, and bursa [✓4th]

727.0 Synovitis and tenosynovitis [✓5th]

727.00 Synovitis and tenosynovitis, unspecified
Synovitis NOS
Tenosynovitis NOS
M65.9 Synovitis and tenosynovitis unspecified [I-10]

N Newborn Age: 0 | P Pediatric Age: 0-17 | M Maternity Age: 12-55 | A Adult Age: 15-124

727.01 Synovitis and tenosynovitis in diseases classified elsewhere

Code first underlying disease as:
tuberculosis (015.0-015.9)

EXCLUDES crystal-induced (275.4)
gonococcal (098.51)
gout (274.00-274.03)
syphilitic (095.7)

727.02 Giant cell tumor of tendon sheath

727.03 Trigger finger (acquired)

DEF: Stenosing tenosynovitis or nodule in flexor tendon; cessation of flexion or extension movement in finger, followed by snapping into place.

727.04 Radial styloid tenosynovitis
de Quervain's disease

727.05 Other tenosynovitis of hand and wrist

727.06 Tenosynovitis of foot and ankle

727.09 Other

727.1 Bunion

DEF: Enlarged first metatarsal head due to inflamed bursa; results in laterally displaced great toe.

727.2 Specific bursitides often of occupational origin

Beat: Chronic crepitant synovitis of wrist
elbow   Miners':
hand   elbow
knee   knee

727.3 Other bursitis
Bursitis NOS

EXCLUDES bursitis:
gonococcal (098.52)
subacromial (726.19)
subcoracoid (726.19)
subdeltoid (726.19)
syphilitic (095.7)
"frozen shoulder" (726.0)

√5ᵗʰ 727.4 Ganglion and cyst of synovium, tendon, and bursa

727.40 Synovial cyst, unspecified

EXCLUDES that of popliteal space (727.51)
AHA: 2Q, '97, 6

727.41 Ganglion of joint

727.42 Ganglion of tendon sheath

Bunion

Normal metatarsophalangeal joint

Exostosis

Ganglia

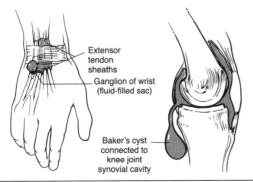

Extensor tendon sheaths

Ganglion of wrist (fluid-filled sac)

Baker's cyst connected to knee joint synovial cavity

727.43 Ganglion, unspecified

727.49 Other
Cyst of bursa

√5ᵗʰ 727.5 Rupture of synovium

727.50 Rupture of synovium, unspecified

727.51 Synovial cyst of popliteal space
Baker's cyst (knee)

727.59 Other

√5ᵗʰ 727.6 Rupture of tendon, nontraumatic

727.60 Nontraumatic rupture of unspecified tendon

727.61 Complete rupture of rotator cuff

727.62 Tendons of biceps (long head)

727.63 Extensor tendons of hand and wrist

727.64 Flexor tendons of hand and wrist

727.65 Quadriceps tendon

727.66 Patellar tendon

727.67 Achilles tendon

727.68 Other tendons of foot and ankle

727.69 Other

√5ᵗʰ 727.8 Other disorders of synovium, tendon, and bursa

727.81 Contracture of tendon (sheath)
Short Achilles tendon (acquired)

727.82 Calcium deposits in tendon and bursa
Calcification of tendon NOS
Calcific tendinitis NOS

EXCLUDES peripheral ligamentous or muscular attachments (726.0-726.9)

727.83 Plica syndrome
Plica knee

DEF: A fold in the synovial tissue formed before birth, creating a septum between two pockets of synovial tissue; most common are the medial patellar plica and the suprapatellar plica. Plica syndrome, or plica knee, refers to symptomatic plica.
AHA: 4Q, '00, 44

727.89 Other
Abscess of bursa or tendon

EXCLUDES xanthomatosis localized to tendons (272.7)
AHA: 2Q, '89, 15

727.9 Unspecified disorder of synovium, tendon, and bursa

√4ᵗʰ 728 Disorders of muscle, ligament, and fascia

EXCLUDES enthesopathies (726.0-726.9)
muscular dystrophies (359.0-359.1)
myoneural disorders (358.00-358.9)
myopathies (359.2-359.9)
nontraumatic hematoma of muscle (729.92)
old disruption of ligaments of knee (717.81-717.89)

728.0 Infective myositis
Myositis:
purulent
suppurative

EXCLUDES myositis:
epidemic (074.1)
interstitial (728.81)
syphilitic (095.6)
tropical (040.81)

DEF: Inflamed connective septal tissue of muscle.

√5ᵗʰ 728.1 Muscular calcification and ossification

728.10 Calcification and ossification, unspecified
Massive calcification (paraplegic)

728.11 Progressive myositis ossificans

DEF: Progressive myositic disease; marked by bony tissue formed by voluntary muscle; occurs among very young.

728.12 Traumatic myositis ossificans
Myositis ossificans (circumscripta)

√4ᵗʰ√5ᵗʰ Additional Digit Required   Unspecified Code   Other Specified Code   Manifestation Code   ▶◀ Revised Text   ● New Code   ▲ Revised Code Title

2011 ICD-9-CM   **Volume 1 – 227**

Diseases of the Musculoskeletal System and Connective Tissue (side margin)

728.13–729.6 (side margin)

728.13 Postoperative heterotopic calcification
DEF: Abnormal formation of calcium deposits in muscular tissue after surgery, marked by a corresponding loss of muscle tone and tension.

728.19 Other
Polymyositis ossificans

728.2 Muscular wasting and disuse atrophy, not elsewhere classified
Amyotrophia NOS
Myofibrosis
> EXCLUDES neuralgic amyotrophy (353.5)
> pelvic muscle wasting and disuse atrophy (618.83)
> progressive muscular atrophy (335.0-335.9)

728.3 Other specific muscle disorders
Arthrogryposis
Immobility syndrome (paraplegic)
> EXCLUDES arthrogryposis multiplex congenita (754.89)
> stiff-man syndrome (333.91)

728.4 Laxity of ligament

728.5 Hypermobility syndrome

728.6 Contracture of palmar fascia   A
Dupuytren's contracture
DEF: Dupuytren's contracture: flexion deformity of finger, due to shortened, thickened fibrosing of palmar fascia; cause unknown; associated with long-standing epilepsy.

√5th 728.7 Other fibromatoses

728.71 Plantar fascial fibromatosis
Contracture of plantar fascia
Plantar fasciitis (traumatic)
DEF: Plantar fascia fibromatosis; causes nodular swelling and pain; not associated with contractures.

728.79 Other
Garrod's or knuckle pads
Nodular fasciitis
Pseudosarcomatous fibromatosis (proliferative) (subcutaneous)
DEF: Knuckle pads: Pea-size nodules on dorsal surface of interphalangeal joints; new growth of fibrous tissue with thickened dermis and epidermis.

√5th 728.8 Other disorders of muscle, ligament, and fascia

728.81 Interstitial myositis
DEF: Inflammation of septal connective parts of muscle tissue.

728.82 Foreign body granuloma of muscle
Talc granuloma of muscle
▶Use additional code to identify foreign body (V90.01-V90.9)◀

728.83 Rupture of muscle, nontraumatic

728.84 Diastasis of muscle
Diastasis recti (abdomen)
> EXCLUDES diastasis recti complicating pregnancy, labor, and delivery (665.8)
DEF: Muscle separation, such as recti abdominis after repeated pregnancies.

728.85 Spasm of muscle
M62.838 Other muscle spasm   I-10

728.86 Necrotizing fasciitis
Use additional code to identify:
    infectious organism (041.00-041.89)
    gangrene (785.4), if applicable
DEF: Fulminating infection begins with extensive cellulitis, spreads to superficial and deep fascia; causes thrombosis of subcutaneous vessels, and gangrene of underlying tissue.
AHA: 4Q, '95, 54

728.87 Muscle weakness (generalized)
> EXCLUDES generalized weakness (780.79)
AHA: 1Q, '05, 13; 4Q, '03, 66
TIP: Assign an additional code from category 438 if the weakness is a result of a CVA.

728.88 Rhabdomyolysis
DEF: A disintegration or destruction of muscle; an acute disease characterized by the excretion of myoglobin into the urine.
AHA: 4Q, '03, 66

728.89 Other
Eosinophilic fasciitis
Use additional E code to identify drug, if drug induced
DEF: Eosinophilic fasciitis: inflammation of fascia of extremities associated with eosinophilia, edema, and swelling; occurs alone or as part of myalgia syndrome.
AHA: 3Q, '06, 13; 3Q, '02, 28; 2Q, '01, 14, 15

728.9 Unspecified disorder of muscle, ligament, and fascia

√4th 729 Other disorders of soft tissues
> EXCLUDES acroparesthesia (443.89)
> carpal tunnel syndrome (354.0)
> disorders of the back (720.0-724.9)
> entrapment syndromes (354.0-355.9)
> palindromic rheumatism (719.3)
> periarthritis (726.0-726.9)
> psychogenic rheumatism (306.0)

729.0 Rheumatism, unspecified and fibrositis
DEF: General term describes diseases of muscle, tendon, nerve, joint, or bone; symptoms include pain and stiffness.

729.1 Myalgia and myositis, unspecified
Fibromyositis NOS
DEF: Myalgia: muscle pain.
DEF: Myositis: inflamed voluntary muscle.
DEF: Fibromyositis: inflamed fibromuscular tissue.
M79.1 Myalgia   I-10

729.2 Neuralgia, neuritis, and radiculitis, unspecified
> EXCLUDES brachial radiculitis (723.4)
> cervical radiculitis (723.4)
> lumbosacral radiculitis (724.4)
> mononeuritis (354.0-355.9)
> radiculitis due to intervertebral disc involvement (722.0-722.2, 722.7)
> sciatica (724.3)
DEF: Neuralgia: paroxysmal pain along nerve; symptoms include brief pain and tenderness at point nerve exits.
DEF: Neuritis: inflamed nerve, symptoms include paresthesia, paralysis and loss of reflexes at nerve site.
DEF: Radiculitis: inflamed nerve root.

√5th 729.3 Panniculitis, unspecified
DEF: Inflammatory reaction of subcutaneous fat; causes nodules; often develops in abdominal region.

729.30 Panniculitis, unspecified site
Weber-Christian disease
DEF: Febrile, nodular, nonsuppurative, relapsing inflammation of subcutaneous fat.

729.31 Hypertrophy of fat pad, knee
Hypertrophy of infrapatellar fat pad

729.39 Other site
> EXCLUDES panniculitis specified as (affecting):
> back (724.8)
> neck (723.6)
> sacral (724.8)

729.4 Fasciitis, unspecified
> EXCLUDES necrotizing fasciitis (728.86)
> nodular fasciitis (728.79)
AHA: 2Q, '94, 13

729.5 Pain in limb
AHA: 2Q, '07, 11
M79.609 Pain in unspecified limb   I-10

729.6 Residual foreign body in soft tissue
▶Use additional code to identify foreign body (V90.01-V90.9)◀
> EXCLUDES foreign body granuloma:
> muscle (728.82)
> skin and subcutaneous tissue (709.4)

N Newborn Age: 0   P Pediatric Age: 0-17   M Maternity Age: 12-55   A Adult Age: 15-124

√5ᵗʰ **729.7 Nontraumatic compartment syndrome**

Code first, if applicable, postprocedural complication (998.89)

EXCLUDES *compartment syndrome NOS (958.90)*
traumatic compartment syndrome (958.90-958.99)

DEF: Compression of nerves and blood vessels within an enclosed space, leading to impaired blood flow and muscle and nerve damage.

729.71 Nontraumatic compartment syndrome of upper extremity

Nontraumatic compartment syndrome of shoulder, arm, forearm, wrist, hand, and fingers

AHA: 4Q, '06, 100-102

729.72 Nontraumatic compartment syndrome of lower extremity

Nontraumatic compartment syndrome of hip, buttock, thigh, leg, foot, and toes

AHA: 4Q, '06, 100-102

729.73 Nontraumatic compartment syndrome of abdomen

AHA: 4Q, '06, 100-102

729.79 Nontraumatic compartment syndrome of other sites

AHA: 4Q, '06, 100-102

√5ᵗʰ **729.8 Other musculoskeletal symptoms referable to limbs**

TIP: Assign for pseudothrombophlebitis, which involves painful swelling of the lower extremity and mimics deep vein thrombosis (DVT).

729.81 Swelling of limb

AHA: 4Q, '88, 6

TIP: Assign for pseudothrombophlebitis, which involves painful swelling of the lower extremity and mimics deep vein thrombosis (DVT).

729.82 Cramp

729.89 Other

EXCLUDES *abnormality of gait (781.2)*
tetany (781.7)
transient paralysis of limb (781.4)

AHA: 4Q, '88, 12

R29.898 Oth symptoms & signs involv musculo sys   I-10

√5ᵗʰ **729.9 Other and unspecified disorders of soft tissue**

AHA: 4Q, '08, 134-136

729.90 Disorders of soft tissue, unspecified

729.91 Post-traumatic seroma

EXCLUDES *seroma complicating a procedure (998.13)*

729.92 Nontraumatic hematoma of soft tissue

Nontraumatic hematoma of muscle

AHA: 4Q, '08, 135

TIP: Assign an additional E code for a drug adverse effect if caused by Coumadin or other anticoagulants.

729.99 Other disorders of soft tissue

Polyalgia

Osteopathies, Chondropathies, and Acquired Musculoskeletal Deformities (730-739)

√4ᵗʰ **730 Osteomyelitis, periostitis, and other infections involving bone**

EXCLUDES *jaw (526.4-526.5)*
petrous bone (383.2)

Use additional code to identify organism, such as Staphylococcus (041.1)

The following fifth-digit subclassification is for use with category 730; valid digits are in [brackets] under each code. See list at beginning of chapter for definitions.

  0   site unspecified
  1   shoulder region
  2   upper arm
  3   forearm
  4   hand
  5   pelvic region and thigh
  6   lower leg
  7   ankle and foot
  8   other specified sites
  9   multiple sites

DEF: Osteomyelitis: bacterial inflammation of bone tissue and marrow.

DEF: Periostitis: inflammation of specialized connective tissue; causes swelling of bone and aching pain.

AHA: 4Q, '97, 43

§ √5ᵗʰ **730.0 Acute osteomyelitis**
[0-9]

Abscess of any bone except accessory sinus, jaw, or mastoid

Acute or subacute osteomyelitis, with or without mention of periostitis

Use additional code to identify major osseous defect, if applicable (731.3)

AHA: 4Q, '06, 103; **For code 730.06:** 1Q, '02, 4; **For code 730.07:** 1Q, '04, 14

§ √5ᵗʰ **730.1 Chronic osteomyelitis**
[0-9]

Brodie's abscess

Chronic or old osteomyelitis, with or without mention of periostitis

Sequestrum of bone

Sclerosing osteomyelitis of Garré

Use additional code to identify major osseous defect, if applicable (731.3)

EXCLUDES *aseptic necrosis of bone (733.40-733.49)*

AHA: 4Q, '06, 103; **For code 730.17:** 3Q, '00, 4

§ √5ᵗʰ **730.2 Unspecified osteomyelitis**
[0-9]

Osteitis or osteomyelitis NOS, with or without mention of periostitis

Use additional code to identify major osseous defect, if applicable (731.3)

AHA: 4Q, '06, 103

M86.9 Osteomyelitis unspecified   I-10

§ √5ᵗʰ **730.3 Periostitis without mention of osteomyelitis**
[0-9]

Abscess of periosteum } without mention of
Periostosis   osteomyelitis

EXCLUDES *that in secondary syphilis (091.61)*

§ √5ᵗʰ **730.7 Osteopathy resulting from poliomyelitis**
[0-9]

Code first underlying disease (045.0-045.9)

§ √5ᵗʰ **730.8 Other infections involving bone in diseases classified elsewhere**
[0-9]

Code first underlying disease as:
tuberculosis (015.0-015.9)
typhoid fever (002.0)

EXCLUDES *syphilis of bone NOS (095.5)*

AHA: 2Q, '97, 16; 3Q, '91, 10

§ √5ᵗʰ **730.9 Unspecified infection of bone**
[0-9]

§   Requires fifth digit. Valid digits are in [brackets] under each code. See beginning of section 710-739 for codes and defintions.

√4ᵗʰ / √5ᵗʰ   Additional Digit Required   Unspecified Code   Other Specified Code   Manifestation Code   ►◄ Revised Text   ● New Code   ▲ Revised Code Title

2011 ICD-9-CM   **Volume 1 – 229**

✓4ᵗʰ 731 Osteitis deformans and osteopathies associated with other disorders classified elsewhere

DEF: Osteitis deformans: Bone disease marked by episodes of increased bone loss, excessive repair attempts; causes weakened, deformed bones with increased mass, bowed long bones, deformed flat bones, pain and pathological fractures; may be fatal if associated with congestive heart failure, giant cell tumors or bone sarcoma; also called Paget's disease.

731.0 Osteitis deformans without mention of bone tumor
Paget's disease of bone

731.1 Osteitis deformans in diseases classified elsewhere
Code first underlying disease as:
malignant neoplasm of bone (170.0-170.9)

731.2 Hypertrophic pulmonary osteoarthropathy
Bamberger-Marie disease
DEF: Clubbing of fingers and toes; related to enlarged ends of long bones, due to chronic lung and heart disease.

731.3 Major osseous defects
Code first underlying disease, if known, such as:
aseptic necrosis (733.40-733.49)
malignant neoplasm of bone (170.0-170.9)
osteomyelitis (730.00-730.29)
osteoporosis (733.00-733.09)
peri-prosthetic osteolysis (996.45)
AHA: 4Q, '06, 103

731.8 Other bone involvement in diseases classified elsewhere
Code first underlying disease as:
diabetes mellitus (249.8, 250.8)

Use additional code to specify bone condition, such as:
acute osteomyelitis (730.00-730.09)
AHA: 1Q, '04, 14; 4Q, '97, 43; 2Q, '97, 16
TIP: For diabetic osteomyelitis, assign a total of three codes: 250.8X, 731.8, and a code from category 730.
M90.89 Osteopathy dz classified elsewhere multiple site　I-10

✓4ᵗʰ 732 Osteochondropathies

DEF: Conditions related to both bone and cartilage, or conditions in which cartilage is converted to bone (enchondral ossification).

732.0 Juvenile osteochondrosis of spine
Juvenile osteochondrosis (of):
marginal or vertebral epiphysis (of Scheuermann)
spine NOS
Vertebral epiphysitis
EXCLUDES adolescent postural kyphosis (737.0)

732.1 Juvenile osteochondrosis of hip and pelvis
Coxa plana
Ischiopubic synchondrosis (of van Neck)
Osteochondrosis (juvenile) of:
acetabulum
head of femur (of Legg-Calvé-Perthes)
iliac crest (of Buchanan)
symphysis pubis (of Pierson)
Pseudocoxalgia

732.2 Nontraumatic slipped upper femoral epiphysis
Slipped upper femoral epiphysis NOS

732.3 Juvenile osteochondrosis of upper extremity
Osteochondrosis (juvenile) of:
capitulum of humerus (of Panner)
carpal lunate (of Kienbock)
hand NOS
head of humerus (of Haas)
heads of metacarpals (of Mauclaire)
lower ulna (of Burns)
radial head (of Brailsford)
upper extremity NOS

732.4 Juvenile osteochondrosis of lower extremity, excluding foot
Osteochondrosis (juvenile) of:
lower extremity NOS
primary patellar center (of Köhler)
proximal tibia (of Blount)
secondary patellar center (of Sinding-Larsen)
tibial tubercle (of Osgood-Schlatter)
Tibia vara

Slipped Femoral Epiphysis

Kline's line — Normal epiphysis — Femoral neck — Pinned fixation — Kline's line — Slipped epiphysis

732.5 Juvenile osteochondrosis of foot
Calcaneal apophysitis
Epiphysitis, os calcis
Osteochondrosis (juvenile) of:
astragalus (of Diaz)
calcaneum (of Sever)
foot NOS
metatarsal
second (of Freiberg)
fifth (of Iselin)
os tibiale externum (of Haglund)
tarsal navicular (of Köhler)

732.6 Other juvenile osteochondrosis
Apophysitis
Epiphysitis　} specified as juvenile, of other
Osteochondritis　site, or site NOS
Osteochondrosis

732.7 Osteochondritis dissecans

732.8 Other specified forms of osteochondropathy
Adult osteochondrosis of spine

732.9 Unspecified osteochondropathy
Apophysitis　} NOS
Epiphysitis　not specified as adult or juvenile, of
Osteochondritis　unspecified site
Osteochondrosis

✓4ᵗʰ 733 Other disorders of bone and cartilage

EXCLUDES bone spur (726.91)
cartilage of, or loose body in, joint (717.0-717.9, 718.0-718.9)
giant cell granuloma of jaw (526.3)
osteitis fibrosa cystica generalisata (252.01)
osteomalacia (268.2)
polyostotic fibrous dysplasia of bone (756.54)
prognathism, retrognathism (524.1)
xanthomatosis localized to bone (272.7)

✓5ᵗʰ 733.0 Osteoporosis
Use additional code to identify major osseous defect, if applicable (731.3)
Use additional code to identify personal history of pathologic (healed) fracture (V13.51)
DEF: Bone mass reduction that ultimately results in fractures after minimal trauma; dorsal kyphosis or loss of height often occur.
AHA: 4Q, '06, 103

733.00 Osteoporosis, unspecified
Wedging of vertebra NOS
AHA: 4Q, '07, 92;1Q, '07, 22; 3Q, '01, 19; 2Q, '98, 12
M81.8 Other osteoporosis w/o current pathological fx　I-10

733.01 Senile osteoporosis
Postmenopausal osteoporosis
AHA: 1Q, '07, 5, 6
M81.0 Age-related osteoporosis without current pathological fracture　I-10

733.02 Idiopathic osteoporosis

733.03 Disuse osteoporosis

733.09 Other
Drug-induced osteoporosis
Use additional E code to identify drug
AHA: 4Q, '03, 108
M81.6 Localized osteoporosis [Lequesne]   `I-10`

√5ᵗʰ **733.1 Pathologic fracture**
Chronic fracture
Spontaneous fracture
EXCLUDES *stress fracture (733.93-733.95)*
traumatic fracture (800-829)
DEF: Fracture due to bone structure weakening by pathological processes (e.g., osteoporosis, neoplasms and osteomalacia).
AHA: 4Q, '08, 158; 1Q, '07, 3-4; 4Q, '93, 25; N-D, '86, 10; N-D, '85, 16
TIP: Assign only for newly diagnosed fractures; refer to V code aftercare categories if patient is receiving routine care during healing or recovery phase.

733.10 Pathologic fracture, unspecified site

733.11 Pathologic fracture of humerus

733.12 Pathologic fracture of distal radius and ulna
Wrist NOS

733.13 Pathologic fracture of vertebrae
Collapse of vertebra NOS
AHA: 3Q, '08, 4; 1Q, '07, 5, 6, 22; 3Q, '99, 5
TIP: Assign for a chronic vertebral pathological fracture for which the patient is receiving medication.
M48.53xA Collapsed vertebra NEC cervicothorac   `I-10`
initial enc

733.14 Pathologic fracture of neck of femur
Femur NOS
Hip NOS
AHA: 1Q, '01, 1; 1Q, '96, 16

733.15 Pathologic fracture of other specified part of femur
AHA: 2Q, '98, 12
M84.453A Pathological fracture, unspec femur,   `I-10`
initial encounter for fx

733.16 Pathologic fracture of tibia or fibula
Ankle NOS

733.19 Pathologic fracture of other specified site

√5ᵗʰ **733.2 Cyst of bone**

733.20 Cyst of bone (localized), unspecified

733.21 Solitary bone cyst
Unicameral bone cyst

733.22 Aneurysmal bone cyst
DEF: Solitary bone lesion, bulges into periosteum; marked by calcified rim.

733.29 Other
Fibrous dysplasia (monostotic)
EXCLUDES *cyst of jaw (526.0-526.2, 526.89)*
osteitis fibrosa cystica (252.01)
polyostotic fibrousdysplasia of bone (756.54)

733.3 Hyperostosis of skull
Hyperostosis interna frontalis
Leontiasis ossium
DEF: Abnormal bone growth on inner aspect of cranial bones.

√5ᵗʰ **733.4 Aseptic necrosis of bone**
Use additional code to identify major osseous defect, if applicable (731.3)
EXCLUDES *osteochondropathies (732.0-732.9)*
DEF: Infarction of bone tissue due to a noninfectious etiology, such as a fracture, ischemic disorder or administration of immunosuppressive drugs; leads to degenerative joint disease or nonunion of fractures.
AHA: 4Q, '06, 103

733.40 Aseptic necrosis of bone, site unspecified

733.41 Head of humerus

733.42 Head and neck of femur
Femur NOS
EXCLUDES *Legg-Calvé-Perthes disease (732.1)*
M87.256 Osteonecrosis due to previous   `I-10`
trauma uns femur

733.43 Medial femoral condyle

733.44 Talus

733.45 Jaw
Use additional E code to identify drug, if drug-induced
EXCLUDES *osteoradionecrosis of jaw (526.89)*
AHA: 4Q, '07, 91

733.49 Other

733.5 Osteitis condensans
Piriform sclerosis of ilium
DEF: Idiopathic condition marked by low back pain; associated with oval or triangular sclerotic, opaque bone next to sacroiliac joints in the ileum.

733.6 Tietze's disease
Costochondral junction syndrome
Costochondritis
DEF: Painful, idiopathic, nonsuppurative, swollen costal cartilage sometimes confused with cardiac symptoms because the anterior chest pain resembles that of coronary artery disease.
M94.0 Chondrocostal junction syndrome (Tietze dz)   `I-10`

733.7 Algoneurodystrophy
Disuse atrophy of bone
Sudeck's atrophy
DEF: Painful, idiopathic complex reflex sympathetic dystrophy, a chronic progressive disease characterized by severe pain, swelling, and changes in the skin.

√5ᵗʰ **733.8 Malunion and nonunion of fracture**
AHA: 2Q, '94, 5

733.81 Malunion of fracture

733.82 Nonunion of fracture
Pseudoarthrosis (bone)

√5ᵗʰ **733.9 Other unspecified disorders of bone and cartilage**
AHA: 4Q, '08, 136-137

733.90 Disorder of bone and cartilage unspecified
M89.9 Disorder of bone, unspecified   `I-10`

733.91 Arrest of bone development or growth
Epiphyseal arrest

733.92 Chondromalacia
Chondromalacia:
NOS
localized, except patella
systemic
tibial plateau
EXCLUDES *chondromalacia of patella (717.7)*
DEF: Articular cartilage softening.

733.93 Stress fracture of tibia or fibula
Stress reaction of tibia or fibula
Use additional external cause code(s) to identify the cause of the stress fracture
AHA: 4Q, '08, 158; 4Q, '01, 48

733.94 Stress fracture of the metatarsals
Stress reaction of metatarsals
Use additional external cause code(s) to identify the cause of the stress fracture
AHA: 4Q, '08, 158; 4Q, '01, 48

733.95 Stress fracture of other bone
Stress reaction of other bone
Use additional external cause code(s) to identify the cause of the stress fracture
EXCLUDES *stress fracture of:*
femoral neck (733.96)
fibula (733.93)
metatarsals (733.94)
pelvis (733.98)
shaft of femur (733.97)
tibia (733.93)
AHA: 4Q, '08, 158; 4Q, '01, 48

733.96 Stress fracture of femoral neck
Stress reaction of femoral neck

Use additional external cause code(s) to identify the cause of the stress fracture

AHA: 4Q, '08, 158

733.97 Stress fracture of shaft of femur
Stress reaction of shaft of femur

Use additional external cause code(s) to identify the cause of the stress fracture

AHA: 4Q, '08, 158

733.98 Stress fracture of pelvis
Stress reaction of pelvis

Use additional external cause code(s) to identify the cause of the stress fracture

AHA: 4Q, '08, 158

733.99 Other
Diaphysitis
Hypertrophy of bone
Relapsing polychondritis

AHA: J-F, '87, 14

734 Flat foot
Pes planus (acquired)
Talipes planus (acquired)

EXCLUDES   congenital (754.61)
rigid flat foot (754.61)
spastic (everted) flat foot (754.61)

√4th 735 Acquired deformities of toe

EXCLUDES   congenital (754.60-754.69, 755.65-755.66)

735.0 Hallux valgus (acquired)
DEF: Angled displacement of the great toe, causing it to ride over or under other toes.

735.1 Hallux varus (acquired)
DEF: Angled displacement of the great toe toward the body midline, away from the other toes.

735.2 Hallux rigidus
DEF: Limited flexion movement at metatarsophalangeal joint of great toe; due to degenerative joint disease.

735.3 Hallux malleus
DEF: Extended proximal phalanx, flexed distal phalanges of great toe; foot resembles claw or hammer.

735.4 Other hammer toe (acquired)

735.5 Claw toe (acquired)
DEF: Hyperextended proximal phalanges, flexed middle and distal phalanges.

735.8 Other acquired deformities of toe
AHA: 4Q, '07, 123

TIP: Assign for hallux limitus, a deformity of the first metatarsophalangeal joint, which restricts the range of motion and can lead to stiffness and pain in the joint.

735.9 Unspecified acquired deformity of toe

√4th 736 Other acquired deformities of limbs

EXCLUDES   congenital (754.3-755.9)

√5th 736.0 Acquired deformities of forearm, excluding fingers

736.00 Unspecified deformity
Deformity of elbow, forearm, hand, or wrist (acquired) NOS

736.01 Cubitus valgus (acquired)
DEF: Deviation of the elbow away from the body midline upon extension; it occurs when the palm is turning outward.

736.02 Cubitus varus (acquired)
DEF: Elbow joint displacement angled laterally; when the forearm is extended, it is deviated toward the midline of the body; also called "gun stock" deformity.

736.03 Valgus deformity of wrist (acquired)
DEF: Abnormal angulation away from the body midline.

736.04 Varus deformity of wrist (acquired)
DEF: Abnormal angulation toward the body midline.

Acquired Deformities of Toe

Hallux valgus

Hallux varus

Hallux malleus (hammer of big toe)

Hammertoe

Acquired Deformities of Forearm

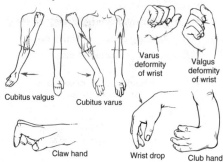

Varus deformity of wrist

Valgus deformity of wrist

Cubitus valgus   Cubitus varus

Claw hand   Wrist drop   Club hand

736.05 Wrist drop (acquired)
DEF: Inability to extend the hand at the wrist due to extensor muscle paralysis.

736.06 Claw hand (acquired)
DEF: Flexion and atrophy of the hand and fingers; found in ulnar nerve lesions, syringomyelia, and leprosy.

736.07 Club hand, acquired
DEF: Twisting of the hand out of shape or position; caused by the congenital absence of the ulna or radius.

736.09 Other

736.1 Mallet finger
DEF: Permanently flexed distal phalanx.

√5th 736.2 Other acquired deformities of finger

736.20 Unspecified deformity
Deformity of finger (acquired) NOS

736.21 Boutonniere deformity
DEF: A deformity of the finger caused by flexion of the proximal interphalangeal joint and hyperextension of the distal joint; also called buttonhole deformity.

736.22 Swan-neck deformity
DEF: Flexed distal and hyperextended proximal interphalangeal joint.

736.29 Other

EXCLUDES   trigger finger (727.03)

AHA: 2Q, '05, 7; 2Q, '89, 13

√5th 736.3 Acquired deformities of hip

736.30 Unspecified deformity
Deformity of hip (acquired) NOS

736.31 Coxa valga (acquired)
DEF: Increase of at least 140 degrees in the angle formed by the axis of the head and the neck of the femur, and the axis of its shaft.

736.32 Coxa vara (acquired)
DEF: The bending downward of the neck of the femur, causing difficulty in movement; a right angle or less may be formed by the axis of the head and neck of the femur, and the axis of its shaft.

736.39 Other
AHA: 2Q, '08, 4; 2Q, '91, 18

TIP: Assign as principal diagnosis for follow-up visit for patient with hip methylmethacrylate cement spacer, following removal of infected joint prosthesis.

Deformities of Lower Limb

√5ᵗʰ **736.4 Genu valgum or varum (acquired)**

  736.41 Genu valgum (acquired)
    DEF: Abnormally close together and an abnormally large space between the ankles; also called "knock-knees."

  736.42 Genu varum (acquired)
    DEF: Abnormally separated knees and the inward bowing of the legs; it is also called "bowlegs."

736.5 Genu recurvatum (acquired)
  DEF: Hyperextended knees; also called "backknee."

736.6 Other acquired deformities of knee
  Deformity of knee (acquired) NOS

√5ᵗʰ **736.7 Other acquired deformities of ankle and foot**
  EXCLUDES deformities of toe (acquired) (735.0-735.9)
           pes planus (acquired) (734)

  736.70 Unspecified deformity of ankle and foot, acquired

  736.71 Acquired equinovarus deformity
    Clubfoot, acquired
    EXCLUDES clubfoot not specified as acquired (754.5-754.7)

  736.72 Equinus deformity of foot, acquired
    DEF: A plantar flexion deformity that forces people to walk on their toes.

  736.73 Cavus deformity of foot
    EXCLUDES that with claw foot (736.74)
    DEF: Abnormally high longitudinal arch of the foot.

  736.74 Claw foot, acquired
    DEF: High foot arch with hyperextended toes at metatarsophalangeal joint and flexed toes at distal joints; also called "main en griffe."

  736.75 Cavovarus deformity of foot, acquired
    DEF: Inward turning of the heel from the midline of the leg and an abnormally high longitudinal arch.

  736.76 Other calcaneus deformity

  736.79 Other
    Acquired:
      pes
      talipes } not elsewhere classified

√5ᵗʰ **736.8 Acquired deformities of other parts of limbs**

  736.81 Unequal leg length (acquired)

  736.89 Other
    Deformity (acquired):
      arm or leg, not elsewhere classified
      shoulder
    AHA: 2Q, '08, 5
    TIP: Assign as principal diagnosis for follow-up visit for patient with humeral methylmethacrylate cement spacer, following removal of infected joint prosthesis.

736.9 Acquired deformity of limb, site unspecified

Kyphosis and Lordosis

√4ᵗʰ **737 Curvature of spine**
  EXCLUDES congenital (754.2)

  737.0 Adolescent postural kyphosis
    EXCLUDES osteochondrosis of spine (juvenile) (732.0)
             adult (732.8)

√5ᵗʰ **737.1 Kyphosis (acquired)**

  737.10 Kyphosis (acquired) (postural)
    M40.05 Postural kyphosis thoracolumbar region   I-10

  737.11 Kyphosis due to radiation

  737.12 Kyphosis, postlaminectomy
    AHA: J-F, '87, 7
    M96.3 Postlaminectomy kyphosis   I-10

  737.19 Other
    EXCLUDES that associated with conditions classifiable elsewhere (737.41)
    AHA: 1Q, '07, 20

√5ᵗʰ **737.2 Lordosis (acquired)**
  DEF: Swayback appearance created by an abnormally increased spinal curvature; it is also referred to as "hollow back" or "saddle back."

  737.20 Lordosis (acquired) (postural)

  737.21 Lordosis, postlaminectomy

  737.22 Other postsurgical lordosis

  737.29 Other
    EXCLUDES that associated with conditions classifiable elsewhere (737.42)

√5ᵗʰ **737.3 Kyphoscoliosis and scoliosis**
  DEF: Kyphoscoliosis: backward and lateral curvature of the spinal column; it is found in vertebral osteochondrosis.
  DEF: Scoliosis: an abnormal deviation of the spine to the left or right of the midline.

  737.30 Scoliosis [and kyphoscoliosis], idiopathic
    AHA: 3Q, '03, 19
    M41.115 Juvenile idiopathic scoliosis thoracolumbar region   I-10

  737.31 Resolving infantile idiopathic scoliosis

  737.32 Progressive infantile idiopathic scoliosis
    AHA: 3Q, '02, 12

Scoliosis and Kyphoscoliosis

Scoliosis   Kyphoscoliosis

√4ᵗʰ√5ᵗʰ Additional Digit Required   Unspecified Code   Other Specified Code   Manifestation Code   ►◄ Revised Text   ● New Code   ▲ Revised Code Title

2011 ICD-9-CM   **Volume 1 – 233**

737.33 Scoliosis due to radiation

737.34 Thoracogenic scoliosis

737.39 Other

> *EXCLUDES* *that associated with conditions classifiable*
> *elsewhere (737.43)*
> *that in kyphoscoliotic heart disease (416.1)*
> AHA: 2Q, '02, 16

√5ᵗʰ 737.4 Curvature of spine associated with other conditions

Code first associated condition as:
Charcôt-Marie-Tooth disease (356.1)
mucopolysaccharidosis (277.5)
neurofibromatosis ▶(237.70-237.79)◀
osteitis deformans (731.0)
osteitis fibrosa cystica (252.01)
osteoporosis (733.00-733.09)
poliomyelitis (138)
tuberculosis [Pott's curvature] (015.0)

737.40 Curvature of spine, unspecified

737.41 Kyphosis

737.42 Lordosis

737.43 Scoliosis

737.8 Other curvatures of spine

737.9 Unspecified curvature of spine
Curvature of spine (acquired) (idiopathic) NOS
Hunchback, acquired
> *EXCLUDES* *deformity of spine NOS (738.5)*

√4ᵗʰ 738 Other acquired deformity
> *EXCLUDES* *congenital (754.0-756.9, 758.0-759.9)*
> *dentofacial anomalies (524.0-524.9)*

738.0 Acquired deformity of nose
Deformity of nose (acquired)
Overdevelopment of nasal bones
> *EXCLUDES* *deflected or deviated nasal septum (470)*

√5ᵗʰ 738.1 Other acquired deformity of head

738.10 Unspecified deformity

738.11 Zygomatic hyperplasia
> DEF: Abnormal enlargement of the zygoma (processus
> zygomaticus temporalis).

738.12 Zygomatic hypoplasia
> DEF: Underdevelopment of the zygoma (processus
> zygomaticus temporalis).

738.19 Other specified deformity
> AHA: 1Q, '06, 8; 2Q, '03, 13

738.2 Acquired deformity of neck

738.3 Acquired deformity of chest and rib
Deformity:
chest (acquired)
rib (acquired)
Pectus:
carinatum, acquired
excavatum, acquired

738.4 Acquired spondylolisthesis
Degenerative spondylolisthesis
Spondylolysis, acquired
> *EXCLUDES* *congenital (756.12)*
> DEF: Vertebra displaced forward over another; due to bilateral defect
> in vertebral arch, eroded articular surface of posterior facets and
> elongated pedicle between fifth lumbar vertebra and sacrum.
> AHA: 4Q, '07, 120; 1Q, '07, 10
> **M43.10** Spondylolisthesis site unspecified   I-10

738.5 Other acquired deformity of back or spine
Deformity of spine NOS
> *EXCLUDES* *curvature of spine (737.0-737.9)*
> AHA: 1Q, '08, 11
> TIP: Assign for post procedural flat back syndrome, which may be the
> result of a previous spinal fusion surgery. Do not assign a surgical
> complication code.

738.6 Acquired deformity of pelvis
Pelvic obliquity
> *EXCLUDES* *intrapelvic protrusion of acetabulum (718.6)*
> *that in relation to labor and delivery (653.0-653.4,*
> *653.8-653.9)*
> DEF: Pelvic obliquity: slanting or inclination of the pelvis at an angle
> between 55 and 60 degrees between the plane of the pelvis and the
> horizontal plane.

738.7 Cauliflower ear
> DEF: Abnormal external ear; due to injury, subsequent perichondritis.

738.8 Acquired deformity of other specified site
Deformity of clavicle
> AHA: 2Q, '01, 15

738.9 Acquired deformity of unspecified site

√4ᵗʰ 739 Nonallopathic lesions, not elsewhere classified
> *INCLUDES* segmental dysfunction
> somatic dysfunction
> DEF: Disability, loss of function or abnormality of a body part that is neither
> classifiable to a particular system nor brought about therapeutically to
> counteract another disease.

739.0 Head region
Occipitocervical region

739.1 Cervical region
Cervicothoracic region

739.2 Thoracic region
Thoracolumbar region

739.3 Lumbar region
Lumbosacral region

739.4 Sacral region
Sacrococcygeal region
Sacroiliac region

739.5 Pelvic region
Hip region
Pubic region

739.6 Lower extremities

739.7 Upper extremities
Acromioclavicular region
Sternoclavicular region

739.8 Rib cage
Costochondral region
Costovertebral region
Sternochondral region

739.9 Abdomen and other
> AHA: 2Q, '89, 14

14. Congenital Anomalies (740-759)

TIP: Codes from chapter 14 may be assigned throughout the life of the patient, whenever the congenital anomaly is diagnosed.

✓4ᵗʰ 740 Anencephalus and similar anomalies

740.0 Anencephalus
Acrania
Amyelencephalus
Hemicephaly
Hemianencephaly
DEF: Fetus without cerebrum, cerebellum and flat bones of skull.

740.1 Craniorachischisis
DEF: Congenital slit in cranium and vertebral column.

740.2 Iniencephaly
DEF: Spinal cord passes through enlarged occipital bone (foramen magnum); absent vertebral bone layer and spinal processes; resulting in both reduction in number and proper fusion of the vertebrae.

✓4ᵗʰ 741 Spina bifida

EXCLUDES *spina bifida occulta (756.17)*

The following fifth-digit subclassification is for use with category 741:
0 **unspecified region**
1 **cervical region**
2 **dorsal [thoracic] region**
3 **lumbar region**

DEF: Lack of closure of spinal cord's bony encasement; marked by cord protrusion into lumbosacral area; evident by elevated alpha-fetoprotein of amniotic fluid.
AHA: 3Q, '94, 7
TIP: For Arnold-Chiari syndrome, Type I, refer to code 348.4.

§ ✓5ᵗʰ **741.0 With hydrocephalus**
[0-3]   Arnold-Chiari syndrome, type II
Chiari malformation, type II
Any condition classifiable to 741.9 with any condition classifiable to 742.3
AHA: 4Q, '97, 51; 4Q, '94, 37; S-O, '87, 10
Q05.4 Unspecified spina bifida with hydrocephalus   I-10

§ ✓5ᵗʰ **741.9 Without mention of hydrocephalus**
[0-3]   Hydromeningocele (spinal)
Hydromyelocele
Meningocele (spinal)
Meningomyelocele
Myelocele
Myelocystocele
Rachischisis
Spina bifida (aperta)
Syringomyelocele
Q05.8 Sacral spina bifida without hydrocephalus   I-10

✓4ᵗʰ 742 Other congenital anomalies of nervous system

EXCLUDES *congenital central alveolar hypoventilation syndrome (327.25)*

742.0 Encephalocele
Encephalocystocele
Encephalomyelocele
Hydroencephalocele
Hydromeningocele, cranial
Meningocele, cerebral
Meningoencephalocele
DEF: Brain tissue protrudes through skull defect.
AHA: 4Q, '94, 37

742.1 Microcephalus
Hydromicrocephaly
Micrencephaly
DEF: Extremely small head or brain.

Spina Bifida

742.2 Reduction deformities of brain
Absence ⎤
Agenesis ⎥ of part of brain
Aplasia ⎥
Hypoplasia ⎦
Agyria
Arhinencephaly
Holoprosencephaly
Microgyria
AHA: 3Q, '03, 15; 4Q, '94, 37
TIP: Assign for septo-optic dysplasia.

742.3 Congenital hydrocephalus
Aqueduct of Sylvius:
anomaly
obstruction, congenital
stenosis
Atresia of foramina of Magendie and Luschka
Hydrocephalus in newborn
EXCLUDES *hydrocephalus:*
acquired (331.3-331.4)
due to congenital toxoplasmosis (771.2)
with any condition classifiable to 741.9 (741.0)
DEF: Fluid accumulation within the skull; involves subarachnoid (external) or ventricular (internal) brain spaces.
AHA: 4Q, '05, 83
Q03.9 Congenital hydrocephalus unspecified   I-10

742.4 Other specified anomalies of brain
Congenital cerebral cyst   Multiple anomalies of brain NOS
Macroencephaly   Porencephaly
Macrogyria   Ulegyria
Megalencephaly
AHA: 1Q, '99, 9; 3Q, '92, 12

Normal Ventricles and Hydrocephalus

---

§ Requires fifth digit. Valid digits are in [brackets] under each code. See category 741 for codes and defintions.

Congenital Anomalies

742.5–743.59

√5ᵗʰ **742.5 Other specified anomalies of spinal cord**

  742.51 Diastematomyelia

    DEF: Congenital anomaly often associated with spina bifida; the spinal cord is separated into halves by a bony tissue resembling a "spike" (a spicule), each half surrounded by a dural sac.

  742.53 Hydromyelia

    Hydrorhachis

    DEF: Dilated central spinal cord canal; characterized by increased fluid accumulation.

  742.59 Other

    Amyelia
    Atelomyelia
    Congenital anomaly of spinal meninges
    Defective development of cauda equina
    Hypoplasia of spinal cord
    Myelatelia
    Myelodysplasia

    AHA: 2Q, '91, 14; 1Q, '89, 10

    TIP: Assign for tethered spinal cord syndrome, regardless of when it is diagnosed.

742.8 Other specified anomalies of nervous system

  Agenesis of nerve
  Displacement of brachial plexus
  Familial dysautonomia
  Jaw-winking syndrome
  Marcus-Gunn syndrome
  Riley-Day syndrome

  EXCLUDES *neurofibromatosis* ▶*(237.70-237.79)*◀

742.9 Unspecified anomaly of brain, spinal cord, and nervous system

  Anomaly
  Congenital:
    disease   of: brain / nervous system / spinal cord
    lesion
  Deformity

√4ᵗʰ **743 Congenital anomalies of eye**

√5ᵗʰ **743.0 Anophthalmos**

  DEF: Complete absence of the eyes or the presence of vestigial eyes.

  743.00 Clinical anophthalmos, unspecified

    Agenesis
    Cogenital absence   of eye
    Anophthalmos NOS

  743.03 Cystic eyeball, congenital

  743.06 Cryptophthalmos

    DEF: Skin is continuous over eyeball, results in apparent absence of eyelids.

√5ᵗʰ **743.1 Microphthalmos**

  Dysplasia
  Hypoplasia   of eye

  Rudimentary eye

  DEF: Abnormally small eyeballs, may be opacities of cornea and lens, scarring of choroid and retina.

  743.10 Microphthalmos, unspecified

  743.11 Simple microphthalmos

  743.12 Microphthalmos associated with other anomalies of eye and adnexa

√5ᵗʰ **743.2 Buphthalmos**

  Glaucoma:
    congenital
    newborn
  Hydrophthalmos

  EXCLUDES *glaucoma of childhood (365.14)*
    traumatic glaucoma due to birth injury (767.8)

  DEF: Distended, enlarged fibrous coats of eye; due to intraocular pressure of congenital glaucoma.

  743.20 Buphthalmos, unspecified

  743.21 Simple buphthalmos

  743.22 Buphthalmos associated with other ocular anomalies

    Keratoglobus, cogenital ⎫
      ⎬ associated with buphthalmos
    Megalocornea ⎭

√5ᵗʰ **743.3 Congenital cataract and lens anomalies**

  EXCLUDES *infantile cataract (366.00-366.09)*

  DEF: Opaque eye lens.

  743.30 Congenital cataract, unspecified

  743.31 Capsular and subcapsular cataract

  743.32 Cortical and zonular cataract

  743.33 Nuclear cataract

  743.34 Total and subtotal cataract, congenital

  743.35 Congenital aphakia

    Congenital absence of lens

  743.36 Anomalies of lens shape

    Microphakia
    Spherophakia

  743.37 Congenital ectopic lens

  743.39 Other

√5ᵗʰ **743.4 Coloboma and other anomalies of anterior segment**

  DEF: Coloboma: ocular tissue defect associated with defect of ocular fetal intraocular fissure; may cause small pit on optic disk, major defects of iris, ciliary body, choroid, and retina.

  743.41 Anomalies of corneal size and shape

    Microcornea

    EXCLUDES *that associated with buphthalmos (743.22)*

  743.42 Corneal opacities, interfering with vision, congenital

  743.43 Other corneal opacities, congenital

  743.44 Specified anomalies of anterior chamber, chamber angle, and related structures

    Anomaly:
      Axenfeld's
      Peters'
      Rieger's

  743.45 Aniridia

    DEF: Incompletely formed or absent iris; affects both eyes; dominant trait; also called congenital hyperplasia of iris.

    AHA: 3Q, '02, 20

  743.46 Other specified anomalies of iris and ciliary body

    Anisocoria, congenital
    Atresia of pupil
    Coloboma of iris
    Corectopia

  743.47 Specified anomalies of sclera

  743.48 Multiple and combined anomalies of anterior segment

  743.49 Other

√5ᵗʰ **743.5 Congenital anomalies of posterior segment**

  743.51 Vitreous anomalies

    Congenital vitreous opacity

  743.52 Fundus coloboma

    DEF: Absent retinal and choroidal tissue; occurs in lower fundus; a bright white ectatic zone of exposed sclera extends into and changes the optic disk.

  743.53 Chorioretinal degeneration, congenital

  743.54 Congenital folds and cysts of posterior segment

  743.55 Congenital macular changes

  743.56 Other retinal changes, congenital

    AHA: 3Q, '99, 12

  743.57 Specified anomalies of optic disc

    Coloboma of optic disc (congenital)

  743.58 Vascular anomalies

    Congenital retinal aneurysm

  743.59 Other

N Newborn Age: 0   P Pediatric Age: 0-17   M Maternity Age: 12-55   A Adult Age: 15-124

√5ᵗʰ **743.6 Congenital anomalies of eyelids, lacrimal system, and orbit**

743.61 Congenital ptosis
DEF: Drooping of eyelid.

743.62 Congenital deformities of eyelids
Ablepharon
Absence of eyelid
Accessory eyelid
Congenital:
  ectropion
  entropion
AHA: 1Q, '00, 22
TIP: Assign for epiblepharon, in which a redundant horizontal skin fold under the eyelid causes an abnormal vertical orientation of the eyelashes; may result in the eyelashes touching the eyeball.

743.63 Other specified congenital anomalies of eyelid
Absence, agenesis, of cilia

743.64 Specified congenital anomalies of lacrimal gland

743.65 Specified congenital anomalies of lacrimal passages
Absence, agenesis of:
  lacrimal apparatus
  punctum lacrimale
  Accessory lacrimal canal

743.66 Specified congenital anomalies of orbit

743.69 Other
Accessory eye muscles

743.8 Other specified anomalies of eye
EXCLUDES congenital nystagmus (379.51)
  ocular albinism (270.2)
  optic nerve hypoplasia (377.43)
  retinitis pigmentosa (362.74)

743.9 Unspecified anomaly of eye
Congenital:
  anomaly NOS } of eye (any part)
  deformity NOS

√4ᵗʰ **744 Congenital anomalies of ear, face, and neck**
EXCLUDES anomaly of:
  cervical spine (754.2, 756.10-756.19)
  larynx (748.2-748.3)
  nose (748.0-748.1)
  parathyroid gland (759.2)
  thyroid gland (759.2)
  cleft lip (749.10-749.25)

√5ᵗʰ **744.0 Anomalies of ear causing impairment of hearing**
EXCLUDES congenital deafness without mention of cause (389.0-389.9)

744.00 Unspecified anomaly of ear with impairment of hearing

744.01 Absence of external ear
Absence of:
  auditory canal (external)
  auricle (ear) (with stenosis or atresia of auditory canal)

744.02 Other anomalies of external ear with impairment of hearing
Atresia or stricture of auditory canal (external)

744.03 Anomaly of middle ear, except ossicles
Atresia or stricture of osseous meatus (ear)

744.04 Anomalies of ear ossicles
Fusion of ear ossicles

744.05 Anomalies of inner ear
Congenital anomaly of:
  membranous labyrinth
  organ of Corti

744.09 Other
Absence of ear, congenital

744.1 Accessory auricle
Accessory tragus   Supernumerary:
Polyotia   ear
Preauricular appendage   lobule
DEF: Redundant tissue or structures of ear.

√5ᵗʰ **744.2 Other specified anomalies of ear**
EXCLUDES that with impairment of hearing (744.00-744.09)

744.21 Absence of ear lobe, congenital

744.22 Macrotia
DEF: Abnormally large pinna of ear.

744.23 Microtia
DEF: Hypoplasia of pinna; associated with absent or closed auditory canal.

744.24 Specified anomalies of Eustachian tube
Absence of Eustachian tube

744.29 Other
Bat ear
Darwin's tubercle
Pointed ear
Prominence of auricle
Ridge ear
EXCLUDES preauricular sinus (744.46)

744.3 Unspecified anomaly of ear
Congenital:
  anomaly NOS } of ear, not elsewhere
  deformity NOS }   classified

√5ᵗʰ **744.4 Branchial cleft cyst or fistula; preauricular sinus**

744.41 Branchial cleft sinus or fistula
Branchial:
  sinus (external) (internal)
  vestige
DEF: Cyst due to failed closure of embryonic branchial cleft.

744.42 Branchial cleft cyst

744.43 Cervical auricle

744.46 Preauricular sinus or fistula

744.47 Preauricular cyst

744.49 Other
Fistula (of):
  auricle, congenital
  cervicoaural

744.5 Webbing of neck
Pterygium colli
DEF: Thick, triangular skinfold, stretches from lateral side of neck across shoulder; associated with Turner's and Noonan's syndromes.

√5ᵗʰ **744.8 Other specified anomalies of face and neck**

744.81 Macrocheilia
Hypertrophy of lip, congenital
DEF: Abnormally large lips.

744.82 Microcheilia
DEF: Abnormally small lips.

744.83 Macrostomia
DEF: Bilateral or unilateral anomaly of mouth due to malformed maxillary and mandibular processes; results in mouth extending toward ear.

744.84 Microstomia
DEF: Abnormally small mouth.

744.89 Other
EXCLUDES congenital fistula of lip (750.25)
  musculoskeletal anomalies (754.0-754.1, 756.0)

744.9 Unspecified anomalies of face and neck
Congenital:
  anomaly NOS } of face [any part] or neck [any
  deformity NOS }   part]

Congenital Anomalies

743.6–744.9

Congenital Anomalies

745–746.7

√4ᵗʰ **745   Bulbus cordis anomalies and anomalies of cardiac septal closure**

745.0   Common truncus
Absent septum ⎫ between aorta and
Communication (abnormal) ⎬ pulmonary artery
Aortic septal defect
Common aortopulmonary trunk
Persistent truncus arteriosus

√5ᵗʰ **745.1   Transposition of great vessels**

745.10   Complete transposition of great vessels
Transposition of great vessels:
    NOS
    classical

745.11   Double outlet right ventricle
Dextratransposition of aorta
Incomplete transposition of great vessels
Origin of both great vessels from right ventricle
Taussig-Bing syndrome or defect

745.12   Corrected transposition of great vessels

745.19   Other

745.2   Tetralogy of Fallot
Fallot's pentalogy
Ventricular septal defect with pulmonary stenosis or atresia, dextraposition of aorta, and hypertrophy of right ventricle
EXCLUDES Fallot's triad (746.09)
DEF: Obstructed cardiac outflow causes pulmonary stenosis, interventricular septal defect and right ventricular hypertrophy.

745.3   Common ventricle
Cor triloculare biatriatum
Single ventricle

745.4   Ventricular septal defect
Eisenmenger's defect or complex
Gerbo dedefect
Interventricular septal defect
Left ventricular-right atrial communication
Roger's disease
EXCLUDES common atrioventricular canal type (745.69)
single ventricle (745.3)
Q21.0 Ventricular septal defect   I-10

745.5   Ostium secundum type atrial septal defect
Defect: Patent or persistent:
   atrium secundum   foramen ovale
   fossa ovalis   ostium secundum
Lutembacher's syndrome
DEF: Opening in atrial septum due to failure of the septum secundum and the endocardial cushions to fuse; there is a rim of septum surrounding the defect.
AHA: ▶3Q, '09, 17;◄ 3Q, '09, 17
Q21.1 Atrial septal defect   I-10

√5ᵗʰ **745.6   Endocardial cushion defects**
DEF: Atrial and/or ventricular septal defects causing abnormal fusion of cushions in atrioventricular canal.

745.60   Endocardial cushion defect, unspecified type
DEF: Septal defect due to imperfect fusion of endocardial cushions.

Heart Defects

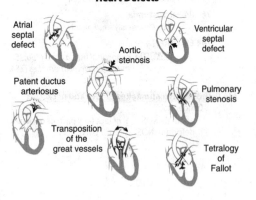

Atrial septal defect

Aortic stenosis

Ventricular septal defect

Patent ductus arteriosus

Pulmonary stenosis

Transposition of the great vessels

Tetralogy of Fallot

745.61   Ostium primum defect
Persistent ostium primum
DEF: Opening in low, posterior septum primum; causes cleft in basal portion of atrial septum; associated with cleft mitral valve.

745.69   Other
Absence of atrial septum
Atrioventricular canal type ventricular septal defect
Common atrioventricular canal
Common atrium

745.7   Cor biloculare
Absence of atrial and ventricular septa
DEF: Atrial and ventricular septal defect; marked by heart with two cardiac chambers (one atrium, one ventricle), and one atrioventricular valve.

745.8   Other

745.9   Unspecified defect of septal closure
Septal defect NOS

√4ᵗʰ **746   Other congenital anomalies of heart**
EXCLUDES endocardial fibroelastosis (425.3)

√5ᵗʰ **746.0   Anomalies of pulmonary valve**
EXCLUDES infundibular or subvalvular pulmonic stenosis (746.83)
tetralogy of Fallot (745.2)

746.00   Pulmonary valve anomaly, unspecified

746.01   Atresia, congenital
Congenital absence of pulmonary valve

746.02   Stenosis, congenital
DEF: Stenosis of opening between pulmonary artery and right ventricle; causes obstructed blood outflow from right ventricle.

746.09   Other
Congenital insufficiency of pulmonary valve
Fallot's triad or trilogy

746.1   Tricuspid atresia and stenosis, congenital
Absence of tricuspid valve

746.2   Ebstein's anomaly
DEF: Malformation of the tricuspid valve characterized by septal and posterior leaflets attaching to the wall of the right ventricle; causing the right ventricle to fuse with the atrium into a large right atrium and a small ventricle; causes heart failure and abnormal cardiac rhythm.

746.3   Congenital stenosis of aortic valve
Congenital aortic stenosis
EXCLUDES congenital:
subaortic stenosis (746.81)
supravalvular aortic stenosis (747.22)
DEF: Stenosis of orifice of aortic valve; obstructs blood outflow from left ventricle.
AHA: 4Q, '88, 8

746.4   Congenital insufficiency of aortic valve
Bicuspid aortic valve
Congenital aortic insufficiency
DEF: Impaired functioning of aortic valve due to incomplete closure; causes backflow (regurgitation) of blood from aorta to left ventricle.
Q23.1 Congenital insufficiency of aortic valve   I-10

746.5   Congenital mitral stenosis
Fused commissure ⎫
Parachute deformity ⎬ of mitral valve
Supernumerary cusps ⎭
DEF: Stenosis of left atrioventricular orifice.
AHA: 3Q, '07, 3

746.6   Congenital mitral insufficiency
DEF: Impaired functioning of mitral valve due to incomplete closure; causes backflow of blood from left ventricle to left atrium.

746.7   Hypoplastic left heart syndrome
Atresia, or marked hypoplasia, of aortic orifice or valve, with hypoplasia of ascending aorta and defective development of left ventricle (with mitral valve atresia)

Ⓝ Newborn Age: 0   Ⓟ Pediatric Age: 0-17   Ⓜ Maternity Age: 12-55   Ⓐ Adult Age: 15-124

✓5ᵗʰ 746.8 Other specified anomalies of heart

746.81 Subaortic stenosis
DEF: Stenosis, of left ventricular outflow tract due to fibrous tissue ring or septal hypertrophy below aortic valve.
AHA: 3Q, '07, 3

746.82 Cor triatriatum
DEF: Transverse septum divides left atrium due to failed resorption of embryonic common pulmonary vein; results in three atrial chambers.

746.83 Infundibular pulmonic stenosis
Subvalvular pulmonic stenosis
DEF: Stenosis of right ventricle outflow tract within infundibulum due to fibrous diaphragm below valve or long, narrow fibromuscular channel.

746.84 Obstructive anomalies of heart, not elsewhere classified
Shone's syndrome
Uhl's disease
Use additional code for associated anomalies, such as:
coarctation of aorta (747.10)
congenital mitral stenosis (746.5)
subaortic stenosis (746.81)

746.85 Coronary artery anomaly
Anomalous origin or communication of coronary artery
Arteriovenous malformation of coronary artery
Coronary artery:
absence
arising from aorta or pulmonary trunk
single
AHA: N-D, '85, 3

746.86 Congenital heart block
Complete or incomplete atrioventricular [AV] block
DEF: Impaired conduction of electrical impulses; due to maldeveloped junctional tissue.

746.87 Malposition of heart and cardiac apex
Abdominal heart
Dextrocardia
Ectopia cordis
Levocardia (isolated)
Mesocardia
EXCLUDES dextrocardia with complete transposition of viscera (759.3)

746.89 Other
Atresia ⎫
Hypoplasia ⎭ of cardiac vein

Congenital:
cardiomegaly
diverticulum, left ventricle
pericardial defect
AHA: 3Q, '00, 3; 1Q, '99, 11; J-F, '85, 3
TIP: Assign for Brugada syndrome, and also for congenital long QT syndrome. Additional codes may be required.
Q24.8 Oth specified congenital malformations of heart I-10

746.9 Unspecified anomaly of heart
Congenital:
anomaly of heart NOS
heart disease NOS

✓4ᵗʰ 747 Other congenital anomalies of circulatory system

747.0 Patent ductus arteriosus
Patent ductus Botalli
Persistent ductus arteriosus
DEF: Open lumen in ductus arteriosus causes arterial blood recirculation in lungs; inhibits blood supply to aorta; symptoms such as shortness of breath more noticeable upon activity.
AHA: ▶3Q, '09, 17◀
Q25.0 Patent ductus arteriosus I-10

✓5ᵗʰ 747.1 Coarctation of aorta
DEF: Localized deformity of aortic media seen as a severe constriction of the vessel lumen; major symptom is high blood pressure in the arms and low pressure in the legs; may result in a CVA, rupture of the aorta, bacterial endocarditis or congestive heart failure.

747.10 Coarctation of aorta (preductal) (postductal)
Hypoplasia of aortic arch
AHA: 3Q, '07, 3; 1Q, '99, 11; 4Q, '88, 8

747.11 Interruption of aortic arch

✓5ᵗʰ 747.2 Other anomalies of aorta

747.20 Anomaly of aorta, unspecified

747.21 Anomalies of aortic arch
Anomalous origin, right subclavian artery
Dextraposition of aorta
Double aortic arch
Kommerell's diverticulum
Overriding aorta
Persistent:
convolutions, aortic arch
right aortic arch
Vascular ring
EXCLUDES hypoplasia of aortic arch (747.10)
AHA: 1Q, '03, 15

747.22 Atresia and stenosis of aorta
Absence ⎫
Aplasia ⎪
Hypoplasia ⎬ of aorta
Stricture ⎭

Supra (valvular)-aortic stenosis
EXCLUDES congenital aortic (valvular) stenosis or stricture, so stated (746.3)
hypoplasia of aorta in hypoplastic left heart syndrome (746.7)

747.29 Other
Aneurysm of sinus of Valsalva
Congenital:
aneurysm ⎫
dilation ⎭ of aorta

747.3 Anomalies of pulmonary artery
Agenesis ⎫
Anomaly ⎪
Atresia ⎪
Coarctation ⎬ of pulmonary artery
Hypoplasia ⎪
Stenosis ⎭

Pulmonary arteriovenous aneurysm
AHA: ▶3Q, '09, 17, 18;◀ 1Q, '04, 16; 1Q, '94, 15; 4Q, '88, 8
TIP: ▶Assign for peripheral pulmonary stenosis (PPS) murmur.◀
Q25.7 Oth congenital malformations of pulmonary artery I-10

✓5ᵗʰ 747.4 Anomalies of great veins

747.40 Anomaly of great veins, unspecified
Anomaly NOS of:
pulmonary veins
vena cava

747.41 Total anomalous pulmonary venous connection
Total anomalous pulmonary venous return [TAPVR]:
subdiaphragmatic
supradiaphragmatic

747.42 Partial anomalous pulmonary venous connection
Partial anomalous pulmonary venous return

747.49 Other anomalies of great veins
Absence ⎫
Congenital ⎬ of vena cava (inferior)
stenosis ⎭ (superior)

Persistent:
left posterior cardinal vein
left superior vena cava
Scimitar syndrome
Transposition of pulmonary veins NOS

747.5 Absence or hypoplasia of umbilical artery
Single umbilical artery

Congenital Anomalies

747.6–748.4

√5ᵗʰ **747.6 Other anomalies of peripheral vascular system**

Absence   ⎫
Anomaly   ⎬ of artery or vein, NEC
Atresia   ⎭

Arteriovenous aneurysm (peripheral)
Arteriovenous malformation of the peripheral vascular system
Congenital:
   aneurysm (peripheral)
   phlebectasia
   stricture, artery
   varix
Multiple renal arteries

   EXCLUDES *anomalies of:*
      cerebral vessels (747.81)
      pulmonary artery (747.3)
      congenital retinal aneurysm (743.58)
      hemangioma (228.00-228.09)
      lymphangioma (228.1)

747.60 Anomaly of the peripheral vascular system, unspecified site

747.61 Gastrointestinal vessel anomaly
   AHA: 3Q, '96, 10
   TIP: Do not assign for gastric or intestinal AV malformation or angiodysplasia not stated to be congenital. See instead code 537.82, 537.83, 569.84, or 569.85.

747.62 Renal vessel anomaly

747.63 Upper limb vessel anomaly

747.64 Lower limb vessel anomaly

747.69 Anomalies of other specified sites of peripheral vascular system

√5ᵗʰ **747.8 Other specified anomalies of circulatory system**

747.81 Anomalies of cerebrovascular system
   Arteriovenous malformation of brain
   Cerebral arteriovenous aneurysm, congenital
   Congenital anomalies of cerebral vessels
   EXCLUDES *ruptured cerebral (arteriovenous) aneurysm (430)*
   Q28.3 Other malformations of cerebral vessels   I-10

747.82 Spinal vessel anomaly
   Arteriovenous malformation of spinal vessel
   AHA: 3Q, '95, 5

747.83 Persistent fetal circulation   N
   Persistent pulmonary hypertension
   Primary pulmonary hypertension of newborn
   DEF: A return to fetal circulation due to constriction of pulmonary arterioles and opening of the ductus arteriosus and foramen ovale, right-to-left shunting, oxygenation of the blood does not occur, and the lungs remain constricted after birth; is seen in term or post-term infants; causes include asphyxiation, meconium aspiration syndrome, acidosis, sepsis, and developmental immaturity.
   AHA: 4Q, '02, 62

Persistent Fetal Circulation

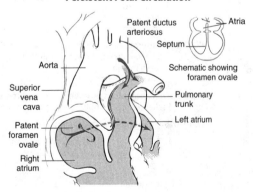

747.89 Other
   Aneurysm, congenital, specified site not elsewhere classified
   EXCLUDES *congenital aneurysm:*
      coronary (746.85)
      peripheral (747.6)
      pulmonary (747.3)
      retinal (743.58)
   AHA: 4Q, '02, 63

747.9 Unspecified anomaly of circulatory system

√4ᵗʰ **748 Congenital anomalies of respiratory system**
   EXCLUDES *congenital central alveolar hypoventilation syndrome (327.25)*
      congenital defect of diaphragm (756.6)

748.0 Choanal atresia
   Atresia   ⎫
   Congenital stenosis ⎬ of nares (anterior) (posterior)
   DEF: Occluded posterior nares (choana), bony or membranous due to failure of embryonic bucconasal membrane to rupture.

748.1 Other anomalies of nose
   Absent nose
   Accessory nose
   Cleft nose
   Congenital:
      deformity of nose
      notching of tip of nose
      perforation of wall of nasal sinus
   Deformity of wall of nasal sinus
   EXCLUDES *congenital deviation of nasal septum (754.0)*

748.2 Web of larynx
   Web of larynx:
      NOS
      glottic
      subglottic
   DEF: Malformed larynx; marked by thin, translucent, or thick, fibrotic spread between vocal folds; affects speech.

748.3 Other anomalies of larynx, trachea, and bronchus
   Absence or agenesis of:
      bronchus
      larynx
      trachea
   Anomaly (of):
      cricoid cartilage
      epiglottis
      thyroid cartilage
      tracheal cartilage
   Atresia (of):
      epiglottis
      glottis
      larynx
      trachea
   Cleft thyroid, cartilage, congenital
   Congenital:
      dilation, trachea
      stenosis:
         larynx
         trachea
      tracheocele
   Diverticulum:
      bronchus
      trachea
   Fissure of epiglottis
   Laryngocele
   Posterior cleft of cricoid cartilage (congenital)
   Rudimentary tracheal bronchus
   Stridor, laryngeal, congenital
   AHA: 1Q, '99, 14
   Q32.4 Other congenital malformations of bronchus   I-10

748.4 Congenital cystic lung
   Disease, lung:
      cystic, congenital
      polycystic, congenital
   Honeycomb lung, congenital
   EXCLUDES *acquired or unspecified cystic lung (518.89)*
   DEF: Enlarged air spaces of lung parenchyma.

N Newborn Age: 0   P Pediatric Age: 0-17   M Maternity Age: 12-55   A Adult Age: 15-124

748.5 Agenesis, hypoplasia, and dysplasia of lung
Absence of lung (fissures) (lobe) (lobe)
Aplasia of lung
Hypoplasia of lung
Sequestration of lung

√5ᵗʰ **748.6 Other anomalies of lung**

748.60 Anomaly of lung, unspecified

748.61 Congenital bronchiectasis

748.69 Other
Accessory lung (lobe)
Azygos lobe (fissure), lung

748.8 Other specified anomalies of respiratory system
Abnormal communication between pericardial and pleural sacs
Anomaly, pleural folds
Atresia of nasopharynx
Congenital cyst of mediastinum

748.9 Unspecified anomaly of respiratory system
Anomaly of respiratory system NOS

√4ᵗʰ **749 Cleft palate and cleft lip**

√5ᵗʰ **749.0 Cleft palate**

749.00 Cleft palate, unspecified

749.01 Unilateral, complete

749.02 Unilateral, incomplete
Cleft uvula

749.03 Bilateral, complete

749.04 Bilateral, incomplete

√5ᵗʰ **749.1 Cleft lip**
Cheiloschisis
Congenital fissure of lip
Harelip
Labium leporinum

749.10 Cleft lip, unspecified

749.11 Unilateral, complete

749.12 Unilateral, incomplete

749.13 Bilateral, complete

749.14 Bilateral, incomplete

√5ᵗʰ **749.2 Cleft palate with cleft lip**
Cheilopalatoschisis

749.20 Cleft palate with cleft lip, unspecified

749.21 Unilateral, complete

749.22 Unilateral, incomplete

Cleft Lip and Palate

Unilateral cleft lip

No cleft palate

Cleft lip with cleft alveolar ridge

No cleft palate

Unilateral cleft lip and cleft palate

Alveolar ridge

Cleft palate

Prolabium

Bilateral cleft lip and cleft palate

Isolated cleft palate

749.23 Bilateral, complete
AHA: 1Q, '96, 14

749.24 Bilateral, incomplete

749.25 Other combinations

√4ᵗʰ **750 Other congenital anomalies of upper alimentary tract**
EXCLUDES dentofacial anomalies (524.0-524.9)

750.0 Tongue tie
Ankyloglossia
DEF: Restricted tongue movement due to lingual frenum extending toward tip of tongue. Tongue may be fused to mouth floor affecting speech.

√5ᵗʰ **750.1 Other anomalies of tongue**

750.10 Anomaly of tongue, unspecified

750.11 Aglossia
DEF: Absence of tongue.

750.12 Congenital adhesions of tongue

750.13 Fissure of tongue
Bifid tongue
Double tongue

750.15 Macroglossia
Congenital hypertrophy of tongue

750.16 Microglossia
Hypoplasia of tongue

750.19 Other

√5ᵗʰ **750.2 Other specified anomalies of mouth and pharynx**

750.21 Absence of salivary gland

750.22 Accessory salivary gland

750.23 Atresia, salivary duct
Imperforate salivary duct

750.24 Congenital fistula of salivary gland

750.25 Congenital fistula of lip
Congenital (mucus) lip pits

750.26 Other specified anomalies of mouth
Absence of uvula

750.27 Diverticulum of pharynx
Pharyngeal pouch

750.29 Other specified anomalies of pharynx
Imperforate pharynx

750.3 Tracheoesophageal fistula, esophageal atresia and stenosis
Absent esophagus
Atresia of esophagus
Congenital:
   esophageal ring
   stenosis of esophagus
   stricture of esophagus
Congenital fistula:
   esophagobronchial
   esophagotracheal
Imperforate esophagus
Webbed esophagus

750.4 Other specified anomalies of esophagus
Dilatation, congenital
Displacement, congenital
Diverticulum   } (of) esophagus
Duplication
Giant

Esophageal pouch
EXCLUDES congenital hiatus hernia (750.6)
AHA: J-F, '85, 3

√4ᵗʰ
√5ᵗʰ   Additional Digit Required   Unspecified Code   Other Specified Code   Manifestation Code   ▶◀ Revised Text   ● New Code   ▲ Revised Code Title

750.5 Congenital hypertrophic pyloric stenosis
Congenital or infantile:
constriction
hypertrophy
spasm } of pylorus
stenosis
stricture

DEF: Obstructed pylorus due to overgrowth of pyloric muscle.
Q40.0 Congenital hypertrophic pyloric stenosis [I-10]

750.6 Congenital hiatus hernia
Displacement of cardia through esophageal hiatus
EXCLUDES congenital diaphragmatic hernia (756.6)

750.7 Other specified anomalies of stomach
Congenital:
cardiospasm
hourglass stomach
Displacement of stomach
Diverticulum of stomach, congenital
Duplication of stomach
Megalogastria
Microgastria
Transposition of stomach

750.8 Other specified anomalies of upper alimentary tract

750.9 Unspecified anomaly of upper alimentary tract
Congenital:
anomaly NOS } of upper alimentary tract [any
deformity NOS } part, except tongue]

✓4ᵗʰ **751 Other congenital anomalies of digestive system**

751.0 Meckel's diverticulum
Meckel's diverticulum (displaced) (hypertrophic)
Persistent:
omphalomesenteric duct
vitelline duct

DEF: Malformed sacs or appendages of ileum of small intestine; can cause strangulation, volvulus and intussusception.
AHA: 1Q, '04, 10

TIP: Assign for mesodiverticular band, a fibrous band connecting the tip of the diverticulum to the mesentery; can cause small bowel herniation and obstruction.

751.1 Atresia and stenosis of small intestine [P]
Atresia of:
duodenum
ileum
intestine NOS
Congenital:
absence
obstruction } of small intestine or intestine
stenosis } NOS
stricture

Imperforate jejunum

751.2 Atresia and stenosis of large intestine rectum, and anal canal [P]
Absence:
anus (congenital)
appendix, congenital
large intestine, congenital
rectum
Atresia of:
anus
colon
rectum
Congenital or infantile:
obstruction of large intestine
occlusion of anus
stricture of anus
Imperforate:
anus
rectum
Stricture of rectum, congenital
AHA: 2Q, '98, 16

751.3 Hirschsprung's disease and other congenital functional disorders of colon
Aganglionosis
Congenital dilation of colon
Congenital megacolon
Macrocolon
DEF: Hirschsprung's disease: enlarged or dilated colon (megacolon), with absence of ganglion cells in the narrowed wall distally; causes inability to defecate.

751.4 Anomalies of intestinal fixation
Congenital adhesions:
omental, anomalous
peritoneal
Jackson's membrane
Malrotation of colon
Rotation of cecum or colon:
failure of
incomplete
insufficient
Universal mesentery

751.5 Other anomalies of intestine
Congenital diverticulum, colon
Dolichocolon
Duplication of:
anus
appendix
cecum
intestine
Ectopic anus
Megaloappendix
Megaloduodenum
Microcolon
Persistent cloaca
Transposition of:
appendix
colon
intestine
AHA: 3Q, '02, 11; 3Q, '01, 8
Q43.9 Congenital malformation of intestine unspecified [I-10]

✓5ᵗʰ **751.6 Anomalies of gallbladder, bile ducts, and liver**

751.60 Unspecified anomaly of gallbladder, bile ducts, and liver

751.61 Biliary atresia [P]
Congenital:
absence } of bile duct
hypoplasia } (common) of
obstruction } passage
stricture
AHA: S-O, '87, 8

751.62 Congenital cystic disease of liver
Congenital polycystic disease of liver
Fibrocystic disease of liver

751.69 Other anomalies of gallbladder, bile ducts, and liver
Absence of:
gallbladder, congenital
liver (lobe)
Accessory:
hepatic ducts
liver
Congenital:
choledochal cyst
hepatomegaly
Duplication of:
biliary duct
cystic duct
gallbladder
liver
Floating:
gallbladder
liver
Intrahepatic gallbladder
AHA: S-O, '87, 8

751.7 Anomalies of pancreas

Absence
Accessory
Agenesis } (of) pancreas
Annular
Hypoplasia

Ectopic pancreatic tissue
Pancreatic heterotopia

> **EXCLUDES** *diabetes mellitus (249.0-249.9, 250.0-250.9)*
> *fibrocystic disease of pancreas*
> *(277.00-277.09)*
> *neonatal diabetes mellitus (775.1)*

751.8 Other specified anomalies of digestive system

Absence (complete) (partial) of alimentary tract NOS
Duplication } of digestive organs NOS
Malposition, congenital

> **EXCLUDES** *congenital diaphragmatic hernia (756.6)*
> *congenital hiatus hernia (750.6)*

751.9 Unspecified anomaly of digestive system

Congenital:
  anomaly NOS } of digestive system NOS
  deformity NOS

√4ᵗʰ 752 Congenital anomalies of genital organs

> **EXCLUDES** *syndromes associated with anomalies in the number and*
> *form of chromosomes (758.0-758.9)*

752.0 Anomalies of ovaries ♀

Absence, congenital
Accessory } (of) ovary
Ectopic
Streak

√5ᵗʰ 752.1 Anomalies of fallopian tubes and broad ligaments

752.10 Unspecified anomaly of fallopian ♀
tubes and broad ligaments

752.11 Embryonic cyst of fallopian tubes ♀
and broad ligaments

Cyst: Cyst:
  epoophoron   parovarian
  fimbrial

  AHA: S-O, '85, 13

752.19 Other ♀

Absence
Accessory } (of) fallopian tube or broad
Atresia   ligament

752.2 Doubling of uterus ♀

Didelphic uterus
Doubling of uterus [any degree] (associated with doubling of
  cervix and vagina)

√5ᵗʰ 752.3 Other anomalies of uterus

  AHA: 3Q, '06, 18

● **752.31 Agenesis of uterus** ♀
Congenital absence of uterus
  Q51.0 Congenital absence of uterus   I-10

● **752.32 Hypoplasia of uterus** ♀

● **752.33 Unicornuate uterus** ♀
Unicornuate uterus with or without a separate
  uterine horn
Uterus with only one functioning horn
  Q51.4 Unicornuate uterus   I-10

● **752.34 Bicornuate uterus** ♀
Bicornuate uterus, complete or partial
  Q51.3 Bicornuate uterus   I-10

● **752.35 Septate uterus** ♀
Septate uterus, complete or partial

● **752.36 Arcuate uterus** ♀

● **752.39 Other anomalies of uterus** ♀
Aplasia of uterus NOS
Müllerian anomaly of the uterus, NEC

> **EXCLUDES** *anomaly of uterus due to exposure to*
> *diethylstilbestrol [DES] in utero*
> *(760.76)*
> *didelphic uterus (752.2)*
> *doubling of uterus (752.2)*

Hypospadias and Epispadias

Hypospadias (ventral view)   Epispadias (dorsal view)

√5ᵗʰ 752.4 Anomalies of cervix, vagina, and external female genitalia

752.40 Unspecified anomaly of cervix, vagina, ♀
and external female genitalia

752.41 Embryonic cyst of cervix, vagina, and ♀
external female genitalia
Cyst of:
  canal of Nuck, congenital
  Gartner's duct
  vagina, embryonal
  vulva, congenital
DEF: Embryonic fluid-filled cysts of cervix, vagina or
external female genitalia.

752.42 Imperforate hymen ♀
DEF: Complete closure of membranous fold around external
opening of vagina.

● **752.43 Cervical agenesis** ♀
Cervical hypoplasia
  Q51.5 Agenesis and aplasia of cervix   I-10

● **752.44 Cervical duplication** ♀

● **752.45 Vaginal agenesis** ♀
Agenesis of vagina, total or partial
  Q52.0 Congenital absence of vagina   I-10

● **752.46 Transverse vaginal septum** ♀

● **752.47 Longitudinal vaginal septum** ♀
Longitudinal vaginal septum with or without
  obstruction

752.49 Other anomalies of cervix, vagina, and ♀
external female genitalia
►Absence of clitoris or vulva
Agenesis of clitoris or vulva
Anomalies of cervix, NEC
Anomalies of hymen, NEC◄
Congenital stenosis or stricture of:
  cervical canal
  vagina
►Müllerian anomalies of the cervix and vagina, NEC◄

> **EXCLUDES** *double vagina associated with total*
> *duplication (752.2)*

  AHA: 3Q, '06, 18

√5ᵗʰ 752.5 Undescended and retractile testicle

  AHA: 4Q, '96, 33

752.51 Undescended testis ♂
Cryptorchism   Ectopic testis
  Q53.20 Undescended testicle unspecified bilateral   I-10

752.52 Retractile testis ♂

√5ᵗʰ 752.6 Hypospadias and epispadias and other penile anomalies

  AHA: 4Q, '96, 34, 35

752.61 Hypospadias ♂
DEF: Abnormal opening of urethra on the ventral surface of
the penis or perineum.
  AHA: 4Q, '03, 67-68; 3Q, '97, 6
  Q54.1 Hypospadias penile   I-10

752.62 Epispadias ♂
Anaspadias
DEF: Urethra opening on dorsal surface of penis.

√4ᵗʰ / √5ᵗʰ Additional Digit Required   Unspecified Code   Other Specified Code   Manifestation Code   ►◄ Revised Text   ● New Code   ▲ Revised Code Title

2011 ICD-9-CM   **October 2010 • Volume 1 – 243**

Congenital Anomalies

752.63–753.8

752.63 Congenital chordee ♂
> **DEF:** Ventral bowing of penis due to fibrous band along corpus spongiosum; occurs with hypospadias.

752.64 Micropenis ♂

752.65 Hidden penis ♂

752.69 Other penile anomalies ♂

752.7 Indeterminate sex and pseudohermaphroditism
Gynandrism
Hermaphroditism
Ovotestis
Pseudohermaphroditism (male) (female)
Pure gonadal dysgenesis
> **EXCLUDES** androgen insensitivity (259.50-259.52)
> pseudohermaphroditism:
> female, with adrenocortical disorder (255.2)
> male, with gonadal disorder (257.8)
> with specified chromosomal anomaly
> (758.0-758.9)
> testicular feminization syndrome (259.50-259.52)
> **DEF:** Pseudohermaphroditism: presence of gonads of one sex and external genitalia of other sex.

√5ᵗʰ 752.8 Other specified anomalies of genital organs
> **EXCLUDES** congenital hydrocele (778.6)
> penile anomalies (752.61-752.69)
> phimosis or paraphimosis (605)

752.81 Scrotal transposition ♂
> **AHA:** 4Q, '03, 67-68

752.89 Other specified anomalies of genital organs
Absence of:
  prostate
  spermatic cord
  vas deferens
Anorchism
Aplasia (congenital) of:
  prostate
  round ligament
  testicle
Atresia of:
  ejaculatory duct
  vas deferens
Fusion of testes
Hypoplasia of testis
Monorchism
Polyorchism

752.9 Unspecified anomaly of genital organs
Congenital:
  anomaly NOS } of genital organ, not
  deformity NOS } elsewhere classified

√4ᵗʰ 753 Congenital anomalies of urinary system

753.0 Renal agenesis and dysgenesis
Atrophy of kidney:
  congenital
  infantile
Congenital absence of kidney(s)
Hypoplasia of kidney(s)
> **Q60.2** Renal agenesis unspecified   I-10

√5ᵗʰ 753.1 Cystic kidney disease
> **EXCLUDES** acquired cyst of kidney (593.2)
> **AHA:** 4Q, '90, 3

753.10 Cystic kidney disease, unspecified
> **Q61.9** Cystic kidney disease unspecified   I-10

753.11 Congenital single renal cyst

753.12 Polycystic kidney, unspecified type
> **Q61.3** Polycystic kidney unspecified   I-10

753.13 Polycystic kidney, autosomal dominant
> **DEF:** Slow progressive disease characterized by bilateral cysts causing increased kidney size and impaired function.

753.14 Polycystic kidney, autosomal recessive
> **DEF:** Rare disease characterized by multiple cysts involving kidneys and liver, producing renal and hepatic failure in childhood or adolescence.

753.15 Renal dysplasia

753.16 Medullary cystic kidney
Nephronopthisis
> **DEF:** Diffuse kidney disease results in uremia onset prior to age 20.

753.17 Medullary sponge kidney
> **DEF:** Dilated collecting tubules; usually asymptomatic but calcinosis in tubules may cause renal insufficiency.

753.19 Other specified cystic kidney disease
Multicystic kidney

√5ᵗʰ 753.2 Obstructive defects of renal pelvis and ureter
> **AHA:** 4Q, '96, 35

753.20 Unspecified obstructive defect of renal pelvis and ureter

753.21 Congenital obstruction of ureteropelvic junction
> **DEF:** Stricture at junction of ureter and renal pelvis.

753.22 Congenital obstruction of ureterovesical junction
Adynamic ureter
Congenital hydroureter
> **DEF:** Stricture at junction of ureter and bladder.

753.23 Congenital ureterocele

753.29 Other
> **Q62.39** Other obstructive defects renal pelvis & ureter   I-10

753.3 Other specified anomalies of kidney
Accessory kidney
Congenital:
  calculus of kidney
  displaced kidney
Discoid kidney
Double kidney with
  double pelvis
Ectopic kidney
Fusion of kidneys
Giant kidney
Horseshoe kidney
Hyperplasia of kidney
Lobulation of kidney
Malrotation of kidney
Trifid kidney (pelvis)
> **AHA:** 1Q, '07, 23
> **TIP:** Assign for Finnish-type congenital nephrosis, along with code 581.3 Nephrotic syndrome.
> **Q63.8** Oth specified congenital malformations of kidney   I-10

753.4 Other specified anomalies of ureter
Absent ureter
Accessory ureter
Deviation of ureter
Displaced ureteric orifice
Double ureter
Ectopic ureter
Implantation, anomalous of ureter

753.5 Exstrophy of urinary bladder
Ectopia vesicae
Extroversion of bladder
> **DEF:** Absence of lower abdominal and anterior bladder walls with posterior bladder wall protrusion.

753.6 Atresia and stenosis of urethra and bladder neck
Congenital obstruction:
  bladder neck
  urethra
Congenital stricture of:
  urethra (valvular)
  urinary meatus
  vesicourethral orifice
Imperforate urinary meatus
Impervious urethra
Urethral valve formation

753.7 Anomalies of urachus
Cyst
Fistula } (of) urachussinus
Patent
Persistent umbilical sinus

753.8 Other specified anomalies of bladder and urethra
Absence, congenital of:
  bladder
  urethra
Accessory:
  bladder
  urethra
Congenital:
  diverticulum of bladder
  hernia of bladder
  prolapse of:
    bladder (mucosa)
    urethra
  urethrorectal fistula
Double:
  urethra
  urinary meatus

Ⓝ Newborn Age: 0   Ⓟ Pediatric Age: 0-17   Ⓜ Maternity Age: 12-55   Ⓐ Adult Age: 15-124

753.9 Unspecified anomaly of urinary system
Congenital:
anomaly NOS } of urinary system [any part,
deformity NOS }   except urachus]

✓4ᵗʰ **754 Certain congenital musculoskeletal deformities**
[INCLUDES] nonteratogenic deformities which are considered to be
due to intrauterine malposition and pressure

754.0 Of skull, face, and jaw
Asymmetry of face
Compression facies
Depressions in skull
Deviation of nasal septum, congenital
Dolichocephaly
Plagiocephaly
Potter's facies
Squashed or bent nose, congenital
[EXCLUDES] dentofacial anomalies (524.0-524.9)
syphilitic saddle nose (090.5)

754.1 Of sternocleidomastoid muscle
Congenital sternomastoid torticollis
Congenital wryneck
Contracture of sternocleidomastoid (muscle)
Sternomastoid tumor

754.2 Of spine
Congenital postural:
lordosis
scoliosis

✓5ᵗʰ **754.3 Congenital dislocation of hip**

754.30 Congenital dislocation of hip, unilateral
Congenital dislocation of hip NOS

754.31 Congenital dislocation of hip, bilateral

754.32 Congenital subluxation of hip, unilateral
Congenital flexion deformity, hip or thigh
Predislocation status of hip at birth
Preluxation of hip, congenital

754.33 Congenital subluxation of hip, bilateral

**754.35 Congenital dislocation of one hip with subluxation
of other hip**

✓5ᵗʰ **754.4 Congenital genu recurvatum and bowing of long bones of
leg**

754.40 Genu recurvatum
DEF: Backward curving of knee joint.

**754.41 Congenital dislocation of knee (with genu
recurvatum)**

754.42 Congenital bowing of femur

754.43 Congenital bowing of tibia and fibula

**754.44 Congenital bowing of unspecified long
bones of leg**

✓5ᵗʰ **754.5 Varus deformities of feet**
[EXCLUDES] acquired (736.71, 736.75, 736.79)

754.50 Talipes varus
Congenital varus deformity of foot, unspecified
Pes varus
DEF: Inverted foot marked by outer sole resting on ground.

754.51 Talipes equinovarus
Equinovarus (congenital)
DEF: Elevated, outward rotation of heel; also called
clubfoot.

754.52 Metatarsus primus varus
DEF: Malformed first metatarsal bone, with bone angled
toward body.

754.53 Metatarsus varus

754.59 Other
Talipes calcaneovarus

✓5ᵗʰ **754.6 Valgus deformities of feet**
[EXCLUDES] valgus deformity of foot (acquired) (736.79)

754.60 Talipes valgus
Congenital valgus deformity of foot, unspecified

754.61 Congenital pes planus
Congenital rocker bottom flat foot
Flat foot, congenital
[EXCLUDES] pes planus (acquired) (734)

754.62 Talipes calcaneovalgus

754.69 Other
Talipes:
equinovalgus
planovalgus

✓5ᵗʰ **754.7 Other deformities of feet**
[EXCLUDES] acquired (736.70-736.79)

754.70 Talipes, unspecified
Congenital deformity of foot NOS

754.71 Talipes cavus
Cavus foot (congenital)

754.79 Other
Asymmetric talipes
Talipes:
calcaneus
equinus

✓5ᵗʰ **754.8 Other specified nonteratogenic anomalies**

754.81 Pectus excavatum
Congenital funnel chest

754.82 Pectus carinatum
Congenital pigeon chest [breast]

754.89 Other
Club hand (congenital)
Congenital:
deformity of chest wall
dislocation of elbow
Generalized flexion contractures of lower limb joints,
congenital
Spade-like hand (congenital)

✓4ᵗʰ **755 Other congenital anomalies of limbs**
[EXCLUDES] those deformities classifiable to 754.0-754.8

✓5ᵗʰ **755.0 Polydactyly**

755.00 Polydactyly, unspecified digits
Supernumerary digits

755.01 Of fingers
Accessory fingers

755.02 Of toes
Accessory toes

✓5ᵗʰ **755.1 Syndactyly**
Symphalangy
Webbing of digits

755.10 Of multiple and unspecified sites

755.11 Of fingers without fusion of bone

755.12 Of fingers with fusion of bone

755.13 Of toes without fusion of bone

755.14 Of toes with fusion of bone

✓5ᵗʰ **755.2 Reduction deformities of upper limb**

755.20 Unspecified reduction deformity of upper limb
Ectromelia NOS } of upper limb
Hemimelia NOS }

Shortening of arm, congenital

755.21 Transverse deficiency of upper limb
Amelia of upper limb
Congenital absence of:
fingers, all (complete or partial)
forearm, including hand and fingers
upper limb, complete
Congenital amputation of upper limb
Transverse hemimelia of upper limb

**755.22 Longitudinal deficiency of upper limb, not
elsewhere classified**
Phocomelia NOS of upper limb
Rudimentary arm

✓4ᵗʰ
✓5ᵗʰ Additional Digit Required   Unspecified Code   Other Specified Code   Manifestation Code   ▶◀ Revised Text   ● New Code   ▲ Revised Code Title

2011 ICD-9-CM   **Volume 1 – 245**

755.23 Longitudinal deficiency, combined, involving humerus, radius, and ulna (complete or incomplete)
Congenital absence of arm and forearm (complete or incomplete) with or without metacarpal deficiency and/or phalangeal deficiency, incomplete
Phocomelia, complete, of upper limb

755.24 Longitudinal deficiency, humeral, complete or partial (with or without distal deficiencies, incomplete)
Congenital absence of humerus (with or without absence of some [but not all] distal elements)
Proximal phocomelia of upper limb

755.25 Longitudinal deficiency, radioulnar, complete or partial (with or without distal deficiencies, incomplete)
Congenital absence of radius and ulna (with or without absence of some [but not all] distal elements)
Distal phocomelia of upper limb

755.26 Longitudinal deficiency, radial, complete or partial (with or without distal deficiencies, incomplete)
Agenesis of radius
Congenital absence of radius (with or without absence of some [but not all] distal elements)

755.27 Longitudinal deficiency, ulnar, complete or partial (with or without distal deficiencies, incomplete)
Agenesis of ulna
Congenital absence of ulna (with or without absence of some [but not all] distal elements)

755.28 Longitudinal deficiency, carpals or metacarpals, complete or partial (with or without incomplete phalangeal deficiency)

755.29 Longitudinal deficiency, phalanges, complete or partial
Absence of finger, congenital
Aphalangia of upper limb, terminal, complete or partial
EXCLUDES *terminal deficiency of all five digits (755.21)*
transverse deficiency of phalanges (755.21)

√5ᵗʰ **755.3 Reduction deformities of lower limb**

755.30 Unspecified reduction deformity of lower limb
Ectromelia NOS   } of lower limb
Hemimelia NOS
Shortening of leg, congenital

755.31 Transverse deficiency of lower limb
Amelia of lower limb
Congenital absence of:
   foot
   leg, including foot and toes
   lower limb, complete
   toes, all, complete
Transverse hemimelia of lower limb

755.32 Longitudinal deficiency of lower limb, not elsewhere classified
Phocomelia NOS of lower limb

755.33 Longitudinal deficiency, combined, involving femur, tibia, and fibula (complete or incomplete)
Congenital absence of thigh and (lower) leg (complete or incomplete) with or without metacarpal deficiency and/or phalangeal deficiency, incomplete
Phocomelia, complete, of lower limb

755.34 Longitudinal deficiency, femoral, complete or partial (with or without distal deficiencies, incomplete)
Congenital absence of femur (with or without absence of some [but not all] distal elements)
Proximal phocomelia of lower limb

755.35 Longitudinal deficiency, tibiofibular, complete or partial (with or without distal deficiencies, incomplete)
Congenital absence of tibia and fibula (with or without absence of some [but not all] distal elements)
Distal phocomelia of lower limb

755.36 Longitudinal deficiency, tibia, complete or partial (with or without distal deficiencies, incomplete)
Agenesis of tibia
Congenital absence of tibia (with or without absence of some [but not all] distal elements)

755.37 Longitudinal deficiency, fibular, complete or partial (with or without distal deficiencies, incomplete)
Agenesis of fibula
Congenital absence of fibula (with or without absence of some [but not all] distal elements)

755.38 Longitudinal deficiency, tarsals or metatarsals, complete or partial (with or without incomplete phalangeal deficiency)

755.39 Longitudinal deficiency, phalanges, complete or partial
Absence of toe, congenital
Aphalangia of lower limb, terminal, complete or partial
EXCLUDES *terminal deficiency of all five digits (755.31)*
transverse deficiency of phalanges (755.31)

755.4 Reduction deformities, unspecified limb
Absence, congenital (complete or partial) of limb NOS
Amelia
Ectromelia   } of unspecified limb
Hemimelia
Phocomelia

√5ᵗʰ **755.5 Other anomalies of upper limb, including shoulder girdle**

755.50 Unspecified anomaly of upper limb

755.51 Congenital deformity of clavicle

755.52 Congenital elevation of scapula
Sprengel's deformity

755.53 Radioulnar synostosis
DEF: Osseous adhesion of radius and ulna.

755.54 Madelung's deformity
DEF: Distal ulnar overgrowth or radial shortening; also called carpus curvus.

755.55 Acrocephalosyndactyly
Apert's syndrome
DEF: Premature cranial suture fusion (craniostenosis); marked by cone-shaped or pointed (acrocephaly) head and webbing of the fingers (syndactyly); similar to craniofacial dysostosis.

755.56 Accessory carpal bones

755.57 Macrodactylia (fingers)
DEF: Abnormally large fingers, toes.

755.58 Cleft hand, congenital
Lobster-claw hand
DEF: Extended separation between fingers into metacarpus; also may refer to large fingers and absent middle fingers of hand.

755.59 Other
Cleidocranial dysostosis
Cubitus:
   valgus, congenital
   varus, congenital
EXCLUDES *club hand (congenital) (754.89)*
congenital dislocation of elbow (754.89)

√5ᵗʰ **755.6 Other anomalies of lower limb, including pelvic girdle**

755.60 Unspecified anomaly of lower limb

755.61 Coxa valga, congenital
DEF: Abnormally wide angle between the neck and shaft of the femur.

755.62 Coxa vara, congenital
DEF: Diminished angle between neck and shaft of femur.

755.63 Other congenital deformity of hip (joint)
Congenital anteversion of femur (neck)
EXCLUDES *congenital dislocation of hip (754.30-754.35)*
AHA: 1Q, '94, 15; S-O, '84, 15
Q65.9 Congenital deformity of hip unspecified   I-10

755.64 Congenital deformity of knee (joint)
Congenital:
absence of patella
genu valgum [knock-knee]
genu varum [bowleg]
Rudimentary patella

755.65 Macrodactylia of toes
DEF: Abnormally large toes.

755.66 Other anomalies of toes
Congenital:
hallux valgus
hallux varus
hammer toe

755.67 Anomalies of foot, not elsewhere classified
Astragaloscaphoid synostosis
Calcaneonavicular bar
Coalition of calcaneus
Talonavicular synostosis
Tarsal coalitions

755.69 Other
Congenital:
angulation of tibia
deformity (of):
ankle (joint)
sacroiliac (joint)
fusion of sacroiliac joint

755.8 Other specified anomalies of unspecified limb

755.9 Unspecified anomaly of unspecified limb
Congenital:
anomaly NOS ⎫
deformity NOS ⎭ of unspecified limb
EXCLUDES *reduction deformity of unspecified limb (755.4)*

√4ᵗʰ **756 Other congenital musculoskeletal anomalies**
EXCLUDES *congenital myotonic chondrodystrophy (359.23)*
those deformities classifiable to 754.0-754.8

756.0 Anomalies of skull and face bones
Absence of skull bones
Acrocephaly
Congenital deformity of forehead
Craniosynostosis
Crouzon's disease
Hypertelorism
Imperfect fusion of skull
Oxycephaly
Platybasia
Premature closure of cranial sutures
Tower skull
Trigonocephaly
EXCLUDES *acrocephalosyndactyly [Apert's syndrome] (755.55)*
dentofacial anomalies (524.0-524.9)
skull defects associated with brain anomalies, such as:
anencephalus (740.0)
encephalocele (742.0)
hydrocephalus (742.3)
microcephalus (742.1)
AHA: 3Q, '98, 9; 3Q, '96, 15
TIP: Assign for Nager syndrome (preaxial acrofacial dysostosis), along with codes for any additional features that are not captured in the code.
Q75.8 Other spec cong malformations skull & face bones   I-10

√5ᵗʰ **756.1 Anomalies of spine**

756.10 Anomaly of spine, unspecified

756.11 Spondylolysis, lumbosacral region
Prespondylolisthesis (lumbosacral)
DEF: Bilateral or unilateral defect through the pars interarticularis of a vertebra causes spondylolisthesis.

756.12 Spondylolisthesis
DEF: Downward slipping of lumbar vertebra over next vertebra; usually related to pelvic deformity.
Q76.2 Congenital spondylolisthesis   I-10

756.13 Absence of vertebra, congenital

756.14 Hemivertebra
DEF: Incomplete development of one side of a vertebra.

756.15 Fusion of spine [vertebra], congenital

756.16 Klippel-Feil syndrome
DEF: Short, wide neck; limits range of motion due to abnormal number of cervical vertebra or fused hemivertebrae.

756.17 Spina bifida occulta
EXCLUDES *spina bifida (aperta) (741.0-741.9)*
DEF: Spina bifida marked by a bony spinal canal defect without a protrusion of the cord or meninges; it is diagnosed by radiography and has no symptoms.

756.19 Other
Platyspondylia
Supernumerary vertebra

756.2 Cervical rib
Supernumerary rib in the cervical region
DEF: Costa cervicalis: extra rib attached to cervical vertebra.

756.3 Other anomalies of ribs and sternum
Congenital absence of:
rib
sternum
Congenital:
fissure of sternum
fusion of ribs
Sternum bifidum
EXCLUDES *nonteratogenic deformity of chest wall (754.81-754.89)*

756.4 Chondrodystrophy
Achondroplasia   Enchondromatosis
Chondrodystrophia (fetalis)   Ollier's disease
Dyschondroplasia
EXCLUDES *congenital myotonic chondrodystrophy (359.23)*
lipochondrodystrophy [Hurler's syndrome] (277.5)
Morquio's disease (277.5)
DEF: Abnormal development of cartilage.
AHA: 2Q, '02, 16; S-O, '87, 10
TIP: Assign for Jeune's syndrome, and also for cartilage-hair syndrome (cartilage-hair hypoplasia).

√5ᵗʰ **756.5 Osteodystrophies**

756.50 Osteodystrophy, unspecified

756.51 Osteogenesis imperfecta
Fragilitas ossium
Osteopsathyrosis
DEF: A collagen disorder commonly characterized by brittle, osteoporotic, easily fractured bones, hypermobility of joints, blue sclerae, and a tendency to hemorrhage.

756.52 Osteopetrosis
DEF: Abnormally dense bone, optic atrophy, hepatosplenomegaly, deafness; sclerosing depletes bone marrow and nerve foramina of skull; often fatal.

756.53 Osteopoikilosis
DEF: Multiple sclerotic foci on ends of long bones, stippling in round, flat bones; identified by x-ray.

756.54 Polyostotic fibrous dysplasia of bone
DEF: Fibrous tissue displaces bone results in segmented ragged-edge café-au-lait spots; occurs in girls of early puberty.

756.55 Chondroectodermal dysplasia
Ellis-van Creveld syndrome
DEF: Inadequate enchondral bone formation; impaired development of hair and teeth, polydactyly, and cardiac septum defects.

756.56 Multiple epiphyseal dysplasia

756.59 Other
Albright (-McCune)-Sternberg syndrome

√4ᵗʰ
√5ᵗʰ Additional Digit Required   Unspecified Code   Other Specified Code   Manifestation Code   ▶◀ Revised Text   ● New Code   ▲ Revised Code Title
2011 ICD-9-CM   **Volume 1 – 247**

Omphalocele

756.6 Anomalies of diaphragm
Absence of diaphragm
Congenital hernia:
  diaphragmatic
  foramen of Morgagni
Eventration of diaphragm
EXCLUDES congenital hiatus hernia (750.6)

√5ᵗʰ 756.7 Anomalies of abdominal wall

756.70 Anomaly of abdominal wall, unspecified

756.71 Prune belly syndrome
Eagle-Barrett syndrome
Prolapse of bladder mucosa
DEF: Prune belly syndrome: absence of lower rectus abdominis muscle and lower and medial oblique muscles; results in dilated bladder and ureters, dysplastic kidneys and hydronephrosis; common in male infants with undescended testicles.
AHA: 4Q, '97, 44

756.72 Omphalocele
Exomphalos
DEF: Exomphalos: umbilical hernia prominent navel.
DEF: Omphalocele: hernia of umbilicus due to impaired abdominal wall; results in membrane-covered intestine protruding through peritoneum and amnion.
AHA: 4Q, '09, 98-99

756.73 Gastroschisis
DEF: Fissure of abdominal wall, results in protruding small or large intestine.
AHA: 4Q, '09, 98-99

756.79 Other congenital anomalies of abdominal wall
EXCLUDES umbilical hernia (551-553 with .1)

√5ᵗʰ 756.8 Other specified anomalies of muscle, tendon, fascia, and connective tissue

756.81 Absence of muscle and tendon
Absence of muscle (pectoral)
AHA: ▶1Q, '10, 13◀

756.82 Accessory muscle

756.83 Ehlers-Danlos syndrome
DEF: Danlos syndrome: connective tissue disorder causes hyperextended skin and joints; results in fragile blood vessels with bleeding, poor wound healing and subcutaneous pseudotumors.

Gastroschisis

756.89 Other
Amyotrophia congenita
Congenital shortening of tendon
AHA: 3Q, '99, 16
TIP: Assign for Stickler's syndrome, a hereditary progressive arthro-ophthalmopathy, along with codes for the specific manifestations.

756.9 Other and unspecified anomalies of musculoskeletal system
Congenital:
  anomaly NOS } of musculoskeletal system, not
  deformity NOS } elsewhere classified

√4ᵗʰ 757 Congenital anomalies of the integument
INCLUDES anomalies of skin, subcutaneous tissue, hair, nails, and breast
EXCLUDES hemangioma (228.00-228.09)
  pigmented nevus (216.0-216.9)

757.0 Hereditary edema of legs
Congenital lymphedema
Hereditary trophedema
Milroy's disease

757.1 Ichthyosis congenita
Congenital ichthyosis
Harlequin fetus
Ichthyosiform erythroderma
DEF: Overproduction of skin cells causes scaling of skin; may result in stillborn fetus or death soon after birth.

757.2 Dermatoglyphic anomalies
Abnormal palmar creases
DEF: Abnormal skin-line patterns of fingers, palms, toes and soles; initial finding of possible chromosomal abnormalities.

√5ᵗʰ 757.3 Other specified anomalies of skin

757.31 Congenital ectodermal dysplasia
DEF: Tissues and structures originate in embryonic ectoderm; includes anhidrotic and hidrotic ectodermal dysplasia and EEC syndrome.

757.32 Vascular hamartomas
Birthmarks   Strawberry nevus
Port-wine stain
DEF: Benign tumor of blood vessels; due to malformed angioblastic tissues.
Q82.5 Congenital non-neoplastic nevus   I-10

757.33 Congenital pigmentary anomalies of skin
Congenital poikiloderma
Urticaria pigmentosa
Xeroderma pigmentosum
EXCLUDES albinism (270.2)
Q82.2 Mastocytosis   I-10

757.39 Other
Accessory skin tags, congenital
Congenital scar
Epidermolysis bullosa
Keratoderma (congenital)
EXCLUDES pilonidal cyst (685.0-685.1)
Q82.8 Other specified congenital malformations of skin   I-10

757.4 Specified anomalies of hair
Congenital: Congenital:
  alopecia   hypertrichosis
  atrichosis   monilethrix
  beaded hair   Persistent lanugo

757.5 Specified anomalies of nails
Anonychia   Congenital:
Congenital: leukonychia
  clubnail   onychauxis
  koilonychia   pachyonychia

757.6 Specified congenital anomalies of breast
Accessory
Congenital absent } breast or nipple
Supernumerary
EXCLUDES absence of pectoral muscle (756.81)
  hypoplasia of breast (611.82)
  micromastia (611.82)

757.8 Other specified anomalies of the integument

757.9　Unspecified anomaly of the integument
　　　Congenital:
　　　anomaly NOS ⎫
　　　deformity NOS ⎬ of integument
　　　　　　　　　⎭

✓4ᵗʰ **758　Chromosomal anomalies**
　　　INCLUDES　syndromes associated with anomalies in the number and
　　　　　　　　form of chromosomes
　　　Use additional codes for conditions associated with the
　　　　chromosomal anomalies

　　758.0　Down syndrome
　　　　Mongolism
　　　　Translocation Down syndrome
　　　　Trisomy:
　　　　　21 or 22
　　　　　G
　　　　Q90.9 Down syndrome unspecified　　　　　　　　I-10

　　758.1　Patau's syndrome
　　　　Trisomy:
　　　　　13
　　　　　D₁
　　　　DEF: Trisomy of 13th chromosome; characteristic failure to thrive,
　　　　severe mental impairment, seizures, abnormal eyes, low-set ears
　　　　and sloped forehead.

　　758.2　Edwards' syndrome
　　　　Trisomy:
　　　　　18
　　　　　E₃
　　　　DEF: Trisomy of 18th chromosome; characteristic mental and
　　　　physical impairments; mainly affects females.

✓5ᵗʰ　**758.3　Autosomal deletion syndromes**

　　　　758.31　Cri-du-chat syndrome
　　　　　　Deletion 5p
　　　　　　DEF: Hereditary congenital syndrome caused by a
　　　　　　microdeletion of short arm of chromosome 5; characterized
　　　　　　by catlike cry in newborn, microcephaly, severe mental
　　　　　　deficiency, and hypertelorism.

　　　　758.32　Velo-cardio-facial syndrome
　　　　　　Deletion 22q11.2
　　　　　　DEF: Microdeletion syndrome affecting multiple organs;
　　　　　　characteristic cleft palate, heart defects, elongated face
　　　　　　with almond-shaped eyes, wide nose, small ears, weak
　　　　　　immune systems, weak musculature, hypothyroidism,
　　　　　　short stature, and scoliosis; deletion at q11.2 on the long
　　　　　　arm of the chromosome 22.

　　　　758.33　Other microdeletions
　　　　　　Miller-Dieker syndrome
　　　　　　Smith-Magenis syndrome
　　　　　　DEF: Miller-Dieker syndrome: deletion from the short arm of
　　　　　　chromosome 17; characteristic mental retardation, speech
　　　　　　and motor development delays, neurological
　　　　　　complications, and multiple abnormalities affecting the
　　　　　　kidneys, heart, gastrointestinal tract; death in infancy or
　　　　　　early childhood.
　　　　　　DEF: Smith-Magenis syndrome: deletion in a certain area of
　　　　　　chromosome 17 that results in craniofacial changes,
　　　　　　speech delay, hoarse voice, hearing loss and behavioral
　　　　　　problems, such as self-destructive head banging, wrist
　　　　　　biting, and tearing at nails.

　　　　758.39　Other autosomal deletions

　　758.4　Balanced autosomal translocation in normal individual

　　758.5　Other conditions due to autosomal anomalies
　　　　Accessory autosomes NEC

　　758.6　Gonadal dysgenesis
　　　　Ovarian dysgenesis　　　　XO syndrome
　　　　Turner's syndrome
　　　　EXCLUDES　pure gonadal dysgenesis (752.7)

　　758.7　Klinefelter's syndrome　　　　　　　　　♂
　　　　XXY syndrome
　　　　DEF: Impaired embryonic development of seminiferous tubes;
　　　　results in small testes, azoospermia, infertility and enlarged
　　　　mammary glands.

✓5ᵗʰ　**758.8　Other conditions due to chromosome anomalies**

　　　　**758.81　Other conditions due to sex
　　　　　　　chromosome anomalies**

　　758.89　Other
　　　　Q99.8 Other specified chromosome abnormalities　　I-10

　**758.9　Conditions due to anomaly of unspecified
　　　chromosome**

✓4ᵗʰ **759　Other and unspecified congenital anomalies**

　　759.0　Anomalies of spleen
　　　　Aberrant ⎫
　　　　Absent　 ⎬ spleen
　　　　Accessory⎭
　　　　Congenital splenomegaly
　　　　Ectopic spleen
　　　　Lobulation of spleen

　　759.1　Anomalies of adrenal gland
　　　　Aberrant ⎫
　　　　Absent　 ⎬ adrenal gland
　　　　Accessory⎭
　　　　EXCLUDES　adrenogenital disorders (255.2)
　　　　　　　　　congenital disorders of steroid metabolism (255.2)

　　759.2　Anomalies of other endocrine glands
　　　　Absent parathyroid gland
　　　　Accessory thyroid gland
　　　　Persistent thyroglossal or thyrolingual duct
　　　　Thyroglossal (duct) cyst
　　　　EXCLUDES　congenital:
　　　　　　　　　goiter (246.1)
　　　　　　　　　hypothyroidism (243)

　　759.3　Situs inversus
　　　　Situs inversus or transversus:
　　　　　abdominalis
　　　　　thoracis
　　　　Transposition of viscera:
　　　　　abdominal
　　　　　thoracic
　　　　EXCLUDES　dextrocardia without mention of complete
　　　　　　　　　transposition (746.87)
　　　　DEF: Laterally transposed thoracic and abdominal viscera.

　　759.4　Conjoined twins
　　　　Craniopagus　　　　Thoracopagus
　　　　Dicephalus　　　　　Xiphopagus
　　　　Pygopagus

　　759.5　Tuberous sclerosis
　　　　Bourneville's disease
　　　　Epiloia
　　　　DEF: Hamartomas of brain, retina and viscera, impaired mental
　　　　ability, seizures and adenoma sebaceum.

　　759.6　Other hamartoses, not elsewhere classified
　　　　Syndrome:
　　　　　Peutz-Jeghers
　　　　　Sturge-Weber (-Dimitri)
　　　　　von Hippel-Lindau
　　　　EXCLUDES　neurofibromatosis ▶(237.70-237.79)◀
　　　　DEF: Peutz-Jeghers: hereditary syndrome characterized by
　　　　hamartomas of small intestine.
　　　　DEF: Sturge-Weber: congenital syndrome characterized by unilateral
　　　　port-wine stain over trigeminal nerve, underlying meninges and
　　　　cerebral cortex.
　　　　DEF: von Hippel-Lindau: hereditary syndrome of congenital
　　　　angiomatosis of the retina and cerebellum.
　　　　AHA: 3Q, '92, 12

　　759.7　Multiple congenital anomalies, so described
　　　　Congenital:
　　　　　anomaly, multiple NOS
　　　　　deformity, multiple NOS

✓5ᵗʰ　**759.8　Other specified anomalies**
　　　　AHA: S-O, '87, 9; S-O, '85, 11

　　　　759.81　Prader-Willi syndrome

　　　　759.82　Marfan syndrome
　　　　　　AHA: 3Q, '93, 11

　　　　759.83　Fragile X syndrome
　　　　　　AHA: 4Q, '94, 41

Congenital Anomalies

759.89–759.9

759.89 Other

Congenital malformation syndromes affecting
  multiple systems, not elsewhere classified
Laurence-Moon-Biedl syndrome

AHA: 3Q, '08, 3; 3Q, '06, 21; 2Q, '05, 17; 2Q, '04, 12; 1Q, '01, 3;
3Q, '99, 17, 18; 3Q, '98, 8

TIP: Assign for the following syndromes:
cardiofaciocutaneous (CFC), Borjeson-Forssman-Lehmann
syndrome (BFLS), Alagille syndrome, startle disease,
Alport's syndrome, branchio-oto-renal (BOR) syndrome,
Costello syndrome, Williams syndrome, Antley-Bixler
syndrome, and multiple pterygium syndrome. Assign
additional codes for any documented manifestations.

759.9 Congenital anomaly, unspecified

15. Certain Conditions Originating in the Perinatal Period (760-779)

INCLUDES conditions which have their origin in the perinatal period, before birth through the first 28 days after birth, even though death or morbidity occurs later

Use additional code(s) to further specify condition

Maternal Causes of Perinatal Morbidity and Mortality (760-763)

AHA: 2Q, '89, 14; 3Q, '90, 5

TIP: A newborn condition is clinically significant when it has implications for the newborn's *future* health care. This is an exception to the UHDDS guidelines.

√4ᵗʰ 760 Fetus or newborn affected by maternal conditions which may be unrelated to present pregnancy

     INCLUDES the listed maternal conditions only when specified as a cause of mortality or morbidity of the fetus or newborn

     EXCLUDES *maternal endocrine and metabolic disorders affecting fetus or newborn (775.0-775.9)*

     AHA: 1Q, '94, 8; 2Q, '92, 12; N-D, '84, 11

     TIP: Do not assign unless the mother's condition has actually affected the fetus or newborn.

760.0 Maternal hypertensive disorders
     Fetus or newborn affected by maternal conditions classifiable to 642

760.1 Maternal renal and urinary tract diseases
     Fetus or newborn affected by maternal conditions classifiable to 580-599

760.2 Maternal infections
     Fetus or newborn affected by maternal infectious disease classifiable to 001-136 and 487, but fetus or newborn not manifesting that disease
     EXCLUDES *congenital infectious diseases (771.0-771.8)*
         maternal genital tract and other localized infections (760.8)

760.3 Other chronic maternal circulatory and respiratory diseases
     Fetus or newborn affected by chronic maternal conditions classifiable to 390-459, 490-519, 745-748

760.4 Maternal nutritional disorders
     Fetus or newborn affected by:
       maternal disorders classifiable to 260-269
       maternal malnutrition NOS
     EXCLUDES *fetal malnutrition (764.10-764.29)*

760.5 Maternal injury
     Fetus or newborn affected by maternal conditions classifiable to 800-995

√5ᵗʰ 760.6 Surgical operation on mother and fetus
     EXCLUDES *cesarean section for present delivery (763.4)*
         damage to placenta from amniocentesis, cesarean section, or surgical induction (762.1)
     AHA: 4Q, '08, 137-138
     TIP: These codes include existing conditions present at the time of birth that are related to procedures performed before the time of delivery.

760.61 Newborn affected by amniocentesis
     EXCLUDES *fetal complications from amniocentesis (679.1)*

760.62 Newborn affected by other in utero procedure
     EXCLUDES *fetal complications of in utero procedure (679.1)*

760.63 Newborn affected by other surgical operations on mother during pregnancy
     EXCLUDES *newborn affected by previous surgical procedure on mother not associated with pregnancy (760.64)*

760.64 Newborn affected by previous surgical procedure on mother not associated with pregnancy

√5ᵗʰ 760.7 Noxious influences affecting fetus or newborn via placenta or breast milk
     Fetus or newborn affected by noxious substance transmitted via placenta or breast milk
     EXCLUDES *anesthetic and analgesic drugs administered during labor and delivery (763.5)*
         drug withdrawal syndrome in newborn (779.5)
     AHA: 3Q, '91, 21

760.70 Unspecified noxious substance
     Fetus or newborn affected by:
       Drug NEC

760.71 Alcohol
     Fetal alcohol syndrome

760.72 Narcotics

760.73 Hallucinogenic agents

760.74 Anti-infectives
     Antibiotics
     Antifungals

760.75 Cocaine
     AHA: 3Q, '94, 6; 2Q, '92, 12; 4Q, '91, 26
     TIP: If documentation indicates drug withdrawal in the newborn, also assign code 779.5 Drug withdrawal syndrome in newborn.

760.76 Diethylstilbestrol [DES]
     AHA: 4Q, '94, 45

760.77 Anticonvulsants   N
     Carbamazepine
     Phenobarbital
     Phenytoin
     Valproic acid
     AHA: 4Q, '05, 82

760.78 Antimetabolic agents   N
     Methotrexate
     Retinoic acid
     Statins
     AHA: 4Q, '05, 82-83

760.79 Other
     Fetus or newborn affected by:
       immune sera   ⎫ transmitted via
       medicinal agents NEC   ⎬ placenta
       toxic substance NEC   ⎭ or breast
     AHA: ▶1Q, '10, 14;◀ 3Q, '09, 21
     P04.8 Newborn (suspected) affected by oth   I-10
     maternl noxious subst

760.8 Other specified maternal conditions affecting fetus or newborn
     Maternal genital tract and other localized infection affecting fetus or newborn, but fetus or newborn not manifesting that disease
     EXCLUDES *maternal urinary tract infection affecting fetus or newborn (760.1)*

760.9 Unspecified maternal condition affecting fetus or newborn

√4ᵗʰ 761 Fetus or newborn affected by maternal complications of pregnancy
     INCLUDES the listed maternal conditions only when specified as a cause of mortality or morbidity of the fetus or newborn

761.0 Incompetent cervix
     DEF: Inadequate functioning of uterine cervix.

761.1 Premature rupture of membranes

761.2 Oligohydramnios
     EXCLUDES *that due to premature rupture of membranes (761.1)*
     DEF: Deficient amniotic fluid.

761.3 Polyhydramnios
     Hydramnios (acute) (chronic)
     DEF: Excess amniotic fluid.

761.4 Ectopic pregnancy
     Pregnancy:
       abdominal
       intraperitoneal
       tubal

√4ᵗʰ / √5ᵗʰ Additional Digit Required   Unspecified Code   Other Specified Code   Manifestation Code   ▶◀ Revised Text   ● New Code   ▲ Revised Code Title

2011 ICD-9-CM   **October 2010 · Volume 1 – 251**

Certain Conditions Originating in the Perinatal Period

761.5–763.84

761.5 Multiple pregnancy
Triplet (pregnancy)
Twin (pregnancy)

761.6 Maternal death

761.7 Malpresentation before labor
Breech presentation
External version
Oblique lie } before labor
Transverse lie
Unstable lie

761.8 Other specified maternal complications of pregnancy affecting fetus or newborn
Spontaneous abortion, fetus

761.9 Unspecified maternal complication of pregnancy affecting fetus or newborn

✓4ᵗʰ **762 Fetus or newborn affected by complications of placenta, cord, and membranes**
INCLUDES the listed maternal conditions only when specified as a cause of mortality or morbidity in the fetus or newborn
AHA: 1Q, '94, 8

762.0 Placenta previa ℕ
DEF: Placenta developed in lower segment of uterus; causes hemorrhaging in last trimester.

762.1 Other forms of placental separation and hemorrhage ℕ
Abruptio placentae
Antepartum hemorrhage
Damage to placenta from amniocentesis, cesarean section, or surgical induction
Maternal blood loss
Premature separation of placenta
Rupture of marginal sinus

762.2 Other and unspecified morphological and functional abnormalities of placenta ℕ
Placental:
dysfunction
infarction
insufficiency

762.3 Placental transfusion syndromes ℕ
Placental and cord abnormality resulting in twin-to-twin or other transplacental transfusion
Use additional code to indicate resultant condition in newborn:
fetal blood loss (772.0)
polycythemia neonatorum (776.4)

762.4 Prolapsed cord ℕ
Cord presentation

762.5 Other compression of umbilical cord ℕ
Cord around neck
Entanglement of cord
Knot in cord
Torsion of cord
AHA: 2Q, '03, 9
TIP: Assign only if the cord compression or entanglement was documented as having affected the fetus/newborn.
P02.5 Newborn (suspected) affected by oth compression umb cord I-10

762.6 Other and unspecified conditions of umbilical cord ℕ
Short cord
Thrombosis
Varices } of umbilical cord
Velamentous insertion
Vasa previa
EXCLUDES infection of umbilical cord (771.4)
single umbilical artery (747.5)
P02.69 Newborn (suspected) affected by oth cond umbil cord I-10

762.7 Chorioamnionitis ℕ
Amnionitis
Membranitis
Placentitis
DEF: Inflamed fetal membrane.

762.8 Other specified abnormalities of chorion and amnion ℕ

762.9 Unspecified abnormality of chorion and amnion ℕ

✓4ᵗʰ **763 Fetus or newborn affected by other complications of labor and delivery**
INCLUDES the listed conditions only when specified as a cause of mortality or morbidity in the fetus or newborn
EXCLUDES newborn affected by surgical procedures on mother (760.61-760.64)
AHA: 1Q, '94, 8

763.0 Breech delivery and extraction ℕ

763.1 Other malpresentation, malposition, and disproportion during labor and delivery ℕ
Fetus or newborn affected by:
abnormality of bony pelvis
contracted pelvis
persistent occipitoposterior position
shoulder presentation
transverse lie
Fetus or newborn affected by conditions classifiable to 652, 653, and 660

763.2 Forceps delivery ℕ
Fetus or newborn affected by forceps extraction

763.3 Delivery by vacuum extractor ℕ

763.4 Cesarean delivery ℕ
EXCLUDES placental separation or hemorrhage from cesarean section (762.1)

763.5 Maternal anesthesia and analgesia ℕ
Reactions and intoxications from maternal opiates and tranquilizers during labor and delivery
EXCLUDES drug withdrawal syndrome in newborn (779.5)

763.6 Precipitate delivery ℕ
Rapid second stage

763.7 Abnormal uterine contractions ℕ
Fetus or newborn affected by:
contraction ring
hypertonic labor
hypotonic uterine dysfunction
uterine inertia or dysfunction
Fetus or newborn affected by conditions classifiable to 661, except 661.3

✓5ᵗʰ **763.8 Other specified complications of labor and delivery affecting fetus or newborn**
AHA: 4Q, '98, 46

763.81 Abnormality in fetal heart rate or rhythm before the onset of labor ℕ

763.82 Abnormality in fetal heart rate or rhythm during labor ℕ
AHA: 4Q, '98, 46

763.83 Abnormality in fetal heart rate or rhythm, unspecified as to time of onset ℕ

763.84 Meconium passage during delivery ℕ
EXCLUDES meconium aspiration (770.11, 770.12)
meconium staining (779.84)
DEF: Fetal intestinal activity that increases in response to a distressed state during delivery; anal sphincter relaxes, and meconium is passed into the amniotic fluid.
AHA: 4Q, '05, 83
TIP: If the meconium was documented as aspirated or had any effect on the newborn, see codes 770.11 and 770.12.

ℕ Newborn Age: 0   ℙ Pediatric Age: 0-17   Ⓜ Maternity Age: 12-55   Ⓐ Adult Age: 15-124

763.89 Other specified complications of labor and delivery affecting fetus or newborn [N]
> Fetus or newborn affected by:
>> abnormality of maternal soft tissues
>> destructive operation on live fetus to facilitate delivery
>> induction of labor (medical)
>> other procedures used in labor and delivery
> Fetus or newborn affected by other conditions classifiable to 650-669

763.9 Unspecified complication of labor and delivery affecting fetus or newborn [N]

Other Conditions Originating in the Perinatal Period (764-779)

The following fifth-digit subclassification is for use with category 764 and codes 765.0-765.1 to denote birthweight:
- **0 unspecified [weight]**
- **1 less than 500 grams**
- **2 500-749 grams**
- **3 750-999 grams**
- **4 1,000-1,249 grams**
- **5 1,250-1,499 grams**
- **6 1,500-1,749 grams**
- **7 1,750-1,999 grams**
- **8 2,000-2,499 grams**
- **9 2,500 grams and over**

✓4th **764 Slow fetal growth and fetal malnutrition**
> AHA: 1Q, '09, 13; 3Q, '04, 4; 4Q, '02, 63; 1Q,'94, 8; 2Q, '91, 19; 2Q, '89, 15

§ ✓5th **764.0 "Light-for-dates" without mention of fetal malnutrition** [N]
[0-9]
> Infants underweight for gestational age
> "Small-for-dates"
> P07.18 Other low birth weight newborn 2000-2499 grams [I-10]

§ ✓5th **764.1 "Light-for-dates" with signs of fetal malnutrition** [N]
[0-9]
> Infants "light-for-dates" classifiable to 764.0, who in addition show signs of fetal malnutrition, such as dry peeling skin and loss of subcutaneous tissue

§ ✓5th **764.2 Fetal malnutrition without mention of "light-for-dates"** [N]
[0-9]
> Infants, not underweight for gestational age, showing signs of fetal malnutrition, such as dry peeling skin and loss of subcutaneous tissue
> Intrauterine malnutrition

§ ✓5th **764.9 Fetal growth retardation, unspecified** [N]
[0-9]
> Intrauterine growth retardation
> AHA: For code 764.97: 1Q, '97, 6

✓4th **765 Disorders relating to short gestation and low birthweight**
> INCLUDES the listed conditions, without further specification, as causes of mortality, morbidity, or additional care, in fetus or newborn
> AHA: 1Q, '97, 6; 1Q, '94, 8; 2Q, '91, 19; 2Q, '89, 15

§ ✓5th **765.0 Extreme immaturity** [N]
[0-9]
> NOTE Usually implies a birthweight of less than 1000 grams.
> Use additional code for weeks of gestation (765.20-765.29)
> AHA: 1Q, '09, 13; 3Q, '04, 4; 4Q, '02, 63; For code 765.03: 4Q, '01, 51

§ ✓5th **765.1 Other preterm infants** [N]
[0-9]
> NOTE Usually implies a birthweight of 1000-2499 grams.
> Prematurity NOS
> Prematurity or small size, not classifiable to 765.0 or as "light-for-dates" in 764
> Use additional code for weeks of gestation (765.20-765.29)
> AHA: 1Q, '09, 13; 3Q, '04, 4; 4Q, '02, 63; For code 765.10: 1Q, '09, 15; 1Q, '94, 14; For code 765.17: 4Q, '08, 139; 1Q, '97, 6; For code 765.18: 4Q, '02, 64
> P07.10 Other low birth weight newborn uns weight [I-10]

✓5th **765.2 Weeks of gestation**
> AHA: 3Q, '04, 4; 4Q, '02, 63
> TIP: Assign as an additional code with category 764 and codes from 765.0 and 765.1, as documented by the provider.

765.20 Unspecified weeks of gestation [N]

765.21 Less than 24 completed weeks of gestation [N]

765.22 24 completed weeks of gestation [N]

765.23 25-26 completed weeks of gestation [N]
> AHA: 1Q, '09, 14

765.24 27-28 completed weeks of gestation [N]

765.25 29-30 completed weeks of gestation [N]
> P07.31 Other preterm newborn 28-31 complete weeks [I-10]

765.26 31-32 completed weeks of gestation [N]
> AHA: 1Q, '09, 14; 4Q, '08, 139

765.27 33-34 completed weeks of gestation [N]

765.28 35-36 completed weeks of gestation [N]
> AHA: 4Q, '02, 64
> P07.32 Other preterm newborn 32-36 complete weeks [I-10]

765.29 37 or more completed weeks of gestation [N]

✓4th **766 Disorders relating to long gestation and high birthweight**
> INCLUDES the listed conditions, without further specification, as causes of mortality, morbidity, or additional care, in fetus or newborn

766.0 Exceptionally large baby [N]
> NOTE Usually implies a birthweight of 4500 grams or more.

766.1 Other "heavy-for-dates" infants [N]
> Other fetus or infant "heavy-" or "large-for-dates" regardless of period of gestation
> P08.1 Other heavy for gestational age newborn [I-10]

✓5th **766.2 Late infant, not "heavy-for-dates"**
> AHA: 2Q, '06, 12; 4Q, '03, 69
> TIP: May be assigned based on gestational age alone, without documentation of any related specific condition or disorder.

766.21 Post-term infant [N]
> Infant with gestation period over 40 completed weeks to 42 completed weeks
> AHA: 1Q, '09, 12;
> P08.21 Post-term newborn [I-10]

766.22 Prolonged gestation of infant [N]
> Infant with gestation period over 42 completed weeks
> Postmaturity NOS
> AHA: 1Q, '09, 12

✓4th **767 Birth trauma**

767.0 Subdural and cerebral hemorrhage [N]
> Subdural and cerebral hemorrhage, whether described as due to birth trauma or to intrapartum anoxia or hypoxia
> Subdural hematoma (localized)
> Tentorial tear
> Use additional code to identify cause
> EXCLUDES intraventricular hemorrhage (772.10-772.14)
>> subarachnoid hemorrhage (772.2)

✓5th **767.1 Injuries to scalp**
> AHA: 4Q, '03, 69

767.11 Epicranial subaponeurotic hemorrhage (massive) [N]
> Subgaleal hemorrhage
> DEF: A hemorrhage that occurs within the space between the galea aponeurotica, or epicranial aponeurosis, a thin tendinous structure that is attached to the skull laterally, and the periosteum of the skull.

767.19 Other injuries to scalp [N]
> Caput succedaneum
> Cephalhematoma
> Chignon (from vacuum extraction)
> P12.89 Other birth injuries to scalp [I-10]

767.2 Fracture of clavicle [N]

767.3 Other injuries to skeleton [N]
> Fracture of:
>> long bones
>> skull
> EXCLUDES congenital dislocation of hip (754.30-754.35)
>> fracture of spine, congenital (767.4)

---

§ Requires fifth digit. Valid digits are in [brackets] under each code. See beginning of section 764-779 for codes and definitions.

✓4th ✓5th Additional Digit Required | Unspecified Code | Other Specified Code | Manifestation Code | ►◄ Revised Text | ● New Code | ▲ Revised Code Title
2011 ICD-9-CM | **Volume 1 – 253**

Epicranial Aponeurosis

767.4 Injury to spine and spinal cord   N
Dislocation
Fracture   } of spine or spinal cord due to
Laceration   } birth trauma
Rupture

767.5 Facial nerve injury   N
Facial palsy

767.6 Injury to brachial plexus   N
Palsy or paralysis:
  brachial
  Erb (-Duchenne)
  Klumpke (-Déjérine)

767.7 Other cranial and peripheral nerve injuries   N
Phrenic nerve paralysis

767.8 Other specified birth trauma   N
Eye damage   Rupture of:
Hematoma of: liver
  liver (subcapsular)   spleen
  testes   Scalpel wound
  vulva   Traumatic glaucoma
    EXCLUDES *hemorrhage classifiable to 772.0-772.9*

767.9 Birth trauma, unspecified   N
Birth injury NOS

√4th **768 Intrauterine hypoxia and birth asphyxia**
NOTE Use only when associated with newborn morbidity classifiable elsewhere
EXCLUDES *acidemia NOS of newborn (775.81)*
acidosis NOS of newborn (775.81)
cerebral ischemia NOS (779.2)
hypoxia NOS of newborn (770.88)
mixed metabolic and respiratory acidosis of newborn (775.81)
respiratory arrest of newborn (770.87)
DEF: Oxygen intake insufficiency due to interrupted placental circulation or premature separation of placenta.
AHA: 4Q, '92, 20

768.0 Fetal death from asphyxia or anoxia before onset of labor or at unspecified time   N

768.1 Fetal death from asphyxia or anoxia during labor   N

768.2 Fetal distress before onset of labor, in liveborn infant   N
Fetal metabolic acidemia before onset of labor, in liveborn infant

768.3 Fetal distress first noted during labor and delivery, in liveborn infant   N
Fetal metabolic acidemia first noted during labor and delivery, in liveborn infant

768.4 Fetal distress, unspecified as to time of onset, in liveborn infant   N
Fetal metabolic acidemia unspecified as to time of onset, in liveborn infant
AHA: N-D, '86, 10

768.5 Severe birth asphyxia   N
Birth asphyxia with neurologic involvement
EXCLUDES *hypoxic-ischemic encephalopathy [HIE] (768.70-768.73)*
AHA: N-D, '86, 3

768.6 Mild or moderate birth asphyxia   N
Other specified birth asphyxia (without mention of neurologic involvement)
EXCLUDES *hypoxic-ischemic encephalopathy [HIE] (768.70-768.73)*
AHA: N-D, '86, 3

√5th **768.7 Hypoxic-ischemic encephalopathy [HIE]**
AHA: ▶4Q, '09, 99-101;◀ 4Q, '06, 104

768.70 Hypoxic-ischemic encephalopathy, unspecified   N

768.71 Mild hypoxic-ischemic encephalopathy   N

768.72 Moderate hypoxic-ischemic encephalopathy   N
AHA: ▶4Q, '09, 101◀

768.73 Severe hypoxic-ischemic encephalopathy   N

768.9 Unspecified birth asphyxia in liveborn infant   N
Anoxia   } NOS, in liveborn infant
Asphyxia   }

769 Respiratory distress syndrome   N
Cardiorespiratory distress syndrome of newborn
Hyaline membrane disease (pulmonary)
Idiopathic respiratory distress syndrome [IRDS or RDS] of newborn
Pulmonary hypoperfusion syndrome
EXCLUDES *transient tachypnea of newborn (770.6)*
DEF: Severe chest contractions upon air intake and expiratory grunting; infant appears blue due to oxygen deficiency and has rapid respiratory rate; formerly called hyaline membrane disease.
AHA: 1Q, '89, 10; N-D, '86, 6
TIP: Do not assign if documentation specifies Type II respiratory distress syndrome, which usually resolves within six to 24 hours after birth; see instead 770.6.
P22.0 Respiratory distress syndrome of newborn   I-10

√4th **770 Other respiratory conditions of fetus and newborn**

770.0 Congenital pneumonia   N
Infective pneumonia acquired prenatally
EXCLUDES *pneumonia from infection acquired after birth (480.0-486)*
AHA: 1Q, '05, 10

√5th **770.1 Fetal and newborn aspiration**
EXCLUDES *aspiration of postnatal stomach contents (770.85, 770.86)*
meconium passage during delivery (763.84)
meconium staining (779.84)
AHA: 4Q, '05, 83

770.10 Fetal and newborn aspiration, unspecified   N

770.11 Meconium aspiration without respiratory symptoms   N
Meconium aspiration NOS

770.12 Meconium aspiration with respiratory symptoms   N
Meconium aspiration pneumonia
Meconium aspiration pneumonitis
Meconium aspiration syndrome NOS
Use additional code to identify any secondary pulmonary hypertension (416.8), if applicable
DEF: Meconium aspiration syndrome: aspiration of fetal intestinal material during or prior to delivery, usually a complication of placental insufficiency, causing pneumonitis and bronchial obstruction (inflammatory reaction of lungs).

770.13 Aspiration of clear amniotic fluid without respiratory symptoms   N
Aspiration of clear amniotic fluid NOS

770.14 Aspiration of clear amniotic fluid with respiratory symptoms   N
Aspiration of clear amniotic fluid with pneumonia
Aspiration of clear amniotic fluid with pneumonitis
Use additional code to identify any secondary pulmonary hypertension (416.8), if applicable

770.15 Aspiration of blood without respiratory symptoms   N
Aspiration of blood NOS

N Newborn Age: 0   P Pediatric Age: 0-17   M Maternity Age: 12-55   A Adult Age: 15-124

770.16 Aspiration of blood with respiratory symptoms N
Aspiration of blood with pneumonia
Aspiration of blood with pneumonitis

Use additional code to identify any secondary
pulmonary hypertension (416.8), if applicable

**770.17 Other fetal and newborn aspiration
without respiratory symptoms** N

**770.18 Other fetal and newborn aspiration
with respiratory symptoms** N
Other aspiration pneumonia
Other aspiration pneumonitis

Use additional code to identify any secondary
pulmonary hypertension (416.8), if applicable

770.2 Interstitial emphysema and related conditions N
Pneumomediastinum }
Pneumopericardium } originating in the perinatal
Pneumothorax } period

P25.0 Interstitial emphysema origin perinatal period I-10

770.3 Pulmonary hemorrhage N
Hemorrhage:
alveolar (lung) }
intra-alveolar (lung) } originating in the
massive pulmonary } perinatal period

770.4 Primary atelectasis N
Pulmonary immaturity NOS
DEF: Alveoli fail to expand causing insufficient air intake by newborn.

770.5 Other and unspecified atelectasis N
Atelectasis:
NOS }
partial } originating in the perinatal
secondary } period
Pulmonary collapse

770.6 Transitory tachypnea of newborn N
Idiopathic tachypnea of newborn
Wet lung syndrome
EXCLUDES respiratory distress syndrome (769)
DEF: Quick, shallow breathing of newborn; short-term problem.
AHA: 4Q, '95, 4; 1Q, '94, 12; 3Q, '93, 7; 1Q, '89, 10; N-D, '86, 6
P22.1 Transient tachypnea of newborn I-10

770.7 Chronic respiratory disease arising in the perinatal period N
Bronchopulmonary dysplasia
Interstitial pulmonary fibrosis of prematurity
Wilson-Mikity syndrome
AHA: 2Q, '91, 19; N-D, '86, 11
P27.8 Other chronic resp dz origin perinatal period I-10

√5ᵗʰ **770.8 Other respiratory problems after birth**
EXCLUDES mixed metabolic and respiratory acidosis of newborn
(775.81)
AHA: 4Q, '02, 65; 2Q, '98, 10; 2Q, '96, 10

770.81 Primary apnea of newborn N
Apneic spells of newborn NOS
Essential apnea of newborn
Sleep apnea of newborn
DEF: Cessation of breathing when a neonate makes no
respiratory effort for 15 seconds, resulting in cyanosis and
bradycardia.
P28.3 Primary sleep apnea of newborn I-10

770.82 Other apnea of newborn N
Obstructive apnea of newborn

770.83 Cyanotic attacks of newborn N

770.84 Respiratory failure of newborn N
EXCLUDES respiratory distress syndrome (769)
AHA: 4Q, '08, 99

**770.85 Aspiration of postnatal stomach
contents without respiratory symptoms** N
Aspiration of postnatal stomach contents NOS
AHA: 4Q, '05, 83

**770.86 Aspiration of postnatal stomach
contents with respiratory symptoms** N
Aspiration of postnatal stomach contents with
pneumonia
Aspiration of postnatal stomach contents with
pneumonitis

Use additional code to identify any secondary
pulmonary hypertension (416.8), if applicable
AHA: 4Q, '05, 83

770.87 Respiratory arrest of newborn N
AHA: 4Q, '06, 104-106

770.88 Hypoxemia of newborn N
Hypoxia NOS of newborn
AHA: 4Q, '06, 104-106

770.89 Other respiratory problems after birth N
AHA: ▶3Q, '09, 20◀
P28.89 Oth specified respiratory conditions I-10
of newborn

**770.9 Unspecified respiratory condition of fetus
and newborn** N

√4ᵗʰ **771 Infections specific to the perinatal period**
INCLUDES infections acquired before or during birth or via the
umbilicus or during the first 28 days after birth
EXCLUDES congenital pneumonia (770.0)
congenital syphilis (090.0-090.9)
infant botulism (040.41)
maternal infectious disease as a cause of mortality or
morbidity in fetus or newborn, but fetus or newborn
not manifesting the disease (760.2)
ophthalmia neonatorum due to gonococcus (098.40)
other infections not specifically classified to this category
AHA: N-D, '85, 4

771.0 Congenital rubella N
Congenital rubella pneumonitis

771.1 Congenital cytomegalovirus infection N
Congenital cytomegalic inclusion disease

771.2 Other congenital infections N
Congenital:
herpes simplex
listeriosis
malaria
toxoplasmosis
tuberculosis

771.3 Tetanus neonatorum N
Tetanus omphalitis
EXCLUDES hypocalcemic tetany (775.4)
DEF: Severe infection of central nervous system; due to exotoxin of
tetanus bacillus from navel infection prompted by nonsterile
technique during umbilical ligation.

771.4 Omphalitis of the newborn N
Infection:
navel cord
umbilical stump
EXCLUDES tetanus omphalitis (771.3)
DEF: Inflamed umbilicus.
AHA: ▶4Q, '09, 102◀

771.5 Neonatal infective mastitis N
EXCLUDES noninfective neonatal mastitis (778.7)

771.6 Neonatal conjunctivitis and dacryocystitis N
Ophthalmia neonatorum NOS
EXCLUDES ophthalmia neonatorum due to gonococcus (098.40)

771.7 Neonatal Candida infection N
Neonatal moniliasis
Thrush in newborn

√5ᵗʰ **771.8 Other infection specific to the perinatal period**
▶Use additional code to identify organism or specific infection◀
AHA: 4Q, '02, 66

771.81 Septicemia [sepsis] of newborn   N
Use additional codes to identify severe sepsis (995.92) and any associated acute organ dysfunction, if applicable
AHA: 4Q, '08, 99
TIP: Assign instead of 038 or 995.91. Assign also a code to identify severe sepsis (995.92) or any acute organ dysfunction, or a code from category 041 to specify the organism.
P36.9 Bacterial sepsis newborn unspecified   I-10

771.82 Urinary tract infection of newborn   N

771.83 Bacteremia of newborn   N

771.89 Other infections specific to the perinatal period   N
Intra-amniotic infection of fetus NOS
Infection of newborn NOS

√4ᵗʰ **772 Fetal and neonatal hemorrhage**
EXCLUDES   fetal hematologic conditions complicating pregnancy (678.0)
hematological disorders of fetus and newborn (776.0-776.9)

772.0 Fetal blood loss affecting newborn   N
Fetal blood loss from:
cut end of co-twin's cord
placenta
ruptured cord
vasa previa
Fetal exsanguination
Fetal hemorrhage into:
co-twin
mother's circulation

√5ᵗʰ **772.1 Intraventricular hemorrhage**
Intraventricular hemorrhage from any perinatal cause
AHA: 4Q, '01, 49; 3Q, '92, 8; 4Q, '88, 8

772.10 Unspecified grade   N

772.11 Grade I   N
Bleeding into germinal matrix

772.12 Grade II   N
Bleeding into ventricle

772.13 Grade III   N
Bleeding with enlargement of ventricle
AHA: 4Q, '01, 51

772.14 Grade IV   N
Bleeding into cerebral cortex

772.2 Subarachnoid hemorrhage   N
Subarachnoid hemorrhage from any perinatal cause
EXCLUDES   subdural and cerebral hemorrhage (767.0)

772.3 Umbilical hemorrhage after birth   N
Slipped umbilical ligature

772.4 Gastrointestinal hemorrhage   N
EXCLUDES   swallowed maternal blood (777.3)

772.5 Adrenal hemorrhage   N

772.6 Cutaneous hemorrhage   N
Bruising
Ecchymoses
Petechiae } in fetus or newborn
Superficial hematoma
P54.5 Neonatal cutaneous hemorrhage   I-10

772.8 Other specified hemorrhage of fetus or newborn   N
EXCLUDES   hemorrhagic disease of newborn (776.0)
pulmonary hemorrhage (770.3)

772.9 Unspecified hemorrhage of newborn   N

√4ᵗʰ **773 Hemolytic disease of fetus or newborn, due to isoimmunization**
DEF: Hemolytic anemia of fetus or newborn due to maternal antibody formation against fetal erythrocytes; infant blood contains nonmaternal antigen.
TIP: Do not assign unless the physician substantiates confirmation by a positive Coomb's (direct antibody or direct antiglobulin) test.

773.0 Hemolytic disease due to Rh isoimmunization   N
Anemia | due to RH:
Erythroblastosis (fetalis) | antibodies
Hemolytic disease (fetus) | isoimmunization
(newborn) | maternal/fetal
Jaundice | incompatibility
Rh hemolytic disease
Rh isoimmunization

773.1 Hemolytic disease due to ABO isoimmunization   N
ABO hemolytic disease
ABO isoimmunization
Anemia | due to ABO:
Erythroblastosis (fetalis) | antibodies
Hemolytic disease (fetus) | isoimmunization
(newborn) | maternal/fetal
Jaundice | incompatibility
DEF: Incompatible Rh fetal-maternal blood grouping; prematurely destroys red blood cells; detected by Coombs test.
AHA: 3Q, '92, 8
P55.1 ABO isoimmunization of newborn   I-10

773.2 Hemolytic disease due to other and unspecified isoimmunization   N
Eythroblastosis (fetalis) (neonatorum) NOS
Hemolytic disease (fetus) (newborn) NOS
Jaundice or anemia due to other and unspecified blood-group incompatibility
AHA: 1Q, '94, 13
P55.9 Hemolytic disease of newborn unspecified   I-10

773.3 Hydrops fetalis due to isoimmunization   N
Use additional code to identify type of isoimmunization (773.0-773.2)
DEF: Massive edema of entire body and severe anemia; may result in fetal death or stillbirth.

773.4 Kernicterus due to isoimmunization   N
Use additional code to identify type of isoimmunization (773.0-773.2)
DEF: Complication of erythroblastosis fetalis associated with severe neural symptoms, high blood bilirubin levels and nerve cell destruction; results in bilirubin-pigmented gray matter of central nervous system.

773.5 Late anemia due to isoimmunization   N

√4ᵗʰ **774 Other perinatal jaundice**

774.0 Perinatal jaundice from hereditary hemolytic anemias   N
Code first underlying disease (282.0-282.9)

774.1 Perinatal jaundice from other excessive hemolysis   N
Fetal or neonatal jaundice from:
bruising
drugs or toxins transmitted from mother
infection
polycythemia
swallowed maternal blood
Use additional code to identify cause
EXCLUDES   jaundice due to isoimmunization (773.0-773.2)

774.2 Neonatal jaundice associated with preterm delivery   N
Hyperbilirubinemia of prematurity
Jaundice due to delayed conjugation associated with preterm delivery
AHA: 3Q, '91, 21
P59.0 Neonatal jaundice associated w/preterm delivery   I-10

√5ᵗʰ **774.3 Neonatal jaundice due to delayed conjugation from other causes**

774.30 Neonatal jaundice due to delayed conjugation, cause unspecified   N
DEF: Jaundice of newborn with abnormal bilirubin metabolism; causes excess accumulated unconjugated bilirubin in blood.

774.31 *Neonatal jaundice due to delayed conjugation in diseases classified elsewhere* N

Code first underlying diseases as:
congenital hypothyroidism (243)
Crigler-Najjar syndrome (277.4)
Gilbert's syndrome (277.4)

774.39 Other N

Jaundice due to delayed conjugation from causes, such as:
breast milk inhibitors
delayed development of conjugating system

774.4 Perinatal jaundice due to hepatocellular damage N

Fetal or neonatal hepatitis
Giant cell hepatitis
Inspissated bile syndrome

774.5 *Perinatal jaundice from other causes* N

Code first underlying cause as:
congenital obstruction of bile duct (751.61)
galactosemia (271.1)
mucoviscidosis (277.00-277.09)

774.6 Unspecified fetal and neonatal jaundice N

Icterus neonatorum
Neonatal hyperbilirubinemia (transient)
Physiologic jaundice NOS in newborn

EXCLUDES *that in preterm infants (774.2)*

AHA: 1Q, '94, 13; 2Q, '89, 15

P59.9 Neonatal jaundice unspecified   I-10

774.7 Kernicterus not due to isoimmunization N

Bilirubin encephalopathy
Kernicterus of newborn NOS

EXCLUDES *kernicterus due to isoimmunization (773.4)*

√4ᵗʰ 775 Endocrine and metabolic disturbances specific to the fetus and newborn

INCLUDES transitory endocrine and metabolic disturbances caused by the infant's response to maternal endocrine and metabolic factors, its removal from them, or its adjustment to extrauterine existence

775.0 Syndrome of "infant of a diabetic mother" N

Maternal diabetes mellitus affecting fetus or newborn (with hypoglycemia)

AHA: 1Q, '04, 7-8; 3Q, '91, 5

TIP: Do not assign if the infant has no manifestations or symptoms of the syndrome; refer instead to code V18.0 Family history, diabetes mellitus.

P70.1 Syndrome of infant of diabetic mother   I-10

775.1 Neonatal diabetes mellitus N

Diabetes mellitus syndrome in newborn infant

AHA: 3Q, '91, 6

775.2 Neonatal myasthenia gravis N

775.3 Neonatal thyrotoxicosis N

Neonatal hyperthydroidism (transient)

775.4 Hypocalcemia and hypomagnesemia of newborn N

Cow's milk hypocalcemia
Hypocalcemic tetany, neonatal
Neonatal hypoparathyroidism
Phosphate-loading hypocalcemia

775.5 Other transitory neonatal electrolyte disturbances N

Dehydration, neonatal

AHA: ▶1Q, '10, 14;◀ 3Q, '09, 21; 1Q, '05, 9

TIP: If the patient has neonatal hyperkalemia, assign also code 276.7 Hyperpotassemia.

P74.1 Dehydration of newborn   I-10

775.6 Neonatal hypoglycemia N

EXCLUDES *infant of mother with diabetes mellitus (775.0)*

AHA: 1Q '94, 8

P70.4 Other neonatal hypoglycemia   I-10

775.7 Late metabolic acidosis of newborn N

√5ᵗʰ 775.8 Other neonatal endocrine and metabolic disturbances

775.81 Other acidosis of newborn N

Acidemia NOS of newborn
Acidosis of newborn NOS
Mixed metabolic and respiratory acidosis of newborn

AHA: 4Q, '06, 104-106

775.89 Other neonatal endocrine and metabolic disturbances N

Amino-acid metabolic disorders described as transitory

AHA: 4Q, '06, 104-106

775.9 Unspecified endocrine and metabolic disturbances specific to the fetus and newborn N

√4ᵗʰ 776 Hematological disorders of newborn

INCLUDES disorders specific to the newborn though possibly originating in utero

EXCLUDES *fetal hematologic conditions (678.0)*

776.0 Hemorrhagic disease of newborn N

Hemorrhagic diathesis of newborn
Vitamin K deficiency of newborn

EXCLUDES *fetal or neonatal hemorrhage (772.0-772.9)*

776.1 Transient neonatal thrombocytopenia N

Neonatal thrombocytopenia due to:
exchange transfusion
idiopathic maternal thrombocytopenia
isoimmunization

DEF: Temporary decrease in blood platelets of newborn.

P61.0 Transient neonatal thrombocytopenia   I-10

776.2 Disseminated intravascular coagulation in newborn N

DEF: Disseminated intravascular coagulation of newborn: clotting disorder due to excess thromboplastic agents in blood as a result of disease or trauma; causes blood clotting within vessels and reduces available elements necessary for blood coagulation.

776.3 Other transient neonatal disorders of coagulation N

Transient coagulation defect, newborn

776.4 Polycythemia neonatorum N

Plethora of newborn
Polycythemia due to:
donor twin transfusion
maternal-fetal transfusion

DEF: Abnormal increase of total red blood cells of newborn.

776.5 Congenital anemia N

Anemia following fetal blood loss

EXCLUDES *anemia due to isoimmunization (773.0-773.2, 773.5)*
hereditary hemolytic anemias (282.0-282.9)

776.6 Anemia of prematurity N

P61.2 Anemia of prematurity   I-10

776.7 Transient neonatal neutropenia N

Isoimmune neutropenia
Maternal transfer neutropenia

EXCLUDES *congenital neutropenia (nontransient) (288.01)*

DEF: Decreased neutrophilic leukocytes in blood of newborn.

776.8 Other specified transient hematological disorders N

776.9 Unspecified hematological disorder specific to newborn N

√4ᵗʰ 777 Perinatal disorders of digestive system

INCLUDES disorders specific to the fetus and newborn

EXCLUDES *intestinal obstruction classifiable to 560.0-560.9*

777.1 Meconium obstruction N

Congenital fecaliths
Delayed passage of meconium
Meconium ileus NOS
Meconium plug syndrome

EXCLUDES *meconium ileus in cystic fibrosis (277.01)*

DEF: Meconium blocked digestive tract of newborn.

777.2 Intestinal obstruction due to inspissated milk N

777.3 Hematemesis and melena due to swallowed maternal blood N

Swallowed blood syndrome in newborn

EXCLUDES *that not due to swallowed maternal blood (772.4)*

√4ᵗʰ √5ᵗʰ Additional Digit Required   Unspecified Code   Other Specified Code   Manifestation Code   ▶◀ Revised Text   ● New Code   ▲ Revised Code Title

Certain Conditions Originating in the Perinatal Period

777.4–779.81

777.4 Transitory ileus of newborn   N
> *EXCLUDES*   *Hirschsprung's disease (751.3)*

√5ᵗʰ 777.5 Necrotizing enterocolitis in newborn
> **DEF:** Serious intestinal infection and inflammation in preterm infants; severity is measured by stages and may progress to life-threatening perforation or peritonitis; resection surgical treatment may be necessary.
> **AHA:** 4Q, '08, 138-140

> **777.50 Necrotizing enterocolitis in newborn, unspecified**   N
> Necrotizing enterocolitis in newborn, NOS

> **777.51 Stage I necrotizing enterocolitis in newborn**   N
> Necrotizing enterocolitis without pneumatosis, without perforation
> **DEF:** Broad-spectrum symptoms with non-specific signs including feeding intolerance, sepsis, gastroenteritis, ileus, metabolic abnormalities.

> **777.52 Stage II necrotizing enterocolitis in newborn**   N
> Necrotizing enterocolitis with pneumatosis, without perforation
> **DEF:** Radiographic confirmation of necrotizing enterocolitis showing intestinal dilatation, fixed loops of bowels, pneumatosis intestinalis, metabolic acidosis, and thrombocytopenia.

> **777.53 Stage III necrotizing enterocolitis in newborn**   N
> Necrotizing enterocolitis with perforation
> Necrotizing enterocolitis with pneumatosis and perforation
> **DEF:** Advanced stage in which infant demonstrates signs of bowel perforation, septic shock, metabolic acidosis, ascites, disseminated intravascular coagulopathy, neutropenia.
> **AHA:** 4Q, '08, 139

777.6 Perinatal intestinal perforation   N
> Meconium peritonitis

777.8 Other specified perinatal disorders of digestive system   N

777.9 Unspecified perinatal disorder of digestive system   N

778 Conditions involving the integument and temperature regulation of fetus and newborn

778.0 Hydrops fetalis not due to isoimmunization   N
> Idiopathic hydrops
> *EXCLUDES*   *hydrops fetalis due to isoimmunization (773.3)*
> **DEF:** Edema of entire body, unrelated to immune response.

778.1 Sclerema neonatorum   N
> Subcutaneous fat necrosis
> **DEF:** Diffuse, rapidly progressing white, waxy, nonpitting hardening of tissue, usually of legs and feet, life-threatening; found in preterm or debilitated infants; unknown etiology.

778.2 Cold injury syndrome of newborn   N

778.3 Other hypothermia of newborn   N

778.4 Other disturbances of temperature regulation of newborn   N
> Dehydration fever in newborn
> Environmentally-induced pyrexia
> Hyperthermia in newborn
> Transitory fever of newborn
> **P81.9** Disturbance of temp regulation newborn uns   I-10

778.5 Other and unspecified edema of newborn   N
> Edema neonatorum

778.6 Congenital hydrocele   N
> Congenital hydrocele of tunica vaginalis
> **P83.5** Congenital hydrocele   I-10

778.7 Breast engorgement in newborn   N
> Noninfective mastitis of newborn
> *EXCLUDES*   *infective mastitis of newborn (771.5)*

778.8 Other specified conditions involving the integument of fetus and newborn   N
> Urticaria neonatorum
> *EXCLUDES*   *impetigo neonatorum (684)*
>   *pemphigus neonatorum (684)*
> **P83.8** Oth spec conditions integument specific newborn   I-10

778.9 Unspecified condition involving the integument and temperature regulation of fetus and newborn   N

√4ᵗʰ 779 Other and ill-defined conditions originating in the perinatal period

779.0 Convulsions in newborn   N
> Fits } in newborn
> Seizures
> **AHA:** N-D, '84, 11
> **TIP:** Clarify with the physician that convulsions are not actually infantile spasms; if so, refer to subcategory 345.6.

779.1 Other and unspecified cerebral irritability in newborn   N

779.2 Cerebral depression, coma, and other abnormal cerebral signs   N
> Cerebral ischemia NOS of newborn
> CNS dysfunction in newborn NOS
> *EXCLUDES*   *cerebral ischemia due to birth trauma (767.0)*
>   *intrauterine cerebral ischemia (768.2-768.9)*
>   *intraventricular hemorrhage (772.10-772.14)*

√5ᵗʰ 779.3 Disorder of stomach function and feeding problems in newborn
> **AHA:** 2Q, '89, 15

> **779.31 Feeding problems in newborn**   N
> Slow feeding in newborn
> *EXCLUDES*   *feeding problem in child over 28 days old (783.3)*
> **AHA:** ▶4Q, '09, 102◄
> **P92.9** Feeding problem of newborn unspecified   I-10

> **779.32 Bilious vomiting in newborn**   N
> *EXCLUDES*   *bilious vomiting in child over 28 days old (787.04)*

> **779.33 Other vomiting in newborn**   N
> Regurgitation of food in newborn
> *EXCLUDES*   *vomiting in child over 28 days old (536.2, 787.01-787.04)*

> **779.34 Failure to thrive in newborn**   N
> *EXCLUDES*   *failure to thrive in child over 28 days old (783.41)*

779.4 Drug reactions and intoxications specific to newborn   N
> Gray syndrome from chloramphenicol administration in newborn
> *EXCLUDES*   *fetal alcohol syndrome (760.71)*
>   *reactions and intoxications from maternal opiates and tranquilizers (763.5)*

779.5 Drug withdrawal syndrome in newborn   N
> Drug withdrawal syndrome in infant of dependent mother
> *EXCLUDES*   *fetal alcohol syndrome (760.71)*
> **AHA:** 3Q, '94, 6
> **TIP:** If the infant is asymptomatic but has a positive drug screen (e.g., for cocaine), assign instead 760.75.

779.6 Termination of pregnancy (fetus)   N
> Fetal death due to:
>   induced abortion
>   termination of pregnancy
> *EXCLUDES*   *spontaneous abortion (fetus) (761.8)*

779.7 Periventricular leukomalacia
> **DEF:** Necrosis of white matter adjacent to lateral ventricles with the formation of cysts; cause of PVL has not been firmly established, but thought to be related to inadequate blood flow in certain areas of the brain.
> **AHA:** 4Q, '01, 50, 51

√5ᵗʰ 779.8 Other specified conditions originating in the perinatal period
> **AHA:** 4Q, '02, 67; 1Q, '94, 15

> **779.81 Neonatal bradycardia**   N
> *EXCLUDES*   *abnormality in fetal heart rate or rhythm complicating labor and delivery (763.81-763.83)*
>   *bradycardia due to birth asphyxia (768.5-768.9)*
> **P29.12** Neonatal bradycardia   I-10

N Newborn Age: 0   P Pediatric Age: 0-17   M Maternity Age: 12-55   A Adult Age: 15-124

779.82 Neonatal tachycardia   N

     EXCLUDES *abnormality in fetal heart rate or rhythm complicating labor and delivery (763.81-763.83)*

779.83 Delayed separation of umbilical cord   N

     AHA: 4Q, '03, 71

779.84 Meconium staining   N

     EXCLUDES *meconium aspiration (770.11, 770.12) meconium passage during delivery (763.84)*

     AHA: 4Q, '05, 83, 88

     P96.83 Meconium staining   I-10

779.85 Cardiac arrest of newborn   N

     AHA: 4Q, '06, 104-106

779.89 Other specified conditions originating in the perinatal period   N

     Use additional code to specify condition

     AHA: 1Q, '06, 18; 2Q, '05, 15; 1Q, '05, 9

     P96.89 Oth spec conditions originating perinatal period   I-10

779.9 Unspecified condition originating in the perinatal period   N

     Congenital debility NOS

     Stillbirth NEC

√4th √5th Additional Digit Required   Unspecified Code   Other Specified Code   Manifestation Code   ▶◀ Revised Text   ● New Code   ▲ Revised Code Title

2011 ICD-9-CM   **Volume 1 – 259**

16. Symptoms, Signs, and Ill-Defined Conditions (780-799)

This section includes symptoms, signs, abnormal results of laboratory or other investigative procedures, and ill-defined conditions regarding which no diagnosis classifiable elsewhere is recorded.

Signs and symptoms that point rather definitely to a given diagnosis are assigned to some category in the preceding part of the classification. In general, categories 780-796 include the more ill-defined conditions and symptoms that point with perhaps equal suspicion to two or more diseases or to two or more systems of the body, and without the necessary study of the case to make a final diagnosis. Practically all categories in this group could be designated as "not otherwise specified," or as "unknown etiology," or as "transient." The Alphabetic Index should be consulted to determine which symptoms and signs are to be allocated here and which to more specific sections of the classification; the residual subcategories numbered .9 are provided for other relevant symptoms which cannot be allocated elsewhere in the classification.

The conditions and signs or symptoms included in categories 780-796 consist of: (a) cases for which no more specific diagnosis can be made even after all facts bearing on the case have been investigated; (b) signs or symptoms existing at the time of initial encounter that proved to be transient and whose causes could not be determined; (c) provisional diagnoses in a patient who failed to return for further investigation or care; (d) cases referred elsewhere for investigation or treatment before the diagnosis was made; (e) cases in which a more precise diagnosis was not available for any other reason; (f) certain symptoms which represent important problems in medical care and which it might be desired to classify in addition to a known cause.

Symptoms (780-789)

AHA: 1Q, '91, 12; 2Q, '90, 3; 2Q, '90, 5; 2Q, '90, 15; M-A, '85, 3

780 General symptoms

780.0 Alteration of consciousness

> EXCLUDES *alteration of consciousness due to:*
> *intracranial injuries (850.0-854.19)*
> *skull fractures (800.00-801.99, 803.00-804.99)*
> *coma:*
> *diabetic (249.2-249.3, 250.2-250.3)*
> *hepatic (572.2)*
> *originating in the perinatal period (779.2)*
>
> AHA: 4Q, '92, 20

780.01 Coma

> DEF: State of unconsciousness from which the patient cannot be awakened.
> AHA: 3Q, '96, 16

780.02 Transient alteration of awareness

> DEF: Temporary, recurring spells of reduced consciousness.

780.03 Persistent vegetative state

> DEF: Persistent wakefulness without consciousness due to nonfunctioning cerebral cortex.

780.09 Other

> Drowsiness
> Semicoma
> Somnolence
> Stupor
> Unconsciousness
> R40.1 Stupor   I-10

780.1 Hallucinations

> Hallucinations:
> NOS
> auditory
> gustatory
> olfactory
> tactile
>
> EXCLUDES *those associated with mental disorders, as functional*
> *psychoses (295.0-298.9)*
> *organic brain syndromes (290.0-294.9, 310.0-310.9)*
> *visual hallucinations (368.16)*
>
> DEF: Perception of external stimulus in absence of stimulus; inability to distinguish between real and imagined.

780.2 Syncope and collapse

> Blackout
> Fainting
> (Near) (Pre) syncope
> Vasovagal attack
>
> EXCLUDES *carotid sinus syncope (337.0)*
> *heat syncope (992.1)*
> *neurocirculatory asthenia (306.2)*
> *orthostatic hypotension (458.0)*
> *shock NOS (785.50)*
>
> DEF: Sudden unconsciousness due to reduced blood flow to brain.
> AHA: 1Q, '02, 6; 3Q, '00, 12; 4Q, '95, 42; 3Q, '95, 14; N-D, '85, 12
> R55 Syncope and collapse   I-10

780.3 Convulsions

> EXCLUDES *convulsions:*
> *epileptic (345.10-345.91)*
> *in newborn (779.0)*
>
> DEF: Sudden, involuntary contractions of the muscles.
> AHA: 2Q, '97, 8; 1Q, '97, 12; 3Q, '94, 9; 1Q, '93, 24; 4Q, '92, 23; N-D, '87, 12

780.31 Febrile convulsions (simple), unspecified

> Febrile seizure NOS
> AHA: 4Q, '97, 45

780.32 Complex febrile convulsions

> Febrile seizure:
> atypical
> complex
> complicated
>
> EXCLUDES *status epilepticus (345.3)*
> AHA: 4Q, '06, 106

780.33 Post traumatic seizures

> EXCLUDES *post traumatic epilepsy (345.00-345.91)*

780.39 Other convulsions

> Convulsive disorder NOS
> Fit NOS
> Recurrent convulsions NOS
> Seizure NOS
> AHA: 1Q, '08, 17; 3Q, '06, 22; 4Q, '04, 51; 1Q, '03, 7; 2Q, '99, 17; 4Q, '98, 39
> R56.9 Unspecified convulsions   I-10

780.4 Dizziness and giddiness

> Light-headedness
> Vertigo NOS
>
> EXCLUDES *Ménière's disease and other specified vertiginous*
> *syndromes (386.0-386.9)*
>
> DEF: Whirling sensations in head with feeling of falling.
> AHA: 2Q, '03, 11; 3Q, '00, 12; 2Q, '97, 9; 2Q, '91, 17
> R42 Dizziness and giddiness   I-10

780.5 Sleep disturbances

> EXCLUDES *circadian rhythm sleep disorders (327.30-327.39)*
> *organic hypersomnia (327.10-327.19)*
> *organic insomnia (327.00-327.09)*
> *organic sleep apnea (327.20-327.29)*
> *organic sleep related movement disorders*
> *(327.51-327.59)*
> *parasomnias (327.40-327.49)*
> *that of nonorganic origin (307.40-307.49)*
>
> AHA: 4Q, '05, 59

780.50 Sleep disturbance, unspecified

780.51 Insomnia with sleep apnea, unspecified

> DEF: Transient cessation of breathing disturbing sleep.

780.52 Insomnia, unspecified

> DEF: Inability to maintain adequate sleep cycle.
> G47.00 Insomnia unspecified   I-10

780.53 Hypersomnia with sleep apnea, unspecified

> DEF: Autonomic response inhibited during sleep; causes insufficient oxygen intake, acidosis and pulmonary hypertension.
> AHA: 1Q, '93, 28; N-D, '85, 4

780.54 Hypersomnia, unspecified

> DEF: Prolonged sleep cycle.

780.55 Disruptions of 24 hour sleep wake cycle, unspecified

780.56 Dysfunctions associated with sleep stages or arousal from sleep

780.57 Unspecified sleep apnea
> AHA: 1Q, '01, 6 ; 1Q, '97, 5; 1Q, '93, 28
> **G47.30** Sleep apnea unspecified   [I-10]

780.58 Sleep related movement disorder, unspecified
> EXCLUDES   restless legs syndrome (333.94)
> AHA: 4Q, '04, 95

780.59 Other

√5ᵗʰ **780.6 Fever and other physiologic disturbances of temperature regulation**
> EXCLUDES   effects of reduced environmental temperature (991.0-991.9)
> effects of heat and light (992.0-992.9)
> fever, chills or hypothermia associated with confirmed infection — code to infection
> AHA: 4Q, '08,140-142; 3Q, '05, 16; 3Q, '00,13; 4Q, '99, 26; 2Q, '91, 8

780.60 Fever, unspecified
> Chills with fever
> Fever NOS
> Fever of unknown origin (FUO)
> Hyperpyrexia NOS
> Pyrexia NOS
> Pyrexia of unknown origin
> EXCLUDES   chills without fever (780.64)
> neonatal fever (778.4)
> pyrexia of unknown origin (during):
>   in newborn (778.4)
>   labor (659.2)
>   the puerperium (672)
> **R50.9** Fever unspecified   [I-10]

780.61 Fever presenting with conditions classified elsewhere
> Code first underlying condition when associated fever is present, such as with:
> leukemia (conditions classifiable to 204-208)
> neutropenia (288.00-288.09)
> sickle-cell disease (282.60-282.69)
> AHA: 4Q, '08, 142

780.62 Postprocedural fever
> EXCLUDES   ▶posttransfusion fever (780.66)◀
> postvaccination fever (780.63)
> TIP: Do not assign a code from category 998 for post-procedural fever.

780.63 Postvaccination fever
> Postimmunization fever

780.64 Chills (without fever)
> Chills NOS
> EXCLUDES   chills with fever (780.60)

780.65 Hypothermia not associated with low environmental temperature
> EXCLUDES   hypothermia:
>   associated with low environmental temperature (991.6)
>   due to anesthesia (995.89)
>   of newborn (778.2, 778.3)

780.66 Febrile nonhemolytic transfusion reaction
> FNHTR
> Posttransfusion fever

√5ᵗʰ **780.7 Malaise and fatigue**
> EXCLUDES   debility, unspecified (799.3)
> fatigue (during):
>   combat (308.0-308.9)
>   heat (992.6)
>   pregnancy (646.8)
> neurasthenia (300.5)
> senile asthenia (797)
> AHA: 4Q, '88, 12; M-A, '87, 8

780.71 Chronic fatigue syndrome
> DEF: Persistent fatigue, symptoms include weak muscles, sore throat, lymphadenitis, headache, depression and mild fever; no known cause; also called chronic mononucleosis, benign myalgic encephalomyelitis, Iceland disease and neurosthenia.
> AHA: 4Q, '98, 48

780.72 Functional quadriplegia
> Complete immobility due to severe physical disability or frailty
> EXCLUDES   hysterical paralysis (300.11)
> immobility syndrome (728.3)
> neurologic quadriplegia (344.00-344.09)
> quadriplegia NOS (344.00)
> DEF: Inability to move due to another condition such as dementia, severe contractures, or arthritis, not a physiologic one; no mental ability to move independently; typically found in severely demented patients.
> AHA: 4Q, '08, 143
> TIP: The functional quadriplegic patient typically has severe dementia and the quadriplegia will be due to a nonneurologic condition.

780.79 Other malaise and fatigue
> Asthenia NOS
> Lethargy
> Postviral (asthenic) syndrome
> Tiredness
> DEF: Asthenia: Any weakness, lack of strength or loss of energy, especially neuromuscular.
> DEF: Lethargy: Listlessness, drowsiness, stupor and apathy.
> DEF: Malaise: Vague feeling of debility or lack of good health.
> DEF: Postviral (asthenic) syndrome: Listlessness, drowsiness, stupor and apathy; follows acute viral infection.
> DEF: Tiredness: General exhaustion or fatigue.
> AHA: 4Q, '04, 78; 1Q, '00, 6; 4Q, '99, 26
> **R53.83** Other fatigue   [I-10]

780.8 Generalized hyperhidrosis
> Diaphoresis   Secondary hyperhidrosis
> Excessive sweating
> EXCLUDES   focal (localized) (primary) (secondary) hyperhidrosis (705.21-705.22)
> Frey's syndrome (705.22)
> DEF: Excessive sweating, appears as droplets on skin; general or localized.
> TIP: Do not assign if documentation indicates a specific diagnosis of focal hyperhidrosis (primary or secondary); see subcategory 705.2.

√5ᵗʰ **780.9 Other general symptoms**
> EXCLUDES   hypothermia:
>   NOS (accidental) (991.6)
>   due to anesthesia (995.89)
>   of newborn (778.2-778.3)
> memory disturbance as part of a pattern of mental disorder
> AHA: 4Q, '02, 67; 4Q, '99, 10; 3Q, '93, 11; N-D, '85, 12

780.91 Fussy infant (baby)   [P]

780.92 Excessive crying of infant (baby)   [N]
> EXCLUDES   excessive crying of child, adolescent or adult (780.95)

780.93 Memory loss
> Amnesia (retrograde)
> Memory loss NOS
> EXCLUDES   memory loss due to:
>   intracranial injuries (850.0-854.19)
>   skull fractures (800.00-801.99, 803.00-804.99)
>   mild memory disturbance due to organic brain damage (310.8)
>   transient global amnesia (437.7)
> AHA: 4Q, '03, 71

780.94 Early satiety
> DEF: The premature feeling of being full; mechanism of satiety is multifactorial.
> AHA: 4Q, '03, 72

780.95 Excessive crying of child, adolescent, or adult
> EXCLUDES   excessive crying of infant (baby) (780.92)
> AHA: 4Q, '05, 89

[N] Newborn Age: 0   [P] Pediatric Age: 0-17   [M] Maternity Age: 12-55   [A] Adult Age: 15-124

780.96 Generalized pain
Pain NOS
AHA: 4Q, '06, 79-81
TIP: For pain syndromes, refer to category 338; if site is specified, refer to index.

780.97 Altered mental status
Change in mental status
EXCLUDES *altered level of consciousness (780.01-780.09)*
altered mental status due to known condition — code to condition
delirium NOS (780.09)
AHA: 4Q, '06, 107
R41.82 Altered mental status unspecified `I-10`

780.99 Other general symptoms
AHA: 4Q, '03, 103

√4ᵗʰ 781 Symptoms involving nervous and musculoskeletal systems
EXCLUDES *depression NOS (311)*
disorders specifically relating to:
back (724.0-724.9)
hearing (388.0-389.9)
joint (718.0-719.9)
limb (729.0-729.9)
neck (723.0-723.9)
vision (368.0-369.9)
pain in limb (729.5)

781.0 Abnormal involuntary movements
Abnormal head movements   Spasms NOS
Fasciculation   Tremor NOS
EXCLUDES *abnormal reflex (796.1)*
chorea NOS (333.5)
infantile spasms (345.60-345.61)
spastic paralysis (342.1, 343.0-344.9)
specified movement disorders classifiable to 333 (333.0-333.9)
that of nonorganic origin (307.2-307.3)
R25.9 Unspecified abnormal involuntary movements `I-10`

781.1 Disturbances of sensation of smell and taste
Anosmia   Parosmia
Parageusia
DEF: Anosmia: loss of sense of smell due to organic factors, including loss of olfactory nerve conductivity, cerebral disease, nasal fossae formation and peripheral olfactory nerve diseases; can also be psychological disorder.
DEF: Parageusia: distorted sense of taste, or bad taste in mouth.
DEF: Parosmia: distorted sense of smell.

781.2 Abnormality of gait
Gait: Gait:
  ataxic   spastic
  paralytic   staggering
EXCLUDES *ataxia:*
NOS (781.3)
locomotor (progressive) (094.0)
difficulty in walking (719.7)
DEF: Abnormal, asymmetric gait.
AHA: 2Q, '05, 6; 2Q, '04, 15
TIP: If the patient's gait abnormality is due to a joint problem, refer to code 719.7 Difficulty in walking.
R26.9 Unspecified abnormalities of gait and mobility `I-10`

781.3 Lack of coordination
Ataxia NOS
Muscular incoordination
EXCLUDES *ataxic gait (781.2)*
cerebellar ataxia (334.0-334.9)
difficulty in walking (719.7)
vertigo NOS (780.4)
AHA: 4Q, '04, 51; 3Q, '97, 12

781.4 Transient paralysis of limb
Monoplegia, transient NOS
EXCLUDES *paralysis (342.0-344.9)*

781.5 Clubbing of fingers
DEF: Enlarged soft tissue of distal fingers.

781.6 Meningismus
Dupré's syndrome
Meningism
DEF: Condition with signs and symptoms that resemble meningeal irritation; it is associated with febrile illness and dehydration with no evidence of infection.
AHA: 3Q, '00,13; J-F, '87, 7

781.7 Tetany
Carpopedal spasm
EXCLUDES *tetanus neonatorum (771.3)*
tetany:
hysterical (300.11)
newborn (hypocalcemic) (775.4)
parathyroid (252.1)
psychogenic (306.0)
DEF: Nerve and muscle hyperexcitability; symptoms include muscle spasms, twitching, cramps, laryngospasm with inspiratory stridor, hyperreflexia and choreiform movements.

781.8 Neurologic neglect syndrome
Asomatognosia   Left-sided neglect
Hemi-akinesia   Sensory extinction
Hemi-inattention   Sensory neglect
Hemispatial neglect   Visuospatial neglect
EXCLUDES ►*visuospatial deficit (799.53)*◄
AHA: 4Q, '94, 37
TIP: If documented as sequelae of a CVA, assign also a code from category 438.

√5ᵗʰ 781.9 Other symptoms involving nervous and musculoskeletal systems
AHA: 4Q, '00, 45

781.91 Loss of height
EXCLUDES *osteoporosis (733.00-733.09)*

781.92 Abnormal posture

781.93 Ocular torticollis
DEF: Abnormal head posture as a result of a contracted state of cervical muscles to correct a visual disturbance; either double vision or a visual field defect.
AHA: 4Q, '02, 68

781.94 Facial weakness
Facial droop
EXCLUDES *facial weakness due to late effect of cerebrovascular accident (438.83)*
AHA: 4Q, '03, 72
TIP: Do not assign if facial droop or weakness is due to Bell's palsy; see instead code 351.0.
R29.810 Facial weakness `I-10`

781.99 Other symptoms involving nervous and musculoskeletal systems

√4ᵗʰ 782 Symptoms involving skin and other integumentary tissue
EXCLUDES *symptoms relating to breast (611.71-611.79)*

782.0 Disturbance of skin sensation
Anesthesia of skin   Hypoesthesia
Burning or prickling   Numbness
  sensation   Paresthesia
Hyperesthesia   Tingling
R20.9 Unspecified disturbances of skin sensation `I-10`

782.1 Rash and other nonspecific skin eruption
Exanthem
EXCLUDES *vesicular eruption (709.8)*
AHA: 4Q, '08, 99

782.2 Localized superficial swelling, mass, or lump
Subcutaneous nodules
EXCLUDES *localized adiposity (278.1)*

782.3 Edema
Anasarca   Localized edema NOS
Dropsy
> **EXCLUDES** *ascites (789.51-789.59)*
> *edema of:*
>   *newborn NOS (778.5)*
>   *pregnancy (642.0-642.9, 646.1)*
> *fluid retention ▶(276.69)◀*
> *hydrops fetalis (773.3, 778.0)*
> *hydrothorax (511.81-511.89)*
> *nutritional edema (260, 262)*

DEF: Edema: excess fluid in intercellular body tissue.
DEF: Anasarca: massive edema in all body tissues.
DEF: Dropsy: serous fluid accumulated in body cavity or cellular tissue.
DEF: Localized edema: edema in specific body areas.
AHA: 2Q, '00, 18
R60.9 Edema unspecified   I-10

782.4 Jaundice, unspecified, not of newborn
Cholemia NOS
Icterus NOS
> **EXCLUDES** *jaundice in newborn (774.0-774.7)*
>   *due to isoimmunization (773.0-773.2, 773.4)*

DEF: Bilirubin deposits of skin, causing yellow cast.
R17 Unspecified jaundice   I-10

782.5 Cyanosis
> **EXCLUDES** *newborn (770.83)*

DEF: Deficient oxygen of blood; causes blue cast to skin.

√5ᵗʰ 782.6 Pallor and flushing

782.61 Pallor

782.62 Flushing
Excessive blushing

782.7 Spontaneous ecchymoses
Petechiae
> **EXCLUDES** *ecchymosis in fetus or newborn (772.6)*
> *purpura (287.0-287.9)*

DEF: Hemorrhagic spots of skin; resemble freckles.

782.8 Changes in skin texture
Induration ⎫
Thickening ⎭ of skin

782.9 Other symptoms involving skin and integumentary tissues

√4ᵗʰ 783 Symptoms concerning nutrition, metabolism, and development

783.0 Anorexia
Loss of appetite
> **EXCLUDES** *anorexia nervosa (307.1)*
> *loss of appetite of nonorganic origin (307.59)*

R63.0 Anorexia   I-10

783.1 Abnormal weight gain
> **EXCLUDES** *excessive weight gain in pregnancy (646.1)*
> *obesity (278.00)*
>   *morbid (278.01)*

√5ᵗʰ 783.2 Abnormal loss of weight and underweight
Use additional code to identify Body Mass Index (BMI), if known (V85.0-V85.54)
AHA: 4Q, '00, 45

783.21 Loss of weight
AHA: 4Q, '05, 96
R63.4 Abnormal weight loss   I-10

783.22 Underweight
AHA: 4Q, '05, 96

783.3 Feeding difficulties and mismanagement
Feeding problem (elderly) (infant)
> **EXCLUDES** *feeding disturbance or problems:*
>   *in newborn (779.31-779.34)*
>   *of nonorganic origin (307.50-307.59)*

AHA: 3Q, '97, 12

√5ᵗʰ 783.4 Lack of expected normal physiological development in childhood
> **EXCLUDES** *delay in sexual development and puberty (259.0)*
> *gonadal dysgenesis (758.6)*
> *pituitary dwarfism (253.3)*
> *slow fetal growth and fetal malnutrition (764.00-764.99)*
> *specific delays in mental development (315.0-315.9)*

AHA: 4Q, '00, 45; 3Q, '97, 4

783.40 Lack of normal physiological development, unspecified
Inadequate development
Lack of development

783.41 Failure to thrive   P
Failure to gain weight
> **EXCLUDES** *failure to thrive in newborn (779.34)*

DEF: Organic failure to thrive: acute or chronic illness that interferes with nutritional intake, absorption, metabolism excretion and energy requirements. Nonorganic FTT is symptom of neglect or abuse.
AHA: 1Q, '03, 12

783.42 Delayed milestones   P
Late talker
Late walker

783.43 Short stature
Growth failure   Lack of growth
Growth retardation   Physical retardation
DEF: Constitutional short stature: stature inconsistent with chronological age. Genetic short stature is when skeletal maturation matches chronological age.

783.5 Polydipsia
Excessive thirst

783.6 Polyphagia
Excessive eating
Hyperalimentation NOS
> **EXCLUDES** *disorders of eating of nonorganic origin (307.50-307.59)*

783.7 Adult failure to thrive   A
R62.7 Adult failure to thrive   I-10

783.9 Other symptoms concerning nutrition, metabolism, and development
Hypometabolism
> **EXCLUDES** *abnormal basal metabolic rate (794.7)*
> *dehydration (276.51)*
> *other disorders of fluid, electrolyte, and acid-base balance (276.0-276.9)*

AHA: 2Q, '04, 3

√4ᵗʰ 784 Symptoms involving head and neck
> **EXCLUDES** *encephalopathy NOS (348.30)*
> *specific symptoms involving neck classifiable to 723 (723.0-723.9)*

784.0 Headache
Facial pain
Pain in head NOS
> **EXCLUDES** *atypical face pain (350.2)*
> *migraine (346.0-346.9)*
> *tension headache (307.81)*

AHA: 3Q, '06, 22; 2Q, '06, 17; 3Q, '00, 13; 1Q, '90, 4; 3Q, '92, 14
TIP: Do not assign if headache syndrome has been diagnosed, refer to category 339.
R51 Headache   I-10

784.1 Throat pain
> **EXCLUDES** *dysphagia (787.20-787.29)*
> *neck pain (723.1)*
> *sore throat (462)*
>   *chronic (472.1)*

784.2 Swelling, mass, or lump in head and neck
Space-occupying lesion, intracranial NOS
AHA: 1Q, '03, 8

784.3 Aphasia

> **EXCLUDES** aphasia due to late effects of cerebrovascular disease (438.11)
> developmental aphasia (315.31)

DEF: Inability to communicate through speech, written word, or sign language.

AHA: 4Q, '04, 78; 4Q, '98, 87; 3Q, '97, 12

R47.01 Aphasia   `I-10`

√5ᵗʰ 784.4 Voice and resonance disorders

AHA: 4Q, '09, 102-103

784.40 Voice and resonance disorder, unspecified

784.41 Aphonia
Loss of voice

784.42 Dysphonia
Hoarseness

784.43 Hypernasality

784.44 Hyponasality

784.49 Other voice and resonance disorders
Change in voice

√5ᵗʰ 784.5 Other speech disturbance

> **EXCLUDES** speech disorder due to late effect of cerebrovascular accident (438.10-438.19)
> ▶stuttering (315.35)◀

AHA: 4Q, '09, 87-88

TIP: For speech disturbances as a late effect of cerebrovascular disease see subcategory 438.1.

784.51 Dysarthria

> **EXCLUDES** dysarthria due to late effect of cerebrovascular accident (438.13)

● **784.52 Fluency disorder in conditions classified elsewhere**
Stuttering in conditions classified elsewhere
Code first underlying disease or condition, such as: Parkinson's disease (332.0)

> **EXCLUDES** adult onset fluency disorder (307.0)
> childhood onset fluency disorder (315.35)
> fluency disorder due to late effect of cerebrovascular accident (438.14)

784.59 Other speech disturbance
Dysphasia
Slurred speech
Speech disturbance NOS
R47.89 Other speech disturbances   `I-10`

√5ᵗʰ 784.6 Other symbolic dysfunction

> **EXCLUDES** developmental learning delays (315.0-315.9)

784.60 Symbolic dysfunction, unspecified

784.61 Alexia and dyslexia
Alexia (with agraphia)
DEF: Alexia: Inability to understand written word due to central brain lesion.
DEF: Dyslexia: Ability to recognize letters but inability to read, spell, and write words; genetic.

784.69 Other

Acalculia	Agraphia NOS
Agnosia	Apraxia

784.7 Epistaxis
Hemorrhage from nose
Nosebleed
AHA: 3Q, '04, 7
R04.0 Epistaxis   `I-10`

784.8 Hemorrhage from throat

> **EXCLUDES** hemoptysis ▶(786.30-786.39)◀

√5ᵗʰ 784.9 Other symptoms involving head and neck

784.91 Postnasal drip
AHA: 4Q, '06, 108

● **784.92 Jaw pain**
Mandibular pain
Maxilla pain

> **EXCLUDES** temporomandibular joint arthralgia (524.62)

784.99 Other symptoms involving head and neck
Choking sensation
Feeling of foreign body in throat
Halitosis
Mouth breathing
Sneezing

> **EXCLUDES** foreign body in throat (933.0)

AHA: 4Q, '06, 108

√4ᵗʰ 785 Symptoms involving cardiovascular system

> **EXCLUDES** heart failure NOS (428.9)

785.0 Tachycardia, unspecified
Rapid heart beat

> **EXCLUDES** neonatal tachycardia (779.82)
> paroxysmal tachycardia (427.0-427.2)

DEF: Excessively rapid heart rate.
AHA: 2Q, '03, 11
R00.0 Tachycardia unspecified   `I-10`

785.1 Palpitations
Awareness of heart beat

> **EXCLUDES** specified dysrhythmias (427.0-427.9)

R00.2 Palpitations   `I-10`

785.2 Undiagnosed cardiac murmurs
Heart murmurs NOS
AHA: 4Q, '92, 16
R01.1 Cardiac murmur unspecified   `I-10`

785.3 Other abnormal heart sounds
Cardiac dullness, increased or decreased
Friction fremitus, cardiac
Precordial friction

785.4 Gangrene

Gangrene:	Gangrenous cellulitis
NOS	Phagedena
spreading cutaneous	

Code first any associated underlying condition

> **EXCLUDES** gangrene of certain sites — see Alphabetic Index
> gangrene with atherosclerosis of the extremities (440.24)
> gas gangrene (040.0)

DEF: Gangrene: necrosis of skin tissue due to bacterial infection, diabetes, embolus and vascular supply loss.
DEF: Gangrenous cellulitis: group A streptococcal infection; begins with severe cellulitis, spreads to superficial and deep fascia; produces gangrene of underlying tissues.
AHA: 1Q, '04, 14; 3Q, '91, 12; 3Q, '90, 15; M-A, '86, 12
I96 Gangrene not elsewhere classified   `I-10`

√5ᵗʰ 785.5 Shock without mention of trauma

785.50 Shock, unspecified
Failure of peripheral circulation
DEF: Peripheral circulatory failure due to heart insufficiencies.
AHA: 2Q, '96, 10

785.51 Cardiogenic shock
DEF: Shock syndrome: associated with myocardial infarction, cardiac tamponade and massive pulmonary embolism; symptoms include mental confusion, reduced blood pressure, tachycardia, pallor and cold, clammy skin.
AHA: 4Q, '08, 182; 3Q, '05, 14
R57.0 Cardiogenic shock   `I-10`

785.52 Septic shock
Shock:
endotoxic
gram-negative
Code first:
systemic inflammatory response syndrome due to infectious process with organ dysfunction (995.92)
AHA: 4Q, '08, 99; 4Q, '06, 113; 2Q, '05, 18-19; 4Q, '03, 73, 79
TIP: The diagnosis of septic shock indicates the presence of severe sepsis; code 785.52 should not be assigned without first assigning code 995.92.

✓4ᵗʰ / ✓5ᵗʰ Additional Digit Required   Unspecified Code   Other Specified Code   Manifestation Code   ▶◀ Revised Text   ● New Code   ▲ Revised Code Title

2011 ICD-9-CM   **October 2010 · Volume 1 – 265**

785.59 Other

Shock:

hypovolemic

EXCLUDES shock (due to):

anesthetic (995.4)

anaphylactic (995.0)

due to serum (999.4)

electric (994.8)

following abortion (639.5)

lightning (994.0)

obstetrical (669.1)

postoperative (998.0)

traumatic (958.4)

AHA: 2Q, '00, 3

785.6 Enlargement of lymph nodes

Lymphadenopathy

"Swollen glands"

EXCLUDES lymphadenitis (chronic) (289.1-289.3)

acute (683)

R59.9 Enlarged lymph nodes unspecified   `I-10`

785.9 Other symptoms involving cardiovascular system

Bruit (arterial)

Weak pulse

`√4th` **786 Symptoms involving respiratory system and other chest symptoms**

`√5th` **786.0 Dyspnea and respiratory abnormalities**

786.00 Respiratory abnormality, unspecified

786.01 Hyperventilation

EXCLUDES hyperventilation, psychogenic (306.1)

DEF: Rapid breathing causes carbon dioxide loss from blood.

786.02 Orthopnea

DEF: Difficulty breathing except in upright position.

786.03 Apnea

EXCLUDES apnea of newborn (770.81, 770.82)

sleep apnea (780.51, 780.53, 780.57)

DEF: Cessation of breathing.

AHA: 4Q, '98, 50

786.04 Cheyne-Stokes respiration

DEF: Rhythmic increase of depth and frequency of breathing with apnea; occurs in frontal lobe and diencephalic dysfunction.

AHA: 4Q, '98, 50

786.05 Shortness of breath

DEF: Inability to take in sufficient oxygen.

AHA: 4Q, '99, 25; 1Q, '99, 6; 4Q, '98, 50

R06.02 Shortness of breath   `I-10`

786.06 Tachypnea

EXCLUDES transitory tachypnea of newborn (770.6)

DEF: Abnormal rapid respiratory rate; called hyperventilation.

AHA: 4Q, '98, 50

786.07 Wheezing

EXCLUDES asthma (493.00-493.92)

DEF: Stenosis of respiratory passageway; causes whistling sound; due to asthma, coryza, croup, emphysema, hay fever, edema, and pleural effusion.

AHA: 4Q, '98, 50

786.09 Other

Respiratory:

distress

insufficiency

EXCLUDES respiratory distress:

following trauma and surgery (518.5)

newborn (770.89)

syndrome (newborn) (769)

adult (518.5)

respiratory failure (518.81, 518.83-518.84)

newborn (770.84)

AHA: 4Q, '05, 90; 2Q, '98, 10; 1Q, '97, 7; 1Q, '90, 9

R06.82 Tachypnea not elsewhere classified   `I-10`

786.1 Stridor

EXCLUDES congenital laryngeal stridor (748.3)

DEF: Obstructed airway causes harsh sound.

786.2 Cough

EXCLUDES cough:

psychogenic (306.1)

smokers' (491.0)

with hemorrhage ▶(786.39)◀

AHA: 4Q, '99, 26

R05 Cough   `I-10`

`√5th` **786.3 Hemoptysis**

DEF: Coughing up blood or blood-stained sputum.

AHA: 2Q, '06, 17; 4Q, '90, 26

● **786.30 Hemoptysis, unspecified**

Pulmonary hemorrhage NOS

R04.8 Hemorr from other sites of respir passages   `I-10`

● **786.31 Acute idiopathic pulmonary hemorrhage in infants [AIPHI]**

Acute idiopathic pulmonary hemorrhage in infant over 28 days old

EXCLUDES pulmonary hemorrhage of newborn under 28 days old (770.3)

von Willebrand's disease (286.4)

● **786.39 Other hemoptysis**

Cough with hemorrhage

R04.2 Hemoptysis   `I-10`

786.4 Abnormal sputum

Abnormal:

amount

color   } (of) sputum

odor

Excessive

`√5th` **786.5 Chest pain**

786.50 Chest pain, unspecified

AHA: 1Q, '07, 19; 2Q, '06, 7; 1Q, '03, 6; 1Q, '02, 4; 4Q, '99, 25

R07.9 Chest pain unspecified   `I-10`

786.51 Precordial pain

DEF: Chest pain over heart and lower thorax.

786.52 Painful respiration

Pain:

anterior chest wall

pleuritic

Pleurodynia

EXCLUDES epidemic pleurodynia (074.1)

AHA: N-D, '84, 17

R07.1 Chest pain on breathing   `I-10`

786.59 Other

Discomfort

Pressure   } in chest

Tightness

EXCLUDES pain in breast (611.71)

AHA: 1Q, '02, 6

TIP: Assign for chest pain due to anxiety, along with an additional code for anxiety. Chest pain is not integral to the diagnosis of anxiety.

R07.89 Other chest pain   `I-10`

786.6 Swelling, mass, or lump in chest

EXCLUDES lump in breast (611.72)

R22.2 Localized swelling, mass, lump, trunk   `I-10`

786.7 Abnormal chest sounds

Abnormal percussion, chest

Friction sounds, chest

Rales

Tympany, chest

EXCLUDES wheezing (786.07)

786.8 Hiccough

EXCLUDES psychogenic hiccough (306.1)

786.9 Other symptoms involving respiratory system and chest

Breath-holding spell

`N` Newborn Age: 0   `P` Pediatric Age: 0-17   `M` Maternity Age: 12-55   `A` Adult Age: 15-124

☑4ᵗʰ **787　Symptoms involving digestive system**
　　　EXCLUDES *constipation (564.00-564.09)*
　　　　　　pylorospasm (537.81)
　　　　　　congenital (750.5)

☑5ᵗʰ **787.0　Nausea and vomiting**
　　　Emesis
　　　EXCLUDES *hematemesis NOS (578.0)*
　　　　　　vomiting:
　　　　　　　bilious, following gastrointestinal surgery (564.3)
　　　　　　　cyclical (536.2)
　　　　　　　　associated with migraine (346.2)
　　　　　　　　psychogenic (306.4)
　　　　　　　excessive, in pregnancy (643.0-643.9)
　　　　　　　fecal matter (569.87)
　　　　　　　habit (536.2)
　　　　　　　of newborn (779.32, 779.33)
　　　　　　　persistent (536.2)
　　　　　　　psychogenic NOS (307.54)
　　　AHA: M-A, '85, 11

　　787.01　Nausea with vomiting
　　　AHA: 1Q, '03, 5
　　　R11.0 Nausea with vomiting　　I-10

　　787.02　Nausea alone
　　　AHA: 3Q, '00, 12; 2Q, '97, 9
　　　R11.1 Nausea alone　　I-10

　　787.03　Vomiting alone

　　787.04　Bilious emesis
　　　Bilious vomiting
　　　EXCLUDES *bilious emesis (vomiting) in newborn (779.32)*
　　　AHA: 4Q, '09, 103-104

787.1　Heartburn
　　Pyrosis　　　　　　Waterbrash
　　EXCLUDES *dyspepsia or indigestion (536.8)*
　　AHA: 2Q, '01, 6

☑5ᵗʰ **787.2　Dysphagia**
　　Code first, if applicable, dysphagia due to late effect of cerebrovascular accident (438.82)
　　AHA: 4Q, '07, 92-94; 3Q, '07, 7; 4Q, '03, 103, 109; 2Q, '01, 4

　　787.20　Dysphagia, unspecified
　　　Difficulty in swallowing NOS

　　787.21　Dysphagia, oral phase

　　787.22　Dysphagia, oropharyngeal phase
　　　AHA: 4Q, '07, 94

　　787.23　Dysphagia, pharyngeal phase

　　787.24　Dysphagia, pharyngoesophageal phase

　　787.29　Other dysphagia
　　　Cervical dysphagia
　　　Neurogenic dysphagia
　　　R13.19 Other dysphagia　　I-10

Phases of Swallowing

Oral phase

Oropharyngeal phase

Pharyngeal phase　　Pharyngeoesophageal phase

787.3　Flatulence, eructation, and gas pain
　　Abdominal distention (gaseous)
　　Bloating
　　Tympanites (abdominal) (intestinal)
　　EXCLUDES *aerophagy (306.4)*
　　DEF: Flatulence: excess air or gas in intestine or stomach.
　　DEF: Eructation: belching, expelling gas through mouth.
　　DEF: Gas pain: gaseous pressure affecting gastrointestinal system.

787.4　Visible peristalsis
　　Hyperperistalsis
　　DEF: Increase in involuntary movements of intestines.

787.5　Abnormal bowel sounds
　　Absent bowel sounds
　　Hyperactive bowel sounds

☑5ᵗʰ **787.6　Incontinence of feces**
　　Encopresis NOS
　　Incontinence of sphincter ani
　　EXCLUDES *that of nonorganic origin (307.7)*
　　AHA: 1Q, '97, 9

●　　**787.60　Full incontinence of feces**
　　　Fecal incontinence NOS
　　　R15 Fecal incontinence　　I-10

●　　**787.61　Incomplete defecation**
　　　EXCLUDES *constipation (564.00-564.09)*
　　　　　　fecal impaction (560.32)

●　　**787.62　Fecal smearing**
　　　Fecal soiling

●　　**787.63　Fecal urgency**

787.7　Abnormal feces
　　Bulky stools
　　EXCLUDES *abnormal stool content (792.1)*
　　　　　　melena:
　　　　　　　NOS (578.1)
　　　　　　　newborn (772.4, 777.3)

☑5ᵗʰ **787.9　Other symptoms involving digestive system**
　　EXCLUDES *gastrointestinal hemorrhage (578.0-578.9)*
　　　　　　intestinal obstruction (560.0-560.9)
　　　　　　specific functional digestive disorders:
　　　　　　　esophagus (530.0-530.9)
　　　　　　　stomach and duodenum (536.0-536.9)
　　　　　　　those not elsewhere classified (564.00-564.9)

　　787.91　Diarrhea
　　　Diarrhea NOS
　　　AHA: 4Q, '08, 99; 4Q, '95, 54
　　　R19.7 Diarrhea unspecified　　I-10

　　787.99　Other
　　　Change in bowel habits
　　　Tenesmus (rectal)
　　　DEF: Tenesmus: Painful, ineffective straining at the rectum with limited passage of fecal matter.

☑4ᵗʰ **788　Symptoms involving urinary system**
　　EXCLUDES *hematuria (599.70-599.72)*
　　　　　　nonspecific findings on examination of the urine (791.0-791.9)
　　　　　　small kidney of unknown cause (589.0-589.9)
　　　　　　uremia NOS (586)
　　　　　　urinary obstruction (599.60, 599.69)

788.0　Renal colic
　　Colic (recurrent) of:
　　　kidney
　　　ureter
　　DEF: Kidney pain.
　　AHA: 3Q, '04, 8
　　TIP: Do not assign if renal colic is due to calculus; see category 592.

788.1　Dysuria
　　Painful urination
　　Strangury

Symptoms, Signs, and Ill-Defined Conditions

788.2–789.0

√5ᵗʰ **788.2 Retention of urine**

Code, if applicable, any causal condition first, such as:
hyperplasia of prostate (600.0-600.9 with fifth-digit 1)
DEF: Accumulation of urine in the bladder due to inability to void.

788.20 Retention of urine, unspecified
AHA: 4Q, '06, 93, 95; 2Q, '04, 18; 3Q, '03, 12-13; 1Q, '03, 6; 3Q, '96, 10
R33.9 Retention of urine unspecified   I-10

788.21 Incomplete bladder emptying
AHA: 4Q, '06, 93

788.29 Other specified retention of urine

√5ᵗʰ **788.3 Urinary incontinence**

Code, if applicable, any causal condition first, such as:
congenital ureterocele (753.23)
genital prolapse (618.00-618.9)
hyperplasia of prostate (600.0-600.9 with fifth-digit 1)
EXCLUDES functional urinary incontinence (788.91)
that of nonorganic origin (307.6)
urinary incontinence associated with cognitive
impairment (788.91)
AHA: 4Q, '06, 93; 4Q, '92, 22

788.30 Urinary incontinence, unspecified
Enuresis NOS
AHA: 1Q, '09, 15
R32 Unspecified urinary incontinence   I-10

788.31 Urge incontinence
DEF: Inability to control urination, upon urge to urinate.
AHA: 1Q, '00, 19

788.32 Stress incontinence, male   ♂
EXCLUDES stress incontinence, female (625.6)
DEF: Inability to control urination associated with weak
sphincter in males.

788.33 Mixed incontinence, (male) (female)
Urge and stress
DEF: Urge, stress incontinence: involuntary discharge of
urine due to anatomic displacement.

788.34 Incontinence without sensory awareness
DEF: Involuntary discharge of urine without sensory
warning.

788.35 Post-void dribbling
DEF: Involuntary discharge of residual urine after voiding.

788.36 Nocturnal enuresis
DEF: Involuntary discharge of urine during the night.

788.37 Continuous leakage
DEF: Continuous, involuntary urine seepage.

788.38 Overflow incontinence
DEF: Leakage caused by pressure of retained urine in the
bladder after the bladder has fully contracted due to
weakened bladder muscles or an obstruction of the
urethra.

788.39 Other urinary incontinence

√5ᵗʰ **788.4 Frequency of urination and polyuria**

Code, if applicable, any causal condition first, such as:
hyperplasia of prostate (600.0-600.9 with fifth-digit 1)

788.41 Urinary frequency
Frequency of micturition
AHA: 4Q, '06, 93

788.42 Polyuria
DEF: Excessive urination.

788.43 Nocturia
DEF: Urination affecting sleep patterns.
AHA: 4Q, '06, 93

788.5 Oliguria and anuria
Deficient secretion of urine
Suppression of urinary secretion
EXCLUDES that complicating:
abortion (634-638 with .3, 639.3)
ectopic or molar pregnancy (639.3)
pregnancy, childbirth, or the puerperium
(642.0-642.9, 646.2)
DEF: Oliguria: diminished urinary secretion related to fluid intake.
DEF: Anuria: lack of urinary secretion due to renal failure or
obstructed urinary tract.

√5ᵗʰ **788.6 Other abnormality of urination**

Code, if applicable, any causal condition first, such as:
hyperplasia of prostate (600.0-600.9 with fifth-digit 1)

788.61 Splitting of urinary stream
Intermittent urinary stream

788.62 Slowing of urinary stream
Weak stream
AHA: 4Q, '06, 93

788.63 Urgency of urination
EXCLUDES urge incontinence (788.31, 788.33)
DEF: Feeling of intense need to urinate; abrupt sensation of
imminent urination.
AHA: 4Q, '06, 93; 4Q, '03, 74

788.64 Urinary hesitancy
AHA: 4Q, '06, 93, 109

788.65 Straining on urination
AHA: 4Q, '06, 93, 109

788.69 Other

788.7 Urethral discharge
Penile discharge
Urethrorrhea

788.8 Extravasation of urine
DEF: Leaking or infiltration of urine into tissues.

√5ᵗʰ **788.9 Other symptoms involving urinary system**
AHA: 1Q, '05, 12; 4Q, '88, 1

788.91 Functional urinary incontinence
Urinary incontinence due to cognitive impairment, or
severe physical disability or immobility
EXCLUDES urinary incontinence due to physiologic
condition (788.30-788.39)
AHA: 4Q, '08, 144-145

788.99 Other symptoms involving urinary system
Extrarenal uremia
Vesical:
pain
tenesmus

√4ᵗʰ **789 Other symptoms involving abdomen and pelvis**
EXCLUDES symptoms referable to genital organs:
female (625.0-625.9)
male (607.0-608.9)
psychogenic (302.70-302.79)

The following fifth-digit subclassification is to be used for codes 789.0,
789.3, 789.4, 789.6:
0 unspecified site
1 right upper quadrant
2 left upper quadrant
3 right lower quadrant
4 left lower quadrant
5 periumbilic
6 epigastric
7 generalized
9 other specified site
Multiple sites

§ √5ᵗʰ **789.0 Abdominal pain**
[0-7, 9]   Cramps, abdominal
AHA: 1Q, '95, 3; **For code 789.06:** 1Q, '02, 5
R10.9 Unspecified abdominal pain   I-10
R10.31 Right lower quadrant pain   I-10
R10.13 Epigastric pain   I-10
R10.84 Generalized abdominal pain   I-10

§   Requires fifth digit. Valid digits are in [brackets] under each code. See category 789 for codes and definitions.

N   Newborn Age: 0   P   Pediatric Age: 0-17   M   Maternity Age: 12-55   A   Adult Age: 15-124

789.1 Hepatomegaly
　Enlargement of liver

789.2 Splenomegaly
　Enlargement of spleen

§ √5ᵗʰ **789.3 Abdominal or pelvic swelling, mass, or lump**
　[0-7, 9]　Diffuse or generalized swelling or mass:
　　　abdominal NOS
　　　umbilical
　　EXCLUDES abdominal distention (gaseous) (787.3)
　　　　　　ascites (789.51-789.59)

§ √5ᵗʰ **789.4 Abdominal rigidity**
　[0-7, 9]

√5ᵗʰ **789.5 Ascites**
　Fluid in peritoneal cavity
　DEF: Serous fluid effusion and accumulation in abdominal cavity.
　AHA: 4Q, '07, 95; 2Q, '05, 8; 4Q, '89, 11

　789.51 Malignant ascites
　　Code first malignancy, such as:
　　　malignant neoplasm of ovary (183.0)
　　　secondary malignant neoplasm of retroperitoneum
　　　　and peritoneum (197.6)
　　AHA: 4Q, '07, 96
　　R18.0 Malignant ascites　　　　　　　　I-10

　789.59 Other ascites
　　AHA: 4Q, '08, 99
　　R18.8 Other ascites　　　　　　　　　　I-10

§ √5ᵗʰ **789.6 Abdominal tenderness**
　[0-7, 9]　Rebound tenderness

789.7 Colic
　Colic NOS　　　　Infantile colic
　　EXCLUDES colic in adult and child over 12 months old (789.0)
　　　　　　renal colic (788.0)
　　DEF: ▶Inconsolable crying in an otherwise well-fed and healthy
　　infant for more than three hours a day, three days a week, for more
　　than three weeks.◀
　　AHA: ▶4Q, '09, 104-105◀

789.9 Other symtoms involving abdomen and pelvis
　Umbilical:
　　bleeding
　　discharge

Nonspecific Abnormal Findings (790-796)
　AHA: 2Q, '90, 16

√4ᵗʰ **790 Nonspecific findings on examination of blood**
　　EXCLUDES abnormality of:
　　　　platelets (287.0-287.9)
　　　　thrombocytes (287.0-287.9)
　　　　white blood cells (288.00-288.9)

√5ᵗʰ **790.0 Abnormality of red blood cells**
　　EXCLUDES anemia:
　　　　congenital (776.5)
　　　　newborn, due to isoimmunization (773.0-773.2,
　　　　　773.5)
　　　　of premature infant (776.6)
　　　　other specified types (280.0-285.9)
　　　hemoglobin disorders (282.5-282.7)
　　　polycythemia:
　　　　familial (289.6)
　　　　neonatorum (776.4)
　　　　secondary (289.0)
　　　　vera (238.4)
　　AHA: 4Q, '00, 46

　790.01 Precipitous drop in hematocrit
　　Drop in hematocritDrop in hemoglobin
　　TIP: Typically reported as a reason for encounter at a dialysis
　　center.

　790.09 Other abnormality of red blood cells
　　Abnormal red cell morphology NOS
　　Abnormal red cell volume NOS
　　Anisocytosis
　　Poikilocytosis

790.1 Elevated sedimentation rate

√5ᵗʰ **790.2 Abnormal glucose**
　　EXCLUDES diabetes mellitus (249.00-249.91, 250.00-250.93)
　　　　dysmetabolic syndrome X (277.7)
　　　　gestational diabetes (648.8)
　　　　glycosuria (791.5)
　　　　hypoglycemia (251.2)
　　　　that complicating pregnancy, childbirth, or
　　　　　puerperium (648.8)
　　AHA: 4Q, '03, 74; 3Q, '91, 5
　　TIP: These codes are typically assigned on encounters before a
　　patient is diagnosed with diabetes mellitus.

　790.21 Impaired fasting glucose
　　Elevated fasting glucose

　790.22 Impaired glucose tolerance test (oral)
　　Elevated glucose tolerance test

　790.29 Other abnormal glucose
　　Abnormal glucose NOS
　　Abnormal non-fasting glucose
　　Hyperglycemia NOS
　　Pre-diabetes NOS
　　AHA: ▶3Q, '09, 5; ◀2Q, '05, 21
　　TIP: ▶Assign for any stress hyperglycemia for which no
　　causal condition is determined including postoperative
　　hyperglycemia that is not specifically documented as a
　　complication of the procedure.◀
　　R73.09 Other abnormal glucose　　　　I-10

790.3 Excessive blood level of alcohol
　Elevated blood-alcohol
　AHA: S-O, '86, 3

**790.4 Nonspecific elevation of levels of transaminase or lactic
　acid dehydrogenase [LDH]**
　R74.0 Nonspecific elevation levels transaminase & LDH　I-10

790.5 Other nonspecific abnormal serum enzyme levels
　Abnormal serum level of:
　　acid phosphatase
　　alkaline phosphatase
　　amylase
　　lipase
　　EXCLUDES deficiency of circulating enzymes (277.6)
　　R74.8 Abnormal levels of other serum enzymes　I-10

790.6 Other abnormal blood chemistry
　Abnormal blood level of:
　　cobalt
　　copper
　　iron
　　lead
　　lithium
　　magnesium
　　mineral
　　zinc
　　EXCLUDES abnormality of electrolyte or acid-base balance
　　　　　(276.0-276.9)
　　　　hypoglycemia NOS (251.2)
　　　　lead poisoning (984.0-984.9)
　　　　specific finding indicating abnormality of:
　　　　　amino-acid transport and metabolism
　　　　　　(270.0-270.9)
　　　　　carbohydrate transport and metabolism
　　　　　　(271.0-271.9)
　　　　　lipid metabolism (272.0-272.9)
　　　　uremia NOS (586)
　　AHA: 4Q, '88, 1
　　TIP: If only azotemia is documented (indexed to 790.6), clarify with
　　physician; if due to uremia or renal failure, code to those conditions
　　instead.
　　R78.89 Finding oth spec substances not norm found blood　I-10

---

§　Requires fifth digit. Valid digits are in [brackets] under each code. See category 789 for codes and definitions.

Symptoms, Signs, and Ill-Defined Conditions

790.7 Bacteremia

EXCLUDES   *bacteremia of newborn (771.83)*
          septicemia (038)

Use additional code to identify organism (041)

DEF: Laboratory finding of bacteria in the blood in the absence of two or more signs of sepsis; transient in nature, progresses to septicemia with severe infectious process.

AHA: 2Q, '03, 7; 4Q, '93, 29; 3Q, '88, 12

TIP: If clinical signs or symptoms indicating systemic disease exist, query physician for the presence of sepsis; code to category 038 if documented.

790.8 Viremia, unspecified

DEF: Presence of a virus in the blood stream.

AHA: 4Q, '88, 10

√5ᵗʰ 790.9 Other nonspecific findings on examination of blood

AHA: 4Q, '93, 29

790.91 Abnormal arterial blood gases

790.92 Abnormal coagulation profile
Abnormal or prolonged:
    bleeding time
    coagulation time
    partial thromboplastin time [PTT]
    prothrombin time [PT]

EXCLUDES   *coagulation (hemorrhagic) disorders (286.0-286.9)*

R79.1 Abnormal coagulaton profile   I-10

790.93 Elevated prostate specific antigen, [PSA]   A♂

790.94 Euthyroid sick syndrome

DEF: Transient alteration of thyroid hormone metabolism due to nonthyroid illness or stress.

AHA: 4Q, '97, 45

790.95 Elevated C-reactive protein [CRP]

DEF: Inflammation in an arterial wall results in elevated C-reactive protein (CRP) in the blood; CRP is a recognized risk factor in cardiovascular disease.

790.99 Other

AHA: 2Q, '03, 14

√4ᵗʰ 791 Nonspecific findings on examination of urine

EXCLUDES   *hematuria NOS (599.70-599.72)*
          specific findings indicating abnormality of:
             amino-acid transport and metabolism (270.0-270.9)
             carbohydrate transport and metabolism (271.0-271.9)

791.0 Proteinuria
Albuminuria
Bence-Jones proteinuria

EXCLUDES   *postural proteinuria (593.6)*
          that arising during pregnancy or the puerperium (642.0-642.9, 646.2)

DEF: Excess protein in urine.

AHA: 3Q, '91, 8

791.1 Chyluria

EXCLUDES   *filarial (125.0-125.9)*

DEF: Excess chyle in urine.

791.2 Hemoglobinuria

DEF: Free hemoglobin in blood due to rapid hemolysis of red blood cells.

791.3 Myoglobinuria

DEF: Myoglobin (oxygen-transporting pigment) in urine.

791.4 Biliuria

DEF: Bile pigments in urine.

791.5 Glycosuria

EXCLUDES   *renal glycosuria (271.4)*

DEF: Sugar in urine.

791.6 Acetonuria
Ketonuria

DEF: Excess acetone in urine.

791.7 Other cells and casts in urine

791.9 Other nonspecific findings on examination of urine
Crystalluria
Elevated urine levels of:
    17-ketosteroids
    catecholamines
    indolacetic acid
    vanillylmandelic acid [VMA]
Melanuria

AHA: 1Q, '05, 12

√4ᵗʰ 792 Nonspecific abnormal findings in other body substances

EXCLUDES   *that in chromosomal analysis (795.2)*

792.0 Cerebrospinal fluid

792.1 Stool contents
Abnormal stool color   Occult stool
Fat in stool   Pus in stool
Mucus in stool

EXCLUDES   *blood in stool [melena] (578.1)*
          newborn (772.4, 777.3)

AHA: 2Q, '92, 9

792.2 Semen   ♂
Abnormal spermatozoa

EXCLUDES   *azoospermia (606.0)*
          oligospermia (606.1)

792.3 Amniotic fluid   M♀

DEF: Nonspecific abnormal findings in amniotic fluid.

AHA: N-D, '86, 4

792.4 Saliva

EXCLUDES   *that in chromosomal analysis (795.2)*

792.5 Cloudy (hemodialysis) (peritoneal) dialysis effluent

AHA: 4Q, '00, 46

792.9 Other nonspecific abnormal findings in body substances
Peritoneal fluid
Pleural fluid
Synovial fluid
Vaginal fluids

√4ᵗʰ 793 Nonspecific (abnormal) findings on radiological and other examination of body structure

INCLUDES   nonspecific abnormal findings of:
          thermography
          ultrasound examination [echogram]
          x-ray examination

EXCLUDES   *abnormal results of function studies and radioisotope scans (794.0-794.9)*

793.0 Skull and head

EXCLUDES   *nonspecific abnormal echoencephalogram (794.01)*

AHA: 3Q, '06, 22

793.1 Lung field
Coin lesion
Shadow   } (of) lung

DEF: Coin lesion of lung: coin-shaped, solitary pulmonary nodule.

793.2 Other intrathoracic organ
Abnormal:
    echocardiogram
    heart shadow
    ultrasound cardiogram
Mediastinal shift

793.3 Biliary tract
Nonvisualization of gallbladder

793.4 Gastrointestinal tract

793.5 Genitourinary organs
Filling defect:
    bladder
    kidney
    ureter

793.6 Abdominal area, including retroperitoneum

793.7 Musculoskeletal system

N   Newborn Age: 0   P   Pediatric Age: 0-17   M   Maternity Age: 12-55   A   Adult Age: 15-124

√5ᵗʰ **793.8 Breast**
AHA: 4Q, '01, 51

793.80 Abnormal mammogram, unspecified

793.81 Mammographic microcalcification
EXCLUDES *mammographic calcification (793.89)*
mammographic calculus (793.89)
DEF: Calcium and cellular debris deposits in the breast that cannot be felt but can be detected on a mammogram; can be a sign of cancer, benign conditions, or changes in the breast tissue as a result of inflammation, injury, or obstructed duct.

793.82 Inconclusive mammogram
Dense breasts NOS
Inconclusive mammogram NEC
Inconclusive mammography due to dense breasts
Inconclusive mammography NEC
AHA: ►4Q, '09, 105-106◄

793.89 Other (abnormal) findings on radiological examination of breast
Mammographic calcification
Mammographic calculus

√5ᵗʰ **793.9 Other**
EXCLUDES *abnormal finding by radioisotope localization of placenta (794.9)*
TIP: Sequence a code for the sign or symptom that was the reason for the imaging or radiological test first.

793.91 Image test inconclusive due to excess body fat
Use additional code to identify Body Mass Index (BMI), if known (V85.0-V85.54)
AHA: 4Q, '06, 109

793.99 Other nonspecific (abnormal) findings on radiological and other examinations of body structure
Abnormal:
placental finding by x-ray or ultrasound method
radiological findings in skin and subcutaneous tissue
AHA: 4Q, '06, 109

√4ᵗʰ **794 Nonspecific abnormal results of function studies**
INCLUDES radioisotope:
scans
uptake studies
scintiphotography

√5ᵗʰ **794.0 Brain and central nervous system**

794.00 Abnormal function study, unspecified

794.01 Abnormal echoencephalogram

794.02 Abnormal electroencephalogram [EEG]

794.09 Other
Abnormal brain scan

√5ᵗʰ **794.1 Peripheral nervous system and special senses**

794.10 Abnormal response to nerve stimulation, unspecified

794.11 Abnormal retinal function studies
Abnormal electroretinogram [ERG]

794.12 Abnormal electro-oculogram [EOG]

794.13 Abnormal visually evoked potential

794.14 Abnormal oculomotor studies

794.15 Abnormal auditory function studies
AHA: 1Q, '04, 15-16
TIP: If the reason for the encounter was for a hearing examination, sequence a code from subcategory V72.1 first. When nonspecific hearing loss is documented, assign 389.9 instead of 794.15.

794.16 Abnormal vestibular function studies

794.17 Abnormal electromyogram [EMG]
EXCLUDES *that of eye (794.14)*

794.19 Other

794.2 Pulmonary
Abnormal lung scan
Reduced:
ventilatory capacity
vital capacity

√5ᵗʰ **794.3 Cardiovascular**

794.30 Abnormal function study, unspecified

794.31 Abnormal electrocardiogram [ECG] [EKG]
EXCLUDES *long QT syndrome (426.82)*
R94.31 Abnormal electrocardiogram [ECG] [EKG] I-10

794.39 Other
Abnormal:
ballistocardiogram
phonocardiogram
vectorcardiogram
R94.39 Abnormal result oth cardiovasculr function study I-10

794.4 Kidney
Abnormal renal function test

794.5 Thyroid
Abnormal thyroid:
scan
uptake

794.6 Other endocrine function study

794.7 Basal metabolism
Abnormal basal metabolic rate [BMR]

794.8 Liver
Abnormal liver scan
R94.5 Abnormal results of liver function studies I-10

794.9 Other
Bladder   Placenta
Pancreas   Spleen

√4ᵗʰ **795 Other and nonspecific abnormal cytological, histological, immunological and DNA test findings**
EXCLUDES *abnormal cytologic smear of anus and anal HPV (796.70-796.79)*
nonspecific abnormalities of red blood cells (790.01-790.09)

√5ᵗʰ **795.0 Abnormal Papanicolaou smear of cervix and cervical HPV**
Abnormal thin preparation smear of cervix
Abnormal cervical cytology
EXCLUDES *abnormal cytologic smear of vagina and vaginal HPV (795.10-795.19)*
carcinoma in situ of cervix (233.1)
cervical intraepithelial neoplasia I (CIN I) (622.11)
cervical intraepithelial neoplasia II (CIN II) (622.12)
cervical intraepithelial neoplasia III (CIN III) (233.1)
dysplasia (histologically confirmed) of cervix (uteri) NOS (622.10)
mild cervical dysplasia (histologically confirmed) (622.11)
moderate cervical dysplasia (histologically confirmed) (622.12)
severe cervical dysplasia (histologically confirmed) (233.1)
AHA: 4Q, '08, 145-146; 4Q, '02, 69

795.00 Abnormal glandular Papanicolaou smear of cervix ♀
Atypical endocervical cells NOS
Atypical endometrial cells NOS
Atypical cervical glandular cells NOS

795.01 Papanicolaou smear of cervix with atypical squamous cells of undetermined significance [ASC-US] ♀
AHA: 2Q, '06, 4

795.02 Papanicolaou smear of cervix with atypical squamous cells cannot exclude high grade squamous intraepithelial lesion [ASC-H] ♀

795.03 Papanicolaou smear of cervix with low grade squamous intraepithelial lesion [LGSIL] ♀

795.04 Papanicolaou smear of cervix with high grade squamous intraepithelial lesion [HGSIL] ♀

√4ᵗʰ
√5ᵗʰ Additional Digit Required   Unspecified Code   Other Specified Code   Manifestation Code   ►◄ Revised Text   ● New Code   ▲ Revised Code Title

Symptoms, Signs, and Ill-Defined Conditions

795.05–795.89

795.05 Cervical high risk human papillomavirus [HPV] DNA test positive ♀

795.06 Papanicolaou smear of cervix with cytologic evidence of malignancy ♀
AHA: 4Q, '06, 110

795.07 Satisfactory cervical smear but lacking transformation zone ♀

795.08 Unsatisfactory cervical cytology smear ♀
Inadequate cervical cytology sample
AHA: 2Q, '06, 4

795.09 Other abnormal Papanicolaou smear of cervix and cervical HPV ♀
Cervical low risk human papillomavirus (HPV) DNA test positive
Use additional code for associated human papillomavirus (079.4)
EXCLUDES *encounter for Papanicolaou cervical smear to confirm findings of recent normal smear following initial abnormal smear (V72.32)*

√5ᵗʰ **795.1 Abnormal Papanicolaou smear of vagina and vaginal HPV**
Abnormal thin preparation smear of vagina NOS
Abnormal vaginal cytology NOS
Use additional code to identify acquired absence of uterus and cervix, if applicable (V88.01-V88.03)
EXCLUDES *abnormal cytologic smear of cervix and cervical HPV (795.00-795.09)*
carcinoma in situ of vagina (233.31)
carcinoma in situ of vulva (233.32)
dysplasia (histologically confirmed) of vagina NOS (623.0, 233.31)
dysplasia (histologically confirmed) of vulva NOS (624.01, 624.02, 233.32)
mild vaginal dysplasia (histologically confirmed) (623.0)
mild vulvar dysplasia (histologically confirmed) (624.01)
moderate vaginal dysplasia (histologically confirmed) (623.0)
moderate vulvar dysplasia (histologically confirmed) (624.02)
severe vaginal dysplasia (histologically confirmed) (233.31)
severe vulvar dysplasia (histologically confirmed) (233.32)
vaginal intraepithelial neoplasia I (VAIN I) (623.0)
vaginal intraepithelial neoplasia II (VAIN II) (623.0)
vaginal intraepithelial neoplasia III (VAIN III) (233.31)
vulvar intraepithelial neoplasia I (VIN I) (624.01)
vulvar intraepithelial neoplasia II (VIN II) (624.02)
vulvar intraepithelial neoplasia III (VIN III) (233.32)
AHA: 4Q, '08, 145-148

795.10 Abnormal glandular Papanicolaou smear of vagina ♀
Atypical vaginal glandular cells NOS

795.11 Papanicolaou smear of vagina with atypical squamous cells of undetermined significance [ASC-US] ♀

795.12 Papanicolaou smear of vagina with atypical squamous cells cannot exclude high grade squamous intraepithelial lesion [ASC-H] ♀

795.13 Papanicolaou smear of vagina with low grade squamous intraepithelial lesion [LGSIL] ♀

795.14 Papanicolaou smear of vagina with high grade squamous intraepithelial lesion [HGSIL] ♀

795.15 Vaginal high risk human papillomavirus [HPV] DNA test positive ♀
EXCLUDES *condyloma acuminatum (078.11)*
genital warts (078.11)

795.16 Papanicolaou smear of vagina with cytologic evidence of malignancy ♀

795.18 Unsatisfactory vaginal cytology smear ♀
Inadequate vaginal cytology sample

795.19 Other abnormal Papanicolaou smear of vagina and vaginal HPV ♀
Vaginal low risk human papillomavirus (HPV) DNA test positive
Use additional code for associated human papillomavirus (079.4)

795.2 Nonspecific abnormal findings on chromosomal analysis
Abnormal karyotype

√5ᵗʰ **795.3 Nonspecific positive culture findings**
Positive culture findings in:
nose   sputum
throat   wound
EXCLUDES *that of:*
blood (790.7-790.8)
urine (791.9)

795.31 Nonspecific positive findings for anthrax
Positive findings by nasal swab
AHA: 4Q, '02, 70
TIP: If the patient has been exposed only to anthrax, assign instead V01.81. If a patient has not been exposed but fears anthrax and tests negative, assign instead V71.82.

795.39 Other nonspecific positive culture findings
EXCLUDES *colonization status (V02.0-V02.9)*

795.4 Other nonspecific abnormal histological findings

795.5 Nonspecific reaction to tuberculin skin test without active tuberculosis
Abnormal result of Mantoux test
PPD positive
Tuberculin (skin test):
positive
reactor

795.6 False positive serological test for syphilis
False positive Wassermann reaction

√5ᵗʰ **795.7 Other nonspecific immunological findings**
EXCLUDES *abnormal tumor markers (795.81-795.89)*
elevated prostate specific antigen [PSA] (790.93)
elevated tumor associated antigens (795.81-795.89)
isoimmunization, in pregnancy (656.1-656.2)
affecting fetus or newborn (773.0-773.2)
AHA: 2Q, '93, 6

795.71 Nonspecific serologic evidence of human immunodeficiency virus [HIV]
Inclusive human immunodeficiency [HIV] test (adult) (infant)
NOTE This code is **only** to be used when a test finding is reported as nonspecific. Asymptomatic positive findings are coded to V08. If any HIV infection symptom or condition is present, see code 042. Negative findings are not coded.
EXCLUDES *acquired immunodeficiency syndrome [AIDS] (042)*
asymptomatic human immunodeficiency virus, [HIV] infection status (V08)
HIV infection, symptomatic (042)
human immunodeficiency virus [HIV] disease (042)
positive (status) NOS (V08)
AHA: 2Q, '04, 11; 1Q, '93, 21; 1Q, '93, 22; 2Q, '92, 11; J-A, '87, 24

795.79 Other and unspecified nonspecific immunological findings
Raised antibody titer
Raised level of immunoglobulins

√5ᵗʰ **795.8 Abnormal tumor markers**
Elevated tumor associated antigens [TAA]
Elevated tumor specific antigens [TSA]
EXCLUDES *elevated prostate specific antigen [PSA] (790.93)*

795.81 Elevated carcinoembryonic antigen [CEA]
AHA: 4Q, '06, 111

795.82 Elevated cancer antigen 125 [CA 125] ♀
AHA: 4Q, '06, 111

795.89 Other abnormal tumor markers
AHA: 4Q, '06, 111

√4ᵗʰ 796 Other nonspecific abnormal findings

796.0 Nonspecific abnormal toxicological findings
Abnormal levels of heavy metals or drugs in blood, urine, or other tissue
▶Use additional code for retained foreign body, if applicable, (V90.01-V90.9)◄
EXCLUDES *excessive blood level of alcohol (790.3)*
AHA: 1Q, '97, 16

796.1 Abnormal reflex

796.2 Elevated blood pressure reading without diagnosis of hypertension
NOTE This category is to be used to record an episode of elevated blood pressure in a patient in whom no formal diagnosis of hypertension has been made, or as an incidental finding.
AHA: 2Q, '03, 11; 3Q, '90, 4; J-A, '84, 12
TIP: Assign an additional E code for poisoning or adverse effect of a drug if the documentation indicates it's the underlying cause of the elevated blood pressure.
R03.0 Elevated blood-pressure reading without dx HTN   I-10

796.3 Nonspecific low blood pressure reading

796.4 Other abnormal clinical findings
AHA: 1Q, '97, 16

796.5 Abnormal finding on antenatal screening   ♀ M
AHA: 4Q, '97, 46

796.6 Abnormal findings on neonatal screening   N
EXCLUDES *nonspecific serologic evidence of human immunodeficiency virus [HIV] (795.71)*
AHA: 4Q, '04, 99

√5ᵗʰ 796.7 Abnormal cytologic smear of anus and anal HPV
EXCLUDES *abnormal cytologic smear of cervix and cervical HPV (795.00-795.09)*
abnormal cytologic smear of vagina and vaginal HPV (795.10-795.19)
anal intraepithelial neoplasia I (AIN I) (569.44)
anal intraepithelial neoplasia II (AIN II) (569.44)
anal intraepithelial neoplasia III (AIN III) (230.5, 230.6)
carcinoma in situ of anus (230.5, 230.6)
dysplasia (histologically confirmed) of anus NOS (569.44)
mild anal dysplasia (histologically confirmed) (569.44)
moderate anal dysplasia (histologically confirmed) (569.44)
severe anal dysplasia (histologically confirmed) (230.5, 230.6)
AHA: 4Q, '08, 117-119

796.70 Abnormal glandular Papanicolaou smear of anus
Atypical anal glandular cells NOS

796.71 Papanicolaou smear of anus with atypical squamous cells of undetermined significance [ASC-US]

796.72 Papanicolaou smear of anus with atypical squamous cells cannot exclude high grade squamous intraepithelial lesion [ASC-H]

796.73 Papanicolaou smear of anus with low grade squamous intraepithelial lesion [LGSIL]

796.74 Papanicolaou smear of anus with high grade squamous intraepithelial lesion [HGSIL]

796.75 Anal high risk human papillomavirus [HPV] DNA test positive

796.76 Papanicolaou smear of anus with cytologic evidence of malignancy

796.77 Satisfactory anal smear but lacking transformation zone

796.78 Unsatisfactory anal cytology smear
Inadequate anal cytology sample

796.79 Other abnormal Papanicolaou smear of anus and anal HPV
Anal low risk human papillomavirus (HPV) DNA test positive
Use additional code for associated human papillomavirus (079.4)

796.9 Other

Ill-Defined and Unknown Causes of Morbidity and Mortality (797-799)

797 Senility without mention of psychosis
Frailty   Senile asthenia
Old age   Senile:
Senescence   debility
           exhaustion
EXCLUDES *senile psychoses (290.0-290.9)*

√4ᵗʰ 798 Sudden death, cause unknown

798.0 Sudden infant death syndrome   P
Cot death
Crib death
Sudden death of nonspecific cause in infancy
DEF: Death of infant under age one due to nonspecific cause.

798.1 Instantaneous death

798.2 Death occurring in less than 24 hours from onset of symptoms, not otherwise explained
Death known not to be violent or instantaneous, for which no cause could be discovered
Died without sign of disease

798.9 Unattended death
Death in circumstances where the body of the deceased was found and no cause could be discovered
Found dead

√4ᵗʰ 799 Other ill-defined and unknown causes of morbidity and mortality

√5ᵗʰ 799.0 Asphyxia and hypoxemia
EXCLUDES *asphyxia and hypoxemia (due to):*
carbon monoxide (986)
hypercapnia (786.09)
inhalation of food or foreign body (932-934.9)
newborn (768.0-768.9)
traumatic (994.7)

799.01 Asphyxia
DEF: Lack of oxygen in inspired air, causing a deficiency of oxygen in tissues (hypoxia) and elevated levels of arterial carbon dioxide (hypercapnia).
AHA: 4Q, '05, 90

799.02 Hypoxemia
DEF: Deficient oxygenation of the blood.
AHA: 3Q, '09, 20; 2Q, '06, 24, 25; 4Q, '05, 90
TIP: Hypoxia is not inherent in COPD (496) and may be assigned in addition, if applicable.
R09.02 Hypoxemia   I-10

799.1 Respiratory arrest
Cardiorespiratory failure
EXCLUDES *cardiac arrest (427.5)*
failure of peripheral circulation (785.50)
respiratory distress:
NOS (786.09)
acute (518.82)
following trauma and surgery (518.5)
newborn (770.89)
syndrome (newborn) (769)
adult (following trauma and surgery) (518.5)
other (518.82)
respiratory failure (518.81, 518.83-518.84)
newborn (770.84)
respiratory insufficiency (786.09)
acute (518.82)

√4ᵗʰ √5ᵗʰ Additional Digit Required   Unspecified Code   Other Specified Code   Manifestation Code   ▶◄ Revised Text   ● New Code   ▲ Revised Code Title

Symptoms, Signs, and Ill-Defined Conditions

799.2–799.9

√5ᵗʰ **799.2 Signs and symptoms involving emotional state**
     EXCLUDES   anxiety (293.84, 300.00-300.09)
                   depression (311)
     AHA: 4Q, '09,107
     TIP: If associated with underlying history of traumatic brain injury (TBI), assign in addition to a code for the late effect of TBI (e.g., 905.0 or 907.0).

     799.21 Nervousness
          Nervous
          AHA: 4Q, '09,108

     799.22 Irritability
          Irritable
          AHA: 4Q, '09,108

     799.23 Impulsiveness
          Impulsive
          EXCLUDES   impulsive neurosis (300.3)

     799.24 Emotional lability

     799.25 Demoralization and apathy
          Apathetic

     799.29 Other signs and symptoms involving emotional state

799.3 Debility, unspecified
     EXCLUDES   asthenia (780.79)
                   nervous debility (300.5)
                   neurasthenia (300.5)
                   senile asthenia (797)

799.4 Cachexia
     Wasting disease
     Code first underlying condition, if known
     DEF: General ill health and poor nutrition.
     AHA: 3Q, '06, 14, 15; 3Q, '90, 17
     TIP: Assign an additional code for any associated malnutrition, if documented.
     R64 Cachexia   `I-10`

√5ᵗʰ **799.5 Signs and symptoms involving cognition**
     EXCLUDES   amnesia (780.93)
                   amnestic syndrome (294.0)
                   attention deficit disorder (314.00-314.01)
                   late effects of cerebrovascular disease (438.0)
                   memory loss (780.93)
                   mild cognitive impairment, so stated (331.83)
                   specific problems in developmental delay (315.00-315.9)
                   transient global amnesia (437.7)
                   visuospatial neglect (781.8)

     799.51 Attention or concentration deficit

     799.52 Cognitive communication deficit

     799.53 Visuospatial deficit

     799.54 Psychomotor deficit

     799.55 Frontal lobe and executive function deficit

     799.59 Other signs and symptoms involving cognition

√5ᵗʰ **799.8 Other ill-defined conditions**

     799.81 Decreased libido   A
          Decreased sexual desire
          EXCLUDES   psychosexual dysfunction with inhibited sexual desire (302.71)
          AHA: 4Q, '03, 75

     799.82 Apparent life threatening event in infant   P
          ALTE
          Apparent life threatening event in newborn and infant
          ▶Code first confirmed diagnosis, if known◀
          ▶Use additional code(s) for associated signs and symptoms if no confirmed diagnosis established, or if signs and symptoms are not associated routinely with confirmed diagnosis, or provide additional information for cause of ALTE◀
          AHA: 4Q, '09, 109
          TIP: Assign this code only when no underlying diagnosis has been identified.

     799.89 Other ill-defined conditions

799.9 Other unknown and unspecified cause
     Undiagnosed disease, not specified as to site or system involved
     Unknown cause of morbidity or mortality
     AHA: 1Q, '98,.4; 1Q, '90, 20

---

17. Injury and Poisoning (800-999)

▶Use additional code for retained foreign body, if applicable, (V90.01-V90.9)◀

Use E code(s) to identify the cause and intent of the injury or poisoning (E800-E999)

NOTE

1. The principle of multiple coding of injuries should be followed wherever possible. Combination categories for multiple injuries are provided for use when there is insufficient detail as to the nature of the individual conditions, or for primary tabulation purposes when it is more convenient to record a single code; otherwise, the component injuries should be coded separately.

    Where multiple sites of injury are specified in the titles, the word "with" indicates involvement of both sites, and the word "and" indicates involvement of either or both sites. The word "finger" includes thumb.

2. Categories for "late effect" of injuries are to be found at 905-909.

FRACTURES (800-829)

EXCLUDES malunion (733.81)
nonunion (733.82)
pathological or spontaneous fracture (733.10-733.19)
stress fractures (733.93-733.95)

NOTE The terms "condyle," "coronoid process," "ramus," and "symphysis" indicate the portion of the bone fractured, not the name of the bone involved.

The descriptions "closed" and "open" used in the fourth-digit subdivisions include the following terms:

closed (with or without delayed healing):

comminuted	impacted
depressed	linear
elevated	simple
fissured	slipped epiphysis
fracture NOS	spiral
greenstick	

open (with or without delayed healing):

compound	puncture
infected	with foreign body
missile	

NOTE A fracture not indicated as closed or open should be classified as closed.

AHA: 4Q, '08, 158; 1Q, '07, 3-4; 4Q, '90, 26; 3Q, '90, 5; 3Q, '90, 13; 2Q, '90, 7; 2Q, '89, 15, S-O, '85, 3

TIP: Assign the acute fracture codes only while the patient is receiving active treatment for the fracture, such as during surgical care, an ED encounter, or evaluation and treatment by a new physician. Otherwise, refer to aftercare category V54.

Fracture of Skull (800-804)

INCLUDES traumatic brain injury due to fracture of skull

The following fifth-digit subclassification is for use with the appropriate codes in category 800, 801, 803, and 804:

0   unspecified state of consciousness
1   with no loss of consciousness
2   with brief [less than one hour] loss of consciousness
3   with moderate [1-24 hours] loss of consciousness
4   with prolonged [more than 24 hours] loss of consciousness and return to pre-existing conscious level
5   with prolonged [more than 24 hours] loss of consciousness, without return to pre-existing conscious level
     Use fifth-digit 5 to designate when a patient is unconscious and dies before regaining consciousness, regardless of the duration of the loss of consciousness
6   with loss of consciousness of unspecified duration
9   with concussion, unspecified

√4ᵗʰ **800**   **Fracture of vault of skull**

     INCLUDES   frontal bone
                parietal bone

     DEF: Fracture of bone that forms skull dome and protects brain.
     AHA: 4Q,'96, 36

§ √5ᵗʰ **800.0**   **Closed without mention of intracranial injury**
                 [0-6, 9]

§ √5ᵗʰ **800.1**   **Closed with cerebral laceration and contusion**
                 [0-6, 9]

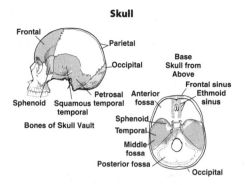

Skull

Frontal — Parietal — Occipital — Base Skull from Above — Frontal sinus — Ethmoid sinus — Petrosal — Anterior fossa — Sphenoid — Squamous temporal — temporal — Sphenoid — Temporal — Middle fossa — Posterior fossa — Occipital

Bones of Skull Vault

§ √5ᵗʰ **800.2**   **Closed with subarachnoid, subdural, and extradural** [0-6, 9]**hemorrhage**

§ √5ᵗʰ **800.3**   **Closed with other and unspecified intracranial** [0-6, 9]**hemorrhage**

§ √5ᵗʰ **800.4**   **Closed with intracranial injury of other and** [0-6, 9]**unspecified nature**

§ √5ᵗʰ **800.5**   **Open without mention of intracranial injury** [0-6, 9]

§ √5ᵗʰ **800.6**   **Open with cerebral laceration and contusion** [0-6, 9]

§ √5ᵗʰ **800.7**   **Open with subarachnoid, subdural, and** [0-6, 9]**extradural hemorrhage**

§ √5ᵗʰ **800.8**   **Open with other and unspecified intracranial** [0-6, 9]**hemorrhage**

§ √5ᵗʰ **800.9**   **Open with intracranial injury of other and** [0-6, 9]**unspecified nature**

√4ᵗʰ **801**   **Fracture of base of skull**

     INCLUDES   fossa:
                anterior
                middle
                posterior
             occiput bone
             orbital roof
             sinus:
                ethmoid
                frontal
             sphenoid bone
             temporal bone

     DEF: Fracture of bone that forms skull floor.
     AHA: 4Q, '96, 36

§ √5ᵗʰ **801.0**   **Closed without mention of intracranial injury** [0-6, 9]

§ √5ᵗʰ **801.1**   **Closed with cerebral laceration and contusion** [0-6, 9]   **AHA:** For code 801.15: 4Q, '96, 36

§ √5ᵗʰ **801.2**   **Closed with subarachnoid, subdural, and** [0-6, 9]**extradural hemorrhage**

§ √5ᵗʰ **801.3**   **Closed with other and unspecified intracranial** [0-6, 9]**hemorrhage**

§ √5ᵗʰ **801.4**   **Closed with intracranial injury of other and** [0-6, 9]**unspecified nature**

§ √5ᵗʰ **801.5**   **Open without mention of intracranial injury** [0-6, 9]

§ √5ᵗʰ **801.6**   **Open with cerebral laceration and contusion** [0-6, 9]

§ √5ᵗʰ **801.7**   **Open with subarachnoid, subdural, and** [0-6, 9]**extradural hemorrhage**

§ √5ᵗʰ **801.8**   **Open with other and unspecified intracranial** [0-6, 9]**hemorrhage**

§ √5ᵗʰ **801.9**   **Open with intracranial injury of other and** [0-6, 9]**unspecified nature**

---

§   Requires fifth digit. Valid digits are in [brackets] under each code. See beginning of section 800-804 for codes and definitions.

√4ᵗʰ / √5ᵗʰ   Additional Digit Required   Unspecified Code   Other Specified Code   Manifestation Code   ▶◀ Revised Text   ● New Code   ▲ Revised Code Title

Injury and Poisoning

802–804.9

Fractures

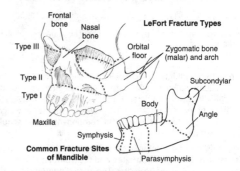

Avulsion · Fracture-dislocation · Impacted · Linear (fissured)

Greenstick

Open (skin broken) · Oblique · Closed spiral

Epiphyseal · Depressed

March · Comminuted

Facial Fracture

Frontal bone · Nasal bone · Orbital floor · Zygomatic bone (malar) and arch

LeFort Fracture Types

Type III · Type II · Type I · Subcondylar · Body · Angle

Maxilla · Symphysis · Parasymphysis

Common Fracture Sites of Mandible

√4ᵗʰ **802 Fracture of face bones**
AHA: 4Q, '96, 36

802.0 Nasal bones, closed
S02.2xxA Fracture nasal bones initial encounter closed fx   I-10

802.1 Nasal bones, open

√5ᵗʰ **802.2 Mandible, closed**
Inferior maxilla   Lower jaw (bone)

    802.20 Unspecified site

    802.21 Condylar process

    802.22 Subcondylar

    802.23 Coronoid process

    802.24 Ramus, unspecified

    802.25 Angle of jaw

    802.26 Symphysis of body

    802.27 Alveolar border of body

    802.28 Body, other and unspecified

    802.29 Multiple sites

√5ᵗʰ **802.3 Mandible, open**

    802.30 Unspecified site

    802.31 Condylar process

    802.32 Subcondylar

    802.33 Coronoid process

    802.34 Ramus, unspecified

    802.35 Angle of jaw

    802.36 Symphysis of body

    802.37 Alveolar border of body

    802.38 Body, other and unspecified

    802.39 Multiple sites

802.4 Malar and maxillary bones, closed
Superior maxilla
Upper jaw (bone)
Zygoma
Zygomatic arch
S02.40xA Fx malar max & zygoma uns initial enc closed fx   I-10

802.5 Malar and maxillary bones, open

802.6 Orbital floor (blow-out), closed
S02.3xxA Fracture orbital floor initial encounter clos fx   I-10

802.7 Orbital floor (blow-out), open

802.8 Other facial bones, closed
Alveolus
Orbit:
    NOS
    part other than roof or floor
Palate
   EXCLUDES   orbital:
       floor (802.6)
       roof (801.0-801.9)
S02.89xA Fx oth skull & face bones initial enc closed fx   I-10

802.9 Other facial bones, open

√4ᵗʰ **803 Other and unqualified skull fractures**
   INCLUDES   skull NOS
             skull multiple NOS
AHA: 4Q, '96, 36

§ √5ᵗʰ **803.0 Closed without mention of intracranial injury**
[0-6, 9]

§ √5ᵗʰ **803.1 Closed with cerebral laceration and contusion**
[0-6, 9]

§ √5ᵗʰ **803.2 Closed with subarachnoid, subdural, and**
[0-6, 9] **extradural hemorrhage**

§ √5ᵗʰ **803.3 Closed with other and unspecified intracranial**
[0-6, 9] **hemorrhage**

§ √5ᵗʰ **803.4 Closed with intracranial injury of other and**
[0-6, 9] **unspecified nature**

§ √5ᵗʰ **803.5 Open without mention of intracranial injury**
[0-6, 9]

§ √5ᵗʰ **803.6 Open with cerebral laceration and contusion**
[0-6, 9]

§ √5ᵗʰ **803.7 Open with subarachnoid, subdural, and**
[0-6, 9] **extradural hemorrhage**

§ √5ᵗʰ **803.8 Open with other and unspecified intracranial**
[0-6, 9] **hemorrhage**

§ √5ᵗʰ **803.9 Open with intracranial injury of other and**
[0-6, 9] **unspecified nature**

√4ᵗʰ **804 Multiple fractures involving skull or face with other bones**
AHA: 4Q, '96, 36

§ √5ᵗʰ **804.0 Closed without mention of intracranial injury**
[0-6, 9]

§ √5ᵗʰ **804.1 Closed with cerebral laceration and contusion**
[0-6, 9]   AHA: For code 804.10: 1Q, '06, 6

§ √5ᵗʰ **804.2 Closed with subarachnoid, subdural, and**
[0-6, 9] **extradural hemorrhage**

§ √5ᵗʰ **804.3 Closed with other and unspecified intracranial**
[0-6, 9] **hemorrhage**

§ √5ᵗʰ **804.4 Closed with intracranial injury of other and**
[0-6, 9] **unspecified nature**

§ √5ᵗʰ **804.5 Open without mention of intracranial injury**
[0-6, 9]

§ √5ᵗʰ **804.6 Open with cerebral laceration and contusion**
[0-6, 9]

§ √5ᵗʰ **804.7 Open with subarachnoid, subdural, and**
[0-6, 9] **extradural hemorrage**

§ √5ᵗʰ **804.8 Open with other and unspecified intracranial**
[0-6, 9] **hemorrhage**

§ √5ᵗʰ **804.9 Open with intracranial injury of other and**
[0-6, 9] **unspecified nature**

§   Requires fifth digit. Valid digits are in [brackets] under each code. See beginning of section 800-804 for codes and definitions.

Fracture of Neck and Trunk (805-809)

✓4ᵗʰ 805 Fracture of vertebral column without mention of spinal cord injury

> INCLUDES neural arch
> spine
> spinous process
> transverse process
> vertebra

> The following fifth-digit subclassification is for use with codes 805.0-805.1:
> **0 cervical vertebra, unspecified level**
> **1 first cervical vertebra**
> **2 second cervical vertebra**
> **3 third cervical vertebra**
> **4 fourth cervical vertebra**
> **5 fifth cervical vertebra**
> **6 sixth cervical vertebra**
> **7 seventh cervical vertebra**
> **8 multiple cervical vertebrae**

§ ✓5ᵗʰ **805.0 Cervical, closed**
[0-8]   Atlas
  Axis
    S12.101A Uns nondisplcd fx 2nd cerv vert initial enc closed fx   I-10

§ ✓5ᵗʰ **805.1 Cervical, open**
[0-8]

805.2 Dorsal [thoracic], closed
    S22.008A Oth fx uns thoracic vertebra initial enc clos fx   I-10

805.3 Dorsal [thoracic], open

805.4 Lumbar, closed
    AHA: 1Q, '07, 7; 4Q, '99, 12
    S32.008A Oth fx uns lumbar vertebra initial enc closed fx   I-10

805.5 Lumbar, open

805.6 Sacrum and coccyx, closed
    S32.19xA Other fx of sacrum initial encounter closed fx   I-10

805.7 Sacrum and coccyx, open

805.8 Unspecified, closed

805.9 Unspecified, open

Vertebral Column

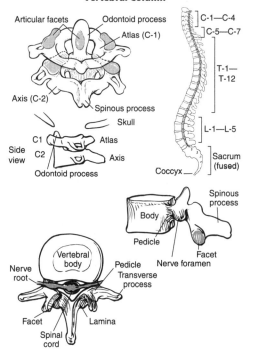

✓4ᵗʰ 806 Fracture of vertebral column with spinal cord injury

> INCLUDES any condition classifiable to 805 with:
> complete or incomplete transverse lesion (of cord)
> hematomyelia
> injury to:
>   cauda equina
>   nerve
> paralysis
> paraplegia
> quadriplegia
> spinal concussion

✓5ᵗʰ **806.0 Cervical, closed**

  806.00 C_1-C_4 level with unspecified spinal cord injury
    Cervical region NOS with spinal cord injury NOS

  806.01 C_1-C_4 level with complete lesion of cord

  806.02 C_1-C_4 level with anterior cord syndrome

  806.03 C_1-C_4 level with central cord syndrome

  806.04 C_1-C_4 level with other specified spinal cord injury
    C_1-C_4 level with:
      incomplete spinal cord lesion NOS
      posterior cord syndrome

  806.05 C_5-C_7 level with unspecified spinal cord injury

  806.06 C_5-C_7 level with complete lesion of cord

  806.07 C_5-C_7 level with anterior cord syndrome

  806.08 C_5-C_7 level with central cord syndrome

  806.09 C_5-C_7 level with other specified spinal cord injury
    C_5-C_7 level with:
      incomplete spinal cord lesion NOS
      posterior cord syndrome

✓5ᵗʰ **806.1 Cervical, open**

  806.10 C_1-C_4 level with unspecified spinal cord injury

  806.11 C_1-C_4 level with complete lesion of cord

  806.12 C_1-C_4 level with anterior cord syndrome

  806.13 C_1-C_4 level with central cord syndrome

  806.14 C_1-C_4 level with other specified spinal cord injury
    C_1-C_4 level with:
      incomplete spinal cord lesion NOS
      posterior cord syndrome

  806.15 C_5-C_7 level with unspecified spinal cord injury

  806.16 C_5-C_7 level with complete lesion of cord

  806.17 C_5-C_7 level with anterior cord syndrome

  806.18 C_5-C_7 level with central cord syndrome

  806.19 C_5-C_7 level with other specified spinal cord injury
    C_5-C_7 level with:
      incomplete spinal cord lesion NOS
      posterior cord syndrome

✓5ᵗʰ **806.2 Dorsal [thoracic], closed**

  806.20 T_1-T_6 level with unspecified spinal cord injury
    Thoracic region NOS with spinal cord injury NOS

  806.21 T_1-T_6 level with complete lesion of cord

  806.22 T_1-T_6 level with anterior cord syndrome

  806.23 T_1-T_6 level with central cord syndrome

  806.24 T_1-T_6 level with other specified spinal cord injury
    T_1-T_6 level with:
      incomplete spinal cord lesion NOS
      posterior cord syndrome

  806.25 T_7-T_{12} level with unspecified spinal cord injury

  806.26 T_7-T_{12} level with complete lesion of cord

  806.27 T_7-T_{12} level with anterior cord syndrome

  806.28 T_7-T_{12} level with central cord syndrome

  806.29 T_7-T_{12} level with other specified spinal cord injury
    T_7-T_{12} level with:
      incomplete spinal cord lesion NOS
      posterior cord syndrome

---

§ Requires fifth digit. Valid digits are in [brackets] under each code. See category 805 for codes and definitions.

✓5th **806.3 Dorsal [thoracic], open**

    806.30 T_1-T_6 level with unspecified spinal cord injury

    806.31 T_1-T_6 level with complete lesion of cord

    806.32 T_1-T_6 level with anterior cord syndrome

    806.33 T_1-T_6 level with central cord syndrome

    806.34 T_1-T_6 level with other specified spinal cord injury
        T_1-T_6 level with:
          incomplete spinal cord lesion NOS
          posterior cord syndrome

    806.35 T_7-T_{12} level with unspecified spinal cord injury

    806.36 T_7-T_{12} level with complete lesion of cord

    806.37 T_7-T_{12} level with anterior cord syndrome

    806.38 T_7-T_{12} level with central cord syndrome

    806.39 T_7-T_{12} level with other specified spinal cord injury
        T_7-T_{12} level with:
          incomplete spinal cord lesion NOS
          posterior cord syndrome

806.4 Lumbar, closed
    AHA: 4Q, '99, 11, 13

806.5 Lumbar, open

✓5th **806.6 Sacrum and coccyx, closed**

    806.60 With unspecified spinal cord injury

    806.61 With complete cauda equina lesion

    806.62 With other cauda equina injury

    806.69 With other spinal cord injury

✓5th **806.7 Sacrum and coccyx, open**

    806.70 With unspecified spinal cord injury

    806.71 With complete cauda equina lesion

    806.72 With other cauda equina injury

    806.79 With other spinal cord injury

806.8 Unspecified, closed

806.9 Unspecified, open

✓4th **807 Fracture of rib(s), sternum, larynx, and trachea**

    The following fifth-digit subclassification is for use with codes 807.0-807.1:

    0 rib(s) unspecifed
    1 one rib
    2 two ribs
    3 three ribs
    4 four ribs
    5 five ribs
    6 six ribs
    7 seven ribs
    8 eight or more ribs
    9 multiple ribs, unspecified

§ ✓5th **807.0 Rib(s), closed**
    [0-9]   S22.31xA Fracture rib right initial encounter closed fx   I-10
            S22.43xG Mx fx ribs bilat subseqnt enc fx delayed healing   I-10

§ ✓5th **807.1 Rib(s), open**
    [0-9]

Ribs, Sternum, Larynx, and Trachea

807.2 Sternum, closed
    DEF: Break in flat bone (breast bone) in anterior thorax.

807.3 Sternum, open
    DEF: Break, with open wound, in flat bone in mid anterior thorax.

807.4 Flail chest

807.5 Larynx and trachea, closed
    Hyoid bone
    Thyroid cartilage
    Trachea

807.6 Larynx and trachea, open

✓4th **808 Fracture of pelvis**

808.0 Acetabulum, closed

808.1 Acetabulum, open

808.2 Pubis, closed
    AHA: 1Q, '08, 9
    S32.50xA Fracture pubis initial encounter closed fracture   I-10

808.3 Pubis, open

✓5th **808.4 Other specified part, closed**

    808.41 Ilium

    808.42 Ischium

    808.43 Multiple pelvic fractures with disruption of pelvic circle
        AHA: 1Q, '08, 9
        TIP: To assign, documentation must indicate multiple pelvic fractures with complete disruption of the pelvic circle.

    808.49 Other
        Innominate bone
        Pelvic rim

✓5th **808.5 Other specified part, open**

    808.51 Ilium

    808.52 Ischium

    808.53 Multiple pelvic fractures with disruption of pelvic circle

    808.59 Other

808.8 Unspecified, closed

808.9 Unspecified, open

✓4th **809 Ill-defined fractures of bones of trunk**

    INCLUDES bones of trunk with other bones except those of skull and face
               multiple bones of trunk

    EXCLUDES *multiple fractures of:*
        pelvic bones alone (808.0-808.9)
        ribs alone (807.0-807.1, 807.4)
        ribs or sternum with limb bones (819.0-819.1, 828.0-828.1)
        skull or face with other bones (804.0-804.9)

809.0 Fracture of bones of trunk, closed

809.1 Fracture of bones of trunk, open

Pelvis and Pelvic Fractures

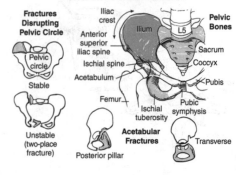

---

§ Requires fifth digit. Valid digits are in [brackets] under each code. See category 807 for codes and definitions.

N Newborn Age: 0   P Pediatric Age: 0-17   M Maternity Age: 12-55   A Adult Age: 15-124

Fracture of Upper Limb (810-819)

☑4ᵗʰ **810 Fracture of clavicle**

| INCLUDES | collar bone
interligamentous part of clavicle

The following fifth-digit subclassification is for use with category 810:
0 **unspecified part**
Clavicle NOS
1 **sternal end of clavicle**
2 **shaft of clavicle**
3 **acromial end of clavicle**

§ ☑5ᵗʰ **810.0 Closed**
[0-3]

§ ☑5ᵗʰ **810.1 Open**
[0-3]

☑4ᵗʰ **811 Fracture of scapula**

| INCLUDES | shoulder blade

The following fifth-digit subclassification is for use with category 811:
0 **unspecified part**
1 **acromial process**
Acromion (process)
2 **coracoid process**
3 **glenoid cavity and neck of scapula**
9 **other**

§ ☑5ᵗʰ **811.0 Closed**
[0-3, 9]

§ ☑5ᵗʰ **811.1 Open**
[0-3, 9]

☑4ᵗʰ **812 Fracture of humerus**

☑5ᵗʰ **812.0 Upper end, closed**

812.00 Upper end, unspecified part
Proximal end   Shoulder

812.01 Surgical neck
Neck of humerus NOS
S42.214A Uns nondsplcd fx surg neck rt I-10
humerus inital enc closed fx

812.02 Anatomical neck

812.03 Greater tuberosity

812.09 Other
Head
Lesser tuberosity
Upper epiphysis
S42.294A Oth nondsplcd fx up end rt humerus I-10
initial enc clos fx

☑5ᵗʰ **812.1 Upper end, open**

812.10 Upper end, unspecified part

812.11 Surgical neck

812.12 Anatomical neck

812.13 Greater tuberosity

812.19 Other

Right Humerus, Anterior View

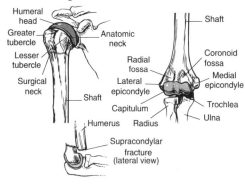

☑5ᵗʰ **812.2 Shaft or unspecified part, closed**

812.20 Unspecified part of humerus
Humerus NOS   Upper arm NOS

812.21 Shaft of humerus
AHA: 4Q, '05, 129; 3Q, '99, 14

☑5ᵗʰ **812.3 Shaft or unspecified part, open**

812.30 Unspecified part of humerus

812.31 Shaft of humerus

☑5ᵗʰ **812.4 Lower end, closed**
Distal end of humerus
Elbow

812.40 Lower end, unspecified part

812.41 Supracondylar fracture of humerus

812.42 Lateral condyle
External condyle

812.43 Medial condyle
Internal epicondyle

812.44 Lower end, unspecified part
Articular process NOS
Lower epiphysis NOS

812.49 Other
Multiple fractures of lower end
Trochlea

☑5ᵗʰ **812.5 Lower end, open**

812.50 Lower end, unspecified part

812.51 Supracondylar fracture of humerus

812.52 Lateral condyle

812.53 Medial condyle

812.54 Condyle(s), unspecified

812.59 Other

☑4ᵗʰ **813 Fracture of radius and ulna**

☑5ᵗʰ **813.0 Upper end, closed**
Proximal end

813.00 Upper end of forearm, unspecified

813.01 Olecranon process of ulna

813.02 Coronoid process of ulna

813.03 Monteggia's fracture
DEF: Fracture near the head of the ulnar shaft, causing
dislocation of the radial head.

**813.04 Other and unspecified fractures of
proximal end of ulna (alone)**
Multiple fractures of ulna, upper end

813.05 Head of radius

813.06 Neck of radius

**813.07 Other and unspecified fractures of
proximal end of radius (alone)**
Multiple fractures of radius, upper end

813.08 Radius with ulna, upper end [any part]

Right Clavicle and Scapula, Anterior View

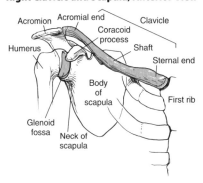

§   Requires fifth digit. Valid digits are In [brackets] under each code. See appropriate category for codes and definitions.

☑4ᵗʰ/☑5ᵗʰ Additional Digit Required   Unspecified Code   Other Specified Code   Manifestation Code   ▶◀ Revised Text   ● New Code   ▲ Revised Code Title

2011 ICD-9-CM   **Volume 1 – 279**

Injury and Poisoning

813.1–815.1

Right Radius and Ulna, Anterior View

√5ᵗʰ **813.1 Upper end, open**

　　813.10 Upper end of forearm, unspecified

　　813.11 Olecranon process of ulna

　　813.12 Coronoid process of ulna

　　813.13 Monteggia's fracture

　　813.14 Other and unspecified fractures of proximal end of ulna (alone)

　　813.15 Head of radius

　　813.16 Neck of radius

　　813.17 Other and unspecified fractures of proximal end of radius (alone)

　　813.18 Radius with ulna, upper end [any part]

√5ᵗʰ **813.2 Shaft, closed**

　　813.20 Shaft, unspecified

　　813.21 Radius (alone)

　　813.22 Ulna (alone)

　　813.23 Radius with ulna
　　　　AHA: ▶4Q, '09, 120◀

√5ᵗʰ **813.3 Shaft, open**

　　813.30 Shaft, unspecified

　　813.31 Radius (alone)

　　813.32 Ulna (alone)

　　813.33 Radius with ulna

√5ᵗʰ **813.4 Lower end, closed**
　　Distal end

　　813.40 Lower end of forearm, unspecified

　　813.41 Colles' fracture
　　　　Smith's fracture
　　　　DEF: Break of lower end of radius; associated with backward movement of the radius lower section.

　　813.42 Other fractures of distal end of radius (alone)
　　　　Dupuytren's fracture, radius
　　　　Radius, lower end
　　　　DEF: Dupuytren's fracture: fracture and dislocation of the forearm; the fracture is of the radius above the wrist, and the dislocation is of the ulna at the lower end.
　　　　S52.501A Uns fx lower end rt radius initial enc closed fx　　I-10

　　813.43 Distal end of ulna (alone)
　　　　Ulna:　　　　　Ulna:
　　　　　head　　　　　lower epiphysis
　　　　　lower end　　　styloid process

　　813.44 Radius with ulna, lower end
　　　　AHA: 1Q, '07, 7

　　813.45 Torus fracture of radius (alone)
　　　　EXCLUDES　torus fracture of radius and ulna (813.47)
　　　　AHA: 4Q, '02, 70

　　813.46 Torus fracture of ulna (alone)
　　　　EXCLUDES　torus fracture of radius and ulna (813.47)
　　　　AHA: ▶4Q, '09, 110◀

　　813.47 Torus fracture of radius and ulna
　　　　AHA: ▶4Q, '09, 110◀

√5ᵗʰ **813.5 Lower end, open**

　　813.50 Lower end of forearm, unspecified

　　813.51 Colles' fracture

　　813.52 Other fractures of distal end of radius (alone)

　　813.53 Distal end of ulna (alone)

　　813.54 Radius with ulna, lower end

√5ᵗʰ **813.8 Unspecified part, closed**

　　813.80 Forearm, unspecified

　　813.81 Radius (alone)
　　　　AHA: 2Q, '98, 19

　　813.82 Ulna (alone)

　　813.83 Radius with ulna

√5ᵗʰ **813.9 Unspecified part, open**

　　813.90 Forearm, unspecified

　　813.91 Radius (alone)

　　813.92 Ulna (alone)

　　813.93 Radius with ulna

√4ᵗʰ **814 Fracture of carpal bone(s)**

The following fifth-digit subclassification is for use with category 814:
　　0　carpal bone, unspecified
　　　　Wrist NOS
　　1　navicular [scaphoid] of wrist
　　2　lunate [semilunar] bone of wrist
　　3　triquetral [cuneiform] bone of wrist
　　4　pisiform
　　5　trapezium bone [larger multangular]
　　6　trapezoid bone [smaller multangular]
　　7　capitate bone [os magnum]
　　8　hamate [unciform] bone
　　9　other

§ √5ᵗʰ **814.0 Closed**
　　[0-9]

§ √5ᵗʰ **814.1 Open**
　　[0-9]

√4ᵗʰ **815 Fracture of metacarpal bone(s)**

INCLUDES　hand [except finger]
　　　　　　metacarpus

The following fifth-digit subclassification is for use with category 815:
　　0　metacarpal bone(s), site unspecified
　　1　base of thumb [first] metacarpal
　　　　Bennett's fracture
　　2　base of other metacarpal bone(s)
　　3　shaft of metacarpal bone(s)
　　4　neck of metacarpal bone(s)
　　9　multiple sites of metacarpus

§ √5ᵗʰ **815.0 Closed**
　　[0-4, 9]

§ √5ᵗʰ **815.1 Open**
　　[0-4, 9]

---

§ Requires fifth digit. Valid digits are in [brackets] under each code. See appropriate category for codes and definitions.

N Newborn Age: 0　　　P Pediatric Age: 0-17　　　M Maternity Age: 12-55　　　A Adult Age: 15-124

Hand Fractures

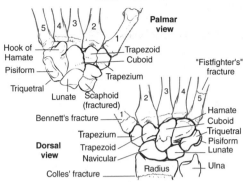

Palmar view

Hook of Hamate
Pisiform
Triquetral
Lunate
Scaphoid (fractured)
Bennett's fracture
Trapezium
Trapezoid
Navicular
Colles' fracture
Radius
Trapezoid
Cuboid
Trapezium
"Fistfighter's" fracture
Hamate
Cuboid
Triquetral
Pisiform
Lunate
Ulna

Dorsal view

✓4ᵗʰ **816 Fracture of one or more phalanges of hand**

INCLUDES finger(s)
thumb

The following fifth-digit subclassification is for use with category 816:
0 phalanx or phalanges, unspecified
1 middle or proximal phalanx or phalanges
2 distal phalanx or phalanges
3 multiple sites

TIP: If phalangeal fracture(s) are due to crushing injury, sequence that code (927.3) first.

§ ✓5ᵗʰ **816.0 Closed**
[0-3]

§ ✓5ᵗʰ **816.1 Open**
[0-3] AHA: For code 816.12: 4Q, '03, 77

✓4ᵗʰ **817 Multiple fractures of hand bones**

INCLUDES metacarpal bone(s) with phalanx or phalanges of same hand

817.0 Closed

817.1 Open

✓4ᵗʰ **818 Ill-defined fractures of upper limb**

INCLUDES arm NOS
multiple bones of same upper limb

EXCLUDES multiple fractures of:
metacarpal bone(s) with phalanx or phalanges (817.0-817.1)
phalanges of hand alone (816.0-816.1)
radius with ulna (813.0-813.9)

818.0 Closed

818.1 Open

✓4ᵗʰ **819 Multiple fractures involving both upper limbs, and upper limb with rib(s) and sternum**

INCLUDES arm(s) with rib(s) or sternum
both arms [any bones]

819.0 Closed

819.1 Open

Fracture of Lower Limb (820-829)

✓4ᵗʰ **820 Fracture of neck of femur**

✓5ᵗʰ **820.0 Transcervical fracture, closed**

820.00 Intracapsular section, unspecified

820.01 Epiphysis (separation) (upper)
Transepiphyseal

820.02 Midcervical section
Transcervical NOS
AHA: 3Q, '03, 12

820.03 Base of neck
Cervicotrochanteric section

820.09 Other
Head of femur   Subcapital
S72.064A Nondsplcd art fx head rt femur initial enc closed fx ▐I-10▌

✓5ᵗʰ **820.1 Transcervical fracture, open**

820.10 Intracapsular section, unspecified

820.11 Epiphysis (separation) (upper)

820.12 Midcervical section

820.13 Base of neck

820.19 Other

✓5ᵗʰ **820.2 Pertrochanteric fracture, closed**

820.20 Trochanteric section, unspecified
Trochanter:
NOS
greater
lesser

820.21 Intertrochanteric section

820.22 Subtrochanteric section
S72.25xA Nondsplcd subtrochant fx lt femur inital enc closed fx ▐I-10▌

✓5ᵗʰ **820.3 Pertrochanteric fracture, open**

820.30 Trochanteric section, unspecified

820.31 Intertrochanteric section

820.32 Subtrochanteric section

820.8 Unspecified part of neck of femur, closed
Hip NOS
Neck of femur NOS
S72.002A Fx uns part neck left femur initial enc clos fx ▐I-10▌

820.9 Unspecified part of neck of femur, open

✓4ᵗʰ **821 Fracture of other and unspecified parts of femur**

✓5ᵗʰ **821.0 Shaft or unspecified part, closed**

821.00 Unspecified part of femur
Thigh
Upper leg
EXCLUDES hip NOS (820.8)

821.01 Shaft
AHA: 1Q, '07, 4; 1Q, '99, 5
S72.331A Displaced obl fx shaft rt femur initial enc clos fx ▐I-10▌

✓5ᵗʰ **821.1 Shaft or unspecified part, open**

821.10 Unspecified part of femur

821.11 Shaft

✓5ᵗʰ **821.2 Lower end, closed**
Distal end

821.20 Lower end, unspecified part

821.21 Condyle, femoral

821.22 Epiphysis, lower (separation)

821.23 Supracondylar fracture of femur

821.29 Other
Multiple fractures of lower end

Right Femur, Anterior View

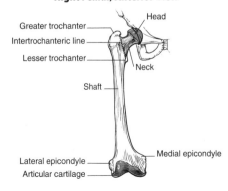

Greater trochanter
Intertrochanteric line
Lesser trochanter
Shaft
Lateral epicondyle
Articular cartilage
Head
Neck
Medial epicondyle

---

§ Requires fifth digit. Valid digits are in [brackets] under each code. See category 816 for codes and definitions.

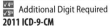

✓4ᵗʰ/✓5ᵗʰ Additional Digit Required   Unspecified Code   Other Specified Code   Manifestation Code   ▶◀ Revised Text   ● New Code   ▲ Revised Code Title

Injury and Poisoning

821.3–825.24

Right Tibia and Fibula, Anterior View

§ ✓5ᵗʰ **823.8 Unspecified part, closed**
[0-2]   Lower leg NOS
AHA: For code 823.82: 1Q, '97, 8

§ ✓5ᵗʰ **823.9 Unspecified part, open**
[0-2]

✓4ᵗʰ **824 Fracture of ankle**
TIP: If ankle fracture also includes syndesmotic injury, assign also code 845.03 Sprains and strains of tibiofibular (ligament), distal.

824.0 Medial malleolus, closed
Tibia involving:
ankle
malleolus
AHA: 1Q, '04, 9

824.1 Medial malleolus, open

824.2 Lateral malleolus, closed
Fibula involving:
ankle
malleolus
AHA: 2Q, '02, 3

824.3 Lateral malleolus, open

824.4 Bimalleolar, closed
Dupuytren's fracture, fibula
Pott's fracture
DEF: Bimalleolar, closed: Breaking of both nodules (malleoli) on either side of ankle joint, without an open wound.
DEF: Dupuytren's fracture (Pott's fracture): The breaking of the farthest end of the lower leg bone (fibula), with injury to the farthest end joint of the other lower leg bone (tibia).
S82.841A Displcd bimalleolar fx rt lw leg intial enc clos fx ⏹I-10

824.5 Bimalleolar, open

824.6 Trimalleolar, closed
Lateral and medial malleolus with anterior or posterior lip of tibia
S82.855G Nondsplcd trimalleolr fx lt lw leg subsq clo delay healing ⏹I-10

824.7 Trimalleolar, open

824.8 Unspecified, closed
Ankle NOS
AHA: 3Q, '00, 12
S89.302A Uns physeal fx low end lt fibula initial enc clo fx ⏹I-10

824.9 Unspecified, open

✓4ᵗʰ **825 Fracture of one or more tarsal and metatarsal bones**

825.0 Fracture of calcaneus, closed
Heel bone
Os calcis

825.1 Fracture of calcaneus, open

✓5ᵗʰ **825.2 Fracture of other tarsal and metatarsal bones, closed**

825.20 Unspecified bone(s) of foot [except toes]
Instep

825.21 Astragalus
Talus

825.22 Navicular [scaphoid], foot

825.23 Cuboid

825.24 Cuneiform, foot

✓5ᵗʰ **821.3 Lower end, open**

821.30 Lower end, unspecified part

821.31 Condyle, femoral

821.32 Epiphysis, lower (separation)

821.33 Supracondylar fracture of femur

821.39 Other

✓4ᵗʰ **822 Fracture of patella**

822.0 Closed
S82.001A Uns fx right patella initial encounter closed fx ⏹I-10

822.1 Open

✓4ᵗʰ **823 Fracture of tibia and fibula**
EXCLUDES Dupuytren's fracture (824.4-824.5)
ankle (824.4-824.5)
radius (813.42, 813.52)
Pott's fracture (824.4-824.5)
that involving ankle (824.0-824.9)

The following fifth-digit subclassification is for use with category 823:
0 tibia alone
1 fibula alone
2 fibula with tibia

§ ✓5ᵗʰ **823.0 Upper end, closed**
[0-2]   Head
Proximal end
Tibia:
condyles
tuberosity
S82.121A Displcd fx lat condyle rt tibia initial enc clos fx ⏹I-10

§ ✓5ᵗʰ **823.1 Upper end, open**
[0-2]

§ ✓5ᵗʰ **823.2 Shaft, closed**
[0-2]

§ ✓5ᵗʰ **823.3 Shaft, open**
[0-2]

§ ✓5ᵗʰ **823.4 Torus fracture**
[0-2]   **DEF:** A bone deformity in children, occurring commonly in the tibia and fibula, in which the bone bends and buckles but does not fracture.
AHA: 4Q, '02, 70

Torus Fracture

Right Foot, Dorsal

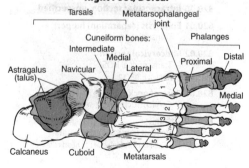

---

§   Requires fifth digit. Valid digits are in [brackets] under each code. See category 823 for codes and definitions.

825.25 Metatarsal bone(s)

825.29 Other
> Tarsal with metatarsal bone(s) only
> EXCLUDES *calcaneus (825.0)*

√5th **825.3 Fracture of other tarsal and metatarsal bones, open**

825.30 Unspecified bone(s) of foot [except toes]

825.31 Astragalus

825.32 Navicular [scaphoid], foot

825.33 Cuboid

825.34 Cuneiform, foot

825.35 Metatarsal bone(s)

825.39 Other

√4th **826 Fracture of one or more phalanges of foot**
> INCLUDES toe(s)

826.0 Closed

826.1 Open

√4th **827 Other, multiple, and ill-defined fractures of lower limb**
> INCLUDES leg NOS
> multiple bones of same lower limb
> EXCLUDES *multiple fractures of:*
> *ankle bones alone (824.4-824.9)*
> *phalanges of foot alone (826.0-826.1)*
> *tarsal with metatarsal bones (825.29, 825.39)*
> *tibia with fibula (823.0-823.9 with fifth-digit 2)*

827.0 Closed

827.1 Open

√4th **828 Multiple fractures involving both lower limbs, lower with upper limb, and lower limb(s) with rib(s) and sternum**
> INCLUDES arm(s) with leg(s) [any bones]
> both legs [any bones]
> leg(s) with rib(s) or sternum

828.0 Closed

828.1 Open

√4th **829 Fracture of unspecified bones**

829.0 Unspecified bone, closed

829.1 Unspecified bone, open

Dislocation (830-839)

> INCLUDES displacement
> subluxation
> EXCLUDES *congenital dislocation (754.0-755.8)*
> *pathological dislocation (718.2)*
> *recurrent dislocation (718.3)*

NOTE The descriptions "closed" and "open," used in the fourth-digit subdivisions, include the following terms:

closed:	open:
complete	compound
dislocation NOS	infected
partial	with foreign body
simple	
uncomplicated	

A dislocation not indicated as closed or open should be classified as closed.

AHA: 3Q, '90, 12

TIP: Do not assign if documentation indicates developmental dislocation; see instead subcategory 718.7.

√4th **830 Dislocation of jaw**
> INCLUDES jaw (cartilage) (meniscus)
> mandible
> maxilla (inferior)
> temporomandibular (joint)

830.0 Closed dislocation

830.1 Open dislocation

√4th **831 Dislocation of shoulder**
> EXCLUDES *sternoclavicular joint (839.61, 839.71)*
> *sternum (839.61, 839.71)*

The following fifth-digit subclassification is for use with category 831:
- 0 **shoulder, unspecified**
  - Humerus NOS
- 1 **anterior dislocation of humerus**
- 2 **posterior dislocation of humerus**
- 3 **inferior dislocation of humerus**
- 4 **acromioclavicular (joint)**
  - Clavicle
- 9 **other**
  - Scapula

TIP: Do not assign if documentation indicates recurrent shoulder dislocation; see instead code 718.31.

§ √5th **831.0 Closed dislocation**
[0-4, 9]

§ √5th **831.1 Open dislocation**
[0-4, 9]

√4th **832 Dislocation of elbow**

The following fifth-digit subclassification is for use with subcategories 832.0 and 832.1:
- 0 **elbow, unspecified**
- 1 **anterior dislocation of elbow**
- 2 **posterior dislocation of elbow**
- 3 **medial dislocation of elbow**
- 4 **lateral dislocation of elbow**
- 9 **other**

§ √5th **832.0 Closed dislocation**
[0-4, 9]

§ √5th **832.1 Open dislocation**
[0-4, 9]

832.2 Nursemaid's elbow
> Subluxation of radial head
> AHA: 4Q, '09, 110-111

√4th **833 Dislocation of wrist**

The following fifth-digit subclassification is for use with category 833:
- 0 **wrist unspecified part**
  - Carpal (bone)
  - Radius, distal end
- 1 **radioulnar (joint), distal**
- 2 **radiocarpal (joint)**
- 3 **midcarpal (joint)**
- 4 **carpometacarpal (joint)**
- 5 **metacarpal (bone), proximal end**
- 9 **other**
  - Ulna, distal end

§ √5th **833.0 Closed dislocation**
[0-5, 9]

§ √5th **833.1 Open dislocation**
[0-5, 9]

√4th **834 Dislocation of finger**
> INCLUDES finger(s)
> phalanx of hand
> thumb

The following fifth-digit subclassification is for use with category 834:
- 0 **finger unspecified part**
- 1 **metacarpophalangeal (joint)**
  - Metacarpal (bone), distal end
- 2 **interphalangeal (joint), hand**

§ √5th **834.0 Closed dislocation**
[0-2]

§ √5th **834.1 Open dislocation**
[0-2]

§ Requires fifth digit. Valid digits are in [brackets] under each code. See appropriate category for codes and definitions.

√4th √5th Additional Digit Required   Unspecified Code   Other Specified Code   Manifestation Code   ►◄ Revised Text   ● New Code   ▲ Revised Code Title

2011 ICD-9-CM   **February 2010 · Volume 1 – 283**

Injury and Poisoning

835–839.59

✓4ᵗʰ **835 Dislocation of hip**

The following fifth-digit subclassification is for use with category 835:
- 0 dislocation of hip, unspecified
- 1 posterior dislocation
- 2 obturator dislocation
- 3 other anterior dislocation

§ ✓5ᵗʰ **835.0 Closed dislocation**
[0-3]

§ ✓5ᵗʰ **835.1 Open dislocation**
[0-3]

✓4ᵗʰ **836 Dislocation of knee**

EXCLUDES   dislocation of knee:
old or pathological (718.2)
recurrent (718.3)
internal derangement of knee joint (717.0-717.5, 717.8-717.9)
old tear of cartilage or meniscus of knee (717.0-717.5, 717.8-717.9)

836.0 Tear of medial cartilage or meniscus of knee, current
Bucket handle tear:
NOS
medial meniscus
} current injury

836.1 Tear of lateral cartilage or meniscus of knee, current

836.2 Other tear of cartilage or meniscus of knee, current
Tear of:

cartilage (semilunar)
meniscus
} current injury, not specified as medial or lateral

836.3 Dislocation of patella, closed

836.4 Dislocation of patella, open

✓5ᵗʰ **836.5 Other dislocation of knee, closed**

836.50 Dislocation of knee, unspecified

836.51 Anterior dislocation of tibia, proximal end
▶Posterior dislocation of femur, distal end, closed◀

836.52 Posterior dislocation of tibia, proximal end
▶Anterior dislocation of femur, distal end, closed◀

836.53 Medial dislocation of tibia, proximal end

836.54 Lateral dislocation of tibia, proximal end

836.59 Other

✓5ᵗʰ **836.6 Other dislocation of knee, open**

836.60 Dislocation of knee, unspecified

836.61 Anterior dislocation of tibia, proximal end
▶Posterior dislocation of femur, distal end, open◀

836.62 Posterior dislocation of tibia, proximal end
▶Anterior dislocation of femur, distal end, open◀

836.63 Medial dislocation of tibia, proximal end

836.64 Lateral dislocation of tibia, proximal end

836.69 Other

✓4ᵗʰ **837 Dislocation of ankle**

INCLUDES   astragalus
fibula, distal end
navicular, foot
scaphoid, foot
tibia, distal end

837.0 Closed dislocation

837.1 Open dislocation

✓4ᵗʰ **838 Dislocation of foot**

The following fifth-digit subclassification is for use with category 838:
- 0 foot unspecified
- 1 tarsal (bone), joint unspecified
- 2 midtarsal (joint)
- 3 tarsometatarsal (joint)
- 4 metatarsal (bone), joint unspecified
- 5 metatarsophalangeal (joint)
- 6 interphalangeal (joint), foot
- 9 other
  Phalanx of foot
  Toe(s)

§ ✓5ᵗʰ **838.0 Closed dislocation**
[0-6, 9]

§ ✓5ᵗʰ **838.1 Open dislocation**
[0-6, 9]

✓4ᵗʰ **839 Other, multiple, and ill-defined dislocations**

✓5ᵗʰ **839.0 Cervical vertebra, closed**
Cervical spine
Neck

839.00 Cervical vertebra, unspecified

839.01 First cervical vertebra

839.02 Second cervical vertebra

839.03 Third cervical vertebra

839.04 Fourth cervical vertebra

839.05 Fifth cervical vertebra

839.06 Sixth cervical vertebra

839.07 Seventh cervical vertebra

839.08 Multiple cervical vertebrae

✓5ᵗʰ **839.1 Cervical vertebra, open**

839.10 Cervical vertebra, unspecified

839.11 First cervical vertebra

839.12 Second cervical vertebra

839.13 Third cervical vertebra

839.14 Fourth cervical vertebra

839.15 Fifth cervical vertebra

839.16 Sixth cervical vertebra

839.17 Seventh cervical vertebra

839.18 Multiple cervical vertebrae

✓5ᵗʰ **839.2 Thoracic and lumbar vertebra, closed**

839.20 Lumbar vertebra

839.21 Thoracic vertebra
Dorsal [thoracic] vertebra

✓5ᵗʰ **839.3 Thoracic and lumbar vertebra, open**

839.30 Lumbar vertebra

839.31 Thoracic vertebra

✓5ᵗʰ **839.4 Other vertebra, closed**

839.40 Vertebra, unspecified site
Spine NOS

839.41 Coccyx

839.42 Sacrum
Sacroiliac (joint)

839.49 Other

✓5ᵗʰ **839.5 Other vertebra, open**

839.50 Vertebra, unspecified site

839.51 Coccyx

839.52 Sacrum

839.59 Other

---

§ Requires fifth digit. Valid digits are in [brackets] under each code. See appropriate category for codes and definitions.

Ⓝ Newborn Age: 0   Ⓟ Pediatric Age: 0-17   Ⓜ Maternity Age: 12-55   Ⓐ Adult Age: 15-124

√5ᵗʰ **839.6 Other location, closed**

839.61 Sternum
Sternoclavicular joint

839.69 Other
Pelvis

√5ᵗʰ **839.7 Other location, open**

839.71 Sternum

839.79 Other

839.8 Multiple and ill-defined, closed
Arm
Back
Hand
Multiple locations, except fingers or toes alone
Other ill-defined locations
Unspecified location

839.9 Multiple and ill-defined, open

Sprains and Strains of Joints and Adjacent Muscles (840-848)

INCLUDES avulsion
hemarthrosis
laceration   of:
rupture   joint capsule
sprain   ligament
strain   muscle
tear   tendon

EXCLUDES *laceration of tendon in open wounds (880-884 and 890-894 with .2)*

√4ᵗʰ **840 Sprains and strains of shoulder and upper arm**

840.0 Acromioclavicular (joint) (ligament)

840.1 Coracoclavicular (ligament)

840.2 Coracohumeral (ligament)

840.3 Infraspinatus (muscle) (tendon)

840.4 Rotator cuff (capsule)
EXCLUDES *complete rupture of rotator cuff, nontraumatic (727.61)*

840.5 Subscapularis (muscle)

840.6 Supraspinatus (muscle) (tendon)

840.7 Superior glenoid labrum lesion
SLAP lesion
AHA: 4Q,'01, 52
DEF: Detachment injury of the superior aspect of the glenoid labrum which is the ring of fibrocartilage attached to the rim of the glenoid cavity of the scapula.

840.8 Other specified sites of shoulder and upper arm

840.9 Unspecified site of shoulder and upper arm
Arm NOS
Shoulder NOS

√4ᵗʰ **841 Sprains and strains of elbow and forearm**

841.0 Radial collateral ligament

841.1 Ulnar collateral ligament

841.2 Radiohumeral (joint)

841.3 Ulnohumeral (joint)

841.8 Other specified sites of elbow and forearm

841.9 Unspecified site of elbow and forearm
Elbow NOS

√4ᵗʰ **842 Sprains and strains of wrist and hand**

√5ᵗʰ **842.0 Wrist**

842.00 Unspecified site

842.01 Carpal (joint)

842.02 Radiocarpal (joint) (ligament)

842.09 Other
Radioulnar joint, distal

√5ᵗʰ **842.1 Hand**

842.10 Unspecified site

842.11 Carpometacarpal (joint)

842.12 Metacarpophalangeal (joint)

842.13 Interphalangeal (joint)

842.19 Other
Midcarpal (joint)

√4ᵗʰ **843 Sprains and strains of hip and thigh**

843.0 Iliofemoral (ligament)

843.1 Ischiocapsular (ligament)

843.8 Other specified sites of hip and thigh

843.9 Unspecified site of hip and thigh
Hip NOS   Thigh NOS

√4ᵗʰ **844 Sprains and strains of knee and leg**

844.0 Lateral collateral ligament of knee

844.1 Medial collateral ligament of knee

844.2 Cruciate ligament of knee

844.3 Tibiofibular (joint) (ligament), superior

844.8 Other specified sites of knee and leg

844.9 Unspecified site of knee and leg
Knee NOS   Leg NOS

√4ᵗʰ **845 Sprains and strains of ankle and foot**

√5ᵗʰ **845.0 Ankle**

845.00 Unspecified site
AHA: 2Q, '02, 3

845.01 Deltoid (ligament), ankle
Internal collateral (ligament), ankle

845.02 Calcaneofibular (ligament)

845.03 Tibiofibular (ligament), distal
AHA: 1Q, '04, 9

845.09 Other
Achilles tendon

√5ᵗʰ **845.1 Foot**

845.10 Unspecified site

845.11 Tarsometatarsal (joint) (ligament)

845.12 Metatarsophalangeal (joint)

845.13 Interphalangeal (joint), toe

845.19 Other

√4ᵗʰ **846 Sprains and strains of sacroiliac region**

846.0 Lumbosacral (joint) (ligament)

846.1 Sacroiliac ligament

846.2 Sacrospinatus (ligament)

846.3 Sacrotuberous (ligament)

846.8 Other specified sites of sacroiliac region

846.9 Unspecified site of sacroiliac region

√4ᵗʰ **847 Sprains and strains of other and unspecified parts of back**
EXCLUDES *lumbosacral (846.0)*

847.0 Neck
Anterior longitudinal (ligament), cervical
Atlanto-axial (joints)
Atlanto-occipital (joints)
Whiplash injury
EXCLUDES *neck injury NOS (959.0)*
thyroid region (848.2)
S13.4xxA Sprain ligaments cervical spine initial encounter   I-10

847.1 Thoracic

847.2 Lumbar

847.3 Sacrum
Sacrococcygeal (ligament)

847.4 Coccyx

Injury and Poisoning

847.9–852.5

847.9 Unspecified site of back
Back NOS

✓4ᵗʰ **848 Other and ill-defined sprains and strains**

848.0 Septal cartilage of nose

848.1 Jaw
Temporomandibular (joint) (ligament)

848.2 Thyroid region
Cricoarytenoid (joint) (ligament)   Thyroid cartilage
Cricothyroid (joint) (ligament)

848.3 Ribs
Chondrocostal (joint)   ⎫ without mention of injury
Costal cartilage   ⎭   to sternum

✓5ᵗʰ **848.4 Sternum**

848.40 Unspecified site

848.41 Sternoclavicular (joint) (ligament)

848.42 Chondrosternal (joint)

848.49 Other
Xiphoid cartilage

848.5 Pelvis
Symphysis pubis
EXCLUDES *that in childbirth (665.6)*

848.8 Other specified sites of sprains and strains

848.9 Unspecified site of sprain and strain

Intracranial Injury, Excluding those with Skull Fracture (850-854)

INCLUDES traumatic brain injury without skull fracture
EXCLUDES *intracranial injury with skull fracture (800-801 and 803-804, except .0 and .5)*
open wound of head without intracranial injury (870.0-873.9)
skull fracture alone (800-801 and 803-804 with .0, .5)

NOTE The description "with open intracranial wound," used in the fourth-digit subdivisions, includes those specified as open or with mention of infection or foreign body.

The following fifth-digit subclassification is for use with categories 851-854:
0 unspecified state of consciousness
1 with no loss of consciousness
2 with brief [less than one hour] loss of consciousness
3 with moderate [1-24 hours] loss of consciousness
4 with prolonged [more than 24 hours] loss of consciousness and return to pre-existing conscious level
5 with prolonged [more than 24 hours] loss of consciousness without return to pre-existing conscious level
  Use fifth-digit 5 to designate when a patient is unconscious and dies before regaining consciousness, regardless of the duration of the loss of consciousness
6 with loss of consciousness of unspecified duration
9 with concussion, unspecified

AHA: 1Q, '93, 22
TIP: If documentation specifies only "head injury," with no further specificity, and is self-limiting, assign instead code 959.01 Head injury, unspecified.

850 Concussion
INCLUDES commotio cerebri
EXCLUDES *concussion with:*
cerebral laceration or contusion (851.0-851.9)
cerebral hemorrhage (852-853)
head injury NOS (959.01)
AHA: 2Q, '96, 6; 4Q, '90, 24
TIP: When a patient is treated for symptoms within 24 to 48 hours of the concussion, clarify with the physician whether the concussion is still in the acute phase or is a postconcussion syndrome; if so, assign instead code 310.2.

850.0 With no loss of consciousness
Concussion with mental confusion or disorientation, without loss of consciousness

✓5ᵗʰ **850.1 With brief loss of consciousness**
Loss of consciousness for less than one hour
AHA: 4Q, '03, 76; 1Q, '99, 10; 2Q, '92, 5

850.11 With loss of consciousness of 30 minutes or less
S06.0x1A Concussion w/loc 30 min/less initial encounter I-10

850.12 With loss of consciousness from 31 to 59 minutes

850.2 With moderate loss of consciousness
Loss of consciousness for 1-24 hours

850.3 With prolonged loss of consciousness and return to pre-existing conscious level
Loss of consciousness for more than 24 hours with complete recovery

850.4 With prolonged loss of consciousness, without return to pre-existing conscious level

850.5 With loss of consciousness of unspecified duration
S06.0x9A Concussion w/loc uns duration initial encounter   I-10

850.9 Concussion, unspecified

✓4ᵗʰ **851 Cerebral laceration and contusion**
AHA: 4Q, '96, 36; 1Q, '93, 22; 4Q, '90, 24

§ ✓5ᵗʰ **851.0 Cortex (cerebral) contusion without mention of**
[0-6, 9]**open intracranial wound**

§ ✓5ᵗʰ **851.1 Cortex (cerebral) contusion with open**
[0-6, 9]**intracranial wound**
AHA: 1Q, '92, 9

§ ✓5ᵗʰ **851.2 Cortex (cerebral) laceration without mention of**
[0-6, 9]**open intracranial wound**
S06.5x0A Traumatic subdurl hemorrhage w/o loc initial enc   I-10

§ ✓5ᵗʰ **851.3 Cortex (cerebral) laceration with open intracranial wound**
[0-6, 9]

§ ✓5ᵗʰ **851.4 Cerebellar or brain stem contusion without mention of**
[0-6, 9]**open intracranial wound**

§ ✓5ᵗʰ **851.5 Cerebellar or brain stem contusion with open**
[0-6, 9]**intracranial wound**

§ ✓5ᵗʰ **851.6 Cerebellar or brain stem laceration without**
[0-6, 9]**mention of open intracranial wound**

§ ✓5ᵗʰ **851.7 Cerebellar or brain stem laceration with open**
[0-6, 9]**intracranial wound**

§ ✓5ᵗʰ **851.8 Other and unspecified cerebral laceration and**
[0-6, 9]**contusion, without mention of open intracranial wound**
Brain (membrane) NOS
AHA: 4Q, '96, 37

§ ✓5ᵗʰ **851.9 Other and unspecified cerebral laceration and**
[0-6, 9]**contusion, with open intracranial wound**

✓4ᵗʰ **852 Subarachnoid, subdural, and extradural hemorrhage, following injury**
EXCLUDES *cerebral contusion or laceration (with hemorrhage) (851.0-851.9)*
DEF: Bleeding from lining of brain; due to injury.

§ ✓5ᵗʰ **852.0 Subarachnoid hemorrhage following injury**
[0-6, 9]**without mention of open intracranial wound**
Middle meningeal hemorrhage following injury

§ ✓5ᵗʰ **852.1 Subarachnoid hemorrhage following injury with**
[0-6, 9]**open intracranial wound**

§ ✓5ᵗʰ **852.2 Subdural hemorrhage following injury without**
[0-6, 9]**mention of open intracranial wound**
AHA: 4Q, '96, 43; For codes 852.21-852.29: 4Q, '07, 107

§ ✓5ᵗʰ **852.3 Subdural hemorrhage following injury with**
[0-6, 9]**open intracranial wound**

§ ✓5ᵗʰ **852.4 Extradural hemorrhage following injury without**
[0-6, 9]**mention of open intracranial wound**
Epidural hematoma following injury

§ ✓5ᵗʰ **852.5 Extradural hemorrhage following injury with**
[0-6, 9]**open intracranial wound**

---

§   Requires fifth digit. Valid digits are in [brackets] under each code. See beginning of section 850-854 for codes and definitions.

Brain

✓4ᵗʰ **853 Other and unspecified intracranial hemorrhage following injury**

§ ✓5ᵗʰ **853.0 Without mention of open intracranial wound**
[0-6, 9]   Cerebral compression due to injury
Intracranial hematoma following injury
Traumatic cerebral hemorrhage
AHA: 3Q, '90, 14

§ ✓5ᵗʰ **853.1 With open intracranial wound**
[0-6, 9]

✓4ᵗʰ **854 Intracranial injury of other and unspecified nature**
INCLUDES injury:
brain NOS
cavernous sinus
intracranial
traumatic brain NOS

EXCLUDES any condition classifiable to 850-853
head injury NOS (959.01)

AHA: 1Q, '99, 10; 2Q, '92, 6
TIP: Assign a code from category 854 for traumatic brain injury (TBI) with diffuse axonal injury (DAI), also known as a shear injury.

§ ✓5ᵗʰ **854.0 Without mention of open intracranial wound**
[0-6, 9]   AHA: For code 854.00: ▶4Q, '09, 108;◀ 2Q, '05, 6

§ ✓5ᵗʰ **854.1 With open intracranial wound**
[0-6, 9]

Internal Injury of Thorax, Abdomen, and Pelvis (860-869)

INCLUDES blast injuries
blunt trauma
bruise
concussion injuries (except cerebral)
crushing   of internal
hematoma   organs
laceration
puncture
tear
traumatic rupture

EXCLUDES concussion NOS (850.0-850.9)
flail chest (807.4)
foreign body entering through orifice (930.0-939.9)
injury to blood vessels (901.0-902.9)

NOTE The description "with open wound," used in the fourth-digit subdivisions, includes those with mention of infection or foreign body.

✓4ᵗʰ **860 Traumatic pneumothorax and hemothorax**
DEF: Traumatic pneumothorax: air or gas leaking into pleural space of lung due to trauma.
DEF: Traumatic hemothorax: blood buildup in pleural space of lung due to trauma.
AHA: 2Q, '93, 4
TIP: If there's no mention of trauma associated with pneumothorax, see instead category 512.

860.0 Pneumothorax without mention of open wound into thorax
S27.0xxA Traumatic pneumothorax initial encounter   I-10

860.1 Pneumothorax with open wound into thorax

860.2 Hemothorax without mention of open wound into thorax

860.3 Hemothorax with open wound into thorax

860.4 Pneumohemothorax without mention of open wound into thorax

860.5 Pneumohemothorax with open wound into thorax

✓4ᵗʰ **861 Injury to heart and lung**
EXCLUDES injury to blood vessels of thorax (901.0-901.9)

✓5ᵗʰ **861.0 Heart, without mention of open wound into thorax**
AHA: 1Q, '92, 9

861.00 Unspecified injury

861.01 Contusion
Cardiac contusion
Myocardial contusion
DEF: Bruising within the pericardium with no mention of open wound.

861.02 Laceration without penetration of heart chambers
DEF: Tearing injury of heart tissue, without penetration of chambers; no open wound.

861.03 Laceration with penetration of heart chambers

✓5ᵗʰ **861.1 Heart, with open wound into thorax**

861.10 Unspecified injury

861.11 Contusion

861.12 Laceration without penetration of heart chambers

861.13 Laceration with penetration of heart chambers

✓5ᵗʰ **861.2 Lung, without mention of open wound into thorax**

861.20 Unspecified injury

861.21 Contusion
DEF: Bruising of lung without mention of open wound.
S27.321A Contusion of lung unilateral initial encounter   I-10

861.22 Laceration

✓5ᵗʰ **861.3 Lung, with open wound into thorax**

861.30 Unspecified injury

861.31 Contusion

861.32 Laceration

✓4ᵗʰ **862 Injury to other and unspecified intrathoracic organs**
EXCLUDES injury to blood vessels of thorax (901.0-901.9)

862.0 Diaphragm, without mention of open wound into cavity

862.1 Diaphragm, with open wound into cavity

✓5ᵗʰ **862.2 Other specified intrathoracic organs, without mention of open wound into cavity**

862.21 Bronchus

862.22 Esophagus

862.29 Other
Pleura
Thymus gland

✓5ᵗʰ **862.3 Other specified intrathoracic organs, with open wound into cavity**

862.31 Bronchus

862.32 Esophagus

§ Requires fifth digit. Valid digits are in [brackets] under each code. See beginning of section 850-854 for codes and definitions.

✓4ᵗʰ ✓5ᵗʰ Additional Digit Required   Unspecified Code   Other Specified Code   Manifestation Code   ▶◀ Revised Text   ● New Code   ▲ Revised Code Title

Injury and Poisoning

862.39–867.6

862.39 **Other**

862.8 **Multiple and unspecified intrathoracic organs, without mention of open wound into cavity**
Crushed chest
Multiple intrathoracic organs

862.9 **Multiple and unspecified intrathoracic organs, with open wound into cavity**

√4ᵗʰ 863 **Injury to gastrointestinal tract**

EXCLUDES *anal sphincter laceration during delivery (664.2)*
bile duct (868.0-868.1 with fifth-digit 2)
gallbladder (868.0-868.1 with fifth-digit 2)

863.0 **Stomach, without mention of open wound into cavity**

863.1 **Stomach, with open wound into cavity**

√5ᵗʰ 863.2 **Small intestine, without mention of open wound into cavity**

863.20 **Small intestine, unspecified site**

863.21 **Duodenum**

863.29 **Other**

√5ᵗʰ 863.3 **Small intestine, with open wound into cavity**

863.30 **Small intestine, unspecified site**

863.31 **Duodenum**

863.39 **Other**

√5ᵗʰ 863.4 **Colon or rectum, without mention of open wound into cavity**

863.40 **Colon, unspecified site**

863.41 **Ascending [right] colon**

863.42 **Transverse colon**

863.43 **Descending [left] colon**

863.44 **Sigmoid colon**

863.45 **Rectum**

863.46 **Multiple sites in colon and rectum**

863.49 **Other**

√5ᵗʰ 863.5 **Colon or rectum, with open wound into cavity**

863.50 **Colon, unspecified site**

863.51 **Ascending [right] colon**

863.52 **Transverse colon**

863.53 **Descending [left] colon**

863.54 **Sigmoid colon**

863.55 **Rectum**

863.56 **Multiple sites in colon and rectum**

863.59 **Other**

√5ᵗʰ 863.8 **Other and unspecified gastrointestinal sites, without mention of open wound into cavity**

863.80 **Gastrointestinal tract, unspecified site**

863.81 **Pancreas, head**

863.82 **Pancreas, body**

863.83 **Pancreas, tail**

863.84 **Pancreas, multiple and unspecified sites**

863.85 **Appendix**

863.89 **Other**
Intestine NOS

√5ᵗʰ 863.9 **Other and unspecified gastrointestinal sites, with open wound into cavity**

863.90 **Gastrointestinal tract, unspecified site**

863.91 **Pancreas, head**

863.92 **Pancreas, body**

863.93 **Pancreas, tail**

863.94 **Pancreas, multiple and unspecified sites**

863.95 **Appendix**

863.99 **Other**

√4ᵗʰ 864 **Injury to liver**

The following fifth-digit subclassification is for use with category 864:
0 **unspecified injury**
1 **hematoma and contusion**
2 **laceration, minor**
Laceration involving capsule only, or without significant involvement of hepatic parenchyma [i.e., less than 1 cm deep]
3 **laceration, moderate**
Laceration involving parenchyma but without major disruption of parenchyma [i.e., less than 10 cm long and less than 3 cm deep]
4 **laceration, major**
Laceration with significant disruption of hepatic parenchyma [i.e., 10 cm long and 3 cm deep]
Multiple moderate lacerations, with or without hematoma
Stellate lacerations of liver
5 **laceration, unspecified**
9 **other**

§ √5ᵗʰ 864.0 **Without mention of open wound into cavity**
[0-5, 9]

§ √5ᵗʰ 864.1 **With open wound into cavity**
[0-5, 9]

√4ᵗʰ 865 **Injury to spleen**

The following fifth-digit subclassification is for use with category 865:
0 **unspecified injury**
1 **hematoma without rupture of capsule**
2 **capsular tears, without major disruption of parenchyma**
3 **laceration extending into parenchyma**
4 **massive parenchymal disruption**
9 **other**

§ √5ᵗʰ 865.0 **Without mention of wound into cavity**
[0-4, 9]

§ √5ᵗʰ 865.1 **With open wound into cavity**
[0-4, 9]

√4ᵗʰ 866 **Injury to kidney**

EXCLUDES *acute kidney injury (nontraumatic) (584.9)*

The following fifth-digit subclassification is for use with category 866:
0 **unspecified injury**
1 **hematoma without rupture of capsule**
2 **laceration**
3 **complete disruption of kidney parenchyma**

AHA: 4Q, '08, 192

§ √5ᵗʰ 866.0 **Without mention of open wound into cavity**
[0-3]

§ √5ᵗʰ 866.1 **With open wound into cavity**
[0-3]

√4ᵗʰ 867 **Injury to pelvic organs**

EXCLUDES *injury during delivery (664.0-665.9)*

867.0 **Bladder and urethra, without mention of open wound into cavity**

AHA: N-D, '85, 15
TIP: Assign for urethral injury due to senile patient's pulling out indwelling urinary catheter.
S37.20xA Unspecified injury of bladder initial encounter   I-10

867.1 **Bladder and urethra, with open wound into cavity**

867.2 **Ureter, without mention of open wound into cavity**

867.3 **Ureter, with open wound into cavity**

867.4 **Uterus, without mention of open wound into cavity**   ♀

867.5 **Uterus, with open wound into cavity**   ♀

867.6 **Other specified pelvic organs, without mention of open wound into cavity**
Fallopian tube
Ovary
Prostate
Seminal vesicle
Vas deferens

---

§   Requires fifth digit. Valid digits are in [brackets] under each code. See appropriate category for codes and definitions.

867.7 Other specified pelvic organs, with open wound into cavity

867.8 Unspecified pelvic organ, without mention of open wound into cavity

867.9 Unspecified pelvic organ, with open wound into cavity

✓4ᵗʰ **868 Injury to other intra-abdominal organs**

The following fifth-digit subclassification is for use with category 868:
0 unspecified intra-abdominal organ
1 adrenal gland
2 bile duct and gallbladder
3 peritoneum
4 retroperitoneum
9 other and multiple intra-abdominal organs

§ ✓5ᵗʰ **868.0 Without mention of open wound into cavity**
[0-4, 9]

§ ✓5ᵗʰ **868.1 With open wound into cavity**
[0-4, 9]

✓4ᵗʰ **869 Internal injury to unspecified or ill-defined organs**
INCLUDES   internal injury NOS
multiple internal injury NOS

869.0 Without mention of open wound into cavity

869.1 With open wound into cavity
AHA: 2Q, '89, 15

Open Wound (870-897)

INCLUDES   animal bite
avulsion
cut
laceration
puncture wound
traumatic amputation
EXCLUDES   burn (940.0-949.5)
crushing (925-929.9)
puncture of internal organs (860.0-869.1)
superficial injury (910.0-919.9)
that incidental to:
dislocation (830.0-839.9)
fracture (800.0-829.1)
internal injury (860.0-869.1)
intracranial injury (851.0-854.1)

NOTE The description "complicated" used in the fourth-digit subdivisions includes those with mention of delayed healing, delayed treatment, foreign body, or infection.
AHA: 4Q, '01, 52
TIP: Do not assign a code designated as "complicated" based only on physician documentation of complicated. For coding purposes, there must be indications of delayed healing, delayed treatment, infection, or foreign body.

Open Wound of Head, Neck, and Trunk (870-879)

✓4ᵗʰ **870 Open wound of ocular adnexa**

870.0 Laceration of skin of eyelid and periocular area

870.1 Laceration of eyelid, full-thickness, not involving lacrimal passages

870.2 Laceration of eyelld Involving lacrimal passages

870.3 Penetrating wound of orbit, without mention of foreign body

870.4 Penetrating wound of orbit with foreign body
EXCLUDES   retained (old) foreign body in orbit (376.6)

870.8 Other specified open wounds of ocular adnexa

870.9 Unspecified open wound of ocular adnexa

✓4ᵗʰ **871 Open wound of eyeball**
EXCLUDES   2nd cranial nerve [optic] injury (950.0-950.9)
3rd cranial nerve [oculomotor] injury (951.0)

871.0 Ocular laceration without prolapse of intraocular tissue
DEF: Tear in ocular tissue without displacing structures.
AHA: 3Q, '96, 7

871.1 Ocular laceration with prolapse or exposure of intraocular tissue

871.2 Rupture of eye with partial loss of intraocular tissue
DEF: Forcible tearing of eyeball, with tissue loss.

871.3 Avulsion of eye
Traumatic enucleation
DEF: Traumatic extraction of eyeball from socket.

871.4 Unspecified laceration of eye

871.5 Penetration of eyeball with magnetic foreign body
EXCLUDES   retained (old) magnetic foreign body in globe (360.50-360.59)

871.6 Penetration of eyeball with (nonmagnetic) foreign body
EXCLUDES   retained (old) (nonmagnetic) foreign body in globe (360.60-360.69)

871.7 Unspecified ocular penetration

871.9 Unspecified open wound of eyeball

✓4ᵗʰ **872 Open wound of ear**

✓5ᵗʰ **872.0 External ear, without mention of complication**

872.00 External ear, unspecified site

872.01 Auricle, ear
Pinna
DEF: Open wound of fleshy, outer ear.

872.02 Auditory canal
DEF: Open wound of passage from external ear to eardrum.

✓5ᵗʰ **872.1 External ear, complicated**

872.10 External ear, unspecified site

872.11 Auricle, ear

872.12 Auditory canal

✓5ᵗʰ **872.6 Other specified parts of ear, without mention of complication**

872.61 Ear drum
Drumhead
Tympanic membrane

872.62 Ossicles

872.63 Eustachian tube
DEF: Open wound of channel between nasopharynx and tympanic cavity.

872.64 Cochlea
DEF: Open wound of snail shell shaped tube of inner ear.

872.69 Other and multiple sites

✓5ᵗʰ **872.7 Other specified parts of ear, complicated**

872.71 Ear drum

872.72 Ossicles

872.73 Eustachian tube

872.74 Cochlea

872.79 Other and multiple sites

872.8 Ear, part unspecified, without mention of complication
Ear NOS

872.9 Ear, part unspecified, complicated

✓4ᵗʰ **873 Other open wound of head**

873.0 Scalp, without mention of complication
S01.01xA Laceration w/o foreign body scalp initial enc   I-10

873.1 Scalp, complicated

✓5ᵗʰ **873.2 Nose, without mention of complication**

873.20 Nose, unspecified site

873.21 Nasal septum
DEF: Open wound between nasal passages.

873.22 Nasal cavity
DEF: Open wound of nostrils.

---

§   Requires fifth digit. Valid digits are in [brackets] under each code. See appropriate category for codes and definitions.

Injury and Poisoning

873.23–879.3

873.23 Nasal sinus
DEF: Open wound of mucous-lined respiratory cavities.

873.29 Multiple sites

√5th **873.3 Nose, complicated**

    873.30 Nose, unspecified site

    873.31 Nasal septum

    873.32 Nasal cavity

    873.33 Nasal sinus

    873.39 Multiple sites

√5th **873.4 Face, without mention of complication**

    873.40 Face, unspecified site

    873.41 Cheek

    873.42 Forehead
        Eyebrow
        AHA: 4Q, '96, 43
        S01.81xA Laceration w/o FB other part head   I-10
        initial enc

    873.43 Lip

    873.44 Jaw

    873.49 Other and multiple sites

√5th **873.5 Face, complicated**

    873.50 Face, unspecified site

    873.51 Cheek

    873.52 Forehead

    873.53 Lip

    873.54 Jaw

    873.59 Other and multiple sites

√5th **873.6 Internal structures of mouth, without mention of complication**

    873.60 Mouth, unspecified site

    873.61 Buccal mucosa
        DEF: Open wound of inside of cheek.

    873.62 Gum (alveolar process)

    873.63 Tooth (broken) (fractured) (due to trauma)
        EXCLUDES cracked tooth (521.81)
        AHA: 1Q, '04, 17

    873.64 Tongue and floor of mouth

    873.65 Palate
        DEF: Open wound of roof of mouth.

    873.69 Other and multiple sites

√5th **873.7 Internal structures of mouth, complicated**

    873.70 Mouth, unspecified site

    873.71 Buccal mucosa

    873.72 Gum (alveolar process)

    873.73 Tooth (broken) (fractured) (due to trauma)
        EXCLUDES cracked tooth (521.81)
        AHA: 1Q, '04, 17

    873.74 Tongue and floor of mouth

    873.75 Palate

    873.79 Other and multiple sites

873.8 Other and unspecified open wound of head without mention of complication
    Head NOS

873.9 Other and unspecified complicated open wound of head

√4th **874 Open wound of neck**

√5th **874.0 Larynx and trachea, without mention of complication**

    874.00 Larynx with trachea

    874.01 Larynx

    874.02 Trachea

√5th **874.1 Larynx and trachea, complicated**

    874.10 Larynx with trachea

    874.11 Larynx

    874.12 Trachea

874.2 Thyroid gland, without mention of complication

874.3 Thyroid gland, complicated

874.4 Pharynx, without mention of complication
    Cervical esophagus

874.5 Pharynx, complicated

874.8 Other and unspecified parts, without mention of complication
    Nape of neck
    Supraclavicular region
    Throat NOS

874.9 Other and unspecified parts, complicated

√4th **875 Open wound of chest (wall)**
    EXCLUDES open wound into thoracic cavity (860.0-862.9)
        traumatic pneumothorax and hemothorax (860.1, 860.3, 860.5)
    AHA: 3Q, '95, 17; 3Q, '93, 17

875.0 Without mention of complication

875.1 Complicated

√4th **876 Open wound of back**
    INCLUDES loin
        lumbar region
    EXCLUDES open wound into thoracic cavity (860.0-862.9)
        traumatic pneumothorax and hemothorax (860.1, 860.3, 860.5)

876.0 Without mention of complication

876.1 Complicated

√4th **877 Open wound of buttock**
    INCLUDES sacroiliac region

877.0 Without mention of complication

877.1 Complicated

√4th **878 Open wound of genital organs (external), including traumatic amputation**
    EXCLUDES injury during delivery (664.0-665.9)
        internal genital organs (867.0-867.9)

878.0 Penis, without mention of complication   ♂

878.1 Penis, complicated   ♂

878.2 Scrotum and testes, without mention of complication   ♂

878.3 Scrotum and testes, complicated   ♂

878.4 Vulva, without mention of complication   ♀
    Labium (majus) (minus)

878.5 Vulva, complicated   ♀

878.6 Vagina, without mention of complication   ♀

878.7 Vagina, complicated   ♀

878.8 Other and unspecified parts, without mention of complication

878.9 Other and unspecified parts, complicated

√4th **879 Open wound of other and unspecified sites, except limbs**

879.0 Breast, without mention of complication

879.1 Breast, complicated

879.2 Abdominal wall, anterior, without mention of complication
    Abdominal wall NOS
    Epigastric region
    Hypogastric region
    Pubic region
    Umbilical region
    AHA: 2Q, '91, 22; 3Q, '90, 5
    TIP: If the abdominal wall open wound results in aortic rupture, sequence code 902.0 first.

879.3 Abdominal wall, anterior, complicated

879.4 Abdominal wall, lateral, without mention of complication
Flank
Groin
Hypochondrium
Iliac (region)
Inguinal region

879.5 Abdominal wall, lateral, complicated

879.6 Other and unspecified parts of trunk, without mention of complication
Pelvic region
Perineum
Trunk NOS

879.7 Other and unspecified parts of trunk, complicated

879.8 Open wound(s) (multiple) of unspecified site(s) without mention of complication
Multiple open wounds NOS
Open wound NOS

879.9 Open wound(s) (multiple) of unspecified site(s), complicated

Open Wound of Upper Limb (880-887)

AHA: N-D, '85, 5
TIP: For degloving injuries, assign code for open wound of the specified site, most often involving extremities.

√4ᵗʰ **880 Open wound of shoulder and upper arm**
The following fifth-digit subclassification is for use with category 880:
    0 shoulder region
    1 scapular region
    2 axillary region
    3 upper arm
    9 multiple sites

§ √5ᵗʰ **880.0 Without mention of complication**
[0-3, 9]

§ √5ᵗʰ **880.1 Complicated**
[0-3, 9] **AHA:** For code 880.13: 2Q, '06, 7

§ √5ᵗʰ **880.2 With tendon involvement**
[0-3, 9]

√4ᵗʰ **881 Open wound of elbow, forearm, and wrist**
The following fifth-digit subclassification is for use with category 881:
    0 forearm
    1 elbow
    2 wrist

§ √5ᵗʰ **881.0 Without mention of complication**
[0-2]

§ √5ᵗʰ **881.1 Complicated**
[0-2]

§ √5ᵗʰ **881.2 With tendon involvement**
[0-2]

√4ᵗʰ **882 Open wound of hand except finger(s) alone**

882.0 Without mention of complication

882.1 Complicated
AHA: 4Q, '08, 152

882.2 With tendon involvement

√4ᵗʰ **883 Open wound of finger(s)**
INCLUDES fingernail
thumb (nail)

883.0 Without mention of complication

883.1 Complicated

883.2 With tendon involvement

√4ᵗʰ **884 Multiple and unspecified open wound of upper limb**
INCLUDES arm NOS
multiple sites of one upper limb
upper limb NOS

884.0 Without mention of complication

884.1 Complicated

884.2 With tendon involvement

√4ᵗʰ **885 Traumatic amputation of thumb (complete) (partial)**
INCLUDES thumb(s) (with finger(s) of either hand)

885.0 Without mention of complication
AHA: 1Q, '03, 7

885.1 Complicated

√4ᵗʰ **886 Traumatic amputation of other finger(s) (complete) (partial)**
INCLUDES finger(s) of one or both hands, without mention of thumb(s)

886.0 Without mention of complication

886.1 Complicated

√4ᵗʰ **887 Traumatic amputation of arm and hand (complete) (partial)**

887.0 Unilateral, below elbow, without mention of complication

887.1 Unilateral, below elbow, complicated

887.2 Unilateral, at or above elbow, without mention of complication

887.3 Unilateral, at or above elbow, complicated

887.4 Unilateral, level not specified, without mention of complication

887.5 Unilateral, level not specified, complicated

887.6 Bilateral [any level], without mention of complication
One hand and other arm

887.7 Bilateral [any level], complicated

Open Wound of Lower Limb (890-897)

AHA: N-D, '85, 5

√4ᵗʰ **890 Open wound of hip and thigh**

890.0 Without mention of complication

890.1 Complicated

890.2 With tendon involvement

√4ᵗʰ **891 Open wound of knee, leg [except thigh], and ankle**
INCLUDES leg NOS
multiple sites of leg, except thigh
EXCLUDES that of thigh (890.0-890.2)
with multiple sites of lower limb (894.0-894.2)

891.0 Without mention of complication
S81.031A Puncture wound w/o FB rt knee initial encounter   I-10

891.1 Complicated

891.2 With tendon involvement

√4ᵗʰ **892 Open wound of foot except toe(s) alone**
INCLUDES heel

892.0 Without mention of complication

892.1 Complicated

892.2 With tendon involvement

√4ᵗʰ **893 Open wound of toe(s)**
INCLUDES toenail

893.0 Without mention of complication

893.1 Complicated
AHA: 4Q, '08, 73

893.2 With tendon involvement

√4ᵗʰ **894 Multiple and unspecified open wound of lower limb**
INCLUDES lower limb NOS
multiple sites of one lower limb, with thigh

894.0 Without mention of complication

894.1 Complicated

894.2 With tendon involvement

§ Requires fifth digit. Valid digits are in [brackets] under each code. See appropriate category for codes and definitions.

Injury and Poisoning

895–903.01

☑4ᵗʰ **895 Traumatic amputation of toe(s) (complete) (partial)**
INCLUDES toe(s) of one or both feet

895.0 Without mention of complication

895.1 Complicated

☑4ᵗʰ **896 Traumatic amputation of foot (complete) (partial)**

896.0 Unilateral, without mention of complication

896.1 Unilateral, complicated

896.2 Bilateral, without mention of complication
EXCLUDES one foot and other leg (897.6-897.7)

896.3 Bilateral, complicated

☑4ᵗʰ **897 Traumatic amputation of leg(s) (complete) (partial)**

897.0 Unilateral, below knee, without mention of complication

897.1 Unilateral, below knee, complicated

897.2 Unilateral, at or above knee, without mention of complication

897.3 Unilateral, at or above knee, complicated

897.4 Unilateral, level not specified, without mention of complication

897.5 Unilateral, level not specified, complicated

897.6 Bilateral [any level], without mention of complication
One foot and other leg

897.7 Bilateral [any level], complicated
AHA: 3Q, '90, 5

Injury to Blood Vessels (900-904)

INCLUDES arterial hematoma
        avulsion
        cut   of blood vessel
        laceration   secondary to other
        rupture   injuries, e.g.;
        traumatic aneurysm or fistula   fracture or open
          (arteriovenous)   wound

EXCLUDES accidental puncture or laceration during medical procedure (998.2)
           intracranial hemorrhage following injury (851.0-854.1)
AHA: 3Q, '90, 5

☑4ᵗʰ **900 Injury to blood vessels of head and neck**

☑5ᵗʰ **900.0 Carotid artery**

900.00 Carotid artery, unspecified

900.01 Common carotid artery

900.02 External carotid artery

900.03 Internal carotid artery

900.1 Internal jugular vein

☑5ᵗʰ **900.8 Other specified blood vessels of head and neck**

900.81 External jugular vein
Jugular vein NOS

900.82 Multiple blood vessels of head and neck

900.89 Other

900.9 Unspecified blood vessel of head and neck

☑4ᵗʰ **901 Injury to blood vessels of thorax**
EXCLUDES traumatic hemothorax (860.2-860.5)

901.0 Thoracic aorta

901.1 Innominate and subclavian arteries

901.2 Superior vena cava

901.3 Innominate and subclavian veins

☑5ᵗʰ **901.4 Pulmonary blood vessels**

901.40 Pulmonary vessel(s), unspecified

901.41 Pulmonary artery

901.42 Pulmonary vein

☑5ᵗʰ **901.8 Other specified blood vessels of thorax**

901.81 Intercostal artery or vein

901.82 Internal mammary artery or vein

901.83 Multiple blood vessels of thorax

901.89 Other
Azygos vein
Hemiazygos vein

901.9 Unspecified blood vessel of thorax

☑4ᵗʰ **902 Injury to blood vessels of abdomen and pelvis**

902.0 Abdominal aorta

☑5ᵗʰ **902.1 Inferior vena cava**

902.10 Inferior vena cava, unspecified

902.11 Hepatic veins

902.19 Other

☑5ᵗʰ **902.2 Celiac and mesenteric arteries**

902.20 Celiac and mesenteric arteries, unspecified

902.21 Gastric artery

902.22 Hepatic artery

902.23 Splenic artery

902.24 Other specified branches of celiac axis

902.25 Superior mesenteric artery (trunk)

902.26 Primary branches of superior mesenteric artery
Ileocolic artery

902.27 Inferior mesenteric artery

902.29 Other

☑5ᵗʰ **902.3 Portal and splenic veins**

902.31 Superior mesenteric vein and primary subdivisions
Ileocolic vein

902.32 Inferior mesenteric vein

902.33 Portal vein

902.34 Splenic vein

902.39 Other
Cystic vein
Gastric vein

☑5ᵗʰ **902.4 Renal blood vessels**

902.40 Renal vessel(s), unspecified

902.41 Renal artery

902.42 Renal vein

902.49 Other
Suprarenal arteries

☑5ᵗʰ **902.5 Iliac blood vessels**

902.50 Iliac vessel(s), unspecified

902.51 Hypogastric artery

902.52 Hypogastric vein

902.53 Iliac artery

902.54 Iliac vein

902.55 Uterine artery   ♀

902.56 Uterine vein   ♀

902.59 Other

☑5ᵗʰ **902.8 Other specified blood vessels of abdomen and pelvis**

902.81 Ovarian artery   ♀

902.82 Ovarian vein   ♀

902.87 Multiple blood vessels of abdomen and pelvis

902.89 Other

902.9 Unspecified blood vessel of abdomen and pelvis

☑4ᵗʰ **903 Injury to blood vessels of upper extremity**

☑5ᵗʰ **903.0 Axillary blood vessels**

903.00 Axillary vessel(s), unspecified

903.01 Axillary artery

903.02 Axillary vein

903.1 Brachial blood vessels

903.2 Radial blood vessels

903.3 Ulnar blood vessels

903.4 Palmar artery

903.5 Digital blood vessels

903.8 Other specified blood vessels of upper extremity
> Multiple blood vessels of upper extremity

903.9 Unspecified blood vessel of upper extremity

√4ᵗʰ **904 Injury to blood vessels of lower extremity and unspecified sites**

904.0 Common femoral artery
> Femoral artery above profunda origin

904.1 Superficial femoral artery

904.2 Femoral veins

904.3 Saphenous veins
> Saphenous vein (greater) (lesser)

√5ᵗʰ **904.4 Popliteal blood vessels**

904.40 Popliteal vessel(s), unspecified

904.41 Popliteal artery

904.42 Popliteal vein

√5ᵗʰ **904.5 Tibial blood vessels**

904.50 Tibial vessel(s), unspecified

904.51 Anterior tibial artery

904.52 Anterior tibial vein

904.53 Posterior tibial artery

904.54 Posterior tibial vein

904.6 Deep plantar blood vessels

904.7 Other specified blood vessels of lower extremity
> Multiple blood vessels of lower extremity

904.8 Unspecified blood vessel of lower extremity

904.9 Unspecified site
> Injury to blood vessel NOS

Late Effects of Injuries, Poisonings, Toxic Effects, and Other External Causes (905-909)

> **NOTE** These categories are to be used to indicate conditions classifiable to 800-999 as the cause of late effects, which are themselves classified elsewhere. The "late effects" include those specified as such, or as sequelae, which may occur at any time after the acute injury.

√4ᵗʰ **905 Late effects of musculoskeletal and connective tissue injuries**
> AHA: 1Q, '95, 10; 2Q, '94, 3

905.0 Late effect of fracture of skull and face bones
> Late effect of injury classifiable to 800-804
> AHA: 3Q, '97, 12

905.1 Late effect of fracture of spine and trunk without mention of spinal cord lesion
> Late effect of injury classifiable to 805, 807-809
> AHA: 1Q, '07, 20

905.2 Late effect of fracture of upper extremities
> Late effect of injury classifiable to 810-819

905.3 Late effect of fracture of neck of femur
> Late effect of injury classifiable to 820

905.4 Late effect of fracture of lower extremities
> Late effect of injury classifiable to 821-827
> S79.001S Uns physeal fx upper end right femur sequela   I-10

905.5 Late effect of fracture of multiple and unspecified bones
> Late effect of injury classifiable to 828-829

905.6 Late effect of dislocation
> Late effect of injury classifiable to 830-839

905.7 Late effect of sprain and strain without mention of tendon injury
> Late effect of injury classifiable to 840-848, except tendon injury

905.8 Late effect of tendon injury
> Late effect of tendon injury due to:
>> open wound [injury classifiable to 880-884 with .2, 890-894 with .2]
>> sprain and strain [injury classifiable to 840-848]
> AHA: 2Q, '89, 13; 2Q, '89, 15

905.9 Late effect of traumatic amputation
> Late effect of injury classifiable to 885-887, 895-897
> **EXCLUDES** *late amputation stump complication (997.60-997.69)*

√4ᵗʰ **906 Late effects of injuries to skin and subcutaneous tissues**

906.0 Late effect of open wound of head, neck, and trunk
> Late effect of injury classifiable to 870-879

906.1 Late effect of open wound of extremities without mention of tendon injury
> Late effect of injury classifiable to 880-884, 890-894 except .2

906.2 Late effect of superficial injury
> Late effect of injury classifiable to 910-919

906.3 Late effect of contusion
> Late effect of injury classifiable to 920-924

906.4 Late effect of crushing
> Late effect of injury classifiable to 925-929

906.5 Late effect of burn of eye, face, head, and neck
> Late effect of injury classifiable to 940-941
> AHA: 4Q, '04, 76

906.6 Late effect of burn of wrist and hand
> Late effect of injury classifiable to 944
> AHA: 4Q, '94, 22

906.7 Late effect of burn of other extremities
> Late effect of injury classifiable to 943 or 945
> AHA: 4Q, '94, 22

906.8 Late effect of burns of other specified sites
> Late effect of injury classifiable to 942, 946-947
> AHA: 4Q, '94, 22

906.9 Late effect of burn of unspecified site
> Late effect of injury classifiable to 948-949
> AHA: 4Q, '94, 22

√4ᵗʰ **907 Late effects of injuries to the nervous system**

907.0 Late effect of intracranial injury without mention of skull fracture
> Late effect of injury classifiable to 850-854
> AHA: ▶4Q, '09, 108;◀ 4Q, '08, 108; 4Q, '03, 103; 3Q, '90, 14
> S06.2x1S Diffuse traumatic brain inj loc 30 min/less sequela   I-10

907.1 Late effect of injury to cranial nerve
> Late effect of injury classifiable to 950-951

907.2 Late effect of spinal cord injury
> Late effect of injury classifiable to 806, 952
> AHA: 4Q, '03, 103; 4Q, '98, 38
> S34.114S Complete lesion L4 of lumbar spinal cord sequela   I-10

907.3 Late effect of injury to nerve root(s), spinal plexus(es), and other nerves of trunk
> Late effect of injury classifiable to 953-954
> AHA: 2Q, '07, 11

907.4 Late effect of injury to peripheral nerve of shoulder girdle and upper limb
> Late effect of injury classifiable to 955

907.5 Late effect of injury to peripheral nerve of pelvic girdle and lower limb
> Late effect of injury classifiable to 956

907.9 Late effect of injury to other and unspecified nerve
> Late effect of injury classifiable to 957

√4ᵗʰ **908 Late effects of other and unspecified injuries**

908.0 Late effect of internal injury to chest
> Late effect of injury classifiable to 860-862

908.1 Late effect of internal injury to intra-abdominal organs
> Late effect of injury classifiable to 863-866, 868

√4ᵗʰ√5ᵗʰ Additional Digit Required   Unspecified Code   Other Specified Code   Manifestation Code   ▶◀ Revised Text   ● New Code   ▲ Revised Code Title

2011 ICD-9-CM   **February 2010 · Volume 1 – 293**

908.2 Late effect of internal injury to other internal organs
Late effect of injury classifiable to 867 or 869

908.3 Late effect of injury to blood vessel of head, neck, and extremities
Late effect of injury classifiable to 900, 903-904

908.4 Late effect of injury to blood vessel of thorax, abdomen, and pelvis
Late effect of injury classifiable to 901-902

908.5 Late effect of foreign body in orifice
Late effect of injury classifiable to 930-939

908.6 Late effect of certain complications of trauma
Late effect of complications classifiable to 958

908.9 Late effect of unspecified injury
Late effect of injury classifiable to 959
AHA: 3Q, '00, 4

✓4ᵗʰ **909 Late effects of other and unspecified external causes**

909.0 Late effect of poisoning due to drug, medicinal or biological substance
Late effect of conditions classifiable to 960-979
EXCLUDES late effect of adverse effect of drug, medicinal or biological substance (909.5)
AHA: 4Q, '03, 103

909.1 Late effect of toxic effects of nonmedical substances
Late effect of conditions classifiable to 980-989

909.2 Late effect of radiation
Late effect of conditions classifiable to 990

909.3 Late effect of complications of surgical and medical care
Late effect of conditions classifiable to 996-999
AHA: 1Q, '93, 29

909.4 Late effect of certain other external causes
Late effect of conditions classifiable to 991-994

909.5 Late effect of adverse effect of drug, medical or biological substance
EXCLUDES late effect of poisoning due to drug, medicinal or biological substance (909.0)
AHA: 4Q, '94, 48

909.9 Late effect of other and unspecified external causes

Superficial Injury (910-919)

EXCLUDES burn (blisters) (940.0-949.5)
contusion (920-924.9)
foreign body:
granuloma (728.82)
inadvertently left in operative wound (998.4)
residual in soft tissue (729.6)
insect bite, venomous (989.5)
open wound with incidental foreign body (870.0-897.7)
AHA: 2Q, '89, 15
TIP: Do not code separately when associated with more severe injuries of the same site.

✓4ᵗʰ **910 Superficial injury of face, neck, and scalp except eye**
INCLUDES cheek
ear
gum
lip
nose
throat
EXCLUDES eye and adnexa (918.0-918.9)

910.0 Abrasion or friction burn without mention of infection
S00.01xA Abrasion of scalp initial encounter   I-10

910.1 Abrasion or friction burn, infected

910.2 Blister without mention of infection

910.3 Blister, infected

910.4 Insect bite, nonvenomous, without mention of infection

910.5 Insect bite, nonvenomous, infected

910.6 Superficial foreign body (splinter) without major open wound and without mention of infection

910.7 Superficial foreign body (splinter) without major open wound, infected

910.8 Other and unspecified superficial injury of face, neck, and scalp without mention of infection

910.9 Other and unspecified superficial injury of face, neck, and scalp, infected

✓4ᵗʰ **911 Superficial injury of trunk**
INCLUDES
abdominal wall	interscapular region
anus	labium (majus) (minus)
back	penis
breast	perineum
buttock	scrotum
chest wall	testis
flank	vagina
groin	vulva

EXCLUDES hip (916.0-916.9)
scapular region (912.0-912.9)

911.0 Abrasion or friction burn without mention of infection
AHA: 3Q, '01, 10

911.1 Abrasion or friction burn, infected

911.2 Blister without mention of infection

911.3 Blister, infected

911.4 Insect bite, nonvenomous, without mention of infection

911.5 Insect bite, nonvenomous, infected

911.6 Superficial foreign body (splinter) without major open wound and without mention of infection

911.7 Superficial foreign body (splinter) without major open wound, infected

911.8 Other and unspecified superficial injury of trunk without mention of infection

911.9 Other and unspecified superficial injury of trunk, infected

✓4ᵗʰ **912 Superficial injury of shoulder and upper arm**
INCLUDES axilla
scapular region

912.0 Abrasion or friction burn without mention of infection

912.1 Abrasion or friction burn, infected

912.2 Blister without mention of infection

912.3 Blister, infected

912.4 Insect bite, nonvenomous, without mention of infection

912.5 Insect bite, nonvenomous, infected

912.6 Superficial foreign body (splinter) without major open wound and without mention of infection

912.7 Superficial foreign body (splinter) without major open wound, infected

912.8 Other and unspecified superficial injury of shoulder and upper arm without mention of infection

912.9 Other and unspecified superficial injury of shoulder and upper arm infected

✓4ᵗʰ **913 Superficial injury of elbow, forearm, and wrist**

913.0 Abrasion or friction burn without mention of infection

913.1 Abrasion or friction burn, infected

913.2 Blister without mention of infection

913.3 Blister, infected

913.4 Insect bite, nonvenomous, without mention of infection

913.5 Insect bite, nonvenomous, infected

913.6 Superficial foreign body (splinter) without major open wound and without mention of infection

913.7 Superficial foreign body (splinter) without major open wound, infected

913.8 Other and unspecified superficial injury of elbow, forearm, and wrist without mention of infection

913.9 Other and unspecified superficial injury of elbow, forearm, and wrist, infected

☑4ᵗʰ **914 Superficial injury of hand(s) except finger(s) alone**

    914.0 Abrasion or friction burn without mention of infection

    914.1 Abrasion or friction burn, infected

    914.2 Blister without mention of infection

    914.3 Blister, infected

    914.4 Insect bite, nonvenomous, without mention of infection

    914.5 Insect bite, nonvenomous, infected

    914.6 Superficial foreign body (splinter) without major open wound and without mention of infection

    914.7 Superficial foreign body (splinter) without major open wound, infected

    914.8 **Other and unspecified superficial injury of hand without mention of infection**

    914.9 **Other and unspecified superficial injury of hand, infected**

☑4ᵗʰ **915 Superficial injury of finger(s)**

    INCLUDES   fingernail
                  thumb (nail)

    915.0 Abrasion or friction burn without mention of infection

    915.1 Abrasion or friction burn, infected

    915.2 Blister without mention of infection

    915.3 Blister, infected

    915.4 Insect bite, nonvenomous, without mention of infection

    915.5 Insect bite, nonvenomous, infected

    915.6 Superficial foreign body (splinter) without major open wound and without mention of infection

    915.7 Superficial foreign body (splinter) without major open wound, infected

    915.8 **Other and unspecified superficial injury of fingers without mention of infection**

        AHA: 3Q, '01, 10

    915.9 **Other and unspecified superficial injury of fingers, infected**

☑4ᵗʰ **916 Superficial injury of hip, thigh, leg, and ankle**

    916.0 Abrasion or friction burn without mention of infection
        S80.812A Abrasion left lower leg initial encounter   I-10

    916.1 Abrasion or friction burn, infected

    916.2 Blister without mention of infection

    916.3 Blister, infected

    916.4 Insect bite, nonvenomous, without mention of infection

    916.5 Insect bite, nonvenomous, infected

    916.6 Superficial foreign body (splinter) without major open wound and without mention of infection

    916.7 Superficial foreign body (splinter) without major open wound, infected

    916.8 **Other and unspecified superficial injury of hip, thigh, leg, and ankle without mention of infection**

    916.9 **Other and unspecified superficial injury of hip, thigh, leg, and ankle, infected**

☑4ᵗʰ **917 Superficial injury of foot and toe(s)**

    INCLUDES   heel
                  toenail

    917.0 Abrasion or friction burn without mention of infection

    917.1 Abrasion or friction burn, infected

    917.2 Blister without mention of infection

    917.3 Blister, infected

    917.4 Insect bite, nonvenomous, without mention of infection

    917.5 Insect bite, nonvenomous, infected

    917.6 Superficial foreign body (splinter) without major open wound and without mention of infection

    917.7 Superficial foreign body (splinter) without major open wound, infected

    917.8 **Other and unspecified superficial injury of foot and toes without mention of infection**
        AHA: 1Q, '03, 13

    917.9 **Other and unspecified superficial injury of foot and toes infected**
        AHA: 1Q, '03, 13
        TIP: Assign for hair strangulation of toe, with infection.

☑4ᵗʰ **918 Superficial injury of eye and adnexa**

    EXCLUDES   burn (940.0-940.9)
                  foreign body on external eye (930.0-930.9)

    918.0 Eyelids and periocular area
        Abrasion
        Insect bite
        Superficial foreign body (splinter)

    918.1 Cornea
        Corneal abrasion
        Superficial laceration
        EXCLUDES   corneal injury due to contact lens (371.82)

    918.2 Conjunctiva

    918.9 **Other and unspecified superficial injuries of eye**
        Eye (ball) NOS

☑4ᵗʰ **919 Superficial injury of other, multiple, and unspecified sites**

    EXCLUDES   multiple sites classifiable to the same three-digit category (910.0-918.9)

    919.0 Abrasion or friction burn without mention of infection

    919.1 Abrasion or friction burn, infected

    919.2 Blister without mention of infection

    919.3 Blister, infected

    919.4 Insect bite, nonvenomous, without mention of infection

    919.5 Insect bite, nonvenomous, infected

    919.6 Superficial foreign body (splinter) without major open wound and without mention of infection

    919.7 Superficial foreign body (splinter) without major open wound, infected

    919.8 **Other and unspecified superficial injuries without mention of infection**

    919.9 **Other and unspecified superficial injury, infected**

Contusion with Intact Skin Surface (920-924)

    INCLUDES   bruise   } without fracture or open
                 hematoma }   wound

    EXCLUDES   concussion (850.0-850.9)
                  hemarthrosis (840.0-848.9)
                  internal organs (860.0-869.1)
                  that incidental to:
                      crushing injury (925-929.9)
                      dislocation (830.0-839.9)
                      fracture (800.0-829.1)
                      internal injury (860.0-869.1)
                      intracranial injury (850.0-854.1)
                      nerve injury (950.0-957.9)
                      open wound (870.0-897.7)

    920 Contusion of face, scalp, and neck except eye(s)
        Cheek
        Ear (auricle)
        Gum
        Lip
        Mandibular joint area
        Nose
        Throat
        S00.33xA Contusion of nose initial encounter   I-10

☑4ᵗʰ **921 Contusion of eye and adnexa**

    921.0 **Black eye, not otherwise specified**

    921.1 **Contusion of eyelids and periocular area**

    921.2 **Contusion of orbital tissues**

☑4ᵗʰ☑5ᵗʰ Additional Digit Required   Unspecified Code   Other Specified Code   Manifestation Code   ►◄ Revised Text   ● New Code   ▲ Revised Code Title

921.3 Contusion of eyeball

TIP: If iridodialysis (rupture of the root of the iris) is present and is due to the eyeball contusion, assign also code 364.76.

921.9 Unspecified contusion of eye
Injury of eye NOS

☑4th **922 Contusion of trunk**

922.0 Breast

922.1 Chest wall
S20.212A Contusion left front wall thorax initial enc   I-10

922.2 Abdominal wall
Flank
Groin

☑5th **922.3 Back**
AHA: 4Q, '96, 39

922.31 Back
EXCLUDES *interscapular region (922.33)*
AHA: 3Q, '99, 14

922.32 Buttock

922.33 Interscapular region

922.4 Genital organs
Labium (majus) (minus)
Penis
Perineum
Scrotum
Testis
Vagina
Vulva

922.8 Multiple sites of trunk

922.9 Unspecified part
Trunk NOS

☑4th **923 Contusion of upper limb**

☑5th **923.0 Shoulder and upper arm**

923.00 Shoulder region

923.01 Scapular region

923.02 Axillary region

923.03 Upper arm

923.09 Multiple sites

☑5th **923.1 Elbow and forearm**

923.10 Forearm

923.11 Elbow

☑5th **923.2 Wrist and hand(s), except finger(s) alone**

923.20 Hand(s)

923.21 Wrist

923.3 Finger
Fingernail
Thumb (nail)

923.8 Multiple sites of upper limb

923.9 Unspecified part of upper limb
Arm NOS

☑4th **924 Contusion of lower limb and of other and unspecified sites**

☑5th **924.0 Hip and thigh**

924.00 Thigh
AHA: 1Q, '09, 10

924.01 Hip
S70.02xA Contusion of left hip initial encounter   I-10

☑5th **924.1 Knee and lower leg**

924.10 Lower leg

924.11 Knee

☑5th **924.2 Ankle and foot, excluding toe(s)**

924.20 Foot
Heel

924.21 Ankle

924.3 Toe
Toenail

924.4 Multiple sites of lower limb

924.5 Unspecified part of lower limb
Leg NOS

924.8 Multiple sites, not elsewhere classified
AHA: 1Q, '03, 7
S70.10xA Contusion of unspecified thigh initial encounter   I-10

924.9 Unspecified site

Crushing Injury (925-929)

Use additional code to identify any associated injuries, such as:
fractures (800-829)
internal injuries (860.0-869.1)
intracranial injuries (850.0-854.1)
AHA: 4Q, '03, 77; 2Q, '93, 7

☑4th **925 Crushing injury of face, scalp, and neck**
Cheek   Pharynx
Ear   Throat
Larynx

925.1 Crushing injury of face and scalp
Cheek
Ear

925.2 Crushing injury of neck
Larynx
Pharynx
Throat

☑4th **926 Crushing injury of trunk**

926.0 External genitalia
Labium (majus) (minus)
Penis
Scrotum
Testis
Vulva

☑5th **926.1 Other specified sites**

926.11 Back

926.12 Buttock

926.19 Other
Breast

926.8 Multiple sites of trunk

926.9 Unspecified site
Trunk NOS

☑4th **927 Crushing injury of upper limb**

☑5th **927.0 Shoulder and upper arm**

927.00 Shoulder region

927.01 Scapular region

927.02 Axillary region

927.03 Upper arm

927.09 Multiple sites

☑5th **927.1 Elbow and forearm**

927.10 Forearm

927.11 Elbow

☑5th **927.2 Wrist and hand(s), except finger(s) alone**

927.20 Hand(s)

927.21 Wrist

927.3 Finger(s)
AHA: 4Q, '03, 77

927.8 Multiple sites of upper limb

927.9 Unspecified site
Arm NOS

☑4th **928 Crushing injury of lower limb**

☑5th **928.0 Hip and thigh**

928.00 Thigh

N Newborn Age: 0   P Pediatric Age: 0-17   M Maternity Age: 12-55   A Adult Age: 15-124

928.01 Hip

√5ᵗʰ **928.1 Knee and lower leg**

928.10 Lower leg

928.11 Knee

√5ᵗʰ **928.2 Ankle and foot, excluding toe(s) alone**

928.20 Foot
Heel

928.21 Ankle

928.3 Toe(s)

928.8 Multiple sites of lower limb

928.9 Unspecified site
Leg NOS

√4ᵗʰ **929 Crushing injury of multiple and unspecified sites**

929.0 Multiple sites, not elsewhere classified

929.9 Unspecified site

Effects Of Foreign Body Entering Through Orifice (930-939)

EXCLUDES *foreign body:*
granuloma (728.82)
inadvertently left in operative wound (998.4, 998.7)
in open wound (800-839, 851-897)
residual in soft tissues (729.6)
superficial without major open wound (910-919
with .6 or .7)

√4ᵗʰ **930 Foreign body on external eye**

EXCLUDES *foreign body in penetrating wound of:*
eyeball (871.5-871.6)
retained (old) (360.5-360.6)
ocular adnexa (870.4)
retained (old) (376.6)

930.0 Corneal foreign body

930.1 Foreign body in conjunctival sac

930.2 Foreign body in lacrimal punctum

930.8 Other and combined sites

930.9 Unspecified site
External eye NOS

931 Foreign body in ear
Auditory canal   Auricle

932 Foreign body in nose
Nasal sinus   Nostril

√4ᵗʰ **933 Foreign body in pharynx and larynx**

933.0 Pharynx
Nasopharynx
Throat NOS

933.1 Larynx
Asphyxia due to foreign body
Choking due to:
food (regurgitated)
phlegm
TIP: Assign for mucous plug causing asphyxia; otherwise, for tracheobronchial, refer to code 519.19 Other diseases of trachea and bronchus.

√4ᵗʰ **934 Foreign body in trachea, bronchus, and lung**

934.0 Trachea

934.1 Main bronchus
AHA: 3Q, '02, 18

934.8 Other specified parts
Bronchioles
Lung

934.9 Respiratory tree, unspecified
Inhalation of liquid or vomitus, lower respiratory tract NOS

√4ᵗʰ **935 Foreign body in mouth, esophagus, and stomach**

935.0 Mouth

935.1 Esophagus
AHA: 1Q, '88, 13
TIP: If esophageal obstruction is due to stenosis, caustic stricture (e.g., lye ingestion), or tumor, assign instead code 530.3.

935.2 Stomach

936 Foreign body in intestine and colon

937 Foreign body in anus and rectum
Rectosigmoid (junction)

938 Foreign body in digestive system, unspecified
Alimentary tract NOS
Swallowed foreign body

√4ᵗʰ **939 Foreign body in genitourinary tract**

939.0 Bladder and urethra

939.1 Uterus, any part   ♀
EXCLUDES *intrauterine contraceptive device:*
complications from (996.32, 996.65)
presence of (V45.51)

939.2 Vulva and vagina   ♀

939.3 Penis   ♂

939.9 Unspecified site

Burns (940-949)

INCLUDES burns from:
electrical heating appliance
electricity
flame
hot object
lightning
radiation
chemical burns (external) (internal)
scalds
EXCLUDES *friction burns (910-919 with .0, .1)*
sunburn (692.71, 692.76-692.77)
AHA: 4Q, 94, 22; 2Q, '90, 7; 4Q, '88, 3; M-A, '86, 9
TIP: Nonhealing burns are coded as acute burns, as is necrosis of burned skin. Assign code 958.3 for any documented infected burn site.

√4ᵗʰ **940 Burn confined to eye and adnexa**

940.0 Chemical burn of eyelids and periocular area

940.1 Other burns of eyelids and periocular area

940.2 Alkaline chemical burn of cornea and conjunctival sac

940.3 Acid chemical burn of cornea and conjunctival sac

940.4 Other burn of cornea and conjunctival sac

940.5 Burn with resulting rupture and destruction of eyeball

940.9 Unspecified burn of eye and adnexa

√4ᵗʰ **941 Burn of face, head, and neck**
EXCLUDES *mouth (947.0)*

The following fifth-digit subclassification is for use with category 941:
0 face and head, unspecified site
1 ear [any part]
2 eye (with other parts of face, head, and neck)
3 lip(s)
4 chin
5 nose (septum)
6 scalp [any part]
Temple (region)
7 forehead and cheek
8 neck
9 multiple sites [except with eye] of face, head and neck

AHA: 4Q, '94, 22; M-A, '86, 9

§ √5ᵗʰ **941.0 Unspecified degree**
[0-9]

§ √5ᵗʰ **941.1 Erythema [first degree]**
[0-9]   **AHA:** For code 941.19: 3Q, '05, 10

§ √5ᵗʰ **941.2 Blisters, epidermal loss [second degree]**
[0-9]

§ √5ᵗʰ **941.3 Full-thickness skin loss [third degree NOS]**
[0-9]

---

§ Requires fifth digit. Valid digits are in [brackets] under each code. See category 941 for codes and definitions.

§ ✓5ᵗʰ **941.4 Deep necrosis of underlying tissues [deep third**
[0-9]   **degree] without mention of loss of a body part**

§ ✓5ᵗʰ **941.5 Deep necrosis of underlying tissues [deep third**
[0-9]   **degree] with loss of a body part**

✓4ᵗʰ **942 Burn of trunk**

> EXCLUDES *scapular region (943.0-943.5 with fifth-digit 6)*

The following fifth-digit subclassificaiton is for use with category 942:
0 **trunk, unspecified site**
1 **breast**
2 **chest wall, excluding breast and nipple**
3 **abdominal wall**
    Flank
    Groin
4 **back [any part]**
    Buttock
    Interscapular region
5 **genitalia**
    Labium (majus) (minus
    Penis
    Perineum
    Scrotum
    Testis
    Vulva
9 **other and multiple sites of trunk**

AHA: 4Q, '94, 22; M-A, '86, 9

§ ✓5ᵗʰ **942.0 Unspecified degree**
[0-5, 9]

§ ✓5ᵗʰ **942.1 Erythema [first degree]**
[0-5, 9]

§ ✓5ᵗʰ **942.2 Blisters, epidermal loss [second degree]**
[0-5, 9]

§ ✓5ᵗʰ **942.3 Full-thickness skin loss [third degree NOS]**
[0-5, 9]

§ ✓5ᵗʰ **942.4 Deep necrosis of underlying tissues [deep third**
[0-5, 9]**degree] without mention of loss of a body part**

§ ✓5ᵗʰ **942.5 Deep necrosis of underlying tissues [deep third**
[0-5, 9]**degree] with loss of a body part**

✓4ᵗʰ **943 Burn of upper limb, except wrist and hand**

The following fifth-digit subclassificaiton is for use with category 943:
0 **upper limb, unspecified site**
1 **forearm**
2 **elbow**
3 **upper arm**
4 **axilla**
5 **shoulder**
6 **scapular region**
9 **multiple sites of upper limb, except wrist and hand**

AHA: 4Q, '94, 22; M-A, '86, 9

§ ✓5ᵗʰ **943.0 Unspecified degree**
[0-6, 9]

§ ✓5ᵗʰ **943.1 Erythema [first degree]**
[0-6, 9]

§ ✓5ᵗʰ **943.2 Blisters, epidermal loss [second degree]**
[0-6, 9]

§ ✓5ᵗʰ **943.3 Full-thickness skin loss [third degree NOS]**
[0-6, 9]

§ ✓5ᵗʰ **943.4 Deep necrosis of underlying tissues [deep third**
[0-6, 9]**degree] without mention of loss of a body part**

§ ✓5ᵗʰ **943.5 Deep necrosis of underlying tissues [deep third**
[0-6, 9]**degree] with loss of a body part**

✓4ᵗʰ **944 Burn of wrist(s) and hand(s)**

The following fifth-digit subclassification is for use with category 944:
0 **hand, unspecified site**
1 **single digit [finger (nail)] other than thumb**
2 **thumb (nail)**
3 **two or more digits, not including thumb**
4 **two or more digits including thumb**
5 **palm**
6 **back of hand**
7 **wrist**
8 **multiple sites of wrist(s) and hand(s)**

§ ✓5ᵗʰ **944.0 Unspecified degree**
[0-8]

§ ✓5ᵗʰ **944.1 Erythema [first degree]**
[0-8]

§ ✓5ᵗʰ **944.2 Blisters, epidermal loss [second degree]**
[0-8]

§ ✓5ᵗʰ **944.3 Full-thickness skin loss [third degree NOS]**
[0-8]

§ ✓5ᵗʰ **944.4 Deep necrosis of underlying tissues [deep third**
[0-8]   **degree] without mention of loss of a body part**

§ ✓5ᵗʰ **944.5 Deep necrosis of underlying tissues [deep third**
[0-8]   **degree] with loss of a body part**

✓4ᵗʰ **945 Burn of lower limb(s)**

The following fifth-digit subclassification is for use with category 945:
0 **lower limb [leg], unspecified site**
1 **toe(s) (nail)**
2 **foot**
3 **ankle**
4 **lower leg**
5 **knee**
6 **thigh [any part]**
9 **multiple sites of lower limb(s)**

AHA: 4Q, '94, 22; M-A, '86, 9

§ ✓5ᵗʰ **945.0 Unspecified degree**
[0-6, 9]

§ ✓5ᵗʰ **945.1 Erythema [first degree]**
[0-6, 9]

§ ✓5ᵗʰ **945.2 Blisters, epidermal loss [second degree]**
[0-6, 9]

§ ✓5ᵗʰ **945.3 Full-thickness skin loss [third degree NOS]**
[0-6, 9]

§ ✓5ᵗʰ **945.4 Deep necrosis of underlying tissues [deep third**
[0-6, 9]**degree] without mention of loss of a body part**

§ ✓5ᵗʰ **945.5 Deep necrosis of underlying tissues [deep third**
[0-6, 9]**degree] with loss of a body part**

✓4ᵗʰ **946 Burns of multiple specified sites**

> INCLUDES   burns of sites classifiable to more than one three-digit category in 940-945

> EXCLUDES *multiple burns NOS (949.0-949.5)*

AHA: 4Q, '94, 22; M-A, '86, 9
TIP: Only assign if the specific sites of the multiple burns are not specified.

946.0 Unspecified degree

946.1 Erythema [first degree]

946.2 Blisters, epidermal loss [second degree]

946.3 Full-thickness skin loss [third degree NOS]

946.4 Deep necrosis of underlying tissues [deep third degree]
without mention of loss of a body part

946.5 Deep necrosis of underlying tissues [deep third degree]
with loss of a body part

✓4ᵗʰ **947 Burn of internal organs**

> INCLUDES   burns from chemical agents (ingested)

AHA: 4Q, '94, 22; M-A, '86, 9

947.0 Mouth and pharynx
    Gum
    Tongue

---

§   Requires fifth digit. Valid digits are in [brackets] under each code. See appropriate category for codes and definitions.

Burns
Degrees of Burns

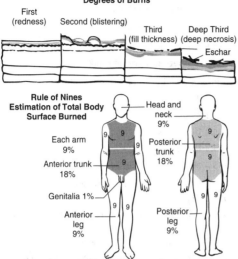

Rule of Nines
Estimation of Total Body Surface Burned

Head and neck 9%

Each arm 9%

Posterior trunk 18%

Anterior trunk 18%

Genitalia 1%

Anterior leg 9%

Posterior leg 9%

947.1 Larynx, trachea, and lung

947.2 Esophagus

947.3 Gastrointestinal tract
Colon   Small intestine
Rectum   Stomach

947.4 Vagina and uterus   ♀

947.8 Other specified sites

947.9 Unspecified site

√4ᵗʰ **948 Burns classified according to extent of body surface involved**
> **NOTE** This category is to be used when the site of the burn is unspecified, or with categories 940-947 when the site is specified.
>
> **EXCLUDES** sunburn (692.71, 692.76-692.77)

The following fifth-digit subclassification is for use with category 948 to indicate the percent of body surface with third degree burn; valid digits are in [brackets] under each code:
  0 less than 10 percent or unspecified
  1 10-19%
  2 20-29%
  3 30-39%
  4 40-49%
  5 50-59%
  6 60-69%
  7 70-79%
  8 80-89%
  9 90% or more of body surface

AHA: 4Q, '94, 22; 4Q, '88, 3; M-A, '86, 9; N-D, '84, 13

§ √5ᵗʰ **948.0 Burn [any degree] involving less than 10**
[0]   **percent of body surface**
> **T31.0** Burns involving less than 10% of body surface   I-10

§ √5ᵗʰ **948.1 10-19 percent of body surface**
[0-1]

§ √5ᵗʰ **948.2 20-29 percent of body surface**
[0-2]

§ √5ᵗʰ **948.3 30-39 percent of body surface**
[0-3]

§ √5ᵗʰ **948.4 40-49 percent of body surface**
[0-4]

§ √5ᵗʰ **948.5 50-59 percent of body surface**
[0-5]

§ √5ᵗʰ **948.6 60-69 percent of body surface**
[0-6]

§ √5ᵗʰ **948.7 70-79 percent of body surface**
[0-7]

§ √5ᵗʰ **948.8 80-89 percent of body surface**
[0-8]

§ √5ᵗʰ **948.9 90 percent or more of body surface**
[0-9]

√4ᵗʰ **949 Burn, unspecified**
> **INCLUDES** burn NOS
>   multiple burns NOS
>
> **EXCLUDES** burn of unspecified site but with statement of the extent of body surface involved (948.0-948.9)

AHA: 4Q, '94, 22; M-A, '86, 9

949.0 Unspecified degree

949.1 Erythema [first degree]

949.2 Blisters, epidermal loss [second degree]

949.3 Full-thickness skin loss [third degree NOS]

949.4 Deep necrosis of underlying tissues [deep third degree] without mention of loss of a body part

949.5 Deep necrosis of underlying tissues [deep third degree] with loss of a body part

Injury to Nerves and Spinal Cord (950-957)
> **INCLUDES** division of nerve
>   lesion in continuity   } (with open
>   traumatic neuroma   wound)
>   traumatic transient paralysis
>
> **EXCLUDES** accidental puncture or laceration during medical procedure (998.2)

√4ᵗʰ **950 Injury to optic nerve and pathways**

950.0 Optic nerve injury
Second cranial nerve

950.1 Injury to optic chiasm

950.2 Injury to optic pathways

950.3 Injury to visual cortex

950.9 Unspecified
Traumatic blindness NOS

√4ᵗʰ **951 Injury to other cranial nerve(s)**

951.0 Injury to oculomotor nerve
Third cranial nerve

951.1 Injury to trochlear nerve
Fourth cranial nerve

951.2 Injury to trigeminal nerve
Fifth cranial nerve

951.3 Injury to abducens nerve
Sixth cranial nerve

951.4 Injury to facial nerve
Seventh cranial nerve

951.5 Injury to acoustic nerve
Auditory nerve
Eighth cranial nerve
Traumatic deafness NOS

951.6 Injury to accessory nerve
Eleventh cranial nerve

951.7 Injury to hypoglossal nerve
Twelfth cranial nerve

951.8 Injury to other specified cranial nerves
Glossopharyngeal [9th cranial] nerve
Olfactory [1st cranial] nerve
Pneumogastric [10th cranial] nerve
Traumatic anosmia NOS
Vagus [10th cranial] nerve

951.9 Injury to unspecified cranial nerve

√4ᵗʰ **952 Spinal cord injury without evidence of spinal bone injury**

√5ᵗʰ **952.0 Cervical**

952.00 C_1-C_4 level with unspecified spinal cord injury
Spinal cord injury, cervical region NOS

952.01 C_1-C_4 level with complete lesion of spinal cord

952.02 C_1-C_4 level with anterior cord syndrome

---

§ Requires fifth digit. Valid digits are in [brackets] under each code. See category 948 for codes and definitions.

Spinal Nerve Roots

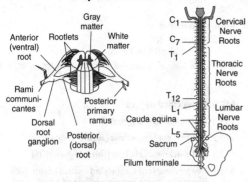

952.03 C$_1$-C$_4$ level with central cord syndrome

952.04 C$_1$-C$_4$ level with other specified spinal cord injury
Incomplete spinal cord lesion at C$_1$-C$_4$ level:
NOS
with posterior cord syndrome

952.05 C$_5$-C$_7$ level with unspecified spinal cord injury

952.06 C$_5$-C$_7$ level with complete lesion of spinal cord

952.07 C$_5$-C$_7$ level with anterior cord syndrome

952.08 C$_5$-C$_7$ level with central cord syndrome

952.09 C$_5$-C$_7$ level with other specified spinal cord injury
Incomplete spinal cord lesion at C$_5$-C$_7$ level:
NOS
with posterior cord syndrome

√5ᵗʰ **952.1 Dorsal [thoracic]**

952.10 T$_1$-T$_6$ level with unspecified spinal cord injury
Spinal cord injury, thoracic region NOS

952.11 T$_1$-T$_6$ level with complete lesion of spinal cord

952.12 T$_1$-T$_6$ level with anterior cord syndrome

952.13 T$_1$-T$_6$ level with central cord syndrome

952.14 T$_1$-T$_6$ level with other specified spinal cord injury
Incomplete spinal cord lesion at T$_1$-T$_6$ level:
NOS
with posterior cord syndrome

952.15 T$_7$-T$_{12}$ level with unspecified spinal cord injury

952.16 T$_7$-T$_{12}$ level with complete lesion of spinal cord

952.17 T$_7$-T$_{12}$ level with anterior cord syndrome

952.18 T$_7$-T$_{12}$ level with central cord syndrome

952.19 T$_7$-T$_{12}$ level with other specified spinal cord injury
Incomplete spinal cord lesion at T$_7$-T$_{12}$ level:
NOS
with posterior cord syndrome

952.2 Lumbar

952.3 Sacral

952.4 Cauda equina

952.8 Multiple sites of spinal cord

952.9 Unspecified site of spinal cord

√4ᵗʰ **953 Injury to nerve roots and spinal plexus**

953.0 Cervical root

953.1 Dorsal root

953.2 Lumbar root

953.3 Sacral root

953.4 Brachial plexus

953.5 Lumbosacral plexus

953.8 Multiple sites

953.9 Unspecified site

√4ᵗʰ **954 Injury to other nerve(s) of trunk, excluding shoulder and pelvic girdles**

954.0 Cervical sympathetic

954.1 Other sympathetic
Celiac ganglion or plexus
Inferior mesenteric plexus
Splanchnic nerve(s)
Stellate ganglion

954.8 Other specified nerve(s) of trunk

954.9 Unspecified nerve of trunk

√4ᵗʰ **955 Injury to peripheral nerve(s) of shoulder girdle and upper limb**

955.0 Axillary nerve

955.1 Median nerve

955.2 Ulnar nerve

955.3 Radial nerve

955.4 Musculocutaneous nerve

955.5 Cutaneous sensory nerve, upper limb

955.6 Digital nerve

955.7 Other specified nerve(s) of shoulder girdle and upper limb

955.8 Multiple nerves of shoulder girdle and upper limb

955.9 Unspecified nerve of shoulder girdle and upper limb

√4ᵗʰ **956 Injury to peripheral nerve(s) of pelvic girdle and lower limb**

956.0 Sciatic nerve

956.1 Femoral nerve

956.2 Posterior tibial nerve

956.3 Peroneal nerve

956.4 Cutaneous sensory nerve, lower limb

956.5 Other specified nerve(s) of pelvic girdle and lower limb

956.8 Multiple nerves of pelvic girdle and lower limb

956.9 Unspecified nerve of pelvic girdle and lower limb

√4ᵗʰ **957 Injury to other and unspecified nerves**

957.0 Superficial nerves of head and neck

957.1 Other specified nerve(s)

957.8 Multiple nerves in several parts
Multiple nerve injury NOS

957.9 Unspecified site
Nerve injury NOS

Certain Traumatic Complications and Unspecified Injuries (958-959)

√4ᵗʰ **958 Certain early complications of trauma**
EXCLUDES *adult respiratory distress syndrome (518.5)*
flail chest (807.4)
post-traumatic seroma (729.91)
shock lung (518.5)
that occurring during or following medical procedures (996.0-999.9)

958.0 Air embolism
Pneumathemia
EXCLUDES *that complicating:*
abortion (634-638 with .6, 639.6)
ectopic or molar pregnancy (639.6)
pregnancy, childbirth, or the puerperium (673.0)
DEF: Arterial obstruction due to introduction of air bubbles into the veins following surgery or trauma.

958.1 Fat embolism
EXCLUDES *that complicating:*
abortion (634-638 with .6, 639.6)
pregnancy, childbirth, or the puerperium (673.8)
DEF: Arterial blockage due to the entrance of fat in circulatory system, after fracture of large bones or administration of corticosteroids.

958.2 Secondary and recurrent hemorrhage

Ⓝ Newborn Age: 0   Ⓟ Pediatric Age: 0-17   Ⓜ Maternity Age: 12-55   Ⓐ Adult Age: 15-124

958.3 Posttraumatic wound infection, not elsewhere classified

> **EXCLUDES** infected open wounds — code to complicated open wound of site
>
> **AHA:** 4Q, '01, 53; S-O, '85, 10
>
> **TIP:** Do not assign if the infection is documented as due to cellulitis; see instead categories 681 and 682 and complicated wound codes.

958.4 Traumatic shock

Shock (immediate) (delayed) following injury

> **EXCLUDES** shock:
> anaphylactic (995.0)
> due to serum (999.4)
> anesthetic (995.4)
> electric (994.8)
> following abortion (639.5)
> lightning (994.0)
> nontraumatic NOS (785.50)
> obstetric (669.1)
> postoperative (998.0)
>
> **DEF:** Shock, immediate or delayed following injury.

958.5 Traumatic anuria

Crush syndrome
Renal failure following crushing

> **EXCLUDES** that due to a medical procedure (997.5)
>
> **DEF:** Complete suppression of urinary secretion by kidneys due to trauma.

958.6 Volkmann's ischemic contracture

Posttraumatic muscle contracture

> **DEF:** Muscle deterioration due to loss of blood supply from injury or tourniquet; causes muscle contraction and results in inability to extend the muscles fully.

958.7 Traumatic subcutaneous emphysema

> **EXCLUDES** subcutaneous emphysema resulting from a procedure (998.81)

958.8 Other early complications of trauma

> **AHA:** 2Q, '92, 13

√5ᵗʰ 958.9 Traumatic compartment syndrome

> **EXCLUDES** nontraumatic compartment syndrome (729.71-729.79)
>
> **DEF:** Compression of nerves and blood vessels within an enclosed space due to previous trauma, which leads to impaired blood flow and muscle and nerve damage.
>
> **TIP:** If the compartment syndrome is specified as chronic or exercise-induced, see instead subcategory 729.7.

> **958.90 Compartment syndrome, unspecified**
>
> > **AHA:** 4Q, '06, 100-102

> **958.91 Traumatic compartment syndrome of upper extremity**
>
> > Traumatic compartment syndrome of shoulder, arm, forearm, wrist, hand, and fingers
> >
> > **AHA:** 4Q, '06, 100-102

> **958.92 Traumatic compartment syndrome of lower extremity**
>
> > Traumatic compartment syndrome of hip, buttock, thigh, leg, foot, and toes
> >
> > **AHA:** 4Q, '06, 100-102

> **958.93 Traumatic compartment syndrome of abdomen**
>
> > **AHA:** 4Q, '06, 100-102

> **958.99 Traumatic compartment syndrome of other sites**
>
> > **AHA:** 4Q, '06, 100-102

√4ᵗʰ 959 Injury, other and unspecified

> **INCLUDES** injury NOS
>
> **EXCLUDES** injury NOS of:
> blood vessels (900.0-904.9)
> eye (921.0-921.9)
> internal organs (860.0-869.1)
> intracranial sites (854.0-854.1)
> nerves (950.0-951.9, 953.0-957.9)
> spinal cord (952.0-952.9)

√5ᵗʰ 959.0 Head, face and neck

> **959.01 Head injury, unspecified**
>
> > **EXCLUDES** concussion (850.1-850.9)
> > with head injury NOS (850.1-850.9)
> > head injury NOS with loss of consciousness (850.1-850.5)
> > specified head injuries (850.0-854.1)
> >
> > **AHA:** 4Q, '08, 108; 4Q, '97, 46
> >
> > **S09.90xA** Unspecified injury of head initial encounter   **I-10**

> **959.09 Injury of face and neck**
>
> > Cheek
> > Ear
> > Eyebrow
> > Lip
> > Mouth
> > Nose
> > Throat
> >
> > **AHA:** 4Q, '97, 46

√5ᵗʰ 959.1 Trunk

> **EXCLUDES** scapular region (959.2)
>
> **AHA:** 4Q, '03, 78; 1Q, '99, 10

> **959.11 Other injury of chest wall**

> **959.12 Other injury of abdomen**

> **959.13 Fracture of corpus cavernosum penis**   ♂

> **959.14 Other injury of external genitals**

> **959.19 Other injury of other sites of trunk**
>
> > Injury of trunk NOS

959.2 Shoulder and upper arm

Axilla
Scapular region

959.3 Elbow, forearm, and wrist

> **AHA:** 1Q, '97, 8

959.4 Hand, except finger

959.5 Finger

Fingernail
Thumb (nail)

959.6 Hip and thigh

Upper leg

959.7 Knee, leg, ankle, and foot

959.8 Other specified sites, including multiple

> **EXCLUDES** multiple sites classifiable to the same four-digit category (959.0-959.7)

959.9 Unspecified site

√4ᵗʰ √5ᵗʰ Additional Digit Required   Unspecified Code   Other Specified Code   Manifestation Code   ►◄ Revised Text   ● New Code   ▲ Revised Code Title

2011 ICD-9-CM   **Volume 1 – 301**

Injury and Poisoning

Poisoning by Drugs, Medicinal and Biological Substances (960-979)

INCLUDES   overdose of these substances
         wrong substance given or taken in error

Use additional code to specify the effects of the poisoning

EXCLUDES   adverse effects ["hypersensitivity," "reaction," etc.] of correct substance properly administered. Such cases are to be classified according to the nature of the adverse effect, such as:
     adverse effect NOS (995.20)
     allergic lymphadenitis (289.3)
     aspirin gastritis (535.4)
     blood disorders (280.0-289.9)
     dermatitis:
         contact (692.0-692.9)
         due to ingestion (693.0-693.9)
     nephropathy (583.9)
     [The drug giving rise to the adverse effect may be identified by use of categories E930-E949.]
     drug dependence (304.0-304.9)
     drug reaction and poisoning affecting the newborn (760.0-779.9)
     nondependent abuse of drugs (305.0-305.9)
     pathological drug intoxication (292.2)

AHA: 2Q, '90, 11

TIP: Assign a poisoning code for interaction between prescribed drug and alcohol or prescribed drug and other nonprescribed drug or medicinal agent. Sequence poisoning code first, then code for manifestation of poisoning.

If respiratory failure is due to a poisoning, the poisoning code must be sequenced first.

✓4ᵗʰ 960 Poisoning by antibiotics

EXCLUDES   antibiotics:
     ear, nose, and throat (976.6)
     eye (976.5)
     local (976.0)

960.0 Penicillins
     Ampicillin
     Carbenicillin
     Cloxacillin
     Penicillin G

960.1 Antifungal antibiotics
     Amphotericin B
     Griseofulvin
     Nystatin
     Trichomycin
     EXCLUDES   preparations intended for topical use (976.0-976.9)

960.2 Chloramphenicol group
     Chloramphenicol
     Thiamphenicol

960.3 Erythromycin and other macrolides
     Oleandomycin
     Spiramycin

960.4 Tetracycline group
     Doxycycline
     Minocycline
     Oxytetracycline

960.5 Cephalosporin group
     Cephalexin
     Cephaloglycin
     Cephaloridine
     Cephalothin

960.6 Antimycobacterial antibiotics
     Cycloserine
     Kanamycin
     Rifampin
     Streptomycin

960.7 Antineoplastic antibiotics
     Actinomycin such as:
         Bleomycin
         Cactinomycin
         Dactinomycin
         Daunorubicin
         Mitomycin

960.8 Other specified antibiotics

960.9 Unspecified antibiotic

✓4ᵗʰ 961 Poisoning by other anti-infectives

EXCLUDES   anti-infectives:
     ear, nose, and throat (976.6)
     eye (976.5)
     local (976.0)

961.0 Sulfonamides
     Sulfadiazine
     Sulfafurazole
     Sulfamethoxazole

961.1 Arsenical anti-infectives

961.2 Heavy metal anti-infectives
     Compounds of:
         antimony
         bismuth
         lead
         mercury
     EXCLUDES   mercurial diuretics (974.0)

961.3 Quinoline and hydroxyquinoline derivatives
     Chiniofon
     Diiodohydroxyquin
     EXCLUDES   antimalarial drugs (961.4)

961.4 Antimalarials and drugs acting on other blood protozoa
     Chloroquine
     Cycloguanil
     Primaquine
     Proguanil [chloroguanide]
     Pyrimethamine
     Quinine

961.5 Other antiprotozoal drugs
     Emetine

961.6 Anthelmintics
     Hexylresorcinol
     Piperazine
     Thiabendazole

961.7 Antiviral drugs
     Methisazone
     EXCLUDES   amantadine (966.4)
         cytarabine (963.1)
         idoxuridine (976.5)

961.8 Other antimycobacterial drugs
     Ethambutol
     Ethionamide
     Isoniazid
     Para-aminosalicylic acid derivatives
     Sulfones

961.9 Other and unspecified anti-infectives
     Flucytosine
     Nitrofuran derivatives

✓4ᵗʰ 962 Poisoning by hormones and synthetic substitutes

EXCLUDES   oxytocic hormones (975.0)

962.0 Adrenal cortical steroids
     Cortisone derivatives
     Desoxycorticosterone derivatives
     Fluorinated corticosteroids

962.1 Androgens and anabolic congeners
     Methandriol
     Nandrolone
     Oxymetholone
     Testosterone

962.2 Ovarian hormones and synthetic substitutes
     Contraceptives, oral
     Estrogens
     Estrogens and progestogens, combined
     Progestogens

962.3 Insulins and antidiabetic agents
Acetohexamide
Biguanide derivatives, oral
Chlorpropamide
Glucagon
Insulin
Phenformin
Sulfonylurea derivatives, oral
Tolbutamide
AHA: 4Q, '93, 19; M-A, '85, 8
TIP: Assign only if documentation indicates overdose of insulin; if due to diabetic adjusting dosage, assign instead 250.8X or 249.8X and E932.3 for adverse reaction to insulin, if applicable.

962.4 Anterior pituitary hormones
Corticotropin
Gonadotropin
Somatotropin [growth hormone]

962.5 Posterior pituitary hormones
Vasopressin
EXCLUDES *oxytocic hormones (975.0)*

962.6 Parathyroid and parathyroid derivatives

962.7 Thyroid and thyroid derivatives
Dextrothyroxin
Levothyroxine sodium
Liothyronine
Thyroglobulin

962.8 Antithyroid agents
Iodides
Thiouracil
Thiourea

962.9 Other and unspecified hormones and synthetic substitutes

√4ᵗʰ **963 Poisoning by primarily systemic agents**

963.0 Antiallergic and antiemetic drugs
Antihistamines
Chlorpheniramine
Diphenhydramine
Diphenylpyraline
Thonzylamine
Tripelennamine
EXCLUDES *phenothiazine-based tranquilizers (969.1)*

963.1 Antineoplastic and immunosuppressive drugs
Azathioprine
Busulfan
Chlorambucil
Cyclophosphamide
Cytarabine
Fluorouracil
Mercaptopurine
thio-TEPA
EXCLUDES *antineoplastic antibiotics (960.7)*

963.2 Acidifying agents

963.3 Alkalizing agents

963.4 Enzymes, not elsewhere classified
Penicillinase

963.5 Vitamins, not elsewhere classified
Vitamin A
Vitamin D
EXCLUDES *nicotinic acid (972.2)*
vitamin K (964.3)

963.8 Other specified systemic agents
Heavy metal antagonists

963.9 Unspecified systemic agent

√4ᵗʰ **964 Poisoning by agents primarily affecting blood constituents**

964.0 Iron and its compounds
Ferric salts
Ferrous sulfate and other ferrous salts

964.1 Liver preparations and other antianemic agents
Folic acid

964.2 Anticoagulants
Coumarin
Heparin
Phenindione
Warfarin sodium
AHA: 1Q, '94, 22
TIP: If documentation indicates an adverse reaction to Coumadin, assign instead manifestation (e.g., hematuria or epistaxis), code 790.92 if abnormal coagulation profile is documented, and E934.2.

964.3 Vitamin K [phytonadione]

964.4 Fibrinolysis-affecting drugs
Aminocaproic acid
Streptodornase
Streptokinase
Urokinase

964.5 Anticoagulant antagonists and other coagulants
Hexadimethrine
Protamine sulfate

964.6 Gamma globulin

964.7 Natural blood and blood products
Blood plasma
Human fibrinogen
Packed red cells
Whole blood
EXCLUDES *transfusion reactions (999.4-999.8)*

964.8 Other specified agents affecting blood constituents
Macromolecular blood substitutes
Plasma expanders

964.9 Unspecified agent affecting blood constituents

√4ᵗʰ **965 Poisoning by analgesics, antipyretics, and antirheumatics**
EXCLUDES *drug dependence (304.0-304.9)*
nondependent abuse (305.0-305.9)

√5ᵗʰ **965.0 Opiates and related narcotics**

965.00 Opium (alkaloids), unspecified
AHA: 3Q, '07, 6

965.01 Heroin
Diacetylmorphine

965.02 Methadone

965.09 Other
Codeine [methylmorphine]
Meperidine [pethidine]
Morphine
AHA: 3Q, '07, 6
T40.4x1A Poisoning oth synthetic narc accidnt initial enc **I-10**

965.1 Salicylates
Acetylsalicylic acid [aspirin]
Salicylic acid salts
AHA: N-D, '94, 15

965.4 Aromatic analgesics, not elsewhere classified
Acetanilid
Paracetamol [acetaminophen]
Phenacetin [acetophenetidin]

965.5 Pyrazole derivatives
Aminophenazone [aminopyrine]
Phenylbutazone

√5ᵗʰ **965.6 Antirheumatics [antiphlogistics]**
EXCLUDES *salicylates (965.1)*
steroids (962.0-962.9)
AHA: 4Q, '98, 50

965.61 Propionic acid derivatives
Fenoprofen
Flurbiprofen
Ibuprofen
Ketoprofen
Naproxen
Oxaprozin
AHA: 4Q, '98, 50

965.69 Other antirheumatics
Gold salts
Indomethacin

Injury and Poisoning

965.7–969.72

965.7 Other non-narcotic analgesics
Pyrabital

965.8 Other specified analgesics and antipyretics
Pentazocine

965.9 Unspecified analgesic and antipyretic

☑4ᵗʰ **966 Poisoning by anticonvulsants and anti-Parkinsonism drugs**

966.0 Oxazolidine derivatives
Paramethadione
Trimethadione

966.1 Hydantoin derivatives
Phenytoin

966.2 Succinimides
Ethosuximide
Phensuximide

966.3 Other and unspecified anticonvulsants
Primidone
EXCLUDES *barbiturates (967.0)*
sulfonamides (961.0)

966.4 Anti-Parkinsonism drugs
Amantadine
Ethopropazine [profenamine]
Levodopa [L-dopa]

☑4ᵗʰ **967 Poisoning by sedatives and hypnotics**
EXCLUDES *drug dependence (304.0-304.9)*
nondependent abuse (305.0-305.9)

967.0 Barbiturates
Amobarbital [amylobarbitone]
Barbital [barbitone]
Butabarbital [butabarbitone]
Pentobarbital [pentobarbitone]
Phenobarbital [phenobarbitone]
Secobarbital [quinalbarbitone]
EXCLUDES *thiobarbiturate anesthetics (968.3)*

967.1 Chloral hydrate group

967.2 Paraldehyde

967.3 Bromine compounds
Bromide
Carbromal (derivatives)

967.4 Methaqualone compounds

967.5 Glutethimide group

967.6 Mixed sedatives, not elsewhere classified

967.8 Other sedatives and hypnotics

967.9 Unspecified sedative or hypnotic
Sleeping:
drug
pill } NOS
tablet

☑4ᵗʰ **968 Poisoning by other central nervous system depressants and anesthetics**
EXCLUDES *drug dependence (304.0-304.9)*
nondependent abuse (305.0-305.9)

968.0 Central nervous system muscle-tone depressants
Chlorphenesin (carbamate)
Mephenesin
Methocarbamol

968.1 Halothane

968.2 Other gaseous anesthetics
Ether
Halogenated hydrocarbon derivatives, except halothane
Nitrous oxide

968.3 Intravenous anesthetics
Ketamine
Methohexital [methohexitone]
Thiobarbiturates, such as thiopental sodium

968.4 Other and unspecified general anesthetics

968.5 Surface [topical] and infiltration anesthetics
Cocaine
Lidocaine [lignocaine]
Procaine
Tetracaine
AHA: 1Q, '93, 25

968.6 Peripheral nerve- and plexus-blocking anesthetics

968.7 Spinal anesthetics

968.9 Other and unspecified local anesthetics
T41.44xA Poisoning uns anesthetic undetermind initial enc   I-10

☑4ᵗʰ **969 Poisoning by psychotropic agents**
EXCLUDES *drug dependence (304.0-304.9)*
nondependent abuse (305.0-305.9)

☑5ᵗʰ **969.0 Antidepressants**
AHA: ▶4Q, '09, 111-112◀

969.00 Antidepressant, unspecified
AHA: 3Q, '07, 6; #5, '94, 9; 3Q, '91, 14; N-D, '84, 14

969.01 Monoamine oxidase inhibitors
MAOI

969.02 Selective serotonin and norepinephrine reuptake inhibitors
SSNRI antidepressants
TIP: Assign for serotonin syndrome due to poisoning, along with 333.99 and E854.0, for accidental poisoning.

969.03 Selective serotonin reuptake inhibitors
SSRI antidepressants
TIP: Assign for serotonin syndrome due to poisoning, along with 333.99 and E854.0, for accidental poisoning.

969.04 Tetracyclic antidepressants

969.05 Tricyclic antidepressants
AHA: ▶4Q, '09, 112◀

969.09 Other antidepressants

969.1 Phenothiazine-based tranquilizers
Chlorpromazine
Fluphenazine
Prochlorperazine
Promazine

969.2 Butyrophenone-based tranquilizers
Haloperidol
Spiperone
Trifluperidol

969.3 Other antipsychotics, neuroleptics, and major tranquilizers

969.4 Benzodiazepine-based tranquilizers
Chlordiazepoxide
Diazepam
Flurazepam
Lorazepam
Medazepam
Nitrazepam
AHA: ▶4Q, '09, 112◀
T42.4x1D Poisoning benzodiazepines accidental subseq enc   I-10

969.5 Other tranquilizers
Hydroxyzine
Meprobamate

969.6 Psychodysleptics [hallucinogens]
Cannabis (derivatives)
Lysergide [LSD]
Marihuana (derivatives)
Mescaline
Psilocin
Psilocybin

☑5ᵗʰ **969.7 Psychostimulants**
EXCLUDES *central appetite depressants (977.0)*
AHA: ▶4Q, '09, 113-114◀

969.70 Psychostimulant, unspecified
AHA: 2Q, '03, 11

969.71 Caffeine

969.72 Amphetamines
Methamphetamines
TIP: Assign for overdose and poisoning by the club drug ecstasy.

Ⓝ Newborn Age: 0   Ⓟ Pediatric Age: 0-17   Ⓜ Maternity Age: 12-55   Ⓐ Adult Age: 15-124

969.73 Methylphenidate

969.79 Other psychostimulants

969.8 Other specified psychotropic agents

969.9 Unspecified psychotropic agent

✓4ᵗʰ **970 Poisoning by central nervous system stimulants**

970.0 Analeptics
Lobeline
Nikethamide

970.1 Opiate antagonists
Levallorphan
Nalorphine
Naloxone

✓5ᵗʰ **970.8 Other specified central nervous system stimulants**
AHA: 1Q, '05, 6

● **970.81 Cocaine**
Crack

● **970.89 Other central nervous system stimulants**

970.9 Unspecified central nervous system stimulant

✓4ᵗʰ **971 Poisoning by drugs primarily affecting the autonomic nervous system**

971.0 Parasympathomimetics [cholinergics]
Acetylcholine
Anticholinesterase:
   organophosphorus
   reversible
Pilocarpine

971.1 Parasympatholytics [anticholinergics and antimuscarinics] and spasmolytics
Atropine
Homatropine
Hyoscine [scopamine]
Quaternary ammonium derivatives
EXCLUDES *papaverine (972.5)*

971.2 Sympathomimetics [adrenergics]
Epinephrine [adrenalin]
Levarterenol [noradrenalin]

971.3 Sympatholytics [antiadrenergics]
Phenoxybenzamine
Tolazoline hydrochloride

971.9 Unspecified drug primarily affecting autonomic nervous system

✓4ᵗʰ **972 Poisoning by agents primarily affecting the cardiovascular system**

972.0 Cardiac rhythm regulators
Practolol
Procainamide
Propranolol
Quinidine
EXCLUDES *lidocaine (968.5)*

972.1 Cardiotonic glycosides and drugs of similar action
Digitalis glycosides
Digoxin
Strophanthins

972.2 Antilipemic and antiarteriosclerotic drugs
Clofibrate
Nicotinic acid derivatives

972.3 Ganglion-blocking agents
Pentamethonium bromide

972.4 Coronary vasodilators
Dipyridamole
Nitrates [nitroglycerin]
Nitrites

972.5 Other vasodilators
Cyclandelate
Diazoxide
Papaverine
EXCLUDES *nicotinic acid (972.2)*

972.6 Other antihypertensive agents
Clonidine
Guanethidine
Rauwolfia alkaloids
Reserpine

972.7 Antivaricose drugs, including sclerosing agents
Sodium morrhuate
Zinc salts

972.8 Capillary-active drugs
Adrenochrome derivatives
Metaraminol

972.9 Other and unspecified agents primarily affecting the cardiovascular system

✓4ᵗʰ **973 Poisoning by agents primarily affecting the gastrointestinal system**

973.0 Antacids and antigastric secretion drugs
Aluminum hydroxide
Magnesium trisilicate
AHA: 1Q, '03, 19

973.1 Irritant cathartics
Bisacodyl
Castor oil
Phenolphthalein

973.2 Emollient cathartics
Dioctyl sulfosuccinates

973.3 Other cathartics, including intestinal atonia drugs
Magnesium sulfate

973.4 Digestants
Pancreatin
Papain
Pepsin

973.5 Antidiarrheal drugs
Kaolin
Pectin
EXCLUDES *anti-infectives (960.0-961.9)*

973.6 Emetics

973.8 Other specified agents primarily affecting the gastrointestinal system

973.9 Unspecified agent primarily affecting the gastrointestinal system

✓4ᵗʰ **974 Poisoning by water, mineral, and uric acid metabolism drugs**

974.0 Mercurial diuretics
Chlormerodrin
Mercaptomerin
Mersalyl

974.1 Purine derivative diuretics
Theobromine
Theophylline
EXCLUDES *aminophylline [theophylline ethylenediamine] (975.7)*
   caffeine (969.71)

974.2 Carbonic acid anhydrase inhibitors
Acetazolamide

974.3 Saluretics
Benzothiadiazides
Chlorothiazide group

974.4 Other diuretics
Ethacrynic acid
Furosemide

974.5 Electrolytic, caloric, and water-balance agents

974.6 Other mineral salts, not elsewhere classified

974.7 Uric acid metabolism drugs
Allopurinol
Colchicine
Probenecid

Injury and Poisoning

975–982.2

√4ᵗʰ **975 Poisoning by agents primarily acting on the smooth and skeletal muscles and respiratory system**

975.0 Oxytocic agents
Ergot alkaloids
Oxytocin
Prostaglandins

975.1 Smooth muscle relaxants
Adiphenine
Metaproterenol [orciprenaline]
EXCLUDES *papaverine (972.5)*

975.2 Skeletal muscle relaxants

975.3 Other and unspecified drugs acting on muscles

975.4 Antitussives
Dextromethorphan
Pipazethate

975.5 Expectorants
Acetylcysteine
Guaifenesin
Terpin hydrate

975.6 Anti-common cold drugs

975.7 Antiasthmatics
Aminophylline [theophylline ethylenediamine]

975.8 Other and unspecified respiratory drugs

√4ᵗʰ **976 Poisoning by agents primarily affecting skin and mucous membrane, ophthalmological, otorhinolaryngological, and dental drugs**

976.0 Local anti-infectives and anti-inflammatory drugs

976.1 Antipruritics

976.2 Local astringents and local detergents

976.3 Emollients, demulcents, and protectants

976.4 Keratolytics, keratoplastics, other hair treatment drugs and preparations

976.5 Eye anti-infectives and other eye drugs
Idoxuridine

976.6 Anti-infectives and other drugs and preparations for ear, nose, and throat

976.7 Dental drugs topically applied
EXCLUDES *anti-infectives (976.0)*
local anesthetics (968.5)

976.8 Other agents primarily affecting skin and mucous membrane
Spermicides [vaginal contraceptives]

976.9 Unspecified agent primarily affecting skin and mucous membrane

√4ᵗʰ **977 Poisoning by other and unspecified drugs and medicinal substances**

977.0 Dietetics
Central appetite depressants

977.1 Lipotropic drugs

977.2 Antidotes and chelating agents, not elsewhere classified

977.3 Alcohol deterrents

977.4 Pharmaceutical excipients
Pharmaceutical adjuncts

977.8 Other specified drugs and medicinal substances
Contrast media used for diagnostic x-ray procedures
Diagnostic agents and kits

977.9 Unspecified drug or medicinal substance

√4ᵗʰ **978 Poisoning by bacterial vaccines**

978.0 BCG

978.1 Typhoid and paratyphoid

978.2 Cholera

978.3 Plague

978.4 Tetanus

978.5 Diphtheria

978.6 Pertussis vaccine, including combinations with a pertussis component

978.8 Other and unspecified bacterial vaccines

978.9 Mixed bacterial vaccines, except combinations with a pertussis component

√4ᵗʰ **979 Poisoning by other vaccines and biological substances**
EXCLUDES *gamma globulin (964.6)*

979.0 Smallpox vaccine

979.1 Rabies vaccine

979.2 Typhus vaccine

979.3 Yellow fever vaccine

979.4 Measles vaccine

979.5 Poliomyelitis vaccine

979.6 Other and unspecified viral and rickettsial vaccines
Mumps vaccine

979.7 Mixed viral-rickettsial and bacterial vaccines, except combinations with a pertussis component
EXCLUDES *combinations with a pertussis component (978.6)*

979.9 Other and unspecified vaccines and biological substances

Toxic Effects of Substances Chiefly Nonmedicinal as to Source (980-989)

▶Use additional code to identify:
personal history of retained foreign body fully removed (V15.53)
retained foreign body status, if applicable, (V90.01-V90.9)◀

Use additional code to specify the nature of the toxic effect

EXCLUDES *burns from chemical agents (ingested) (947.0-947.9)*
localized toxic effects indexed elsewhere (001.0-799.9)
respiratory conditions due to external agents (506.0-508.9)

√4ᵗʰ **980 Toxic effect of alcohol**

980.0 Ethyl alcohol
Denatured alcohol   Grain alcohol
Ethanol

Use additional code to identify any associated:
acute alcohol intoxication (305.0)
in alcoholism (303.0)
drunkenness (simple) (305.0)
pathological (291.4)
AHA: 4Q, '09, 112; 3Q, '96, 16
T51.0x1A Toxic effect ethanol accidental initial encountr   I-10

980.1 Methyl alcohol
Methanol
Wood alcohol

980.2 Isopropyl alcohol
Dimethyl carbinol
Isopropanol
Rubbing alcohol

980.3 Fusel oil
Alcohol:
amyl
butyl
propyl

980.8 Other specified alcohols

980.9 Unspecified alcohol

981 Toxic effect of petroleum products
Benzine   Petroleum:
Gasoline   ether
Kerosene   naphtha
Paraffin wax   spirit

√4ᵗʰ **982 Toxic effect of solvents other than petroleum-based**

982.0 Benzene and homologues

982.1 Carbon tetrachloride

982.2 Carbon disulfide
Carbon bisulfide

Ⓝ Newborn Age: 0   Ⓟ Pediatric Age: 0-17   Ⓜ Maternity Age: 12-55   Ⓐ Adult Age: 15-124

982.3 Other chlorinated hydrocarbon solvents
Tetrachloroethylene
Trichloroethylene
EXCLUDES *chlorinated hydrocarbon preparations other than*
solvents (989.2)
AHA: 3Q, '08, 6-7

982.4 Nitroglycol

982.8 Other nonpetroleum-based solvents
Acetone

✓4ᵗʰ **983 Toxic effect of corrosive aromatics, acids, and caustic alkalis**

983.0 Corrosive aromatics
Carbolic acid or phenol
Cresol

983.1 Acids
Acid:
hydrochloric
nitric
sulfuric

983.2 Caustic alkalis
Lye
Potassium hydroxide
Sodium hydroxide

983.9 Caustic, unspecified

✓4ᵗʰ **984 Toxic effect of lead and its compounds (including fumes)**
INCLUDES that from all sources except medicinal substances

984.0 Inorganic lead compounds
Lead dioxide
Lead salts

984.1 Organic lead compounds
Lead acetate
Tetraethyl lead

984.8 Other lead compounds

984.9 Unspecified lead compound

✓4ᵗʰ **985 Toxic effect of other metals**
INCLUDES that from all sources except medicinal substances

985.0 Mercury and its compounds
Minamata disease

985.1 Arsenic and its compounds

985.2 Manganese and its compounds

985.3 Beryllium and its compounds

985.4 Antimony and its compounds

985.5 Cadmium and its compounds

985.6 Chromium

985.8 Other specified metals
Brass fumes
Copper salts
Iron compounds
Nickel compounds
AHA: 1Q, '88, 5
TIP: Assign for aluminum overloading or excessive concentration of
aluminum in the body, along with E879.1 if due to renal dialysis and
E879.8 if due to total parenteral nutrition.

985.9 Unspecified metal

986 Toxic effect of carbon monoxide
Carbon monoxide from any source

✓4ᵗʰ **987 Toxic effect of other gases, fumes, or vapors**

987.0 Liquefied petroleum gases
Butane
Propane

987.1 Other hydrocarbon gas

987.2 Nitrogen oxides
Nitrogen dioxide
Nitrous fumes

987.3 Sulfur dioxide

987.4 Freon
Dichloromonofluoromethane

987.5 Lacrimogenic gas
Bromobenzyl cyanide
Chloroacetophenone
Ethyliodoacetate

987.6 Chlorine gas

987.7 Hydrocyanic acid gas

987.8 Other specified gases, fumes, or vapors
Phosgene
Polyester fumes

987.9 Unspecified gas, fume, or vapor
AHA: 3Q, '05, 10
TIP: Assign for smoke inhalation, along with the appropriate E code
describing the source of the smoke and fumes.

✓4ᵗʰ **988 Toxic effect of noxious substances eaten as food**
EXCLUDES *allergic reaction to food, such as:*
gastroenteritis (558.3)
rash (692.5, 693.1)
food poisoning (bacterial) (005.0-005.9)
toxic effects of food contaminants, such as:
aflatoxin and other mycotoxin (989.7)
mercury (985.0)

988.0 Fish and shellfish

988.1 Mushrooms

988.2 Berries and other plants

988.8 Other specified noxious substances eaten as food

988.9 Unspecified noxious substance eaten as food

✓4ᵗʰ **989 Toxic effect of other substances, chiefly nonmedicinal as to source**

989.0 Hydrocyanic acid and cyanides
Potassium cyanide
Sodium cyanide
EXCLUDES *gas and fumes (987.7)*

989.1 Strychnine and salts

989.2 Chlorinated hydrocarbons
Aldrin
Chlordane
DDT
Dieldrin
EXCLUDES *chlorinated hydrocarbon solvents (982.0-982.3)*

989.3 Organophosphate and carbamate
Carbaryl
Dichlorvos
Malathion
Parathion
Phorate
Phosdrin

989.4 Other pesticides, not elsewhere classified
Mixtures of insecticides

989.5 Venom
Bites of venomous snakes, lizards, and spiders
Tick paralysis

989.6 Soaps and detergents

989.7 Aflatoxin and other mycotoxin [food contaminants]

✓5ᵗʰ **989.8 Other substances, chiefly nonmedicinal as to source**
AHA: 4Q, '95, 60

989.81 Asbestos
EXCLUDES *asbestosis (501)*
exposure to asbestos (V15.84)

989.82 Latex

989.83 Silicone
EXCLUDES *silicone used in medical devices, implants*
and grafts (996.00-996.79)

989.84 Tobacco

989.89 Other

989.9 Unspecified substance, chiefly nonmedicinal as to source

Injury and Poisoning

990–994.9

Other and Unspecified Effects of External Causes (990-995)

990 Effects of radiation, unspecified
Complication of:
 phototherapy
 radiation therapy
Radiation sickness

[The type of radiation giving rise to the adverse effect may be identified by use of the E codes.]

EXCLUDES *specified adverse effects of radiation. Such conditions are to be classified according to the nature of the adverse effect, as:*
 burns (940.0-949.5)
 dermatitis (692.7-692.8)
 leukemia (204.0-208.9)
 pneumonia (508.0)
 sunburn (692.71, 692.76-692.77)

✓4ᵗʰ **991 Effects of reduced temperature**

991.0 Frostbite of face

991.1 Frostbite of hand

991.2 Frostbite of foot

991.3 Frostbite of other and unspecified sites

991.4 Immersion foot
Trench foot
DEF: Paresthesia, edema, blotchy cyanosis of foot, the skin is soft (macerated), pale and wrinkled, and the sole is swollen with surface ridging and following sustained immersion in water.

991.5 Chilblains
Erythema pernio
Perniosis
DEF: Red, swollen, itchy skin; follows damp cold exposure; also associated with pruritus and a burning feeling in hands, feet, ears, and face in children, legs and toes in women, and hands and fingers in men.

991.6 Hypothermia
Hypothermia (accidental)
EXCLUDES *hypothermia following anesthesia (995.89)*
 hypothermia not associated with low environmental temperature (780.65)
DEF: Reduced body temperature due to low environmental temperatures.

991.8 Other specified effects of reduced temperature

991.9 Unspecified effect of reduced temperature
Effects of freezing or excessive cold NOS

✓4ᵗʰ **992 Effects of heat and light**
EXCLUDES *burns (940.0-949.5)*
 diseases of sweat glands due to heat (705.0-705.9)
 malignant hyperpyrexia following anesthesia (995.86)
 sunburn (692.71, 692.76-692.77)

992.0 Heat stroke and sunstroke
Heat apoplexy Siriasis
Heat pyrexia   Thermoplegia
Ictus solaris
▶Use additional code(s) to identify any associated complication of heat stroke, such as:
 alterations of consciousness (780.01-780.09)
 systemic inflammatory response syndrome (995.93-995.94)◀
DEF: Headache, vertigo, cramps and elevated body temperature due to high environmental temperatures.

992.1 Heat syncope
Heat collapse

992.2 Heat cramps

992.3 Heat exhaustion, anhydrotic
Heat prostration due to water depletion
EXCLUDES *that associated with salt depletion (992.4)*

992.4 Heat exhaustion due to salt depletion
Heat prostration due to salt (and water) depletion

992.5 Heat exhaustion, unspecified
Heat prostration NOS

992.6 Heat fatigue, transient

992.7 Heat edema
DEF: Fluid retention due to high environmental temperatures.

992.8 Other specified heat effects

992.9 Unspecified

✓4ᵗʰ **993 Effects of air pressure**

993.0 Barotrauma, otitic
Aero-otitis media
Effects of high altitude on ears
DEF: Ringing ears, deafness, pain and vertigo due to air pressure changes.

993.1 Barotrauma, sinus
Aerosinusitis
Effects of high altitude on sinuses

993.2 Other and unspecified effects of high altitude
Alpine sickness   Hypobaropathy
Andes disease   Mountain sickness
Anoxia due to high altitude
AHA: 3Q, '88, 4

993.3 Caisson disease
Bends
Compressed-air disease
Decompression sickness
Divers' palsy or paralysis
DEF: Rapid reduction in air pressure while breathing compressed air; symptoms include skin lesions, joint pains, respiratory and neurological problems.

993.4 Effects of air pressure caused by explosion

993.8 Other specified effects of air pressure

993.9 Unspecified effect of air pressure

✓4ᵗʰ **994 Effects of other external causes**
EXCLUDES *certain adverse effects not elsewhere classified (995.0-995.8)*

994.0 Effects of lightning
Shock from lightning
Struck by lightning NOS
EXCLUDES *burns (940.0-949.5)*

994.1 Drowning and nonfatal submersion
Bathing cramp
Immersion
AHA: 3Q, '09, 14; 3Q, '88, 4
TIP: When near-drowning results in acute respiratory edema, assign also code 518.5 Post-traumatic pulmonary insufficiency.

994.2 Effects of hunger
Deprivation of food
Starvation

994.3 Effects of thirst
Deprivation of water

994.4 Exhaustion due to exposure

994.5 Exhaustion due to excessive exertion
Exhaustion due to overexertion

994.6 Motion sickness
Air sickness   Travel sickness
Seasickness

994.7 Asphyxiation and strangulation
Suffocation (by): Suffocation (by):
 bedclothes   plastic bag
 cave-in   pressure
 constriction   strangulation
 mechanical
EXCLUDES *asphyxia from:*
 carbon monoxide (986)
 inhalation of food or foreign body (932-934.9)
 other gases, fumes, and vapors (987.0-987.9)

994.8 Electrocution and nonfatal effects of electric current
Shock from electric current
Shock from electroshock gun (taser)
EXCLUDES *electric burns (940.0-949.5)*

994.9 Other effects of external causes
Effects of:
 abnormal gravitational [G] forces or states
 weightlessness

☑4ᵗʰ 995 Certain adverse effects not elsewhere classified

     EXCLUDES *complications of surgical and medical care (996.0-999.9)*

995.0 Other anaphylactic shock

Allergic shock ⎫ NOS or due to adverse effect
Anaphylactic   ⎬ of correct medicinal
    reaction   ⎬ substance properly
Anaphylaxis   ⎭ administered

Use additional E code to identify external cause, such as:
adverse effects of correct medicinal substance properly
administered [E930-E949]

     EXCLUDES *anaphylactic reaction to serum (999.4)*
               anaphylactic shock due to adverse food reaction (995.60-995.69)

DEF: Immediate sensitivity response after exposure to specific antigen; results in life-threatening respiratory distress; usually followed by vascular collapse, shock, urticaria, angioedema and pruritus.

AHA: 4Q, '93, 30

995.1 Angioneurotic edema

Giant urticaria

     EXCLUDES *urticaria:*
               due to serum (999.5)
               other specified (698.2, 708.0-708.9, 757.33)

DEF: Circulatory response of deep dermis, subcutaneous or submucosal tissues; causes localized edema and wheals.

▲   ☑5ᵗʰ **995.2 Other and unspecified adverse effect of drug, medicinal and biological substance**

     EXCLUDES *pathological drug intoxication (292.2)*

AHA: 2Q, '97, 12; 3Q, '95, 13; 3Q, '92, 16

TIP: Codes from this subcategory should not be assigned for inpatient cases; their use is limited to certain outpatient cases in which there is no documentation of specific symptoms associated with the adverse effect.

995.20 Unspecified adverse effect of unspecified drug, medicinal and biological substance

▶Unspecified adverse effect of unspecified medicinal substance properly administered◀

AHA: 4Q, '06, 112

995.21 Arthus phenomenon

Arthus reaction

AHA: 4Q, '06, 112

995.22 Unspecified adverse effect of anesthesia

AHA: 4Q, '06, 112

995.23 Unspecified adverse effect of insulin

AHA: 4Q, '06, 112

995.24 Failed moderate sedation during procedure

Failed conscious sedation during procedure

AHA: 4Q, '09, 114

TIP: If documentation indicates a personal history of failed moderate sedation, assign instead code V15.80 History of failed moderate sedation.

995.27 Other drug allergy

▶Allergic reaction NEC (due) to correct medical substance properly administered◀
Drug allergy NOS
Drug hypersensitivity NOS
▶Hypersensitivity (due) to correct medical substance properly administered◀

AHA: 4Q, '06, 112

995.29 Unspecified adverse effect of other drug, medicinal and biological substance

▶Unspecified adverse effect of medicinal substance NEC properly administered◀

AHA: 4Q, '06, 112

995.3 Allergy, unspecified

Allergic reaction NOS   Idiosyncrasy NOS
Hypersensitivity NOS

     EXCLUDES *allergic reaction NOS to correct medicinal substance properly administered (995.27)*
               allergy to existing dental restorative materials (525.66)
               specific types of allergic reaction, such as:
                   allergic diarrhea (558.3)
                   dermatitis (691.0-693.9)
                   hayfever (477.0-477.9)

995.4 Shock due to anesthesia

Shock due to anesthesia in which the correct substance was properly administered

     EXCLUDES *complications of anesthesia in labor or delivery (668.0-668.9)*
               overdose or wrong substance given (968.0-969.9)
               postoperative shock NOS (998.0)
               specified adverse effects of anesthesia classified elsewhere, such as:
                   anoxic brain damage (348.1)
                   hepatitis (070.0-070.9), etc.
               unspecified adverse effect of anesthesia (995.22)

☑5ᵗʰ **995.5 Child maltreatment syndrome**

Use additional code(s), if applicable, to identify any associated injuries

Use additional E code to identify:
nature of abuse (E960-E968)
perpetrator (E967.0-E967.9)

AHA: 1Q, '98, 11

TIP: Although separate codes for any associated injuries should be assigned, codes from this subcategory may be assigned alone if there are no documented injuries or associated conditions.

995.50 Child abuse, unspecified   **P**

995.51 Child emotional/psychological abuse   **P**

AHA: 4Q, '96, 38, 40

995.52 Child neglect (nutritional)   **P**

AHA: 4Q, '96, 38, 40

995.53 Child sexual abuse   **P**

AHA: 4Q, '96, 39, 40

995.54 Child physical abuse   **P**

Battered baby or child syndrome

     EXCLUDES *shaken infant syndrome (995.55)*

AHA: 3Q, '99, 14; 4Q, '96, 39, 40

995.55 Shaken infant syndrome   **P**

Use additional code(s) to identify any associated injuries

AHA: 4Q, '96, 40, 43

995.59 Other child abuse and neglect   **P**

Multiple forms of abuse

☑5ᵗʰ **995.6 Anaphylactic shock due to adverse food reaction**

Anaphylactic reaction due to food
Anaphylactic shock due to nonpoisonous foods

AHA: 4Q, '93, 30

TIP: Codes from this subcategory may be assigned not only for anaphylactic shock, but also for any documentation of anaphylactic reaction to food.

995.60 Due to unspecified food

995.61 Due to peanuts

995.62 Due to crustaceans

995.63 Due to fruits and vegetables

995.64 Due to tree nuts and seeds

AHA: 1Q, '08, 12

995.65 Due to fish

995.66 Due to food additives

995.67 Due to milk products

995.68 Due to eggs

995.69 Due to other specified food

995.7 Other adverse food reactions, not elsewhere classified

Use additional code to identify the type of reaction, such as:
hives (708.0)
wheezing (786.07)

     EXCLUDES *anaphylactic shock due to adverse food reaction (995.60-995.69)*
               asthma (493.0, 493.9)
               dermatitis due to food (693.1)
                 in contact with skin (692.5)
               gastroenteritis and colitis due to food (558.3)
               rhinitis due to food (477.1)

☑4ᵗʰ ☑5ᵗʰ Additional Digit Required   Unspecified Code   Other Specified Code   Manifestation Code   ▶◀ Revised Text   ● New Code   ▲ Revised Code Title

2011 ICD-9-CM   **October 2010 · Volume 1 – 309**

Injury and Poisoning

995.8–995.94

Continuum of Illness Due to Infection

Bacteremia ➡ Septicemia ➡ Sepsis

Severe Sepsis with Septic Shock ⬅ Severe Sepsis ⬅

⬇

MODS (Multiple Organ Dysfunction Syndrome) ➡ Death

✓5ᵗʰ **995.8 Other specified adverse effects, not elsewhere classified**

995.80 Adult maltreatment, unspecified Ⓐ
Abused person NOS
Use additional code to identify:
any associated injury
perpetrator (E967.0-E967.9)
AHA: 4Q, '96, 41, 43

995.81 Adult physical abuse Ⓐ
Battered:
person syndrome NEC
man
spouse
woman
Use additional code to identify:
any association injury
nature of abuse (E960-E968)
perpetrator (E967.0-E967.9)
AHA: 4Q, '96, 42, 43

995.82 Adult emotional/psychological abuse Ⓐ
Use additional E code to identify perpetrator (E967.0-E967.9)

995.83 Adult sexual abuse Ⓐ
Use additional code(s) to identify:
any associated injury
perpetrator (E967.0-E967.9)

995.84 Adult neglect (nutritional) Ⓐ
Use additional code(s) to identify:
intent of neglect (E904.0, E968.4)
perpetrator (E967.0-E967.9)

995.85 Other adult abuse and neglect Ⓐ
Multiple forms of abuse and neglect
Use additional code(s) to identify
any associated injury
intent of neglect (E904.0, E968.4)
nature of abuse (E960-E968)
perpetrator (E967.0-E967.9)

995.86 Malignant hyperthermia
Malignant hyperpyrexia due to anesthesia
AHA: 4Q, '98, 51

995.89 Other
Hypothermia due to anesthesia
AHA: 2Q, '04, 18; 3Q, '03, 12

✓5ᵗʰ **995.9 Systemic inflammatory response syndrome (SIRS)**
DEF: Clinical response to infection or trauma that can trigger an acute inflammatory reaction and progresses to coagulation, impaired fibrinolysis, and organ failure; manifested by two or more of the following symptoms: fever, tachycardia, tachypnea, leukocytosis or leukopenia.
AHA: 4Q, '06, 113-116; 2Q, '04, 16; 4Q, '02, 71
TIP: Coding these conditions requires a minimum of two codes: the underlying cause (e.g., Infection or trauma) is sequenced first, followed by a code from subcategory 995.9.

995.90 Systemic inflammatory response syndrome, unspecified
SIRS NOS

995.91 Sepsis
Systemic inflammatory response syndrome due to infectious process without acute organ dysfunction
Code first underlying infection
EXCLUDES sepsis with acute organ dysfunction (995.92)
sepsis with multiple organ dysfunction (995.92)
severe sepsis (995.92)
AHA: 4Q, '08, 72; 4Q, '07, 86; 4Q, '06, 113-116; 2Q, '04, 16; 4Q, '03, 79

995.92 Severe sepsis
Sepsis with acute organ dysfunction
Sepsis with multiple organ dysfunction (MOD)
Systemic inflammatory response syndrome due to infectious process with acute organ dysfunction
Code first underlying infection
Use additional code to specify acute organ dysfunction, such as:
acute kidney failure (584.5-584.9)
acute respiratory failure (518.81)
critical illness myopathy (359.81)
critical illness polyneuropathy (357.82)
disseminated intravascular coagulopathy [DIC] (286.6)
encephalopathy (348.31)
hepatic failure (570)
septic shock (785.52)
AHA: 4Q, '09, 98; 4Q, '08, 99; 4Q, '07, 97; 4Q, '06, 113-116; 2Q, '05, 18-19; 1Q, '05, 7; 1Q, '05, 7; 2Q, '04, 16; 4Q, '03, 73, 79
R65.21 Severe sepsis with septic shock   I-10

995.93 Systemic inflammatory response syndrome due to noninfectious process without acute organ dysfunction
Code first underlying conditions, such as:
acute pancreatitis (577.0)
trauma
EXCLUDES systemic inflammatory response syndrome due to noninfectious process with acute organ dysfunction (995.94)
AHA: ▶1Q, '10, 10-11;◀ 4Q, '06, 113-116

995.94 Systemic inflammatory response syndrome due to noninfectious process with acute organ dysfunction
Code first underlying conditions, such as:
acute pancreatitis (577.0)
▶heat stroke (992.0)◀
trauma
Use additional code to specify acute organ dysfunction, such as:
acute kidney failure (584.5-584.9)
acute respiratory failure (518.81)
critical illness myopathy (359.81)
critical illness polyneuropathy (357.82)
disseminated intravascular coagulopathy [DIC] syndrome (286.6)
encephalopathy (348.31)
hepatic failure (570)
EXCLUDES severe sepsis (995.92)
AHA: ▶1Q, '10, 10;◀ 4Q, '06, 113-116; 4Q, '03, 79

Ⓝ Newborn Age: 0   Ⓟ Pediatric Age: 0-17   Ⓜ Maternity Age: 12-55   Ⓐ Adult Age: 15-124

Complications of Surgical and Medical Care, Not Elsewhere Classified (996-999)

EXCLUDES *adverse effects of medicinal agents (001.0-799.9, 995.0-995.8)*
burns from local applications and irradiation (940.0-949.5)
complications of:
    conditions for which the procedure was performed
    surgical procedures during abortion, labor, and delivery (630-676.9)
poisoning and toxic effects of drugs and chemicals (960.0-989.9)
postoperative conditions in which no complications are present, such as:
    artificial opening status (V44.0-V44.9)
    closure of external stoma (V55.0-V55.9)
    fitting of prosthetic device (V52.0-V52.9)
specified complications classified elsewhere
    anesthetic shock (995.4)
    electrolyte imbalance (276.0-276.9)
    postlaminectomy syndrome (722.80-722.83)
    postmastectomy lymphedema syndrome (457.0)
    postoperative psychosis (293.0-293.9)
    any other condition classified elsewhere in the Alphabetic Index when described as due to a procedure

√4ᵗʰ **996 Complications peculiar to certain specified procedures**

INCLUDES complications, not elsewhere classified, in the use of artificial substitutes [e.g., Dacron, metal, Silastic, Teflon] or natural sources [e.g., bone] involving:
anastomosis (internal)
graft (bypass) (patch)
implant
internal device:
    catheter
    electronic
    fixation
    prosthetic
reimplant
transplant

EXCLUDES *accidental puncture or laceration during procedure (998.2)*
capsular contracture of breast implant (611.83)
complications of internal anastomosis of:
    gastrointestinal tract (997.4)
    urinary tract (997.5)
endosseous dental implant failures (525.71-525.79)
intraoperative floppy iris syndrome [IFIS] (364.81)
mechanical complication of respirator (V46.14)
other specified complications classified elsewhere, such as:
    hemolytic anemia (283.1)
    functional cardiac disturbances (429.4)
    serum hepatitis (070.2-070.3)

AHA: 1Q, '94, 3

√5ᵗʰ **996.0 Mechanical complication of cardiac device, implant, and graft**

Breakdown (mechanical)   Obstruction, mechanical
Displacement   Perforation
Leakage   Protrusion

AHA: 2Q, '08, 9; 2Q, '93, 9

TIP: If the documentation indicates that the cardiac device (e.g., pacemaker, heart valve prosthesis) has reached its normally occurring end of life, do not assign a complication code; see instead subcategory V53.3.

996.00 Unspecified device, implant, and graft

996.01 Due to cardiac pacemaker (electrode)
AHA: 2Q, '06, 15; 2Q, '99, 11
T82.120A Displacement cardiac electrode initial encounter   I-10

996.02 Due to heart valve prosthesis

996.03 Due to coronary bypass graft
EXCLUDES *atherosclerosis of graft (414.02, 414.03)*
embolism [occlusion NOS] [thrombus] of graft (996.72)
AHA: 2Q, '95, 17; N-D, '86, 5

996.04 Due to automatic implantable cardiac defibrillator
AHA: 2Q, '05, 3

996.09 Other
AHA: 2Q, '93, 9

996.1 Mechanical complication of other vascular device, implant, and graft
Mechanical complications involving:
aortic (bifurcation) graft (replacement)
arteriovenous:
    dialysis catheter ⎫
    fistula   ⎬ surgically created
    shunt   ⎭
balloon (counterpulsation) device, intra-aortic
carotid artery bypass graft
femoral-popliteal bypass graft
umbrella device, vena cava

EXCLUDES *atherosclerosis of biological graft (440.30-440.32)*
embolism [occlusion NOS] [thrombus] of (biological) (synthetic) graft (996.74)
peritoneal dialysis catheter (996.56)
AHA: 1Q, '06, 10; 2Q, '05, 8; 1Q, '02, 13; 1Q, '95, 3
TIP: Assign for a nonmaturing AV fistula and also for postprocedural reduction in transjugular intrahepatic portosystemic shunt flow in a patient with a TIPS catheter.
T82.330A Leakage aortic bifurcation graft initial enc   I-10

996.2 Mechanical complication of nervous system device, implant, and graft
Mechanical complications involving:
dorsal column stimulator
electrodes implanted in brain [brain "pacemaker"]
peripheral nerve graft
ventricular (communicating) shunt
AHA: 2Q, '99, 4; S-O, '87, 10

√5ᵗʰ **996.3 Mechanical complication of genitourinary device, implant, and graft**
AHA: 3Q, '01, 13; S-O, '85, 3

996.30 Unspecified device, implant, and graft

996.31 Due to urethral [indwelling] catheter

996.32 Due to intrauterine contraceptive device   ♀

996.39 Other
Cystostomy catheter
Prosthetic reconstruction of vas deferens
Repair (graft) of ureter without mention of resection
EXCLUDES *complications due to:*
    external stoma of urinary tract (997.5)
    internal anastomosis of urinary tract (997.5)

√5ᵗʰ **996.4 Mechanical complication of internal orthopedic device, implant, and graft**
Mechanical complications involving:
external (fixation) device utilizing internal screw(s), pin(s) or other methods of fixation
grafts of bone, cartilage, muscle, or tendon
internal (fixation) device such as nail, plate, rod, etc.
Use additional code to identify prosthetic joint with mechanical complication (V43.60-V43.69)
EXCLUDES *complications of external orthopedic device, such as: pressure ulcer due to cast (707.00-707.09)*
AHA: 4Q, '05, 91; 2Q, '99, 10; 2Q, '98, 19; 2Q, '96, 11; 3Q, '95, 16; N-D, '85, 11
TIP: Since these codes may be used for any joint device complications, assign an additional code from subcategory V43.6 to specify the joint involved.

996.40 Unspecified mechanical complication of internal orthopedic device, implant, and graft

996.41 Mechanical loosening of prosthetic joint
Aseptic loosening
AHA: 4Q, '05, 112
T84.031A Mech loosening int lt hip prosth jnt initial enc   I-10

996.42 Dislocation of prosthetic joint
Instability of prosthetic joint
Subluxation of prosthetic joint
T84.020D Displacment internal right hip prosth subsqt enc   I-10

996.43 Broken prosthetic joint implant
Breakage (fracture) of prosthetic joint

√4ᵗʰ √5ᵗʰ Additional Digit Required   **Unspecified Code**   **Other Specified Code**   **Manifestation Code**   ▶◀ Revised Text   ● New Code   ▲ Revised Code Title

2011 ICD-9-CM   **Volume 1 – 311**

Injury and Poisoning

996.44–996.68

996.44 Peri-prosthetic fracture around prosthetic joint
AHA: 4Q, '05, 93

996.45 Peri-prosthetic osteolysis
Use additional code to identify major osseous defect, if applicable (731.3)
AHA: 4Q, '06, 103

996.46 Articular bearing surface wear of prosthetic joint

996.47 Other mechanical complication of prosthetic joint implant
Mechanical complication of prosthetic joint NOS
Prosthetic joint implant failure NOS

996.49 Other mechanical complication of other internal orthopedic device, implant, and graft
Breakage of internal fixation device in bone
Dislocation of internal fixation device in bone
EXCLUDES mechanical complication of prosthetic joint implant (996.41-996.47)
AHA: ▶1Q, '10, 7◀

√5ᵗʰ **996.5 Mechanical complication of other specified prosthetic device, implant, and graft**
Mechanical complications involving:
nonabsorbable surgical material NOS
other graft, implant, and internal device, not elsewhere classified
prosthetic implant in:
bile duct
breast
chin
orbit of eye
AHA: 1Q, '98, 11

996.51 Due to corneal graft

996.52 Due to graft of other tissue, not elsewhere classified
Skin graft failure or rejection
EXCLUDES failure of artificial skin graft (996.55)
failure of decellularized allodermis (996.55)
sloughing of temporary skin allografts or xenografts (pigskin) — omit code
AHA: 1Q, '96, 10

996.53 Due to ocular lens prosthesis
EXCLUDES contact lenses — code to condition
AHA: 1Q, '00, 9

996.54 Due to breast prosthesis
Breast capsule (prosthesis)
Mammary implant
AHA: 2Q, '98, 14; 3Q, '92, 4
TIP: If documentation indicates capsular contracture of breast implant, see instead code 611.83.

996.55 Due to artificial skin graft and decellularized allodermis
Dislodgement
Displacement
Failure
Non-adherence
Poor incorporation
Shearing
AHA: 4Q, '98, 52

996.56 Due to peritoneal dialysis catheter
EXCLUDES mechanical complication of arteriovenous dialysis catheter (996.1)
AHA: 4Q, '98, 54

996.57 Due to insulin pump
AHA: 4Q, '03, 81-82

996.59 Due to other implant and internal device, not elsewhere classified
Nonabsorbable surgical material NOS
Prosthetic implant in:
bile duct
chin
orbit of eye
AHA: 2Q, '99, 13; 3Q, '94, 7
TIP: Assign for clogged biliary stent and also for nonfunctioning pressure equalization (PE) tubes.

√5ᵗʰ **996.6 Infection and inflammatory reaction due to internal prosthetic device, implant, and graft**
Infection (causing obstruction) ⎱ due to (presence of) any device,
Inflammation ⎰ implant, and graft classifiable to 996.0-996.5
Use additional code to identify specified infections
AHA: 2Q, '89, 16; J-F, '87, 14

996.60 Due to unspecified device, implant, and graft

996.61 Due to cardiac device, implant, and graft
Cardiac pacemaker or defibrillator:
electrode(s), lead(s)
pulse generator
subcutaneous pocket
Coronary artery bypass graft
Heart valve prosthesis

996.62 Due to other vascular device, implant, and graft
Arterial graft
Arteriovenous fistula or shunt
Infusion pump
Vascular catheter (arterial) (dialysis) (peripheral venous)
EXCLUDES infection due to:
central venous catheter (999.31)
Hickman catheter (999.31)
peripherally inserted central catheter [PICC] (999.31)
portacath (port-a-cath) (999.31)
triple lumen catheter (999.31)
umbilical venous catheter (999.31)
AHA: 4Q, '07, 86; 2Q, '04, 16; 1Q, '04, 5; 4Q, '03, 107, 111; 2Q, '03, 7; 2Q, '94, 13
T82.7xxA Inf & inflam react oth card vasc dev gft initial enc   [I-10]

996.63 Due to nervous system device, implant, and graft
Electrodes implanted in brain
Peripheral nerve graft
Spinal canal catheter
Ventricular (communicating) shunt (catheter)

996.64 Due to indwelling urinary catheter
Use additional code to identify specified infections, such as:
cystitis (595.0-595.9)
sepsis (038.0-038.9)
AHA: 3Q, '09, 10-11; 3Q, '93, 6
TIP: Assign for documented infection due to the presence of an indwelling urinary catheter, whether Foley, suprapubic, or other type.
T83.51xD Inf & inflam react indwll urinary cath subsq enc   [I-10]

996.65 Due to other genitourinary device implant, and graft
Intrauterine contraceptive device
AHA: 1Q, '00, 15

996.66 Due to internal joint prosthesis
Use additional code to identify infected prosthetic joint (V43.60-V43.69)
AHA: 2Q, '08, 3-5; 2Q, '07, 7; 4Q, '05, 91, 113; 2Q, '91, 18
TIP: Do not assign for the second admission of a staged procedure whereby the infected prosthesis has been previously removed and the patient now returns for placement of a new prosthesis; see instead codes from category 736.
T84.51xA Inf & inflam reaction int rt hip pros initial enc   [I-10]

996.67 Due to other internal orthopedic device, implant, and graft
Bone growth stimulator (electrode)
Internal fixation device (pin) (rod) (screw)

996.68 Due to peritoneal dialysis catheter
Exit-site infection or inflammation
AHA: 4Q, '98, 54

N Newborn Age: 0   P Pediatric Age: 0-17   M Maternity Age: 12-55   A Adult Age: 15-124

996.69 Due to other internal prosthetic device, implant, and graft
Breast prosthesis
Ocular lens prosthesis
Prosthetic orbital implant
AHA: 2Q, '08, 11; 4Q, '03, 108; 4Q, '98, 52

√5ᵗʰ **996.7 Other complications of internal (biological) (synthetic) prosthetic device, implant, and graft**
Complication NOS
Occlusion NOS
Embolism
Fibrosis   } due to (presence of) any device,
Hemorrhage   implant, and graft
Pain   classifiable to 996.0-996.5
Stenosis
Thrombus

Use additional code to identify complication, such as:
pain due to presence of device, implant or graft (338.18-338.19, 338.28-338.29)
venous embolism and thrombosis (453.2-453.9)
EXCLUDES *disruption (dehiscence) of internal suture material (998.31)*
transplant rejection (996.8)
AHA: 2Q, '07, 12; 4Q, '05, 94; 1Q, '89, 9; N-D, '86, 5

996.70 Due to unspecified device, implant, and graft

996.71 Due to heart valve prosthesis

996.72 Due to other cardiac device, implant, and graft
Cardiac pacemaker or defibrillator:
electrode(s), lead(s)
subcutaneous pocket
Coronary artery bypass (graft)
EXCLUDES *occlusion due to atherosclerosis (414.02-414.06)*
AHA: 3Q, '08, 10; 3Q, '06, 8, 25; 3Q, '01, 20
TIP: Assign for in-stent stenosis of previously placed coronary artery stent.
T82.847A Pain cardiac prosth devc impl graft initial enc `I-10`

996.73 Due to renal dialysis device, implant, and graft
AHA: 2Q, '91, 18
T82.858A Stenosis vasc prosth devc impl graft initial enc `I-10`

996.74 Due to other vascular device, implant, and graft
EXCLUDES *occlusion of biological graft due to atherosclerosis (440.30-440.32)*
AHA: 1Q, '03, 16, 17

996.75 Due to nervous system device, implant, and graft

996.76 Due to genitourinary device, implant, and graft
AHA: 1Q, '09, 15; 1Q, '00, 15
T83.83xA Hemorrhage GU prosth devc impl graft initial enc `I-10`

996.77 Due to internal joint prosthesis
Use additional code to identify prosthetic joint (V43.60-V43.69)
AHA: 4Q, '05, 91
T84.84xA Pain int ortho prosth devc impl gft initial enc `I-10`

996.78 Due to other internal orthopedic device, implant, and graft
AHA: 2Q, '03, 14

996.79 Due to other internal prosthetic device, implant, and graft
AHA: 2Q, '04, 7; 1Q,'01, 8; 3Q, '95, 14; 3Q, '92, 4

√5ᵗʰ **996.8 Complications of transplanted organ**
Transplant failure or rejection
Use additional code to identify nature of complication, such as:
cytomegalovirus (CMV) infection (078.5)
graft-versus-host disease (279.50-279.53)
malignancy associated with organ transplant (199.2)
post-transplant lymphoproliferative disorder (PTLD) (238.77)
AHA: 4Q, '08, 82-83; 3Q, '01, 12; 3Q, '93, 3, 4; 2Q, '93, 11; 1Q, '93, 24
TIP: Assign only if the complication affects the function of the transplanted organ. Assign also a code for the specific complication.

996.80 Transplanted organ, unspecified

996.81 Kidney
AHA: ►1Q, '10, 9;◄ 4Q, '08, 83; 3Q, '03, 16; 3Q, '98, 6, 7; 3Q, '94, 8; 2Q, '94, 9; 1Q, '93, 24
TIP: Do not assign for chronic kidney disease (CKD) status following kidney transplant. The provider must indicate transplant failure, rejection, or other complication to support assignment of this code.
T86.11 Kidney transplant rejection `I-10`

996.82 Liver
AHA: 4Q, '08, 82, 99; 3Q, '03, 17; 3Q, '98, 3, 4

996.83 Heart
AHA: 3Q, '03, 16; 4Q, '02, 53; 3Q, '98, 5

996.84 Lung
AHA: 2Q, '03, 12; 3Q, '98, 5

996.85 Bone marrow
AHA: 4Q, '08, 91; 4Q, '90, 4

996.86 Pancreas

996.87 Intestine

996.89 Other specified transplanted organ
AHA: 3Q, '94, 5

√5ᵗʰ **996.9 Complications of reattached extremity or body part**

996.90 Unspecified extremity

996.91 Forearm

996.92 Hand

996.93 Finger(s)

996.94 Upper extremity, other and unspecified

996.95 Foot and toe(s)

996.96 Lower extremity, other and unspecified

996.99 Other specified body part

√4ᵗʰ **997 Complications affecting specified body systems, not elsewhere classified**
Use additional code to identify complications
EXCLUDES *the listed conditions when specified as:*
causing shock (998.0)
complications of:
anesthesia:
adverse effect (001.0-799.9, 995.0-995.8)
in labor or delivery (668.0-668.9)
poisoning (968.0-969.9)
implanted device or graft (996.0-996.9)
obstetrical procedures (669.0-669.4)
reattached extremity (996.90-996.96)
transplanted organ (996.80-996.89)
AHA: 1Q, '94, 4; 1Q, '93, 26

√5ᵗʰ **997.0 Nervous system complications**

997.00 Nervous system complication, unspecified

997.01 Central nervous system complication
Anoxic brain damage
Cerebral hypoxia
EXCLUDES *cerebrovascular hemorrhage or infarction (997.02)*
AHA: 1Q, '07, 22; 1Q, '06, 15
TIP: Assign for hyperperfusion syndrome, a complication of carotid endarterectomy.

Injury and Poisoning

997.02–997.79

997.02 Iatrogenic cerebrovascular infarction or hemorrhage
Postoperative stroke
AHA: 3Q, '06, 6; 2Q, '04, 8; 4Q, '95, 57
TIP: Assign an additional code to specify the type of postoperative stroke involved.
I97.810 Intraop cerebrvascular infarct during card surg `I-10`

997.09 Other nervous system complications
G97.0 Cerebrospinal fluid leak from spinal puncture `I-10`

997.1 Cardiac complications
Cardiac:
  arrest
  insufficiency   } during or resulting from a procedure
Cardiorespiratory failure
Heart failure
EXCLUDES *the listed conditions as long-term effects of cardiac surgery or due to the presence of cardiac prosthetic device (429.4)*
AHA: 4Q, '08, 179; 2Q, '02, 12
I97.711 Intraoperative cardiac arrest during oth surgery `I-10`

997.2 Peripheral vascular complications
Phlebitis or thrombophlebitis during or resulting from a procedure
EXCLUDES *the listed conditions due to:*
  implant or catheter device (996.62)
  infusion, perfusion, or transfusion (999.2)
  complications affecting blood vessels (997.71-997.79)
AHA: 1Q, '03, 6; 3Q, '02, 24-26
T81.72xA Complication of vein following a procedure NEC init. enc `I-10`

✓5ᵗʰ **997.3 Respiratory complications**
EXCLUDES *iatrogenic [postoperative] pneumothorax (512.1)*
  iatrogenic pulmonary embolism (415.11)
  Mendelson's syndrome in labor and delivery (668.0)
  specified complications classified elsewhere, such as:
    adult respiratory distress syndrome (518.5)
    pulmonary edema, postoperative (518.4)
    respiratory insufficiency, acute, postoperative (518.5)
    shock lung (518.5)
    tracheostomy complications (519.00-519.09)
    transfusion related acute lung injury [TRALI] (518.7)
AHA: 1Q, '97, 10; 2Q, '93, 3; 2Q, '93, 9; 4Q, '90, 25

997.31 Ventilator associated pneumonia
Ventilator associated pneumonitis
Use additional code to identify organism
AHA: 4Q, '08, 148-149
TIP: Do not assign unless the provider has documented the relationship between the pneumonia and ventilation status.

997.39 Other respiratory complications
Mendelson's syndrome resulting from a procedure
Pneumonia (aspiration) resulting from a procedure
DEF: Mendelson's syndrome: acid pneumonitis due to aspiration of gastric acids, may occur after anesthesia or sedation.
J95.4 Chem pneumonitis d/t anesthesia [Mendelson syndrm] `I-10`

997.4 Digestive system complications
Complications of:
  intestinal (internal) anastomosis and bypass, not elsewhere classified, except that involving urinary tract
Hepatic failure
Hepatorenal syndrome   } specified as due to a procedure
Intestinal obstruction NOS
EXCLUDES *gastrostomy complications (536.40-536.49)*
  specified gastrointestinal complications classified elsewhere, such as:
    blind loop syndrome (579.2)
    colostomy and enterostomy complications (569.60-569.69)
    complications of intestinal pouch (569.71-569.79)
    gastrojejunal ulcer (534.0-534.9)
    infection of esophagostomy (530.86)
    infection of external stoma (569.61)
    mechanical complication of esophagostomy (530.87)
    pelvic peritoneal adhesions, female (614.6)
    peritoneal adhesions (568.0)
    peritoneal adhesions with obstruction (560.81)
    postcholecystectomy syndrome (576.0)
    postgastric surgery syndromes (564.2)
    pouchitis (569.71)
    vomiting following gastrointestinal surgery (564.3)
AHA: 2Q, '01, 4-6; 3Q, '99, 4; 2Q, '99, 14; 3Q, '97, 7; 1Q, '97, 11; 2Q, '95, 7; 1Q, '93, 26; 3Q, '92, 15; 2Q, '89, 15; 1Q, '88, 14
K91.3 Postprocedural intestinal obstruction `I-10`

997.5 Urinary complications
Complications of:
  external stoma of urinary tract
  internal anastomosis and bypass of urinary tract, including that involving intestinal tract
Oliguria or anuria
Renal (kidney):   } specified as due to procedure
  failure (acute)
  insufficiency (acute)
Tubular necrosis (acute)
EXCLUDES *specified complications classified elsewhere, such as:*
  postoperative stricture of:
    ureter (593.3)
    urethra (598.2)
AHA: 3Q, '03, 13; 3Q, '96, 10, 15; 4Q, '95, 73; 1Q, '92, 13; 2Q, '89, 16; M-A, '87, 10; S-O, '85, 3
TIP: If a urinary tract infection is specified as a postoperative complication, assign both 997.5 and 599.0.
N99.0 Postprocedural (acute) (chronic) renal failure `I-10`

✓5ᵗʰ **997.6 Amputation stump complication**
EXCLUDES *admission for treatment for a current traumatic amputation — code to complicated traumatic amputation*
  phantom limb (syndrome) (353.6)
AHA: 4Q, '95, 82

997.60 Unspecified complication

997.61 Neuroma of amputation stump
DEF: Hyperplasia generated nerve cell mass following amputation.

997.62 Infection (chronic)
Use additional code to identify the organism
AHA: 1Q, '05, 15 4Q, '96, 46
TIP: If cellulitis is specified as a manifestation of the infection, assign an additional code from category 681 or 682.
T87.43 Infection amputation stump right lower extremity `I-10`

997.69 Other
AHA: 1Q, '05, 15

✓5ᵗʰ **997.7 Vascular complications of other vessels**
EXCLUDES *peripheral vascular complications (997.2)*

997.71 Vascular complications of mesenteric artery
AHA: 4Q, '01, 53
TIP: For postoperative mesenteric artery embolism, assign also code 557.0 Acute vascular insufficiency of intestine.

997.72 Vascular complications of renal artery

997.79 Vascular complications of other vessels

| N | Newborn Age: 0 | P | Pediatric Age: 0-17 | M | Maternity Age: 12-55 | A | Adult Age: 15-124 |

√5ᵗʰ **997.9 Complications affecting other specified body systems, not elsewhere classified**

> **EXCLUDES** *specified complications classified elsewhere, such as:*
> *broad ligament laceration syndrome (620.6)*
> *postartificial menopause syndrome (627.4)*
> *postoperative stricture of vagina (623.2)*

997.91 Hypertension

> **EXCLUDES** *essential hypertension (401.0-401.9)*
> **AHA:** 4Q, '95, 57

997.99 Other

Vitreous touch syndrome

DEF: Vitreous touch syndrome: vitreous protruding through pupil and attaches to corneal epithelium; causes aqueous fluid in vitreous body; marked by corneal edema, loss of lucidity; complication of cataract surgery.
AHA: 2Q, '94, 12; 1Q, '94, 17

√4ᵗʰ **998 Other complications of procedures, not elsewhere classified**

> **EXCLUDES** ▶*fluid overload due to transfusion (blood) (276.61)*
> *TACO (276.61)*
> *transfusion associated circulatory overload (276.61)*◀
> **AHA:** 1Q, '94, 4

998.0 Postoperative shock

Collapse NOS ⎫ during or resulting from
Shock (endotoxic) ⎬ a surgical
  (hypovolemic septic) ⎭ procedure

> **EXCLUDES** *shock:*
> *anaphylactic due to serum (999.4)*
> *anesthetic (995.4)*
> *electric (994.8)*
> *following abortion (639.5)*
> *obstetric (669.1)*
> *traumatic (958.4)*

√5ᵗʰ **998.1 Hemorrhage or hematoma or seroma complicating a procedure**

> **EXCLUDES** *hemorrhage, hematoma, or seroma:*
> *complicating cesarean section or puerperal perineal wound (674.3)*
> *due to implanted device or graft (996.70-996.79)*

998.11 Hemorrhage complicating a procedure

AHA: 3Q '03, 13; 1Q, '03, 4; 4Q, '97, 52; 1Q, '97, 10
I97.410 Intraop hemorrhage circ sys organ comp card cath   `I-10`

998.12 Hematoma complicating a procedure

AHA: 3Q, '06, 12; 1Q, '03, 6; 3Q, '02, 24, 26

998.13 Seroma complicating a procedure

AHA: 4Q, '96, 46; 1Q, '93, 26; 2Q, '92, 15; S-O, '87, 8

998.2 Accidental puncture or laceration during a procedure

Accidental perforation by catheter or other instrument during a procedure on:
blood vessel
nerve
organ

> **EXCLUDES** *iatrogenic [postoperative] pneumothorax (512.1)*
> *puncture or laceration caused by implanted device intentionally left in operation wound (996.0-996.5)*
> *specified complications classified elsewhere, such as:*
> *broad ligament laceration syndrome (620.6)*
> *dural tear (349.31)*
> *incidental durotomy (349.31)*
> *trauma from instruments during delivery (664.0-665.9)*

AHA: ▶1Q, '10, 8, 11;◀ 2Q, '07, 9; 1Q, '06, 15; 3Q, '02, 24, 26; 3Q, '94, 6; 3Q, '90, 17; 3Q, '90, 18
I97.51 Accidentl punct lac circ sys organ dur circ proc   `I-10`

√5ᵗʰ **998.3 Disruption of wound**

Dehiscence ⎫
Rupture ⎬ of operation wound

Disruption of any suture materials or other closure method

> **EXCLUDES** *disruption of:*
> *cesarean wound (674.1)*
> *perineal wound, puerperal (674.2)*
> **AHA:** 4Q, '08, 149-152; 4Q, '02, 73; 1Q, '93, 19

998.30 Disruption of wound, unspecified

Disruption of wound NOS

998.31 Disruption of internal operation (surgical) wound

Disruption or dehiscence of closure of:
  fascia, superficial or muscular
  internal organ
  muscle or muscle flap
  ribs or rib cage
  skull or craniotomy
  sternum or sternotomy
  tendon or ligament
Deep disruption or dehiscence of operation wound NOS

> **EXCLUDES** *complications of internal anastomosis of:*
> *gastrointestinal tract (997.4)*
> *urinary tract (997.5)*

998.32 Disruption of external operation (surgical) wound

Disruption of operation wound NOS
Disruption or dehiscence of closure of:
  cornea
  mucosa
  skin
  subcutaneous tissue
Full-thickness skin disruption or dehiscence
Superficial disruption or dehiscence of operation wound

AHA: 1Q, '06, 8; 1Q, '05, 11; 4Q, '03, 104, 106
T81.31xA Disruption ext operation wound NEC initial enc   `I-10`

998.33 Disruption of traumatic injury wound repair

Disruption or dehiscence of closure of traumatic laceration (external) (internal)
AHA: 4Q, '08, 151, 152

998.4 Foreign body accidentally left during a procedure

Adhesions ⎫ due to foreign body accidentally left in
Obstruction ⎬ operative wound or body cavity
Perforation ⎭ during a procedure

> **EXCLUDES** *obstruction or perforation caused by implanted device intentionally left in body (996.0-996.5)*
> **AHA:** 1Q, '09,18; 1Q, '89, 9

√5ᵗʰ **998.5 Postoperative infection**

> **EXCLUDES** *bleb associated endophthalmitis (379.63)*
> *infection due to:*
> *implanted device (996.60-996.69)*
> *infusion, perfusion, or transfusion (999.31-999.39)*
> *postoperative obstetrical wound infection (674.3)*

998.51 Infected postoperative seroma

Use additional code to identify organism
AHA: 4Q, '96, 46

998.59 Other postoperative infection

Abscess: ⎫
  intra-abdominal ⎪
  stitch ⎬ postoperative
  subphrenic ⎪
  wound ⎪
Septicemia ⎭

Use additional code to identify infection
AHA: 2Q, '06, 23; 4Q, '04, 76; 4Q, '03, 104, 106-107; 3Q, '98, 3; 3Q, '95, 5; 2Q, '95, 7; 3Q, '94, 6; 1Q, '93, 19; J-F, '87, 14
TIP: Do not assign if the infection is related to an internal prosthetic device, implant, or graft; see instead subcategory 996.6.
T81.4xxA Infection following procedure initl encounter   `I-10`

998.6 Persistent postoperative fistula

AHA: J-F, '87, 14
T81.83xD Persistent postprocedural fistula subsequent enc   `I-10`

998.7 Acute reaction to foreign substance accidentally left during a procedure

Peritonitis:
  aseptic
  chemical

Injury and Poisoning

998.8–999.60

✓5ᵗʰ **998.8 Other specified complications of procedures, not elsewhere classified**

AHA: 4Q, '94, 46; 1Q, '89, 9

998.81 Emphysema (subcutaneous) (surgical) resulting from a procedure

998.82 Cataract fragments in eye following cataract surgery

998.83 Non-healing surgical wound

AHA: 4Q, '96, 47

998.89 Other specified complications

AHA: 2Q, '09, 11; 3Q, '06, 9; 3Q, '05, 16; 3Q, '99, 13; 2Q, '98, 16

TIP: Assign for cases in which a procedure is performed on the wrong body site (e.g., right leg versus left leg), along with E876.5-E876.7.

T81.89 Other complications of procedures NEC   I-10

998.9 Unspecified complication of procedure, not elsewhere classified

Postoperative complication NOS

EXCLUDES *complication NOS of obstetrical, surgery or procedure (669.4)*

AHA: 4Q, '93, 37

✓4ᵗʰ **999 Complications of medical care, not elsewhere classified**

INCLUDES complications, not elsewhere classified, of:
     dialysis (hemodialysis) (peritoneal) (renal)
     extracorporeal circulation
     hyperalimentation therapy
     immunization
     infusion
     inhalation therapy
     injection
     inoculation
     perfusion
     transfusion
     vaccination
     ventilation therapy

Use additional code, where applicable, to identify specific complication

EXCLUDES *specified complications classified elsewhere such as:*
     complications of implanted device (996.0-996.9)
     contact dermatitis due to drugs (692.3)
     dementia dialysis (294.8)
     transient (293.9)
     dialysis disequilibrium syndrome (276.0-276.9)
     poisoning and toxic effects of drugs and chemicals (960.0-989.9)
     postvaccinal encephalitis (323.51)
     water and electrolyte imbalance (276.0-276.9)

999.0 Generalized vaccinia

EXCLUDES *vaccinia not from vaccine (051.02)*

DEF: Skin eruption, self-limiting; follows vaccination; due to transient viremia with virus localized in skin.

999.1 Air embolism

Air embolism to any site following infusion, perfusion, or transfusion

EXCLUDES *embolism specified as:*
     complicating:
        abortion (634-638 with .6, 639.6)
        ectopic or molar pregnancy (639.6)
        pregnancy, childbirth, or the puerperium (673.0)
     due to implanted device (996.7)
     traumatic (958.0)

999.2 Other vascular complications

Phlebitis
Thromboembolism   } following infusion, perfusion, or transfusion
Thrombophlebitis

EXCLUDES *extravasation of vesicant drugs (999.81, 999.82)*
     the listed conditions when specified as:
        due to implanted device (996.61-996.62. 996.72-996.74)
        postoperative NOS (997.2, 997.71-997.79)

AHA: 2Q, '97, 5

TIP: Do not assign for IV infiltration; if the infiltration is severe enough to cause other complications, a code for the specific complication should be assigned. For chemotherapy extravasation, see code 999.81.

T80.1xxA Vasc comp follw inf transfusn tx inj initial enc   I-10

✓5ᵗʰ **999.3 Other infection**

Infection
Sepsis   } following infusion, injection, transfusion, or vaccination
Septicemia

Use additional code to identify the specified infection, such as:
     septicemia (038.0-038.9)

EXCLUDES *the listed conditions when specified as:*
     due to implanted device (996.60-996.69)
     postoperative NOS (998.51-998.59)

AHA: 4Q, '07, 96; 2Q, '01, 11, 12; 2Q, '97, 5; J-F, '87, 14

999.31 Infection due to central venous catheter

Catheter-related bloodstream infection (CRBSI) NOS
Infection due to:
     Hickman catheter
     peripherally inserted central catheter (PICC)
     portacath (port-a-cath)
     triple lumen catheter
     umbilical venous catheter

EXCLUDES *infection due to:*
     arterial catheter (996.62)
     catheter NOS (996.69)
     peripheral venous catheter (996.62)
     urinary catheter (996.64)

AHA: 4Q, '08, 72, 193; 4Q, '07, 97

T80.21xD Inf due to central venous cath subsequent enc   I-10

999.39 Infection following other infusion, injection, transfusion, or vaccination

AHA: 4Q, '08, 99

999.4 Anaphylactic shock due to serum

Anaphylactic reaction due to serum

EXCLUDES *shock:*
     allergic NOS (995.0)
     anaphylactic:
        NOS (995.0)
        due to drugs and chemicals (995.0)

DEF: Life-threatening hypersensitivity to foreign serum; causes respiratory distress, vascular collapse, and shock.

999.5 Other serum reaction

Intoxication by serum
Protein sickness
Serum rash
Serum sickness
Urticaria due to serum

EXCLUDES *serum hepatitis (070.2-070.3)*

DEF: Serum sickness: Hypersensitivity to foreign serum; causes fever, hives, swelling, and lymphadenopathy.

▲ ✓5ᵗʰ **999.6 ABO incompatibility reaction due to transfusion of blood or blood products**

EXCLUDES *minor blood group antigens reactions (Duffy) (E) (K(ell)) (Kidd) (Lewis) (M) (N) (P) (S) (999.75-999.79)*

● **999.60 ABO incompatibility reaction, unspecified**

ABO incompatible blood transfusion NOS
Reaction to ABO incompatibility from transfusion NOS

Ⓝ Newborn Age: 0   Ⓟ Pediatric Age: 0-17   Ⓜ Maternity Age: 12-55   Ⓐ Adult Age: 15-124

Injury and Poisoning

● 999.61 **ABO incompatibility with hemolytic transfusion reaction not specified as acute or delayed**
ABO incompatibility with hemolytic transfusion reaction at unspecified time after transfusion
Hemolytic transfusion reaction (HTR) due to ABO incompatibility

● 999.62 **ABO incompatibility with acute hemolytic transfusion reaction**
ABO incompatibility with hemolytic transfusion reaction less than 24 hours after transfusion
Acute hemolytic transfusion reaction (AHTR) due to ABO incompatibility

● 999.63 **ABO incompatibility with delayed hemolytic transfusion reaction**
ABO incompatibility with hemolytic transfusion reaction 24 hours or more after transfusion
Delayed hemolytic transfusion reaction (DHTR) due to ABO incompatibility

● 999.69 **Other ABO incompatibility reaction**
Delayed serologic transfusion reaction (DSTR) from ABO incompatibility
Other ABO incompatible blood transfusion
Other reaction to ABO incompatibility from transfusion

▲ √5ᵗʰ 999.7 **Rh and other non-ABO incompatibility reaction due to transfusion of blood or blood products**
Elevation of Rh titer

● 999.70 **Rh incompatibility reaction, unspecified**
Reaction due to Rh factor in transfusion NOS
Rh incompatible blood transfusion NOS
Unspecified reaction due to incompatibility related to Rh antigens (C) (c) (D) (E) (e)
Unspecified reaction to Rh incompatibility

● 999.71 **Rh incompatibility with hemolytic transfusion reaction not specified as acute or delayed**
Hemolytic transfusion reaction (HTR) due to Rh incompatibility
HTR due to incompatibility related to Rh antigens (C) (c) (D) (E) (e), not specified as acute or delayed
Rh incompatibility with hemolytic transfusion reaction at unspecified time after transfusion

● 999.72 **Rh incompatibility with acute hemolytic transfusion reaction**
Acute hemolytic transfusion reaction (AHTR) due to Rh incompatibility
AHTR due to incompatibility related to Rh antigens (C) (c) (D) (E) (e)
Rh incompatibility with hemolytic transfusion reaction less than 24 hours after transfusion

● 999.73 **Rh incompatibility with delayed hemolytic transfusion reaction**
Delayed hemolytic transfusion reaction (DHTR) due to Rh incompatibility
DHTR due to incompatibility related to Rh antigens (C) (c) (D) (E) (e)
Rh incompatibility with hemolytic transfusion reaction 24 hours or more after transfusion

● 999.74 **Other Rh incompatibility reaction**
Delayed serologic transfusion reaction (DSTR) from Rh incompatibility
Other reaction due to incompatibility related to Rh antigens (C) (c) (D) (E) (e)
Other reaction to Rh incompatible blood transfusion

● 999.75 **Non-ABO incompatibility reaction, unspecified**
Non-ABO incompatible blood transfusion NOS
Reaction to non-ABO antigen incompatibility from transfusion NOS
Unspecified reaction due to incompatibility related to minor antigens (Duffy) (Kell) (Kidd) (Lewis) (M) (N) (P) (S)

● 999.76 **Non-ABO incompatibility with hemolytic transfusion reaction not specified as acute or delayed**
Hemolytic transfusion reaction (HTR) due to non-ABO incompatibility
HTR from incompatibility related to minor antigens (Duffy) (Kell) (Kidd) (Lewis) (M) (N) (P) (S)
Non-ABO incompatibility with hemolytic transfusion reaction at unspecified time after transfusion

● 999.77 **Non-ABO incompatibility with acute hemolytic transfusion reaction**
Acute hemolytic transfusion reaction (AHTR) due to non-ABO incompatibility
AHTR from incompatibility related to minor antigens (Duffy) (Kell) (Kidd) (Lewis) (M) (N) (P) (S)
Non-ABO incompatibility with hemolytic transfusion reaction less than 24 hours after transfusion

● 999.78 **Non-ABO incompatibility with delayed hemolytic transfusion reaction**
Delayed hemolytic transfusion reaction (DHTR) due to non-ABO incompatibility
DHTR from incompatibility related to minor antigens (Duffy) (Kell) (Kidd) (Lewis) (M) (N) (P) (S)
Non-ABO incompatibility with hemolytic transfusion reaction 24 hours or more after transfusion

● 999.79 **Other non-ABO incompatibility reaction**
Delayed serologic transfusion reaction (DSTR) from non-ABO incompatibility
Other non-ABO incompatible blood transfusion
Other reaction due to incompatibility related to minor antigens (Duffy) (Kell) (Kidd) (Lewis) (M) (N) (P) (S)
Other reaction to non-ABO incompatibility from transfusion

▲ √5ᵗʰ 999.8 **Other and unspecified infusion and transfusion reaction**
EXCLUDES ►◄ *ABO incompatibility reactions (999.60-999.69)*
febrile nonhemolytic transfusion reaction (FNHTR) (780.66)
hemochromatosis due to repeated red blood cell transfusions (275.02)
non-ABO incompatibility reactions (999.75-999.79)◄
postoperative shock (998.0)
►*posttransfusion purpura (287.41)*
Rh incompatibility reactions (999.70-999.74)
transfusion associated circulatory overload (TACO) (276.61)◄
transfusion related acute lung injury [TRALI] (518.7)
AHA: 4Q, '08, 152-155; 3Q, '00, 9

● 999.80 **Transfusion reaction, unspecified**
Incompatible blood transfusion NOS
Reaction to blood group incompatibility in infusion or transfusion NOS

999.81 **Extravasation of vesicant chemotherapy**
Infiltration of vesicant chemotherapy
AHA: 4Q, '08, 155

999.82 **Extravasation of other vesicant agent**
Infiltration of other vesicant agent

● 999.83 **Hemolytic transfusion reaction, incompatibility unspecified**
Hemolytic transfusion reaction (HTR) with antigen incompatibility unspecified, not specified as acute or delayed
HTR with incompatibility unspecified at unspecified time after transfusion

● 999.84 **Acute hemolytic transfusion reaction, incompatibility unspecified**
Acute hemolytic transfusion reaction (AHTR) with antigen incompatibility unspecified
AHTR, incompatibility unspecified

● 999.85 **Delayed hemolytic transfusion reaction, incompatibility unspecified**
Delayed hemolytic transfusion reaction (DHTR) with antigen incompatibility unspecified
DHTR, incompatibility unspecified

999.88 **Other infusion reaction**

Injury and Poisoning

999.89–999.9

999.89 **Other transfusion reaction**
> ►Delayed serologic transfusion reaction (DSTR), incompatibility unspecified◄

Use additional code to identify graft-versus-host reaction (279.5)

AHA: 4Q, '08, 99, 154

999.9 **Other and unspecified complications of medical care, not elsewhere classified**

Complications, not elsewhere classified, of:

electroshock
inhalation
ultrasound } therapy
ventilation

Unspecified misadventure of medical care

EXCLUDES *unspecified complication of:*
phototherapy (990)
radiation therapy (999)
ventilator associated pneumonia (997.31)

AHA: 3Q, '06, 25; 1Q, '03, 19; 2Q, '97, 5

N   Newborn Age: 0   P   Pediatric Age: 0-17   M   Maternity Age: 12-55   A   Adult Age: 15-124

Supplementary Classification Of Factors Influencing Health Status and Contact with Health Services ▶(V01-V91)◀

This classification is provided to deal with occasions when circumstances other than a disease or injury classifiable to categories 001-999 (the main part of ICD) are recorded as "diagnoses" or "problems." This can arise mainly in three ways:

a) When a person who is not currently sick encounters the health services for some specific purpose, such as to act as a donor of an organ or tissue, to receive prophylactic vaccination, or to discuss a problem which is in itself not a disease or injury. This will be a fairly rare occurrence among hospital inpatients, but will be relatively more common among hospital outpatients and patients of family practitioners, health clinics, etc.

b) When a person with a known disease or injury, whether it is current or resolving, encounters the health care system for a specific treatment of that disease or injury (e.g., dialysis for renal disease; chemotherapy for malignancy; cast change).

c) When some circumstance or problem is present which influences the person's health status but is not in itself a current illness or injury. Such factors may be elicited during population surveys, when the person may or may not be currently sick, or be recorded as an additional factor to be borne in mind when the person is receiving care for some current illness or injury classifiable to categories 001-999.

In the latter circumstances the V code should be used only as a supplementary code and should not be the one selected for use in primary, single cause tabulations. Examples of these circumstances are a personal history of certain diseases, or a person with an artificial heart valve in situ.

AHA: J-F, '87, 8

Persons with Potential Health Hazards Related to Communicable Diseases (V01-V06)

EXCLUDES *family history of infectious and parasitic diseases (V18.8)*
personal history of infectious and parasitic diseases (V12.0)

V01 Contact with or exposure to communicable diseases
TIP: Do not assign if the patient shows signs or symptoms of the disease to which he or she was exposed.

V01.0 Cholera
Conditions classifiable to 001

V01.1 Tuberculosis
Conditions classifiable to 010-018

V01.2 Poliomyelitis
Conditions classifiable to 045

V01.3 Smallpox
Conditions classifiable to 050

V01.4 Rubella
Conditions classifiable to 056

V01.5 Rabies
Conditions classifiable to 071

V01.6 Venereal diseases
Conditions classifiable to 090-099
AHA: 4Q, '07, 125

V01.7 Other viral diseases
Conditions classifiable to 042-078 and V08, except as above
AHA: 2Q, '92, 11

V01.71 Varicella

V01.79 Other viral diseases

V01.8 Other communicable diseases
Conditions classifiable to 001-136, except as above
AHA: J-A, '87, 24

V01.81 Anthrax
AHA: 4Q, '02, 70, 78

V01.82 Exposure to SARS-associated coronavirus
AHA: 4Q, '03, 46-47

V01.83 Escherichia coli (E. coli)

V01.84 Meningococcus
Z20.811 Contact with and exposure to meningococcus   I-10

V01.89 Other communicable diseases

V01.9 Unspecified communicable diseases

V02 Carrier or suspected carrier of infectious diseases
INCLUDES colonization status
AHA: 3Q, '95, 18; 3Q, '94, 4

V02.0 Cholera

V02.1 Typhoid

V02.2 Amebiasis

V02.3 Other gastrointestinal pathogens

V02.4 Diphtheria

V02.5 Other specified bacterial diseases

V02.51 Group B streptococcus
AHA: 3Q, '06, 14; 1Q, '02, 14; 4Q, '98, 56

V02.52 Other streptococcus

V02.53 Methicillin susceptible Staphylococcus aureus
MSSA colonization
AHA: 4Q, '08, 69, 71, 156

V02.54 Methicillin resistant Staphylococcus aureus
MRSA colonization
AHA: 4Q, '08, 69, 71, 72, 156

V02.59 Other specified bacterial diseases
Meningococcal
Staphylococcal

V02.6 Viral hepatitis
Hepatitis Australian-antigen [HAA] [SH] carrier
Serum hepatitis carrier

V02.60 Viral hepatitis carrier, unspecified
AHA: 4Q, '97, 47

V02.61 Hepatitis B carrier
AHA: 4Q, '97, 47
Z22.51 Carrier of viral hepatitis B   I-10

V02.62 Hepatitis C carrier
AHA: 4Q, '97, 47

V02.69 Other viral hepatitis carrier
AHA: 4Q, '97, 47

V02.7 Gonorrhea

V02.8 Other venereal diseases

V02.9 Other specified infectious organism
AHA: 3Q, '95, 18; 1Q, '93, 22; J-A, '87, 24

V03 Need for prophylactic vaccination and inoculation against bacterial diseases
EXCLUDES *vaccination not carried out (V64.00-V64.09)*
vaccines against combinations of diseases (V06.0-V06.9)

V03.0 Cholera alone

V03.1 Typhoid-paratyphoid alone [TAB]

V03.2 Tuberculosis [BCG]

V03.3 Plague

V03.4 Tularemia

V03.5 Diphtheria alone

V03.6 Pertussis alone

V03.7 Tetanus toxoid alone

V03.8 Other specified vaccinations against single bacterial diseases

V03.81 Hemophilus influenza, type B [Hib]

V03.82 Streptococcus pneumoniae [pneumococcus]

V03.89 Other specified vaccination
AHA: 2Q, '00, 9
TIP: Assign for vaccination against Lyme disease.

V03.9 Unspecified single bacterial disease

V04 Need for prophylactic vaccination and inoculation against certain viral diseases
EXCLUDES *vaccines against combinations of diseases (V06.0-V06.9)*

V04.0 Poliomyelitis

V04.1 Smallpox

Additional Digit Required   Unspecified Code   Other Specified Code   Manifestation Code   ▶◀ Revised Text   ● New Code   ▲ Revised Code Title

2011 ICD-9-CM   October 2010 • Volume 1 – 319

V Codes

V04.2 Measles alone

V04.3 Rubella alone

V04.4 Yellow fever

V04.5 Rabies

V04.6 Mumps alone

V04.7 Common cold

☑5ᵗʰ **V04.8** Other viral diseases
AHA: 4Q, '03, 83

V04.81 Influenza

V04.82 Respiratory syncytial virus (RSV)
AHA: 1Q, '09, 14

V04.89 Other viral diseases
AHA: 2Q, '07, 9
TIP: Assign for vaccination against human papilloma virus (HPV).

☑4ᵗʰ **V05** Need for other prophylactic vaccination and inoculation against single diseases
EXCLUDES vaccines against combinations of diseases (V06.0-V06.9)

V05.0 Athropod-borne viral encephalitis

V05.1 Other arthropod-borne viral diseases

V05.2 Leshmaniasis

V05.3 Viral hepatitis

V05.4 Varicella
Chickenpox

V05.8 Other specified disease
AHA: 1Q, '01, 4; 3Q, '91, 20

V05.9 Unspecified single disease

☑4ᵗʰ **V06** Need for prophylactic vaccination and inoculation against combinations of diseases
NOTE Use additional single vaccination codes from categories V03-V05 to identify any vaccinations not included in a combination code.

V06.0 Cholera with typhoid-paratyphoid [cholera+TAB]

V06.1 Diphtheia-tetanus-pertussis, combined [DTP] [DTaP]
AHA: 4Q, '03, 83; 3Q, '98, 13

V06.2 Diphtheria-tetanus-pertussis with typhoid-paratyphoid [DTP+TAB]

V06.3 Diphtheria-tetanus-pertussis with poliomyelitis [DTP+polio]

V06.4 Measles-mumps-rubella [MMR]

V06.5 Tetanus-diphtheria [Td] [DT]
AHA: 4Q, '03, 83

V06.6 Streptococcus pneumoniae [pneumococcus] and influenza

V06.8 Other combinations
EXCLUDES multiple single vaccination codes (V03.0-V05.9)
AHA: 1Q, '94, 19

V06.9 Unspecified combined vaccine

Persons with Need for Isolation, Other Potential Health Hazards and Prophylactic Measures (V07-V09)

▲ ☑4ᵗʰ **V07** Need for isolation and other prophylactic or treatment measures
EXCLUDES ► long-term (current) (prophylactic) use of certain specific drugs (V58.61-V58.69) ◄
prophylactic organ removal (V50.41-V50.49)

V07.0 Isolation
Admission to protect the individual from his surroundings or for isolation of individual after contact with infectious diseases

V07.1 Desensitization to allergens

V07.2 Prophylactic immunotherapy
Administration of:
antivenin
immune sera [gamma globulin]
RhoGAM
tetanus antitoxin

☑5ᵗʰ **V07.3** Other prophylactic chemotherapy

V07.31 Prophylactic fluoride administration

V07.39 Other prophylactic chemotherapy
EXCLUDES maintenance chemotherapy following disease (V58.11)

V07.4 Hormone replacement therapy (postmenopausal) ♀
Z79.890 Hormone replacement therapy postmenopausal   I-10

▲ ☑5ᵗʰ **V07.5** Use of agents affecting estrogen receptors and estrogen levels
Code first, if applicable:
malignant neoplasm of breast (174.0-174.9, 175.0-175.9)
malignant neoplasm of prostate (185)
Use additional code, if applicable, to identify:
estrogen receptor positive status (V86.0)
family history of breast cancer (V16.3)
genetic susceptibility to cancer (V84.01-V84.09)
personal history of breast cancer (V10.3)
personal history of prostate cancer (V10.46)
postmenopausal status (V49.81)
EXCLUDES hormone replacement therapy (postmenopausal) (V07.4)
AHA: 4Q, '08, 156

▲ **V07.51** Use of selective estrogen receptor modulators [SERMs]
Use of:
raloxifene (Evista)
tamoxifen (Nolvadex)
toremifene (Fareston)
Z79.81 Long term (current) use agent affecting   I-10
estrogen receptors

▲ **V07.52** Use of aromatase inhibitors
Use of:
anastrozole (Arimidex)
exemestane (Aromasin)
letrozole (Femara)

▲ **V07.59** Use of other agents affecting estrogen receptors and estrogen levels
Use of:
estrogen receptor downregulators
fulvestrant (Faslodex)
gonadotropin-releasing hormone (GnRH) agonist
goserelin acetate (Zoladex)
leuprolide acetate (leuprorelin) (Lupron)
megestrol acetate (Megace)

▲ **V07.8** Other specified prophylactic or treatment measure
AHA: 1Q, '92, 11
TIP: Assign for patients having prophylactic breast removal because of a strong family history of breast cancer, along with code V16.3 Family history of breast cancer.

▲ **V07.9** Unspecified prophylactic or treatment measure

V08 Asymptomatic human immunodeficiency virus [HIV] infection status
HIV positive NOS
NOTE This code is only to be used when no HIV infection symptoms or conditions are present. If any HIV infection symptoms or conditions are present, see code 042.
EXCLUDES AIDS (042)
human immunodeficiency virus [HIV] disease (042)
exposure to HIV (V01.79)
nonspecific serologic evidence of HIV (795.71)
symptomatic human immunodeficiency virus [HIV] infection (042)
AHA: 2Q, '04, 11; 2Q, '99, 8; 3Q, '95, 18
Z21 Asymptomatic HIV infection status   I-10

√4th V09 Infection with drug-resistant microorganisms
NOTE This category is intended for use as an additional code for infectious conditions classified elsewhere to indicate the presence of drug-resistance of the infectious organism.
AHA: 3Q, '94, 4; 4Q, '93, 22

V09.0 Infection with microorganisms resistant to penicillins
AHA: 2Q, '06, 16; 4Q, '03, 104, 106

V09.1 Infection with microorganisms resistant to cephalosporins and other B-lactam antibiotics

V09.2 Infection with microorganisms resistant to macrolides

V09.3 Infection with microorganisms resistant to tetracyclines

V09.4 Infection with microorganisms resistant to aminoglycosides

√5th V09.5 Infection with microorganisms resistant to quinolones and fluoroquinolones

V09.50 Without mention of resistance to multiple quinolones and fluoroquinoles

V09.51 With resistance to multiple quinolones and fluoroquinoles

V09.6 Infection with microorganisms resistant to sulfonamides

√5th V09.7 Infection with microorganisms resistant to other specified antimycobacterial agents
EXCLUDES Amikacin (V09.4)
Kanamycin (V09.4)
Streptomycin [SM] (V09.4)

V09.70 Without mention of resistance to multiple antimycobacterial agents

V09.71 With resistance to multiple antimycobacterial agents

√5th V09.8 Infection with microorganisms resistant to other specified drugs
Vancomycin (glycopeptide) intermediate staphylococcus aureus (VISA/GISA)
Vancomycin (glycopeptide) resistant enterococcus (VRE)
Vancomycin (glycopeptide) resistant staphylococcus aureus (VRSA/GRSA)

V09.80 Without mention of resistance to multiple drugs

V09.81 With resistance to multiple drugs

√5th V09.9 Infection with drug-resistant microorganisms, unspecified
Drug resistance, NOS

V09.90 Without mention of multiple drug resistance
Z16 Infection with drug resistant microorganisms   I-10

V09.91 With multiple drug resistance
Multiple drug resistance NOS

Persons with Potential Health Hazards Related to Personal and Family History (V10-V19)

EXCLUDES obstetric patients where the possibility that the fetus might be affected is the reason for observation or management during pregnancy (655.0-655.9)
AHA: J-F, '87, 1

√4th V10 Personal history of malignant neoplasm
AHA: 4Q, '02, 80; 4Q, '98, 69; 1Q, '95, 4; 3Q, '92, 5; M-J, '85, 10; 2Q, '90, 9
TIP: Assign the codes in this category only for a personal history of primary malignancy (not metastatic malignancies).

√5th V10.0 Gastrointestinal tract
History of conditions classifiable to 140-159
EXCLUDES personal history of malignant carcinoid tumor (V10.91)
personal history of malignant neuroendocrine tumor (V10.91)

V10.00 Gastrointestinal tract, unspecified

V10.01 Tongue

V10.02 Other and unspecified oral cavity and pharynx

V10.03 Esophagus

V10.04 Stomach

V10.05 Large intestine
Z85.03 Personal hx prim malig neoplasm large intestine   I-10
AHA: 3Q, '99, 7; 1Q, '95, 4

V10.06 Rectum, rectosigmoid junction, and anus

V10.07 Liver

V10.09 Other
AHA: 4Q, '03, 111

√5th V10.1 Trachea, bronchus, and lung
History of conditions classifiable to 162
EXCLUDES personal history of malignant carcinoid tumor (V10.91)
personal history of malignant neuroendocrine tumor (V10.91)

V10.11 Bronchus and lung

V10.12 Trachea

√5th V10.2 Other respiratory and intrathoracic organs
History of conditions classifiable to 160, 161, 163-165

V10.20 Respiratory organ, unspecified

V10.21 Larynx
AHA: 4Q, '03, 108, 110

V10.22 Nasal cavities, middle ear, and accessory sinuses

V10.29 Other

V10.3 Breast
History of conditions classifiable to 174 and 175
AHA: 3Q, '07, 4; 1Q, '07, 6; 2Q, '03, 5; 4Q, '01, 66; 4Q, '98, 65; 4Q, '97, 50; 1Q, '91, 16; 1Q, '90, 21
Z85.3 Personal history primary malig neoplasm breast   I-10

√5th V10.4 Genital organs
History of conditions classifiable to 179-187

V10.40 Female genital organ, unspecfied   ♀

V10.41 Cervix uteri   ♀
AHA: 4Q, '07, 99

V10.42 Other parts of uterus   ♀

V10.43 Ovary   ♀

V10.44 Other female genital organs   ♀

V10.45 Male genital organ, unspecfied   ♂

V10.46 Prostate   ♂
AHA: 1Q, '09, 15

V10.47 Testis   ♂
Z85.47 Personal history primary malig neoplasm testis   I-10

V10.48 Epididymis   ♂

V Codes

V10.49–V12.53

    V10.49 Other male genital organs ♂

✓5ᵗʰ **V10.5 Urinary organs**
    History of conditions classifiable to 188 and 189
    EXCLUDES ▸ *personal history of malignant carcinoid tumor (V10.91)*
    personal history of malignant neuroendocrine tumor (V10.91)◂

    V10.50 Urinary organ, unspecified

    V10.51 Bladder

    V10.52 Kidney
      EXCLUDES *renal pelvis (V10.53)*
      AHA: 2Q, '04, 4

    V10.53 Renal pelvis
      AHA: 4Q, '01, 55

    V10.59 Other

✓5ᵗʰ **V10.6 Leukemia**
    Conditions classifiable to 204-208
    EXCLUDES *leukemia in remission (204-208)*
    AHA: 2Q, '92, 13; 4Q, '91, 26; 4Q, '90, 3

    V10.60 Leukemia, unspecified

    V10.61 Lymphoid leukemia

    V10.62 Myeloid leukemia

    V10.63 Monocytic leukemia

    V10.69 Other

✓5ᵗʰ **V10.7 Other lymphatic and hematopoietic neoplasms**
    Conditions classifiable to 200-203
    EXCLUDES *listed conditions in 200-203 in remission*
    AHA: M-J, '85, 18

    V10.71 Lymphosarcoma and reticulosarcoma

    V10.72 Hodgkin's disease

    V10.79 Other

✓5ᵗʰ **V10.8 Personal history of malignant neoplasm of other sites**
    History of conditions classifiable to 170-173, 190-195
    EXCLUDES *personal history of malignant carcinoid tumor (V10.91)*
    personal history of malignant neuroendocrine tumor (V10.91)

    V10.81 Bone
      AHA: 2Q, '03, 13

    V10.82 Malignant melanoma of skin

    V10.83 Other malignant neoplasm of skin

    V10.84 Eye

    V10.85 Brain
      AHA: 1Q, '01, 6

    V10.86 Other parts of the nervous system
      EXCLUDES *peripheral sympathetic, and parasympathetic nerves (V10.89)*

    V10.87 Thyroid

    V10.88 Other endocrine glands and related structures

    V10.89 Other

✓5ᵗʰ **V10.9 Other and unspecified personal history of malignant neoplasm**
    AHA: 4Q, '09, 115

    V10.90 Personal history of unspecified malignant neoplasm
    Personal history of malignant neoplasm NOS
    EXCLUDES *personal history of malignant carcinoid tumor (V10.91)*
    personal history of malignant neuroendocrine tumor (V10.91)
    personal history of Merkel cell carcinoma (V10.91)

    V10.91 Personal history of malignant neuroendocrine tumor
    Personal history of malignant carcinoid tumor NOS
    Personal history of malignant neuroendocrine tumor NOS
    Personal history of Merkel cell carcinoma NOS
    Code first any continuing functional activity, such as: carcinoid syndrome (259.2)

✓4ᵗʰ **V11 Personal history of mental disorder**

    V11.0 Schizophrenia
      EXCLUDES *that in remission (295.0-295.9 with fifth-digit 5)*

    V11.1 Affective disorders
    Personal history of manic-depressive psychosis
      EXCLUDES *that in remission (296.0-296.6 with fifth-digit 5, 6)*

    V11.2 Neurosis

    V11.3 Alcoholism

●   **V11.4 Combat and operational stress reaction**

    V11.8 Other mental disorders

    V11.9 Unspecified mental disorder

✓4ᵗʰ **V12 Personal history of certain other diseases**
    AHA: 3Q, '92, 11

✓5ᵗʰ **V12.0 Infectious and parasitic diseases**
    EXCLUDES *personal history of infectious diseases specific to a body system*

    V12.00 Unspecified infectious and parasitic disease

    V12.01 Tuberculosis

    V12.02 Poliomyelitis
      Z86.12 Personal history of poliomyelitis   I-10

    V12.03 Malaria

    V12.04 Methicillin resistant Staphylococcus aureus
    MRSA
      AHA: 4Q, '08, 69, 71

    V12.09 Other

    V12.1 Nutritional deficiency

    V12.2 Endocrine, metabolic, and immunity disorders
      EXCLUDES *history of allergy (V14.0-V14.9, 80 .01-V15.09)*
      AHA: 3Q, '07, 5

    V12.3 Diseases of blood and blood-forming organs

✓5ᵗʰ **V12.4 Disorders of nervous system and sense organs**

    V12.40 Unspecified disorder of nervous system and sense organs

    V12.41 Benign neoplasm of the brain
      AHA: 4Q, '97, 48
      TIP: Benign neoplasms of the brain are tracked separately because, besides being potentially life-threatening, they often recur and can be difficult to treat.

    V12.42 Infections of the central nervous system
    Encephalitis   Meningitis
      AHA: 4Q, '05, 95

    V12.49 Other disorders of nervous system and sense organs
      AHA: 4Q, '98, 59

✓5ᵗʰ **V12.5 Diseases of circulatory system**
    EXCLUDES *old myocardial infarction (412)*
    postmyocardial infarction syndrome (411.0)
    AHA: 4Q, '95, 61

    V12.50 Unspecified circulatory disease

    V12.51 Venous thrombosis and embolism
    Pulmonary embolism
      AHA: 3Q, '06, 12; 4Q, '03, 108; 1Q, '02, 15

    V12.52 Thrombophlebitis

    V12.53 Sudden cardiac arrest
    Sudden cardiac death successfully resuscitated
      AHA: 4Q, '07, 98

V12.54 Transient ischemic attack [TIA], and cerebral infarction without residual deficits
　　Prolonged reversible ischemic neurological deficit [PRIND]
　　Reversible ischemic neurologic deficit [RIND]
　　Stroke NOS without residual deficits
　　EXCLUDES *history of traumatic brain injury (V15.52)*
　　　　late effects of cerebrovascular disease (438.0-438.9)
　　AHA: 4Q, '07, 98
　　TIP: Assign for old CVA for which the patient has no residual deficits; if deficits are present, see category 438.
　　Z86.73 Personal hx TIA & cerebral infarct w/o deficits [I-10]

V12.59 Other
　　AHA: 2Q, '07, 3; 4Q, '99, 4; 4Q, '98, 88; 4Q, '97, 37

√5ᵗʰ **V12.6 Diseases of respiratory system**
　　EXCLUDES *tuberculosis (V12.01)*

V12.60 Unspecified disease of respiratory system

V12.61 Pneumonia (recurrent)
　　AHA: 4Q, '05, 95

V12.69 Other diseases of respiratory system

√5ᵗʰ **V12.7 Diseases of digestive system**
　　AHA: 1Q, '95, 3; 2Q, '89, 16

V12.70 Unspecified digestive disease

V12.71 Peptic ulcer disease

V12.72 Colonic polyps
　　AHA: 3Q, '02, 15
　　Z86.010 Personal history of colonic polyps [I-10]

V12.79 Other

√4ᵗʰ **V13 Personal history of other diseases**

√5ᵗʰ **V13.0 Disorders of urinary system**

V13.00 Unspecified urinary disorder

V13.01 Urinary calculi

V13.02 Urinary (tract) infection
　　AHA: 4Q, '05, 95

V13.03 Nephrotic syndrome
　　AHA: 4Q, '05, 95

V13.09 Other

V13.1 Trophoblastic disease ♀
　　EXCLUDES *supervision during a current pregnancy (V23.1)*

√5ᵗʰ **V13.2 Other genital system and obstetric disorders**
　　EXCLUDES ▶*recurrent pregnancy loss (646.3)*◀
　　　　without current pregnancy (629.81)
　　　　supervision during a current pregnancy of a woman with poor obstetric history (V23.0-V23.9)

V13.21 Personal history of pre-term labor ♀
　　EXCLUDES *current pregnancy with history of pre-term labor (V23.41)*
　　AHA: 4Q, '02, 78

V13.22 Personal history of cervical dysplasia ♀
　　Personal history of conditions classifiable to 622.10-622.12
　　EXCLUDES *personal history of malignant neoplasm of cervix uteri (V10.41)*
　　AHA: 4Q, '07, 98

● **V13.23 Personal history of vaginal dysplasia** ♀
　　Personal history of conditions classifiable to 623.0
　　EXCLUDES *personal history of malignant neoplasm of vagina (V10.44)*

● **V13.24 Personal history of vulvar dysplasia** ♀
　　Personal history of conditions classifiable to 624.01-624.02
　　EXCLUDES *personal history of malignant neoplasm of vulva (V10.44)*

V13.29 Other genital system and obstetric disorders ♀

V13.3 Diseases of skin and subcutaneous tissue

V13.4 Arthritis

√5ᵗʰ **V13.5 Other musculoskeletal disorders**
　　AHA: 4Q, '08, 158
　　TIP: Personal histories of pathological, stress, or traumatic fractures are separately classified because a patient with such a history is at much higher risk of refracture of the same site.

V13.51 Pathologic fracture
　　Healed pathologic fracture
　　EXCLUDES *personal history of traumatic fracture (V15.51)*

V13.52 Stress fracture
　　Healed stress fracture
　　EXCLUDES *personal history of traumatic fracture (V15.51)*

V13.59 Other musculoskeletal disorders

▲ √5ᵗʰ **V13.6 Congenital (corrected) malformations**
　　AHA: 4Q, '98, 63

▲ **V13.61 Personal history of (corrected) hypospadias** ♂

● **V13.62 Personal history of other (corrected) congenital malformations of genitourinary system**

● **V13.63 Personal history of (corrected) congenital malformations of nervous system**

● **V13.64 Personal history of (corrected) congenital malformations of eye, ear, face and neck**
　　Corrected cleft lip and palate

● **V13.65 Personal history of (corrected) congenital malformations of heart and circulatory system**

● **V13.66 Personal history of (corrected) congenital malformations of respiratory system**

● **V13.67 Personal history of (corrected) congenital malformations of digestive system**

● **V13.68 Personal history of (corrected) congenital malformations of integument, limbs, and musculoskeletal systems**

▲ **V13.69 Personal history of other (corrected) congenital malformations**
　　AHA: 1Q, '04, 16

V13.7 Perinatal problems
　　EXCLUDES *low birth weight status (V21.30-V21.35)*

V13.8 Other specified diseases

V13.9 Unspecified disease
　　AHA: 4Q, '06, 117

√4ᵗʰ **V14 Personal history of allergy to medicinal agents**

V14.0 Penicillin
　　Z88.0 Allergy status to penicillin [I-10]

V14.1 Other antibiotic agent

V14.2 Sulfonamides

V14.3 Other anti-infective agent

V14.4 Anesthetic agent

V14.5 Narcotic agent

V14.6 Analgesic agent

V14.7 Serum or vaccine

V14.8 Other specified medicinal agents

V14.9 Unspecified medicinal agent

√4ᵗʰ **V15 Other personal history presenting hazards to health**
　　EXCLUDES *personal history of drug therapy (V87.41-V87.49)*

√5ᵗʰ **V15.0 Allergy, other than to medicinal agents**
　　EXCLUDES *allergy to food substance used as base for medicinal agent (V14.0-V14.9)*
　　AHA: 4Q, '00, 42, 49
　　TIP: A person who has had an allergic episode to a substance in the past should always be considered allergic to the substance.

V15.01 Allergy to peanuts
　　Z91.010 Allergy to peanuts [I-10]

√4ᵗʰ
√5ᵗʰ Additional Digit Required　　Unspecified Code　　Other Specified Code　　Manifestation Code　　▶◀ Revised Text　　● New Code　　▲ Revised Code Title

2011 ICD-9-CM　　　　　　　　　　　　　　　　　　　　　　　　　　**October 2010 · Volume 1 – 323**

V12.54–V15.01

V15.02 Allergy to milk products
> **EXCLUDES** *lactose intolerance (271.3)*
> AHA: 1Q, '03, 12

V15.03 Allergy to eggs

V15.04 Allergy to seafood
Seafood (octopus) (squid) ink
Shellfish

V15.05 Allergy to other foods
Food additives
Nuts other than peanuts

V15.06 Allergy to insects and arachnids
Bugs
Insect bites and stings
Spiders

V15.07 Allergy to latex
Latex sensitivity

V15.08 Allergy to radiographic dye
Contrast media used for diagnostic x-ray procedures

V15.09 Other allergy, other than to medicinal agents

V15.1 Surgery to heart and great vessels
> **EXCLUDES** *replacement by transplant or other means*
> *(V42.1-V42.2, V43.2-V43.4)*
> AHA: 1Q, '04, 16

√5ᵗʰ **V15.2 Surgery to other organs**
> **EXCLUDES** *replacement by transplant or other means*
> *(V42.0-V43.8)*
> AHA: 4Q, '08, 158

V15.21 Personal history of undergoing in utero ♀
procedure during pregnancy
> AHA: 4Q, '08, 158

V15.22 Personal history of undergoing in utero procedure
while a fetus
> AHA: 4Q, '08, 158

V15.29 Surgery to other organs

V15.3 Irradiation
Previous exposure to therapeutic or other ionizing radiation

√5ᵗʰ **V15.4 Psychological trauma**
> **EXCLUDES** *history of condition classifiable to 290-316*
> *(V11.0-V11.9)*

V15.41 History of physical abuse
Rape
> AHA: 3Q, '99, 15

V15.42 History of emotional abuse
Neglect
> AHA: 3Q, '99, 15

V15.49 Other
> AHA: 3Q, '99, 15

√5ᵗʰ **V15.5 Injury**
> AHA: 4Q, '08, 158

V15.51 Traumatic fracture
Healed traumatic fracture
> **EXCLUDES** *personal history of pathologic and stress*
> *fracture (V13.51, V13.52)*
> **TIP:** Personal histories of pathological, stress, or traumatic
> fractures are separately classified because a patient with
> such a history is at much higher risk of refracture of the
> same site.

V15.52 History of traumatic brain injury
> **EXCLUDES** *personal history of cerebrovascular accident*
> *(cerebral infarction) without residual*
> *deficits (V12.54)*
> AHA: 4Q, '09, 115

● **V15.53 Personal history of retained foreign body fully**
removed

V15.59 Other injury

V15.6 Poisoning

V15.7 Contraception
> **EXCLUDES** *current contraceptive management (V25.0-V25.4)*
> *presence of intrauterine contraceptive device as*
> *incidental finding (V45.5)*

√5ᵗʰ **V15.8 Other specified personal history presenting hazards to**
health
> **EXCLUDES** *contact with and (suspected) exposure to:*
> *aromatic compounds and dyes (V87.11-V87.19)*
> *arsenic and other metals (V87.01-V87.09)*
> *molds (V87.31)*
> AHA: 4Q, '95, 62

V15.80 History of failed moderate sedation
History of failed conscious sedation
> AHA: 4Q, '09, 115

V15.81 Noncompliance with medical treatment
> **EXCLUDES** *noncompliance with renal dialysis (V45.12)*
> AHA: 3Q, '07, 9; 4Q, '06, 136; 2Q, '03, 7; 2Q, '01, 11, 12, 13; 2Q,
> '99, 17; 2Q, '97, 11; 1Q, '97, 12; 3Q, '96, 9

V15.82 History of tobacco use
> **EXCLUDES** *tobacco dependence (305.1)*
> AHA: 1Q, '09, 17
> **Z87.82** Personal history of nicotine dependence   I-10

V15.83 Underimmunization status
Delinquent immunization status
Lapsed immunization schedule status
> AHA: 4Q, '09, 115

V15.84 Contact with and (suspected) exposure to asbestos
> AHA: 4Q, '09, 116

V15.85 Contact with and (suspected) exposure to
potentially hazardous body fluids
> AHA: 4Q, '09, 116

V15.86 Contact with and (suspected) exposure to lead
> AHA: 4Q, '09, 116

V15.87 History of extracorporeal membrane oxygenation
[ECMO]
> AHA: 4Q, '03, 84

V15.88 History of fall
At risk for falling
> AHA: 4Q, '05, 95
> **Z91.81** History of falling   I-10

V15.89 Other
> **EXCLUDES** *contact with and (suspected) exposure to*
> *other potentially hazardous:*
> *chemicals (V87.2)*
> *substances (V87.39)*
> AHA: 3Q, '08, 7; 3Q, '07, 5; 1Q, '90, 21; N-D, '84, 12

V15.9 Unspecified personal history presenting
hazards to health

√4ᵗʰ **V16 Family history of malignant neoplasm**

V16.0 Gastrointestinal tract
Family history of condition classifiable to 140-159
> AHA: 1Q, '99, 4
> **TIP:** Family history of colon cancer is a condition that meets the
> criteria of "high risk" for a screening colonoscopy.

V16.1 Trachea, bronchus, and lung
Family history of condition classifiable to 162

V16.2 Other respiratory and intrathoracic organs
Family history of condition classifiable to 160-161, 163-165

V16.3 Breast
Family history of condition classifiable to 174
> AHA: 4Q, '04, 107; 2Q, '03, 4; 2Q, '00, 8; 1Q, '92, 11
> **Z80.3** Family history of malignant neoplasm of breast   I-10

√5ᵗʰ **V16.4 Genital organs**
Family history of condition classifiable to 179-187
> AHA: 4Q, '97, 48

V16.40 Genital organ, unspecified

V16.41 Ovary
> AHA: 3Q, '09, 5

V16.42 Prostate
> **Z80.42** Family history of malignant neoplasm   I-10
> of prostate

V16.43 Testis
V16.49 Other
AHA: 2Q, '06, 2

√5ᵗʰ **V16.5 Urinary organs**
Family history of condition classifiable to 188-189

V16.51 Kidney

V16.52 Bladder
AHA: 4Q, '07, 98

V16.59 Other

V16.6 Leukemia
Family history of condition classifiable to 204-208

V16.7 Other lymphatic and hematopoietic neoplasms
Family history of condition classifiable to 200-203

V16.8 Other specified malignant neoplasm
Family history of other condition classifiable to 140-199

V16.9 Unspecified malignant neoplasm

√4ᵗʰ **V17 Family history of certain chronic disabling diseases**

V17.0 Psychiatric condition
EXCLUDES *family history of mental retardation (V18.4)*

V17.1 Stroke (cerebrovascular)
Z82.3 Family history of stroke   I-10

V17.2 Other neurological diseases
Epilepsy
Huntington's chorea

V17.3 Ischemic heart disease

√5ᵗʰ **V17.4 Other cardiovascular diseases**
AHA: 1Q, '04, 6

V17.41 Family history of sudden cardiac death [SCD]
EXCLUDES *family history of ischemic heart disease (V17.3)*
family history of myocardial infarction (V17.3)
AHA: 4Q, '07, 98

V17.49 Family history of other cardiovascular diseases
Family history of cardiovascular disease NOS

V17.5 Asthma

V17.6 Other chronic respiratory conditions

V17.7 Arthritis

√5ᵗʰ **V17.8 Other musculoskeletal diseases**

V17.81 Osteoporosis
AHA: 4Q, '05, 95

V17.89 Other musculoskeletal diseases

√4ᵗʰ **V18 Family history of certain other specific conditions**

V18.0 Diabetes mellitus
AHA: 1Q, '04, 8
TIP: Assign for a normal infant born to a diabetic mother who presents with no manifestations of the syndrome.

√5ᵗʰ **V18.1 Other endocrine and metabolic diseases**

V18.11 Multiple endocrine neoplasia [MEN] syndrome
AHA: 4Q, '07, 98, 100

V18.19 Other endocrine and metabolic diseases

V18.2 Anemia

V18.3 Other blood disorders

V18.4 Mental retardation

√5ᵗʰ **V18.5 Digestive disorders**

V18.51 Colonic polyps
EXCLUDES *family history of malignant neoplasm of gastrointestinal tract (V16.0)*
AHA: 4Q, '06, 117
Z83.71 Family history of colonic polyps   I-10

V18.59 Other digestive disorders

√5ᵗʰ **V18.6 Kidney diseases**

V18.61 Polycystic kidney

V18.69 Other kidney diseases

V18.7 Other genitourinary diseases

V18.8 Infectious and parasitic diseases

V18.9 Genetic disease carrier
AHA: 4Q, '05, 95

√4ᵗʰ **V19 Family history of other conditions**

V19.0 Blindness or visual loss

V19.1 Other eye disorders

V19.2 Deafness or hearing loss

V19.3 Other ear disorders

V19.4 Skin conditions

V19.5 Congenital anomalies

V19.6 Allergic disorders

V19.7 Consanguinity

V19.8 Other condition

Persons Encountering Health Services in Circumstances Related to Reproduction and Development (V20-V29)

√4ᵗʰ **V20 Health supervision of infant or child**

V20.0 Foundling   PDx P

V20.1 Other healthy infant or child receiving care   PDx P
Medical or nursing care supervision of healthy infant in cases of:
maternal illness, physical or psychiatric
socioeconomic adverse condition at home
too many children at home preventing or interfering with normal care
AHA: 1Q, '00, 25; 3Q, '89, 14

V20.2 Routine infant or child health check   PDx P
Developmental testing of infant or child
Health check for child over 28 days old
Immunizations appropriate for age
Routine vision and hearing testing
Use additional code(s) to identify:
special screening examination(s) performed (V73.0-V82.9)
EXCLUDES *health check for child under 29 days old (V20.31-V20.32)*
newborn health supervision (V20.31-V20.32)
special screening for developmental handicaps (V79.3)
AHA: ▶4Q, '09, 115;◀ 1Q, '09, 15; 1Q, '04, 15

√5ᵗʰ **V20.3 Newborn health supervision**
Health check for child under 29 days old
EXCLUDES *health check for child over 28 days old (V20.2)*
AHA: ▶4Q, '09, 117◀

V20.31 Health supervision for newborn under 8 days old   N PDx
Health check for newborn under 8 days old

V20.32 Health supervision for newborn 8 to 28 days old   N PDx
Health check for newborn 8 to 28 days old
Newborn weight check
AHA: ▶4Q, '09, 102,117◀

√4ᵗʰ **V21 Constitutional states in development**

V21.0 Period of rapid growth in childhood

V21.1 Puberty

V21.2 Other adolecsence

√5ᵗʰ **V21.3 Low birth weight status**
EXCLUDES *history of perinatal problems*
AHA: 4Q, '00, 51
TIP: There are no age restrictions on these V codes after the perinatal period; assign for patients without the initial condition who may continue to manifest the consequences of it.

V21.30 Low birth weight status, unspecified

√4ᵗʰ
√5ᵗʰ Additional Digit Required   Unspecified Code   Other Specified Code   Manifestation Code   ▶◀ Revised Text   ● New Code   ▲ Revised Code Title
2011 ICD-9-CM   **February 2010 · Volume 1 – 325**

V16.43–V21.30

V Codes

V21.31–V25.41

V21.31 Low birth weight status, less than 500 grams

V21.32 Low birth weight status, 500-999 grams

V21.33 Low birth weight status, 1000-1499 grams

V21.34 Low birth weight status, 1500-1999 grams

V21.35 Low birth weight status, 2000-2500 grams

V21.8 Other specified constitutional states in development

V21.9 Unspecified constitutional state in development

√4ᵗʰ **V22 Normal pregnancy**

> EXCLUDES *pregnancy examination or test, pregnancy unconfirmed (V72.40)*
>
> AHA: 4Q, '07, 125
>
> **TIP:** Do not assign with any code from chapter 11, "Complications of Pregnancy, Childbirth, and the Puerperium."

V22.0 Supervision of normal first pregnancy   PDx ♀

> AHA: 3Q, '99, 16
>
> **Z34.00** Encounter suprvisn norm 1 pregnancy uns trimestr   I-10

V22.1 Supervision of other normal pregnancy   PDx ♀

> AHA: 3Q, '99, 16

V22.2 Pregnant state, incidental   ♀

> Pregnant state NOS

√4ᵗʰ **V23 Supervision of high-risk pregnancy**

> AHA: 1Q, '90, 10

V23.0 Pregnancy with history of infertility   M ♀

V23.1 Pregnancy with history of trophoblastic disease   M ♀

> Pregnancy with history of:
> hydatidiform mole
> vesicular mole
>
> EXCLUDES *that without current pregnancy (V13.1)*

V23.2 Pregnancy with history of abortion   M ♀

> Pregnancy with history of conditions classifiable to 634-638
>
> EXCLUDES ▶*recurrent pregnancy loss:*◀
> *care during pregnancy (646.3)*
> *that without current pregnancy (629.81)*

V23.3 Grand multiparity   M ♀

> EXCLUDES *care in relation to labor and delivery (659.4)*
> *that without current pregnancy (V61.5)*

√5ᵗʰ **V23.4 Pregnancy with other poor obstetric history**

> Pregnancy with history of other conditions classifiable to 630-676

V23.41 Pregnancy with history of labor pre-term   M ♀

> AHA: 4Q, '02, 79

V23.49 Pregnancy with other poor obstetric history   M ♀

V23.5 Pregnancy with other poor reproductive history   M ♀

> Pregnancy with history of stillbirth or neonatal death

V23.7 Insufficient prenatal care   M ♀

> History of little or no prenatal care

√5ᵗʰ **V23.8 Other high-risk pregnancy**

> AHA: 4Q, '08, 158; 4Q, '98, 56, 63

V23.81 Elderly primigravida   M ♀

> First pregnancy in a woman who will be 35 years of age or older at expected date of delivery
>
> EXCLUDES *elderly primigravida complicating pregnancy (659.5)*

V23.82 Elderly multigravida   M ♀

> Second or more pregnancy in a woman who will be 35 years of age or older at expected date of delivery
>
> EXCLUDES *elderly multigravida complicating pregnancy (659.6)*

V23.83 Young primigravida   M ♀

> First pregnancy in a female less than 16 years old at expected date of delivery
>
> EXCLUDES *young primigravida complicating pregnancy (659.8)*

V23.84 Young multigravida   M ♀

> Second or more pregnancy in a female less than 16 years old at expected date of delivery
>
> EXCLUDES *young multigravida complicating pregnancy (659.8)*

V23.85 Pregnancy resulting from assisted reproductive technology   M ♀

> Pregnancy resulting from in vitro fertilization
>
> AHA: 4Q, '08, 160

V23.86 Pregnancy with history of in utero procedure during previous pregnancy   M ♀

> EXCLUDES *management of pregnancy affected by in utero procedure during current pregnancy (679.0-679.1)*
>
> AHA: 4Q, '08, 158, 160

V23.89 Other high-risk pregnancy   M ♀

> AHA: 3Q, '06, 14

V23.9 Unspecified high-risk pregnancy   M ♀

√4ᵗʰ **V24 Postpartum care and examination**

V24.0 Immediately after delivery   PDx M ♀

> Care and observation in uncomplicated cases
>
> AHA: 3Q, '06, 11

V24.1 Lactating mother   PDx ♀

> Supervision of lactation

V24.2 Routine postpartum follow-up   PDx ♀

√4ᵗʰ **V25 Encounter for contraceptive management**

> AHA: 4Q, '92, 24

√5ᵗʰ **V25.0 General counseling and advice**

V25.01 Prescription of oral contraceptives   ♀

V25.02 Initiation of other contraceptive measures

> Fitting of diaphragm
> Prescription of foams, creams, or other agents
>
> AHA: 3Q, '97, 7

V25.03 Encounter for emergency contraceptive counseling and prescription

> Encounter for postcoital contraceptive counseling and prescription
>
> AHA: 4Q, '03, 84

V25.04 Counseling and instruction in natural family planning to avoid pregnancy

> AHA: 4Q, '07, 99
>
> **Z30.02** Counsel & instruct natural family plan avoid pg   I-10

V25.09 Other

> Family planning advice

▲ √5ᵗʰ **V25.1 Encounter for insertion or removal of intrauterine contraceptive device**

> EXCLUDES ▶*encounter for routine checking of intrauterine contraceptive device (V25.42)*◀

● **V25.11 Encounter for insertion of intrauterine contraceptive device**   ♀

● **V25.12 Encounter for removal of intrauterine contraceptive device**   ♀

● **V25.13 Encounter for removal and reinsertion of intrauterine contraceptive device**   ♀

> Encounter for replacement of intrauterine contraceptive device

V25.2 Sterilization

> Admission for interruption of fallopian tubes or vas deferens

V25.3 Menstrual extraction   ♀

> Menstrual regulation

√5ᵗʰ **V25.4 Surveillance of previously prescribed contraceptive methods**

> Checking, reinsertion, or removal of contraceptive device
> Repeat prescription for contraceptive method
> Routine examination in connection with contraceptive maintenance

V25.40 Contraceptive surveillance, unspecified

V25.41 Contraceptive pill   ♀

N Newborn Age: 0   P Pediatric Age: 0-17   M Maternity Age: 12-55   A Adult Age: 15-124   PDx Primary Diagnosis

V25.42 Intrauterine contraceptive device ♀
▶Checking of intrauterine device◄
EXCLUDES ▶insertion or removal of intrauterine contraceptive device (V25.11-V25.13)
presence of intrauterine contraceptive device as incidental finding (V45.51)◄

V25.43 Implantable subdermal contraceptive ♀

V25.49 Other contraceptive method
AHA: 3Q, '97, 7

V25.5 Insertion of implantable subdermal contraceptive ♀
AHA: 3Q, '92, 9

V25.8 Other specified contraceptive management
Postvasectomy sperm count
EXCLUDES sperm count following sterilization reversal (V26.22)
sperm count for fertility testing (V26.21)
AHA: 3Q, '96, 9

V25.9 Unspecified contraceptive management

√4ᵗʰ **V26 Procreative management**

V26.0 Tuboplasty or vasoplasty after previous sterilization
AHA: 2Q, '95, 10
TIP: Assign for encounters for tubal ligation or vasectomy reversal procedures.

V26.1 Artificial insemination ♀

√5ᵗʰ **V26.2 Investigation and testing**
EXCLUDES postvasectomy sperm count (V25.8)
AHA: 4Q, '00, 56

V26.21 Fertility testing
Fallopian insufflation
Sperm count for fertility testing
EXCLUDES genetic counseling and testing (V26.31-V26.39)

V26.22 Aftercare following sterilization reversal
Fallopian insufflation following sterilization reversal
Sperm count following sterilization reversal

V26.29 Other investigation and testing
AHA: 2Q, '96, 9; N-D, '85, 15

√5ᵗʰ **V26.3 Genetic counseling and testing**
EXCLUDES fertility testing (V26.21)
nonprocreative genetic screening (V82.71, V82.79)
AHA: 4Q, '05, 96

V26.31 Testing of female for genetic disease carrier status ♀
AHA: 4Q, '06, 117

V26.32 Other genetic testing of female ♀
▶Use additional code to identify recurrent pregnancy loss (629.81, 646.3)◄
AHA: 4Q, '06, 117
Z31.438 Encounter oth genetic test female procreative mngmnt   I-10

V26.33 Genetic counseling

V26.34 Testing of male for genetic disease carrier status ♂
AHA: 4Q, '06, 117

▲ **V26.35 Encounter for testing of male partner of female with recurrent pregnancy loss** ♂
AHA: 4Q, '06, 117

V26.39 Other genetic testing of male ♂
AHA: 4Q, '06, 117

√5ᵗʰ **V26.4 General counseling and advice**

V26.41 Procreative counseling and advice using natural family planning
AHA: 4Q, '07, 99

V26.42 Encounter for fertility preservation counseling
Encounter for fertility preservation counseling prior to cancer therapy
Encounter for fertility preservation counseling prior to surgical removal of gonads
AHA: 4Q, '09, 117

V26.49 Other procreative management, counseling and advice

√5ᵗʰ **V26.5 Sterilization status**

V26.51 Tubal ligation status ♀
EXCLUDES infertility not due to previous tubal ligation (628.0-628.9)
Z98.51 Tubal ligation status   I-10

V26.52 Vasectomy status ♂

√5ᵗʰ **V26.8 Other specified procreative management**

V26.81 Encounter for assisted reproductive fertility procedure cycle   PDx ♀
Patient undergoing in vitro fertilization cycle
Use additional code to identify the type of infertility
EXCLUDES pre-cycle diagnosis and testing — code to reason for encounter
AHA: 4Q, '07, 99

V26.82 Encounter for fertility preservation procedure   PDx
Encounter for fertility preservation procedure prior to cancer therapy
Encounter for fertility preservation procedure prior to surgical removal of gonads
AHA: 4Q, '09, 117

V26.89 Other specified procreative management

V26.9 Unspecified procreative management

√4ᵗʰ **V27 Outcome of delivery**
NOTE This category is intended for the coding of the outcome of delivery on the mother's record.
AHA: 2Q, '91, 16
TIP: Assign on the maternal chart for every admission during which a delivery occurs.

V27.0 Single liveborn   M ♀
AHA: 4Q, '08, 192; 4Q, '05, 81; 2Q, '03, 9; 2Q, '02, 10; 1Q, '01, 10; 3Q, '00, 5; 4Q, '98, 77; 4Q, '95, 59; 1Q, '92, 9
Z37.0 Single live birth   I-10

V27.1 Single stillborn   M ♀

V27.2 Twins, both liveborn   M ♀
Z37.2 Twins both liveborn   I-10

V27.3 Twins, one liveborn and one stillborn   M ♀

V27.4 Twins, both stillborn   M ♀

V27.5 Other multiple birth, all liveborn   M ♀

V27.6 Other multiple birth, some liveborn   M ♀

V27.7 Other multiple birth, all stillborn   M ♀

V27.9 Unspecified outcome of delivery   M ♀
Single birth }
Multiple birth } outcome to infant unspecified

√4ᵗʰ **V28 Encounter for antenatal screening of mother**
EXCLUDES abnormal findings on screening — code to findings
routine prenatal care (V22.0-V23.9)
suspected fetal conditions affecting management of pregnancy (655.00-655.93, 656.00- 656.93, 657.00-657.03, 658.00-658.93)
suspected fetal conditions not found (V89.01-V89.09)
AHA: 4Q, '06, 117; 1Q, '04, 11

V28.0 Screening for chromosomal anomalies by amniocentesis   M ♀

V28.1 Screening for raised alpha-fetoprotein levels in amniotic fluid   M ♀

V28.2 Other screening based on amniocentesis   M ♀

V28.3 Encounter for routine screening for malformation using ultrasonics ♀
Encounter for routine fetal ultrasound NOS
EXCLUDES encounter for fetal anatomic survey (V28.81)
genetic counseling and testing (V26.31-V26.39)

V28.4 Screening for fetal growth retardation using ultrasonics ♀

V28.5 Screening for isoimmunization ♀

√4ᵗʰ
√5ᵗʰ Additional Digit Required   Unspecified Code   Other Specified Code   Manifestation Code   ▶◄ Revised Text   ● New Code   ▲ Revised Code Title

V28.6–V42.84

V28.6 Screening for Streptococcus B Ⓜ♀
    AHA: 4Q, '97, 46

✓5ᵗʰ **V28.8 Other specified antenatal screening**
    AHA: 4Q, '08, 159; 3Q, '99, 16

    V28.81 Encounter for fetal anatomic survey Ⓜ♀

    V28.82 Encounter for screening for risk Ⓜ♀
        of pre-term labor

    V28.89 Other specified antenatal screening Ⓜ♀
        Chorionic villus sampling
        Genomic screening
        Nuchal translucency testing
        Proteomic screening

    V28.9 Unspecified antenatal screening ♀

✓4ᵗʰ **V29 Observation and evaluation of newborns and infants for suspected condition not found**
    NOTE This category is to be used for newborns, within the neonatal period, (the first 28 days of life) who are suspected of having an abnormal condition resulting from exposure from the mother or the birth process, but without signs or symptoms, and, which after examination and observation, is found not to exist.
    EXCLUDES suspected fetal conditions not found (V89.01-V89.09)
    AHA: 1Q, '00, 25; 4Q, '94, 47; 1Q, '94, 9; 4Q, '92, 21
    TIP: Do not assign if the infant shows any signs or symptoms.

¹ **V29.0 Observation for suspected infectious condition** Ⓝ
    AHA: 1Q, '01, 10

¹ **V29.1 Observation for suspected neurological condition** Ⓝ

¹ **V29.2 Observation for suspected respiratory condition** Ⓝ

¹ **V29.3 Observation for suspected genetic** Ⓝ
    or metabolic condition
    AHA: 2Q, '05, 21; 4Q, '98, 59, 68

¹ **V29.8 Observation for other specified suspected** Ⓝ
    condition
    AHA: 2Q, '03, 15

¹ **V29.9 Observation for unspecified suspected** Ⓝ
    condition
    AHA: 1Q, '02, 6

Liveborn Infants According to Type of Birth (V30-V39)

    NOTE These categories are intended for the coding of liveborn infants who are consuming health care [e.g., crib or bassinet occupancy].

    The following fourth-digit subdivisions are for use with categories V30-V39

    ✓5ᵗʰ 0 **Born in hospital** Ⓝ
        1 **Born before admission to hospital** Ⓝ
        2 **Born outside hospital and not hospitalized**
    The following two fifth-digits are for use with the fourth-digit .0, Born in hospital:
        0 **delivered without mention of cesarean delivery**
        1 **delivered by cesarean delivery**

    AHA: 1Q, '01, 10

§ ✓4ᵗʰ **V30 Single liveborn** PDx
    AHA: 2Q, '03, 9; 4Q, '98, 46, 59; 1Q, '94, 9; For code V30.00: 1Q, '04, 8, 16; 4Q, '03, 68; For code V30.01: ▶4Q, '09, 101;◀ 4Q, '05, 88; For code V30.10: 3Q, '06, 10
    Z38.00 Single liveborn infant delivered vaginally I-10

§ ✓4ᵗʰ **V31 Twin, mate liveborn** PDx
    AHA: 3Q, '92, 10
    Z38.31 Twin liveborn infant delivered by cesarean I-10

§ ✓4ᵗʰ **V32 Twin, mate stillborn** PDx

§ ✓4ᵗʰ **V33 Twin, unspecified** PDx

§ ✓4ᵗʰ **V34 Other multiple, mates all liveborn** PDx

§ ✓4ᵗʰ **V35 Other multiple, mates all stillborn** PDx

§ ✓4ᵗʰ **V36 Other multiple, mates live and stillborn** PDx

§ ✓4ᵗʰ **V37 Other multiple, unspecified** PDx

§ ✓4ᵗʰ **V39 Unspecified** PDx

Persons with a Condition Influencing Their Health Status (V40-V49)

    NOTE These categories are intended for use when these conditions are recorded as "diagnoses" or "problems."
    TIP: Includes patients with a carrier status or who have sequelae or residual of a past condition or disease, which may affect current or future treatment.

✓4ᵗʰ **V40 Mental and behavioral problems**

    V40.0 Problems with learning

    V40.1 Problems with communication [including speech]

    V40.2 Other mental problems

    V40.3 Other behavioral problems

    V40.9 Unspecified mental or behavioral problem

✓4ᵗʰ **V41 Problems with special senses and other special functions**

    V41.0 Problems with sight

    V41.1 Other eye problems

    V41.2 Problems with hearing

    V41.3 Other ear problems

    V41.4 Problems with voice production

    V41.5 Problems with smell and taste

    V41.6 Problems with swallowing and mastication

    V41.7 Problems with sexual function
        EXCLUDES marital problems (V61.10)
                psychosexual disorders (302.0-302.9)

    V41.8 Other problems with special functions

    V41.9 Unspecified problem with special functions

✓4ᵗʰ **V42 Organ or tissue replaced by transplant**
    INCLUDES homologous or heterologous (animal) (human) transplant organ status
    AHA: 3Q, '98, 3, 4
    TIP: Do not assign if the patient has a complication of the transplanted organ; the code from subcategory 996.8 provides the information.

    V42.0 Kidney
        AHA: 1Q, '08, 10; 1Q, '03, 10; 3Q, '01, 12
        Z94.0 Kidney transplant status I-10

    V42.1 Heart
        AHA: 3Q, '03, 16; 3Q, '01, 13

    V42.2 Heart valve

    V42.3 Skin

    V42.4 Bone

    V42.5 Cornea

    V42.6 Lung

    V42.7 Liver
        Z94.4 Liver transplant status I-10

    ✓5ᵗʰ **V42.8 Other specified organ or tissue**
        AHA: 4Q, '98, 64; 4Q, '97, 49

        V42.81 Bone marrow

        V42.82 Peripheral stem cells

        V42.83 Pancreas
            AHA: 1Q, '03, 10; 2Q, '01, 16

        V42.84 Intestines
            AHA: 4Q, '00, 48, 50

¹ A code from the V30–V39 series may be sequenced before the V29 on the newborn medical record.
§ Require fourth and fifth digits. See beginning of section V30-V39 for codes and definitions.

V42.89 Other

V42.9 Unspecified organ or tissue

☑4ᵗʰ **V43 Organ or tissue replaced by other means**

     INCLUDES   organ or tissue assisted by other means
                 replacement of organ by:
                      artificial device
                      mechanical device
                      prosthesis

     EXCLUDES   *cardiac pacemaker in situ (V45.01)*
                 fitting and adjustment of prosthetic device (V52.0-V52.9)
                 renal dialysis status (V45.11)

     V43.0 Eye globe

     V43.1 Lens
         Pseudophakos
         AHA: 4Q, '98, 65

☑5ᵗʰ   **V43.2 Heart**
         Fully implantable artificial heart
         Heart assist device
         AHA: 4Q, '03, 85

         V43.21 Heart assist device

         V43.22 Fully implantable artificial heart

     V43.3 Heart valve
         AHA: 3Q, '06, 7; 3Q, '02, 13, 14
         TIP: If the status post heart valve replacement information includes "porcine" or mention of other homologous or heterologous tissue, assign instead V42.2.
         Z95.2 Presence of prosthetic heart valve   I-10

     V43.4 Blood vessel

     V43.5 Bladder

☑5ᵗʰ   **V43.6 Joint**
         AHA: 4Q, '05, 91

         V43.60 Unspecified joint

         V43.61 Shoulder

         V43.62 Elbow

         V43.63 Wrist

         V43.64 Hip
             AHA: 1Q, '09, 6; 2Q, '08, 3-5; 3Q, '06, 4, 5; 4Q, '05, 93, 112; 2Q, '04, 15
             Z96.641 Presence of right artificial hip joint   I-10

         V43.65 Knee
             AHA: 3Q, '06, 5

         V43.66 Ankle

         V43.69 Other

     V43.7 Limb

☑5ᵗʰ   **V43.8 Other organ or tissue**
         V43.81 Larynx
             AHA: 4Q, '95, 55

         V43.82 Breast
             AHA: 4Q, '95, 55
             Z98.82 Breast implant status   I-10

         V43.83 Artificial skin

         V43.89 Other

☑4ᵗʰ **V44 Artificial opening status**
         EXCLUDES   *artificial openings requiring attention or management (V55.0-V55.9)*
     TIP: Do not assign if the patient has a complication of the artificial opening, such as infection or obstruction; assign only the complication code.

     V44.0 Tracheostomy
         AHA: 4Q, '03, 103, 107, 111; 1Q, '01, 6

     V44.1 Gastrostomy
         AHA: 4Q, '03, 103, 107-108, 110; 1Q, '01, 12; 3Q, '97, 12; 1Q, '93, 26

     V44.2 Ileostomy

     V44.3 Colostomy
         AHA: 4Q, '03, 110
         Z93.3 Colostomy status   I-10

     V44.4 Other artificial opening of gastrointestinal tract

☑5ᵗʰ   **V44.5 Cystostomy**

         V44.50 Cystostomy, unspecified

         V44.51 Cutaneous-vesicostomy

         V44.52 Appendico-vesicostomy

         V44.59 Other cystostomy

     V44.6 Other artificial opening of urinary tract
         Nephrostomy   Urethrostomy
         Ureterostomy

     V44.7 Artificial vagina

     V44.8 Other artificial opening status

     V44.9 Unspecified artificial opening status

☑4ᵗʰ **V45 Other postprocedural states**
     EXCLUDES   *aftercare management (V51-V58.9)*
                malfunction or other complication — code to condition
     AHA: 4Q, '03, 85

☑5ᵗʰ   **V45.0 Cardiac device in situ**
         EXCLUDES   *artificial heart (V43.22)*
                   heart assist device (V43.21)

         V45.00 Unspecified cardiac device

         V45.01 Cardiac pacemaker
             EXCLUDES   ►*cardiac defibrillator with synchronous cardiac pacemaker (V45.02)*◄

         V45.02 Automatic implantable cardiac defibrillator
             ►With synchronous cardiac pacemaker◄
             Z95.810 Presence auto implantable cardiac defibrillator   I-10

         V45.09 Other specified cardiac device
             Carotid sinus pacemaker in situ

☑5ᵗʰ   **V45.1 Renal dialysis status**
         EXCLUDES   *admission for dialysis treatment or session (V56.0)*
         AHA: 4Q, '08, 157; 1Q, '08, 7; 4Q, '07, 86; 3Q, '07, 9; 4Q, '06, 136; 4Q, '05, 96; 2Q, '03, 7; 2Q, '01, 12, 13

         V45.11 Renal dialysis status
             Hemodialysis status
             Patient requiring intermittent renal dialysis
             Peritoneal dialysis status
             Presence of arterial-venous shunt (for dialysis)
             AHA: 4Q, '08, 157, 193
             Z99.2 Dependence on renal dialysis   I-10

         V45.12 Noncompliance with renal dialysis

     V45.2 Presence of cerebrospinal fluid drainage device
         Cerebral ventricle (communicating) shunt, valve, or device in situ
         EXCLUDES   *malfunction (996.2)*
         AHA: 4Q, '03, 106

     V45.3 Intestinal bypass or anastomosis status
         EXCLUDES   *bariatric surgery status (V45.86)*
                   gastric bypass status (V45.86)
                   obesity surgery status (V45.86)

     V45.4 Arthrodesis status
         AHA: N-D, '84, 18
         TIP: If there is a complication of the fusion graft site that requires refusion or revision, assign instead a code from subcategory 996.4.

☑5ᵗʰ   **V45.5 Presence of contraceptive device**
         V45.51 Intrauterine contraceptive device   ♀
             EXCLUDES   ►*checking of device (V25.42)*
                       complication from device (996.32)
                       insertion and removal of device (V25.11-V25.13)◄
             Z97.5 Presence of intrauterine contraceptive device   I-10

         V45.52 Subdermal contraceptive implant

         V45.59 Other

2011 ICD-9-CM   ☑4ᵗʰ ☑5ᵗʰ Additional Digit Required   Unspecified Code   Other Specified Code   Manifestation Code   ►◄ Revised Text   ● New Code   ▲ Revised Code Title

October 2010 · Volume 1 – 329

V42.89–V45.59

V Codes

V45.6–V47.9

✓5ᵗʰ **V45.6 States following surgery of eye and adnexa**

Cataract extraction
Filtering bleb   } state following eye
Surgical eyelid adhesion   surgery

EXCLUDES *aphakia (379.31)*
artificial eye globe (V43.0)

AHA: 4Q, '98, 65; 4Q, '97, 49

V45.61 Cataract extraction status
Use additional code for associated artificial
lens status (V43.1)

**V45.69 Other states following surgery of eye
and adnexa**
AHA: 2Q, '01, 16; 1Q, '98, 10; 4Q, '97, 19

✓5ᵗʰ **V45.7 Acquired absence of organ**
AHA: 4Q, '98, 65; 4Q, '97, 50

V45.71 Acquired absence of breast and nipple
EXCLUDES *congenital absence of breast and nipple
(757.6)*
AHA: 4Q, '08, 159; 4Q, '01, 66

V45.72 Acquired absence of intestine (large)(small)

V45.73 Acquired absence of kidney

V45.74 Other parts of urinary tract
Bladder
AHA: 4Q, '00, 51

V45.75 Stomach
AHA: 4Q, '00, 51

V45.76 Lung
AHA: 4Q, '00, 51

V45.77 Genital organs
EXCLUDES *acquired absence of cervix and uterus
(V88.01-V88.03)*
*female genital mutilation status
(629.20-629.29)*
AHA: 1Q, '03, 13, 14; 4Q, '00, 51

V45.78 Eye
AHA: 4Q, '00, 51

V45.79 Other acquired absence of organ
EXCLUDES ► *acquired absence of pancreas
(V88.11-V88.12)* ◄
AHA: 4Q, '00, 51

✓5ᵗʰ **V45.8 Other postprocedural status**

V45.81 Aortocoronary bypass status
AHA: 4Q, '03, 105; 3Q, '01, 15; 3Q, '97, 16

**V45.82 Percutaneous transluminal coronary angioplasty
status**

V45.83 Breast implant removal status
AHA: 4Q, '95, 55

V45.84 Dental restoration status
Dental crowns status
Dental fillings status
AHA: 4Q, '01, 54

V45.85 Insulin pump status

V45.86 Bariatric surgery status
Gastric banding status
Gastric bypass status for obesity
Obesity surgery status
EXCLUDES *bariatric surgery status complicating
pregnancy, childbirth or the
puerperium (649.2)*
*intestinal bypass or anastomosis status
(V45.3)*
AHA: 2Q, '09, 10; 4Q, '06, 118
Z98.84 Bariatric surgery status   I-10

V45.87 Transplanted organ removal status
Transplanted organ previously removed due to
complication, failure, rejection or infection
EXCLUDES *encounter for removal of transplanted organ
— code to complication of
transplanted organ (996.80-996.89)*
AHA: 4Q, '08, 157

**V45.88 Status post administration of tPA (rtPA) in a
different facility within the last 24 hours prior to
admission to current facility**
Code first condition requiring tPA administration,
such as:
acute cerebral infarction (433.0-433.9
with fifth-digit 1, 434.0-434.9 with fifth
digit 1)
acute myocardial infarction (410.00-410.92)
AHA: 4Q, '08, 157
TIP: Assign only on receiving facility record; assign even if
the patient is still receiving tPA at the time of transfer.

V45.89 Other
Presence of neuropacemaker or other electronic
device
EXCLUDES *artificial heart valve in situ (V43.3)*
vascular prosthesis in situ (V43.4)
AHA: 1Q, '95, 11

✓4ᵗʰ **V46 Other dependence on machines and devices**

V46.0 Aspirator

✓5ᵗʰ **V46.1 Respirator [Ventilator]**
Iron lung
AHA: 4Q, '05, 96; 4Q, '03, 103; 1Q, '01, 12; J-F, '87, 7 3

V46.11 Dependence on respirator, status
AHA: 4Q, '04, 100
Z99.11 Dependence on respirator ventilator status   I-10

**V46.12 Encounter for respirator dependence   PDx
during power failure**
AHA: 4Q, '04, 100

**V46.13 Encounter for weaning from respirator   PDx
[ventilator]**

V46.14 Mechanical complication of respirator [ventilator]
Mechanical failure of respirator [ventilator]

V46.2 Supplemental oxygen
Long-term oxygen therapy
AHA: 4Q, '03, 108; 4Q, '02, 79

V46.3 Wheelchair dependence
Wheelchair confinement status
Code first cause of dependence, such as:
muscular dystrophy (359.1)
obesity ► (278.00-278.03) ◄
AHA: 4Q, '08, 157

V46.8 Other enabling machines
Hyperbaric chamber
Possum [Patient-Operated-Selector-Mechanism]
EXCLUDES *cardiac pacemaker (V45.0)*
kidney dialysis machine (V45.11)

V46.9 Unspecified machine dependence
AHA: 4Q, '06, 117

✓4ᵗʰ **V47 Other problems with internal organs**

V47.0 Deficiencies of internal organs

V47.1 Mechanical and motor problems with internal organs

V47.2 Other cardiorespiratory problems
Cardiovascular exercise intolerance with pain (with):
at rest
less than ordinary activity
ordinary activity

V47.3 Other digestive problems

V47.4 Other urinary problems

V47.5 Other genital problems

V47.9 Unspecified

N Newborn Age: 0   P Pediatric Age: 0-17   M Maternity Age: 12-55   A Adult Age: 15-124   PDx Primary Diagnosis

✓4ᵗʰ **V48 Problems with head, neck, and trunk**

V48.0 Deficiencies of head
> EXCLUDES deficiencies of ears, eyelids, and nose (V48.8)

V48.1 Deficiencies of neck and trunk

V48.2 Mechanical and motor problems with head

V48.3 Mechanical and motor problems with neck and trunk

V48.4 Sensory problem with head

V48.5 Sensory problem with neck and trunk

V48.6 Disfigurements of head

V48.7 Disfigurements of neck and trunk

V48.8 Other problems with head, neck, and trunk

V48.9 Unspecified problem with head, neck, or trunk

✓4ᵗʰ **V49 Other conditions influencing health status**

V49.0 Deficiencies of limbs

V49.1 Mechanical problems with limbs

V49.2 Motor problems with limbs

V49.3 Sensory problems with limbs

V49.4 Disfigurements of limbs

V49.5 Other problems of limbs

✓5ᵗʰ **V49.6 Upper limb amputation status**
> AHA: 4Q, '05, 94; 4Q, '98, 42; 4Q, '94, 39

V49.60 Unspecified level
> Z89.201 Acquired absence of right upper limb I-10
> uns level

V49.61 Thumb

V49.62 Other finger(s)
> AHA: 2Q, '05, 7

V49.63 Hand

V49.64 Wrist
> Disarticulation of wrist

V49.65 Below elbow

V49.66 Above elbow
> Disarticulation of elbow

V49.67 Shoulder
> Disarticulation of shoulder

✓5ᵗʰ **V49.7 Lower limb amputation status**
> AHA: 3Q, '06, 5; 4Q, '05, 94; 4Q, '98, 42; 4Q, '94, 39

V49.70 Unspecified level

V49.71 Great toe

V49.72 Other toe(s)

V49.73 Foot

V49.74 Ankle
> Disarticulation of ankle

V49.75 Below knee
> Z89.52 Acquired absence of left leg below I-10
> knee

V49.76 Above knee
> Disarticulation of knee

V49.77 Hip
> Disarticulation of hip

✓5ᵗʰ **V49.8 Other specified conditions influencing health status**
> AHA: 4Q, '00, 51

V49.81 Asymptomatic postmenopausal status A ♀
(age-related) (natural)
> EXCLUDES menopausal and premenopausal disorder
> (627.0-627.9)
> postsurgical menopause (256.2)
> premature menopause (256.31)
> symptomatic menopause (627.0-627.9)
> AHA: 4Q, '09, 106; 4Q, '02, 79; 4Q, '00, 54

V49.82 Dental sealant status
> AHA: 4Q, '01, 54

V49.83 Awaiting organ transplant status

V49.84 Bed confinement status
> AHA: 4Q, '05, 96

V49.85 Dual sensory impairment
> Blindness with deafness
> Combined visual hearing impairment
> Code first:
> hearing impairment (389.00-389.9)
> visual impairment (369.00-369.9)
> AHA: 4Q, '07, 100

● **V49.86 Do not resuscitate status**
> Z66 Do not resuscitate I-10

● **V49.87 Physical restraints status**
> EXCLUDES restraint due to a procedure – omit code

V49.89 Other specified conditions influencing health status
> AHA: 4Q, '05, 94

V49.9 Unspecified

Persons Encountering Health Services for Specific Procedures and Aftercare (V50-V59)

> NOTE Categories V51-V59 are intended for use to indicate a reason
> for care in patients who may have already been treated for
> some disease or injury not now present, or who are receiving
> care to consolidate the treatment, to deal with residual states,
> or to prevent recurrence.
> EXCLUDES follow-up examination for medical surveillance following
> treatment (V67.0-V67.9)

✓4ᵗʰ **V50 Elective surgery for purposes other than remedying health states**

V50.0 Hair transplant

V50.1 Other plastic surgery for unacceptable cosmetic appearance
> Breast augmentation or reduction
> Face-lift
> EXCLUDES encounter for breast reduction (611.1)
> plastic surgery following healed injury or operation
> (V51.0-V51.8)

V50.2 Routine or ritual circumcision ♂
> Circumcision in the absence of significant medical indication

V50.3 Ear piercing

✓5ᵗʰ **V50.4 Prophylactic organ removal**
> EXCLUDES organ donations (V59.0-V59.9)
> therapeutic organ removal — code to condition
> AHA: 4Q, '94, 44
> TIP: Assign an additional code, such as one from category V16 Family
> history of malignant neoplasm, to indicate the reason for the
> prophylactic organ removal.

V50.41 Breast
> AHA: 4Q, '04, 107

V50.42 Ovary ♀
> AHA: 3Q, '09, 5

V50.49 Other
> AHA: 3Q, '09, 5

V50.8 Other
> Z40.8 Encounter for other prophylactic surgery I-10

V50.9 Unspecified

✓4ᵗʰ **V51 Aftercare involving the use of plastic surgery**
> Plastic surgery following healed injury or operation
> EXCLUDES cosmetic plastic surgery (V50.2)
> plastic surgery as treatment for current condition or injury —
> code to condition or injury
> repair of scarred tissue — code to scar
> AHA: 4Q, '08, 159

V51.0 Encounter for breast reconstruction PDx A
following mastectomy
> EXCLUDES deformity and disproportion of reconstructed breast
> (612.0-612.1)
> AHA: 4Q, '08, 159-160

V51.8 Other aftercare involving the use of plastic surgery

✓4ᵗʰ / ✓5ᵗʰ Additional Digit Required   Unspecified Code   Other Specified Code   Manifestation Code   ►◄ Revised Text   ● New Code   ▲ Revised Code Title

2011 ICD-9-CM   **October 2010 · Volume 1 – 331**

✓4ᵗʰ V52 Fitting and adjustment of prosthetic device and implant

INCLUDES removal of device

EXCLUDES malfunction or complication of prosthetic device (996.0-996.7)
status only, without need for care (V43.0-V43.8)

AHA: 4Q, '05, 94; 4Q, '95, 55 ; 1Q, '90, 7

V52.0 Artificial arm (complete) (partial)

V52.1 Artificial leg (complete) (partial)

V52.2 Artificial eye

V52.3 Dental prosthetic device

V52.4 Breast prosthesis and implant ♀

Elective implant exchange (different material) (different size)
Removal of tissue expander without synchronous insertion of permanent implant

EXCLUDES admission for initial breast implant insertion for breast augmentation (V50.1)
complications of breast implant (996.54, 996.69, 996.79)
encounter for breast reconstruction following mastectomy (V51.0)

AHA: 4Q, '95, 80, 81

V52.8 Other specified prosthetic device

AHA: 2Q, '02, 12, 16

V52.9 Unspecified prosthetic device

✓4ᵗʰ V53 Fitting and adjustment of other device

INCLUDES removal of device
replacement of device

EXCLUDES status only, without need for care (V45.0-V45.8)

✓6ᵗʰ V53.0 Devices related to nervous system and special senses

AHA: 4Q, '98, 66; 4Q, '97, 51

V53.01 Fitting and adjustment of cerebral ventricular (communicating) shunt

AHA: 4Q, '97, 51

V53.02 Neuropacemaker (brain) (peripheral nerve) (spinal cord)

V53.09 Fitting and adjustment of other devices related to nervous system and special senses

Auditory substitution device
Visual substitution device

AHA: 2Q, '99, 4

V53.1 Spectacles and contact lenses

V53.2 Hearing aid

✓5ᵗʰ V53.3 Cardiac device

Reprogramming

AHA: 3Q, '92, 3; 1Q, '90, 7; M-J, '87, 8 ; N-D, '84, 18

TIP: Assign for cardiac device replacement when the device has reached normal end-of-life parameters.

V53.31 Cardiac pacemaker

EXCLUDES ►automatic implantable cardiac defibrillator with synchronous cardiac pacemaker (V53.32)◄
mechanical complication of cardiac pacemaker (996.01)

AHA: 1Q, '02, 3

V53.32 Automatic implantable cardiac defibrillator

►With synchronous cardiac pacemaker◄

AHA: 3Q, '05, 8

V53.39 Other cardiac device

AHA: 2Q, '08, 9; 1Q, '07, 20

V53.4 Orthodontic devices

✓5ᵗʰ V53.5 Other gastrointestinal appliance and device

EXCLUDES colostomy (V55.3)
ileostomy (V55.2)
other artificial opening of digestive tract (V55.4)

AHA: 4Q, '09, 116

V53.50 Fitting and adjustment of intestinal appliance and device

V53.51 Fitting and adjustment of gastric lap band

V53.59 Fitting and adjustment of other gastrointestinal appliance and device

V53.6 Urinary devices

Urinary catheter

EXCLUDES cystostomy (V55.5)
nephrostomy (V55.6)
ureterostomy (V55.6)
urethrostomy (V55.6)

V53.7 Orthopedic devices

Orthopedic: Orthopedic:
  brace   corset
  cast   shoes

EXCLUDES other orthopedic aftercare (V54)

V53.8 Wheelchair

✓5ᵗʰ V53.9 Other and unspecified device

AHA: 2Q, '03, 6

V53.90 Unspecified device

V53.91 Fitting and adjustment of insulin pump

Insulin pump titration

V53.99 Other device

AHA: 2Q, '09, 10

✓4ᵗʰ V54 Other orthopedic aftercare

EXCLUDES fitting and adjustment of orthopedic devices (V53.7)
malfunction of internal orthopedic device (996.40-996.49)
other complication of nonmechanical nature (996.60-996.79)

AHA: 4Q, '08, 158; 1Q, '07, 3-4; 3Q, '95, 3

✓5ᵗʰ V54.0 Aftercare involving internal fixation device

EXCLUDES malfunction of internal orthopedic device (996.40-996.49)
other complication of nonmechanical nature (996.60-996.79)
removal of external fixation device (V54.89)

AHA: 4Q, '03, 87

V54.01 Encounter for removal of internal fixation device

V54.02 Encounter for lengthening/adjustment of growth rod

V54.09 Other aftercare involving internal fixation device

✓5ᵗʰ V54.1 Aftercare for healing traumatic fracture

EXCLUDES aftercare following joint replacement (V54.81)
aftercare for amputation stump (V54.89)

AHA: 4Q, '02, 80

TIP: Assign for follow-up and treatment during the healing phase of the fracture; an aftercare code should be used for all subsequent encounters after the initial encounter for care of a fracture.

V54.10 Aftercare for healing traumatic fracture of arm, unspecified

V54.11 Aftercare for healing traumatic fracture of upper arm

V54.12 Aftercare for healing traumatic fracture of lower arm

AHA: 1Q, '07, 7

V54.13 Aftercare for healing traumatic fracture of hip

AHA: 1Q, '09, 6; 4Q, '03, 103, 105; 2Q, '03, 16

V54.14 Aftercare for healing traumatic fracture of leg, unspecified

V54.15 Aftercare for healing traumatic fracture of upper leg

EXCLUDES aftercare for healing traumatic fracture of hip (V54.13)

AHA: 3Q, '06, 6

V54.16 Aftercare for healing traumatic fracture of lower leg

V54.17 Aftercare for healing traumatic fracture of vertebrae

V54.19 Aftercare for healing traumatic fracture of other bone

AHA: 1Q, '05, 13; 4Q, '02, 80

N Newborn Age: 0   P Pediatric Age: 0-17   M Maternity Age: 12-55   A Adult Age: 15-124   PDx Primary Diagnosis

☑5ᵗʰ V54.2 Aftercare for healing pathologic fracture

> **EXCLUDES** *aftercare following joint replacement (V54.81)*
> AHA: 4Q, '02, 80

V54.20 Aftercare for healing pathologic fracture of arm, unspecified

V54.21 Aftercare for healing pathologic fracture of upper arm

V54.22 Aftercare for healing pathologic fracture of lower arm

V54.23 Aftercare for healing pathologic fracture of hip

V54.24 Aftercare for healing pathologic fracture of leg, unspecified

V54.25 Aftercare for healing pathologic fracture of upper leg

> **EXCLUDES** *aftercare for healing pathologic fracture of hip (V54.23)*

V54.26 Aftercare for healing pathologic fracture of lower leg

V54.27 Aftercare for healing pathologic fracture of vertebrae

> AHA: 1Q, '07, 6; 4Q, '03, 108

V54.29 Aftercare for healing pathologic fracture of other bone

> AHA: 4Q, '02, 80

☑5ᵗʰ V54.8 Other orthopedic aftercare

> AHA: 3Q, '01, 19; 4Q, '99, 5

V54.81 Aftercare following joint replacement

> Use additional code to identify joint replacement site (V43.60-V43.69)
> AHA: 1Q, '09, 6; 3Q, '06, 4; 2Q, '04, 15; 4Q, '02, 80

V54.89 Other orthopedic aftercare

> Aftercare for healing fracture NOS

V54.9 Unspecified orthopedic aftercare

☑4ᵗʰ V55 Attention to artificial openings

> **INCLUDES** adjustment or repositioning of catheter
> closure
> passage of sounds or bougies
> reforming
> removal or replacement of catheter
> toilet or cleansing
>
> **EXCLUDES** *complications of external stoma ▶(519.00-519.09, 569.60-569.69, 997.5)◀*
> *status only, without need for care (V44.0-V44.9)*

V55.0 Tracheostomy

V55.1 Gastrostomy

> AHA: 4Q, '99, 9; 3Q, '97, 7, 8; 1Q, '96, 14; 3Q, '95, 13
> TIP: Assign for gastrostomy or PEG tube that has been dislodged or clogged, for which simple irrigation or replacement is performed.

V55.2 Ileostomy

V55.3 Colostomy

> AHA: 1Q, '09, 5; 2Q, '05, 4; 3Q, '97, 9
> Z43.3 Encounter for attention to colostomy　　　　I-10

V55.4 Other artificial opening of digestive tract

> AHA: 2Q, '05, 14; 1Q, '03, 10

V55.5 Cystostomy

V55.6 Other artificial opening of urinary tract

> Nephrostomy　　　　Urethrostomy
> Ureterostomy

V55.7 Artificial vagina

V55.8 Other specified artificial opening

V55.9 Unspecified artificial opening

☑4ᵗʰ V56 Encounter for dialysis and dialysis catheter care

> Use additional code to identify the associated condition
> **EXCLUDES** *dialysis preparation — code to condition*
> AHA: 4Q, '98, 66; 1Q, '93, 29

V56.0 Extracorporeal dialysis　　　　　　　PDx

> Dialysis (renal) NOS
> **EXCLUDES** *dialysis status (V45.11)*
> AHA: 4Q, '05, 79; 1Q, '04, 23; 4Q, '00, 40; 3Q, '98, 6; 2Q, '98, 20

V56.1 Fitting and adjustment of extracorporeal dialysis catheter

> Removal or replacement of catheter
> Toilet or cleansing
> Use additional code for any concurrent extracorporeal dialysis (V56.0)
> AHA: 2Q, '98, 20

V56.2 Fitting and adjustment of peritoneal dialysis catheter

> Use additional code for any concurrent peritoneal dialysis (V56.8)
> AHA: 4Q, '98, 55

☑5ᵗʰ V56.3 Encounter for adequacy testing for dialysis

> AHA: 4Q, '00, 55

V56.31 Encounter for adequacy testing for hemodialysis

V56.32 Encounter for adequacy testing for peritoneal dialysis

> Peritoneal equilibration test

V56.8 Other dialysis

> Peritoneal dialysis
> AHA: 4Q, '98, 55

☑4ᵗʰ V57 Care involving use of rehabilitation procedures

> Use additional code to identify underlying condition
> AHA: 3Q, '06, 3; 1Q, '02, 19; 3Q, '97, 12; 1Q, '90, 6; S-O, '86, 3
> TIP: Assign codes from this category for episodes of care related to rehabilitation.

V57.0 Breathing exercises　　　　　　　　PDx

V57.1 Other physical therapy　　　　　　　PDx

> Therapeutic and remedial exercises, except breathing
> AHA: 3Q, '06, 4; 2Q, '04, 15; 4Q, '02, 56; 4Q, '99, 5

☑5ᵗʰ V57.2 Occupational therapy and vocational rehabilitation

V57.21 Encounter for occupational therapy　PDx

> AHA: 4Q, '99, 7

V57.22 Encounter for vocational therapy　　PDx

V57.3 Speech-language therapy　　　　　　PDx

> AHA: 4Q, '97, 36

V57.4 Orthoptic training　　　　　　　　　PDx

☑5ᵗʰ V57.8 Other specified rehabilitation procedure

V57.81 Orthotic training　　　　　　　　　PDx

> Gait training in the use of artificial limbs

V57.89 Other　　　　　　　　　　　　　　PDx

> Multiple training or therapy
> AHA: 4Q, '07, 94; 3Q, '06, 6; 4Q, '03, 105-106, 108; 2Q, '03, 16; 1Q '02, 16; 3Q, '01, 21; 3Q, '97, 11, 12; S-O, '86, 4

V57.9 Unspecified rehabilitation procedure　PDx

☑4ᵗʰ V58 Encounter for other and unspecified procedures and aftercare

> **EXCLUDES** *convalescence and palliative care (V66)*
> TIP: If a patient is admitted for both radiation therapy and chemotherapy, either code V58.0 or V58.11 may be sequenced as the principal diagnosis.

V58.0 Radiotherapy　　　　　　　　　　　PDx

> Encounter or admission for radiotherapy
> **EXCLUDES** *encounter for radioactive implant — code to condition*
> *radioactive iodine therapy — code to condition*
> AHA: 3Q, '92, 5; 2Q, '90, 7; J-F, '87, 13
> Z51.0 Encounter for antineoplastic radiation therapy　　I-10

☑4ᵗʰ/☑5ᵗʰ Additional Digit Required　　Unspecified Code　　Other Specified Code　　Manifestation Code　　▶◀ Revised Text　　● New Code　　▲ Revised Code Title

2011 ICD-9-CM　　　　　　　　　　　　　　　　　　　　　　**October 2010 · Volume 1 – 333**

√5ᵗʰ **V58.1 Encounter for antineoplastic chemotherapy and immunotherapy**

Encounter or admission for chemotherapy

EXCLUDES *chemotherapy and immunotherapy for nonneoplastic conditions — code to condition*

AHA: 1Q, '04, 13; 2Q, '03, 16; 3Q, '93, 4; 2Q, '92, 6; 2Q, '91, 17; 2Q, '90, 7; S-O, '84, 5

V58.11 Encounter for antineoplastic chemotherapy `PDx`

AHA: 4Q, '09, 79; 4Q, '08, 82, 155; 4Q, '07, 104; 2Q, '06, 20-21; 4Q, '05, 98

Z51.11 Encounter for antineoplastic chemotherapy `I-10`

V58.12 Encounter for antineoplastic immunotherapy `PDx`

AHA: 4Q, '05, 98

V58.2 Blood transfusion, without reported diagnosis

√5ᵗʰ **V58.3 Attention to dressings and sutures**

Change or removal of wound packing

EXCLUDES *attention to drains (V58.49)*
planned postoperative wound closure (V58.41)

AHA: 2Q, '05, 14

V58.30 Encounter for change or removal of nonsurgical wound dressing

Encounter for change or removal of wound dressing NOS

AHA: 4Q, '09, 150; 4Q, '06, 117

V58.31 Encounter for change or removal of surgical wound dressing

AHA: 4Q, '06, 117

Z48.01 Encounter change/removal surgical wound dressing `I-10`

V58.32 Encounter for removal of sutures

Encounter for removal of staples

AHA: 4Q, '06, 117

Z48.02 Encounter for removal of sutures `I-10`

√5ᵗʰ **V58.4 Other aftercare following surgery**

NOTE Codes from this subcategory should be used in conjunction with other aftercare codes to fully identify the reason for the aftercare encounter

EXCLUDES *aftercare following sterilization reversal surgery (V26.22)*
attention to artificial openings (V55.0-V55.9)
orthopedic aftercare (V54.0-V54.9)

AHA: 4Q, '99, 9; N-D, '87, 9

V58.41 Encounter for planned postoperative wound closure

EXCLUDES *disruption of operative wound (998.31-998.32)*
encounter for dressings and suture aftercare (V58.30-V58.32)

AHA: 4Q, '99, 15

V58.42 Aftercare following surgery for neoplasm

Conditions classifiable to 140-239

AHA: 4Q, '02, 80

V58.43 Aftercare following surgery for injury and trauma

Conditions classifiable to 800-999

EXCLUDES *aftercare for healing traumatic fracture (V54.10-V54.19)*

AHA: 4Q, '02, 80

V58.44 Aftercare following organ transplant

Use additional code to identify the organ transplanted (V42.0-V42.9)

AHA: 4Q, '04, 101

V58.49 Other specified aftercare following surgery

Change or removal of drains

AHA: 1Q, '96, 8, 9

V58.5 Orthodontics

EXCLUDES *fitting and adjustment of orthodontic device (V53.4)*

√5ᵗʰ **V58.6 Long-term (current) drug use**

▶Long-term (current) prophylactic drug use◀

EXCLUDES *drug abuse and dependence complicating pregnancy (648.3-648.4)*
drug abuse (305.00-305.93)
drug dependence (304.00-304.93)
hormone replacement therapy (postmenopausal) (V07.4)
▶*use of agents affecting estrogen receptors and estrogen levels (V07.51-V07.59)*◀

AHA: 4Q, '08, 159; 4Q, '03, 85; 4Q, '02, 84; 3Q, '02, 15; 4Q, '95, 61

TIP: Do not assign for patients on detoxification drugs or maintenance programs to prevent withdrawal symptoms related to drug dependence; assign instead drug dependence code(s).

V58.61 Long-term (current) use of anticoagulants

EXCLUDES *long-term (current) use of aspirin (V58.66)*

AHA: 4Q, '08, 135; 3Q, '06, 13; 3Q, '04, 7; 4Q, '03, 108; 3Q, '02, 13-16; 1Q, '02, 15, 16

Z79.01 Long term (current) use of anticoagulants `I-10`

V58.62 Long-term (current) use of antibiotics

AHA: 4Q, '98, 59

V58.63 Long-term (current) use of antiplatelets/antithrombotics

EXCLUDES *long-term (current) use of aspirin (V58.66)*

V58.64 Long-term (current) use of non-steroidal anti-inflammatories (NSAID)

EXCLUDES *long-term (current) use of aspirin (V58.66)*

V58.65 Long-term (current) use of steroids

Z79.5 Long term (current) use of steroids `I-10`

V58.66 Long-term (current) use of aspirin

AHA: 4Q, '04, 102

V58.67 Long-term (current) use of insulin

AHA: 4Q, '04, 55-56, 103

Z79.4 Long term (current) use of insulin `I-10`

V58.69 Long-term (current) use of other medications

Other high-risk medications
Long term current use of methadone
Long term current use of opiate analgesic

AHA: 4Q, '09, 83; 3Q, '09, 3; 4Q, '08, 156; 2Q, '04, 10; 1Q, '04, 13; 1Q, '03, 11; 2Q, '00, 8; 3Q, '99, 13; 2Q, '99, 17; 1Q, '97, 12; 2Q, '96, 7

√5ᵗʰ **V58.7 Aftercare following surgery to specified body systems, not elsewhere classified**

NOTE Codes from this subcategory should be used in conjunction with other aftercare codes to fully identify the reason for the aftercare encounter

EXCLUDES *aftercare following organ transplant (V58.44)*
aftercare following surgery for neoplasm (V58.42)

AHA: 4Q, '03, 104; 4Q, '02, 80

V58.71 Aftercare following surgery of the sense organs, NEC

Conditions classifiable to 360-379, 380-389

V58.72 Aftercare following surgery of the nervous system, NEC

Conditions classifiable to 320-359

EXCLUDES *aftercare following surgery of the sense organs, NEC (V58.71)*

V58.73 Aftercare following surgery of the circulatory system, NEC

Conditions classifiable to 390-459

AHA: 2Q, '09, 12; 4Q, '03, 105

V58.74 Aftercare following surgery of the respiratory system, NEC

Conditions classifiable to 460-519

V58.75 Aftercare following surgery of the teeth, oral cavity and digestive system, NEC

Conditions classifiable to 520-579

AHA: 2Q, '05, 14

N Newborn Age: 0   **P** Pediatric Age: 0-17   **M** Maternity Age: 12-55   **A** Adult Age: 15-124   **PDx** Primary Diagnosis

334 – Volume 1 · October 2010   **2011 ICD-9-CM**

V58.76 Aftercare following surgery of the genitourinary system, NEC
Conditions classifiable to 580-629
> **EXCLUDES** *aftercare following sterilization reversal (V26.22)*
AHA: 1Q, '05, 11-12

V58.77 Aftercare following surgery of the skin and subcutaneous tissue, NEC
Conditions classifiable to 680-709

V58.78 Aftercare following surgery of the musculoskeletal system, NEC
Conditions classifiable to 710-739
> **EXCLUDES** *orthopedic aftercare (V54.01-V54.9)*

✓5ᵗʰ **V58.8 Other specified procedures and aftercare**
AHA: 4Q, '94, 45; 2Q, '94, 8

V58.81 Fitting and adjustment of vascular catheter
Removal or replacement of catheter
Toilet or cleansing
> **EXCLUDES** *complication of renal dialysis (996.73)*
> *complication of vascular catheter (996.74)*
> *dialysis preparation — code to condition*
> *encounter for dialysis (V56.0-V56.8)*
> *fitting and adjustment of dialysis catheter (V56.1)*

V58.82 Fitting and adjustment of nonvascular catheter, NEC
Removal or replacement of catheter
Toilet or cleansing
> **EXCLUDES** *fitting and adjustment of peritoneal dialysis catheter (V56.2)*
> *fitting and adjustment of urinary catheter (V53.6)*

V58.83 Encounter for therapeutic drug monitoring
Use additional code for any associated long- term (current) drug use (V58.61-V58.69)
> **EXCLUDES** *blood-drug testing for medico- legal reasons (V70.4)*
DEF: Drug monitoring: Measurement of the level of a specific drug in the body or measurement of a specific function to assess effectiveness of a drug.
AHA: 4Q, '08, 156; 2Q, '04, 10; 1Q, '04, 13;4Q, '03, 85; 4Q, '02, 84; 3Q, '02, 13-16

V58.89 Other specified aftercare
AHA: 4Q, '98, 59

V58.9 Unspecified aftercare

✓4ᵗʰ **V59 Donors**
> **EXCLUDES** *examination of potential donor (V70.8)*
> *self-donation of organ or tissue — code to condition*
AHA: 4Q, '95, 62; 1Q, '90, 10; N-D, '84,
TIP: Assign only for living donations to other individuals, not for self-donation or for cadaveric donations.

✓5ᵗʰ **V59.0 Blood**

V59.01 Whole blood `PDx`

V59.02 Stem cells `PDx`

V59.09 Other `PDx`

V59.1 Skin `PDx`

V59.2 Bone `PDx`

V59.3 Bone marrow `PDx`

V59.4 Kidney `PDx`

V59.5 Cornea `PDx`

V59.6 Liver `PDx`

✓5ᵗʰ **V59.7 Egg (oocyte) (ovum)**
AHA: 4Q, '05, 99

V59.70 Egg (oocyte) (ovum) donor, unspecified `PDx` ♀

V59.71 Egg (oocyte) (ovum) donor, under age 35, anonymous recipient `PDx` ♀
Egg donor, under age 35 NOS

V59.72 Egg (oocyte) (ovum) donor, under age 35, designated recipient `PDx` ♀

V59.73 Egg (oocyte) (ovum) donor, age 35 and over, anonymous recipient `PDx` ♀
Egg donor, age 35 and over NOS

V59.74 Egg (oocyte) (ovum) donor, age 35 and over, designated recipient `PDx` ♀

V59.8 Other specified organ or tissue `PDx`
AHA: 3Q, '02, 20

V59.9 Unspecified organ or tissue `PDx`

Persons Encountering Health Services in Other Circumstances (V60-V69)

✓4ᵗʰ **V60 Housing, household, and economic circumstances**

V60.0 Lack of housing
Hobos	Transients
Social migrants	Vagabonds
Tramps	

V60.1 Inadequate housing
Lack of heating
Restriction of space
Technical defects in home preventing adequate care

V60.2 Inadequate material resources
Economic problem   Poverty NOS

V60.3 Person living alone

V60.4 No other household member able to render care
Person requiring care (has) (is):
family member too handicapped, ill, or otherwise unsuited to render care
partner temporarily away from home
temporarily away from usual place of abode
> **EXCLUDES** *holiday relief care (V60.5)*

V60.5 Holiday relief care
Provision of health care facilities to a person normally cared for at home, to enable relatives to take a vacation

V60.6 Person living in residential institution
Boarding school resident

✓5ᵗʰ **V60.8 Other specified housing or economic circumstances**
AHA: ▶4Q, '09, 118◀

V60.81 Foster care (status)

V60.89 Other specified housing or economic circumstances

V60.9 Unspecified housing or economic circumstance

✓4ᵗʰ **V61 Other family circumstances**
> **INCLUDES** *when these circumstances or fear of them, affecting the person directly involved or others, are mentioned as the reason, justified or not, for seeking or receiving medical advice or care*
AHA: 1Q, '90, 9

✓5ᵗʰ **V61.0 Family disruption**
AHA: 4Q, '08, 160

V61.01 Family disruption due to family member on military deployment
Individual or family affected by other family member being on deployment
> **EXCLUDES** *family disruption due to family member on non-military extended absence from home (V61.08)*

V61.02 Family disruption due to return of family member from military deployment
Individual or family affected by other family member having returned from deployment (current or past conflict)

V61.03 Family disruption due to divorce or legal separation

V61.04 Family disruption due to parent-child estrangement
> **EXCLUDES** *other family estrangement (V61.09)*

V61.05 Family disruption due to child in welfare custody

V61.06 Family disruption due to child in foster care or in care of non-parental family member

V Codes

V61.07–V62.89

V61.07 Family disruption due to death of family member
> EXCLUDES *bereavement (V62.82)*
> AHA: 4Q, '09, 117

V61.08 Family disruption due to other extended absence of family member
> EXCLUDES *family disruption due to family member on military deployment (V61.01)*
> AHA: 4Q, '09, 117

V61.09 Other family disruption
Family estrangement NOS

√5th V61.1 Counseling for marital and partner problems
> EXCLUDES *problems related to:*
> *psychosexual disorders (302.0-302.9)*
> *sexual function (V41.7)*

V61.10 Counseling for marital and partner problems, unspecified
Marital conflict
Marital relationship problem
Partner conflict
Partner relationship problem

V61.11 Counseling for victim of spousal and partner abuse
> EXCLUDES *encounter for treatment of current injuries due to abuse (995.80-995.85)*

V61.12 Counseling for perpetrator of spousal and partner abuse

√5th V61.2 Parent-child problems

V61.20 Counseling for parent-child problem, unspecified
Concern about behavior of child
Parent-child conflict
Parent-child relationship problem

V61.21 Counseling for victim of child abuse
Child battering   Child neglect
> EXCLUDES *current injuries due to abuse (995.50-995.59)*

V61.22 Counseling for perpetrator of parental child abuse
> EXCLUDES *counseling for non-parental abuser (V62.83)*

V61.23 Counseling for parent-biological child problem
Concern about behavior of biological child
Parent-biological child conflict
Parent-biological child relationship problem
> AHA: 4Q, '09, 117

V61.24 Counseling for parent-adopted child problem
Concern about behavior of adopted child
Parent-adopted child conflict
Parent-adopted child relationship problem
> AHA: 4Q, '09, 117

V61.25 Counseling for parent (guardian)-foster child problem
Concern about behavior of foster child
Parent (guardian)-foster child conflict
Parent (guardian)-foster child relationship problem
> AHA: 4Q, '09, 117

V61.29 Other parent-child problems
> AHA: 3Q, '99, 16

V61.3 Problems with aged parents or in-laws

√5th V61.4 Health problems within family

V61.41 Alcoholism in family

V61.42 Substance abuse in family
> AHA: 4Q, '09, 117

V61.49 Other
Care of   } sick or handicapped person
Presence of } in family or household

V61.5 Multiparity

V61.6 Illegitimacy or illegitimate pregnancy   M ♀

V61.7 Other unwanted pregnancy   M ♀

V61.8 Other specified family circumstances
Problems with family members NEC
Sibling relationship problem

V61.9 Unspecified family circumstance

√4th V62 Other psychosocial circumstances
> INCLUDES *those circumstances or fear of them, affecting the person directly involved or others, mentioned as the reason, justified or not, for seeking or receiving medical advice or care*
> EXCLUDES *previous psychological trauma (V15.41-V15.49)*

V62.0 Unemployment
> EXCLUDES *circumstances when main problem is economic inadequacy or poverty (V60.2)*

V62.1 Adverse effects of work environment

√5th V62.2 Other occupational circumstances or maladjustment
> AHA: 4Q, '08, 160

V62.21 Personal current military deployment status   A
Individual (civilian or military) currently deployed in theater or in support of military war, peacekeeping and humanitarian operations

V62.22 Personal history of return from military deployment   A
Individual (civilian or military) with past history of military war, peacekeeping and humanitarian deployment (current or past conflict)

V62.29 Other occupational circumstances or maladjustment   A
Career choice problem
Dissatisfaction with employment
Occupational problem

V62.3 Educational circumstances
Academic problem
Dissatisfaction with school environment
Educational handicap

V62.4 Social maladjustment
Acculturation problem
Cultural deprivation
Political, religious, or sex discrimination
Social:
   isolation
   persecution

V62.5 Legal circumstances
Imprisonment   Litigation
Legal investigation   Prosecution

V62.6 Refusal of treatment for reasons of religion or conscience

√5th V62.8 Other psychological or physical stress, not elsewhere classified

V62.81 Interpersonal problems, not elsewhere classified
Relational problem NOS

V62.82 Bereavement, uncomplicated
> EXCLUDES *bereavement as adjustment reaction (309.0)*
> *family disruption due to death of family member (V61.07)*

V62.83 Counseling for perpetrator of physical/sexual abuse
> EXCLUDES *counseling for perpetrator of parental child abuse (V61.22)*
> *counseling for perpetrator of spousal and partner abuse (V61.12)*

V62.84 Suicidal ideation
> EXCLUDES *suicidal tendencies (300.9)*
> DEF: Thoughts of committing suicide; no actual attempt of suicide has been made.
> AHA: 4Q, '05, 96
> TIP: Assign as a secondary diagnosis for patients who have not attempted suicide, and who may not be considered a suicide risk, but who have indicated thoughts about suicide.
> R45.85 Suicidal ideation   I-10

V62.85 Homicidal ideation

V62.89 Other
Borderline intellectual functioning
Life circumstance problems
Phase of life problems
Religious or spiritual problem

V62.9 Unspecified psychosocial circumstance

✓4ᵗʰ **V63 Unavailability of other medical facilities for care**
AHA: 1Q, '91, 21

V63.0 Residence remote from hospital or other health care facility

V63.1 Medical services in home not available
EXCLUDES *no other household member able to render care (V60.4)*
AHA: 4Q, '01, 67; 1Q, '01, 12

V63.2 Person awaiting admission to adequate facility elsewhere

V63.8 Other specified reasons for unavailability of medical facilities
Person on waiting list undergoing social agency investigation

V63.9 Unspecified reason for unavailability of medical facilities

✓4ᵗʰ **V64 Persons encountering health services for specific procedures, not carried out**

✓5ᵗʰ **V64.0 Vaccination not carried out**
AHA: 4Q, '05, 99

V64.00 Vaccination not carried out, unspecified reason

V64.01 Vaccination not carried out because of acute illness

V64.02 Vaccination not carried out because of chronic illness or condition

V64.03 Vaccination not carried out because of immune compromised state

V64.04 Vaccination not carried out because of allergy to vaccine or component
Z28.04 Immunization not carried out pt allergy vaccine I-10

V64.05 Vaccination not carried out because of caregiver refusal
Guardian refusal   Parent refusal
EXCLUDES *vaccination not carried out because of caregiver refusal for religious reasons (V64.07)*
AHA: ▶4Q, '09, 115;◀ 1Q, '07, 12

V64.06 Vaccination not carried out because of patient refusal

V64.07 Vaccination not carried out for religious reasons

V64.08 Vaccination not carried out because patient had disease being vaccinated against

V64.09 Vaccination not carried out for other reason

V64.1 Surgical or other procedure not carried out because of contraindication
TIP: Assign an additional code to indicate the contraindication (reason the surgery or other procedure was canceled).

V64.2 Surgical or other procedure not carried out because of patient's decision
AHA: 2Q, '01, 8

V64.3 Procedure not carried out for other reasons

✓5ᵗʰ **V64.4 Closed surgical procedure converted to open procedure**
AHA: 4Q, '03, 87; 4Q, '98, 68; 4Q, '97, 52

V64.41 Laparoscopic surgical procedure converted to open procedure

V64.42 Thoracoscopic surgical procedure converted to open procedure

V64.43 Arthroscopic surgical procedure converted to open procedure

✓4ᵗʰ **V65 Other persons seeking consultation**

V65.0 Healthy person accompanying sick person
Boarder

✓5ᵗʰ **V65.1 Person consulting on behalf of another person**
Advice or treatment for nonattending third party
EXCLUDES *concern (normal) about sick person in family (V61.41-V61.49)*
AHA: 4Q, '03, 84

V65.11 Pediatric pre-birth visit for expectant parent(s)
Pre-adoption visit for adoptive parent(s)

V65.19 Other person consulting on behalf of another person

V65.2 Person feigning illness
Malingerer   Peregrinating patient
AHA: 3Q, '99, 20
TIP: Assign for patients engaged in what is documented as "drug-seeking behavior."

V65.3 Dietary surveillance and counseling
Dietary surveillance and counseling (in):
NOS
colitis
diabetes mellitus
food allergies or intolerance
gastritis
hypercholesterolemia
hypoglycemia
obesity
Use additional code to identify Body Mass Index (BMI), if known (V85.0-V85.54)
AHA: 4Q, '05, 96

✓5ᵗʰ **V65.4 Other counseling, not elsewhere classified**
Health:
advice
education
instruction
EXCLUDES *counseling (for):*
contraception (V25.40-V25.49)
genetic (V26.31-V26.39)
on behalf of third party (V65.11-V65.19)
procreative management (V26.41-V26.49)

V65.40 Counseling NOS

V65.41 Exercise counseling

V65.42 Counseling on substance use and abuse
Z71.6 Tobacco abuse counseling I-10

V65.43 Counseling on injury prevention

V65.44 Human immunodeficiency virus [HIV] counseling

V65.45 Counseling on other sexually transmitted diseases

V65.46 Encounter for insulin pump training
Z71.82 Insulin pump counseling and training I-10

V65.49 Other specified counseling
AHA: 4Q, '08, 156; 2Q, '00, 8

V65.5 Person with feared complaint in whom no diagnosis was made
Feared condition not demonstrated
Problem was normal state
"Worried well"

V65.8 Other reasons for seeking consultation
EXCLUDES *specified symptoms*
AHA: 3Q, '92, 4

V65.9 Unspecified reason for consultation

✓4ᵗʰ **V66 Convalescence and palliative care**

V66.0 Following surgery   PDx

V66.1 Following radiotherapy   PDx

V66.2 Following chemotherapy   PDx

V66.3 Following psychotherapy and other treatment for mental disorder   PDx

V66.4 Following treatment of fracture   PDx

✓4ᵗʰ ✓5ᵗʰ Additional Digit Required   Unspecified Code   Other Specified Code   Manifestation Code   ▶◀ Revised Text   ● New Code   ▲ Revised Code Title

V Codes

V66.5–V70.2

V66.5 Following other treatment `PDx`

V66.6 Following combined treatment `PDx`

V66.7 Encounter for palliative care
End of life care
Hospice care
Terminal care
Code first underlying disease
AHA: 3Q, '08, 13; 2Q, '05, 9; 4Q, '03, 107; 1Q, '98, 11; 4Q, '96, 47, 48
TIP: Assign as secondary diagnosis when treatment is focused on management of pain and symptoms in a patient with an incurable disease.
Z51.5 Encounter for palliative care `I-10`

V66.9 Unspecified convalescence `PDx`
AHA: 4Q, '99, 8

✓4th **V67 Follow-up examination**
INCLUDES surveillance only following completed treatment
EXCLUDES surveillance of contraception (V25.40-V25.49)
AHA: 4Q, '08, 157; 2Q, '03, 5; 4Q, '94, 98

✓5th **V67.0 Following surgery**
AHA: 4Q, '00, 56; 4Q, '98, 69; 4Q, '97, 50; 2Q, '95, 8;1Q, '95, 4; 3Q, '92, 11

V67.00 Following surgery, unspecified

V67.01 Follow-up vaginal pap smear ♀
Vaginal pap-smear, status-post hysterectomy for malignant condition
Use additional code to identify:
acquired absence of uterus (V88.01-V88.03)
personal history of malignant neoplasm (V10.40-V10.44)
EXCLUDES vaginal pap smear status-post hysterectomy for non-malignant condition (V76.47)
AHA: 4Q, '08, 157

V67.09 Following other surgery
EXCLUDES sperm count following sterilization reversal (V26.22)
sperm count for fertility testing (V26.21)
AHA: 3Q, '08, 6; 3Q, '03, 16; 3Q, '02, 15

V67.1 Following radiotherapy

V67.2 Following chemotherapy
Cancer chemotherapy follow-up

V67.3 Following psychotherapy and other treatment for mental disorder

V67.4 Following treatment of healed fracture
EXCLUDES current (healing) fracture aftercare (V54.0-V54.9)
AHA: 1Q, '09, 6; 1Q, '90, 7

✓5th **V67.5 Following other treatment**

V67.51 Following completed treatment with high-risk medications, not elsewhere classified
EXCLUDES long-term (current) drug use (V58.61-V58.69)
AHA: 1Q, '99, 5, 6;4Q, '95, 61 ; 1Q, '90, 18

V67.59 Other

V67.6 Following combined treatment

V67.9 Unspecified follow-up examination

✓4th **V68 Encounters for administrative purposes**

✓5th **V68.0 Issue of medical certificates**
EXCLUDES encounter for general medical examination (V70.0-V70.9)

V68.01 Disability examination `PDx`
Use additional code(s) to identify specific examination(s), screening and testing performed (V72.0-V82.9)
AHA: 4Q, '07, 101

V68.09 Other issue of medical certificates `PDx`

V68.1 Issue of repeat prescriptions `PDx`
Issue of repeat prescription for:
appliance
glasses
medications
EXCLUDES repeat prescription for contraceptives (V25.41-V25.49)

V68.2 Request for expert evidence `PDx`

✓5th **V68.8 Other specified administrative purpose**

V68.81 Referral of patient without examination or treatment `PDx`

V68.89 Other `PDx`

V68.9 Unspecified administrative purpose `PDx`

✓4th **V69 Problems related to lifestyle**
AHA: 4Q, '94, 48

V69.0 Lack of physical exercise

V69.1 Inappropriate diet and eating habits
EXCLUDES anorexia nervosa (307.1)
bulimia (783.6)
malnutrition and other nutritional deficiencies (260-269.9)
other and unspecified eating disorders (307.50-307.59)

V69.2 High-risk sexual behavior

V69.3 Gambling and betting
EXCLUDES pathological gambling (312.31)

V69.4 Lack of adequate sleep
Sleep deprivation
EXCLUDES insomnia (780.52)

V69.5 Behavioral insomnia of childhood `P`
DEF: Behaviors on the part of the child or caregivers that cause negative compliance with a child's sleep schedule; results in lack of adequate sleep.
AHA: 4Q, '05, 99

V69.8 Other problems related to lifestyle
Self-damaging behavior

V69.9 Problem related to lifestyle, unspecified

Persons Without Reported Diagnosis Encountered During Examination and Investigation of Individuals and Populations (V70-V82)

NOTE Nonspecific abnormal findings disclosed at the time of these examinations are classifiable to categories 790-796.

✓4th **V70 General medical examination**
Use additional code(s) to identify any special screening examination(s) performed (V73.0-V82.9)

V70.0 Routine general medical examination at a health care facility `PDx`
Health checkup
EXCLUDES health checkup of infant or child over 28 days old (V20.2)
health supervision of newborn 8 to 28 days old (V20.32)
health supervision of newborn under 8 days old (V20.31)
pre-procedural general physical examination (V72.83)

V70.1 General psychiatric examination, requested by the authority `PDx`

V70.2 General psychiatric examination, other and unspecified `PDx`

V70.3 Other medical examination for administrative purposes `PDx`
General medical examination for:
  admission to old age home
  adoption
  camp
  driving license
  immigration and naturalization
  insurance certification
  marriage
  prison
  school admission
  sports competition
> **EXCLUDES** *attendance for issue of medical certificates (V68.0)*
> *pre-employment screening (V70.5)*

AHA: 3Q, '08, 6; 1Q, '90, 6
Z02.6 Encounter for exam for insurance purposes `I-10`

V70.4 Examination for medicolegal reasons `PDx`
Blood-alcohol tests   Paternity testing
Blood-drug tests
> **EXCLUDES** *examination and observation following:*
> *accidents (V71.3, V71.4)*
> *assault (V71.6)*
> *rape (V71.5)*

V70.5 Health examination of defined subpopulations `PDx`
Armed forces personnel
Inhabitants of institutions
Occupational healthexaminations
Pre-employment screening
Preschool children
Prisoners
Prostitutes
Refugees
School children
Students

V70.6 Health examination in population surveys `PDx`
> **EXCLUDES** *special screening (V73.0-V82.9)*

V70.7 Examination of participant in clinical trial
Examination of participant or control in clinical research
AHA: 2Q, '06, 5-6; 4Q, '01, 55

V70.8 Other specified general medical examinations `PDx`
Examination of potential donor of organ or tissue

V70.9 Unspecified general medical examination `PDx`

`√4th` **V71 Observation and evaluation for suspected conditions not found**
> **INCLUDES** This category is to be used when persons without a diagnosis are suspected of having an abnormal condition, without signs or symptoms, which requires study, but after examination and observation, is found not to exist. This category is also for use for administrative and legal observation status.
> **EXCLUDES** *suspected maternal and fetal conditions not found (V89.01-V89.09)*

AHA: 4Q, '94, 47; 2Q, '90, 5; M-A, '87, 1
TIP: Assign observation codes only as principal/first-listed diagnosis and only if there is no documentation of any signs or symptoms.

`√5th` **V71.0 Observation for suspected mental condition**

V71.01 Adult antisocial behavior `A` `PDx`
Dyssocial behavior or gang activity in adult without manifest psychiatric disorder

V71.02 Childhood or adolescent antisocial behavior `PDx`
Dyssocial behavior or gang activity in child or adolescent without manifest psychiatric disorder

V71.09 Other suspected mental condition `PDx`

V71.1 Observation for suspected malignant neoplasm `PDx`

V71.2 Observation for suspected tuberculosis `PDx`

V71.3 Observation following accident at work `PDx`

V71.4 Observation following other accident `PDx`
Examination of individual involved in motor vehicle traffic accident
AHA: 1Q, '06, 9

V71.5 Observation following alleged rape or seduction `PDx`
Examination of victim or culprit

V71.6 Observation following other inflicted injury `PDx`
Examination of victim or culprit

V71.7 Observation for suspected cardiovascular disease `PDx`
AHA: 1Q, '04, 6; 3Q, '90, 10; S-O, '87, 10

`√5th` **V71.8 Observation and evaluation for other specified suspected conditions**
> **EXCLUDES** *contact with and (suspected) exposure to (potentially) hazardous substances (V15.84-V15.86, V87.0-V87.31)*

AHA: 4Q, '00, 54 ; 1Q, '90, 19

V71.81 Abuse and neglect `PDx`
> **EXCLUDES** *adult abuse and neglect (995.80-995.85)*
> *child abuse and neglect (995.50-995.59)*

AHA: 4Q, '00, 55

V71.82 Observation and evaluation for suspected exposure to anthrax `PDx`
AHA: 4Q, '02, 70, 85

V71.83 Observation and evaluation for suspected exposure to other biological agent `PDx`
AHA: 4Q, '03, 47

V71.89 Other specified suspected conditions `PDx`
AHA: 3Q, '08, 7; 2Q, '03, 15

V71.9 Observation for unspecified suspected condition `PDx`
AHA: 1Q, '02, 6

`√4th` **V72 Special investigations and examinations**
> **INCLUDES** routine examination of specific system
Use additional code(s) to identify any special screening examination(s) performed (V73.0-V82.9)
> **EXCLUDES** *general medical examination (V70.0-V70.4)*
> *general screening examination of defined population groups (V70.5, V70.6, V70.7)*
> *health supervision of newborn 8 to 28 days old (V20.32)*
> *health supervision of newborn under 8 days old (V20.31)*
> *routine examination of infant or child over 28 days old (V20.2)*

V72.0 Examination of eyes and vision
AHA: 1Q, '04, 15

`√5th` **V72.1 Examination of ears and hearing**
AHA: 1Q, '04, 15

V72.11 Encounter for hearing examination following failed hearing screening
AHA: 4Q, '06, 118
Z01.110 Encounter hearing exam follow failed hearing scr `I-10`

V72.12 Encounter for hearing conservation and treatment
AHA: 4Q, '07, 100

V72.19 Other examination of ears and hearing

V72.2 Dental examination

`√5th` **V72.3 Gynecological examination**
> **EXCLUDES** *cervical Papanicolaou smear without general gynecological examination (V76.2)*
> *routine examination in contraceptive management (V25.40-V25.49)*

V72.31 Routine gynecological examination ♀
General gynecological examination with or without Papanicolaou cervical smear
Pelvic examination (annual) (periodic)
Use additional code to identify:
  human papillomavirus (HPV) screening (V73.81)
  routine vaginal Papanicolaou smear (V76.47)
AHA: 2Q, '06, 2-3; 4Q, '05, 98

`√4th` `√6th` Additional Digit Required   Unspecified Code   Other Specified Code   Manifestation Code   ►◄ Revised Text   ● New Code   ▲ Revised Code Title

2011 ICD-9-CM   **Volume 1 – 339**

V72.32 Encounter for Papanicolaou cervical smear to confirm findings of recent normal smear following initial abnormal smear ♀
> AHA: 2Q, '06, 4

√5ᵗʰ **V72.4 Pregnancy examination or test**
> AHA: 4Q, '05, 98

V72.40 Pregnancy examination or test, pregnancy unconfirmed ♀
> Possible pregnancy, not (yet) confirmed

V72.41 Pregnancy examination or test, negative result ♀

V72.42 Pregnancy examination or test, positive result ♀ Ⓜ

V72.5 Radiological examination, not elsewhere classified
> Routine chest x-ray
> EXCLUDES radiologic examinations as part of pre-procedural testing (V72.81-V72.84)
> AHA: 1Q, '90, 19

√5ᵗʰ **V72.6 Laboratory examination**
> Encounters for blood and urine testing
> AHA: 4Q, '09, 117-118; 2Q, '06, 4; 1Q, '90, 22

V72.60 Laboratory examination, unspecified

V72.61 Antibody response examination
> Immunity status testing
> EXCLUDES encounter for allergy testing (V72.7)

V72.62 Laboratory examination ordered as part of a routine general medical examination
> Blood tests for routine general physical examination

V72.63 Pre-procedural laboratory examination
> Blood tests prior to treatment or procedure
> Pre-operative laboratory examination

V72.69 Other laboratory examination

V72.7 Diagnostic skin and sensitization tests
> Allergy tests
> Skin tests for hypersensitivity
> EXCLUDES diagnostic skin tests for bacterial diseases (V74.0-V74.9)

√5ᵗʰ **V72.8 Other specified examinations**
> EXCLUDES pre-procedural laboratory examinations (V72.63)

V72.81 Pre-operative cardiovascular examination
> Pre-procedural cardiovascular examination
> Z01.810 Encounter for preprocedural cardiovascular exam   Ⓘ₁₀

V72.82 Pre-operative respiratory examination
> Pre-procedural respiratory examination
> AHA: 3Q, '96, 14

V72.83 Other specified pre-operative examination
> Examination prior to chemotherapy
> Other pre-procedural examination
> Pre-procedural general physical examination
> EXCLUDES routine general medical examination (V70.0)
> AHA: 3Q, '96, 14

V72.84 Pre-operative examination, unspecified
> Pre-procedural examination, unspecified

V72.85 Other specified examination
> AHA: 4Q, '05, 96; 1Q, '04, 12

V72.86 Encounter for blood typing

V72.9 Unspecified examination
> AHA: 4Q, '06, 117

√4ᵗʰ **V73 Special screening examination for viral and chlamydial diseases**
> AHA: 1Q, '04, 11

V73.0 Poliomyelitis

V73.1 Smallpox

V73.2 Measles

V73.3 Rubella

V73.4 Yellow fever

V73.5 Other arthropod-borne viral diseases
> Dengue fever
> Hemorrhagic fever
> Viral encephalitis:
>   mosquito-borne
>   tick-borne

V73.6 Trachoma

√5ᵗʰ **V73.8 Other specified viral and chlamydial diseases**

V73.81 Human papillomavirus [HPV]
> AHA: 4Q, '07, 100

V73.88 Other specified chlamydial diseases
> AHA: 4Q, '07, 124

V73.89 Other specified viral diseases

√5ᵗʰ **V73.9 Unspecified viral and chlamydial disease**

V73.98 Unspecified chlamydial disease

V73.99 Unspecified viral disease

√4ᵗʰ **V74 Special screening examination for bacterial and spirochetal diseases**
> INCLUDES diagnostic skin tests for these diseases
> AHA: 1Q, '04, 11

V74.0 Cholera

V74.1 Pulmonary tuberculosis

V74.2 Leprosy [Hansen's disease]

V74.3 Diphtheria

V74.4 Bacterial conjunctivitis

V74.5 Venereal disease
> Screening for bacterial and spirochetal sexually transmitted diseases
> Screening for sexually transmitted diseases NOS
> EXCLUDES special screening for nonbacterial sexually transmitted diseases (V73.81-V73.89, V75.4, V75.8)
> AHA: 4Q, '07, 124

V74.6 Yaws

V74.8 Other specified bacterial and spirochetal diseases
> Brucellosis
> Leptospirosis
> Plague
> Tetanus
> Whooping cough

V74.9 Unspecified bacterial and spirochetal disease

√4ᵗʰ **V75 Special screening examination for other infectious diseases**
> AHA: 1Q, '04, 11

V75.0 Rickettsial diseases

V75.1 Malaria

V75.2 Leishmaniasis

V75.3 Trypanosomiasis
> Chagas' disease
> Sleeping sickness

V75.4 Mycotic infections

V75.5 Schistosomiasis

V75.6 Filariasis

V75.7 Intestinal helminthiasis

V75.8 Other specified parasitic infections

V75.9 Unspecified infectious disease

√4ᵗʰ **V76 Special screening for malignant neoplasms**
> AHA: 1Q, '04, 11
> TIP: Whenever a screening examination is performed, the screening code is the first-listed code, regardless of the findings or any procedure that is performed as a result of the findings.

V76.0 Respiratory organs

√5ᵗʰ **V76.1 Breast**
> AHA: 4Q, '98, 67

V76.10 Breast screening, unspecified

Ⓝ Newborn Age: 0   Ⓟ Pediatric Age: 0-17   Ⓜ Maternity Age: 12-55   Ⓐ Adult Age: 15-124   PDx Primary Diagnosis

V76.11 Screening mammogram for high-risk patient ♀
AHA: 2Q, '03, 4

V76.12 Other screening mammogram
AHA: 4Q, '09, 106; 2Q, '06, 10; 2Q, '03, 3-4

V76.19 Other screening breast examination

V76.2 Cervix ♀
Routine cervical Papanicolaou smear
EXCLUDES *special screening for human papillomavirus (V73.81)*
that as part of a general gynecological examination
(V72.31)

V76.3 Bladder

√5ᵗʰ **V76.4 Other sites**

V76.41 Rectum

V76.42 Oral cavity

V76.43 Skin

V76.44 Prostate ♂
Z12.5 Encounter screening malignant neoplasm I-10
prostate

V76.45 Testis ♂

V76.46 Ovary ♀
AHA: 4Q, '00, 52

V76.47 Vagina ♀
Vaginal pap smear status-post hysterectomy for
non-malignant condition
Use additional code to identify acquired absence of
uterus (V88.01-V88.03)
EXCLUDES *vaginal pap smear status-post hysterectomy*
for malignant condition (V67.01)
AHA: 4Q, '08, 157; 4Q, '00, 52

V76.49 Other sites
AHA: 1Q, '99, 4

√5ᵗʰ **V76.5 Intestine**
AHA: 4Q, '00, 52

V76.50 Intestine, unspecified

V76.51 Colon
▶Screening colonoscopy NOS◀
EXCLUDES *rectum (V76.41)*
AHA: 4Q, '01, 56
Z12.11 Encounter screening malignant neoplasm I-10
of colon

V76.52 Small intestine

√5ᵗʰ **V76.8 Other neoplasm**
AHA: 4Q, '00, 52

V76.81 Nervous system

V76.89 Other neoplasm

V76.9 Unspecified

√4ᵗʰ **V77 Special screening for endocrine, nutritional, metabolic, and**
immunity disorders
AHA: 1Q, '04, 11

V77.0 Thyroid disorders

V77.1 Diabetes mellitus

V77.2 Malnutrition

V77.3 Phenylketonuria [PKU]

V77.4 Galactosemia

V77.5 Gout

V77.6 Cystic fibrosis
Screening for mucoviscidosis

V77.7 Other inborn errors of metabolism

V77.8 Obesity

√5ᵗʰ **V77.9 Other and unspecified endocrine, nutritional, metabolic,**
and immunity disorders
AHA: 4Q, '00, 53

V77.91 Screening for lipoid disorders
Screening for cholesterol level
Screening for hypercholesterolemia
Screening for hyperlipidemia

V77.99 Other and unspecified endocrine nutritional
metabolic and immunity disorders

√4ᵗʰ **V78 Special screening for disorders of blood and blood-forming**
organs
AHA: 1Q, '04, 11

V78.0 Iron deficiency anemia

V78.1 Other and unspecified deficiency anemia

V78.2 Sickle cell disease or trait

V78.3 Other hemoglobinopathies

V78.8 Other disorders of blood and blood-forming organs

V78.9 Unspecified disorder of blood and blood-forming organs

√4ᵗʰ **V79 Special screening for mental disorders and developmental**
handicaps
AHA: 1Q, '04, 11

V79.0 Depression

V79.1 Alcoholism

V79.2 Mental retardation

V79.3 Developmental handicaps in early childhood

V79.8 Other specified mental disorders and
developmental handicaps

V79.9 Unspecified mental disorder and
developmental handicap

√4ᵗʰ **V80 Special screening for neurological, eye, and ear diseases**
AHA: 1Q, '04, 11

√5ᵗʰ **V80.0 Neurological conditions**
AHA: 4Q, '09, 116

V80.01 Traumatic brain injury

V80.09 Other neurological conditions

V80.1 Glaucoma

V80.2 Other eye conditions
Screening for:
cataract
congenital anomaly of eye
senile macular lesions
EXCLUDES *general vision examination (V72.0)*

V80.3 Ear diseases
EXCLUDES *general hearing examination (V72.11-V72.19)*

√4ᵗʰ **V81 Special screening for cardiovascular, respiratory, and**
genitourinary diseases
AHA: 1Q, '04, 11

V81.0 Ischemic heart disease

V81.1 Hypertension

V81.2 Other and unspecified cardiovascular conditions

V81.3 Chronic bronchitis and emphysema

V81.4 Other and unspecified respiratory conditions
EXCLUDES *screening for:*
lung neoplasm (V76.0)
pulmonary tuberculosis (V74.1)

V81.5 Nephropathy
Screening for asymptomatic bacteriuria

V81.6 Other and unspecified genitourinary conditions

√4ᵗʰ **V82 Special screening for other conditions**
AHA: 1Q, '04, 11

V82.0 Skin conditions

V82.1 Rheumatoid arthritis

V82.2 Other rheumatic disorders

√4ᵗʰ/√5ᵗʰ Additional Digit Required   Unspecified Code   Other Specified Code   Manifestation Code   ▶◀ Revised Text   ● New Code   ▲ Revised Code Title
2011 ICD-9-CM   **October 2010 • Volume 1 – 341**

V76.11–V82.2

V Codes

V82.3–V86.1

V82.3 Congenital dislocation of hip

V82.4 Maternal postnatal screening for chromosomal anomalies ♀

> EXCLUDES *antenatal screening by amniocentesis (V28.0)*

V82.5 Chemical poisoning and other contamination

> Screening for:
> heavy metal poisoning
> ingestion of radioactive substance
> poisoning from contaminated water supply
> radiation exposure

V82.6 Multiphasic screening

✓5th **V82.7 Genetic screening**

> EXCLUDES *genetic testing for procreative management (V26.31-V26.39)*

V82.71 Screening for genetic disease carrier status
> AHA: 4Q, '06, 118

V82.79 Other genetic screening
> AHA: 4Q, '06, 118

✓5th **V82.8 Other specified conditions**
> AHA: 4Q, '00, 53

V82.81 Osteoporosis
> Use additional code to identify:
> hormone replacement therapy (postmenopausal) status (V07.4)
> postmenopausal (age-related) (natural) status (V49.81)
> AHA: 4Q, '00, 54

V82.89 Other specified conditions

V82.9 Unspecified condition

Genetics (V83-V84)

✓4th **V83 Genetic carrier status**
> AHA: 4Q, '02, 79; 4Q, '01, 54
> TIP: The patient does not have the disease or carry a risk of developing it, but may genetically pass it to offspring who then may develop it.

✓5th **V83.0 Hemophilia A carrier**

V83.01 Asymptomatic hemophilia A carrier

V83.02 Symptomatic hemophilia A carrier

✓5th **V83.8 Other genetic carrier status**

V83.81 Cystic fibrosis gene carrier

V83.89 Other genetic carrier status

✓4th **V84 Genetic susceptibility to disease**
> INCLUDES confirmed abnormal gene
> Use additional code, if applicable, for any associated family history of the disease (V16-V19)
> AHA: 4Q, '04, 106
> TIP: The patient has a gene that increases the risk of developing a specific disease; assign only as a secondary condition.

✓5th **V84.0 Genetic susceptibility to malignant neoplasm**
> Code first, if applicable, any current malignant neoplasms (140.0-195.8, 200.0-208.9, 230.0-234.9)
> Use additional code, if applicable, for any personal history of malignant neoplasm (V10.0-V10.9)

V84.01 Genetic susceptibility to malignant neoplasm of breast
> AHA: 4Q, '04, 107
> Z15.01 Genetic susceptibility malignant neoplasm breast   [I-10]

V84.02 Genetic susceptibility to malignant neoplasm of ovary ♀

V84.03 Genetic susceptibility to malignant neoplasm of prostate ♂

V84.04 Genetic susceptibility to malignant neoplasm of endometrium ♀

V84.09 Genetic susceptibility to other malignant neoplasm

✓5th **V84.8 Genetic susceptibility to other disease**

V84.81 Genetic susceptibility to multiple endocrine neoplasia [MEN]
> AHA: 4Q, '07, 100

V84.89 Genetic susceptibility to other disease

Body Mass Index (V85)

✓4th **V85 Body Mass Index [BMI]**
> Kilograms per meters squared
> NOTE BMI adult codes are for use for persons over 20 years old
> AHA: 4Q, '08, 191; 4Q, '05, 97
> TIP: While BMI may be coded from dietician or other caregiver documentation, the diagnosis of being overweight or obese must be coded from physician documentation.

V85.0 Body Mass Index less than 19, adult [A]

V85.1 Body Mass Index between 19-24, adult [A]

✓5th **V85.2 Body Mass Index between 25-29, adult**

V85.21 Body Mass Index 25.0-25.9, adult [A]

V85.22 Body Mass Index 26.0-26.9, adult [A]

V85.23 Body Mass Index 27.0-27.9, adult [A]

V85.24 Body Mass Index 28.0-28.9, adult [A]

V85.25 Body Mass Index 29.0-29.9, adult [A]

✓5th **V85.3 Body Mass Index between 30-39, adult**

V85.30 Body Mass Index 30.0-30.9, adult [A]

V85.31 Body Mass Index 31.0-31.9, adult [A]

V85.32 Body Mass Index 32.0-32.9, adult [A]

V85.33 Body Mass Index 33.0-33.9, adult [A]

V85.34 Body Mass Index 34.0-34.9, adult [A]

V85.35 Body Mass Index 35.0-35.9, adult [A]

V85.36 Body Mass Index 36.0-36.9, adult [A]

V85.37 Body Mass Index 37.0-37.9, adult [A]

V85.38 Body Mass Index 38.0-38.9, adult [A]

V85.39 Body Mass Index 39.0-39.9, adult [A]

✓5th **V85.4 Body Mass Index 40 and over, adult**

● **V85.41 Body Mass Index 40.0-44.9, adult** [A]

● **V85.42 Body Mass Index 45.0-49.9, adult** [A]

● **V85.43 Body Mass Index 50.0-59.9, adult** [A]

● **V85.44 Body Mass Index 60.0-69.9, adult** [A]

● **V85.45 Body Mass Index 70 and over, adult** [A]

✓5th **V85.5 Body Mass Index, pediatric**
> NOTE BMI pediatric codes are for use for persons age 2-20 years old. These percentiles are based on the growth charts published by the Centers for Disease Control and Prevention (CDC)
> AHA: 4Q, '06, 118

V85.51 Body Mass Index, pediatric, less than 5th percentile for age [P]

V85.52 Body Mass Index, pediatric, 5th percentile to less than 85th percentile for age [P]

V85.53 Body Mass Index, pediatric, 85th percentile to less than 95th percentile for age [P]

V85.54 Body Mass Index, pediatric, greater than or equal to 95th percentile for age [P]
> Z68.54 Body mass index (BMI) ≥ 95% for age   [I-10]

Estrogen Receptor Status (V86)

✓4th **V86 Estrogen receptor status**
> Code first malignant neoplasm of breast (174.0-174.9, 175.0-175.9)
> AHA: 4Q, '06, 118

V86.0 Estrogen receptor positive status [ER+]

V86.1 Estrogen receptor negative status [ER-]

Other Specified Personal Exposures and History Presenting Hazards to Health (V87)

☑4ᵗʰ V87 Other specified personal exposures and history presenting hazards to health

☑5ᵗʰ **V87.0 Contact with and (suspected) exposure to hazardous metals**
> **EXCLUDES** exposure to lead (V15.86)
> toxic effect of metals (984.0-985.9)
> AHA: 4Q, '08, 158

V87.01 Arsenic

V87.09 Other hazardous metals
Chromium compounds
Nickel dust

☑5ᵗʰ **V87.1 Contact with and (suspected) exposure to hazardous aromatic compounds**
> **EXCLUDES** toxic effects of aromatic compounds (982.0, 983.0)
> AHA: 4Q, '08, 158

V87.11 Aromatic amines

V87.12 Benzene

V87.19 Other hazardous aromatic compounds
Aromatic dyes NOS
Polycyclic aromatic hydrocarbons

V87.2 Contact with and (suspected) exposure to other potentially hazardous chemicals
Dyes NOS
> **EXCLUDES** exposure to asbestos (V15.84)
> toxic effect of chemicals (980-989)
> AHA: 4Q, '08, 158

☑5ᵗʰ **V87.3 Contact with and (suspected) exposure to other potentially hazardous substances**
> **EXCLUDES** contact with and (suspected) exposure to potentially hazardous body fluids (V15.85)
> ▶personal history of retained foreign body fully removed (V15.53)◀
> toxic effect of substances (980-989)

V87.31 Exposure to mold

V87.32 Contact with and (suspected) exposure to algae bloom
> AHA: 4Q, '09, 116

V87.39 Contact with and (suspected) exposure to other potentially hazardous substances

☑5ᵗʰ **V87.4 Personal history of drug therapy**
> **EXCLUDES** long-term (current) drug use (V58.61-V58.69)
> AHA: 4Q, '09, 116; 4Q, '08, 159

V87.41 Personal history of antineoplastic chemotherapy
Z92.6 Personal hx chemotherapy for neoplastic disease   I-10

V87.42 Personal history of monoclonal drug therapy

V87.43 Personal history of estrogen therapy

V87.44 Personal history of inhaled steroid therapy

V87.45 Personal history of systemic steroid therapy
Personal history of steroid therapy NOS

V87.46 Personal history of immunosuppression therapy
> **EXCLUDES** personal history of steroid therapy (V87.44, V87.45)

V87.49 Personal history of other drug therapy

Acquired Absence of Other Organs and Tissue (V88)

☑4ᵗʰ V88 Acquired absence of other organs and tissue

☑5ᵗʰ **V88.0 Acquired absence of cervix and uterus**
> AHA: 4Q, '08, 157

V88.01 Acquired absence of both cervix and uterus ♀
Acquired absence of uterus NOS
Status post total hysterectomy

V88.02 Acquired absence of uterus with remaining cervical stump ♀
Status post partial hysterectomy with remaining cervical stump

V88.03 Acquired absence of cervix with remaining uterus ♀

● ☑5ᵗʰ **V88.1 Acquired absence of pancreas**
Use additional code to identify any associated:
insulin use (V58.67)
secondary diabetes mellitus (249.00-249.91)

● **V88.11 Acquired total absence of pancreas**
Acquired absence of pancreas NOS

● **V88.12 Acquired partial absence of pancreas**

Other Suspected Conditions Not Found (V89)

☑4ᵗʰ V89 Other suspected conditions not found

☑5ᵗʰ **V89.0 Suspected maternal and fetal conditions not found**
> **EXCLUDES** known or suspected fetal anomalies affecting management of mother, not ruled out (655.00, 655.93, 656.00-656.93, 657.00-657.03, 658.00-658.93)
> newborn and perinatal conditions — code to condition
> AHA: 4Q, '08, 159
> **TIP:** These investigations are performed while the fetus is in utero; the codes should be assigned only on the mother's medical record.

V89.01 Suspected problem with amniotic cavity and membrane not found Ⓜ♀
Suspected oligohydramnios not found
Suspected polyhydramnios not found

V89.02 Suspected placental problem not found Ⓜ♀

V89.03 Suspected fetal anomaly not found Ⓜ♀

V89.04 Suspected problem with fetal growth not found Ⓜ♀

V89.05 Suspected cervical shortening not found Ⓜ♀

V89.09 Other suspected maternal and fetal condition not found Ⓜ♀

▶Retained Foreign Body (V90)◀

● **☑4ᵗʰ V90 Retained foreign body**
Embedded fragment (status)
Embedded splinter (status)
Retained foreign body status
> **EXCLUDES** artificial joint prosthesis status (V43.60-V43.69)
> foreign body accidentally left during a procedure (998.4)
> foreign body entering through orifice (930.0-939.9)
> in situ cardiac devices (V45.00-V45.09)
> organ or tissue replaced by other means (V43.0-V43.89)
> organ or tissue replaced by transplant (V42.0-V42.9)
> personal history of retained foreign body removed (V15.53)
> superficial foreign body (splinter) (categories 910-917 and 919 with 4ᵗʰ character 6 or 7, 918.0)

● ☑5ᵗʰ **V90.0 Retained radioactive fragment**

● **V90.01 Retained depleted uranium fragments**

● **V90.09 Other retained radioactive fragments**
Other retained depleted isotope fragments
Retained nontherapeutic radioactive fragments

● ☑5ᵗʰ **V90.1 Retained metal fragments**
> **EXCLUDES** retained radioactive metal fragments (V90.01-V90.09)

● **V90.10 Retained metal fragments, unspecified**
Retained metal fragment NOS

● **V90.11 Retained magnetic metal fragments**

● **V90.12 Retained nonmagnetic metal fragments**

● ☑5ᵗʰ **V90.2 Retained plastic fragments**
Acrylics fragments
Diethylhexylphthalates fragments
Isocyanate fragments

● ☑5ᵗʰ **V90.3 Retained organic fragments**

● **V90.31 Retained animal quills or spines**

● **V90.32 Retained tooth**

● **V90.33 Retained wood fragments**

● **V90.39 Other retained organic fragments**

☑4ᵗʰ ☑5ᵗʰ Additional Digit Required   Unspecified Code   Other Specified Code   Manifestation Code   ▶◀ Revised Text   ● New Code   ▲ Revised Code Title

2011 ICD-9-CM   **October 2010 · Volume 1 – 343**

V87–V90.39

- ☑5ᵗʰ **V90.8 Other specified retained foreign body**
- **V90.81 Retained glass fragments**
- **V90.83 Retained stone or crystalline fragments**
  Retained concrete or cement fragments
- **V90.89 Other specified retained foreign body**
- ☑5ᵗʰ **V90.9 Retained foreign body, unspecified material**

►Multiple Gestation Placenta Status (V91)◄

- ☑4ᵗʰ **V91 Multiple gestation placenta status**
  Code first multiple gestation (651.0-651.9)

- ☑5ᵗʰ **V91.0 Twin gestation placenta status**
- **V91.00 Twin gestation, unspecified number of placenta, unspecified number of amniotic sacs**
- **V91.01 Twin gestation, monochorionic/monoamniotic (one placenta, one amniotic sac)**
- **V91.02 Twin gestation, monochorionic/diamniotic (one placenta, two amniotic sacs)**
- **V91.03 Twin gestation, dichorionic/diamniotic (two placentae, two amniotic sacs)**
- **V91.09 Twin gestation, unable to determine number of placenta and number of amniotic sacs**

- ☑5ᵗʰ **V91.1 Triplet gestation placenta status**
- **V91.10 Triplet gestation, unspecified number of placenta and unspecified number of amniotic sacs**
- **V91.11 Triplet gestation, with two or more monochorionic fetuses**
- **V91.12 Triplet gestation, with two or more monoamniotic fetuses**

- **V91.19 Triplet gestation, unable to determine number of placenta and number of amniotic sacs**

- ☑5ᵗʰ **V91.2 Quadruplet gestation placenta status**
- **V91.20 Quadruplet gestation, unspecified number of placenta and unspecified number of amniotic sacs**
- **V91.21 Quadruplet gestation, with two or more monochorionic fetuses**
- **V91.22 Quadruplet gestation, with two or more monoamniotic fetuses**
- **V91.29 Quadruplet gestation, unable to determine number of placenta and number of amniotic sacs**

- ☑5ᵗʰ **V91.9 Other specified multiple gestation placenta status**
  Placenta status for multiple gestations greater than quadruplets
- **V91.90 Other specified multiple gestation, unspecified number of placenta and unspecified number of amniotic sacs**
- **V91.91 Other specified multiple gestation, with two or more monochorionic fetuses**
- **V91.92 Other specified multiple gestation, with two or more monoamniotic fetuses**
- **V91.99 Other specified multiple gestation, unable to determine number of placenta and number of amniotic sacs**

N Newborn Age: 0   **P** Pediatric Age: 0-17   **M** Maternity Age: 12-55   **A** Adult Age: 15-124   **PDx** Primary Diagnosis

Supplementary Classification of External Causes of Injury and Poisoning (E000-E999)

This section is provided to permit the classification of environmental events, circumstances, and conditions as the cause of injury, poisoning, and other adverse effects. Where a code from this section is applicable, it is intended that it shall be used in addition to a code from one of the main chapters of ICD-9-CM, indicating the nature of the condition. Certain other conditions which may be stated to be due to external causes are classified in Chapters 1 to 16 of ICD-9-CM. For these, the "E" code classification should be used as an additional code for more detailed analysis.

Machinery accidents [other than those connected with transport] are classifiable to category E919, in which the fourth digit allows a broad classification of the type of machinery involved.

Categories for "late effects" of accidents and other external causes are to be found at E929, E959, E969, E977, E989, and E999.

External Cause Status (E000)

NOTE A code from category E000 may be used in conjunction with the external cause code(s) assigned to a record to indicate the status of the person at the time the event occurred. A single code from category E000 should be assigned for an encounter.

√4ᵗʰ **E000** **External cause status**

E000.0 **Civilian activity done for income or pay**
Civilian activity done for financial or other compensation
EXCLUDES *military activity (E000.1)*

E000.2 **Volunteer activity**
EXCLUDES *activity of child or other family member assisting in compensated work of other family member (E000.8)*

E000.1 **Military activity**
EXCLUDES *activity of off-duty military personnel (E000.8)*

E000.8 **Other external cause status**
►Activity of child or other family member assisting in compensated work of other family member◄
Activity NEC
Hobby not done for income
Leisure activity
Off-duty activity of military personnel
Recreation or sport not for income or while a student
Student activity
EXCLUDES *civilian activity done for income or compensation (E000.0)*
military activity (E000.1)

E000.9 **Unspecified external cause status**

Activity (E001-E030)

NOTE Categories E001 to E030 are provided for use to indicate the activity of the person seeking healthcare for an injury or health condition, such as a heart attack while shoveling snow, which resulted from, or was contributed to, by the activity. These codes are appropriate for use for both acute injuries, such as those from chapter 17, and conditions that are due to the long-term, cumulative affects of an activity, such as those from chapter 13. They are also appropriate for use with external cause codes for cause and intent if identifying the activity provides additional information on the event.

These codes should be used in conjunction with other external cause codes for external cause status (E000) and place of occurrence (E849).

This section contains the following broad activity categories:

E001   Activities involving walking and running
E002   Activities involving water and water craft
E003   Activities involving ice and snow
E004   Activities involving climbing, rappelling, and jumping off
E005   Activities involving dancing and other rhythmic movement
E006   Activities involving other sports and athletics played individually
E007   Activities involving other sports and athletics played as a team or group
E008   Activities involving other specified sports and athletics
E009   Activity involving other cardiorespiratory exercise
E010   Activity involving other muscle strengthening exercises
E011   Activities involving computer technology and electronic devices
E012   Activities involving arts and handcrafts
E013   Activities involving personal hygiene and household maintenance
E014   Activities involving person providing caregiving
E015   Activities involving food preparation, cooking and grilling
E016   Activities involving property and land maintenance, building and construction
E017   Activities involving roller coasters and other types of external motion
E018   Activities involving playing musical instrument
E019   Activities involving animal care
E029   Other activity
E030   Unspecified activity

√4ᵗʰ **E001** **Activities involving walking and running**
EXCLUDES *walking an animal (E019.0)*
walking or running on a treadmill (E009.0)

E001.0 **Walking, marching and hiking**
Walking, marching and hiking on level or elevated terrain
EXCLUDES *mountain climbing (E004.0)*

E001.1 **Running**

√4ᵗʰ **E002** **Activities involving water and water craft**
EXCLUDES *activities involving ice (E003.0-E003.9)*
boating and other watercraft transport accidents (E830-E838)

E002.0 **Swimming**

E002.1 **Springboard and platform diving**

E002.2 **Water polo**

E002.3 **Water aerobics and water exercise**

E002.4 **Underwater diving and snorkeling**
SCUBA diving

E002.5 **Rowing, canoeing, kayaking, rafting and tubing**
Canoeing, kayaking, rafting and tubing in calm and turbulent water

E002.6 **Water skiing and wake boarding**

E002.7 **Surfing, windsurfing and boogie boarding**

E002.8 **Water sliding**

E002.9 **Other activity involving water and watercraft**
Activity involving water NOS
Parasailing
Water survival training and testing

√4ᵗʰ **E003** **Activities involving ice and snow**
EXCLUDES *shoveling ice and snow (E016.0)*

E003.0 **Ice skating**
Figure skating (singles) (pairs)
Ice dancing
EXCLUDES *ice hockey (E003.1)*

E003.1 **Ice hockey**

E003.2 **Snow (alpine) (downhill) skiing, snow boarding, sledding, tobogganing and snow tubing**
EXCLUDES *cross country skiing (E003.3)*

E003.3 **Cross country skiing**
Nordic skiing

E003.9 **Other activity involving ice and snow**
Activity involving ice and snow NOS

√4ᵗʰ **E004** **Activities involving climbing, rappelling, and jumping off**
EXCLUDES *hiking on level or elevated terrain (E001.0)*
jumping rope (E006.5)
sky diving (E840-E844)
trampoline jumping (E005.3)

E004.0 **Mountain climbing, rock climbing and wall climbing**

E004.1 **Rappelling**

E004.2 **BASE jumping**
Building, Antenna, Span, Earth jumping

E004.3 **Bungee jumping**

E004.4 **Hang gliding**

E004.9 **Other activity involving climbing, rappelling and jumping off**

√4ᵗʰ **E005 Activities involving dancing and other rhythmic movement**
> *EXCLUDES martial arts (E008.4)*

E005.0 Dancing

E005.1 Yoga

E005.2 Gymnastics
Rhythmic gymnastics
> *EXCLUDES trampoline (E005.3)*

E005.3 Trampoline

E005.4 Cheerleading

E005.9 Other activity involving dancing and other rhythmic movements

√4ᵗʰ **E006 Activities involving other sports and athletics played individually**
> *EXCLUDES dancing (E005.0)*
> *gymnastic (E005.2)*
> *trampoline (E005.3)*
> *yoga (E005.1)*

E006.0 Roller skating (inline) and skateboarding

E006.1 Horseback riding

E006.2 Golf

E006.3 Bowling

E006.4 Bike riding
> *EXCLUDES transport accident involving bike riding (E800-E829)*

E006.5 Jumping rope

E006.6 Non-running track and field events
> *EXCLUDES running (any form) (E001.1)*

E006.9 Other activity involving other sports and athletics played individually
> *EXCLUDES activities involving climbing, rappelling, and jumping (E004.0-E004.9)*
> *activities involving ice and snow (E003.0-E003.9)*
> *activities involving walking and running (E001.0-E001.9)*
> *activities involving water and watercraft (E002.0-E002.9)*

√4ᵗʰ **E007 Activities involving other sports and athletics played as a team or group**
> *EXCLUDES ice hockey (E003.1)*
> *water polo (E002.2)*

E007.0 American tackle football
Football NOS

E007.1 American flag or touch football

E007.2 Rugby

E007.3 Baseball
Softball

E007.4 Lacrosse and field hockey

E007.5 Soccer

E007.6 Basketball

E007.7 Volleyball (beach) (court)

E007.8 Physical games generally associated with school recess, summer camp and children
Capture the flag
Dodge ball
Four square
Kickball

E007.9 Other activity involving other sports and athletics played as a team or group
Cricket

√4ᵗʰ **E008 Activities involving other specified sports and athletics**

E008.0 Boxing

E008.1 Wrestling

E008.2 Racquet and hand sports
Handball
Racquetball
Squash
Tennis

E008.3 Frisbee
Ultimate frisbee

E008.4 Martial arts
Combatives

E008.9 Other specified sports and athletics activity
> *EXCLUDES sports and athletics activities specified in categories E001-E007*

√4ᵗʰ **E009 Activity involving other cardiorespiratory exercise**
Activity involving physical training

E009.0 Exercise machines primarily for cardiorespiratory conditioning
Elliptical and stepper machines
Stationary bike
Treadmill

E009.1 Calisthenics
Jumping jacks
Warm up and cool down

E009.2 Aerobic and step exercise

E009.3 Circuit training

E009.4 Obstacle course
Challenge course
Confidence course

E009.5 Grass drills
Guerilla drills

E009.9 Other activity involving cardiorespiratory exercise
> *EXCLUDES activities involving cardiorespiratory exercise specified in categories E001-E008*

√4ᵗʰ **E010 Activity involving other muscle strengthening exercises**

E010.0 Exercise machines primarily for muscle strengthening

E010.1 Push-ups, pull-ups, sit-ups

E010.2 Free weights
Barbells
Dumbbells

E010.3 Pilates

E010.9 Other activity involving other muscle strengthening exercises
> *EXCLUDES activities involving muscle strengthening specified in categories E001-E009*

√4ᵗʰ **E011 Activities involving computer technology and electronic devices**
> *EXCLUDES electronic musical keyboard or instruments (E018.0)*

E011.0 Computer keyboarding
Electronic game playing using keyboard or other stationary device

E011.1 Hand held interactive electronic device
Cellular telephone and communication device
Electronic game playing using interactive device
> *EXCLUDES electronic game playing using keyboard or other stationary device (E011.0)*

E011.9 Other activity involving computer technology and electronic devices

√4ᵗʰ **E012 Activities involving arts and handcrafts**
> *EXCLUDES activities involving playing musical instrument (E018.0-E018.3)*

E012.0 Knitting and crocheting

E012.1 Sewing

E012.2 Furniture building and finishing
Furniture repair

E012.9 Activity involving other arts and handcrafts

√4ᵗʰ Fourth-digit Required   ▶◀ Revised Text   ● New Code   ▲ Revised Code TitleDx

✅4ᵗʰ **E013 Activities involving personal hygiene and household maintenance**

> **EXCLUDES** *activities involving cooking and grilling (E015.0-E015.9)*
> *activities involving property and land maintenance, building and construction (E016.0-E016.9)*
> *activity involving persons providing caregiving (E014.0-E014.9)*
> *dishwashing (E015.0)*
> *food preparation (E015.0)*
> *gardening (E016.1)*

E013.0 Personal bathing and showering

E013.1 Laundry

E013.2 Vacuuming

E013.3 Ironing

E013.4 Floor mopping and cleaning

E013.5 Residential relocation
> Packing up and unpacking involved in moving to a new residence

E013.8 Other personal hygiene activity

E013.9 Other household maintenance

✅4ᵗʰ **E014 Activities involving person providing caregiving**

E014.0 Caregiving involving bathing

E014.1 Caregiving involving lifting

E014.9 Other activity involving person providing caregiving

✅4ᵗʰ **E015 Activities involving food preparation, cooking and grilling**

E015.0 Food preparation and clean up
> Dishwasing

E015.1 Grilling and smoking food

E015.2 Cooking and baking
> Use of stove, oven and microwave oven

E015.9 Other activity involving cooking and grilling

✅4ᵗʰ **E016 Activities involving property and land maintenance, building and construction**

E016.0 Digging, shoveling and raking
> Dirt digging
> Raking leaves
> Snow shoveling

E016.1 Gardening and landscaping
> Pruning, trimming shrubs, weeding

E016.2 Building and construction

E016.9 Other activity involving property and land maintenance, building and construction

✅4ᵗʰ **E017 Activities involving roller coasters and other types of external motion**

E017.0 Roller coaster riding

E017.9 Other activity involving external motion

✅4ᵗʰ **E018 Activities involving playing musical instrument**
> Activity involving playing electric musical instrument

E018.0 Piano playing
> Musical keyboard (electronic) playing

E018.1 Drum and other percussion instrument playing

E018.2 String instrument playing

E018.3 Wind and brass instrument playing

✅4ᵗʰ **E019 Activities involving animal care**
> **EXCLUDES** *horseback riding (E006.1)*

E019.0 Walking an animal

E019.1 Milking an animal

E019.2 Grooming and shearing an animal

E019.9 Other activity involving animal care

✅4ᵗʰ **E029 Other activity**

E029.0 Refereeing a sports activity

E029.1 Spectator at an event

E029.2 Rough housing and horseplay

E029.9 Other activity

E030 Unspecified activity

Transport Accidents (E800-E848)

Definitions and Examples Related to Transport Accidents

(a) A **transport accident** (E800-E848) is any accident involving a device designed primarily for, or being used at the time primarily for, conveying persons or goods from one place to another.

> **INCLUDES** accidents involving:
> aircraft and spacecraft (E840-E845)
> watercraft (E830-E838)
> motor vehicle (E810-E825)
> railway (E800-E807)
> other road vehicles (E826-E829)

In classifying accidents which involve more than one kind of transport, the above order of precedence of transport accidents should be used.

Accidents involving agricultural and construction machines, such as tractors, cranes, and bulldozers, are regarded as transport accidents only when these vehicles are under their own power on a highway [otherwise the vehicles are regarded as machinery]. Vehicles which can travel on land or water, such as hovercraft and other amphibious vehicles, are regarded as watercraft when on the water, as motor vehicles when on the highway, and as off-road motor vehicles when on land, but off the highway.

> **EXCLUDES** *accidents:*
> *in sports which involve the use of transport but where the transport vehicle itself was not involved in the accident*
> *involving vehicles which are part of industrial equipment used entirely on industrial premises*
> *occurring during transportation but unrelated to the hazards associated with the means of transportation [e.g., injuries received in a fight on board ship; transport vehicle involved in a cataclysm such as an earthquake]*
> *to persons engaged in the maintenance or repair of transport equipment or vehicle not in motion, unlesss injured by another vehicle in motion*

(b) A **railway accident** is a transport accident involving a railway train or other railway vehicle operated on rails, whether in motion or not.

> **EXCLUDES** *accidents:*
> *in repair shops*
> *in roundhouse or on turntable*
> *on railway premises but not involving a train or other railway vehicle*

(c) A **railway train** or **railway vehicle** is any device with or without cars coupled to it, desiged for traffic on a railway.

> **INCLUDES** interurban:
> electric car ⎫ (operated chiefly on its own
> street car ⎬ right-of-way, not open to
> ⎭ other traffic)
> railway train, any power [diesel] [electric] [steam]:
> funicular
> monorail or two-rail
> subterranean or elevated
> other vehicle designed to run on a railway track
>
> **EXCLUDES** *interurban electric cars [streetcars] specified to be operating on a right-of-way that forms part of the public street or highway [definition (h)]*

(d) A **railway** or **railroad** is a right-of-way designed for traffic on rails, which is used by carriages or wagons transporting passengers or freight, and by other rolling stock, and which is not open to other public vehicular traffic.

(e) A **motor vehicle accident** is a transport accident involving a motor vehicle. It is defined as a motor vehicle traffic accident or as a motor vehicle nontraffic accident according to whether the accident occurs on a public highway or elsewhere.

> **EXCLUDES** *injury or damage due to cataclysm*
> *injury or damage while a motor vehicle, not under its own power, is being loaded on, or unloaded from, another conveyance*

(f) A **motor vehicle traffic accident** is any motor vehicle accident occurring on a public highway [i.e., originating, terminating, or involving a vehicle partially on the highway]. A motor vehicle accident is assumed to have occurred on the highway unless another place is specified, except in the case of accidents involving only off-road motor vehicles which are classified as nontraffic accidents unless the contrary is stated.

✅4ᵗʰ Fourth-digit Required   ▶◀ Revised Text   ● New Code   ▲ Revised Code TitleDx

(g) A **motor vehicle nontraffic accident** is any motor vehicle accident which occurs entirely in any place other than a public highway.

(h) A **public highway [trafficway]** or **street** is the entire width between property lines [or other boundary lines] of every way or place, of which any part is open to the use of the public for purposes of vehicular traffic as a matter of right or custom. A **roadway** is that part of the public highway designed, improved, and ordinarily used, for vehicular travel.

> INCLUDES approaches (public) to:
>> docks
>> public building
>> station
>
> EXCLUDES driveway (private)
>> parking lot
>> ramp
>> roads in:
>>> airfield
>>> farm
>>> industrial premises
>>> mine
>>> private grounds
>>> quarry

(i) A **motor vehicle** is any mechanically or electrically powered device, not operated on rails, upon which any person or property may be transported or drawn upon a highway. Any object such as a trailer, coaster, sled, or wagon being towed by a motor vehicle is considered a part of the motor vehicle.

> INCLUDES automobile [any type]
>> bus
>> construction machinery, farm and industrial machinery, steam roller, tractor, army tank, highway grader, or similar vehicle on wheels or treads, while in transport under own power
>> fire engine (motorized)
>> motorcycle
>> motorized bicycle [moped] or scooter
>> trolley bus not operating on rails
>> truck
>> van
>
> EXCLUDES devices used solely to move persons or materials within the confines of a building and its premises, such as:
>> building elevator
>> coal car in mine
>> electric baggage or mail truck used solely within a railroad station
>> electric truck used solely within an industrial plant
>> moving overhead crane

(j) A **motorcycle** is a two-wheeled motor vehicle having one or two riding saddles and sometimes having a third wheel for the support of a sidecar. The sidecar is considered part of the motorcycle.

> INCLUDES motorized:
>> bicycle [moped]
>> scooter
>> tricycle

(k) An **off-road motor vehicle** is a motor vehicle of special design, to enable it to negotiate rough or soft terrain or snow. Examples of special design are high construction, special wheels and tires, driven by treads, or support on a cushion of air.

> INCLUDES all terrain vehicle [ATV]
>> army tank
>> hovercraft, on land or swamp
>> snowmobile

(l) A **driver** of a motor vehicle is the occupant of the motor vehicle operating it or intending to operate it. A **motorcyclist** is the driver of a motorcycle. Other authorized occupants of a motor vehicle are **passengers**.

(m) An **other road vehicle** is any device, except a motor vehicle, in, on, or by which any person or property may be transported on a highway.

> INCLUDES animal carrying a person or goods
>> animal-drawn vehicles
>> animal harnessed to conveyance
>> bicycle [pedal cycle]
>> streetcar
>> tricycle (pedal)
>
> EXCLUDES pedestrian conveyance [definition (q)]

(n) A **streetcar** is a device designed and used primarily for transporting persons within a municipality, running on rails, usually subject to normal traffic control signals, and operated principally on a right-of-way that forms part of the traffic way. A trailer being towed by a streetcar is considered a part of the streetcar.

> INCLUDES interurban or intraurban electric or streetcar, when specified to be operating on a street or public highway
>> tram (car)
>> trolley (car)

(o) A **pedal cycle** is any road transport vehicle operated solely by pedals.

> INCLUDES bicycle
>> pedal cycle
>> tricycle
>
> EXCLUDES motorized bicycle [definition (j)]

(p) A **pedal cyclist** is any person riding on a pedal cycle or in a sidecar attached to such a vehicle.

(q) A **pedestrian conveyance** is any human powered device by which a pedestrian may move other than by walking or by which a walking person may move another pedestrian.

> INCLUDES baby carriage
>> coaster wagon
>> heelies, wheelies
>> ice skates
>> ►motorized mobility scooter◄
>> perambulator
>> pushcart
>> pushchair
>> roller skates
>> scooter
>> skateboard
>> skis
>> sled
>> wheelchair ►(electric)◄

(r) A **pedestrian** is any person involved in an accident who was not at the time of the accident riding in or on a motor vehicle, railroad train, streetcar, animal-drawn or other vehicle, or on a bicycle or animal.

> INCLUDES person:
>> changing tire of vehicle
>> in or operating a pedestrian conveyance
>> making adjustment to motor of vehicle
>> on foot

(s) A **watercraft** is any device for transporting passengers or goods on the water.

(t) A **small boat** is any watercraft propelled by paddle, oars, or small motor, with a passenger capacity of less than ten.

> INCLUDES boat NOS
>> canoe
>> coble
>> dinghy
>> punt
>> raft
>> rowboat
>> rowing shell
>> scull
>> skiff
>> small motorboat
>
> EXCLUDES barge
>> lifeboat (used after abandoning ship)
>> raft (anchored) being used as a diving platform
>> yacht

(u) An **aircraft** is any device for transporting passengers or goods in the air.

> INCLUDES airplane [any type]
>> balloon
>> bomber
>> dirigible
>> glider (hang)
>> military aircraft
>> parachute

(v) A **commercial transport aircraft** is any device for collective passenger or freight transportation by air, whether run on commercial lines for profit or by government authorities, with the exception of military craft.

✔4ᵗʰ Fourth-digit Required   ►◄ Revised Text   ● New Code   ▲ Revised Code TitleDx

Railway Accidents (E800-E807)

NOTE For definitions of railway accident and related terms see definitions (a) to (d).

EXCLUDES accidents involving railway train and:
aircraft (E840.0-E845.9)
motor vehicle (E810.0-E825.9)
watercraft (E830.0-E838.9)

The following fourth-digit subdivisions are for use with categories E800-E807 to identify the injured person:

.0 Railway employee
Any person who by virtue of his employment in connection with a railway, whether by the railway company or not, is at increased risk of involvement in a railway accident, such as:
catering staff of train
driver
guard
porter
postal staff on train
railway fireman
shunter
sleeping car attendant

.1 Passenger on railway
Any authorized person traveling on a train, except a railway employee.
EXCLUDES *intending passenger waiting at station (.8)*
unauthorized rider on railway vehicle (.8)

.2 Pedestrian
See definition (r)

.3 Pedal cyclist
See definition (p)

.8 Other specified person
Intending passenger or bystander waiting at station
Unauthorized rider on railway vehicle

.9 Unspecified person

§ ✓4ᵗʰ **E800 Railway accident involving collision with rolling stock**
INCLUDES collision between railway trains or railway vehicles, any kind
collision NOS on railway
derailment with antecedent collision with rolling stock or NOS

§ ✓4ᵗʰ **E801 Railway accident involving collision with other object**
INCLUDES collision of railway train with:
buffers
fallen tree on railway
gates
platform
rock on railway
streetcar
other nonmotor vehicle
other object
EXCLUDES *collision with:*
aircraft (E840.0-E842.9)
motor vehicle (E810.0-E810.9, E820.0-E822.9)

§ ✓4ᵗʰ **E802 Railway accident involving derailment without antecedent collision**

§ ✓4ᵗʰ **E803 Railway accident involving explosion, fire, or burning**
EXCLUDES *explosion or fire, with antecedent derailment (E802.0-E802.9)*
explosion or fire, with mention of antecedent collision (E800.0-E801.9)

§ ✓4ᵗʰ **E804 Fall in, on, or from railway train**
INCLUDES fall while alighting from or boarding railway train
EXCLUDES *fall related to collision, derailment, or explosion of railway train (E800.0-E803.9)*

§ ✓4ᵗʰ **E805 Hit by rolling stock**
INCLUDES crushed
injured
killed } by railway train or part
knocked down
run over
EXCLUDES *pedestrian hit by object set in motion by railway train (E806.0-E806.9)*

§ ✓4ᵗʰ **E806 Other specified railway accident**
INCLUDES hit by object falling in railway train
injured by door or window on railway train
nonmotor road vehicle or pedestrian hit by object set in motion by railway train
railway train hit by falling:
earth NOS
rock
tree
other object
EXCLUDES *railway accident due to cataclysm (E908-E909)*

§ ✓4ᵗʰ **E807 Railway accident of unspecified nature**
INCLUDES found dead
injured } on railway right-of-way NOS
railway accident NOS

Motor Vehicle Traffic Accidents (E810-E819)

NOTE For definitions of motor vehicle traffic accident, and related terms, see definitions (e) to (k).

EXCLUDES accidents involving motor vehicle and aircraft *(E840.0-E845.9)*

The following fourth-digit subdivisions are for use with categories E810-E819 to identify the injured person:

.0 Driver of motor vehicle other than motorcycle
See definition (l)

.1 Passenger in motor vehicle other than motorcycle
See definition (l)

.2 Motorcyclist
See definition (l)

.3 Passenger on motorcycle
See definition (l)

.4 Occupant of streetcar

.5 Rider of animal; occupant of animal-drawn vehicle

.6 Pedal cyclist
See definition (p)

.7 Pedestrian
See definition (r)

.8 Other specified person
Occupant of vehicle other than above
Person in railway train involved in accident
Unauthorized rider of motor vehicle

.9 Unspecified person

§ ✓4ᵗʰ **E810 Motor vehicle traffic accident involving collision with train**
EXCLUDES *motor vehicle collision with object set in motion by railway train (E815.0-E815.9)*
railway train hit by object set in motion by motor vehicle (E818.0-E818.9)

§ ✓4ᵗʰ **E811 Motor vehicle traffic accident involving re-entrant collision with another motor vehicle**
INCLUDES collision between motor vehicle which accidentally leaves the roadway then re-enters the same roadway, or the opposite roadway on a divided highway, and another motor vehicle
EXCLUDES *collision on the same roadway when none of the motor vehicles involved have left and re-entered the highway (E812.0-E812.9)*

§ ✓4ᵗʰ **E812 Other motor vehicle traffic accident involving collision with motor vehicle**
INCLUDES collision with another motor vehicle parked, stopped, stalled, disabled, or abandoned on the highway
motor vehicle collision NOS
EXCLUDES *collision with object set in motion by another motor vehicle (E815.0-E815.9)*
re-entrant collision with another motor vehicle (E811.0-E811.9)

---

§ Requires fourth-digit. See beginning of appropriate section for codes and definitions.

§ ✓4ᵗʰ **E813 Motor vehicle traffic accident involving collision with other vehicle**

    INCLUDES   collision between motor vehicle, any kind, and:
        other road (nonmotor transport) vehicle, such as:
           animal carrying a person
           animal-drawn vehicle
           pedal cycle
           streetcar

    EXCLUDES   collision with:
        object set in motion by nonmotor road vehicle (E815.0-E815.9)
        pedestrian (E814.0-E814.9)
      nonmotor road vehicle hit by object set in motion by motor vehicle (E818.0-E818.9)

§ ✓4ᵗʰ **E814 Motor vehicle traffic accident involving collision with pedestrian**

    INCLUDES   collision between motor vehicle, any kind, and pedestrian
      pedestrian dragged, hit, or run over by motor vehicle, any kind

    EXCLUDES   *pedestrian hit by object set in motion by motor vehicle (E818.0-E818.9)*

§ ✓4ᵗʰ **E815 Other motor vehicle traffic accident involving collision on the highway**

    INCLUDES   collision (due to loss of control) (on highway) between motor vehicle, any kind, and:
      abutment (bridge) (overpass)
      animal (herded) (unattended)
      fallen stone, traffic sign, tree, utility pole
      guard rail or boundary fence
      interhighway divider
      landslide (not moving)
      object set in motion by railway train or road vehicle (motor) (nonmotor)
      object thrown in front of motor vehicle
      other object, fixed, movable, or moving
      safety island
      temporary traffic sign or marker
      wall of cut made for road

    EXCLUDES   collision with:
        any object off the highway (resulting from loss of control) (E816.0-E816.9)
        any object which normally would have been off the highway and is not stated to have been on it (E816.0-E816.9)
        motor vehicle parked, stopped, stalled, disabled, or abandoned on highway (E812.0-E812.9)
        moving landslide (E909)
      motor vehicle hit by object:
        set in motion by railway train or road vehicle (motor) (nonmotor) (E818.0-E818.9)
        thrown into or on vehicle (E818.0-E818.9)

§ ✓4ᵗʰ **E816 Motor vehicle traffic accident due to loss of control, without collision on the highway**

    INCLUDES   motor vehicle:
      failing to make curve
      going out of control (due to):   and:
        blowout   coliding with object off the highway
        burst tire   overturning
        driver falling asleep   stopping abruptly off the highway
        drive inattention
        excessive speed
        failure of mechanical part

    EXCLUDES   *collision on highway following loss of control (E810.0-E815.9)*
      loss of control of motor vehicle following collision on the highway (E810.0-E815.9)

§ ✓4ᵗʰ **E817 Noncollision motor vehicle traffic accident while boarding or alighting**

    INCLUDES   fall down stairs of motor bus
      fall from car in street   } while boarding or alighting
      injured by moving part of the vehicle
      trapped by door of motor bus

§ ✓4ᵗʰ **E818 Other noncollision motor vehicle traffic accident**

    INCLUDES   accidental poisoning from exhaust gas generated by
      breakage of any part of
      explosion of any part of
      fall, jump, or being accidentally pushed from   } motor vehicle while in motion
      fire starting in
      hit by object thrown into or on
      injured by being thrown against some part of, or object in
      injury from moving part of
      object falling in or on
      object thrown on
      collision of railway train or road vehicle except motor vehicle, with object set in motion by motor vehicle
      motor vehicle hit by object set in motion by railway train or road vehicle (motor) (nonmotor)
      pedestrian, railway train, or road vehicle (motor) (nonmotor) hit by object set in motion by motor vehicle

    EXCLUDES   collision between motor vehicle and:
        object set in motion by railway train or road vehicle (motor) (nonmotor) (E815.0-E815.9)
        object thrown towards the motor vehicle (E815.0-E815.9)
      person overcome by carbon monoxide generated by stationary motor vehicle off the roadway with motor running (E868.2)

§ ✓4ᵗʰ **E819 Motor vehicle traffic accident of unspecified nature**

    INCLUDES   motor vehicle traffic accident NOS
      traffic accident NOS

Motor Vehicle Nontraffic Accidents (E820-E825)

    NOTE   For definitions of motor vehicle nontraffic accident and related terms see definition (a) to (k).

    INCLUDES   accidents involving motor vehicles being used in recreational or sporting activities off the highway
      collision and noncollision motor vehicle accidents occurring entirely off the highway

    EXCLUDES   accidents involving motor vehicle and:
        aircraft (E840.0-E845.9)
        watercraft (E830.0-E838.9)
      accidents, not on the public highway, involving agricultural and construction machinery but not involving another motor vehicle (E919.0, E919.2, E919.7)

The following fourth-digit subdivisions are for use with categories E820-E825 to identify the injured person:

.0 Driver of motor vehicle other than motorcycle
    See definition (l)
.1 Passenger in motor vehicle other than motorcycle
    See definition (l)
.2 Motorcyclist
    See definition (l)
.3 Passenger on motorcycle
    See definition (l)
.4 Occupant of streetcar
.5 Rider of animal; occupant of animal-drawn vehicle
.6 Pedal cyclist
    See definition (p)
.7 Pedestrian
    See definition (r)
.8 Other specified person
    Occupant of vehicle other than above
    Person in railway train involved in accident
    Unauthorized rider of motor vehicle
.9 Unspecified person

---

§   Requires fourth-digit. See beginning of appropriate section for codes and definitions.

✓4ᵗʰ Fourth-digit Required   ▶◀ Revised Text   ● New Code   ▲ Revised Code TitleDx

§ ✓4ᵗʰ **E820 Nontraffic accident involving motor-driven snow vehicle**

     INCLUDES breakage of part of
     fall from
     hit by   } motor-driven snow
     overturning of   vehicle (not on
     run over or dragged by   public highway)

     collision of motor-driven snow vehicle with:
       animal (being ridden) (-drawn vehicle)
       another off-road motor vehicle
       other motor vehicle, not on public highway
       railway train
       other object, fixed or movable
     injury caused by rough landing of motor-driven snow
       vehicle (after leaving ground on rough terrain)

     EXCLUDES *accident on the public highway involving motor driven*
       snow vehicle (E810.0-E819.9)

§ ✓4ᵗʰ **E821 Nontraffic accident involving other off-road motor vehicle**

     INCLUDES breakage of part of
     fall from
     hit by   } off-road motorvehicle
     overturning of   except snow
     run over or dragged by   vehicle (not on
     thrown against some part   public highway
       of or object in

     collision with:
       animal (being ridden) (-drawn vehicle)
       another off-road motor vehicle, except snow vehicle
       other motor vehicle, not on public highway
       other object, fixed or movable

     EXCLUDES *accident on public highway involving off-road motor*
       vehicle (E810.0-E819.9)
       collision between motor driven snow vehicle and other
       off-road motor vehicle (E820.0-E820.9)
       hovercraft accident on water (E830.0-E838.9)

§ ✓4ᵗʰ **E822 Other motor vehicle nontraffic accident involving collision with moving object**

     INCLUDES collision, not on public highway, between motor vehicle,
       except off-road motor vehicle and:
       animal
       nonmotor vehicle
       other motor vehicle, except off-road motor vehicle
       pedestrian
       railway train
       other moving object

     EXCLUDES *collision with:*
       motor-driven snow vehicle (E820.0-E820.9)
       other off-road motor vehicle (E821.0-E821.9)

§ ✓4ᵗʰ **E823 Other motor vehicle nontraffic accident involving collision with stationary object**

     INCLUDES collision, not on public highway, between motor vehicle,
       except off-road motor vehicle, and any object,
       fixed or movable, but not in motion

§ ✓4ᵗʰ **E824 Other motor vehicle nontraffic accident while boarding and alighting**

     INCLUDES fall
     injury from oving part   while boarding or alighting
       of motor   from motor vehicle,
       vehicle   } except off-road motor
        vehicle, not on public
     trapped by door of   highway
       motor vehhicle

§ ✓4ᵗʰ **E825 Other motor vehicle nontraffic accident of other and unspecified nature**

     INCLUDES accidental poisoning from carbon
       monoxide generated by
     breakage of any part of
     explosion of any part of
     fall, jump, or being accidentally   motor vehicle
       pushed from   while in
     fire starting in   } motion, not
     hit by object thrown into, towards,   on public
       or on   highway
     injured by being thrown against
       some part of, or object in
     injury from moving part of
     object falling in or on
     motor vehicle nontraffic accident NOS

     EXCLUDES *fall from or in stationary motor vehicle (E884.9, E885.9)*
       overcome by carbon monoxide or exhaust gas generated by
       stationary motor vehicle off the roadway with motor
       running (E868.2)
       struck by falling object from or in stationary motor vehicle
       (E916)

Other Road Vehicle Accidents (E826-E829)

NOTE Other road vehicle accidents are transport accidents involving road
     vehicles other than motor vehicles. For definitions of other road
     vehicle and related terms see definitions (m) to (o).

INCLUDES accidents involving other road vehicles being used in recreational
     or sporting activities

EXCLUDES *collision of other road vehicle [any] with:*
     aircraft (E840.0-E845.9)
     motor vehicle (E813.0-E813.9, E820.0-E822.9)
     railway train (E801.0-E801.9))

The following fourth-digit subdivisions are for use with categories E826-E829
to identify the injured person:
   .0 Pedestrian
     See definition (r)
   .1 Pedal cyclist
     See definition (p)
   .2 Rider of animal
   .3 Occupant of animal-drawn vehicle
   .4 Occupant of streetcar
   .8 Other specified person
   .9 Unspecified person

§ ✓4ᵗʰ **E826 Pedal cycle accident**

   [0-9]   INCLUDES breakage of any part of pedal cycle
     collision between pedal cycle and:
       animal (being ridden) (herded) (unattended)
       another pedal cycle
       any pedestrian
       nonmotor road vehicle
       other object, fixed, movable, or moving, not set in
         motion by motor vehicle, railway train, or aircraft
     entanglement in wheel of pedal cycle
     fall from pedal cycle
     hit by object falling or thrown on the pedal cycle
     pedal cycle accident NOS
     pedal cycle overturned

§ ✓4ᵗʰ **E827 Animal-drawn vehicle accident**

   [0,2,4,8,9]   INCLUDES breakage of any part of vehicle
     collision between animal-drawn vehicle and:
       animal (being ridden) (herded) (unattended)
       nonmotor road vehicle, except pedal cycle
       pedestrian, pedestrian conveyance, or pedestrian
         vehicle
       other object, fixed, movable, or moving, not set in
         motion by motor vehicle, railway train, or aircraft

     fall from
     knocked down by
     overturning of   } animal drawn vehicle
     running over by
     thrown from

     EXCLUDES *collision of animal-drawn vehicle with pedal cycle*
       (E826.0-E826.9)

§   Requires fourth-digit. See beginning of appropriate section for codes and definitions.

✓4ᵗʰ Fourth-digit Required   ►◄ Revised Text   ● New Code   ▲ Revised Code TitleDx

2011 ICD-9-CM   **E Codes – 7**

E820–E827

§ ✓4ᵗʰ **E828 Accident involving animal being ridden**

[0,2,4,8,9] INCLUDES collision between animal being ridden and:

        another animal

        nonmotor road vehicle, except pedal cycle, and animal-drawn vehicle

        pedestrian, pedestrian conveyance, or pedestrian vehicle

        other object, fixed, movable, or moving, not set in motion by motor vehicle, railway train, or aircraft

        fall from

        knocked down by ⎫

        thrown from   ⎬ animal being ridden

        trampled by   ⎭

    ridden animal stumbled and fell

EXCLUDES *collision of animal being ridden with:*

    animal-drawn vehicle (E827.0-E827.9)

    pedal cycle (E826.0-E826.9)

§ ✓4ᵗʰ **E829 Other road vehicle accidents**

[0,4,8,9] INCLUDES accident while boarding ⎫

    or alighting from   ⎪

    blow from object in   ⎪ streetcar

    breakage of any part of ⎬ nonmotor road vehicle

    caught in door of   ⎪   not classifiable to

    derailment of   ⎪   E826-E828

    fall in, on, or from   ⎪

    fire in   ⎭

    collision between streetcar or nonmotor road vehicle, except as in E826-E828, and:

        animal (not being ridden)

        another nonmotor road vehicle not classifiable to E826-E828

        pedestrian

        other object, fixed, movable, or moving, not set in motion by motor vehicle, railway train, or aircraft

    nonmotor road vehicle accident NOS

    streetcar accident NOS

EXCLUDES *collision with:*

    animal being ridden (E828.0-E828.9)

    animal-drawn vehicle (E827.0-E827.9)

    pedal cycle (E826.0-E826.9)

Water Transport Accidents (E830-E838)

NOTE For definitions of water transport accident and related terms see definitions (a), (s), and (t).

INCLUDES watercraft accidents in the course of recreational activities

EXCLUDES *accidents involving both aircraft, including objects set in motion by aircraft, and watercraft (E840.0-E845.9)*

The following fourth-digit subdivisions are for use with categories E830-E838 to identify the injured person:

.0 Occupant of small boat, unpowered

.1 Occupant of small boat, powered

    See definition (t)

    EXCLUDES *water skier (.4)*

.2 Occupant of other watercraft — crew

    Persons:

        engaged in operation of watercraft

        providing passenger services [cabin attendants, ship's physician, catering personnel]

        working on ship during voyage in other capacity [musician in band, operators of shops and beauty parlors

.3 Occupant of other watercraft — other than crew

    Passenger

    Occupant of lifeboat, other than crew, after abandoning ship

.4 Water skier

.5 Swimmer

.6 Dockers, stevedores

    Longshoreman employed on the dock in loading and unloading ships

.7 Occupant of military watercraft, any type

.8 Other specified person

    Immigration and custom officials on board ship

    Person:

        accompanying passenger or member of crew visiting boat

    Pilot (guiding ship into port)

.9 Unspecified person

§ ✓4ᵗʰ **E830 Accident to watercraft causing submersion**

INCLUDES submersion and drowning due to:

    boat overturning

    boat submerging

    falling or jumping from burning ship

    falling or jumping from crushed watercraft

    ship sinking

    other accident to watercraft

§ ✓4ᵗʰ **E831 Accident to watercraft causing other injury**

INCLUDES any injury, except submersion and drowning, as a result of an accident to watercraft

    burned while ship on fire

    crushed between ships in collision

    crushed by lifeboat after abandoning ship

    fall due to collision or other accident to watercraft

    hit by falling object due to accident to watercraft

    injured in watercraft accident involving collision

    struck by boat or part thereof after fall or jump from damaged boat

EXCLUDES *burns from localized fire or explosion on board ship (E837.0-E837.9)*

§ ✓4ᵗʰ **E832 Other accidental submersion or drowning in water transport accident**

INCLUDES submersion or drowning as a result of an accident other than accident to the watercraft, such as:

    fall:

        from gangplank

        from ship

        overboard

    thrown overboard by motion of ship

    washed overboard

EXCLUDES *submersion or drowning of swimmer or diver who voluntarily jumps from boat not involved in an accident (E910.0-E910.9)*

§ ✓4ᵗʰ **E833 Fall on stairs or ladders in water transport**

EXCLUDES *fall due to accident to watercraft (E831.0-E831.9)*

§ ✓4ᵗʰ **E834 Other fall from one level to another in water transport**

EXCLUDES *fall due to accident to watercraft (E831.0-E831.9)*

§ ✓4ᵗʰ **E835 Other and unspecified fall in water transport**

EXCLUDES *fall due to accident to watercraft (E831.0-E831.9)*

§ ✓4ᵗʰ **E836 Machinery accident in water transport**

INCLUDES injuries in water transport caused by:

    deck   ⎫

    engine room ⎪

    galley   ⎬ machinery

    laundry   ⎪

    loading   ⎭

§ ✓4ᵗʰ **E837 Explosion, fire, or burning in watercraft**

INCLUDES explosion of boiler on steamship

    localized fire on ship

EXCLUDES *burning ship (due to collision or explosion) resulting in:*

    submersion or drowning (E830.0-E830.9)

    other injury (E831.0-E831.9)

§ ✓4ᵗʰ **E838 Other and unspecified water transport accident**

INCLUDES accidental poisoning by gases or fumes on ship

    atomic power plant malfunction in watercraft

    crushed between ship and stationary object [wharf]

    crushed between ships without accident to watercraft

    crushed by falling object on ship or while loading or unloading

    hit by boat while water skiing

    struck by boat or part thereof (after fall from boat)

    watercraft accident NOS

---

§ Requires fourth-digit. Valid digits are in [brackets] under each code. See beginning of appropriate section for codes and definitions.

✓4ᵗʰ Fourth-digit Required   ▶◀ Revised Text   ● New Code   ▲ Revised Code TitleDx

Air and Space Transport Accidents (E840-E845)

NOTE For definition of aircraft and related terms see definitions (u) and (v).

The following fourth-digit subdivisions are for use with categories E840-E845 to identify the injured person. Valid fourth digits are in [brackets] under codes E842-E845:

.0 Occupant of spacecraft

.1 Occupant of military aircraft, any
Crew in military aircraft [air force] [army] [national guard] [navy]
Passenger (civilian) (military) in military aircraft [air force] [army] [national guard] [navy]
Troops in military aircraft [air force] [army] [national guard] [navy]
EXCLUDES *occupants of aircraft operated under jurisdiction of police departments (.5)*
parachutist (.7)

.2 Crew of commercial aircraft (powered) in surface to surface transport

.3 Other occupant of commercial aircraft (powered) in surface to surface transport
Flight personnel:
not part of crew
on familiarization flight
Passenger on aircraft (powered) NOS

.4 Occupant of commercial aircraft (powered) in surface to air transport
Occupant [crew] [passenger] of aircraft (powered) engaged in activities, such as:
aerial spraying (crops) (fire retardants)
air drops of emergency supplies
air drops of parachutists, except from military craft
crop dusting
lowering of construction material [bridge or telephone pole]
sky writing

.5 Occupant of other powered aircraft
Occupant [crew] [passenger] of aircraft (powered) engaged in activities, such as:
aerobatic flying
aircraft racing
rescue operation
storm surveillance
traffic surveillance
Occupant of private plane NOS

.6 Occupant of unpowered aircraft, except parachutist
Occupant of aircraft classifiable to E842

.7 Parachutist (military) (other)
Person making voluntary descent
EXCLUDES *person making descent after accident to aircraft (.1-.6)*

.8 Ground crew, airline employee
Persons employed at airfields (civil) (military) or launching pads, not occupants of aircraft

.9 Other person

§ ✓4ᵗʰ **E840 Accident to powered aircraft at takeoff or landing**
[INCLUDES] collision of aircraft with any object, fixed, movable, or moving
crash
explosion on aircraft } while taking off or landing
fire on aircraft
forced landing

§ ✓4ᵗʰ **E841 Accident to powered aircraft, other and unspecified**
[INCLUDES] aircraft accident NOS
aircraft crash or wreck NOS
any accident to powered aircraft while in transit or when not specified whether in transit, taking off, or landing
collision of aircraft with another aircraft, bird, or any object, while in transit
explosion on aircraft while in transit
fire on aircraft while in transit

§ ✓4ᵗʰ **E842 Accident to unpowered aircraft**
[6-9] [INCLUDES] any accident, except collision with powered aircraft, to:
balloon
glider
hang glider
kite carrying a person
hit by object falling from unpowered aircraft

§ ✓4ᵗʰ **E843 Fall in, on, or from aircraft**
[0-9] [INCLUDES] accident in boarding or alighting from aircraft, any kind
fall in, on, or from aircraft [any kind], while in transit, taking off, or landing, except when as a result of an accident to aircraft

§ ✓4ᵗʰ **E844 Other specified air transport accidents**
[0-9] [INCLUDES] hit by:
aircraft
object falling from aircraft
injury by or from:
machinery of aircraft } without
rotating propellar } accident
voluntary parachute descent } to aircraft
poisoning by carbon monoxide from aircraft while in transit
sucked into jet
any accident involving other transport vehicle (motor) (nonmotor) due to being hit by object set in motion by aircraft (powered)
EXCLUDES *air sickness (E903)*
effects of:
high altitude (E902.0-E902.1)
pressure change (E902.0-E902.1)
injury in parachute descent due to accident to aircraft (E840.0-E842-9)

§ ✓4ᵗʰ **E845 Accident involving spacecraft**
[0,8,9] [INCLUDES] launching pad accident
EXCLUDES *effects of weightlessness in spacecraft (E928.0)*

Vehicle Accidents Not Elsewhere Classifiable (E846-E848)

E846 Accidents involving powered vehicles used solely within the buildings and premises of industrial or commercial establishment
Accident to, on, or involving:
battery powered airport passenger vehicle
battery powered trucks (baggage) (mail)
coal car in mine
logging car
self propelled truck, industrial
station baggage truck (powered)
tram, truck, or tub (powered) in mine or quarry
Collision with:
pedestrian
other vehicle or object within premises
Explosion of
Fall from } powered vehicle, industrial or
Overturning of } commercial
Struck by
EXCLUDES *accidental poisoning by exhaust gas from vehicle not elsewhere classifiable (E868.2)*
injury by crane, lift (fork), or elevator (E919.2)

E847 Accidents involving cable cars not running on rails
Accident to, on, or involving:
cable car, not on rails
ski chair-lift
ski-lift with gondola
téléférique
Breakage of cable
Caught or dragged by
Fall or jump from } cable car, not on rails
Object thrown from or in

E848 Accidents involving other vehicles, not elsewhere classifiable
Accident to, on, or involving:
ice yacht
land yacht
nonmotor, nonroad vehicle NOS

§ Requires fourth-digit. See beginning of appropriate section for codes and definitions.

Place of Occurrence (E849)

✓4ᵗʰ **E849** **Place of Occurrence**

NOTE The following category is for use to denote the place where the injury or poisoning occurred.

E849.0 Home
  Apartment
  Boarding house
  Farm house
  Home premises
  House (residential)
  Noninstitutional place of residence
  Private:
    driveway
    garage
    garden
    home
    walk
  Swimming pool in private house or garden
  Yard of home
  EXCLUDES *home under construction but not yet occupied (E849.3)*
        institutional place of residence (E849.7)

E849.1 Farm
  Farm:
    buildings
    land under cultivation
  EXCLUDES *farm house and home premises of farm (E849.0)*

E849.2 Mine and quarry
  Gravel pit
  Sand pit
  Tunnel under construction

E849.3 Industrial place and premises
  Building under construction
  Dockyard
  Dry dock
  Factory
    building
    premises
  Garage (place of work)
  Industrial yard
  Loading platform (factory) (store)
  Plant, industrial
  Railway yard
  Shop (place of work)
  Warehouse
  Workhouse

E849.4 Place for recreation and sport
  Amusement park   *Playground, including school*
  Baseball field   *playground*
  Basketball court   *Public park*
  Beach resort   *Racecourse*
  Cricket ground   *Resort NOS*
  Fives court   *Riding school*
  Football field   *Rifle range*
  Golf course   *Seashore resort*
  Gymnasium   *Skating rink*
  Hockey field   *Sports palace*
  Holiday camp   *Stadium*
  Ice palace   *Swimming pool, public*
  Lake resort   *Tennis court*
  Mountain resort   *Vacation resort*
  EXCLUDES *that in private house or garden (E849.0)*

E849.5 Street and highway

E849.6 Public building
  Building (including adjacent grounds) used by the general public or by a particular group of the public, such as:
  airport
  bank
  café
  casino
  church
  cinema
  clubhouse
  courthouse
  dance hall
  garage building (for car storage)
  hotel
  market (grocery or other commodity)
  movie house
  music hall
  nightclub
  office
  office building
  opera house
  post office
  public hall
  radio broadcasting station
  restaurant
  school (state) (public) (private)
  shop, commercial
  station (bus) (railway)
  store
  theater
  EXCLUDES *home garage (E849.0)*
        industrial building or workplace (E849.3)

E849.7 Residential institution
  Children's home
  Dormitory
  Hospital
  Jail
  Old people's home
  Orphanage
  Prison
  Reform school

E849.8 Other specified places
  Beach NOS   *Pond or pool (natural)*
  Canal   *Prairie*
  Caravan site NOS   *Public place NOS*
  Derelict house   *Railway line*
  Desert   *Reservoir*
  Dock   *River*
  Forest   *Sea*
  Harbor   *Seashore NOS*
  Hill   *Stream*
  Lake NOS   *Swamp*
  Mountain   *Trailer court*
  Parking lot   *Woods*
  Parking place

E849.9 Unspecified place

Accidental Poisoning by Drugs, Medicinal Substances, and Biologicals (E850-E858)

INCLUDES　accidental overdose of drug, wrong drug given or taken in error, and drug taken inadvertently

accidents in the use of drugs and biologicals in medical and surgical procedures

EXCLUDES　*administration with suicidal or homicidal intent or intent to harm, or in circumstances classifiable to E980-E989 (E950.0-E950.5, E962.0, E980.0-E980.5)*

correct drug properly administered in therapeutic or prophylactic dosage, as the cause of adverse effect (E930.0-E949.9)

NOTE　See Alphabetic Index for more complete list of specific drugs to be classified under the fourth-digit subdivisions. The American Hospital Formulary numbers can be used to classify new drugs listed by the American Hospital Formulary Service (AHFS). See Appendix C.

✓4ᵗʰ E850　Accidental poisoning by analgesics, antipyretics, and antirheumatics

E850.0　Heroin
Diacetylmorphine

E850.1　Methadone

E850.2　Other opiates and related narcotics
Codeine [methylmorphine]
Meperidine [pethidine]
Morphine
Opium (alkaloids)

E850.3　Salicylates
Acetylsalicylic acid [aspirin]
Amino derivatives of salicylic acid
Salicylic acid salts

E850.4　Aromatic analgesics, not elsewhere classified
Acetanilid
Paracetamol [acetaminophen]
Phenacetin [acetophenetidin]

E850.5　Pyrazole derivatives
Aminophenazone [amidopyrine]
Phenylbutazone

E850.6　Antirheumatics [antiphlogistics]
Gold salts
Indomethacin
EXCLUDES　*salicylates (E850.3)*
steroids (E858.0)

E850.7　Other non-narcotic analgesics
Pyrabital

E850.8　Other specified analgesics and antipyretics
Pentazocine

E850.9　Unspecified analgesic or antipyretic

E851　Accidental poisoning by barbiturates
Amobarbital [amylobarbitone]
Barbital [barbitone]
Butabarbital [butabarbitone]
Pentobarbital [pentobarbitone]
Phenobarbital [phenobarbitone]
Secobarbital [quinalbarbitone]
EXCLUDES　*thiobarbiturates (E855.1)*

✓4ᵗʰ E852　Accidental poisoning by other sedatives and hypnotics

E852.0　Chloral hydrate group

E852.1　Paraldehyde

E852.2　Bromine compounds
Bromides
Carbromal (derivatives)

E852.3　Methaqualone compounds

E852.4　Glutethimide group

E852.5　Mixed sedatives, not elsewhere classified

E852.8　Other specified sedatives and hypnotics

E852.9　Unspecified sedative or hypnotic
Sleeping:
drug ⎫
pill ⎬ NOS
tablet ⎭

✓4ᵗʰ E853　Accidental poisoning by tranquilizers

E853.0　Phenothiazine-based tranquilizers
Chlorpromazine　　Prochlorperazine
Fluphenazine　　　Promazine

E853.1　Butyrophenone-based tranquilizers
Haloperidol　　　Trifluperidol
Spiperone

E853.2　Benzodiazepine-based tranquilizers
Chlordiazepoxide　Lorazepam
Diazepam　　　　Medazepam
Flurazepam　　　Nitrazepam

E853.8　Other specified tranquilizers
Hydroxyzine　　　Meprobamate

E853.9　Unspecified tranquilizer

✓4ᵗʰ E854　Accidental poisoning by other psychotropic agents

E854.0　Antidepressants
Amitriptyline
Imipramine
Monoamine oxidase [MAO] inhibitors

E854.1　Psychodysleptics [hallucinogens]
Cannabis derivatives　　Mescaline
Lysergide [LSD]　　　　Psilocin
Marihuana (derivatives)　Psilocybin

E854.2　Psychostimulants
Amphetamine
Caffeine
EXCLUDES　*central appetite depressants (E858.8)*

E854.3　Central nervous system stimulants
Analeptics
Opiate antagonists

E854.8　Other psychotropic agents

✓4ᵗʰ E855　Accidental poisoning by other drugs acting on central and autonomic nervous system

E855.0　Anticonvulsant and anti-Parkinsonism drugs
Amantadine
Hydantoin derivatives
Levodopa [L-dopa]
Oxazolidine derivatives [paramethadione] [trimethadione]
Succinimides

E855.1　Other central nervous system depressants
Ether
Gaseous anesthetics
Halogenated hydrocarbon derivatives
Intravenous anesthetics
Thiobarbiturates, such as thiopental sodium

E855.2　Local anesthetics
Cocaine　　　　　　Procaine
Lidocaine [lignocaine]　Tetracaine

E855.3　Parasympathomimetics [cholinergics]
Acetylcholine　　　　　Anticholinesterase:
Anticholinesterase:　　　reversible
organophosphorus　　Pilocarpine

E855.4　Parasympatholytics [anticholinergics and antimuscarinics] and spasmolytics
Atropine　　　　Hyoscine [scopolamine]
Homatropine　　Quaternary ammonium derivatives

E855.5　Sympathomimetics [adrenergics]
Epinephrine [adrenalin]
Levarterenol [noradrenalin]

E855.6　Sympatholytics [antiadrenergics]
Phenoxybenzamine
Tolazoline hydrochloride

E855.8　Other specified drugs acting on central and autonomic nervous systems

E855.9 **Unspecified drug acting on central and autonomic nervous systems**

E856 **Accidental poisoning by antibiotics**

E857 **Accidental poisoning by other anti-infectives**

√4ᵗʰ E858 **Accidental poisoning by other drugs**

E858.0 **Hormones and synthetic substitutes**

E858.1 **Primarily systemic agents**

E858.2 **Agents primarily affecting blood constituents**

E858.3 **Agents primarily affecting cardiovascular system**

E858.4 **Agents primarily affecting gastrointestinal system**

E858.5 **Water, mineral, and uric acid metabolism drugs**

E858.6 **Agents primarily acting on the smooth and skeletal muscles and respiratory system**

E858.7 **Agents primarily affecting skin and mucous membrane, ophthalmological, otorhinolaryngological, and dental drugs**

E858.8 **Other specified drugs**
   Central appetite depressants

E858.9 **Unspecified drug**

Accidental Poisoning by Other Solid and Liquid Substances, Gases, and Vapors (E860-E869)

NOTE Categories in this section are intended primarily to indicate the external cause of poisoning states classifiable to 980-989. They may also be used to indicate external causes of localized effects classifiable to 001-799.

√4ᵗʰ E860 **Accidental poisoning by alcohol, not elsewhere classified**

E860.0 **Alcoholic beverages**
   Alcohol in preparations intended for consumption

E860.1 **Other and unspecified ethyl alcohol and its products**
   Denatured alcohol   Grain alcohol NOS
   Ethanol NOS   Methylated spirit

E860.2 **Methyl alcohol**
   Methanol   Wood alcohol

E860.3 **Isopropyl alcohol**
   Dimethyl carbinol   Rubbing alcohol subsitute
   Isopropanol   Secondary propyl alcohol

E860.4 **Fusel oil**
   Alcohol: Alcohol:
     amyl   propyl
     butyl

E860.8 **Other specified alcohols**

E860.9 **Unspecified alcohol**

√4ᵗʰ E861 **Accidental poisoning by cleansing and polishing agents, disinfectants, paints, and varnishes**

E861.0 **Synthetic detergents and shampoos**

E861.1 **Soap products**

E861.2 **Polishes**

E861.3 **Other cleansing and polishing agents**
   Scouring powders

E861.4 **Disinfectants**
   Household and other disinfectants not ordinarily used on the person
   EXCLUDES carbolic acid or phenol (E864.0)

E861.5 **Lead paints**

E861.6 **Other paints and varnishes**
   Lacquers   Paints, other than lead
   Oil colors   White washes

E861.9 **Unspecified**

√4ᵗʰ E862 **Accidental poisoning by petroleum products, other solvents and their vapors, not elsewhere classified**

E862.0 **Petroleum solvents**
   Petroleum: Petroleum:
     ether   naphtha
     benzine

E862.1 **Petroleum fuels and cleaners**
   Antiknock additives to petroleum fuels
   Gas oils
   Gasoline or petrol
   Kerosene
   EXCLUDES kerosene insecticides (E863.4)

E862.2 **Lubricating oils**

E862.3 **Petroleum solids**
   Paraffin wax

E862.4 **Other specified solvents**
   Benzene

E862.9 **Unspecified solvent**

√4ᵗʰ E863 **Accidental poisoning by agricultural and horticultural chemical and pharmaceutical preparations other than plant foods and fertilizers**
   EXCLUDES plant foods and fertilizers (E866.5)

E863.0 **Insecticides of organochlorine compounds**
   Benzene hexachloride   Dieldrin
   Chlordane   Endrine
   DDT   Toxaphene

E863.1 **Insecticides of organophosphorus compounds**
   Demeton   Parathion
   Diazinon   Phenylsulphthion
   Dichlorvos   Phorate
   Malathion   Phosdrin
   Methyl parathion

E863.2 **Carbamates**
   Aldicarb   Propoxur
   Carbaryl

E863.3 **Mixtures of insecticides**

E863.4 **Other and unspecified insecticides**
   Kerosene insecticides

E863.5 **Herbicides**
   2, 4-Dichlorophenoxyacetic acid [2, 4-D]
   2, 4, 5-Trichlorophenoxyacetic acid [2, 4, 5-T]
   Chlorates
   Diquat
   Mixtures of plant foods and fertilizers with herbicides
   Paraquat

E863.6 **Fungicides**
   Organic mercurials (used in seed dressing)
   Pentachlorophenols

E863.7 **Rodenticides**
   Fluoroacetates   Warfarin
   Squill and derivatives   Zinc phosphide
   Thallium

E863.8 **Fumigants**
   Cyanides   Phosphine
   Methyl bromide

E863.9 **Other and unspecified**

√4ᵗʰ E864 **Accidental poisoning by corrosives and caustics, not elsewhere classified**
   EXCLUDES those as components of disinfectants (E861.4)

E864.0 **Corrosive aromatics**
   Carbolic acid or phenol

E864.1 **Acids**
   Acid:
     hydrochloric
     nitric
     sulfuric

E864.2 **Caustic alkalis**
   Lye

E864.3 **Other specified corrosives and caustics**

E864.4 **Unspecified corrosives and caustics**

☑4ᵗʰ E865 Accidental poisoning from poisonous foodstuffs and poisonous plants
> **INCLUDES** any meat, fish, or shellfish
> plants, berries, and fungi eaten as, or in mistake for, food, or by a child
>
> **EXCLUDES** *anaphylactic shock due to adverse food reaction (995.60-995.69)*
> *food poisoning (bacterial) (005.0-005.9)*
> *poisoning and toxic reactions to venomous plants (E905.6-E905.7)*

E865.0 Meat

E865.1 Shellfish

E865.2 Other fish

E865.3 Berries and seeds

E865.4 Other specified plants

E865.5 Mushrooms and other fungi

E865.8 Other specified foods

E865.9 Unspecified foodstuff or poisonous plant

☑4ᵗʰ E866 Accidental poisoning by other and unspecified solid and liquid substances
> **EXCLUDES** *these substances as a component of:*
> *medicines (E850.0-E858.9)*
> *paints (E861.5-E861.6)*
> *pesticides (E863.0-E863.9)*
> *petroleum fuels (E862.1)*

E866.0 Lead and its compounds and fumes

E866.1 Mercury and its compounds and fumes

E866.2 Antimony and its compounds and fumes

E866.3 Arsenic and its compounds and fumes

E866.4 Other metals and their compounds and fumes
> Beryllium (compounds)
> Brass fumes
> Cadmium (compounds)
> Copper salts
> Iron (compounds)
> Manganese (compounds)
> Nickel (compounds)
> Thallium (compounds)

E866.5 Plant foods and fertilizers
> **EXCLUDES** *mixtures with herbicides (E863.5)*

E866.6 Glues and adhesives

E866.7 Cosmetics

E866.8 Other specified solid or liquid substances

E866.9 Unspecified solid or liquid substance

E867 Accidental poisoning by gas distributed by pipeline
> Carbon monoxide from incomplete combustion of piped gas
> Coal gas NOS
> Liquefied petroleum gas distributed through pipes (pure or mixed with air)
> Piped gas (natural) (manufactured)

☑4ᵗʰ E868 Accidental poisoning by other utility gas and other carbon monoxide

E868.0 Liquefied petroleum gas distributed in mobile containers

Butane	or carbon monoxide
Liquefied hydrocarbon gas NOS	from incomplete conbustion of
Propane	these gases

E868.1 Other and unspecified utility gas

Acetylene	or carbon monoxide
Gas NOS used for lighting, heating, or cooking	from incomplete conbustion of
Water gas	these gases

E868.2 Motor vehicle exhaust gas
> Exhaust gas from:
> any type of combustion engine not in watercraft
> farm tractor, not in transit
> gas engine
> motor pump
> motor vehicle, not in transit
>
> **EXCLUDES** *poisoning by carbon monoxide from:*
> *aircraft while in transit (E844.0-E844.9)*
> *motor vehicle while in transit (E818.0-E818.9)*
> *watercraft whether or not in transit (E838.0-E838.9)*

E868.3 Carbon monoxide from incomplete combustion of other domestic fuels
> Carbon monoxide from incomplete combustion of:
> coal
> coke ⎱ in domestic stove or fireplace
> kerosene ⎰
> wood
>
> **EXCLUDES** *carbon monoxide from smoke and fumes due to conflagration (E890.0-E893.9)*

E868.8 Carbon monoxide from other sources
> Carbon monoxide from:
> blast furnace gas
> incomplete combustion of fuels in industrial use
> kiln vapor

E868.9 Unspecified carbon monoxide

☑4ᵗʰ E869 Accidental poisoning by other gases and vapors
> **EXCLUDES** *effects of gases used as anesthetics (E855.1, E938.2)*
> *fumes from heavy metals (E866.0-E866.4)*
> *smoke and fumes due to conflagration or explosion (E890.0-E899)*

E869.0 Nitrogen oxides

E869.1 Sulfur dioxide

E869.2 Freon

E869.3 Lacrimogenic gas [tear gas]
> Bromobenzyl cyanide
> Chloroacetophenone
> Ethyliodoacetate

E869.4 Second-hand tobacco smoke

E869.8 Other specified gases and vapors
> Chlorine
> Hydrocyanic acid gas

E869.9 Unspecified gases and vapors

Misadventures to Patients During Surgical and Medical Care (E870-E876)

> **EXCLUDES** *accidental overdose of drug and wrong drug given in error (E850.0-E858.9)*
> *surgical and medical procedures as the cause of abnormal reaction by the patient, without mention of misadventure at the time of procedure (E878.0-E879.9)*

☑4ᵗʰ E870 Accidental cut, puncture, perforation, or hemorrhage during medical care

E870.0 Surgical operation

E870.1 Infusion or transfusion

E870.2 Kidney dialysis or other perfusion

E870.3 Injection or vaccination

E870.4 Endoscopic examination

E870.5 Aspiration of fluid or tissue, puncture, and catheterization
> Abdominal paracentesis
> Aspirating needle biopsy
> Blood sampling
> Lumbar puncture
> Thoracentesis
>
> **EXCLUDES** *heart catheterization (E870.6)*

E870.6 Heart catheterization

E870.7 Administration of enema

E870.8 Other specified medical care

E870.9 Unspecified medical care

✓4ᵗʰ E871 Foreign object left in body during procedure

E871.0 Surgical operation

E871.1 Infusion or transfusion

E871.2 Kidney dialysis or other perfusion

E871.3 Injection or vaccination

E871.4 Endoscopic examination

E871.5 Aspiration of fluid or tissue, puncture, and catheterization
Abdominal paracentesis
Aspiration needle biopsy
Blood sampling
Lumbar puncture
Thoracentesis
EXCLUDES heart catheterization (E871.6)

E871.6 Heart catheterization

E871.7 Removal of catheter or packing

E871.8 Other specified procedures

E871.9 Unspecified procedure

✓4ᵗʰ E872 Failure of sterile precautions during procedure

E872.0 Surgical operation

E872.1 Infusion or transfusion

E872.2 Kidney dialysis and other perfusion

E872.3 Injection or vaccination

E872.4 Endoscopic examination

E872.5 Aspiration of fluid or tissue, puncture, and catheterization
Abdominal paracentesis
Aspiration needle biopsy
Blood sampling
Lumbar puncture
Thoracentesis
EXCLUDES heart catheterization (E872.6)

E872.6 Heart catheterization

E872.8 Other specified procedures

E872.9 Unspecified procedure

✓4ᵗʰ E873 Failure in dosage
EXCLUDES accidental overdose of drug, medicinal or biological substance (E850.0-E858.9)

E873.0 Excessive amount of blood or other fluid during transfusion or infusion

E873.1 Incorrect dilution of fluid during infusion

E873.2 Overdose of radiation in therapy

E873.3 Inadvertent exposure of patient to radiation during medical care

E873.4 Failure in dosage in electroshock or insulin-shock therapy

E873.5 Inappropriate [too hot or too cold] temperature in local application and packing

E873.6 Nonadministration of necessary drug or medicinal substance

E873.8 Other specified failure in dosage

E873.9 Unspecified failure in dosage

✓4ᵗʰ E874 Mechanical failure of instrument or apparatus during procedure

E874.0 Surgical operation

E874.1 Infusion and transfusion
Air in system

E874.2 Kidney dialysis and other perfusion

E874.3 Endoscopic examination

E874.4 Aspiration of fluid or tissue, puncture, and catheterization
Abdominal paracentesis   Lumbar puncture
Aspiration needle biopsy   Thoracentesis
Blood sampling
EXCLUDES heart catheterization (E874.5)

E874.5 Heart catheterization

E874.8 Other specified procedures

E874.9 Unspecified procedure

✓4ᵗʰ E875 Contaminated or infected blood, other fluid, drug, or biological substance
INCLUDES presence of:
bacterial pyrogens
endotoxin-producing bacteria
serum hepatitis-producing agent

E875.0 Contaminated substance transfused or infused

E875.1 Contaminated substance injected or used for vaccination

E875.2 Contaminated drug or biological substance administered by other means

E875.8 Other

E875.9 Unspecified

✓4ᵗʰ E876 Other and unspecified misadventures during medical care

E876.0 Mismatched blood in transfusion

E876.1 Wrong fluid in infusion

E876.2 Failure in suture and ligature during surgical operation

E876.3 Endotracheal tube wrongly placed during anesthetic procedure

E876.4 Failure to introduce or to remove other tube or instrument
EXCLUDES foreign object left in body during procedure (E871.0-E871.9)

* **E876.5 Performance of wrong operation (procedure) on correct patient**
Wrong device implanted into correct surgical site
EXCLUDES correct operation (procedure) performed on wrong body part (E876.7)

* **E876.6 Performance of operation (procedure) on patient not scheduled for surgery**
Performance of operation (procedure) intended for another patient
Performance of operation (procedure) on wrong patient

* **E876.7 Performance of correct operation (procedure) on wrong side/body part**
Performance of correct operation (procedure) on wrong side
Performance of correct operation (procedure) on wrong site

E876.8 Other specified misadventures during medical care
Performance of inappropriate treatment NEC

E876.9 Unspecified misadventure during medical care

---

* Wrong surgery edit applies.

Surgical and Medical Procedures as the Cause of Abnormal Reaction of Patient or Later Complication, Without Mention of Misadventure at the Time of Procedure (E878-E879)

INCLUDES　procedures as the cause of abnormal reaction, such as:
　　displacement or malfunction of prosthetic device
　　hepatorenal failure, postoperative
　　malfunction of external stoma
　　postoperative intestinal obstruction
　　rejection of transplanted organ

EXCLUDES　*anesthetic management properly carried out as the cause of adverse effect (E937.0-E938.9)*
　　infusion and transfusion, without mention of misadventure in the technique of procedure (E930.0-E949.9)

☑4ᵗʰ **E878　Surgical operation and other surgical procedures as the cause of abnormal reaction of patient, or of later complication, without mention of misadventure at the time of operation**

E878.0　Surgical operation with transplant of whole organ
　　Transplantation of:
　　　heart
　　　kidney
　　　liver

E878.1　Surgical operation with implant of artificial internal device
　　Cardiac pacemaker
　　Electrodes implanted in brain
　　Heart valve prosthesis
　　Internal orthopedic device

E878.2　Surgical operation with anastomosis, bypass, or graft, with natural or artificial tissues used as implant
　　Anastomosis:
　　　arteriovenous
　　　gastrojejunal
　　Graft of blood vessel, tendon, or skin
　　EXCLUDES　*external stoma (E878.3)*

E878.3　Surgical operation with formation of external stoma
　　Colostomy　　　　Gastrostomy
　　Cystostomy　　　Ureterostomy
　　Duodenostomy

E878.4　Other restorative surgery

E878.5　Amputation of limb(s)

E878.6　Removal of other organ (partial) (total)

E878.8　Other specified surgical operations and procedures

E878.9　Unspecified surgical operations and procedures

☑4ᵗʰ **E879　Other procedures, without mention of misadventure at the time of procedure, as the cause of abnormal reaction of patient, or of later complication**

E879.0　Cardiac catheterization

E879.1　Kidney dialysis

E879.2　Radiological procedure and radiotherapy
　　EXCLUDES　*radio-opaque dyes for diagnostic x-ray procedures (E947.8)*

E879.3　Shock therapy
　　Electroshock therapy
　　Insulin-shock therapy

E879.4　Aspiration of fluid
　　Lumbar puncture
　　Thoracentesis

E879.5　Insertion of gastric or duodenal sound

E879.6　Urinary catheterization

E879.7　Blood sampling

E879.8　Other specified procedures
　　Blood transfusion

E879.9　Unspecified procedure

Accidental Falls (E880-E888)

EXCLUDES　*falls (in or from):*
　　burning building (E890.8, E891.8)
　　into fire (E890.0-E899)
　　into water (with submersion or drowning) (E910.0-E910.9)
　　machinery (in operation) (E919.0-E919.9)
　　on edged, pointed, or sharp object (E920.0-E920.9)
　　transport vehicle (E800.0-E845.9)
　　vehicle not elsewhere classifiable (E846-E848)

☑4ᵗʰ **E880　Fall on or from stairs or steps**

E880.0　Escalator

E880.1　Fall on or from sidewalk curb
　　EXCLUDES　*fall from moving sidewalk (E885.9)*

E880.9　Other stairs or steps

☑4ᵗʰ **E881　Fall on or from ladders or scaffolding**

E881.0　Fall from ladder

E881.1　Fall from scaffolding

E882　Fall from or out of building or other structure
　　Fall from:　　　　　Fall from:
　　　balcony　　　　　　turret
　　　bridge　　　　　　viaduct
　　　building　　　　　wall
　　　flagpole　　　　　window
　　　tower　　　　　　Fall through roof
　　EXCLUDES　*collapse of a building or structure (E916)*
　　　fall or jump from burning building (E890.8, E891.8)

☑4ᵗʰ **E883　Fall into hole or other opening in surface**
　　INCLUDES　fall into:　　　　fall into:
　　　cavity　　　　　　shaft
　　　dock　　　　　　swimming pool
　　　hole　　　　　　tank
　　　pit　　　　　　　well
　　　quarry
　　EXCLUDES　*fall into water NOS (E910.9)*
　　　that resulting in drowning or submersion without mention of injury (E910.0-E910.9)

E883.0　Accident from diving or jumping into water [swimming pool]
　　Strike or hit:
　　　against bottom when jumping or diving into water
　　　wall or board of swimming pool
　　　water surface
　　EXCLUDES　*diving with insufficient air supply (E913.2)*
　　　effects of air pressure from diving (E902.2)

E883.1　Accidental fall into well

E883.2　Accidental fall into storm drain or manhole

E883.9　Fall into other hole or other opening in surface

☑4ᵗʰ **E884　Other fall from one level to another**

E884.0　Fall from playground equipment
　　EXCLUDES　*recreational machinery (E919.8)*

E884.1　Fall from cliff

E884.2　Fall from chair

E884.3　Fall from wheelchair
　　►Fall from motorized mobility scooter
　　Fall from motorized wheelchair◄

E884.4　Fall from bed

E884.5　Fall from other furniture

E884.6　Fall from commode
　　Toilet

E884.9　Other fall from one level to another
　　Fall from:　　　　　Fall from:
　　　embankment　　　stationary vehicle
　　　haystack　　　　tree

☑4ᵗʰ **E885　Fall on same level from slipping, tripping, or stumbling**

E885.0　Fall from (nonmotorized) scooter
　　EXCLUDES　►*fall from motorized mobility scooter (E884.3)*◄

E885.1 Fall from roller skates
Heelies
In-line skates
Wheelies

E885.2 Fall from skateboard

E885.3 Fall from skis

E885.4 Fall from snowboard

E885.9 Fall from other slipping, tripping, or stumbling
Fall on moving sidewalk

☑4ᵗʰ **E886 Fall on same level from collision, pushing, or shoving, by or with other person**

> EXCLUDES *crushed or pushed by a crowd or human stampede (E917.1, E917.6)*

E886.0 In sports
Tackles in sports

> EXCLUDES *kicked, stepped on, struck by object, in sports (E917.0, E917.5)*

E886.9 Other and unspecified
Fall from collision of pedestrian (conveyance) with another pedestrian (conveyance)

E887 Fracture, cause unspecified

☑4ᵗʰ **E888 Other and unspecified fall**
Accidental fall NOS
Fall on same level NOS

E888.0 Fall resulting in striking against sharp object
Use additional external cause code to identify object (E920)

E888.1 Fall resulting in striking against other object

E888.8 Other fall

E888.9 Unspecified fall
Fall NOS

Accidents Caused by Fire and Flames (E890-E899)

> INCLUDES asphyxia or poisoning due to conflagration or ignition
> burning by fire
> secondary fires resulting from explosion

> EXCLUDES *arson (E968.0)*
> *fire in or on:*
> *machinery (in operation) (E919.0-E919.9)*
> *transport vehicle other than stationary vehicle (E800.0-E845.9)*
> *vehicle not elsewhere classifiable (E846-E848)*

☑4ᵗʰ **E890 Conflagration in private dwelling**

> INCLUDES conflagration in:
> apartment
> boarding house
> camping place
> caravan
> farmhouse
> house
> lodging house
> mobile home
> private garage
> rooming house
> tenement
> conflagration originating from sources classifiable to E893-E898 in the above buildings

E890.0 Explosion caused by conflagration

E890.1 Fumes from combustion of polyvinylchloride [PVC] and similar material in conflagration

E890.2 Other smoke and fumes from conflagration
Carbon monoxide ⎫
Fumes NOS ⎬ from conflagration in private building
Smoke NOS ⎭

E890.3 Burning caused by conflagration

E890.8 Other accident resulting from conflagration
Collapse of ⎫
Fall from ⎬ burning private building
Hit by object falling from ⎪
Jump from ⎭

E890.9 Unspecified accident resulting from conflagration in private dwelling

☑4ᵗʰ **E891 Conflagration in other and unspecified building or structure**
Conflagration in:
barn
church
convalescent and other residential home
dormitory of educational institution
factory
farm outbuildings
hospital
hotel
school
store
theater
Conflagration originating from sources classifiable to E893-E898, in the above buildings

E891.0 Explosion caused by conflagration

E891.1 Fumes from combustion of polyvinylchloride [PVC] and similar material in conflagration

E891.2 Other smoke and fumes from conflagration
Carbon monoxide ⎫
Fumes NOS ⎬ from conflagration in private building or structure
Smoke NOS ⎭

E891.3 Burning caused by conflagration

E891.8 Other accident resulting from conflagration
Collapse of ⎫
Fall from ⎬ burning private building or structure
Hit by object falling from ⎪
Jump from ⎭

E891.9 Unspecified accident resulting from conflagration of other and unspecified building or structure

E892 Conflagration not in building or structure
Fire (uncontrolled) (in) (of):
forest
grass
hay
lumber
mine
prairie
transport vehicle [any], except while in transit
tunnel

☑4ᵗʰ **E893 Accident caused by ignition of clothing**

> EXCLUDES *ignition of clothing:*
> *from highly inflammable material (E894)*
> *with conflagration (E890.0-E892)*

E893.0 From controlled fire in private dwelling
Ignition of clothing from:
normal fire (charcoal) (coal) ⎫
(electric) (gas) (wood) in: ⎪
brazier ⎬ in private dwelling (as listed in E890)
fireplace ⎪
furnace ⎪
stove ⎭

E893.1 From controlled fire in other building or structure
Ignition of clothing from:
normal fire (charcoal) (coal) ⎫
(electric) (gas) (wood) in: ⎪
brazier ⎬ in other building or structure (as listed in E891)
fireplace ⎪
furnace ⎪
stove ⎭

E893.2 From controlled fire not in building or structure
Ignition of clothing from:
bonfire (controlled)
brazier fire (controlled), not in building or structure
trash fire (controlled)

> EXCLUDES *conflagration not in building (E892)*
> *trash fire out of control (E892)*

E893.8 From other specified sources

Ignition of clothing from:	Ignition of clothing from:
blowlamp	cigarette
blowtorch	lighter
burning bedspread	matches
candle	pipe
cigar	welding torch

E893.9 Unspecified source
Ignition of clothing (from controlled fire NOS) (in building NOS) NOS

E894 Ignition of highly inflammable material
Ignition of:
benzine
gasoline
fat
kerosene } (with ignition of clothing)
paraffin
petrol

EXCLUDES *ignition of highly inflammable material with:*
conflagration (E890.0-E892)
explosion (E923.0-E923.9)

E895 Accident caused by controlled fire in private dwelling
Burning by (flame of) normal fire (charcoal) (coal) (electric) (gas) (wood) in:
brazier
fireplace } in private dwelling (as listed in E890)
furnace
stove

EXCLUDES *burning by hot objects not producing fire or flames (E924.0-E924.9)*
ignition of clothing from these sources (E893.0)
poisoning by carbon monoxide from incomplete combustion of fuel (E867-E868.9)
that with conflagration (E890.0-E890.9)

E896 Accident caused by controlled fire in other and unspecified building or structure
Burning by (flame of) normal fire (charcoal) (coal)(electric)(gas)(wood) in:
brazier
fireplace } in other building or structure (as
furnace   listed in E891)
stove

EXCLUDES *burning by hot objects not producing fire or flames (E924.0-E924.9)*
ignition of clothing from these sources (E893.1)
poisoning by carbon monoxide from incomplete combustion of fuel (E867-E868.9)
that with conflagration (E891.0-E891.9)

E897 Accident caused by controlled fire not in building or structure
Burns from flame of:
bonfire
brazier fire, not in building or structure } controlled
trash fire

EXCLUDES *ignition of clothing from these sources (E893.2)*
trash fire out of control (E892)
that with conflagration (E892)

☑4ᵗʰ **E898 Accident caused by other specified fire and flames**

EXCLUDES *conflagration (E890.0-E892)*
that with ignition of:
clothing (E893.0-E893.9)
highly inflammable material (E894)

E898.0 Burning bedclothes
Bed set on fire NOS

E898.1 Other

Burning by:	Burning by:
blowlamp	lamp
blowtorch	lighter
candle	matches
cigar	pipe
cigarette	welding torch
fire in room NOS	

E899 Accident caused by unspecified fire
Burning NOS

Accidents Due to Natural and Environmental Factors (E900-E909)

☑4ᵗʰ **E900 Excessive heat**

E900.0 Due to weather conditions
Excessive heat as the external cause of:
ictus solaris
siriasis
sunstroke

E900.1 Of man-made origin
Heat (in):
boiler room
drying room
factory
furnace room
generated in transport vehicle
kitchen

E900.9 Of unspecified origin

☑4ᵗʰ **E901 Excessive cold**

E901.0 Due to weather conditions
Excessive cold as the cause of:
chilblains NOS
immersion foot

E901.1 Of man-made origin

Contact with or inhalation of:	Prolonged exposure in:
dry ice	deep freeze unit
liquid air	refrigerator
liquid hydrogen	
liquid nitrogen	

E901.8 Other specified origin

E901.9 Of unspecified origin

☑4ᵗʰ **E902 High and low air pressure and changes in air pressure**

E902.0 Residence or prolonged visit at high altitude
Residence or prolonged visit at high altitude as the cause of:
Acosta syndrome
Alpine sickness
altitude sickness
Andes disease
anoxia, hypoxia
barotitis, barodontalgia, barosinusitis, otitic barotrauma
hypobarism, hypobaropathy
mountain sickness
range disease

E902.1 In aircraft
Sudden change in air pressure in aircraft during ascent or descent as the cause of:
aeroneurosis
aviators' disease

E902.2 Due to diving
High air pressure from rapid descent in water
Reduction in atmospheric pressure while surfacing from deep water diving } as the cause of:
caisson disease
divers' disease
divers' palsy or paralysis

E902.8 Due to other specified causes
Reduction in atmospheric pressure while surfacing from underground

E902.9 Unspecified cause

E903 Travel and motion

E Codes

E904–E909.3

✓4ᵗʰ **E904 Hunger, thirst, exposure, and neglect**

> *EXCLUDES*   *any condition resulting from homicidal intent (E968.0-E968.9)*
> *hunger, thirst, and exposure resulting from accidents connected with transport (E800.0-E848)*

E904.0 Abandonment or neglect of infants and helpless persons

Exposure to weather conditions ⎤
Hunger or thirst   ⎦ resulting from abandonment or neglect

Desertion of newborn
Inattention at or after birth
Lack of care (helpless person) (infant)

> *EXCLUDES*   *criminal [purposeful] neglect (E968.4)*

E904.1 Lack of food

Lack of food as the cause of:
    inanition
    insufficient nourishment
    starvation

> *EXCLUDES*   *hunger resulting from abandonment or neglect (E904.0)*

E904.2 Lack of water

Lack of water as the cause of:
    dehydration
    inanition

> *EXCLUDES*   *dehydration due to acute fluid loss (276.51)*

E904.3 Exposure (to weather conditions), not elsewhere classifiable

Exposure NOS
Humidity
Struck by hailstones

> *EXCLUDES*   *struck by lightning (E907)*

E904.9 Privation, unqualified

Destitution

✓4ᵗʰ **E905 Venomous animals and plants as the cause of poisoning and toxic reactions**

> *INCLUDES*   *chemical released by animal*
> *insects*
> *release of venom through fangs, hairs, spines, tentacles, and other venom apparatus*

> *EXCLUDES*   *eating of poisonous animals or plants (E865.0-E865.9)*

E905.0 Venomous snakes and lizards

Cobra	Mamba
Copperhead snake	Rattlesnake
Coral snake	Sea snake
Fer de lance	Snake (venomous)
Gila monster	Viper
Krait	Water moccasin

> *EXCLUDES*   *bites of snakes and lizards known to be nonvenomous (E906.2)*

E905.1 Venomous spiders

Black widow spider
Brown spider
Tarantula (venomous)

E905.2 Scorpion

E905.3 Hornets, wasps, and bees

Yellow jacket

E905.4 Centipede and venomous millipede (tropical)

E905.5 Other venomous arthropods

Sting of:
    ant
    caterpillar

E905.6 Venomous marine animals and plants

Puncture by sea urchin spine
Sting of:
    coral
    jelly fish
    nematocysts
    sea anemone
    sea cucumber
    other marine animal or plant

> *EXCLUDES*   *bites and other injuries caused by nonvenomous marine animal (E906.2-E906.8)*
> *bite of sea snake (venomous) (E905.0)*

E905.7 Poisoning and toxic reactions caused by other plants

Injection of poisons or toxins into or through skin by plant thorns, spines, or other mechanisms

> *EXCLUDES*   *puncture wound NOS by plant thorns or spines (E920.8)*

E905.8 Other specified

E905.9 Unspecified

Sting NOS
Venomous bite NOS

✓4ᵗʰ **E906 Other injury caused by animals**

> *EXCLUDES*   *poisoning and toxic reactions caused by venomous animals and insects (E905.0-E905.9)*
> *road vehicle accident involving animals (E827.0-E828.9)*
> *tripping or falling over an animal (E885.9)*

E906.0 Dog bite

E906.1 Rat bite

E906.2 Bite of nonvenomous snakes and lizards

E906.3 Bite of other animal except arthropod

Cats	Rodents, except rats
Moray eel	Shark

E906.4 Bite of nonvenomous arthropod

Insect bite NOS

E906.5 Bite by unspecified animal

Animal bite NOS

E906.8 Other specified injury caused by animal

Butted by animal
Fallen on by horse or other animal, not being ridden
Gored by animal
Implantation of quills of porcupine
Pecked by bird
Run over by animal, not being ridden
Stepped on by animal, not being ridden

> *EXCLUDES*   *injury by animal being ridden (E828.0-E828.9)*

E906.9 Unspecified injury caused by animal

E907 Lightning

> *EXCLUDES*   *injury from:*
> *fall of tree or other object caused by lightning (E916)*
> *fire caused by lightning (E890.0-E892)*

✓4ᵗʰ **E908 Cataclysmic storms, and floods resulting from storms**

> *EXCLUDES*   *collapse of dam or man-made structure causing flood (E909.3)*

E908.0 Hurricane

Storm surge
"Tidal wave" caused by storm action
Typhoon

E908.1 Tornado

Cyclone
Twisters

E908.2 Floods

Torrential rainfall
Flash flood

> *EXCLUDES*   *collapse of dam or man-made structure causing flood (E909.3)*

E908.3 Blizzard (snow)(ice)

E908.4 Dust storm

E908.8 Other cataclysmic storms

Cloudburst

E908.9 Unspecified cataclysmic storms, and floods resulting from storms

Storm NOS

✓4ᵗʰ **E909 Cataclysmic earth surface movements and eruptions**

E909.0 Earthquakes

E909.1 Volcanic eruptions

Burns from lava
Ash inhalation

E909.2 Avalanche, landslide, or mudslide

E909.3 Collapse of dam or man-made structure

✓4ᵗʰ Fourth-digit Required   ▶◀ Revised Text   ● New Code   ▲ Revised Code TitleDx

E909.4 Tidalwave caused by earthquake
Tidalwave NOS
Tsunami
> *EXCLUDES*   *tidalwave caused by tropical storm (E908.0)*

E909.8 Other cataclysmic earth surface movements and eruptions

E909.9 Unspecified cataclysmic earth surface movements and eruptions

Accidents Caused by Submersion, Suffocation, and Foreign Bodies (E910-E915)

✓4ᵗʰ E910 Accidental drowning and submersion
> *INCLUDES*   immersion
> swimmers' cramp
> *EXCLUDES*   *diving accident (NOS) (resulting in injury except drowning)*
> *(E883.0)*
> *diving with insufficient air supply (E913.2)*
> *drowning and submersion due to:*
> *cataclysm (E908-E909)*
> *machinery accident (E919.0-E919.9)*
> *transport accident (E800.0-E845.9)*
> *effect of high and low air pressure (E902.2)*
> *injury from striking against objects while in running water*
> *(E917.2)*

E910.0 While water-skiing
Fall from water skis with submersion or drowning
> *EXCLUDES*   *accident to water-skier involving a watercraft and*
> *resulting in submersion or other injury*
> *(E830.4, E831.4)*

E910.1 While engaged in other sport or recreational activity with diving equipment
Scuba diving NOS
Skin diving NOS
Underwater spear fishing NOS

E910.2 While engaged in other sport or recreational activity without diving equipment
Fishing or hunting, except from boat or with diving equipment
Ice skating
Playing in water
Surfboarding
Swimming NOS
Voluntarily jumping from boat, not involved in accident, for swim NOS
Wading in water
> *EXCLUDES*   *jumping into water to rescue another person*
> *(E910.3)*

E910.3 While swimming or diving for purposes other than recreation or sport
Marine salvage
Pearl diving
Placement of fishing nets   (with diving equipment)
Rescue (attempt) of another person
Underwater construction or repairs

E910.4 In bathtub

E910.8 Other accidental drowning or submersion
Drowning in:
quenching tank
swimming pool

E910.9 Unspecified accidental drowning or submersion
Accidental fall into water NOS
Drowning NOS

E911 Inhalation and ingestion of food causing obstruction of respiratory tract or suffocation
Aspiration and inhalation of food [any] (into respiratory tract) NOS
Asphyxia by
Choked on   food [including bone, seed in food, regurgitated food]
Suffocation by
Compression of trachea
Interruption of respiration   by food lodged in esophagus
Obstruction of respiration
Obstruction of pharynx by food (bolus)
> *EXCLUDES*   *injury, except asphyxia and obstruction of respiratory*
> *passage, caused by food (E915)*
> *obstruction of esophagus by food without mention of*
> *asphyxia or obstruction of respiratory passage (E915)*

E912 Inhalation and ingestion of other object causing obstruction of respiratory tract or suffocation
Aspiration and inhalation of foreign body except food (into respiratory tract) NOS
Foreign object [bean] [marble] in nose
Obstruction of pharynx by foreign body
Compression
Interruption of respiration   by foreign body in esophagus
Obstruction of respiration
> *EXCLUDES*   *injury, except asphyxia and obstruction of respiratory*
> *passage, caused by foreign body (E915)*
> *obstruction of esophagus by foreign body without mention*
> *of asphyxia or obstruction in respiratory passage*
> *(E915)*

✓4ᵗʰ E913 Accidental mechanical suffocation
> *EXCLUDES*   *mechanical suffocation from or by:*
> *accidental inhalation or ingestion of:*
> *food (E911)*
> *foreign object (E912)*
> *cataclysm (E908-E909)*
> *explosion (E921.0-E921.9, E923.0-E923.9)*
> *machinery accident (E919.0-E919.9)*

E913.0 In bed or cradle
> *EXCLUDES*   *suffocation by plastic bag (E913.1)*

E913.1 By plastic bag

E913.2 Due to lack of air (in closed place)
Accidentally closed up in refrigerator or other airtight enclosed space
Diving with insufficient air supply
> *EXCLUDES*   *suffocation by plastic bag (E913.1)*

E913.3 By falling earth or other substance
Cave-in NOS
> *EXCLUDES*   *cave-in caused by cataclysmic earth surface*
> *movements and eruptions (E909)*
> *struck by cave-in without asphyxiation or*
> *suffocation (E916)*

E913.8 Other specified means
Accidental hanging, except in bed or cradle

E913.9 Unspecified means
Asphyxia, mechanical NOS
Strangulation NOS
Suffocation NOS

E914 Foreign body accidentally entering eye and adnexa
> *EXCLUDES*   *corrosive liquid (E924.1)*

E915 Foreign body accidentally entering other orifice
> *EXCLUDES*   *aspiration and inhalation of foreign body, any, (into*
> *respiratory tract) NOS (E911-E912)*

Other Accidents (E916-E928)

E916 Struck accidentally by falling object
    Collapse of building, except on fire
    Falling:
        rock
        snowslide NOS
        stone
        tree
    Object falling from:
        machine, not in operation
        stationary vehicle

    Code first:
        collapse of building on fire (E890.0-E891.9)
        falling object in:
            cataclysm (E908-E909)
            machinery accidents (E919.0-E919.9)
            transport accidents (E800.0-E845.9)
            vehicle accidents not elsewhere classifiable (E846-E848)
        object set in motion by:
            explosion (E921.0-E921.9, E923.0-E923.9)
            firearm (E922.0-E922.9)
            projected object (E917.0-E917.9)

✓4ᵗʰ E917 Striking against or struck accidentally by objects or persons
    INCLUDES   bumping into or
                against   object (moving) (projected)
          colliding with   (stationary)
          kicking against   pedestrian conveyance
          stepping on   person
          struck by
    EXCLUDES *fall from:*
        collision with another person, except when caused by a
            crowd (E886.0-E886.9)
        stumbling over object (E885.9)
        fall resulting in striking against object (E888.0, E888.1)
        injury caused by:
            assault (E960.0-E960.1, E967.0-E967.9)
            cutting or piercing instrument (E920.0-E920.9)
            explosion (E921.0-E921.9, E923.0-E923.9)
            firearm (E922.0-E922.9)
            machinery (E919.0-E919.9)
            transport vehicle (E800.0-E845.9)
            vehicle not elsewhere classifiable (E846-E848)

E917.0 In sports without subsequent fall
    Kicked or stepped on during game (football) (rugby)
    Struck by hit or thrown ball
    Struck by hockey stick or puck

E917.1 Caused by a crowd, by collective fear or panic without subsequent fall
    Crushed
    Pushed   by crowd or human
    Stepped on   stampede

E917.2 In running water without subsequent fall
    EXCLUDES *drowning or submersion (E910.0-E910.9)*
            that in sports (E917.0, E917.5)

E917.3 Furniture without subsequent fall
    EXCLUDES *fall from furniture (E884.2, E884.4-E884.5)*

E917.4 Other stationary object without subsequent fall
    Bath tub
    Fence
    Lamp-post

E917.5 Object in sports with subsequent fall
    Knocked down while boxing

E917.6 Caused by a crowd, by collective fear or panic with subsequent fall

E917.7 Furniture with subsequent fall
    EXCLUDES *fall from furniture (E884.2, E884.4-E884.5)*

E917.8 Other stationary object with subsequent fall
    Bath tub
    Fence
    Lamp-post

E917.9 Other striking against with or without subsequent fall

E918 Caught accidentally in or between objects
    Caught, crushed, jammed, or pinched in or between moving or
        stationary objects, such as:
    escalator
    folding object
    hand tools, appliances, or implements
    sliding door and door frame
    under packing crate
    washing machine wringer
    EXCLUDES *injury caused by:*
        cutting or piercing instrument (E920.0-E920.9)
        machinery (E919.0-E919.9)
        mechanism or component of firearm and air gun
            (E928.7)
        transport vehicle (E800.0-E845.9)
        vehicle not elsewhere classifiable (E846-E848)
        struck accidentally by:
            falling object (E916)
            object (moving) (projected) (E917.0-E917.9)

✓4ᵗʰ E919 Accidents caused by machinery
    INCLUDES   burned by
        caught in (moving parts of)
        collapse of
        crushed by
        cut or pierced by
        drowning or submersion caused by
        explosion of, on, in
        fall from or into moving part of   machinery
        fire starting in or on   (accident)
        mechanical suffocation caused by
        object falling from, on, in motion
            by
        overturning of
        pinned under
        run over by
        struck by
        thrown from

    caught between machinery and other object
    machinery accident NOS
    EXCLUDES *accidents involving machinery, not in operation (E884.9,*
        E916-E918)
        injury caused by:
        electric current in connection with machinery
            (E925.0-E925.9)
        escalator (E880.0, E918)
        explosion of pressure vessel in connection with
            machinery (E921.0-E921.9)
        mechanism or component of firearm and air gun
            (E928.7)
        moving sidewalk (E885.9)
        powered hand tools, appliances, and implements
            (E916-E918, E920.0-E921.9, E923.0-E926.9)
        transport vehicle accidents involving machinery
            (E800.0-E848)
        poisoning by carbon monoxide generated by machine
            (E868.8)

E919.0 Agricultural machines

Animal-powered	Farm tractor
agricultural machine	Harvester
Combine	Hay mower or rake
Derrick, hay	Reaper
Farm machinery NOS	Thresher

    EXCLUDES *that in transport under own power on the highway*
        (E810.0-E819.9)
        that being towed by another vehicle on the
            highway (E810.0-E819.9, E827.0-E827.9,
            E829.0-E829.9)
        that involved in accident classifiable to E820-E829
            (E820.0-E829.9)

E919.1 Mining and earth-drilling machinery
    Bore or drill (land) (seabed)
    Shaft hoist
    Shaft lift
    Under-cutter
    EXCLUDES *coal car, tram, truck, and tub in mine (E846)*

    ✓4ᵗʰ Fourth-digit Required   ▶◀ Revised Text   ● New Code   ▲ Revised Code TitleDx

E919.2 Lifting machines and appliances

Chain hoist
Crane
Derrick
Elevator (building) (grain)   except in agricultural
Forklift truck   or mining
Lift   operations
Pulley block
Winch

EXCLUDES that being towed by another vehicle on the highway (E810.0-E819.9, E827.0-E827.9, E829.0-829.9)
that in transport under own power on the highway (E810.0-E819.9)
that involved in accident classifiable to E820-E829 (E820-E829.9)

E919.3 Metalworking machines

Abrasive wheel   Metal:
Forging machine   milling machine
Lathe   power press
Mechanical shears   rolling-mill
Metal: sawing machine
   drilling machine

E919.4 Woodworking and forming machines

Band saw   Overhead plane
Bench saw   Powered saw
Circular saw   Radial saw
Molding machine   Sander

EXCLUDES hand saw (E920.1)

E919.5 Prime movers, except electrical motors

Gas turbine
Internal combustion engine
Steam engine
Water driven turbine

EXCLUDES that being towed by other vehicle on the highway (E810.0-E819.9, E827.0-E827.9, E829.0-E829.9)
that in transport under own power on the highway (E810.0-E819.9)

E919.6 Transmission machinery

Transmission: Transmission:
belt   pinion
cable   pulley
chain   shaft
gear

E919.7 Earth moving, scraping, and other excavating machines

Bulldozer   Steam shovel
Road scraper

EXCLUDES that being towed by other vehicle on the highway (E810.0-E819.9, E827.0-E827.9, E829.0-E829.9)
that in transport under own power on the highway (E810.0-E819.9)

E919.8 Other specified machinery

Machines for manufacture of:
   clothing
   foodstuffs and beverages
   paper
Printing machine
Recreational machinery
Spinning, weaving, and textile machines

E919.9 Unspecified machinery

✓4ᵗʰ E920 Accidents caused by cutting and piercing instruments or objects

INCLUDES
                                    edged
accidental injury (by) object   pointed
                                    sharp

EXCLUDES injury caused by mechanism or component of firearm and air gun (E928.7)

E920.0 Powered lawn mower

E920.1 Other powered hand tools

Any powered hand tool [compressed air] [electric] [explosive cartridge] [hydraulic power], such as:
drill
hand saw
hedge clipper
rivet gun
snow blower
staple gun

EXCLUDES band saw (E919.4)
bench saw (E919.4)

E920.2 Powered household appliances and implements

Blender   Electric:
Electric: knife
   beater or mixer   sewing machine
   can opener   Garbage disposal appliance
   fan

E920.3 Knives, swords, and daggers

E920.4 Other hand tools and implements

Axe   Paper cutter
Can opener NOS   Pitchfork
Chisel   Rake
Fork   Scissors
Hand saw   Screwdriver
Hoe   Sewing machine, not powered
Ice pick   Shovel
Needle (sewing)

E920.5 Hypodermic needle

Contaminated needle
Needle stick

E920.8 Other specified cutting and piercing instruments or objects

Arrow   Nail
Broken glass   Plant thorn
Dart   Splinter
Edge of stiff paper Tin can lid
Lathe turnings

EXCLUDES animal spines or quills (E906.8)
flying glass due to explosion (E921.0-E923.9)

E920.9 Unspecified cutting and piercing instrument or object

✓4ᵗʰ E921 Accident caused by explosion of pressure vessel

INCLUDES accidental explosion of pressure vessels, whether or not part of machinery

EXCLUDES explosion of pressure vessel on transport vehicle (E800.0-E845.9)

E921.0 Boilers

E921.1 Gas cylinders

Air tank   Pressure gas tank

E921.8 Other specified pressure vessels

Aerosol can   Tin can lid
Automobile tire

E921.9 Unspecified pressure vessel

✓4ᵗʰ E922 Accident caused by firearm, and air gun missile

EXCLUDES injury caused by mechanism or component of firearm and air gun (E928./)

E922.0 Handgun

Pistol   Revolver

EXCLUDES Verey pistol (E922.8)

E922.1 Shotgun (automatic)

E922.2 Hunting rifle

E922.3 Military firearms

Army rifle   Machine gun

E922.4 Air gun

BB gun   Pellet gun

E922.5 Paintball gun

E922.8 Other specified firearm missile

Verey pistol [flare]

E922.9 Unspecified firearm missile

Gunshot wound NOS
Shot NOS

E Codes

E923–E926.5

✓4ᵗʰ E923   Accident caused by explosive material

> INCLUDES flash burns and other injuries resulting from explosion of
>   explosive material
>   ignition of highly explosive material with explosion
>
> EXCLUDES *explosion:*
>   *in or on machinery (E919.0-E919.9)*
>   *on any transport vehicle, except stationary motor vehicle*
>   *(E800.0-E848)*
>   *with conflagration (E890.0, E891.0,E892)*
>   *injury caused by mechanism or component of firearm and*
>   *air gun (E928.7)*
>   *secondary fires resulting from explosion (E890.0-E899)*

E923.0   Fireworks

E923.1   Blasting materials
>   Blasting cap   Dynamite
>   Detonator   Explosive [any] used in blasting
>   operations

E923.2   Explosive gases
>   Acetylene   Fire damp
>   Butane   Gasoline fumes
>   Coal gas   Methane
>   Explosion in mine NOS   Propane

E923.8   Other explosive materials
>   Bomb   Torpedo
>   Explosive missile   Explosion in munitions:
>   Grenade   dump
>   Mine   factory
>   Shell

E923.9   Unspecified explosive material
>   Explosion NOS

**✓4ᵗʰ E924   Accident caused by hot substance or object, caustic or
corrosive material, and steam**

> EXCLUDES *burning NOS (E899)*
>   *chemical burn resulting from swallowing a corrosive*
>   *substance (E860.0-E864.4)*
>   *fire caused by these substances and objects (E890.0-E894)*
>   *radiation burns (E926.0-E926.9)*
>   *therapeutic misadventures (E870.0-E876.9)*

E924.0   Hot liquids and vapors, including steam
>   Burning or scalding by:
>   boiling water
>   hot or boiling liquids not primarily caustic or corrosive
>   liquid metal
>   steam
>   other hot vapor
>   EXCLUDES *hot (boiling) tap water (E924.2)*

E924.1   Caustic and corrosive substances
>   Burning by:
>   acid [any kind]
>   ammonia
>   caustic oven cleaner or other substance
>   corrosive substance
>   lye
>   vitriol

E924.2   Hot (boiling) tap water

E924.8   Other
>   Burning by:
>   heat from electric heating appliance
>   hot object NOS
>   light bulb
>   steam pipe

E924.9   Unspecified

✓4ᵗʰ E925   Accident caused by electric current

> INCLUDES electric current from exposed wire, faulty appliance, high
>   voltage cable, live rail, or open electric socket as
>   the cause of:
>   burn
>   cardiac fibrillation
>   convulsion
>   electric shock
>   electrocution
>   puncture wound
>   respiratory paralysis
>
> EXCLUDES *burn by heat from electrical appliance (E924.8)*
>   *lightning (E907)*

E925.0   Domestic wiring and appliances

**E925.1   Electric power generating plants, distribution stations,
transmission lines**
>   Broken power line

E925.2   Industrial wiring, appliances, and electrical machinery
>   Conductors
>   Control apparatus
>   Electrical equipment and machinery
>   Transformers

E925.8   Other electric current
>   Wiring and appliances in or on:
>   farm [not farmhouse]
>   outdoors
>   public building
>   residential institutions
>   schools

E925.9   Unspecified electric current
>   Burns or other injury from electric current NOS
>   Electric shock NOS
>   Electrocution NOS

✓4ᵗʰ E926   Exposure to radiation

> EXCLUDES *abnormal reaction to or complication of treatment without*
>   *mention of misadventure (E879.2)*
>   *atomic power plant malfunction in water transport*
>   *(E838.0-E838.9)*
>   *misadventure to patient in surgical and medical procedures*
>   *(E873.2-E873.3)*
>   *use of radiation in war operations (E996-E997.9)*

E926.0   Radiofrequency radiation

Overexposure to:	from:
microwave radiation	high-powered radio and
radar radiation	television transmitters
radiofrequency	industrial radiofrequency
radiofrequency	induction heaters
radiation [any]	radar installations

E926.1   Infrared heaters and lamps
>   Exposure to infrared radiation from heaters and lamps as
>   the cause of:
>   blistering
>   burning
>   charring
>   inflammatory change
>   EXCLUDES *physical contact with heater or lamp (E924.8)*

E926.2   Visible and ultraviolet light sources
>   Arc lamps
>   Black light sources
>   Electrical welding arc
>   Oxygas welding torch
>   Sun rays
>   Tanning bed
>   EXCLUDES *excessive heat from these sources (E900.1-E900.9)*

E926.3   X-rays and other electromagnetic ionizing radiation
>   Gamma rays
>   X-rays (hard) (soft)

E926.4   Lasers

E926.5   Radioactive isotopes
>   Radiobiologicals
>   Radiopharmaceuticals

E926.8 Other specified radiation
Artificially accelerated beams of ionized particles generated by:
betatrons
synchrotrons

E926.9 Unspecified radiation
Radiation NOS

☑4ᵗʰ **E927 Overexertion and strenuous and repetitive movements or loads**
Use additional code to identify activity (E001-E030)

E927.0 Overexertion from sudden strenuous movement
Sudden trauma from strenuous movement

E927.1 Overexertion from prolonged static position
Overexertion from maintaining prolonged positions, such as:
holding
sitting
standing

E927.2 Excessive physical exertion from prolonged activity

E927.3 Cumulative trauma from repetitive motion
Cumulative trauma from repetitive movements

E927.4 Cumulative trauma from repetitive impact

E927.8 Other overexertion and strenuous and repetitive movements or loads

E927.9 Unspecified overexertion and strenuous and repetitive movements or loads

☑4ᵗʰ **E928 Other and unspecified environmental and accidental causes**

E928.0 Prolonged stay in weightless environment
Weightlessness in spacecraft (simulator)

E928.1 Exposure to noise
Noise (pollution)
Sound waves
Supersonic waves

E928.2 Vibration

E928.3 Human bite

E928.4 External constriction caused by hair

E928.5 External constriction caused by other object

E928.6 Environmental exposure to harmful algae and toxins
Algae bloom NOS
Blue-green algae bloom
Brown tide
Cyanobacteria bloom
Florida red tide
Harmful algae bloom
Pfiesteria piscicida
Red tide

E928.7 Mechanism or component of firearm and air gun
Injury due to:
explosion of gun parts
recoil
Pierced, cut, crushed, or pinched by slide, trigger mechanism, scope, or other gun part
Powder burn from firearm or air gun
EXCLUDES accident caused by firearm and air gun missile (E922.0-E922.9)

E928.8 Other

E928.9 Unspecified accident
Accident NOS
Blow NOS
Casualty (not due to war)
Decapitation
} stated as accidentally inflicted

Knocked down
Killed
Injury [any part of body, or unspecified]
Mangled
Wound
} stated as accidentally inflicted, but not otherwise specified

*EXCLUDES fracture, cause unspecified (E887)
injuries undetermined whether accidentally or purposely inflicted (E980.0-E989)*

Late Effects Of Accidental Injury (E929)

NOTE This category is to be used to indicate accidental injury as the cause of death or disability from late effects, which are themselves classifiable elsewhere. The "late effects" include conditions reported as such, or as sequelae which may occur at any time after the attempted suicide or self-inflicted injury.

☑4ᵗʰ **E929 Late effects of accidental injury**
*EXCLUDES late effects of:
surgical and medical procedures (E870.0-E879.9)
therapeutic use of drugs and medicines (E930.0-E949.9)*

E929.0 Late effects of motor vehicle accident
Late effects of accidents classifiable to E810-E825

E929.1 Late effects of other transport accident
Late effects of accidents classifiable to E800-E807, E826-E838, E840-E848

E929.2 Late effects of accidental poisoning
Late effects of accidents classifiable to E850-E858, E860-E869

E929.3 Late effects of accidental fall
Late effects of accidents classifiable to E880-E888

E929.4 Late effects of accident caused by fire
Late effects of accidents classifiable to E890-E899

E929.5 Late effects of accident due to natural and environmental factors
Late effects of accidents classifiable to E900-E909

E929.8 Late effects of other accidents
Late effects of accidents classifiable to E910-E928.8

E929.9 Late effects of unspecified accident
Late effects of accidents classifiable to E928.9

Drugs, Medicinal And Biological Substances Causing Adverse Effects In Therapeutic Use (E930-E949)

INCLUDES correct drug properly administered in therapeutic or prophylactic dosage, as the cause of any adverse effect including allergic or hypersensitivity reactions

*EXCLUDES accidental overdose of drug and wrong drug given or taken in error (E850.0-E858.9)
accidents in the technique of administration of drug or biological substance, such as accidental puncture during injection, or contamination of drug (E870.0-E876.9)
administration with suicidal or homicidal intent or intent to harm, or in circumstances classifiable to E950.0-E950.5, E962.0, E980.0-E980.5*

NOTE See Alphabetic Index for more complete list of specific drugs to be classified under the fourth-digit subdivisions. The American Hospital Formulary numbers can be used to classify new drugs listed by the American Hospital Formulary Service (AHFS). See Appendix C.

☑4ᵗʰ **E930 Antibiotics**
EXCLUDES that used as eye, ear, nose, and throat [ENT], and local anti-infectives (E946.0-E946.9)

E930.0 Penicillins
Natural
Synthetic
Semisynthetic, such as:
ampicillin
Semisynthetic, such as:
cloxacillin
nafcillin
oxacillin

E930.1 Antifungal antibiotics
Amphotericin B
Griseofulvin
Hachimycin [trichomycin]
Nystatin

E930.2 Chloramphenicol group
Chloramphenicol
Thiamphenicol

E930.3 Erythromycin and other macrolides
Oleandomycin
Spiramycin

E930.4 Tetracycline group
Doxycycline
Minocycline
Oxytetracycline

E930.5 Cephalosporin group
Cephalexin
Cephaloglycin
Cephaloridine
Cephalothin

E930.6 Antimycobacterial antibiotics
Cycloserine
Kanamycin
Rifampin
Streptomycin

E Codes

E930.7–E934.1

E930.7 Antineoplastic antibiotics
Actinomycins, such as:
Bleomycin
Cactinomycin
Dactinomycin
Daunorubicin
Mitomycin
EXCLUDES *other antineoplastic drugs (E933.1)*

E930.8 Other specified antibiotics

E930.9 Unspecified antibiotic

✓4ᵗʰ **E931 Other anti-infectives**
EXCLUDES *ENT, and local anti-infectives (E946.0-E946.9)*

E931.0 Sulfonamides
Sulfadiazine
Sulfafurazole
Sulfamethoxazole

E931.1 Arsenical anti-infectives

E931.2 Heavy metal anti-infectives
Compounds of:
antimony
bismuth
lead
mercury
EXCLUDES *mercurial diuretics (E944.0)*

E931.3 Quinoline and hydroxyquinoline derivatives
Chiniofon
Diiodohydroxyquin
EXCLUDES *antimalarial drugs (E931.4)*

E931.4 Antimalarials and drugs acting on other blood protozoa
Chloroquine phosphate   Proguanil [chloroguanide]
Cycloguanil   Pyrimethamine
Primaquine   Quinine (sulphate)

E931.5 Other antiprotozoal drugs
Emetine

E931.6 Anthelmintics
Hexylresorcinol   Piperazine
Male fern oleoresin   Thiabendazole

E931.7 Antiviral drugs
Methisazone
EXCLUDES *amantadine (E936.4)*
cytarabine (E933.1)
idoxuridine (E946.5)

E931.8 Other antimycobacterial drugs
Ethambutol
Ethionamide
Isoniazid
Para-aminosalicylic acid derivatives
Sulfones

E931.9 Other and unspecified anti-infectives
Flucytosine
Nitrofuranderivatives

✓4ᵗʰ **E932 Hormones and synthetic substitutes**

E932.0 Adrenal cortical steroids
Cortisone derivatives
Desoxycorticosterone derivatives
Fluorinated corticosteroid

E932.1 Androgens and anabolic congeners
Nandrolone phenpropionate
Oxymetholone
Testosterone and preparations

E932.2 Ovarian hormones and synthetic substitutes
Contraceptives, oral
Estrogens
Estrogens and progestogens combined
Progestogens

E932.3 Insulins and antidiabetic agents
Acetohexamide
Biguanide derivatives, oral
Chlorpropamide
Glucagon
Insulin
Phenformin
Sulfonylurea derivatives, oral
Tolbutamide
EXCLUDES *adverse effect of insulin administered for shock therapy (E879.3)*

E932.4 Anterior pituitary hormones
Corticotropin
Gonadotropin
Somatotropin [growth hormone]

E932.5 Posterior pituitary hormones
Vasopressin
EXCLUDES *oxytocic agents (E945.0)*

E932.6 Parathyroid and parathyroid derivatives

E932.7 Thyroid and thyroid derivatives
Dextrothyroxine
Levothyroxine sodium
Liothyronine
Thyroglobulin

E932.8 Antithyroid agents
Iodides
Thiouracil
Thiourea

E932.9 Other and unspecified hormones and synthetic substitutes

✓4ᵗʰ **E933 Primarily systemic agents**

E933.0 Antiallergic and antiemetic drugs
Antihistamines   Diphenylpyraline
Chlorpheniramine   Thonzylamine
Diphenhydramine   Tripelennamine
EXCLUDES *phenothiazine-based tranquilizers (E939.1)*

E933.1 Antineoplastic and immunosuppressive drugs
Azathioprine
Busulfan
Chlorambucil
Cyclophosphamide
Cytarabine
Fluorouracil
Mechlorethamine hydrochloride
Mercaptopurine
Triethylenethiophosphoramide [thio-TEPA]
EXCLUDES *antineoplastic antibiotics (E930.7)*

E933.2 Acidifying agents

E933.3 Alkalizing agents

E933.4 Enzymes, not elsewhere classified
Penicillinase

E933.5 Vitamins, not elsewhere classified
Vitamin A
Vitamin D
EXCLUDES *nicotinic acid (E942.2)*
vitamin K (E934.3)

E933.6 Oral bisphosphonates

E933.7 Intravenous bisphosphonates

E933.8 Other systemic agents, not elsewhere classified
Heavy metal antagonists

E933.9 Unspecified systemic agent

✓4ᵗʰ **E934 Agents primarily affecting blood constituents**

E934.0 Iron and its compounds
Ferric salts
Ferrous sulphate and other ferrous salts

E934.1 Liver preparations and other antianemic agents
Folic acid

✓4ᵗʰ Fourth-digit Required   ►◄ Revised Text   ● New Code   ▲ Revised Code TitleDx

E934.2 Anticoagulants
Coumarin
Heparin
Phenindione
Prothrombin synthesis inhibitor
Warfarin sodium

E934.3 Vitamin K [phytonadione]

E934.4 Fibrinolysis-affecting drugs
Aminocaproic acid   Streptokinase
Streptodornase   Urokinase

E934.5 Anticoagulant antagonists and other coagulants
Hexadimethrine bromide
Protamine sulfate

E934.6 Gamma globulin

E934.7 Natural blood and blood products
Blood plasma
Human fibrinogen
Packed red cells
Whole blood

E934.8 Other agents affecting blood constituents
Macromolecular blood substitutes

E934.9 Unspecified agent affecting blood constituents

✓4ᵗʰ **E935 Analgesics, antipyretics, and antirheumatics**

E935.0 Heroin
Diacetylmorphine

E935.1 Methadone

E935.2 Other opiates and related narcotics
Codeine [methylmorphine]
Meperidine [pethidine]
Morphine
Opium (alkaloids)

E935.3 Salicylates
Acetylsalicylic acid [aspirin]
Amino derivatives of salicylic acid
Salicylic acid salts

E935.4 Aromatic analgesics, not elsewhere classified
Acetanilid
Paracetamol [acetaminophen]
Phenacetin [acetophenetidin]

E935.5 Pyrazole derivatives
Aminophenazone [aminopyrine]
Phenylbutazone

E935.6 Antirheumatics [antiphlogistics]
Gold salts
Indomethacin
EXCLUDES *salicylates (E935.3)*
steroids (E932.0)

E935.7 Other non-narcotic analgesics
Pyrabital

E935.8 Other specified analgesics and antipyretics
Pentazocine

E935.9 Unspecified analgesic and antipyretic

✓4ᵗʰ **E936 Anticonvulsants and anti-Parkinsonism drugs**

E936.0 Oxazolidine derivatives
Paramethadione
Trimethadione

E936.1 Hydantoin derivatives
Phenytoin

E936.2 Succinimides
Ethosuximide
Phensuximide

E936.3 Other and unspecified anticonvulsants
Beclamide
Primidone

E936.4 Anti-Parkinsonism drugs
Amantadine
Ethopropazine [profenamine]
Levodopa [L-dopa]

✓4ᵗʰ **E937 Sedatives and hypnotics**

E937.0 Barbiturates
Amobarbital [amylobarbitone]
Barbital [barbitone]
Butabarbital [butabarbitone]
Pentobarbital [pentobarbitone]
Phenobarbital [phenobarbitone]
Secobarbital [quinalbarbitone]
EXCLUDES *thiobarbiturates (E938.3)*

E937.1 Chloral hydrate group

E937.2 Paraldehyde

E937.3 Bromine compounds
Bromide
Carbromal (derivatives)

E937.4 Methaqualone compounds

E937.5 Glutethimide group

E937.6 Mixed sedatives, not elsewhere classified

E937.8 Other sedatives and hypnotics

E937.9 Unspecified
Sleeping:
drug ⎫
pill ⎬ NOS
tablet ⎭

✓4ᵗʰ **E938 Other central nervous system depressants and anesthetics**

E938.0 Central nervous system muscle-tone depressants
Chlorphenesin (carbamate)
Mephenesin
Methocarbamol

E938.1 Halothane

E938.2 Other gaseous anesthetics
Ether
Halogenated hydrocarbon derivatives, except halothane
Nitrous oxide

E938.3 Intravenous anesthetics
Ketamine
Methohexital [methohexitone]
Thiobarbiturates, such as thiopental sodium

E938.4 Other and unspecified general anesthetics

E938.5 Surface and infiltration anesthetics
Cocaine
Lidocaine [lignocaine]
Procaine
Tetracaine

E938.6 Peripheral nerve- and plexus-blocking anesthetics

E938.7 Spinal anesthetics

E938.9 Other and unspecified local anesthetics

✓4ᵗʰ **E939 Psychotropic agents**

E939.0 Antidepressants
Amitriptyline
Imipramine
Monoamine oxidase [MAO] Inhibitors

E939.1 Phenothiazine-based tranquilizers
Chlorpromazine   Prochlorperazine
Fluphenazine   Promazine
Phenothiazine

E939.2 Butyrophenone-based tranquilizers
Haloperidol
Spiperone
Trifluperidol

E939.3 Other antipsychotics, neuroleptics, and major tranquilizers

E939.4 Benzodiazepine-based tranquilizers
Chlordiazepoxide   Lorazepam
Diazepam   Medazepam
Flurazepam   Nitrazepam

E939.5 Other tranquilizers
Hydroxyzine
Meprobamate

✓4ᵗʰ Fourth-digit Required   ▶◀ Revised Text   ● New Code   ▲ Revised Code TitleDx

E939.6 Psychodysleptics [hallucinogens]
Cannabis (derivatives)   Mescaline
Lysergide [LSD]   Psilocin
Marihuana (derivatives)   Psilocybin

E939.7 Psychostimulants
Amphetamine
Caffeine
> **EXCLUDES** *central appetite depressants (E947.0)*

E939.8 Other psychotropic agents

E939.9 Unspecified psychotropic agent

☑4ᵗʰ **E940 Central nervous system stimulants**

E940.0 Analeptics
Lobeline
Nikethamide

E940.1 Opiate antagonists
Levallorphan
Nalorphine
Naloxone

E940.8 Other specified central nervous system stimulants

E940.9 Unspecified central nervous system stimulant

☑4ᵗʰ **E941 Drugs primarily affecting the autonomic nervous system**

E941.0 Parasympathomimetics [cholinergics]
Acetylcholine
Anticholinesterase:
   organophosphorus
   reversible
Pilocarpine

E941.1 Parasympatholytics [anticholinergics and antimuscarinics] and spasmolytics
Atropine
Homatropine
Hyoscine [scopolamine]
Quaternary ammonium derivatives
> **EXCLUDES** *papaverine (E942.5)*

E941.2 Sympathomimetics [adrenergics]
Epinephrine [adrenalin]
Levarterenol [noradrenalin]

E941.3 Sympatholytics [antiadrenergics]
Phenoxybenzamine
Tolazolinehydrochloride

E941.9 Unspecified drug primarily affecting the autonomic nervous system

☑4ᵗʰ **E942 Agents primarily affecting the cardiovascular system**

E942.0 Cardiac rhythm regulators
Practolol   Propranolol
Procainamide   Quinidine

E942.1 Cardiotonic glycosides and drugs of similar action
Digitalis glycosides   Strophanthins
Digoxin

E942.2 Antilipemic and antiarteriosclerotic drugs
Cholestyramine   Nicotinic acid derivatives
Clofibrate   Sitosterols
> **EXCLUDES** *dextrothyroxine (E932.7)*

E942.3 Ganglion-blocking agents
Pentamethonium bromide

E942.4 Coronary vasodilators
Dipyridamole   Nitrites
Nitrates [nitroglycerin]   Prenylamine

E942.5 Other vasodilators
Cyclandelate   Hydralazine
Diazoxide   Papaverine

E942.6 Other antihypertensive agents
Clonidine   Rauwolfia alkaloids
Guanethidine   Reserpine

E942.7 Antivaricose drugs, including sclerosing agents
Monoethanolamine
Zinc salts

E942.8 Capillary-active drugs
Adrenochrome derivatives
Bioflavonoids
Metaraminol

E942.9 Other and unspecified agents primarily affecting the cardiovascular system

☑4ᵗʰ **E943 Agents primarily affecting gastrointestinal system**

E943.0 Antacids and antigastric secretion drugs
Aluminum hydroxide
Magnesium trisilicate

E943.1 Irritant cathartics
Bisacodyl
Castor oil
Phenolphthalein

E943.2 Emollient cathartics
Sodium dioctyl sulfosuccinate

E943.3 Other cathartics, including intestinal atonia drugs
Magnesium sulfate

E943.4 Digestants
Pancreatin
Papain
Pepsin

E943.5 Antidiarrheal drugs
Bismuth subcarbonate
Pectin
Kaolin
> **EXCLUDES** *anti-infectives (E930.0-E931.9)*

E943.6 Emetics

E943.8 Other specified agents primarily affecting the gastrointestinal system

E943.9 Unspecified agent primarily affecting the gastrointestinal system

☑4ᵗʰ **E944 Water, mineral, and uric acid metabolism drugs**

E944.0 Mercurial diuretics
Chlormerodrin   Mercurophylline
Mercaptomerin   Mersalyl

E944.1 Purine derivative diuretics
Theobromine
Theophylline
> **EXCLUDES** *aminophylline [theophylline ethylenediamine] (E945.7)*

E944.2 Carbonic acid anhydrase inhibitors
Acetazolamide

E944.3 Saluretics
Benzothiadiazides
Chlorothiazide group

E944.4 Other diuretics
Ethacrynic acid   Furosemide

E944.5 Electrolytic, caloric, and water-balance agents

E944.6 Other mineral salts, not elsewhere classified

E944.7 Uric acid metabolism drugs
Cinchophen and congeners
Colchicine
Phenoquin
Probenecid

☑4ᵗʰ **E945 Agents primarily acting on the smooth and skeletal muscles and respiratory system**

E945.0 Oxytocic agents
Ergot alkaloids
Prostaglandins

E945.1 Smooth muscle relaxants
Adiphenine
Metaproterenol [orciprenaline]
> **EXCLUDES** *papaverine (E942.5)*

E945.2 Skeletal muscle relaxants
Alcuronium chloride
Suxamethonium chloride

E945.3 Other and unspecified drugs acting on muscles

☑4ᵗʰ Fourth-digit Required   ►◄ Revised Text   ● New Code   ▲ Revised Code TitleDx

E945.4 Antitussives
Dextromethorphan
Pipazethate hydrochloride

E945.5 Expectorants
Acetylcysteine
Cocillana
Guaifenesin [glyceryl guaiacolate]
Ipecacuanha
Terpin hydrate

E945.6 Anti-common cold drugs

E945.7 Antiasthmatics
Aminophylline [theophylline ethylenediamine]

E945.8 Other and unspecified respiratory drugs

☑4ᵗʰ **E946 Agents primarily affecting skin and mucous membrane, ophthalmological, otorhinolaryngological, and dental drugs**

E946.0 Local anti-infectives and anti-inflammatory drugs

E946.1 Antipruritics

E946.2 Local astringents and local detergents

E946.3 Emollients, demulcents, and protectants

E946.4 Keratolytics, kerstoplastics, other hair treatment drugs and preparations

E946.5 Eye anti-infectives and other eye drugs
Idoxuridine

E946.6 Anti-infectives and other drugs and preparations for ear, nose, and throat

E946.7 Dental drugs topically applied

E946.8 Other agents primarily affecting skin and mucous membrane
Spermicides

E946.9 Unspecified agent primarily affecting skin and mucous membrane

☑4ᵗʰ **E947 Other and unspecified drugs and medicinal substances**

E947.0 Dietetics

E947.1 Lipotropic drugs

E947.2 Antidotes and chelating agents, not elsewhere classified

E947.3 Alcohol deterrents

E947.4 Pharmaceutical excipients

E947.8 Other drugs and medicinal substances
Contrast media used for diagnostic x-ray procedures
Diagnostic agents and kits

E947.9 Unspecified drug or medicinal substance

☑4ᵗʰ **E948 Bacterial vaccines**

E948.0 BCG vaccine

E948.1 Typhoid and paratyphoid

E948.2 Cholera

E948.3 Plague

E948.4 Tetanus

E948.5 Diphtheria

E948.6 Pertussis vaccine, including combinations with a pertussis component

E948.8 Other and unspecified bacterial vaccines

E948.9 Mixed bacterial vaccines, except combinations with a pertussis component

☑4ᵗʰ **E949 Other vaccines and biological substances**
EXCLUDES *gamma globulin (E934.6)*

E949.0 Smallpox vaccine

E949.1 Rabies vaccine

E949.2 Typhus vaccine

E949.3 Yellow fever vaccine

E949.4 Measles vaccine

E949.5 Poliomyelitis vaccine

E949.6 Other and unspecified viral and rickettsial vaccines
Mumps vaccine

E949.7 Mixed viral-rickettsial and bacterial vaccines, except combinations with a pertussis component
EXCLUDES *combinations with a pertussis component (E948.6)*

E949.9 Other and unspecified vaccines and biological substances

Suicide and Self-inflicted Injury (E950-E959)

INCLUDES injuries in suicide and attempted suicide
self-inflicted injuries specified as intentional

☑4ᵗʰ **E950 Suicide and self-inflicted poisoning by solid or liquid substances**

E950.0 Analgesics, antipyretics, and antirheumatics

E950.1 Barbiturates

E950.2 Other sedatives and hypnotics

E950.3 Tranquilizers and other psychotropic agents

E950.4 Other specified drugs and medicinal substances

E950.5 Unspecified drug or medicinal substance

E950.6 Agricultural and horticultural chemical and pharmaceutical preparations other than plant foods and fertilizers

E950.7 Corrosive and caustic substances
Suicide and self-inflicted poisoning by substances classifiable to E864

E950.8 Arsenic and its compounds

E950.9 Other and unspecified solid and liquid substances

☑4ᵗʰ **E951 Suicide and self-inflicted poisoning by gases in domestic use**

E951.0 Gas distributed by pipeline

E951.1 Liquefied petroleum gas distributed in mobile containers

E951.8 Other utility gas

☑4ᵗʰ **E952 Suicide and self-inflicted poisoning by other gases and vapors**

E952.0 Motor vehicle exhaust gas

E952.1 Other carbon monoxide

E952.8 Other specified gases and vapors

E952.9 Unspecified gases and vapors

☑4ᵗʰ **E953 Suicide and self-inflicted injury by hanging, strangulation, and suffocation**

E953.0 Hanging

E953.1 Suffocation by plastic bag

E953.8 Other specified means

E953.9 Unspecified means

E954 Suicide and self-inflicted injury by submersion [drowning]

☑4ᵗʰ **E955 Suicide and self-inflicted injury by firearms, air guns and explosives**

E955.0 Handgun

E955.1 Shotgun

E955.2 Hunting rifle

E955.3 Military firearms

E955.4 Other and unspecified firearm
Gunshot NOS
Shot NOS

E955.5 Explosives

E955.6 Air gun
BB gun
Pellet gun

E955.7 Paintball gun

E955.9 Unspecified

E956 Suicide and self-inflicted injury by cutting and piercing instrument

---

☑4ᵗʰ Fourth-digit Required   ▶◀ Revised Text   ● New Code   ▲ Revised Code TitleDx

E Codes

E957–E968.8

☑4ᵗʰ **E957 Suicide and self-inflicted injuries by jumping from high place**

    E957.0 Residential premises

    E957.1 Other man-made structures

    E957.2 Natural sites

    E957.9 Unspecified

☑4ᵗʰ **E958 Suicide and self-inflicted injury by other and unspecified means**

    E958.0 Jumping or lying before moving object

    E958.1 Burns, fire

    E958.2 Scald

    E958.3 Extremes of cold

    E958.4 Electrocution

    E958.5 Crashing of motor vehicle

    E958.6 Crashing of aircraft

    E958.7 Caustic substances, except poisoning

         EXCLUDES *poisoning by caustic substance (E950.7)*

    E958.8 Other specified means

    E958.9 Unspecified means

E959 Late effects of self-inflicted injury

    NOTE This category is to be used to indicate circumstances classifiable to E950-E958 as the cause of death or disability from late effects, which are themselves classifiable elsewhere. The "late effects" include conditions reported as such, or as sequelae which may occur at any time after the attempted suicide or self-inflicted injury.

Homicide and Injury Purposely Inflicted by Other Persons (E960-E969)

    INCLUDES injuries inflicted by another person with intent to injure or kill, by any means

    EXCLUDES *injuries due to:*
            legal intervention (E970-E978)
            operations of war (E990-E999)
            terrorism (E979)

☑4ᵗʰ **E960 Fight, brawl, rape**

    E960.0 Unarmed fight or brawl
        Beatings NOS
        Brawl or fight with hands, fists, feet
        Injured or killed in fight NOS
        EXCLUDES *homicidal:*
            injury by weapons (E965.0-E966, E969)
            strangulation (E963)
            submersion (E964)

    E960.1 Rape

E961 Assault by corrosive or caustic substance, except poisoning
    Injury or death purposely caused by corrosive or caustic substance, such as:
        acid [any]
        corrosive substance
        vitriol
    EXCLUDES *burns from hot liquid (E968.3)*
         chemical burns from swallowing a corrosive substance (E962.0-E962.9)

☑4ᵗʰ **E962 Assault by poisoning**

    E962.0 Drugs and medicinal substances
        Homicidal poisoning by any drug or medicinal substance

    E962.1 Other solid and liquid substances

    E962.2 Other gases and vapors

    E962.9 Unspecified poisoning

E963 Assault by hanging and strangulation
    Homicidal (attempt):
        garrotting or ligature
        hanging
        strangulation
        suffocation

E964 Assault by submersion [drowning]

☑4ᵗʰ **E965 Assault by firearms and explosives**

    E965.0 Handgun
        Pistol
        Revolver

    E965.1 Shotgun

    E965.2 Hunting rifle

    E965.3 Military firearms

    E965.4 Other and unspecified firearm

    E965.5 Antipersonnel bomb

    E965.6 Gasoline bomb

    E965.7 Letter bomb

    E965.8 Other specified explosive
        Bomb NOS (placed in):
            car
            house
        Dynamite

    E965.9 Unspecified explosive

E966 Assault by cutting and piercing instrument
    Assassination (attempt), homicide (attempt) by any instrument classifiable under E920
    Homicidal:
        cut
        puncture } any part of the body
        stab
    Stabbed any part of the body

☑4ᵗʰ **E967 Perpetrator of child and adult abuse**

    NOTE Selection of the correct perpetrator code is based on the relationship between the perpetrator and the victim

    E967.0 By father, stepfather, or boyfriend
        Male partner of child's parent or guardian

    E967.1 By other specified person

    E967.2 By mother, stepmother, or girlfriend
        Female partner of child's parent or guardian

    E967.3 By spouse or partner
        Abuse of spouse or partner by ex-spouse or ex-partner

    E967.4 By child

    E967.5 By sibling

    E967.6 By grandparent

    E967.7 By other relative

    E967.8 By non-related caregiver

    E967.9 By unspecified person

☑4ᵗʰ **E968 Assault by other and unspecified means**

    E968.0 Fire
        Arson
        Homicidal burns NOS
        EXCLUDES *burns from hot liquid (E968.3)*

    E968.1 Pushing from a high place

    E968.2 Striking by blunt or thrown object

    E968.3 Hot liquid
        Homicidal burns by scalding

    E968.4 Criminal neglect
        Abandonment of child, infant, or other helpless person with intent to injure or kill

    E968.5 Transport vehicle
        Being struck by other vehicle or run down with intent to injure
        Pushed in front of, thrown from, or dragged by moving vehicle with intent to injure

    E968.6 Air gun
        BB gun
        Pellet gun

    E968.7 Human bite

    E968.8 Other specified means

☑4ᵗʰ Fourth-digit Required   ▶◀ Revised Text   ● New Code   ▲ Revised Code TitleDx

E968.9 Unspecified means
　　　Assassination (attempt) NOS
　　　Homicidal (attempt):
　　　　injury NOS
　　　　wound NOS
　　　Manslaughter (nonaccidental)
　　　Murder (attempt) NOS
　　　Violence, non-accidental

E969 Late effects of injury purposely inflicted by other person
　　　NOTE This category is to be used to indicate circumstances classifiable to E960-E968 as the cause of death or disability from late effects, which are themselves classifiable elsewhere. The "late effects" include conditions reported as such, or as sequelae which may occur at any time after injury purposely inflicted by another person.

Legal Intervention (E970-E978)

　　　INCLUDES injuries inflicted by the police or other law-enforcing agents, including military on duty, in the course of arresting or attempting to arrest lawbreakers, suppressing disturbances, maintaining order, and other legal action
　　　　legal execution
　　　EXCLUDES injuries caused by civil insurrections (E990.0-E999)

E970 Injury due to legal intervention by firearms
　　　Gunshot wound
　　　Injury by:
　　　　machine gun
　　　　revolver
　　　　rifle pellet or rubber bullet
　　　　shot NOS

E971 Injury due to legal intervention by explosives
　　　Injury by:
　　　　dynamite
　　　　explosive shell
　　　　grenade
　　　　mortar bomb

E972 Injury due to legal intervention by gas
　　　Asphyxiation by gas
　　　Injury by tear gas
　　　Poisoning by gas

E973 Injury due to legal intervention by blunt object
　　　Hit, struck by:
　　　　baton (nightstick)
　　　　blunt object
　　　　stave

E974 Injury due to legal intervention by cutting and piercing instrument
　　　Cut
　　　Incised wound
　　　Injured by bayonet
　　　Stab wound

E975 Injury due to legal intervention by other specified means
　　　Blow
　　　Manhandling

E976 Injury due to legal intervention by unspecified means

E977 Late effects of injuries due to legal intervention
　　　NOTE This category is to be used to indicate circumstances classifiable to E970-E976 as the cause of death or disability from late effects, which are themselves classifiable elsewhere. The "late effects" include conditions reported as such, or as sequelae, which may occur at any time after the injury due to legal intervention.

E978 Legal execution
　　　All executions performed at the behest of the judiciary or ruling authority [whether permanent or temporary] as:
　　　asphyxiation by gas
　　　beheading, decapitation (by guillotine)
　　　capital punishment
　　　electrocution
　　　hanging
　　　poisoning
　　　shooting
　　　other specified means

Terrorism (E979)

　☑⁴ᵗʰ **E979 Terrorism**
　　　Injuries resulting from the unlawful use of force or violence against persons or property to intimidate or coerce a Government, the civilian population, or any segment thereof, in furtherance of political or social objective

E979.0 Terrorism involving explosion of marine weapons
　　　Depth-charge
　　　Marine mine
　　　Mine NOS, at sea or in harbour
　　　Sea-based artillery shell
　　　Torpedo
　　　Underwater blast

E979.1 Terrorism involving destruction of aircraft
　　　Aircraft used as a weapon
　　　Aircraft:
　　　　burned
　　　　exploded
　　　　shot down
　　　Crushed by falling aircraft

E979.2 Terrorism involving other explosions and fragments
　　　Antipersonnel bomb (fragments)
　　　Blast NOS
　　　Explosion (of):
　　　　artillery shell
　　　　breech-block
　　　　cannon block
　　　　mortar bomb
　　　　munitions being used in terrorism
　　　　NOS
　　　Fragments from:
　　　　artillery shell
　　　　bomb
　　　　grenade
　　　　guided missile
　　　　land-mine
　　　　rocket
　　　　shell
　　　　shrapnel
　　　Mine NOS

E979.3 Terrorism involving fires, conflagration and hot substances
　　　Burning building or structure:
　　　　collapse of
　　　　fall from
　　　　hit by falling object in
　　　　jump from
　　　Conflagration NOS
　　　Fire (causing):
　　　　Asphyxia
　　　　Burns
　　　　NOS
　　　　Other injury
　　　Melting of fittings and furniture in burning
　　　Petrol bomb
　　　Smouldering building or structure

E979.4 Terrorism involving firearms
　　　Bullet:
　　　　carbine
　　　　machine gun
　　　　pistol
　　　　rifle
　　　　rubber (rifle)
　　　Pellets (shotgun)

E979.5 Terrorism involving nuclear weapons
　　　Blast effects
　　　Exposure to ionizing radiation from nuclear weapon
　　　Fireball effects
　　　Heat from nuclear weapon
　　　Other direct and secondary effects of nuclear weapons

E979.6 Terrorism involving biological weapons
　　　Anthrax
　　　Cholera
　　　Smallpox

☑⁴ Fourth-digit Required　　　►◄ Revised Text　　　● New Code　　　▲ Revised Code TitleDx

E979.7 Terrorism involving chemical weapons
Gases, fumes, chemicals
Hydrogen cyanide
Phosgene
Sarin

E979.8 Terrorism involving other means
Drowning and submersion
Lasers
Piercing or stabbing instruments
Terrorism NOS

E979.9 Terrorism, secondary effects
NOTE This code is for use to identify conditions occurring subsequent to a terrorist attack not those that are due to the initial terrorist act
EXCLUDES *late effect of terrorist attack (E999.1)*

Injury Undetermined Whether Accidentally or Purposely Inflicted (E980-E989)

NOTE Categories E980-E989 are for use when it is unspecified or it cannot be determined whether the injuries are accidental (unintentional), suicide (attempted), or assault.

√4ᵗʰ **E980 Poisoning by solid or liquid substances, undetermined whether accidentally or purposely inflicted**

E980.0 Analgesics, antipyretics, and antirheumatics

E980.1 Barbiturates

E980.2 Other sedatives and hypnotics

E980.3 Tranquilizers and other psychotropic agents

E980.4 Other specified drugs and medicinal substances

E980.5 Unspecified drug or medicinal substance

E980.6 Corrosive and caustic substances
Poisoning, undetermined whether accidental or purposeful, by substances classifiable to E864

E980.7 Agricultural and horticultural chemical and pharmaceutical preparations other than plant foods and fertilizers

E980.8 Arsenic and its compounds

E980.9 Other and unspecified solid and liquid substances

√4ᵗʰ **E981 Poisoning by gases in domestic use, undetermined whether accidentally or purposely inflicted**

E981.0 Gas distributed by pipeline

E981.1 Liquefied petroleum gas distributed in mobile containers

E981.8 Other utility gas

√4ᵗʰ **E982 Poisoning by other gases, undetermined whether accidentally or purposely inflicted**

E982.0 Motor vehicle exhaust gas

E982.1 Other carbon monoxide

E982.8 Other specified gases and vapors

E982.9 Unspecified gases and vapors

√4ᵗʰ **E983 Hanging, strangulation, or suffocation, undetermined whether accidentally or purposely inflicted**

E983.0 Hanging

E983.1 Suffocation by plastic bag

E983.8 Other specified means

E983.9 Unspecified means

E984 Submersion [drowning], undetermined whether accidentally or purposely inflicted

√4ᵗʰ **E985 Injury by firearms, air guns and explosives, undetermined whether accidentally or purposely inflicted**

E985.0 Handgun

E985.1 Shotgun

E985.2 Hunting rifle

E985.3 Military firearms

E985.4 Other and unspecified firearm

E985.5 Explosives

E985.6 Air gun
BB gun   Pellet gun

E985.7 Paintball gun

E986 Injury by cutting and piercing instruments, undetermined whether accidentally or purposely inflicted

√4ᵗʰ **E987 Falling from high place, undetermined whether accidentally or purposely inflicted**

E987.0 Residential premises

E987.1 Other man-made structures

E987.2 Natural sites

E987.9 Unspecified site

√4ᵗʰ **E988 Injury by other and unspecified means, undetermined whether accidentally or purposely inflicted**

E988.0 Jumping or lying before moving object

E988.1 Burns, fire

E988.2 Scald

E988.3 Extremes of cold

E988.4 Electrocution

E988.5 Crashing of motor vehicle

E988.6 Crashing of aircraft

E988.7 Caustic substances, except poisoning

E988.8 Other specified means

E988.9 Unspecified means

E989 Late effects of injury, undetermined whether accidentally or purposely inflicted
NOTE This category is to be used to indicate circumstances classifiable to E980-E988 as the cause of death or disability from late effects, which are themselves classifiable elsewhere. The "late effects" include conditions reported as such, or as sequelae, which may occur at any time after injury, undetermined whether accidentally or purposely inflicted.

Injury Resulting from Operations of War (E990-E999)

INCLUDES injuries to military personnel and civilians caused by war and civil insurrections and occurring during the time of war and insurrection, and peacekeeping missions

EXCLUDES *accidents during training of military personnel manufacture of war material and transport, unless attributable to enemy action*

√4ᵗʰ **E990 Injury due to war operations by fires and conflagrations**
INCLUDES asphyxia, burns, or other injury originating from fire caused by a fire-producing device or indirectly by any conventional weapon

E990.0 From gasoline bomb
Incendiary bomb

E990.1 From flamethrower

E990.2 From incendiary bullet

E990.3 From fire caused indirectly from conventional weapon
EXCLUDES *fire aboard military aircraft (E994.3)*

E990.9 From other and unspecified source

√4ᵗʰ **E991 Injury due to war operations by bullets and fragments**
EXCLUDES *injury due to bullets and fragments due to war operations, but occurring after cessation of hostilities (E998.0)*
injury due to explosion of artillery shells and mortars (E993.2)
injury due to explosion of improvised explosive device [IED] (E993.3-E993.5)
injury due to sea-based artillery shell (E992.3)

E991.0 Rubber bullets (rifle)

E991.1 Pellets (rifle)

E991.2 Other bullets
    Bullet [any, except rubber bullets and pellets]:
      carbine
      machine gun
      pistol
      rifle
      shotgun

E991.3 Antipersonnel bomb (fragments)

E991.4 Fragments from munitions
    Fragments from:
      artillery shell
      bombs, except antipersonnel
      detonation of unexploded ordnance [UXO]
      grenade
      guided missile
      land mine
      rockets
      shell

E991.5 Fragments from person-borne improvised explosive device [IED]

E991.6 Fragments from vehicle-borne improvised explosive device [IED]
    IED borne by land, air, or water transport vehicle

E991.7 Fragments from other improvised explosive device [IED]
    Roadside IED

E991.8 Fragments from weapons
    Fragments from:
      artillery
      autocannons
      automatic grenade launchers
      missile launchers
      mortars
      small arms

E991.9 Other and unspecified fragments
    Shrapnel NOS

√4ᵗʰ **E992 Injury due to war operations by explosion of marine weapons**

E992.0 Torpedo

E992.1 Depth charge

E992.2 Marine mines
    Marine mines at sea or in harbor

E992.3 Sea-based artillery shell

E992.8 Other marine weapons

E992.9 Unspecified marine weapon
    Underwater blast NOS

√4ᵗʰ **E993 Injury due to war operations by other explosion**
    Injuries due to direct or indirect pressure or air blast of an explosion occurring during war operations
    EXCLUDES *injury due to fragments resulting from an explosion (E991.0-E991.9)*
        injury due to detonation of unexploded ordnance but occurring after cessation of hostilities (E998.0-E998.9)
        injury due to nuclear weapons (E996.0-E996.9)

E993.0 Aerial bomb

E993.1 Guided missile

E993.2 Mortar
    Artillery shell

E993.3 Person-borne improvised explosive device [IED]

E993.4 Vehicle-borne improvised explosive device [IED]
    IED borne by land, air, or water transport vehicle

E993.5 Other improvised explosive device [IED]
    Roadside IED

E993.6 Unintentional detonation of own munitions
    Unintentional detonation of own ammunition (artillery) (mortars)

E993.7 Unintentional discharge of own munitions launch device
    Unintentional explosion of own:
      autocannons
      automatic grenade launchers
      missile launchers
      small arms

E993.8 Other specified explosion
    Bomb
    Grenade
    Land mine

E993.9 Unspecified explosion
    Air blast NOS
    Blast NOS
    Blast wave NOS
    Blast wind NOS
    Explosion NOS

√4ᵗʰ **E994 Injury due to war operations by destruction of aircraft**

E994.0 Destruction of aircraft due to enemy fire or explosives
    Air to air missile
    Explosive device placed on aircraft
    Rocket propelled grenade [RPG]
    Small arms fire
    Surface to air missile

E994.1 Unintentional destruction of aircraft due to own onboard explosives

E994.2 Destruction of aircraft due to collision with other aircraft

E994.3 Destruction of aircraft due to onboard fire

E994.8 Other destruction of aircraft

E994.9 Unspecified destruction of aircraft

√4ᵗʰ **E995 Injury due to war operations by other and unspecified forms of conventional warfare**

E995.0 Unarmed hand-to-hand combat
    EXCLUDES *intentional restriction of airway (E995.3)*

E995.1 Struck by blunt object
    Baton (nightstick)
    Stave

E995.2 Piercing object
    Bayonet
    Knife
    Sword

E995.3 Intentional restriction of air and airway
    Intentional submersion
    Strangulation
    Suffocation

E995.4 Unintentional drowning due to inability to surface or obtain air
    Submersion

E995.8 Other forms of conventional warfare

E995.9 Unspecified form of conventional warfare

√4ᵗʰ **E996 Injury due to war operations by nuclear weapons**
    Dirty bomb NOS
    EXCLUDES *late effects of injury due to nuclear weapons (E999.0, E999.1)*

E996.0 Direct blast effect of nuclear weapon
    Injury to bodily organs due to blast pressure

E996.1 Indirect blast effect of nuclear weapon
    Injury due to being thrown by blast
    Injury due to being struck or crushed by blast debris

E996.2 Thermal radiation effect of nuclear weapon
    Burns due to thermal radiation
    Fireball effects
    Flash burns
    Heat effects

E996.3 Nuclear radiation effects
    Acute radiation exposure
    Beta burns
    Fallout exposure
    Radiation sickness
    Secondary effects of nuclear weapons

E996.8 Other effects of nuclear weapons

E996.9 Unspecified effect of nuclear weapon

E991.2–E996.9

√4ᵗʰ Fourth-digit Required   ►◄ Revised Text   ● New Code   ▲ Revised Code TitleDx

√4ᵗʰ **E997** **Injury due to war operations by other forms of unconventional warfare**

E997.0 **Lasers**

E997.1 **Biological warfare**

E997.2 **Gases, fumes, and chemicals**

E997.3 **Weapon of mass destruction [WMD], unspecified**

E997.8 **Other specified forms of unconventional warfare**

E997.9 **Unspecified form of unconventional warfare**

√4ᵗʰ **E998** **Injury due to war operations but occurring after cessation of hostilities**

Injuries due to operations of war but occurring after cessation of hostilities by any means classifiable under E990-E997

Injuries by explosion of bombs or mines placed in the course of operations of war, if the explosion occurred after cessation of hostilities

E998.0 **Explosion of mines**

E998.1 **Explosion of bombs**

E998.8 **Injury due to other war operations but occurring after cessation of hostilities**

E998.9 **Injury due to unspecified war operations but occurring after cessation of hostilities**

√4ᵗʰ **E999** **Late effect of injury due to war operations and terrorism**

NOTE This category is to be used to indicate circumstances classifiable to E979, E990-E998 as the cause of death or disability from late effects, which are themselves classifiable elsewhere. The "late effects" include conditions reported as such, or as sequelae, which may occur at any time after the injury, resulting from operations of war or terrorism

E999.0 **Late effect of injury due to war operations**

E999.1 **Late effect of injury due to terrorism**

√4ᵗʰ Fourth-digit Required   ▶◀ Revised Text   ● New Code   ▲ Revised Code TitleDx

Appendix A: Morphology of Neoplasms

The World Health Organization has published an adaptation of the International Classification of Diseases for oncology (ICD-O). It contains a coded nomenclature for the morphology of neoplasms, which is reproduced here for those who wish to use it in conjunction with Chapter 2 of the International Classification of Diseases, 9th Revision, Clinical Modification.

The morphology code numbers consist of five digits; the first four identify the histological type of the neoplasm and the fifth indicates its behavior. The one-digit behavior code is as follows:

/0	Benign
/1	Uncertain whether benign or malignant
	Borderline malignancy
/2	Carcinoma in situ
	Intraepithelial
	Noninfiltrating
	Noninvasive
/3	Malignant, primary site
/6	Malignant, metastatic site
	Secondary site
/9	Malignant, uncertain whether primary or metastatic site

In the nomenclature below, the morphology code numbers include the behavior code appropriate to the histological type of neoplasm, but this behavior code should be changed if other reported information makes this necessary. For example, "chordoma (M9370/3)" is assumed to be malignant; the term "benign chordoma" should be coded M9370/0. Similarly, "superficial spreading adenocarcinoma (M8143/3)" described as "noninvasive" should be coded M8143/2 and "melanoma (M8720/3)" described as "secondary" should be coded M8720/6.

The following table shows the correspondence between the morphology code and the different sections of Chapter 2:

Morphology Code Histology/Behavior		ICD-9-CM Chapter 2	
Any	0	210-229	Benign neoplasms
M8000-M8004	1	239	Neoplasms of unspecified nature
M8010+	1	235-238	Neoplasms of uncertain behavior
Any	2	230-234	Carcinoma in situ
Any	3	140-195 200-208	Malignant neoplasms, stated or presumed to be primary
Any	6	196-198	Malignant neoplasms, stated or presumed to be secondary

The ICD-O behavior digit /9 is inapplicable in an ICD context, since all malignant neoplasms are presumed to be primary (/3) or secondary (/6) according to other information on the medical record.the first-listed term of the full ICD-O morphology nomenclature appears against each code number in the list below. The ICD-9-CM Alphabetical Index (Volume 2), however, includes all the ICD-O synonyms as well as a number of other morphological names still likely to be encountered on medical records but omitted from ICD-O as outdated or otherwise undesirable.

A coding difficulty sometimes arises where a morphological diagnosis contains two qualifying adjectives that have different code numbers. An example is "transitional cell epidermoid carcinoma." "Transitional cell carcinoma NOS" is M8120/3 and "epidermoid carcinoma NOS" is M8070/3. In such circumstances, the higher number (M8120/3 in this example) should be used, as it is usually more specific.

Coded Nomenclature for Morphology of Neoplasms

M800	**Neoplasms NOS**
M8000/0	Neoplasm, benign
M8000/1	Neoplasm, uncertain whether benign or malignant
M8000/3	Neoplasm, malignant
M8000/6	Neoplasm, metastatic
M8000/9	Neoplasm, malignant, uncertain whether primary or metastatic
M8001/0	Tumor cells, benign
M8001/1	Tumor cells, uncertain whether benign or malignant
M8001/3	Tumor cells, malignant
M8002/3	Malignant tumor, small cell type
M8003/3	Malignant tumor, giant cell type
M8004/3	Malignant tumor, fusiform cell type
M801-M804	**Epithelial neoplasms NOS**
M8010/0	Epithelial tumor, benign
M8010/2	Carcinoma in situ NOS
M8010/3	Carcinoma NOS
M8010/6	Carcinoma, metastatic NOS
M8010/9	Carcinomatosis
M8011/0	Epithelioma, benign
M8011/3	Epithelioma, malignant
M8012/3	Large cell carcinoma NOS
M8020/3	Carcinoma, undifferentiated type NOS
M8021/3	Carcinoma, anaplastic type NOS
M8022/3	Pleomorphic carcinoma
M8030/3	Giant cell and spindle cell carcinoma
M8031/3	Giant cell carcinoma
M8032/3	Spindle cell carcinoma
M8033/3	Pseudosarcomatous carcinoma
M8034/3	Polygonal cell carcinoma
M8035/3	Spheroidal cell carcinoma
M8040/1	Tumorlet
M8041/3	Small cell carcinoma NOS
M8042/3	Oat cell carcinoma
M8043/3	Small cell carcinoma, fusiform cell type
M805-M808	**Papillary and squamous cell neoplasms**
M8050/0	Papilloma NOS (except Papilloma of urinary bladder M8120/1)
M8050/2	Papillary carcinoma in situ
M8050/3	Papillary carcinoma NOS
M8051/0	Verrucous papilloma
M8051/3	Verrucous carcinoma NOS
M8052/0	Squamous cell papilloma
M8052/3	Papillary squamous cell carcinoma
M8053/0	Inverted papilloma
M8060/0	Papillomatosis NOS
M8070/2	Squamous cell carcinoma in situ NOS
M8070/3	Squamous cell carcinoma NOS
M8070/6	Squamous cell carcinoma, metastatic NOS
M8071/3	Squamous cell carcinoma, keratinizing type NOS
M8072/3	Squamous cell carcinoma, large cell, nonkeratinizing type
M8073/3	Squamous cell carcinoma, small cell, nonkeratinizing type
M8074/3	Squamous cell carcinoma, spindle cell type
M8075/3	Adenoid squamous cell carcinoma
M8076/2	Squamous cell carcinoma in situ with questionable stromal invasion
M8076/3	Squamous cell carcinoma, microinvasive
M8080/2	Queyrat's erythroplasia
M8081/2	Bowen's disease
M8082/3	Lymphoepithelial carcinoma
M809-M811	**Basal cell neoplasms**
M8090/1	Basal cell tumor
M8090/3	Basal cell carcinoma NOS
M8091/3	Multicentric basal cell carcinoma
M8092/3	Basal cell carcinoma, morphea type
M8093/3	Basal cell carcinoma, fibroepithelial type
M8094/3	Basosquamous carcinoma
M8095/3	Metatypical carcinoma
M8096/0	Intraepidermal epithelioma of Jadassohn
M8100/0	Trichoepithelioma
M8101/0	Trichofolliculoma
M8102/0	Tricholemmoma
M8110/0	Pilomatrixoma
M812-M813	**Transitional cell papillomas and carcinomas**
M8120/0	Transitional cell papilloma NOS
M8120/1	Urothelial papilloma
M8120/2	Transitional cell carcinoma in situ
M8120/3	Transitional cell carcinoma NOS
M8121/0	Schneiderian papilloma
M8121/1	Transitional cell papilloma, inverted type
M8121/3	Schneiderian carcinoma
M8122/3	Transitional cell carcinoma, spindle cell type
M8123/3	Basaloid carcinoma
M8124/3	Cloacogenic carcinoma
M8130/3	Papillary transitional cell carcinoma
M814-M838	**Adenomas and adenocarcinomas**
M8140/0	Adenoma NOS
M8140/1	Bronchial adenoma NOS
M8140/2	Adenocarcinoma in situ
M8140/3	Adenocarcinoma NOS
M8140/6	Adenocarcinoma, metastatic NOS
M8141/3	Scirrhous adenocarcinoma
M8142/3	Linitis plastica
M8143/3	Superficial spreading adenocarcinoma
M8144/3	Adenocarcinoma, intestinal type
M8145/3	Carcinoma, diffuse type
M8146/0	Monomorphic adenoma
M8147/0	Basal cell adenoma
M8150/0	Islet cell adenoma
M8150/3	Islet cell carcinoma
M8151/0	Insulinoma NOS
M8151/3	Insulinoma, malignant
M8152/0	Glucagonoma NOS
M8152/3	Glucagonoma, malignant
M8153/1	Gastrinoma NOS
M8153/3	Gastrinoma, malignant
M8154/3	Mixed islet cell and exocrine adenocarcinoma
M8160/0	Bile duct adenoma
M8160/3	Cholangiocarcinoma

M8161/0	Bile duct cystadenoma
M8161/3	Bile duct cystadenocarcinoma
M8170/0	Liver cell adenoma
M8170/3	Hepatocellular carcinoma NOS
M8180/0	Hepatocholangioma, benign
M8180/3	Combined hepatocellular carcinoma and cholangiocarcinoma
M8190/0	Trabecular adenoma
M8190/3	Trabecular adenocarcinoma
M8191/0	Embryonal adenoma
M8200/0	Eccrine dermal cylindroma
M8200/3	Adenoid cystic carcinoma
M8201/3	Cribriform carcinoma
M8210/0	Adenomatous polyp NOS
M8210/3	Adenocarcinoma in adenomatous polyp
M8211/0	Tubular adenoma NOS
M8211/3	Tubular adenocarcinoma
M8220/0	Adenomatous polyposis coli
M8220/3	Adenocarcinoma in adenomatous polyposis coli
M8221/0	Multiple adenomatous polyps
M8230/3	Solid carcinoma NOS
M8231/3	Carcinoma simplex
M8240/1	Carcinoid tumor NOS
M8240/3	Carcinoid tumor, malignant
M8241/1	Carcinoid tumor, argentaffin NOS
M8241/3	Carcinoid tumor, argentaffin, malignant
M8242/1	Carcinoid tumor, nonargentaffin NOS
M8242/3	Carcinoid tumor, nonargentaffin, malignant
M8243/3	Mucocarcinoid tumor, malignant
M8244/3	Composite carcinoid
M8250/1	Pulmonary adenomatosis
M8250/3	Bronchiolo-alveolar adenocarcinoma
M8251/0	Alveolar adenoma
M8251/3	Alveolar adenocarcinoma
M8260/0	Papillary adenoma NOS
M8260/3	Papillary adenocarcinoma NOS
M8261/1	Villous adenoma NOS
M8261/3	Adenocarcinoma in villous adenoma
M8262/3	Villous adenocarcinoma
M8263/0	Tubulovillous adenoma
M8270/0	Chromophobe adenoma
M8270/3	Chromophobe carcinoma
M8280/0	Acidophil adenoma
M8280/3	Acidophil carcinoma
M8281/0	Mixed acidophil-basophil adenoma
M8281/3	Mixed acidophil-basophil carcinoma
M8290/0	Oxyphilic adenoma
M8290/3	Oxyphilic adenocarcinoma
M8300/0	Basophil adenoma
M8300/3	Basophil carcinoma
M8310/0	Clear cell adenoma
M8310/3	Clear cell adenocarcinoma NOS
M8311/1	Hypernephroid tumor
M8312/3	Renal cell carcinoma
M8313/0	Clear cell adenofibroma
M8320/3	Granular cell carcinoma
M8321/0	Chief cell adenoma
M8322/0	Water-clear cell adenoma
M8322/3	Water-clear cell adenocarcinoma
M8323/0	Mixed cell adenoma
M8323/3	Mixed cell adenocarcinoma
M8324/0	Lipoadenoma
M8330/0	Follicular adenoma
M8330/3	Follicular adenocarcinoma NOS
M8331/3	Follicular adenocarcinoma, well differentiated type
M8332/3	Follicular adenocarcinoma, trabecular type

M8333/0	Microfollicular adenoma
M8334/0	Macrofollicular adenoma
M8340/3	Papillary and follicular adenocarcinoma
M8350/3	Nonencapsulated sclerosing carcinoma
M8360/1	Multiple endocrine adenomas
M8361/1	Juxtaglomerular tumor
M8370/0	Adrenal cortical adenoma NOS
M8370/3	Adrenal cortical carcinoma
M8371/0	Adrenal cortical adenoma, compact cell type
M8372/0	Adrenal cortical adenoma, heavily pigmented variant
M8373/0	Adrenal cortical adenoma, clear cell type
M8374/0	Adrenal cortical adenoma, glomerulosa cell type
M8375/0	Adrenal cortical adenoma, mixed cell type
M8380/0	Endometrioid adenoma NOS
M8380/1	Endometrioid adenoma, borderline malignancy
M8380/3	Endometrioid carcinoma
M8381/0	Endometrioid adenofibroma NOS
M8381/1	Endometrioid adenofibroma, borderline malignancy
M8381/3	Endometrioid adenofibroma, malignant

M839-M842 Adnexal and skin appendage neoplasms

M8390/0	Skin appendage adenoma
M8390/3	Skin appendage carcinoma
M8400/0	Sweat gland adenoma
M8400/1	Sweat gland tumor NOS
M8400/3	Sweat gland adenocarcinoma
M8401/0	Apocrine adenoma
M8401/3	Apocrine adenocarcinoma
M8402/0	Eccrine acrospiroma
M8403/0	Eccrine spiradenoma
M8404/0	Hidrocystoma
M8405/0	Papillary hydradenoma
M8406/0	Papillary syringadenoma
M8407/0	Syringoma NOS
M8410/0	Sebaceous adenoma
M8410/3	Sebaceous adenocarcinoma
M8420/0	Ceruminous adenoma
M8420/3	Ceruminous adenocarcinoma

M843 Mucoepidermoid neoplasms

M8430/1	Mucoepidermoid tumor
M8430/3	Mucoepidermoid carcinoma

M844-M849 Cystic, mucinous, and serous neoplasms

M8440/0	Cystadenoma NOS
M8440/3	Cystadenocarcinoma NOS
M8441/0	Serous cystadenoma NOS
M8441/1	Serous cystadenoma, borderline malignancy
M8441/3	Serous cystadenocarcinoma NOS
M8450/0	Papillary cystadenoma NOS
M8450/1	Papillary cystadenoma, borderline malignancy
M8450/3	Papillary cystadenocarcinoma NOS
M8460/0	Papillary serous cystadenoma NOS
M8460/1	Papillary serous cystadenoma, borderline malignancy
M8460/3	Papillary serous cystadenocarcinoma
M8461/0	Serous surface papilloma NOS
M8461/1	Serous surface papilloma, borderline malignancy
M8461/3	Serous surface papillary carcinoma
M8470/0	Mucinous cystadenoma NOS
M8470/1	Mucinous cystadenoma, borderline malignancy

M8470/3	Mucinous cystadenocarcinoma NOS
M8471/0	Papillary mucinous cystadenoma NOS
M8471/1	Papillary mucinous cystadenoma, borderline malignancy
M8471/3	Papillary mucinous cystadenocarcinoma
M8480/0	Mucinous adenoma
M8480/3	Mucinous adenocarcinoma
M8480/6	Pseudomyxoma peritonei
M8481/3	Mucin-producing adenocarcinoma
M8490/3	Signet ring cell carcinoma
M8490/6	Metastatic signet ring cell carcinoma

M850-M854 Ductal, lobular, and medullary neoplasms

M8500/2	Intraductal carcinoma, noninfiltrating NOS
M8500/3	Infiltrating duct carcinoma
M8501/2	Comedocarcinoma, noninfiltrating
M8501/3	Comedocarcinoma NOS
M8502/3	Juvenile carcinoma of the breast
M8503/0	Intraductal papilloma
M8503/2	Noninfiltrating intraductal papillary adenocarcinoma
M8504/0	Intracystic papillary adenoma
M8504/2	Noninfiltrating intracystic carcinoma
M8505/0	Intraductal papillomatosis NOS
M8506/0	Subareolar duct papillomatosis
M8510/3	Medullary carcinoma NOS
M8511/3	Medullary carcinoma with amyloid stroma
M8512/3	Medullary carcinoma with lymphoid stroma
M8520/2	Lobular carcinoma in situ
M8520/3	Lobular carcinoma NOS
M8521/3	Infiltrating ductular carcinoma
M8530/3	Inflammatory carcinoma
M8540/3	Paget's disease, mammary
M8541/3	Paget's disease and infiltrating duct carcinoma of breast
M8542/3	Paget's disease, extramammary (except Paget's disease of bone)

M855 Acinar cell neoplasms

M8550/0	Acinar cell adenoma
M8550/1	Acinar cell tumor
M8550/3	Acinar cell carcinoma

M856-M858 Complex epithelial neoplasms

M8560/3	Adenosquamous carcinoma
M8561/0	Adenolymphoma
M8570/3	Adenocarcinoma with squamous metaplasia
M8571/3	Adenocarcinoma with cartilaginous and osseous metaplasia
M8572/3	Adenocarcinoma with spindle cell metaplasia
M8573/3	Adenocarcinoma with apocrine metaplasia
M8580/0	Thymoma, benign
M8580/3	Thymoma, malignant

M859-M867 Specialized gonadal neoplasms

M8590/1	Sex cord-stromal tumor
M8600/0	Thecoma NOS
M8600/3	Theca cell carcinoma
M8610/0	Luteoma NOS
M8620/1	Granulosa cell tumor NOS
M8620/3	Granulosa cell tumor, malignant
M8621/1	Granulosa cell-theca cell tumor
M8630/0	Androblastoma, benign
M8630/1	Androblastoma NOS
M8630/3	Androblastoma, malignant
M8631/0	Sertoli-Leydig cell tumor

M8632/1	Gynandroblastoma
M8640/0	Tubular androblastoma NOS
M8640/3	Sertoli cell carcinoma
M8641/0	Tubular androblastoma with lipid storage
M8650/0	Leydig cell tumor, benign
M8650/1	Leydig cell tumor NOS
M8650/3	Leydig cell tumor, malignant
M8660/0	Hilar cell tumor
M8670/0	Lipid cell tumor of ovary
M8671/0	Adrenal rest tumor

M868-M871 Paragangliomas and glomus tumors

M8680/1	Paraganglioma NOS
M8680/3	Paraganglioma, malignant
M8681/1	Sympathetic paraganglioma
M8682/1	Parasympathetic paraganglioma
M8690/1	Glomus jugulare tumor
M8691/1	Aortic body tumor
M8692/1	Carotid body tumor
M8693/1	Extra-adrenal paraganglioma NOS
M8693/3	Extra-adrenal paraganglioma, malignant
M8700/0	Pheochromocytoma NOS
M8700/3	Pheochromocytoma, malignant
M8710/3	Glomangiosarcoma
M8711/0	Glomus tumor
M8712/0	Glomangioma

M872-M879 Nevi and melanomas

M8720/0	Pigmented nevus NOS
M8720/3	Malignant melanoma NOS
M8721/3	Nodular melanoma
M8722/0	Balloon cell nevus
M8722/3	Balloon cell melanoma
M8723/0	Halo nevus
M8724/0	Fibrous papule of the nose
M8725/0	Neuronevus
M8726/0	Magnocellular nevus
M8730/0	Nonpigmented nevus
M8730/3	Amelanotic melanoma
M8740/0	Junctional nevus
M8740/3	Malignant melanoma in junctional nevus
M8741/2	Precancerous melanosis NOS
M8741/3	Malignant melanoma in precancerous melanosis
M8742/2	Hutchinson's melanotic freckle
M8742/3	Malignant melanoma in Hutchinson's melanotic freckle
M8743/3	Superficial spreading melanoma
M8750/0	Intradermal nevus
M8760/0	Compound nevus
M8761/1	Giant pigmented nevus
M8761/3	Malignant melanoma in giant pigmented nevus
M8770/0	Epithelioid and spindle cell nevus
M8771/3	Epithelioid cell melanoma
M8772/3	Spindle cell melanoma NOS
M8773/3	Spindle cell melanoma, type A
M8774/3	Spindle cell melanoma, type B
M8775/3	Mixed epithelioid and spindle cell melanoma
M8780/0	Blue nevus NOS
M8780/3	Blue nevus, malignant
M8790/0	Cellular blue nevus

M880 Soft tissue tumors and sarcomas NOS

M8800/0	Soft tissue tumor, benign
M8800/3	Sarcoma NOS
M8800/9	Sarcomatosis NOS
M8801/3	Spindle cell sarcoma
M8802/3	Giant cell sarcoma (except of bone M9250/3)

M8803/3	Small cell sarcoma
M8804/3	Epithelioid cell sarcoma

M881-M883 Fibromatous neoplasms

M8810/0	Fibroma NOS
M8810/3	Fibrosarcoma NOS
M8811/0	Fibromyxoma
M8811/3	Fibromyxosarcoma
M8812/0	Periosteal fibroma
M8812/3	Periosteal fibrosarcoma
M8813/0	Fascial fibroma
M8813/3	Fascial fibrosarcoma
M8814/3	Infantile fibrosarcoma
M8820/0	Elastofibroma
M8821/1	Aggressive fibromatosis
M8822/1	Abdominal fibromatosis
M8823/1	Desmoplastic fibroma
M8830/0	Fibrous histiocytoma NOS
M8830/1	Atypical fibrous histiocytoma
M8830/3	Fibrous histiocytoma, malignant
M8831/0	Fibroxanthoma NOS
M8831/1	Atypical fibroxanthoma
M8831/3	Fibroxanthoma, malignant
M8832/0	Dermatofibroma NOS
M8832/1	Dermatofibroma protuberans
M8832/3	Dermatofibrosarcoma NOS

M884 Myxomatous neoplasms

M8840/0	Myxoma NOS
M8840/3	Myxosarcoma

M885-M888 Lipomatous neoplasms

M8850/0	Lipoma NOS
M8850/3	Liposarcoma NOS
M8851/0	Fibrolipoma
M8851/3	Liposarcoma, well differentiated type
M8852/0	Fibromyxolipoma
M8852/3	Myxoid liposarcoma
M8853/3	Round cell liposarcoma
M8854/3	Pleomorphic liposarcoma
M8855/3	Mixed type liposarcoma
M8856/0	Intramuscular lipoma
M8857/0	Spindle cell lipoma
M8860/0	Angiomyolipoma
M8860/3	Angiomyoliposarcoma
M8861/0	Angiolipoma NOS
M8861/1	Angiolipoma, infiltrating
M8870/0	Myelolipoma
M8880/0	Hibernoma
M8881/0	Lipoblastomatosis

M889-M892 Myomatous neoplasms

M8890/0	Leiomyoma NOS
M8890/1	Intravascular leiomyomatosis
M8890/3	Leiomyosarcoma NOS
M8891/1	Epithelioid leiomyoma
M8891/3	Epithelioid leiomyosarcoma
M8892/1	Cellular leiomyoma
M8893/0	Bizarre leiomyoma
M8894/0	Angiomyoma
M8894/3	Angiomyosarcoma
M8895/0	Myoma
M8895/3	Myosarcoma
M8900/0	Rhabdomyoma NOS
M8900/3	Rhabdomyosarcoma NOS
M8901/3	Pleomorphic rhabdomyosarcoma
M8902/3	Mixed type rhabdomyosarcoma
M8903/0	Fetal rhabdomyoma
M8904/0	Adult rhabdomyoma
M8910/3	Embryonal rhabdomyosarcoma
M8920/3	Alveolar rhabdomyosarcoma

M893-M899 Complex mixed and stromal neoplasms

M8930/3	Endometrial stromal sarcoma
M8931/1	Endolymphatic stromal myosis
M8932/0	Adenomyoma
M8940/0	Pleomorphic adenoma
M8940/3	Mixed tumor, malignant NOS
M8950/3	Mullerian mixed tumor
M8951/3	Mesodermal mixed tumor
M8960/1	Mesoblastic nephroma
M8960/3	Nephroblastoma NOS
M8961/3	Epithelial nephroblastoma
M8962/3	Mesenchymal nephroblastoma
M8970/3	Hepatoblastoma
M8980/3	Carcinosarcoma NOS
M8981/3	Carcinosarcoma, embryonal type
M8982/0	Myoepithelioma
M8990/0	Mesenchymoma, benign
M8990/1	Mesenchymoma NOS
M8990/3	Mesenchymoma, malignant
M8991/3	Embryonal sarcoma

M900-M903 Fibroepithelial neoplasms

M9000/0	Brenner tumor NOS
M9000/1	Brenner tumor, borderline malignancy
M9000/3	Brenner tumor, malignant
M9010/0	Fibroadenoma NOS
M9011/0	Intracanalicular fibroadenoma NOS
M9012/0	Pericanalicular fibroadenoma
M9013/0	Adenofibroma NOS
M9014/0	Serous adenofibroma
M9015/0	Mucinous adenofibroma
M9020/0	Cellular intracanalicular fibroadenoma
M9020/1	Cystosarcoma phyllodes NOS
M9020/3	Cystosarcoma phyllodes, malignant
M9030/0	Juvenile fibroadenoma

M904 Synovial neoplasms

M9040/0	Synovioma, benign
M9040/3	Synovial sarcoma NOS
M9041/3	Synovial sarcoma, spindle cell type
M9042/3	Synovial sarcoma, epithelioid cell type
M9043/3	Synovial sarcoma, biphasic type
M9044/3	Clear cell sarcoma of tendons and aponeuroses

M905 Mesothelial neoplasms

M9050/0	Mesothelioma, benign
M9050/3	Mesothelioma, malignant
M9051/0	Fibrous mesothelioma, benign
M9051/3	Fibrous mesothelioma, malignant
M9052/0	Epithelioid mesothelioma, benign
M9052/3	Epithelioid mesothelioma, malignant
M9053/0	Mesothelioma, biphasic type, benign
M9053/3	Mesothelioma, biphasic type, malignant
M9054/0	Adenomatoid tumor NOS

M906-M909 Germ cell neoplasms

M9060/3	Dysgerminoma
M9061/3	Seminoma NOS
M9062/3	Seminoma, anaplastic type
M9063/3	Spermatocytic seminoma
M9064/3	Germinoma
M9070/3	Embryonal carcinoma NOS
M9071/3	Endodermal sinus tumor
M9072/3	Polyembryoma
M9073/1	Gonadoblastoma
M9080/0	Teratoma, benign
M9080/1	Teratoma NOS
M9080/3	Teratoma, malignant NOS
M9081/3	Teratocarcinoma

Appendix A: Morphology of Neoplasms

M9082/3	Malignant teratoma, undifferentiated type
M9083/3	Malignant teratoma, intermediate type
M9084/0	Dermoid cyst
M9084/3	Dermoid cyst with malignant transformation
M9090/0	Struma ovarii NOS
M9090/3	Struma ovarii, malignant
M9091/1	Strumal carcinoid

M910   **Trophoblastic neoplasms**

M9100/0	Hydatidiform mole NOS
M9100/1	Invasive hydatidiform mole
M9100/3	Choriocarcinoma
M9101/3	Choriocarcinoma combined with teratoma
M9102/3	Malignant teratoma, trophoblastic

M911   **Mesonephromas**

M9110/0	Mesonephroma, benign
M9110/1	Mesonephric tumor
M9110/3	Mesonephroma, malignant
M9111/1	Endosalpingioma

M912-M916   **Blood vessel tumors**

M9120/0	Hemangioma NOS
M9120/3	Hemangiosarcoma
M9121/0	Cavernous hemangioma
M9122/0	Venous hemangioma
M9123/0	Racemose hemangioma
M9124/3	Kupffer cell sarcoma
M9130/0	Hemangioendothelioma, benign
M9130/1	Hemangioendothelioma NOS
M9130/3	Hemangioendothelioma, malignant
M9131/0	Capillary hemangioma
M9132/0	Intramuscular hemangioma
M9140/3	Kaposi's sarcoma
M9141/0	Angiokeratoma
M9142/0	Verrucous keratotic hemangioma
M9150/0	Hemangiopericytoma, benign
M9150/1	Hemangiopericytoma NOS
M9150/3	Hemangiopericytoma, malignant
M9160/0	Angiofibroma NOS
M9161/1	Hemangioblastoma

M917   **Lymphatic vessel tumors**

M9170/0	Lymphangioma NOS
M9170/3	Lymphangiosarcoma
M9171/0	Capillary lymphangioma
M9172/0	Cavernous lymphangioma
M9173/0	Cystic lymphangioma
M9174/0	Lymphangiomyoma
M9174/1	Lymphangiomyomatosis
M9175/0	Hemolymphangioma

M918-M920   **Osteomas and osteosarcomas**

M9180/0	Osteoma NOS
M9180/3	Osteosarcoma NOS
M9181/3	Chondroblastic osteosarcoma
M9182/3	Fibroblastic osteosarcoma
M9183/3	Telangiectatic osteosarcoma
M9184/3	Osteosarcoma in Paget's disease of bone
M9190/3	Juxtacortical osteosarcoma
M9191/0	Osteoid osteoma NOS
M9200/0	Osteoblastoma

M921-M924   **Chondromatous neoplasms**

M9210/0	Osteochondroma
M9210/1	Osteochondromatosis NOS
M9220/0	Chondroma NOS
M9220/1	Chondromatosis NOS
M9220/3	Chondrosarcoma NOS
M9221/0	Juxtacortical chondroma
M9221/3	Juxtacortical chondrosarcoma
M9230/0	Chondroblastoma NOS
M9230/3	Chondroblastoma, malignant
M9240/3	Mesenchymal chondrosarcoma
M9241/0	Chondromyxoid fibroma

M925   **Giant cell tumors**

M9250/1	Giant cell tumor of bone NOS
M9250/3	Giant cell tumor of bone, malignant
M9251/1	Giant cell tumor of soft parts NOS
M9251/3	Malignant giant cell tumor of soft parts

M926   **Miscellaneous bone tumors**

M9260/3	Ewing's sarcoma
M9261/3	Adamantinoma of long bones
M9262/0	Ossifying fibroma

M927-M934   **Odontogenic tumors**

M9270/0	Odontogenic tumor, benign
M9270/1	Odontogenic tumor NOS
M9270/3	Odontogenic tumor, malignant
M9271/0	Dentinoma
M9272/0	Cementoma NOS
M9273/0	Cementoblastoma, benign
M9274/0	Cementifying fibroma
M9275/0	Gigantiform cementoma
M9280/0	Odontoma NOS
M9281/0	Compound odontoma
M9282/0	Complex odontoma
M9290/0	Ameloblastic fibro-odontoma
M9290/3	Ameloblastic odontosarcoma
M9300/0	Adenomatoid odontogenic tumor
M9301/0	Calcifying odontogenic cyst
M9310/0	Ameloblastoma NOS
M9310/3	Ameloblastoma, malignant
M9311/0	Odontoameloblastoma
M9312/0	Squamous odontogenic tumor
M9320/0	Odontogenic myxoma
M9321/0	Odontogenic fibroma NOS
M9330/0	Ameloblastic fibroma
M9330/3	Ameloblastic fibrosarcoma
M9340/0	Calcifying epithelial odontogenic tumor

M935-M937   **Miscellaneous tumors**

M9350/1	Craniopharyngioma
M9360/1	Pinealoma
M9361/1	Pineocytoma
M9362/3	Pineoblastoma
M9363/0	Melanotic neuroectodermal tumor
M9370/3	Chordoma

M938-M948   **Gliomas**

M9380/3	Glioma, malignant
M9381/3	Gliomatosis cerebri
M9382/3	Mixed glioma
M9383/1	Subependymal glioma
M9384/1	Subependymal giant cell astrocytoma
M9390/0	Choroid plexus papilloma NOS
M9390/3	Choroid plexus papilloma, malignant
M9391/3	Ependymoma NOS
M9392/3	Ependymoma, anaplastic type
M9393/1	Papillary ependymoma
M9394/1	Myxopapillary ependymoma
M9400/3	Astrocytoma NOS
M9401/3	Astrocytoma, anaplastic type
M9410/3	Protoplasmic astrocytoma
M9411/3	Gemistocytic astrocytoma
M9420/3	Fibrillary astrocytoma
M9421/3	Pilocytic astrocytoma
M9422/3	Spongioblastoma NOS
M9423/3	Spongioblastoma polare
M9430/3	Astroblastoma

M9440/3	Glioblastoma NOS
M9441/3	Giant cell glioblastoma
M9442/3	Glioblastoma with sarcomatous component
M9443/3	Primitive polar spongioblastoma
M9450/3	Oligodendroglioma NOS
M9451/3	Oligodendroglioma, anaplastic type
M9460/3	Oligodendroblastoma
M9470/3	Medulloblastoma NOS
M9471/3	Desmoplastic medulloblastoma
M9472/3	Medullomyoblastoma
M9480/3	Cerebellar sarcoma NOS
M9481/3	Monstrocellular sarcoma

M949-M952   **Neuroepitheliomatous neoplasms**

M9490/0	Ganglioneuroma
M9490/3	Ganglioneuroblastoma
M9491/0	Ganglioneuromatosis
M9500/3	Neuroblastoma NOS
M9501/3	Medulloepithelioma NOS
M9502/3	Teratoid medulloepithelioma
M9503/3	Neuroepithelioma NOS
M9504/3	Spongioneuroblastoma
M9505/1	Ganglioglioma
M9506/0	Neurocytoma
M9507/0	Pacinian tumor
M9510/3	Retinoblastoma NOS
M9511/3	Retinoblastoma, differentiated type
M9512/3	Retinoblastoma, undifferentiated type
M9520/3	Olfactory neurogenic tumor
M9521/3	Esthesioneurocytoma
M9522/3	Esthesioneuroblastoma
M9523/3	Esthesioneuroepithelioma

M953   **Meningiomas**

M9530/0	Meningioma NOS
M9530/1	Meningiomatosis NOS
M9530/3	Meningioma, malignant
M9531/0	Meningotheliomatous meningioma
M9532/0	Fibrous meningioma
M9533/0	Psammomatous meningioma
M9534/0	Angiomatous meningioma
M9535/0	Hemangioblastic meningioma
M9536/0	Hemangiopericytic meningioma
M9537/0	Transitional meningioma
M9538/1	Papillary meningioma
M9539/3	Meningeal sarcomatosis

M954-M957   **Nerve sheath tumor**

M9540/0	Neurofibroma NOS
M9540/1	Neurofibromatosis NOS
M9540/3	Neurofibrosarcoma
M9541/0	Melanotic neurofibroma
M9550/0	Plexiform neurofibroma
M9560/0	Neurilemmoma NOS
M9560/1	Neurinomatosis
M9560/3	Neurilemmoma, malignant
M9570/0	Neuroma NOS

M958   **Granular cell tumors and alveolar soft part sarcoma**

M9580/0	Granular cell tumor NOS
M9580/3	Granular cell tumor, malignant
M9581/3	Alveolar soft part sarcoma

M959-M963   **Lymphomas, NOS or diffuse**

M9590/0	Lymphomatous tumor, benign
M9590/3	Malignant lymphoma NOS
M9591/3	Malignant lymphoma, non Hodgkin's type
M9600/3	Malignant lymphoma, undifferentiated cell type NOS
M9601/3	Malignant lymphoma, stem cell type

M9602/3	Malignant lymphoma, convoluted cell type NOS
M9610/3	Lymphosarcoma NOS
M9611/3	Malignant lymphoma, lymphoplasmacytoid type
M9612/3	Malignant lymphoma, immunoblastic type
M9613/3	Malignant lymphoma, mixed lymphocytic-histiocytic NOS
M9614/3	Malignant lymphoma, centroblastic-centrocytic, diffuse
M9615/3	Malignant lymphoma, follicular center cell NOS
M9620/3	Malignant lymphoma, lymphocytic, well differentiated NOS
M9621/3	Malignant lymphoma, lymphocytic, intermediate differentiation NOS
M9622/3	Malignant lymphoma, centrocytic
M9623/3	Malignant lymphoma, follicular center cell, cleaved NOS
M9630/3	Malignant lymphoma, lymphocytic, poorly differentiated NOS
M9631/3	Prolymphocytic lymphosarcoma
M9632/3	Malignant lymphoma, centroblastic type NOS
M9633/3	Malignant lymphoma, follicular center cell, noncleaved NOS

M964   *Reticulosarcomas*

M9640/3	Reticulosarcoma NOS
M9641/3	Reticulosarcoma, pleomorphic cell type
M9642/3	Reticulosarcoma, nodular

M965-M966   *Hodgkin's disease*

M9650/3	Hodgkin's disease NOS
M9651/3	Hodgkin's disease, lymphocytic predominance
M9652/3	Hodgkin's disease, mixed cellularity
M9653/3	Hodgkin's disease, lymphocytic depletion NOS
M9654/3	Hodgkin's disease, lymphocytic depletion, diffuse fibrosis
M9655/3	Hodgkin's disease, lymphocytic depletion, reticular type
M9656/3	Hodgkin's disease, nodular sclerosis NOS
M9657/3	Hodgkin's disease, nodular sclerosis, cellular phase
M9660/3	Hodgkin's paragranuloma
M9661/3	Hodgkin's granuloma
M9662/3	Hodgkin's sarcoma

M969   **Lymphomas, nodular or follicular**

M9690/3	Malignant lymphoma, nodular NOS

M9691/3	Malignant lymphoma, mixed lymphocytic-histiocytic, nodular
M9692/3	Malignant lymphoma, centroblastic-centrocytic, follicular
M9693/3	Malignant lymphoma, lymphocytic, well differentiated, nodular
M9694/3	Malignant lymphoma, lymphocytic, intermediate differentiation, nodular
M9695/3	Malignant lymphoma, follicular center cell, cleaved, follicular
M9696/3	Malignant lymphoma, lymphocytic, poorly differentiated, nodular
M9697/3	Malignant lymphoma, centroblastic type, follicular
M9698/3	Malignant lymphoma, follicular center cell, noncleaved, follicular

M970   **Mycosis fungoides**

M9700/3	Mycosis fungoides
M9701/3	Sezary's disease

M971-M972   **Miscellaneous reticuloendothelial neoplasms**

M9710/3	Microglioma
M9720/3	Malignant histiocytosis
M9721/3	Histiocytic medullary reticulosis
M9722/3	Letterer-Siwe's disease

M973   **Plasma cell tumors**

M9730/3	Plasma cell myeloma
M9731/0	Plasma cell tumor, benign
M9731/1	Plasmacytoma NOS
M9731/3	Plasma cell tumor, malignant

M974   **Mast cell tumors**

M9740/1	Mastocytoma NOS
M9740/3	Mast cell sarcoma
M9741/3	Malignant mastocytosis

M975   **Burkitt's tumor**

M9750/3	Burkitt's tumor

M980-M994   **Leukemias NOS**

M9800/3	Leukemias NOS
M9800/3	Leukemia NOS
M9801/3	Acute leukemia NOS
M9802/3	Subacute leukemia NOS
M9803/3	Chronic leukemia NOS
M9804/3	Aleukemic leukemia NOS

M981   **Compound leukemias**

M9810/3	Compound leukemia

M982   **Lymphoid leukemias**

M9820/3	Lymphoid leukemia NOS

M9821/3	Acute lymphoid leukemia
M9822/3	Subacute lymphoid leukemia
M9823/3	Chronic lymphoid leukemia
M9824/3	Aleukemic lymphoid leukemia
M9825/3	Prolymphocytic leukemia

M983   **Plasma cell leukemias**

M9830/3	Plasma cell leukemia

M984   **Erythroleukemias**

M9840/3	Erythroleukemia
M9841/3	Acute erythremia
M9842/3	Chronic erythremia

M985   **Lymphosarcoma cell leukemias**

M9850/3	Lymphosarcoma cell leukemia

M986   **Myeloid leukemias**

M9860/3	Myeloid leukemia NOS
M9861/3	Acute myeloid leukemia
M9862/3	Subacute myeloid leukemia
M9863/3	Chronic myeloid leukemia
M9864/3	Aleukemic myeloid leukemia
M9865/3	Neutrophilic leukemia
M9866/3	Acute promyelocytic leukemia

M987   **Basophilic leukemias**

M9870/3	Basophilic leukemia

M988   **Eosinophilic leukemias**

M9880/3	Eosinophilic leukemia

M989   **Monocytic leukemias**

M9890/3	Monocytic leukemia NOS
M9891/3	Acute monocytic leukemia
M9892/3	Subacute monocytic leukemia
M9893/3	Chronic monocytic leukemia
M9894/3	Aleukemic monocytic leukemia

M990-M994   **Miscellaneous leukemias**

M9900/3	Mast cell leukemia
M9910/3	Megakaryocytic leukemia
M9920/3	Megakaryocytic myelosis
M9930/3	Myeloid sarcoma
M9940/3	Hairy cell leukemia

M995-M997   **Miscellaneous myeloproliferative and lymphoproliferative disorders**

M9950/1	Polycythemia vera
M9951/1	Acute panmyelosis
M9960/1	Chronic myeloproliferative disease
M9961/1	Myelosclerosis with myeloid metaplasia
M9962/1	Idiopathic thrombocythemia
M9970/1	Chronic lymphoproliferative disease

Appendix B: Glossary of Mental Disorders

was officially deleted October 1, 2004

Appendix C: Classification of Drugs by American Hospital Formulary Service List Number and Their ICD-9-CM Equivalents

The coding of adverse effects of drugs is keyed to the continually revised Hospital Formulary of the American Hospital Formulary Service (AHFS) published under the direction of the American Society of Hospital Pharmacists.

The following section gives the ICD-9-CM diagnosis code for each AHFS list.

AHFS* List		ICD-9-CM Dx Code
4:00	ANTIHISTAMINE DRUGS	963.0
8:00	ANTI-INFECTIVE AGENTS	
8:04	Amebacides	961.5
	hydroxyquinoline derivatives	961.3
	arsenical anti-infectives	961.1
	quinoline derivatives	961.3
8:12.04	Antifungal Antibiotics	960.1
	nonantibiotics	961.9
8:12.06	Cephalosporins	960.5
8:12.08	Chloramphenicol	960.2
8:12.12	The Erythromycins	960.3
8:12.16	The Penicillins	960.0
8:12.20	The Streptomycins	960.6
8:12.24	The Tetracyclines	960.4
8:12.28	Other Antibiotics	960.8
	antimycobacterial antibiotics	960.6
	macrolides	960.3
8:16	Antituberculars	961.8
	antibiotics	960.6
8:18	Antivirals	961.7
8:20	Plasmodicides (antimalarials)	961.4
8:24	Sulfonamides	961.0
8:26	The Sulfones	961.8
8:28	Treponemicides	961.2
8:32	Trichomonacides	961.5
	hydroxyquinoline derivatives	961.3
	nitrofuran derivatives	961.9
8:36	Urinary Germicides	961.9
	quinoline derivatives	961.3
8:40	Other Anti-Infectives	961.9
10:00	ANTINEOPLASTIC AGENTS	963.1
	antibiotics	960.7
	progestogens	962.2
12:00	AUTONOMIC DRUGS	
12:04	Parasympathomimetic (Cholinergic) Agents	971.0
12:08	Parasympatholytic (Cholinergic Blocking Agents	971.1
12:12	Sympathomimetic (Adrenergic) Agents	971.2
12:16	Sympatholytic (Adrenergic Blocking) Agents	971.3
12:20	Skeletal Muscle Relaxants	975.2
	central nervous system muscle-tone depressants	968.0
16:00	BLOOD DERIVATIVES	964.7
20:00	BLOOD FORMATION AND COAGULATION	
20:04	Antianemia Drugs	964.1
20:04.04	Iron Preparations	964.0
20:04.08	Liver and Stomach Preparations	964.1
20:12.04	Anticoagulants	964.2
20:12.08	Antiheparin Agents	964.5
20:12.12	Coagulants	964.5
20:12.16	Hemostatics	964.5
	capillary-active drugs	972.8
	fibrinolysis-affecting agents	964.4
	natural products	964.7
24:00	CARDIOVASCULAR DRUGS	
24:04	Cardiac Drugs	972.9
	cardiotonic agents	972.1
	rhythm regulators	972.0
24:06	Antilipemic Agents	972.2
	thyroid derivatives	962.7

AHFS* List		ICD-9-CM Dx Code
24:08	Hypotensive Agents	972.6
	adrenergic blocking agents	971.3
	ganglion-blocking agents	972.3
	vasodilators	972.5
24:12	Vasodilating Agents	972.5
	coronary	972.4
	nicotinic acid derivatives	972.2
24:16	Sclerosing Agents	972.7
28:00	CENTRAL NERVOUS SYSTEM DRUGS	
28:04	General Anesthetics	968.4
	gaseous anesthetics	968.2
	halothane	968.1
	intravenous anesthetics	968.3
28:08	Analgesics and Antipyretics	965.9
	antirheumatics	965.61-965.69
	aromatic analgesics	965.4
	non-narcotics NEC	965.7
	opium alkaloids	965.00
	heroin	965.01
	methadone	965.02
	specified type NEC	965.09
	pyrazole derivatives	965.5
	salicylates	965.1
	specified type NEC	965.8
28:10	Narcotic Antagonists	970.1
28:12	Anticonvulsants	966.3
	barbiturates	967.0
	benzodiazepine-based tranquilizers	969.4
	bromides	967.3
	hydantoin derivatives	966.1
	oxazolidine derivative	966.0
	succinimides	966.2
28:16.04	Antidepressants	969.00-969.09
28:16.08	Tranquilizers	969.5
	benzodiazepine-based	969.4
	butyrophenone-based	969.2
	major NEC	969.3
	phenothiazine-based	969.1
28:16.12	Other Psychotherapeutic Agents	969.8
28:20	Respiratory and Cerebral Stimulants	970.9
	analeptics	970.0
	anorexigenic agents	977.0
	psychostimulants	969.70-969.79
	specified type NEC	970.8
28:24	Sedatives and Hypnotics	967.9
	barbiturates	967.0
	benzodiazepine-based tranquilizers	969.4
	chloral hydrate group	967.1
	glutethamide group	967.5
	intravenous anesthetics	968.3
	methaqualone	967.4
	paraldehyde	967.2
	phenothiazine-based tranquilizers	969.1
	specified type NEC	967.8
	thiobarbiturates	968.3
	tranquilizer NEC	969.5
36:00	DIAGNOSTIC AGENTS	977.8
40:00	ELECTROLYTE, CALORIC, AND WATER BALANCE AGENTS NEC	974.5
40:04	Acidifying Agents	963.2
40:08	Alkalinizing Agents	963.3
40:10	Ammonia Detoxicants	974.5
40:12	Replacement Solutions NEC	974.5
	plasma volume expanders	964.8
40:16	Sodium-Removing Resins	974.5
40:18	Potassium-Removing Resins	974.5
40:20	Caloric Agents	974.5
40:24	Salt and Sugar Substitutes	974.5

AHFS* List		ICD-9-CM Dx Code
40:28	Diuretics NEC	974.4
	carbonic acid anhydrase inhibitors	974.2
	mercurials	974.0
	purine derivatives	974.1
	saluretics	974.3
40:36	Irrigating Solutions	974.5
40:40	Uricosuric Agents	974.7
44:00	ENZYMES NEC	963.4
	fibrinolysis-affecting agents	964.4
	gastric agents	973.4
48:00	EXPECTORANTS AND COUGH PREPARATIONS	
	antihistamine agents	963.0
	antitussives	975.4
	codeine derivatives	965.09
	expectorants	975.5
	narcotic agents NEC	965.09
52:00	EYE, EAR, NOSE, AND THROAT PREPARATIONS	
52:04	Anti-Infectives	
	ENT	976.6
	ophthalmic	976.5
52:04.04	Antibiotics	
	ENT	976.6
	ophthalmic	976.5
52:04.06	Antivirals	
	ENT	976.6
	ophthalmic	976.5
52:04.08	Sulfonamides	
	ENT	976.6
	ophthalmic	976.5
52:04.12	Miscellaneous Anti-Infectives	
	ENT	976.6
	ophthalmic	976.5
52:08	Anti-Inflammatory Agents	
	ENT	976.6
	ophthalmic	976.5
52:10	Carbonic Anhydrase Inhibitors	974.2
52:12	Contact Lens Solutions	976.5
52:16	Local Anesthetics	968.5
52:20	Miotics	971.0
52:24	Mydriatics	
	adrenergics	971.2
	anticholinergics	971.1
	antimuscarinics	971.1
	parasympatholytics	971.1
	spasmolytics	971.1
	sympathomimetics	971.2
52:28	Mouth Washes and Gargles	976.6
52:32	Vasoconstrictors	971.2
52:36	Unclassified Agents	
	ENT	976.6
	ophthalmic	976.5
56:00	GASTROINTESTINAL DRUGS	
56:04	Antacids and Absorbents	973.0
56:08	Anti-Diarrhea Agents	973.5
56:10	Antiflatulents	973.8
56:12	Cathartics NEC	973.3
	emollients	973.2
	irritants	973.1
56:16	Digestants	973.4
56:20	Emetics and Antiemetics	
	antiemetics	963.0
	emetics	973.6
56:24	Lipotropic Agents	977.1
60:00	GOLD COMPOUNDS	965.69
64:00	HEAVY METAL ANTAGONISTS	963.8
68:00	HORMONES AND SYNTHETIC SUBSTITUTES	
68:04	Adrenals	962.0
68:08	Androgens	962.1
68:12	Contraceptives	962.2
68:16	Estrogens	962.2
68:18	Gonadotropins	962.4

AHFS* List		ICD-9-CM Dx Code
68:20	Insulins and Antidiabetic Agents	962.3
68:20.08	Insulins	962.3
68:24	Parathyroid	962.6
68:28	Pituitary	
	anterior	962.4
	posterior	962.5
68:32	Progestogens	962.2
68:34	Other Corpus Luteum Hormones	962.2
68:36	Thyroid and Antithyroid	
	antithyroid	962.8
	thyroid	962.7
72:00	LOCAL ANESTHETICS NEC	968.9
	topical (surface) agents	968.5
	infiltrating agents (intradermal) (subcutaneous) (submucosal)	968.5
	nerve blocking agents (peripheral) (plexus) (regional)	968.6
	spinal	968.7
76:00	OXYTOCICS	975.0
78:00	RADIOACTIVE AGENTS	990
80:00	SERUMS, TOXOIDS, AND VACCINES	
80:04	Serums	979.9
	immune globulin (gamma) (human)	964.6
80:08	Toxoids NEC	978.8
	diphtheria	978.5
	and tetanus	978.9
	with pertussis component	978.6
	tetanus	978.4
	and diphtheria	978.9
	with pertussis component	978.6
80:12	Vaccines NEC	979.9
	bacterial NEC	978.8
	with other bacterial component	978.9
	pertussis component	978.6
	viral and rickettsial component	979.7
	rickettsial NEC	979.6
	with bacterial component	979.7
	pertussis component	978.6
	viral component	979.7
	viral NEC	979.6
	with bacterial component	979.7
	pertussis component	978.6
	rickettsial component	979.7
84:00	SKIN AND MUCOUS MEMBRANE PREPARATIONS	
84:04	Anti-Infectives	976.0
84:04.04	Antibiotics	976.0
84:04.08	Fungicides	976.0
84:04.12	Scabicides and Pediculicides	976.0
84:04.16	Miscellaneous Local Anti-Infectives	976.0
84:06	Anti-Inflammatory Agents	976.0
84:08	Antipruritics and Local Anesthetics	
	antipruritics	976.1
	local anesthetics	968.5
84:12	Astringents	976.2
84:16	Cell Stimulants and Proliferants	976.8
84:20	Detergents	976.2
84:24	Emollients, Demulcents, and Protectants	976.3
84:28	Keratolytic Agents	976.4
84:32	Keratoplastic Agents	976.4
84:36	Miscellaneous Agents	976.8
86:00	SPASMOLYTIC AGENTS	975.1
	antiasthmatics	975.7
	papaverine	972.5
	theophyllin	974.1
88:00	VITAMINS	
88:04	Vitamin A	963.5
88:08	Vitamin B Complex	963.5
	hematopoietic vitamin	964.1
	nicotinic acid derivatives	972.2
88:12	Vitamin C	963.5

	AHFS* List	ICD-9-CM Dx Code
88:16	Vitamin D	963.5
88:20	Vitamin E	963.5
88:24	Vitamin K Activity	964.3
88:28	Multivitamin Preparations	963.5
92:00	UNCLASSIFIED THERAPEUTIC AGENTS	977.8

* American Hospital Formulary Service

Appendix D: Classification of Industrial Accidents According to Agency

Annex B to the Resolution concerning Statistics of Employment Injuries adopted by the Tenth International Conference of Labor Statisticians on 12 October 1962

1 Machines

11	*Prime-Movers, except Electrical Motors*
111	*Steam engines*
112	*Internal combustion engines*
119	*Others*
12	*Transmission Machinery*
121	*Transmission shafts*
122	*Transmission belts, cables, pulleys, pinions, chains, gears*
129	*Others*
13	*Metalworking Machines*
131	*Power presses*
132	*Lathes*
133	*Milling machines*
134	*Abrasive wheels*
135	*Mechanical shears*
136	*Forging machines*
137	*Rolling-mills*
139	*Others*
14	*Wood and Assimilated Machines*
141	*Circular saws*
142	*Other saws*
143	*Molding machines*
144	*Overhand planes*
149	*Others*
15	*Agricultural Machines*
151	*Reapers (including combine reapers)*
152	*Threshers*
159	*Others*
16	*Mining Machinery*
161	*Under-cutters*
169	*Others*
19	*Other Machines Not Elsewhere Classified*
191	*Earth-moving machines, excavating and scraping machines, except means of transport*
192	*Spinning, weaving and other textile machines*
193	*Machines for the manufacture of food-stuffs and beverages*
194	*Machines for the manufacture of paper*
195	*Printing machines*
199	*Others*

2 Means of Transport and Lifting Equipment

21	*Lifting Machines and Appliances*
211	*Cranes*
212	*Lifts and elevators*
213	*Winches*
214	*Pulley blocks*
219	*Others*
22	*Means of Rail Transport*
221	*Inter-urban railways*
222	*Rail transport in mines, tunnels, quarries, industrial establishments, docks, etc.*
229	*Others*
23	*Other Wheeled Means of Transport, Excluding Rail Transport*
231	*Tractors*
232	*Lorries*
233	*Trucks*
234	*Motor vehicles, not elsewhere classified*
235	*Animal-drawn vehicles*
236	*Hand-drawn vehicles*
239	*Others*
24	*Means of Air Transport*
25	*Means of Water Transport*
251	*Motorized means of water transport*
252	*Non-motorized means of water transport*
26	*Other Means of Transport*
261	*Cable-cars*
262	*Mechanical conveyors, except cable-cars*
269	*Others*

3 Other Equipment

31	*Pressure Vessels*
311	*Boilers*
312	*Pressurized containers*
313	*Pressurized piping and accessories*
314	*Gas cylinders*
315	*Caissons, diving equipment*
319	*Others*
32	*Furnaces, Ovens, Kilns*
321	*Blast furnaces*
322	*Refining furnaces*
323	*Other furnaces*
324	*Kilns*
325	*Ovens*
33	*Refrigerating Plants*
34	*Electrical Installations, Including Electric Motors, but Excluding Electric Hand Tools*
341	*Rotating machines*
342	*Conductors*
343	*Transformers*
344	*Control apparatus*
349	*Others*
35	*Electric Hand Tools*
36	*Tools, Implements, and Appliances, Except Electric Hand Tools*
361	*Power-driven hand tools, except electrichand tools*
362	*Hand tools, not power-driven*
369	*Others*
37	*Ladders, Mobile Ramps*
38	*Scaffolding*
39	*Other Equipment, Not Elsewhere Classified*

4 Materials, Substances and Radiations

41	*Explosives*
42	*Dusts, Gases, Liquids and Chemicals, Excluding Explosives*
421	*Dusts*
422	*Gases, vapors, fumes*
423	*Liquids, not elsewhere classified*
424	*Chemicals, not elsewhere classified*
43	*Flying Fragments*
44	*Radiations*
441	*Ionizing radiations*
449	*Others*
49	*Other Materials and Substances Not Elsewhere Classified*

5 Working Environment

51	*Outdoor*
511	*Weather*
512	*Traffic and working surfaces*
513	*Water*
519	*Others*
52	*Indoor*
521	*Floors*
522	*Confined quarters*
523	*Stairs*
524	*Other traffic and working surfaces*
525	*Floor openings and wall openings*
526	*Environmental factors (lighting, ventilation, temperature, noise, etc.)*
529	*Others*
53	*Underground*
531	*Roofs and faces of mine roads and tunnels, etc.*
532	*Floors of mine roads and tunnels, etc.*
533	*Working-faces of mines, tunnels, etc.*
534	*Mine shafts*
535	*Fire*
536	*Water*
539	*Others*

6 Other Agencies, Not Elsewhere Classified

61	*Animals*
611	*Live animals*
612	*Animal products*
69	*Other Agencies, Not Elsewhere Classified*

7 Agencies Not Classified for Lack of Sufficient Data

Appendix E: List of Three-digit Categories

1. Infectious and Parasitic Diseases

Intestinal infectious diseases (001-009)
001 Cholera
002 Typhoid and paratyphoid fevers
003 Other salmonella infections
004 Shigellosis
005 Other food poisoning (bacterial)
006 Amebiasis
007 Other protozoal intestinal diseases
008 Intestinal infections due to other organisms
009 Ill-defined intestinal infections

Tuberculosis (010-018)
010 Primary tuberculous infection
011 Pulmonary tuberculosis
012 Other respiratory tuberculosis
013 Tuberculosis of meninges and central nervous system
014 Tuberculosis of intestines, peritoneum, and mesenteric glands
015 Tuberculosis of bones and joints
016 Tuberculosis of genitourinary system
017 Tuberculosis of other organs
018 Miliary tuberculosis

Zoonotic bacterial diseases (020-027)
020 Plague
021 Tularemia
022 Anthrax
023 Brucellosis
024 Glanders
025 Melioidosis
026 Rat-bite fever
027 Other zoonotic bacterial diseases

Other bacterial diseases (030-042)
030 Leprosy
031 Diseases due to other mycobacteria
032 Diphtheria
033 Whooping cough
034 Streptococcal sore throat and scarlatina
035 Erysipelas
036 Meningococcal infection
037 Tetanus
038 Septicemia
039 Actinomycotic infections
040 Other bacterial diseases
041 Bacterial infection in conditions classified elsewhere and of unspecified site

Human immunodeficiency virus (042)
042 Human immunodeficiency virus [HIV] disease

Poliomyelitis and other non-arthropod-borne viral diseases and prion diseases of central nervous system (045-049)
045 Acute poliomyelitis
046 Slow virus infections and prion diseases of central nervous system
047 Meningitis due to enterovirus
048 Other enterovirus diseases of central nervous system
049 Other non-arthropod-borne viral diseases of central nervous system

Viral diseases generally accompanied by exanthem (050-058)
050 Smallpox
051 Cowpox and paravaccinia
052 Chickenpox
053 Herpes zoster
054 Herpes simplex
055 Measles
056 Rubella
057 Other viral exanthemata
058 Other human herpesvirus
059 Other poxvirus infections

Arthropod-borne viral diseases (060-066)
060 Yellow fever
061 Dengue
062 Mosquito-borne viral encephalitis
063 Tick-borne viral encephalitis
064 Viral encephalitis transmitted by other and unspecified arthropods
065 Arthropod-borne hemorrhagic fever
066 Other arthropod-borne viral diseases

Other diseases due to viruses and Chlamydiae (070-079)
070 Viral hepatitis
071 Rabies
072 Mumps
073 Ornithosis
074 Specific diseases due to Coxsackievirus
075 Infectious mononucleosis
076 Trachoma
077 Other diseases of conjunctiva due to viruses and Chlamydiae
078 Other diseases due to viruses and Chlamydiae
079 Viral infection in conditions classified elsewhere and of unspecified site

Rickettsioses and other arthropod-borne diseases (080-088)
080 Louse-borne [epidemic] typhus
081 Other typhus
082 Tick-borne rickettsioses
083 Other rickettsioses
084 Malaria
085 Leishmaniasis
086 Trypanosomiasis
087 Relapsing fever
088 Other arthropod-borne diseases

Syphilis and other venereal diseases (090-099)
090 Congenital syphilis
091 Early syphilis, symptomatic
092 Early syphilis, latent
093 Cardiovascular syphilis
094 Neurosyphilis
095 Other forms of late syphilis, with symptoms
096 Late syphilis, latent
097 Other and unspecified syphilis
098 Gonococcal infections
099 Other venereal diseases

Other spirochetal diseases (100-104)
100 Leptospirosis
101 Vincent's angina
102 Yaws
103 Pinta
104 Other spirochetal infection

Mycoses (110-118)
110 Dermatophytosis
111 Dermatomycosis, other and unspecified
112 Candidiasis
114 Coccidioidomycosis
115 Histoplasmosis
116 Blastomycotic infection
117 Other mycoses
118 Opportunistic mycoses

Helminthiases (120-129)
120 Schistosomiasis [bilharziasis]
121 Other trematode infections
122 Echinococcosis
123 Other cestode infection
124 Trichinosis
125 Filarial infection and dracontiasis
126 Ancylostomiasis and necatoriasis
127 Other intestinal helminthiases
128 Other and unspecified helminthiases
129 Intestinal parasitism, unspecified

Other infectious and parasitic diseases (130-136)
130 Toxoplasmosis
131 Trichomoniasis
132 Pediculosis and phthirus infestation
133 Acariasis
134 Other infestation
135 Sarcoidosis
136 Other and unspecified infectious and parasitic diseases

Late effects of infectious and parasitic diseases (137-139)
137 Late effects of tuberculosis
138 Late effects of acute poliomyelitis
139 Late effects of other infectious and parasitic diseases

2. Neoplasms

Malignant neoplasm of lip, oral cavity, and pharynx (140-149)
140 Malignant neoplasm of lip
141 Malignant neoplasm of tongue
142 Malignant neoplasm of major salivary glands
143 Malignant neoplasm of gum
144 Malignant neoplasm of floor of mouth
145 Malignant neoplasm of other and unspecified parts of mouth
146 Malignant neoplasm of oropharynx
147 Malignant neoplasm of nasopharynx
148 Malignant neoplasm of hypopharynx
149 Malignant neoplasm of other and ill-defined sites within the lip, oral cavity, and pharynx

Malignant neoplasm of digestive organs and peritoneum (150-159)
150 Malignant neoplasm of esophagus
151 Malignant neoplasm of stomach
152 Malignant neoplasm of small intestine, including duodenum
153 Malignant neoplasm of colon
154 Malignant neoplasm of rectum, rectosigmoid junction, and anus
155 Malignant neoplasm of liver and intrahepatic bile ducts
156 Malignant neoplasm of gallbladder and extrahepatic bile ducts
157 Malignant neoplasm of pancreas
158 Malignant neoplasm of retroperitoneum and peritoneum
159 Malignant neoplasm of other and ill-defined sites within the digestive organs and peritoneum

Malignant neoplasm of respiratory and intrathoracic organs (160-165)
160 Malignant neoplasm of nasal cavities, middle ear, and accessory sinuses
161 Malignant neoplasm of larynx
162 Malignant neoplasm of trachea, bronchus, and lung
163 Malignant neoplasm of pleura
164 Malignant neoplasm of thymus, heart, and mediastinum
165 Malignant neoplasm of other and ill-defined sites within the respiratory system and intrathoracic organs

Malignant neoplasm of bone, connective tissue, skin, and breast (170-176)
170 Malignant neoplasm of bone and articular cartilage
171 Malignant neoplasm of connective and other soft tissue
172 Malignant melanoma of skin
173 Other malignant neoplasm of skin
174 Malignant neoplasm of female breast
175 Malignant neoplasm of male breast
176 Kaposi's sarcoma

Appendix E: List of Three-digit Categories

Malignant neoplasm of genitourinary organs (179-189)
179 Malignant neoplasm of uterus, part unspecified
180 Malignant neoplasm of cervix uteri
181 Malignant neoplasm of placenta
182 Malignant neoplasm of body of uterus
183 Malignant neoplasm of ovary and other uterine adnexa
184 Malignant neoplasm of other and unspecified female genital organs
185 Malignant neoplasm of prostate
186 Malignant neoplasm of testis
187 Malignant neoplasm of penis and other male genital organs
188 Malignant neoplasm of bladder
189 Malignant neoplasm of kidney and other unspecified urinary organs

Malignant neoplasm of other and unspecified sites (190-199)
190 Malignant neoplasm of eye
191 Malignant neoplasm of brain
192 Malignant neoplasm of other and unspecified parts of nervous system
193 Malignant neoplasm of thyroid gland
194 Malignant neoplasm of other endocrine glands and related structures
195 Malignant neoplasm of other and ill-defined sites
196 Secondary and unspecified malignant neoplasm of lymph nodes
197 Secondary malignant neoplasm of respiratory and digestive systems
198 Secondary malignant neoplasm of other specified sites
199 Malignant neoplasm without specification of site

Malignant neoplasm of lymphatic and hematopoietic tissue (200-208)
200 Lymphosarcoma and reticulosar-coma and other specified malignant tumors of lymphatic tissue
201 Hodgkin's disease
202 Other malignant neoplasm of lymphoid and histiocytic tissue
203 Multiple myeloma and immunoproliferative neoplasms
204 Lymphoid leukemia
205 Myeloid leukemia
206 Monocytic leukemia
207 Other specified leukemia
208 Leukemia of unspecified cell type

Neuroendocrine tumors (209)
209 Neuroendocrine tumors

Benign neoplasms (210-229)
210 Benign neoplasm of lip, oral cavity, and pharynx
211 Benign neoplasm of other parts of digestive system
212 Benign neoplasm of respiratory and intrathoracic organs
213 Benign neoplasm of bone and articular cartilage
214 Lipoma
215 Other benign neoplasm of connective and other soft tissue
216 Benign neoplasm of skin
217 Benign neoplasm of breast
218 Uterine leiomyoma
219 Other benign neoplasm of uterus
220 Benign neoplasm of ovary
221 Benign neoplasm of other female genital organs
222 Benign neoplasm of male genital organs
223 Benign neoplasm of kidney and other urinary organs
224 Benign neoplasm of eye
225 Benign neoplasm of brain and other parts of nervous system

226 Benign neoplasm of thyroid gland
227 Benign neoplasm of other endocrine glands and related structures
228 Hemangioma and lymphangioma, any site
229 Benign neoplasm of other and unspecified sites

Carcinoma in situ (230-234)
230 Carcinoma in situ of digestive organs
231 Carcinoma in situ of respiratory system
232 Carcinoma in situ of skin
233 Carcinoma in situ of breast and genitourinary system
234 Carcinoma in situ of other and unspecified sites

Neoplasms of uncertain behavior (235-238)
235 Neoplasm of uncertain behavior of digestive and respiratory systems
236 Neoplasm of uncertain behavior of genitourinary organs
237 Neoplasm of uncertain behavior of endocrine glands and nervous system
238 Neoplasm of uncertain behavior of other and unspecified sites and tissues

Neoplasms of unspecified nature (239)
239 Neoplasm of unspecified nature

3. Endocrine, Nutritional and Metabolic Diseases, and Immunity Disorders

Disorders of thyroid gland (240-246)
240 Simple and unspecified goiter
241 Nontoxic nodular goiter
242 Thyrotoxicosis with or without goiter
243 Congenital hypothyroidism
244 Acquired hypothyroidism
245 Thyroiditis
246 Other disorders of thyroid

Diseases of other endocrine glands (249-259)
249 Secondary diabetes mellitus
250 Diabetes mellitus
251 Other disorders of pancreatic internal secretion
252 Disorders of parathyroid gland
253 Disorders of the pituitary gland and its hypothalamic control
254 Diseases of thymus gland
255 Disorders of adrenal glands
256 Ovarian dysfunction
257 Testicular dysfunction
258 Polyglandular dysfunction and related disorders
259 Other endocrine disorders

Nutritional deficiencies (260-269)
260 Kwashiorkor
261 Nutritional marasmus
262 Other severe protein-calorie malnutrition
263 Other and unspecified protein-calorie malnutrition
264 Vitamin A deficiency
265 Thiamine and niacin deficiency states
266 Deficiency of B-complex components
267 Ascorbic acid deficiency
268 Vitamin D deficiency
269 Other nutritional deficiencies

Other metabolic disorders and immnity disorders (270-279)
270 Disorders of amino-acid transport and metabolism
271 Disorders of carbohydrate transport and metabolism
272 Disorders of lipoid metabolism
273 Disorders of plasma protein metabolism
274 Gout
275 Disorders of mineral metabolism
276 Disorders of fluid, electrolyte, and acid-base balance
277 Other and unspecified disorders of metabolism

278 Overweight, obesity and other hyperalimentation
279 Disorders involving the immune mechanism

4. Diseases of Blood and Blood-forming Organs (280-289)
280 Iron deficiency anemias
281 Other deficiency anemias
282 Hereditary hemolytic anemias
283 Acquired hemolytic anemias
284 Aplastic anemia
285 Other and unspecified anemias
286 Coagulation defects
287 Purpura and other hemorrhagic conditions
288 Diseases of white blood cells
289 Other diseases of blood and blood-forming organs

5. Mental Disorders

Organic psychotic conditions (290-294)
290 Senile and presenile organic psychotic conditions
291 Alcoholic psychoses
292 Drug psychoses
293 Transient organic psychotic conditions
294 Other organic psychotic conditions (chronic)

Other psychoses (295-299)
295 Schizophrenic psychoses
296 Affective psychoses
297 Paranoid states
298 Other nonorganic psychoses
299 Psychoses with origin specific to childhood

Neurotic disorders, personality disorders, and other nonpsychotic mental disorders (300-316)
300 Neurotic disorders
301 Personality disorders
302 Sexual and gender identity disorders
303 Alcohol dependence syndrome
304 Drug dependence
305 Nondependent abuse of drugs
306 Physiological malfunction arising from mental factors
307 Special symptoms or syndromes, not elsewhere classified
308 Acute reaction to stress
309 Adjustment reaction
310 Specific nonpsychotic mental disorders following organic brain damage
311 Depressive disorder, not elsewhereclassified
312 Disturbance of conduct, not elsewhere classified
313 Disturbance of emotions specific tochildhood and adolescence
314 Hyperkinetic syndrome of childhood
315 Specific delays in development
316 Psychic factors associated with diseases classified elsewhere

Mental retardation (317-319)
317 Mild mental retardation
318 Other specified mental retardation
319 Unspecified mental retardation

6. Diseases of the Nervous System and Sense Organs

Inflammatory diseases of the central nervous system (320-326)
320 Bacterial meningitis
321 Meningitis due to other organisms
322 Meningitis of unspecified cause
323 Encephalitis, myelitis, and encephalomyelitis
324 Intracranial and intraspinal abscess
325 Phlebitis and thrombophlebitis of intracranial venous sinuses

326   Late effects of intracranial abscess or pyogenic infection

Organic Sleep Disorders (327)
327   Organic sleep disorders

Hereditary and degenerative diseases of the central nervous system (330-337)
330   Cerebral degenerations usually manifest in childhood
331   Other cerebral degenerations
332   Parkinson's disease
333   Other extrapyramidal diseases and abnormal movement disorders
334   Spinocerebellar disease
335   Anterior horn cell disease
336   Other diseases of spinal cord
337   Disorders of the autonomic nervous system

Pain (338)
338   Pain, not elsewhere classified

Other headache syndromes (339)
339   Other headache syndromes

Other disorders of the central nervous system (340-349)
340   Multiple sclerosis
341   Other demyelinating diseases of central nervous system
342   Hemiplegia and hemiparesis
343   Infantile cerebral palsy
344   Other paralytic syndromes
345   Epilepsy and recurrent seizures
346   Migraine
347   Cataplexy and narcolepsy
348   Other conditions of brain
349   Other and unspecified disorders of the nervous system

Disorders of the peripheral nervous system (350-359)
350   Trigeminal nerve disorders
351   Facial nerve disorders
352   Disorders of other cranial nerves
353   Nerve root and plexus disorders
354   Mononeuritis of upper limb and mononeuritis multiplex
355   Mononeuritis of lower limb
356   Hereditary and idiopathic peripheral neuropathy
357   Inflammatory and toxic neuropathy
358   Myoneural disorders
359   Muscular dystrophies and other myopathies

Disorders of the eye and adnexa (360-379)
360   Disorders of the globe
361   Retinal detachments and defects
362   Other retinal disorders
363   Chorioretinal inflammations and scars and other disorders of choroid
364   Disorders of iris and ciliary body
365   Glaucoma
366   Cataract
367   Disorders of refraction and accommodation
368   Visual disturbances
369   Blindness and low vision
370   Keratitis
371   Corneal opacity and other disorders of cornea
372   Disorders of conjunctiva
373   Inflammation of eyelids
374   Other disorders of eyelids
375   Disorders of lacrimal system
376   Disorders of the orbit
377   Disorders of optic nerve and visual pathways
378   Strabismus and other disorders of binocular eye movements
379   Other disorders of eye

Diseases of the ear and mastoid process (380-389)
380   Disorders of external ear

381   Nonsuppurative otitis media and Eustachian tube disorders
382   Suppurative and unspecified otitis media
383   Mastoiditis and related conditions
384   Other disorders of tympanic membrane
385   Other disorders of middle ear and mastoid
386   Vertiginous syndromes and other disorders of vestibular system
387   Otosclerosis
388   Other disorders of ear
389   Hearing loss

7. Diseases of the Circulatory System

Acute rheumatic fever (390-392)
390   Rheumatic fever without mention of heart involvement
391   Rheumatic fever with heart involvement
392   Rheumatic chorea

Chronic rheumatic heart disease (393-398)
393   Chronic rheumatic pericarditis
394   Diseases of mitral valve
395   Diseases of aortic valve
396   Diseases of mitral and aortic valves
397   Diseases of other endocardial structures
398   Other rheumatic heart disease

Hypertensive disease (401-405)
401   Essential hypertension
402   Hypertensive heart disease
403   Hypertensive kidney disease
404   Hypertensive heart and kidney disease
405   Secondary hypertension

Ischemic heart disease (410-414)
410   Acute myocardial infarction
411   Other acute and subacute form of ischemic heart disease
412   Old myocardial infarction
413   Angina pectoris
414   Other forms of chronic ischemic heart disease

Diseases of pulmonary circulation (415-417)
415   Acute pulmonary heart disease
416   Chronic pulmonary heart disease
417   Other diseases of pulmonary circulation

Other forms of heart disease (420-429)
420   Acute pericarditis
421   Acute and subacute endocarditis
422   Acute myocarditis
423   Other diseases of pericardium
424   Other diseases of endocardium
425   Cardiomyopathy
426   Conduction disorders
427   Cardiac dysrhythmias
428   Heart failure
429   Ill-defined descriptions and complications of heart disease

Cerebrovascular disease (430-438)
430   Subarachnoid hemorrhage
431   Intracerebral hemorrhage
432   Other and unspecified intracranial hemorrhage
433   Occlusion and stenosis of precerebral arteries
434   Occlusion of cerebral arteries
435   Transient cerebral ischemia
436   Acute but ill-defined cerebrovascular disease
437   Other and ill-defined cerebrovascular disease
438   Late effects of cerebrovascular disease

Diseases of arteries, arterioles, and capillaries (440-449)
440   Atherosclerosis
441   Aortic aneurysm and dissection
442   Other aneurysm
443   Other peripheral vascular disease
444   Arterial embolism and thrombosis
445   Atheroembolism
446   Polyarteritis nodosa and allied conditions

447   Other disorders of arteries and arterioles
448   Diseases of capillaries
449   Septic arterial embolism

Diseases of veins and lymphatics, and other diseases of circulatory system (451-459)
451   Phlebitis and thrombophlebitis
452   Portal vein thrombosis
453   Other venous embolism and thrombosis
454   Varicose veins of lower extremities
455   Hemorrhoids
456   Varicose veins of other sites
457   Noninfective disorders of lymphatic channels
458   Hypotension
459   Other disorders of circulatory system

8. Diseases of the Respiratory System

Acute respiratory infections (460-466)
460   Acute nasopharyngitis [common cold]
461   Acute sinusitis
462   Acute pharyngitis
463   Acute tonsillitis
464   Acute laryngitis and tracheitis
465   Acute upper respiratory infections of multiple or unspecified sites
466   Acute bronchitis and bronchiolitis

Other diseases of upper respiratory tract (470-478)
470   Deviated nasal septum
471   Nasal polyps
472   Chronic pharyngitis and nasopharyngitis
473   Chronic sinusitis
474   Chronic disease of tonsils and adenoids
475   Peritonsillar abscess
476   Chronic laryngitis and aryngotracheitis
477   Allergic rhinitis
478   Other diseases of upper respiratory tract

Pneumonia and influenza (480-488)
480   Viral pneumonia
481   Pneumococcal pneumonia [Streptococcus pneumoniae pneumonia]
482   Other bacterial pneumonia
483   Pneumonia due to other specified organism
484   Pneumonia in infectious diseases classified elsewhere
485   Bronchopneumonia, organism unspecified
486   Pneumonia, organism unspecified
487   Influenza
488   Influenza due to certain identified influenza viruses

Chronic obstructive pulmonary disease and allied conditions (490-496)
490   Bronchitis, not specified as acute or chronic
491   Chronic bronchitis
492   Emphysema
493   Asthma
494   Bronchiectasis
495   Extrinsic allergic alveolitis
496   Chronic airways obstruction, not elsewhere classified

Pneumoconioses and other lung diseases due to external agents (500-508)
500   Coal workers' pneumoconiosis
501   Asbestosis
502   Pneumoconiosis due to other silica or silicates
503   Pneumoconiosis due to other inorganic dust
504   Pneumopathy due to inhalation of other dust
505   Pneumoconiosis, unspecified
506   Respiratory conditions due to chemical fumes and vapors
507   Pneumonitis due to solids and liquids
508   Respiratory conditions due to other and unspecified external agents

Other diseases of respiratory system (510-519)

510 Empyema
511 Pleurisy
512 Pneumothorax
513 Abscess of lung and mediastinum
514 Pulmonary congestion and hypostasis
515 Postinflammatory pulmonary fibrosis
516 Other alveolar and parietoalveolar pneumopathy
517 Lung involvement in conditions classified elsewhere
518 Other diseases of lung
519 Other diseases of respiratory system

9. Diseases of the Digestive System

Diseases of oral cavity, salivary glands, and jaws (520-529)

520 Disorders of tooth development and eruption
521 Diseases of hard tissues of teeth
522 Diseases of pulp and periapical tissues
523 Gingival and periodontal diseases
524 Dentofacial anomalies, including malocclusion
525 Other diseases and conditions of the teeth and supporting structures
526 Diseases of the jaws
527 Diseases of the salivary glands
528 Diseases of the oral soft tissues, excluding lesions specific for gingiva and tongue
529 Diseases and other conditions of the tongue

Diseases of esophagus, stomach, and duodenum (530-538)

530 Diseases of esophagus
531 Gastric ulcer
532 Duodenal ulcer
533 Peptic ulcer, site unspecified
534 Gastrojejunal ulcer
535 Gastritis and duodenitis
536 Disorders of function of stomach
537 Other disorders of stomach and duodenum
538 Gastrointestinal mucositis (ulcerative)

Appendicitis (540-543)

540 Acute appendicitis
541 Appendicitis, unqualified
542 Other appendicitis
543 Other diseases of appendix

Hernia of abdominal cavity (550-553)

550 Inguinal hernia
551 Other hernia of abdominal cavity, with gangrene
552 Other hernia of abdominal cavity, with ob-struction, but without mention of gangrene
553 Other hernia of abdominal cavity without mention of obstruction or gangrene

Noninfective enteritis and colitis (555-558)

555 Regional enteritis
556 Ulcerative colitis
557 Vascular insufficiency of intestine
558 Other noninfective gastroenteritis and colitis

Other diseases of intestines and peritoneum (560-569)

560 Intestinal obstruction without mention of hernia
562 Diverticula of intestine
564 Functional digestive disorders, not elsewhere classified
565 Anal fissure and fistula
566 Abscess of anal and rectal regions
567 Peritonitis and retroperitoneal infections
568 Other disorders of peritoneum
569 Other disorders of intestine

Other diseases of digestive system (570-579)

570 Acute and subacute necrosis of liver
571 Chronic liver disease and cirrhosis
572 Liver abscess and sequelae of chronic liver disease
573 Other disorders of liver
574 Cholelithiasis
575 Other disorders of gallbladder
576 Other disorders of biliary tract
577 Diseases of pancreas
578 Gastrointestinal hemorrhage
579 Intestinal Malabsorption

10. Diseases of the Genitourinary System

Nephritis, nephrotic syndrome, and nephrosis (580-589)

580 Acute gloerulonephritis
581 Nephrotic syndrome
582 Chronic glomerulonephritis
583 Nephritis and nephropathy, not specified as acute or chronic
584 Acute kidney failure
585 Chronic kidney disease (CKD)
586 Renal failure, unspecified
587 Renal sclerosis, unspecified
588 Disorders resulting from impaired renal function
589 Small kidney of unknown cause

Other diseases of urinary system (590-599)

590 Infections of kidney
591 Hydronephrosis
592 Calculus of kidney and ureter
593 Other disorders of kidney and ureter
594 Calculus of lower urinary tract
595 Cystitis
596 Other disorders of bladder
597 Urethritis, not sexually transmitted, and urethral syndrome
598 Urethral stricture
599 Other disorders of urethra and urinary tract

Diseases of male genital organs (600-608)

600 Hyperplasia of prostate
601 Inflammatory diseases of prostate
602 Other disorders of prostate
603 Hydrocele
604 Orchitis and epididymitis
605 Redundant prepuce and phimosis
606 Infertility, male
607 Disorders of penis
608 Other disorders of male genital organs

Disorders of breast (610-612)

610 Benign mammary dysplasias
611 Other disorders of breast
612 Deformity and disproportion of reconstructed breast

Inflammatory disease of female pelvic organs (614-616)

614 Inflammatory disease of ovary, fallopian tube, pelvic cellular tissue, and peritoneum
615 Inflammatory diseases of uterus, except cervix
616 Inflammatory disease of cervix, vagina, and vulva

Other disorders of female genital tract (617-629)

617 Endometriosis
618 Genital prolapse
619 Fistula involving female genital tract
620 Noninflammatory disorders of ovary, fallopian tube, and broad ligament
621 Disorders of uterus, not elsewhere classified
622 Noninflammatory disorders of cervix
623 Noninflammatory disorders of vagina
624 Noninflammatory disorders of vulva and perineum
625 Pain and other symptoms associated with female genital organs
626 Disorders of menstruation and other abnormal bleeding from female genital tract
627 Menopausal and postmenopausal disorders
628 Infertility, female
629 Other disorders of female genital organs

11. Complications of Pregnancy, Childbirth and the Puerperium

Ectopic and molar pregnancy and other pregnancy with abortive outcome (630-639)

630 Hydatidiform mole
631 Other abnormal product of conception
632 Missed abortion
633 Ectopic pregnancy
634 Spontaneous abortion
635 Legally induced abortion
636 Illegally induced abortion
637 Unspecified abortion
638 Failed attempted abortion
639 Complications following abortion and ectopic and molar pregnancies

Complications mainly related to pregnancy (640-649)

640 Hemorrhage in early pregnancy
641 Antepartum hemorrhage, abruptio placentae, and placenta previa
642 Hypertension complicating pregnancy, childbirth, and the puerperium
643 Excessive vomiting in pregnancy
644 Early or threatened labor
645 Prolonged pregnancy
646 Other complications of pregnancy, not elsewhere classified
647 Infective and parasitic conditions in the mother classifiable elsewhere but complicating pregnancy, childbirth, and the puerperium
648 Other current conditions in the mother classifiable elsewhere but complicating pregnancy, childbirth, and the puerperium
649 Other conditions or status of the mother complicating pregnancy, childbirth, or puerperium

Normal delivery, and other indications for care in pregnancy, labor, and delivery (650-659)

650 Normal delivery
651 Multiple gestation
652 Malposition and malpresentation of fetus
653 Disproportion
654 Abnormality of organs and soft tissues of pelvis
655 Known or suspected fetal abnormality affecting management of mother
656 Other fetal and placental problems affecting management of mother
657 Polyhydramnios
658 Other problems associated with amniotic cavity and membranes
659 Other indications for care or intervention related to labor and delivery and not elsewhere classified

Complications occurring mainly in the course of labor and delivery (660-669)

660 Obstructed labor
661 Abnormality of forces of labor
662 Long labor
663 Umbilical cord complications
664 Trauma to perineum and vulva during delivery
665 Other obstetrical trauma
666 Postpartum hemorrhage
667 Retained placenta or membranes, without hemorrhage
668 Complications of the administration of anesthetic or other sedation in labor and delivery
669 Other complications of labor and delivery, not elsewhere classified

Complications of the puerperium (670-679)
670   Major puerperal infection
671   Venous complications in pregnancy and the puerperium
672   Pyrexia of unknown origin during the puerperium
673   Obstetrical pulmonary embolism
674   Other and unspecified complications of the puerperium, not elsewhere classified
675   Infections of the breast and nipple associated with childbirth
676   Other disorders of the breast associated with childbirth, and disorders of lactation
677   Late effect of complication of pregnancy, childbirth, and the puerperium
678   Other fetal conditions
679   Complications of in utero procedures

12. Diseases of the Skin and Subcutaneous Tissue

Infections of skin and subcutaneous tissue (680-686)
680   Carbuncle and furuncle
681   Cellulitis and abscess of finger and toe
682   Other cellulitis and abscess
683   Acute lymphadenitis
684   Impetigo
685   Pilonidal cyst
686   Other local infections of skin and subcutaneous tissue

Inflammatory conditions of skin and subcutaneous tissue (690-698)
690   Erythematosquamous dermatosis
691   Atopic dermatitis and related conditions
692   Contact dermatitis and other eczema
693   Dermatitis due to substances taken internally
694   Bullous dermatoses
695   Erythematous conditions
696   Psoriasis and similar disorders
697   Lichen
698   Pruritus and related conditions

Other diseases of skin and subcutaneous tissue (700-709)
700   Corns and callosities
701   Other hypertrophic and atrophic conditions of skin
702   Other dermatoses
703   Diseases of nail
704   Diseases of hair and hair follicles
705   Disorders of sweat glands
706   Diseases of sebaceous glands
707   Chronic ulcer of skin
708   Urticaria
709   Other disorders of skin and subcutaneous tissue

13. Diseases of the Musculoskeletal System and Connective Tissue

Arthropathies and related disorders (710-719)
710   Diffuse diseases of connective tissue
711   Arthropathy associated with infections
712   Crystal arthropathies
713   Arthropathy associated with other disorders classified elsewhere
714   Rheumatoid arthritis and other inflammatory polyarthropathies
715   Osteoarthrosis and allied disorders
716   Other and unspecified arthropathies
717   Internal derangement of knee
718   Other derangement of joint
719   Other and unspecified disorder of joint

Dorsopathies (720-724)
720   Ankylosing spondylitis and other inflammatory spondylopathies

721   Spondylosis and allied disorders
722   Intervertebral disc disorders
723   Other disorders of cervical region
724   Other and unspecified disorders of back

Rheumatism, excluding the back (725-729)
725   Polymyalgia rheumatica
726   Peripheral enthesopathies and allied syndromes
727   Other disorders of synovium, tendon, and bursa
728   Disorders of muscle, ligament, and fascia
729   Other disorders of soft tissues

Osteopathies, chondropathies, and acquired musculoskeletal deformities (730-739)
730   Osteomyelitis, periostitis, and other infections involving bone
731   Osteitis deformans and osteopathies associated with other disorders classified elsewhere
732   Osteochondropathies
733   Other disorders of bone and cartilage
734   Flat foot
735   Acquired deformities of toe
736   Other acquired deformities of limbs
737   Curvature of spine
738   Other acquired deformity
739   Nonallopathic lesions, not elsewhere classified

14. Congenital Anomalies

740   Anencephalus and similar anomalies
741   Spina bifida
742   Other congenital anomalies of nervous system
743   Congenital anomalies of eye
744   Congenital anomalies of ear, face, and neck
745   Bulbus cordis anomalies and anomalies of cardiac septal closure
746   Other congenital anomalies of heart
747   Other congenital anomalies of circulatory system
748   Congenital anomalies of respiratory system
749   Cleft palate and cleft lip
750   Other congenital anomalies of upper alimentary tract
751   Other congenital anomalies of digestive system
752   Congenital anomalies of genital organs
753   Congenital anomalies of urinary system
754   Certain congenital musculoskeletal deformities
755   Other congenital anomalies of limbs
756   Other congenital musculoskeletal anomalies
757   Congenital anomalies of the integument
758   Chromosomal anomalies
759   Other and unspecified congenital anomalies

15. Certain Conditions Originating in the Perinatal Period

Maternal causes of perinatal morbidity and mortality (760-763)
760   Fetus or newborn affected by maternal conditions which may be unrelated to present pregnancy
761   Fetus or newborn affected by maternal complications of pregnancy
762   Fetus or newborn affected by complications of placenta, cord, and membranes
763   Fetus or newborn affected by other complications of labor and delivery

Other conditions originating in the perinatal period (764-779)
764   Slow fetal growth and fetal malnutrition
765   Disorders relating to short gestation and unspecified low birthweight
766   Disorders relating to long gestation and high birthweight
767   Birth trauma
768   Intrauterine hypoxia and birth asphyxia
769   Respiratory distress syndrome

770   Other respiratory conditions of fetus and newborn
771   Infections specific to the perinatal period
772   Fetal and neonatal hemorrhage
773   Hemolytic disease of fetus or newborn, due to isoimmunization
774   Other perinatal jaundice
775   Endocrine and metabolic disturbances specific to the fetus and newborn
776   Hematological disorders of newborn
777   Perinatal disorders of digestive system
778   Conditions involving the integument and temperature regulation of fetus and newborn
779   Other and ill-defined conditions originating in the perinatal period

16. Symptoms, Signs, and Ill-defined Conditions

Symptoms (780-789)
780   General symptoms
781   Symptoms involving nervous and musculoskeletal systems
782   Symptoms involving skin and other integumentary tissue
783   Symptoms concerning nutrition, metabolism, and development
784   Symptoms involving head and neck
785   Symptoms involving cardiovascular system
786   Symptoms involving respiratory system and other chest symptoms
787   Symptoms involving digestive system
788   Symptoms involving urinary system
789   Other symptoms involving abdomen and pelvis

Nonspecific abnormal findings (790-796)
790   Nonspecific findings on examination of blood
791   Nonspecific findings on examination of urine
792   Nonspecific abnormal findings in other body substances
793   Nonspecific (abnormal) findings on radiological and other examination of body structure
794   Nonspecific abnormal results of function studies
795   Nonspecific abnormal histological and immunological findings
796   Other nonspecific abnormal findings

Ill-defined and unknown causes of morbidity and mortality (797-799)
797   Senility without mention of psychosis
798   Sudden death, cause unknown
799   Other ill-defined and unknown causes of morbidity and mortality

17. Injury and Poisoning

Fracture of skull (800-804)
800   Fracture of vault of skull
801   Fracture of base of skull
802   Fracture of face bones
803   Other and unqualified skull fractures
804   Multiple fractures involving skull or face with other bones

Fracture of spine and trunk (805-809)
805   Fracture of vertebral column without mention of spinal cord lesion
806   Fracture of vertebral column with spinal cord lesion
807   Fracture of rib(s), sternum, larynx, and trachea
808   Fracture of pelvis
809   Ill-defined fractures of bones of trunk

Fracture of upper limb (810-819)
810   Fracture of clavicle
811   Fracture of scapula
812   Fracture of humerus
813   Fracture of radius and ulna
814   Fracture of carpal bone(s)

815 Fracture of metacarpal bone(s)
816 Fracture of one or more phalanges of hand
817 Multiple fractures of hand bones
818 Ill-defined fractures of upper limb
819 Multiple fractures involving both upper limbs, and upper limb with rib(s) and sternum

Fracture of lower limb (820-829)
820 Fracture of neck of femur
821 Fracture of other and unspecified parts of femur
822 Fracture of patella
823 Fracture of tibia and fibula
824 Fracture of ankle
825 Fracture of one or more tarsal and metatarsal bones
826 Fracture of one or more phalanges of foot
827 Other, multiple, and ill-defined fractures of lower limb
828 Multiple fractures involving both lower limbs, lower with upper limb, and lower limb(s) with rib(s) and sternum
829 Fracture of unspecified bones

Dislocation (830-839)
830 Dislocation of jaw
831 Dislocation of shoulder
832 Dislocation of elbow
833 Dislocation of wrist
834 Dislocation of finger
835 Dislocation of hip
836 Dislocation of knee
837 Dislocation of ankle
838 Dislocation of foot
839 Other, multiple, and ill-defined dislocations

Sprains and strains of joints and adjacent muscles (840-848)
840 Sprains and strains of shoulder and upper arm
841 Sprains and strains of elbow and forearm
842 Sprains and strains of wrist and hand
843 Sprains and strains of hip and thigh
844 Sprains and strains of knee and leg
845 Sprains and strains of ankle and foot
846 Sprains and strains of sacroiliac region
847 Sprains and strains of other and unspecified parts of back
848 Other and ill-defined sprains and strains

Intracranial injury, excluding those with skull fracture (850-854)
850 Concussion
851 Cerebral laceration and contusion
852 Subarachnoid, subdural, and extradural hemorrhage, following injury
853 Other and unspecified intracranial hemorrhage following injury
854 Intracranial injury of other and unspecified nature

Internal injury of chest, abdomen, and pelvis (860-869)
860 Traumatic pneumothorax and hemothorax
861 Injury to heart and lung
862 Injury to other and unspecified intrathoracic organs
863 Injury to gastrointestinal tract
864 Injury to liver
865 Injury to spleen
866 Injury to kidney
867 Injury to pelvic organs
868 Injury to other intra-abdominal organs
869 Internal injury to unspecified or ill-defined organs

Open wound of head, neck, and trunk (870-879)
870 Open wound of ocular adnexa
871 Open wound of eyeball
872 Open wound of ear
873 Other open wound of head
874 Open wound of neck

875 Open wound of chest (wall)
876 Open wound of back
877 Open wound of buttock
878 Open wound of genital organs (external), including traumatic amputation
879 Open wound of other and unspecified sites, except limbs

Open wound of upper limb (880-887)
880 Open wound of shoulder and upper arm
881 Open wound of elbow, forearm, and wrist
882 Open wound of hand except finger(s) alone
883 Open wound of finger(s)
884 Multiple and unspecified open wound of upper limb
885 Traumatic amputation of thumb (complete) (partial)
886 Traumatic amputation of other finger(s) (complete) (partial)
887 Traumatic amputation of arm and hand (complete) (partial)

Open wound of lower limb (890-897)
890 Open wound of hip and thigh
891 Open wound of knee, leg [except thigh], and ankle
892 Open wound of foot except toe(s) alone
893 Open wound of toe(s)
894 Multiple and unspecified open wound of lower limb
895 Traumatic amputation of toe(s) (complete) (partial)
896 Traumatic amputation of foot (complete) (partial)
897 Traumatic amputation of leg(s) (complete) (partial)

Injury to blood vessels (900-904)
900 Injury to blood vessels of head and neck
901 Injury to blood vessels of thorax
902 Injury to blood vessels of abdomen and pelvis
903 Injury to blood vessels of upper extremity
904 Injury to blood vessels of lower extremity and unspecified sites

Late effects of injuries, poisonings, toxic effects, and other external causes (905-909)
905 Late effects of musculoskeletal and connective tissue injuries
906 Late effects of injuries to skin and subcutaneous tissues
907 Late effects of injuries to the nervous system
908 Late effects of other and unspecified injuries
909 Late effects of other and unspecified external causes

Superficial injury (910-919)
910 Superficial injury of face, neck, and scalp except eye
911 Superficial injury of trunk
912 Superficial injury of shoulder and upper arm
913 Superficial injury of elbow, forearm, and wrist
914 Superficial injury of hand(s) except finger(s) alone
915 Superficial injury of finger(s)
916 Superficial injury of hip, thigh, leg, and ankle
917 Superficial injury of foot and toe(s)
918 Superficial injury of eye and adnexa
919 Superficial injury of other, multiple, and unspecified sites

Contusion with intact skin surface (920-924)
920 Contusion of face, scalp, and neck except eye(s)
921 Contusion of eye and adnexa
922 Contusion of trunk
923 Contusion of upper limb
924 Contusion of lower limb and of other and unspecified sites

Crushing injury (925-929)
925 Crushing injury of face, scalp, and neck

926 Crushing injury of trunk
927 Crushing injury of upper limb
928 Crushing injury of lower limb
929 Crushing injury of multiple and unspecified sites

Effects of foreign body entering through orifice (930-939)
930 Foreign body on external eye
931 Foreign body in ear
932 Foreign body in nose
933 Foreign body in pharynx and larynx
934 Foreign body in trachea, bronchus, and lung
935 Foreign body in mouth, esophagus, and stomach
936 Foreign body in intestine and colon
937 Foreign body in anus and rectum
938 Foreign body in digestive system, unspecified
939 Foreign body in genitourinary tract

Burns (940-949)
940 Burn confined to eye and adnexa
941 Burn of face, head, and neck
942 Burn of trunk
943 Burn of upper limb, except wrist and hand
944 Burn of wrist(s) and hand(s)
945 Burn of lower limb(s)
946 Burns of multiple specified sites
947 Burn of internal organs
948 Burns classified according to extent of body surface involved
949 Burn, unspecified

Injury to nerves and spinal cord (950-957)
950 Injury to optic nerve and pathways
951 Injury to other cranial nerve(s)
952 Spinal cord injury without evidence of spinal bone injury
953 Injury to nerve roots and spinal plexus
954 Injury to other nerve(s) of trunk excluding shoulder and pelvic girdles
955 Injury to peripheral nerve(s) of shoulder girdle and upper limb
956 Injury to peripheral nerve(s) of pelvic girdle and lower limb
957 Injury to other and unspecified nerves

Certain traumatic complications and unspecified injuries (958-959)
958 Certain early complications of trauma
959 Injury, other and unspecified

Poisoning by drugs, medicinals and biological substances (960-979)
960 Poisoning by antibiotics
961 Poisoning by other anti-infectives
962 Poisoning by hormones and synthetic substitutes
963 Poisoning by primarily systemic agents
964 Poisoning by agents primarily affecting blood constituents
965 Poisoning by analgesics, antipyretics, and antirheumatics
966 Poisoning by anticonvulsants and anti-Parkinsonism drugs
967 Poisoning by sedatives and hypnotics
968 Poisoning by other central nervous system depressants and anesthetics
969 Poisoning by psychotropic agents
970 Poisoning by central nervous system stimulants
971 Poisoning by drugs primarily affecting the autonomic nervous system
972 Poisoning by agents primarily affecting the cardiovascular system
973 Poisoning by agents primarily affecting the gastrointestinal system
974 Poisoning by water, mineral, and uric acid metabolism drugs
975 Poisoning by agents primarily acting on the smooth and skeletal muscles and respiratory system

976 Poisoning by agents primarily affecting skin and mucous membrane, ophthalmological, otorhinolaryngological, and dental drugs
977 Poisoning by other and unspecified drugs and medicinals
978 Poisoning by bacterial vaccines
979 Poisoning by other vaccines and biological substances

Toxic effects of substances chiefly nonmedicinal as to source (980-989)
980 Toxic effect of alcohol
981 Toxic effect of petroleum products
982 Toxic effect of solvents other than petroleum-based
983 Toxic effect of corrosive aromatics, acids, and caustic alkalis
984 Toxic effect of lead and its compounds (including fumes)
985 Toxic effect of other metals
986 Toxic effect of carbon monoxide
987 Toxic effect of other gases, fumes, or vapors
988 Effect of noxious substances eaten as food
989 Toxic effect of other substances, chiefly nonmedicinal as to source

Other and unspecified effects of external causes (990-995)
990 Effects of radiation, unspecified
991 Effects of reduced temperature
992 Effects of heat and light
993 Effects of air pressure
994 Effects of other external causes
995 Certain adverse effects, not elsewhere classified

Complications of surgical and medical care, not elsewhere classified (996-999)
996 Complications peculiar to certain specified procedures
997 Complications affecting specified body systems, not elsewhere classified
998 Other complications of procedures, not elsewhere classified
999 Complications of medical care, not elsewhere classified

Supplementary Classification of Factors Influencing Health Status and Contact With Health Services

Persons with potential health hazards related to communicable diseases (V01-V09)
V01 Contact with or exposure to communicable diseases
V02 Carrier or suspected carrier of infectious diseases
V03 Need for prophylactic vaccination and inoculation against bacterial diseases
V04 Need for prophylactic vaccination and inoculation against certain viral diseases
V05 Need for other prophylactic vaccination and inoculation against single diseases
V06 Need for prophylactic vaccination and inoculation against combinations of diseases
V07 Need for isolation and other prophylactic or treatment measures
V08 Asymptomatic human immunodeficiency virus [HIV] infection status
V09 Infection with drug-resistant microorganisms

Persons with potential health hazards related to personal and family history (V10-V19)
V10 Personal history of malignant neoplasm
V11 Personal history of mental disorder
V12 Personal history of certain other diseases
V13 Personal history of other diseases
V14 Personal history of allergy to medicinal agents

V15 Other personal history presenting hazards to health
V16 Family history of malignant neoplasm
V17 Family history of certain chronic disabling diseases
V18 Family history of certain other specific conditions
V19 Family history of other conditions

Persons encountering health services in circumstances related to reproduction and development (V20-V29)
V20 Health supervision of infant or child
V21 Constitutional states in development
V22 Normal pregnancy
V23 Supervision of high-risk pregnancy
V24 Postpartum care and examination
V25 Encounter for contraceptive management
V26 Procreative management
V27 Outcome of delivery
V28 Antenatal screening
V29 Observation and evaluation of newborns and infants for suspected condition not found

Liveborn infants according to type of birth (V30-V39)
V30 Single liveborn
V31 mate liveborn
V32 Twin, mate stillborn
V33 Twin, unspecified
V34 Other multiple, mates all liveborn
V35 Other multiple, mates all stillborn
V36 Other multiple, mates live- and stillborn
V37 Other multiple, unspecified
V39 Unspecified

Persons with a condition influencing their health status (V40-V49)
V40 Mental and behavioral problems
V41 Problems with special senses and other special functions
V42 Organ or tissue replaced by transplant
V43 Organ or tissue replaced by other means
V44 Artificial opening status
V45 Other postprocedural states
V46 Other dependence on machines
V47 Other problems with internal organs
V48 Problems with head, neck, and trunk
V49 Other conditions influencing health status

Persons encountering health services for specific procedures and aftercare (V50-V59)
V50 Elective surgery for purposes other than remedying health states
V51 Aftercare involving the use of plastic surgery
V52 Fitting and adjustment of prosthetic device
V53 Fitting and adjustment of other device
V54 Other orthopedic aftercare
V55 Attention to artificial openings
V56 Encounter for dialysis and dialysis catheter care
V57 Care involving use of rehabilitation procedures
V58 Encounter for other and unspecified procedures and aftercare
V59 Donors

Persons encountering health services in other circumstances (V60-V69)
V60 Housing, household, and economic circumstances
V61 Other family circumstances
V62 Other psychosocial circumstances
V63 Unavailability of other medical facilities for care
V64 Persons encountering health services for specific procedures, not carried out
V65 Other persons seeking consultation
V66 Convalescence and palliative care
V67 Follow-up examination
V68 Encounters for administrative purposes
V69 Problems related to lifestyle

Persons without reported diagnosis encountered during examination and investigation of individuals and populations (V70-V82)
V70 General medical examination
V71 Observation and evaluation for suspected conditions not found
V72 Special investigations and examinations
V73 Special screening examination for viral and chlamydial diseases
V74 Special screening examination for bacterial and spirochetal diseases
V75 Special screening examination for other infectious diseases
V76 Special screening for malignant neoplasms
V77 Special screening for endocrine, nutritional, metabolic, and immunity disorders
V78 Special screening for disorders of blood and blood-forming organs
V79 Special screening for mental disorders and developmental handicaps
V80 Special screening for neurological, eye, and ear diseases
V81 Special screening for cardiovascular, respiratory, and genitourinary diseases
V82 Special screening for other conditions

Genetics (V83-V84)
V83 Genetic carrier status
V84 Genetic susceptibility to disease

Body mass index (V85)
V85 Body Mass Index [BMI]

Estrogen receptor status (V86)
V86 Estrogen receptor status

Other specified personal exposures and history presenting hazards to health (V87)
V87 Other specified personal exposures and history presenting hazards to health

Acquired absence of other organs and tissue (V88)
V88 Acquired absence of other organs and tissue

Other suspected conditions not found (V89)
V89 Other suspected conditions not found

Retained Foreign Body (V90)
V90 Retained foreign body

Multiple Gestation Placenta Status (V91)
V91 Multiple gestation placenta status

Supplementary Classification of External Causes of Injury and Poisoning

External Cause Status (E000)
E000 External cause status

Activity (E001-E030)
E001 Activities involving walking and running
E002 Activities involving water and water craft
E003 Activities involving ice and snow
E004 Activities involving climbing, rappelling, and jumping off
E005 Activities involving dancing and other rhythmic movement
E006 Activities involving other sports and athletics played individually
E007 Activities involving other sports and athletics played as a team or group
E008 Activities involving other specified sports and athletics
E009 Activity involving other cardiorespiratory exercise
E010 Activity involving other muscle strengthening exercises
E011 Activities involving computer technology and electronic devices
E012 Activities involving arts and handcrafts

E013   Activities involving personal hygiene and household maintenance
E014   Activities involving person providing caregiving
E015   Activities involving food preparation, cooking and grilling
E016   Activities involving property and land maintenance, building and construction
E017   Activities involving roller coasters and other types of external motion
E018   Activities involving playing musical instrument
E019   Activities involving animal care
E029   Other activity
E030   Unspecified activity

Transport Accidents (E800-E848)

Railway accidents (E800-E807)
E800   Railway accident involving collision with roling stock
E801   Railway accident involving collision with other object
E802   Railway accident involving derailment without antecedent collision
E803   Railway accident involving explosion, fire, or burning
E804   Fall in, on, or from railway train
E805   Hit by rolling stock
E806   Other specified railway accident
E807   Railway accident of unspecified nature

Motor vehicle traffic accidents (E810-E819)
E810   Motor vehicle traffic accident involving collision with train
E811   Motor vehicle traffic accident involving re-entrant collision with another motor vehicle
E812   Other motor vehicle traffic accident involving collision with another motor vehicle
E813   Motor vehicle traffic accident involving collision with other vehicle
E814   Motor vehicle traffic accident involving collision with pedestrian
E815   Other motor vehicle traffic accident involving collision on the highway
E816   Motor vehicle traffic accident due to loss of control, without collision on the highway
E817   Noncollision motor vehicle traffic accident while boarding or alighting
E818   Other noncollision motor vehicle traffic accident
E819   Motor vehicle traffic accident of unspecified nature

Motor vehicle nontraffic accidents (E820-E825)
E820   Nontraffic accident involving motor-driven snow vehicle
E821   Nontraffic accident involving other off-road motor vehicle
E822   Other motor vehicle nontraffic accident involving collision with moving object
E823   Other motor vehicle nontraffic accident involving collision with stationary object
E824   Other motor vehicle nontraffic accident while boarding and alighting
E825   Other motor vehicle nontraffic accident of other and unspecified nature

Other road vehicle accidents (E826-E829)
E826   Pedal cycle accident
E827   Animal-drawn vehicle accident
E828   Accident involving animal being ridden
E829   Other road vehicle accidents

Water transport accidents (E830-E838)
E830   Accident to watercraft causing submersion
E831   Accident to watercraft causing other injury
E832   Other accidental submersion or drowning in water transport accident
E833   Fall on stairs or ladders in water transport
E834   Other fall from one level to another in water transport

E835   Other and unspecified fall in water transport
E836   Machinery accident in water transport
E837   Explosion, fire, or burning in watercraft
E838   Other and unspecified water transport accident

Air and space transport accidents (E840-E845)
E840   Accident to powered aircraft at takeoff or landing
E841   Accident to powered aircraft, other and unspecified
E842   Accident to unpowered aircraft
E843   Fall in, on, or from aircraft
E844   Other specified air transport accidents
E845   Other involving spacecraft

Vehicle accidents, not elsewhere classfiable (E846-E849)
E846   Accidents involving powered vehicles used solely within the buildings and premises of an industrial or commercial establishment
E847   Accidents involving cable cars not running on rails
E848   Accidents involving other vehicles, not elsewhere classifiable
E849   Place of occurrence

Accidental poisoning by drugs, medicinal substances, and biologicals (E850-E858)
E850   Accidental poisoning by analgesics, antipyretics, and antirheumatics
E851   Accidental poisoning by barbiturates
E852   Accidental poisoning by other sedatives and hypnotics
E853   Accidental poisoning by tranquilizers
E854   Accidental poisoning by other psychotropic agents
E855   Accidental poisoning by other drugs acting on central and autonomic nervous systems
E856   Accidental poisoning by antibiotics
E857   Accidental poisoning by anti-infectives
E858   Accidental poisoning by other drugs

Accidental poisoning by other solid and liquid substances, gases, and vapors (E860-E869)
E860   Accidental poisoning by alcohol, not elsewhere classified
E861   Accidental poisoning by cleansing and polishing agents, disinfectants, paints, and varnishes
E862   Accidental poisoning by petroleum products, other solvents and their vapors, not elsewhere classified
E863   Accidental poisoning by agricultural and horticultural chemical and pharmaceutical preparations other than plant foods and fertilizers
E864   Accidental poisoning by corrosives and caustics, not elsewhere classified
E865   Accidental poisoning from poisonous foodstuffs and poisonous plants
E866   Accidental poisoning by other and unspecified solid and liquid substances
E867   Accidental poisoning by gas distributed by pipeline
E868   Accidental poisoning by other utility gas and other carbon monoxide
E869   Accidental poisoning by other gases and vapors

Misadventures to patients during surgical and medical care (E870-E876)
E870   Accidental cut, puncture, perforation, or hemorrhage during medical care
E871   Foreign object left in body during procedure
E872   Failure of sterile precautions during procedure
E873   Failure in dosage
E874   Mechanical failure of instrument or apparatus during procedure
E875   Contaminated or infected blood, other fluid, drug, or biological substance
E876   Other and unspecified misadventures during medical care

Surgical and medical procedures as the cause of abnormal reaction of patient or later complication, without mention of misadventure at the time of procedure (E878-E879)
E878   Surgical operation and other surgical procedures as the cause of abnormal reaction of patient, or of later complication, without mention of misadventure at the time of operation
E879   Other procedures, without mention of misadventure at the time of procedure, as the cause of abnormal reaction of patient, or of later complication

Accidental falls (E880-E888)
E880   Fall on or from stairs or steps
E881   Fall on or from ladders or scaffolding
E882   Fall from or out of building or other structure
E883   Fall into hole or other opening in surface
E884   Other fall from one level to another
E885   Fall on same level from slipping, tripping, or stumbling
E886   Fall on same level from collision, pushing or shoving, by or with other person
E887   Fracture, cause unspecified
E888   Other and unspecified fall

Accidents caused by fire and flames (E890-E899)
E890   Conflagration in private dwelling
E891   Conflagration in other and unspecified building or structure
E892   Conflagration not in building or structure
E893   Accident caused by ignition of clothing
E894   Ignition of highly inflammable material
E895   Accident caused by controlled fire in private dwelling
E896   Accident caused by controlled fire in other and unspecified building or structure
E897   Accident caused by controlled fire not in building or structure
E898   Accident caused by other specified fire and flames
E899   Accident caused by unspecified fire

Accidents due to natural and environmental factors (E900-E909)
E900   Excessive heat
E901   Excessive cold
E902   High and low air pressure and changes in air pressure
E903   Travel and motion
E904   Hunger, thirst, exposure, and neglect
E905   Venomous animals and plants as the cause of poisoning and toxic reactions
E906   Other injury caused by animals
E907   Lightning
E908   Cataclysmic storms, and floods resulting from storms
E909   Cataclysmic earth surface movements and eruptions

Accidents caused by submersion, suffocation, and foreign bodies (E910-E915)
E910   Accidental drowning and submersion
E911   Inhalation and ingestion of food causing obstruction of respiratory tract or suffocation
E912   Inhalation and ingestion of other object causing obstruction of respiratory tract or suffocation
E913   Accidental mechanical suffocation
E914   Foreign body accidentally entering eye and adnexa
E915   Foreign body accidentally entering other orifice

Other accidents (E916-E928)
E916   Struck accidentally by falling object
E917   Striking against or struck accidentally by objects or persons
E918   Caught accidentally in or between objects
E919   Accidents caused by machinery

E920   Accidents caused by cutting and piercing instruments or objects
E921   Accident caused by explosion of pressure vessel
E922   Accident caused by firearm missile
E923   Accident caused by explosive material
E924   Accident caused by hot substance or object, caustic or corrosive material, and steam
E925   Accident caused by electric current
E926   Exposure to radiation
E927   Overexertion and strenuous movements
E928   Other and unspecified environmental and accidental causes

Late effects of accidental injury (E929)
E929   Late effects of accidental injury

Drugs, medicinal and biological substances causing adverse effects in therapeutic use (E930-E949)
E930   Antibiotics
E931   Other anti-infectives
E932   Hormones and synthetic substitutes
E933   Primarily systemic agents
E934   Agents primarily affecting blood constituents
E935   Analgesics, antipyretics, and antirheumatics
E936   Anticonvulsants and anti-Parkinsonism drugs
E937   Sedatives and hypnotics
E938   Other central nervous system depressants and anesthetics
E939   Psychotropic agents
E940   Central nervous system stimulants
E941   Drugs primarily affecting the autonomic nervous system
E942   Agents primarily affecting the cardiovascular system
E943   Agents primarily affecting gastrointestinal system
E944   Water, mineral, and uric acid metabolism drugs
E945   Agents primarily acting on the smooth and skeletal muscles and respiratory system
E946   Agents primarily affecting skin and mucous membrane, ophthalmological, otorhinolaryngological, and dental drugs
E947   Other and unspecified drugs and medicinal substances
E948   Bacterial vaccines
E949   Other vaccines and biological substances

Suicide and self-inflicted injury (E950-E959)
E950   Suicide and self-inflicted poisoning by solid or liquid substances
E951   Suicide and self-inflicted poisoning by gases in domestic use
E952   Suicide and self-inflicted poisoning by other gases and vapors
E953   Suicide and self-inflicted injury by hanging, strangulation, and suffocation
E954   Suicide and self-inflicted injury by submersion [drowning]
E955   Suicide and self-inflicted injury by firearms and explosives
E956   Suicide and self-inflicted injury by cutting and piercing instruments
E957   Suicide and self-inflicted injuries by jumping from high place
E958   Suicide and self-inflicted injury by other and unspecified means
E959   Late effects of self-inflicted injury

Homicide and injury purposely inflicted by other persons (E960-E969)
E960   Fight, brawl, and rape
E961   Assault by corrosive or caustic substance, except poisoning
E962   Assault by poisoning
E963   Assault by hanging and strangulation
E964   Assault by submersion [drowning]
E965   Assault by firearms and explosives
E966   Assault by cutting and piercing instrument
E967   Child and adult battering and other maltreatment
E968   Assault by other and unspecified means
E969   Late effects of injury purposely inflicted by other person

Legal intervention (E970-E978)
E970   Injury due to legal intervention by firearms
E971   Injury due to legal intervention by explosives
E972   Injury due to legal intervention by gas
E973   Injury due to legal intervention by blunt object
E974   Injury due to legal intervention by cutting and piercing instruments
E975   Injury due to legal intervention by other specified means
E976   Injury due to legal intervention by unspecified means
E977   Late effects of injuries due to legal intervention
E978   Legal execution

Terrorism (E979)
E979   Terrorism

Injury undetermined whether accidentally or purposely inflicted (E980-E989)
E980   Poisoning by solid or liquid substances, undetermined whether accidentally or purposely inflicted
E981   Poisoning by gases in domestic use, undetermined whether accidentally or purposely inflicted
E982   Poisoning by other gases, undetermined whether accidentally or purposely inflicted
E983   Hanging, strangulation, or suffocation, undetermined whether accidentally or purposely inflicted
E984   Submersion [drowning], undetermined whether accidentally or purposely inflicted
E985   Injury by firearms and explosives, undetermined whether accidentally or purposely inflicted
E986   Injury by cutting and piercing instruments, undetermined whether accidentally or purposely inflicted
E987   Falling from high place, undetermined whether accidentally or purposely inflicted
E988   Injury by other and unspecified means, undetermined whether accidentally or purposely inflicted
E989   Late effects of injury, undetermined whether accidentally or purposely inflicted

Injury resulting from operations of war (E990-E999)
E990   Injury due to war operations by fires and conflagrations
E991   Injury due to war operations by bullets and fragments
E992   Injury due to war operations by explosion of marine weapons
E993   Injury due to war operations by other explosion
E994   Injury due to war operations by destruction of aircraft
E995   Injury due to war operations by other and unspecified forms of conventional warfare
E996   Injury due to war operations by nuclear weapons
E997   Injury due to war operations by other forms of unconventional warfare
E998   Injury due to war operations but occurring after cessation of hostilities
E999   Late effects of injury due to war operations